Davidson's
Principles and Practice of
Medicine

Sir Stanley Davidson (1894–1981)

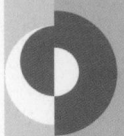

This famous textbook was the brainchild of one of the great Professors of Medicine of the 20th century. Stanley Davidson was born in Sri Lanka and began his medical undergraduate training at Trinity College, Cambridge; this was interrupted by World War I and later resumed in Edinburgh. He was seriously wounded in battle, and the carnage and shocking waste of young life that he encountered at that time had a profound effect on his subsequent attitudes and values.

In 1930 Stanley Davidson was appointed Professor of Medicine at the University of Aberdeen, one of the first full-time Chairs of Medicine anywhere and the first in Scotland. In 1938 he took up the Chair of Medicine at Edinburgh and was to remain in this post until retirement in 1959. He was a renowned educator and a particularly gifted teacher at the bedside, where he taught that everything had to be questioned and explained. He himself gave most of the systematic lectures in Medicine, which were made available as typewritten notes that emphasised the essentials and far surpassed any textbook available at the time.

Principles and Practice of Medicine was conceived in the late 1940s with its origins in those lecture notes. The first edition, published in 1952, was a masterpiece of clarity and uniformity of style. It was of modest size and price, but sufficiently comprehensive and up to date to provide students with the main elements of sound medical practice. Although the format and presentation have seen many changes in 19 subsequent editions, Sir Stanley's original vision and objectives remain. More than half a century after its first publication, his book continues to inform and educate students, doctors and health professionals all over the world.

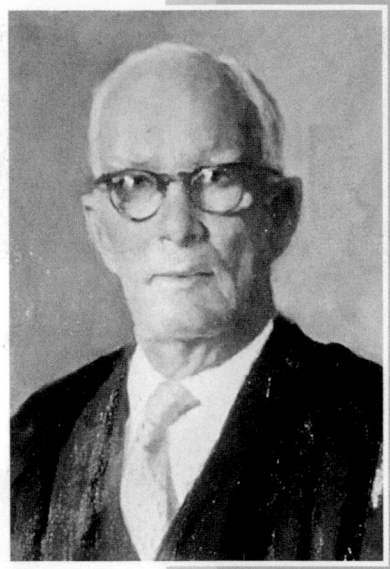

Portrait reproduced by courtesy of the Royal College of Physicians of Edinburgh

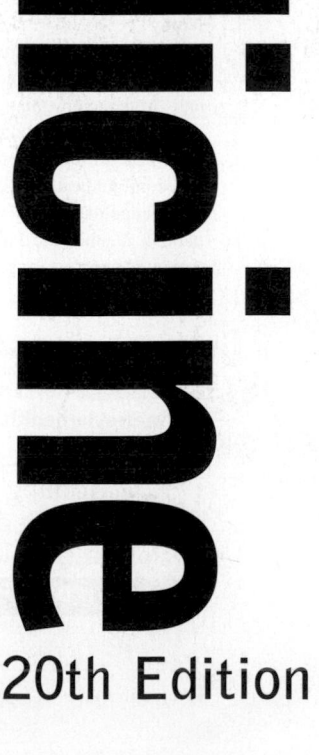

Davidson

Davidson's
Principles & Practice of

Medicine

The Editors

Nicholas A. Boon MA MD FRCP(Ed) FESC
Consultant Cardiologist, Royal Infirmary of Edinburgh;
Honorary Reader, University of Edinburgh

Nicki R. Colledge BSc FRCP(Ed)
Consultant Geriatrician, Liberton Hospital, Edinburgh
and Royal Infirmary of Edinburgh;
Honorary Senior Lecturer in Geriatric Medicine,
University of Edinburgh

Brian R. Walker BSc MD FRCP(Ed)
Professor of Endocrinology,
University of Edinburgh

John A.A. Hunter *OBE* BA MD FRCP(Ed)
Professor Emeritus of Dermatology,
University of Edinburgh

Illustrated by **Robert Britton**

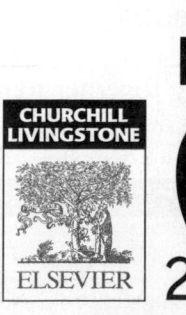

CHURCHILL
LIVINGSTONE

ELSEVIER

20th Edition

Edinburgh London New York Oxford Philadelphia St Louis Sydney Toronto 2006

CHURCHILL
LIVINGSTONE
ELSEVIER

An imprint of Elsevier Limited

First edition 1952
Second edition 1954
Third edition 1956
Fourth edition 1958
Fifth edition 1960
Sixth edition 1962
Seventh edition 1964
Eighth edition 1966
Ninth edition 1968
Tenth edition 1971

Eleventh edition 1974
Twelfth edition 1977
Thirteenth edition 1981
Fourteenth edition 1984
Fifteenth edition 1987
Sixteenth edition 1991
Seventeenth edition 1995
Eighteenth edition 1999
Nineteenth edition 2002
Twentieth edition 2006

Main Edition
ISBN-13: 978-0-443-10057-4
ISBN-10: 0-443-10057-8

International Edition
ISBN-13: 978-0-443-10133-5
ISBN-10: 0-443-10133-7

Reprinted 2006

British Library Cataloguing in Publication Data
A catalogue record for this book is available from the British Library

Library of Congress Cataloging in Publication Data
A catalog record for this book is available from the Library of Congress

Note
Medical knowledge is constantly changing. Standard safety precautions must be followed, but as new research and clinical experience broaden our knowledge, changes in treatment and drug therapy may become necessary or appropriate. Readers are advised to check the most current product information provided by the manufacturer of each drug to be administered to verify the recommended dose, the method and duration of administration, and contraindications. It is the responsibility of the practitioner, relying on experience and knowledge of the patient, to determine dosages and the best treatment for each individual patient. Neither the Publisher nor the editors assume any liability for any injury and/or damage to persons or property arising from this publication.

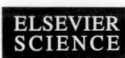
Commissioning Editor:
Laurence Hunter

Editorial Project Manager:
Wendy Lee

Project Manager:
Nancy Arnott

Cover Designer:
Stewart Larking

Illustration Manager:
Bruce Hogarth

Medical Illustrator:
Robert Britton

Charts:
Hard Lines Agency

Printed in India

Contents

CONTENTS

Preface

Davidson's Principles and Practice of Medicine was first published in 1952 and has one of the longest pedigrees of any textbook of medicine. At least two million copies have been sold and the book has acquired a large following of medical students, doctors and other health professionals all over the world. It has been translated into many languages and has won numerous prizes. Like all successful textbooks, *Davidson* has only endured because it has evolved to meet the changing needs of its readership. The comments that we receive from readers, expert reviewers and International Advisory Board have a major impact on how each edition of the book is revised. In the 20th edition a wealth of new material has been included, yet the book continues to provide an easily read, concise and up-to-date account of clinical medicine.

In recent editions the layout and style of *Davidson* have been overhauled dramatically. The feedback we receive suggests that these innovations have been warmly welcomed so in this edition we have concentrated on content and substance. The depth and breadth of coverage have been increased to meet the needs of candidates preparing for Membership of the Royal College of Physicians or its equivalent. The book's global perspective has also been enhanced through the excellent work of the International Advisory Board and the input of distinguished new authors from outside the UK. Both SI and non-SI units are now quoted in the text.

Since its first edition, *Davidson* has sought to explain the basis for medical practice. The integration of 'pre-clinical' science with clinical practice is now a feature of many undergraduate medical curricula, and many students use *Davidson* from the outset of their medical course. The first part of the book, 'Principles of Medicine', has therefore been extensively revised. To highlight the professional and ethical principles underlying medical practice, the book begins with a new chapter, 'Good Medical Practice'. To enhance coverage of the mechanisms of health and disease, there are new chapters on 'Molecular Mechanisms of Disease', 'Immunological Factors in Disease', 'Environmental and Nutritional Factors in Disease' and 'Principles of Infectious Disease'. Many examples of relevant clinical problems have been included within these chapters to help bring the medical sciences to life for the new student and rejuvenate the interest of the experienced clinician. The second part of the book, 'Practice of Medicine', covers the important medical specialties. Each of these chapters has been rewritten and there are new chapters on 'HIV and AIDS', 'Sexually Transmitted Infections' and 'Clinical Biochemistry and Metabolism'.

A popular innovation for the last edition of *Davidson* was the website, which gave the reader online access to the text, illustrations and many other features. For this edition, the website has been enhanced using the Student Consult platform and will provide integrated links to selected parts of our sister books, *Macleod's Clinical Examination* (now in its 11th edition) and *Principles and Practice of Surgery*. The website also offers a convenient way of searching for information, and more than 750 new self-testing questions with detailed answers linked to the online text.

Professor Brian Walker has joined the editorial team and 24 new authors have contributed material to this edition. Their input has helped to refresh and energise the book and the whole team has striven to produce an outstanding, clear and modern edition of *Davidson's Principles and Practice of Medicine*. Finally, we would like to acknowledge the enormous contribution of Sir Stanley Davidson and all the previous editors and authors, who laid the foundations for what remains one of the world's leading textbooks of medicine.

Edinburgh
2006

N.A.B., N.R.C., B.R.W., J.A.A.H.

Acknowledgements

Following the publication of the 19th edition of *Davidson's Principles and Practice of Medicine*, Professor Christopher Haslett and Professor Edwin Chilvers, who played a huge part in the recent development of the book, retired as editors. We are deeply indebted to them and to those authors who have stepped down from this edition. They include Dr Peter B. Carey, Professor Paul A. Corris, Dr Marie T. Fallon, Professor Keith A.A. Fox, Professor O. James Garden, Dr Andrew Haynes, Dr Geoffrey G. Lloyd, Dr Fred Nye, Dr William D. Plant, Professor Ian Power, Dr Lance N. Sandle, Professor John Savill, Professor Prakash Shetty, Dr Kenneth J. Simpson, Professor John F. Smyth, Dr Anthony D. Toft and Dr Stephen J. Watt.

We would like to thank the following for their valuable role in shaping the 20th edition: Professor Kenneth Boyd for his assistance with Chapter 1; Colonel Timothy Hodgetts for reviewing the environmental disease sections in Chapter 5; Dr Stephen Lawrie for reviewing sections of Chapter 10; Dr Craig Ferguson for his advice on infective endocarditis in Chapter 18; and Dr Paul Dodson and Dr Robert Lindsay for helping update parts of Chapter 21.

Detailed chapter reviews were commissioned to help plan this new edition and we are grateful to Dr J. Bennison, Dr J. Din, Dr D. Errington, Dr M. Field, Dr N. Finer, Dr N. Hirani, Dr F.E. Karet, Dr E. McDonald, Dr D. Nathwani, Dr P. Rae, Dr A. Shand and Dr P. Shepherd for these.

As part of the publishers' review, students from several medical schools supplied many innovative ideas on how to enhance the book. We are especially indebted to the following for their enthusiastic support: Chun Bong, Geoff Cross, Sommit Dan, Victoria Ferguson, Michael Hunter, Ify Mordi, C.L. Nwaneri, Ee Ting Ooi, Jennifer Price, Michael Reschen, Yee Ting Sim, Kate Thompson and Grace Yang.

We would like to express our gratitude to the many readers who have used the email feedback address to contact us with suggestions for improvements. Their input has been invaluable and is much appreciated; they are unfortunately too numerous to mention individually.

As part of the Student Consult website there are 750 'best of five' self-testing questions available. We are very grateful to Dr Alan Japp, Dr Sunil Adwani, Dr Kenneth Baillie and Dr Sarah Walsh for their expertise and enthusiasm in compiling these.

We thank colleagues who have generously provided many of the illustrations that appear in this edition. They are acknowledged on pages 1325–1326.

We are especially grateful to all those working for Churchill Livingstone, in particular Laurence Hunter, Wendy Lee, Ruth Swan, Jim Killgore and Robert Britton, for their expertise in the shaping, collation and illustration of this edition. We would also like to thank Anne McCarthy for her labours in compiling the extensive index and Ian Ross for expert proofreading.

Edinburgh   N.A.B., N.R.C., B.R.W., J.A.A.H.
2006

Contributors

Chris Allen MA MD FRCP
Consultant Neurologist, Addenbrooke's Hospital,
Cambridge, UK

Jeffrey K. Aronson MA MBChB DPhil FRCP FBPharmacolS
Reader in Clinical Pharmacology, University of
Oxford, UK

Peter Bloomfield MD FRCP FACC
Consultant Cardiologist, Royal Infirmary of Edinburgh;
Honorary Senior Lecturer, University of Edinburgh, UK

Nicholas A. Boon MD FRCP(Ed) FESC
Consultant Cardiologist, Royal Infirmary of Edinburgh;
Honorary Reader, University of Edinburgh, UK

Andrew W. Bradbury BSc MB ChB MD MBA FRCS(Ed)
Head of Surgery and Professor of Vascular Surgery,
University of Birmingham; Consultant Vascular Surgeon
and Director of Research and Development, Heart of
England NHS Foundation Trust, UK

Leslie Burnett MB BS BSc(Med) PhD FRCPA MAACB FHGSA
Director, Pacific Laboratory Medicine Services, Royal
North Shore Hospital of Sydney; Clinical Professor in
Pathology, Northern Clinical School, University of
Sydney; Adjunct Professor in Science and Technology,
University of Technology, Sydney, Australia

Mark Byers MRCGP DA DipIMC
Lieutenant-Colonel, 3 Close Support Medical
Regiment, Catterick Garrison, North Yorkshire, UK

David Allan Cameron MA MSc MD FRCP
Consultant Medical Oncologist, Western General
Hospital, Edinburgh; part-time Senior Lecturer in
Medical Oncology, University of Edinburgh, UK

Roger William Chapman BSc MD(Lond) FRCP(Lond)
Consultant Gastroenterologist/Hepatologist, John
Radcliffe Hospital, Oxford; Honorary Senior Lecturer
in Medicine, Oxford University Clinical Medical
School, Oxford, UK

Nicki Colledge BSc FRCP(Ed)
Consultant Geriatrician, Liberton Hospital, Edinburgh
and Royal Infirmary of Edinburgh; Honorary Senior
Lecturer in Geriatric Medicine, University of
Edinburgh, UK

Jane Collier MD FRCP
Consultant Hepatologist, John Radcliffe Hospital,
Oxford, UK

Jenny I.O. Craig MD FRCP(Ed) FRCPath
Consultant Haematologist, Addenbrooke's Hospital,
Cambridge, UK

Allan D. Cumming MD FRCP
Director of Undergraduate Learning and Teaching and
Professor of Medical Education, University of
Edinburgh; Consultant Renal Physician, Royal Infirmary
of Edinburgh, UK

Martin Dennis MD FRCP(Ed)
Professor of Stroke Medicine, University of
Edinburgh, UK

Michael Doherty MA MD FRCP
Professor of Rheumatology, University of Nottingham;
Consultant Rheumatologist, City Hospital,
Nottingham, UK

Michael John Field MD BS BSc FRACP
Professor of Medicine, University of Sydney; Associate
Dean and Head, Northern Clinical School, Royal
North Shore Hospital of Sydney, Australia

Miles Fisher MD FRCP(Glas) FRCP(Ed)
Consultant Physician, Glasgow Royal Infirmary;
Honorary Clinical Senior Lecturer, University of Glasgow,
UK

Brian M. Frier BSc(Hons) MD FRCP(Ed) FRCP(Glas)
Consultant Physician, Department of Diabetes, Royal
Infirmary of Edinburgh; Honorary Professor of
Diabetes, University of Edinburgh, UK

Jane Goddard PhD FRCP(Ed)
Consultant Nephrologist, Royal Infirmary of Edinburgh;
Honorary Senior Lecturer, University of Edinburgh, UK

Ian S. Grant FRCP(Ed) FRCP(Glas) FFARCSI
Consultant in Intensive Care Medicine and Anaesthesia,
Western General Hospital, Edinburgh, UK

Neil Grubb MD MRCP
Consultant in Cardiac Electrophysiology, Royal
Infirmary of Edinburgh; Honorary Senior Lecturer,
University of Edinburgh, UK

Phil Hanlon MD FRCP FFPH MRCGP
Professor of Public Health, University of Glasgow, UK

Peter Clive Hayes MD PhD FRCP
Professor of Hepatology and Honorary Consultant
Gastroenterologist, Scottish Liver Transplant Unit and
Gastroenterology and Liver Unit, Royal Infirmary of
Edinburgh, UK

Grahame Charles William Howard BSc(Hons) MD
FRCP(Ed) FRCR
Consultant Clinical Oncologist, Edinburgh Cancer
Centre; Honorary Senior Lecturer, University of
Edinburgh, UK

J. Alastair Innes PhD FRCP(Ed)
Consultant Physician and Honorary Reader in
Respiratory Medicine, Western General Hospital,
Edinburgh, UK

George John MD FRACP FJFICM
Professor of Medicine, Christian Medical College,
Vellore, Tamil Nadu, India

Alison L. Jones BSc(Hons) MD FRCP(Ed) FRCP FiBiol
Consultant Physician and Clinical Toxicologist, Director
of Guy's and St Thomas' Poisons Unit, Medical
Toxicology Unit, Guy's and St Thomas' NHS
Foundation Trust, London, UK

Lakshman Karalliedde MBBS DA FRCA
Consultant, Chemical Hazards and Poisons Division
(London), Health Protection Agency, UK

Peter C. Lanyon DM FRCP MRCGP
Consultant Rheumatologist, University Hospital,
Queen's Medical Centre, Nottingham, UK

Diana N.J. Lockwood BSc MD FRCP
Reader in Tropical Medicine, London School of
Hygiene and Tropical Medicine; Consultant Physician
and Leprologist, Hospital for Tropical Diseases,
London, UK

Christopher A. Ludlam MBChB BSc PhD FRCP FRCPath
Professor of Haematology and Coagulation Medicine,
University of Edinburgh; Director, Haemophilia and
Thrombosis Centre, Royal Infirmary of Edinburgh, UK

Christian J. Lueck PhD FRCP FRCP(Ed) FRACP
Head, Department of Neurology, Canberra Hospital;
Associate Professor, Australian National University
Medical School, Canberra, Australia

D.B.L. McClelland PhD(Leiden) FRCP FRCPath
Consultant, Scottish National Blood Transfusion
Service, Edinburgh, UK

Sara Marshall MRCP(Eire) FRCPath(UK) PhD
Senior Lecturer in Immunology, Imperial College,
London; Honorary Consultant in Immunology, Chelsea
and Westminster Hospital, London, UK

David E. Newby PhD DM FRCP
Professor of Cardiology, University of Edinburgh, UK

David Richard Oxenham FRCP(Ed) FAChPM
Medical Director, Marie Curie Hospice, Edinburgh;
Honorary Senior Lecturer, University of Edinburgh, UK

Kelvin R. Palmer MD FRCP(Ed) FRCP(Lond) FRCS(Ed)
Consultant Gastroenterologist, Western General
Hospital, Edinburgh, UK

Simon Paterson-Brown MS MPhil FRCS
Consultant General and Upper Gastrointestinal
Surgeon, Royal Infirmary of Edinburgh, UK

Ian D. Penman MD FRCP(Ed)
Consultant Gastroenterologist, Western General
Hospital, Edinburgh; part-time Senior Lecturer,
University of Edinburgh, UK

Stephen Potts MA MRCPsych
Consultant Liaison Psychiatrist, Royal Infirmary of
Edinburgh; Honorary Senior Clinical Lecturer,
University of Edinburgh, UK

Stuart H. Ralston MD FRCP FMedSci FRSE
ARC Professor of Rheumatology, University of
Edinburgh; Honorary Consultant Rheumatologist,
NHS Lothian, Edinburgh, UK

Jonathan L. Rees BMedSci FRCP FRCP(Ed) FMedSci
Grant Chair of Dermatology, University of Edinburgh;
Honorary Consultant, Lothian Health, University
Hospitals Division, Edinburgh, UK

Peter T. Reid MD FRCP(Ed)
Consultant Physician and Honorary Senior Lecturer in
Respiratory Medicine, Western General Hospital,
Edinburgh, UK

Richard N. Sandford PhD FRCP
Wellcome Trust Senior Fellow in Clinical Research,
University Reader in Renal Genetics and Honorary
Consultant in Medical Genetics, Addenbrooke's
Hospital, Cambridge, UK

Olivia M.V. Schofield FRCP(Ed)
Consultant Dermatologist, Royal Infirmary of
Edinburgh, UK

Gordon R. Scott BSc FRCP
Consultant in Genitourinary Medicine and Honorary
Senior Lecturer, University of Edinburgh, UK

Jonathan Robert Seckl BSc PhD FRCP(Ed) FMedSci FRSE
Moncrieff–Arnott Professor of Molecular Medicine,
University of Edinburgh; Honorary Consultant
Physician, Lothian Health, UK

Michael C. Sharpe MA MD FRCP FRCP(Ed) FRCPsych
Professor of Psychological Medicine and Symptoms
Research, University of Edinburgh, UK

Laurence H. Stewart MD FRCS(Ed) FRCS(Urol)
Consultant Urological Surgeon, Western General
Hospital, Edinburgh, UK

Peter Stewart FRACP FRCPA MBA
Clinical Director, Sydney South West Pathology
Service; Associate Professor of Biochemistry, University
of Sydney, Australia

Mark W.J. Strachan BSc(Hons) MD FRCP(Ed)
Consultant Physician, Western General Hospital,
Edinburgh; Honorary Senior Lecturer, University of
Edinburgh, UK

David Richmond Sullivan FRACP FRCPA
Senior Staff Specialist, Royal Prince Alfred Hospital,
Camperdown, New South Wales; Clinical Associate
Professor, University of Sydney, Australia

Christopher B. Summerton MA MD FRCP FRCP(Ed)
Consultant in Gastroenterology and General
Medicine, Trafford Healthcare NHS Trust,
Manchester, UK

Shyam Sundar MD FRCP(Lond) FAMS FNA
Professor of Medicine, Institute of Medical Sciences,
Banaras Hindu University, India

W.T. Andrew Todd BSc FRCP FRCPS(Glas)
Consultant Physician, Lanarkshire Area Infectious
Diseases Unit, Monklands Hospital, Airdrie; Honorary
Senior Lecturer, University of Glasgow, UK

David F. Treacher MA FRCP
Consultant Physician in Intensive Care, Guy's and
St Thomas' NHS Trust, London, UK

Neil Turner PhD FRCP
Professor of Nephrology, University of Edinburgh;
Honorary Consultant Nephrologist, Royal Infirmary of
Edinburgh, UK

Brian R. Walker BSc MD FRCP(Ed)
Professor of Endocrinology, University of Edinburgh, UK

Simon Walker MB BS(Lond) MA DM(Oxon)
Senior Lecturer and Honorary Consultant in Clinical
Biochemistry, University of Edinburgh, UK

Ed Wilkins FRCP FRCPath
Consultant Physician in Infectious Diseases, North
Manchester General Hospital, Manchester, UK

International Advisory Board

INTERNATIONAL EDITOR'S PREFACE

It is always most gratifying for *Davidson*'s authors and editors to learn how highly our book is rated by students and teachers around the world. Not only is it encouraging for us to know that our efforts are valued in lands far away from our desks, but it also provides us with a stimulus to write a text that has true global application.

An International Advisory Board was established in 2000, with a specific remit to advise on the relevance of the book's content in an international setting. No fewer than 32 experienced clinicians and teachers from a total of 13 countries now make up this Board. Its members continue to provide an invaluable insight into the day-to-day practice of medicine overseas, for which the editors are most grateful.

For this 20th edition the editors also wished to have a more international author base. The chapters on 'Good Medical Practice', 'Poisoning' and 'Infectious Diseases', in particular, have benefited greatly from the input of doctors with a wealth of experience overseas, while a team of Australian contributors has taken a refreshing approach to the new chapter on 'Clinical Biochemistry and Metabolism'.

On a visit to the Indian subcontinent in 2004, the publishers and I had the opportunity to meet teachers and students from medical colleges in India, Bangladesh and Sri Lanka. We listened to their suggestions as to how *Davidson* could be improved and have taken many of these ideas on board, including, for example, extra detail on rheumatic fever and more specialised coverage of conditions as diverse as snake bites, dengue and leishmaniasis. When they read this edition, we trust that it will be obvious to those whom we met that our visit was not simply a public relations exercise!

We sincerely hope that our readers all over the world will appreciate the enhanced international flavour of this latest edition, and once again look forward to receiving their comments.

Edinburgh   J.A.A.H.
2006

MEMBERS OF THE INTERNATIONAL ADVISORY BOARD

An introduction to *Davidson's Principles and Practice of Medicine*

The first section of this book, 'Principles of Medicine', describes the basis on which medicine is practised and the fundamental mechanisms determining health and disease, which are relevant to all medical specialties. The second section, 'Practice of Medicine', is devoted to individual medical specialties. While each chapter has been written by experts in the field, a uniform approach has been adopted and great care taken to avoid unnecessary duplication.

The system-based chapters follow a standard format, beginning with an overview of relevant clinical examination, followed by an account of functional anatomy, physiology and investigations, then describing the common presentations of disease, and finishing with details of the individual diseases of that system. In this edition, where appropriate, the chapters in the first section follow a similar format; the introduction of a problem-based approach in chapters which describe the immunological, cell and molecular basis of disease brings the close links between modern medical science and clinical practice into sharp focus.

The methods used to present information in a uniform style throughout the book are described below.

CLINICAL EXAMINATION OVERVIEWS

The value of good clinical skills is highlighted by a two-page overview of the important elements of the clinical examination at the beginning of each system-based chapter. The left-hand page of these sections uses a manikin to illustrate the key steps in the examination of the relevant system, beginning with simple observations and progressing in a logical sequence around the body. The right-hand page expands on selected themes and includes useful tips on examination technique and the interpretation of physical signs. These overviews are intended to act as an aide-mémoire and not as a replacement for a detailed text on clinical examination. This can be found in our sister title, *Macleod's Clinical Examination*.

PRESENTING PROBLEMS

Medical students and junior doctors are expected not only to learn a bewildering mix of facts about various disorders, but also to develop an analytical, problem-based approach to formulating a differential diagnosis and a plan of investiga-tion for patients who present with particular symptoms or signs of disease. In *Davidson* this is addressed by incorporating a 'Presenting Problems' section (signalled by red headings) into all system-based chapters. Under their previous name of 'Major Manifestations', these were a popular feature of the last three editions. They have now been expanded to include over 200 presentations, represent-ing the most common reasons for referral to each medical specialty. The same approach has been used in several of the chapters in the 'Principles of Medicine' section, to reinforce the close connection between clinical problems and fundamental mechanisms of disease. Many patients present with symptoms such as weight loss, dizziness or breath-lessness, which are not specific to a particular system; these are described in one chapter and cross-referenced elsewhere. An index of presenting problems may be found on the inside back cover.

CLASSIFICATION OF BOXES AND TABLES

Boxes and tables are a popular and efficient way of present-ing information, and are particularly useful for revision. They are classified by the type of information they contain using the following symbols:

 Causes

 Clinical features/complications

 Investigations

 Treatment/adverse effects

 Evidence-based medicine

 In old age

 Other information

ISSUES IN OLD AGE

In most developed countries, older people comprise 20% of the population and are the chief users of health care. Older people contract the same diseases as those who are younger but there are often important differences in the way they present and how they are best managed.

Chapter 7, 'Ageing and Disease', concentrates on the principles of managing the frailest group who suffer from multiple pathology and disability, and who tend to present with non-specific problems such as falls. However, many older people suffer from specific single-organ pathology that will be managed by appropriate specialists. This is recognised in *Davidson* by incorporation of 'In Old Age' boxes into each chapter. These describe common presentations, implications of physiological changes of ageing, effects of age on investigations, problems of treatment in old age, and the benefits and risks of intervention in older people. This provides an insight into the care of older people wherever they may present.

EVIDENCE-BASED MEDICINE

Clinicians must base their practice on the best available evidence. This needs to be up to date, relevant, authoritative and easily accessible. In this edition of *Davidson* we have incorporated over 150 evidence-based medicine (EBM) panels that summarise the results of the most recent systematic reviews (SRs) or randomised controlled trials (RCTs) in key therapeutic areas. These panels also provide details of the landmark trials in each area and, when available, a website address which gives the reader access to additional references and more detailed management guidelines.

The EBM panels contain recommendations that are supported by evidence obtained from meta-analysis of several RCTs or one (or more) high-quality RCT. Recommendations conform to 'Grade A' criteria as described and used by the Scottish Intercollegiate Guidelines Network (SIGN; see www.sign.ac.uk).

Certain EBM panels incorporate data on the numbers needed to treat for benefit (NNT_B); 'NNT_B' defines the number of people you would need to treat for a given period of time to prevent one additional adverse outcome or to achieve one additional beneficial outcome. Likewise, the absolute risk reduction (ARR) values quoted refer to the difference in risk between the experimental and control groups in the trial. A detailed account of evidence-based medicine in drug therapy, including details of the calculation of NNT_B, risk ratios and odds ratios, can be found in Chapter 2, 'Good Prescribing' (pp. 17–35). Further guidance on applying research evidence to clinical practice is available at www.clinicalevidence.org.

New evidence is being provided all the time. Resources for up-to-date information on systematic reviews include www.cochrane.org. Additional specialist websites are provided in the 'Further Information' sections at the end of each chapter.

TERMINOLOGY

A recent European Community Directive requires member states to use Recommended International Non-proprietary Names (rINNs) for drugs. This terminology, with the exception of adrenaline and noradrenaline, is therefore used throughout the book; however, British spellings have been retained for drug classes and groups (e.g. amphetamines not amfetamines).

UNITS OF MEASUREMENT

The International System of Units (SI units) is the recommended means for presentation of laboratory data and has been used throughout *Davidson*. However, we recognise that many laboratories around the world continue to provide data in non-SI units. In this edition values in non-SI units have been included in the text for the commonly measured analytes. Both SI and non-SI units are also given in the Appendix, which describes the reference ranges used in Edinburgh's laboratories. It is important to appreciate that these reference ranges may vary from those used in other laboratories.

FINDING WHAT YOU ARE LOOKING FOR

A detailed contents list is given on the opening page of each chapter. In addition, the book contains numerous cross-references to help readers find their way around, along with an extensive index of over 10 000 subject entries. The online text on Student Consult (www.studentconsult.com) allows for detailed searches of the content by keyword. A list of up-to-date reviews and useful websites with links to management guidelines appears at the end of each chapter.

ONLINE SELF-ASSESSMENT QUESTIONS

'Best of five' questions are now widely used for examination purposes as a reliable and discriminatory test of factual knowledge. To help readers to acquire the knowledge necessary for good medical practice, 750 brand new questions based on the content of this edition of *Davidson* are provided at www.studentconsult.com. Answers are provided with explanatory text and direct links to the online text.

Online contents

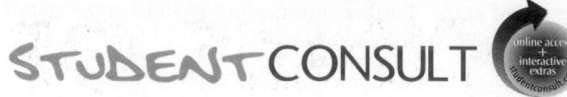

This 20th edition of *Davidson's Principles and Practice of Medicine* is accompanied by an online version, accessed via **www.studentconsult.com**. To use this invaluable online companion, simply follow the instructions on the inside front cover of this book.

Features of the online version
- The fully searchable text of all 28 chapters, approachable via keywords, subject headings or index
- Over 1000 illustrations, to view online or download
- Sophisticated on-screen navigation showing you where you are within the book
- Hypertext-linked cross-references
- A practical drug therapy formulary.

Future enhancement of the online version with additional new features will take place.

Integration links
Integration links will guide you towards bonus content from other textbooks, including our sister publication, *Macleod's Clinical Examination*. These links constitute an extra user-friendly layer of information wrapped around your textbook. Curriculum-based and high-yield, they are designed to improve your chances of success in medical school examinations by collecting relevant information together for you.

'Best of Five' self-testing questions
Prepare for examinations or refresh your knowledge of *Davidson*'s content with 750 'best of five' self-testing questions.

This unique new feature will enhance your learning experience and has been designed to test your understanding and assist you in acquiring the knowledge you will need to practise as a clinician. Specifically written for this edition of *Davidson*, these questions provide a comprehensive review of the topics of greatest importance that are most likely to feature in student examinations. Corresponding to each of the book's chapters, the questions are enhanced by answers linked to the online text for in-depth exploration of a specific topic. The detailed explanations will help clarify why a particular answer is right or wrong, and the links will point you towards appropriate areas for revision. Many of the answers link to the evidence-based medicine content of the text. The questions are suitable for all levels, and range in difficulty from core knowledge to more advanced topics.

Authors

Alan G. Japp MBChB(Hons) BSc(Hons) MRCP
Clinical Research Fellow in Cardiology, Royal Infirmary of Edinburgh, UK

Sunil Adwani MBChB(Hons) BSc(Hons) MRCP
Senior House Officer in Medicine, Victoria Hospital, Kirkcaldy, UK

J. Kenneth Baillie BSc(Hons) MBChB MRCP
Senior House Officer, Department of Anaesthesia, Critical Care and Pain Medicine, Royal Infirmary of Edinburgh, UK

Sarah Walsh MB BCh BAO BMedSci MRCP
Dermatology Registrar, Royal Infirmary of Edinburgh, UK

ADDED VALUE WITH DAVIDSON

Cecil Textbook of Medicine online

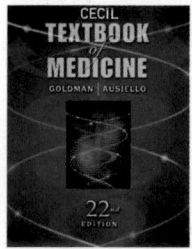

As a purchaser of *Davidson's Principles and Practice of Medicine*, you are entitled to a year's free access to the online version of the 22nd edition of *Cecil Textbook of Medicine*. This feature provides a powerful extra resource and will give you the opportunity to become acquainted with an outstanding medical reference work, consulted by students, practitioners and researchers all over the world. To access *Cecil Textbook of Medicine*, please follow the link under 'My E-ditions' after activating your book on Student Consult.

Medicine

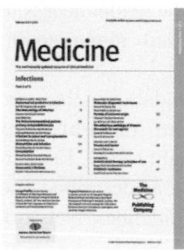

You are also eligible for a one-year, half-price personal subscription to *Medicine* as a special extra feature of the Student Consult website. This unique journal provides comprehensive and systematic coverage of the principles and practice of internal medicine and will be particularly useful for physicians in training. Both specialist physicians and general practitioners will find it an indispensable resource for reading and reference, while students will find much of value in each issue. Designed for easy reading and fast assimilation of information, *Medicine* will be a trusted cornerstone of your reference library. To take up this offer, please follow the link on the *Davidson* 'Welcome' page after activating your book on Student Consult.

This offer is only open to non-subscribers to *Medicine*.

Feedback
The editors and publisher hope that you will find this edition of *Davidson's Principles and Practice of Medicine* informative and easy to use. We would be delighted to hear from you if you have any comments or suggestions to make for future editions of the book. Please e-mail us at:

davidson.feedback@elsevier.com

Part 1
PRINCIPLES OF
MEDICINE

1

N.A. BOON
A.D. CUMMING
G. JOHN

Good medical practice

Patients (and doctors) differ in their beliefs, attitudes and expectations. Good medical practice, or the art of medicine, hinges on the ability to recognise and respect these differences and to treat every patient as an individual. This chapter will describe how to provide the patient, and their family, with relevant but complex information, discuss management options, and reach appropriate ethical decisions that are commensurate with the available resources.

THE DOCTOR–PATIENT RELATIONSHIP

The contents of this book are not all based on indisputable contemporary evidence; many reflect wisdom and understanding distilled over hundreds of years and passed from generation to generation of doctors. This perceived wisdom lies at the heart of the way that doctors and patients interact;

it demands respect, and if the doctor also displays compassion, sets the scene for the development of trust.

The doctor–patient relationship is in itself therapeutic; a successful consultation with a trusted and respected practitioner will therefore have beneficial effects irrespective of any other therapy given. The doctor–patient relationship is also multi-layered, dynamic and bilateral. Figure 1.1 illustrates how it may be influenced by differences in attitudes or beliefs, and behaviours or roles, with some exemplar statements that can be attributed to either the doctor or the patient.

Health care is increasingly provided by a multi-disciplinary team; patients with chronic diseases like renal failure will therefore interact with a wide array of health professionals. The doctor usually takes the lead in determining the overall direction of care but must also guide the patient through the unfamiliar landscape, language and

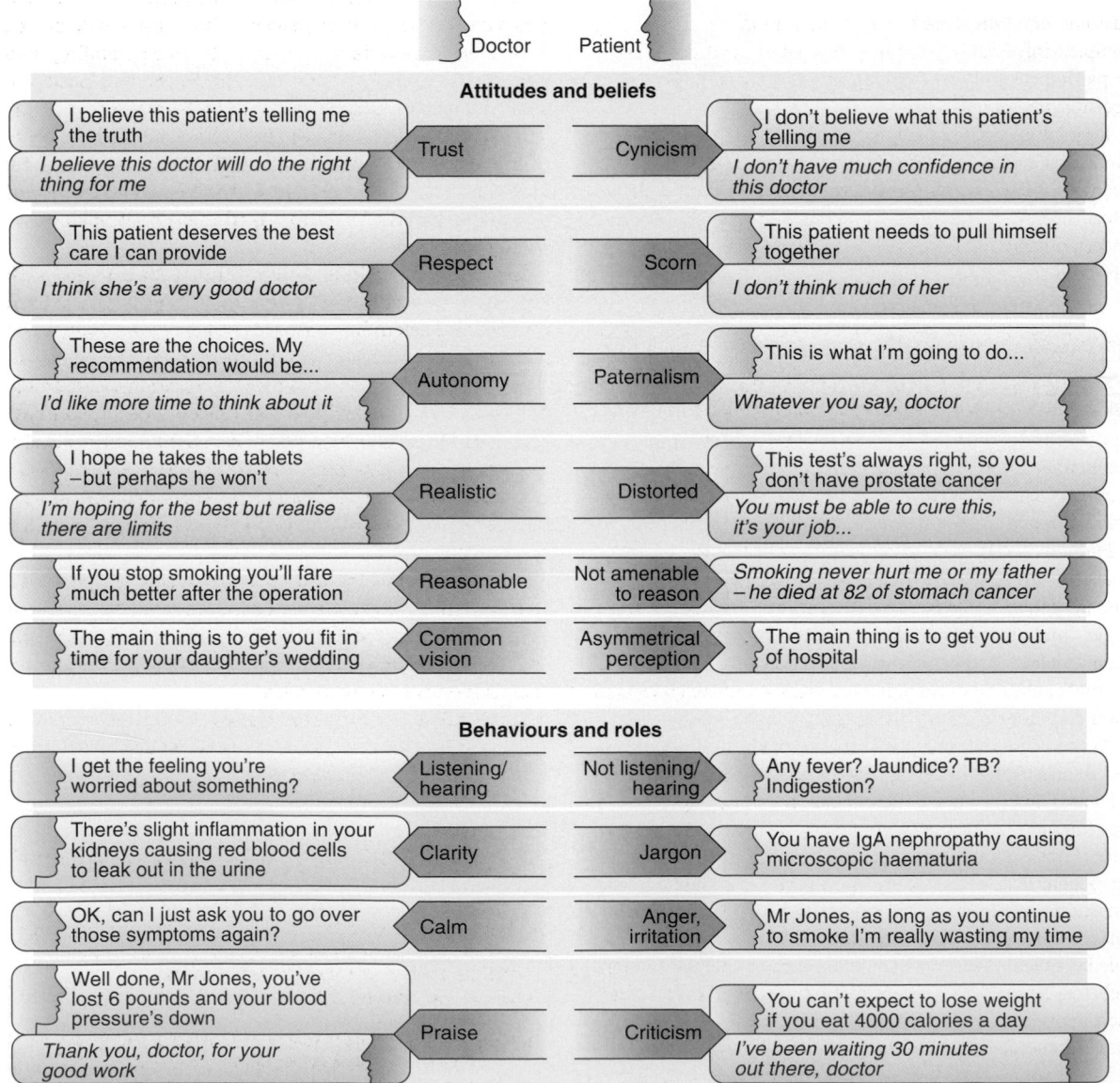

Fig. 1.1 The doctor–patient relationship.

1.1 THE DUTIES OF A DOCTOR REGISTERED WITH THE UK GENERAL MEDICAL COUNCIL

- Make the care of your patient your first concern
- Treat every patient politely and considerately
- Respect the patient's dignity and privacy
- Listen to patients and respect their views
- Give patients information in a way they can understand
- Respect the rights of patients to be fully involved in decisions about their care
- Keep your professional knowledge and skills up to date
- Recognise the limits of your professional competence
- Be honest and trustworthy
- Respect and protect confidential information
- Make sure that your personal beliefs do not prejudice your patient's care
- Act quickly to protect patients from risk if you have good reason to believe that you or a colleague may not be fit to practise
- Avoid abusing your position as a doctor
- Work with colleagues in the ways that best serve patients' interests

1.2 SOME BARRIERS TO GOOD COMMUNICATION IN HEALTH CARE

The clinician

- Authoritarian or dismissive attitude
- Hurried approach
- Use of jargon
- Unable to speak first language of patient
- No experience of patient's cultural background

The patient

- Anxiety
- Reluctance to discuss sensitive or seemingly trivial issues
- Misconceptions
- Conflicting sources of information
- Cognitive impairment
- Hearing/speech/visual impediment

customs of clinical care; interpret, synthesise and convey complex information; and help the patient and their family to participate fully in thinking about their care and in the decision-making process.

Regulatory bodies such as the United Kingdom General Medical Council seek to define the medical side of the doctor–patient relationship in terms of the duties of a doctor (Box 1.1). It is common for medical schools to require undergraduate students to sign an ethical code of conduct based on statements like this.

CLINICAL AND COMMUNICATION SKILLS

Good communication is the single most important component of good medical practice because it identifies problems quickly and clearly, defines expectations, and helps to establish trust between the clinician and patient.

Failures in communication lead to poor health outcomes, strained working relations, widespread dissatisfaction among patients, their families and health professionals, anger and litigation. Sadly, poor communication is commonplace in most health-care systems and has become the root cause of most complaints. Some common barriers to good communication are listed in Box 1.2.

At the beginning of a medical consultation many patients feel ill and most will be apprehensive. Their distress will be enhanced and effective communication will be impossible if the clinician appears indifferent, unsympathetic and short of time. First impressions are critical and it is essential that the patient be put at ease by appropriate introductions and a friendly greeting (get up, shake hands or say namaste (or whatever is culturally appropriate) and look at the patient, *not* the notes). The clinician must ensure that the patient feels that he or she is the centre of interest, and should begin each interview by outlining the likely course of events and agreeing the objectives of the consultation.

The main aim of a medical interview is to establish a factual account of the patient's illness. However, this is not enough; the clinician must also explore the patient's own feelings, determine how they interpret their symptoms, and unearth all their concerns and fears before suggesting and agreeing a plan of management. These goals will not be met unless clinicians demonstrate understanding and empathy (i.e. imagine themselves in the patient's position). Empathy is not the same as sympathy (feeling sorry for the patient), which is rarely helpful. Most patients have more than one concern and will be reluctant to discuss potentially important issues if they feel that the clinician is not interested, or is likely to dismiss their complaints as irrational or trivial.

Listening and talking to the patient with care and skill will usually lead to a provisional diagnosis, establish rapport, and determine which investigations are likely to be most productive. The clinician must allow the patient to describe their problems without overbearing questioning, but should try to facilitate the process with appropriate questions (Box 1.3). Non-verbal communication is equally important. The patient's facial expressions and body language may betray hidden fears. The clinician can help the patient to talk more freely by smiling or nodding appropriately.

The doctor must also ensure that dignity is preserved and that the patient feels comfortable throughout the examination; this may entail the presence of a chaperone and always requires explanation in advance of whatever examination is to be performed.

A detailed account of history-taking and clinical examination can be found in Davidson's sister title, *MacLeod's Clinical Examination*.

1.3 THE MEDICAL INTERVIEW: QUESTION TYPES

- **Open questions** allow the patient to express their own thoughts and feelings, e.g. 'How have you been since we last saw you?', 'Is there anything else that you want to mention?'
- **Closed questions** are requests for factual information, e.g. 'When did this pain start?'
- **Leading questions** invite specific responses and suggest options, e.g. 'You'll be glad when this treatment is over, won't you?'
- **Reflecting questions** help to develop or expand topics, e.g. 'Can you tell me more about your family?'

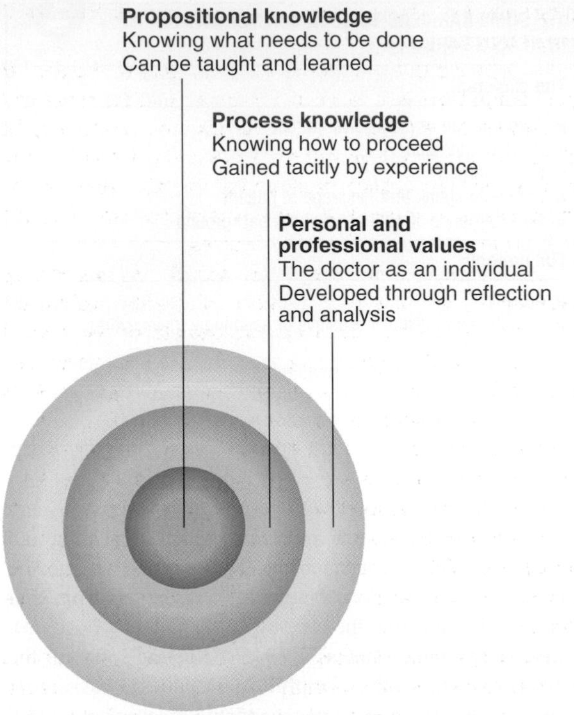

Propositional knowledge
Knowing what needs to be done
Can be taught and learned

Process knowledge
Knowing how to proceed
Gained tacitly by experience

**Personal and
professional values**
The doctor as an individual
Developed through reflection
and analysis

Fig. 1.2 **The personal and professional development of a doctor.**

1.5 SOME APPRAISAL TECHNIQUES

- Formal, structured assessment (e.g. postgraduate examinations)
- 360-degree assessment (surveying colleagues from medicine and other disciplines who work alongside the practitioner)
- Educational supervision and mentoring (a specific colleague has nominated responsibility to guide, and also assess, the practitioner)
- Logbooks (records of work undertaken and outcomes)
- Portfolio-based assessment (the practitioner accumulates a record of educational and clinical experiences together with evidence of reflective practice)

1.4 THE NOVICE–EXPERT SHIFT

- **Novices** use pre-determined methods which they learn
- **Advanced beginners** recognise that these methods are not effective in all circumstances and can adapt them according to context
- **Competent professionals** are able to make conscious independent choices and can manage and regulate their own practice
- **Proficient professionals** make use of intuition based on experience; integrate multiple aspects of practice in a holistic model
- **Experts** function largely through 'unconscious competence' and are inseparable from the tasks they undertake

---

PERSONAL AND PROFESSIONAL DEVELOPMENT

Good doctors never stop learning, and continue to develop their knowledge, skills and attributes throughout their working lives, to the benefit of their patients and themselves. Personal and professional development (PPD) requires a reflective and self-directed approach to the study and practice of medicine (Fig. 1.2), and will maximise both life-long effectiveness and personal satisfaction. Linked to this is the concept of the novice–expert shift (Box 1.4).

PPD begins in the first days at medical school and continues through postgraduate training and subsequent professional practice; maintaining competence and expertise requires continuous professional development (CPD). In the UK this is formally regulated by professional bodies such as the Royal Colleges, and is linked to processes of appraisal (Box 1.5) and re-accreditation for established practitioners.

To support this process, outcomes and competences for PPD are being defined at all levels of medical training, including undergraduate and postgraduate study. These sit alongside and complement curricula that focus on discipline-based knowledge and skills.

AUDIT

An important element of reflective learning is audit of clinical practice against recognised standards, many of which are now published as guidelines.

Guidelines

A large number of local and national bodies (e.g. in the UK, SIGN—Scottish Intercollegiate Guidelines Network; NICE—National Institute for Clinical Excellence), as well as international ones (e.g. the World Health Organisation), have produced treatment guidelines based on rigorous and systematic reviews of the medical literature. Although these guidelines are authoritative they are only applicable to certain well-defined situations and do not substitute for good clinical judgement.

INVESTIGATIONS

Modern medical practice has become dominated by sophisticated and often expensive investigations. It is easy to forget that the judicious use of these tools, and the interpretation of the data that they provide, is crucially dependent on good basic clinical skills. Indeed, a test should only be ordered if it is clear that the result will influence the patient's management and the perceived value of the resulting information exceeds the anticipated discomfort, risk and cost of the procedure. Clinicians should therefore analyse their patient's condition carefully and draw up a provisional management plan before requesting any investigations.

THE 'NORMAL' RANGE

Although some tests provide qualitative results (present or absent, e.g. faecal occult blood testing, p. 869), most

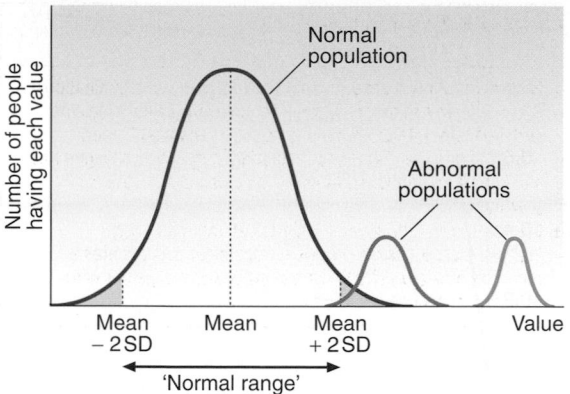

Fig. 1.3 Normal distribution and normal range. For many tests, the frequency distribution of results in the normal healthy population (red line) is a symmetrical bell-shaped curve. The mean ± 2 standard deviations (SD) encompasses 95% of the normal population and usually defines the 'normal range'; 2.5% of the normal population have values above, and 2.5% below, the normal range (shaded areas). For some diseases (blue line), test results overlap with the normal population, or even with the normal range. For other diseases, tests may be more reliable because there is no overlap between the normal and abnormal population (green line).

provide quantitative results (i.e. a value on a continuous numeric scale). In order to classify quantitative results as normal or abnormal, it is necessary to define a 'normal range'. Many quantitative measurements in populations exhibit a bell-shaped, or Gaussian, frequency distribution (Fig. 1.3); this is called a 'normal distribution' and is characteristic of biological variables determined by a complex mixture of genetic and environmental factors (e.g. height) and of test results (e.g. plasma sodium concentration). A normal distribution can be described by the mean value (which places the centre of the bell-shaped curve on the x axis) and the standard deviation (SD, which describes the width of the bell-shaped curve). Within each SD away from the mean there is a fixed percentage of the population. By convention, the 'normal range' is usually defined as those values which encompass 95% of the population, i.e. the values within 2 SDs above and below the mean. If this convention is used, however, 2.5% of the normal population will have values above, and 2.5% will have values below, the normal range.

'Abnormal' results, i.e. those lying beyond 2 SDs from the mean, may occur either because the person is one of the 2.5% of the normal population whose test result is outside the normal range, or because they have a disease characterised by a different result from the test. Test results in 'abnormal' populations also have a bell-shaped distribution with a different mean and SD (Fig. 1.3). In some diseases, there is typically no overlap between results from the normal and abnormal population (e.g. elevated serum creatinine in renal failure, p. 461). In many diseases, however, there is overlap, sometimes extending into the normal range (e.g. elevated serum thyroxine in toxic multinodular goitre, p. 759). In these circumstances, the greater the difference between the test result and the limits of the normal range, the higher the chance that the person has a disease, but there is a risk that results within the normal range may be 'false negatives' and results outside the normal range may be 'false positives'.

Each time a test is performed in a member of the normal population there is a 5% (1 in 20) chance that the result will be outside the 'normal range'. If two tests are performed, the chance that one of them will be 'abnormal' is 10% (2 in 20), and so on; the chance of detecting an 'abnormal' result increases the more tests are performed, so multiple indiscriminate testing should be avoided.

In practice, normal ranges are usually established by performing the test in a number of healthy volunteers who are assumed to be a random sample of the normal population. Not all populations are the same, however, and while it is common to have different normal ranges for tests in men and women, or in children and adults, clinicians need to be aware that normal ranges defined either by test manufacturers or even within the local laboratory may have been established in small numbers of young healthy people who are not necessarily representative of their patient population. This is another reason to recognise that 'normal ranges' do not discriminate perfectly between health and disease.

For some tests, the clinical decision does not depend on whether or not the patient is a member of the normal population. This commonly applies to quantitative risk factors for future disease. For example, higher plasma total cholesterol levels are associated with a higher risk of future myocardial infarction (p. 580 and the Appendix) within the normal population. Although a 'normal range' for cholesterol can be calculated, cholesterol-lowering therapy is commonly recommended for people with values within the normal range; the 'cut-off' value at which therapy is recommended depends upon the presence of other risk factors for cardiovascular disease. The 'normal range' for plasma cholesterol is therefore redundant and the phrase 'normal plasma cholesterol level' is unhelpful. Similar arguments apply for interpretation of values of blood pressure (p. 580), blood glucose (p. 580), bone mineral density (p. 1123) etc.

Some quantitative test results are not normally distributed, usually because a substantial proportion of the normal population will have an unrecordably low result (e.g. serum prostate-specific antigen, p. 511, and serum troponin, p. 525), and the distribution cannot be described by mean and SDs. Alternative statistical procedures can be used to calculate 95th centiles, but it is common in these circumstances to use information from normal and abnormal people to identify 'cut-off' values which are associated with a certain risk of disease, as described below.

SENSITIVITY AND SPECIFICITY

Many tests are potentially hazardous and none is completely reliable. All diagnostic tests can produce false positives (an abnormal result in the absence of disease) and false negatives (a normal test in a patient with disease). The diagnostic accuracy of a test can be expressed in terms of its sensitivity and its specificity (Box 1.6).

Sensitivity is defined as the percentage of the test population who are affected by the index condition and test

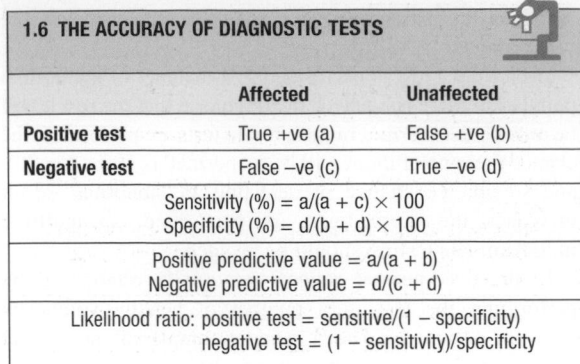

1.6 THE ACCURACY OF DIAGNOSTIC TESTS

	Affected	Unaffected
Positive test	True +ve (a)	False +ve (b)
Negative test	False −ve (c)	True −ve (d)

Sensitivity (%) = a/(a + c) × 100
Specificity (%) = d/(b + d) × 100

Positive predictive value = a/(a + b)
Negative predictive value = d/(c + d)

Likelihood ratio: positive test = sensitive/(1 − specificity)
negative test = (1 − sensitivity)/specificity

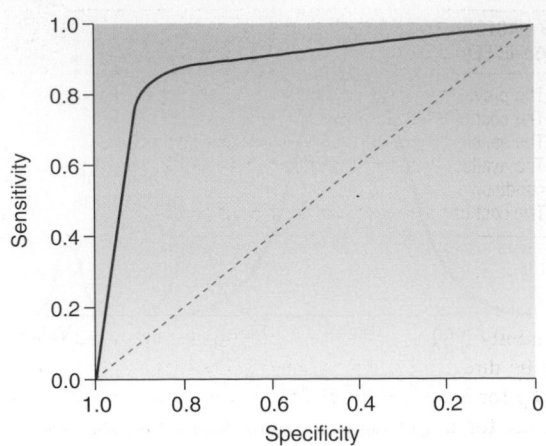

Fig. 1.4   A receiver operating characteristic graph illustrating the trade-off between sensitivity and specificity for a given test. The closer the curve lies to the top left-hand corner, the more useful the test.

positive for it. In contrast, specificity is defined as the percentage of the test population who are healthy and test negative. A very sensitive test will detect most disease but may generate abnormal findings in healthy people. A negative result will therefore reliably exclude disease but a positive test is likely to require further evaluation. On the other hand, a very specific test may miss significant pathology but is likely to establish the diagnosis, beyond doubt, when the result is positive.

In choosing how a test is used to guide decision-making there will be an inevitable trade-off between emphasising sensitivity as opposed to specificity. For example, defining an exercise electrocardiogram (p. 528) as abnormal if there is ≥ 0.5 mm ST depression will ensure that very few cases of coronary artery disease are missed, but will generate a lot of false positive tests (high sensitivity, low specificity). On the other hand, using a cut-off point of ≥ 2.0 mm ST depression will detect most cases of important coronary disease with far fewer false positive results. This trade-off can be illustrated by the receiver operating characteristic curve of the test (Fig. 1.4).

PREDICTIVE VALUE

The predictive value of a test is determined by its sensitivity and specificity, and can be expressed in several ways. The positive predictive value (Box 1.6) is the probability that a patient with a positive test has the index condition, whilst the negative predictive value (Box 1.6) is the probability that a patient with a negative test does not have the condition. The likelihood ratio (Box 1.6) expresses the odds that a given finding would occur in a patient with, as opposed to a patient without, the index condition (as the odds rise above 1 the probability that disease is present rises).

The interpretation, and therefore the utility, of a test is critically dependent on the circumstances in which it is used. For example, 2 mm ST elevation in leads V_2 and V_3 of a 12-lead ECG is likely to represent acute myocardial infarction if the subject is a 54-year-old male with multiple cardiovascular risk factors and severe crushing central chest pain, but will probably be a normal variant if the subject is an 18-year-old asymptomatic Afro-Caribbean man.

The value of a diagnostic test is determined by the prevalence of the condition in the test population (Bayes' theorem). Indeed, the probability that a subject has a particular condition (the post-test probability) can be

1.7 BAYES' THEOREM: POST-TEST LIKELIHOOD OF DISEASE

Positive test
Post-test probability of disease $= \dfrac{pre \times sens}{(pre \times sens) + ((1 - sens) \times (1 - spec))}$

Negative test
Post-test probability of disease $= \dfrac{pre \times (1 - sens)}{(pre \times (1 - sens)) + ((1 - pre) \times spec)}$

(pre = pre-test probability of disease; sens = sensitivity; spec = specificity)

EXAMPLE
Assume: Exercise tolerance testing for the diagnosis of coronary artery disease (CAD) (using cut-off of 2 mm ST depression) has 70% sensitivity (0.7) and 90% specificity (0.9)
The pre-test odds of significant CAD in a 65-year-old woman with atypical angina on effort are 50% (0.5)

Post-test odds of significant CAD will be:

Positive test $\dfrac{0.5 \times 0.7}{(0.5 \times 0.7) + (0.3 \times 0.1)} = 92\%$

Negative test $\dfrac{0.5 \times 0.3}{(0.5 \times 0.3) + (0.5 \times 0.9)} = 25\%$

In contrast, the pre-test probability of significant coronary disease in a 45-year-old man with typical angina on effort would be 90%, with post-test odds of 95% in the event of a positive exercise test and 75% in the event of a negative test.

calculated if the pre-test probability and the sensitivity and specificity of the test are known (Box 1.7). Bayesian analysis dictates that a test is most valuable when there is an intermediate pre-test probability of disease. Clinicians seldom have access to such precise information but must appreciate the importance of integrating clinical and laboratory data.

SCREENING

Many health-care systems run screening programmes in order to detect important (and treatable) disease in

1

1.8 FACTORS THAT INFLUENCE THE COST-EFFECTIVENESS OF HEALTH SCREENING

- The prevalence of the index condition in the target population
- The cost of the screening test
- The sensitivity and specificity of the screening test
- The availability and effectiveness of treatment for the index condition
- The cost of not detecting and treating the condition

1.9 EXPLAINING THE RISKS AND BENEFITS OF THERAPY

Would you take a drug once a day for a year to prevent stroke if:
- it reduced your risk of having a stroke by 47%?
- it reduced your chance of suffering a stroke from 0.26% to 0.14%?
- there was one chance in 850 that it would prevent you having a stroke?
- 849 out of 850 patients derived no benefit from the treatment?
- there was a 99.7% chance that you would not have a stroke anyway?

All these statements are derived from the same data* and describe an equivalent effect.

* MRC trial of treatment of mild hypertension (bendroflumethiazide vs placebo). BMJ 1985; 291:97–104.

1

apparently healthy but at-risk individuals. These initiatives may be directed towards a single pathology (e.g. mammography for breast cancer, p. 255) or may comprise a battery of tests for a wide range of conditions. For the reasons outlined above, screening will inevitably generate a number of false-positive results that require further, potentially expensive and sometimes risky, investigation. This can engender a good deal of unnecessary anxiety for the patient and may create difficult dilemmas for the clinician; for example, it may be difficult to determine how to evaluate minor abnormalities of the liver function tests in an otherwise healthy person (p. 942).

Some of the criteria that must be considered before deciding if the wider costs of a screening programme can be justified are listed in Box 1.8.

ESTIMATING AND COMMUNICATING RISK

Medical management decisions are usually made by weighing up the anticipated benefits of a particular procedure or treatment against the potential risks. Health professionals are increasingly encouraged to involve patients, and their families, in the decision-making process and must therefore be able to explain risk in an accurate and understandable way.

Providing the relevant biomedical facts is seldom sufficient to guide decision-making because a patient's perception of risk is often coloured by emotional, and sometimes irrational, factors. Building trust is the first and most crucial step in establishing good communication and will only be possible if the doctor or health professional displays both care and competence. Most patients will have access to information from a wide variety of sometimes conflicting sources including the Internet, books, magazines, self-help groups, other health-care professionals, friends and family. The clinician must therefore be aware of and sensitive to the way in which these resources influence the patient.

The next step in the decision-making process is to clarify the problem and present the evidence base. Statistics and probabilities can be confusing and data can be presented in many ways (Box 1.9). Relative risk describes the proportional increase in risk; it is a useful measure of the size of an effect. In contrast, absolute risk describes the actual chance of an event, and is what matters to most patients. Terms such as 'common', 'rare', 'probable' and 'unlikely' are elastic. Whenever possible, the clinician should quote numerical

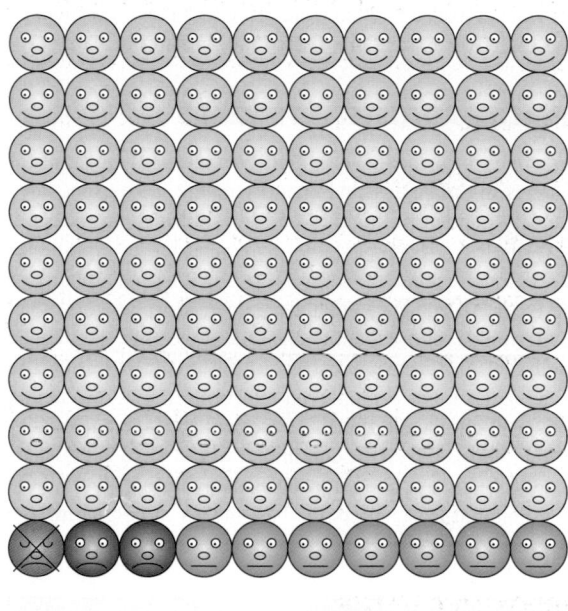

Feel better No difference Stroke Dead

Fig. 1.5 Visual portrayal of benefit and risks of an operation that is expected to relieve symptoms in 90% of patients, but cause stroke in 2% and death in 1%.

information using consistent denominators (e.g. '90 of every 100 patients who have this operation feel much better, 1 will die during the operation and 2 will suffer a stroke'). Positive framing ('There is a 99% chance of survival') and negative framing ('There is a 1% chance of death') may both be appropriate. A variety of visual aids can be used to present complex statistical information in a digestible way (Fig. 1.5).

Finally, it is essential to allow the patient to place their own weighting on the potential benefits and adverse effects of each course of action. Thus, some patients may choose to sacrifice a good chance of pain relief because they are not prepared to run even a small risk of paralysis, whilst others may opt to proceed with very high-risk spinal surgery because they find their current circumstances intolerable.

1

RESOURCES

COST-EFFECTIVENESS

The best available health care can be expensive. No country can now afford to provide unlimited state-of-the-art medicine for all its citizens. Health-care systems must therefore take account of the cost-effectiveness of the treatments they provide. This can create difficult dilemmas for clinicians who may be asked to withhold expensive but effective therapies (e.g. implantable cardioverter defibrillators) from individual patients on the basis that the money will do more good for more patients if it is spent elsewhere.

Whenever possible, funding decisions should be based on evidence rather than anecdote and opinion. The principles of evidence-based medicine are critical to the assessment of cost-effectiveness and are discussed in detail in Chapter 2.

QUALITY-ADJUSTED LIFE YEARS

Outcomes from health care can be measured in terms of changes in the quality and quantity of life. Life expectancy is easily defined but quality of life is difficult to measure. Nevertheless, it is possible to construct a continuum between perfect health (score 1), survival with no quality of life (score 0) and states that are perceived to be worse than death (minus score). Quality and quantity of life can then be combined in a measure known as the quality-adjusted life year (QALY). For example, an intervention that results in a patient living an additional 4 years with an average quality of life rated as 0.6 on the continuum would yield 2.4 QALYs (4×0.6). This sort of approach has many failings but, for the time being at least, offers the best means of comparing the cost-effectiveness of a wide range of treatments.

PRACTISING MEDICINE IN LOW-RESOURCE SETTINGS

The problems associated with medical care in low-resource areas cluster in four domains:

- *Prevention versus cure.* Prevention is easier, cheaper and more effective than cure for many diseases. On the other hand, curative medicine is immediate, highly visible and glamorous. This tension is most evident when a disease is common and the benefits of prevention have yet to be realised. The allocation of adequate resources for long-term prevention needs both political will and social acceptance.
- *Acute versus chronic care.* Acute medical care produces immediate and often gratifying results whilst treating chronic illness can be time-consuming and less rewarding. Facilities for chronic care are therefore accorded a low priority in many health-care systems. Unfortunately, this often results in patients who require long-term care being denied treatment altogether or being managed inappropriately (at high cost) in the acute sector.

- *The ideal versus the possible.* Most medical management guidelines are derived from studies that were conducted in well-resourced health-care systems. In trying to apply this knowledge to the developing world, there are tensions between best practice and what is possible. For example, anticoagulant therapy may pose risks that were not evident in the studies that underpin guidelines if it is prescribed in areas where reliable laboratories are not available and medications that interact with warfarin are commonly purchased 'over the counter'.
- *Channels of health-care provision.* In developing countries health care may be delivered through government-run public clinics (usually free or subsidised services) or non-governmental organisations (sometimes subsidised but usually privately funded services). Many of the available services are too costly for the average patient so, for the benefit of the community as a whole, there is a need for constructive cooperation between all health-care sectors.

The best possible practice is that which can be delivered within the available resources in a specific setting. Compassionate care given with empathy, understanding and good communication is always within the physician's reach, even when physical resources are inadequate.

ETHICS

Ethics is the 'science' of morality. Medical ethics is concerned both with the standards of conduct and competence expected of members of the medical profession, and with the study of ethical problems raised by the practice of medicine. Recent advances in biomedical science and their application to clinical care have thrown up many difficult ethical problems. These include human cloning, the human genome project, eugenics, women's health, new reproductive technologies, antenatal screening, abortion, priority-setting, global medicine, underserved populations, brain death, organ transplantation, end-of-life issues, assisted suicide and advance directives. Detailed discussion of these is beyond the scope of this chapter, but a framework for the application of ethics to medical practice will be described.

In general, ethical problems relate to the intentions or motives of those involved, their actions, the consequences of their actions, and the context in which their actions take place. Ethical problems can be analysed in a variety of ways, and different analytical approaches may lead to different conclusions. To find the best solution, it may be necessary to apply several different analytical approaches and attempt to reconcile the conclusions. In modern medical practice there is not always time to do this systematically. However, the process of applying an ethical framework to a given situation is a key element in clinical decision-making and helps to ensure that a decision is both morally acceptable and legally defensible.

- *Virtue ethics* is concerned with the character of the persons involved and with their actions. Are my intentions (what my actions aim at) and my motives (what moves me to act) good or bad, wise or unwise, sensible or unrealistic, patient-centred or self-centred etc.? Is the course of action I propose to take one which would be considered appropriate by a prudent doctor—or by a prudent patient? The focus here is on the characteristics of a virtuous person. Right action flows from the nature of that person.

- *Deontological ethics* is concerned with whether a proposed action or course of action, in itself and regardless of its consequences, is right or wrong. Is it ever right or always wrong to kill, to tell a lie, to break a promise? Deontological (from the Greek for 'duty') considerations include rights as well as duties, and omissions as well as acts. An action is right if it is in accordance with an established moral rule or principle.
- *Teleological ethics* (or consequentialism) is concerned with the consequences of a proposed action or course of action. Are they likely to be good or bad, in the short term and long term, for the patient, doctor, family and society? What will promote a net balance of good over harm for the individual as well as 'the greatest good of the greatest number'? Who decides (or can predict) what is the 'best' outcome?

An ethical problem can therefore be addressed by trying to decide what a virtuous person would do, whether an action or course of action is right or wrong in itself, or what its consequences might be. Yet the circumstances in which any decision is made will vary, and what may be right in one context may be wrong in another. *Situation ethics* recognises this, emphasising the need to consider carefully the context (or situation) in which a course of action is chosen.

Ethics are applied to the practice of medicine in three broad areas.

- *Clinical ethics* deal with the relationship between clinicians and individual patients.
- *Public health ethics* deal with the health issues of groups of people—the community.
- *Research ethics* deal with issues related to clinical research.

CLINICAL ETHICS

KEY PRINCIPLES OF CLINICAL ETHICS

In clinical ethics, four key principles are frequently used to underpin the analysis of a problem, and are often abbreviated to 'autonomy, beneficence, non-maleficence and justice'.

Respect for persons and their autonomy

This respect is a significant aspect of the relationship between patient and physician. The patient seeks out a physician based on a desire to attain freedom from a disability or disease which limits their ability to exercise their autonomy (the power or right of self-determination). Unless the patient is a child, is unconscious or is mentally incapacitated, it is the patient's choice to seek advice. The

physician must therefore respect the patient's autonomy. This includes the patient's right to refuse therapy. The physician must also actively seek to empower the patient with adequate information. Respect for persons and their autonomy has important implications for truth-telling, informed consent and confidentiality.

Truth-telling

Telling the truth is essential to generating and maintaining trust between the physician and the patient. This includes providing information about the nature of the illness, expected outcome and therapeutic alternatives, and answering questions honestly. The facts should not be given 'brutally' but with due sensitivity to appropriate timing and to the patient's capacity to cope with bad news. There are two rare situations where the truth may, at least for a time, be withheld:

- if it will cause real harm to the patient (e.g. a depressed patient likely to commit suicide who has to be told they have cancer). This is sometimes called therapeutic privilege, since it should be exercised only in the patient's vital interests and for very serious clinical reasons.
- if the patient makes it clear that they do not want to hear the bad news (but always bearing in mind that this may be a stage in the patient's adjustment to their condition).

In no case should false information be given, and the physician should always be prepared to justify any decision to withhold relevant information.

Informed consent

This term describes the participation of a patient in decisions about their health care. In order to facilitate this, the clinician must provide the patient with an adequate explanation of the nature of the decision, and details of the relevant risks, benefits and uncertainties of each possible course of action. The amount of information to provide will vary, depending on the patient's condition and the complexity of the treatment, and on the physician's assessment of the patient's understanding of the situation. Not all options need be explained, but those that a 'prudent patient' would consider significant should be explored—for example, by open questioning (Box 1.3, p. 5).

From both a legal and an ethical perspective the patient retains the right to decide what is in his or her best interests. All adults have decision-making capacity if they can understand the relevant information (which may have to be explained in simple terms), consider the implications of the relevant options, and make a communicable decision. If a patient makes choices that seem irrational or are at variance with professional advice, that does not mean that they lack capacity.

When the patient does lack decision-making capacity, the clinician should always act in the best interests of the patient. In an emergency, consent may be presumed, but only for treatment immediately necessary to preserve the patient's life and health, and if there is no clear evidence that this would be against the previous settled wishes of the patient when competent (for example, blood transfusion in the case of an adult Jehovah's Witness). If the patient has a

1

legally entitled surrogate decision-maker, the consent of the latter should be sought wherever possible. It is also good practice to involve close relatives in decision-making, but the hierarchy of surrogate decision-makers will depend on local laws and culture.

Confidentiality

Confidentiality in relation to the appropriate management of patient-specific information is important in generating and maintaining trust in the physician–patient relationship. Health-care teams must take precautions to prevent un-authorised access to patient records, and may disclose patient-identifying information only when the patient has given consent or when required by law. Where such information is shared with other health-care professionals in order to optimise individual patient care, this should be done on a strictly 'need-to-know' basis.

Beneficence

This is the principle of doing good, or acting in another person's best interests. In clinical ethics, the term refers to the good of the individual patient. It means considering the patient's view of their own best interests as well as their medical best interests. Situations may arise where there is a conflict between what is good for the individual and what is best for society, but the traditional medical approach is that stated in the Declaration of Geneva (World Medical Association): 'The health of my patient will be my first consideration.'

Non-maleficence

This is the principle of doing no harm: in medicine, the traditional *primum non nocere*. In balancing beneficence and non-maleficence (benefit versus risk), the relevant information must be shared with the patient, who can then be helped to make an informed decision.

Justice

Justice relates to the distribution of medical care and allocation of resources. In order to distribute health resources justly, the concept of utility—'greatest good for the greatest number'—must be considered. In the case of individual patients, however, justice is also equated with 'being fair' and 'even-handed'. The concept of fair delivery of health care can be viewed from three perspectives:

- Respect for the *needs* of the individual. Health care is delivered first to those who need it most. This perspective is particularly relevant when need must be assessed by some kind of triage.
- Respect for the *rights* of a person. Everyone who needs health care is entitled to a fair share of the resources available. This perspective is particularly relevant when local or global economic, social, educational or other inequalities prevent or reduce equitable access to health care.
- Respect for *merit*. Health care is delivered on the basis of value judgements, based on financial, political, social or other factors relating to the value of the individual to society. The relevance of this perspective to health care is widely disputed, not least because such value

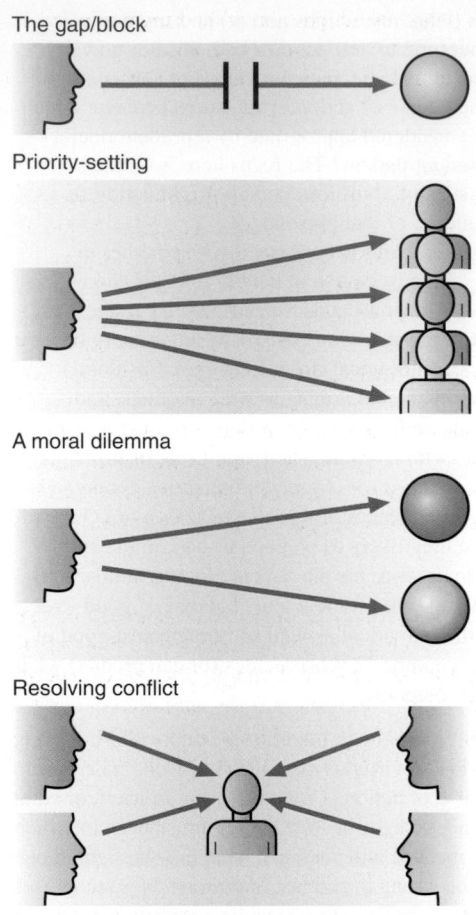

The gap/block

Priority-setting

A moral dilemma

Resolving conflict

Fig. 1.6   A classification of ethical problems.

judgements are difficult to make in practice and to defend ethically.

TYPES OF ETHICAL PROBLEM

When faced with an ethical problem, it is often helpful to characterise it in terms of certain patterns which can be recognised (Fig. 1.6).

A gap or block

The ideal goal is clearly seen but there are major obstacles to achieving it. The obstacles may be economic or social, or in the belief system of the patient. The obvious answer—to bridge the gap or remove the block—may not be possible within the available time frame and resources. A young boy from a poor family in a developing country who has Wilson's disease and needs a liver transplant, is an example of an economic block. Some problems of this kind cannot be resolved satisfactorily in the clinical context until or unless they are resolved in the economic or political context.

Priority-setting

The right course of action is clear, but prioritisation is necessary and the principles to guide that process have to be defined. A decision to allot the last bed in intensive care to either an 80-year-old patient with pneumonia or a 20-year-old with advanced lymphoma is an example. While it is not possible to cover all eventualities, guidelines agreed in advance with relevant stakeholders are often helpful.

A moral dilemma

Acting in accordance with one ethical principle may conflict with another ethical principle. This can create a moral dilemma—a choice between two alternatives, neither of which is ethically satisfactory. For example, a physician may decide that a particular mode of therapy is best (principle of beneficence) while the patient makes a different choice (principle of respect for autonomy). In theory the dilemma can be resolved only if one of the ethical principles is given priority; ethical analysis (see below) can help to achieve this. True moral dilemmas are less common in practice than in theory; apparent dilemmas can often be resolved by good physician–patient communication.

Resolving conflict

A conflict of opinion may arise between members of the team responsible for care of the patient. Differing views should normally be resolved through discussion, but if this does not work, decision-making authority allocated in advance may have to be invoked. The challenge then is to ensure consistent and accurate implementation of the decision.

ETHICAL ANALYSIS

Ethical analysis (or moral reasoning) is the process of thinking through ethical problems and reaching a conclusion. It helps the decision-maker to grow personally and professionally, allows communication of the process by which a decision is made, and permits the process to be constructively criticised. It can be used systematically: for example, in retrospective review of difficult cases. When, in everyday practice, time for reflection is limited, knowledge of methods of moral reasoning provides a useful back-ground and aid for decision-making, and is often employed in ways analogous to those of 'the novice–expert shift' (Box 1.4, p. 6). Some approaches that can be applied are:

- *A principles approach*. This involves analysing an ethical problem in terms of the principles of respect for autonomy, beneficence, non-maleficence and justice. If all of these principles support a particular course of action, then that course of action is probably correct, and there may in fact no longer be an ethical problem. If, however, different principles suggest different courses of action, this approach has no intrinsic mechanism for deciding which principle has priority. On the other hand, analysing the problem in terms of these principles can help to clarify the nature of the ethical problem and the issues which need to be addressed if the problem is to be resolved.
- *A casuistry (cases) approach*. This uses precedent as a guide to what to do. A case is recalled or imagined which is similar to that under discussion, but where the right choice of action/behaviour was obvious. Then the

features which make the present case different, if any, are analysed and considered to see if and why they lead to a different conclusion. A variation on this approach, related to virtue ethics, is to imagine what a physician who was particularly skilled or experienced in this type of situation would do, or how a previous patient might have viewed the problem.

- *A perspectives (or narrative) approach*. This involves considering the views of all the stakeholders—the patient, their family or carers, the health-care team, the health service, and society. The greater the degree of concordance of these views on a particular outcome, the more likely it is that the decision leading to that outcome is right. A narrative approach is similar to this, but involves listening attentively to the different 'stories' told by the stakeholders about the problem and how they perceive it in their own experience. Where these stories differ can provide clues to a more nuanced understanding of the problem and how, if possible, it might be resolved.
- *A counter-argument approach*. A particular course of action is chosen and the best ethical arguments against it are then marshalled and evaluated. This may or may not cause the decision to be reconsidered.
- *Application of rules*. In certain common and clearly defined situations, externally imposed rules (including the law) may require, or guide towards, a specific course of action. This does not obviate the need for ethical analysis. Moreover, any such rules must be reviewed regularly.

While all of these approaches may be useful, it is important to remember that none of them removes the need on the one hand for the exercise of judgement, and on the other for good communication and consensus decision-making. No less important is the need for all of this to be based on sound and shared information about the clinical and human facts of the case. In this respect a useful, integrated way of addressing ethical problems is provided by what has been called:

- *An onion-peel approach*. This uses a layered framework to analyse the problem systematically (Box 1.10).

Discussion with colleagues and others is crucial in reaching ethical decisions. Many hospitals have a Clinical Ethics Committee to review difficult decisions. Up-to-date, accurate, valid and reliable data should inform the decision-making progress. Local legal issues must be considered. Once a conclusion has been reached, a strategy to complete the action must be implemented. Post-hoc evaluation of decisions is important, and again is best carried out collectively by an Ethics Committee or other means of retrospective review.

A CLINICAL ETHICS SCENARIO

A 70-year-old man who has chronic obstructive pulmonary disease, hypertension and diabetes mellitus is admitted to hospital with pneumonia. His memory has been deteriorating for 3 years with a rapid decline in cognition

1

over the last 3 months and he now needs help to carry out his activities of daily living. A neurologist has evaluated him and has excluded reversible causes of dementia. The patient deteriorates and needs mechanical ventilation. His wife states that he told her (when he was well) that he did not want to be put on 'life support machines' and is therefore opposed to mechanical ventilation. Two of his children fail to confirm this and request active treatment. What care should be given?

On the one hand, considered mainly in teleological terms:

The patient is incapable of making an autonomous decision. The closest surrogate indicates that he would have preferred to forego life-sustaining therapy at this stage. (Respect for autonomy might support this.) The consequences of ventilation would probably be to prolong the process of dying (which non-maleficence could argue against) rather than increase his chances of recovery to a good quality of life. Beneficence requires that he receive general care and symptom relief immediately. An appropriate action therefore is not to ventilate the patient but to continue basic medical (fluids, oxygen and antibiotics) and nursing care in a general ward setting in order to optimise patient comfort.

On the other hand, considered in deontological as well as teleological terms:

The present illness is due to a potentially reversible infection. The patient's real preference is uncertain and his family, who have difficulty in looking after him, have expressed different views. In terms of the duty of a physician to make the patient's health the first consideration, and of the patient's right to appropriate health care

regardless of his age or mental condition, it would therefore be appropriate to institute all possible care including ventilation on an intensive care unit.

In practice:

The physician responsible for the patient's care should consider the different courses of action suggested, but not determined, by these ethical analyses, explain the reasons for and against each course of action to the patient's family and, if one of them is the patient's legal surrogate, help that person come to a decision. Where there is no legal surrogate, the physician will have to come to a judgement about what is in the patient's best interests, recognising that, while judgement is always fallible, whatever decision is made must be defensible if challenged on legal or ethical grounds. Decisions that are reached on the basis of ethical and moral reasoning will be relatively easy to defend.

In this case, further discussion of the relevant issues with the relatives and other members of the health-care team led to concordance. The patient was treated by artificial ventilation in the intensive care unit for 3 days. He made a good recovery and appeared grateful for the care he had received.

Some basic concepts related to end-of-life care are discussed in Chapter 12.

PUBLIC HEALTH ETHICS

In public health, there is no equivalent to the patient seeking out a doctor. Educating the public to choose desired (healthy) behaviours is important and a wide range of strategies can be used (Ch. 5). In certain circumstances, an element of coercion, at the expense of autonomy, may be allowable for the public good; for example, in epidemics such as severe acute respiratory syndrome (SARS), travel restrictions may be necessary to prevent spread of the disease. Ethical issues related to lifestyle may also create potential conflict between public health imperatives and the activities of profit-motivated companies (e.g. the tobacco and alcohol industries). Resolution of these conflicts depends on good communication and a political and social will to prioritise health considerations in a legislative framework.

RESEARCH ETHICS

This is primarily concerned with the regulation of clinical studies involving patients or healthy volunteers. Often, patients agree to participate in studies because the evidence of benefit for available therapies, or the superiority of one over another, is inconclusive. In so doing, they may be treated with a therapy that ultimately proves to be inferior to the alternate form being tested. Fully informed consent is therefore essential. Mechanisms of recruitment are crucial. Any degree of coercion or pressure to participate must be avoided. Compensation and reimbursement to subjects, and to investigators, should be proportionate to the effort involved and must not act as an inducement. Mechanisms to compensate subjects in the event of harm must be put in place and made explicit to the subject, and should not rely on the subject having to prove negligence. Subjects should not be enrolled in multiple studies. Formal Research Ethics Committees should scrutinise all proposals to carry out clinical research and monitor the process to its conclusion.

Patients in the control arm of a trial should be offered a universal standard of care for the disease being studied. This may not always be possible and, when trials are carried out in underdeveloped areas by institutions in well-developed countries, the minimum standard of care offered to the control group should be the best intervention available for that disease in that country.

COMPLEMENTARY AND ALTERNATIVE MEDICINE

Complementary and alternative medicine (CAM) refers to a group of medical and health-care systems, practices and products that are not considered to be part of conventional medicine. It covers an enormous and ever-changing range of activities, from well-established physical therapies such as osteopathy to spiritual measures such as prayer specifically for health. Proponents suggest that CAM focuses on the whole person—their lifestyle, environment, diet, and their mental, emotional and spiritual health, as well as their physical complaints.

'Complementary medicine' is the term used to describe the use of these treatments in conjunction with conventional medicine (e.g. acupuncture to reduce pain after surgery). 'Alternative medicine' describes their use in place of conventional medicine (e.g. reflexology instead of anti-inflammatory drugs for arthritis). Clearly most forms of treatment can be used in either way, so the term CAM is often used generically. 'Integrative medicine' describes the use of conventional therapy in combination with one or more complementary therapies for which there is evidence of efficacy and safety.

A variety of different taxonomies are used for CAM therapies. The National Center for Complementary and Alternative Medicine in the USA uses the following classification:

- *Alternative medical systems.* These have their own constructs of theory and practice, often based on ancient historical beliefs. Examples are homeopathy, naturopathy, traditional Chinese medicine and Ayurveda.
- *Mind–body interactions.* These rely on the mind's capacity to influence physical function. Examples are meditation, prayer, mental healing, music therapy and dance.
- *Biologically based therapies.* These involve the use or regulation of an extraneous agent or preparation. Examples include herbal medicine, dietary supplementation and nutritional medicine.
- *Manipulative and body-based methods.* These are based on manipulation or movement of parts of the body. They include osteopathy, chiropractic, reflexology and massage (which is often combined with aromatherapy).
- *Energy therapies.* These involve use of energy fields. Examples include gi gong, reiki and therapeutic touch.

Some forms of CAM are embedded in the cultural norms of particular social and ethnic groups, e.g. traditional Chinese medicine. In Western society, the use of CAM is extensive and growing. For example, in 2002 in the United States, at any one time 36% of the population were using some form of CAM. If prayer for health reasons was included this figure rose to 62%. The most common medical conditions involved were back, neck, head or joint pain, upper respiratory tract infections, anxiety or depression, gastrointestinal symptoms and sleep disturbance.

The popularity of CAM may reflect a lack of confidence in conventional medicine, particularly a belief that it will not help the condition or may cause harm. In contrast, CAM is often perceived to be completely safe; patients may therefore be willing to experiment with it as a 'no-lose' measure. Moreover, many forms of CAM are, regardless of any therapeutic benefit, inherently pleasurable.

SAFETY

Not all CAM therapies are safe; some are toxic in their own right (e.g. dietary supplements containing ephedrine alkaloids—now banned in the USA) and others are harmful if used in combination with conventional treatment (e.g. garlic supplements that interfere with the action of anti-HIV chemotherapy).

There is also potential for harm when alternative medicine is used to treat serious or life-threatening medical conditions if the resultant delay in seeking conventional treatment compromises clinical outcome, in a way that the patient would not have chosen had they been fully informed at the outset.

EVIDENCE

In an era where evidence-based medicine (Ch. 2) is the norm, practitioners and advocates of CAM are increasingly challenged to justify these treatments through independent, well-conducted, randomised controlled clinical trials. In some cases this may be difficult (e.g. the placebo arm of a double-blind trial of acupuncture). In addition, it can be argued that different types and standards of evidence, focusing on patient satisfaction and subjective benefit rather than measurable clinical outcomes, are more appropriate for CAM. The literature in this area is growing rapidly but, at present, only a minority of CAM therapies are supported by evidence that would be acceptable for conventional medicine. These are primarily the 'big five' CAM therapies—homeopathy, osteopathy, chiropractic, acupuncture and herbal medicine. Moreover, where evidence does exist it is often limited to a small subset of the clinical conditions for which the treatment is used.

REGULATION

The 'big five' CAM therapies have professional regulatory frameworks in place, and others are following suit. Nevertheless, for many CAM therapies, there is no established

1

structure of training, certification and accreditation, and practice is effectively open to all. Set against the demanding training and life-long continuous professional development that pertains to conventional medicine, this constitutes an important barrier to integrative medicine.

INTEGRATED HEALTH CARE

There is a considerable popular and political impetus behind moves to integrate CAM with conventional medicine and health care at the level of resource allocation, service design, clinical practice, education and research. Almost 50% of general practices in the UK now offer some form of access to CAM, and this is an increasing trend in hospitals. Historically, patients using both types of therapy have often experienced conflicting advice and value judgements, poor or absent communication between practitioners, and even hostility or ridicule. They often revert to secrecy—an inherently undesirable and potentially dangerous outcome. Integrated healthcare aims to understand and remove the barriers that create such dilemmas for patients. It aims to let them exercise their choice of treatment in an open environment characterised by good communication, respect, and due consideration of autonomy, efficacy and risk.

FURTHER INFORMATION

Books and journal articles
Bligh J. Learning about science is still important. Medical Education 2003; 37:944–945.
BMA Ethics Department. Medical ethics today: the BMA's handbook of ethics and law. 2nd edn. London: BMJ Publishing; 2004.
Boyd KM, Higgs R, Pinching AJ. The new dictionary of medical ethics. London: BMJ Publishing; 1997.
Eisenberg DM, Davis RB, Ettner SL et al. Trends in alternative medicine use in the United States, 1990–1997: results of a follow-up national survey. JAMA 1998; 280(18):1569–1575.
Paling J. Strategies to help patients understand risks. Br J Med 2003; 327:745–748.
Rawlins MD. NICE work—providing guidance to the British National Health Service. New Engl J Med 2004; 351:1383–1385.
Williams JR. Medical ethics manual. Ferney-Voltaire Cedex: World Medical Association; 2005.

Websites
www.gmc-uk.org *UK General Medical Council. The following are available here: Tomorrow's doctors—reports from the UK General Medical Council Education Committee, 1993 and 2002; Good medical practice, May 2001; The new doctor, April 1997.*
www.nice.org.uk *National Institute for Health and Clinical Excellence.*
www.sign.ac.uk *Scottish Intercollegiate Guidelines Network.*
www.who.int *World Health Organization.*

2

J.K. ARONSON

Good prescribing

The purpose of drug therapy is to cure or ameliorate disease or to alleviate symptoms. However, all drugs have adverse effects to a greater or lesser extent. Before prescribing, the potential benefit of therapy should be weighed against the potential harm (the benefit to harm balance, often called the benefit to risk ratio).

WHAT MAKES A GOOD PRESCRIBER?

A good prescriber:

- prescribes only when necessary; this requires assessment of when the balance of benefit to harm is favourable
- chooses medicines that are appropriate to the pathophysiology of the disease; this implies a thorough understanding of that pathophysiology and the pharmacology of the relevant drugs
- chooses a dosage regimen that is appropriate to the disease and the patient; this implies a thorough understanding of drug formulations, their handling by the body, their actions, and the sources of variability in patient responsiveness
- continues therapy for an appropriate time and alters doses during therapy when necessary; this implies careful monitoring of the effects of drugs.

In this chapter the basic principles that the doctor will need to become a good prescriber are outlined.

THE BALANCE OF BENEFIT AND HARM IN DRUG THERAPY

The balance of benefit and harm in drug therapy can be assessed by considering various factors (Box 2.1).

The balance of benefit and harm will be favourable if the disease is life-threatening, the drug highly effective and the only one available, and the risk of serious adverse effects negligible. For example, acetylcysteine is highly effective in preventing liver damage after paracetamol overdose (p. 208), its adverse effects are uncommon and usually mild, and no other agent is as effective.

2.1 FACTORS THAT DETERMINE THE BALANCE OF BENEFIT AND HARM IN DRUG THERAPY		
	Balance of benefit and harm	
Factor	Favourable	Unfavourable
Seriousness of the problem	Life-threatening	Trivial
Efficacy of the drug	High	Low
Seriousness of adverse effects	Trivial	Serious
Frequency of adverse effects	Rare	Frequent
Efficacy of therapeutic alternatives	Poor	Good
Safety of therapeutic alternatives	Poor	Good

The balance of benefit and harm will be unfavourable if the disease is trivial, the drug poorly effective with more effective and safer competitors, and the risk of serious adverse effects high. For example, aminophenazone, used in some countries to treat headache, can cause severe bone-marrow depression, and there are much safer and equally effective alternatives.

Most cases lie somewhere between these two extremes.

When assessing the balance of benefit to harm remember that some drugs can cause adverse effects when given in dosages that are within or only a little above the usual therapeutic range; these drugs are said to have a low therapeutic index (Box 2.2).

Assessment of the balance of benefit and harm is best made by using the tenets that are collectively known as evidence-based medicine.

2.2 SOME DRUGS WITH A LOW THERAPEUTIC INDEX

- Aminoglycoside antibiotics
- Anticoagulants
- Anticonvulsants
- Antihypertensive drugs
- Cardiac glycosides
- Cytotoxic and immunosuppressant drugs
- Drugs that act on the central nervous system
- Oral contraceptives

EVIDENCE-BASED MEDICINE IN DRUG THERAPY

For many years doctors have tried to use the available evidence when making decisions about the use of drugs or other therapeutic measures; this started happening as long ago as the 18th century and perhaps before. However, in the early 1990s it was pointed out that the ways in which they did so were somewhat haphazard. For example, treatment strategies would often be formulated in unsystematic reviews of the published data, using selected pieces of evidence that experts in the field judged to be the most valuable or relevant. Inevitably, bias crept in when such judgements were made. The discipline of evidence-based medicine was therefore invented in order to introduce a more systematic approach to the use of evidence in making therapeutic and other decisions.

This was made possible by:

- the development of statistical techniques for the systematic analysis of data
- the realisation that it was important to analyse all the available data, both published and unpublished
- the development of computerised databases of relevant information, linked to methods by which that information could be traced.

The tenets of evidence-based medicine are that well-formulated questions about medical management, including diagnosis and therapy, can be answered by:

2

- carrying out high-quality, randomised, controlled clinical trials
- tracing all the available evidence
- analysing the evidence systematically
- determining how valid and useful the evidence is
- applying the evidence to the management of the individual patient.

Although there are well-established methods for carrying out the first four of these procedures, it is the last that is the most important and the most difficult. This is because the evidence on which decisions are made is usually derived from large populations, which may not have included patients like those the prescriber wants to treat; even if the trials were representative of such patients, there is so much interindividual variability that mean values taken from studies of populations may not be applicable to individuals. Methods for dealing with this are available, but are not as well developed or easily applied as the methods for obtaining the evidence. In addition, there are many therapeutic problems for which adequate evidence is not available at all; in such cases one uses what evidence there is, indifferent though it may be.

This chapter deals with the ways in which evidence-based medicine can inform drug therapy. However, the principles apply equally well to other forms of patient care, including examination, investigation and other forms of treatment.

BENEFICIAL EFFECTS AND THE NUMBER NEEDED TO TREAT (NNT$_B$)

Benefit in drug therapy is often expressed as the so-called number needed to treat (NNT or NNT$_B$), which is the number of patients that would need to be treated in order to prevent one clinical event (for example, a stroke or a pregnancy). A simple example illustrates how this is calculated. Of 239 patients with the acute pain of third molar extraction, 122 were given placebo, of whom nine (7.4%) had at least 50% pain relief by 6 hours, compared with 65 (55.6%) of the 117 patients who were given ibuprofen; the difference was therefore 55.6–7.4 = 48.2%, or an effect size of 0.482. This is known as the absolute risk reduction, and the NNT$_B$ is the inverse of this: 1/0.482 = 2.1. In other words one out of every two people who take a single dose of ibuprofen will have better than 50% pain relief in the 6 hours after the dose. The 95% confidence interval of this estimate (the calculation of which is more complicated) was 1.7 to 2.6; in other words, the mean estimate of the NNT$_B$ was 2.1 and there was a 95% chance that the true value lay between 1.7 and 2.6.

When a drug is given repeatedly, rather than as a single dose, the duration of therapy also has to be stated. For example, in a systematic analysis of the use of warfarin to prevent strokes in patients with atrial fibrillation there were 53 strokes in 1450 patients who took warfarin (3.66%) and 133 in 1450 patients who took placebo (9.17%). The effect size was thus 9.17–3.66 = 5.51% (0.0551) and the NNT$_B$ was 18 (1/0.0551). The confidence interval was 14 to 27. So, on the basis of these results, if 18 patients are treated with warfarin for 1 year, one stroke will be prevented. Note that these numbers cannot be multiplied up to longer durations of treatment; in other words, this analysis does not imply that if 18 patients have treated for 2 years, two strokes will be prevented; a longer trial would be needed to find out what the actual value was.

For a further perspective on the meaning of the NNT$_B$, consider oral contraception. On average a woman who has unprotected sex for 1 year has a 40% chance of becoming pregnant, while a woman who takes some form of oral contraception has a 3% chance; this 37% difference translates into an NNT$_B$ of 2.7 (1/0.37). Now because oral contraception is so effective it might be expected that the NNT$_B$ would be very close to 1, but that is not so, since the NNT$_B$ takes into account the rate that occurs without treatment. In other words if 100 women are treated for a year with an oral contraceptive 37 (100/2.7) pregnancies will be prevented. But 97 of the women taking the treatment do not become pregnant; that is because the other 60 women would not have become pregnant anyway, even without treatment. Of course, that means that they have taken the treatment without benefit and may have had adverse effects as well; however, it would not have been possible to identify the women likely to benefit, either in advance or even retrospectively.

ADVERSE EFFECTS AND THE NUMBER NEEDED TO TREAT FOR HARM (NNT$_H$)

The other side of the coin, the number needed to treat for harm to occur (NNH or NNT$_H$), can be similarly calculated from data on adverse effects of drugs. For example, in a meta-analysis of 13 trials of the effect of thiazide diuretics in essential hypertension, 205 out of 3275 patients taking a thiazide had erectile impotence, compared with 67 out of 5295 patients taking placebo; the NNT$_H$ for this effect is 20 (Box 2.3).

THE BALANCE OF BENEFIT AND HARM ASSESSED FROM THE NNT$_B$ AND NNT$_H$

Although one might expect to be able to express the balance of benefit to harm as the simple ratio of the NNT$_B$ to the NNT$_H$, the comparison is not straightforward, since the quality of the benefit and the severity of the harm also need to be considered. How, for example, can we compare the benefit of long-term oral anticoagulation in patients with atrial fibrillation (the prevention of embolic stroke) with the harm that anticoagulation can cause (gastrointestinal haemorrhage)?

However, knowing the numbers can help. Consider, for instance, tamoxifen, which prolongs survival in breast cancer (by an anti-oestrogenic action) and reduces the risk of myocardial infarction (by an oestrogenic effect on blood lipids), but can cause endometrial cancer and venous thromboembolism:

- NNT$_B$ to prevent one death = 17
- NNT$_B$ to prevent one myocardial infarction = 29

2

2.3 CALCULATION OF NNT$_H$, RISK RATIO AND ODDS RATIO

(A) A THEORETICAL CASE				(B) A REAL CASE*			
Group	Number with adverse event	Number without adverse event	Total	Group	Number with adverse event	Number without adverse event	Total
Active treatment	a	b	a+b	Drug	205	3070	3275
Placebo	c	d	c+d	Placebo	67	5228	5295
Total	a+c	b+d	a+b+c+d	Total	272	8298	8570

1. Calculation of number needed to treat for harm (NNT$_H$)
Rate of event in treated group = a/(a+b)
Rate of event in placebo group = c/(c+d)
Difference (absolute harm increase) = a/(a+b) − c/(c+d) = A
NNT$_H$ = 1/A

2. Calculation of relative risk (RR)
Rate of event in treated group = a/(a+b)
Rate of event in placebo group = c/(c+d)
Relative risk = [a/(a+b)]/[c/(c+d)]

3. Calculation of odds ratio (OR)
Odds of event in treated group = a/b
Odds of event in placebo group = c/d
Odds ratio = (a/b)/(c/d)

1. Calculation of number needed to treat for harm (NNT$_H$)
Rate of event in treated group = 205/3275
Rate of event in placebo group = 67/5295
Difference (absolute harm increase) = 205/3275 − 67/5295 = 0.0499
$$NNT_H = \frac{1}{0.0499} = 20$$

2. Calculation of risk ratio (RR)
Rate of event in treated group = 205/3275
Rate of event in placebo group = 67/5295
Relative risk = [205/3275]/[67/5295] = 5.0 (i.e. a five-fold risk)

3. Calculation of odds ratio (OR)
Odds of event in treated group = 205/3070
Odds of event in placebo group = 67/5228
Odds ratio = [205/3070]/[67/5228] = 5.2 (i.e. relative odds of about 5 to 1 on)

* Erectile impotence with thiazide diuretics in hypertension over a mean of 4 years, a meta-analysis of 13 RCTs (Hypertension 1999; 34:710).

- NNT$_H$ for one case of endometrial cancer = 143
- NNT$_H$ for one venous thromboembolism = 130

These figures suggest that treating 1000 women with breast cancer for 2–5 years will prevent about 60 deaths and 34 myocardial infarctions, at the cost of 7 cases of endometrial cancer and 7 cases of venous thrombo-embolism, clearly a favourable benefit to harm balance. Of course, calculations of this sort yield probabilities that relate to the patients that have been studied in clinical trials. They do not necessarily apply to the whole population and they certainly do not predict what the outcome will be in the individual case.

There are other ways of expressing results of this kind. For example, it is possible to calculate the risk ratio (RR) or odds ratio (OR), each with its confidence interval (Box 2.3). The larger the effect, the higher the odds ratio is relative to the risk ratio—at incidences of up to about 15% the risk ratio and odds ratio are very similar, but at higher incidences the odds ratio starts to overestimate the risk ratio considerably. Note that two treatments can have exactly the same risk ratio but different values of NNT$_H$. For example, a treatment that increased the risk of an adverse event from 1% to 2% would have a risk ratio of 2 but an NNT$_H$ of 100 (1/0.01), while a treatment that increased the risk of an adverse event from 25% to 50% would also have a risk ratio of 2 but an NNT$_H$ of 4 (1/0.25), a much more important effect. When it was reported that third-generation progestogens approximately doubled the risk of deep venous thrombosis compared with older progestogens, the announcement caused some women to panic; what they did not appreciate was that the baseline risk was very low and the NNT$_H$ therefore very high.

OBTAINING THE BEST EVIDENCE

Although the well-designed, large, randomised clinical trial (RCT), preferably placebo-controlled, is the gold standard for obtaining the best evidence, there are other ways. Some of these are listed in Box 2.4, roughly in the order of the quality of evidence they yield. This order is slightly different from the order that others have proposed, because in the author's view a well-designed RCT is more reliable than a meta-analysis of the same size; however, a very large meta-analysis (i.e. one that is much bigger than the largest RCT) may provide better evidence. Furthermore, depending on

2.4 SOME METHODS OF OBTAINING EVIDENCE IN DRUG THERAPY

- Prospective, randomised, double-blind, placebo-controlled trial*
- Prospective, randomised, double-blind, comparative trial (drug vs. drug)*
- Systematic review (meta-analysis)*
- Systematic review (other types of analysis)*
- Cohort study*
- Case-control study*
- Point prevalence study*
- Subgroup analysis of a large trial (generates hypotheses for further trials)
- N-of-one trial
- Other trials (e.g. non-randomised, non-controlled, historical controls, retrospective analysis)
- Non-systematic review
- Case report

* All assumed to be of the same size.

the quality of the design and conduct, the evidence that any of these forms of study provides can vary; for instance, a well-conducted cohort study may provide better evidence than a poorly designed RCT. This hierarchy should not therefore be taken as an absolute measure of the quality of evidence, because in different circumstances one form of evidence may be better than another. For example, in studies of drugs that lower the serum cholesterol concentration, large randomised controlled trials will indicate whether a drug works or not, but observational studies, such as case-control studies, are much better for elucidating dose-response relations.

One of these methods is worthy of brief further mention, the N-of-one (or controlled single-patient) trial. As mentioned above, it can be difficult to extrapolate from the results of large randomised clinical trials to the practical application of drug therapy in the individual patient. In some cases, evidence from large RCTs may not even be available (if, for example, the disease is rare). In such cases an N-of-one trial may help. Here the patient is given either the active drug or a matching placebo at different times and double-blind, and the response to each is noted; thus, in N-of-one trials patients act as their own controls. This type of trial can provide useful information about the effect of a drug in the symptomatic treatment of chronic stable conditions in an individual only if the course of the disease is predictable, if the treatment has a rapid and easily measured therapeutic effect, and if the effect of a single dose of the drug is not long-lasting.

DRUG DISCOVERY AND DEVELOPMENT

Most drug discovery nowadays is carried out by pharmaceutical companies, although they rely heavily on research done in academic institutions. Governments in developed countries spend about twice as much on drug research as pharmaceutical companies. Current estimates of the costs to a company of developing a new drug range from $200 million to $800 million.

DRUG DISCOVERY

There are several ways in which drugs are discovered:

- *Herbal or traditional remedies*: for example, morphine from the opium poppy (*Papaver somniferum*), atropine from deadly nightshade (*Atropa belladonna*), digitoxin and digoxin from foxgloves (*Digitalis purpurea* and *Digitalis lanata* respectively) and new antimalarial drugs from the *Artemisia* species.
- *From studying endogenous agents in animals*: for example, insulin from dog pancreas and the anticoagulant hirudin from the medicinal leech (*Hirudo medicinalis*).
- *Serendipity*: for example, penicillins from Alexander Fleming's chance observation of the effect of *Penicillium* mould on bacterial growth, the sulphonylureas from observations of the hypoglycaemic

effects of sulphonamides in patients being treated for typhoid fever, and the observation that sildenafil, which was developed for angina, caused penile erection.
- *Metabolites of existing drugs*: for example, paracetamol (the main metabolite of phenacetin), oxazepam (a metabolite of chlordiazepoxide) and mesalazine (the active metabolite of sulfasalazine).
- *Empirical chemistry plus applied pharmacology*, to date the most productive process. The structures of existing compounds with known effects (for example, through endogenous pharmacology or action in some screening test) are modified until active compounds are found; examples include the development of β-blockers based on isoprenaline and histamine H_2-receptor antagonists based on histamine.
- *Rational design based on pharmacology*: for example, the development of levodopa for Parkinson's disease after the discovery of dopamine in the brain and its role as a neurotransmitter and the synthesis of monoclonal antibodies specific to receptors that have been identified as suitable targets.
- *Rational design based on the human genome*; this has been trumpeted as a future method of drug discovery, but has so far been disappointing.

DRUG DEVELOPMENT

When a new drug has been discovered it goes through a defined developmental process, after which it is licensed for use and marketed.

Preclinical pharmacology and toxicology

Preclinical studies include extensive pharmacological testing in vitro and in animals, including short-term and long-term toxicity testing.

Clinical testing (volunteer studies)

Next, the drug's pharmacokinetics are studied after single and multiple doses. If it has measurable effects in healthy people its human pharmacology is studied, adverse effects are recorded, and clinical, biochemical and haematological toxicity are assessed. In some cases (for example, drugs for AIDS or cancer) healthy volunteer studies are not possible and the drug is tried immediately in patients.

Phase I studies

Phase I studies in patients or healthy volunteers concentrate on the clinical pharmacology of the drug, its short-term safety, its likely efficacy, its pharmacological effects and its pharmacokinetics in disease. These early studies also provide information about the likely effective dose.

Phase II studies

In phase II studies further evidence of safety and efficacy is obtained in larger numbers of patients, with further attention to dose-ranging and adverse effects.

Phase III studies

Phase III studies are full-scale clinial trials.

MARKETING AND POST-MARKETING SURVEILLANCE

If the regulatory authorities are convinced about quality, safety and efficacy, the drug will be formulated as a medicinal product, which will receive a product licence and be marketed for approved indications.

Surveillance of the effects of a new drug continues after marketing, both formally and informally. There is a post-marketing surveillance scheme in the UK, in which research into adverse drug reactions after marketing is performed, and doctors are encouraged to report suspected adverse effects informally to regulatory agencies (for example, the yellow card scheme in the UK and Medwatch in the USA). If new serious adverse effects are noted the drug may be withdrawn or its licensed indications may be changed. Examples in the UK include:

- aspirin, which is now restricted to those over 16 years of age, because of the risk of Reye's syndrome
- clozapine, for which a blood monitoring scheme is mandatory, in order to detect agranulocytosis as soon as it occurs
- thalidomide, which, having been withdrawn, has been reintroduced into therapy for different indications, although it has not been relicensed and is contraindicated in premenopausal women
- cisapride, which was suspended in 2000 pending further information on the risk of cardiac arrhythmias; it was subsequently withdrawn by the manufacturers
- rofecoxib, which was withdrawn from the market by the manufacturers in 2004 because of an increased risk of stroke.

PRACTICAL PRESCRIBING

WHEN TO PRESCRIBE A DRUG

Drug therapy is not always necessary. For example, a mild tremor in Parkinson's disease may not be unduly troublesome; even though drug treatment can alleviate it, it may also cause unwanted effects, outweighing the benefit. Do not be tempted to prescribe a drug simply to end a consultation. If a patient expects drug therapy, discuss the pros and cons. Try to estimate the balance of benefit and harm and prescribe only if it seems favourable.

HOW TO CHOOSE A DRUG TO PRESCRIBE

If the decision is made to prescribe a drug, the first step will be to choose the therapeutic class. Sometimes the choice is restricted, sometimes wide, as a few examples illustrate (Box 2.5).

Having chosen the class of drug, the next step is to choose the group of drugs within that class. Again the choice may be restricted or wide (Box 2.6). The choice of an anti-

2.5 EXAMPLES OF CHOOSING A THERAPEUTIC CLASS OF DRUG

Indication	Therapeutic class
Infection	Antibiotic
Depression	Antidepressant
Acute attack of asthma	Bronchodilators
Diabetes mellitus	Oral hypoglycaemic drugs Insulin
Congestive cardiac failure	Diuretics ACE inhibitors Vasodilators
Hypertension	Diuretics ACE inhibitors β-adrenoceptor antagonists Calcium antagonists

2.6 EXAMPLES OF CHOOSING A GROUP OF DRUGS FROM WITHIN A CLASS

Therapeutic class	Therapeutic group
Anticoagulants	Coumarin anticoagulants Heparins Thrombin inhibitors
Diuretics	Thiazides Loop diuretics Potassium-sparing diuretics
Antibiotics	Penicillins Cephalosporins Tetracyclines Aminoglycosides Macrolides Quinolones

2.7 EXAMPLES OF CONTRAINDICATIONS TO ANTIBIOTICS

Antibiotic	Example of contraindication
Penicillins	Allergy
Quinolones	Pregnancy and children (teratogenic in animals)
Sulphonamides	Late pregnancy (risk of kernicterus in neonate)
Tetracyclines	Children (affects growing bones and teeth) Renal impairment (e.g. elderly people)

coagulant depends on whether short-term or long-term treatment is indicated. The choice of a diuretic in the treatment of cardiac failure depends on the severity of the problem, whether acute or chronic therapy is indicated, the convenience of the timing of the diuresis, and potassium balance. The choice of an antibiotic depends on the sensitivities of the infecting organism, the site of infection and contraindications, as some examples show (Box 2.7).

Drug interactions can also affect therapy, as in the case of antibiotics (Box 2.8).

The last step is to choose a particular drug from within the class. In some cases the choice is unimportant. For example, all thiazide diuretics have equal efficacy and adverse effects.

2.8 EXAMPLES OF DRUG INTERACTIONS WITH ANTIBIOTICS

Antibiotic	Interacting drug	Mechanism	Effect
Gentamicin	Furosemide	Additive	Ototoxicity
Metronidazole	Alcohol	Inhibition of aldehyde dehydrogenase	'Disulfiram reaction'
Metronidazole	Warfarin	Inhibition of metabolism	Potentiation of anticoagulation
Rifampicin	Oestrogens (oral contraceptives)	Induction of metabolism	Reduced contraceptive effect
Rifampicin	Warfarin	Induction of metabolism	Reduced effect of warfarin
Tetracycline	Antacids	Chelation	Reduced effect of tetracycline
Tetracycline	Warfarin	Altered clotting factor activity	Potentiation of anticoagulation

2

2.9 EXAMPLES OF CHOOSING A PARTICULAR DRUG FROM WITHIN A GROUP

Therapeutic group	Drug
Thiazide diuretics	Bendroflumethiazide Chlorothiazide Cyclopenthiazide Hydrochlorothiazide Hydroflumethiazide Polythiazide
Penicillins	Benzylpenicillin (penicillin G) Phenoxymethylpenicillin (penicillin V) Amoxicillin Co-amoxiclav (amoxicillin + clavulanic acid) Ampicillin Flucloxacillin Azlocillin Ticarcillin

In contrast, the choice of a specific penicillin is important and will depend on the infection and the organism causing it (Box 2.9).

HOW TO MAKE A RATIONAL CHOICE

Many factors dictate the choice of a particular drug:

- *Absorption.* Generally try to choose drugs that are well absorbed. Bumetanide is better absorbed than furosemide, particularly when the gut is congested in heart failure, in which oral bumetanide may be effective if oral furosemide has failed; alternatively use intravenous furosemide.
- *Distribution.* The distribution of a drug to a particular tissue sometimes dictates choice; for example, tetracyclines are concentrated in the bile, and lincomycin and clindamycin in bones.
- *Metabolism.* In severe liver disease try to avoid drugs that are extensively metabolised (for example, opiate analgesics). Genetic factors can influence the extent of metabolism of a drug. Although many examples of such variability have been described, these factors do not make a large impact on drug prescribing; however, some important examples are listed in Box 2.10.
- *Excretion.* In renal insufficiency try to avoid drugs that are extensively excreted; for example, avoid the aminoglycoside antibiotics if alternative antibiotics are suitable.
- *Efficacy.* One would generally choose drugs that have the highest efficacy, although that is not always necessary if the less efficacious drug is adequate and easier or safer to use. Insulin is more efficacious at lowering the blood sugar than the oral hypoglycaemic drugs, but the latter can often be satisfactorily used in type 2 diabetes.
- *Features of the disease.* Choose an antibiotic to match the known or suspected sensitivity of the infective organism; for example, amoxicillin for a patient with a community-acquired bronchopneumonia (p. 691), since the likeliest organisms will be the pneumococcus (*Streptococcus pneumoniae*) or *Haemophilus influenzae*; sputum culture, with identification of the organism and its sensitivity to different antibiotics, will help.
- *Severity of disease.* Mild pain will generally respond to aspirin or paracetamol; more severe pain may require more potent analgesics, such as codeine phosphate or even morphine. Mild hypertension often responds to a single drug, such as a thiazide diuretic or a β-adrenoceptor antagonist (β-blocker); more severe hypertension may require a combination (p. 613).
- *Coexisting diseases.* In hypertension coexisting left ventricular failure would prompt the use of a diuretic combined with an ACE inhibitor whilst coexisting angina pectoris without heart failure would prompt the use of a β-blocker.
- *Avoiding adverse effects.* In asthma avoid β-blockers. In penicillin hypersensitivity choose an alternative drug (for example, a cephalosporin in bronchopneumonia). Genetic factors can increase the risk of an adverse drug reaction; some important examples are listed in Box 2.10.
- *Avoiding adverse drug interactions.* Avoid non-steroidal anti-inflammatory drugs, which can cause gastrointestinal bleeding, in patients taking warfarin. Avoid tetracyclines, sulphonamides, chloramphenicol and the antifungal imidazoles (e.g. ketoconazole) in patients taking warfarin, since they inhibit its metabolism.
- *Patient adherence to therapy.* Atenolol, which can be taken once daily, is often prescribed instead of short-acting β-blockers, in the hope that minimising

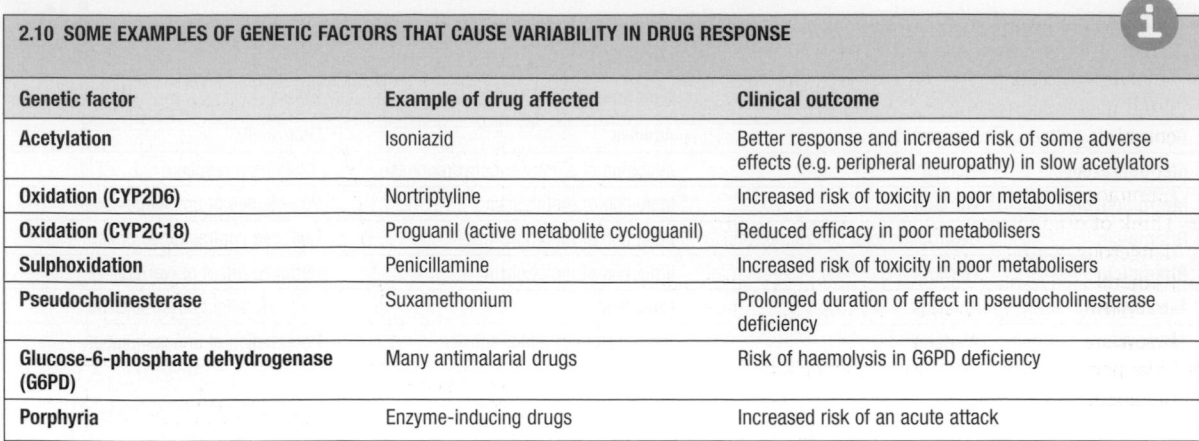

2.10 SOME EXAMPLES OF GENETIC FACTORS THAT CAUSE VARIABILITY IN DRUG RESPONSE

Genetic factor	Example of drug affected	Clinical outcome
Acetylation	Isoniazid	Better response and increased risk of some adverse effects (e.g. peripheral neuropathy) in slow acetylators
Oxidation (CYP2D6)	Nortriptyline	Increased risk of toxicity in poor metabolisers
Oxidation (CYP2C18)	Proguanil (active metabolite cycloguanil)	Reduced efficacy in poor metabolisers
Sulphoxidation	Penicillamine	Increased risk of toxicity in poor metabolisers
Pseudocholinesterase	Suxamethonium	Prolonged duration of effect in pseudocholinesterase deficiency
Glucose-6-phosphate dehydrogenase (G6PD)	Many antimalarial drugs	Risk of haemolysis in G6PD deficiency
Porphyria	Enzyme-inducing drugs	Increased risk of an acute attack

the frequency of drug administration will improve patient adherence.

- *Cost.* If two drugs are of equal efficacy and safety, one would generally choose the cheaper. However, pharmacoeconomics (beyond the scope of this text) is a complicated subject, and the true costs of drug therapy cannot always be calculated merely on the basis of the relative costs of two drugs.

CHOOSING THE ROUTE OF ADMINISTRATION

There are several reasons for choosing a particular route of administration, as some examples illustrate (Box 2.11).

2.11 REASONS FOR CHOOSING A PARTICULAR ROUTE OF ADMINISTRATION

Reason	Example
Only one route possible	Dopamine (intravenous) Glibenclamide (oral)
Patient adherence	Phenothiazines and thioxanthenes (intramuscular depot injections in schizophrenia)
Poor absorption	Furosemide (intravenous, in severe heart failure)
Vomiting	Phenothiazines (rectal) Sumatriptan (nasal spray)
Avoiding first-pass metabolism	Glyceryl trinitrate (sublingual)
Rapid action	Glyceryl trinitrate (sublingual) Sumatriptan (nasal spray)
Direct access to the site of action	Bronchodilators (inhalation, in asthma) Corticosteroids (rectal, in ulcerative colitis) Local application to skin, eyes, etc.
Ease of access	Benzodiazepines (rectal diazepam if intravenous access is difficult in status epilepticus) Subcutaneous fluids (hypodermoclysis)
Controlled release	Insulin (subcutaneous)

CHOOSING A FORMULATION

Oral formulations include tablets, capsules, granules, elixirs and suspensions. Drugs for injection come as lyophilised powders for reconstitution before injection, or as solutions ready for injection; solutions come in single-dose ampoules, single-dose or multiple-dose vials, and half-litre or litre bottles for infusion. Some examples show how the choice of formulation can be important.

Lithium salts and theophylline come in several different ordinary and modified-release formulations, each with different absorption characteristics. A formulation that produces adequate serum lithium or theophylline concentrations in one patient may not be suitable for another, and it is sometimes worth changing the formulation if serum concentrations are suboptimal. These are examples of drugs that should be prescribed by specific brand name rather than the non-proprietary name.

Iron salts are available as tablets for twice- or thrice-daily administration or as modified-release formulations for once-daily administration. Adverse effects are fewer with the modified-release formulations, but the iron is more erratically absorbed. It is usual to start with an ordinary formulation of iron and change to a modified-release formulation if adverse effects are intolerable.

CHOOSING A DOSAGE REGIMEN

The dose of the drug, and the frequency and timing of its administration constitute the dosage regimen. Each prescription should be treated as an experiment to try to find the regimen that produces the best therapeutic effect with minimal adverse effects, according to some simple principles:

- Generally, start with a dosage at the lower end of the recommended dosage range. Exceptions to this rule include glucocorticoids and carbimazole, which are begun in high dosages and then reduced to maintenance dosages. Some drugs are given in a loading dose (for example, digoxin, warfarin and amiodarone), followed by a maintenance dose.

2

- Increase the dosage slowly, monitoring the therapeutic effect at regular intervals and looking for adverse effects.
- If adverse effects occur, reduce the dosage or try another drug; in some cases lower dosages may be possible by combining drugs (for example, azathioprine reduces glucocorticoid dosage requirements in immunosuppression).
- Think of drug interactions and avoid potentially dangerous combinations.
- Remember that pharmacokinetic and pharmacodynamic variability can alter dosage requirements, as discussed below.
- Take particular care with drugs that have a low therapeutic index.

PHARMACOKINETIC VARIABILITY

Because absorption, distribution and elimination of drugs vary from patient to patient, flexibility in dosages is necessary. The examples in Box 2.12 show how to respond to differences or changes in pharmacokinetics.

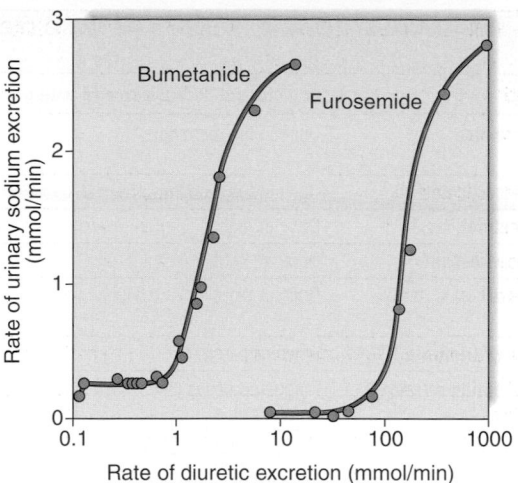

Fig. 2.1 **Dose-response curves for bumetanide and furosemide.** The two drugs have different potencies (the doses required to produce the same effect differ) but the same efficacy (the maximal effect is the same).

2.12 THERAPEUTIC APPROACHES TO PHARMACOKINETIC PROBLEMS

Pharmacokinetic problem	Therapeutic approach
Poor absorption	Increase the dose Choose another route of administration Use another drug
Altered tissue distribution	One-off doses may have to be altered Usually does not affect chronic therapy, unless distribution to the target tissue is altered; may have to choose a different drug
Altered protein binding	Usually does not affect long-term doses (but does alter steady-state total plasma drug concentration)
Reduced renal elimination	Reduce dosage (use creatinine clearance as a guide)
Reduced hepatic elimination	Low-clearance drugs*: reduce oral and intravenous doses High-clearance drugs*: reduce oral (but not intravenous) doses
* Box 2.15.	

PHARMACODYNAMIC VARIABILITY

Pharmacological responses are usually governed by the dose-response curve. An example is seen in Figure 2.1, which shows the effects of two loop diuretics, bumetanide and furosemide, on urinary sodium excretion. The two diuretics have different potencies, which can be dealt with by using different dosages; however, they both have the same efficacy, so that comparable dosages should produce the same diuretic effect.

Variability in dose-responsiveness dictates flexibility in prescribing. If a therapeutic effect does not occur with the first dosage chosen, an effect may be achieved by making small increases within the therapeutic dosage range. Of course, increasing the dosage will also increase the risk of adverse effects. Certain diseases can alter a dose-response curve (for example, there is resistance to digoxin in hyperthyroidism) and the pharmacodynamics of a drug can be affected by another drug.

CHOOSING THE FREQUENCY OF DRUG ADMINISTRATION

It is thought that patient adherence to therapy is improved if drugs are given only once or twice daily, rather than three or four times, although the evidence that this is true is scanty. However, it makes sense to simplify the therapeutic regimen. In general, therefore, try to choose drugs that can be given no more than twice daily. A modified-release formulation can be useful in this respect. In some special cases the frequency of drug administration is an important consideration in therapy (Box 2.13).

CHOOSING THE TIME OF DRUG ADMINISTRATION

For many drugs the time of administration is unimportant. However, there are occasionally pharmacokinetic or therapeutic reasons for giving drugs at particular times (Box 2.13). Meal times do not usually affect drug administration, since although food may reduce the speed of absorption of a drug it generally does not reduce the extent of absorption; tetracyclines are an exception—their absorption is greatly reduced by divalent and trivalent cations, and they should not be taken with food or antacids. Food sometimes helps to reduce adverse gastrointestinal effects; for instance, the effects of aspirin on the stomach are partly reduced by taking it with food.

2.13 SOME SPECIAL EXAMPLES OF FREQUENCY AND TIMING OF DRUG ADMINISTRATION

Drug	Recommended frequency or timing	Reasons
Furosemide	Once in the morning	Kidney refractory to a second dose within 6 hours; night-time diuresis undesirable
Glucocorticoids	Once in the morning	Minimises inhibitory effects on adrenal function
Salmeterol	Once at night	Prevents early morning symptoms
Antidepressants	Once at night	Allows adverse effects to occur during sleep
Digoxin	Once at night	So that when blood samples for plasma concentration measurement are taken it is at least 6 hours after the last dose
Glyceryl trinitrate	When required	Relief of acute symptoms
Long-acting nitrates	Staggered doses (see *British National Formulary*)	To avoid tolerance
Tetracyclines	2 hours before or after food	Divalent and trivalent cations chelate tetracyclines
Opiates	In anticipation of pain	Better relief in chronic pain
Levodopa	Several times a day	Dictated by the duration of action (often wears off quickly during long-term therapy)
Statins	Once at night	Inhibition of HMG CoA reductase is greater at night

ALTERING DRUG DOSAGES IN SPECIAL CIRCUMSTANCES

ALTERING DOSAGES IN RENAL INSUFFICIENCY

If a drug is more than 50% eliminated unchanged by the kidneys or has active metabolites that are eliminated by the kidneys, the maintenance dosage must be altered in renal insufficiency; it is not usually necessary to alter a one-off dose. Creatinine clearance can be used as a guide to reducing maintenance dosages; the serum creatinine concentration can also be used, but it is a less reliable indicator of renal function and does not rise above the reference range until renal function is impaired by at least 50%.

In some cases dosages should be reduced because the pharmacological effects interact with renal impairment (for example, ACE inhibitors worsen potassium retention). Some drugs should be avoided entirely in renal insufficiency, for either pharmacokinetic or pharmacodynamic reasons (Box 2.14).

Diuretics are relatively ineffective in severe renal insufficiency, partly because they cannot gain access to their site of action, the luminal epithelium. Thiazide diuretics should therefore not be used, and high dosages of loop diuretics may be required for efficacy. Potassium-sparing diuretics should not be used, because of the increased risk of hyperkalaemia.

ALTERING DOSAGES IN HEPATIC FAILURE

The liver has a large functional capacity, and chronic hepatic insufficiency usually has to be considerable before it affects drug dosages. In chronic liver disease, jaundice, ascites, a prolonged prothrombin time, hypoalbuminaemia, malnutrition and encephalopathy all make clinically important impairment of drug metabolism more likely. Hepatic drug clearance may be reduced in acute hepatitis, in hepatic

congestion due to cardiac failure, and if there is intrahepatic arteriovenous shunting (for example, in hepatic cirrhosis).

In contrast to renal insufficiency there is no easy way of calculating changes in dosage in patients with impaired hepatic function; this is because there are no good tests of hepatic drug-metabolising capacity, even by a single metabolic route, or of biliary excretion. Dosages of drugs that are metabolised by the liver should therefore be altered according to the therapeutic response, and with careful clinical monitoring for signs of adverse effects.

If a drug has a high rate of hepatic clearance (Box 2.15) it will be mostly cleared during its first passage through the liver (so-called 'first-pass' metabolism). In such cases hepatic impairment increases the amount of drug that escapes metabolism in the liver after oral administration, reducing oral dosage requirements but not altering intravenous dosage requirements. For example, clomethiazole is normally extensively metabolised presystemically by the liver, and this is reduced by chronic liver disease, such as alcoholic cirrhosis. When using oral clomethiazole in a patient with cirrhosis, take care to ensure that overdosage, with the risk of respiratory depression, does not occur.

The pharmacological effects of some drugs are altered in liver disease, with increased risks of adverse effects (Box 2.16).

ALTERING DOSAGES IN OLDER PEOPLE

Both drug handling and responses to drugs change as people age, and there is much more variability in drug response in elderly people than in younger people, because people age at different rates. This means that responses to drugs are much less predictable, and so dosage regimens of some drugs are different. Adverse drug reactions are more likely in old people; frail old people are particularly at risk, partly because they tend to have poorer renal function and smaller livers and partly because they are less able to maintain their homoeostatic control mechanisms than younger people or fit old people.

2.14 SOME DRUGS WHOSE DOSAGES ARE AFFECTED BY RENAL INSUFFICIENCY*

Mild renal insufficiency (creatinine clearance 20–50 ml/min or serum creatinine 150–300 µmol/l)

- ACE inhibitors (monitor carefully; increase dosages if renal function does not worsen with low doses)
- Aminoglycosides
- Chlorpropamide
- Digoxin
- Fibrates
- Lithium
- Zidovudine

Moderate renal insufficiency (creatinine clearance 10–20 ml/min or serum creatinine 300–700 µmol/l)

- Some β-blockers (e.g. atenolol, sotalol)
- Opioid analgesics

Severe renal insufficiency (creatinine clearance < 10 ml/min or serum creatinine > 700 µmol/l; many of these patients receive renal replacement therapy, which can affect drug pharmacokinetics)

- Azathioprine
- Cephalosporins
- Cimetidine
- Isoniazid
- Penicillins
- Sulphonylurea hypoglycaemic drugs (gliclazide, glipizide, gliquidone)

Drugs to avoid in renal insufficiency

Any degree of renal insufficiency
- Mesalazine
- Metformin
- Non-steroidal anti-inflammatory drugs
- Tetracyclines (except doxycycline and minocycline)

Moderate or severe renal insufficiency
- Lithium
- Methotrexate

Severe renal insufficiency
- Chloramphenicol
- Chloroquine
- Fibrates
- Sulphonylurea hypoglycaemic drugs (chlorpropamide, glibenclamide)

* These guidelines mirror those recommended in the *British National Formulary*.

2.15 SOME DRUGS OF LOW AND HIGH HEPATIC CLEARANCE RATES

Low

- Aspirin
- Codeine
- Diazepam
- Isoniazid
- Nortriptyline
- Paracetamol
- Phenobarbital
- Phenytoin
- Procainamide
- Quinidine
- Theophylline
- Warfarin

High

- Clomethiazole
- Glyceryl trinitrate
- Labetalol
- Lidocaine
- Morphine
- Pethidine
- Propranolol
- Simvastatin

2.16 SOME DRUGS WHOSE ACTIONS ARE INCREASED IN LIVER DISEASE

Drug	Adverse effect
Oral anticoagulants	Increased anticoagulation (reduced clotting factor synthesis)
Metformin	Lactic acidosis
Chloramphenicol	Bone-marrow suppression
Non-steroidal anti-inflammatory drugs	Gastrointestinal bleeding
Sulphonylureas	Hypoglycaemia

Inappropriate polypharmacy is common in old people and the scope for drug interactions is large (p. 167); in patients over 60 years of age the error rate in taking drugs is about 60%, and the rate of errors increases markedly if more than three drugs are prescribed.

Many old people find it difficult to swallow tablets, and the more frail and the more ill they are, the more difficult it becomes. For example, many potassium tablets are large and can be difficult to swallow. Tablets or capsules can adhere to the oesophageal mucosa, and tablets should be swilled down with at least 60 ml of water to avoid hold-up. Elixirs may be preferable, but not all drugs are available as elixirs, and they can have their own problems. For example, the taste of a potassium elixir may not be acceptable.

Drug distribution is sometimes altered in old people. Dosages should be adjusted for body weight, particularly for drugs with a low therapeutic index.

Old people have an increased proportion of body fat, and lipid-soluble drugs tend to accumulate to a greater extent than in younger patients.

The metabolism of some drugs is reduced in old people—for example, clomethiazole, lidocaine, nifedipine, phenobarbital, propranolol and theophylline. Dosages of these drugs should therefore be reduced.

Renal function falls with age, and drugs that are mainly excreted in the urine, or that have active metabolites that are excreted, may require dosage reductions (see above). Serum creatinine may be deceptively reassuring because of reduced muscle mass in old age; in the frail, creatinine clearance should therefore always be calculated using an equation such as Cockroft–Gault (p. 462).

Some drugs are best avoided in old people. For example, tetracyclines accumulate when renal function is poor, causing nausea and vomiting, which in turn cause dehydration and further deterioration in renal function, and may lead to unsteadiness and falls (p. 166).

Drug sensitivity is sometimes altered (usually increased) in old age. Old people are more sensitive to the effects of digoxin, probably because of increased sensitivity of their sodium/potassium pump. This, combined with reduced renal function and an increased susceptibility to potassium loss due to diuretics, makes them more liable to digoxin toxicity. In contrast, there is reduced sensitivity of β-adrenoceptors in old people, and this may reduce some of the pharmacological effects of β-adrenoceptor agonists and antagonists. Altered sensitivity to drugs in old people can be due to altered physiological responses. For example, reduced baroreceptor function can lead to increased hypo-tension after the administration of antihypertensive drugs. Other examples include increased sensitivity to the anti-coagulant effects of warfarin and increased responsiveness of the brain to centrally active drugs—for example, anti-depressants, hypnotics, neuroleptic drugs, sedatives and tranquillisers.

Some of these principles are illustrated in Figure 2.2, which shows the difference in nifedipine pharmacokinetics and pharmacodynamic responses between young and old men. After an intravenous dose of nifedipine (2.5 mg) the old men had higher plasma nifedipine concentrations and a fall in blood pressure; the difference in blood pressure response was partly due to the difference in plasma concentration, but was mostly due to a difference in baroreceptor reflexes, as shown by the difference in heart rate response.

In general, when prescribing drugs for old people, try to use as few drugs as possible, start with low dosages, and increase the dosages carefully only if required. Choose easily swallowed formulations, and keep therapy as simple as possible (for example, with once-daily drugs and formulations). Take great care in frail old people.

WHEN TO STOP DRUG TREATMENT

Sometimes a single dose of a drug is sufficient; for example, aspirin to treat a headache or diamorphine to treat the pain of myocardial infarction. In contrast, life-long therapy is usually required for the treatment of diabetes mellitus, essential hypertension, hypothyroidism and pernicious anaemia.

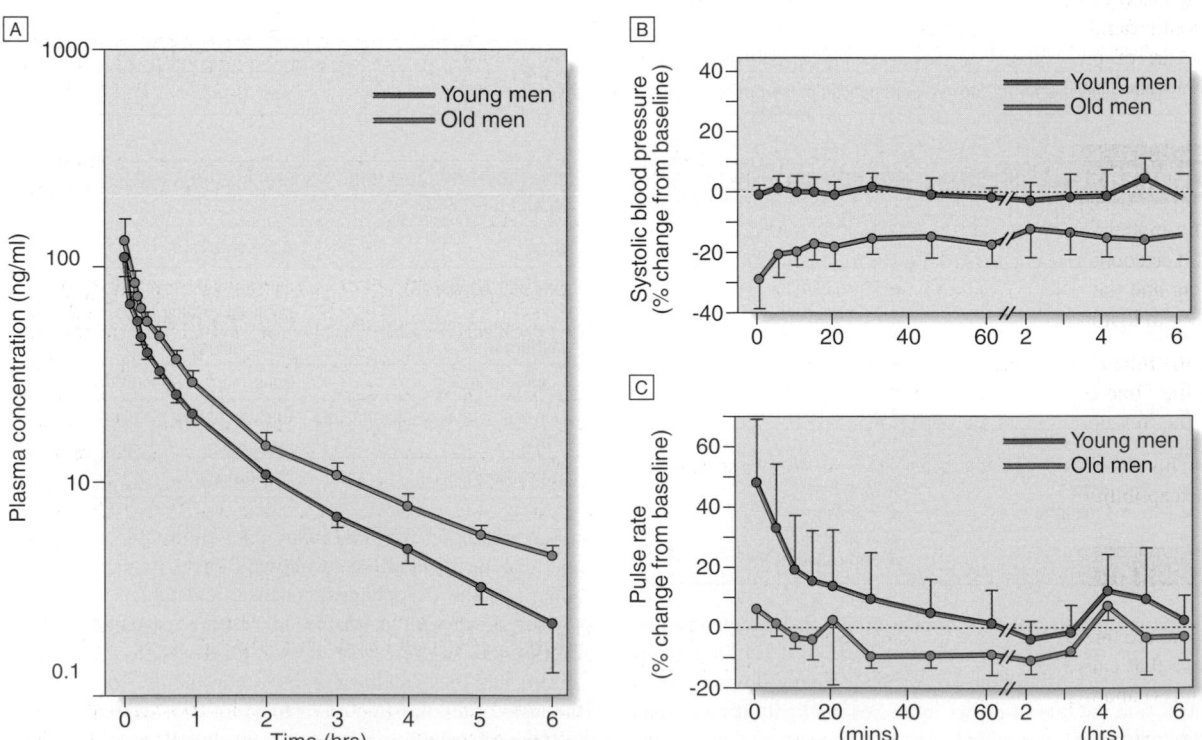

Fig. 2.2 Differences between young men and old men given an intravenous dose of nifedipine. [A] Old men have higher plasma concentrations than young men. [B] and [C] Old men have a greater fall in blood pressure and a smaller rise in heart rate than young men.

Treatments of intermediate duration can pose problems. For example, it is still not clear for how long treatment with warfarin should be continued in the treatment of deep venous thrombosis and pulmonary embolism (p. 728). The duration of treatment of infections with antibiotics varies from infection to infection, and depends on the infecting organism, the site of infection, and the response to treatment. For example, uncomplicated urinary tract infection with cystitis usually requires treatment for only a few days, pyelonephritis requires treatment for 1–2 weeks, and acute prostatitis 4–6 weeks. When a drug treatment is started, it is wise to plan the likely duration of therapy. It is also important to review long-term treatment at regular intervals to assess whether continued treatment is required. A hospital admission is often an opportunity for revising drug therapy, and it is not uncommon for drugs to be withdrawn in the interim or even permanently following an acute severe illness.

PRESCRIBING IN CONSTRAINED CIRCUMSTANCES

When prescribing takes place in a developing country economic constraints may limit the list of drugs available. The World Health Organization has published a so-called Model Formulary, including a list of essential medicines and helpful advice about how to use them.

For a junior doctor (e.g. a pre-registration house officer in the UK) the ability to prescribe will be constrained by limited knowledge and experience. Junior doctors should not be expected to prescribe from a wide range of drugs. A suggested formulary of drugs with which medical students should familiarise themselves as a first step in learning the art of prescribing is listed on the Davidson website (www.studentconsult.com).

ADVERSE DRUG REACTIONS

The modern classification of adverse drug reactions takes into account three aspects of the interaction between the drug and the patient that produces the adverse effect of the drug in that patient:

- the relation of the adverse effect to the Dose of the drug
- the Time-course of the effect
- the Susceptibility of the patient.

This classification is known as DoTS (Dose, Time-course, Susceptibility).

DOSE-RELATEDNESS

There are three types of adverse drug effect in relation to the dose that causes it: toxic effects, collateral effects (or side effects) and hypersusceptibility effects.

- A *toxic effect* is one that occurs as an exaggeration of the desired therapeutic effect and occurs at doses at or near the top of the dose-response curve. For example,

syncope due to a β-blocker is a toxic effect—it occurs by the same mechanism as the therapeutic effect (lowering of the blood pressure).
- *Collateral effects* occur at doses in the middle of the usual dose-response curve but in a tissue other than that in which the therapeutic action is sought, although not necessarily in another organ. They can occur either:
  — through the same pharmacological effect as that whereby the therapeutic action is produced (for example, colour vision disturbance from sildenafil), or
  — through a distinct pharmacological effect (for example, a dry mouth due to an anticholinergic effect of a tricyclic antidepressant).
- *Hypersusceptibility effects* occur at subtherapeutic doses in susceptible patients. Penicillin allergy is a hypersusceptibility effect.

Toxic effects can be avoided by using dosages at the lower end of the recommended range and increasing cautiously, monitoring carefully for therapeutic and adverse effects. Collateral adverse effects may not be avoidable; if they occur despite careful dosage adjustment it may be necessary to use a different drug. Hypersusceptibility effects can be avoided by identifying the susceptibility factors, for example a history of penicillin allergy is a contraindication to the use of any penicillin.

TIME-COURSE OF ADVERSE EFFECTS

The different patterns of time-course of adverse reactions are listed in Box 2.17, with illustrative examples.

SUSCEPTIBILITY TO ADVERSE DRUG REACTIONS

The sources of the various factors that can increase the susceptibility of an individual to an adverse effect of a drug are listed in Box 2.18.

DRUG INTERACTIONS

A drug interaction occurs when the effects of one drug (the object drug) are altered (increased or decreased) by the effects of another drug (the precipitant drug). Although a drug interaction usually results in an adverse effect, in some cases it can prove beneficial—for example, the pharmacodynamic synergy between diuretics and ACE inhibitors in the treatment of hypertension. The classification of drug interactions by mechanism is shown in Box 2.19.

PHARMACEUTICAL INTERACTIONS

Pharmaceutical interactions are physicochemical interactions, either of a drug with an intravenous infusion solution or of two drugs in the same solution, resulting in the loss of activity of the drugs involved. Pharmaceutical

2.17 TIME-RELATED CLASSIFICATION OF ADVERSE DRUG REACTIONS

Type of reaction	Examples	Implications
TIME-INDEPENDENT		
Due to a change in dose or concentration (*pharmaceutical effects*)	Toxicity due to increased systemic availability	Beware of changing formulations of some drugs (e.g. modified-release formulations of lithium)
Due to a change in dose or concentration (*pharmacokinetic effects*)	Digitalis toxicity due to renal insufficiency	Forewarn the patient; monitor carefully throughout treatment; alter dosage when pharmacokinetics change (e.g. renal insufficiency); avoid interacting drugs
Occurs without a change in dose (*pharmacodynamic effects*)	Digitalis toxicity due to hypokalaemia	Forewarn the patient; monitor carefully throughout treatment; avoid precipitating (pharmacodynamic) factors; avoid interacting drugs
TIME-DEPENDENT		
Rapid (due to rapid administration)	Red man syndrome (vancomycin) Hypertension (digitalis) Hypotension (adipiodone)	Administer slowly
First dose (of a course)	Hypotension (α_1-adrenoceptor antagonists and ACE inhibitors) Type I hypersensitivity reactions	Take special precautions for the first dose Careful history taking; if a reaction occurs, avoid re-exposure; counsel the patient
Early (abates with repeated exposure)	Adverse reactions that involve tolerance (e.g. nitrate-induced headache)	Monitor during the early stages; give appropriate reassurance; expect adverse effects if strategies to avoid tolerance are adopted
Intermediate (risk increases at first, then diminishes)	Venous thromboembolism (antipsychotic drugs) Hypersensitivity reactions types II, III and IV	Monitoring not needed after the high-risk period unless susceptibility changes; withdraw drug if a reaction develops
Late (risk increases with time)	Osteoporosis (glucocorticoids) Tardive dyskinesia (dopamine receptor antagonists) Retinopathy (chloroquine) Tissue phospholipid deposition (amiodarone) Withdrawal syndromes: opiates, benzodiazepines, hypertension (clonidine and methyldopa), myocardial infarction (β-blockers)	Assess baseline function; forewarn the patient; monitor periodically during prolonged treatment Withdraw slowly; forewarn the patient; replace with a longer-acting drug if withdrawal is not possible
Delayed	Carcinogenesis (ciclosporin, diethylstilbestrol) Teratogenesis (thalidomide)	Avoid or screen; counsel or forewarn the patient

2.18 SOURCES OF ALTERED SUSCEPTIBILITY TO ADVERSE DRUG REACTIONS

Source of susceptibility	Examples	Implications
Genetic	Porphyria Succinylcholine sensitivity Malignant hyperthermia CYP isozyme polymorphisms	Screen for abnormalities; avoid specific drugs
Age	Neonates (chloramphenicol) Elderly people (hypnotics)	Adjust doses according to age
Sex	Alcohol intoxication Mefloquine, neuropsychiatric effects ACE inhibitors, cough Lupus-like syndrome (e.g. hydralazine)	Use different doses in men and women
Physiology altered	Phenytoin in pregnancy	Alter dose or avoid
Exogenous factors	Drug interactions Interactions with food (e.g. grapefruit juice with drugs cleared by CYP3A4)	Alter dose or avoid co-administration
Disease	Renal insufficiency (e.g. lithium) Hepatic cirrhosis (e.g. morphine)	Screen for abnormalities; avoid specific drugs; use reduced doses

2.19 CLASSIFICATION OF DRUG INTERACTIONS BY MECHANISM

Mechanism	Example		
	Object drug	Precipitant drug	Result
Pharmaceutical	Sodium bicarbonate	Calcium gluconate	Precipitation of insoluble calcium carbonate
Pharmacokinetic			
Reduced absorption	Tetracyclines	Calcium, aluminium, magnesium salts	Reduced tetracycline absorption
Reduced protein binding	Phenytoin	Aspirin	Reduced phenytoin plasma concentration with same therapeutic effect
Reduced metabolism (CYP3A4)	Terfenadine	Grapefruit juice	Cardiac arrhythmias (prolonged QT interval, p. 527)
Reduced metabolism (CYP2C19)	Phenytoin	Ticlopidine	Phenytoin toxicity
Reduced metabolism (CYP2D6)	Clozapine	Paroxetine	Clozapine toxicity
Reduced metabolism (other enzymes)	Azathioprine	Allopurinol	Azathioprine toxicity
Increased metabolism	Ciclosporin	St John's wort	Loss of immunosuppression
Reduced renal elimination	Lithium	Diuretics	Lithium toxicity
Pharmacodynamic			
Direct antagonism	Opiates	Naloxone	Reversal of opiate effects
Direct potentiation	Alcohol	Antidepressants	Increased sedation
Indirect potentiation	Anti-arrhythmic drugs	Diuretics	Cardiac arrhythmias (hypokalaemia)

interactions are too numerous to remember in detail, but they can be simply avoided:

- by giving intravenous drugs via bolus injection or an infusion burette or syringe pump
- by using only dextrose or saline for drug infusion
- by not mixing drugs in the same infusion solution, unless the mixture is known to be safe (e.g. potassium chloride with insulin).

PHARMACOKINETIC INTERACTIONS

Pharmacokinetic interactions occur when the absorption, distribution or elimination (metabolism or excretion) of the object drug is altered by the precipitant drug.

ABSORPTION INTERACTIONS

Absorption interactions are usually not important. Exceptions include impaired absorption of tetracyclines by chelation with divalent and trivalent cations. Metoclopramide increases the rate of gastric emptying and this hastens the absorption of analgesics in the treatment of an acute attack of migraine, a beneficial effect.

DISTRIBUTION INTERACTIONS: PROTEIN-BINDING DISPLACEMENT

Protein-binding displacement causes an increase in the circulating concentration of unbound drug. However, this is only important if the object drug is highly protein-bound (greater than 90%) and is not widely distributed to body tissues. In practice, this limits important interactions of this type to warfarin and phenytoin. When these drugs are displaced their clearance rate increases in proportion to the degree of displacement and so at steady state the total concentration of drug in the plasma falls to a new equilibrium value, and the unbound concentration is the

same as it was before the precipitant drug was introduced, in spite of an increase in the unbound fraction. This means that provided the patient can 'weather' the increase, if any, in unbound concentration of the object drug for as long as it takes to reach the new steady state, such an interaction will not be clinically important.

METABOLISM INTERACTIONS

Drug interactions involving metabolism are important interactions. They occur when the metabolism of an object drug is either inhibited or increased by a precipitant drug. There are two phases of drug metabolism. Phase I metabolic reactions (for example, dealkylation, deamination, hydroxylation, sulphoxidation) are carried out by isoenzymes of the mixed-function oxidase (cytochrome P450) system and are subject to interactions. Phase II reactions are conjugations (for example, acetylation, methylation, glucuronidation, sulphatation), which are not affected by interactions.

Induction of drug metabolism

Induction of the metabolism of a drug reduces the amount of drug in the body, and therefore reduces its effects. This can result, for example, in pregnancy, despite what would otherwise have been adequate oral contraception, if the woman also takes an enzyme inducer, such as carbamazepine, phenytoin or rifampicin.

Inhibition of drug metabolism

Inhibition of drug metabolism occurs through inhibition of either the mixed-function oxidase reactions or other specific metabolic pathways.

Examples of the former include inhibition of warfarin metabolism by chloramphenicol, cimetidine, ketoconazole, metronidazole, and quinolones, inhibition of phenytoin metabolism by isoniazid, and inhibition of theophylline metabolism by quinolone and macrolide antibiotics (for example, erythromycin).

2

Examples of the latter include the inhibition by allopurinol of the metabolism of azathioprine and 6-mercaptopurine by xanthine oxidase and of dietary amines by monoamine oxidase inhibitors.

EXCRETION INTERACTIONS

Competition for renal tubular secretion reduces drug excretion. For example, probenecid inhibits the tubular secretion of penicillin, increasing the blood concentration of penicillin and prolonging its therapeutic effects, a beneficial interaction. Amiodarone, quinidine and verapamil inhibit the tubular secretion of digoxin by inhibiting the transport protein P glycoprotein, increasing plasma digoxin concentrations and potentially causing toxicity. Salicylates inhibit the active secretion of methotrexate. Diuretics inhibit the renal excretion of lithium.

PHARMACODYNAMIC INTERACTIONS

In pharmacodynamic interactions the effect of a drug is altered at its site of action. Such interactions are either direct or indirect.

DIRECT PHARMACODYNAMIC INTERACTIONS

Direct pharmacodynamic interactions occur when two drugs either act on the same site (antagonism or synergism) or act on two different sites with a similar end result. For example, naloxone reverses the effects of opiates and vitamin K reverses the effects of warfarin. The anticoagulant effects of warfarin are increased in direct synergistic interactions with anabolic steroids and tetracyclines. Any drug that has a depressant action on central nervous function can potentiate the effect of another such drug, whether or not the two drugs have effects on the same receptors; for example, alcohol potentiates the action of any other centrally acting drug.

INDIRECT PHARMACODYNAMIC INTERACTIONS

In indirect pharmacodynamic interactions a pharmacological, therapeutic or toxic effect of the precipitant drug in some way alters the therapeutic or toxic effect of the object drug, but the two effects are not themselves related and do not themselves interact.

The effects of anticoagulants can be increased by three indirect effects: reduced platelet aggregation (for example, by salicylates, dipyridamole, clopidogrel and non-steroidal anti-inflammatory drugs) or thrombocytopenia; gastrointestinal ulceration (for example, non-steroidal anti-inflammatory drugs); and increased fibrinolysis (for example, metformin).

Alterations in fluid and electrolyte balance by diuretics increase the effects of cardiac glycosides and class I anti-arrhythmic drugs (for example, lidocaine, quinidine, procainamide and phenytoin).

AVOIDING ADVERSE DRUG INTERACTIONS

The simple way of avoiding adverse drug interactions is to avoid combinations that are known to be dangerous. If that is not possible, the dosage of the object drug should be reduced in advance of starting the precipitant drug and the precipitant drug should be introduced slowly. When a theoretical interaction is anticipated on the basis of the known properties of two drugs, even if it has not been previously described, careful monitoring will help recognise adverse effects early.

WRITING A DRUG PRESCRIPTION

A prescription should be a precise, accurate, clear, readable set of instructions, sufficient for a nurse to administer a drug accurately in hospital, or for a pharmacist to provide a patient with both the correct drug and the instructions on how to take it. The information that should be written on a prescription is given in Box 2.20.

2.20 INFORMATION TO BE GIVEN ON A UK PRESCRIPTION OUTSIDE HOSPITAL

- The date
- The patient's name, initials and address
- The age of a child under 12
- The name of the drug, preferably in capitals (use generic names when possible)
- The formulation to be prescribed
- The strength of the formulation
- The dose
- The frequency of administration
- The route of administration
- The doctor's name, address and signature

WRITING DRUG DOSES

- Quantities of 1 gram or more should be written in grams. For example, write 2 g.
- Quantities less than 1 gram but more than 1 milligram should be written in milligrams. For example, write 100 mg, not 0.1 g.
- Quantities less than 1 milligram should be written in micrograms or nanograms as appropriate. Do not abbreviate micrograms or nanograms. For example, write 100 micrograms, not 0.1 mg, 100 µg, 100 mcg, or 100 ug.
- If a decimal point cannot be avoided for values less than 1, write a zero before it. For example, write 0.5 ml, not .5 ml.
- For liquid medicines given orally the dose should be stated as the number of milligrams in either 5 ml or 10 ml of solution.

PRESCRIBING CONTROLLED DRUGS

Because of the problems of drug addiction and misuse of drugs, in the United Kingdom drugs likely to be abused are

2.21 REQUIREMENTS FOR UK PRESCRIPTIONS FOR CONTROLLED DRUGS

Prescriptions for controlled drugs must:
- be completely written in the prescriber's handwriting in ink
- be signed and dated by the prescriber
- specify the prescriber's address
- specify the name and address of the patient
- state the form and strength (if appropriate) of the drug
- state the total quantity of the drug or the number of dose units to be dispensed in both words and figures
- state the exact size of each dose in both words and figures

the subject of the *Misuse of Drugs Act* (1971), the *Misuse of Drugs (Notification of and Supply to Addicts) Regulations* (1973) and the *Misuse of Drugs Regulations* (1985). The requirements for the prescription of controlled drugs are listed in Box 2.21. Doctors in other countries should make themselves familiar with local regulations.

ABBREVIATIONS

Some abbreviations that are used in prescribing are listed in Box 2.22. Other abbreviations should be avoided and instructions should whenever possible be written in plain English.

2.22 ACCEPTABLE ABBREVIATIONS IN PRESCRIPTIONS

Abbreviation	Latin meaning	English translation
b.d. or b.i.d.	Bis in die	Twice a day
gutt.	Guttae	Drops
i.m.	–	Intramuscular(ly)
i.v.	–	Intravenous(ly)
o.d.	Omni die	(Once) every day
o.m.	Omni mane[1]	(Once) every morning
o.n.	Omni nocte[1]	(Once) every night
p.o.	Per os	By mouth
PR	Per rectum	By the anal route
p.r.n.	Pro re nata	Whenever required
PV	Per vaginam	By the vaginal route
q.d.s.	Quater die sumendum[2]	Four times a day
s.c.	–	Subcutaneous(ly)
stat.	Statim	Immediately
t.d.s.	Ter die sumendum[2]	Three times a day

[1] Sometimes written simply as 'mane' or 'nocte'.
[2] The abbreviations t.i.d. or q.i.d. (ter or quater in die) are sometimes used instead; do not use q.d. to mean once a day.

DRUG NOMENCLATURE

Drugs have different kinds of names:

- the chemical name, whose form generally follows the rules issued by the International Union of Pure and Applied Chemistry (IUPAC).
- the approved (official or generic) name. This is usually the International Nonproprietary Name (INN), either

recommended (rINN) or proposed (pINN) by the WHO, but may be some locally approved name (for example the British Approved Name, BAN, or United States Adopted Name, USAN).
- the proprietary name (brand name or trade name), given to it by a pharmaceutical manufacturer.

For example:

- chemical name: (*R*)-1-(3,4-dihydroxyphenyl)-2-methylaminoethanol
- International Nonproprietary Name: epinephrine; British Approved Name: adrenaline
- proprietary names: Epipen® for intramuscular injection and Eppy® or Simplene® eyedrops.

Since the chemical name is generally, as in this case, unsuitable for routine prescribing, either the approved name or proprietary name is used. Which should one choose? For some drugs the question is trivial, since only one proprietary formulation exists; for example, donepezil is currently available in the UK only as Aricept®.

However, several proprietary formulations of the same chemical entity usually become available when the patent expires on a drug with a previously unique proprietary name. For instance, amoxicillin was first marketed as Amoxil®. When the patent expired the number of proprietary brands multiplied. This can cause prescribing and dispensing problems. For example, in the UK whether the prescriber writes 'donepezil BP' or 'Aricept' the patient will receive Aricept®. However, if the prescriber writes 'amoxicillin BP' the pharmacist may dispense any proprietary formulation, provided that it conforms to the description laid out in the BP (*British Pharmacopoeia*), and will generally dispense the cheapest available.

By writing the proprietary name the prescriber can ensure that a particular formulation of a drug is prescribed. However, in some hospitals (e.g. in the UK) the hospital pharmacy may stock only one formulation, and even if the hospital doctor writes 'Amoxil' on an inpatient prescription chart the pharmacist may dispense some other approved formulation for which the hospital will have negotiated an economic deal with the supplier.

There are advantages and disadvantages to the prescribing of drugs by their generic (non-proprietary) as opposed to their proprietary names. The advantages include:

- *Awareness of the prescription*. The name of the compound often indicates to what class it belongs, usually by virtue of its suffix; e.g. -statin (HMGCoA reductase inhibitors), -olol (β-blockers, although beware stanozolol), -floxacin (quinolone antibiotics).
- *Drug stocks*. If, say, 'Almodan' rather than 'amoxicillin' is prescribed, and an outside pharmacy stocks only Amoxil®, the pharmacist cannot legally dispense the prescription without first consulting the doctor; clearly, this can cause inconvenience to all concerned and might result in delayed treatment.
- *Expense*. It is generally cheaper to prescribe by the approved name, since the pharmacist will dispense the cheapest variant held in stock.

2

The disadvantages of prescribing by non-proprietary name include:

- *Remembering names*. Proprietary names are chosen by pharmaceutical companies because they are catchy, usually easier to remember than the corresponding generic name, and shorter and easier to spell (compare, for example, 'Plavix' with 'clopidogrel'). Furthermore, a single proprietary name will do when the formulation contains two or more drugs (compare, for example, 'Fefol' with 'ferrous sulphate plus folic acid'). In recent years there has been a move in the UK to counteract this problem by giving single approved names to some common combinations of drugs; for example, the combination of dihydrocodeine with paracetamol (acetaminophen) is known as co-dydramol.
- *Quality of product*. For a few drugs a change in tablet excipients has large effects on the absorption of the drug from the formulation. Important examples include lithium salts, nifedipine and theophylline, which should always be prescribed by brand name.
- *Continuity of treatment*. Patients not infrequently become confused if the drug they are being given changes its form with every prescription. Continuity can be achieved by prescribing the same proprietary formulation every time.

In hospital it is usually better to prescribe by approved name, since the pharmacy will dispense whatever formulation is held in stock. The proprietary name can be used when a combination product is prescribed for which no single approved name exists (for example, 'Fefol'). In general practice it is also usually best to prescribe by approved name. However, in some cases (for example, lithium salts, nifedipine and theophylline) the proprietary name should be used. Doctors who make the effort to prescribe when possible by approved name will generally find it just as easy as prescribing by proprietary name.

Countries in the European Community are required to use International Nonproprietary Names, except for adrenaline and noradrenaline (BANs that are permitted instead of the rINNs epinephrine and norepinephrine, primarily for reasons of safety).

MONITORING DRUG THERAPY

There is no space here for a detailed discussion of how to monitor drug therapy, which should be done using (in order of preference) clinical, pharmacodynamic or pharmacokinetic methods. For some drugs whose effects can be monitored by measuring plasma concentrations, target concentrations are given in Box 2.23.

2.23 USUAL THERAPEUTIC AND TOXIC PLASMA CONCENTRATIONS OF COMMONLY MEASURED DRUGS					
Drug	Optimal sampling time	Concentration below which a therapeutic effect is unlikely		Concentration above which a toxic effect is more likely	
		Mass units	Molar units	Mass units	Molar units
Aspirin (salicylate)					
Analgesic	Just before next dose	20 mg/l	0.15 µmol/l	300 mg/l	2.2 µmol/l
Anti-inflammatory	Just before next dose	150 mg/l	1.1 µmol/l	300 mg/l	2.2 µmol/l
Carbamazepine	Just before next dose	4 mg/l	17 µmol/l	10 mg/l	42 µmol/l
Cardiac glycosides					
Digitoxin	Just before next dose	15 µg/l	20 nmol/l	30 µg/l	39 nmol/l
Digoxin	11 hrs after last dose	0.8 µg/l	1.0 nmol/l	2 µg/l	2.6 nmol/l
Ciclosporin*	Just before next dose	125 µg/l	104 nmol/l	200 µg/l	166 nmol/l
Lithium	12 hrs after last dose	—	0.4 mmol/l	—	1.0 mmol/l
Phenytoin	Just before next dose	10 mg/l	40 µmol/l	20 mg/l	80 µmol/l
Theophylline	Just before next dose	10 mg/l	55 µmol/l	20 mg/l	110 µmol/l

* Measured in whole blood by specific radioimmunoassay or HPLC.

Notes
1. Care should be taken in comparing results between different laboratories (particularly with ciclosporin).
2. The concentration below which a therapeutic effect is unlikely and the concentration above which a toxic effect is more likely together constitute a target range within which satisfactory therapy is likely to be achieved; however, dosages should be adjusted according to the clinical response, not the concentration, which should only be used as a guide.
3. Note the units used when interpreting results. Laboratories may report in mass units or molar units or both; µg/l = ng/ml; mg/l = µg/ml.
4. Remember that pharmacokinetics differ from individual to individual; for within-patient comparisons always use the same time after the last dose.
5. Remember that pharmacodynamics differ from individual to individual and that different individuals respond differently to the same concentration of drug; other factors that can alter the individual response should be considered.
6. For paracetamol see Figure 9.3, page 209.
7. For aminoglycosides consult your laboratory.

FURTHER INFORMATION

Books and journal articles

Aronson JK. Where name and image meet—the argument for adrenaline. British Medical Journal 2000; 320:506–509.

Association of the British Pharmaceutical Industry. Compendium of data sheets and summaries of product characteristics. London: Datapharm; new edition every year.

British National Formulary. London: British Medical Association and the Pharmaceutical Society of Great Britain; new edition every 6 months. *Guide to currently available formulations, with notes on dosages, uses, adverse effects and interactions; chapters on prescribing, especially in renal failure, in liver disease, in pregnancy and during breastfeeding, and appendices on drug interactions and intravenous additives. The British National Formulary for Children (BNFC) is specifically designed for paediatric prescribing.*

Grahame-Smith DG, Aronson JK. Oxford textbook of clinical pharmacology and drug therapy. 3rd edn. Oxford: Oxford University Press; 2001. *Contains a more detailed account of the principles outlined here.*

Richards D, Aronson JK. Oxford handbook of practical drug therapy. Oxford: Oxford University Press; 2005. *Contains practical guidance.*

Sackett DL, Richardson WS, Rosenberg W, Haynes RB. Evidence-based medicine: how to practise and teach EBM. Edinburgh: Churchill Livingstone; 2000. *A useful introduction to evidence-based medicine.*

WHO Model Formulary. World Health Organization; 2004. *The equivalent of the British National Formulary for developing countries.*

Websites

http://mednet3.who.int/medicine/organization/par/edl/eml.shtml *The WHO limited list and formulary.*

www.bnf.org *British National Formulary.*

www.clinicalevidence.org *A compendium of best evidence, published by the British Medical Journal.*

www.cochrane.co.uk *The Cochrane Collaboration.*

www.cebm.utoronto.ca *Evidence-based medicine.*

2

J.R. SECKL
R. SANDFORD

Molecular mechanisms of disease

In the half-century since the key discoveries of the cell cycle and the structure of DNA, the new sciences of molecular genetics and cell biology have progressively revolutionised our understanding of the inheritance and molecular basis of disease. These insights have spawned a technological revolution which has provided a wide range of diagnostic and predictive tests for hereditary disease susceptibility. They have also led to entirely new approaches to treatment (gene therapy, stem cell therapy) and the prospect that optimal choices of medicines can be tailored to the individual patient (pharmacogenomics).

This chapter reviews the key principles in molecular genetics and cell biology. The emphasis is on the approach to diseases which are known to have a genetic basis, and on the role and practice of the clinical geneticist. In addition, the chapter highlights how advances in cell and molecular biology may be used in future in this exciting and rapidly developing area of medicine.

Genetic disease is very common. Up to half of all major childhood disability and mortality has a genetic cause. The role of genetic variation in common adult diseases such as hypertension, diabetes mellitus and cancer is becoming much clearer. Thus, clinicians from all medical and surgical specialties will be involved in the management of genetic disease. Genetic and other molecular tests are advancing rapidly, and have the potential not only to provide individuals with a secure diagnosis and accurate information about the consequences of having or developing a disease, but also to indicate the risks of transmitting it to offspring and the choices regarding screening, prevention and treatment. Understanding the use of today's tools in the genetics clinic will be invaluable to tomorrow's doctors, who have to ensure that increasing knowledge of the molecular basis of disease can be used to greatest advantage in the future.

FUNCTIONAL ANATOMY, PATHOPHYSIOLOGY AND INVESTIGATIONS

MOLECULAR BIOLOGY: CHROMOSOMES AND GENES

The anatomy of the human genome

Deoxyribonucleic acid (DNA) is the fundamental building block of life. It contains just four 'bases' (guanine, cytosine, adenine or thymine), which pair up by hydrogen bonding in only two combinations (G–C or A–T) to form a double-stranded helix. The DNA is coiled to form nucleosomes which coil again to form chromosomes.

In 2003 the Human Genome Project was officially completed. This massive international collaboration revealed that there are 3.2 billion (3.2×10^9) bases in the human genome. The DNA is packaged into 22 pairs of autosomal chromosomes and 2 sex chromosomes (XX in females or XY in males), seen in the nuclei of almost all normal human cells; physiological exceptions are gametes (sperm and ova) which, following meiosis, have only one set of chromosomes, and a few anucleate cells lacking the ability to replicate or survive in the longer term (red blood cells and platelets).

Only 2–3% of total chromosomal DNA encodes the unique sequences of active genes and their regulatory regions. A gene is a region of DNA which codes for a specific protein (Fig. 3.1). The Human Genome Project has revealed that there are many fewer than the 10^5 or so genes previously estimated. Currently, around 20 000 genes have been identified as encoding proteins or, more rarely, bioactive ribonucleic acid (e.g. transfer RNA). Not all of the DNA within a gene codes for the eventual protein;

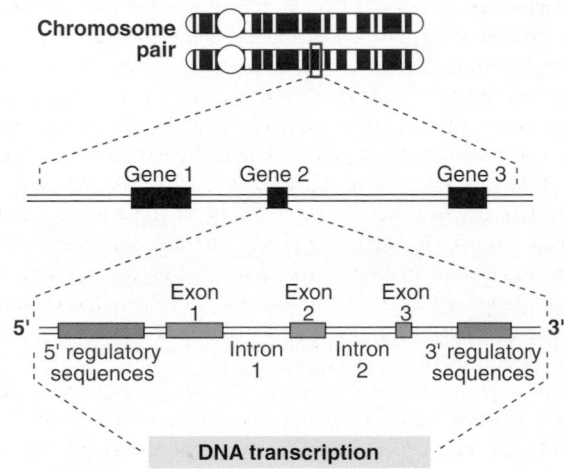

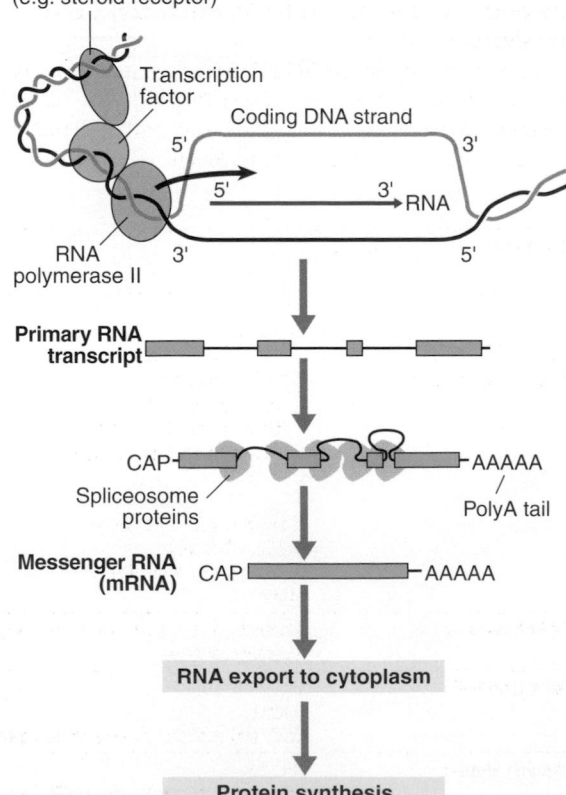

Fig. 3.1 RNA synthesis and its translation into protein.

sequences within the gene include coding regions (exons), non-coding regions (introns) and regulatory sequences. DNA is not decoded directly into protein; during transcription, chromosomal DNA remains in the nucleus, whereas protein synthesis occurs in ribosomes in the cytoplasm. The conversion of DNA sequence to protein is mediated by RNA.

The majority of DNA consists of introns, pseudogenes, transposable elements derived from viral DNA or RNA, and highly repetitive sequences which are often tightly coiled around histone proteins to form nucleosomes (Fig. 3.2). Such elements have, in the main, no clear function. Pseudogenes, which are mutated duplications of genes that cannot be translated into a functional protein, can be important clinically because they may misalign with a neighbouring authentic gene at meiosis. Any crossover may mutate the normal gene. This is a common mechanism of mutation of the gene encoding 21-hydroxylase; its dysfunction causes congenital adrenal hyperplasia (p. 789).

Individuals inherit a unique pattern of DNA sequences. Despite the fact that the sequence of the genome is more than 99.9% identical between individuals, this still enables many millions of different base–pair variations (or 'polymorphisms') to be present. Much of this natural variation in DNA occurs in non-coding regions and is of no direct relevance to function. Other variants may occur within genes, leading to alterations in protein sequence and possibly function. If a particular variation results in sufficient impairment of protein function to bring about a deleterious effect, a genetic disease may result.

Reading the genetic code: transcription and translation

The genetic code by which DNA directs the transcription of RNA and its translation into protein (Fig. 3.1) is a series of codons running 5′ to 3′ along the linear coding strand of DNA. Each codon is a three-nucleotide unit which specifies a particular amino acid to be incorporated into the mature protein, e.g. methionine: ATG. There are 4^3 (64) different triplets; 61 specify one of the 20 amino acids. Three—TAA, TAG and TGA—are 'nonsense' codons which terminate the growing polypeptide chain.

RNA is found in different types, which fulfil different functions. Messenger RNA (mRNA) is the product of transcription of a gene after splicing out of the non-coding (intronic) sequences, capping the mRNA and adding a polyA tail. This carries the genetic code to the cytoplasm and ribosomes, made of ribosomal RNA. Here, specific transfer RNAs (tRNA) attach to the triplet codons via a complementary triplet anticodon. These tRNAs bear the relevant amino acid and, once aligned, allow assembly of the protein.

The combination of transcription and translation is sometimes called, more loosely, expression. Gene transcription is highly regulated. Upstream (5′) of the transcribed region of a gene is the gene promoter. This stretch of DNA, often very long (several 10^4 of bases), contains the gene's key regulatory regions. The promoter is where specific proteins may attach to the double helix to facilitate or repress transcription. Such transcription factors bind to specific sequences of DNA, such as the TATA and CCAAT 'boxes'. Binding to these sites modulates attachment of other proteins including the RNA polymerase II complex which then proceeds along the coding strand of DNA, assembling a strand of mRNA complementary to the DNA template.

Transcription factors are often regulated by signals from outside the cell (steroids and thyroid hormones act directly, whereas other agents such as cytokines, growth factors and peptide hormones act via 'second messenger' signalling pathways). Several broad classes of transcription factor, and their roles in disease, are now recognised (Box 3.1). In addition, alterations within the promoter to which the transcription factors bind may lead to disease. For example, the DNA binding site for the transcription factor SF1 in

3.1 TRANSCRIPTION FACTORS		
Transcription factor classes	**Examples**	**Disorders associated with altered function (mutations/deletions)**
Zinc finger proteins	Steroid receptors	
	Androgen receptor	Testicular feminisation/androgen insensitivity
	Glucocorticoid receptor	Glucocorticoid resistance
	Mineralocorticoid receptor	Pseudohypoaldosteronism type 1 (loss of function mutations)
		Hypertension (gain of function mutations)
	Thyroid hormone receptors	Thyroid resistance
	Vitamin D receptor	Vitamin D-resistant rickets
	Wilms tumour gene (WT1)	Wilms tumour
	BRCA1	Familial breast cancer
Helix turn helix	Homeotic (hox) genes which control pattern formation in embryogenesis	Developmental abnormalities, e.g. synpolydactyly and aniridia (Pax-6)
Helix loop helix	MASH-1	Neuroblastoma
	TWIST	Saethre–Chotzen syndrome
	MITF (microphthalmia-associated transcription factor)	Waardenburg syndrome type 2
Leucine zippers	jun, fos	Oncogenes in various cancers
	Hepatocyte nuclear factor (HNF) 1α	Maturity-onset diabetes of the young (MODY) type 3
	MAF	Abnormal eye development

the promoter of the collagen 1A1 gene is mutated in a proportion of patients with osteoporosis (p. 1121). This mutation leads to subtle over-production of collagen 1A1 strands, causing an imbalance of collagen fibres and fragility of bone structure. Similarly, variation in the promoter of the gene encoding intestinal lactase determines whether or not this is 'shut off' in adulthood (producing lactose intolerance, p. 902).

Downstream (3′) of the start of transcription are a series of exons which code for mRNA, and introns, which are spliced out to reveal the mature RNA and have a poorly understood function. Alternative splicing of some genes allows more than one protein product to be produced, sometimes with entirely distinct function. Thus the calcitonin gene expressed in thyroid C cells produces mRNA molecules with one complement of exons encoding the hormone calcitonin (p. 744), but the same gene is differently spliced in neurons to produce an alternative mRNA encoding the neurotransmitter calcitonin-gene-related peptide. Splice sites are specific sequences at the junctions of exons and introns where the enzymes mediating splicing normally cut mRNA. Splice site mutations are common causes of genetic disease: for example, in many patients with Tay–Sachs disease and in the fibrillin genes in Marfan's syndrome (p. 605).

CELL BIOLOGY

Our bodies are made up of many billions of cells. Each is derived originally from a single fertilised egg or zygote. Many rounds of cell division through embryogenesis and fetal and postnatal development lead to the formation and maturation of differentiated tissues, organs, their supporting structures and associated networks of nerves, blood vessels and lymphatics. Almost all body cells have a nucleus containing chromosomal DNA encoding the proteins necessary to allow differentiated cell development, function and often senescence and programmed death.

The cell is not a static structure but is in a state of continuous flux. Intracellular components move, and the cell changes shape and state, responding to its internal needs and external cues. Moreover, all cellular components continually undergo turnover. Human cells do not exist in isolation but are continually in contact and communication with others. This occurs at the level of communication not only with direct neighbours via physical junctions but also with nearby and remote cells by the secretion of a series of messenger molecules. The classic view of the endocrine system, where these molecules or hormones function in long-range interaction, has been greatly extended by the understanding that many cells have paracrine interactions with cells in the immediate neighbourhood or regulate themselves with their own secretions (autocrine control).

FUNCTIONAL ANATOMY OF CELLS

Cell membrane
The cell (or 'plasma') membrane is crucial for all intercellular communications, representing the site of release of signalling molecules, the point of direct contact between cells, and the site of many of the receptors which respond to signals in the environment. The membrane is a semi-permeable phospholipid bilayer, with hydrophilic surfaces and a hydrophobic core (Fig. 3.2). A series of proteins 'float' in the membrane, some only on one surface (inner or outer), many spanning the membrane. The proteins form a host of receptors, pores, ion channels, pumps, associated energy suppliers and so on, which allow the cell continually to sample the extracellular milieu, take up crucial molecules for function, and exclude or exchange unwanted substances. Many proteins within the cell membrane are highly dynamic in the lateral plane, associating and disassociating rapidly to subserve their functions.

Transport
The cell membrane is freely permeable to water, gases, urea, ethanol and many hydrophobic substances such as steroids and thyroid hormones. It is impermeable to other molecules, including ions, glucose and other fuels, amino acids and peptides. Active transport of these molecules involves either channels or pumps. Channels are relatively non-specific, with passage related to the size and charge of a molecule, driven in or out of the cell along a concentration gradient. Channel proteins are exemplified by ion channels, which permit the rapid, size-selective flux of ions across the cell membrane. Carrier proteins and pumps are highly specific for their substrate and often use energy (adenosine triphosphate, ATP) to drive transport against a concentration gradient.

Such membrane proteins are subject to mutation and dysfunction. For example, mutation of the CFTR chloride channel, highly expressed in lung and the gut, leads to defective chloride transport, producing cystic fibrosis. Most commonly a three-base–pair deletion (ΔF508, Box 3.2, p. 46) leads to a misfolded CFTR protein which fails to reach the membrane.

Endocytosis
In order to take up molecules and matter larger than the size constraints of membrane transport, the cell employs a series of endocytic processes. These involve encapsulating material to be internalised within an invaginated fold of plasma membrane. Such engulfing is typically mediated by specific binding of the particle to surface receptors. This can involve phagocytosis of large particles/whole cells or small molecule uptake; the latter typically takes place via interaction with receptors in specialised regions of the cell membrane called clatharin-coated pits. These then bud off the membrane and sort the engulfed contents for intracellular transport or recycling to the membrane. This is the pathway of uptake of low-density lipoprotein (LDL) cholesterol, which binds to cell membranes via the clatharin-pit LDL receptor. Mutation of the receptor in familial hypercholesterolaemia (p. 446) leads to failure to bind LDL cholesterol. Intriguingly, in some families, mutations in a specific tyrosine in the intracellular tail of the receptor, which normally attaches the protein to clatharin, prevents receptors concentrating in clatharin-coated pits and hence impairs uptake of LDL, even though the receptors are present elsewhere in the cell membrane.

3

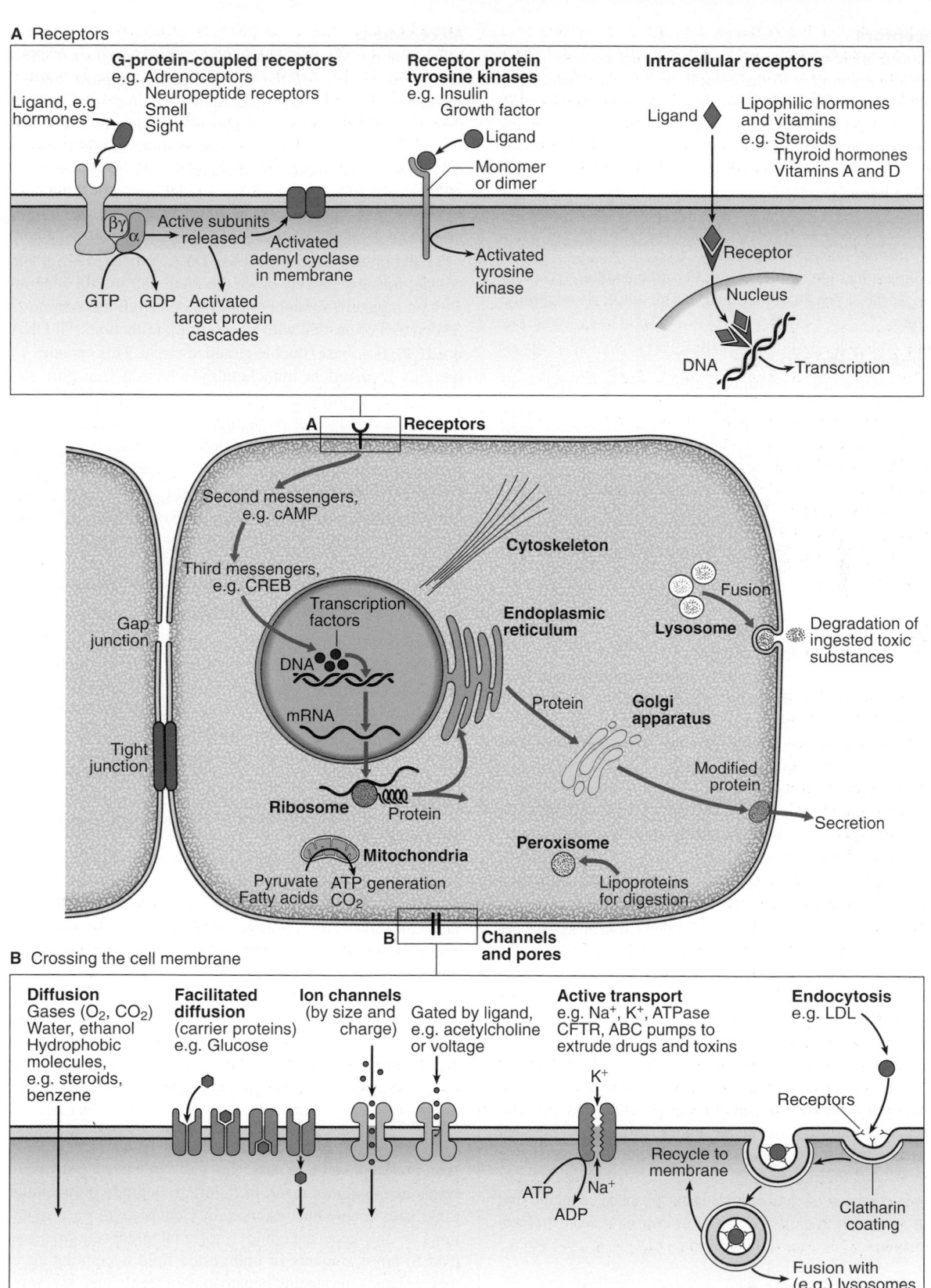

Fig. 3.2 An archetypal human cell showing intracellular organelles. [A] The various types of receptor that receive signals from the extracellular environment and transduce these into intracellular messengers. [B] The cellular mechanism whereby molecules and particles can cross the cell membrane. GDP/GTP = guanine diphosphate/triphosphate; ATP = adenosine triphosphate; cAMP = cyclic adenosine monophosphate; CREB = cAMP response element binding protein; LDL = low-density lipoproteins; ABC = ATP binding cassette transporters.

Receptors

Cell membrane receptors transduce a signal from the extracellular environment to the cytoplasm, typically inducing a second messenger signalling cascade. Membrane receptors can be grouped into ion channel-linked receptors, G-protein-linked receptors and enzyme-linked receptors. In addition, there are nuclear receptors for steroids, sterols, retinoids and thyroid hormones. Receptors, particularly those on the cell surface, are the most common molecular 'targets' for drugs.

Ion channel-linked receptors

Examples include some major neurotransmitter receptors such as those for glutamate and the nicotinic acetylcholine receptor.

G-protein-linked receptors

These are the most common cellular receptor type; over 1000 have been found, binding catecholamines, peptides and prostaglandins, and subserving key sensations such as sight (rhodopsin), smell and taste. G-protein receptors typically have seven transmembrane spans. Once its extracellular domain has been activated by a ligand, the G-protein-coupled receptor changes conformation. Its cytosolic domain then attaches to guanine triphosphate (GTP)-binding proteins (G-proteins) which transmit the signal to a further intracellular messenger, typically an enzyme or ion channel.

Enzyme-linked surface receptors

These directly activate an enzyme activity within the cell. This may be a kinase or phosphatase domain in the intracellular part of the receptor protein. Key examples are the receptor protein-tyrosine kinase, approximately 60 in number, which include the binding sites for insulin and most growth factors. Such receptors dimerise for activity. Mutations which interfere with the dimerisation of the insulin receptor lead to childhood insulin resistance and growth failure. Conversely, mutations in a fibroblast growth factor receptor gene which cause constitutive dimerisation in the absence of ligand produce overgrowth of bone manifesting as an autosomal dominant form of craniosynostosis called Crouzon syndrome.

Intracellular receptors

There are intracellular receptors for steroid and thyroid hormones and vitamins A and D, which either are already present in the nucleus (thyroid and oestrogen receptors) or rapidly enter the nucleus when activated by ligand (glucocorticoid receptors). Activated receptors function as transcription factors to regulate the promoter activity and hence transcription of target genes. Mutations in such receptors lead to loss of function and hormone resistance (Box 3.1). Rare mutations of the mineralocorticoid receptor cause activation of the receptor in the absence of ligand and produce severe hypertension due to excessive renal sodium retention.

Cytoplasm, organelles and the cytoskeleton

Within the cell, the cytoplasm contains a number of specialised organelles as well as the cytoskeleton, a network of structural proteins which maintain the shape of the cell and its ability to traffic intracellular organelles.

Mitochondria

Mitochondria are the cell's key energy producers. The double membrane of the mitochondrion imports energy substrates derived from lipids and carbohydrates. ATP is then generated by oxidative phosphorylation of adenosine via the passage of electrons down an ionic gradient across the inner mitochondrial membrane. Dephosphorylation of ATP releases the energy for most reactions within the cell. Mitochondria are most numerous in cells with high metabolic demands such as muscle.

Mitochondria have their own DNA, inherited from the oöcyte, thus exclusively down the maternal line. In keeping with an organelle thought to have arisen from the symbiotic association of the cell with a bacterium, mitochondrial DNA is a 16 kb (kilobase) double-stranded circle. This encodes 13 proteins involved in mitochondrial electron transport and oxidative phosphorylation. The mutational rate is relatively high due to the lack of protection of mitochondrial DNA by chromatin, although functional defects are usually prevented by the existence of multiple copies of mitochondrial DNA, often 2–10 copies per mitochondrion. When transmitted, mitochondrial gene defects follow the maternal line. Thus Leber's hereditary optic neuropathy, a cause of blindness due to mutations in mitochondrial genes of the electron transport chain, is curiously much more common in males, but is always transmitted by females.

Endoplasmic reticulum (ER)

ER is another internal phospholipid bilayer membrane structure crucial to protein processing and degradation. A specialised form of the endoplasm is the Golgi apparatus, where initially processed polypeptides are matured by post-translational modification, such as glycosylation, into the mature protein which can be exported into the cytoplasm or packaged into vesicles for secretion.

Peroxisomes

Peroxisomes are small, single-membrane bound cytoplasmic organelles containing 50 or more oxidative enzymes such as catalase. Peroxisomes are involved in the metabolism of fatty and bile acids, cholesterol, purines and amino acids. The enzymes are encoded by nuclear genes and need to be transported into peroxisomes. Mutations of these enzymes which affect their transport into peroxisomes result in general peroxisomal diseases with diverse manifestations such as Zellweger's syndrome (cerebrohepatorenal syndrome with developmental delay, fits, hepatomegaly, renal cysts and elevated long-chain fatty acids).

Lysosomes

The acidic pH and enzymes within lysosomes provide protein degradation within the cell. Inherited defects in lysosomal enzymes result in failure to degrade intracellular toxic substances. For instance, in Gaucher's disease mutations of the gene encoding lysosomal glucocerebrosidase lead to large amounts of undigested lipid accumulating in macrophages, producing hepatosplenomegaly and, if severe, deposition in the brain and mental retardation.

Cytoskeleton

A series of actin and intermediate filaments and microtubules underlie the cell membrane and attach to membrane-

3

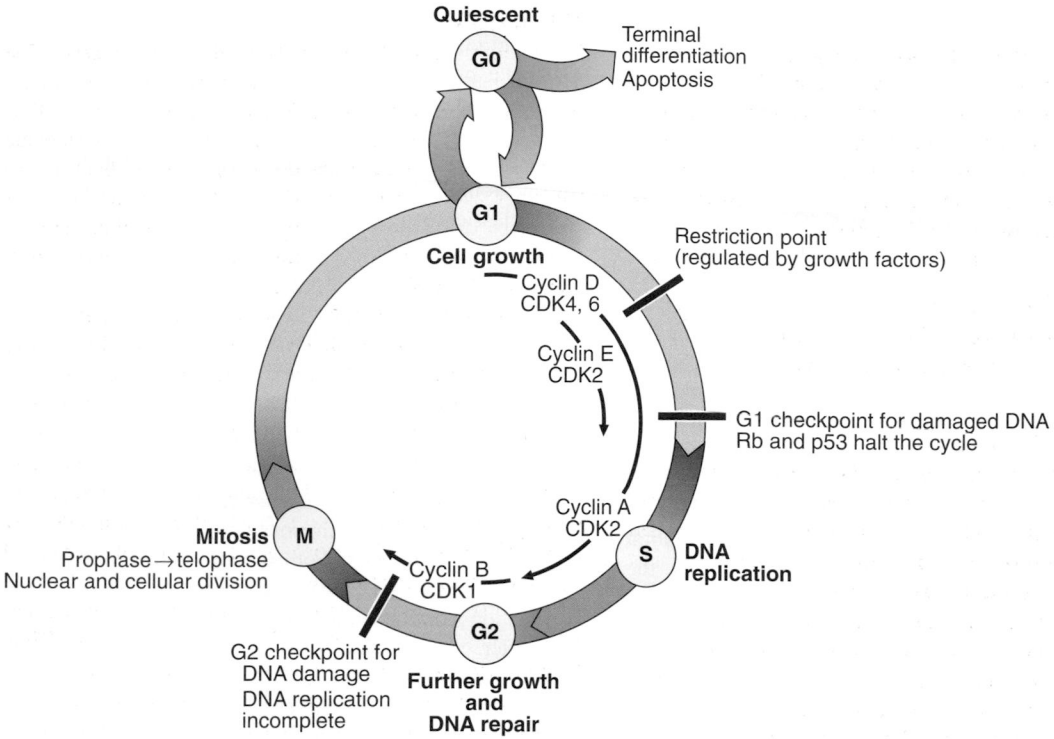

Fig. 3.3 The cell cycle. The various stages of the cell cycle, with the key checkpoints, cyclins and cyclin-dependent kinases (CDKs) that control passage through the cycle. (Rb = retinoblastoma gene product)

bound subcellular organelles. They maintain the cell's shape, and allow movement and intracellular transport. Dysfunction causes a variety of disorders. For instance, some keratin genes encode intermediate filaments in epithelia. In epidermolysis bullosa simplex (p. 1273), mutations in these genes lead to cell fragility, producing the characteristic blistering on mild trauma.

LIFE AND DEATH OF CELLS

Cellular replication is a fundamental key to biology, allowing propagation of germ cells, the zygote, embryonal development, organ growth and maturation, and tissue repair. In adult life most of our cells undergo repeated division. It has recently been recognised that even in organs such as the brain that appear to be terminally differentiated there is an ongoing low rate of birth of neurons in at least some subregions. Conversely, there is also a need for senescent cells to die in order to maintain turnover and remodelling of most organs. Cells must die in a regulated fashion to minimise uncontrolled lysis, local release of lysosomal enzymes and therefore further damage.

The cell cycle

This is the alternation of cell division and interphase (Fig. 3.3). Typically, a cell will spend most of its time in interphase, growing and functioning. Interphase is divided into G1 (gap 1) phase between mitosis (M) and the discrete point (S phase) at which DNA replication begins, and G2 between DNA replication and mitosis. In G1 the cell is

metabolically active, synthesising RNA and protein. If the cell is preparing to divide, it enters S phase to replicate DNA. This involves DNA polymerase enzymes which duplicate the strands of existing DNA in an analogous way to the reading of RNA in Figure 3.1. The cell then enters G2, when the new DNA is repaired before proceeding to mitotic division. The cell cycle takes anything from less than 24 hours to essentially not occurring at all (many neurons and skeletal muscle cells).

The cell cycle must be tightly regulated to prevent uncontrolled cell division or inadequate cell replication. A series of enzymes called cyclin-dependent kinases (CDKs) phosphorylate downstream proteins which control whether a cell enters the cell cycle and, at each point, whether it progresses or not. There are key checkpoints between G1 and S phase, and between G2 and mitosis, ensuring that damaged or misaligned chromosomes and damaged or unreplicated DNA are not passed on but rather are repaired. Failure of these control processes is a crucial factor in cancer. Critical cell cycle checkpoint proteins, such as p53 and ATM (a gene which is mutated in ataxia telangiectasia), are key factors in oncogenesis (see below).

Stem cells

Stem cells are primitive cells with the possibility of both self-renewal and differentiation. Totipotent stem cells (embryonal stem (ES) cells), which can form any tissue type, are typical of the early embryo up to the stage of gastrulation. Stem cells, which are probably less pluripotent (adult stem cells), may still form many cell types within a

3

3

tissue or a related series of tissues, and are also found in many adult organs. Such cells may be exploitable in restorative therapy of degenerative conditions, such as Alzheimer's disease and myocardial infarction, but this area of science is in its infancy (p. 61).

Programmed cell death—apoptosis

To minimise the release of toxic intracellular contents which occurs with necrosis, most cells can undergo 'programmed cell death', a deliberate activation of specific genes producing cell 'suicide'. The process, dubbed 'apoptosis', has a strict order of progression: an initiation event (which is cell type- and stimulus-specific); an effector stage when molecules of the *BCL-2* family act as opposing death agonists (e.g. Bax) and antagonists (e.g. *BCL-2*) to interact with other apoptosis factors; and ultimately a cascade of caspases leading to the degradation phase. Degradation results in chromatin aggregation and nuclear condensation into membrane vesicles (apoptotic bodies), while the integrity of cell membranes is preserved and the apoptotic cell signals to, and is engulfed by, phagocytic cells such as macrophages. Safe disposal of the apoptotic cell is then effected without stimulation of inflammation.

Apoptosis is a crucial feature of all phases of life from early embryogenesis through to senescence. Cell types which depend upon continued growth factor stimulation for survival will undergo apoptosis if they are deprived of growth factors. Usually this occurs at the critical G1–S phase transition, but some cells such as thymocytes can undergo apoptosis anywhere in the cell cycle.

MOLECULAR PATHOPHYSIOLOGY

GENETIC DISEASES

Genetic variations—polymorphisms

Although we all share genome sequences that are 99.9% identical, the remaining 0.1% is crucially responsible for all the genetic diversity between individuals. In fact, compared with other species, human DNA is highly polymorphic. Many of our genes are allelic; in other words, there are differences in the precise base sequence between individuals. Many of these differences are simple polymorphisms either in non-coding regions or, if in translated regions of exons, coding for either the same or a closely related amino acid with consequently little or no effect on the function of the protein. Single nucleotide polymorphisms (SNPs or 'snips') are common; there are $> 10^7$ described so far in the human genome and doubtless more will be reported. SNPs act as allelic markers, helping to track genetic associations with disease across the whole genome. Most SNPs are silent, although some alter the encoded protein sequence or affect the promoter and hence the level of mRNA transcription.

This heterogeneity leads to the subtle variations in phenotypes within the population, including variations in susceptibility to disease.

Mutations

A mutation is an alteration in the DNA sequence which alters the protein product of a gene in such a way as to contribute to or cause a disease (Fig. 3.4). There are around 1500 human genes which bear mutations in the germ line which can be inherited to cause disease, and probably more will be found. Whilst perhaps only 1 in 1000 individuals has a classical single gene disorder (usually inherited as a Mendelian dominant, recessive or X-linked trait; Fig. 3.8, p. 55), the contribution of a pool of genes to multifactorial (polygenic) disorders is being recognised increasingly.

Acquired mutations within somatic cells are also fairly common, but cells have very efficient repair mechanisms to rectify most mutations. Causes of increased mutation rate include:

- *Ionising radiation.* This includes X-rays and nuclear fallout. Ionising radiation generates ions by forcing electrons from atoms; the ions destabilise and break DNA or change bases. For example, there has been an increase in thyroid cancer in children exposed to radiation from the Chernobyl nuclear power plant disaster.
- *Non-ionising radiation.* This does not form charged ions but moves electrons between orbits of an atom which makes it chemically unstable, disrupting DNA. A good example is solar ultraviolet radiation causing skin cancers.
- *Chemical mutagens.* A host of chemicals such as nitrogen mustard, formaldehyde, vinyl chloride and other alkylating agents are powerful chemical mutagens.

DNA repair and its defects

Any error in DNA replication or any somatic mutation is usually repaired highly successfully (over 99% of cases) by a family of DNA repair enzymes. Loss of a specific DNA repair enzyme usually causes multifaceted degenerative disorders including, typically, susceptibility to cancer. A good example is xeroderma pigmentosum (XP). This group of disorders is due to defects in DNA repair genes which deal primarily with the effects of non-ionising radiation. Predictably, such patients develop skin cancers. Werner's syndrome, also known as progeria or the syndrome of premature ageing, is due to mutation of one of a series of DNA repair enzymes and presents with premature skin ageing, degenerative disorders and cancer. Hereditary non-polyposis colorectal cancer (HNPCC) produces proximal colon and other cancers because of a defect in one of a series of DNA mismatch repair enzymes.

Despite these highly efficient repair systems approximately 1 base in a billion per cell division undergoes a mutation that persists. For a particular gene the mutation rate depends on its size and specific sequence. Some genes have mutation 'hot spots': for example, the collagen genes, in which mutations can lead to osteogenesis imperfecta.

Point mutations

Point mutations are single nucleotide changes. The change of one nucleotide for another, also called a substitution, is the most common type of mutation. It may alter a codon,

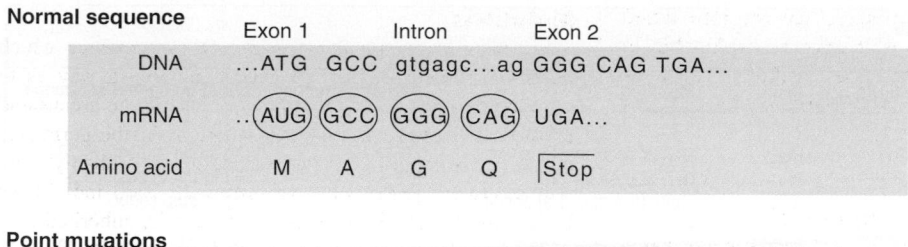

Normal sequence

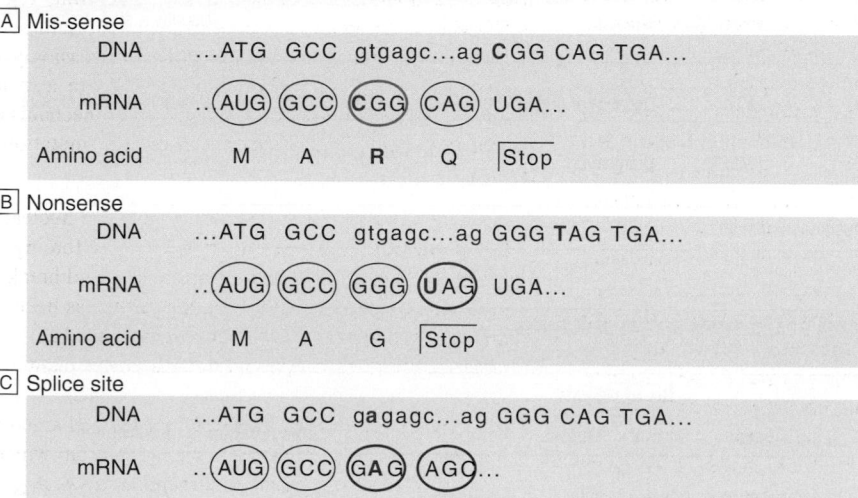

Point mutations

A Mis-sense

B Nonsense

C Splice site

Insertions and deletions

D Insertion

E Deletion

Fig. 3.4 Types of mutation.
Normal genomic DNA spanning two exons and an intervening intron is shown. This is the 'coding strand' sequence; RNA is actually read from the complementary strand (Fig. 3.1, p. 38). After splicing, the intron is removed and the predicted mRNA and protein sequence is shown. Various examples of mutation are illustrated. [A] A mis-sense mutation alters a single amino acid residue to an R. The change to a charged residue would be expected to alter protein function and ligand-binding. [B] A nonsense mutation results in premature termination of the polypeptide chain. This would be expected to result in loss of protein function. [C] A splice site mutation results in retention of the intron. This produces a novel polypeptide sequence that would be predicted to alter protein function. [D] Insertion of a nine base–pair sequence results in two novel amino acids and a premature termination codon. [E] Deletion of a six base–pair sequence results in loss of two amino acid residues which, in a functional region of the protein, would be expected to alter function.

resulting in an amino acid change in the protein (a mis-sense mutation), or introduce a premature stop codon truncating the protein (a nonsense mutation). The premature truncation of a protein is likely to result in loss of function, whereas the change of a single amino acid can have a variety of effects including loss of function or occasionally gain of a novel function. Examples of diseases commonly caused by point mutations are familial adenomatous polyposis coli and autosomal dominant polycystic kidney disease (Box 3.2).

Insertions and deletions

One or more nucleotides may be inserted or deleted in a DNA strand. When this occurs in a gene it may result in abnormal splicing or alteration of the reading frame (frameshift mutation). The insertion or deletion of a single nucleotide will alter the downstream coding sequence. This will cause an abnormal protein to be synthesised and may

also create a premature stop codon. Larger insertions or deletions also occur. Many examples of this type of mutation exist. Perhaps the most common is the ΔF508 mutation in the cystic fibrosis gene, *CFTR* (p. 46).

Duplications

A region of DNA may be duplicated. This may occur due to the presence of repeated similar or identical DNA sequences resulting in misalignment during DNA replication. If an entire gene is duplicated, then the increased amount of gene product may have a deleterious effect. This is the mechanism involved in hereditary motor and sensory neuropathy (HMSN type 1; Box 3.2).

Triplet repeat mutations

This class of mutation has been identified in a variety of inherited diseases, and interestingly results mainly in neurological diseases (Box 3.3). They consist of a variable

3.2 DISEASE-CAUSING MUTATIONS

Disease	Inheritance	Gene	Mutation	Carrier frequency	Effect on coding sequence
Point mutations					
Haemochromatosis	AR	HFE	G–A at position 845	10%	Cys to Tyr at position 282
α_1-antitrypsin deficiency	AR	PI	G–A at position 1197	3%	Glu to Lys at position 342
Familial adenomatous polyposis coli	AD	APC	Multiple, e.g. C–T at position 904	–	Arg to stop codon
Achondroplasia	AD	FGFR3	G–A at position 1138	–	Arg to Gly at position 380
Autosomal dominant polycystic kidney disease	AD	PKD1/PKD2	Multiple	–	Usually a stop codon
Insertion/deletions					
Cystic fibrosis	AR	CFTR	Deletion of codon 508 (TTT)	23%	Deletion of Phe (ΔF508)
Duplications					
Hereditary motor and sensory neuropathy type 1	AD	PMP22	Duplication		

(AR = autosomal recessive; AD = autosomal dominant)

3.3 DISEASES ASSOCIATED WITH TRIPLET AND OTHER REPEAT SEQUENCES

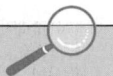

		No. of repeats				
	Repeat	Normal	Mutant	Gene	Gene location	Inheritance
Coding repeat expansion						
Huntington's disease	[CAG]	6–34	> 35	Huntingtin	4p16	AD
Spinocerebellar ataxia (type 1)	[CAG]	6–39	> 40	Ataxin	6p22–23	AD
Spinocerebellar ataxia (types 2, 3, 6, 7)	[CAG]	Various	Various	Various	Various	AD
Dentatorubral-pallidoluysian atrophy	[CAG]	7–25	> 49	Atrophin	12p12–13	AD
Machado–Joseph disease	[CAG]	12–40	> 67	MJD	14q32	AD
Spinobulbar muscular atrophy	[CAG]	11–34	> 40	Androgen receptor	Xq11–12	XL recessive
Non-coding repeat expansion						
Myotonic dystrophy	[CTG]	5–37	> 50	DMPK-3'UTR	19q13	AD
Friedreich's ataxia	[GAA]	7–22	> 200	Frataxin-intronic	9q13	AR
Progressive myoclonic epilepsy	[---]$_{4–6}$	2–3	> 25	Cystatin B-5'UTR	21q	AR
Fragile X mental retardation	[CGG]	5–52	> 200	FMR1-5'UTR	Xq27	XL dominant
Fragile site mental retardation 2 (FRAXE)	[GCC]	6–35	> 200	FMR2	Xq28	XL, probably recessive

The triplet repeat diseases fall into two major groups: those with disease resulting from expansion of $[CAG]_n$ repeats in coding DNA, resulting in multiple adjacent glutamine residues (polyglutamine tracts), and those with non-coding repeats. The latter tend to be longer. Unaffected parents usually display 'pre-mutation' allele lengths that are just above the normal range. (UTR = untranslated region; AD = autosomal dominant; AR = autosomal recessive; XL = X-linked)

length of DNA in which the same triplet of nucleotides is repeated. These are unstable areas and may represent expansions from a normal number of repeats. In normal DNA the triplets may encode amino acids in a gene, may be located in the 5′, 3′ or intronic untranslated region of a gene, or may have a poorly understood role in DNA near to functioning genes. Disease occurs when the number of triplet repeats expands beyond a certain limit. This increase occurs over several generations and is the genetic explanation for the phenomenon of anticipation. Anticipation is when the onset of disease occurs at a younger age or the disease severity increases in subsequent generations.

When triplet expansions exceed a certain size they often give rise to very early onset (apparent in the neonatal period or in childhood) of a disease that usually begins in adults. In some conditions the risk of an expansion increasing in size is influenced by whether it was inherited from the mother or father. In juvenile Huntington's disease (p. 1222) the expansion is usually inherited from the father, whilst in myotonic dystrophy the severe neonatal form usually occurs when the mutation is inherited from the mother (p. 1254). The preponderance of neurological features with expanded triplet repeats within very disparate genes perhaps reflects the sensitivity of long-lived cells such as neurons to damage by abnormal proteins and mRNAs rather than a specific role of the gene in neurons.

Chromosomal abnormalities

This term describes major rearrangements in DNA structure which affect many genes. The most common are shown in Box 3.4. Unlike mutations, which are detected only by sophisticated tests (see below), chromosomal rearrangements are often 'visible' when examining a karyotype under the microscope. These were, therefore, the first genetic disorders to be characterised.

Chromosomal disorders are extremely common and probably affect more than half of all conceptions. However, most affected offspring spontaneously miscarry, so that the

3

3.4 EXAMPLES OF CHROMOSOMAL DISORDERS

Chromosomes	Result
2n (46, XX)	Normal female
2n (46, XY)	Normal male
NUMERICAL ABNORMALITIES	
Triploidy (3n), **tetraploidy** (4n)	Spontaneous abortion
Parthenogenesis (2n from same parent)	Spontaneous abortion
Aneuploidy (2n + specific chromosome)	
Trisomy 21 (47, XY, +21)	Down's syndrome (characteristic facies, IQ usually < 50, congenital heart disease, reduced life expectancy)
Trisomy 18 (47, XY, +18)	Edwards' syndrome (characteristic skull and facies, frequent malformations of heart, kidney and other organs)
Trisomy 13 (47, XY, +13)	Patau's syndrome (cleft lip and palate, polydactyly, small head, frequent congenital heart disease)
Sex chromosome aneuploidies Phenotypically male	
47, XXY	Klinefelter's syndrome (infertility, gynaecomastia, small testes—p. 771)
47, XYY	XYY male (usually asymptomatic, often tall)
Phenotypically female	
47, XXX	Trisomy X (usually asymptomatic, 20% mentally handicapped)
45, XO	Turner's syndrome (short stature, webbed neck, primary amenorrhoea—p. 770)
STRUCTURAL CHROMOSOME ABERRATIONS **Inherited**	
46, XY,del(5p)	Cri du chat syndrome, deletion of short arm of chromosome 5
45, XY,t(14;21)	Fusion of 14 and 21, no essential chromosomal material lost (NORMAL, but balanced carrier of abnormal chromosome)
46, XY,t(14;21)	Fused 14;21 chromosome has segregated into gamete with normal chromosome 21, and fertilisation has generated trisomy 21 (Down's syndrome)
Acquired	*Occur in over 50% of haematological malignancies; also common in other neoplastic cells*
46, XY,t(9,22)	Philadelphia chromosome (chronic myeloid leukaemia)
46, XY,t(2,8) or t(8,14) or t(8,22)	Burkitt's lymphoma

3.5 DISEASES DUE TO CHROMOSOMAL MICRODELETIONS

Disease	Chromosome	Clinical features
DiGeorge syndrome	22	Facial dysmorphism, congenital heart disease (sometimes the only feature), absent parathyroids, palatal abnormalities
Williams' syndrome	7	Supravalvular aortic stenosis, facial dysmorphism, learning difficulties, hypercalcaemia
WAGR	11	**W**ilms tumour, **a**niridia, **g**enitourinary abnormalities, mental **r**etardation
Angelman's/Prader–Willi syndrome	15	Abnormal movements, ataxia, mental retardation, hypotonia, marked obesity

live-born frequency is about 0.6%, of which one-third are clinically serious. Approximately 50% of spontaneous miscarriages are due to chromosome abnormalities. There are two broad types of chromosome aberration: numerical, in which there is an incorrect number of chromosomes in somatic cells, and structural, in which there is an alteration in the structure of one or more chromosomes.

The gain or loss of one or more chromosomes (aneuploidy) usually results in early pregnancy loss, but the presence of certain single extra chromosomes (trisomy) may be compatible with survival and give rise to distinct clinical syndromes. Down's syndrome or trisomy 21 (47, XX/XY, +21) is the most common trisomy seen in live births. The incidence increases with maternal age, rising from 1:1500 at age 20 to 1:50 at age 43. Screening for Down's syndrome during pregnancy is now routinely offered in most developed countries using serum screening, fetal ultrasound and amniocentesis (Box 3.17, p. 57). An additional sex chromosome (X or Y) usually has less severe clinical effects (e.g. XXY Klinefelter's syndrome, p. 771).

Survival with the loss of a chromosome (monosomy) is confined to the X or Y chromosome. 45, X0 causes Turner's syndrome (p. 770).

Abnormal chromosome structure may be due to translocations, deletions, duplications or inversions. Translocations are due to the exchange of genetic material between different chromosomes. The exchange of material between two different chromosomes is referred to as a reciprocal translocation and is balanced if there is no net loss. Such translocations are usually unique to an individual and can be inherited. They are relatively common, being found in about 1:500 individuals. Translocations may cause disease if the chromosome breakpoint disrupts a gene (e.g. the Philadelphia (Ph) chromosome, p. 1044), or if loss of genetic material occurs during meiosis; in the latter case the translocation is said to be unbalanced. Unbalanced translocations frequently give rise to severe developmental defects or early pregnancy loss. A special type of translocation, the Robertsonian translocation, involves two of chromosomes 13, 14, 15, 21 or 22. The involvement of chromosome 21 in this type of translocation may result in a pregnancy with Down's syndrome and a relatively high risk of recurrence. Consequences of smaller deletions within chromosomes, spanning more than one gene, are described in Box 3.5. Subtelomeric deletions, or loss of DNA adjacent to the telomeres which form the ends of a chromosome, are increasingly recognised as a cause of mental handicap.

ONCOGENESIS

There are many examples of disorders of the integrated function of cells throughout the chapters of this book. A key common characteristic of all cells is the ability to regulate the cell cycle (p. 43). The best example of the consequences of abnormal cell replication is in the development of cancer, i.e. oncogenesis. This topic also illustrates the close links between advances in molecular biology and cell biology.

Most tumours are clonal, i.e. they arise from a single starting cell which has escaped from normal growth controls, replicated more frequently and/or failed to undergo programmed death. Cancer cells proliferate and eventually gain the capacity to migrate to distant sites and show further uncontrolled replication (metastasis, Fig. 3.5). Such escape is caused and facilitated by the accumulation of mutations within the DNA of a cancerous cell as a result of inheritance and environmental carcinogens. Clearly, mutations will arise more rapidly if external mutagens are increased (e.g. in smokers) or if the cell is defective in DNA repair systems. Cancer is thus a disease that affects the fundamental processes of molecular and cell biology.

The first step in the typical multistep process to cancer is tumour initiation. This is usually a 'somatic' mutation in a single cell leading to increased proliferation. As the clone of mutated cells increases, one or more may be subject to additional mutations which confer growth advantage, leading to further proliferation of these subclonal lines. Later mutations with 'advantages' of greater growth or invasiveness lead to aggressive and metastasising cancer. Less commonly, germ-line mutations are present which predispose an individual to cancers in several sites; these mutations can be inherited and are the basis for familial cancer syndromes.

Oncogenes

This term refers to a gene which, when mutated or introduced (by an oncogenic virus), facilitates neoplastic proliferation. The normal function of such genes is usually to produce factors involved in growth control, the cell cycle or apoptosis. Oncogenes can be broadly divided into two groups, according to whether their oncogenic effect is gain of a pro-oncogenic gene (i.e. overactivity of a 'proto-oncogene' or gain of an oncogenic virus) or loss of an endogenous anti-oncogenic 'tumour suppressor' function.

Viral oncogenes

Retroviral oncogenes cause a minority of cancers. These DNA sequences are introduced from an exogenous viral infection or, theoretically, have been incorporated into the human genome from viral infections in our ancestors. They cause cancer in many mammalian species. Human T-cell lymphotropic virus type 1 (HTLV-1) causes T-cell leukaemia in regions in which it is endemic (the Far East, Africa and the Caribbean). It achieves this by exploiting the host T cell to express a viral protein which interferes with cell cycle control. Other examples include human papillomavirus E7, which inappropriately phosphorylates pRB (the product of the retinoblastoma gene) leading to cervical carcinoma, and herpes virus 8, which encodes a cyclin that drives the host cell through the G1–S checkpoint. Other viral infections associated with cancers (human immunodeficiency virus (HIV), herpes simplex virus 2 (HSV2), and Epstein–Barr virus (EBV)) usually act by suppressing endogenous immune function and hence cancer surveillance rather than having a direct oncogenic effect.

Proto-oncogenes

The majority of known oncogenes are components of signal transduction pathways in which mutations, or the presence of increased copies of a gene, mimic persistent growth factor stimulation.

An early discovery was the *H-RAS* oncogene in which a single point mutation, which changes a single amino acid, turns an innocuous guanine nucleotide binding protein in the growth factor-signalling pathway into an oncogene stimulating uncontrolled proliferation in a host of cancers. The mutation blocks the ability of *H-RAS* to catalyse removal of GTP; persisting high levels of GTP mimic continuous growth factor stimulation.

In multiple endocrine neoplasia type 2 (MEN 2, p. 802), the *RET* gene is mutated, leading to endogenous activation of a receptor tyrosine kinase normally only active when stimulated by its growth factor ligand, glial cell-derived neurotropic factor. Tumours in neuroendocrine organs result.

Other proto-oncogene examples are genes encoding receptors (e.g. *ERBB* in breast carcinoma, which forms the target for a specific therapeutic monoclonal antibody, herceptin) and transcription factors such as c-myc which is important in gastrointestinal tumours, lymphomas and leukaemias. In Burkitt's lymphoma (Box 3.4), the characteristic translocation of a fragment of chromosome 8 to chromosome 2 inserts c-myc without its normal control sequences in an area which is upstream of an immunoglobulin gene; this leads to inappropriate c-myc expression in lymphocytes and stimulates their proliferation. Similarly, in chronic myeloid leukaemia (CML, p. 1044), with its characteristic translocation of chromosome 9 to chromosome 22 (the Philadelphia chromosome), the *ABL* proto-oncogene from chromosome 9 is fused downstream of the chromosome 22 gene *BCR*. This removes the normal control sequences for *ABL* and leads to unregulated expression of the ABL tyrosine kinase and cancer. Striking exploitation of

3

this knowledge has been achieved with the development of a drug, imatinib, which inhibits ABL tyrosine kinase and is an effective treatment for CML.

Tumour suppressor genes

Tumour suppressor genes usually encode proteins whose normal function is to inhibit the cell cycle or to induce apoptosis to prevent transmission of uncorrectable DNA defects. Direct inhibitors of the cell cycle include *pRb*, which is mutated in retinoblastoma. Other tumour suppressor genes encode components of inhibitory growth factor-signalling pathways, particularly those of transforming growth factor (TGF)-β and its associated cytoplasmic signalling molecules such as Smad2 and Smad4 (the *DPC4* 'deleted in pancreatic carcinoma' gene). *Neurofibromin* encodes a Ras inhibitor which is mutated in neurofibromatosis. *APC*, the gene mutated in familial adenomatous polyposis and 60% of sporadic colon adenomas and carcinomas, is thought to operate as an oncogene by rendering cells less susceptible to apoptosis. A key tumour suppressor gene, *p53*, overrides other signals which would otherwise stimulate cell proliferation. The importance of *p53* is illustrated by the fact that it is inactivated in over 50% of human tumours, including breast and colon carcinomas, and childhood leukaemias.

When an oncogene results from a mutation reducing the activity of a tumour suppressor, a single mutation is usually insufficient to cause cancer unless an additional mutation inactivates the second copy of the gene (Knudson's 'two-hit'

model of tumorigenesis). If, on the other hand, an oncogene results from overactivity of a proto-oncogene, a mutation in only one of the two copies may be sufficient to promote tumorigenesis. This is also true in an important exception to the two-hit rule, the case of the tumour suppressor gene *p53*, since mutations in only one allele may be sufficient to result in a biological effect. This reflects the operation of the protein as a tetramer, so abnormalities in any one of the subunits may derange its overall function. This ability of one allele to disrupt the function of protein from both alleles is called a 'dominant negative' effect.

Multistep carcinogenesis (Fig. 3.5)

The cell's complex self-regulating machinery means that more than one mutation is often required to produce a malignant, metastasising tumour such as a carcinoma. For example, if a cell mutates to produce a growth factor for which it already expresses the receptor (autocrine stimulation), that cell will replicate more frequently but will still be subject to cell cycle checkpoints to promote DNA integrity in its progeny. If an additional mutation overriding a cell cycle checkpoint occurs, that cell and its progeny may go on to accumulate further mutations, some of which may allow it to replicate an unlimited number of times, or to separate from its matrix and cellular attachments without undergoing apoptosis. As deregulated growth continues, cancer cells become increasingly unable to differentiate, fail to respond to the normal local signals in their tissue of origin, and cease to ensure appropriate chromosomal

3

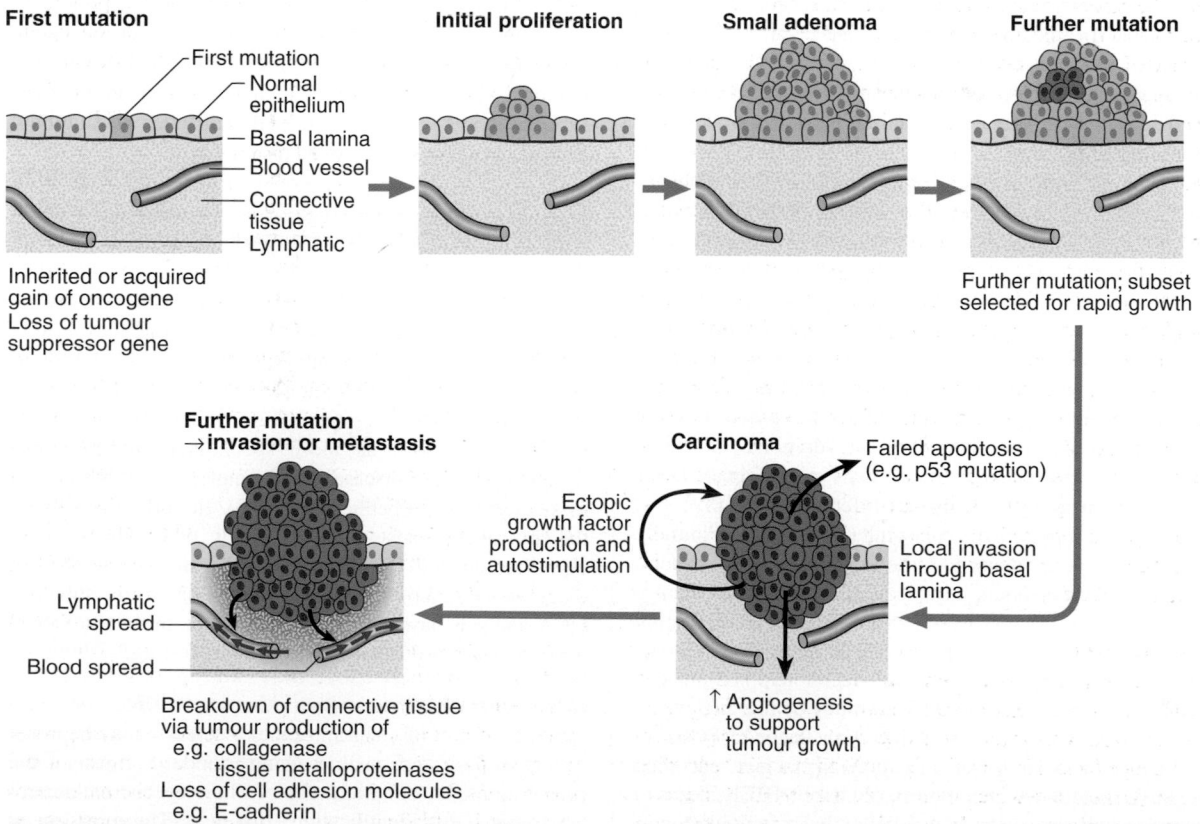

Fig. 3.5 **Oncogenesis.** The multistep origin of cancer, showing events implicated in cancer initiation, progression, invasion and metastasis.

3.6 EXAMPLES OF FAMILIAL CANCER SYNDROMES

Disease	Inheritance	Gene	Tumour(s)	Page reference
Retinoblastoma	AD	RB1	Retinoblastoma, osteosarcoma	–
Familial breast/ovarian cancer	AD	BRCA1 and BRCA2	Breast, ovary	Ch. 8
Hereditary non-polyposis colorectal cancer (HNPCC)	AD	hMSH2, hMLH1, hPMS1, hPMS2	Colorectal, endometrial, stomach, breast, urinary tract	925
Von Hippel–Lindau disease	AD	VHL	CNS haemangioblastoma, renal, phaeochromocytoma	1238
Peutz–Jeghers syndrome	AD	STK11	Gastrointestinal, endometrial, breast, ovary	925
Li–Fraumeni syndrome	AD	p53	Sarcoma, brain, breast, leukaemia, adrenal	–

segregation pre-division, generating the classical malignant pathological appearances of disorganised growth, variable levels of differentiation, and polyploidy.

Inherited basis of cancer

It is important to recognise that most of the mutations described above arise in a somatic cell and are not transmitted to the patient's offspring. Nevertheless, some human families are genetically prone to cancer (Box 3.6). One group of cancer patients, exemplified by XP and HNPCC families, have defects in DNA repair enzymes (see above) so that they accumulate mutations at a faster rate. More commonly, individuals in cancer-prone families inherit a mutation in a particular oncogene, reducing the number of additional mutations a cell from that person requires to become neoplastic. The two-hit model explains why even in members of these cancer-prone families, tumours may not develop for many years. The inherited oncogene may be particularly relevant for a certain cell type, predisposing to a particular form of tumour (e.g. *N-Ras* and neurological tumours), or be able to deregulate growth in a variety of different cell types (e.g. *p53* mutations in Li–Fraumeni syndrome families who are particularly prone to early-onset leukaemias, sarcomas, and breast and brain malignancies).

Other pathological features of solid tumours

Haematological malignancies occur in cells which are already anchorage-independent and circulating. However, additional features are required for a solid tumour to grow and metastasise. The acquisition of additional mutations means that the secondary tumour cells may replicate faster than the primary, or be unable to differentiate as fully.

The blood supply to the enlarging mass of cells is initially rate-limiting, as evidenced by the ischaemic centres to solid tumours. Some tumours may acquire mutations to enhance the secretion of factors which stimulate neovascularisation (angiogenesis), but often physiology suffices since hypoxia, via activation of the transcription factor hypoxia-induced factor 1α (HIF1α), is a potent stimulus of the angiogenic factor vascular endothelial cell growth factor (VEGF). In von Hippel–Lindau disease mutations of the gene encoding the VHL protein, which normally sequesters HIF1α, leads to vascular tumours such as cerebellar haemangioblastomas and retinal haemangiomas, and other cancers.

Metastasis

Metastasis, the cardinal feature of most malignant tumours, requires a cancer cell to have the ability to detach from its surroundings without undergoing apoptosis. Certain mutations result in nuclei receiving signals as if they were anchored to local structures—e.g. mutations in APC. In addition, metastasising cells must acquire the novel abilities to invade through local tissues to reach blood vessels, survive in the circulation, adhere to a blood vessel wall and migrate into the new tissue. Many of these features are facilitated by the synthesis of cellular adhesion molecules or tissue-degradative enzymes such as metalloproteinases. Adherence to the endothelium in the new site cannot simply reflect the fact that the cells adhere to the nearest capillary bed, since metastases display tissue specificity (e.g. thyroid cancer to bone). Specific cellular adhesion mechanisms analogous to those used by inflammatory cells are thought to operate. Also, to escape destruction by cells of the immune system, tumour cells may down-regulate cell-surface expression of recognition molecules or induce a general depression of immune responses.

INVESTIGATIONS IN GENETIC DISEASE

The diagnosis and investigation of genetic disease are no different from those of any other disease in that they require an accurate history, thorough clinical examination and the appropriate use of diagnostic tests. These include haematology, biochemistry, immunology, radiology and histopathology as well as more specialised investigations depending on the disease: for example, electrophysiology in suspected neuropathies (Box 3.7). In addition to these, the clinical geneticist and, increasingly, other clinicians use chromosome and DNA analysis to confirm or exclude a diagnosis (Fig. 3.6). Modern techniques of chromosome and DNA analysis have had a dramatic effect on the number of genetic diseases that can be detected by testing.

Detecting chromosomal abnormalities

The loss of part of a chromosome or deletion may be either 'microscopic' and visible using standard chromosome preparations, or 'submicroscopic' where special techniques are required for identification (Box 3.5). The most useful investigation is fluorescent in situ hybridisation (FISH,

3.7 EXAMPLES OF NON-DNA-BASED INVESTIGATIONS FOR COMMON GENETIC DISEASES

Disease	Investigation	Page
Haemoglobinopathy e.g. sickle cell disease	Haemoglobin electrophoresis	1035
Coagulation disorders e.g. haemophilia	Clotting factor levels	1057
Immune deficiencies e.g. hypogammaglobulinaemia	Ig levels, complement levels	74
Inborn errors of metabolism e.g. phenylketonuria	Enzyme assays, amino acid levels	442
Endocrine disease e.g. congenital adrenal hyperplasia	Hormone levels, enzyme assays	789
Renal disease e.g. autosomal dominant polycystic kidney disease	Radiology, renal biopsy	506
Myopathy e.g. mitochondrial myopathy	Muscle biopsy, enzyme assay	1255
Skeletal dysplasias e.g. osteogenesis imperfecta	Radiology	1131

Fig. 3.6C). Many syndromes due to microscopic and submicroscopic deletions have been identified, usually the result of loss of one copy of several adjacent genes (Box 3.5).

The use of whole genome arrays (DNA 'chips') will revolutionise chromosome analysis in the future and allow the rapid detection of gain or loss of DNA in individuals in whom a karyotype is normal but symptoms and signs suggest an underlying genetic cause (Box 3.11). These chips (also called microarrays) contain thousands of miniature 'probes', i.e. short sequences of DNA which are complementary to known sequences in the normal genome (Fig. 3.6F). Each probe is embedded in one of thousands of miniature 'wells' on the chip. The patient's sample is hybridised to the chip, and positive and negative results for each probe are typically read off using a robot which detects fluorescent 'labels' inserted in the DNA. This allows a map of much of the patient's DNA to be constructed from just one test, and missing sequences to be identified.

Gene 'linkage'

The process of attributing an inherited disease to a specific gene typically begins with investigation of the affected family or families. The polymorphisms in the normal genome (p. 44) can be 'mapped' using SNPs, or variations in the pattern of DNA fragments generated with 'restriction enzymes' (these enzymes cut DNA at specific sequences so that variations in sequence result in restriction fragment length polymorphisms, RFLPs). Comparison of the map in affected and unaffected individuals allows identification of the 'locus' of DNA where the responsible gene resides. The confidence of association ('linkage') with the disease in question is influenced by the number of subjects studied, the strength of the effect of the gene on the disease, and the closeness of the SNP or RFLP to the gene in question. The confidence can be expressed as a LoD (likelihood of disequilibrium) score, which is $-\log_{10}$ of the probability (p value) of linkage; by convention a LoD score of > 3 ($p < 0.001$) is taken to be statistically significant. Once a

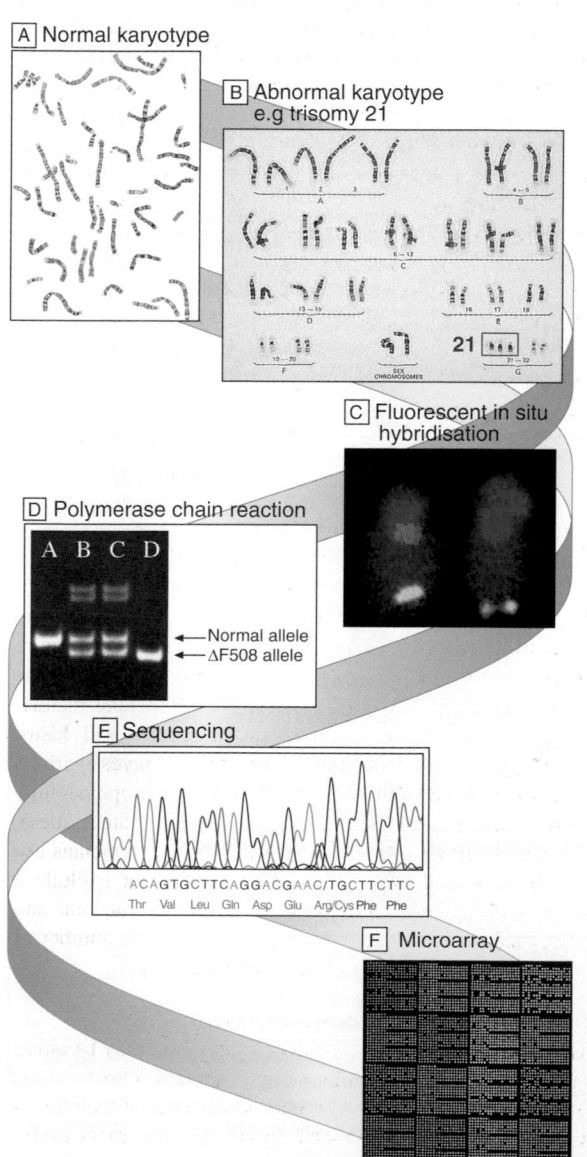

A Normal karyotype

B Abnormal karyotype e.g trisomy 21

C Fluorescent in situ hybridisation

D Polymerase chain reaction

A B C D

← Normal allele
← ΔF508 allele

E Sequencing

ACAGTGCTTCAGGACGAAC/TGCTTCTTC
Thr Val Leu Gln Asp Glu Arg/Cys Phe Phe

F Microarray

Fig. 3.6 Common investigations of DNA in genetic disease. A and B Normal and abnormal chromosome number and structure can be determined by karyotype analysis. C Submicroscopic deletions can be visualised using fluorescent in situ hybridisation (FISH). D Amplification of DNA using the polymerase chain reaction (PCR) can be used to test for many common mutations. A is a normal result for the cystic fibrosis CF ΔF508 test. B and C are carriers (heterozygotes) and D is homozygous and therefore affected with CF. E DNA from polymerase chain reactions can be sequenced directly to identify mutations F Microarray analysis can rapidly identify small regions of DNA loss or gain.

3.8 EXAMPLES OF GENETIC DISEASES FOR WHICH DIRECT GENE TESTING IS ROUTINELY AVAILABLE

Disease	Gene/protein
Point mutations	
Haemochromatosis	HFE
Neurofibromatosis type 1 and 2	NF1 and NF2 (neurofibromin and merlin)
Tuberous sclerosis	TSC1 and TSC2 (hamartin and tuberin)
Von Hippel–Lindau disease	VHL
Achondroplasia	FGFR
Marfan's syndrome	FBN1 (fibrillin)
Familial breast cancer	BRCA1 and BRCA2
Deletions/point mutations	
Cystic fibrosis	CFTR
Incontinentia pigmenti	NEMO
Duchenne/Becker muscular dystrophy	DMD (dystrophin)
Gene duplication	
Hereditary motor and sensory neuropathy type 1	PMP22
Triplet repeat expansion	
Myotonic dystrophy	DMPK
Huntington's disease	Huntingtin
Fragile X syndrome	FMR1
Friedreich's ataxia	FRDA1 (frataxin)
Ataxia-telangiectasia	ATM

3.9 COMMON MONOGENIC DISORDERS AFFECTING MAJOR ORGAN SYSTEMS

System	Disease	Inheritance
Multisystem	Neurofibromatosis	AD
	Tuberous sclerosis	AD
Respiratory	α_1-antitrypsin deficiency	AR
	Cystic fibrosis	AR
	Kartagener's syndrome	AR
Cardiovascular	Hypertrophic cardiomyopathy	AD
	Long QT syndromes	AD and AR
	22q deletion syndrome	AD
Renal	Polycystic kidney disease	AD
	Alport's syndrome	XL
	Finnish nephropathy	AR
	Renal tubular acidosis	AR
	Haemolytic-uraemic syndrome	AR
	Benign familial haematuria	AD
Gastrointestinal	Hereditary pancreatitis	AD
	Cystic fibrosis	AR
	Familial adenomatous polyposis coli	AD
Hepatic	Gilbert's disease	AD
	Haemochromatosis	AR
	Wilson's disease	AR
	α_1-antitrypsin deficiency	AR
	Polycystic liver disease	AD
Metabolic	Phenylketonuria	AR
	Familial hypercholesterolaemia	AD
	Acute intermittent porphyria	AD
	Galactosaemia	AR
	Glycogen storage diseases	AR
	Homocystinuria	AR
Endocrine	Congenital adrenal hyperplasia	AR
	Multiple endocrine neoplasia	AD
	Kallmann's syndrome	XL or AD
Haematological	Sickle-cell disease	AR
	Alpha- and beta-thalassaemia	AR
	Haemophilia A and B	XL
	Glucose-6-phosphate dehydrogenase deficiency	XL
Neuromuscular	Duchenne muscular dystrophy	XL
	Myotonic dystrophy	AD
	Spinal muscular atrophy	AR
	Hereditary motor and sensory neuropathy type 1	AD
Central nervous system	Huntington's disease	AD
	Familial Alzheimer's disease	AD
	Friedreich's ataxia	AR
	Hereditary spastic paraplegia	Mainly AD
Connective tissue	Ehlers–Danlos syndrome	AD
	Marfan's syndrome	AD
	Osteogenesis imperfecta	Mostly AD
	Achondroplasia	AD
Skin	Albinism	AR
	Epidermolysis bullosa	AD
	Neurofibromatosis	AD
	Xeroderma pigmentosum	AR
Eye	Retinitis pigmentosa	AR, AD, XL
	Ocular albinism	XL
	Colour blindness	XL
	Leber's optic atrophy	Mitochondrial

locus has been identified, more detailed mapping within the locus can then be undertaken and the relevant mutation confirmed by sequencing the relevant gene.

DNA sequence analysis

The polymerase chain reaction (PCR) can amplify virtually any gene sequence for analysis by gel electrophoresis or, now almost ubiquitously, by automated DNA sequencing (Fig. 3.6). Despite the identification of the gene or genes responsible for a disorder, it still may not be possible to search routinely for mutations in individuals or families due to outstanding technical challenges. Whilst some diseases such as cystic fibrosis are mainly due to a single common mutation for which a test can readily be developed (Box 3.8), other diseases are due to a wide variety of mutations (in either the same or a different gene), necessitating the screening of all exons and adjacent sequences. Whilst such screening can be undertaken in dedicated research laboratories, this level of investigation is often impossible in hospital diagnostic laboratories. Even with current developments in DNA technology (including high-throughput sequencing and DNA 'chips'), routine laboratory testing for many diseases is not yet available, although technologies are likely to be streamlined and costs should fall.

PRESENTING PROBLEMS IN GENETIC DISEASE

Patterns of presentation

Due to the very varied nature of genetic alterations that underlie clinical disease, genetic disease may present at any

3.10 THE ROLE OF THE CLINICAL GENETICIST

- Diagnosis of all types of genetic disease, birth defects and development abnormalities
- Assessment of genetic risk
- Genetic counselling
- Predictive testing for genetic disease, especially late-onset disorders
- Follow-up and screening for certain genetic disorders
- Provision of genetic services to extended families

3.11 COMMON PRESENTATIONS OF GENETIC DISEASE

- Healthy individuals with a known family history
- Organ-specific disease and recognised genetic diseases, e.g. cancers, dementia, polycystic kidney disease
- Abnormal antenatal scan/pregnancy screening result
- Pregnancy loss/neonatal death associated with severe malformations
- Congenital abnormalities (dysmorphology)
- Developmental delay
- Deafness/blindness

3.12 THE CHROMOSOMAL AND GENETIC BASIS OF DYSMORPHIC SYNDROMES

Syndrome/genetic mechanism/test	Features include
Down's syndrome Trisomy 21 Karyotype	Characteristic facies Mental retardation Single palmar crease Neonatal hypotonia Short stature Congenital heart defects
Turner's syndrome Monosomy X Karyotype	Short stature Streak gonads Primary amenorrhoea Neck webbing Aortic coarctation
Smith–Magenis syndrome 17p microdeletion FISH	Characteristic facies Mental retardation Congenital heart disease Sleep disturbance Self-destructive behaviour
DiGeorge syndrome 22q microdeletion FISH	Characteristic facies Parathyroid hypoplasia Thymic hypoplasia Congenital heart disease Psychiatric illness Cleft lip
Bardet–Biedl syndrome BBS1-8 (AR) Mutation analysis	Mental retardation Retinopathy Polydactyly Obesity Hypogenitalism
Smith–Lemli–Opitz syndrome DHCR (AR) 7-dehydrocholesterol levels	Mental retardation Microcephaly Photosensitivity Heart defects Hypospadias
Van der Woude syndrome IRF6 (AD) Mutation analysis	Cleft lip/palate Lower lip pits/sinuses
Crouzon's syndrome FGFR (AD) Mutation analysis	Craniosynostosis Hypertelorism Exophthalmos Characteristic facies
Orofaciodigital syndrome type I OFD1 (XL) Mutation analysis	Oral frenula Clefting of jaw and tongue Lobulated tongue Malformations of face and skull Polycystic kidney disease Mental retardation

(DHCR = 7-dehydrocholesterol reductase; IRF6 = interferon regulatory factor-6; FGFR = fibroblast growth factor receptor; FISH = fluorescent in situ hybridisation)

age from early development to old age and in any tissue or organ system (Box 3.9). Frequently, several systems are involved, either as a primary feature of the disease or due to secondary complications. It is increasingly important that all clinicians are able to elicit a history suggestive of inherited disease and know when to use the specialist skills of the medical geneticist (Box 3.10). Certain presentations are commonly seen in the medical genetics clinic and these are listed in Box 3.11.

DYSMORPHIC SYNDROMES

A difficult role for the clinical geneticist is the diagnosis of malformation syndromes and birth defects, many of which are rare (dysmorphology). Their recognition has important implications for future management, detection of additional complications and recurrence risks. The use of dysmorphology databases for syndrome identification is now well established but often only complements the diagnostic skill of the experienced clinical geneticist. The chromosomal and genetic basis of a wide range of dysmorphic syndromes has been identified (Box 3.12).

MONOGENIC AND CHROMOSOMAL DISEASE

Clinical assessment

Constructing a pedigree

Collecting a pedigree or family tree is a fundamental part of the approach to genetic disease. The basic symbols and nomenclature used in drawing a pedigree are given in Figure 3.7. The family history taken in a routine medical clerking should be presented in this manner. It will often reveal important genetic risks in a family that otherwise might not have been appreciated. This is especially true when taking a family history relating to cancer.

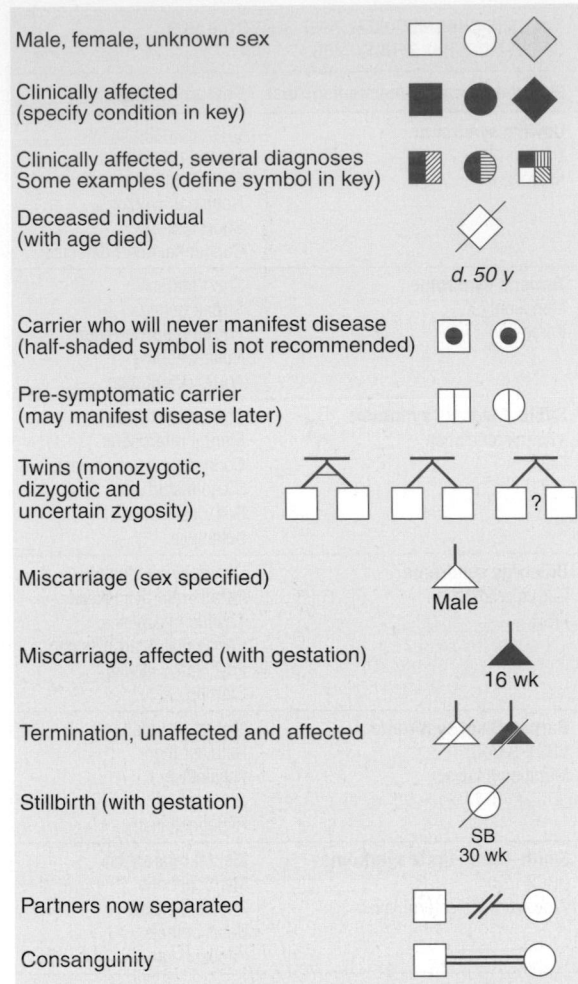

Male, female, unknown sex

Clinically affected
(specify condition in key)

Clinically affected, several diagnoses
Some examples (define symbol in key)

Deceased individual
(with age died)

d. 50 y

Carrier who will never manifest disease
(half-shaded symbol is not recommended)

Pre-symptomatic carrier
(may manifest disease later)

Twins (monozygotic,
dizygotic and
uncertain zygosity)

?

Miscarriage (sex specified)

Male

Miscarriage, affected (with gestation)

16 wk

Termination, unaffected and affected

Stillbirth (with gestation)

SB
30 wk

Partners now separated

Consanguinity

Fig. 3.7 Common symbols used in constructing a pedigree.

A pedigree must include details from both sides of the family, any history of pregnancy loss or infant death, consanguinity, and details of all medical conditions in family members. Other significant information includes dates of birth and age at death.

It is important to be aware that a diagnosis given by a family member, or even obtained from a death certificate, may be wrong. This is often true in cases of cancer where 'stomach' may mean any part of the bowel, and 'brain' may refer to secondary deposits or be used where the primary site has not been identified.

Inheritance patterns

The common modes of inheritance are described in Figure 3.8.

Different individuals who inherit a particular disease mutation rarely demonstrate an identical phenotype, since they may not share the other genetic or environmental factors that unmask the full effect of the mutation. Penetrance is defined as the proportion of individuals who develop the disease phenotype. The mutation is said to be fully penetrant if all individuals who inherit it develop disease phenotype. If additional environmental factors are

needed, the gene may display late-onset penetrance, or may even be non-penetrant if the individual is never exposed to sufficient additional factors (Fig. 3.9). Disease expression describes the degree to which the severity of the disease phenotype may vary. These factors may make it difficult to determine whether some diseases are autosomal dominant, X-linked, mitochondrial or imprinted.

For mutations in some genes the effect depends on whether it is inherited from the mother or father. This is called 'genomic imprinting' (Box 3.13). For example, a critical region on chromosome 15q contains several genes in which only the paternal or maternal allele is transcriptionally active; the other allele is permanently inactivated, typically by methylation of the DNA which prevents transcription. Deletion of these genes on the paternal chromosome causes Prader–Willi syndrome, whereas deletion of the maternal chromosome causes Angelman's syndrome (Box 3.13).

Investigations

The testing modalities described on pages 50–52 may or may not allow routine testing for the suspected inherited disease. Even if they are available, careful consideration must be given to the implications of the results of genetic testing, both for the patient and for other members of their family, before it is undertaken. Where testing is not available, the diagnosis may rely upon information from patient records, from pathology reports or from a detailed clinical examination.

Diagnostic tests

In the presence of the characteristic symptoms or signs of a particular disease a genetic test may be used to confirm the clinical diagnosis.

Predictive tests

In the absence of symptoms or signs of disease in an individual at risk of inheriting a genetic disease, a genetic test can be used to determine whether that individual carries the disease-causing mutation—a presymptomatic or predictive test. Predictive tests are usually carried out for adult-onset disorders such as familial cancer syndromes (Box 3.6, p. 50) and neurodegenerative disorders such as

---

Fig. 3.8 Principles of inheritance. A Mendelian transmission of a single pair of autosomes, where the mother has a single mutant gene (red circle) on the chromosome shown in white. B Pattern of inheritance of a mutant gene using conventional symbol designation, with characteristic features of resulting genetic diseases. (Male = square; female = circle; unaffected = white; affected = black; unaffected carrier = grey; deceased = strike-through; see Fig. 3.7 for full explanation of symbols used in family pedigrees)

Fig. 3.9 The spectrum of genetic disease: how the genotype influences the phenotype. A particular characteristic or disease in an individual may be due to a specific genetic abnormality (monogenic disease), or may reflect several predisposing genes (polygenic disease). In each case, environmental factors may further influence the phenotype; in their absence, genetic factors alone may be insufficient to allow the disease to develop, resulting in non-penetrance (see text).

3

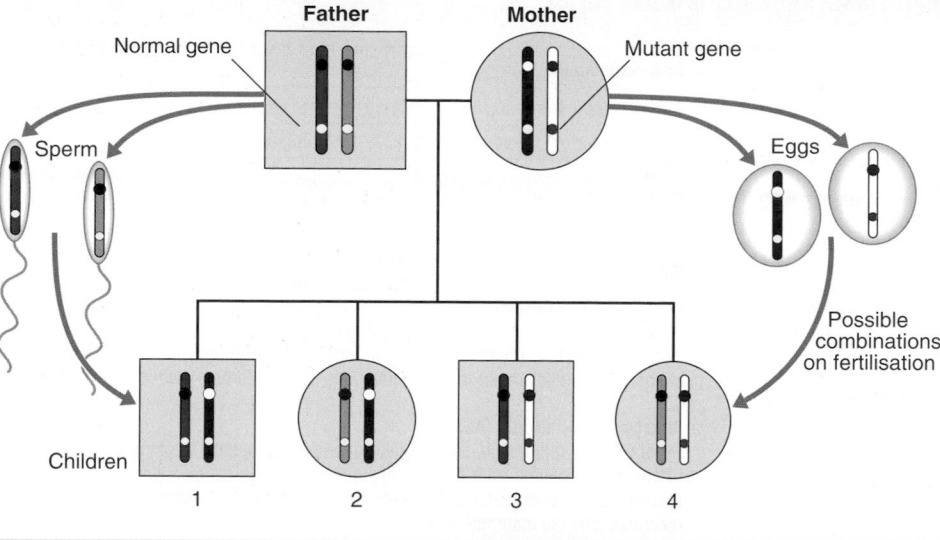

A

3

B

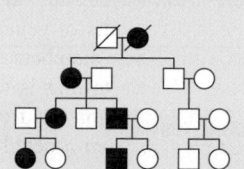

Autosomal inheritance
(gene on chromosome 1–22)

Dominant inheritance

The second copy of the gene on the homologous chromosome cannot compensate for the mutated copy:

- Consecutive generations are affected
- Half of offspring are affected, male = female
- Unaffected individual cannot transmit disease

Assuming full penetrance; see text

Recessive inheritance

The second copy of the gene on the homologous chromosome compensates for the mutated copy:

- Half the children of unaffected carriers will be carriers
- If both parents are carriers, then one-quarter of their offspring are affected, and one-half are carriers
- Usually only one generation is affected

Affected individuals may have two identical mutant copies arising from a common ancestor as shown above, or different in 'compound heterozygotes'

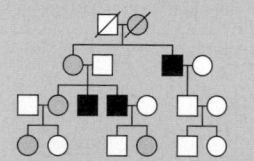

X-linked inheritance
(X chromosome gene)

A second copy of the gene is only present in females. In X-linked recessive disease:

- Only males are affected
- Unaffected female carriers transmit the disease
- Half of carrier female's offspring inherit mutation —males are affected and females are carriers
- Affected males cannot transmit the disease to their sons, but all of their daughters are carriers

X-linked diseases are occasionally dominant

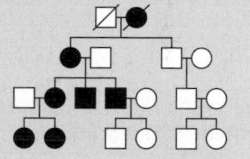

Non-germ line cytoplasmic inheritance
(e.g. gene on mitochondrial DNA)

- Males and females are affected
- No males transmit disease
- Variable proportion of offspring from female are affected

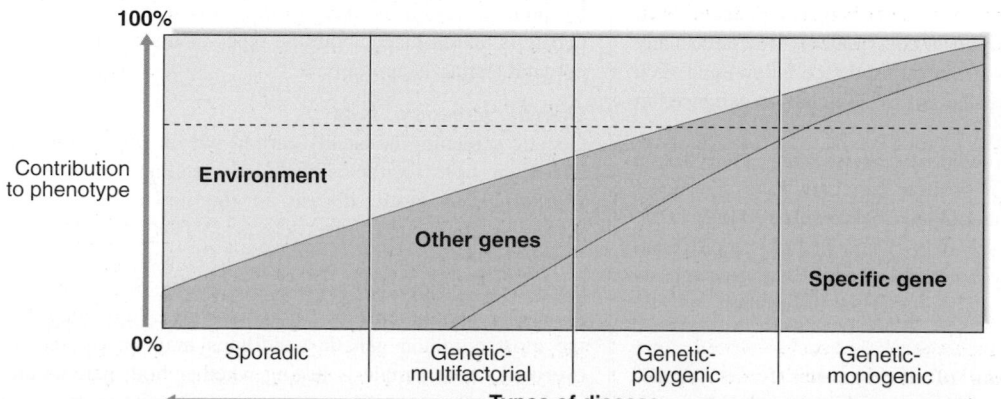

3.13 IMPRINTED GENES IMPLICATED IN HUMAN DISEASE

Chromosome	Gene(s)	Disease example
6q26	IGF2R	Tumour suppressor—inactivated by inappropriate imprinting
11p13	WT1	Wilms tumour: WT1 gene mutated in 10–15% of cases
11p15	p57^{KIP2} HASH2, INS2 IGF2, H19	**Beckwith–Wiederman syndrome** General 'over-growth', advanced ageing and increased childhood tumours. Probably due to mutations in p57^{KIP2}
	WT2	**Wilms tumour**
15q11–q13	SNRPN Necdin and others	**Prader–Willi syndrome** Obesity, hypogonadism and varying degrees of mental retardation. Lack of paternal contribution (due to deletion of paternal 15q11–q13, or inheritance of both chromosome 15q11–q13 regions from the mother). Currently thought to be a contiguous gene syndrome, due to loss of at least SNRPN and necdin
	Ubiquitin protein ligase E3A (UBE3A)	**Angelman's syndrome (AS)** Severe mental retardation, ataxia, epilepsy and inappropriate laughing bouts due to mutations in the UBE3A gene inherited from the patient's mother. The neurological phenotype results because most tissues express both maternal and paternal alleles of UBE3A, whereas the brain expresses predominantly the maternal allele
X chromosome		**Duchenne muscular dystrophy** If, by chance, a sufficient number of the X chromosomes containing the normal gene are inactivated in muscle, even heterozygotes may have symptoms. Conversely, if a higher proportion of the disease gene-carrying chromosome is inactivated, a carrier female may test negative on biochemical screening for elevated creatine kinase levels

3.14 PREDICTIVE TESTING STRATEGY FOR HUNTINGTON'S DISEASE

- Predictive testing is only carried out by experienced genetic counselling centres
- Predictive testing is not offered to children
- Fully informed patient consent is required
- Individuals should be seen on several occasions prior to testing to ensure all information about testing is given and understood. This often includes a home visit. Assessment by a psychiatrist should be considered
- A reasonable interval of several months should be left between the initial counselling and making a decision about testing
- Consent is obtained, a blood sample for DNA testing is taken and a date is agreed for providing the results. The result is only ever given in person
- An individual may withdraw from testing at any time
- Adequate follow-up arrrangements must be made
- The result must not be disclosed to any other person without written consent

3.15 SOME INDICATIONS FOR PRENATAL TESTING

- Advanced maternal age and a high-risk serum screening result
- A previous child with a detectable chromosome abnormality or a parent with a chromosome abnormality such as a balanced translocation
- A parent or child with a genetic disease for which testing is available
- Abnormal antenatal scan

death or severe disability, may be offered after careful explanation of the risks involved where a positive result will be used to decide about termination of pregnancy. Some indications for testing are listed in Box 3.15; methods used are summarised in Box 3.16.

Non-invasive ultrasound scanning is usually offered to all pregnant couples and is particularly important if there is a previous history of serious developmental abnormalities. As the range of tests for genetic diseases increases, demand for prenatal testing is likely to rise. A considerable ethical debate is taking place about the types of disease for which prenatal testing is appropriate.

Genetic 'screening' tests

Genetic screening is usually carried out on populations or at-risk groups. Examples include screening for phenylketonuria and cystic fibrosis in the newborn, prenatal screening for neural tube defects (NTDs) and Down's syndrome in pregnant women (Box 3.17), and screening for carriers of haemoglobinopathies and Tay–Sachs disease in at-risk populations (p. 1035). However, screening for the most common genetic conditions may be offered to everyone. An example is testing whether both parents are carriers for the cystic fibrosis gene in early pregnancy.

Huntington's disease (Box 3.14), or when a positive result in children will affect screening and management, such as in familial polyposis coli (p. 924). However, many complicated ethical issues are raised (see below) and such tests should only be carried out by clinicians experienced in their use.

Whilst a negative predictive test is clearly viewed as a favourable outcome, a positive test may have significant consequences. These should have been explained fully in the counselling process (see below) and include employment discrimination and psychological effects. Evidence suggests that serious psychological sequelae are uncommon.

Prenatal testing

Direct invasive testing of a pregnancy for a specific condition, usually one severe enough to cause early infant

3.16 METHODS USED IN PRENATAL TESTING

Test	Gestation	Comments
Ultrasound	1st trimester onwards	Increased nuchal translucency (an oedematous flap of skin at the base of the neck) for trisomies and Turner's; all major abnormalities such as neural tube defects (NTDs), congenital heart disease
Chorionic villus biopsy	From 11 weeks	2% risk of miscarriage; used for early chromosomal, DNA and biochemical analysis; a specialised test
Amniocentesis	From 14 weeks	<1% risk of miscarriage; used for chromosomal and some biochemical analysis, e.g. α-fetoprotein for NTD
Cordocentesis	From 19 weeks	2–3% risk of miscarriage; a highly specialised test; used for chromosomal and DNA analysis

3.17 SCREENING FOR DOWN'S SYNDROME

EBM

'Antenatal screening in the first and second trimester identifies fetuses at risk of Down's syndrome. Tests which currently have sensitivity > 60% and specificity > 95% include:
  First trimester (11–14 weeks): nuchal translucency; or nuchal translucency, human chorionic gonadotrophin (hCG) and pregnancy-associated plasma protein-A (PAPP-A)
  Second trimester (13–20 weeks): triple test (hCG, α-fetoprotein, unconjugated oestriol, uE3)
Other combinations are available for use from 11–20 weeks.'

For further information: 💻 www.nice.org.uk

Ethical issues in genetic testing

Genetic tests have great value in the diagnosis of disease when clinical features are present. Their use in predictive testing when governed by carefully constructed protocols, e.g. in familial cancer and Huntington's disease (Box 3.14), has also been widely accepted. Their wider use has caused considerable controversy, as illustrated by concerns about the use of genetic test results by the insurance industry. However, certain rules and ethical considerations cover the use of genetic tests and the disclosure of their results to anyone but the individual undergoing the test. These are widely employed and have prevented the inappropriate use of genetic tests, but as with any 'ethical' issue they may be open to different interpretations.

Particular concerns have been raised about the use of genetic tests in children. Testing is clearly appropriate if the condition is present or usually occurs in childhood or when proven treatments are available, e.g. testing a child for cystic fibrosis when early therapy reduces disease progression (p. 685), or for MEN 2 when early thyroidectomy prevents medullary thyroid carcinoma (p. 803). However, testing is not normally carried out for late-onset disorders where the child is healthy and no benefit from early intervention exists. In this situation families should be encouraged to discuss testing openly, with the help of genetic counselling, so that the child can make his or her own informed decision as a young adult, taking into account medical, emotional, family and social consequences.

As genetic tests become available for a wide range of conditions their potential use for prenatal diagnosis and subsequent decisions regarding termination of pregnancy must also be considered. This raises many issues, including what abnormality should be considered severe enough to justify termination, parental rights, the rights of the unborn child and the acceptance of disability in society.

Genetic counselling

An accurate clinical and molecular diagnosis is required for providing information to a family about the risk of developing and transmitting disease and methods for screening, diagnosis and prevention; it also forms the basis for making the often very difficult decisions concerning major life events such as planning a family. This process is usually described as genetic counselling (Box 3.18). It should be considered to be an essential part of the management of individuals and families with genetic disease. The ideal setting is a medical genetics clinic, where counselling is usually provided by a medical geneticist and a specialist nurse counsellor. It may also be provided by a clinician with particular skills in this area, such as an obstetrician or paediatrician.

The key requirement for genetic counselling is the provision of adequate time in a quiet place free of disturbance. This may be hard to achieve in a busy medical outpatient clinic or hospital ward. A 1-hour initial consultation will usually allow most aspects of the counselling process to be carried out. Follow-up visits may be shorter. Contact outside the clinic is also important. This often takes the form of pre-clinic visits or telephone calls to explain the purpose of the appointment and to identify concerns and issues that may not be obvious in the referral letter, as well as follow-up after the clinic visit to obtain further information and samples and to give support. Great value is also placed on providing information in a written form. This may involve the use of information leaflets or, more commonly, a post-clinic letter summarising the important points discussed. This permanent record given to the patient will prevent important information from being forgotten and may also be used to inform other family members.

Strict patient confidentiality should be observed at all times and information from medical records obtained only with prior consent. It is usually the responsibility of the individual (consultand) seeking genetic counselling to obtain further family details or the consent of relatives to provide such information, but help and support for this process are often provided within the framework of the genetics clinic.

3.18 ELEMENTS OF GENETIC COUNSELLING

- Establishing a diagnosis of genetic disease
- Estimation of the risks to the individual and other family members
- Provision of information and support

3

Many special problems may be encountered in genetic counselling, including adoption and the risk of a child having a genetic disorder, consanguinity and the increase in genetic risks, and non-paternity as an incidental finding. These and many other situations require a high degree of skill to manage effectively without causing distress to individuals, couples and families.

Risk calculation

Not only can the calculation of risk in a genetic disease be complicated, but communicating this risk clearly and effectively to a patient may be difficult. A 5% (or 1:20) risk of a child being affected may be perceived by some individuals as low, but to a couple who already have a severely affected child this may be unacceptably high. In a family with a highly penetrant autosomal dominant disorder in which there are many affected individuals, a 50% (1:2) risk may be readily accepted. In the case of a severely affected child born to a very mildly affected parent who was not aware of the diagnosis, a 50% risk for each subsequent child may be devastating. Therefore the concept of high or low risk supported with a precise risk figure will be interpreted very differently by different individuals and will be modified by the severity of the disease and their previous experience of it.

Risk can be calculated in many different ways and the details are beyond the scope of this chapter. Several excellent books describing risk estimation are listed on page 9, and risk is also discussed below). There are pitfalls in providing accurate risks and non-specialists should approach the subject with caution.

An empiric risk (Box 3.19) is based on observational data obtained from a population comparable to the one the patient is from (e.g. the maternal age-related incidence of trisomy 21 in live-born infants, p. 47). Empiric risks have been derived for many conditions which have either multifactorial inheritance (e.g. NTDs) or an identical clinical phenotype without a specific diagnosis (e.g. profound childhood sensorineural hearing loss).

In the case of a fully penetrant Mendelian disorder it may also be possible to give accurate risks. For example, children of a healthy individual who has a sibling with an autosomal recessive disorder will have a very low risk of being affected, although they will have a 33% (1:3) chance

---

3.20 GENETIC DISEASE AND COUNSELLING IN OLD AGE

- **Genetic disease:** may present for the first time in elderly patients, e.g. Huntington's disease.
- **Genetic counselling:** remains essential in the management of genetic disease presenting in old age.
- **Special problems:** many other family members may be identified as being at risk during counselling.

50% risk of being a carrier from one parent ($1/2 \times 2/3$) and from the other who has a population risk. The pregnancy of a couple who have had a child previously affected with an autosomal recessive disorder will have a 25% (1:4) risk of being affected, and the child of an individual affected with an autosomal dominant disorder will be at 50% (1:2) risk.

However, Mendelian risks can be modified. Thus an individual at 50% risk of inheriting an autosomal dominant disease may have a lower risk if he or she is well beyond an age where the majority of affected individuals would be expected to be symptomatic (age-related penetrance). The 50% figure is the prior genetic risk and has to be modified by conditional information to give a new 'modified risk'. It is essential to consider such conditional information if it is available.

Bayes' theorem (p. 8) is commonly used to calculate such modified risks. This enables all information to be used in calculating a risk figure. A very simple Bayesian calculation is illustrated. Consider a woman who is at risk of being a carrier of an X-linked recessive disease. Her grandfather and brother are affected, which makes her mother an obligate gene carrier. Her risk of being a carrier is therefore 50%. However, she has two unaffected sons. This information can be used to modify her risk. The prior probability that she is a carrier is 1:2 and that she is not a carrier also 1:2. The conditional probability that she would have two normal sons if she were a carrier is $1/2 \times 1/2$, i.e. $1/4$. If she were not a carrier, the probability of having normal sons is 1. From this, the joint probability for each outcome can be calculated (the prior risk × the conditional risk): $1/2 \times 1/4$ ($1/8$) for being a carrier and $1/2 \times 1$ ($1/2$) for not being a carrier. The final risk, or relative probability, for each outcome can then be obtained by dividing the joint probability for that outcome by the sum of the joint probabilities. The probability that she is a carrier is therefore $1/8/(1/8 + 1/2) = 1/5$ (20%).

POLYGENIC DISEASE

Susceptibility to many common diseases is influenced by genetic factors. This is often recognised by an increased incidence of the disease in first-degree relatives of affected individuals but not in a pattern typical of single-gene disorders (Fig. 3.8). This risk can be measured by the λ_s value. This is the sibling recurrence risk expressed as a ratio to the population risk (Box 3.21). Examples include congenital malformations, asthma/atopy, ischaemic heart disease, and susceptibility to inflammatory and autoimmune

---

3.19 EMPIRIC SIBLING RECURRENCE RISKS FOR SOME COMMON CLINICAL DISORDERS*

- Bilateral cleft lip and palate — 5.7%
- Severe childhood deafness (unknown cause) — 10%
- Neural tube defects — 3%
- Congenital heart disease — 2–3%
- Severe mental retardation (unknown cause) — 3%
- Vesico-ureteric reflux — 10%
- Epilepsy — 5%
- Schizophrenia — 9%
- Bipolar disorder — 13%
- Type II diabetes mellitus — 10%
- Alzheimer's disease (< 65 years) — 4–12%

*Parents normal.

3.21 RISK TO SIBLINGS OF AFFECTED PATIENTS FOR COMMON POLYGENIC DISEASES

Disease	λ_s
Type I diabetes mellitus	15
Systemic lupus erythematous	10–20
Multiple sclerosis	20–40
Schizophrenia	10
Ischaemic heart disease	4–12

disease. In addition, many 'quantitative traits' have a strong genetic component. These are variables which are continuously distributed in the population, extremes of which often predispose to disease, such as blood pressure, blood glucose, body weight, and blood lipids.

Each of these disease traits is determined by interactions between a number of genes. Detailed knowledge of the human genome should allow identification of these genes using 'linkage' (p. 51), but this is proving a more difficult research task than was anticipated. It appears that very large studies are required to unravel the contributions of individual genes to complex quantitative traits, partly because many of these traits are also influenced by environmental factors. This is also termed multifactorial inheritance. Modification of the traditional linkage-based approach to the identification of disease genes has recently been successful. These studies may utilise twins or affected sibling pairs. Animal models have also been successfully used to identify disease susceptibility genes where breeding experiments can easily be carried out.

A number of monogenic conditions have similar phenotypes: for example, hypertension is caused by loss-of-function mutations in 11β-hydroxylase (a rare form of congenital adrenal hyperplasia, p. 789) and in 11β-hydroxysteroid dehydrogenase type 2 (p. 778). These are therefore 'candidate genes' for hypertension. The investigation of candidate genes has been employed extensively in case-control and population-based research, but results have been somewhat disappointing, often being hard to replicate in different populations.

This area is a key target for current research and is likely to change practice in clinical genetics substantially in the next decade or two.

RESEARCH FRONTIERS IN MOLECULAR MEDICINE

MOLECULAR BASIS OF DISEASE

Molecular medicine aims to take understanding of molecular processes from the genome and gene regulation to the proteome (the whole range of proteins produced from the genome) and beyond, in order to establish how such processes function in health and fail in disease and to offer novel rational diagnostic and therapeutic approaches. The number of proteins is much larger than the number of genes available since genes may show alternate splicing and

proteins can undergo considerable post-translational modification such as glycosylation and acetylation. Typically, this involves many teams of multidisciplinary researchers who can cover the diverse range of relevant techniques and translate the fundamental science 'from bench to bedside'. No one scientist or clinician can be expert in every area but an appreciation of the process is important to all.

A typical molecular medicine research programme that aims to understand a disease with a genetic/molecular basis might be pursued thus:

- The chromosomal locus or loci responsible for a disorder is identified by scrutiny of affected families or by population association studies and SNP analyses (p. 51).
- With luck, an SNP encodes a functional polymorphism/mutation in a gene. More typically, a series of SNPs are co-associated in linkage disequilibrium in sufferers from the disorder to give a 'haplotype' affecting a gene or perhaps several genes in a particular locus.
- 'Data-mining' of the human genome project and other 'bioinformatics' approaches suggest candidate genes which are in the locus for further exploration.
- Function of the candidate gene is examined in relevant cell lines. Mutation or knockout of the genes in such cells is explored using, for instance, small interfering (si)RNAs and cell transfection experiments.
- The gene is examined in animal models. Its pattern of tissue expression, cellular localisation and regulation by, for examples, endocrine, cytokine and developmental factors is documented. Altered expression in animal models of the disease is examined and the possibility of mutations in the gene in such models explored.
- Transgenic animals with tissue-specific over-expression are constructed to explore pathophysiology.
- Knockout mice, in which the gene has been deleted/disrupted by homologous recombination in mouse embryonic stem cells, are made to explore the physiological consequences of the loss of the gene product. Tissue-specific gene knockout mice can be made (for example, using the Cre-Lox recombination system) to dissect the role of the gene in particular tissues.
- Polymorphisms are sought in relevant human populations with attenuated forms of the disorder found in the initial presentation or as indicated by the animal and cellular studies.
- Further models are used to test gene-specific therapies before their extension to humans.
- Structural analysis of the gene product aids computer-based rational drug design.
- Drugs are developed as discussed on page 21.

MOLECULAR THERAPEUTICS

PHARMACOGENOMICS

The science of dissecting the genetic determinants of drug kinetics and effects using information from the human genome is called pharmacogenomics. It has been known for the last 50 years or more that polymorphisms in genes affect

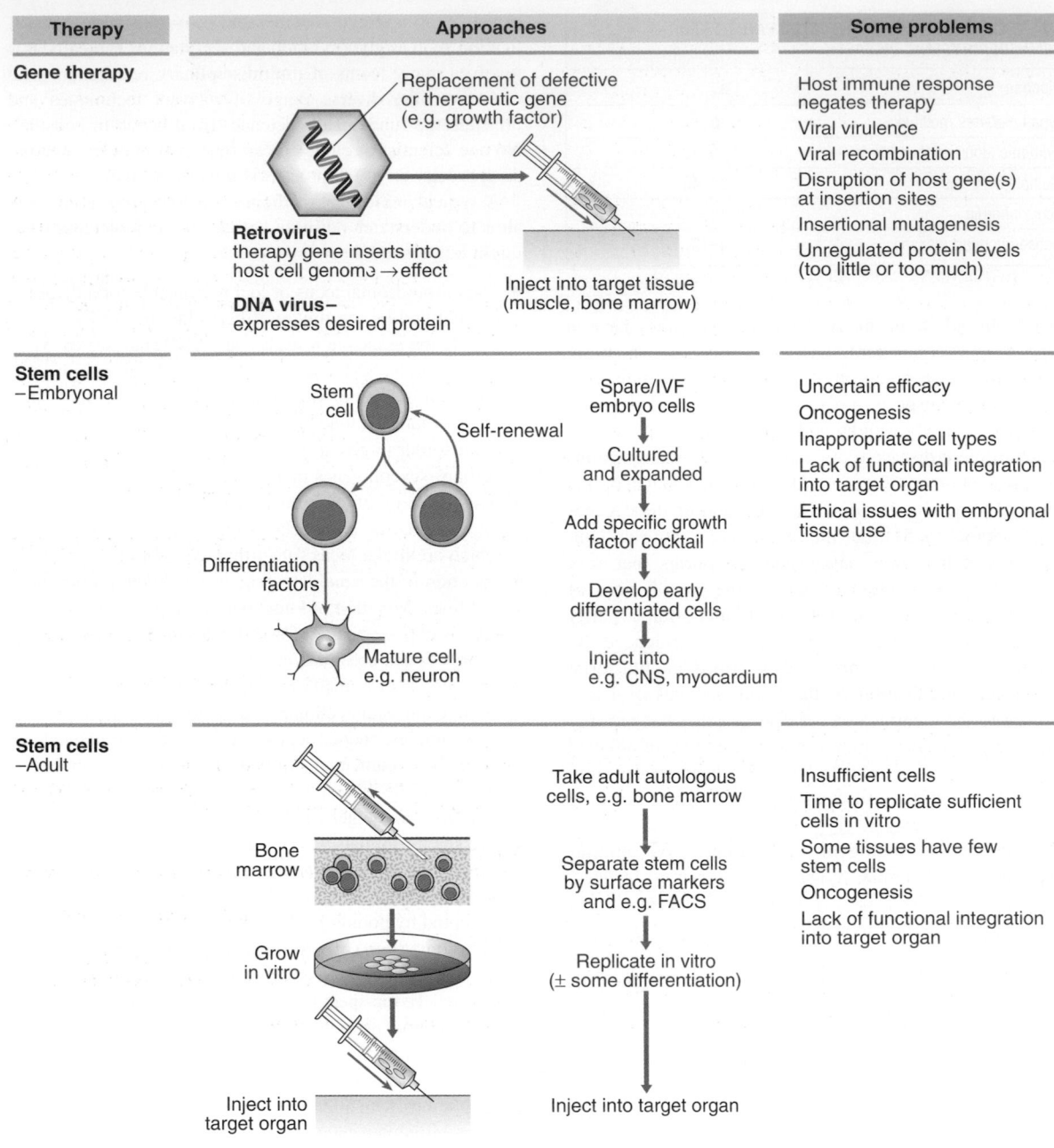

Therapy	Approaches	Some problems

Fig. 3.10 Experimental gene and cell therapies. The general approaches to novel gene and stem cell therapies are shown, with their potential or real problems and current limitations. (FACS = fluorescence-activated cell sorting)

individual responses to some drugs, such as debrisoquine. Recently, it has been recognised that a large series of polymorphic genes are involved in drug absorption, distribution, tissue effects and metabolism. For example, a large family of cytochrome P450 genes, mostly expressed in the liver, determine the metabolism of a host of specific drugs. These genes are highly polymorphic. Thus, polymorphisms in the *CYP2D6* gene determine codeine activation and those in the *CYP2C9* gene affect warfarin inactivation. Polymorphisms in these and other drug metabolic genes determine the persistence of drugs and, therefore, should provide information about dosages and toxicity. Whilst this subject remains in its infancy the

ambition is to use information from the Human Genome Project, particularly from its next phase of sequencing common human polymorphisms and understanding their function, to be able to predict the best specific drugs and dosages for individual patients. It is likely that today's medical students will use pharmacogenomic information increasingly during the course of their careers.

GENE THERAPY

Despite the excitement over the Human Genome Project, the prospects of gene therapy (Fig. 3.10), raised over the last decade or more, have yet to be fully realised. To date experiments to replace or repair mutated genes have met with very limited success. Most notable have been approaches to replace defective genes in inherited human immune deficiency syndromes. Genetic engineering of a patient's bone marrow cells can be undertaken in vitro and the resulting re-engineered bone marrow transplanted back. Initial positive findings in the treatment of severe combined immune deficiency syndrome (p. 72) have been tempered more recently with the development of leukaemia-like conditions in some treated children. Similar trials in haemophilia have been plagued with fears over safety. Problems include the use of viral 'vectors' to introduce the new replacement copies of the defective gene; the viral vector is needed to allow access into cells and integration and/or transcription of the replacement gene construct. Whilst intrinsically non-replicating, viral vectors may recombine with endogenous or acquired viruses to produce a virulent strain or induce an immune response. It has not yet been possible to use non-viral means to introduce sufficient numbers of copies of replacement genes to have significant biological effects. Considerable further development is still required before gene therapy can be fully assessed and either take its place in the pantheon of treatments or be consigned to the dustbin of unfulfilled promise.

STEM CELL THERAPY

Stem cells, primitive cells with the possibility of both self-renewal and differentiation, offer very exciting potential therapies for the future (Fig. 3.10). Broadly these come in two categories: embryonal stem cells derived from the early blastocyst, and adult stem cells present in differentiated tissues.

Much of the excitement (and controversy) surrounds embryonal stem cells which are derived from human embryos left over from in vitro fertilisation programmes. In mammalian model species, such cells can be taken and used to regenerate differentiated tissue cells such as in heart and brain. They have the ability to produce any cell in the body and proliferate rapidly in culture, and so could be used to refashion damaged organs. Such experiments are still in their infancy but are progressing fast.

In contrast, adult stem cells reflect a tiny minority of multipotent cells within normal differentiated tissues which can undergo further division and differentiation. Even some brain neurons show this property. Attempts have already been made to use adult stem cells from bone marrow to treat a variety of conditions, such as myocardial infarction. Although some encouraging functional outcomes have been reported, it is too soon as yet to tell whether these approaches work by the anticipated mechanism of transdifferentiation (cells of one tissue turning into cells of another) or whether bone marrow cells exert other effects (for example, releasing growth factors which stimulate neighbouring cells to replicate). Another concern is whether there will ever be sufficient adult stem cells present in an individual adult to produce enough progeny cells to reverse major degenerative diseases of old age effectively.

3

FURTHER INFORMATION

Books and journal articles

Alberts B. Molecular biology of the cell. 4th edn. New York: Garland Science; 2002.

Cooper GM. The cell: a molecular approach. 3rd edn. Sunderland: Sinauer; 2003.

Harper PS. Practical genetic counselling. 6th edn. London: Arnold; 2004.

Lewin B. Genes VIII. Oxford: Prentice Hall; 2003.

Young ID. Introduction to risk calculation in genetic counselling. 2nd edn. Oxford: Oxford University Press; 1999.

Websites

www.bshg.org.uk *British Society for Human Genetics; has report on genetic testing of children.*

www.ensembl.org *Annotated genome databases from multiple organisms.*

www.ncbi.nlm.nih.gov *Extensive collection of genome databases.*

www.ncbi.nlm.nih.gov/Omim/ *Online Mendelian Inheritance in Man (OMIM).*

www.nhgri.nih.gov *Human Genome Project.*

4

S.E. MARSHALL

Immunological factors in disease

The immune system has evolved to protect the host from pathogens while minimising damage to self tissue. Despite the ancient observation that recovery from a disease frequently results in protection against that condition, the existence of the immune system as a functional entity was not recognised until the end of the 19th century. More recently, it has become clear that the immune system not only protects against infection, but also limits excessive responses that might lead to autoimmune diseases. Dysfunction or deficiency of the immune response leads to a wide variety of diseases, involving every organ system in the body.

The aim of this chapter is to provide a general understanding of immunology and how it contributes to human disease. It reviews the key components of the immune response, followed by five sections that illustrate the clinical presentation of the most common forms of immune dysfunction. More detailed discussion of individual conditions may be found in the relevant organ-specific chapters of this book.

FUNCTIONAL ANATOMY, PHYSIOLOGY AND INVESTIGATIONS

The immune system consists of an intricately linked network of cells, proteins and lymphoid organs which are strategically placed to ensure maximal protection against infection (Fig. 4.1). Immune defences are normally categorised into the innate immune response, which provides immediate protection against an invading pathogen, and the adaptive or acquired immune response, which takes more time to develop but confers exquisite specificity and long-lasting protection. The properties of these two types of immune response are listed in Box 4.1.

4

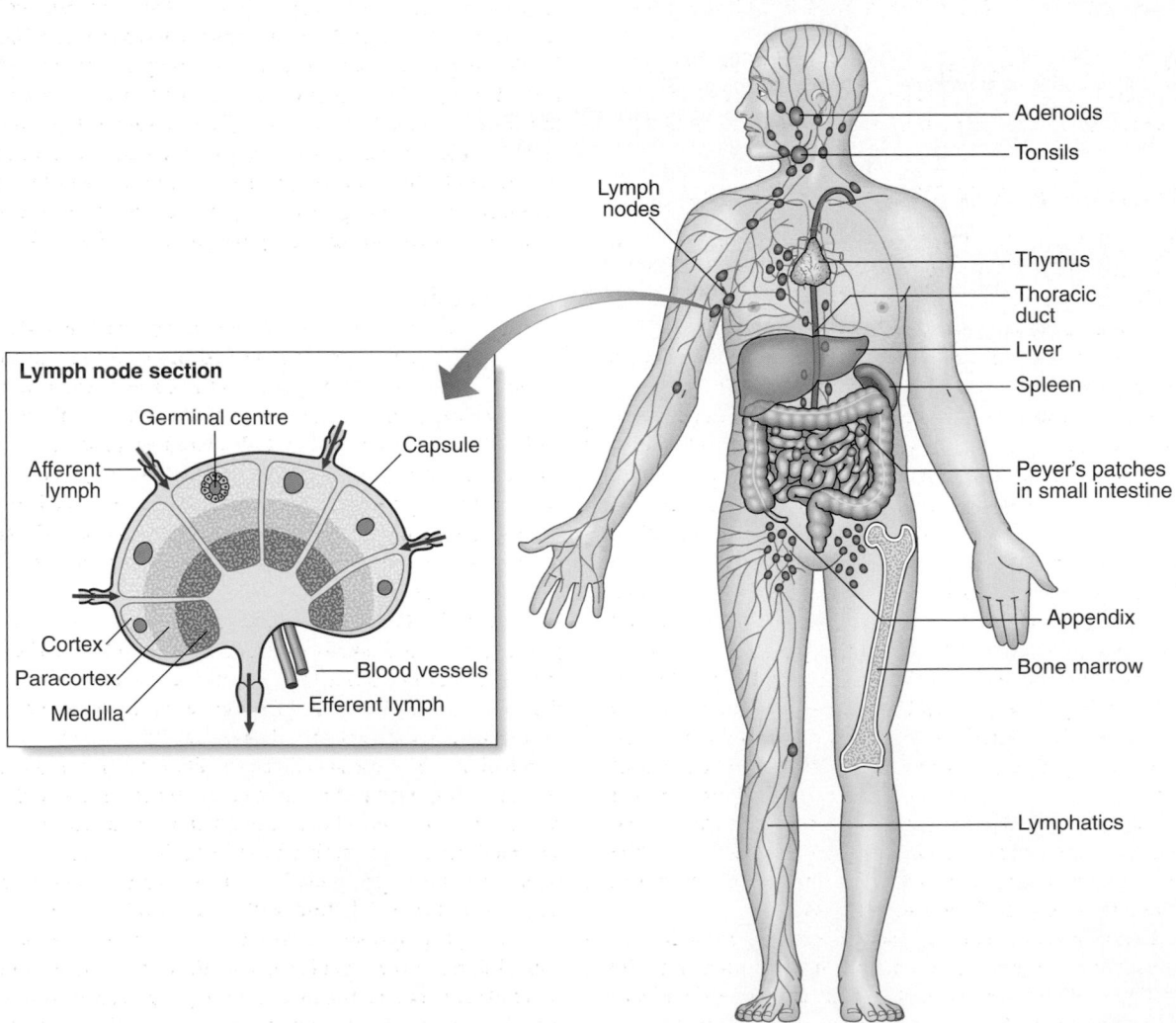

Fig. 4.1 **Anatomy of the acquired immune system.**

4.1 PROPERTIES OF IMMUNE RESPONSES

Innate response	Adaptive response
Characteristics	
Recognises generic microbial structures	Antigen-specific responses
Immediately mobilised (minutes)	Slow response (days)
No memory	Memory
Genetically encoded	Not genetically encoded
Essentially identical responses in all individuals	Acquired as an adaptive response to exposure to antigen
Present in invertebrates and vertebrates	Present in vertebrates only
Immune components	
Constitutive barriers (e.g. skin)	T and B lymphocytes
Phagocytes	
Natural killer cells	
Soluble mediators, e.g. complement	Secreted molecules, e.g. antibody
Pattern recognition molecules	Antigen-specific receptors

THE INNATE IMMUNE SYSTEM

Non-specific defences against infection include anatomical barriers, phagocytic cells, soluble molecules such as complement and acute phase proteins, and natural killer cells.

CONSTITUTIVE BARRIERS TO INFECTION

The tightly packed, highly keratinised cells of the skin constantly undergo renewal and replacement, which physically limits colonisation by microorganisms. Microbial growth is inhibited by physiological factors such as low pH and low oxygen tension, and sebaceous glands secrete hydrophobic oils that further repel water and microorganisms. Sweat also contains lysozyme, an enzyme that destroys the structural integrity of bacterial cell walls; ammonia, which has antibacterial properties; and several antimicrobial peptides such as defensins. Similarly, the mucous membranes of the respiratory, gastrointestinal and genitourinary tract provide a constitutive barrier to infection. Secreted mucus acts as a physical barrier to trap invading pathogens, and secretory IgA prevents bacteria and viruses attaching to and penetrating epithelial cells. As in the skin, lysozyme and antimicrobial peptides can directly kill invading pathogens, and additionally lactoferrin acts to starve invading bacteria of iron. Within the respiratory tract, cilia directly trap pathogens and contribute to removal of mucus, assisted by physical manoeuvres such as sneezing and coughing. In the gastrointestinal tract, hydrochloric acid and salivary amylase chemically destroy bacteria, while normal peristalsis and induced vomiting or diarrhoea promote clearance of invading organisms.

Endogenous commensal bacteria provide an additional constitutive defence against infection. Approximately 100 trillion (10^{14}) bacteria normally reside at epithelial surfaces in symbiosis with the human host. They compete with pathogenic microorganisms for scarce resources, including space and nutrients. In addition, they produce fatty acids and bactericidins that inhibit the growth of many pathogens. Eradication of the normal flora with broad-spectrum antibiotics commonly results in opportunistic infection by organisms which rapidly colonise an undefended ecological niche.

These constitutive barriers are highly effective, but if external defences are breached by a wound or pathogenic organism, the specific soluble proteins and cells of the innate immune system are activated.

PHAGOCYTES

Phagocytes ('eating cells') are specialised cells which ingest and kill microorganisms, scavenge cellular and infectious debris, and produce inflammatory molecules which regulate other components of the immune system. They include neutrophils, monocytes and macrophages, and are crucial for defence against bacterial and fungal infections.

Phagocytes express a wide range of surface receptors that allow them to identify microorganisms. These pattern recognition receptors include the Toll-like receptors and mannose receptors. They recognise generic motifs not present on mammalian cells, such as bacterial cell wall components, bacterial DNA and viral double-stranded RNA. While phagocytes can recognise microorganisms through pattern recognition receptors alone, engulfment of microorganisms is greatly enhanced by opsonisation. Opsonins include acute phase proteins such as C-reactive protein (CRP), antibodies and complement. They bind both to the pathogen and to phagocyte receptors, acting as a bridge between the two and facilitating phagocytosis (Fig. 4.2).

Neutrophils

Neutrophils, also known as polymorphonuclear leucocytes, are derived from the bone marrow and circulate freely in the blood (Fig. 4.5, p. 72). They are short-lived cells with a half-life of 6 hours, and are produced at the rate of 10^{11} cells daily. Their functions are to kill microorganisms directly, facilitate the rapid transit of cells through tissues, and non-specifically amplify the immune response. This is mediated by enzymes contained in granules which also provide an intracellular milieu for the killing and degradation of microorganisms.

Changes in damaged or infected cells trigger the local production of inflammatory molecules and cytokines. These stimulate the production and maturation of neutrophils in the bone marrow. The neutrophils are recruited to the site by chemotactic agents and by changes in the activated local endothelium. The transit of neutrophils through the blood stream is responsible for the rise in leucocyte count that occurs in early infection. Once within infected tissue, activated neutrophils seek out and engulf invading microorganisms. These are initially enclosed within membrane-bound vesicles which fuse with cytoplasmic granules to form the phagolysosome. Within this protected compartment, killing of the organism occurs through a combination of oxidative and non-oxidative killing. Oxidative killing, also known as the respiratory burst, is mediated by the NADPH oxidase enzyme complex, which converts oxygen

4

4

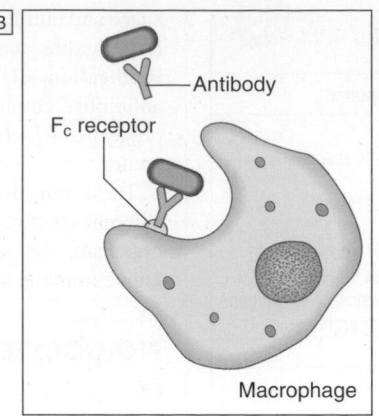

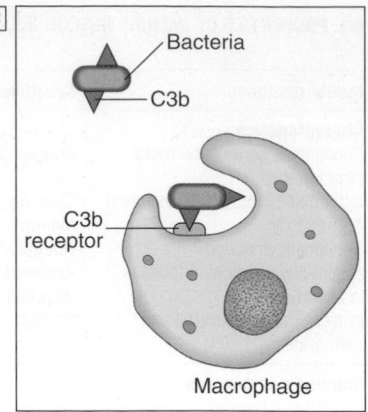

Fig. 4.2 **Opsonisation.** Opsonisation of microbial products may be augmented by several components. ⒶC-reactive protein. ⒷAntibody. ⒸComplement fragments.

into reactive oxygen species such as hydrogen peroxide and superoxide that are lethal to microorganisms. When combined with myeloperoxidase, hypochlorous ions (HOCl⁻, analogous to bleach) are produced, which are highly effective oxidants and antimicrobial agents. Non-oxidative (oxygen-independent) killing occurs through the release of bacteriocidal enzymes into the phagolysosome, including lysozyme and lactoferrin. Each enzyme has a unique antimicrobial spectrum, providing broad coverage against bacteria and fungi.

The process of phagocytosis depletes neutrophil glycogen reserves, and is followed by neutrophil cell death. As the cells die, their contents are released and lysosomal enzymes degrade collagen and other components of the interstitium, causing liquefaction of closely adjacent tissue. The accumulation of dead and dying neutrophils results in the formation of pus which, if extensive, may result in abscess formation.

Monocytes and macrophages

Monocytes are the precursors of tissue macrophages. They are produced in the bone marrow and exported to the circulation, where they constitute about 5% of leucocytes. After 7–10 hours in the blood stream, they migrate to peripheral tissues where they differentiate into tissue macrophages and reside for long periods. Specialised populations of tissue macrophages include Küpffer cells in the liver, alveolar macrophages in the lung, mesangial cells in the kidney, and microglial cells in the brain. Macrophages, like neutrophils, are capable of phagocytosis and killing of microorganisms but also play an important role in the amplification and regulation of the inflammatory response (Box 4.2). Unlike neutrophils, macrophages do not die after killing pathogens.

CYTOKINES

Cytokines are small soluble proteins that act as multipurpose chemical messengers. They can be produced by cells involved in innate and adaptive immune responses and by stromal tissue. More than 100 cytokines have been described, with overlapping, complex roles in modifying the

---

4.2 FUNCTIONS OF MACROPHAGES ⓘ

Initiation and amplification of the inflammatory response

- Stimulate the acute phase response (production of IL-1, TNF-α and IL-6)
- Activate vascular endothelium (IL-1, TNF-α)
- Stimulate neutrophil maturation and chemotaxis (IL-1, IL-8)
- Stimulate monocyte chemotaxis

Killing of microorganisms

- Phagocytosis
- Microbial killing through oxidative and non-oxidative mechanisms

Resolution and repair of inflammation

- Scavenging of necrotic and apoptotic cells and other debris
- Tissue remodelling (elastase, collagenase, matrix proteins)
- Down-regulation of inflammatory cytokines
- Scar formation (IL-1, platelet-derived growth factor, fibroblast growth factor)

Link between innate and adaptive immune system

- Present antigen to T cells
- T cell-derived cytokines increase phagocytosis and microbicidal activity of macrophages in a positive feedback loop

---

immune microenvironment. Subtle differences in cytokine composition, particularly at the initiation of an immune response, may have a major effect on outcome. The most important cytokines are listed in Box 4.3.

COMPLEMENT

The complement system is a group of more than 20 tightly regulated, functionally linked proteins that act to promote inflammation and eliminate invading pathogens. Complement proteins are produced by the liver, and are present in the circulation as inactive molecules. When triggered, they enzymatically activate other proteins in a rapidly amplified biological cascade analogous to the coagulation cascade (p. 1008).

There are three mechanisms by which the complement cascade may be triggered (Fig. 4.3):

4.3 IMPORTANT CYTOKINES IN REGULATION OF THE IMMUNE RESPONSE

Cytokine	Source	Actions
Interferon-alpha (IFN-α)	T cells and NK cells Macrophages	Antiviral activity Activates NK cells, CD8+ T cells and macrophages
Interferon-gamma (IFN-γ)	T cells	Increases antimicrobial and antitumour activity of macrophages Determines cytokine production by T cells and macrophages
Tumour necrosis factor alpha (TNF-α)	Macrophages	Pro-inflammatory Increases apoptosis and expression of cytokines and adhesion molecules Directly cytotoxic
Interleukin-1 (IL-1)	Macrophages and neutrophils	Acute phase reactant Stimulates neutrophil recruitment, fever, T cell and macrophage activation, immunoglobulin production
Interleukin-2 (IL-2)	CD4+ T cells	Stimulates proliferation and differentiation of antigen-specific T lymphocytes
Interleukin-4 (IL-4)	CD4+ T cells and mast cells	Stimulates maturation of B and T cells, and production of IgE antibody
Interleukin-6 (IL-6)	Monocytes and macrophages	Acute phase reactant Stimulates maturation of B cells into plasma cells
Interleukin-12 (IL-12)	Monocytes and macrophages	Stimulates IFN-γ and TNF-α release by T cells, activates natural killer (NK) cells

4

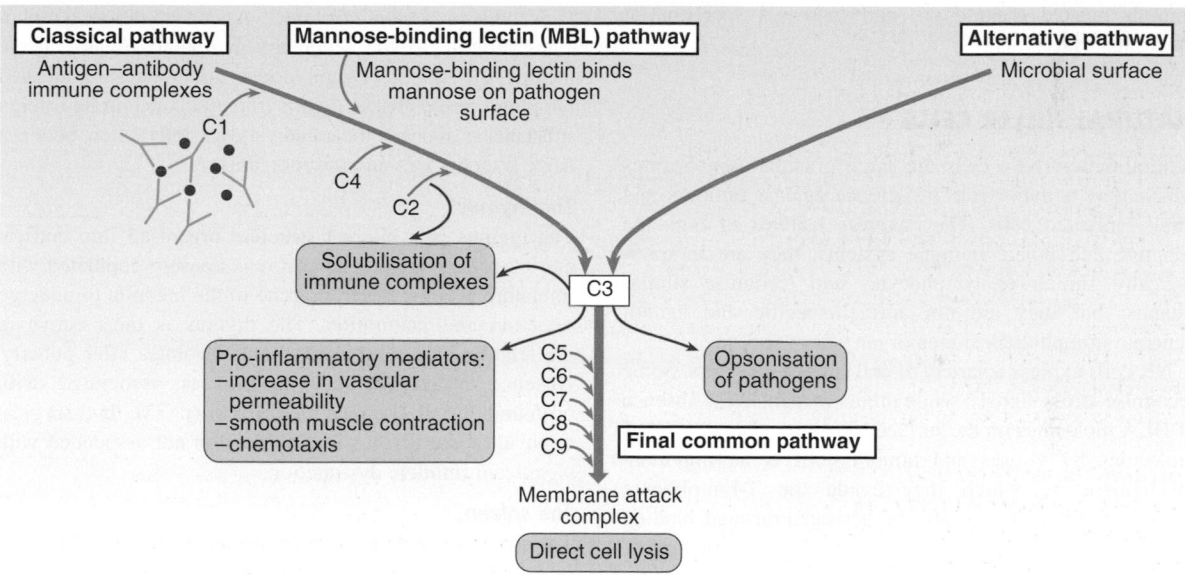

Fig. 4.3   **The complement pathway.** The activation of C3 is central to complement activation.

- *The alternative pathway* is directly triggered by binding of C3 to bacterial cell wall components such as lipopolysaccharide of Gram-negative bacteria and teichoic acid of Gram-positive bacteria.
- *The classical pathway* is initiated when IgM or IgG antibody binds to antigen, forming immune complexes. This induces a conformational change in the antibody, exposing a binding site for the first protein in the classical pathway, C1. Changes in C1 after binding result in activation of the cascade.
- *The lectin pathway* is activated by the direct binding of mannose-binding lectin to microbial cell surface carbohydrates. This mimics the binding of C1 to immune complexes, and directly stimulates the classical pathway, bypassing the need for immune complex formation.

Activation of complement by any of these pathways results in activation of C3, which in turn activates the final common pathway, where the complement proteins C5–C9 assemble together to form the membrane attack complex. This can insert into and puncture target cell walls, leading to osmotic cell lysis. This step is particularly important in the defence against encapsulated bacteria such as *Neisseria* spp. and *Haemophilus influenzae*. The complement fragments generated by activation of the cascade can also act as opsonins, rendering microorganisms more susceptible to phagocytosis by macrophages and neutrophils (Fig. 4.2). In addition, they are chemotactic agents, promoting leucocyte trafficking to sites of inflammation. Some fragments act as anaphylotoxins, binding to complement receptors on mast cells and triggering release of histamine, which increases vascular permeability. The products of complement activation also help to target immune complexes to antigen-presenting cells, providing a link between the innate and the acquired immune systems. Finally, activated complement products dissolve the immune complexes that triggered the cascade, minimising bystander damage to surrounding tissues.

MAST CELLS AND BASOPHILS

Mast cells and basophils are bone marrow-derived cells which play a central role in allergic disorders. Mast cells reside predominantly in tissues exposed to the external environment, such as the skin and gut, while basophils are located in the circulation and are recruited into tissues in response to inflammation. Both contain large cytoplasmic granules which enclose preformed vasoactive substances such as histamine (Fig. 4.9, p. 84). Additional mediators are synthesised de novo after activation, including leukotrienes, prostaglandins and cytokines. Local release of these mediators initiates an inflammatory cascade which increases local blood flow and vascular permeability, stimulates smooth muscle contraction, and increases secretion at mucosal surfaces.

NATURAL KILLER CELLS

Natural killer (NK) cells are large granular lymphocytes which play a major role in defence against tumours and virally infected cells. They express features of both the adaptive and innate immune systems: they are morphologically similar to lymphocytes and recognise similar ligands, but they are not antigen-specific and cannot generate immunological memory.

NK cells express a variety of cell surface receptors. Some recognise stress signals, while others recognise the absence of HLA molecules on the surface (down-regulation of HLA molecules by viruses and tumour cells is an important mechanism by which they evade the T-lymphocyte response). NK cells can also be activated through binding of antigen-bound IgG antibody to surface receptors. This physically links the NK cell to its target in a manner analogous to opsonisation and is known as antibody-dependent cellular cytotoxicity (ADCC).

Activated NK cells can kill their targets in various ways: pore-forming proteins such as perforin induce direct cell lysis, while proteolytic enzymes known as granzymes stimulate apoptosis. In addition, NK cells produce a variety of cytokines such as TNF-α, IL-1, IFN-α and IFN-γ which have direct antiviral and antitumour effects.

THE ADAPTIVE IMMUNE SYSTEM

If the innate immune system fails to provide effective protection against an invading pathogen, the adaptive immune system (Fig. 4.1, p. 64) is mobilised. This possesses three key characteristics:

- it has exquisite specificity and is able to discriminate between very small differences in molecular structure

- it is highly adaptive and can respond to an unlimited number of molecules
- it possesses immunological memory, being able to recall previous encounter with an antigen and respond more effectively than on the first occasion.

There are two major arms of the adaptive immune response: humoral immunity is mediated by antibody, which is produced by B lymphocytes, while cellular immunity is mediated by T lymphocytes, which synthesise and release cytokines that affect other cells. These interact closely with each other and with the components of the innate immune system to maximise the effectiveness of the immune response.

LYMPHOID ORGANS

Primary lymphoid organs. The primary lymphoid organs are involved in lymphocyte development. They include the bone marrow, where both T and B lymphocytes are derived from haemopoietic stem cells and where B lymphocytes also mature, and the thymus, which is the site of T-cell maturation.

Secondary lymphoid organs. After maturation, lymphocytes migrate to the secondary lymphoid organs. These include the spleen, lymph nodes and mucosa-associated lymphoid tissue. These organs trap and concentrate foreign substances, and are the major site of interaction between naïve lymphocytes and microorganisms.

The thymus

The thymus is a bilobed structure organised into cortical and medullary areas. The cortex is densely populated with immature T cells, which migrate to the medulla to undergo selection and maturation. The thymus is most active in the fetal and neonatal period, and involutes after puberty. Absence of thymic development is associated with profound T-cell immune deficiency (p. 73), but surgical removal of the thymus in childhood is not associated with significant immune dysfunction.

The spleen

The spleen is the largest of the secondary lymphoid organs. It is highly effective at filtering the blood, and is an important site of phagocytosis of senescent erythrocytes, bacteria, immune complexes and other debris. It is also a major site of antibody synthesis. The spleen is composed of white pulp which is rich in lymphocytes, and red pulp which contains sinuses filled with large numbers of erythrocytes and macrophages. It is particularly important for defence against encapsulated bacteria, and asplenic individuals are at risk of overwhelming *Streptococcus pneumoniae* and *H. influenzae* infection.

Lymph nodes

Lymph nodes are positioned to maximise exposure to lymph draining from sites of external contact. They are highly organised structures, and four major compartments are recognised (Fig. 4.1, p. 64):

- The cortex contains primary lymphoid follicles which are the site of B-lymphocyte interactions. Germinal centres are formed within the cortex after B cells encounter antigen and undergo intense proliferation.

- The paracortex is rich in T lymphocytes and dendritic cells, a specialised population of antigen-presenting cells.
- The medulla is the major site of antibody-secreting plasma cells.
- Within the medulla there are many sinuses, which contain large numbers of macrophages.

Mucosa-associated lymphoid tissue

These tissues have a similar function and anatomic organisation as lymph nodes. They include Peyer's patches in the small intestine, submucosal lymphoid follicles in the appendix, and tonsils in the pharynx.

Lymphatics

The lymphoid tissue is connected by lymphatics, which have three major functions: they provide access to lymph nodes, return tissue fluid to the venous system, and transport fat from the small intestine to the blood stream. The lymphatics begin as blind-ending capillaries, which come together to form lymphatic ducts. These enter and then leave regional lymph nodes as afferent and efferent ducts respectively. They eventually coalesce and drain into the thoracic duct and subsequently into the superior vena cava. Lymphatics may be either deep or superficial, and in general follow the distribution of major blood vessels.

HUMORAL IMMUNITY

B lymphocytes

These specialised cells arise from haemopoietic bone marrow stem cells, and their major function is to produce antibody. Mature B lymphocytes can be found in the bone marrow, lymphoid tissue, spleen, and to a lesser extent the blood stream. They express a unique immunoglobulin receptor on their cell surface (the B-cell receptor), which binds to soluble antigen. Encounters with antigen usually occur within the lymph nodes, where, if provided with appropriate signals from nearby T lymphocytes, stimulated antigen-specific B cells respond by rapidly proliferating in a process known as clonal expansion. This is accompanied by

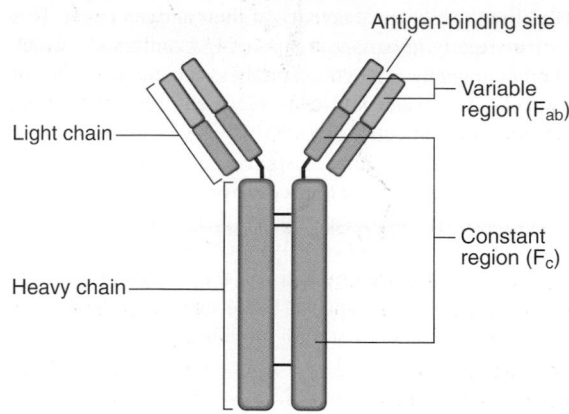

Fig. 4.4   The structure of an immunoglobulin (antibody) molecule.

a highly complex series of genetic rearrangements which generates B-cell populations that express receptors of greater affinity than the original. These cells differentiate into either long-lived memory cells, which reside in the lymph nodes, or plasma cells which produce antibody.

Immunoglobulins

Immunoglobulins (Ig) molecules are soluble proteins made up of two heavy and two light chains (Fig. 4.4). The heavy chain determines the antibody class or isotype, i.e. IgG, IgA, IgM, IgE, IgD. Subclasses of IgG and IgA also occur. The antigen is recognised by the antigen-binding regions (F_{ab}) of both heavy and light chains, while the consequences of antibody-binding are determined by the constant region of the heavy chain (F_c) (Box 4.4).

Antibodies can bring about a number of different actions. Firstly, they facilitate phagocytosis by acting as opsonins (Fig. 4.2, p. 66). A similar bridging mechanism facilitates cell killing by cytotoxic cells, particularly natural killer cells (ADCC, p. 68). Binding of some antibodies to antigen may also trigger activation of the classical complement pathway (Fig. 4.3). In addition, antibodies may act directly to

4.4 CLASSES AND PROPERTIES OF ANTIBODY					
Antibody	Range of concentration in serum	Complement activation ('fixation')	Opsonisation	External secretions	Other properties
IgG	8.0–16.0 g/l	IgG1 +++ IgG2 + IgG3 +++	IgG1 ++ IgG3 ++	++	4 subclasses: IgG1, IgG2, IgG3, IgG4 Distributed equally between blood and extracellular fluid Can be transferred across placenta IgG2 is particularly important in making antibodies against polysaccharides
IgA	1.5–4.0 g/l	–	–	++++	2 subclasses: IgA1, IgA2 Highly effective at neutralising toxins Particularly important at mucosal surfaces
IgM	0.5–2.0 g/l	++++	–	+	Highly effective at agglutinating pathogens
IgE	0.003–0.04 g/l	–	–	–	Majority of IgE is bound to mast cells, basophils and eosinophils Important in allergic disease and defence against parasite infection
IgD	Not detected	–	–	–	Function unknown

4

neutralise the biological activity of their antigen target. This is a particularly important feature of IgA antibodies, which act predominantly at mucosal surfaces; genetic deficiency of IgA may be associated with recurrent respiratory and gastrointestinal infections (p. 74).

The humoral immune response is characterised by memory, i.e. the response to successive exposures to antigen is qualitatively and quantitatively different than on first exposure. When a previously unstimulated (naïve) B lymphocyte is activated by antigen, the first antibody to be produced is IgM, which appears in the serum after 5–10 days. Depending on additional stimuli provided by T lymphocytes, other antibody classes (IgG, IgA and IgE) are produced 3–7 days later. If, some time later, a memory B cell is re-exposed to antigen, the lag time between antigen exposure and the production of antibody is decreased (to 2–3 days), the titre of antibodies produced is greatly increased, and the response is dominated by IgG antibodies of high affinity. Furthermore, in contrast to the initial antibody response, secondary antibody responses are independent of stimuli from T lymphocytes. This allows the rapid generation of highly specific responses on pathogen re-exposure.

CELLULAR IMMUNITY

T lymphocytes mediate cellular immunity, and are particularly important for defence against viruses, fungi and intracellular bacteria. They also play an important immunoregulatory role, orchestrating and regulating the responses of other cells of the immune system. T lymphocyte precursors arise in bone marrow and are exported as immature cells to the thymus. Within the thymus, each cell expresses a T-cell receptor with a unique specificity, and undergoes a stringent selection process to ensure that autoreactive T cells are deleted, mature T lymphocytes leave the thymus and expand to populate other organs of the immune system. It has been estimated that an individual possesses 10^7–10^9 T-cell clones, each with a unique T-cell receptor, ensuring at least partial coverage for any antigen encountered.

T cells respond to protein antigens, but not in their native form. For recognition, intact antigen must be processed into component peptides. These bind to a protein framework known as HLA (human leucocyte antigen). This process is known as antigen processing and presentation. HLA molecules exhibit extreme polymorphism: for example, more than 500 different HLA-B alleles have been identified. As each HLA molecule presents a subtly different peptide repertoire to T lymphocytes, this ensures enormous diversity in recognition of antigens within the population.

T lymphocytes can be segregated into two groups on the basis of function, recognition of HLA molecules and expression of cell surface proteins. Leucocyte cell surface molecules are named systematically by assigning them a cluster of differentiation (CD) antigen number.

CD8+ ('cytotoxic') T lymphocytes

These are specialised cells that recognise antigenic peptides in association with HLA class I (HLA-A, HLA-B, HLA-C). They kill infected cells directly through the production of pore-forming molecules such as perforin, or by triggering apoptosis of the target cell. They also secrete cytokines such as IFN-γ which have antiviral activity.

CD4+ ('helper') T lymphocytes

In contrast, CD4+ T lymphocytes recognise peptides presented on HLA class II molecules (HLA-DR, HLA-DP and HLA-DQ) and have mainly immunoregulatory functions. They produce cytokines and provide co-stimulatory signals that support the activation of CD8+ T lymphocytes and assist the production of mature antibody by B cells. In addition, they interact closely with phagocytes which determines cytokine production by both cell types.

CD4+ lymphocytes can be further subdivided into subsets on the basis of the cytokines they produce:

- Typically, Th1 cells produce IL-2, IFN-γ and TNF-α, and support the development of delayed type hypersensitivity responses (p. 80).
- Th2 cells typically secrete IL-4, IL-5 and IL-10 and promote allergic responses (p. 83).
- A further subset of specialised CD4+ lymphocytes known as regulatory cells are important in the regulation of other CD4+ cells and the prevention of autoimmune disease.

INVESTIGATIONS

Investigations of immune function are outlined in specific sections later in this chapter.

IMMUNE DEFICIENCY

The consequences of deficiencies of the immune system include recurrent infections, autoimmunity and susceptibility to malignancy. Immune deficiency may arise through intrinsic defects in immune function, but is much more commonly due to secondary causes including infection, drug therapy, malignancy and ageing. This chapter gives an overview of the rare primary immune deficiencies. More than 100 such deficiencies have been described, most of which are genetically determined and usually present in childhood or adolescence. The clinical manifestations are dictated by the component of the immune system involved (Box 4.5). However, there is considerable overlap and redundancy in the immune network, and some diseases do not fall easily into this classification.

PRESENTING PROBLEMS IN IMMUNE DEFICIENCY

RECURRENT INFECTIONS

Many patients with an immune deficiency present with recurrent infections. While there is no accepted definition of 'too many' infections, features that may indicate immune deficiency are shown in Box 4.6. Frequent, severe infections or infections caused by unusual organisms or at unusual sites are the most useful indicator.

4.5 IMMUNE DEFICIENCIES AND COMMON PATTERNS OF INFECTION

	Phagocyte deficiency	Complement deficiency	T-lymphocyte deficiency	Antibody deficiency
Bacteria	*Staphylococcus aureus* *Pseudomonas aeruginosa* *Serratia marcescens* *Burkholderia cenocepacia* *Mycobacterium tuberculosis* Atypical mycobacteria	*Neisseria meningitidis* *Neisseria gonorrhoeae* *Haemophilus influenzae* *Streptococcus pneumoniae*	*Mycobacterium tuberculosis* Atypical mycobacteria	*Haemophilus influenzae* *Streptococcus pneumoniae* *Staphylococcus aureus*
Fungi	*Candida* spp *Aspergillus* spp		*Candida* spp *Aspergillus* spp	
Viruses			Cytomegalovirus (CMV) Epstein–Barr virus (EBV) Herpes zoster	Enteroviruses
Protozoa			*Pneumocystis carinii* (now *jirovecii*) *Toxoplasma gondii* *Cryptosporidia*	*Giardia lamblia*

4.6 WARNING SIGNS OF IMMUNE DEFICIENCY

- 8 respiratory tract infections/year in a child, or > 4 respiratory tract infections/year in an adult
- > 1 infection requiring hospital admission or intravenous antibiotics
- Infections with unusual organisms
- Infections at unusual sites
- Chronic infection unresponsive to usual treatment
- Early end-organ damage (e.g. bronchiectasis)
- Family history of immune deficiency

Baseline investigations include full blood count and white cell differential, acute phase reactants (CRP, see below), renal and liver function tests, urine dipstick and serum immunoglobulins with protein electrophoresis. Additional microbiological, virological and radiological tests may be appropriate. At this stage it is often clear which category of immune deficiency is being considered, and specific investigation can be undertaken as described below.

If an immune deficiency is suspected but has not yet been formally characterised, patients should not receive live vaccines because of the risk of vaccine-induced disease. Discussion with specialist teams will help determine whether additional preventative measures such as prophylactic antibiotics are indicated.

PRIMARY PHAGOCYTE DEFICIENCIES

Primary phagocyte deficiencies (Fig. 4.5) usually present with recurrent bacterial and fungal infections, often affecting unusual sites. The majority present in childhood, but milder forms may present in adults.

Leucocyte adhesion deficiencies

These are disorders of phagocyte migration, where failure to express adhesion molecules results in the inability of phagocytes to exit the blood stream. These conditions are characterised by recurrent bacterial infections, and sites of infection lack pus or neutrophil infiltration. Peripheral blood neutrophil counts may be very high during acute infection because of the failure of mobilised neutrophils to exit blood vessels. Specialised tests show reduced or absent expression of adhesion molecules on neutrophils.

Chronic granulomatous disease

This results from mutations in the genes encoding the NADPH oxidase enzyme, causing a failure of oxidative killing. This may be demonstrated using the nitroblue tetrazolium reduction test (NBT), which measures the ability to reduce a colourless intracellular dye to an insoluble blue compound after neutrophil activation. The defect leads to susceptibility to catalase-positive organisms such as *Staphylococcus aureus*, *Burkholderia cenocepacia* and aspergillus. Intracellular killing of mycobacteria in macrophages is also impaired. Infections most commonly involve the lungs, lymph nodes, soft tissues, bone, skin and urinary tract and are characterised histologically by granuloma formation.

Defects in cytokines and cytokine receptors

Defects of cytokines such as IFN-γ, IL-12 or their receptors also result in failure of intracellular killing, and individuals are particularly susceptible to mycobacterial infections. Detailed assessment of cytokine deficiencies is currently only performed in specialised laboratories.

Management

Patients require aggressive management of existing infections, including intravenous antibiotics and surgical drainage of abscesses, and long-term prophylaxis with antifungal agents and trimethoprim–sulfamethoxazole. Specific treatment depends upon the nature of the defect, and stem cell transplantation may be considered.

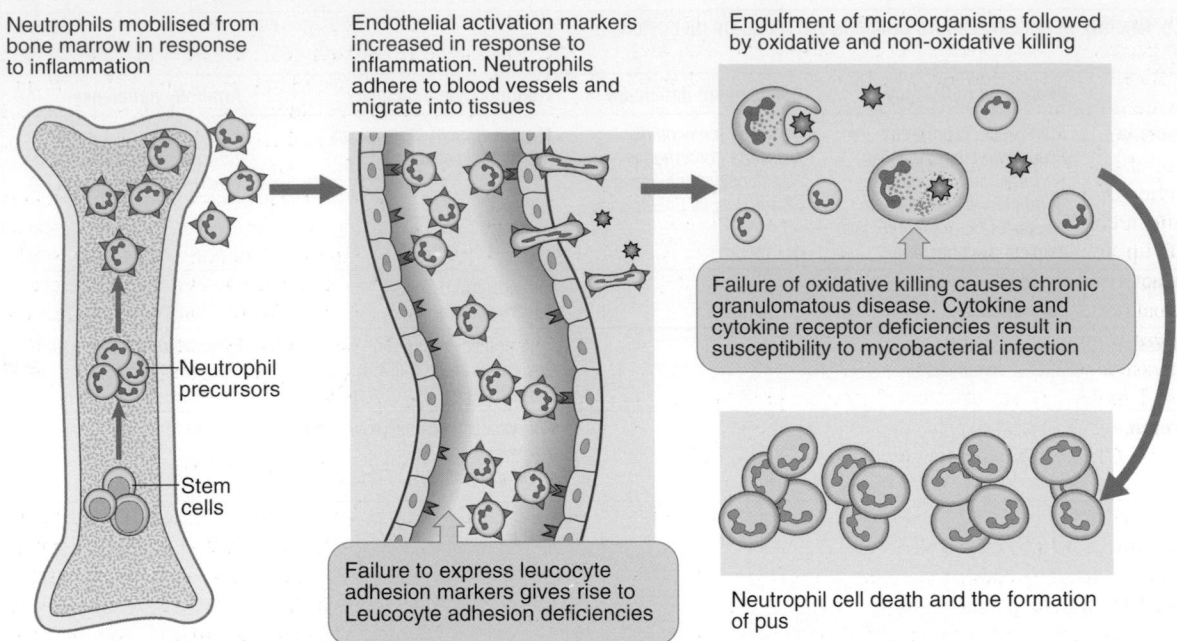

Neutrophils mobilised from bone marrow in response to inflammation

Endothelial activation markers increased in response to inflammation. Neutrophils adhere to blood vessels and migrate into tissues

Engulfment of microorganisms followed by oxidative and non-oxidative killing

Neutrophil precursors

Stem cells

Failure of oxidative killing causes chronic granulomatous disease. Cytokine and cytokine receptor deficiencies result in susceptibility to mycobacterial infection

Failure to express leucocyte adhesion markers gives rise to Leucocyte adhesion deficiencies

Neutrophil cell death and the formation of pus

Fig. 4.5 Neutrophil function and dysfunction (green boxes).

COMPLEMENT PATHWAY DEFICIENCIES

Genetic deficiencies of almost all the complement pathway proteins (Fig. 4.3) have been described. The major feature of deficiencies of the classical and alternative pathway components is recurrent infection with encapsulated bacteria, particularly *Neisseria* species. This reflects the importance of the complement membrane attack complex in defence against these bacteria. In addition, genetic deficiencies of the classical complement pathway (C1, C2 and C4) are associated with a high prevalence of auto-immune disease, particularly severe systemic lupus erythematosus (SLE, p. 1132).

In contrast to other complement deficiencies, mannose-binding lectin deficiency is very common (5% of the population). Individuals with complete mannose-binding lectin deficiency have an increased incidence of bacterial infections if subjected to an additional cause of immune compromise, such as prematurity or chemotherapy. However, the importance of this deficiency in otherwise healthy individuals remains uncertain.

Deficiency of the regulatory protein C1 inhibitor is not associated with recurrent infections, but causes recurrent angioedema. This is discussed on page 87.

Investigations and management

Complement C3 and C4 are the only complement components that are routinely measured. Screening for complement deficiencies is performed using functional tests of the complement pathway. The CH50 (classical haemo-lytic pathway 50, also known as total haemolytic complement THC) involves adding the patient's serum to sheep red blood cells (SRBC) coated with anti-SRBC antibody. If the cells lyse, the serum contains all the components of the classical and membrane attack pathways. Absence of lysis indicates a complement deficiency and should be followed by measurement of individual components. However, complement proteins degrade rapidly at room temperature, and the most common cause of an absent CH50 is delay in transportation of the sample to the laboratory.

There is no definitive treatment of complement deficiencies. Patients are at risk of meningococcal and other infections, and should be vaccinated with meningococcal, pneumococcal and *H. influenzae* B vaccines in order to boost their adaptive immune responses. Life-long prophylactic penicillin to prevent meningococcal infection is also recommended. At-risk family members should be screened for complement deficiencies with functional complement assays.

PRIMARY DEFICIENCIES OF THE ADAPTIVE IMMUNE SYSTEM

COMBINED B- AND T-LYMPHOCYTE IMMUNE DEFICIENCIES

Severe combined immune deficiency is caused by defects in lymphoid precursors and results in the combined failure of B- and T-cell maturation. The absence of an effective adaptive immune response causes recurrent bacterial, fungal and viral infections soon after birth. Stem cell transplantation is the only current treatment option, although specific gene therapy is under investigation.

PRIMARY T-LYMPHOCYTE DEFICIENCIES

These are characterised by recurrent viral, protozoal and fungal infections (Box 4.5). In addition, many T-cell deficiencies are associated with defective antibody production because of the importance of T cells in providing help for B cells. These disorders generally present in childhood and are illustrated in Figure 4.6.

DiGeorge syndrome. This results from failure of development of the 3rd/4th pharyngeal pouch, usually caused by a deletion of 22q11. It is associated with abnormalities of the aortic arch, hypocalcaemia, tracheo-oesophageal fistulae, cleft lip and palate, and absent thymic development. It is characterised by very low numbers of mature T cells despite normal development in the bone marrow.

Bare lymphocyte syndromes. These are caused by absent expression of HLA molecules within the thymus. If HLA class I molecules are affected, CD8+ lymphocytes fail to develop, while absent expression of HLA class II molecules affects CD4+ lymphocyte maturation. In addition to recurrent infections, failure to express HLA class I is associated with systemic vasculitis caused by uncontrolled activation of natural killer cells.

Autoimmune lymphoproliferative syndrome. This is caused by failure of apoptosis (p. 44). It is characterised by accumulation of lymphocytes and persistence of autoreactive cells, and patients develop lymphadenopathy, splenomegaly and a variety of autoimmune diseases.

Investigations and management

The principal tests for T-lymphocyte deficiencies are a total lymphocyte count and quantitation of lymphocyte subpopulations by flow cytometry. Serum immunoglobulins should also be quantified. Functional tests of T-cell activation and proliferation and/or an HIV test may be indicated (p. 76).

Patients with suspected T-cell immune deficiencies should receive anti-*Pneumocystis* and antifungal prophylaxis, and require aggressive management of specific infections. Immunoglobulin replacement may be indicated if disease is associated with defective antibody production. Stem cell transplantation may be appropriate in bare lymphocyte syndromes, and thymic transplantation has been used for DiGeorge syndrome.

PRIMARY ANTIBODY DEFICIENCIES

Primary antibody deficiencies (Fig. 4.7) are characterised by recurrent bacterial infections, particularly of the respiratory and gastrointestinal tract. The most common causative organisms are bacteria such as *S. pneumoniae* and *H. influenzae*. Severe inherited disorders of antibody production are rare and usually present at 5–6 months of age, when the protective benefit of transferred maternal

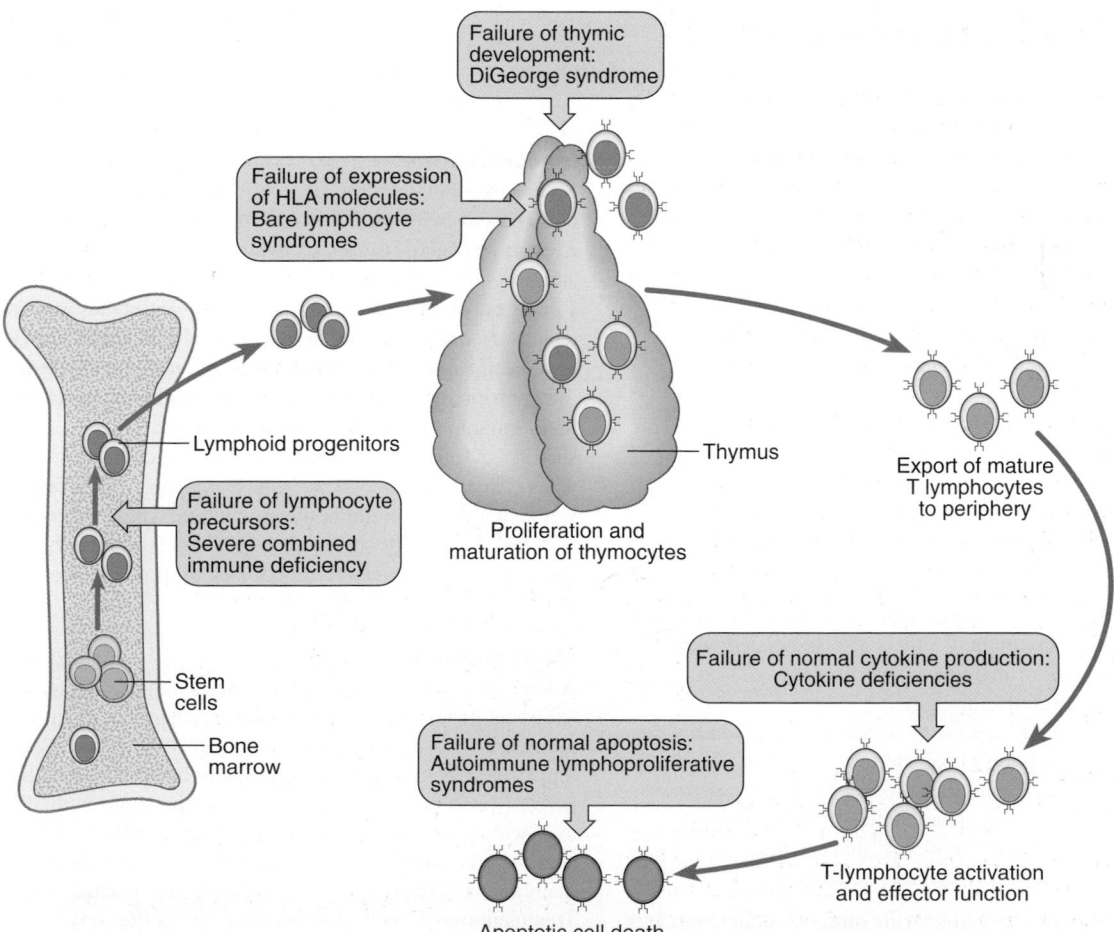

Fig. 4.6   T-lymphocyte function and dysfunction (green boxes).

4

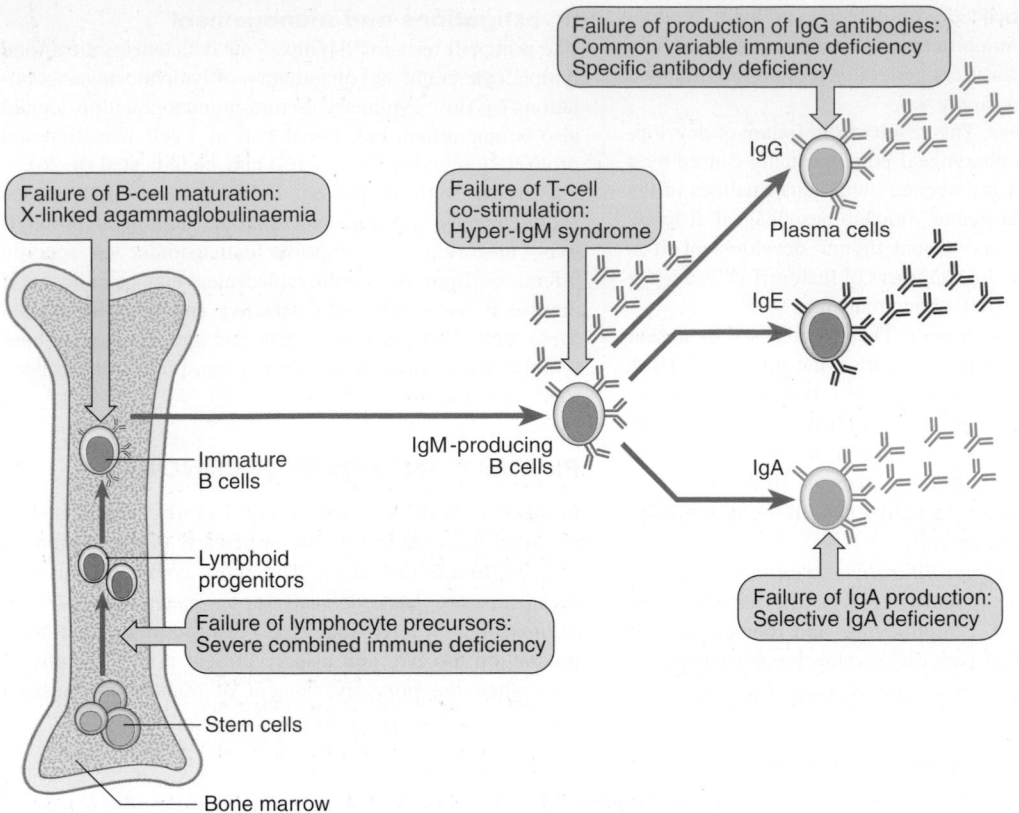

Failure of production of IgG antibodies:
Common variable immune deficiency
Specific antibody deficiency

IgG

Plasma cells

Failure of B-cell maturation:
X-linked agammaglobulinaemia

Failure of T-cell
co-stimulation:
Hyper-IgM syndrome

IgE

Immature
B cells

IgM-producing
B cells

IgA

Lymphoid
progenitors

Failure of lymphocyte precursors:
Severe combined immune deficiency

Failure of IgA production:
Selective IgA deficiency

Stem cells

Bone marrow

Fig. 4.7 B-lymphocyte function and primary antibody deficiencies (green boxes).

immunoglobulin has waned. Three major primary antibody deficiencies present in adulthood:

- *Selective IgA deficiency* is the most common primary immune deficiency, affecting 1:600 Northern Europeans. In most patients, low (< 0.05 g/l) or undetectable IgA is an incidental finding with no clinical sequelae. However, 30% of individuals experience recurrent mild respiratory and gastrointestinal infections. In some patients, there is a compensatory increase in serum IgG levels.
- *Common variable immune deficiency (CVID)* is a heterogeneous adult-onset primary immune deficiency of unknown cause. It is characterised by low serum IgG levels and failure to make antibody responses to exogenous pathogens. Paradoxically, antibody-mediated autoimmune diseases such as idiopathic thrombocytopenic purpura and autoimmune haemolytic anaemia are common. CVID is also associated with an increased risk of malignancy, particularly lymphoproliferative disease.
- *Specific antibody deficiency or functional IgG antibody deficiency* is a poorly characterised condition which causes defective antibody responses to polysaccharide antigens. Some patients are deficient in the antibody subclasses IgG2 and IgG4, and this condition was previously called IgG subclass deficiency.

There is overlap between specific antibody deficiency, IgA deficiency and CVID, and some patients may progress to a more global antibody deficiency over time.

Investigations
Serum immunoglobulins (Box 4.7) should be measured in conjunction with protein and urine electrophoresis to exclude secondary causes of hypogammaglobulinaemia. In addition, specific antibody responses to known pathogens should be assessed by measuring IgG antibodies against tetanus, *H. influenzae* and *S. pneumoniae* (most patients will have been exposed to some of these antigens through either infection or immunisation). If specific antibody levels are low, immunisation with the appropriate killed vaccine should be followed by repeat antibody measurement 6–8 weeks later; failure to mount a response indicates a significant defect in antibody production. These functional tests have generally superseded IgG subclass quantitation. Quantitation of B and T lymphocytes by flow cytometry is also useful.

Management
All patients with antibody deficiencies require aggressive treatment of infections, and prophylactic antibiotics may be indicated. The mainstay of treatment is immunoglobulin replacement (intravenous immunoglobulin, IVIG), which is derived from pooled plasma and contains IgG antibodies to a wide variety of common organisms. IVIG is usually administered intravenously every 3–4 weeks with the aim of maintaining trough IgG levels within the normal range. Treatment may be self-administered, and is life-long.

With the exception of selective IgA deficiency, immunisation is generally not effective because of the defect in IgG

4.7 INVESTIGATION OF PRIMARY ANTIBODY DEFICIENCIES

	Serum immunoglobulins				Circulating lymphocyte numbers		
	IgM	IgG	IgA	IgE	B cells	T cells	Other investigations
Selective IgA deficiency	Normal	Often elevated	Absent	Normal	Normal	Normal	
Common variable immune deficiency	Normal or low	Low	Low	Low	Variable	Variable	Failure to produce specific antibodies after test immunisation
Specific antibody deficiency	Normal	Normal	Normal or low	Normal	Normal	Normal	Failure to produce specific antibodies after test immunisation

antibody production. As with all primary immune deficiencies, live vaccines should be avoided.

SECONDARY IMMUNE DEFICIENCIES

Secondary immune deficiencies are much more common than primary immune deficiencies, and occur if the immune system is compromised by external factors (Box 4.8). Infection is a common cause of secondary immune deficiency, particularly HIV infection, measles and other viral illnesses. Immune deficiency is also an expected side-effect of some drugs, particularly those used in the management of transplantation, autoimmunity and cancer (p. 265). In addition, it may be an idiosyncratic effect of other agents, particularly anti-epileptic medication. Physiological immune deficiency occurs at the extremes of life, and the decline of the immune response in the elderly is known as

4.8 CAUSES OF SECONDARY IMMUNE DEFICIENCY

Physiological immune deficiency

- Ageing
- Prematurity
- Pregnancy

Infection

- Human immunodeficiency virus
- Measles
- Mycobacterial infection

Iatrogenic

- Immunosuppressive therapy
- Antineoplastic agents
- Corticosteroids
- Stem cell transplantation
- Radiation injury

Malignancy

- B-cell malignancies including leukaemia, lymphoma and myeloma
- Solid tumours
- Thymoma

Biochemical and nutritional disorders

- Malnutrition
- Renal insufficiency/dialysis
- Diabetes mellitus
- Specific mineral deficiencies, e.g. iron, zinc

Other conditions

- Burns
- Asplenia/hyposplenism

4.9 IMMUNE SENESCENCE

- **T-cell responses:** decline, with reduced delayed type hypersensitivity responses.
- **Antibody production:** decreased for many exogenous antigens. Although autoantibody production rises, autoimmune disease is less common.
- **Response to vaccination:** reduced, e.g. 30% of healthy older people may not develop protective immunity after influenza vaccination.
- **Allergic disorders and transplant rejection:** less common.
- **Susceptibility to infection:** increased, e.g. community-acquired pneumonia by threefold and urinary tract infection by 20-fold. Latent infections, e.g. tuberculosis and herpes zoster, may be reactivated.
- **Manifestations of infection:** may be absent, e.g. lack of pyrexia or leucocytosis.

immune senescence (Box 4.9). Management of secondary immune deficiency is described in the relevant chapters on HIV (Ch. 14), oncology (Ch. 11) and haematological disorders (Ch. 24).

THE INFLAMMATORY RESPONSE

Inflammation is the response of tissues to injury or infection, and is necessary for normal repair and healing. This section focuses on the generic inflammatory response, and its multisystem manifestations. The role of inflammation in specific diseases is illustrated in many other chapters of this book.

PHYSIOLOGY AND PATHOLOGY

ACUTE INFLAMMATION

Acute inflammation is the result of rapid and complex interplay between the cells and soluble molecules of the innate immune system. The classical external signs include heat, redness, pain and swelling (calor, rubor, dolor and oedema, Fig. 4.8).

The inflammatory process is initiated by local tissue injury or infection, with early infiltration of phagocytic cells and an increase in enzymes within the inflamed tissues such as cyclo-oxygenase and inducible nitric oxide

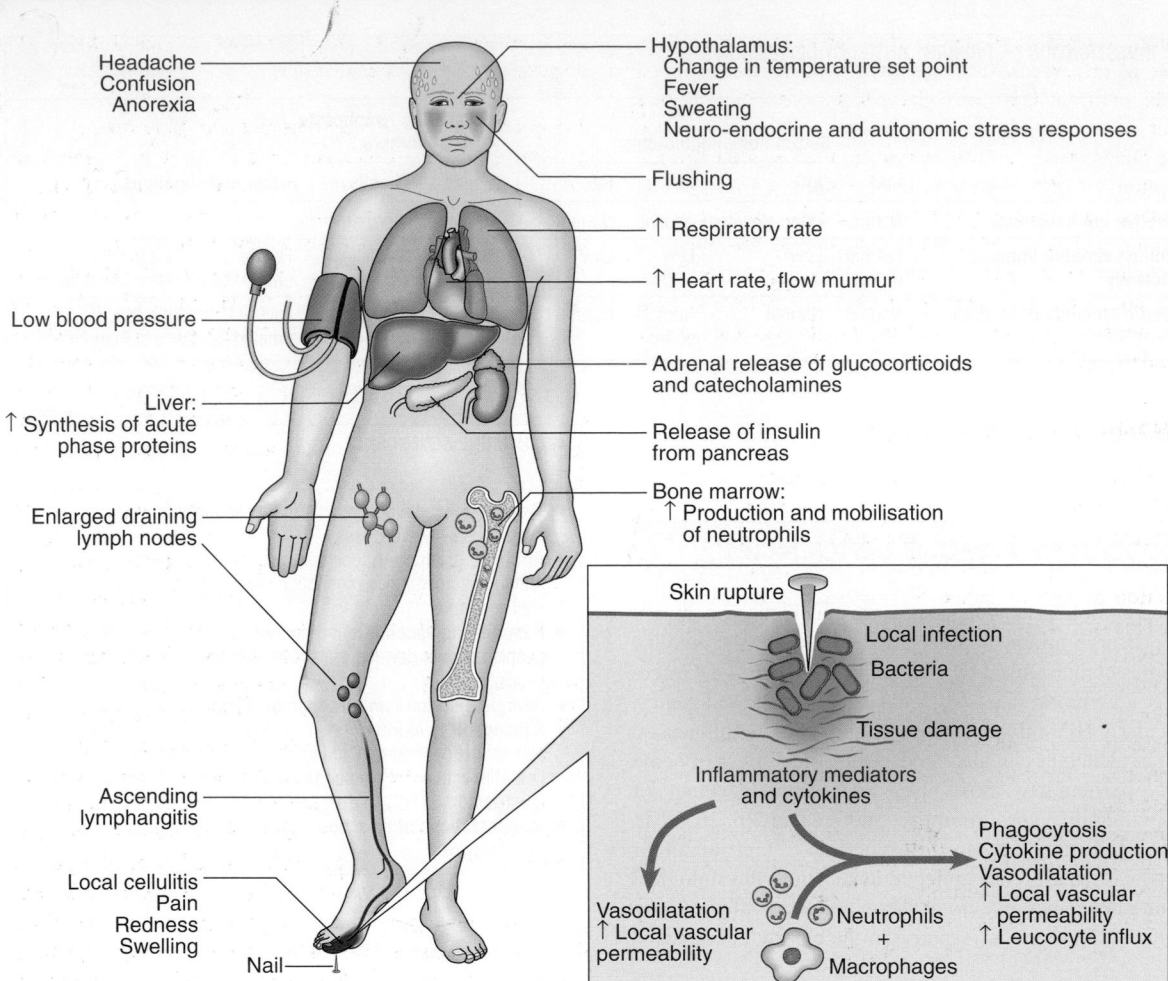

Fig. 4.8 Clinical features of acute inflammation. In this example, the response is to a penetrating injury in the foot.

synthase. As a result, there is release of leukotrienes, prostaglandins, histamine, kinins, anaphylotoxins and nitric oxide. The effect is vasodilatation and increased local vascular permeability, thereby increasing flow of fluid and cells to the affected tissue. In addition, pro-inflammatory cytokines produced at the site of injury have profound systemic effects. IL-1, TNF-α and IL-6 act on the hypothalamus to raise the temperature set-point, and stimulate the production of acute phase proteins by the liver.

Acute phase proteins

Acute phase proteins are produced by the liver in response to inflammatory stimuli and have a wide range of activities. C-reactive protein (CRP) and serum amyloid A may be increased 1000-fold, contributing to host defence and stimulating repair and regeneration. Fibrinogen plays an essential role in wound healing, and α_1-antitrypsin and α_1-antichymotrypsin control the pro-inflammatory cascade by neutralising the enzymes produced by activated neutrophils preventing widespread tissue destruction. In addition, antioxidants such as haptoglobin and manganese superoxide dismutase scavenge for oxygen free radicals, while increased levels of iron-binding proteins such as transferrin, ferritin and lactoferrin decrease the iron

available for uptake by bacteria. Immunoglobulins are not acute phase proteins but are often increased in chronic inflammation.

Resolution of inflammation

Resolution of an inflammatory response is crucial for normal healing. This involves active down-modulation of inflammatory stimuli and repair of bystander damage to local tissues. Extravasated neutrophils undergo apoptosis and are phagocytosed by macrophages, along with the remains of microorganisms. Macrophages also synthesise collagenase and elastase, which break down local connective tissue and aid in the removal of debris. Macrophage-derived cytokines including TGF-β and platelet-derived growth factor attract fibroblasts and promote the synthesis of new collagen, while angiogenic factors stimulate new vessel formation.

Sepsis and septic shock

Septic shock is the clinical manifestation of overwhelming inflammation. Failure of normal inhibitory mechanisms results in excessive production of pro-inflammatory cytokines by macrophages. This results in hypotension, hypovolaemia, decreased perfusion and tissue oedema. In

4

addition, uncontrolled neutrophil activation causes the release of proteases and oxygen free radicals within blood vessels, causing damage to the vascular endothelium and further increasing capillary permeability. Direct activation of the coagulation pathway combines with endothelial cell disruption to form clots within the damaged vessels. The clinical consequences include cardiovascular collapse, acute respiratory distress syndrome, disseminated intravascular coagulation, multiorgan failure, and often death (p. 186). Septic shock most frequently results from infection with Gram-negative bacteria, because lipopolysaccharide is particularly effective at activating the inflammatory cascade.

CHRONIC INFLAMMATION

Failure to remove an inflammatory stimulus results in chronic inflammation. Persisting microorganisms stimulate the ongoing accumulation of neutrophils, macrophages and activated T lymphocytes. If this is associated with local deposition of fibrous connective tissue, a granuloma may form. This is characteristic of infections such as tuberculosis and leprosy, in which the microorganism is protected by a cell wall which shields it from killing, despite phagocytosis.

In most instances, the development of an active immune response is beneficial to the host, and results in either clearance or control of the infection with minimal local damage. However, inappropriately vigorous or prolonged immune responses may cause significant bystander tissue damage. These are known as hypersensitivity responses and may involve either antibody or cell-mediated responses. The Gell and Coombs classification of hypersensitivity responses is discussed on page 80.

INVESTIGATIONS

The changes associated with inflammation are reflected in many laboratory investigations. Leucocytosis is common, and reflects the transit of activated neutrophils and monocytes to the site of infection (p. 65). The platelet count may be increased. Chronic inflammation is frequently associated with normocytic normochromic anaemia. The CRP (see below) is the most widely used clinical measure of acute inflammation, but levels of fibrinogen, ferritin and complement components may also be increased as part of the acute phase response, while albumin levels are reduced.

C-reactive protein

C-reactive protein is an acute phase reactant which opsonises invading pathogens. Levels of CRP increase within 6 hours of an inflammatory stimulus, and may rise up to 1000-fold. Measurement of CRP provides a direct index of acute inflammation, and the plasma half-life of CRP is 19 hours, so levels fall in just a few days once the stimulus is removed. Sequential measurement is useful in monitoring disease activity (Box 4.10). For reasons which remain unclear, some diseases are associated with only minor elevations of CRP concentration despite unequivocal evidence of active inflammation. These include SLE, scleroderma, ulcerative colitis and leukaemia. Importantly,

intercurrent infection does provoke a significant CRP response in these conditions.

Erythrocyte sedimentation rate (ESR)

In contrast to the CRP, the ESR is an indirect measure of the acute phase response. It measures the rate of fall of erythrocytes through plasma, and a major determinant of this is aggregation of red cells. Normally, erythrocytes do not clump together because of their repellent negative charge; plasma proteins are positively charged and act to neutralise the surface charge of erythrocytes. An increase in plasma proteins, particularly fibrinogen, overcomes the repulsive forces of erythrocytes, causing them to stack together like tyres, or rouleaux. Rouleaux have a higher mass/surface area ratio than single red cells, and thus sediment faster.

Thus the ESR is a composite measure of plasma protein composition, concentration, and erythrocyte morphology. The most common cause of an increased ESR is an acute phase response, which causes an increase in plasma protein concentration. This is accompanied by a corresponding increase in circulating CRP levels. However, other conditions that do not affect acute phase proteins may alter plasma protein composition and concentration (Box 4.10). Most importantly, immunoglobulins comprise a significant proportion of plasma proteins, but do not participate in the acute phase response. Thus any condition that causes a monoclonal or polyclonal increase in serum immunoglobulins will increase the ESR. In addition, changes in erythrocyte surface area and density will influence sedimentation, and abnormal red cell morphology can make rouleau formation impossible. For these reasons, an inappropriately low ESR occurs in spherocytosis, sickle cell anaemia, microcytic anaemia and with low plasma protein levels.

As CRP is a simpler and more sensitive early indicator of the acute phase response, it is increasingly used in preference to the ESR. If both ESR and CRP are used, any discrepancy should be resolved by assessing the individual determinants of the ESR, i.e. full blood count and film, serum immunoglobulins (IgG, IgA and IgM) and protein electrophoresis. The IgE concentration in plasma is very low and does not contribute significantly to the ESR.

Plasma viscosity

Plasma viscosity is another surrogate measure of plasma protein concentration. It is affected by the concentration of large plasma proteins, including fibrinogen and immunoglobulins, especially IgM.

PRESENTING PROBLEMS IN INFLAMMATION

In most patients presenting with the manifestations of acute inflammation shown in Figure 4.8, it is possible to rapidly identify the source of the problem, and assess the consequences as discussed in other chapters. Systemic manifestations of inflammation include fever (p. 136), leucocytosis (p. 1014) and shock (p. 186).

4

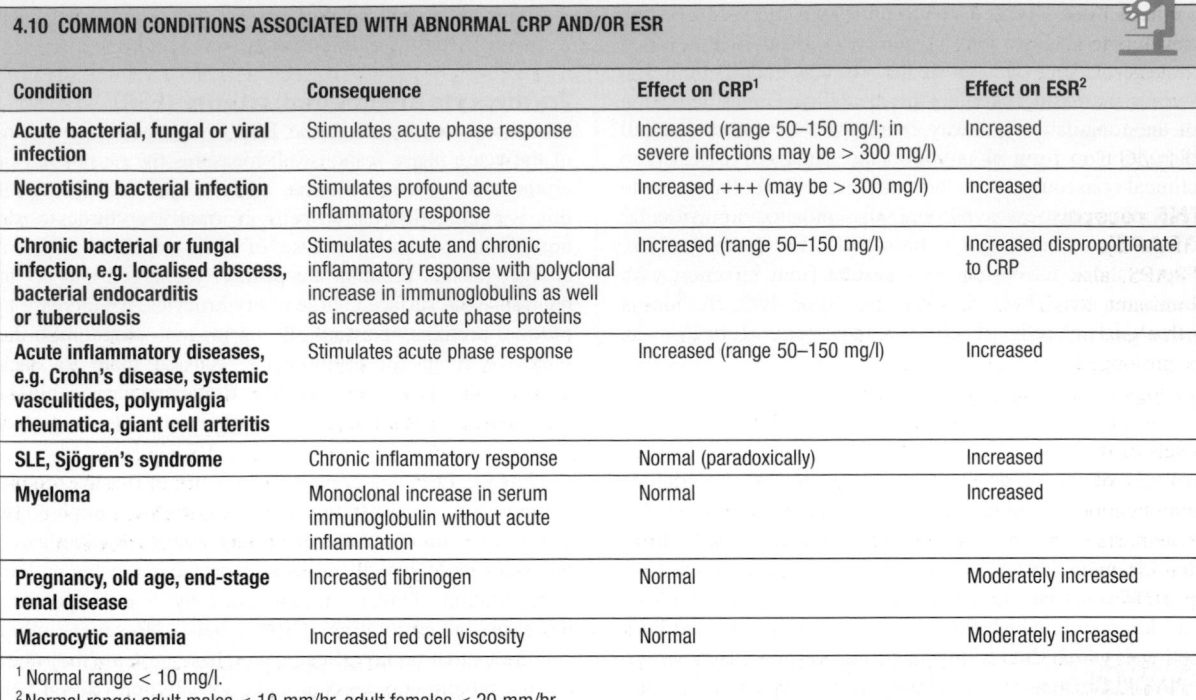

4.10 COMMON CONDITIONS ASSOCIATED WITH ABNORMAL CRP AND/OR ESR

Condition	Consequence	Effect on CRP[1]	Effect on ESR[2]
Acute bacterial, fungal or viral infection	Stimulates acute phase response	Increased (range 50–150 mg/l; in severe infections may be > 300 mg/l)	Increased
Necrotising bacterial infection	Stimulates profound acute inflammatory response	Increased +++ (may be > 300 mg/l)	Increased
Chronic bacterial or fungal infection, e.g. localised abscess, bacterial endocarditis or tuberculosis	Stimulates acute and chronic inflammatory response with polyclonal increase in immunoglobulins as well as increased acute phase proteins	Increased (range 50–150 mg/l)	Increased disproportionate to CRP
Acute inflammatory diseases, e.g. Crohn's disease, systemic vasculitides, polymyalgia rheumatica, giant cell arteritis	Stimulates acute phase response	Increased (range 50–150 mg/l)	Increased
SLE, Sjögren's syndrome	Chronic inflammatory response	Normal (paradoxically)	Increased
Myeloma	Monoclonal increase in serum immunoglobulin without acute inflammation	Normal	Increased
Pregnancy, old age, end-stage renal disease	Increased fibrinogen	Normal	Moderately increased
Macrocytic anaemia	Increased red cell viscosity	Normal	Moderately increased

[1] Normal range < 10 mg/l.
[2] Normal range: adult males < 10 mm/hr, adult females < 20 mm/hr.

UNEXPLAINED RAISED ESR

The ESR should not be used to screen asymptomatic patients for the presence of disease. However, in the era of frequent routine laboratory testing, an unexplained raised ESR is a common problem.

Clinical assessment

A comprehensive history and examination are crucial. Extreme elevations in the ESR (> 100 mm/hr) rarely occur in the absence of significant disease (Box 4.10).

Investigations

Assessing the CRP, serum immunoglobulins and urine electrophoresis will help determine if the elevation in ESR is due to an acute inflammatory process (Box 4.10)

A full blood count may show a normocytic, normochromic anaemia, which occurs in many chronic diseases. Leucocytosis may reflect infection, inflammatory disease or tissue necrosis. Neutrophilia suggests infection or acute inflammation. Atypical lymphocytes may occur in some chronic infections such as CMV and EBV.

Abnormalities in liver function suggest either a local infective process (hepatitis, hepatic abscess or biliary sepsis) or systemic disease including malignancy.

Blood and urine cultures should be performed.

Imaging

A chest X-ray and abdominal CT scan may identify a source of unknown infection or malignancy. An abdominal and pelvic ultrasound may identify hepatic lesions, abdominal nodes, and local intra-abdominal or pelvic abscesses. An MRI scan is more appropriate for the diagnosis of soft tissue or bone/joint infections. Echocardiography is used to look for vegetations and assess valve function in suspected bacterial endocarditis. White cell scans are rarely indicated, but may occasionally be useful in identification of the site of pyogenic infection. An isotope scan may identify evidence of malignancy or focal bone infection.

PERIODIC FEVER SYNDROMES

These rare disorders are characterised by recurrent episodes of fever and organ inflammation associated with an elevated acute phase response.

Familial Mediterranean fever (FMF)

This is the most common of the familial periodic fevers, predominantly affecting Mediterranean people, including Arabs, Turks, Sephardic Jews and Armenians. It results from mutations of the pyrin gene, which is thought to regulate neutrophil-mediated inflammation. FMF is characterised by painful attacks of fever associated with peritonitis, pleuritis and arthritis, and lasts from a few hours to 4 days. During acute episodes, CRP levels are markedly increased. The majority of individuals have their first attack before the age of 20. The major complication of FMF is AA amyloidosis (p. 79). Colchicine significantly reduces the number of febrile episodes in 90% of patients, but does not stop an established attack.

Hyper-IgD syndrome (HIDS)

HIDS is an autosomal recessive disorder that causes recurrent attacks of fever, abdominal pain, diarrhoea, lymphadenopathy, arthralgia, skin lesions and aphthous ulceration. Most patients originate from the Netherlands and northern France. The defect is a mutation in the gene for mevalonate kinase, which is involved in the metabolism of cholesterol, but how this causes an inflammatory periodic fever remains unknown. Serum IgD levels are persistently elevated. No specific treatment is available, although trials of HMG CoA reductase inhibitors are ongoing.

TNF receptor-associated periodic syndrome (TRAPS)

TRAPS, also known as Hibernian fever, is an autosomal dominant syndrome causing recurrent periodic fever, arthralgia, myalgia, serositis and skin rashes. Attacks may be prolonged (> 1 week). During a typical attack, laboratory findings include neutrophilia, increased CRP and elevated IgA levels. The diagnosis can be confirmed by low serum levels of the soluble type 1 TNF receptor and by molecular analysis of the TNFRSF1A gene. As in FMF, the major complication is amyloidosis, and regular screening for proteinuria is advised. TRAPS responds to systemic corticosteroids, and soluble TNF receptor therapy may be effective (p. 1094).

AMYLOIDOSIS

The amyloidoses are a group of acquired and hereditary disorders characterised by the extracellular deposition of insoluble proteins. These complex deposits consist of fibrils of the specific protein involved linked to glycosamino-glycans and proteoglycans, and serum amyloid P (SAP). Protein accumulation may be localised or systemic, and the clinical manifestations depend upon the organ(s) affected. The diagnosis of amyloidosis should be considered in all cases of unexplained nephrotic syndrome (p. 479), cardiomyopathy (p. 641) and peripheral neuropathy (p. 1246).

Amyloid diseases are classified by aetiology and type of protein deposited. Box 4.11 lists the causes and manifestations.

Diagnosis

The diagnosis is established by biopsy, which may be of an affected organ, rectum or subcutaneous fat. The pathognomonic histological feature is apple-green birefringence of amyloid deposits when stained with Congo red dye and viewed under polarised light. Immunohistochemical staining can then identify the type of amyloid fibril present. Quantitative scintigraphy with radiolabelled serum amyloid P is a valuable tool in determining the overall load and distribution of amyloid deposits.

Management

The aims of treatment are to support the function of affected organs, and, in acquired amyloidosis, to prevent further amyloid deposition through treatment of the primary cause. Where the latter is possible, regression of existing amyloid deposits may occur. Liver transplantation may provide definitive treatment in selected patients with hereditary transthyretin amyloidosis.

4

4.11 AMYLOID DISORDERS			
Disorder	**Pathological basis**	**Predisposing conditions**	**Other features**
ACQUIRED SYSTEMIC AMYLOIDOSIS			
Reactive (AA) amyloidosis	Increased production of serum amyloid A as part of prolonged or recurrent acute inflammatory response	Chronic infection (TB, leprosy, bronchiectasis, chronic abscess, osteomyelitis) Chronic inflammatory diseases (rheumatoid arthritis, familial Mediterranean fever)	90% of patients present with non-selective proteinuria or nephrotic syndrome
Light chain amyloidosis (AL)	Increased production of monoclonal light chain	Monoclonal gammopathies, including myeloma, benign gammopathies and plasmacytoma	Restrictive cardiomyopathy, peripheral and autonomic neuropathy, carpal tunnel syndrome, proteinuria, spontaneous purpura, amyloid nodules and plaques Macroglossia occurs rarely but is pathognomonic Poor prognosis
Dialysis-associated (Aβ2M) amyloidosis	Accumulation of circulating β_2-microglobulin due to failure of renal catabolism	Renal dialysis	Carpal tunnel syndrome, chronic arthropathy and pathological fractures secondary to amyloid bone cyst formation Manifestations occur 5–10 years after the start of dialysis
Senile systemic amyloidosis	Normal transthyretin protein deposited in tissues	Age > 70 years	Feature of normal ageing (affects > 90% of 90-year-olds) Usually asymptomatic
HEREDITARY SYSTEMIC AMYLOIDOSIS			
> 20 forms of hereditary systemic amyloidosis	Production of protein with an abnormal structure that predisposes to amyloid fibril formation Most often due to transthyretin mutation	Autosomal dominant inheritance	Peripheral and autonomic neuropathy, cardiomyopathy Renal involvement unusual 10% of gene carriers are asymptomatic throughout life

4

AUTOIMMUNE DISEASE

Autoimmunity can be defined as the presence of immune responses against self-targets, and is to some extent ubiquitous. It may be a harmless phenomenon, identified by the presence of low titre autoantibodies or autoreactive T cells. However, autoimmune diseases occur if these responses cause significant organ damage. These are a major cause of chronic morbidity and disability, affecting up to 1 in 30 adults at some time.

PHYSIOLOGY AND PATHOLOGY

Immunological tolerance

This is the process by which the immune system distinguishes self from foreign tissue.

Central tolerance occurs during lymphocyte development and operates in the thymus and bone marrow. Here, T and B lymphocytes that recognise self antigens are deleted before they develop into fully immunocompetent cells. This process is most active in fetal life, but continues throughout life as immature lymphocytes are generated.

Some autoreactive cells inevitably evade deletion and escape into the peripheral circulation. These cells are controlled through peripheral tolerance mechanisms. These include the suppression of autoreactive cells by 'regulatory' T cells and the generation of hyporesponsiveness ('anergy') in lymphocytes which encounter antigen in the absence of the co-stimulatory signals that accompany inflammation. In addition, some tissues such as the eye are not normally patrolled by lymphocytes. Antigens within these 'immunologically privileged' sites are inaccessible to autoreactive cells.

Failure of any of these tolerance mechanisms may result in the development of autoimmune disease.

Factors predisposing to autoimmune disease

Both genetic and environmental factors contribute to the development of autoimmune disease. The most important genetic determinants of autoimmune susceptibility are the HLA genes, reflecting their importance in shaping lymphocyte responses (Box 4.12). Other genes that contribute to susceptibility to autoimmune disease include genes determining cytokine activity, co-stimulation and cell death.

Several environmental factors can trigger autoimmunity in genetically predisposed individuals. The most widely studied of these is infection, as occurs in acute rheumatic fever following streptococcal infection or reactive arthritis following bacterial infection. A number of mechanisms have been postulated, including cross-reactivity between the infectious pathogen and self determinants (molecular mimicry), and release of sequestered antigens which are not usually visible to the immune system from damaged tissue. Alternatively, infection may result in the production of inflammatory cytokines which overwhelm normal control mechanisms that prevent bystander damage. Occasionally, the development of autoimmune disease is a side-effect of drug treatment. For example, the metabolic products of the anaesthetic agent halothane bind to liver enzymes, resulting in a structurally novel protein. This is recognised as a new (foreign) antigen by the immune system, and the autoantibodies and activated T cells directed against it may cause hepatic necrosis. Autoimmune diseases are much more common in women than in men, for reasons which remain unclear.

Classification of autoimmune diseases

The spectrum of autoimmune diseases is broad (Box 4.13), and these conditions are frequently classified as organ-specific or multisystem. There is considerable overlap and it is also useful to consider the predominant mechanism responsible for tissue damage. The Gell and Coombs classification of hypersensitivity distinguishes four types of immune response which result in bystander tissue damage. These are described in Box 4.14.

Type I hypersensitivity is not associated with autoimmune disease. In type II hypersensitivity, injury is clearly localised to a single tissue or organ. By contrast, in type III hypersensitivity immune complexes aggregate together and are

4.12 HLA ASSOCIATIONS IN AUTOIMMUNE DISEASE

Disease	HLA association	Relative risk
Ankylosing spondylitis	B27	~90:1
Type 1 diabetes	DR3/DR4	~20:1
Rheumatoid arthritis	DR4	~5:1
Graves' disease	DR3	~5:1
Myasthenia gravis	DR3	~3:1

4.13 THE SPECTRUM OF AUTOIMMUNE DISEASE

Type	Disease	Page no.
Organ-specific Immune response directed against localised antigens	Graves' disease	754
	Hashimoto's thyroiditis	757
	Addison's disease	782
	Pernicious anaemia	1028
	Type 1 diabetes	810
	Sympathetic ophthalmoplegia	1197
	Goodpasture's syndrome	502
	Pemphigus vulgaris	1275
	Bullous pemphigoid	1275
	Idiopathic thrombocytopenic purpura	1056
	Autoimmune haemolytic anaemia	1033
	Myasthenia gravis	1252
	Rheumatoid arthritis	1101
	Dermatomyositis	1136
	Primary biliary cirrhosis	978
	Autoimmune hepatitis	977
	Sjögren's syndrome	1137
Multisystem Immune response directed to widespread target antigens	Systemic sclerosis	1134
	Mixed connective tissue disease	1137
	SLE	1132

4.14 GELL AND COOMBS CLASSIFICATION OF HYPERSENSITIVITY DISEASES

Type	Mechanism	Example of disease in response to exogenous agent	Example of autoimmune disease
Type I Immediate hypersensitivity	IgE-mediated mast cell degranulation	Allergic disease	None described
Type II Antibody-mediated	Binding of cytotoxic IgG or IgM antibodies to cell surface causes cell killing	ABO blood transfusion reaction Hyperacute transplant rejection	Autoimmune haemolytic anaemia Idiopathic thrombocytopenic purpura Goodpasture's syndrome
Type III Immune complex-mediated	IgG or IgM bind soluble antigen to form immune complexes which trigger classical complement pathway activation	Serum sickness Farmer's lung	
Type IV Delayed type	Activated T cells, NK cells and phagocytes	Acute cellular rejection Nickel hypersensitivity	Type 1 diabetes Hashimoto's thyroiditis

widely deposited in blood vessel walls, skin, joints and glomeruli where they cause a chronic inflammatory response with triggering of the classical complement cascade and recruitment and activation of phagocytes and CD4$^+$ lymphocytes. The site of immune complex deposition is determined by the relative amount of antibody, size of the immune complexes, nature of the antigen and local haemodynamics. Generalised deposition of immune complexes gives rise to systemic diseases such as SLE. In type IV hypersensitivity activated T cells mediate phagocytosis and NK recruitment. Autoantibodies may occur, but these are not primarily responsible for the tissue damage.

INVESTIGATIONS

AUTOANTIBODIES

An increasing number of autoantibodies can be identified in the laboratory, and are useful in disease diagnosis and monitoring. The usefulness of a specific test increases with prior probability, so the 'shotgun approach' of ordering a number of laboratory tests without reference to clinical context increases the risk of false positive results.

Antibody is quantified either by titre (the minimal dilution at which the antibody can be detected) or by concentration in standardised units. The normal range for a given population may vary depending on the method used.

Rheumatoid factor

A rheumatoid factor is an antibody directed against the common (F$_c$) region of human IgG. Rheumatoid factors may be of any immunoglobulin class but IgM is most commonly tested. In general, a titre > 1:40 or unit value > 20 U is considered positive, although this varies with method.

The name 'rheumatoid factor' is a misnomer, and conveys an undeserved specificity to this test. Only 50% of patients with rheumatoid arthritis are positive for rheumatoid factor at the time of diagnosis; a further 25% will become seropositive in the first 2 years of disease (p. 1074). Thus this test is insufficiently sensitive to rule out rheumatoid arthritis. In addition, rheumatoid factor has low specificity for rheumatoid arthritis, being associated with a wide

4.15 CONDITIONS ASSOCIATED WITH A POSITIVE RHEUMATOID FACTOR

Disease	Frequency (%)
Rheumatoid arthritis with extra-articular manifestations	100
Rheumatoid arthritis (overall)	75
Sjögren's syndrome	90
Mixed essential cryoglobulinaemia	90
Primary biliary cirrhosis	50
Subacute bacterial endocarditis	40
SLE	30
Tuberculosis	15
Elderly (> 65 years)	20

variety of autoimmune and non-autoimmune conditions, and a common finding in the elderly (Box 4.15). The major indication for rheumatoid factor testing is to evaluate prognosis in rheumatoid arthritis, as it is associated with more severe erosive disease and extra-articular disease manifestations such as nodules, vasculitis and Felty's syndrome.

Anti-CCP antibody

Antibodies to cyclic citrullinated peptide (anti-CCP antibodies) bind to peptides in which the amino acid arginine has been converted to citrulline by peptidylarginine deiminase, an enzyme abundant in the inflamed synovium. It is a more specific test for rheumatoid arthritis than rheumatoid factor and a better predictor of an aggressive disease course. In patients with undifferentiated arthritis, anti-CCP antibodies may predict those who are likely to develop rheumatoid arthritis.

Antinuclear antibodies

Antinuclear antibodies (ANA) are a group of antibodies which bind to components of the nucleus. They are detected by applying serum to a human cell line (Hep 2 cells) followed by immunofluorescence microscopy. An antibody titre of > 1:80 is usually considered positive with this method. The pattern of immunofluorescence reflects binding to discrete nuclear components, and specific patterns may be associated with clinical subgroups. For example, a peripheral or rim pattern is primarily associated with SLE, while

4.16 CONDITIONS ASSOCIATED WITH A POSITIVE ANTINUCLEAR ANTIBODY

Disease	Approximate frequency
Diseases for which an ANA is useful in diagnosis	
SLE	~100%
Scleroderma	60–80%
Sjögren's syndrome	40–70%
Dermatomyositis or polymyositis	30–80%
Mixed connective tissue disease	100%
Autoimmune hepatitis	Part of diagnostic criteria
Diseases for which an ANA is not useful in diagnosis	
Rheumatoid arthritis	30–50%
Autoimmune thyroid disease	30–50%
Malignancy	Varies widely
Infectious diseases	Varies widely

N.B. 5% of healthy individuals have an ANA titre > 1:80.

nucleolar staining is seen in association with diffuse scleroderma.

The major indication for ANA testing is in the diagnosis of SLE, where it has a very high sensitivity (almost 100%), and a negative ANA test virtually excludes the diagnosis. However, the specificity is low (Box 4.16), and ANA may be present in low titre in healthy individuals. Repeating ANA tests is rarely useful, and there is no role for serial monitoring of ANA titre as there is no correlation with disease activity.

Antibodies to extractable nuclear antigens

If an ANA test is positive, it is useful to establish which nuclear component is being recognised, although in many cases the precise specificity remains unknown. Some nuclear antigens are soluble and can be extracted from the nucleus ('extractable nuclear antigens'). Antibodies to these antigens have high specificity for individual disease subgroups (Box 4.17), although sensitivity is low. There is little value in testing for antibodies to extractable nuclear antigens if the ANA is negative.

Anti-DNA antibodies

Anti-DNA antibodies bind to double-stranded DNA and are highly specific for SLE (95%). They occur in up to 60% of SLE patients at some time in their disease course. Very high titres are associated with more severe disease, including renal or central nervous system involvement. They are useful in disease monitoring as an increase in antibody titre is associated with disease activity and may precede disease relapse. Antibodies to single-stranded DNA are non-specific and have little clinical utility.

Antiphospholipid antibodies

Antiphospholipid antibodies are associated with the development of venous and arterial thrombosis and recurrent fetal loss. This may occur in isolation (primary antiphospholipid syndrome), or as a complication of SLE (secondary antiphospholipid syndrome). Antiphospholipid antibodies can also be detected in a wide variety of rheumatic, infectious and malignant conditions, although in these situations they are not usually associated with thrombosis.

There are several kinds of antiphospholipid antibodies, but the most commonly measured are anticardiolipin antibodies and lupus anticoagulant. Anticardiolipin antibodies are immunoglobulins directed against phospholipids, particularly β2 glycoprotein-1. The targets of the lupus anticoagulant are prothrombin and occasionally β2 glycoprotein-1. Thus while they have overlapping specificities, these antibodies are discordant in up to 40% of cases. If there is a clinical suspicion of the antiphospholipid syndrome, both tests should be performed. Lupus anticoagulant cannot be assessed if the patient is on anticoagulant therapy.

Anti-neutrophil cytoplasmic antibodies

Anti-neutrophil cytoplasmic antibodies (ANCA) are IgG antibodies to the cytoplasmic constituents of granulocytes. Two common patterns are described in association with vasculitic syndromes: cytoplasmic fluorescence (c-ANCA) is associated with antibodies to proteinase-3 (PR3), and

4.17 CONDITIONS ASSOCIATED WITH ANTIBODIES TO EXTRACTABLE NUCLEAR ANTIGENS

Antibody	Disease association
Anti-centromere antibody	CREST variant of scleroderma (sensitivity 60%, specificity 98%) Also occasionally found in primary Raynaud's syndrome
Anti-histone antibody	Drug-induced lupus
Anti-Jo-1 (anti-histidyl-tRNA synthetase)	Polymyositis, dermatomyositis or polymyositis–scleroderma overlap (20–30%). Particularly associated with interstitial lung disease
Anti-La antibody (anti-SS-B)	Sjögren's syndrome SLE (20–60%)
Anti-ribonucleoprotein antibody (anti-RNP)	Mixed connective tissue disease SLE, usually in conjunction with anti-Sm antibodies
Anti-Ro antibody (anti-SS-A)	SLE (35–60%): associated with photosensitivity, thrombocytopenia and subacute cutaneous lupus Maternal anti-Ro antibodies associated with neonatal lupus and congenital heart block Sjögren's syndrome (40–80%)
Anti-RNA polymerase I	Rapidly progressive diffuse scleroderma
Anti-Smith antibody (Anti-Sm)	Very specific for SLE (15–30%): associated with more benign prognosis
Anti-topoisomerase I antibody (Anti-Scl70)	Diffuse scleroderma: associated with more severe organ involvement, including pulmonary fibrosis

occurs in more than 90% of patients with Wegener's granulomatosis with renal involvement, and with somewhat lower sensitivity in patients with limited Wegener's granulomatosis. A perinuclear staining pattern (p-ANCA) is associated with antibodies to other cytoplasmic enzymes, particularly myeloperoxidase (MPO), lactoferrin and elastase. A positive p-ANCA alone is a non-specific finding, but if due to MPO antibodies is associated with microscopic polyarteritis and Churg–Strauss vasculitis. Atypical p-ANCA, which are not due to anti-myeloperoxidase antibodies, are commonly found in patients with ulcerative colitis and auto-immune liver disease but are not of diagnostic or prognostic significance. Serial measurement of anti-PR3 or anti-MPO antibodies may be useful for disease monitoring.

MEASURES OF COMPLEMENT ACTIVATION

Quantitation of complement components may be useful in the evaluation of immune complex mediated diseases. Classical complement pathway activation leads to a decrease in circulating (unactivated) C4, and is often associated with decreased C3 levels. Serial measurement of C3 and C4 is used in the routine monitoring of SLE.

PRESENTING PROBLEMS IN AUTOIMMUNE DISEASE

Presentations of specific autoimmune diseases are described elsewhere in this book (listed in Box 4.13).

CRYOGLOBULINAEMIA

Cryoglobulins are immunoglobulins that form precipitates in the cold. They are classified into three types on the basis of the properties of the immunoglobulin (Box 4.18).

Testing for cryoglobulins requires the transport of a serum specimen to the laboratory at 37°C. Clinical management includes avoidance of cold and treatment of the underlying pathology. Type II and type III cryoglobulins may respond to immunosuppression and/or plasmapheresis to remove the pathogenic antibody.

ALLERGY

Allergic diseases are a common and increasing cause of illness, affecting between 15% and 20% of the population at some time. They comprise a range of disorders from mild to life-threatening, and affect many organs. Atopy is the tendency to produce an exaggerated IgE immune response to otherwise harmless environmental substances, and an allergic disease may be defined as the clinical manifestation of this inappropriate IgE immune response.

PATHOLOGY

Normally, the immune system does not make detectable responses to the many environmental substances such as foods and inhaled particles to which it is exposed on a daily basis. In an allergic reaction, initial exposure to an otherwise harmless exogenous substance (or allergen) triggers the production of specific IgE antibodies by activated B cells (Fig. 4.9 and Box 4.19). These are bound to the surface of mast cells via high affinity IgE receptors, a step that is not immediately associated with clinical sequelae. However, upon re-exposure, the allergen binds to membrane-bound IgE which activates the mast cells. These release a variety of vasoactive mediators (the early phase response) causing a type I hypersensitivity reaction and the symptoms of allergy. These range from sneezing and rhinorrhoea to anaphylaxis (Box 4.20). Persistent activation of mast cells

4.18 CLASSIFICATION OF CRYOGLOBULINS

	Type I	Type II	Type III
Immunoglobulin isotype and specificity	Monoclonal IgM paraprotein with no particular specificity	Monoclonal IgM paraprotein directed towards constant region of IgG	Polyclonal IgM or IgG directed towards constant region of IgG
Prevalence	25%	25%	50%
Disease association	Lymphoproliferative disease, especially Waldenström macroglobulinaemia (p. 1051)	Infection, particularly hepatitis B and hepatitis C; lymphoproliferative disease	Infection, particularly hepatitis B and C; autoimmune disease including rheumatoid arthritis and SLE
Symptoms	Hyperviscosity: Raynaud's phenomenon Acrocyanosis Retinal vessel occlusion Arterial and venous thrombosis	Small-vessel vasculitis: Purpuric rash Arthralgia Cutaneous ulceration Hepatosplenomegaly Glomerulonephritis Raynaud's phenomenon	Small-vessel vasculitis: Purpuric rash Arthralgia Cutaneous ulceration Hepatosplenomegaly Glomerulonephritis Raynaud's phenomenon
Protein electrophoresis	Monoclonal IgM paraprotein	Monoclonal IgM paraprotein	No monoclonal paraprotein
Rheumatoid factor	Negative	Strongly positive	Strongly positive
Complement	Normal	Decreased C4	Decreased C4
Serum viscosity	Raised	Normal	Normal

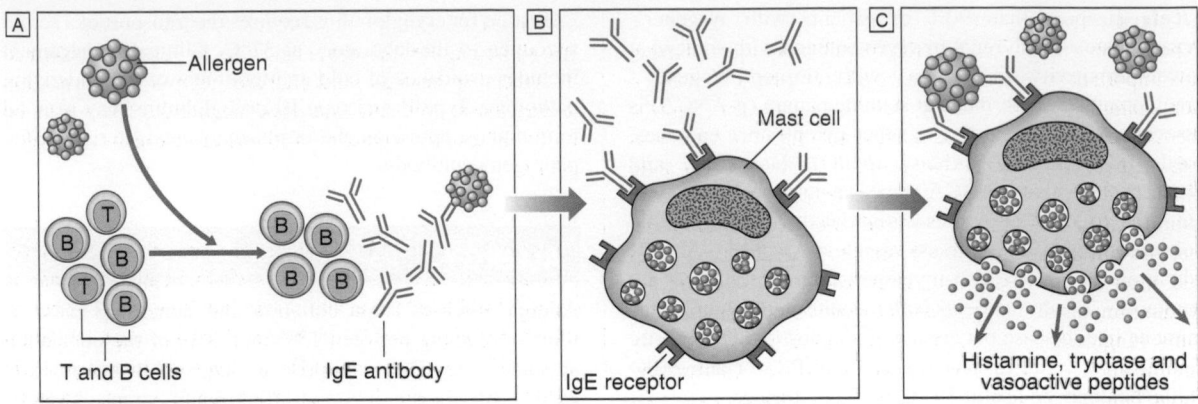

Fig. 4.9 Type I (immediate) hypersensitivity response. Ⓐ After an encounter with allergen, B cells produce IgE antibody against the allergen. Ⓑ Specific IgE antibodies bind to circulating mast cells via high-affinity IgE cell surface receptors. Ⓒ On re-encounter with allergen, the allergen binds to the IgE antibody-coated mast cells. This triggers mast cell activation with release of vasoactive mediators (Box 4.19).

4

4.19 PRODUCTS OF MAST CELL DEGRANULATION ⓘ

Mediator	Biological effects
Preformed and stored within granules	
Histamine	Vasodilatation, chemotaxis, bronchoconstriction and mucus secretion. Increases capillary permeability
Tryptase	Activates C3
Eosinophil chemotactic factor	Eosinophil chemotaxis
Neutrophil chemotactic factor	Neutrophil chemotaxis
Newly synthesised	
Leukotrienes	Increase vascular permeability, chemotaxis and mucus secretion. Smooth muscle contraction
Prostaglandins	Bronchoconstriction, platelet aggregation and vasodilatation
Thromboxanes	Bronchoconstriction
Platelet-activating factor	Bronchoconstriction, chemotaxis of eosinophils and neutrophils

results in the recruitment of other cells to the site of release. In some patients, the early phase response is followed 4–8 hours later by persistent swelling and local inflammation. This is known as the late phase reaction and is mediated by basophils, eosinophils and macrophages. Long-standing or recurrent allergic inflammation may give rise to a chronic inflammatory response characterised by a complex infiltrate of macrophages, eosinophils and T lymphocytes, in addition to mast cells and basophils. Once this has been established, inhibition of mast cell mediators with antihistamines is clinically ineffective. Mast cells may also be non-specifically triggered through a variety of other signals such as neuropeptides, anaphylotoxins and bacterial peptides.

Factors influencing susceptibility to allergic diseases

The incidence of allergic diseases is increasing in both industrialised and non-industrialised countries. The reasons for this are largely unexplained, but one widely held hypothesis is the 'hygiene hypothesis'. This proposes that infections in early life bias the immune system against the development of allergies, and that allergy is the penalty for the decreased incidence of infection that has resulted from improvements in sanitation and health care.

A number of other factors contribute to the development of allergic diseases, the strongest of which is a family history. A number of genes contribute to disease susceptibility including those controlling cytokine production and IgE levels. The expression of a genetic predisposition is governed by environmental factors such as pollutants and cigarette smoke, and the incidence of bacterial and viral infection.

PRESENTING PROBLEMS IN ALLERGY

A GENERAL APPROACH TO THE ALLERGIC PATIENT

Common presentations of allergic disease are shown in Box 4.20, and are discussed in detail in other chapters in this book. This chapter describes the general principles of the approach to the allergic patient and some of the more severe manifestations of allergy.

4.20 COMMON ALLERGIC DISEASES ⓘ

● Urticaria	p. 1270
● Angioedema	p. 87
● Atopic dermatitis	p. 1283
● Allergic conjunctivitis	p. 1108, 1110
● Allergic rhinitis (hay fever)	p. 729
● Allergic asthma	p. 670
● Food allergy	p. 902
● Drug allergy	p. 1310
● Allergy to insect venom	p. 88
● Anaphylaxis	p. 86

Clinical assessment

When assessing a patient with possible allergic disease, it is important to identify what the patient means by allergy. For example, up to 20% of the UK population describe themselves as having a food allergy, although < 1% have an IgE-mediated hypersensitivity reaction confirmed on double blind challenge. Establish the nature of symptoms and identify specific triggers, the predictability of a reaction, and the time lag between exposure to a potential allergen and onset of symptoms. An allergic reaction usually occurs within minutes of exposure and provokes predictable symptoms (angioedema, urticaria, wheezing etc). Specifically enquire about other allergic symptoms, past and present, and about family history of allergic disease. Identify potential allergens in the home and workplace, and always take a detailed drug history, including compliance, side-effects and the use of complementary therapies.

Investigations

Skin prick tests

Skin prick testing is the 'gold standard' of allergy testing. A droplet of diluted standardised allergen solution is placed on the forearm, and the skin is superficially punctured through the droplet with a sterile lancet. After 10 minutes, a positive response is indicated by a local weal and flare response ≥ 2 mm larger than the negative control. A major advantage of skin prick testing is that patients can clearly see the results, which may be useful in gaining compliance with avoidance measures. Disadvantages include the remote risk of a severe allergic reaction, so resuscitation facilities should be available. Antihistamines inhibit the magnitude of the response and should be discontinued for at least 2 days before testing; corticosteroids do not influence test results.

Specific IgE tests

An alternative to skin prick testing is the quantitation of IgE directed against the putative allergen. The sensitivity and specificity of specific IgE tests (previously known as radioallergosorbent tests, RAST) is lower than skin prick tests, but they may be very useful if skin testing is inappropriate (Box 4.21).

There is no indication for routine testing of specific IgG antibodies in the investigation of allergic diseases.

Supervised exposure to allergen (challenge test)

Placebo-controlled allergen challenges are usually performed in specialist centres, and include bronchial provocation testing, nasal challenge and food challenge. These may be useful in the investigation of occupational asthma or food allergy.

Mast cell tryptase

After a systemic allergic reaction, the circulating level of mast cell mediators increases dramatically. Tryptase is the most stable of these, and serum levels peak at 1–2 hours, remaining elevated for 24 hours. Measurement of serum mast cell tryptase is useful in investigating a possible anaphylactic event. Acute samples should be accompanied by a convalescent sample to assist interpretation.

Non-specific markers of atopic disease: total serum IgE and eosinophilia

Peripheral blood eosinophilia is common in atopic individuals. However, eosinophilia greater than 20% or an absolute eosinophil count greater than $1.5 \times 10^9/l$ should initiate a search for a non-atopic cause (p. 296).

Atopy is the most common cause of elevated total IgE in developed countries. However, there are many other causes of raised total IgE, including parasite and helminth infections (p. 360), lymphomas (p. 1047) and Churg–Strauss vasculitis (p. 1141). Moreover, significant allergic disease can occur despite a normal total IgE level. Thus total IgE quantitation is not indicated in the routine investigation of allergic disease.

Management

- *Avoidance of the allergen* should be rigorously attempted, and the advice of specialist dietitians and occupational physicians may be required.
- *Antihistamines* block histamine H_1 tissue receptors, thereby inhibiting the effects of histamine release. Long-acting, non-sedating preparations are particularly useful for prophylaxis against frequent attacks.
- *Corticosteroids* down-regulate proinflammatory cytokine production. They are highly effective in allergic disease, and if used topically their adverse effects may be minimised.

4.21 METHODS OF ALLERGY TESTING		
Tests	**Advantages**	**Disadvantages**
Skin prick tests	More sensitive and specific than specific IgE tests Immediate answer Patient can see the result Cheap	Require experience for accurate interpretation Very rarely may induce anaphylaxis Unreliable in patients with extensive skin disease Unreliable if a patient is taking antihistamines
Specific IgE tests (RAST tests)	Useful if patient is on antihistamines, is uncooperative, or has severe generalised skin disease or dermatographism Useful for testing allergens associated with anaphylactic reactions Can be used post mortem to identify allergens responsible for lethal anaphylaxis Can evaluate cross-reactivity between insect venoms	Expensive Delay in obtaining results Lower sensitivity and specificity than skin tests Accuracy is decreased by very high levels of total IgE

- *Sodium cromoglicate* stabilises the mast cell membrane, inhibiting the release of vasoactive mediators. When inhaled prophylactically, it is partially effective in preventing acute asthma and allergic rhinitis but has no effect if given after allergen exposure. It is poorly absorbed and therefore ineffective in the management of food allergies.
- *Antigen-specific immunotherapy* involves the sequential administration of escalating amounts of dilute allergen over a prolonged period of time. Its mechanism of action is unknown, but it is highly effective in the prevention of insect venom anaphylaxis, and allergic rhinitis secondary to grass pollen. However, it carries a risk of iatrogenic anaphylaxis and should only be performed in specialised centres.
- *Omalizumab*, a monoclonal antibody against IgE, inhibits the binding of IgE to mast cells and basophils. It is effective in moderate and severe allergic asthma and rhinitis, and may also have a role in the management of severe peanut allergy.
- *Preloaded self-injectable adrenaline* (epinephrine) may be life-saving in the acute management of anaphylaxis.

ANAPHYLAXIS

Anaphylaxis is a potentially life-threatening, systemic allergic reaction caused by the release of histamine and other vasoactive mediators.

Clinical assessment

The clinical features are shown in Figure 4.10. Assess the severity of a reaction; the time between allergen exposure and onset of symptoms provides a guide. Enquire about potential triggers; if not immediately obvious, a detailed history of the previous 24 hours may be helpful. The most common allergens are foods, latex, insect venom and drugs (Box 4.22). A history of previous local allergic responses to the offending agent is common. The route of allergen exposure may influence the principal clinical features of a reaction; for example, if an allergen is inhaled, the major symptom is frequently wheezing. Features of anaphylaxis may overlap with the direct toxic effects of drugs and venoms (Ch. 9). Potentiating factors such as exercise or alcohol can lower the threshold for an anaphylactic event.

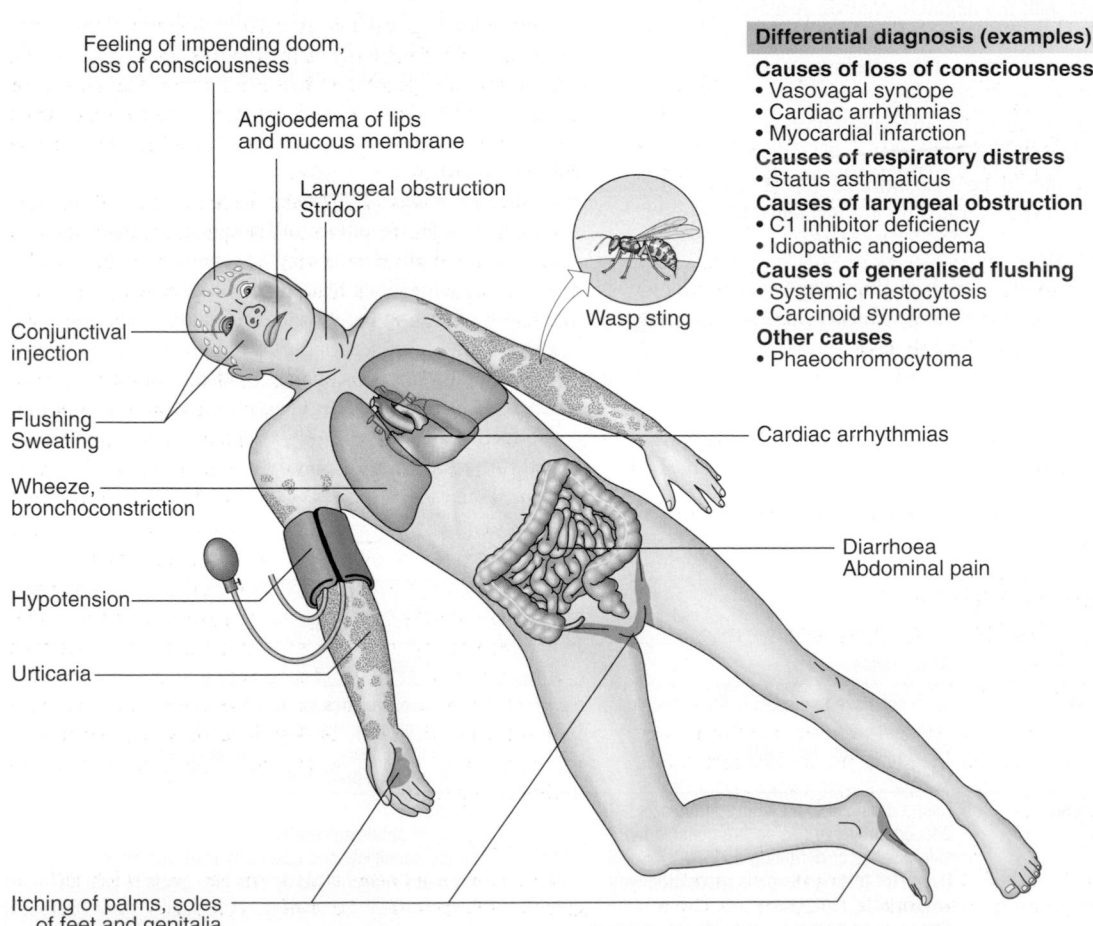

Differential diagnosis (examples)

Causes of loss of consciousness
- Vasovagal syncope
- Cardiac arrhythmias
- Myocardial infarction

Causes of respiratory distress
- Status asthmaticus

Causes of laryngeal obstruction
- C1 inhibitor deficiency
- Idiopathic angioedema

Causes of generalised flushing
- Systemic mastocytosis
- Carcinoid syndrome

Other causes
- Phaeochromocytoma

Feeling of impending doom, loss of consciousness

Angioedema of lips and mucous membrane

Laryngeal obstruction Stridor

Wasp sting

Conjunctival injection

Flushing Sweating

Wheeze, bronchoconstriction

Hypotension

Urticaria

Cardiac arrhythmias

Diarrhoea Abdominal pain

Itching of palms, soles of feet and genitalia

Fig. 4.10 Clinical manifestations of anaphylaxis. In this example, the response is to an insect sting containing venom to which the patient is allergic.

4.22 COMMON CAUSES OF IMMEDIATE GENERALISED REACTIONS

Anaphylaxis: IgE-mediated mast cell degranulation

Foods
- Peanuts
- Tree nuts
- Fish and shellfish
- Milk
- Eggs
- Soy products

Insect stings
- Bee venom
- Wasp venom

Chemicals, drugs and other foreign proteins
- Penicillin and other antibiotics
- Intravenous anaesthetic agents, e.g. suxamethonium, propofol
- Latex

Anaphylactoid, non-IgE-mediated mast cell degranulation

Drugs
- Opiates
- Aspirin
- Radiocontrast media

Physical
- Exercise
- Cold

Idiopathic
- No cause can be identified in 30% of patients with anaphylaxis

Investigations

Measurement of acute and convalescent serum mast cell tryptase concentrations may be useful to confirm the diagnosis.

A number of conditions may mimic anaphylaxis (Fig. 4.10). Anaphylactoid reactions result from the non-specific degranulation of mast cells by drugs, chemicals or other triggers (Box 4.22), and do not involve IgE antibodies. The clinical presentations are indistinguishable, and in the acute situation discriminating between them is unnecessary. However, this may be important in identifying precipitating factors and appropriate avoidance measures. Specific IgE tests may be preferable to skin prick tests when investigating patients with a history of anaphylaxis.

Management

Anaphylaxis is an acute medical emergency. The immediate management includes:

- preventing further contact with the allergen (e.g. removal of bee sting)
- ensuring airway patency
- administration of oxygen
- restoration of blood pressure (laying the patient flat, intravenous fluids)
- prompt administration of adrenaline (epinephrine).

Adrenaline (epinephrine) reverses the action of histamine within minutes. It should be given intramuscularly (adult dose, 0.3–1.0 ml 1:1000 solution) and repeated at 5–10 minute intervals if the initial response is inadequate. This should be followed by intravenous antihistamines (chlorphenamine 10–20 mg i.m. or slow i.v. injection), which limit ongoing inflammation. Corticosteroids (hydro-cortisone 100–300 mg) prevent late-phase symptoms in severely affected patients. Supportive treatments including nebulised β_2-agonists may also be indicated.

Individuals who experience an anaphylactic event should be referred for specialist assessment. The aim is to identify the trigger factor, to educate the patient regarding avoidance and management of subsequent episodes, and to identify whether specific treatment such as immunotherapy is indicated. If the trigger factor cannot be identified or cannot be avoided, recurrence is common. Patients who have previously experienced an anaphylactic event should be prescribed self-injectable adrenaline and they and their families or carers should be instructed on its use. The use of a MedicAlert (or similar) bracelet will increase the likelihood that adrenaline will be administered in an emergency.

ANGIOEDEMA

Angioedema is the episodic, localised, non-pitting swelling of submucous or subcutaneous tissues. It may occur alone or in conjunction with urticaria (p. 1270). Angioedema is most commonly the result of mast cell degranulation, which may be spontaneous or triggered by an allergic IgE-mediated response. However other important causes include drug reactions (e.g. to ACE inhibitors) and C1 inhibitor deficiency.

Aetiology and clinical assessment

Patients with angioedema experience localised soft tissue oedema, most frequently affecting the face (Fig. 4.11), extremities and genitalia. Involvement of the larynx or tongue may cause life-threatening respiratory tract obstruction, and oedema of the intestine may cause abdominal pain and distension.

Angioedema most frequently occurs as part of an IgE-mediated, allergic response and a specific trigger such as food, animal dander or insect venom should be sought. Allergic angioedema is usually accompanied by urticaria, and patients frequently have a history of other allergic symptoms.

Physical stimuli such as heat, cold or vigorous exercise may also cause spontaneous mast cell degranulation and angioedema, which is associated with dermatographism.

Drug-induced angioedema is common. It is most frequently associated with ACE inhibitors, aspirin and non-steroidal anti-inflammatory agents (both topical and systemic), radiocontrast media, opiates and antibiotics.

Hereditary angioedema is characterised by recurrent self-limited attacks involving the skin, subcutaneous tissue, upper respiratory tract or gastrointestinal tract. Attacks may be precipitated by local trauma (e.g. dental procedures) and last from several hours to 2–3 days. An important diagnostic discriminator is that hereditary angioedema is not associated with urticaria and does not respond to antihistamine therapy.

Investigations

If the history implicates a clear trigger, skin prick tests or specific IgE tests may be useful. Frequently, however, no cause is identified, and the aim of investigation is to exclude underlying conditions that may precipitate idiopathic angioedema in susceptible individuals, such as hypothyroid-

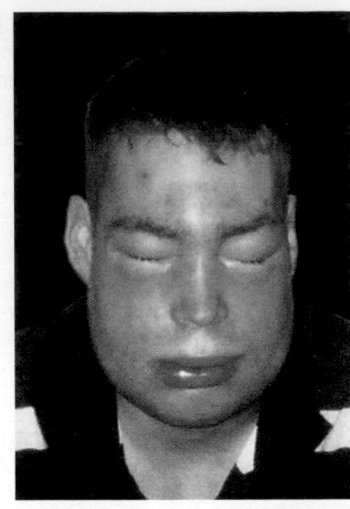

Fig. 4.11 Angioedema. This young man has hereditary angioedema. A Normal appearance. B During an acute attack.

4

ism and underlying infection. Laboratory tests should include a full blood count, thyroid function, CRP and liver function tests. Angioedema without urticaria may indicate hereditary or acquired C1 inhibitor deficiency, and complement studies including C3, C4 and C1 inhibitor levels should be performed.

Management

Oral antihistamines are the mainstay of treatment of allergic or idiopathic angioedema, and may be used prophylactically or after the onset of symptoms. They are ineffective in hereditary angioedema and ACE inhibitor-associated angioedema.

Patients should be advised to seek urgent medical attention if they experience tongue or throat swelling, as this may cause fatal airway obstruction.

SPECIFIC ALLERGIES

INSECT VENOM ALLERGY

Local reactions to insect stings may cause extensive swelling around the site lasting as long as 7 days, but usually do not require specific treatment. Generalised reactions vary from mild to life-threatening. Toxic reactions to venom after multiple (50–100) simultaneous stings may mimic anaphylaxis. In addition, exposure to large amounts of insect venom frequently stimulates the production of IgE antibodies, and thus may be followed by allergic reactions to single stings. Antigen-specific immunotherapy with bee or wasp venom reduces the incidence of recurrent anaphylaxis from 50–60% to 10% after 2 years of treatment (Box 4.23).

PEANUT ALLERGY

Peanut allergy is the most common food-related allergy. More than 50% of patients present before the age of 3 years, and some individuals react to their first known exposure to peanuts, possibly because of sensitisation by topical creams.

4.23 IMMUNOTHERAPY FOR ALLERGY `EBM`

'Immunotherapy is effective for treatment of allergic rhinitis, allergic asthma and stinging insect hypersensitivity. Clinical studies to date do not support the use of allergen immunotherapy for food hypersensitivity, chronic urticaria and/or angioedema.'

• Joint Task Force on Practice Parameters. Ann Allergy Asthma Immunol 2003; 90:1–40.

For further information: 💻 www.cochrane.org

Peanuts are ubiquitous in the Western diet, and every year up to 25% of peanut-allergic individuals will experience a reaction as a result of inadvertent exposure. Peanut allergy rarely resolves, and life-long avoidance is recommended.

BIRCH ORAL ALLERGY SYNDROME

This syndrome is characterised by birch pollen hay fever, and local angioedema after contact with fresh fruit (especially apples), vegetables and nuts. Cooked fruits and vegetables are tolerated without difficulty. It is due to shared or cross-reactive allergens which are destroyed by cooking or digestion, and can be confirmed by skin prick testing using fresh fruit. Severe allergic reactions are unusual.

HEREDITARY ANGIOEDEMA

Hereditary angioedema (HAE, also known as inherited C1 inhibitor deficiency) is an autosomal dominant disorder caused by decreased production of C1 inhibitor protein. This complement regulatory protein inhibits spontaneous activation of the classical complement pathway. C1 inhibitor is also a regulatory protein for the kinin cascade, activation of which gives rise to local pain and swelling.

In HAE, angioedema may be spontaneous or triggered by local trauma or infection. Multiple parts of the body may be involved, especially the face, extremities, upper airway and gastrointestinal tract. Oedema of the intestinal wall causes severe abdominal pain, and many patients with undiagnosed

HAE undergo exploratory laparotomy. The most important complication is laryngeal obstruction, often associated with minor dental procedures, which may be fatal. Episodes of angioedema are self-limiting and usually resolve within 48 hours. Patients with HAE generally present in childhood or adolescence, but may go undiagnosed for many years. A family history can be identified in 80% of cases. HAE is not associated with allergic diseases, and is specifically not associated with urticaria.

Acute episodes are always accompanied by low C4 levels and the diagnosis can be confirmed by C1 inhibitor measurement: the majority of patients have C1 inhibitor levels < 50% of normal. A minority of patients have a dysfunctional protein, which can be assessed with functional assays. Prevention is with attenuated androgens (e.g. danazol) which increase endogenous production of complement proteins. Severe acute attacks should be treated with infusion of purified C1 inhibitor preparations. Alternatively, fresh frozen plasma is a source of C1 inhibitor and may be life-saving.

Acquired C1 inhibitor deficiency

This rare disorder is clinically indistinguishable from HAE but presents in late adulthood. It is associated with autoimmune and lymphoproliferative diseases, and treatment of the underlying disorder may induce remission of angioedema.

TRANSPLANTATION AND GRAFT REJECTION

Transplantation provides the opportunity for definitive treatment of end-stage organ disease. In addition to solid organs, transplantation has extended to pancreatic islet cells, bowel and multi-organ transplants (Box 4.24). The complications after transplantation depend upon the organ transplanted, the genetic disparity between recipient and donor, the primary disease, and drug therapy used. The major complications are graft rejection and infection. Transplant survival has significantly improved over the last twenty years, a result of less toxic immunosuppressive agents and increased understanding of the process of transplant rejection.

Stem cell transplantation and its complications are discussed in Chapter 24.

4.24 NUMBER OF SOLID ORGAN TRANSPLANTS IN UK PER YEAR, 2003[1]

Organ	Number transplanted	Number waiting[2]
Kidney	1697	5072
Liver	625	239
Heart	148	99
Heart and lung	15	59
Lung	135	267
Kidney and pancreas	42	84

[1] From www.uktransplant.org.uk.
[2] Patients actively waiting for a transplant on 31 December 2003.

TRANSPLANT REJECTION

Solid organ transplantation inevitably stimulates an aggressive immune response by the recipient, unless the transplant is between monozygotic twins. The nature of the rejection response is determined by the genetic disparity between the donor and recipient, the immune status of the host and the nature of the tissue transplanted (Box 4.25). The most important genetic determinant is the difference between donor and recipient HLA proteins (p. 70). Their extensive polymorphism means that they are almost invariably recognised as foreign by the recipient immune system, unless an active attempt has been made to minimise incompatibility. Compatibility at all HLA loci decreases acute rejection, improves graft survival, and allows the use of less intense immunosuppressive protocols.

- *Hyperacute rejection* results in rapid and irreversible destruction of the graft. It is mediated by pre-existing recipient antibodies against donor blood group antigens (ABO incompatibility) or donor HLA antigens, which arise as a result of previous exposure through transplantation, blood transfusion or pregnancy. It is very rarely seen in clinical practice as the use of ABO matching, screening for anti-HLA antibodies, and pre-transplant cross-matching ensures the prior identification of recipients with antibodies against a potential donor.
- *Acute vascular rejection* is mediated by antibody formed de novo after transplantation. It is more curtailed than the hyperacute response because of the use of

4.25 CLASSIFICATION OF TRANSPLANT REJECTION

Type	Time	Pathological findings	Mechanism	Treatment
Hyperacute rejection	Minutes to hours	Thrombosis, necrosis	Preformed antibody and complement activation (type II hypersensitivity)	None
Acute vascular rejection	5–30 days	Vasculitis	T and B lymphocytes and antibody	Increase immunosuppression
Acute cellular rejection	5–30 days	Cellular infiltration	CD4 and CD8 T cells (type IV hypersensitivity)	Increase immunosuppression
Chronic allograft failure	> 30 days	Fibrosis, scarring	Immune and non-immune mechanisms	Minimise drug toxicity, control hypertension and hyperlipidaemia

4

intercurrent immunosuppression, but it is also associated with reduced graft survival. Aggressive immunosuppressive therapy is indicated, and physical removal of antibody through plasmapheresis may be effective. Not all post-transplant anti-donor antibodies cause graft damage; their consequences are determined by specificity and ability to trigger the complement cascade.

- *Acute cellular rejection* is the most common form of graft rejection. It is mediated by activated T lymphocytes which recognise donor antigens. This results in deterioration in graft function, and if allowed to progress, may cause fever, pain and tenderness over the graft. Acute cellular rejection is usually amenable to increased immunosuppressive therapy.
- *Chronic allograft failure*, also known as chronic rejection, is a major cause of graft loss. It is associated with proliferation of transplant vascular smooth muscle, interstitial fibrosis and scarring. The pathogenesis is poorly understood, but contributing factors include immunological damage caused by subacute rejection, hypertension, hyperlipidaemia and chronic drug toxicity.

Investigations to avoid rejection

HLA typing
HLA typing using genetic or serological assays determines an individual's HLA polymorphisms, and facilitates donor–recipient matching.

Anti-HLA antibody screening
Potential transplant recipients are screened for the presence of anti-HLA antibodies using either recombinant HLA proteins or a pool of lymphocytes from individuals with broadly representative HLA types. If antibodies are detected, their specificity is further characterised and the recipient is excluded from receiving a transplant which carries these alleles.

Donor–recipient cross-matching
Cross-matching is a functional assay that directly tests whether serum from a recipient (which potentially contains anti-donor antibodies) is able to bind and/or kill donor lymphocytes. It is specific to a prospective donor, and is done immediately prior to transplantation. A positive cross-match is a contraindication to transplantation because of the risk of hyperacute rejection.

C4d staining
C4d is a fragment of the complement protein C4, and deposition of C4d in graft capillaries indicates local activation of the classical complement pathway. This is specific to antibody-mediated damage and is useful in the early diagnosis of vascular rejection.

COMPLICATIONS OF TRANSPLANT IMMUNOSUPPRESSION

The prevention of transplant rejection requires indefinite treatment with immunosuppressive agents. In general, two or more immunosuppressive drugs are used in synergistic combinations in order to minimise drug side-effects (Box 4.26). The major non-specific complications of long-term immunosuppression are infection and malignancy, and their risk increases with increasing level of immunosuppression. The risk of some opportunistic infections may be minimised through the use of prophylactic medication (e.g. ganciclovir for CMV prophylaxis and trimethoprim for *Pneumocystis* prophylaxis). Immunisation with killed vaccines is appropriate although the immune response may be curtailed because of immune suppression. Live vaccines should not be given. Immunosuppression is associated with an increased risk of malignancy, because T-cell suppression results in failure to control viral infections. Virus-associated tumours include lymphoma (associated with Epstein–Barr virus), Kaposi's sarcoma (associated with human herpesvirus 8) and skin tumours (associated with human papillomavirus). Immunosuppression is also associated with a small increase in the incidence of common cancers such as lung, breast or colon cancer.

4.26 IMMUNOSUPPRESSIVE DRUGS USED IN TRANSPLANTATION		
Drug	**Mechanism of action**	**Major adverse effects**
Anti-proliferative agents e.g. azathioprine, mycophenolate mofetil	Inhibit DNA synthesis: block lymphocyte proliferation and cytokine synthesis May be directly cytotoxic at high doses	Increased susceptibility to infection Leucopenia Hepatotoxicity
Calcineurin inhibitors e.g. ciclosporin, tacrolimus	Inhibit T-cell signalling: prevent lymphocyte activation and block cytokine transcription	Increased susceptibility to infection Hypertension Nephrotoxicity Diabetogenic (especially tacrolimus) Gingival hypertrophy, hirsutism (ciclosporin)
Corticosteroids	Decrease phagocytosis and release of proteolytic enzymes; decrease lymphocyte activation and proliferation; decrease cytokine production; decrease antibody production	Increased susceptibility to infection Other complications (p. 778)
Anti-T-cell induction agents e.g. anti-thymocyte globulin (ATG), anti-CD3 monoclonal antibody	Depletion or blockade of T cells by antibodies to cell surface proteins	Profound non-specific immunosuppression Increased susceptibility to infection

LIVING ORGAN DONATION

The major problem in transplantation is the shortage of organ donors (Box 4.24). Cadaveric organ donors are usually previously healthy individuals who experience brain stem death (p. 1186), frequently as a result of road traffic accidents or cerebrovascular events. However, even if all potential donors were to donate their organs, their numbers would be insufficient to meet current needs. An alternative is the use of living donors, and altruistic living donation, usually from close relatives, is widely used in renal transplantation. Living organ donation is inevitably associated with some risk to the donor, and it is highly regulated to ensure appropriate appreciation of the risks involved. Because of concerns about coercion and exploitation, non-altruistic organ donation (the sale of organs) is illegal in most countries.

FURTHER INFORMATION

Books and journal articles

Abbas AK, Lichtman AH. Cellular and molecular immunology. 6th edn. Philadelphia: Saunders; 2005.

Janeway CA, Travers P, Walport M, et al. Immunobiology: the immune system in health and disease. 6th edn. New York: Churchill Livingstone; 2001.

Morris PJ. Transplantation—a medical miracle of the 20th century. New England Journal of Medicine 2004; 351: 2678–2680.

Nairn A, Helbert M. Immunology for medical students. Edinburgh: Mosby; 2002.

Notarangelo L, Casanova JL, Fischer A, et al, for the International Union of Immunological Societies Primary Immunodeficiency Diseases Classification Committee. Primary immunodeficiency diseases: An update. Journal of Allergy and Clinical Immunology 2004; 114: 677–687.

Rich RR, Fleischer TA, Shearer WT, et al. Clinical immunology: Principles and practice. 2nd edn. London: Mosby; 2001.

Websites

www.aaaai.org *Useful resources for the management of patients with allergic disorders.*

www.arc.org.uk *A UK charity dedicated to arthritis research. Contains useful information about the management of systemic autoimmune diseases.*

www.rcpamanual.edu.au *An online manual of pathological investigation published by the Royal College of Pathologists of Australia. It includes comprehensive information about immunology laboratory tests.*

www.ukpin.org.uk *The UK Primary Immunodeficiency Network (UKPIN) is a multidisciplinary organisation of those caring for patients with primary immune deficiencies. It publishes guidelines on the diagnosis and treatment of these conditions.*

www.uktransplant.org.uk, www.eurotransplant.nl and www.unos.org *These sites provide comprehensive information about organ transplantation in the UK, Europe and USA.*

4

5

P. HANLON
M. BYERS
B.R. WALKER
C. SUMMERTON

Environmental and nutritional factors in disease

The molecular and cellular mechanisms of disease which are intrinsic to the individual patient (Chs 3 and 4) are modified by interactions with the external environment; examples are shown in Figure 5.1. Typically, environmental changes affect many physiological systems and do not respect boundaries between medical specialties. All environmental factors affect individuals, but many simultaneously affect families, communities and populations. The investigation and management of health in communities and populations is a defining characteristic of the specialty of 'public health' in the UK, but the principles apply in all specialties.

Exposure to infectious agents is a major environmental determinant of health and is described in Chapter 6. The present chapter describes the approach to other common environmental factors which influence health.

PRINCIPLES AND INVESTIGATION OF ENVIRONMENTAL FACTORS IN DISEASE

5

ENVIRONMENTAL EFFECTS ON HEALTH

The hierarchy of systems

A clinician taking a history and examining a patient subconsciously considers many levels at which problems may be occurring, including molecular, cellular, tissue, organ and body systems. When the environment's influence on health is being considered, this 'hierarchy of systems' extends beyond the individual to include the family, community, population and ecology. An example of the utility of this key concept is shown in Box 5.1, which describes determinants of atheromatous coronary heart disease operating at each level of a hierarchy. It is clearly insufficient for health professionals to consider only one or two levels.

Interactions between people and their environment

The model of a hierarchy of systems demonstrates that it is not sufficient for a clinician to focus too quickly on the disease process without considering the context. More complex models not only take account of the interactions between levels of the hierarchy, but also recognise that individuals and societies influence their environment and their response to ill health (Fig. 5.2). Health status is an emergent quality of a whole system of complex interactions between the determinants of health, including genetic inheritance, the physical circumstances in which people live (e.g. housing, air quality, working environment), the social environment (e.g. levels of friendship, support and trust), personal behaviour (smoking, diet, exercise) and access to money and the other resources that give people control over their lives. Health care is certainly not the only determinant—and is usually not the major determinant—of health status in the population.

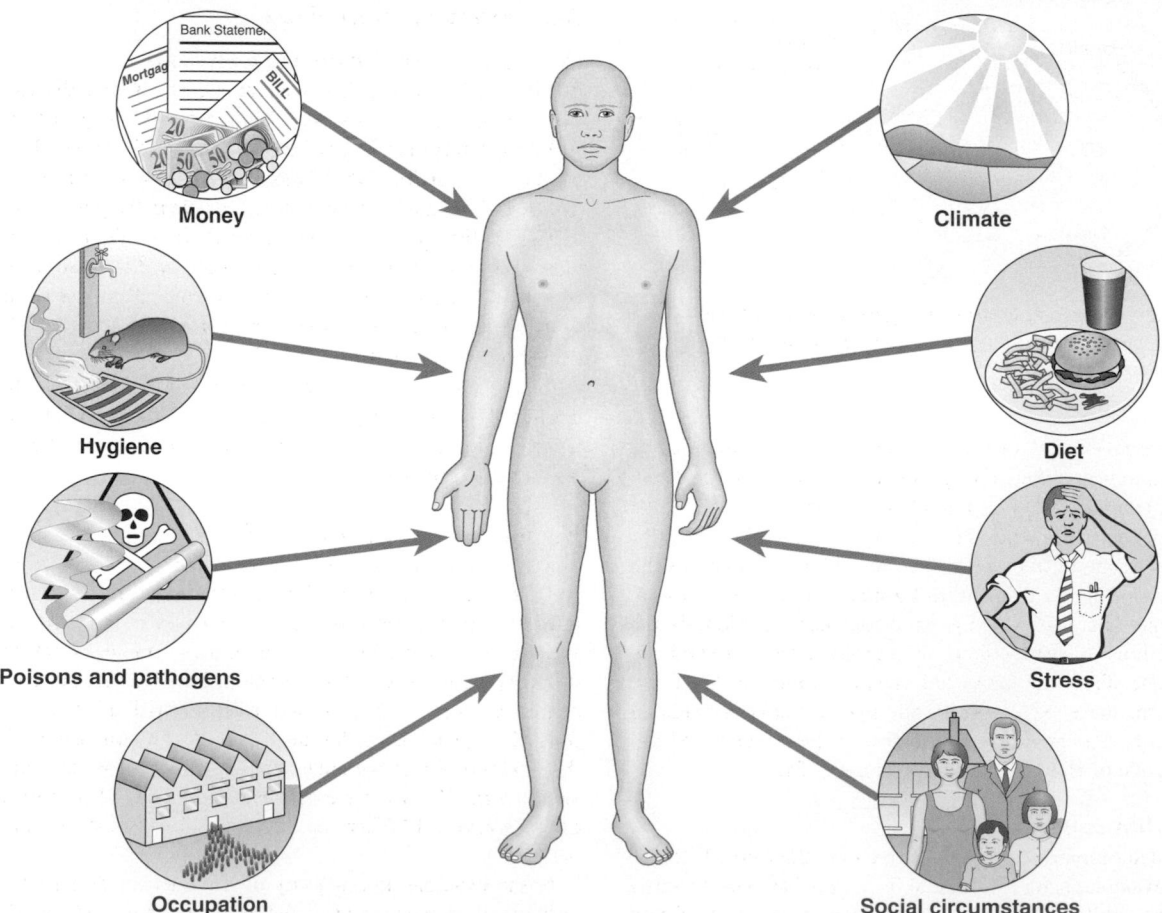

Money

Climate

Hygiene

Diet

Poisons and pathogens

Stress

Occupation

Social circumstances

Fig. 5.1   Examples of environmental factors which influence health.

5.1 'HIERARCHY OF SYSTEMS' APPLIED TO ISCHAEMIC HEART DISEASE

Level in the hierarchy	Example of effect
Molecular	ApoB mutation causing hypercholesterolaemia
Cellular	Foam cells accumulate in vessel wall
Tissue	Atheroma and thrombosis of coronary artery
Organ	Ischaemia and infarction of myocardium
System	Cardiac failure
Person	Limited exercise capacity, impact on employment
Family	Passive smoking, diet
Community	Consumption of health service resources
Population	Major cause of mortality and morbidity
Society	Policies on smoking, screening for risk factors
Ecology	Agriculture influencing fat content in diet

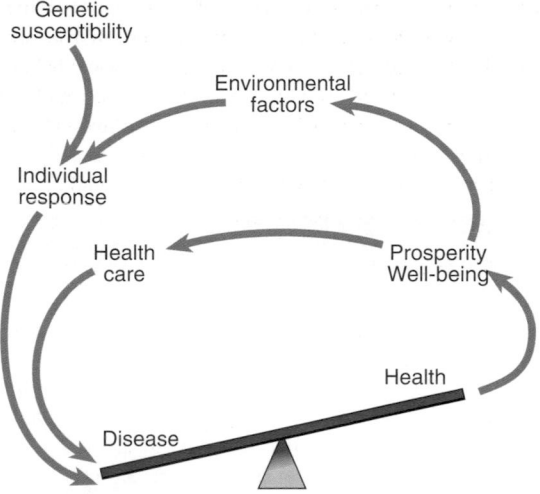

Fig. 5.2 Interactions between the individual and his or her environment in determining the outcome of the balance between health and disease.

These systems do not operate in isolation in separate communities. When one group responds to ill health by manipulating its environment, the consequences may be global. For example, an Afghan farmer who turns to growing opium in order to feed his children influences the environment of a teenager in Europe; in turn, drug abuse in Europe has fostered higher prevalence of blood-borne infectious diseases such as human immunodeficiency virus/acquired immunodeficiency syndrome (HIV/AIDS); in turn, these have spilled out into sexually transmitted disease; this process contributes to the tragedy of the epidemic of HIV/AIDS, particularly in Africa.

The life course

The determinants of health operate over the whole lifespan. For example, habits, values, skills and behaviours acquired during childhood and adolescence have a profound influence on educational outcomes, job prospects and risk

of disease. These attributes (for example, the ability to form empathetic relationships, the ability to assess risk, the ability to be calmly assertive) have a strong influence on whether a young person takes up damaging behaviour like smoking, risky sexual behaviours and drug misuse.

Influences on health can even operate before birth. Individuals with low birth weight have been shown to have higher prevalence of risk factors such as hypertension and type 2 diabetes as young adults and of cardiovascular disease in middle age. It has been suggested that under-nutrition during middle to late gestation permanently 'programmes' cardiovascular and metabolic responses.

The 'life course' perspective highlights the cumulative effect on health of exposures to episodes of illness, adverse environmental conditions and behaviours which damage health. In this way biological and social risk factors at each stage of life link to form pathways to disease.

INVESTIGATIONS IN ENVIRONMENTAL HEALTH

5

A number of 'tools' can be used to explore the effects of the environment on disease. To illustrate these, consider a situation where it is suspected that exposure to a potential risk ('f') is associated with a disease ('d').

Descriptive epidemiology

How common—incidence and prevalence
The first task is to establish accurately how common disease 'd' is within the population. This is usually expressed in one of two ways (Box 5.2). The prevalence of disease 'd' is calculated by dividing the number of people with the disease at a specified time by the number of people in the population at risk at that time. Prevalence tends to be higher if the disease is common (many new cases) and/or if the disease is of longer duration. The incidence of disease 'd' is a measure of the rate at which new cases occur in the population at risk during a defined period of time.

In the example in one town, among 5000 people described below, 1500 new cases of disease 'd' were recorded during 1 year. This gives an incidence rate of 300 per thousand per year.

Variability by person, place and time
'Descriptive epidemiology' may provide clues for causation and will assist in providing health services for those affected. The incidence of disease may vary throughout the year. A longer period of observation may establish whether it is becoming more or less common. Detailed recording of characteristics of the affected patients will address the following questions. Who are the victims of this disease? Are males or females more commonly affected? What is the age pattern? What are the occupations and social positions of those affected? Where do those with the disease live and work?

In the example, the majority of the cases of disease 'd' (300 out of 360) occurred among men and women who work at the local chemical factory.

5.2 CALCULATION OF RISK USING DESCRIPTIVE EPIDEMIOLOGY

Prevalence

- The ratio of the number of people with the disease at a specified time to the number of people in the population who are at risk

Incidence

- The number of new cases occurring in the population at risk during a defined period of time

Attributable risk

- The difference between the risk (or incidence) of disease in exposed and non-exposed populations

Attributable fraction

- The ratio of the attributable risk to the incidence

Relative risk

- The ratio of the risk (or incidence) in the exposed population to the risk (or incidence) in the non-exposed population

5.3 THE WORLD HEALTH ORGANIZATION'S OTTAWA CHARTER

Key components of improving health in the population:
- Build healthy public policy
- Create supportive environments
- Strengthen community action
- Develop personal skills
- Re-orientate health services

Measuring risk

A formal experiment is established to measure risk. The 1000 factory workers are to be followed up for 1 year and compared to a cohort of adults with a similar age and sex distribution but who do not work in a factory.

The incidence (new cases) of disease 'd' in 1000 workers exposed to risk 'f' (factory work) was 300. The incidence (new cases) of disease 'd' in 1000 people not exposed to risk 'f' (factory work) was 60. The relative risk is the incidence in the exposed population (300 per thousand per year) divided by the incidence in the non-exposed population (60 per thousand per year). This was 300/60 = 5, meaning that those working in the factory are 5 times more likely to contract the disease. The attributable risk of exposure 'f' for disease 'd' is the incidence in the exposed population (300) minus the incidence in the non-exposed population (60), which is 240 per thousand per year. The fraction, or proportion, of the disease in the exposed population which can be attributed to risk (f) is called the attributable fraction, in this case (300 – 60)/300 = 0.8. This means that 80% of the disease can be attributed to the exposure.

Establishing cause and effect

Associations between a risk factor and a disease do not prove that the risk factor causes the disease. For example, both multiple sclerosis and blue eyes are more common in the northern hemisphere, but it is implausible that having blue eyes is the cause of multiple sclerosis. Biological plausibility is an important test, but cause and effect can only be proven by more detailed investigation. In infectious diseases, the criteria have been defined in Koch's postulates (p. 130).

PREVENTIVE MEDICINE

The idea that diseases have a single cause and that a single intervention will prevent them is appealing. Environmental factors frequently appear to lend themselves to this

approach. There are many examples of epidemiological associations defining causative factors in disease, e.g. the association between cigarette smoking and lung cancer (p. 705). However, as illustrated in Figure 5.1 and Box 5.1, the complexity of the interactions between physical, social and economic determinants of health means that successful prevention is difficult. For example, more than 20% of the UK population still smokes cigarettes and smoking is increasing amongst some groups of women and in the developing world. Moreover, the life course perspective illustrates that it may be necessary to intervene early in life, or even before birth, to prevent important diseases in later life. Successful preventive interventions are likely to occur at many levels, involving more than just management of health-care services (Box 5.3).

ENVIRONMENTAL DISEASES

This chapter does not aim to be comprehensive in considering the numerous environmental determinants of ill health, many of which are discussed elsewhere in this book. In the following examples it is useful to consider the concept of homeostasis, familiar in cell and whole-body physiology, that describes the capacity to maintain the internal milieu by adapting to increases or decreases in a given environmental factor. However, there are limits to the coping abilities of any system, at which 'too much' or 'too little' of a given environmental factor results in ill health. The capacity to adapt to environmental challenges is typically less robust at extremes of age, so that the youngest and oldest (Box 5.4) in society are most vulnerable.

One of the most important environmental influences on health is nutrition and this is discussed in a separate section later in the chapter.

5.4 ENVIRONMENTAL FACTORS IN DISEASE IN OLD AGE

- **Quality of life:** the major goal of public health policy in the young is to prolong lifespan; in old age, the quality of life is arguably more important than its duration.
- **Life course:** the environmental factors that determine life expectancy operate throughout the lifespan and begin before birth.
- **Susceptibility to risk:** decline in many physiological functions increases risks from cold, pollution, accidents in the home etc.
- **Reliance on support:** in many societies, financial, family and community support for the elderly is declining, with increasing risks of social isolation, poverty, malnutrition and neglect.

CARBON DIOXIDE AND GLOBAL WARMING

In past decades important issues in this chapter might have included lead in water or atmospheric pollution. However, at the beginning of the 21st century, climate change is arguably the most important environmental health issue. This is an idea that has grown from the 'greenhouse gases' theory proposed over a hundred years ago by Swedish scientist Svante Arrhenius, to a demonstrable fact today. Argument continues about the cause but there is an increasing consensus that the temperature of the globe is rising, climate is being affected and, if the trend continues, sea levels will rise and rainfall patterns will be altered with the result that both droughts and floods will become more common.

The health impacts of global warming will include changes in the geographical range of some vector-borne infectious diseases and the effects of adverse weather conditions. Severe storms, floods and droughts have claimed millions of lives during the past 20 years and have adversely affected the lives of many more. It is estimated that ~123 000 people per annum died in weather-related catastrophes between 1972 and 1996, most of them in Africa and the Indian subcontinent. The economic costs of property damage and the impact on agriculture, food supplies and prosperity have also been substantial. The experience of the past three decades will only worsen if climate scientists' predictions for global warming are realised.

Currently, politicians cannot agree on an effective framework of actions to tackle the problem. Meanwhile, the industrialised world continues with lifestyles and waste that are beyond the planet's limits to sustain. Rapidly growing economies in the world's two most populous states, India and China, are going to be a vital part of the unfolding problem or solution.

POVERTY AND AFFLUENCE

The adverse health consequences of poverty and lack of spending by governments are well documented. In recent years adverse health consequences of excessive affluence are also becoming apparent (Box 5.5). Despite experiencing sustained economic growth for the last 50 years, people in many industrialised countries are not getting any happier and the familiar litany of socioeconomic problems—crime, congestion, inequality, etc.—persists. Living in societies that give pride of place to economic growth means that there is constant pressure to contribute by performing ever harder at work and by consuming as much as—or more than—we can afford. Under such constant pressures, people become stressed and ill, and may adopt unhealthy strategies to mitigate their discomfort. So, they overeat, overshop, watch a lot of television, or use sex or drugs (legal and illegal) as 'pain-killers'. These behaviours often lead to obesity, addiction, mental health problems, and alcohol-related and sexually transmitted diseases.

Many countries are now experiencing a 'double burden'. They have large populations still living in poverty who are

5.5 EXAMPLES OF EFFECTS OF FINANCIAL RESOURCES ON HEALTH
Poverty
• Respiratory disease exacerbated or caused by air pollution • Exposure to unnecessary hazards in the workplace or living environment • Poor hygiene causing diarrhoeal diseases and debilitating intestinal parasitic infections • Malnutrition • Cardiovascular disease
Affluence
• Physical inactivity • Alcohol and drug consumption • High rates of suicide, depression, anxiety and stress • Sexually transmitted infection • Obesity

suffering from problems such as diarrhoea and malnutrition, alongside affluent populations (often in cities) who suffer from chronic diseases such as diabetes and heart disease, caused at least in part by the processes described above. Recent research suggests that uneven distribution of wealth is a more important determinant of health than the absolute level of wealth, as measured by gross domestic product (GDP); countries that have a narrower or more even distribution of wealth enjoy longer life expectancies than countries with similar or higher GDPs but wider distributions of wealth. The mechanism is not understood.

ENVIRONMENTAL POISONS

Either involuntarily or deliberately, we expose ourselves to many poisons and hazards. Examples discussed in other chapters include industrial/occupational hazards, such as asbestos (p. 721) and other carcinogens (p. 254), and 'social' poisons, such as alcohol and drugs of misuse (p. 212).

SMOKING

Smoking tobacco dramatically increases the risk of developing many diseases. It is responsible for a substantial majority of cases of lung cancer and chronic obstructive pulmonary disease, and most smokers die either from these respiratory diseases or from ischaemic heart disease. Smoking also causes cancers of the upper respiratory and gastro-intestinal tracts, pancreas, bladder and kidney, and increases risks of peripheral vascular disease, stroke and peptic ulceration. Maternal smoking is an important cause of fetal growth retardation. Moreover, there is increasing evidence that passive (or 'secondhand') smoking has adverse effects on cardiovascular and respiratory health.

When the ill-health effects of smoking were first discovered, doctors imagined that warning people about the dangers of smoking would result in them giving up. An initial decline in smoking rates in the 1960s suggested that these assumptions were correct (Fig. 5.3), but in most countries of the developed world this decline has since slowed or plateaued, while rates are increasing amongst

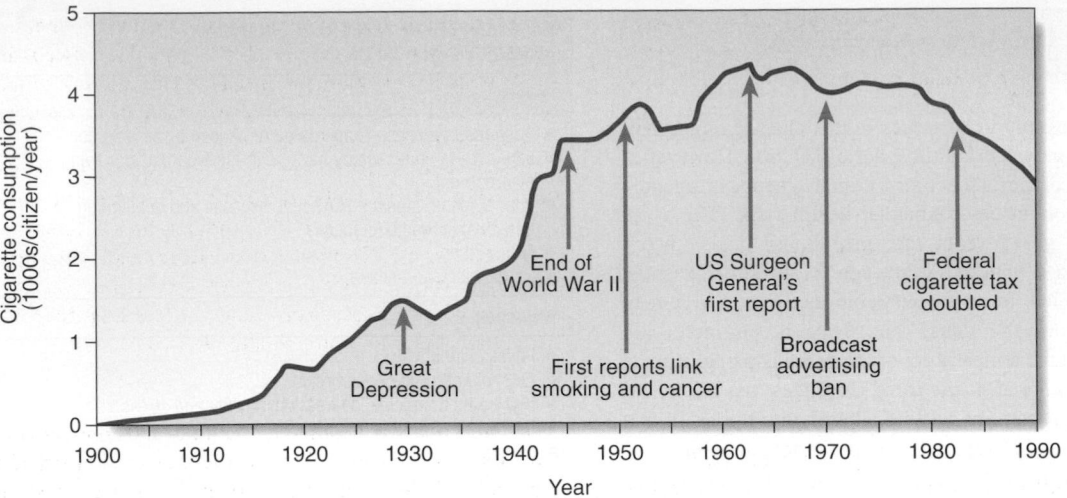

Fig. 5.3   Trends in tobacco consumption in the USA in the 20th century.

young women and in many developing countries where tobacco companies have found new markets. World-wide, there are ~1 billion smokers, and 3 million die prematurely each year as a result of their habit. In the USA, it has been estimated that > 5 million years of potential life and ~$90 billion of productivity are lost each year due to smoking.

In reality, there is a complex hierarchy of systems that interact to cause smokers to initiate and maintain their habit. At the molecular and cellular levels, nicotine acts on the nervous system to create dependence, so that smokers experience unpleasant effects when they attempt to quit. So, even if they know it is harmful, the role of addiction in maintaining the habit is important. Influences at the personal and social level are just as important. For example, research has shown that many individuals bolster their denial of the harmful effects of smoking by focusing on someone they know personally who smoked until he was very old, went to the pub every day and died peacefully in his bed at home. Such strong counter-examples help smokers to maintain internal beliefs that comfort them when presented with statistical evidence. Young female smokers are often motivated more by the desire to 'stay slim' or 'look cool' than to avoid an illness in middle life.

Even if a smoker decides to quit, there are a variety of influences in the wider environment that alter the chances of sustained success, including peer pressure, cigarette advertising, and finding oneself in circumstances where one previously smoked. The tobacco industry works very hard to maintain and expand the smoking habit and its advertising budget is much greater than that available to health promoters.

Helping people to stop smoking

The majority of adult smokers say they would like to give up smoking but only 2% of smokers per year manage by will-power alone. The strategies commonly employed to stop smoking and their impact are shown in Boxes 5.6 and 5.7. Health professionals can work with the individual smoker to understand his or her beliefs and motivations.

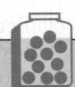

5.6 METHODS FOR SMOKING CESSATION

Smokers who are not motivated to try to stop smoking

- Record smoking status at regular intervals
- Anti-smoking advice
- Encourage change in attitude towards smoking to improve motivation

Motivated light smokers (< 10/day)

- Anti-smoking advice
- Involve in anti-smoking support programme

Motivated heavy smokers (10–15/day)

- As above plus nicotine replacement therapy (NRT) (minimum 8 weeks)

Motivated heavy smokers (> 15/day)

- As above plus bupropion if NRT and behavioural support are unsuccessful and patient remains motivated

EBM

5.7 SMOKING CESSATION

'Placebo or will-power alone has a ~2% chance of abstinence for ≥ 6 months. This can be increased by the percentage shown:
- written self-help materials: 1%
- opportunistic advice from doctor: 2%
- face-to-face behavioural support from specialist: 4–7%
- proactive telephone counselling: 2%
- NRT with limited or intensive behavioural support: 5–12%
- bupropion with intensive behavioural support: 9%.'

- Health Education Board for Scotland, Edinburgh; 2000.

Participation in groups has also been shown to be effective. Nicotine replacement therapies or use of bupropion (an antidepressant which acts centrally) can reduce cravings. If intensive support is combined with pharmacological aids, quit rates are significantly improved. Although the absolute quit rates seem modest, smoking cessation interventions are cost-effective and, if widely available, can contribute to reduction in smoking prevalence.

However, action at the societal level, such as bans on tobacco advertising, increasing taxation on tobacco, regulation of the sale of tobacco, making sure all workplaces and public spaces are smoke-free, and placing clear warnings on cigarette packets, may be more effective. Countries that have adopted these policies are being rewarded by falling smoking rates (Fig. 5.3).

RADIATION EXPOSURE

Radiation includes ionising (Box 5.8) and non-ionising radiations (ultraviolet (UV), visible light, laser, infrared and microwave). It is important to understand their potential toxicity in medical practice because they are used in many investigations and treatments (e.g. ionising radiation in X-rays, computed tomography (CT), and radionucleotide scans and therapies, or non-ionising UV therapy for the skin and in laser therapy for diabetic retinopathy). The sun's rays (including infrared and UV) are also important to health, with increased exposure contributing to burns and skin cancer (p. 1301). Global industrialisation and generation of fluorocarbons has raised concerns about loss of the ozone layer in the upper atmosphere, with increased exposure to UV rays. Man-made disasters, including the Chernobyl nuclear power station explosion and the nuclear bombs at Nagasaki and Hiroshima, have graphically illustrated the potential harm of ionising radiation.

IONISING RADIATIONS

These are high-energy electromagnetic radiations such as X-rays and gamma rays, or consist of subatomic particles such as alpha and beta particles and neutrons. They are characterised by their ability to interact in a physico-chemical manner on contact with matter or tissue. The clinical effects of different forms of radiation depend upon their range in air and tissue penetration (Box 5.8).

Dosage and exposure

The dose of radiation is based upon the energy absorbed by a unit mass of tissue and is measured in grays (Gy), with 1 Gy representing 1 J/kg. This unit is useful in assessing high-dose exposures to specific organ systems. However, to take account of differences between the behaviour of different radiations and in the sensitivity of various tissues, weighting factors are used to produce a unit of effective dose, measured in sieverts (Sv). This value reflects the absorbed dose weighted for the damaging effects of the particular form of radiation and is most valuable in assessing chronic low-dose or whole-body exposures.

'Background radiation' refers to our exposure to the radioactivity of naturally occurring substances on earth (e.g. radon gas) together with cosmic radiation (neutrons from outer space). This produces an average individual dose of approximately 2.4 mSv per year, although it varies—probably within a harmless range—according to local geology and the extent of high-altitude flying.

Effects of radiation exposure

Effects may occur in exposed individuals, and potentially in their offspring through effects on the exposed individual's germ cells. Effects on the individual are classified as either deterministic or stochastic.

Deterministic effects

Deterministic effects show increasing severity as dose increases above a threshold. Tissues with actively dividing cells, such as bone marrow and gastrointestinal mucosa, are particularly sensitive to ionising radiation. Lymphocyte depletion is the most sensitive marker of bone marrow injury and, after exposure to a fatal dose, marrow aplasia is a likely cause of death. However, gastrointestinal mucosal toxicity may cause earlier death due to profound diarrhoea, vomiting, dehydration and sepsis. The gonads are highly radiosensitive and radiation may result in temporary or permanent sterility. Eye exposure can result in cataract. Irradiation of the lung and central nervous system may induce acute inflammatory reactions, sometimes proceeding to pulmonary fibrosis and permanent neurological deficit. The skin is subject to radiation burns. Bone necrosis and lymphatic fibrosis are characteristic following regional irradiation, particularly in therapy of breast cancer. The thyroid gland is not inherently sensitive but its ability to concentrate iodine makes it susceptible to damage after exposure to relatively low doses of radioactive iodine isotopes, such as were released from Chernobyl.

Stochastic effects

Stochastic effects show increasing probability of occurring as dose increases but severity is independent of dose. Carcinogenesis represents a stochastic effect. Epidemiological studies of the appearance of malignancy after radiation exposure, e.g. after Hiroshima and Chernobyl, are used to calculate the predicted risk after exposure. With acute exposures, leukaemia may arise after an interval of about 2 years and solid tumours after an interval of about 10 years. Thereafter the incidence rises with time. An individual's risk depends on the dose received, the time to accumulate the total dose and the interval following exposure.

Management of radiation exposure

This is essentially supportive. Assessment of exposure dose, from which the outcome can be predicted, may be possible with the aid of changes in the peripheral lymphocyte count.

The principal problems after large-dose exposures are maintenance of adequate hydration, control of sepsis and

5.8 PROPERTIES OF IONISING RADIATIONS			
	Range in air	Range in tissue	Protection
Alpha particles	Few centimetres	No penetration	Paper
Beta particles	Few metres	Few millimetres	Aluminium sheet
X-rays/gamma rays	Kilometres	Passes through	Lead
Neutrons	Kilometres	Passes through	Concrete or thick polythene

the management of marrow aplasia which may require transplantation. Associated conventional injuries, such as thermal burns or other trauma, should be managed in the normal way. Exposure to radioisotopes that accumulate in the bone (e.g. ^{90}strontium) should be treated with sodium calcium edetate or other equivalent chelating agents and high doses of oral calcium. Immediate administration of potassium iodide (133 mg/day) is an important intervention in patients with inadvertent radio-iodine contamination as this substantially reduces the extent of radio-iodine uptake by the thyroid gland.

EXTREMES OF TEMPERATURE

THERMOREGULATION

Body heat is generated by basal metabolic activity and muscle movement and lost by conduction (which is more effective in water than in air), convection (which is increased by wind or fanning), evaporation (which is increased by sweating or hyperventilating but decreased in high humidity) and radiation (which is most important at lower temperatures when other mechanisms conserve heat) (Box 5.9). Body temperature is controlled in the hypothalamus, which is directly sensitive to changes in core temperature and indirectly responds to temperature-sensitive neurons in the skin. The normal 'set-point' of core temperature is tightly regulated within $37 \pm 0.5°C$, as required to preserve normal function of many enzymes and other metabolic processes. The temperature set-point is increased in response to infection (p. 136).

In a cold environment, protective mechanisms include cutaneous vasoconstriction (which is effective in the limbs but less so over the trunk and scalp) and shivering. However, any muscle activity which involves movement may promote heat loss by increasing convective loss from the skin and respiratory heat loss by stimulating ventilation. In a hot environment, sweating is the main mechanism for increasing heat loss. This usually occurs when the ambient temperature rises above 32.5°C or during exercise.

5.10 THERMOREGULATION IN OLD AGE

- **Age-associated changes:** in vasomotor function, skeletal muscle response and sweating mean that older people react more slowly to changes in temperature.
- **Increased comorbidity:** thermoregulatory problems are more likely in the presence of pathology, e.g. atherosclerosis and hypothyroidism, and medication, e.g. sedatives and hypnotics.
- **Hypothermia:** may arise as a primary event, but more commonly complicates other diseases, e.g. pneumonia, stroke or fracture.
- **Ambient temperature:** financial pressures and older equipment may lead to inadequate heating during cold weather.

HYPOTHERMIA

Hypothermia exists when the body's normal thermal regulatory mechanisms are unable to maintain heat in a cold environment and core temperature falls below 35°C (Fig. 5.4).

In some circumstances thermoregulatory mechanisms are impaired and core body temperature may fall slowly over many hours or days. The very young are susceptible because they have poor thermoregulation and a high body surface area to weight ratio, but it is the elderly who are at highest risk. Hypothyroidism is often a contributory factor in the elderly, while alcohol or other drugs (e.g. phenothiazines) commonly impede the thermoregulatory response in younger people. More rarely, hypothermia is secondary to glucocorticoid insufficiency, stroke, hepatic failure or hypoglycaemia.

Hypothermia also occurs in normal individuals whose thermoregulatory mechanisms are intact but insufficient to cope with the intensity of the thermal stress. Typical situations include immersion in cold water, when core temperature may fall very rapidly, and exposure to extreme climates (e.g. hill walkers and mountaineers).

Clinical features

Diagnosis is dependent on recognition of the environmental circumstances and measurement of core (rectal) body temperature. It is important that the true core temperature is

5.9 THERMOREGULATION: RESPONSES TO HOT AND COLD ENVIRONMENTS			
	Mechanism	Hot environment	Cold environment
Heat production	Basal metabolic rate	→	↓ in hypothermia
	Muscle activity	↓ by lethargy ↓ in severe hypothermia	↑ by shivering
Heat loss	Conduction*	↑ by vasodilatation	↓ by vasoconstriction ↑↑ in water < 31°C
	Convection*	↑ by vasodilatation ↓ by lethargy	↓ by vasoconstriction ↑ by wind and movement
	Evaporation*	↑↑ by sweating ↓ by high humidity	↑ by hyperventilation
	Radiation	↑ by vasodilatation	↓ by vasoconstriction (but is the major heat loss in dry cold)

*These losses are dependent on the relative ambient and skin temperatures.

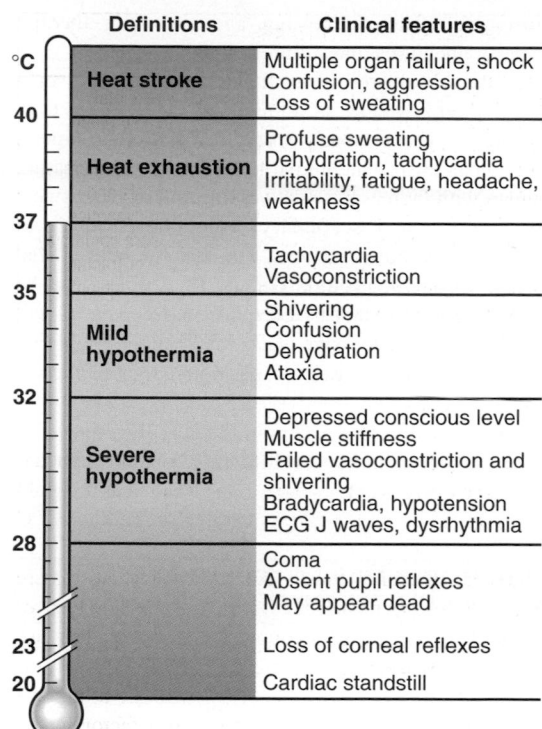

Definitions		Clinical features
°C		
Heat stroke		Multiple organ failure, shock Confusion, aggression Loss of sweating
Heat exhaustion		Profuse sweating Dehydration, tachycardia Irritability, fatigue, headache, weakness
		Tachycardia Vasoconstriction
Mild hypothermia		Shivering Confusion Dehydration Ataxia
Severe hypothermia		Depressed conscious level Muscle stiffness Failed vasoconstriction and shivering Bradycardia, hypotension ECG J waves, dysrhythmia
		Coma Absent pupil reflexes May appear dead
		Loss of corneal reflexes
		Cardiac standstill

Fig. 5.4 Clinical features of abnormal core temperature. The hypothalamus normally maintains core temperature at 37°C but this set-point is altered—for example, in fever (pyrexia, p. 136)—and may be lost in hypothalamic disease (p. 792). In these circumstances the clinical picture at a given core temperature may be different.

recorded (using a low-reading thermometer) since measurement of tympanic membrane temperature is less accurate and cutaneous or oral temperatures can be misleading. Clinical features depend on the degree of hypothermia (Fig. 5.4).

It is very difficult to diagnose death reliably by clinical means in a cold patient. It has been suggested that in extreme environmental conditions irreversible hypothermia is probably present if there is asystole (no carotid pulse for 1 minute), the chest and abdomen are rigid, and the core temperature is below 9°C (the lowest temperature from which a patient has ever recovered). However, in general, resuscitative measures should continue until the core temperature is normal and only then should a diagnosis of brain death be considered (p. 1187).

Investigations

Haemoconcentration and metabolic acidosis are common. The electrocardiogram (ECG) may show characteristic J waves which occur at the junction of the QRS complex and the ST segment (Fig. 5.5). Cardiac dysrhythmias, including ventricular fibrillation, may occur. Although the arterial oxygen tension may be normal when measured at room temperature, the arterial PO_2 in the blood falls by 7% for each °C fall in core temperature. Serum aspartate aminotransferase and creatine kinase may be elevated secondary to muscle damage and the serum amylase is often high due to subclinical pancreatitis. If the cause of hypothermia is not obvious, additional tests should identify

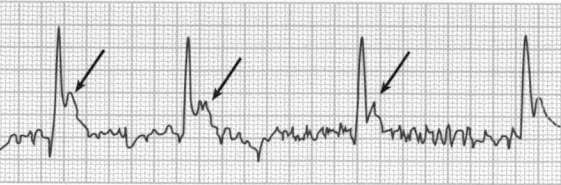

Fig. 5.5 Electrocardiogram showing J waves (arrows) in a hypothermic patient.

thyroid and pituitary dysfunction (p. 743), hypoglycaemia and the possibility of drug intoxication (p. 205).

Management

The objectives of management are to rewarm the patient in a controlled manner while treating the associated hypoxia, fluid and electrolyte disturbance, and cardiovascular abnormalities, particularly dysrhythmias. The most appropriate method depends partly on severity and partly on the circumstances leading to hypothermia.

Mild hypothermia

When core temperature is only modestly reduced (> 32°C) and the patient is conscious, passive rewarming is appropriate. Outdoors, heat loss is prevented by sheltering the patient from the cold, replacing wet clothing, covering the head and insulating him or her from the ground. Once in hospital, patients should be maintained in a warm room, with additional thermal insulation (blankets and/or space film blanket). They should be given warm fluids to drink and an adequate calorie intake. Core temperature will rise slowly over a few hours as a result of normal metabolic heat production. Underlying conditions should be treated promptly (e.g. hypothyroidism with tri-iodothyronine 10 µg i.v. 8-hourly, p. 750).

Severe hypothermia

Severe hypothermia (core temperature < 32°C) is associated with substantial metabolic disturbance, and cardiac dysrhythmias are common. Patients should be handled gently and maintained in a horizontal position to avoid precipitating dysrhythmia. Immersion victims whose core temperature may have fallen rapidly can be rewarmed in a bath of warm water at 40°C. In patients whose temperature has fallen more gradually, rewarming should take place more slowly. The patient should be insulated as above and nursed in a warm room, preferably in an intensive care unit, with the aim of increasing core temperature by 1°C per hour. Surface rewarming (e.g. using warm air jetted through a paper blanket) should be cautious as reperfusion and vasodilatation of surface tissues may precipitate hypotension, increase oxygen demand and contribute to acidosis. In addition to supplementary oxygen, warm intravenous fluids should be given. Monitoring of cardiac rhythm and arterial blood gases, including H⁺ (pH) is essential. Significant acidosis may require correction (p. 437).

Very occasionally, more active rewarming measures are required. These include the administration of warm humidified oxygen, lavage of the stomach, peritoneal cavity or rectum with warm fluid, haemodialysis and cardiac

5

bypass. The latter has the considerable advantage of allowing control of cardiac output despite rhythm disturbance and hence permits very rapid rewarming.

COLD INJURY

Frostbite

This represents the direct freezing of body tissues and usually affects the extremities, in particular the fingers, toes, ears and face. Risk factors include smoking, peripheral vascular disease, dehydration and alcohol consumption. The tissues may become anaesthetised before freezing and as a result the injury is often not recognised until later, e.g. when boots are removed. Frostbitten tissue is initially pale and doughy to the touch and insensitive to pain. Once frozen, the tissue is hard.

Rewarming should not be attempted if there is any further risk of freezing as refreezing substantially increases the ultimate injury. Rewarming may be active using warm water and is associated with considerable pain. Rubbing and direct heat should be avoided as they may exacerbate tissue injury. Thereafter management involves protection of the injured tissue and avoidance of infection. After initial blistering, recovery proceeds over weeks or months. Surgery to remove dead tissue may ultimately be necessary but should be delayed, as surprisingly good recovery may occur over an extended period.

Non-freezing cold injury (trench or immersion foot)

This is a less severe form of cold injury resulting from prolonged exposure to cold and usually damp conditions. Initially the limb (usually foot) appears cold, ischaemic and numb but there is no freezing of the tissue. On rewarming the limb appears mottled and thereafter becomes hyperaemic, swollen and painful. Recovery may take many months, during which there may be chronic pain and sensitivity to cold. The pathology remains uncertain but probably involves endothelial injury. Gradual rewarming is associated with less pain than rapid rewarming. The pain and associated paraesthesia may be difficult to control with normal analgesics and, if persistent, may require the addition of amitriptyline. The patient is at risk of further damage on subsequent exposure to the cold.

Chilblains

Chilblains are tender, red or purplish skin lesions that occur in the cold and wet. They are often seen in horse riders, cyclists and swimmers and are more common in women than men. They are short-lived, and although painful, are not usually serious.

ILLNESSES IN THE HEAT

When generation of heat exceeds the body's capacity for heat loss, core temperature rises. Heat illness occurs either when the environmental temperature is high, or when sweating is impaired or its efficacy as a heat loss mechanism is reduced by high ambient humidity. Susceptibility to heat illness is exacerbated by increased muscular activity, other intercurrent illnesses, increasing age and drug therapy (particularly phenothiazines, diuretics and alcohol).

A considerable degree of acclimatisation occurs over a period of several weeks in individuals who move to a hot climate or who regularly work in a hot environment. Adaptive mechanisms include stimulation of the sweating mechanism with increased sweat volume and reduced sweat sodium content, and secondary hyperaldosteronism to maintain body sodium balance. The risk of heat-related illness falls as acclimatisation occurs. Heat illness can be prevented to a large extent by adequate replacement of salt and water, although excessive water intake alone should be avoided because of the risk of dilutional hyponatraemia (p. 429).

A spectrum of illnesses occurs in the heat (Fig. 5.4). The cause is usually obvious but the differential diagnosis should be considered (Box 5.11).

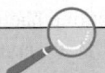

5.11 DIFFERENTIAL DIAGNOSIS IN PATIENTS WITH ELEVATED CORE BODY TEMPERATURE

- Heat illness (heat exhaustion, heat stroke)
- Sepsis, including meningitis
- Malaria
- Drug overdose
- Malignant hyperpyrexia
- Thyroid storm (p. 749)

Heat cramps

These painful muscle contractions occur most commonly in the legs of young people following vigorous exercise and profuse sweating in hot weather. There is no elevation of core temperature. The mechanism is considered to be extracellular sodium depletion as a result of persistent sweating, exacerbated by replacement of water but not salt. Symptoms usually respond rapidly to salt replacement.

Heat syncope

This is similar to a vasovagal faint (p. 553) and is related to peripheral vasodilatation in hot weather.

Heat exhaustion

Heat exhaustion occurs with prolonged exertion in hot and humid weather, profuse sweating and inadequate salt and water replacement. There is an elevation in core (rectal) temperature to between 37°C and 40°C, leading to the clinical features shown in Figure 5.4. Blood analyses may show evidence of dehydration with mild elevation of the blood urea, sodium concentration and haematocrit. Treatment involves removal of the patient from the heat, active cooling using cool sponging, and fluid replacement. This may be achieved by using oral rehydration mixtures containing both salt and water or intravenous isotonic saline. Adult patients may require 5 litres or more positive fluid balance in the first 24 hours. Untreated, heat exhaustion may progress to heat stroke.

Heat stroke

This occurs when the core body temperature rises above 40°C and is a severe and life-threatening condition. The symptoms of heat exhaustion (see above) progress to include headache, nausea and vomiting. Neurological manifestations include a coarse muscle tremor and confusion, aggression or loss of consciousness. The patient's skin feels very hot, and sweating is often absent due to failure of thermoregulatory mechanisms. Complications include hypovolaemic shock, lactic acidosis, disseminated intravascular coagulation, rhabdomyolysis, hepatic and renal failure, and pulmonary and cerebral oedema.

The patient should be managed in an intensive care unit with rapid cooling by spraying with water (to increase evaporation heat loss), fanning (to increase convection heat loss), and ice packs in the axillae and groins (to increase conduction heat loss). Cold crystalloid intravenous fluid replacement is given with appropriate monitoring (p. 179). Sedation with benzodiazepines may be required. Investigations reflect the complications and include coagulation studies and measurement of muscle enzymes in addition to routine haematology and biochemistry.

With appropriate treatment, recovery from heat stroke can be rapid (within 1–2 hours) but patients who have had core temperatures higher than 40°C should be monitored carefully for later onset of rhabdomyolysis and other complications before discharge from hospital. Clear advice to avoid recurrence, and avoidance of heavy exercise during recovery, are important.

HIGH ALTITUDE

Exposure to high altitude has become commonplace as a result of developments within the last century including air travel, extreme altitude mountaineering and even tourism (e.g. in the Andes). The physiological effects of high altitude are very significant. On Everest, the barometric pressure of the atmosphere falls from sea level by ~50% at base camp (5400 m) and ~70% at the summit (8848 m). Since the atmosphere is flattened at the poles, due to the centrifugal effect of the earth's rotation, the atmosphere is thinner at 5800 m on Mount McKinley in Alaska than at the same altitude on Kilimanjaro on the equator. Barometric pressure is also lower in winter than in summer. With the fall in barometric pressure, the proportions of oxygen, nitrogen and carbon dioxide in air do not change, but the pressure of each of these falls in proportion to barometric pressure (Fig. 5.6). Oxygen tension within the pulmonary alveolae is further reduced at altitude because the partial pressure of water vapour is related to body temperature and not barometric pressure, and so is proportionately greater at altitude, accounting for only 6% of barometric pressure at sea level, but 19% at 8848 m.

PHYSIOLOGICAL EFFECTS OF HIGH ALTITUDE

Reduction in oxygen tension results in a fall in arterial oxygen saturation (Fig. 5.6). This varies widely between individuals, depending on the shape of the sigmoid oxygen–haemoglobin dissociation curve (p. 1005) and the ventilatory response. Acclimatisation to hypoxaemia at high

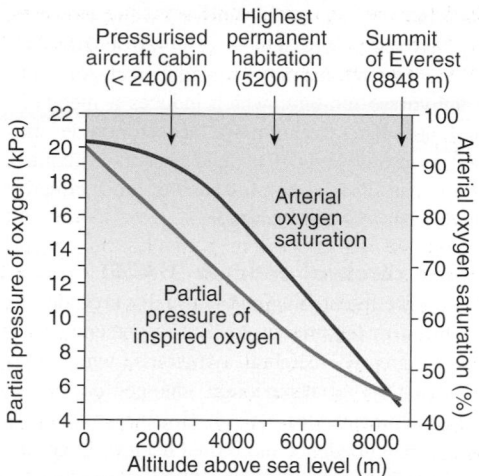

Fig. 5.6 Change in inspired oxygen tension and blood oxygen saturation at altitude. The blue curve shows changes in oxygen availability at altitude and the red curve shows the typical resultant changes in arterial oxygen saturation in a healthy person. Oxygen saturation varies between individuals according to the shape of the oxygen–haemoglobin dissociation curve and the ventilatory response to hypoxaemia. (To convert kPa to mmHg, multiply by 7.5.)

altitude involves a shift in this dissociation curve (dependent on 2,3-DPG), erythropoiesis, polycythaemia, and hyperventilation resulting from hypoxic drive (which is sustained despite hypocapnia by restoration of cerebrospinal fluid pH to normal in prolonged hypoxia). These processes take a few days. Above 3000 m, an ascent rate of no more than 300 m per day should allow acclimatisation and prevent altitude illness, but this rate is too slow for many travellers' plans.

ILLNESSES AT HIGH ALTITUDE

Ascent to altitudes up to 2500 m or travel in a pressurised aircraft cabin is harmless to healthy people. Above 2500 m high-altitude illnesses may occur in previously healthy people, and above 3500 m these become common.

Sudden ascent to altitudes above 6000 m, as experienced by aviators, balloonists and astronauts, may result in decompression illness with the same clinical features as seen in divers (p. 106). Rapid ascent to altitudes above 7000 m may result in loss of consciousness. However, most altitude illness occurs in travellers or mountaineers.

Acute mountain sickness (AMS)

AMS is a syndrome comprising headache (the principal symptom) together with fatigue, anorexia, nausea and vomiting, difficulty sleeping and dizziness. Ataxia and peripheral oedema may be present. Its aetiology is not fully understood but it is thought that hypoxaemia increases cerebral blood flow and hence intracranial pressure. Symptoms occur within 6–12 hours of an ascent and vary in severity from trivial to completely incapacitating. The incidence in travellers to 3000 m may be 40–50%, depending on the rate of ascent.

Treatment of mild cases consists of rest and simple analgesia; symptoms usually resolve after 1–3 days at a stable altitude but may recur with further ascent. However, occasionally there is progression to cerebral oedema (see below). Persistent symptoms may respond to acetazolamide, a carbonic anhydrase inhibitor which induces a metabolic acidosis and stimulates ventilation; acetazolamide may also be used as prophylaxis if a rapid ascent is planned. Corticosteroids can also be helpful but the most effective treatment is descent to a lower altitude.

High-altitude cerebral oedema (HACE)

This is rare and life-threatening and is usually preceded by AMS. In addition to features of AMS, the presentation is with rapidly progressive cerebral symptoms, which may include hallucination or behavioural change, confusion, visual loss and ultimately loss of consciousness. Ataxia is usually present, papilloedema and retinal haemorrhages are common, and focal neurological signs may be found.

Treatment is directed at improving oxygenation. Descent to lower altitude is the single most important intervention but, if this is impossible, nursing the patient with oxygen therapy in a portable pressurised bag may be helpful. High-dose corticosteroids, diuretics and mannitol have all been used but efficacy is difficult to assess as these treatments are usually administered in field conditions.

High-altitude pulmonary oedema (HAPE)

This life-threatening condition usually occurs in the first 4 days after ascent above 2500 m. Unlike HACE, HAPE may occur de novo without the preceding signs of AMS. Presentation is with symptoms of dry cough, breathlessness and extreme fatigue. Later, the cough becomes productive of bloody sputum. It is associated with crepitations in both lung fields, profound hypoxaemia, pulmonary hypertension and radiological evidence of diffuse alveolar oedema. It is not known whether the alveolar oedema is a result of mechanical stress on the pulmonary capillaries associated with the high pulmonary arterial pressure or an effect of hypoxia on capillary permeability. It appears to occur in susceptible subjects and such individuals are at particular risk of further episodes with future ascents. Other predisposing factors include youth, rapidity of ascent, the presence of AMS and heavy exertion.

Treatment is directed at reversal of hypoxia with immediate descent wherever possible and administration of oxygen. Reduction of pulmonary arterial pressure with nifedipine has also proved helpful and this agent has been used for prophylaxis in susceptible subjects.

Other diseases at high altitude

Chronic mountain sickness (Monge's disease)

This occurs on prolonged exposure to altitude and has been reported in residents of Colorado, South America and Tibet. Patients present with headache, poor concentration and other signs of polycythaemia. They are cyanosed and often have finger clubbing.

High-altitude retinal haemorrhage

This occurs in over 30% of trekkers at 5000 m. The haemorrhages are usually asymptomatic and resolve spontaneously. Visual defects can occur with haemorrhage involving the macula, but there is no specific treatment.

Venous thrombosis

This has been reported at altitudes over 6000 m. Risk factors include dehydration, inactivity and the cold. The use of the oral contraceptive pill at high altitude should be considered carefully as this is an additional risk factor.

Refractory cough

A cough at high altitude is common and usually benign. It may be due to breathing dry, cold air and increased mouth breathing, with a consequent dry oral mucosa. Dry cough is also a sign of HAPE. A sore throat and cold-induced rhinorrhoea are also common.

AIR TRAVEL

Commercial aircraft usually cruise at 10 000–12 000 m, with the cabin pressurised to an equivalent of around 2400 m. At this altitude, the partial pressure of oxygen is 16 kPa (120 mmHg), leading to a PaO_2 in healthy people of 7.0–8.5 kPa (53–64 mmHg). Oxygen saturation is also reduced, but to a lesser degree (Fig. 5.6). Although well tolerated by healthy people, in patients with respiratory disease this degree of hypoxia may be dangerous. In addition, the reduction in barometric pressure at altitude leads to increases in gas volume within body cavities.

Advice for patients with respiratory disease

The British Thoracic Society has published guidance on the management of patients with respiratory disease who want to fly. Specialist pre-flight assessment is advised for all patients who have hypoxaemia (oxygen saturation < 95%) at sea level, and includes spirometry and a hypoxic challenge test with 15% oxygen (performed in hospital). Air travel may have to be avoided or be undertaken only with inspired oxygen therapy during the flight. Asthmatic patients should be advised to carry their inhalers in their hand baggage. Following pneumothorax, flying should be avoided while air remains in the pleural cavity, but can be considered after proven resolution or definitive (surgical) treatment.

Advice for other patients

Other circumstances in which patients are more susceptible to hypoxia require individual assessment. These include cardiac dysrhythmia, sickle-cell disease and ischaemic heart disease. Most airlines decline to carry pregnant women after the 36th week of gestation. In complicated pregnancies it may be advisable to avoid air travel at an earlier stage.

Patients who have had recent abdominal surgery, including laparoscopy, should avoid flying until all intraperitoneal gas is reabsorbed. Ear and sinus pain, due to changes in gas volume on flying, is common but usually mild. Patients with chronic sinusitis and otitis media may need specialist assessment, but a healthy mobile tympanic membrane visualised during a Valsalva manoeuvre usually suggests a patent Eustachian tube.

On long-haul flights, patients with diabetes mellitus may need to adjust their insulin or oral hypoglycaemic drug dosing according to the timing of in-flight and subsequent meals (p. 835). Advice is available from Diabetes UK and

5

other websites. It is wise to carry documentary evidence of the need to carry needles and insulin.

Deep venous thrombosis

Air travellers have an increased risk of venous thrombosis (p. 1018), due to a combination of factors including loss of venous emptying because of prolonged immobilisation (lack of muscular activity) and reduced barometric pressure on the tissues, together with haemoconcentration as a result of oedema and perhaps a degree of hypoxia-induced diuresis.

Venous thrombosis can probably be prevented by avoiding dehydration or excess alcohol and exercising muscles during the flight. Without a clear cost–benefit analysis, prophylaxis with aspirin or heparin cannot be recommended routinely, but may be considered in high-risk cases.

ILLNESSES UNDER WATER

DROWNING AND NEAR-DROWNING

Drowning refers to death due to asphyxiation following immersion in water. It remains a common cause of accidental death throughout the world and is particularly common in young children (Box 5.12). In about 10% of cases no water enters the lungs and death follows intense laryngospasm ('dry' drowning). Near-drowning describes the effects of water inhalation on those who survive immersion. Prolonged immersion in cold water, with or without water inhalation, results in a rapid fall in core body temperature and hypothermia (p. 100).

Following inhalation of water, there is a rapid onset of ventilation–perfusion imbalance with hypoxaemia, and the development of diffuse pulmonary oedema. Fresh water is hypotonic and, although rapidly absorbed across alveolar membranes, impairs surfactant function and leads to alveolar collapse and hence right-to-left shunting of un-oxygenated blood. Absorption of large amounts of hypotonic fluid can result in haemolysis. Salty sea water is hypertonic and inhalation provokes alveolar oedema, but the overall clinical effect is similar to that of freshwater drowning. Infection may develop later, particularly after inhalation of contaminated water.

Clinical features

Those rescued alive (near-drowning) are often unconscious and not breathing. Hypoxaemia and a metabolic acidosis are inevitable features. Some rapidly recover spontaneous ventilation and consciousness. The acute lung injury usually resolves rapidly over 48–72 hours unless infection occurs (Fig. 5.7). Early complications include dehydration, hypotension, haemoptysis and cardiac dysrhythmias. A small number of patients, mainly the more severely ill, progress to develop the acute respiratory distress syndrome (ARDS, p. 188).

It is important to recognise that survival may be possible after immersion for periods of up to 30 minutes in very cold water. The rapid development of hypothermia after immersion may be protective and remarkable recoveries have been reported after prolonged immersion, particularly in children. Long-term outcome depends mainly on the severity of the cerebral hypoxic injury and is predicted by the duration of immersion, delay in resuscitation, intensity of acidosis and the presence of cardiac arrest. However, recovery with normal cerebral function is possible despite these poor prognostic indicators.

Management

Initial management requires cardiopulmonary resuscitation with administration of oxygen and maintenance of the circulation (p. 556). It is important to clear the airway of foreign bodies but attempts to drain the lungs physically are misdirected since most inhaled fluid will have been absorbed and such efforts simply delay resuscitation. Continuous positive airways pressure (CPAP, p. 193) is particularly useful in maintaining arterial oxygenation for spontaneously breathing patients. Observation is required for a minimum of 24 hours after the event. Prophylactic antibiotic treatment is only required if exposure was to obviously contaminated water.

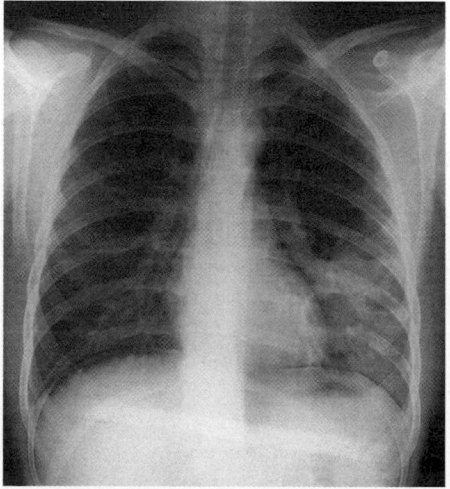

Fig. 5.7 Near-drowning. Chest X-ray of a 39-year-old farmer 2 weeks after immersion in a polluted freshwater ditch for 5 minutes before rescue. The X-ray shows airspace consolidation and cavities in the left lower lobe reflecting secondary staphylococcal pneumonia and abscess formation.

5.12 MOST COMMON CAUSES OF DROWNING BY AGE	
Infants/young children	
• Domestic baths	• Garden pools
Adolescents	
• Swimming pools	• Rivers, other bathing sites
Adults	
• Water sports, boating, fishing etc.	• Occupational
Older people	
• Domestic baths	

DIVING

Recreational scuba diving is becoming increasingly popular. However, the high density of water means that even recreational diving at modest depths takes place under very high barometric pressures, at which gases behave differently. The consequences on the diver's return to lower pressure are the usual reasons for diving-associated illness.

Ambient pressure under water increases by 101 kPa (1 atmosphere) for every 10 metres of seawater (msw) depth. As divers descend, the partial pressures of the gases they are breathing increase (Box 5.13) and the blood and tissue concentrations of dissolved gases increase accordingly. Nitrogen is a weak anaesthetic agent, and if the inspiratory pressure of nitrogen is allowed to increase above ~320 kPa (i.e. a depth of ~30 msw) it produces 'narcosis', resulting in impairment of cognitive function and manual dexterity, not unlike alcohol intoxication. For this reason, compressed air can only be used for shallow diving. Oxygen is also toxic at inspired pressures above ~40 kPa (inducing apprehension, muscle twitching, euphoria, sweating, tinnitus, nausea and vertigo), so 100% oxygen cannot be used as an alternative. For dives deeper than ~30 msw, mixtures of oxygen with helium and/or nitrogen are usually used.

5.13 PHYSICS OF BREATHING COMPRESSED AIR WHILE DIVING IN SEA WATER

Depth	Lung volume	Barometric pressure	PiO_2	PiN_2
Surface	100%	101 kPa (1 atmos)	21 kPa	79 kPa
10 m	50%	202 kPa (2 atmos)	42 kPa	159 kPa
20 m	33%	303 kPa (3 atmos)	63 kPa	239 kPa
30 m	25%	404 kPa (4 atmos)	84 kPa	319 kPa

Diving-related deaths can occur as a result of underwater equipment failure, entrapment or vomiting, leading to water inhalation and drowning. However, an important group of disorders present once the diver has returned to the surface. These occur as a result of the expanding volume of gases within body cavities as pressure is reduced (barotrauma) or as a result of gaseous substances coming out of solution in blood and tissues during decompression, after supersaturation at high pressure.

Clinical features

Decompression illness

Symptoms of decompression illness usually present during or within 4 hours of a dive but can also be provoked by flying; as a result, patients may present to medical services at sites far removed from the dive.

Exposure of individuals to increased partial pressures of nitrogen results in additional nitrogen being dissolved in body tissues; the amount dissolved depends on the depth/ pressure and on the duration of the dive. On ascent, the tissues become supersaturated with nitrogen, and this places the diver at risk of producing a critical quantity of gas (bubbles) in tissues if the ascent is too fast. The gas so formed may cause symptoms locally, by bubbles passing through the pulmonary vascular bed (Box 5.14) or by embolisation elsewhere. Arterial embolisation may occur if the gas load in the venous system exceeds the lungs' abilities to excrete nitrogen, or when bubbles pass through a patent foramen ovale (present asymptomatically in 25–30% of adults, p. 633). It can be difficult to differentiate between arterial gas embolism and decompression illness, but the distinction may be irrelevant as far as treatment is concerned. Although there is often an obvious provoking dive-related factor, decompression illness may occur even after apparently safe and well-conducted dives. The diver's 'buddy' must also be assessed, even if asymptomatic.

5.14 ASSESSMENT OF A PATIENT WITH DECOMPRESSION ILLNESS*

Evolution

- Progressive
- Static
- Relapsing
- Spontaneously improving

Manifestations

- **Pain:** often large joints, e.g. shoulder ('the bends')
- **Neurological:** any deficit is possible
- **Audiovestibular**
  Vertigo, tinnitus, nystagmus
  May mimic inner ear barotrauma
- **Pulmonary**
  Chest pain, cough, haemoptysis, dyspnoea
  May be due to arterial gas embolism
- **Cutaneous:** itching, erythematous rash
- **Lymphatic:** tender lymph nodes, oedema
- **Constitutional:** headache, fatigue, general malaise

Dive profile

- Depth
- Type (gas used)
- Duration of dive

* This information is required by diving specialists to decide appropriate treatment. See contact details on page 127.

Barotrauma

During the ascent phase of a dive, the gas in the diver's lungs expands due to the decreasing pressure. The diver must therefore ascend slowly and breathe regularly; if ascent is rapid or the diver holds his/her breath, the expanding gas may cause lung rupture (pulmonary barotrauma). This can result in pneumomediastinum, pneumothorax or arterial gas embolism due to gas passing directly into the pulmonary venous system. Other air-filled body cavities may be subject to barotrauma, including the middle ear and sinuses.

Management

The patient is nursed in a horizontal position. Treatment is:

- *Intravenous fluid replacement* (with 0.9% saline or Hartmann's solution) to correct the intravascular fluid loss from endothelial bubble injury and the dehydration associated with immersion. Maintenance of an adequate

5

peripheral circulation is important for the excretion of excess dissolved gas.

- *High-flow oxygen*, given by a tight-fitting mask using a rebreathing bag. This assists in the washout of excess inert gas (nitrogen) and may reduce the extent of local tissue hypoxia resulting from focal embolic injury. Nitrous oxide-inhaled analgesic gas should be avoided.
- *Recompression*, requiring transfer of the patient to a recompression chamber facility as soon as is appropriate to the patient's condition. Transfer may be by surface or air, provided that the altitude remains low (< 300 m) and the patient continues to breathe 100% oxygen. Recompression reduces the volume of gas within tissues and puts nitrogen back into solution.

The majority of patients make a complete recovery with treatment. However, a small but significant number are left with neurological disability.

NUTRITIONAL FACTORS IN DISEASE

Obtaining adequate nutrition is a fundamental requirement for survival of every individual and species, and remains the dominant activity in the lives of most animals. The politics of food provision for humans is complex, and is a prominent factor in wars, natural disasters and the global economy. In recent decades, economic success has been rewarded by plentiful nutrition unknown to previous generations, which

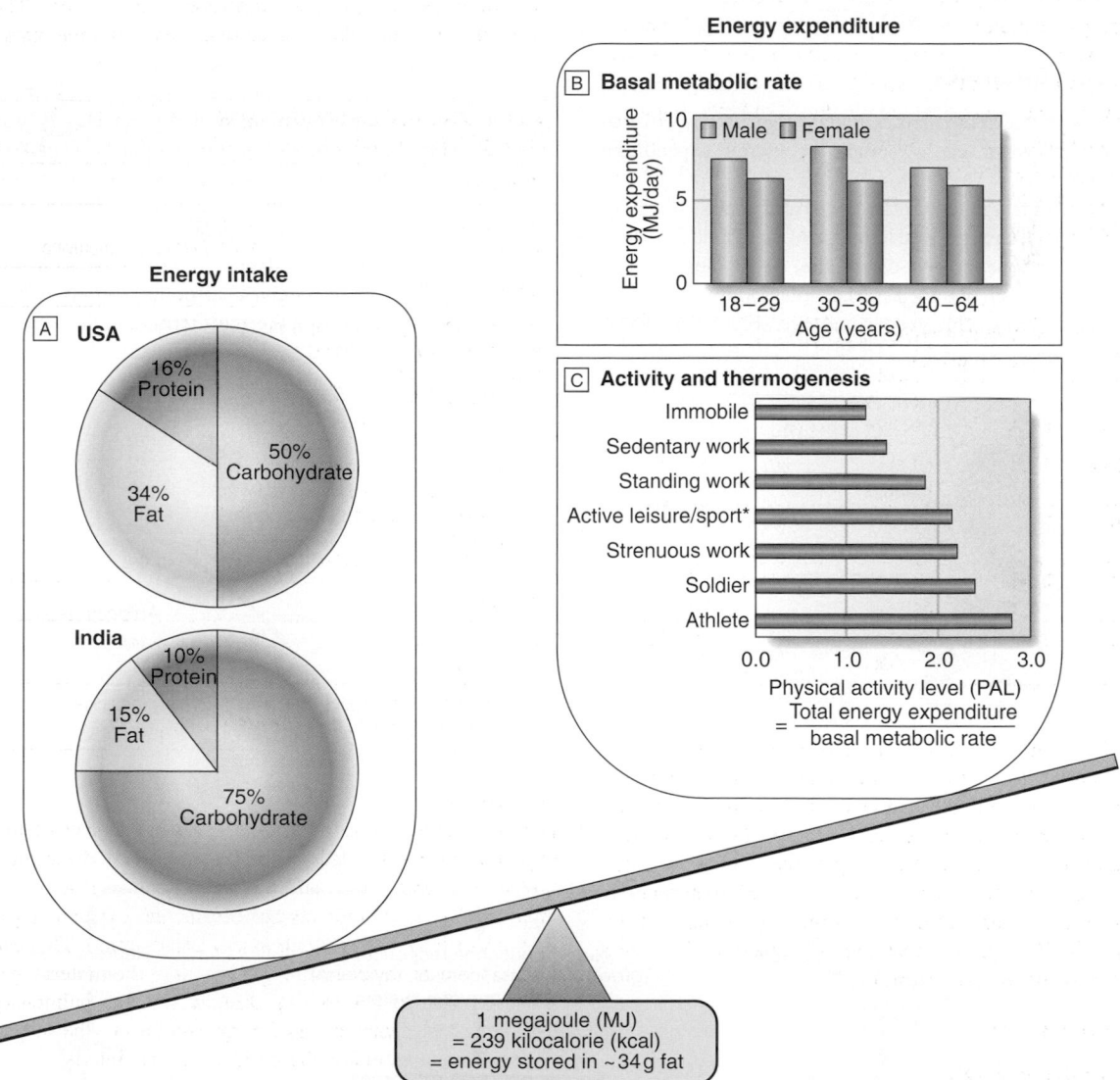

Fig. 5.8 **Determinants of energy balance.** [A] Energy intake is shown as national averages, which obscure substantial regional variations, but emphasise the dramatic differences in total energy consumed and the source of energy in different countries. UK figures are similar to the USA. [B] Data for normal basal metabolic rate (BMR) were obtained in 107 healthy men and 212 healthy women in various countries. Note that BMR declines from middle age and is lower in women, even after adjustment for body size. [C] The influence of activity on energy expenditure can be expressed as physical activity level (PAL), which is the multiple of BMR by which total energy expenditure is increased by activity. The highest recorded PALs have been ~4.0 in participants in the Tour de France and Arctic explorers. * Leisure or sport activity increases PAL by ~0.3 for each 30–60 minutes of moderate exercise performed 4–5 times per week.

has led to a pandemic of obesity with its serious consequences for health. For the less economically successful, famine and malnutrition still present a huge global burden. Quality as well as quantity of food influences health. In developed countries, inappropriate dietary intakes have been linked with diseases such as coronary heart disease and cancer. In other parts of the world, deficiencies of simple vitamins lead to avoidable conditions such as blindness due to vitamin A deficiency. A proper understanding of nutrition is therefore essential in order to deal with the needs of individual patients and to inform the decisions of public policy-makers.

FUNCTIONAL ANATOMY AND PHYSIOLOGY OF NUTRITION

ENERGY BALANCE

The laws of thermodynamics dictate that energy balance is achieved when energy intake = energy expenditure (Fig. 5.8).

The basal metabolic rate (BMR) describes the obligatory energy expenditure required to maintain metabolic functions in tissues and hence to sustain life. It is most closely predicted by lean body mass (i.e. total body mass − fat mass), and varies with gender and age (Fig. 5.8B). Extra

metabolic energy is consumed during growth, pregnancy and lactation, and when febrile. The second component of energy expenditure is determined by the level of muscular activity; this is highly variable according to occupation and lifestyle (Fig. 5.8C). Finally, energy is expended during digestion of food (termed the 'thermic effect of food'), although this is a small component (< 10%) of total energy expenditure.

Energy intake is determined by the 'macronutrient' content of food. Three dietary components can provide fuel for oxidation in the mitochondria to generate energy (as adenosine triphosphate (ATP), p. 1005). These have different energy densities: carbohydrates (4 kcal/g), fat (9 kcal/g) and protein (4 kcal/g).

Regulation of energy balance

In keeping with the fundamental role of maintaining energy balance for survival, energy intake and expenditure are highly regulated (Fig. 5.9). Moreover, they overlap with the control of reproductive function, so that pregnancy is most likely to occur during times of nutritional plenty when both mother and baby have a better chance of survival. Improved nutrition is thought to be the reason for the increasingly early onset of puberty in many societies.

Regulation of energy balance is coordinated in the hypothalamus, which receives afferent signals which indicate nutritional status in the short term (e.g. the stomach

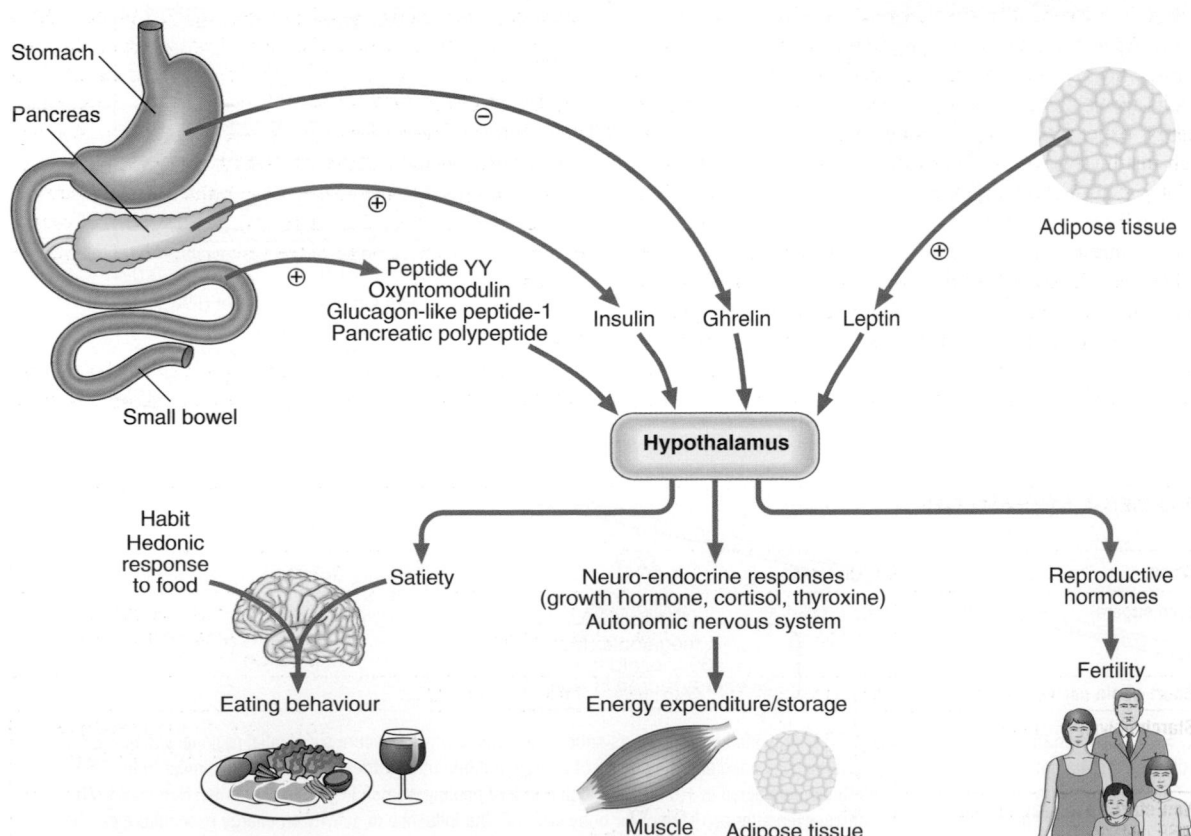

Fig. 5.9 Regulation of energy balance and its link with reproduction. ⊕ indicates factors which are stimulated by eating and induce satiety. ⊖ indicates factors which are suppressed by eating and inhibit satiety.

hormone ghrelin, which falls immediately after eating and rises gradually thereafter to suppress satiety and signal that it is time for the next meal) and long term (e.g. the adipose hormone leptin, which increases with increasing fat mass and stimulates satiety). The hypothalamus responds with changes in many local neurotransmitters (e.g. the peptide POMC, fragments of which stimulate melanocortin receptors; neuropeptide Y; CART; Agouti-related peptide). In turn, these alter activity in numerous efferent pathways which influence energy balance (Fig. 5.9), including hormones controlled by effects of the hypothalamus on the pituitary gland (Fig. 20.2, p. 743), and neural control circuits which connect with the cerebral cortex and autonomic nervous system.

Responses to under- and over-nutrition

These complex regulatory pathways allow adaptation to variations in nutrition. In response to starvation, reproductive function (menstrual cycles in women) is suppressed, BMR is reduced, and there are profound psychological effects including conserving energy through lethargy. These adjustments can 'defend' body weight within certain limits. However, in the low-insulin state of severe starvation (Fig. 21.2, p. 809), fuels are liberated from stores initially in glycogen (in liver and muscle), then in triglyceride (lipolysis in adipose tissue, with excess free fatty acid supply to the liver leading to ketosis) and finally in protein (proteolysis in muscle).

In response to over-nutrition, BMR is increased, and energy is consumed in the work of carrying increased fat stores. As a result, body weight is 'defended' within certain limits, and an increase in energy intake above this limit results in weight gain until a 'plateau' is reached at which energy expenditure is correspondingly increased. In the high-insulin state of over-nutrition, excess energy is invested in fatty acids and stored as triglycerides; these are deposited principally in the adipose tissue but they may also spill over and accumulate in liver (non-alcoholic fatty liver disease, p. 971) and skeletal muscle. In the absence of hypothalamic function (e.g. in a patient with craniopharyngioma, Fig. 20.30, p. 803), or in rare patients with mutations in relevant genes (e.g. in leptin or melanocortin-4 receptors), loss of satiety signals, together with loss of the adaptive changes in energy expenditure, result in relentless weight gain without any plateau.

ENERGY-YIELDING NUTRIENTS (MACRONUTRIENTS)

Carbohydrates

The types of carbohydrate and their dietary sources are listed in Box 5.15. The 'available' carbohydrates (starches and sugars) are broken down to monosaccharides before absorption from the gut (p. 854), and supply a major part of the energy in a normal diet (Fig. 5.8A). No individual carbohydrate is an essential nutrient as carbohydrates can be synthesised de novo from glycerol or protein. However, if the available carbohydrate intake is less than 100 g per day, increased lipolysis leads to ketosis (Fig. 21.5, p. 812).

Intrinsic sugars and the foods that contain them are thought to be more acceptable nutritionally than extrinsic sugars because they are associated with other nutrients naturally present in the food. Moreover, refined extrinsic sugars increase the risk of dental caries. Starches in cereal foods (wheat, rice), root foods (potatoes, cassava) and legumes (lentils, beans, peas) provide the largest proportion of calories in most diets around the world. Although all starches are polymers of glucose, linked by the same 1–4 glycosidic linkages, they do not all behave in the same way when they are eaten. Some starches are digested promptly by salivary and then pancreatic amylase and produce rapid delivery of glucose to the blood. Other starches are more slowly digested either because they are protected in the structure of the food, because of their crystal structure or because the molecule is unbranched (amylose). These differences are the basis for the 'glycaemic index' of foods, which describes the area under the curve of the rise in blood glucose concentration in the 2 hours following ingestion of 50 g carbohydrate, expressed as a percentage of the response to 50 g anhydrous glucose.

Dietary fibre

Dietary fibre can be defined as those parts of food which are not digested by human enzymes. Most dietary fibre is made

5.15 DIETARY CARBOHYDRATES			
Class	**Components**	**Examples**	**Source**
Free sugars	Monosaccharides Disaccharides	Glucose, fructose Sucrose, lactose, maltose	Intrinsic: fruits, milks, vegetables Extrinsic (extracted, refined): beet or cane sucrose
Short-chain carbohydrates	Oligosaccharides	Maltodextrins, fructo-oligosaccharides	
Starch polysaccharides	Rapidly digestible Slowly digestible Resistant		Cereals (wheat, rice), root vegetables (potato), legumes (lentils, beans, peas)
Non-starch polysaccharides (NSP, dietary fibre)	Fibrous Viscous	Cellulose Hemicellulose Pectins Gums	Plants

up of non-starch polysaccharides (NSP), the natural packing of plant foods (Box 5.15). A small percentage of 'resistant' dietary starch may also escape digestion in the small intestine and pass unchanged into the large intestine. These carbohydrates may be fermented by the resident bacteria in the colon, contributing to flatus formation.

Some types of NSP, notably the hemicellulose of wheat, increase the water-holding capacity of colonic contents and the bulk of faeces. They relieve simple constipation, appear to prevent diverticulosis and may reduce the risk of cancer of the colon. Other viscous, indigestible polysaccharides like pectin and guar gum have greater effect in the upper gastrointestinal tract. They slow gastric emptying, contribute to satiety, and reduce bile salt absorption and hence plasma cholesterol concentration.

Fats

Fatty acids have the highest energy density of the macro-nutrients (9 kcal/g) and so are useful to people with a large energy requirement, but may be an insidious cause of obesity in societies where fat consumption is excessive (Fig. 5.8A). Free fatty acids are absorbed in chylomicrons (p. 443), allowing access of complex molecules into the circulation. Fatty acid structures are shown in Figure 5.10. The principal polyunsaturated fatty acid in plant seed oils is linoleic acid (18:2 ω6). This and its elongated ω6 derivatives, γ-linolenic acid (18:3 ω6) and arachidonic acid (20:4 ω6), are the 'essential' fatty acids, which are required in the diet because they are precursors of prostaglandins and eicosanoids and part of the structure of lipid membranes in all cells.

The ω3 series of polyunsaturated fatty acids, e.g. eicosapentaenoic (20:5 ω3) and docosahexaenoic (22:6 ω3), occur in fish oils and in the lipids of the human brain and retina. They are inhibitors of thrombosis and appear to act by competitively antagonising thromboxane A_2 formation. Purified fish oils, e.g. ω3 marine triglycerides, also lower plasma triglyceride levels and may prevent coronary heart disease. In contrast, saturated fats (especially those containing myristic (14:0) and palmitic (16:0) acids) are mainly found in animal fats and may accelerate vascular disease. They increase plasma low-density lipoproteins and total cholesterol.

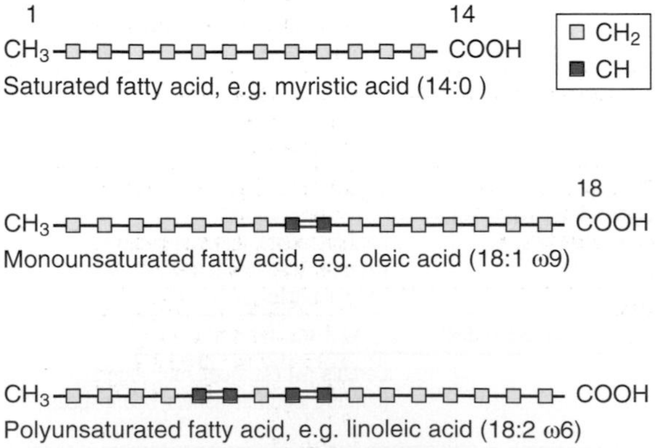

Cholesterol is also absorbed directly from food in chylomicrons and is an important substrate for steroid and sterol synthesis, but it is not an important source of energy.

Proteins

Proteins form the main structural component of body cells and an adequate intake is essential for health. They are made up of some 20 different amino acids, of which nine are 'essential' (Box 5.16), i.e. they cannot be synthesised in humans but are indispensable for synthesis of important proteins. Another group of five amino acids are termed 'conditionally essential', meaning that they can be synthesised from one or more of the essential amino acids provided there is an adequate dietary supply (Box 5.17). The remaining amino acids can be synthesised in the body by transamination, provided there is a sufficient supply of amino groups.

5.16 ESSENTIAL AMINO ACIDS	
• Tryptophan	• Valine
• Histidine	• Phenylalanine
• Methionine	• Lysine
• Threonine	• Leucine
• Isoleucine	

5.17 CONDITIONALLY ESSENTIAL AMINO ACIDS	
Amino acid	Precursors
Cysteine	Methionine, serine
Tyrosine	Phenylalanine
Arginine	Glutamine/glutamate, aspartate
Proline	Glutamate
Glycine	Serine, choline

The nutritive value of different proteins depends on the relative proportions of essential amino acids they contain (sometimes called their 'biological value'). Proteins of animal origin, particularly from eggs, milk and meat, are generally of higher biological value than the proteins of vegetable origin, which are low in one or more of the indispensable amino acids. However, when two different vegetable proteins are eaten together (e.g. a cereal and a legume), their amino acid contents can complement one another and produce a mix of indispensable amino acids with an adequate protein nutritive value. This is the principle of protein supply in a vegan or vegetarian diet.

OTHER NUTRIENTS (MICRONUTRIENTS)

A variety of other molecules are vital components of the diet but do not contribute to energy balance. These include vitamins and inorganic metals and ions. They are discussed in the context of deficiency states on pages 121–127.

1   14
CH₃–□–□–□–□–□–□–□–□–□–□–□–□– COOH   □ CH₂
Saturated fatty acid, e.g. myristic acid (14:0)   ■ CH

                                          18
CH₃–□–□–□–□–□–□–□–■–■–□–□–□–□–□–□–□– COOH
Monounsaturated fatty acid, e.g. oleic acid (18:1 ω9)

CH₃–□–□–□–■–■–□–■–■–□–□–□–□–□–□–□– COOH
Polyunsaturated fatty acid, e.g. linoleic acid (18:2 ω6)

Fig. 5.10   Schematic representation of fatty acids. A standard nomenclature is used whereby the number of carbon atoms is specified and the number and position of the double bond(s) relative to the methyl (–CH₃, ω) end of the molecule are indicated after a colon.

DIETARY RECOMMENDATIONS

Recommendations for calorie intake (Box 5.18) and the proportions of different macronutrients (Box 5.19) have been calculated on the basis of providing a balance of essential nutrients while minimising the risks of excessive refined sugar (dental caries, high glycaemic index) or saturated fat (obesity, coronary heart disease). In addition, recommended dietary fibre intake is based on avoiding risks of colonic disease. The usual recommendation for an adequate protein intake is 10% of the total calories, i.e. about 65 g per day for the average adult. The minimum requirement is around 40 g of protein with a high proportion of indispensable amino acids or a high biological value.

Recommendations for micronutrients are discussed on pages 121–127.

5.18 DAILY ENERGY REQUIREMENTS

Circumstances	Requirements	
	Healthy adult females	Healthy adult males
At rest	6.7 MJ (1600 kcal)	8.4 MJ (2000 kcal)
Light work	8.4 MJ (2000 kcal)	11.3 MJ (2700 kcal)
Heavy work	9.4 MJ (2250 kcal)	14.6 MJ (3500 kcal)

5.19 POPULATION MACRONUTRIENT GOALS

Nutrient	Limits for population average intakes	
	Lower	Upper
Total fat (% of total energy)	15	30
Saturated fatty acids (% total energy)	0	10
Polyunsaturated fatty acids (% total energy)	3	7
Dietary cholesterol (mg/day)	0	300
Total carbohydrate (% total energy)	55	75
Free sugars (% total energy)	0	10
Complex carbohydrate (% total energy)	50	70
Dietary fibre (g/day)		
As non-starch polysaccharides	16	24
As total dietary fibre	27	40
Protein (% total energy)	10	15

PRESENTING PROBLEMS OF ALTERED ENERGY BALANCE

OBESITY

Obesity is widely regarded as a pandemic with potentially disastrous consequences for human health. More than 20% of adults in the UK, and more than 30% in USA, are obese (i.e. body mass index, BMI $\geq$ 30 kg/m^2, see definition on p. 113). The prevalence of obesity has increased ~threefold within the last 20 years and continues to rise. In developing countries, average national rates of obesity are not nearly so high, but these figures disguise alarmingly high rates of obesity in many urban communities.

Complications of obesity

Health consequences of obesity are shown in Box 5.20. Obesity has adverse effects on both mortality and morbidity. Changes in mortality are difficult to analyse due to the confounding effects of lower body weight in cigarette smokers. However, it is clear that the lowest mortality rates are seen in individuals with a BMI of 18.5–24. Data from population studies, such as that in Framingham, USA, show that for individuals aged between 30 and 42 years, the risk of death increases by 1% per annum for each 0.5 kg increase in weight; for those aged 50–62, this figure is 2%. The result is that obesity reduces life expectancy by 7.1 years in men and 5.8 years in women amongst non-smokers, and by 13.7 and 13.3 years respectively amongst smokers. Coronary heart disease (Fig. 5.11) is the major cause of death but cancer rates are also increased in the overweight, especially colorectal cancer in males and cancer of the gallbladder, biliary tract, breast, endometrium and cervix in females. Epidemic obesity is accompanied by an epidemic of type 2 diabetes (p. 813). The only medical benefit of obesity is seen in osteoporosis, where bone density increases in response to increased mechanical stress (p. 1121). Obesity may lead to profound psychological consequences for individuals. Society also suffers from the effects of obesity-related disability and early retirement.

5.20 COMPLICATIONS OF OBESITY

Risk factors	Outcomes

'Metabolic syndrome'
  Type 2 diabetes
  Hypertension
  Hyperlipidaemia
	Coronary heart disease
	Stroke
	Diabetes complications

Liver fat accumulation	Non-alcoholic steatohepatitis Cirrhosis
Restricted ventilation	Exertional dyspnoea Sleep apnoea Respiratory failure (Pickwickian syndrome)
Mechanical effects of weight	Urinary incontinence Osteoarthritis Varicose veins
Increased peripheral steroid interconversion in adipose tissue	Hormone-dependent cancers (breast, uterus) Polycystic ovary syndrome (infertility, hirsutism)
Others	Psychological morbidity (low self-esteem, depression) Socioeconomic disadvantage (lower income, less likely to be promoted) Gallstones Colorectal cancer Skin infections (groin and submammary candidiasis; hidradenitis)

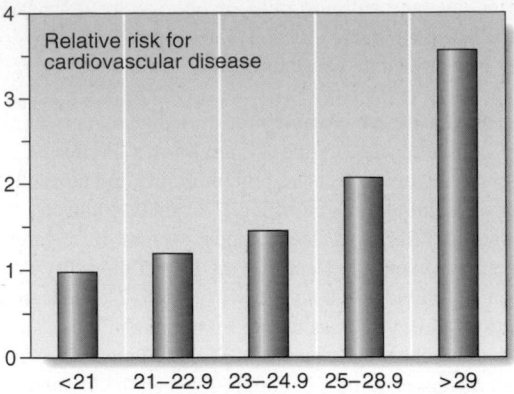

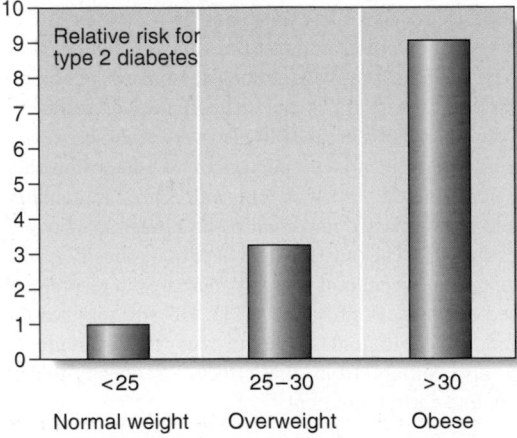

Fig. 5.11 Risks of diabetes and cardiovascular disease in overweight and obese women. Data are from the Nurses' Health Study in the USA, a large survey mostly of Caucasian women. In some ethnic groups (e.g. South Asians, Native Americans) and in people with higher waist circumference, the metabolic complications are even more severe at a given level of BMI.

Body fat distribution

For some complications of obesity, the distribution rather than the absolute amount of excess adipose tissue appears to be important. Increased intra-abdominal fat causes 'central' ('abdominal', 'visceral', 'android' or 'apple-shaped') obesity, which contrasts with subcutaneous fat accumulation causing 'generalised' ('gynoid' or 'pear-shaped') obesity; the former is more common in men and is more closely associated with type 2 diabetes, the metabolic syndrome and cardiovascular disease (Box 5.20). The key difference between these depots of fat probably lies in their vascular anatomy, with intra-abdominal fat draining into the portal vein and thence directly to the liver. Thus many factors which are released from adipose tissue (including free fatty acids; 'adipokines' such as tumour necrosis factor alpha (TNF-α), adiponectin and resistin; and steroid hormones including cortisol) may be at higher concentration in the liver and hence induce insulin resistance and promote type 2 diabetes (p. 813). Other differences in fat metabolism and adipokine release between visceral and subcutaneous adipose tissue have been reported but are of uncertain significance.

Aetiology

Accumulation of fat results from a discrepancy between energy consumption and expenditure over and above that which can be compensated for by hypothalamic regulation of basal metabolic rate (BMR). A small daily excess consumption of only 0.2–0.8 MJ (50–200 kcal; < 10% of intake) can lead to a weight gain of 2–20 kg over a period of 4–10 years. Given the cumulative effects of subtle energy excess, body fat content shows 'tracking' with age, such that individuals are likely to maintain their rank in the age-adjusted population distribution throughout their lives. Thus obese children are very likely to become obese adults. Weight tends to increase throughout adult life, as BMR and physical activity decrease (Fig. 5.8).

The pandemic of obesity reflects changes in both energy intake and energy expenditure (Box 5.21), although both of these are difficult to measure reliably. The estimated average global daily supply of food energy per person increased from ~2350 kcal in the 1960s to ~2800 kcal in the 1990s, but its delivery is unequal. For example, in India it is estimated that 5% of the population receives 40% of the available food energy, leading to obesity in the urban population in parallel with persisting malnutrition in some rural communities. In affluent societies, a significant proportion of this food supply is discarded. However, in the USA, the average daily energy intake of men reportedly rose from 2450 kcal in 1971 to 2618 kcal in 2000. Well-documented increases have occurred in portion sizes, particularly of energy-dense foods such as drinks with high refined sugar content and high-fat snacks. These snacks are less effective at suppressing appetite and their consumption between normal meal times decreases the recognition of food eaten.

Circumstantial evidence suggests that corresponding changes in energy expenditure are important; obesity is correlated positively with the number of hours spent watching television, and inversely with levels of physical activity (including 'non-exercise activity thermogenesis', i.e. fidgeting).

Susceptibility to obesity

Although obese people were ridiculed in the past when they bemoaned their inability to control their weight, today there is little doubt that susceptibility to obesity, and to its

5.21 SOME REASONS FOR THE INCREASING PREVALENCE OF OBESITY—THE 'OBESOGENIC' ENVIRONMENT	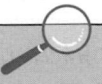
Increasing energy intake	
↑ Portion sizes ↑ Snacking and loss of regular meals ↑ Energy-dense food (mainly fat) ↑ Affluence	
Decreasing energy expenditure	
↑ Car ownership ↓ Walking to school/work ↑ Automation; ↓ manual labour ↓ Sports in schools ↑ Time spent on video games and watching TV ↑ Central heating	

5

adverse consequences, varies between individuals. It is not true that obese subjects have a 'slow metabolism', since their BMR is higher than that of lean subjects, but it can be argued that their metabolism is not increased as much as it needs to be following weight gain. Twin and adoption studies confirm a genetic influence on obesity. The pattern of inheritance suggests a polygenic disorder, with small contributions from a number of different genes, together accounting for 25–70% of variation in weight. Polymorphisms in > 90 genes have been implicated in obesity in single studies, and 15 of these have been replicated in more than five studies; these are genes which might influence appetite, activity levels, rates of lipid oxidation and adipocyte hyperplasia, but a clear picture of their contribution remains elusive.

A few rare single gene disorders cause severe childhood obesity. These include mutations of the melanocortin-4 receptor (MC4R) that accounts for approximately 5% of severe early-onset obesity, defects in the enzymes processing POMC in the hypothalamus, and mutations in the leptin gene (Fig. 5.9). The latter can be effectively treated by leptin injections. Additional genetic conditions in which obesity is a feature include the Prader–Willi (p. 47) and Lawrence–Moon–Biedl syndromes.

Reversible causes of obesity and weight gain

In a few cases presenting with obesity, specific causal factors can be identified and treated (Box 5.22). These patients are distinguished from those with idiopathic obesity by their short history, with a recent marked change in the trajectory of their adult weight.

5.22 POTENTIALLY REVERSIBLE CAUSES OF WEIGHT GAIN	
Endocrine factors	
• Hypothyroidism	• Hypothalamic tumours or injury
• Cushing's syndrome	• Insulinoma
Drug treatments	
• Tricyclic antidepressants	• Corticosteroids
• Sulphonylureas	• Sodium valproate
• Oestrogen-containing contraceptive pill	• β-blockers

Clinical assessment and investigations

In assessing an individual presenting with obesity, the aims are to quantify the problem, exclude an underlying cause, identify complications, and reach a management plan.

Obesity can be quantified conveniently using the body mass index (BMI). BMI is calculated as the person's weight in kilograms divided by the square of his or her height in metres (kg/m^2). For example, an adult weighing 70 kg with a height of 1.75 metres has a BMI of $70/1.75^2 = 22.9$. This adjusts crudely for differences in body habitus, and provides the usual definition of severity of obesity (Box 5.23). A simple measure which reflects the degree of abdominal obesity is the waist circumference, measured at the level of the umbilicus. A waist circumference of > 102 cm in men or > 88 cm in women indicates that the risk of metabolic and

5.23 QUANTIFYING OBESITY WITH BODY MASS INDEX (WEIGHT/HEIGHT²)		
BMI (kg/m^2)	**Classification***	**Risk of obesity comorbidity**
18.5–24.9	Normal range	Negligible
25.0–29.9	Overweight	Mildly increased
> 30.0	**Obese**	
30.0–34.9	Class I	Moderate
35.0–39.9	Class II	Severe
> 40.0	Class III	Very severe

* Classification of the World Health Organization (WHO) and International Obesity Task Force.

cardiovascular complications of obesity is high. More sophisticated measurements of body composition, including percentage body fat estimation by bioimpedance or dual energy X-ray absorptiometry (DEXA) scanning, are available but of uncertain clinical value.

A dietary history, especially if obtained by a specialist dietitian, may be helpful in guiding dietary advice, but is notoriously susceptible to under-reporting of food consumption. It is important, however, to consider 'pathological' eating behaviour (such as binge eating, nocturnal eating or bulimia, p. 248), which may be the most important issue to address in some patients. Alcohol consumption is an important source of energy intake which should be considered in detail.

The history of weight gain is most helpful in considering underlying causes. A patient who has recently begun to gain substantial weight for the first time or at a faster rate than previously, and is not taking relevant drugs (Box 5.22), is more likely to have an underlying disorder such as hypothyroidism (p. 750) or Cushing's syndrome (p. 779). A more detailed history and examination should be performed with these conditions in mind. All obese patients should have thyroid function tests performed on one occasion, and an overnight dexamethasone suppression test or 24-hour urine free cortisol if Cushing's syndrome is suspected. Monogenic and 'syndromic' causes of obesity are usually only relevant in children presenting with severe obesity.

Assessment of the diverse complications of obesity (Box 5.20) requires a thorough history and examination and some screening tests. The impact of obesity on the patient's life and work is a major consideration. Assessment of other cardiovascular risk factors is important. Blood pressure should be measured with a large cuff if required (p. 609). The presence of associated type 2 diabetes and dyslipidaemia can be detected by measuring blood glucose and a serum lipid profile, ideally in a fasting morning sample. Elevated serum transaminases occur in patients with non-alcoholic fatty liver disease (p. 971).

Management

The health risks of obesity are largely reversible. All interventions which have been proven to reduce weight in well-conducted studies in obese patients have also been shown to ameliorate cardiovascular risk factors. Lifestyle advice which lowers body weight and increases physical exercise

5

reduces the incidence of type 2 diabetes (p. 829). Given the high prevalence of obesity and the large magnitude of its risks, population strategies to prevent and reverse obesity are high on the priority list for most health organisations. Initiatives include promoting healthy eating in schools, enhancing walking and cycling options for commuters, and liaising with the food industry to reduce energy and fat content and label foods appropriately. It remains to be seen whether these initiatives will stem the tide of obesity.

The following section considers the management of individual patients. Many will self-refer with obesity, others will present with one of the complications of their obesity, and increasingly patients are being identified during health screening examinations.

Most patients seeking assistance with obesity are motivated to lose weight but will have attempted weight loss previously without long-term success. Often weight will have oscillated between periods of successful weight loss and then regain of weight (often called 'recidivism'). They may hold misconceptions that they have an underlying disease, inaccurate perceptions of their energy intake and expenditure, and an unrealistic view of the target weight which they would regard as a 'success'. An empathetic explanation of energy balance, which recognises that some individuals are more susceptible to obesity than others and therefore require greater deficits in energy balance in order to lose and sustain body weight, is important. Exclusion of underlying 'hormone imbalance' with simple tests is reassuring and shifts the focus on to consideration of energy balance. Appropriate goals for weight loss should be agreed, recognising that the slope of the relationship between obesity and many of its complications becomes steeper with increasing BMI, so that a given amount of weight loss achieves greater risk reduction at higher levels of BMI. A reasonable goal for most patients is to lose 10% of body weight.

The specific management plan will vary according to the severity of the obesity (Box 5.23) and the associated risk factors and complications. It will also be influenced by availability of resources; health-care providers and regulators have generally been careful not to recommend expensive interventions (especially long-term drug therapy and surgery) for everyone who is overweight. Instead most guidelines focus resources on short-term interventions in those who have high health risks and comorbidities associated with their obesity, and who have demonstrated their capacity to alter their lifestyle to achieve weight loss (Fig. 5.12).

Lifestyle advice

Behavioural modification to avoid some of the effects of the 'obesogenic' environment (Box 5.21) is the cornerstone of long-term control of weight. A study of subjects followed up after successful weight loss in Colorado found that the principal predictors of sustained weight loss are the maintenance of high physical activity levels and the regular consumption of breakfast (suggesting a regular eating pattern). All patients should be advised to maximise their physical activity, with reference to the modest extra activity required to increase PAL ratios (Fig. 5.8C, p. 107). Where possible, this should be incorporated in the daily routine (e.g. walking rather than driving to work) since this is more likely to be sustained. Alternative exercise, e.g. swimming, may be necessary if musculoskeletal complications prevent walking. Changes in eating behaviour (including food selection, portion size control, avoidance of snacking, regular meals to encourage satiety, and substitution of sugar with artificial sweeteners) should be discussed. Support from a trained health-care professional (e.g. a dietitian) and participation in a group discussion may be helpful.

Weight loss diets

In overweight people, adherence to the lifestyle advice above may gradually induce weight loss. In obese patients, more active intervention is usually required to lose weight before conversion to 'weight maintenance' advice above. A significant industry has developed marketing diets for weight loss. These vary substantially in their balance of macronutrients (Box 5.24), but there is little evidence that they vary in their medium-term (1 year) efficacy. What they have in common is a reduction in daily total energy intake of ~2.5 MJ (600 kcal) from the patient's normal consumption. The goal is to lose ~0.5 kg/week. Weight loss is highly variable, with patient compliance being the major determinant of success. Compliance is better with moderate relative reductions of ~600 kcal in daily calorie intake than with 'fixed' regimes of 1000 kcal intake per day, which may represent a reduction of > 1500 kcal/day in many patients. There is some evidence that weight loss diets are most effective in their early weeks, and that compliance is improved by novelty of the diet; this provides some justification for switching to a different dietary regime when weight loss slows on the first diet. Vitamin supplementation is wise in those diets in which macronutrient balance is markedly disturbed.

In some patients more rapid weight loss is required, e.g. in preparation for surgery. There is no role for starvation diets which carry a risk of sudden death from heart disease, exacerbated by profound loss in muscle mass and the

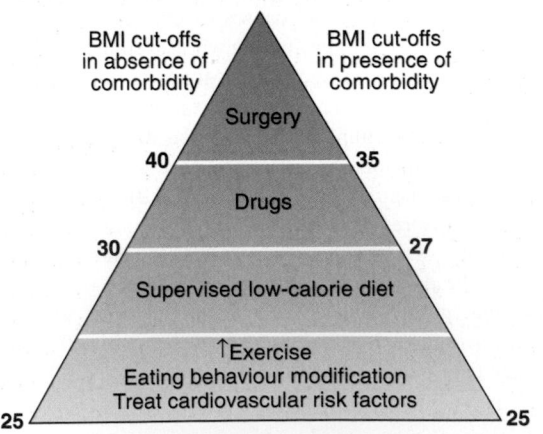

Fig. 5.12 Therapeutic options for obesity. Relevant comorbidities include type 2 diabetes, hypertension, cardiovascular disease, sleep apnoea, and waist circumference > 102 cm in men or 88 cm in women. This is an approximate consensus of the numerous national guidelines which vary slightly in their recommendations and are revised every few years.

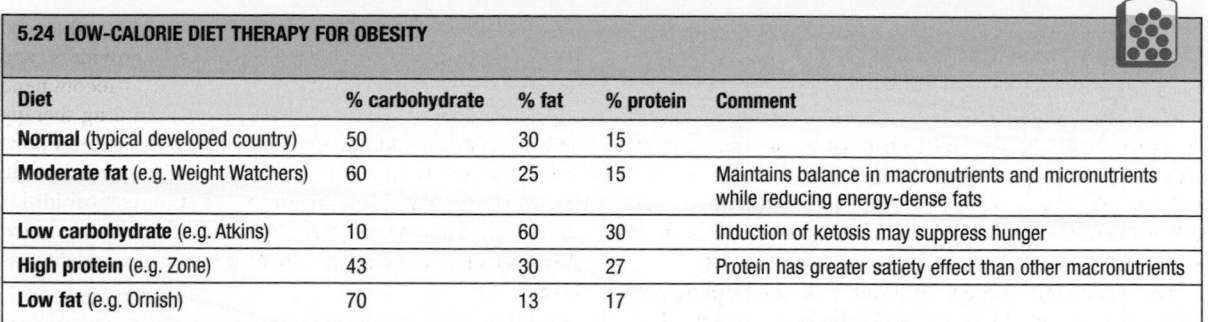

5.24 LOW-CALORIE DIET THERAPY FOR OBESITY

Diet	% carbohydrate	% fat	% protein	Comment
Normal (typical developed country)	50	30	15	
Moderate fat (e.g. Weight Watchers)	60	25	15	Maintains balance in macronutrients and micronutrients while reducing energy-dense fats
Low carbohydrate (e.g. Atkins)	10	60	30	Induction of ketosis may suppress hunger
High protein (e.g. Zone)	43	30	27	Protein has greater satiety effect than other macronutrients
Low fat (e.g. Ornish)	70	13	17	

5.25 DRUGS WHICH LOWER BODY WEIGHT

Status	Drugs	Mechanism of action
Not recommended due to toxicity	Amphetamines Fenfluramine, dexfenfluramine	Catecholaminergic in CNS and periphery Serotonergic in CNS
Not recommended as primary treatment; weight loss a useful minor/temporary effect	Fluoxetine Metformin	Serotonergic in CNS Unknown
Currently recommended	Orlistat Sibutramine	Pancreatic lipase inhibitor Serotonergic in CNS
In advanced development*	Rimonabant	Cannabinoid receptor antagonist

* Many other approaches are in development, several of which have reached clinical trials.

development of arrhythmias secondary to elevated free fatty acids and deranged electrolytes. Very low calorie diets (VLCDs) produce weight losses of 1.5–2.5 kg/week compared to 0.5 kg/week on conventional regimes, and hence require the supervision of an experienced physician and nutritionist. Unfortunately, most patients regain weight after stopping such a diet, so VLCDs are mainly used for short-term rapid weight loss. The composition of the diet should ensure a minimum of 50 g of protein each day for men and 40 g of protein for women to minimise muscle degradation. Energy content should be a minimum of 1.65 MJ (400 kcal) for women of height < 1.73 m, and 2.1 MJ (500 kcal) for all men and for women taller than 1.73 m. Side-effects tend to be a problem in the early stages and include orthostatic hypotension, headache, diarrhoea and nausea.

Support for patients during weight loss is important. This can be achieved by a dietitian or by regular attendance at a weight loss group.

Drugs

A huge investment has been made by the pharmaceutical industry to find drugs for obesity. The side-effect profile has limited the use of many earlier agents, but two drugs are currently available and newer agents are likely to be approved and marketed soon (Box 5.25). There is no role for diuretics, or for thyroxine therapy without biochemical evidence of hypothyroidism.

Orlistat inhibits pancreatic and gastric lipases and thereby decreases the hydrolysis of ingested triglycerides, reducing dietary fat absorption by ~30%. The drug is not absorbed and adverse side-effects relate to the effect of the resultant fat malabsorption on the gut, namely loose stools, oily spotting, faecal urgency, flatus and the potential for

5.26 LONG-TERM USE OF ORLISTAT IN OBESITY **EBM**

'In patients with a BMI > 30 kg/m^2, 4 years of treatment with orlistat + lifestyle advice, in comparison with placebo + lifestyle advice, increased weight loss from 3.0 to 5.8 kg and reduced the incidence of type 2 diabetes from 9.0% to 6.2%. Orlistat also improved blood pressure and serum lipid profile.'

- Torgerson JS, et al. Diabetes Care 2004 27:155–161.

malabsorption of fat-soluble vitamins. Orlistat is taken with each of the three main meals of the day and the dose can be adjusted (60–120 mg) to minimise side-effects. Its efficacy is shown in Box 5.26 and Figure 5.13; these effects may be explained because patients taking orlistat adhere better to low-fat diets in order to avoid unpleasant gastrointestinal side-effects.

Sibutramine reduces food intake through β_1-adrenoceptor and 5-HT$_{2A/2C}$ (5-hydroxytryptamine, serotonin) receptor agonist activity in the central nervous system. Weight loss achieved with this agent is 3–5 kg better than placebo with 6 months' therapy and is associated with an improvement in lipid profile. Side-effects include dry mouth, constipation and insomnia. Unfortunately, noradrenergic effects of the drug can increase heart rate and blood pressure; these effects are especially undesirable in many obese patients, so that this agent is usually a second choice after orlistat and cannot be used in those with hypertension or cardiovascular disease. There is insufficient evidence to recommend co-prescription of orlistat and sibutramine.

Drug therapy is usually reserved for patients with high risk of complications from obesity (Fig. 5.12), and its optimum timing and duration are controversial. Although

5

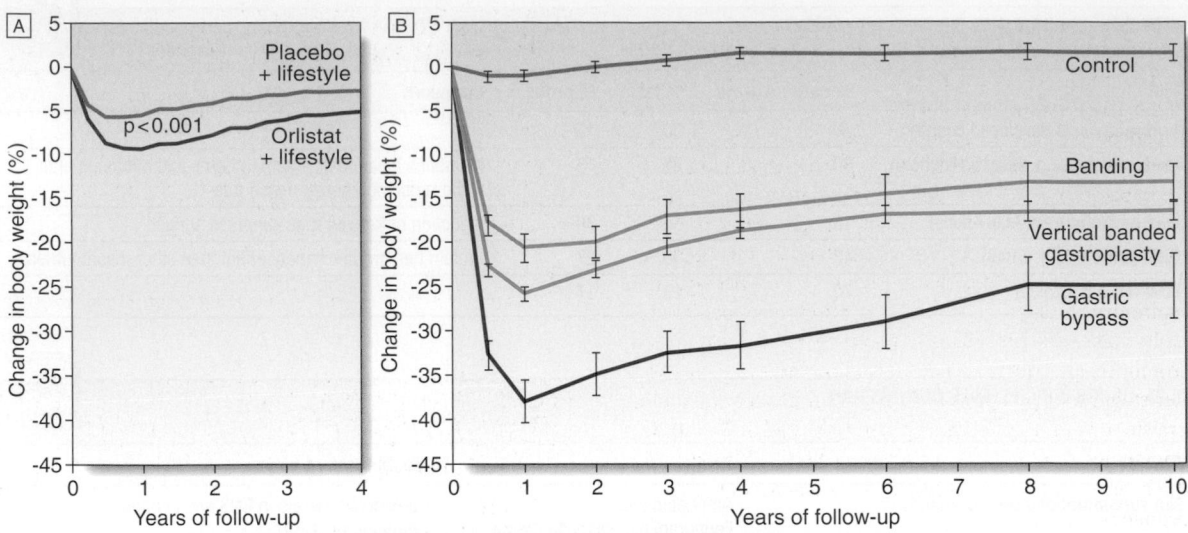

Fig. 5.13   Effects of orlistat and bariatric surgery on weight loss. Ⓐ These data are from the study referenced in Box 5.26. Ⓑ Data for surgery are from Sjostrom L, et al. New Engl J Med 2004; 351:2683–2693. In this study, for each obese subject undergoing surgery a matched control subject was selected whose obesity was 'treated' by standard non-operative interventions. Note that, although orlistat is effective, the maximum weight loss achieved was ~11%; surgery achieves much more substantial and prolonged weight loss.

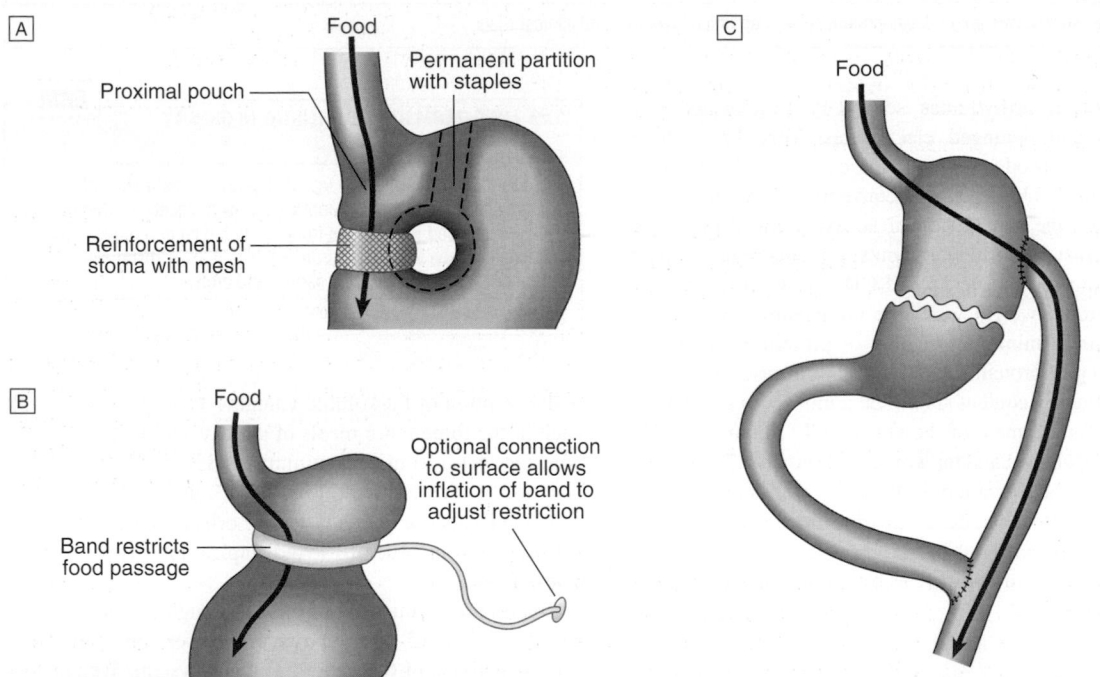

Fig. 5.14   Bariatric surgical procedures. Ⓐ Vertical banded gastroplasty. Ⓑ Laparoscopic banding, with the option of a reservoir band and subcutaneous access to restrict the stomach further after compensatory expansion has occurred. Ⓒ Roux-en-Y gastric bypass.

life-long therapy is advocated for many drugs which reduce risk on the basis of relatively short-term research trials (e.g. drugs for hypertension and osteoporosis), it is notable that patients who continue to take anti-obesity drugs tend to regain weight with time (Fig. 5.13). This observation, together with considerations of optimal use of finite health-care resources, has led to the recommendation in many guidelines that anti-obesity drugs are used in the short term to maximise the weight loss achieved with low calorie diets

(so that inevitable regain of weight starts from a lower baseline), but are not used in the long-term maintenance of weight. It follows that they should only be introduced in patients who are demonstrating their adherence to a low calorie diet by current weight loss (e.g. recent weight loss of at least 2.5 kg) and should only be continued while patients continue to lose weight (e.g. at least 5% every 3 months). This approach is currently standard practice in the UK, but may or may not stand the test of time.

Surgery

'Bariatric' surgery to reduce the size of the stomach is by far the most effective long-term treatment for obesity (Fig. 5.13). Several approaches are used (Fig. 5.14) and all can be performed laparoscopically. The mechanism of weight loss may not relate to limiting the stomach or absorptive capacity per se, but rather in disrupting the release of ghrelin from the stomach, which signals hunger in the hypothalamus. Complications depend upon the approach. Mortality is low in experienced centres but post-operative respiratory problems, wound infection and dehiscence, staple leaks, stomal stenosis, marginal ulcers and venous thrombosis are common. Additional problems may arise at a later stage, such as pouch and distal oesophageal dilatation, persistent vomiting, 'dumping' (p. 888) and micronutrient deficiencies, particularly of folate, vitamin B_{12} and iron, which are of concern especially to women contemplating pregnancy.

Bariatric surgery should be contemplated in patients who have very high risks of complications of obesity (Fig. 5.12), in whom extensive dietary and drug therapy has been ineffective or inadequately effective, and who are motivated to undergo surgery. Only experienced specialist surgeons should undertake these procedures.

Cosmetic surgical procedures may be required in obese patients. Apronectomy is usually advocated to remove an overhang of abdominal skin, especially if infected or ulcerated. This operation is of no value for long-term weight reduction if food intake remains unrestricted.

Treatment of additional risk factors

Obesity must not be treated in isolation and other risk factors must be addressed, including smoking, excess alcohol consumption, diabetes mellitus, hyperlipidaemia and hypertension. Treatment of these risk factors is discussed in the relevant chapters.

MALNUTRITION

STARVATION AND FAMINE

In some parts of the world, malnutrition due to famine remains endemic. WHO figures suggest that malnutrition contributes to 30 000 deaths every day in children under 5 years old. While obesity is a pandemic, there remain regions of the world, particularly in Africa, where the prevalence of BMI < 18.5 (Box 5.27) in adults remains as high as 20% and growth retardation due to malnutrition in children as high as 50%.

In children, starvation (protein-energy malnutrition, PEM) is manifest as the syndromes of kwashiorkor (malnutrition with oedema) and marasmus (malnutrition with marked muscle-wasting). Treatment of these conditions is not discussed in this adult medicine textbook. In adults, the predominant form of PEM is undernutrition, i.e. the result of a sustained negative energy (calorie) balance. Causes are shown in Box 5.28. Causes of weight loss are considered further on page 871.

5.27 CLASSIFICATION OF MALNUTRITION IN ADULTS BY BODY MASS INDEX (WEIGHT/HEIGHT^2)

BMI (kg/m^2)	Classification
> 20	Adequate nutrition
18.5–20	Marginal
< 18.5	**Malnutrition**
17–18.5	Mild
16–17	Moderate
< 16	Severe

5.28 CAUSES OF UNDERNUTRITION AND WEIGHT LOSS IN ADULTS

Decreased energy intake

- Famine
- Persistent regurgitation or vomiting
- Anorexia, including anorexia nervosa
- Malabsorption (e.g. small intestinal disease)
- Maldigestion (e.g. pancreatic exocrine insufficiency)

Increased energy expenditure

- Increased BMR (thyrotoxicosis, trauma, fever, cancer cachexia)
- Excessive physical activity (e.g. marathon runners)
- Energy loss (e.g. glycosuria in diabetes)
- Impaired energy storage (e.g. Addison's disease, phaeochromocytoma)

Clinical assessment

In starvation, the severity of malnutrition can be assessed by anthropometric measurements. Height and weight are used to calculate BMI (Box 5.27). Relative loss of muscle and subcutaneous fat can be estimated by measuring mid-arm circumference (at the middle of the humerus) and skinfold thickness over the triceps (using special callipers); muscle mass is estimated by subtracting triceps skinfold thickness from mid-arm circumference. These measurements are most useful in monitoring progress during treatment. The clinical features of severe undernutrition in adults include:

- loss of weight
- thirst, weakness, feeling cold, nocturia, amenorrhoea or impotence, craving for food
- lax, pale, dry skin with loss of turgor and, occasionally, pigmented patches
- hair thinning or loss (except in adolescents)
- cold and cyanosed extremities, pressure sores
- muscle wasting, best demonstrated by the appearance of the temporalis and periscapular muscles and reduced mid-arm circumference
- loss of subcutaneous fat, reflected in reduced skinfold thickness and mid-arm circumference
- oedema, which may be present without hypoalbuminaemia ('famine oedema')
- subnormal body temperature, slow pulse, low blood pressure and small heart
- distended abdomen, with diarrhoea
- diminished tendon jerks

5.29 INFECTIONS ASSOCIATED WITH PEM

Patients with starvation have increased susceptibility to:
- Gastroenteritis and Gram-negative septicaemia
- Respiratory infections, especially bronchopneumonia
- Certain viral diseases, especially measles and herpes simplex
- Tuberculosis
- Streptococcal and staphylococcal skin infections
- Helminthic infestations

- apathy, loss of initiative, depression, introversion, aggression if food is nearby
- susceptibility to infections (Box 5.29).

Undernutrition often leads to vitamin deficiencies, especially thiamin, folate and vitamin C (pp. 121–125). Diarrhoea is also seen, leading to depletion of sodium, potassium and magnesium. The high mortality rate in famine situations is often due to infections, e.g. typhus or cholera epidemics, but the usual signs of infection may not appear. In advanced starvation, patients become completely inactive and may assume a flexed, fetal position. In the last stage of starvation, death comes quietly and often quite suddenly. The very old are most vulnerable. All organs are atrophied at necropsy, except the brain, which tends to maintain its weight.

Investigations
In a famine, laboratory investigations may be impractical, but will show that plasma free fatty acids are increased and there is ketosis and a mild metabolic acidosis. Plasma glucose is low but albumin concentration is often maintained because the liver still functions normally. Insulin secretion is diminished, glucagon and cortisol tend to increase, and reverse T_3 replaces normal tri-iodothyronine (p. 744). The resting metabolic rate falls, partly because of reduced lean body mass and partly because of hypothalamic compensation (Fig. 5.8, p. 107). The urine has a fixed specific gravity and creatinine excretion becomes low. There may be mild anaemia, leucopenia and thrombocytopenia. The erythrocyte sedimentation rate is normal unless there is infection. Tests of delayed skin hypersensitivity, e.g. to tuberculin, are falsely negative. The electrocardiogram shows sinus brachycardia and low voltage.

Management
Whether in a famine or in wasting secondary to disease, people need to be graded according to BMI (Box 5.27). People with mild starvation are in no danger; those with moderate starvation need extra feeding. People who are severely underweight need hospital care.

In severe starvation there is atrophy of the intestinal epithelium and of the exocrine pancreas, and the bile is dilute. When food becomes available, it should be given in small amounts at first. Food should be palatable and similar to the usual staple meal—for example, a cereal with some sugar, milk powder and oil. Salt should be restricted and micronutrient supplements may be essential (e.g. potassium, magnesium, zinc and multivitamins). Between 6.3 and 8.4 MJ/day (1500–2000 kcal/day) will prevent progressive

undernutrition, but additional calories may be required for regain of weight. The energy deficit can be calculated from the body weight deficit once the patient is rehydrated. Each kg of weight loss corresponds to ~25–29 MJ (~6000–7000 kcal), depending on the proportion of muscle and fat loss. During refeeding, a weight gain of 5% body weight per month indicates satisfactory progress. Other care is supportive, and includes care for the skin, adequate hydration, treatment of infections, and careful monitoring of body temperature since thermoregulation may be impaired.

Circumstances and resources are different in every famine, but many problems are non-medical and concern organisation, infrastructure, liaison, politics, procurement, security and ensuring that food is distributed on the basis of need. Lastly, plans must be made for the future for prevention and/or earlier intervention if similar circumstances prevail.

MALNUTRITION IN HOSPITAL

Malnutrition is a common problem in the hospital setting. Studies in the UK have shown that approximately one-third of patients are affected by moderate or severe malnutrition on admission. The elderly are particularly at risk. Once in hospital, many patients lose weight due to factors such as poor appetite, concurrent illness and even being kept 'nil by mouth' for investigations. Malnutrition is poorly recognised in hospital and has serious consequences, both for the individual patient and for the consumption of medical resources. Significant malnutrition leads to physical effects such as impaired immunity and muscle weakness, which in turn affect cardiac and respiratory function. The malnourished patient is often apathetic and withdrawn. This may be mistaken for a depressive illness and can affect cooperation with treatment. Poor nutrition leads to delayed wound healing after surgery and these patients are also more likely to develop post-operative infection. Thus, malnutrition leads to increased morbidity, mortality and length of hospital stay.

However, this deterioration can be prevented with proper monitoring and with the involvement of an appropriate multidisciplinary team. As a minimum standard, all patients should be weighed on admission to hospital. For those patients undergoing a prolonged admission, weight should be rechecked on a weekly basis. A useful scoring system for

---

5.30 ENERGY BALANCE IN OLD AGE

- **Body composition:** muscle mass is decreased and percentage body fat increased.
- **Energy expenditure:** with the fall in lean body mass, BMR is decreased and energy requirements are reduced.
- **Weight loss:** after weight gain throughout adult life, weight often falls beyond the age of 70 years. This may reflect decreased appetite, loss of smell and taste, and decreased interest and financial resources for food preparation, especially after loss of a partner.
- **BMI:** less reliable in old age as height is lost (due to kyphosis, osteoporotic crush fractures, loss of intervertebral disc spaces). Alternative measurements include arm demispan and knee height, which can be extrapolated to estimate height.

5

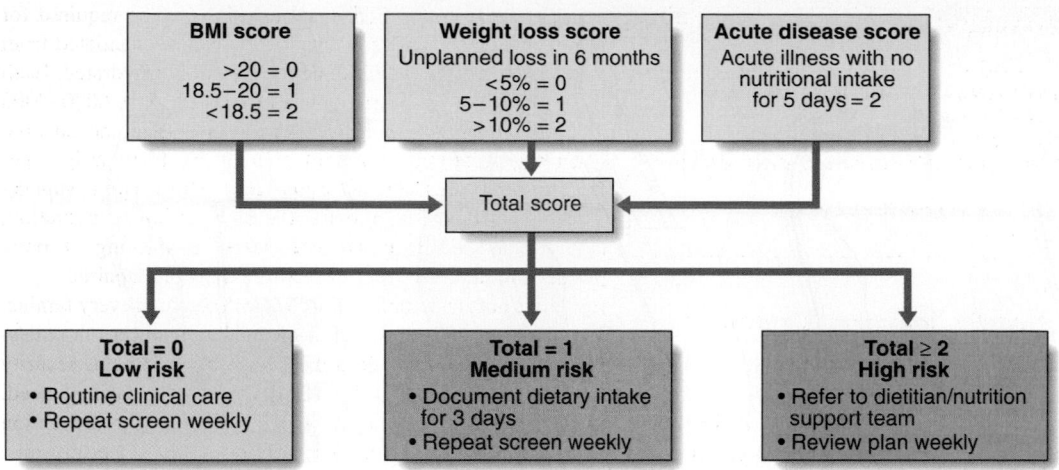

Fig. 5.15 Screening hospitalised patients for risk of malnutrition. Adapted from the British Association of Parenteral and Enteral Nutrition 'Malnutrition Universal Screening Tool' (www.bapen.org.uk).

identifying patients at nutritional risk is shown in Figure 5.15.

Nutritional support of the hospital patient

Normal diet

As a first step, patients should be encouraged to eat a normal and adequate diet. This is often neglected and there is evidence of substantial wastage in hospital food. A significant proportion of patients are able to consume normal food but do not take adequate amounts. Inadequate intake may be due to unpalatability of food, cultural and religious factors requiring patients to follow a specified diet, or simple problems such as difficulty with hand dexterity (arthritis, stroke) or immobility in bed. Patients who have been deemed to be at risk of malnutrition (Fig. 5.15) should be on a regular food chart to record the quantities eaten. Hospital catering departments have an important role in providing acceptable and adequate meals.

Dietary supplements

If a patient is unable to achieve sufficient nutritional intake from normal diet alone, then dietary supplements should be used. These are drinks with high energy and protein content, and are available in cartons as manufactured, flavoured products or made in the hospital kitchen from milk products and egg. To ensure that such supplements are taken regularly, they should be prescribed by the doctor and administered by the nursing staff, rather than simply being placed on the hospital bedside locker. Taking dietary supplements does not significantly affect the patient's consumption of normal food.

Enteral tube feeding

Those patients who are unable to swallow normally may require artificial nutritional support: for example, after acute stroke or throat surgery or with long-term neurological problems such as motor neuron disease and multiple sclerosis. The enteral route should always be used if possible, since feeding via the gastrointestinal tract preserves the integrity of the mucosal barrier. This prevents

bacteraemia and, in intensive care patients, reduces the risk of multi-organ failure.

If the need for artificial nutritional support is thought to be short-term, then feeding is instituted using a fine-bore nasogastric tube. It is crucial that the position of the tube in the stomach is confirmed before any fluid is administered as intrabronchial tube placement is not uncommon and severe respiratory complications can occur if fluid is inadvertently infused into a bronchus. Gastric aspirate has a pH < 4. If there is any doubt about the result of pH testing of the aspirate, then a chest X-ray should be performed to identify the tube below the diaphragm. Once this position is confirmed, specially prepared liquid feeds are administered either by continuous infusion or using a bolus technique. If the patient fails to absorb the administered feed or vomits it up, this may indicate gastric outlet obstruction or gastric stasis. This problem can be overcome by placing a nasojejunal tube or by using an endoscopic or radiological technique.

If there is a need for long-term artificial enteral feeding, a percutaneous endoscopic gastrostomy (PEG) should be sited (Fig. 5.16). A PEG tube is more comfortable for the patient, since there is no irritation to the nasal mucosa. The tube is less likely to become displaced or to be pulled out so the feed can be given more reliably. However, inserting a gastrostomy is an invasive procedure and is associated with complications such as local infection (30%) and inadvertent puncture of other intra-abdominal organs (causing peritonitis and bleeding). It takes approximately 10 days for a fibrous tract to form around the PEG tube. If the PEG is displaced or removed during that time, there is a high risk of peritonitis. If a problem occurs with food absorption, a jejunal extension can be placed through the PEG tube and liquid feed administered directly into the small bowel.

Parenteral nutrition

Intravenous feeding should only be used when enteral feeding is impossible. Parenteral feeding is expensive and carries higher risks of complications. The evidence suggests little benefit if parenteral feeding is required for less than 1 week.

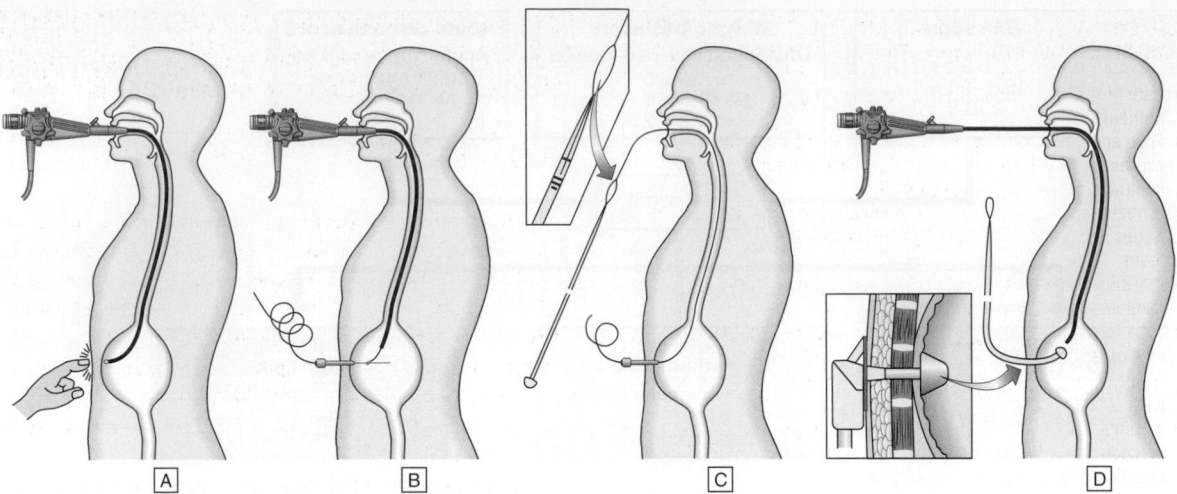

Fig. 5.16 Percutaneous endoscopic gastrostomy (PEG) placement. Ⓐ Finger pressure on anterior abdominal wall noted by endoscopist. Ⓑ Following insertion of a cannula through the anterior abdominal wall into the stomach, a guidewire is threaded through the cannula and grasped by the endoscopic forceps or snare. Ⓒ The endoscope is withdrawn with the guidewire. The gastrostomy tube is then attached to the guidewire. Ⓓ The guidewire and tube are pulled back through the mouth, oesophagus and stomach to exit on the anterior abdominal wall, and the endoscope is repassed to confirm the site of placement of the retention device. The latter closely abuts the gastric mucosa; its position is maintained by an external fixation device (see inset). It is also possible to place PEG tubes using fluoroscopic guidance in patients in whom endoscopy is difficult.

There are a number of possible routes for parenteral nutrition.

Peripheral venous cannula. This can only be used for low osmolality solutions due to the development of thrombophlebitis, and so is unsuitable for patients with high nutritional requirements.

Peripherally inserted cannula (PIC). This involves placing a 20 cm cannula into a mid-arm vein. Once again, hyperosmolar solutions cannot be used.

Peripherally inserted central catheter (PICC). Here, a 60 cm cannula is inserted into a vein in the antecubital fossa. The distal end lies in a central vein, allowing hyperosmolar solutions to be used.

Central line. The subclavian route is preferred to the internal jugular vein, due to lower infection rates. Hyperosmolar solutions can be used without difficulty. Lines need to be handled with strict aseptic technique, and a single lumen tube is preferred, to prevent infection.

If access has been gained to a central vein, nutritional support is usually given as an 'all in one' mixture. The main energy source is provided by carbohydrate, usually as glucose. The solution also contains amino acids, lipid emulsion, electrolytes, trace elements and vitamins. These are normally mixed as a large bag in a sterile environment, with the constituents adjusted according to the results of regular blood monitoring. Relevant tests include:

- daily: urea and electrolytes, glucose
- twice weekly: liver function tests, calcium, phosphate, magnesium
- weekly: full blood count, zinc, triglycerides
- monthly: copper, selenium, manganese.

If the patient develops fever or other features of septicaemia, it should be assumed that there is a line infection. Blood cultures should be taken, the existing line removed, the tip sent for bacteriological analysis, and a new line inserted using a guidewire technique.

Refeeding syndrome

When nutritional support is given to a malnourished patient, bodily mechanisms are shifted from a state of catabolism to one of anabolism. The administration of carbohydrates stimulates the release of insulin, which in turn leads to cellular uptake of phosphate, potassium and magnesium. Falling serum levels can lead to serious consequences, such as cardiac arrhythmias. It is essential that these are measured in blood and corrected before refeeding is commenced. In patients who are thiamin-deficient, Wernicke's encephalopathy might also be precipitated by refeeding with carbohydrates (p. 1218). This can be countered by giving thiamin before starting nutritional support.

Legal and ethical aspects of artificial nutritional support

The ability to intervene with artificial nutritional support raises many legal and ethical dilemmas. Starvation will inevitably lead to death but the inability to eat may be part of the natural course of a disease process. Difficult decisions are raised by situations such as cerebrovascular accidents, where swallowing ability is lost. The institution of feeding may speed recovery and lead to better functional outcome; on the other hand, feeding might prolong the process of dying in severe stroke. There will be different approaches to these decisions, depending on the local availability of resources as well as legal, cultural and religious influences. Some guidelines are given in Box 5.31.

5

5.31 ETHICAL AND LEGAL CONSIDERATIONS IN THE MANAGEMENT OF ARTIFICIAL NUTRITIONAL SUPPORT*

- Care of the sick involves the duty of providing adequate fluid and nutrients
- Food and fluid should not be withheld from a patient who expresses a desire to eat and drink, unless there is a medical contraindication (e.g. risk of aspiration)
- A treatment plan should include consideration of nutritional issues and should be agreed by all members of the health-care team
- In a situation of palliative care, tube feeding should only be instituted if it is needed to relieve symptoms
- Tube feeding is usually regarded in law as a medical treatment. Like other treatments, the need for such support should be reviewed on a regular basis and changes made in the light of clinical circumstances
- A competent adult patient must give consent for any invasive procedures, including the passage of a nasogastric tube or the insertion of a central venous cannula
- If a patient is unable to give consent, the health-care team should act in that person's best interests, taking into account any previously expressed wishes of the patient and the views of family
- Under certain specified circumstances (e.g. anorexia nervosa), it will be appropriate to provide artificial nutritional support to the unwilling patient

* Based on British Association for Parenteral and Enteral Nutrition guidelines (www.bapen.org.uk).

DISEASES OF 'MICRONUTRIENTS'—VITAMINS AND MINERALS

VITAMINS

Vitamins are organic substances with key roles in certain metabolic pathways; they are required in small amounts in food because they are not synthesised in the body (Box 5.32). Vitamins are broadly categorised into those that are fat-soluble (vitamins A, D, E and K) or water-soluble (vitamins of the B complex group and vitamin C). This is an important distinction, since deficiency of fat-soluble vitamins is seen in conditions of fat malabsorption (e.g. biliary obstruction).

Deficiencies of vitamins still occur in developed countries, e.g. of folate, thiamin and vitamins D and C. Older people and alcoholic patients are particularly at risk. Some of these deficiencies are induced by diseases or drugs. In developing countries, vitamin deficiency diseases are more prevalent; for example, vitamin A deficiency is a major cause of blindness in children. Thiamin deficiency and scurvy are seen in situations such as refugee camps.

5

5.32 SUMMARY OF CLINICALLY IMPORTANT VITAMINS

Recommended name (alternative name)	Sources	Deficiency	Excess	Investigations
FAT-SOLUBLE				
Vitamin A	Liver, milk, butter, cheese, fish oils	Xerophthalmia, night blindness, keratomalacia, follicular hyperkeratosis	Liver damage, bone damage, teratogenesis	Serum retinol
Vitamin D	Mainly manufactured in skin under the influence of sunlight	Rickets, osteomalacia	Hypercalcaemia	Plasma 25(OH)D or 1,25(OH)$_2$D
Vitamin E	Vegetables, seed oils	Haemolytic anaemia, ataxia		Plasma vitamin E
Vitamin K	Green vegetables, dairy products	Coagulation disorder		Coagulation assay (e.g. prothrombin time) ± plasma vitamin K
WATER-SOLUBLE				
Thiamin (Vitamin B$_1$)	Cereals, grains, bean, pork	Beri-beri, Wernicke–Korsakoff syndrome		RBC transketolase or whole blood vitamin B$_1$
Riboflavin (Vitamin B$_2$)	Milk	Glossitis, stomatitis		RBC glutathione reductase or whole blood vitamin B$_2$
Niacin (Nicotinic acid, nicotinamide, vitamin B$_3$)	Meat, cereals	Pellagra		Urinary metabolites
Vitamin B$_6$ (Pyridoxine)	Meat, fish, potatoes, bananas	Polyneuropathy	Polyneuropathy	Plasma pyridoxal phosphate or erythrocyte transaminase activation coefficient
Biotin	Liver, egg yolk, cereals, yeast	Dermatitis, alopecia, paraesthesiae		Whole blood or urine biotin
Folate	Liver	Anaemia		RBC folate
Vitamin B$_{12}$ (Cobalamin)	Animal products	Anaemia, neurological degeneration		Plasma B$_{12}$
Vitamin C (Ascorbic acid)	Fresh fruit and vegetables	Scurvy		Plasma ascorbic acid (daily intake) Leucocyte ascorbic acid (tissue stores)

(RBC = erythrocyte, red blood cell)

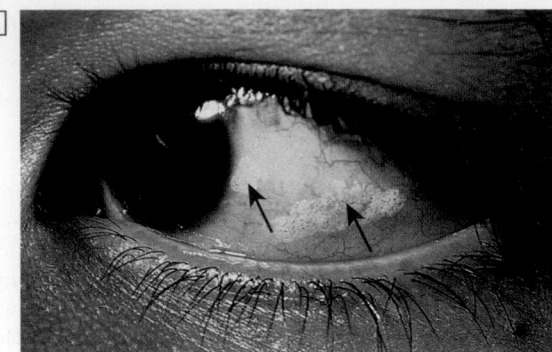

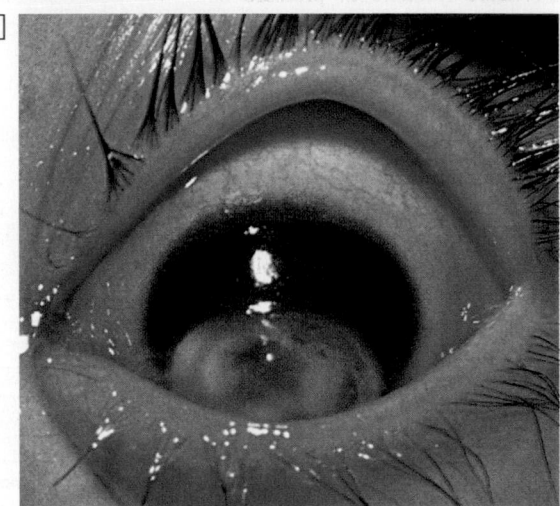

Fig. 5.17 Eye signs of vitamin A deficiency. [A] Bitot's spots showing the white triangular plaques (arrows). [B] Keratomalacia secondary to vitamin A deficiency in a 14-month-old child. There is liquefactive necrosis affecting the greater part of the cornea. The relative sparing of the superior aspect of the cornea is typical.

Some vitamins also have pharmacological actions when given at supraphysiological doses, e.g. the use of vitamin A (with precautions, p. 1300) for acne. Taking vitamin supplements is fashionable in many countries and some patients take very high doses. Side-effects or toxicity are most serious with high dosages of vitamins A, B$_6$ and D.

Investigation of suspected vitamin deficiency or excess may involve direct measurement of vitamin concentrations in plasma or in blood cells in which it is concentrated (Box 5.32). If direct assays are not available, measurement of activity of a metabolic pathway in which the vitamin is involved is an alternative.

FAT-SOLUBLE VITAMINS

Vitamin A (retinol)

Retinol itself is found only in foods of animal origin and liver is the richest source. However, vitamin A is also produced in the intestine by the splitting of carotenes, which are present in green vegetables, carrots and some fruits. Carotenes provide two-thirds of total vitamin A intake in the UK (and all of the intake in vegans). Retinol is metabolised to several other molecules, whose functions are listed below.

- 11-*cis* retinaldehyde is the initial part of the photoreceptor complex in rods of the retina.
- Retinoic acid induces differentiation of epithelial cells by binding to specific nuclear receptors, which turn on responsive genes. In vitamin A deficiency, mucus-secreting cells are replaced by keratin-producing cells.
- Retinoids are necessary for normal growth, fetal development, fertility, haematopoiesis and immune function. Deficient children suffer more severe respiratory infections and gastroenteritis, and morbidity and mortality are increased.

Deficiency

Globally, the most important consequence of vitamin A deficiency is blindness. Each year, approximately 500 000 new cases of blindness occur in young children, mostly in Asia. The WHO is giving high priority to its prevention.

Night blindness is the earliest sign of deficiency and is due to an impairment of the dark adaptation process. The diagnosis is supported by low plasma retinol concentration and is confirmed by marked improvement in dark adaptation following therapeutic doses of retinol. If untreated, the

condition progresses with loss of the normal mucous cells from the cornea, which takes on a dull, hazy, lacklustre appearance due to keratinisation; this is described as xerophthalmia. Bitot's spots may appear as glistening white plaques of desquamated thickened conjunctival epithelium, usually triangular in shape and firmly adherent to the underlying conjunctiva (Fig. 5.17). The final consequence of deficiency is the development of keratomalacia, leading to corneal ulceration, scarring and irreversible blindness.

On diagnosis of vitamin A deficiency a single large dose of 60 mg retinol as palmitate or acetate (200 000 U) should be given orally or, if there is vomiting or severe diarrhoea, by intramuscular injection. The oral dose should be repeated the next day and again prior to discharge or at a follow-up visit. Prevention is also an important issue. In countries where vitamin A deficiency is endemic, pregnant women should be advised to eat dark green leafy vegetables and yellow fruits, to build up stores of retinol in the fetal liver. Babies should also be given such vegetables or locally available carotene-rich fruits. In communities where xerophthalmia occurs, single prophylactic oral doses of 60 mg retinol (200 000 U) as palmitate given to pre-school children significantly reduces mortality from gastroenteritis

5

and respiratory infections; a similar large dose is indicated in any child with measles. Repeated oral administration of these doses to children every 4–6 months is now used in some endemic areas.

Toxicity

Single large doses in children, as described above, are well tolerated. The most serious side-effects of repeated moderate or high doses of retinol are liver damage, hyperostosis and teratogenicity. Women in developed countries who are pregnant are therefore advised not to take vitamin A supplements. Acute overdose leads to nausea and headache, increased intracranial pressure and skin desquamation. Excessive intake of carotene can cause a benign condition in which pigmentation of the skin occurs (hypercarotenosis); this gradually fades when the excessive intake is stopped.

Vitamin D

The natural form of vitamin D, cholecalciferol, is a modified steroid. It is formed in the skin by the action of UV light on 7-dehydrocholesterol, a metabolite of cholesterol. Natural dietary sources include egg yolk, oily fish, butter and milk, but these contribute very little to the body's requirements compared with that generated in skin. Cholecalciferol itself is not biologically active, and is converted in the liver to 25-hydroxycholecalciferol (25(OH)D), which is further hydroxylated in the kidneys to 1,25-dihydroxychole-calciferol (1,25(OH)$_2$D), the active form of vitamin D (Fig. 20.16, p. 772). 1,25(OH)$_2$D activates specific intra-cellular receptors which influence calcium metabolism. The effects of vitamin D deficiency (calcium deficiency, rickets and osteomalacia) are described on pages 772 and 1126.

The pharmaceutical form of pure vitamin D is (ergo)-calciferol, made by the action of UV light on ergosterol (a sterol found in fungi). Ergocalciferol is added (in controlled amounts) to margarines and (in North America) to milk. Excessive doses of ergocalciferol, or the hydroxylated metabolites which are also available, cause hypercalcaemia (p. 772).

Vitamin E

There are eight related fat-soluble substances with vitamin E activity. The most important dietary form is α-tocopherol. Rich sources include vegetable oils, whole-grain cereals and nuts. Vitamin E has many direct metabolic actions. It is an important antioxidant, preventing oxidation of poly-unsaturated fatty acids in cell membranes by free radicals; it plays a role in maintaining cell membrane structure; it affects DNA synthesis and cell signalling; and it is involved in the anti-inflammatory and immune systems.

In animal studies, vitamin E deficiency leads to myopathies, neuropathies and liver necrosis. This results from the effects of cell membrane damage with consequent cell leakage. Human deficiency states are rare and have only been described in premature infants and in malabsorption. The first feature of human deficiency is a mild haemolytic anaemia. In chronic fat malabsorption, ataxia and visual scotomas occur which respond to vitamin E.

Diets rich in vitamin E are consumed in countries with lower rates of coronary heart disease. However, randomised controlled trials have not demonstrated cardioprotective effects of vitamin E and other antioxidants.

Vitamin K

Adequate amounts of vitamin K are normally supplied in the average diet (from leafy vegetables and liver) or synthesised by bacteria in the colon. Vitamin K is a co-factor in the production of an unusual amino acid, γ-carboxyglutamate (gla). Gla residues are part of the protein molecule of four of the coagulation factors (II, VII, IX and X, p. 1008), conferring on these proteins their capacity to bind to phospholipid surfaces in the presence of calcium. For this reason, vitamin K deficiency leads to prolonged coagulation and bleeding.

Vitamin K has important roles in three situations:

- In the newborn, primary deficiency can occur because placental transfer of vitamin K is inefficient, the neonatal bowel has not yet acquired bacteria and breast milk contains little of the vitamin. Vitamin K is given routinely to newborn babies to prevent haemorrhagic disease of the newborn. This remains a significant cause of infant mortality and morbidity on a world-wide basis.
- In obstructive jaundice, dietary vitamin K is not absorbed and it is very important to administer the vitamin in parenteral form before surgery.
- Warfarin and related anticoagulants (p. 1009) act by antagonising vitamin K.

WATER-SOLUBLE VITAMINS

Thiamin (vitamin B$_1$)

Thiamin is widely distributed in foods of both vegetable and animal origin, although cereals are the main sources. Thiamin pyrophosphate (TPP) is involved in carbohydrate metabolism. It is an essential co-enzyme for the decarboxylation of pyruvate to acetyl-co-enzyme A. This is the bridge between glycolysis and the tricarboxylic acid (Krebs) cycle. TPP is also the co-enzyme for transketolase in the hexose monophosphate shunt pathway and for decarboxylation of α-ketoglutarate to succinate in the Krebs cycle. Consequently, when thiamin is deficient:

- Cells cannot metabolise glucose aerobically to generate energy as ATP; this is likely to affect the nervous system first, since it depends largely on glucose for its energy requirements.
- There is accumulation of pyruvic and lactic acids, which produce vasodilatation and increased cardiac output.

Deficiency—beri-beri

In the developed world, thiamin deficiency is mainly encountered in chronic alcoholics. Poor diet, impaired absorption, storage and phosphorylation of thiamin in the liver, and the increased requirements for thiamin due to the high energy in ethanol all contribute to deficiency. In the developing world, deficiency usually arises as a consequence of a diet based on polished rice. The body has very limited stores of thiamin, so deficiency starts after only 1 month on a thiamin-free diet and takes several forms:

- Infantile beri-beri is seen in exclusively breastfed infants of thiamin-deficient mothers, and is invariably fatal.

- Dry (or neurological) beri-beri manifests with chronic peripheral neuropathy, and wrist and/or foot drop, and may cause Korsakoff's psychosis and Wernicke's encephalopathy (pp. 246 and 1217).
- Wet (or cardiac) beri-beri causes generalised oedema due to biventricular heart failure with pulmonary congestion.

In dry beri-beri, response to thiamin is not uniformly good. However, multivitamin therapy seems to produce some improvement, suggesting that other vitamin deficiencies may be involved. Wernicke's encephalopathy and wet beri-beri should be treated without delay with i.v. Pabrinex, as described on pages 246 and 1217. Korsakoff's psychosis is irreversible and does not respond to thiamin treatment.

Riboflavin (vitamin B₂)

Riboflavin is part of the oxidation chain in the mitochondria, acting as a co-enzyme in oxidation reduction reactions. It is widely distributed in animal and vegetable foods, the richest supply coming from milk and its non-fat products. Levels of the vitamin are low in staple cereals but germination increases its content. It is destroyed under alkaline conditions by heat and by exposure to UV light.

Clinical deficiency is rare in developed countries. It mainly affects the tongue and lips and manifests as glossitis, angular stomatitis and cheilosis. The genitals may be affected, as well as the skin areas rich in sebaceous glands, causing nasolabial or facial dyssebacea. Rapid recovery usually follows administration of riboflavin 10 mg daily by mouth.

Niacin (nicotinic acid and nicotinamide)

Nicotinic acid and nicotinamide have equal biological activity and are considered together in foods under the generic term 'niacin'. Nicotinamide is an essential part of the two important pyridine nucleotides, nicotinamide adenine dinucleotide (NAD) and nicotinamide adenine dinucleotide phosphate (NADP), which play a key role as hydrogen acceptors and donors for many enzymes. A special feature of this vitamin is that it can be synthesised in the body in limited amounts from tryptophan, e.g. from eggs and cheese.

Deficiency — pellagra

Pellagra was formerly endemic among the poor who subsisted chiefly on maize; maize contains niacytin, which is a form of niacin that the body is unable to utilise. Pellagra can develop in only 8 weeks in individuals eating diets that are very deficient in niacin and tryptophan. It remains a problem in parts of Africa, and is occasionally seen in alcoholics and in patients with chronic small intestinal disease in developed countries. Pellagra can occur in Hartnup's disease, a genetic disorder characterised by impaired absorption of several amino acids, including tryptophan. It is also seen occasionally in carcinoid syndrome (p. 791), when tryptophan is utilised in the excessive production of 5-HT, rather than being available for the synthesis of niacin.

Pellagra has been called the disease of the three Ds:

- *Dermatitis*. Characteristically, there is erythema resembling severe sunburn, appearing symmetrically

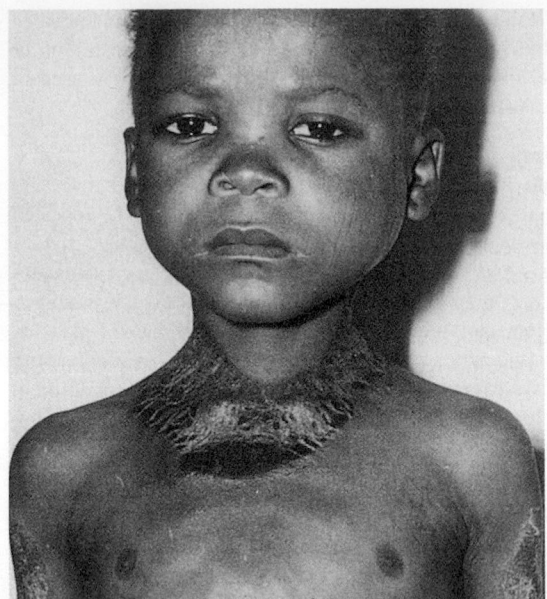

Fig. 5.18 Dermatitis due to pellagra (niacin deficiency). The lesions appear on those parts of the body exposed to sunlight. The classic 'Casal's necklace' can be seen around the neck and upper chest.

over the parts of the body exposed to sunlight, particularly the limbs and especially on the neck, but not the face (Casal's necklace, Fig. 5.18). The skin lesions may progress to vesiculation, cracking, exudation and secondary infection.
- *Diarrhoea*. This is often associated with anorexia, nausea, glossitis and dysphagia, reflecting the presence of a non-infective inflammation that extends throughout the gastrointestinal tract.
- *Dementia*. In severe deficiency, delirium occurs acutely, with dementia developing in chronic cases.

Treatment is with nicotinamide, given in a dose of 100 mg 8-hourly by mouth or by the parenteral route. The response is usually rapid. Within 24 hours, the erythema diminishes, the diarrhoea ceases and a striking improvement occurs in the patient's mental state.

Pyridoxine (vitamin B₆)

Pyridoxine, pyridoxal and pyridoxamine are three closely related compounds with similar physiological actions. The active form of the vitamin in humans is pyridoxal 5-phosphate, the co-enzyme for a large number of enzymes involved in the metabolism of amino acids. Vitamin B₆ is available in most foods, but rich sources include meat, fish, potatoes and bananas.

Dietary deficiency seems to be rare. However, certain drugs, such as isoniazid and penicillamine, act as chemical antagonists to pyridoxine and cause deficiency. Isoniazid causes peripheral neuropathy, which responds to B₆ administration. Some cases of sideroblastic anaemia (p. 1023) also respond to treatment with pyridoxine.

Large doses of vitamin B₆ have an antiemetic effect in radiotherapy-induced nausea. It has become popular to

5

take vitamin B_6 supplements for the treatment of nausea in pregnancy, carpal tunnel syndrome and premenstrual syndrome but there is no convincing evidence of benefit. Very high doses of vitamin B_6 taken for several months can cause a sensory polyneuropathy.

Biotin

Biotin is a co-enzyme in carbohydrate, fatty acid and amino acid metabolism. Biotin deficiency rarely occurs with a natural diet but is occasionally seen in patients consuming raw eggs because avidin in raw eggs binds to biotin in the intestine and inactivates it. The clinical features of deficiency include scaly dermatitis, alopecia and paraesthesia. A form of seborrhoeic dermatitis of infants responds to biotin.

Vitamin B_{12} and folate

These vitamins and the haematological disorders due to their deficiency are discussed on pages 1027–1029.

Vitamin B_{12} deficiency—neurological features

Severe prolonged vitamin B_{12} deficiency may cause megaloblastic anaemia and/or neurological degeneration. In some cases the neurological disease predominates, perhaps because adequate intake of folate maintains erythropoiesis. Vitamin B_{12}, but not folate, is needed for the integrity of myelin. In severe deficiency there is insidious, diffuse and uneven demyelination. It may be clinically manifest as peripheral neuropathy or spinal cord degeneration affecting both posterior and lateral columns ('subacute combined degeneration of the spinal cord', p. 1245) or there may be cerebral manifestations (resembling dementia) or optic atrophy. Treatment with hydroxocobalamin should produce improvement but this may be slow.

Folic acid in the prevention of neural tube defects

Three major birth defects (spina bifida, anencephaly and encephalocele) all result from imperfect closure of the neural tube which takes place 3–4 weeks after conception. Folate is directly involved in DNA and RNA synthesis and a higher than normal level is required during embryonic development. Maternal supplementation with folate reduces the risk of neural tube defects (Box 5.34). The UK Department of Health advises that women who have experienced a pregnancy affected by a neural tube defect should take 5 mg of folic acid daily from before conception and throughout the first trimester. In addition, all women planning a pregnancy are advised to include good sources of folate in their diet. Liver is the richest source of folate but an alternative source (e.g. leafy vegetables) is advised in early pregnancy because of the high vitamin A content of liver (p. 123).

5.34 PERICONCEPTUAL FOLATE SUPPLEMENTATION AND NEURAL TUBE DEFECTS | **EBM**

'Folate supplementation in advance of conception and during the first trimester reduces the incidence of neural tube defects by ~70%.'

- Lumley J, et al. (Cochrane Review). Cochrane Library, issue 3, 2005.

For further information: 💻 www.cochrane.org

Vitamin C (ascorbic acid)

Ascorbic acid is the most active reducing agent in the aqueous phase of living tissues and is involved in intracellular electron transfer. Crucially, it takes part in the hydroxylation of proline and lysine in protocollagen to hydroxyproline and hydroxylysine in mature collagen. Ascorbic acid is present in fresh fruit and vegetables. Unfortunately, it is very easily destroyed by heat, increased pH and light, and is very soluble in water. Hence many traditional cooking methods reduce or eliminate it.

It has been suggested that high-dose vitamin C improves immune function (including resistance to the common cold) and cholesterol turnover but such effects remain unproven in controlled trials. Daily intakes of more than 1 g/day have been reported to cause diarrhoea and the formation of renal oxalate stones.

Deficiency—scurvy

Defective formation of collagen impairs healing of wounds, and causes capillary haemorrhage and reduced platelet adhesiveness (normal platelets are rich in ascorbate). Precipitants and clinical features of scurvy are shown in Box 5.35.

For treatment, a dose of 250 mg vitamin C 8-hourly by mouth should saturate the tissues quickly. The general deficiencies of the patient's former diet also need to be corrected and other vitamin supplements given if necessary.

5.35 SCURVY—VITAMIN C DEFICIENCY

Precipitants

Dietary deficiency
- Lack of dietary fruit and vegetables > 2 months
- Infants fed exclusively on boiled milk

Increased requirement for vitamin C
- Trauma, surgery, burns, infections
- Smoking
- Drugs (corticosteroids, aspirin, indometacin, tetracycline)

Clinical features
- Swollen gums which bleed easily
- Perifollicular and petechial haemorrhages
- Ecchymoses
- Haemarthrosis
- Gastrointestinal bleeding
- Anaemia
- Poor wound healing

INORGANIC NUTRIENTS

Sixteen or more inorganic elements are essential dietary constituents for humans (Box 5.36). Deficiency disease is seen when there is inadequate dietary intake or excessive loss from the body. Toxic effects have also been observed from self-medication and disordered absorption or excretion. Examples of clinical manifestations of toxicity are readily seen with excess of iron (haemochromatosis or haemosiderosis), fluoride (fluorosis seen in India, p. 226), copper (Wilson's disease) and selenium (selenosis seen in parts of China).

5.36 ESSENTIAL INORGANIC NUTRIENTS

- Sodium
- Potassium
- Chloride, magnesium
- Calcium
- Phophorus
- Iron
- Zinc
- Copper
- Chromium
- Selenium
- Manganese
- Molybdenum
- Iodine
- Fluoride
- Cobalt[1]
- Sulphur[2]

[1] Physiologically active in the form of vitamin B_{12}.
[2] Required in the form of the amino acids methionine and cysteine.

Calcium

Calcium is the most abundant cation in the body and powerful homeostatic mechanisms exist for maintaining circulating ionised calcium levels (p. 771). The main dietary sources are listed in Box 5.37. Calcium content in food is rarely inadequate but calcium absorption may be impaired in the following circumstances:

- vitamin D deficiency (pp. 771 and 1126)
- malabsorption secondary to small intestinal disease
- with foods containing oxalate (e.g. spinach) or phytate (whole-grain cereals) that tend to form insoluble salts with calcium.

Calcium deficiency causes impaired bone mineralisation. The potential benefits of a high calcium intake in osteoporosis are discussed on page 1125.

5.37 DIETARY SOURCES OF CALCIUM

- Milks, cheese, yoghurt, eggs
- Fish eaten with bones, e.g. sardines, pilchards
- Some shellfish
- Some nuts, e.g. almonds, peanuts
- Some legumes, e.g. chickpeas, beans
- Bread (if fortified)

Phosphorus

Dietary deficiency of phosphorus is rare since it is present in nearly all foods and phosphates are added to a number of processed foods. Phosphate deficiency occurs:

- in premature infants fed on human milk
- in patients with renal tubular phosphate loss (p. 441)
- due to prolonged high dosage of aluminium hydroxide (p. 490)
- sometimes when alcoholics are fed with high-carbohydrate foods
- in patients receiving parenteral nutrition if inadequate phosphate is provided.

Deficiency causes hypophosphataemia (p. 441) and muscle weakness secondary to ATP deficiency.

Iron

Iron is needed in the synthesis of haemoglobin. It is also involved in the transport of electrons within cells and in a

5.38 DIETARY SOURCES OF IRON

Haem iron	
• Muscle meat (red more than white)	• Organ meat (e.g. liver) • Fish and shellfish

Non-haem iron	
• Oatmeal • Legumes (peas, beans), nuts, dried fruit • Wholemeal bread	• Iron-fortified cereal foods • Red wine • Chocolate

number of enzyme reactions. The major consequence of iron deficiency is anaemia, which is discussed on page 1025. This is one of the most important nutritional causes of ill health in all parts of the world.

There is no physiological mechanism for excretion of iron, so homeostasis depends on the regulation of iron absorption. The normal daily loss of iron is 1 mg, arising from desquamated surface cells and intestinal losses. A regular loss of only 2 ml of blood per day doubles the iron requirement. On average 30 mg of iron is lost during menstruation and hence pre-menopausal women require about twice as much iron as men.

Absorption of haem iron in foods of animal origin is usually high, whereas the non-haem iron in cereals and vegetables is poorly absorbed. Fruits and vegetables with vitamin C content enhance iron absorption, while the tannins in tea reduce it. Foods rich in iron are listed in Box 5.38. Because of the inefficient absorption of iron, the requirement for iron in the diet is about ten times the body's physiological requirements.

Dietary iron overload is occasionally observed and results in iron accumulation in the liver and, rarely, cirrhosis. Haemochromatosis results from an inherited increase in iron absorption and is described on page 974.

Iodine

Iodine is needed for synthesis of thyroid hormones (p. 744). It is present in sea fish, seaweed and most plant foods grown near the sea. The amount of iodine in soil and water influences the iodine content of most foods. Iodine is, however, lacking in the highest mountainous areas of the world (e.g. the Alps and the Himalayas) and in the soil of frequently flooded plains (e.g. Bangladesh). About a billion people in the world are estimated to have an inadequate iodine intake and hence are at risk of iodine deficiency disorder. Goitre is the most common manifestation, affecting 200 million people world-wide (p. 759).

In those areas where most women have endemic goitre, 1% or more of babies are born with cretinism (characterised by mental and physical retardation). There is a higher prevalence than usual of deafness, slowed reflexes and poor learning in the remaining population. The best way of preventing neonatal cretinism is by ensuring adequate levels of iodine during pregnancy. This can be achieved by intramuscular injections with 1–2 ml of iodised poppy seed oil (475–950 mg iodine) to women of child-bearing age every 3–5 years, by administration of iodised oil orally

5

at 6-monthly or yearly intervals to adults and children, or by providing iodised salt for cooking.

Zinc

Zinc is present in most foods of vegetable and animal origin. It is an essential component of many enzymes, including carbonic anhydrase, alcohol dehydrogenase and alkaline phosphatase. Acute zinc deficiency has been reported in patients receiving prolonged zinc-free parenteral nutrition and causes diarrhoea, mental apathy, a moist eczematoid dermatitis especially around the mouth, and loss of hair. Zinc deficiency is responsible for the clinical features seen in the very rare congenital disorder known as acrodermatitis enteropathica (growth retardation, hair loss and chronic diarrhoea). In the Middle East chronic deficiency has been described in association with dwarfism and hypogonadism. Zinc deficiency has also been observed secondary to protein energy malnutrition (PEM), malabsorption syndromes, and alcoholism and associated hepatic cirrhosis. In PEM, associated zinc deficiency causes thymic atrophy, and zinc supplements may accelerate the healing of skin lesions, promote general well-being, improve appetite and reduce the morbidity associated with the malnourished state.

Selenium

There is a family of seleno-enzymes that includes glutathione peroxidase, which helps prevent free radical damage to cells, and monodeiodinase which converts thyroxine to triiodothyronine (p. 744). North American soil has higher selenium content than European and Asian soil, and the decreasing reliance of Europe on imported American food in recent decades has increased the prevalence of selenium deficiency. This can cause hypothyroidism, cardiomyopathy in children (Keshan's disease) and myopathy in adults.

Fluoride

Fluoride has an important influence on the prevention of dental caries, since it increases the resistance of the enamel to acid attack. If the water supply of a locality contains more than 1 part per million (ppm) of fluoride, the incidence of dental caries is low. Soft waters usually contain no fluoride, whilst very hard waters may contain over 10 ppm. The benefit of fluoride is greatest when it is taken before the permanent teeth erupt, while their enamel is being laid down. The addition of traces of fluoride (at 1 ppm) to public water supplies is now a widespread practice.

Chronic fluoride poisoning is occasionally seen where the water supply contains > 10 ppm fluoride. It can also occur in workers handling cryolite (aluminium sodium fluoride), used in smelting aluminium. Features of fluoride poisoning are described on page 226.

Other minerals

The roles of sodium, potassium and magnesium are discussed in Chapter 16.

Copper metabolism is abnormal in Wilson's disease (p. 975). Deficiency occasionally occurs in young children; the main features are microcytic hypochromic anaemia, neutropenia, retarded growth, skeletal rarefaction and dermatosis.

Chromium facilitates the action of insulin. Deficiency presents as hyperglycaemia and has been reported in some children with PEM and as a rare complication of prolonged parenteral nutrition.

FURTHER INFORMATION

Books and journal articles

Ashton J, Seymour H. The new public health. Milton Keynes: Open University; 1995.

Detels R, Breslow L. Current scope and concerns in public health. In: Detels R, McEwen J, Beaglehole R, Tanaka H. Oxford textbook of public health. 4th edn. Oxford: Oxford University Press; 2002.

Evans RG, Barer ML, Marmor TR, eds. Why are some people healthy and others not? The determinants of health of populations. New York: Aldine de Gruyter; 1994.

Greaves I, Porter K, eds. Pre-hospital medicine: the principles and practice of immediate care. London: Arnold; 1999.

Institute of Naval Medicine Report R98013. The prevention and management of diving accidents. Gosport: Undersea Medicine Division, Institute of Naval Medicine; 1998.

Pollard A, Murdoch D, eds. The high altitude medicine handbook. 3rd edn. Oxford: Radcliffe Medical; 2003.

Wilkinson R, Marmot M. The solid facts. Geneva: WHO; 1998.

Websites

www.cdc.gov/nccdphp/dnpa/obesity *The USA Centers for Disease Control statistics and other links.*

www.hpa.org.uk/radiation *The Health Protection Agency provides information and links on all forms of radiation for patients and professionals.*

www.nhlbi.nih.gov/guidelines *The National Heart, Lung and Blood Institute provides several theoretical and practical tools for managing obesity.*

www.who.int/nut *WHO recommendations and intervention programmes for macronutrient and micronutrient-related diseases.*

Telephone numbers

In the UK two organisations provide advice on the clinical management of diving illness and the availability of the nearest recompression facility:

Aberdeen Royal Infirmary +44 (0)1224 681818. *Hyperbaric doctor on call.*

Royal Navy +44 (0)7831 151523.

5

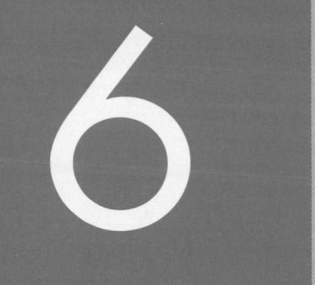

6

W.T.A. TODD
S. SUNDAR
D.N.J. LOCKWOOD

Principles of infectious disease

Infection and the disease that results from it remain the greatest killers of humankind. The pathology of infection differs from all other disease processes in that it comprises an interaction between the human body and another organism, usually microscopic in nature. Infection has been part of our evolution, evident by the development of a complex immune system, the major function of which is to combat and prevent infection. All systems of the body are susceptible to infection, and understanding infection and its management is integral to every medical subspecialty and to every aspect of clinical care.

INFECTIOUS AGENTS

The concept of an infectious agent emerged in the mid-19th century and was eruditely defined by a German physician, Robert Koch (1843–1910), using *Bacillus anthracis* in mice. He demonstrated the isolation of this single microorganism from cases of anthrax, the reproduction of the disease by inoculation of the organism into experimental animals and the re-isolation of the same organism from these experimental cases. The fulfilment of these sequential events has become the standard for the definition of an infectious agent (known as Koch's postulates).

The agents causing infection in man fall into four major classes.

Prions

These are the simplest infectious agents, consisting of a single protein molecule with the ability to catalyse a conformational change in an endogenous protein (PrP). Disease is produced by the structural and functional changes that result (p. 1234).

Viruses

Viruses contain two types of macromolecule: proteins and nucleic acids, the latter of only one type (either DNA or RNA). They cannot reproduce autonomously, needing to enter a prokaryotic or eukaryotic cell and 'divert' the intracellular mechanisms to viral reproduction.

Bacteria

Long known as 'prokaryotes', bacteria share the following essential features: they contain both RNA and DNA, have facilities for protein metabolism and are generally free living, although some (e.g. *Chlamydia* and rickettsiae) are intracellular parasites. Bacteria have no nuclei but reproduce autonomously. They include mycoplasmas, spirochaetes, *Actinomyces*, bacilli and cocci.

Eukaryotes

These organisms exhibit subcellular compartmentalisation with intracellular functions being achieved by specific organelles, e.g. nucleus, chloroplasts, mitochondria and Golgi apparatus.

The eukaryotes involved in human infection include fungi (p. 372), protozoa (unicellular eukaryotes with a flexible cell membrane, p. 342) and parasitic worms (helminths, p. 360).

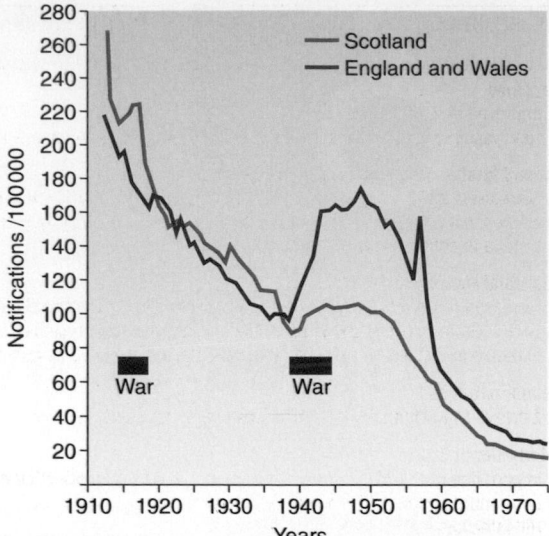

Fig. 6.1 Pulmonary tuberculosis in the UK during the 20th century.

EPIDEMIOLOGY OF INFECTION

PATTERNS OF INFECTION IN DEVELOPED COUNTRIES

During the last 100 years the incidence of communicable diseases in developed countries has fallen dramatically. This has been due to improved nutrition, better sanitation and housing (Fig. 6.1), immunisation and antimicrobial chemotherapy. Infections such as diphtheria, poliomyelitis and tetanus have decreased and in some locations have almost disappeared. Smallpox, a lethal virus infection, has been eradicated from the world while another lethal infection, human immunodeficiency virus (HIV), has emerged in pandemic proportions.

The factors responsible for these changes are summarised in Box 6.1. These include the development of microbial resistance, immunosuppression, foreign travel, altered sexual behaviour, injection drug use, changes in animal husbandry and food production, and the availability and uptake of vaccines. Some infections which had declined or been controlled are now resurgent, e.g. tuberculosis in a multi-resistant form. In addition, the identification of microorganisms as causative agents in conditions previously unrecognised as having an infectious aetiology has opened up new therapeutic avenues: for example, the aetiological role of *Helicobacter pylori* in peptic ulceration.

PATTERNS OF INFECTION IN TROPICAL COUNTRIES

In less developed countries, especially in the tropics, infection remains one of the most common causes of disease

6.1 INFLUENCES ON PATTERNS OF INFECTION IN DEVELOPED COUNTRIES

Vaccines
- Improved uptake of vaccines
- New vaccines, e.g. conjugate vaccines for *Haemophilus influenzae* type B, meningococcal type C disease, pneumococcal vaccine

Animal husbandry and preparation of food
- *Salmonella* and *Campylobacter* infections originating in poultry and eggs
- *Escherichia coli* type O157, causing haemorrhagic colitis and haemolytic uraemic syndrome, associated with beef
- Listeria infections from soft cheeses

Microbial resistance
- Increased resistance in common bacterial pathogens including *Staphylococcus aureus* (meticillin-resistant, MRSA; glycopeptide-resistant, GRSA), Gram-negative bacilli (extended spectrum β-lactamase resistance, ESBL), *Streptococcus pneumoniae* (penicillin), vancomycin-resistant enterococci (VRE) and multidrug-resistant *Mycobacterium tuberculosis* (MDRTB)

Sexual behaviour
- Increase in HIV infection and other sexually transmitted diseases

International travel
- Importation of malaria (average number of cases per annum 2500 to UK, 2000 to France, 1000 to Germany)
- Legionnaires' disease from holiday hotels
- HIV infection

Immunosuppression
- Advances in the treatment of malignant disease and in organ transplantation, leading to infections with opportunistic organisms

Resurgence of infections
- Tuberculosis—world-wide, especially in association with HIV infection
- Poliomyelitis in the Netherlands (in a religious sect refusing vaccines)
- Streptococcal infections in the USA (including rheumatic fever)
- Measles in the USA (mainly in immigrants in inner cities)
- Diphtheria in the former Soviet Union
- Hepatitis A and typhoid fever in the former Yugoslavia

Injection drug addiction

'New' and emerging infections
- West Nile fever in the USA
- Bioterrorism
- Avian/pandemic 'flu

and death, particularly in children, determining the strength of the working man or woman, the health of the mother and the pattern of systemic disease, including neoplasia, in the community (Box 6.2). Multiple disease is common and the clinical patterns of illness differ from those in temperate zones. The complex interaction between chronic parasitism, respiratory and diarrhoeal diseases, tuberculosis, malnutrition and its immunosuppressive effects, and HIV infection has a particularly deleterious effect on the health of children. Up to 40% of children may die before they reach 5 years of age in these situations. Chronic infections can damage important organs: liver and kidneys in schistosomiasis, the heart in trypanosomiasis cruzi, lungs, bones and lymph nodes in tuberculosis, bone marrow reserves in malaria and hookworm infections, the gut in tropical sprue and nerves in leprosy. These organs may then fail under increased demands of work, growth, pregnancy or additional disease. Chronic ill health is thereby imposed on millions of sufferers in the tropics.

Disease control by vaccination (e.g. yellow fever), vector control (e.g. malaria, African trypanosomiasis) and general improvement in living standards (e.g. plague, relapsing fever) has had a significant impact, but remains imperfect and the diseases reappear. Other epidemic diseases, such as cholera in Asia and meningococcal meningitis in Africa, remain largely uncontrolled and kill hundreds of thousands of people annually. Efficient vaccines exist for many

6.2 PATTERNS OF INFECTION IN TROPICAL COUNTRIES

Killers of children, preventable but variably prevalent

• Measles	• Hepatitis B
• Diphtheria	• Gastroenteritis
• Pertussis	• Malaria
• Poliomyelitis	• Meningococcal disease
• Tetanus	• Acute diarrhoeal illness

Chronic disabling infections, widely prevalent

• Leprosy	• Amoebiasis
• Tuberculosis	• Intestinal helminths
• Trachoma	• Schistosomiasis
• Malaria	• Filarial infection
• Trypanosomiasis cruzi	

Epidemic diseases, actual (marked *) and potential

• Louse-borne typhus and relapsing fever	• HIV infection*
• Cholera*	• Tuberculosis*, in association with HIV epidemic
• Malaria	• Influenza
• Visceral leishmaniasis*	• Enteric fevers

Infections liable to focal outbreaks (zoonotic or vector-borne)

• Dengue fever, e.g. Thailand	• Plague, e.g. Vietnam
• Cutaneous leishmaniasis, e.g. Sudan	• Anthrax, e.g. USA (bioterrorism)
• African trypanosomiasis, e.g. Zambia	• Yellow fever, e.g. Kenya, Nigeria

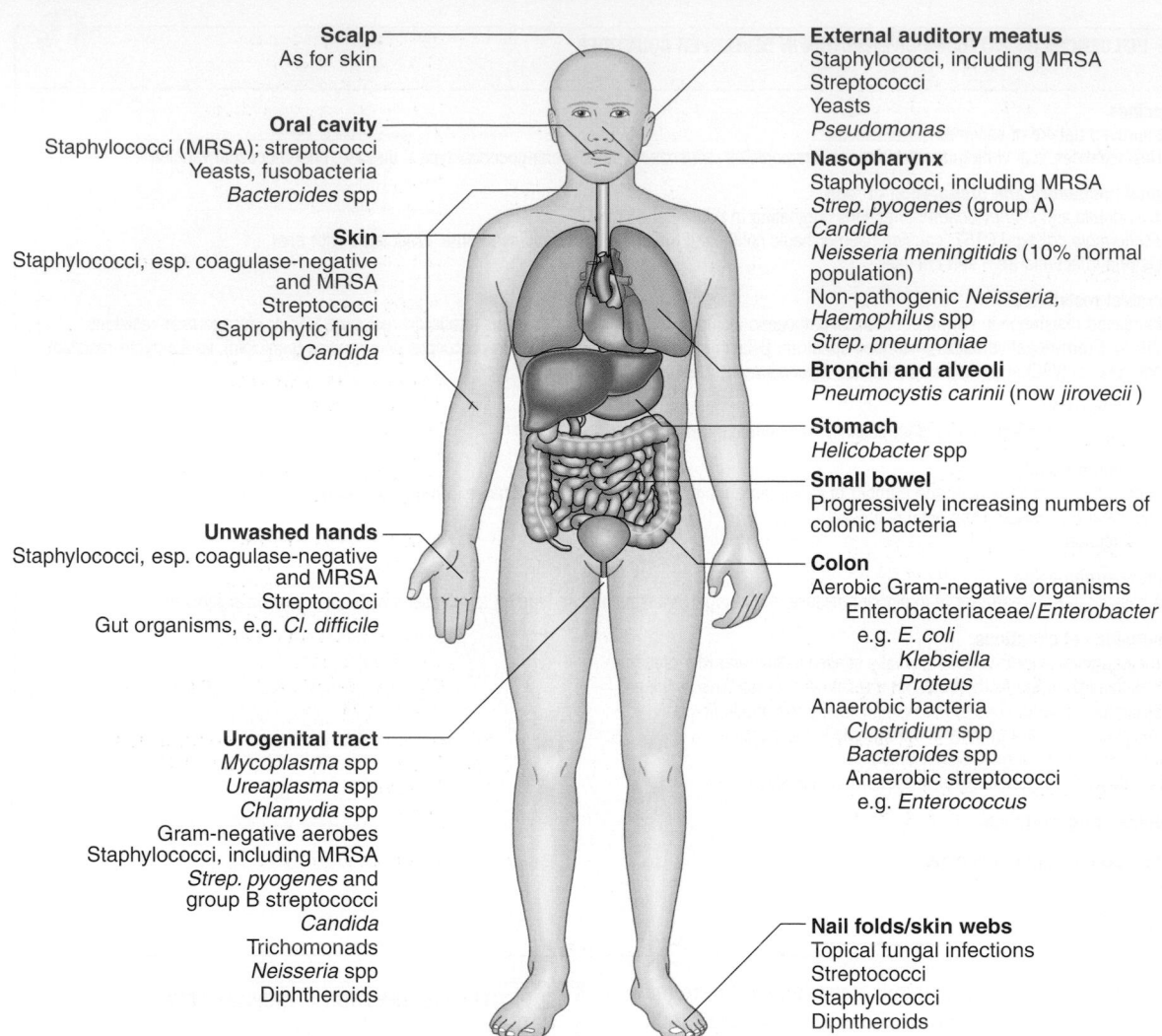

Scalp
As for skin

Oral cavity
Staphylococci (MRSA); streptococci
Yeasts, fusobacteria
Bacteroides spp

Skin
Staphylococci, esp. coagulase-negative
and MRSA
Streptococci
Saprophytic fungi
Candida

Unwashed hands
Staphylococci, esp. coagulase-negative
and MRSA
Streptococci
Gut organisms, e.g. *Cl. difficile*

Urogenital tract
Mycoplasma spp
Ureaplasma spp
Chlamydia spp
Gram-negative aerobes
Staphylococci, including MRSA
Strep. pyogenes and
group B streptococci
Candida
Trichomonads
Neisseria spp
Diphtheroids

External auditory meatus
Staphylococci, including MRSA
Streptococci
Yeasts
Pseudomonas

Nasopharynx
Staphylococci, including MRSA
Strep. pyogenes (group A)
Candida
Neisseria meningitidis (10% normal
population)
Non-pathogenic *Neisseria,*
Haemophilus spp
Strep. pneumoniae

Bronchi and alveoli
Pneumocystis carinii (now *jirovecii*)

Stomach
Helicobacter spp

Small bowel
Progressively increasing numbers of
colonic bacteria

Colon
Aerobic Gram-negative organisms
    Enterobacteriaceae/*Enterobacter*
        e.g. *E. coli*
            Klebsiella
            Proteus
Anaerobic bacteria
    Clostridium spp
    Bacteroides spp
    Anaerobic streptococci
        e.g. *Enterococcus*

Nail folds/skin webs
Topical fungal infections
Streptococci
Staphylococci
Diphtheroids

Fig. 6.2 Endogenous infection: reservoirs of infection in adults.

diseases such as poliomyelitis, measles, rubella, meningitis, tetanus and hepatitis A and B, but in many countries they have made little impact because of cost and the practical difficulties of delivery. Development, especially in the form of dams and irrigation, has often encouraged the spread of vector-borne diseases such as malaria and schistosomiasis, while the exploitation of the Amazonian forests has resulted in mutilating outbreaks of mucocutaneous leishmaniasis. Migration to urban slums increases the risk of gastro-intestinal disease, tuberculosis and 'Western' diseases such as hypertension, and has contributed materially to the acquired immunodeficiency syndrome (AIDS) epidemic which is wreaking havoc in developing countries, especially Africa, the Indian subcontinent and South-east Asia. Lack of material resources has severely limited the availability of therapeutic agents, particularly in the management of HIV disease in the developing world.

Finally, in developing countries, infectious diseases are often associated with natural disasters such as drought, flooding and earthquakes as well as with war and political strife.

SOURCE AND SPREAD OF INFECTION

Major advances have been made over the course of the last 50 years in our understanding of the pathogenicity of microorganisms, the human immune response to them and our ability to treat these infections. Viruses, bacteria, fungi and protozoa all interact with the human body and do so in a relationship that is symbiotic (involving mutually advantageous coexistence), saprophytic (in which organisms consume dead or dying material without causing disease) or parasitic (when the presence of organisms is detrimental to the host).

The symbiotic relationship is by far the most common link between microorganisms and the host, as represented by the vast numbers of colonising organisms (bacteria) in the human gut, upper respiratory tract and lower genital tract, and on the skin and superficial mucous membranes (Fig. 6.2). Often the human body benefits from this type of colonisation, as in the prevention of supervening infection with *Clostridium difficile* by normal gut flora or *Candida*

6

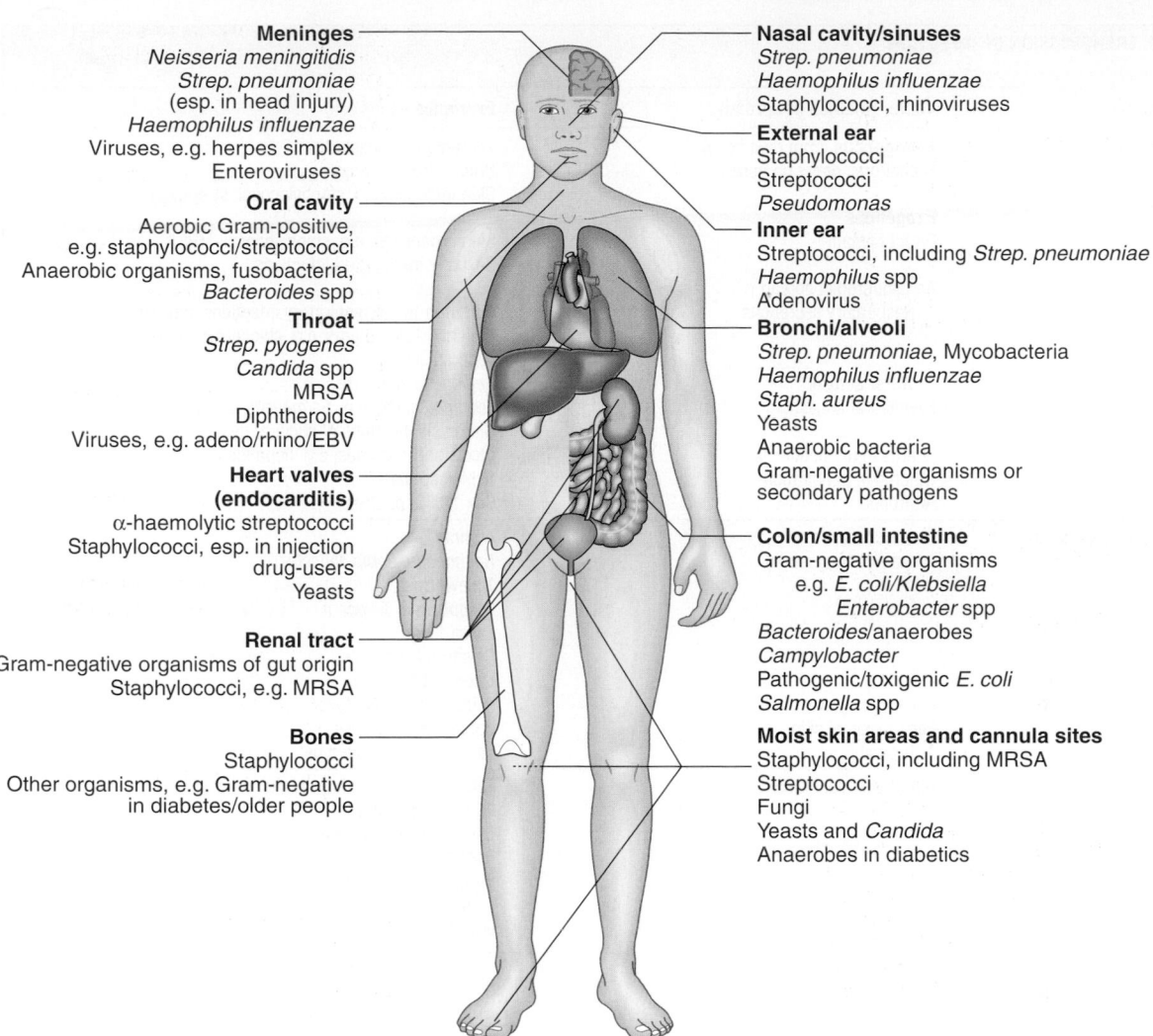

Meninges
Neisseria meningitidis
Strep. pneumoniae
(esp. in head injury)
Haemophilus influenzae
Viruses, e.g. herpes simplex
Enteroviruses

Oral cavity
Aerobic Gram-positive,
e.g. staphylococci/streptococci
Anaerobic organisms, fusobacteria,
Bacteroides spp

Throat
Strep. pyogenes
Candida spp
MRSA
Diphtheroids
Viruses, e.g. adeno/rhino/EBV

**Heart valves
(endocarditis)**
α-haemolytic streptococci
Staphylococci, esp. in injection
drug-users
Yeasts

Renal tract
Gram-negative organisms of gut origin
Staphylococci, e.g. MRSA

Bones
Staphylococci
Other organisms, e.g. Gram-negative
in diabetes/older people

Nasal cavity/sinuses
Strep. pneumoniae
Haemophilus influenzae
Staphylococci, rhinoviruses

External ear
Staphylococci
Streptococci
Pseudomonas

Inner ear
Streptococci, including *Strep. pneumoniae*
Haemophilus spp
Adenovirus

Bronchi/alveoli
Strep. pneumoniae, Mycobacteria
Haemophilus influenzae
Staph. aureus
Yeasts
Anaerobic bacteria
Gram-negative organisms or
secondary pathogens

Colon/small intestine
Gram-negative organisms
e.g. *E. coli/Klebsiella*
Enterobacter spp
Bacteroides/anaerobes
Campylobacter
Pathogenic/toxigenic *E. coli*
Salmonella spp

Moist skin areas and cannula sites
Staphylococci, including MRSA
Streptococci
Fungi
Yeasts and *Candida*
Anaerobes in diabetics

Fig. 6.3 Common infecting organisms.

6

albicans by vaginal lactobacilli. Some exist in a saprophytic relationship such as fungal skin infections with minimal local damage and little or no systemic upset. True infection only occurs when microorganisms upset normal physiology or breach skin and/or mucous membranes and enter the blood stream or normally sterile environments such as connective tissue, bones, muscles and joints or the central nervous system (Fig. 6.3). Subsequent illness is produced in the individual by the interaction of the host immune mechanisms and the infecting organism and its toxic effects.

Human reservoirs

Infection may originate from the patient (endogenous, Fig. 6.2), usually from skin, nasopharynx or bowel, or from outside sources (exogenous), often another person who may be either suffering from an infection or carrying a pathogenic microorganism. Carriers are usually healthy and may harbour the organism in the throat (for example, diphtheria or meningococci), bowel (salmonella) or blood (hepatitis B or cytomegalovirus).

Animal reservoirs

Animals act as a significant source of many infections that transmit directly from animals to man (zoonoses). Examples are:

- contaminated meat/poultry (food poisoning organisms, e.g. *Campylobacter*, *Salmonella* and botulism)
- milk (tuberculosis, brucellosis)
- body fluids, e.g. saliva (rabies), urine (leptospirosis, Lassa fever)
- bird faeces/secretions (psittacosis).

Environmental reservoirs

The environment acts as a source of many infective pathogens, e.g. *Legionella* in air-conditioning or domestic water pipes, and enteropathogens (typhoid, cholera, cryptosporidia or hepatitis A) in water supplies. The soil may harbour spores of clostridia (tetanus) or anthrax.

6.3 TRANSMISSION OF INFECTION

Reservoir	Vector (method of spread)	Examples
Human	**Endogenous** (from own body)	Threadworms, cestodes
	Faecal/oral, direct on hands	Urinary tract infection
		Skin infection, e.g. staphylococci, streptococci
	Exogenous	
	Direct contact	Skin organisms, e.g. staphylococci, MRSA
		Sexually transmitted infections
	Aerosol/droplet spread	
	Respiratory secretions	Common upper respiratory infections, influenza
		Childhood exanthems, e.g. chickenpox, measles
		Tuberculosis
	Water aerosol	*Legionella*, norovirus
	Faecal/oral (ingestion)	Food poisoning, e.g. *Salmonella*, *Campylobacter*
		Giardiasis, hepatitis A, cholera, dysentery
	Sharps injury/needlestick	Blood-borne viruses, e.g. hepatitis B and C, HIV
	Other skin penetration	Schistosomiasis
	Arthropod	Box 13.52, p. 339
Animal (zoonoses)	Direct contact	Anthrax
	Faecal/oral (ingestion)	*Salmonella*, *Campylobacter*
		Tapeworms
		Toxoplasma, *Toxocara*
		Lassa fever
		Bovine tuberculosis
		Listeria, brucellosis
	Aerosol/droplet	Psittacosis, Lassa fever
	Penetration of skin	Rabies, leptospirosis
	Arthropod	Yellow fever (jungle type)
Environmental	Direct/skin penetration	Tetanus, wound botulism, gas gangrene
		Wound diphtheria
		Mycetoma, Buruli ulcer
		Hookworm
	Ingestion	*Toxoplasma*, *Toxocara*
		Listeria
		Giardiasis

TRANSMISSION OF INFECTION

Microorganisms may be transmitted by several routes.

- *Endogenous infection* may develop as a result of local spread, e.g. from bowel to peritoneum, or be spread via the blood stream. An example of the latter type is endocarditis caused by *Strep. sanguis* originating in the patient's mouth and entering the blood during dental procedures.
- *Exogenous infection* may be acquired directly or indirectly by one of the routes shown in Box 6.3.

Health care-acquired infection

Although community-acquired infection represents the bulk of all infection seen both in primary and secondary care, the transmission of infection in or during health care (health care-acquired infection, HAI) has now become extremely important in the ongoing care of patients. Previously known as nosocomial infections, HAIs affect approximately 10% of all hospital admissions and create a significant burden both clinically and economically. The close proximity of compromised patients in the hospital setting, coupled with the concentrated use of antibiotics and the ease of transmission by health-care workers, has led to the selection of multidrug-resistant organisms such as MRSA (p. 313), vancomycin-resistant enterococci (VRE) and extended spectrum β-lactamase resistant (ESBL) Enterobacteriaceae. In addition, the easy spread of organisms such as these, plus infections such as *Clostridium difficile* (p. 329) and norovirus (p. 311), may lead to outbreaks of infection that can only be contained by ward or hospital closure.

MICROORGANISM–HOST INTERACTIONS

Infection has many effects on the body, summarised in Box 6.4. They may be acute, chronic, allergic or toxigenic. Chronic effects are seen especially in children in tropical countries.

Incubation period

The incubation period is the period between the invasion of the tissues by pathogens and the appearance of clinical features of infection. The period of infectivity is the time that the patient is infectious to others. Incubation periods of major infections and periods of infectivity in childhood infectious diseases are shown in Boxes 6.5 and 6.6.

6.4 CLINICAL EFFECTS OF INFECTION ON THE BODY

Acute

- Fever; anorexia, protein catabolism, negative nitrogen balance, acute-phase protein response, hypoalbuminaemia, low serum iron, sequestration of iron, anaemia, neutrophilia
- Inflammation; pain, dysfunction, tissue damage
- Convulsions; especially in children
- Confusion; especially in the elderly
- Shock; sustained fall in circulating blood volume associated with lowered systemic vascular resistance
- Haemorrhage; haemolytic anaemia, intravascular coagulation
- Organ failure; kidneys, liver, lung, heart, brain, necrosis of skin

Chronic

- Weight loss and muscle-wasting
- Malnutrition; especially associated with diarrhoea
- Retardation of growth and intellect in children
- Anaemia; iron sequestration, maturation arrest in marrow, folate deficiency
- Tissue destruction; e.g. lung in pneumonia or tuberculosis, nerves in leprosy, liver in hepatitis B
- Post-infective syndromes; e.g. lactose intolerance, malabsorption, irritable colon, depression, post-viral fatigue syndrome

'Allergic' (immune-mediated)

- Rash; e.g. urticaria with helminths, maculo-papular in typhoid and endocarditis, erythema nodosum in tuberculosis
- Arthritis; e.g. in rheumatic fever, Reiter's syndrome
- Pericarditis; e.g. in meningococcal infection
- Encephalitis; e.g. in measles or following vaccines
- Peripheral neuropathy; e.g. in post-infective polyneuritis
- Haemolytic anaemia; e.g. in infectious mononucleosis
- Nephritis; e.g. in streptococcal infection

'Toxic' (toxin-mediated)

- Erythematous rash in streptococcal infection
- Multisystem disturbance in staphylococcal or streptococcal toxic shock syndrome
- Diarrhoea; e.g. staphylococcal enterotoxin, *Bacillus cereus*
- Organ disturbance; e.g. diphtheria
- Neurological; e.g. tetanus, botulinum, diphtheria

6.5 INCUBATION PERIODS OF IMPORTANT INFECTIONS

Infection	Incubation period	
	Maximum range	Normal range
Short incubation periods (< 7 days)		
Anthrax	2–5 days	
Bacillary dysentery	1–7 days	
Cholera	Hours–5 days	2–3 hours
Diphtheria	2–5 days	
Gonorrhoea	2–5 days	
Meningococcaemia	2–10 days	3–4 days
Scarlet fever	1–3 days	
Intermediate incubation periods (7–21 days)		
Amoebiasis	14 days–months	21 days
Chickenpox	14–21 days	
Lassa fever	7–14 days	
Malaria	8 days–months	
Measles	7–14 days	10 days
Mumps	12–21 days	18 days
Poliomyelitis	3–21 days	7–10 days
Psittacosis	4–14 days	10 days
Rubella	14–21 days	18 days
Trypanosoma rhodesiense infection	14–21 days	
Typhoid fever	7–21 days	
Typhus fever	7–14 days	12 days
Whooping cough	7–10 days	7 days
Long incubation periods (> 21 days)		
Brucellosis	Days–months	
Filariasis	3 months–years	
Hepatitis A	2–6 weeks	4 weeks
Hepatitis B	6 weeks–6 months	12 weeks
Leishmaniasis		
Cutaneous	1 week–months	
Visceral	2 weeks–2 years	2–4 months
Leprosy	Years	2–5 years
Rabies	Variable	2–8 weeks
Schistosomiasis	Weeks–years	
Trypanosoma gambiense infection	Weeks–years	
Tuberculosis	Months–years	

6

PATHOLOGY OF INFECTION

Disease due to infection is the result of interaction between a microorganism and the defence mechanisms of the body. The outcome of this interaction can range from no demonstrable effect to death, and will depend on the number and virulence of the organisms, the physiological and anatomical effects that they induce, and the effectiveness of the body's natural defences. There are strong genetic influences which determine the response to infection. Clear examples of this are the genetic polymorphisms in expression of cytokine release (e.g. tumour necrosis factor-alpha, TNF-α) and cytokine receptor expression (e.g. interferon-gamma, IFN-γ).

Organisms act directly and/or through their toxins. Many of these effects are generalised, but some act at specific anatomical sites: for example, poliomyelitis virus in anterior horn cells, hepatitis virus in hepatocytes, *Pneumococcus* in the lung alveoli, and tetanus and diphtheria toxins at nerve terminals.

6.6 PERIODS OF INFECTIVITY IN CHILDHOOD INFECTIOUS DISEASES

Disease	Infectious period
Chickenpox	5 days before rash to 6 days after last crop
Diphtheria	2–3 weeks (shorter with antibiotic therapy)
Measles	From onset of prodromal symptoms to 4 days after onset of rash
Mumps	3 days before salivary swelling to 7 days after
Rubella	7 days before onset of rash to 4 days after
Scarlet fever	10–21 days after onset of rash (shortened to 1 day by penicillin)
Whooping cough	7 days after exposure to 3 weeks after onset of symptoms (shortened to 7 days by antibiotics)

Shock is a particular problem in severe infections (p. 186). Its aetiology is complex and results from reduced systemic vascular resistance brought about by dilated small vessels and leaky capillaries under the influence of several mediators, including kinins, complement components, histamine, cytokines and endogenous opiates. Endotoxin from Gram-negative bacteria is well known to mediate release of these agents. Shock caused by cell wall components and lipoteichoic acid from Gram-positive bacteria is clinically indistinguishable from Gram-negative shock. The cycle of shock, tissue anoxia and organ failure is difficult to break and may lead to a fatal outcome within hours.

THERMOREGULATION

Human metabolic processes are critically temperature-dependent, and an individual's body temperature rarely varies by more than 1°C from baseline. The peripheral effector mechanisms are sweating (to reduce temperature), shivering (to raise temperature by muscle activity) and vasoregulation (constriction or dilatation). In addition, behavioural changes take place (p. 100). The central thermostat is situated in the hypothalamus. Heat- and cold-sensitive neurons are located in the anterior hypothalamus and pre-optic area. Temperature information from peripheral receptors is integrated, allowing modulation of the body's heat production, conservation and loss. This is controlled by neuronal mechanisms involving the limbic system, lower brain stem, spinal cord and autonomic nerves. Temperature in healthy adults is tightly controlled at a mean of 36.8°C; there is, however, a physiological diurnal variation of approximately 0.5°C, with the maximum occurring between 1600 and 2000 hrs and the minimum between 0200 and 0600 hrs. 'Fever' can be defined as a regulated elevation in body temperature above the customary set point of the hypothalamic thermostat.

THE FEBRILE RESPONSE

The initiation of fever begins when exogenous or endogenous stimuli, including pyrogens, are presented to specialised host cells, principally monocytes and macrophages. This process stimulates the synthesis and release of various pyrogenic cytokines including interleukin-1, TNF-α, interleukin-6 and IFN-γ. After release, these polypeptides can be found in virtually all body fluids. Cytokine–receptor interactions in the pre-optic region of the anterior hypothalamus activate phospholipase A. This enzyme liberates plasma membrane arachidonic acid as substrate for the cyclo-oxygenase pathway. The resulting mediator, prostaglandin E_2, then modifies the responsiveness of thermosensitive neurons in the thermoregulatory centre.

The classic 'rigor' occurs when the body, usually in response to exogenous pyrogens, inappropriately attempts to 'reset' core temperature to a higher level. This latter varies; hence the cyclical shivering followed by sweating, tachycardia and flushing as the body attempts to regain normal temperature control. Exogenous pyrogens are molecules which interact with host cells to induce the secretion of pyrogenic cytokines. Most act directly on monocytes or macrophages.

The best-characterised exogenous pyrogens are found in bacterial cell walls. 'Endotoxin' is a hydrophobic lipopolysaccharide which is a component of the cell walls of Gram-negative bacteria. Biological activity lies in the lipid A moiety, and the most important fatty acid producing fever has been identified as β-hydroxymyristic acid. As well as provoking the febrile response, endotoxin also plays a major role in the induction of septic shock. The molecule is widely distributed in Gram-negative bacteria and is found in non-virulent and weakly virulent species as well as in major pathogens such as salmonellae.

Muramyl dipeptide (MDP) is an exogenous pyrogen found in all bacteria with cell walls (and is therefore absent from mycoplasmas). A constituent of peptidoglycan, MDP is relatively more important in Gram-positive than Gram-negative organisms, as the latter possess only a thin peptidoglycan layer. On a weight-to-weight basis, however, MDP is $10–10^3$ times less active than endotoxins. MDP induces fever by interacting with specific receptors on monocytes and polymorphs.

The role of viruses as pyrogens is complex. Viruses which invade macrophages stimulate cytokine production by a mechanism which probably involves double-stranded RNA. Interferon production by infected non-phagocytic cells also contributes to fever, as does necrosis of tissue brought about by virus invasion.

FEVER AS A DEFENSIVE ADAPTATION?

There is suggestive evidence that, for some microorganisms at least, a febrile host response may assist in curtailing infection and speeding recovery. Experimental data support the notion that raised body temperature interferes with the growth and/or virulence factors of a selection of bacterial and viral pathogens. Conversely, suppression of fever by antipyretics may increase viral shedding and the incidence of complications in infections caused by influenza, measles and rhinoviruses. Nevertheless, the role of the febrile response as a defence mechanism requires further study.

THE MANAGEMENT OF INFECTION

Disease related to microorganisms results from the interaction of the infecting agent and the defences of the

---

EBM

6.7 ANTIBIOTICS AND THE COMMON COLD

'Analysis of seven RCTs comparing antibiotic therapy with placebo in acute upper respiratory infections indicates that there is not enough evidence of important benefits to support such treatment. Moreover, there is a significant increase in adverse effects associated with antibiotic use.'

● Arrol B, et al. (Cochrane Review). Cochrane Library, issue 4, 2000. Oxford: Update Software.

For further information: 💻 www.update-software.com

6.8 ANTIBIOTICS IN PHARYNGITIS ('SORE THROAT')

'In an analysis of 25 studies comprising 11 452 cases of sore throat, antibiotics shortened the duration of symptoms by a mean of 1 day half-way through the illness and by 16 hours overall. They are most effective if a throat swab is positive for *Streptococcus*. By 7 days 90% of treated and untreated cases were symptom-free. Suppurative complications were reduced by antibiotics: otitis media OR = 0.22, acute sinusitis OR = 0.46, quinsy OR = 0.46.'

- Del Mar CB, et al. (Cochrane Review). Cochrane Library, issue 4, 2000. Oxford: Update Software.

For further information: 💻 www.update-software.com

human immune system. The management of infection and its consequences therefore requires a combination of action to reduce or inhibit the infecting agent and limitation of the inflammatory responses in the host. This may involve much more than simple antimicrobial therapy; indeed, antibiotics are not required for all infective processes (Boxes 6.7 and 6.8).

PREVENTION OF INFECTION

Any reduction in the reservoirs of infection will naturally reduce the incidence of disease produced by these organisms. Endogenous reservoirs may be reduced by chemoprophylaxis (Box 6.9) or by physical isolation of cases whilst infective (Box 6.6). Similarly, physical separation of animal sources from human hosts and their

6.9 INDICATIONS FOR CHEMOPROPHYLAXIS IN CONTACTS OF PATIENTS WITH INFECTIOUS DISEASES

Infection to be prevented	Antimicrobiol agent indicated	Adult dose
Diphtheria	Erythromycin	500 mg 6-hourly for 5 days
Meningococcal infection	Rifampicin Ciprofloxacin	600 mg 12-hourly for 2 days 500 mg as single dose
Whooping cough	Erythromycin	500 mg 6-hourly for 7 days
Tuberculosis	Isoniazid	300 mg daily for 6 months

6.10 INDICATIONS FOR PROPHYLACTIC IMMUNOGLOBULINS

Human normal immunoglobulin (pooled immunoglobulin)

- Virus A hepatitis (travellers* and debilitated children)
- Measles (child with heart or lung disease)

Human specific immunoglobulin

- Virus B hepatitis (needlestick injuries, sexual partner)
- Tetanus (susceptible injured patients)
- Rabies (post-exposure protection)
- Chickenpox (immunosuppressed children, adults and pregnant women)
- Respiratory syncytial virus infection (high-risk infants, e.g. premature—investigational use)

*If not protected by active immunisation.

rapid treatment will reduce zoonoses. Blockage of transmission by source isolation, vector control or careful infection control will also halt the spread of infection.

Public health measures control spread of infection and vaccination may improve 'herd immunity' in communities.

Prophylactic immunoglobulin may help some individuals at high risk of infection (Box 6.10).

VACCINATION

The potential to prevent disease by inducing immunity through vaccination remains an important area of clinical medicine. There is a need both to generate vaccines for those conditions where none presently exists, such as HIV and malaria, and to improve the efficacy of other vaccines that are currently in use, e.g. for influenza.

Of the features required for an ideal vaccine (Box 6.11), safety and protection are perhaps the most important.

The design of potential vaccines is greatly influenced by the qualitative nature of the immune response (cell-mediated or humoral immunity) required to mediate protection. Older polysaccharide vaccines, such as pneumococcal polyvalent vaccine, produce an antibody response that is short-lived and without long-lasting memory (lack of T-cell activation). However, conjugation of the polysaccharide moiety to a

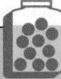

6.11 CHARACTERISTICS OF EFFECTIVE VACCINES

Safety

- No disease must be caused by the vaccine itself

Protection

- Protection must be at the population level (herd immunity) and prevent disease when the infectious agent is encountered in the individual

Long-lasting effects

- Protection must be long-lasting, i.e. induce T- and B-cell memory

Cost

- Inexpensive to produce and deliver

Administration

- Easy to deliver with no side-effects

6.12 GUIDELINES FOR IMMUNISATION AGAINST INFECTIOUS DISEASE

- The principal contraindication to inactivated vaccines is a significant reaction to a previous dose
- Live vaccines should not be given to pregnant women or to the immunosuppressed, or in the presence of an acute infection
- If two live vaccines are required, they should be given either simultaneously in opposite arms or 3 weeks apart
- Live vaccines should not be given for 3 months after an injection of human normal immunoglobulin (HNI)
- HNI should not be given for 2 weeks after a live vaccine
- Hay fever, asthma, eczema, sickle-cell disease, topical corticosteroid therapy, antibiotic therapy, prematurity and chronic heart and lung diseases, including tuberculosis, are not contraindications to immunisation

6.13 VACCINES AND THEIR INDICATIONS	
Live attenuated vaccines	**Inactivated/conjugated vaccines**
Childhood immunisation	
Measles	Pertussis
Mumps	*H. influenzae* type B (HIB)
Rubella	Meningococcal A and C
Poliomyelitis[1]	Poliomyelitis
BCG (tuberculosis)	
MMR (measles, mumps and rubella)	
Travel	
Yellow fever	Cholera
Typhoid[1]	Rabies
	Japanese B encephalitis
	Hepatitis A
	Hepatitis B
	Rabies
	European tick-borne encephalitis
	Diphtheria/tetanus
Special-risk groups	
Influenza	Pneumococcal
Varicella	Hepatitis B
	Meningococcal quadrivalent A,C,Y,W135[2]
	Plague
	Poliomyelitis[1]

[1]Both live and inactivated vaccines available. Vaccinated groups are not exclusive. (Poliomyelitis vaccination in childhood now uses an inactivated virus in the UK.)
[2]This is required for visitors to the Haj (Saudi Arabia).
Note Toxoids (inactivated toxins) immunise against diphtheria and tetanus.

6.14 VACCINATION AND PNEUMOCOCCAL PNEUMONIA	EBM

'Nine-valent pneumococcal vaccination, administered over 3 doses, reduces first episodes of pneumonia, mortality and hospital admissions in Gambian children.'

● Cutts FT, et al. Lancet 2005; 365:1139–1146.

protein, as in haemophilus B conjugate vaccine or meningococcal C vaccine, provides immunological memory and sustained response. New vaccines of this type are becoming available for *Salmonella typhi* and *Strep. pneumoniae* infections. Furthermore, the route of administration may also be important and, where down-regulation of the immune response is required, delivery via the mucosal surfaces of the gastrointestinal and respiratory tracts is an effective way of inducing immunological tolerance. The World Health Organization (WHO) has provided guidelines for the immunisation of children in developing countries. General guidelines and indications for immunisation are shown in Boxes 6.12 and 6.13.

Vaccination has been a very successful means of controlling infection throughout the world (Box 6.14). The world-wide eradication of smallpox (declared by WHO in 1980) is the best example of this. Vaccination becomes successful once the 'herd immunity' of the population reaches the required level to prevent ongoing spread of the wild-type virus. For example, measles, being very infectious, requires over 90% vaccination in susceptible persons before this can be achieved. Significant reductions in notifications of both measles and mumps have followed the introduction of effective vaccination schedules (Figs 13.5 and 13.10, pp. 300 and 303). From the mid-1990s in the UK, public concern about possible links of measles, mumps and rubella (MMR) vaccine to autism and inflammatory bowel disease (IBD) significantly reduced vaccine uptake to levels that allowed reappearance of wild virus activity. In the UK the Medical Research Council set up an expert group that has concluded that there is no scientific evidence to link MMR to autism or IBD. The UK Committee on the Safety of Medicines working party reached a similar conclusion. Following discussion with all major health organisations, the Chief Medical Officers of England, Scotland and Wales have advised that the MMR vaccine is safe, is the best way to protect children against these diseases, and should be given at the appropriate times in the UK vaccination schedule. UK and WHO recommended vaccination schedules are given in Boxes 6.15 and 6.16.

INFECTION CONTROL

HAIs have to be managed by comprehensive antibiotic policies and careful adherence to strict infection control

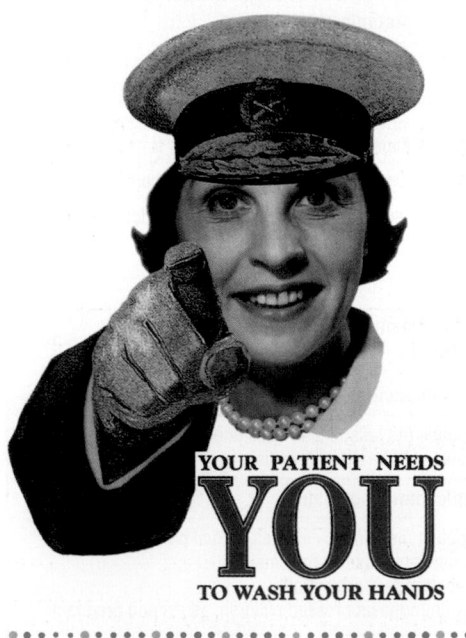

Wash your Hands!

YOUR PATIENT NEEDS
YOU
TO WASH YOUR HANDS

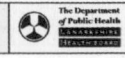

Fig. 6.4 Poster urging health-care workers to wash their hands.

6.15 UK RECOMMENDED VACCINATION SCHEDULE

Age/environment	Vaccination	Notes
2 months or as soon as possible thereafter	**Recommended** Adsorbed diphtheria, pertussis, tetanus (DPT) + *Haemophilus influenzae* type B conjugate (HIB) + Oral polio vaccine (OPV) + Meningococcal group C (Men C) conjugate vaccine	Three doses with 4-week gap between doses
	+ BCG for neonates at risk of tuberculosis	Neonates at risk = immigrants or those with known contact with tuberculosis *One* dose only
2nd year of life	Measles, mumps and rubella (MMR) HIB	If not previously immunised
Pre-school/nursery school entry	Adsorbed DPT OPV MMR	Single booster provided previously immunised
10–14 years	BCG	Only if Mantoux test negative
Pre-school-leaving or pre-employment/further education	Adsorbed DPT OPV	Single booster
	Men C	If not previously immunised
Over 65 or with chronic illness	Annual influenza vaccination Consider pneumococcal multivalent	Chronic heart or respiratory disease, diabetes mellitus, immunocompromised
Travel-related	**Other** Hepatitis A, hepatitis B Typhoid i.v. and oral Yellow fever Cholera Rabies European tick-borne encephalitis Meningococcal quadrivalent	The recommendations for these vaccinations depend on the region to be visited and the risk encountered
Occupational or other risk-related	Hepatitis A Hepatitis B	Exposure to raw sewage/faecal–oral Laboratory staff Injection drug-users; at-risk sexual behaviour Infants born to mothers who are high-risk hepatitis B surface antigen carriers High-risk disease: haemophilia, chronic renal failure Health-care workers and trainees; residents and staff in institutions for severe learning difficulties

6.16 IMMUNISATION SCHEDULE FOR INFANTS RECOMMENDED BY THE WHO EXPANDED PROGRAMME ON IMMUNISATION

Vaccine	Birth	6 weeks	10 weeks	14 weeks	9 months	At appropriate age
BCG	✓					
Oral polio	✓	✓	✓	✓		
Diphtheria, pertussis, tetanus		✓	✓	✓		
Hepatitis B					✓	
Scheme A[1]	✓	✓				
Scheme B[1]		✓	✓	✓		
Haemophilus influenzae type B		✓	✓	✓		
Yellow fever					✓[2]	
Measles					✓[3]	
Japanese B encephalitis						✓[4]
European tick-borne encephalitis						✓[4]

[1] Scheme A is recommended in countries where perinatal transmission of hepatitis B virus is frequent (e.g. South-east Asia). Scheme B may be used in countries where perinatal transmission is less frequent (e.g. countries in sub-Saharan Africa).
[2] In countries where yellow fever poses a risk.
[3] A second opportunity to receive a dose of measles vaccine should be provided, either as part of the routine schedule or as a campaign.
[4] In countries where these infections are endemic.

6

6.17 INFECTION CONTROL STRATEGIES

Type of infection	Strategy
Endogenous	
Post-operative infections	Careful attention to skin antisepsis and operator hand hygiene
	Pre-operative antibiotic prophylaxis
	Pre-operative gut washout
Splenectomy	Pre-operative vaccination (pneumococcal/*Haemophilus*)
Exogenous	
Contact (person to person or from fomites)	Hand hygiene for all patient contact procedures (alcohol liquid)
	Use of disposable protective clothing (gloves/gowns)
	'Tagging' of case records
	Cleaning/disinfection of fomites
Air-borne	Hand hygiene
	Mask use, both preventive (case) and protective (health-care workers)
	Negative pressure isolation (health-care workers)
	Positive pressure isolation (case)
Faecal/oral	Hand hygiene
	Use of protective clothing for health-care workers and food industry workers
	Food hygiene

protocols (Box 6.17). Although environmental cleanliness and clean clothing are cosmetically important, recent evidence has confirmed the absolute importance of hand hygiene in the control of HAI. The use of alcohol hand lotion and its promotion to all health-care workers for use between every patient contact is an effective alternative to soap and water in prevention of HAI (Fig. 6.4).

OUTBREAK CONTROL

An outbreak of infection is defined as two or more linked cases of an infectious disease occurring simultaneously or unexpectedly or the occurrence of any disease clearly in excess of normal expectancy. Different types of outbreak are recognised (Box 6.18). Many countries have systems of compulsory notification of contagious conditions to public health authorities so that outbreaks can be recognised and appropriate measures put in place to control the further spread of the condition (Box 6.19). These measures will depend on the source of the infection, its infectivity and mode of transmission, and may include source isolation, quarantine of sufferers or those incubating the condition (Box 6.5, p. 135) and mass treatment or vaccination programmes.

PRINCIPLES OF FOOD HYGIENE

An understanding of the temperatures at which spoilage and pathogenic bacteria are inhibited and destroyed underpins the essentials of food hygiene (Fig. 6.5). Following high-profile outbreaks such as the Central Scotland *E. coli* O157 outbreak of 1996, UK butchers' premises and food preparation establishments have had to be licensed and registered respectively; all proprietors are now required to have gained certification in food hygiene. An essential element of this is an understanding of hazard analysis of critical control points (HACCP) in the process of food

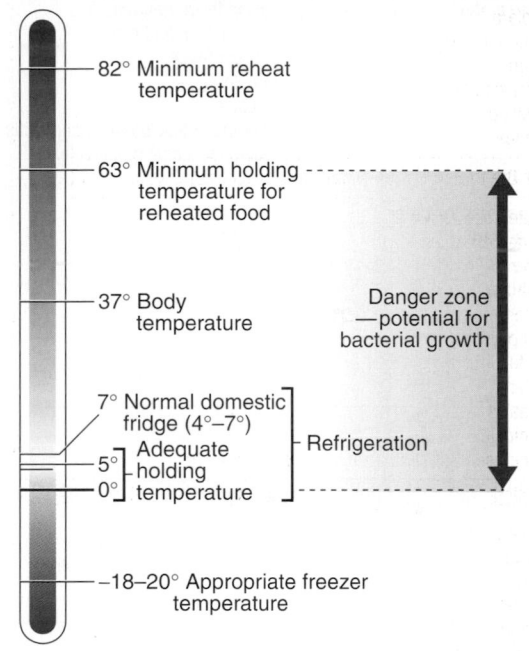

Fig. 6.5 Important temperatures (°C) in food hygiene.

82° Minimum reheat temperature

63° Minimum holding temperature for reheated food

37° Body temperature

Danger zone —potential for bacterial growth

7° Normal domestic fridge (4°–7°)

5° Adequate holding temperature

0°

Refrigeration

−18–20° Appropriate freezer temperature

preparation. National systems of surveillance, based on compulsory notification of food poisoning and recommendations for the setting up of outbreak control teams, allow for the rapid recognition of outbreaks and their speedy control.

CASE MANAGEMENT

The management of individuals with established infection combines non-specific measures to combat the symptoms of the body's reaction to invasion by microorganisms, e.g.

6.18 OUTBREAK CLASSIFICATION

Type of outbreak	Description	Characteristics
Point source	Exposure to a single source of infection at a defined time point, e.g. consumption of contaminated food at a social function	All exposed will develop symptoms at or around expected incubation period for that illness
Common source	Exposure to a single source of infection over a period of time, e.g. asymptomatic carrier of infection in a retail food outlet	Large numbers of people may be exposed over a prolonged period of time National and international food distribution networks and extensive national and international travel have expanded the possibilities of this type of outbreak
Person-to-person	Chain of infection from one infected individual to another, e.g. a child infected at a party then infects family members and school friends	Clusters of infection are separated by the incubation period of the infection
Epidemic	Widespread, increased, unusual incidence of a disease in the community, e.g. a new antigenic variation of influenza	Waves of infection spread through communities affecting all those with no active immunity to that infection

6.19 NOTIFIABLE INFECTIOUS DISEASES IN BRITAIN

Under the Public Health (Control of Diseases) Act 1984

- Cholera
- Food poisoning
- Plague
- Relapsing fever
- Smallpox
- Typhus

Under the Public Health (Infectious Diseases) Regulations 1988

- Acute encephalitis
- Acute poliomyelitis
- Anthrax
- Diphtheria
- Dysentery (amoebic or bacillary)
- Leprosy
- Leptospirosis
- Malaria
- Measles
- Meningitis
- Meningococcal septicaemia (without meningitis)
- Mumps
- Ophthalmia neonatorum
- Paratyphoid fever
- Rabies
- Rubella
- Scarlet fever
- Tetanus
- Tuberculosis
- Typhoid fever
- Viral haemorrhagic fever

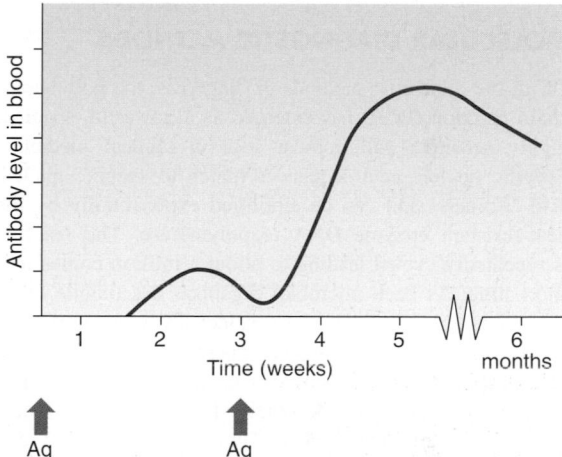

Fig. 6.6   Typical antibody response (IgG) after exposure to a specific antigen.

methods and appropriate use of the laboratory by the clinician.

Exact microbiological diagnosis can only be established by direct demonstration of the organism, its antigen or nucleic acid sequences. Indirect evidence of infection is indicated by an immune response to a specific microbe. An acute rise in antibody titres is especially helpful in establishing the diagnosis. This occurs 10–14 days after initial infection (Fig. 6.6) with an IgM response preceding an IgG one.

DIRECT DEMONSTRATION

Direct demonstration of the microbes in the tissue or body fluid of relevance is the most specific way to demonstrate a causative organism. Various methods are employed, as follows:

- *Microscopic examination of biological fluids or tissue slides with appropriate stains*. For example, Gram staining of CSF to demonstrate Gram-negative diplococci of meningococcal meningitis, or

fever, headache and myalgia, with the treatment of complications of infection such as shock, organ failure and haemorrhage and with specific antimicrobial therapy to kill or inhibit the growth of causative microorganisms.

MICROBIOLOGICAL INVESTIGATION OF INFECTION

An essential component in the management of infection is an understanding of the basic microbiological investigation

Ziehl–Neelson staining of acid-fast bacilli in sputum in tuberculosis or in skin slit-smears in leprosy infections.

- *In vitro culture.* Culturing the relevant body fluid in appropriate media is an excellent and highly sensitive method for recovering causative organisms, e.g. urinary tract infections and pneumonias. However, long incubation (6–8 weeks) may be required with slow-growing bacteria (e.g. tuberculosis). An automated radiometric/non-radiometric CO_2 detection system (BACTEC) enables early detection of bacterial growth including tuberculosis and allows evaluation of antibiotic sensitivity (by demonstration of inhibition of growth at different drug concentrations).
- *Animal inoculation.* Inoculating susceptible animals with infected material is now rarely used in diagnosis.

MOLECULAR DIAGNOSTIC METHODS

Of all the molecular methods of diagnosis, the polymerase chain reaction (PCR) has emerged as a powerful, specific, highly sensitive and popular tool in clinical medicine. Specific nucleic acid sequences match to specific nucleic acid 'primers' and can be amplified exponentially by the heat-resistant enzyme DNA taqpolymerase. The reaction is repeatedly cycled leading to about a million copies in a short time. As each microbial organism has unique DNA sequences, it is possible to select PCR primers that specifically identify pathogenic microorganisms. Presence of multiple microorganisms can be tested in one clinical sample and results can be obtained usually within a few hours using 'multiplex' PCR. Fluorescent dyes with different emission spectrums may be attached to the different primers and the final nucleic acid polymers examined by light spectroscopy. Reverse transcriptase (RT)-PCR can be used to quantify mRNA levels from much smaller samples. This technique is sensitive enough to enable quantification of RNA from a single cell. RT-PCR amplifies very small amounts of any kind of RNA (mRNA, rRNA) and makes complementary DNA, which is then amplified with conventional PCR. HIV viral copies are estimated through this method.

Real-time PCR is used to quantify the organisms and is employed in estimation of HIV viral load. Similarly, instead of gel-electrophoretic detection, principles of ELISA (see below) may be applied for detection of PCR amplification (PCR-ELISA).

In general, PCR methodology has become the standard and most sensitive for the detection of pathogens in body fluids. Two major disadvantages prevent its universal acceptance:

- Firstly, its cost is prohibitive in many resource-poor situations.
- Secondly, its sensitivity is such that any contamination from laboratory or other sources renders it potentially dangerous in producing false positive results. Absolute standards of purity and laboratory control are therefore required before the technique can be validated for routine use.

IMMUNODIAGNOSIS

Immunological methods in the aetiological diagnosis of diseases involve in vitro examination of an antigen–antibody reaction in body fluids, including blood. Most of the immunodiagnostic methods for infectious disease have been based on the detection of specific antibodies, although specific antigens and whole infective agents can also be detected.

Enzyme-linked immunosorbent assay (ELISA)

In this method either microbial proteins or antibodies are detected. Microwells in ELISA plates are coated with antibodies to the target proteins (antibodies or antigens), which are then 'captured' from clinical material by these coated antibodies. A second antibody, conjugated with an enzyme, is then captured by the target protein. A chromogenic substrate (to the enzyme) is then added. Colour intensity is measured by the operator and indicates the presence of the appropriate protein.

Depending on the type of capturing protein, various generations of ELISA have been developed. In first-generation ELISAs either crude antigen or single antigen is used for the test. But in second- and third-generation ELISAs either multiple antigens or recombinant antigen or/and specific peptides are used, which leads to improvement in sensitivity and specificity.

Sometimes, for antigen demonstration, a sandwich ELISA is performed, in which another step is added so that the antigen is sandwiched between two layers of antibodies. Occasionally, cross-reactivity with ELISA can occur, although with improvement in techniques, specificity has improved.

Rapid immunochromatographic test

Adaptation of the ELISA technique, by embedding it in a nitrocellulose membrane of a test strip, allows rapid detection of antigen or antibodies in patient's body fluids, most commonly blood or serum. The presence of these specific proteins is indicated by the development of coloured bands on the strip. These diagnostic strip tests are simple, rapid, cheap and reliable.

Western blot (immunoblot) test

In Western blot, antibodies to multiple specific protein ligands are detected, and high specificity is the characteristic of this method. Microbial protein is run on polyacrylamide gel electrophoresis to separate the ligands, which are then transferred on to a nitrocellulose membrane strip. This is then incubated with the patient's sera, leading to binding of specific antibodies to discrete protein bands. Enzymatically labelled anti-immunoglobulins bind to these antibodies and may be visualised by the addition of an enzyme substrate to produce coloured bands.

6

Immunofluorescence

Direct immunofluorescence

Specific antibodies labelled with a fluorescent dye combine with the antigen present in the patient's specimen. This is a highly sensitive and specific method.

Indirect immunofluorescence test

This is used for detection of specific antibodies. Microbial antigen is incubated with patients' sera, and if specific antibodies are present, these combine with the antigen. Antigen–antibody complexes are detected with fluorescent-labelled antisera to human gammaglobulin, observed under ultraviolet light.

Complement fixation test

The complement fixation test (CFT) has traditionally been used for determination of antimicrobial antibodies in the patient's sera. It is based on the ability of the patient's antibodies to form complement-activating immune complexes upon binding to their antigens. This is a very versatile and sensitive test. The patient's serum is heat-treated to remove native complement and then added to specific antigen. Sheep blood is added and, if antigen-specific antibodies are present, complement is used in the antigen–antibody reaction. The sheep erythrocytes, coated with receptor, haemolyse in the presence of free complement; absence of haemolysis indicates presence of specific antibodies, i.e. a positive complement fixation test.

Agglutination test

When a particulate antigen is mixed with its specific IgM antibody, it leads to agglutination in optimal conditions and concentrations. Incomplete or monovalent antibodies do not cause agglutination.

Direct agglutination

The Weil–Felix test, now seldom used in the diagnosis of typhus fever, utilises a heterophile agglutination test based on a shared common antigen between rickettsiae, typhus and some strains of *Proteus*. In the direct agglutination test (DAT) for visceral leishmaniasis, fixed and stained promastigotes are mixed with the patient's serum and the presence of antibodies leads to agglutination.

Indirect (passive) agglutination test

A soluble antigen is attached to the surface of a carrier particle, and these particles agglutinate when incubated with patient's sera containing antibodies. It is more convenient and more sensitive for detection of antibodies. When, instead of Ag, the Ab is adsorbed to a carrier particle to detect Ag, this technique is known as reversed passive agglutination.

Latex agglutination

Latex particles, coated with specific antibody, can demonstrate the presence of bacterial toxins such as those produced by *Vibrio cholerae* in cholera and by staphylococci in the toxic shock syndrome, or viral antigens (e.g. rotavirus, adenovirus and herpes simplex). Presence of the particular antigen will cause agglutination of the latex particles.

Haemagglutination test

In this test, soluble antigens are coupled to red blood cells, which act as carrier particles. If mixed with sera containing antibodies, agglutination is detected. This is used in the diagnosis of syphilis and herpes virus infections.

Immunodiffusion

Antigen–antibody precipitation in pre-formed gel is utilised in this method. Depending on the aims of the test, either antigen or antibody is incorporated in the gel. The patient's serum is added to wells made in the gel and antigen–antibody precipitation is observed. Antibodies against *Histoplasma*, *Blastomyces*, *Coccidioides*, *Paracoccidioides* and some opportunistic fungi are routinely detected by radial immunodiffusion.

In counter-current immunoelectrophoresis (CIE), specific antisera and patient's body fluid are placed in separate wells and electronically driven together (thus speeding the test). Precipitation lines, as in the simple gel diffusion test, indicate the presence of the antigen (pathogen) in the sample. This is used for detection of various antigens such as HBsAg and specific antigens for *Cryptococcus* in cerebrospinal fluid.

CLINICIAN–LABORATORY INTERFACE

Regular, active interaction between the clinician and the microbiology laboratory is vital in the best management of infectious diseases. The process should be a dynamic one where the clinician, knowledgeable about available tests and their clinical application, can, after discussion with laboratory experts, institute management appropriate to the patient's current clinical status. This is best seen in antibiotic management when, perhaps after initial empirical therapy (see below), treatment can be tailored, taking into account the microbiological results and clinical state. Similarly, close liaison between the clinician and laboratory expert should determine appropriate investigations of a patient with a fever of unknown origin (p. 286).

PRINCIPLES OF ANTIMICROBIAL THERAPY

Antimicrobial drugs constitute one of the most important and successful groups of therapeutic agents. Best antimicrobial prescribing requires an understanding of the pharmacokinetics of the drugs, their mode of action and their spectrum of activity against infecting organisms, coupled with the clinical skills to diagnose the body system affected and most likely infecting organism. The potential for continual mutation and evolution of the microorganisms involved in infectious diseases means that effective antimicrobial therapy is a dynamic process which must account for developing resistance and changing pathogenicity in infecting agents.

ANTIMICROBIAL RESISTANCE

Although effective antimicrobial therapy is potentially available for all infections, the ongoing use of antimicrobials has potentiated high levels of resistance. Some organisms are becoming resistant to all known antimicrobials. Meticillin-resistant *Staph. aureus* (MRSA) and now glycopeptide-resistant *Staph. aureus* and enterococci (GRSA, GRSE) are examples. Multidrug-resistant *M. tuberculosis* (MDRTB, p. 702) is a similar serious threat. The recent history of antiretroviral therapy has demonstrated that this phenomenon is applicable to viral infections as well as traditional bacterial diseases (p. 400). A number of factors, individually or in combination, have led to the enhanced resistance now seen in some circumstances:

- *inappropriate prescription* for non-specific febrile illness or common viral infections
- *inadequate dosage* or treatment length to achieve eradication of infection
- poor compliance/adherence to regimens by patients
- *use of 'broad-spectrum' antimicrobials* for specific infections, exposing non-pathogenic commensals to antibiotic pressure
- 'over the counter' availability of antibiotics
- use in the food industry as 'growth promoters' in animal husbandry.

MECHANISMS OF ACTION AND RESISTANCE TO ANTIMICROBIALS

The mechanisms of action and of microbial resistance for the major classes of antimicrobial are shown in Box 6.20. These genetically coded resistance mutations are highly transmissible and the ability of resistant commensal bacteria, selected under antibiotic pressure, to exchange genetic material across species barriers has resulted in resistance to multiple antimicrobials being passed to pathogenic organisms in the gut lumen and other body sites.

DEVELOPMENT OF REFINED AND NEW ANTIMICROBIALS

Since the introduction of antibiotic and antimicrobial therapy in the mid-20th century many pharmacological refinements have allowed the development of antimicrobials with improved pharmacokinetics and enhanced activity against resistant organisms. It is salutary, however, that over recent years the development of new antibacterial agents has declined. The approval of the US Food and Drug Administration (FDA) of new antimicrobials has declined by 56% over the last 20 years. Of the nine new antibacterial agents approved by the FDA since 1998, only two have a

6.20 MECHANISMS OF ACTION AND RESISTANCE OF COMMON CLASSES OF ANTIMICROBIAL

Class of antimicrobial	Mechanisms of action	Mechanisms of resistance
Beta-lactams	Inhibit cell wall synthesis. Competitively block transpeptidases, penicillin-binding proteins and peptidoglycan synthesis. Periplasmic space in Gram-positive organisms. Intracellular in Gram-negative. Only act on dividing bacteria	Altered Gram-negative porin channels. Modification of penicillin-binding proteins (MRSA). Production of hydrolysing β-lactamase enzymes (chromosomal or plasmid-mediated)
Glycopeptides	Inhibit late stages of cell wall peptidoglycan synthesis at two stages	Large molecules; cannot penetrate Gram-negative porins so Gram-negative intrinsically resistant. Chemical substitution to prevent binding to transpeptidase
Aminoglycosides	Bind to 30S subunit of bacterial ribosomes (Require specific transport mechanism across Gram-negative outer/inner membranes). Disrupt bacterial protein synthesis	Membrane impermeability. Enzyme inactivation of active sites (Multiple enzymes now involved, specific for different aminoglycosides)
Macrolides, lincosamides and streptogramins	Reversibly bind to 50S subunit of bacterial ribosomes, block peptide bond formation and disrupt protein synthesis	Modification of bacterial target (cross-resistance to all macrolides/lincosamides/streptogramins)
Tetracyclines	Inhibit protein synthesis by preventing tRNA binding to ribosomes and modify ribosomal subunits. pH-dependent accumulation in cells	Active efflux of antibiotic from cells
Chloramphenicol	Competitively inhibits transfer of tRNA-binding to 50S ribosomal subunit	Specific enzyme (acyltransferase) that inactivates the antibiotic often plasmid-mediated. Reduced entry of drug through modified porins
Quinolones	Inhibit topoisomerases (DNA gyrase) and topoisomerase IV to prevent supercoiling or uncoiling of DNA, so effectively preventing DNA replication and causing cell death	Mutation of topoisomerases. Porin impermeability. Active efflux
Imidazoles	Under aerobic conditions form superoxide-damaging proteins, nuclear acids and lipids	
Sulphonamides	Inhibit dihydrofolate and tetrahydrofolate reductase, so inhibit folic acid synthesis from para-aminobenzoic acid (PABA)	Hyperproduction of PABA enzyme mutation

novel mode of action, i.e. have significant activity against already resistant organisms. There is therefore a pressing need to take extreme care in the use of antimicrobials to preserve their activity for future generations.

SCIENCE OF ANTIMICROBIAL THERAPY

Effective antimicrobial therapy requires an understanding of a number of principles:

- *Minimal inhibitory concentration (MIC)*, expressed as a percentage (MIC_{90}), is defined as the lowest concentration of antibiotic required to inhibit 90% of the colonies of a particular organism. The lower the MIC, the more sensitive the organism to that agent. As an in vitro measurement the MIC does not always accurately predict clinical outcome. Roxithromycin has in vitro MICs much lower than those in vivo due to a marked inhibitory effect of serum.
- *Co-administration of certain antimicrobials*, e.g. aminoglycosides and β-lactams, produces a synergistic effect greater than their combined MICs. This can be harnessed clinically in the management of difficult infections such as bacterial endocarditis (p. 629).
- *Drug absorption and elimination*, e.g. phenoxymethylpenicillin is erratically absorbed orally, and antacids or iron compounds in the stomach reduce the absorption of quinolones and tetracyclines. Antibiotics are most commonly eliminated from the body via renal or hepatic pathways. Disordered renal or hepatic function may compromise excretion and requires dosage modification.
- *Protein-binding* determines the availability of the drug and may produce side-effects due to competition with other drugs, e.g. warfarin.
- *Lipophilic drugs*, e.g. quinolones, cross cell membranes well whilst hydrophilic drugs, e.g. aminoglycosides, remain in the extracellular fluid space.
- *The plasma half-life* ($t_{1/2}$) of the drug allows recommendations on the timing of dosing schedules.
- Certain classes of antimicrobial, e.g. aminoglycosides and macrolides, exhibit a clinically useful '*post-antibiotic effect*' (PAE) with inhibition of microbial multiplication beyond the time when the MIC is reached in plasma. This allows modification of dosing schedules.
- Some antibiotics have efficacy reduced by the '*inoculum effect*', where the presence of large numbers of organisms inhibits the antibiotic despite apparent (MIC-based) sensitivity.

Details of individual compounds should be available in the manufacturer's data sheet or publications such as the *British National Formulary*.

SELECTION OF APPROPRIATE ANTIBIOTIC THERAPY

The selection of antibiotic therapy for an infection requires a knowledge of:

- the infecting organism, including the pathogen most likely to be present in given clinical or geographical circumstances
- the local patterns of antimicrobial resistance in common pathogens
- an understanding of the pharmacokinetics of the antimicrobials selected
- the physiology of the patient, metabolic upset, renal or hepatic dysfunction, age and available routes of administration.

The human body is in contact with many potentially infectious agents: bacteria, viruses, fungi or protozoa. Most are harmless colonisers causing no clinical upset but forming a natural reservoir of potential infection in the human host (Fig. 6.2, p. 132).

The clinical history should determine the systems of the body most likely to be involved in disease. Figure 6.3 (p. 133) shows common pathogens found in different systems.

EMPIRICAL 'BLIND' ANTIBIOTIC CHOICE

Once the body system involved and likely pathogens have been identified and appropriate laboratory specimens sent to confirm their presence, the most appropriate antibiotic should be selected. Most hospitals now have antibiotic policies or 'sepsis protocols', devised, using local sensitivity patterns, to guide initial antimicrobial therapy. These aim to prevent inappropriate therapy, and limit resistance development whilst maximising effectiveness. They require regular review and updating according to local resistance patterns and prescribing practice. It is standard practice that in severe infection preference should be given to bactericidal therapy rather than bacteriostatic; however, there is no clear evidence of differing effectiveness. The dosage and duration of therapy depend on the nature of the infection and the severity of the illness. A simple urinary tract infection in an adult female may only require 3 days of oral therapy, but deep-seated infections like osteomyelitis or endocarditis will require prolonged parenteral therapy for 6 weeks or more. The aim is to maintain the antibiotic concentration above the MIC in the given body compartment (Fig. 6.7).

An algorithm for the selection of antibiotics is given in Figure 6.8.

ROUTE OF ADMINISTRATION

Some antibiotics, e.g. aminoglycosides, are only available intravenously. Others, such as metronidazole and chloramphenicol, are as well distributed after oral administration as intravenously. In general, parenteral administration should

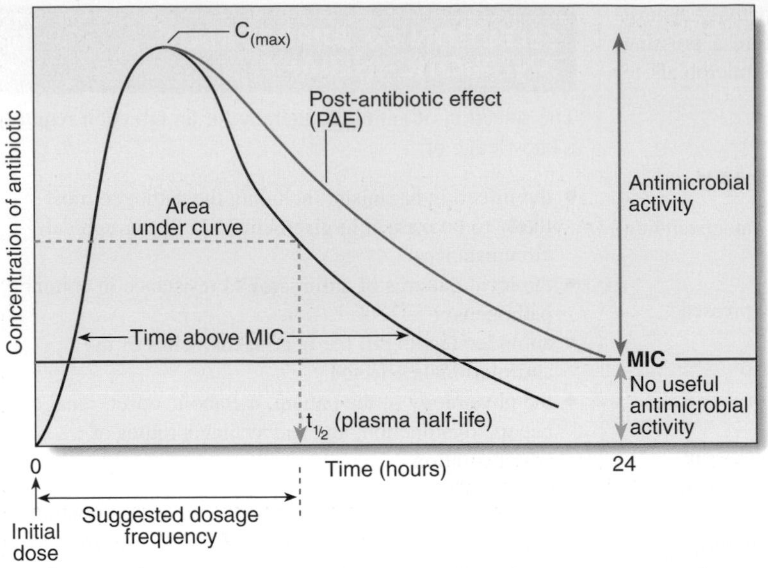

Fig. 6.7   Antimicrobial pharmacokinetics.
(MIC = minimal inhibitory concentration)

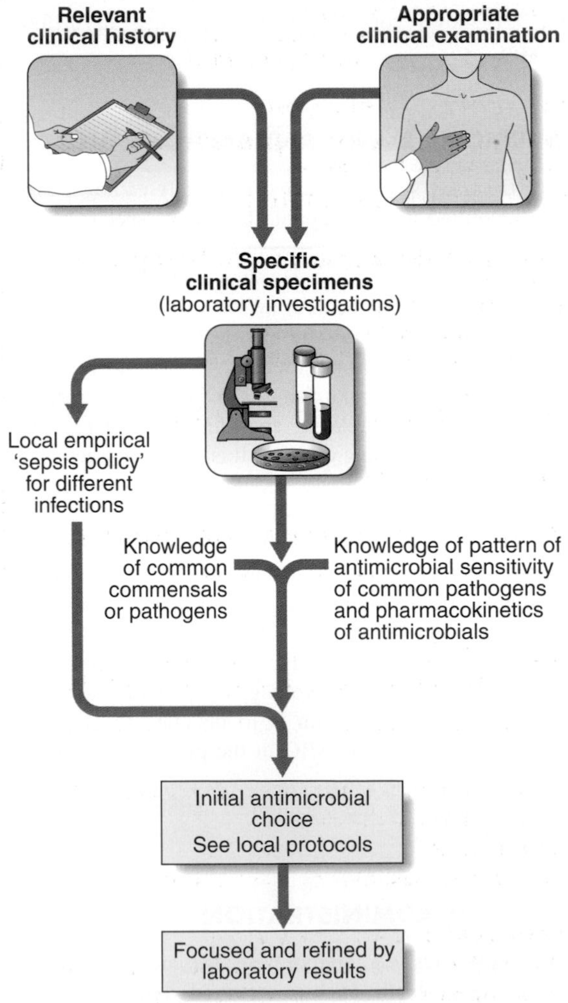

6

Fig. 6.8   Selection of appropriate antimicrobial agents.

be reserved for the patient who is severely ill and/or unable to take medication orally. Provided a satisfactory response to therapy is evident and no deep-seated or septicaemic infection is evident, the 'switch' to appropriate oral therapy should be made as soon as possible. Most authorities accept 48 hours free of fever following the start of antimicrobial therapy as an indication that 'i.v. to oral switch' may take place.

MONITORING ANTIBIOTIC THERAPY

When potentially toxic antibiotics such as aminoglycosides are used it is standard practice to monitor drug levels immediately before (trough) and, usually, 1 hour after (peak) administration and to adjust dosage accordingly, both to prevent accumulation of the drug and to check that the dose is reaching required levels in the body (Box 6.23, p. 151). In serious infections where the level of antibiotic must exceed the MIC over time, serum antibacterial levels should be measured (serum bactericidal or bacteriostatic levels) and the dosage adjusted to achieve satisfactory kill.

ANTIBIOTIC CHEMOPROPHYLAXIS

Knowledge of the pathogenesis of infection and the host susceptibility to certain organisms has led to the development of guidelines for the prevention of disease in certain clearly defined circumstances. A selection of these is shown in Box 6.21.

ANTIMICROBIAL AGENTS

BETA-LACTAM ANTIBIOTICS

These antibiotics have a β-lactam ring structure and exert a bactericidal action by disrupting cell wall synthesis in

6.21 SYSTEMIC PROPHYLAXIS WITH ANTIMICROBIAL AND IMMUNOLOGICAL THERAPY*

Disease/circumstance	Management
VIRAL	
Hepatitis B	
Sharps exposure, unprotected sexual exposure	Immediate hepatitis B immune globulin (HBIG); commence rapid vaccination course: 0.1 month, 6 months
Birth to HBV-positive mother	Immediate HBIG; commence rapid vaccination course
HIV	
Sharps exposure, unprotected sexual exposure	Commence 6 weeks highly activated antiretroviral therapy
Pregnancy/birth to HIV-positive mother	From week 28 zidovudine + lopinavir/ritonavir
	I.v. zidovudine during delivery; 6 weeks oral zidovudine to infant
Influenza A	Amantidine or rimantadine 100 mg daily p.o.
Respiratory syncytial virus	Palivizumab 15 mg/kg commencing before season
Varicella zoster	
Post-exposure prophylaxis in susceptible immunocompromised	Varicella immune globulin
Perinatally exposed newborn infants	Varicella immune globulin
BACTERIAL	
Bacterial endocarditis prevention	
Dental procedures	Amoxicillin 2 g (child 50 mg/kg) oral 1 hour pre-procedure (i.v. 30 mins before)
	Alternative: clindamycin 600 mg (child 20 mg/kg)
Gastrointestinal/genitourinary procedures	Ampicillin 2 g + gentamicin 1.5 mg/kg i.v. 30 mins before, ampicillin 2 g 6 hours later
	Alternative: vancomycin 1 g over 1 hour + gentamicin 1.5 mg/kg
Neonatal group B streptococcal diseases	(Assuming adequate prenatal screening etc.)
Pre-term or premature rupture of membranes in positive mother	Ampicillin 2 g 6-hourly + erythromycin 250 mg 6-hourly, 48 hours, 5 days × amoxicillin 250 mg 8-hourly and erythromycin 250 mg 6-hourly
Milroy's disease	
Streptococcal invasion of lymphoedema	I.v. benzathine penicillin 1.2 MU every 4 weeks
Spontaneous bacterial peritonitis (in ascites and cirrhosis)	Daily norfloxacin 400 mg (reduces Gram-negative bacteraemia from 27% to 3% but increases Gram-positive infections)
Post-splenectomy bacteraemia	Adults phenoxymethylpenicillin 250 mg 12-hourly
Rheumatic fever (group A streptococci)	
Primary (after group A streptococci pharyngitis)	Penicillin for 10 days prevents rheumatic fever, even if started late in initial disease
Secondary (after documented rheumatic fever)	Phenoxymethylpenicillin 250 mg 12-hourly
	(with carditis—10 years or until 25 years old)
	(without carditis—5 years or until 18 years old)
Abdominal/pelvic sepsis	
After colonic/gynaecological surgery	Gentamicin or cephalosporin + metronidazole (single dose)
Tetanus	
Wound or injury	Erythromycin 500 mg 6-hourly for 7 days
Gas gangrene	
Wound or injury	Penicillin 600 mg 6-hourly for 5 days or metronidazole 500 mg 8-hourly for 5 days
PROTOZOAL	
Malaria	
Travel to malarious countries	Depends on country (p. 347)

* Knowledge of the pathogenesis of infection and the host susceptibility to certain organisms has led to the development of guidelines for the prevention of disease in certain clearly defined circumstances.

rapidly dividing organisms. Generally, they achieve good levels in lung, kidney, bone, muscle and liver, and in pleural, synovial, pericardial and peritoneal fluids. They are classified into eight groups:

- natural penicillins: benzylpenicillin, phenoxymethylpenicillin
- penicillinase-resistant penicillins: meticillin, flucloxacillin
- aminopenicillins: ampicillin, amoxicillin
- carboxy- and ureidopenicillins: ticarcillin, piperacillin
- cephalosporins: first–fourth-generation compounds
- monobactams: aztreonam
- carbapenems: imipenem, meropenem
- β-lactamase inhibitors, e.g. clavulanic acid.

Pharmacokinetics: key points
- Not inhibited by abscess environment (low pH, low O_2, high protein and polymorphonuclear cells).
- Poor penetration to monocytes, low cerebrospinal fluid levels except in the presence of inflammation.

- Inoculum effect reduces activity.
- Generally safe in pregnancy (except imipenem/cilastatin).

Adverse reactions

Generalised allergy to penicillin occurs in 0.7–10% of cases and anaphylaxis in 0.004–0.015%. Over 90% of patients with infectious mononucleosis develop a rash if given aminopenicillins; this does not imply lasting allergy. Established penicillin allergy does not imply allergy to other classes, particularly the cephalosporins. The second- and third-generation cephalosporins have a low incidence of allergy and an almost negligible rate of anaphylaxis, even in the presence of established penicillin allergy.

Adverse effects

Gastrointestinal upset and diarrhoea are common side-effects, and a mild reversible hepatitis is well recognised with many of the drugs in this class. Leucopenia, thrombo-cytopenia and coagulation deficiencies can occur. Interstitial nephritis and increased renal damage in combination with aminoglycosides are also well recognised (p. 504). Seizures and encephalopathy have been reported, particularly with high doses in the presence of renal insufficiency. Direct intrathecal injection of a β-lactam is contraindicated. Thrombophlebitis occurs in up to 5% of patients receiving parenteral therapy with these agents.

Drug interactions

Synergism occurs in combination with aminoglycosides. Simultaneous dual β-lactam administration is unpredictable, either synergy or antagonism resulting. Ampicillin decreases the biological effect of oral contraceptives and the whole class is significantly affected by concurrent administration of probenecid, producing a 2–4-fold increase in the peak serum concentration.

In practice, penicillins are very cheap, well-tolerated, safe and easy-to-use antibiotics. The potential for synergy with aminoglycosides can be put to therapeutic advantage. Oral absorption is, however, poor or unreliable, major adverse/allergic reactions can occur, and resistance is increasing. Broad-spectrum drugs are only available intravenously.

NATURAL PENICILLINS (BENZYLPENICILLIN, PHENOXYMETHYLPENICILLIN)

Benzylpenicillin (dose: 1.2–2.4 g i.v. 6-hourly), phenoxy-methylpenicillin (250–500 mg oral 6-hourly). Natural penicillins are primarily effective against Gram-positive organisms (except staphylococci) and anaerobic organisms. *Strep. pyogenes* has remained sensitive to natural penicillins world-wide (Fig. 6.9) but penicillin resistance in *Strep. pneumoniae* has steadily increased world-wide, reaching over 30% in USA and 50–60% in parts of Asia in 1999.

METICILLIN/FLUCLOXACILLIN

Flucloxacillin (500 mg–1 g 6-hourly oral or i.v.). These are the mainstay of treatment for staphylococcal infections and other Gram-positive organisms, being resistant to staphylococcal penicillinase (Fig. 6.10).

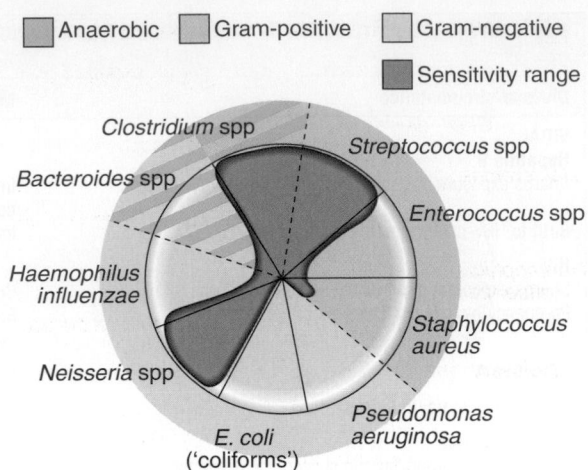

Fig. 6.9   Natural penicillin: spectrum of activity.

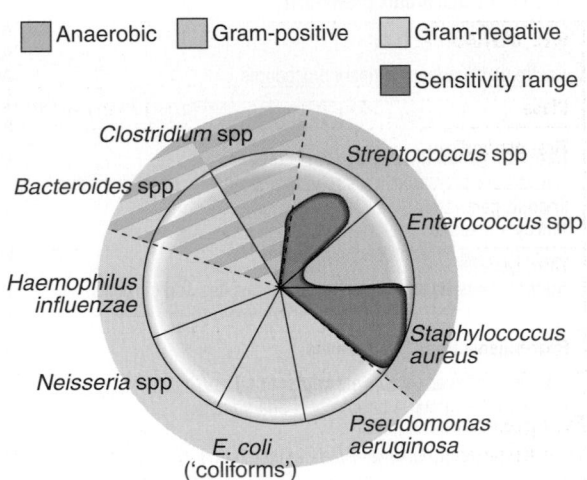

Fig. 6.10   Flucloxacillin: spectrum of activity.

THE AMINOPENICILLINS

Ampicillin (500 mg 6-hourly), amoxicillin (500 mg–1 g 8-hourly oral or i.v.). Ampicillin and amoxicillin have the same spectrum of activity as the natural penicillins with additional Gram-negative cover against Enterobacteriaceae. Amoxicillin has much better oral absorption than ampicillin. Many organisms are resistant due to β-lactamase production but the addition of β-lactam inhibitors (e.g. clavulanic acid, producing co-amoxiclav) to aminopenicillins has improved clinical usefulness (Fig. 6.11).

CARBOXYPENICILLINS (TICARCILLIN) AND UREIDOPENICILLINS (PIPERACILLIN)

These are particularly active against Gram-negative organisms, especially *Pseudomonas* spp, resistant to the aminopenicillins. Beta-lactamase inhibitors may also be used to extend their spectrum of activity.

CEPHALOSPORINS

These are arranged in 'generations' (Box 6.22).

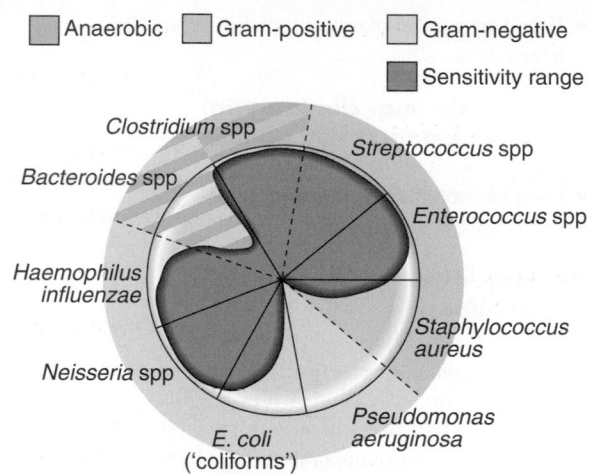

Fig. 6.11 **Amoxicillin: spectrum of activity.**

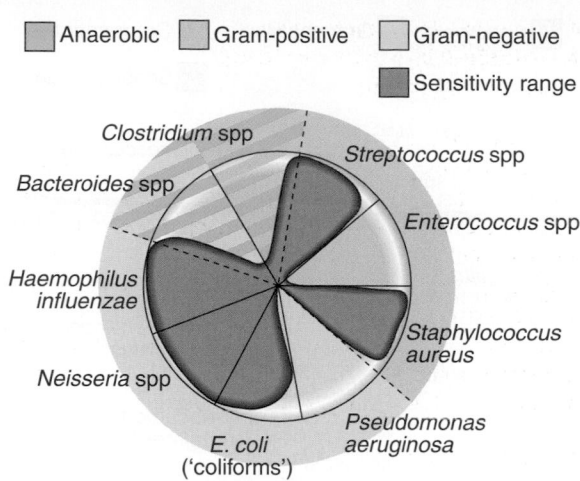

Fig. 6.12 **Cefuroxime: spectrum of activity.**

6.22 CEPHALOSPORINS		
Class	**Examples**	**Route of administration**
First generation	Cefalexin	Oral
	Cefazolin	I.v.
Second generation	Cefuroxime	Oral/i.v.
	Cefoxitin	
Third generation	Cefixime	Oral
	Ceftriaxone	I.v.
	Ceftazidime	I.v.
Fourth generation	Cefepime	I.v.

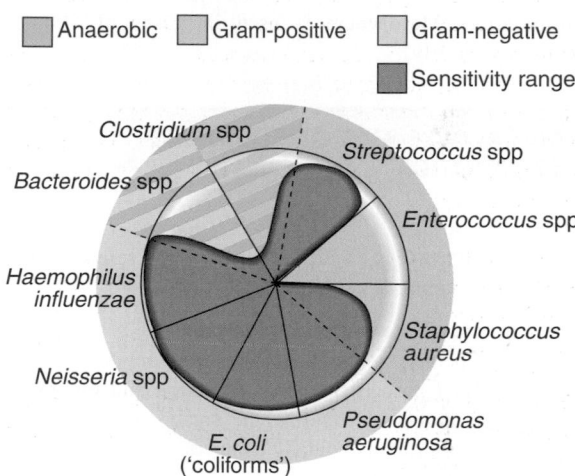

Fig. 6.13 **Ceftazidime: spectrum of activity.**

First generation

The first-generation compounds, e.g. cefalexin (250 mg 6-hourly), show excellent activity against Gram-positive organisms, with some activity against Gram-negative organisms. Many of them are potentially nephrotoxic.

Second generation

Second-generation cephalosporins retain Gram-positive activity but have extended Gram-negative activity and some anti-anaerobic activity. Cefuroxime, usually given i.v. 750 mg–1.5 g 8-hourly, is the best-known example (Fig. 6.12).

Third generation

Third-generation cephalosporins further improve anti-Gram-negative cover but some, such as ceftazidime, have particularly good antipseudomonal activity whilst losing some of their Gram-positive effectiveness. Ceftriaxone has excellent Gram-negative activity and retains good activity against *Strep. pyogenes*, haemolytic streptococci and many staphylococci. They are only available intravenously and, although effective (Fig. 6.13), are very expensive.

Fourth generation

Fourth-generation cephalosporins retain excellent broad-spectrum activity.

Cephalosporins are safe and reliable antibiotics, have a broad spectrum of activity and show some synergy with aminoglycosides. The more active compounds are only available in intravenous form. They are significantly associated with *Cl. difficile* enteritis (p. 329). The group shows little anti-anaerobic activity and none against *Enterococcus* spp. Oral formulations of the third- and fourth-generation compounds are expensive and poorly absorbed and unreliable therapeutically.

MONOBACTAMS

Aztreonam (1–2 g 12-hourly) is the only agent available in this class. It has excellent anti-Gram-negative antibiotic activity but no useful activity against Gram-positive organisms or anaerobes. It is only available as a parenteral preparation.

CARBAPENEMS

These have the broadest antibiotic activity of the β-lactam antibiotics and include activity against anaerobes (Fig. 6.14). They are very expensive and only available in intravenous

149

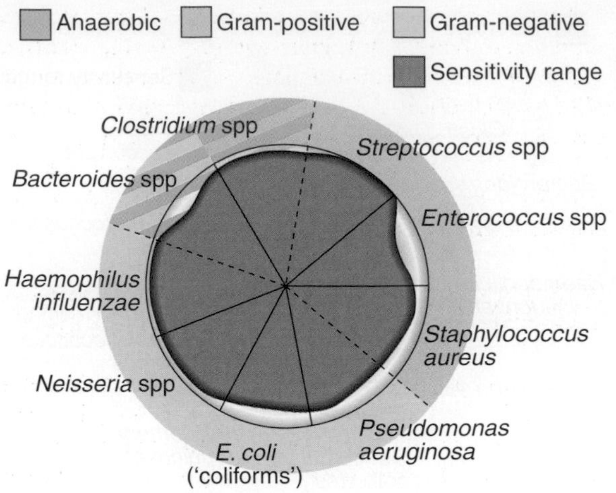

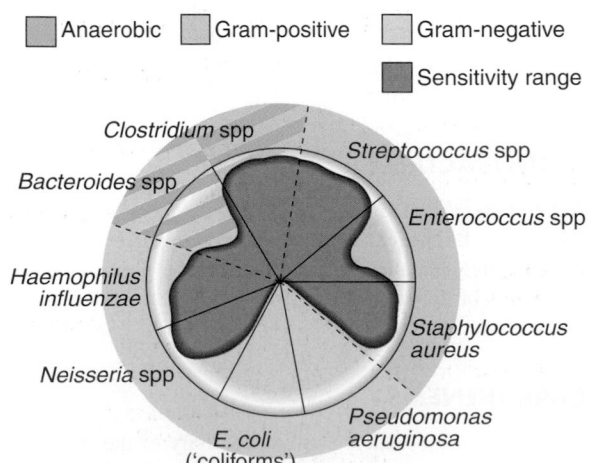

Anaerobic   Gram-positive   Gram-negative

Sensitivity range

Clostridium spp

Bacteroides spp

Haemophilus influenzae

Neisseria spp

E. coli ('coliforms')

Streptococcus spp

Enterococcus spp

Staphylococcus aureus

Pseudomonas aeruginosa

Fig. 6.14 Meropenem: spectrum of activity.

formulation. Meropenem is used in doses of 500 mg infusion 8-hourly.

MACROLIDE AND LINCOSAMIDE ANTIBIOTICS

Erythromycin

First launched in 1952, erythromycin remains the 'reference' macrolide antibiotic (Fig. 6.15).

Lincosamides (lincomycin, clindamycin)

Although chemically unrelated, the lincosamides possess closely related properties, modes of action and resistance patterns. Both classes bind to the same element of the ribosome so they are potentially competitive and should not be administered together.

Macrolide pharmacokinetics: key points
- Poorly absorbed orally.
- Short half-life (except azithromycin).
- High protein binding.

Anaerobic   Gram-positive   Gram-negative

Sensitivity range

Clostridium spp

Bacteroides spp

Haemophilus influenzae

Neisseria spp

E. coli ('coliforms')

Streptococcus spp

Enterococcus spp

Staphylococcus aureus

Pseudomonas aeruginosa

Fig. 6.15 Erythromycin: spectrum of activity.

- Excellent intracellular accumulation, good CSF penetration.

Lincosamide (e.g. clindamycin) pharmacokinetics: key points
- Good bioavailability.
- Food has no effect on absorption.
- Limited CSF penetration.

Adverse effects (macrolides and lincosamides)
- Generally very safe.
- Gastrointestinal upset, especially in young adults (erythromycin 30%, clindamycin 10–30%).
- Cholestatic jaundice with erythromycin estolate.
- Prolongation of QT interval on ECG, potential for torsades de pointes.
- Clindamycin—diarrhoea in 2–30% linked to *Cl. difficile* (Fig. 6.15).

The macrolides are used in the clinical management of Gram-positive infections where penicillin allergy occurs. Erythromycin is given in a dose of 250–500 mg 6-hourly, clarithromycin 250–500 mg 12-hourly. They are also particularly useful in the treatment of *Mycoplasma*, *Chlamydia* and rickettsial infections. The long intracellular half-life of azithromycin allows single-dose/short-course therapy (500 mg daily for 3 days) for genitourinary infections caused by these organisms.

KETOLIDES

The rapid development of penicillin and macrolide resistance amongst respiratory pathogens over the last decade has stimulated the development of this new class of antimicrobials. By molecular reconstruction the class is endowed with the ability to overcome the most common form of macrolide resistance amongst pathogens plus the theoretical property of lower resistance development.

Telithromycin is the first antibiotic of this class to reach the market. For management of respiratory tract infections a dose of 800 mg daily for 5 days is recommended. As for the macrolides, it has useful activity against atypical organisms in addition to the common bacterial causes of respiratory infection.

AMINOGLYCOSIDES

Aminoglycosides are very effective anti-Gram-negative antibiotics. It was thought they would become obsolete due to their marked oto- and nephrotoxicity; however, careful monitoring of renal function and drug levels and short treatment regimens minimise these problems. Aminoglycosides are particularly useful where β-lactam or quinolone resistance occurs in health care-acquired infections. They are not subject to an inoculum effect (reduced activity in the presence of a high concentration of bacteria) and they all exhibit a post-antibiotic effect (PAE) and synergism with β-lactam antibiotics.

6

6.23 THE AMINOGLYCOSIDES: DOSAGES

Aminoglycoside	Max. daily dose (mg/kg/24 hrs)	Maximum plasma levels	
		Peak level	Pre-dose level
Gentamicin	5	10 mg/l	2 mg/l
Tobramycin	5	10 mg/l	2 mg/l
Netilmicin	6	12 mg/l	2 mg/l
Amikacin	15	30 mg/l	10 mg/l

Notes
1. Plasma levels should be monitored in all patients if possible and must be measured in the elderly, in infants, and if high doses are given or if renal function is impaired.
2. Gentamicin, tobramycin and netilmicin are usually given 8- or 12-hourly if renal function is normal. Single daily dosage is also effective and less nephro- and ototoxic.
3. 60–80 mg 12-hourly of gentamicin is recommended for synergistic activity with β-lactams.

Pharmacokinetics: key points

- Negligible oral absorption (unless significant renal impairment).
- Hydrophilic so excellent penetration to body cavities and serosal fluids (distribution matches extracellular fluid).
- Very poor intracellular penetration (except hair cells in cochlea and renal cortical cells).
- Negligible CSF and corneal penetration.
- Peak plasma levels 30 minutes after infusion.
- Post-antibiotic effect allows once-daily administration (except in endocarditis, pregnancy, chronic renal disease and ascites).
- Monitoring of therapeutic levels required (Box 6.23).

Adverse reactions

- Renal toxicity (usually reversible), worse with concomitant vancomycin, cisplatin, amphotericin B, contrast media.
- Cochlear toxicity (permanent) more likely in older people.
- Neuromuscular blockade after rapid intravenous infusion (increased with calcium channel blockers, myasthenia gravis and hypomagnesaemia).

Aminoglycosides are very effective in Gram-negative sepsis and body fluid infection (Fig. 6.16), exerting synergism with β-lactam antibiotics. The post-antibiotic effect can be utilised to reduce toxicity and allow once-daily dosing. They cause very little local irritation at injection sites and negligible allergic responses. Intravenous therapy and close monitoring of blood levels are required. As a rule, courses should be limited to 10 days or less.

QUINOLONES

Of these synthetic agents (Box 6.24), the early quinolones had purely anti-Gram-negative activity, fluoroquinolones (e.g. ciprofloxacin) have 10–100 times greater activity against Gram-negative organisms (Fig. 6.17), and newer drugs, such as levo-, moxi-, spar-, gemi- and gati-floxacin, have improved anti-Gram-positive and anti-anaerobic capability. These antibiotics may now be used against respiratory pathogens in an empirical manner. Resistance has emerged since the early 1990s. In Spain, other European countries and the USA, resistance to ciprofloxacin of up to 10–20% in *E. coli* has been demonstrated.

Pharmacokinetics: key points

- Well absorbed after oral administration but delayed by food, antacids, ferrous sulphate and multivitamins.

6.24 QUINOLONES

Compound	Route of administration
Nalidixic acid	Oral
Fluoroquinolones	
Norfloxacin	Oral
Ciprofloxacin	I.v./oral
Ofloxacin	I.v./oral
Levofloxacin (L-isomer of ofloxacin)	I.v./oral
Sparfloxacin	Awaiting UK licence
Moxifloxacin	Oral

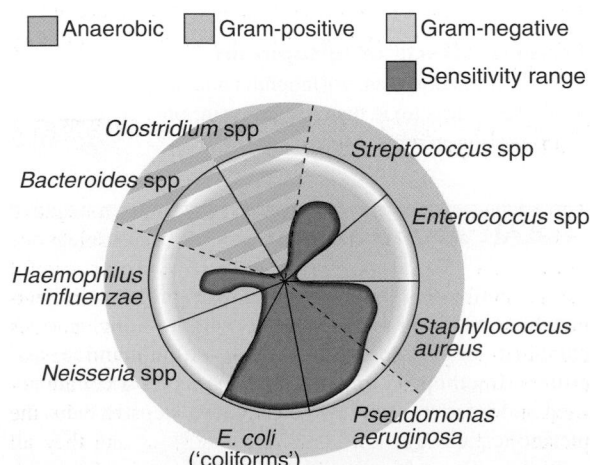

Fig. 6.16 Gentamicin: spectrum of activity.

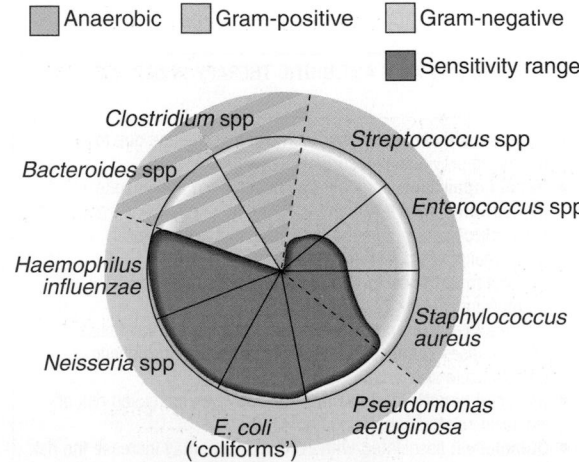

Fig. 6.17 Ciprofloxacin: spectrum of activity.

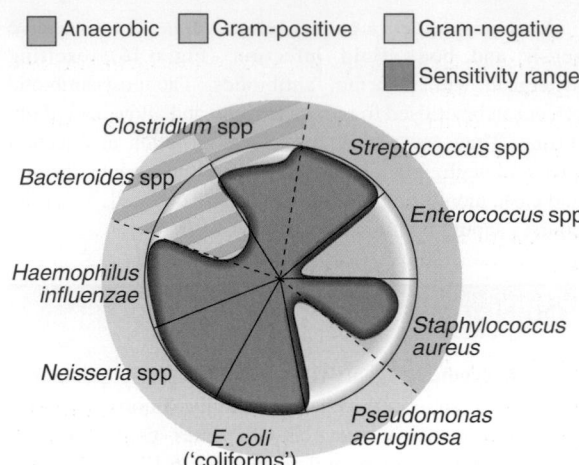

Fig. 6.18 **The newer quinolones (moxifloxacin): spectrum of activity.**

- Wide volume of distribution.
- Good intracellular penetration concentrating in phagocytes with high bioavailability.
- Tissue concentration twice that of serum.

Adverse reactions
- Very few side-effects.
- Rare skin reactions (phototoxicity).
- Gastrointestinal side-effects in 1–5%, tremor, dizziness and occasional seizures in 5–12% (Box 6.25).
- Coadministration with xanthines and theophyllines reduces clearance of these drugs so may produce insomnia and increases seizure potential.
- Bone and joint disease in animal studies limits use in children.
- Central nervous system effects such as confusion and seizures occur especially in the elderly.

The quinolones allow excellent anti-Gram-negative activity from oral dosing and have useful activity against atypical or intracellular organisms, e.g. *Mycoplasma* and *Chlamydia*. Other than recent additions to the class, they have poor Gram-positive activity and little action against

anaerobic infections (Fig. 6.18). Normal doses: ciprofloxacin 250–750 mg 12-hourly orally or 200–400 mg 12-hourly i.v.; levofloxacin 250–500 mg daily orally or 500 mg daily/ 12-hourly i.v.; moxifloxacin 400 mg once daily orally.

GLYCOPEPTIDES (VANCOMYCIN AND TEICOPLANIN)

Vancomycin is effective against Gram-positive organisms and, with teicoplanin, remains useful against MRSA and resistant enterococci. Some coagulase-negative staphylococci, enterococci and MRSA demonstrate levels of intermediate sensitivity or resistance to it (glycopeptide intermediate—GISA). The inappropriate use of vancomycin should be limited, particularly in the management of *Cl. difficile* infections, to prevent further resistance development. Gram-negative organisms are not sensitive to glycopeptides. (Dose: vancomycin 500 mg–1 g i.v. 12-hourly, 125 mg 6-hourly orally for *Cl. difficile*.) Teicoplanin has greater in vitro activity than vancomycin against Gram-positive organisms and can be used in a once-daily regimen (200–400 mg daily i.v.). It is not approved by the FDA for use in the USA. Neither drug has any activity against Gram-negative organisms or achieves any useful oral absorption.

Pharmacokinetics of vancomycin: key points
- Must be given by slow intravenous infusion with good tissue distribution and has a short half-life.
- Only enters CSF in the presence of inflammation.

Pharmacokinetics of teicoplanin: key points
- Long half-life allows once-daily dosing.
- More lipophilic than vancomycin, with good tissue penetration.

Adverse effects of vancomycin
- Histamine release due to rapid infusion produces the 'red-man' anaphylactoid reaction.
- Nephrotoxicity enhanced by concomitant aminoglycosides.
- Requires therapeutic monitoring.

Adverse effects of teicoplanin
- Rash, bronchospasm, eosinophilia and anaphylaxis.
- Markedly less toxic than vancomycin; only requires monitoring in renal impairment.

FOLATE ANTAGONISTS

These antibiotics interfere with the prokaryotic cell metabolism of para-aminobenzoic acid to folic acid. A combination of two antibiotics (a sulphonamide and either trimethoprim or pyrimethamine) is most commonly used and interferes with two consecutive steps in the same metabolic pathway.

Resistance to these antibiotics and the risk of adverse effects have limited their clinical usefulness over the years.

6.25 PROBLEMS WITH ANTIBIOTIC THERAPY IN OLD AGE

- **Hypersensitivity reactions:** increase in incidence due to increased previous exposure.
- **Renal impairment:** may be significant in old age despite 'normal' creatinine levels (p. 461)
  — **nephrotoxicity** is more likely, e.g. first-generation cephalosporins, aminoglycosides
  — **accumulation of β-lactam antibiotics:** may result in myoclonus, seizures or coma.
- **Reduced gastric acid production:** gastric pH is increased, which causes increased penicillin absorption and reduced ketoconazole absorption.
- **Reduced hepatic metabolism:** results in an increased risk of isoniazid-related hepatotoxicity.
- **Quinolones:** associated with confusion and may increase the risk of seizures.

Two combinations—trimethoprim/sulfamethoxazole (co-trimoxazole) and pyrimethamine/sulfadoxine (Fansidar)—remain important. Co-trimoxazole in high dosage (120 mg/kg) is the first-line drug for *Pneumocystis pneumoniae* infection in HIV disease.

Pharmacokinetics: key points
- Well absorbed orally with good bioavailability.
- Displace bilirubin from albumin so predispose to kernicterus in infants.
- Sulphonamides are hydrophilic, distributing well to the extracellular fluid.
- Trimethoprim is lipophilic with high tissue concentrations.

Adverse reactions
- Most are dose- and time-related (therapy for urinary tract infection should be no more than 3 days).
- Fatal marrow dysplasia and haemolysis in glucose-6-phosphate deficiency more common in the elderly.
- Skin and mucocutaneous reactions especially common and related to sulphonamide component.
- All reactions more common in high-dose therapy in HIV disease.

TETRACYCLINES AND CHLORAMPHENICOL

TETRACYCLINES

Of this mainly bacteriostatic class, the newer drugs doxycycline and minocycline show better absorption and distribution than older ones. Most streptococci, *Haemophilus*, *Moraxella*, *E. coli* and *Proteus* species are now resistant and tetracyclines are mostly used against *Mycoplasma*, *Chlamydia* and *Rickettsia*, plus *Borrelia* and other spirochaetes.

They have been used widely in veterinary practice therapeutically and as growth promoters. This practice, now banned in the European Union, is still prevalent in the USA and may account for much enterobacterial resistance.

Tigecycline
Chemical modification of the tetracycline molecule produced the semi-synthetic tetracycline analogue glycylcycline. The FDA licensed this antibiotic in the USA in 2005. It is a broad-spectrum parenteral-only antibiotic that is probably most valuable against resistant Gram-positive and Gram-negative pathogens such as MRSA and ESBL. It is only available for adult use in intravenous form, dose 100 mg by infusion followed by 50 mg 12-hourly. It has prominent gastrointestinal side-effects and all the limitations of the tetracycline group.

Pharmacokinetics: key points
- Best oral absorption in the fasting state (doxycycline 100% absorbed unless gastric pH rises).
- CSF levels increased in chronic inflammation (useful in Lyme disease).

Adverse reactions
- All tetracyclines except doxycycline are contraindicated in renal failure.
- Marked effect on bowel flora, causing side-effects of nausea and diarrhoea.
- Bind to metallic ions in bones and teeth, causing discoloration (avoid in children and pregnancy).
- Phototoxic skin reactions.
- Hypernatraemia (p. 431—used therapeutically in hyponatraemia).

CHLORAMPHENICOL

This widely used but potentially toxic antibiotic is bacteriostatic to most organisms but apparently bactericidal to *H. influenzae*, *Strep. pneumoniae* and *Neisseria meningitidis*. It has a very broad spectrum of activity against aerobic and anaerobic organisms, spirochaetes, *Rickettsia*, *Chlamydia* and *Mycoplasma*. It also has quite useful clinical activity against anaerobes such as *Bacteroides fragilis* (dose 50 mg/kg, divided 6-hourly).

Pharmacokinetics: key points
- Well absorbed after i.v. or oral dose (not i.m.). Good tissue distribution and levels.
- Good CSF levels.
- Crosses placenta and reaches breast milk.
- Competes for binding site with macrolides and lincosamides.

Adverse reactions
- Dose-dependent 'grey baby' syndrome in infants (cyanosis and circulatory collapse due to inability to conjugate drug and excrete active form in urine).
- Reversible dose-dependent bone marrow depression (adults) if > 4 g per day administered or cumulative dose > 25 g.
- Severe idiopathic aplastic anaemia in 1:25 000–40 000 treatment regimens (unrelated to dose, duration of therapy or route of administration).

Chloramphenicol remains a potent and cheap antibiotic, widely used throughout the world. Its use, however, is increasingly reserved for severe and life-threatening infections where other antibiotics are either unavailable or impractical. In the developed world its use is now confined to bacterial meningitis from *N. meningitidis* or *H. influenzae* (B) and to enteric fever or other life-threatening conditions without alternative therapy.

NITROIMIDAZOLES (METRONIDAZOLE, TINIDAZOLE)

The main clinical use of nitroimidazoles is in anaerobic infections, being highly active against strictly anaerobic bacteria, especially *B. fragilis*, *Cl. difficile* and other *Clostridia* species (metronidazole 400 mg 8-hourly). They retain significant antiprotozoal activity against amoebae and *Giardia*. They can be used as radiosensitising agents in some solid tumours.

Pharmacokinetics: key points
- Almost completely absorbed after oral administration (60% after rectal administration).
- Well distributed, especially brain and CSF.
- Safe in pregnancy.

Adverse effects
- Metallic taste (dose-dependent).
- Severe vomiting if taken with alcohol—'antabuse effect'.

OTHER ANTIMICROBIALS

OXAZOLIDINONES

These are organically synthesised antibiotics and show excellent oral absorption with activity similar to vancomycin against Gram-positive organisms such as streptococci, staphylococci and MRSA. They are competitively inhibited by coadministration of chloramphenicol and vancomycin/clindamycin.

Linezolid
This is the only oxazolidinone currently available for clinical use. It is rapidly absorbed, is approximately 30% protein-bound and appears very safe. Some 60% of patients taking this drug complain of some mild gastrointestinal side-effects and tongue discoloration.

STREPTOGRAMINS

These recently introduced antibiotics are active against highly resistant *Strep. faecium* or resistant MRSA infections. They are only available in intravenous formulations and show good tissue penetration but do not cross the blood–brain barrier or the placenta. Significant phlebitis occurs at injection sites and a raised creatinine and eosinophilia are recognised. They should be reserved for these resistant organisms.

QUINUPRISTIN/DALFOPRISTIN (3:7 RATIO) COMBINATION

This drug has recently been licensed in the UK for the treatment of serious Gram-positive infections which are resistant to standard therapies. Dose: 7.5 mg/kg 8-hourly.

FUSIDIC ACID

This antibiotic, active against Gram-positive bacteria including Gram-positive anaerobes, is available in intravenous, oral or topical formulations. It is lipid-soluble and efficiently distributed to peripheral compartments, including brain tissue. It demonstrates unpredictable antibacterial activity when combined with other antibiotics, so reducing its usefulness. It can be combined with clindamycin and rifampicin in the treatment of MRSA. It interacts with coumarin derivatives and oral contraceptives.

NITROFURANTOIN

This drug has very rapid renal elimination and is active against aerobic Gram-negative and Gram-positive bacteria including enterococci. It is used only as a urinary tract antibiotic, being safe in pregnancy and childhood. It can produce eosinophilic lung infiltrates, fever, pulmonary fibrosis, nerve disease, hepatitis and haemolytic anaemia.

SPECTINOMYCIN

Chemically similar to the aminoglycosides and given intramuscularly, spectinomycin is rapidly and completely absorbed. It was developed to treat strains of *N. gonorrhoeae* resistant to β-lactam antibiotics. Unfortunately, resistance to spectinomycin is very common and its only indication is the treatment of gonococcal urethritis in pregnancy or when the patient is allergic to β-lactam antibiotics.

ANTIFUNGAL AGENTS

See Box 6.26.

POLYENES (AMPHOTERICIN B)

Amphotericin B is the most important antifungal agent available and has been so since 1960. It is useful in the treatment of severe candidiasis, aspergillosis, cryptococcosis and the endemic mycoses of the Americas. It is also

6.26 ANTIFUNGAL DRUGS	
Drug	**Dose**
For topical application	
Nystatin	
Clotrimazole	
Econazole	
Amphotericin B	
For oral administration	
Ketoconazole	200 mg daily
Fluconazole	50–400 mg daily (max. 14 days)*
Itraconazole	100–200 mg daily
Voriconazole	200–400 mg 12-hourly (see literature)
Flucytosine	20 mg/kg daily
Griseofulvin	500 mg daily
Terbinafine	250 mg daily
For intravenous infusion	
Amphotericin B (also a liposomal preparation)	Initially 1 mg/kg/day (consult expert)
Flucytosine	200 mg/kg daily
Fluconazole	200–400 mg daily
Voriconazole	6 mg/kg 12-hourly (adults)
Caspofungin	70 mg daily, reducing to 50 mg/day

* Up to 400 mg daily for several weeks may be necessary in severely immunocompromised patients with invasive fungal infections. Invasive fungal infections requiring high doses and prolonged therapy should be treated by physicians with experience of these diseases. In an immunocompromised host (HIV) chronic antifungal secondary prophylaxis may be required.

6

frequently used as empirical therapy in patients with neutropenic fever (p. 1014) where fungal infections are common.

Pharmacokinetics of amphotericin B: key points

- Parent compound extremely lipophilic, insoluble in water.
- Very poor oral absorption.
- Long half-life in serum allows once-daily administration.
- Poor penetration to CSF (but still useful in the management of fungal meningitis).
- Lozenge form for mucocutaneous infections.

Adverse reactions

- Danger of insoluble emboli during therapy (in-line filter should always be used).
- Immediate rare anaphylaxis on infusion; test dose should always be given.
- Infusion-related problems in 50% of cases.
- Renal toxicity occurs rapidly in 80% of those treated (reversible and ameliorated by concomitant fluid infusion).

Lipid formulations of amphotericin B

Lipid formulations of amphotericin B have been developed to maximise the antifungal spectrum but reduce the toxicity of the parent compound. These are either a mixture of amphotericin B complexed with two phospholipids or an encapsulated formulation in unilamellar liposomes.

The drug becomes active when it dissociates from its lipid component following administration. It is only available intravenously. Adverse reactions are similar to but considerably less frequent than with amphotericin B.

FLUCYTOSINE

This drug has particular activity against yeasts (*Candida* spp and *Cryptococcus*). Although it is effective alone, the target organisms develop resistance fairly rapidly. Flucytosine should always be administered in combination with another antifungal agent.

The oral dose provides 90% of the predicted intravenous levels and is so effective that in the USA the intravenous formulation of this drug is no longer available.

Adverse reactions

These include neutropenia, anaemia, thrombocytopenia or profound pancytopenia; there may be slow recovery on withdrawal of the drug and asymptomatic disturbance of liver transaminases.

ECHINOCANDINS

This new class of antifungals acts to inhibit glucan synthesis in the fungal cell wall. This novel mode of action differentiates them from existing antifungals and potentially provides a safer, more potent alternative to amphotericin B in the management of severe/systemic fungal infections. There is little likelihood of cross-resistance from azoles or polyenes. Currently, echinocandins are active against

Candida (plus non-*albicans Candida*) and *Aspergillus* species.

Caspofungin is the first echinocandin licensed for use in the UK (70 mg i.v. by infusion on the first day, 50 mg thereafter). It remains very expensive and is therefore reserved for severe/resistant infections unresponsive to other antifungals.

AZOLE ANTIFUNGALS

These include miconazole, clotrimazole, ketoconazole, fluconazole and itraconazole. New agents voriconazole (200–400 mg 12-hourly dependent upon body weight) and posaconazole have an extended spectrum of activity and excellent efficacy via oral administration. They are particularly indicated as alternatives to amphotericin B in serious invasive fungal disease, e.g. aspergillosis, or resistant candidal infection.

Miconazole and clotrimazole are used solely for cutaneous and mucosal infections. Ketoconazole has a broad spectrum as the first oral antifungal agent with reasonable activity against *Candida* and *Aspergillus* spp. It is relatively cheap and cost-effective but has significant hepatic side-effects.

Fluconazole

Dose: 50–400 mg daily or 150 mg as single dose for vaginal candidiasis. This has ease of administration, an excellent safety profile and wide efficacy in *Candida* syndromes. The drug is highly water-soluble and distributes widely to all body sites and tissues, including CSF, where 89% of plasma levels can be recorded. It is well absorbed orally and has a long half-life of 30 hours, but lacks activity against *Aspergillus* spp.

Itraconazole

Dose: 100–200 mg daily dependent on infecting organism and host immune status. This is the only other oral antifungal agent active against *Aspergillus*. It is similar to fluconazole except for poor absorption orally, requiring a low gastric pH. It is lipophilic and distributes extensively, particularly to toe nails and fingernails; CSF penetration is poor.

OTHER ANTIFUNGAL AGENTS

Nystatin

Nystatin has a broad antifungal spectrum. Due to renal toxicity it is only available in topical formulation. It is particularly useful against mucosal candidiasis. The azole antifungals have gradually replaced nystatin but remain considerably more expensive. It may find a resurgence of use in azole-resistant candidiasis in HIV/AIDS.

Griseofulvin

For many years the standard therapy in the treatment of tinea unguium, griseofulvin has been largely superseded by other agents. It remains a cheap and effective agent; 50% is absorbed in fasting patients with virtually 100% bioavailability. Absorption is maximised by a fatty meal. It is deposited in keratin precursor cells, which then become virtually impervious to fungal invasion. The duration of

6

treatment depends on the response and is 2–4 weeks for tinea corporis or capitis, 4–8 weeks for tinea pedis and 4–6 months for tinea unguium.

Terbinafine

This has largely replaced griseofulvin as the major agent available against dermatophytes, yeasts, moulds and dimorphic fungi. It is well absorbed orally with minimal improvement with food. It can be given once daily and distributes with high concentration to sebum and skin with a long half-life of greater than 1 week. It is used for nail and skin infections, and topical therapy is reserved for the tinea infections. The major adverse reaction is hepatic toxicity. Terbinafine is not recommended for breastfeeding mothers and should not be applied vaginally.

ANTIVIRAL AGENTS

Most viral infections resolve without intervention in immunocompetent individuals. Antiviral therapy is available for a limited number of viral infections (Boxes 6.27 and 14.22, p. 397).

ANTIRETROVIRAL AGENTS

These agents, used predominantly against HIV, are discussed fully in Chapter 14.

DRUGS ACTIVE AGAINST THE HERPES GROUP OF ORGANISMS

Aciclovir, valaciclovir, famciclovir, ganciclovir and foscarnet

These drugs are predominantly acyclic analogues of guanosine. They are phosphorylated by virus-derived thymidine kinase (TK) enzymes and disrupt viral DNA metabolism. Aciclovir and its pro-drug valaciclovir, and penciclovir and its pro-drug famciclovir have activity against herpes simplex and varicella zoster virus but very little or no activity against cytomegalovirus. Aciclovir is slowly and incompletely absorbed by oral dosing; much better levels are achieved intravenously or by use of the pro-drug valaciclovir.

These drugs are extremely well tolerated with very few side-effects. Renal dysfunction may occur after rapid infusion of very large doses. CNS disturbance (agitation, hallucination, disorientation, tremors and mild clonus) have also been described. Famciclovir has good bioavailability orally and very rare adverse effects.

These drugs are extremely useful in the treatment of oral or genital herpes simplex infections and in larger dose against either acute chickenpox or herpes zoster infections (Box 13.30, p. 304). In varicella zoster pneumonitis the intravenous formulation of aciclovir should be used (dose 10 mg/kg 8-hourly).

Ganciclovir

By chemical modification of the aciclovir molecule, enhanced activity against cytomegalovirus is produced at the expense of increased toxicity. Although ganciclovir has the same activity as aciclovir against HSV-1 and 2 and varicella zoster virus, its toxicity limits its use. Despite very poor oral absorption, an oral formulation is available allowing maintenance therapy following intravenous medication for cytomegalovirus infection in HIV disease.

Adverse effects
- Bone marrow suppression (thrombocytopenia, neutropenia).
- Azoospermia.
- Mutually antagonistic antiviral with zidovudine (ZDV).
- Nephrotoxicity with ciclosporin or amphotericin B.

6.27 ANTIVIRAL DRUGS

Drug	Routes of administration	Indications	Side-effects
Aciclovir Valaciclovir	Topical Oral Intravenous	Herpes zoster Chickenpox (esp. in immunosuppressed) Herpes simplex infection: encephalitis, genital tract, eye	Rash, headache, gastrointestinal toxicity, neurotoxicity (i.v. only) Increase in urea and creatinine
Famciclovir Penciclovir	Oral Topical or systemic	Herpes zoster and genital herpes simplex infection Herpes zoster	Rash, headache Local irritation Herpes simplex keratitis
Amantadine	Oral	Prophylaxis of influenza A	CNS symptoms, nausea
Zanamivir	Inhalation	Influenza A and B	Bronchospasm, gastrointestinal side-effects, rash
Oseltamivir	Oral	Influenza A and B	Gastrointestinal side-effects, rash, rarely hepatitis
Ribavirin	Oral	Lassa fever Respiratory syncytial virus infection in infants (inhalation) Chronic hepatitis C infection (with interferons)	Reticulocytosis Respiratory depression
Ganciclovir	Intravenous/oral	Cytomegalovirus infection in immunosuppressed	Leucopenia, thrombocytopenia
HAART (p. 397)	Oral	HIV infection (including AIDS)	CNS symptoms, anaemia Lipodystrophy

Cidofovir

This is a newly formulated agent with potent activity against cytomegalovirus. It retains its activity against most cytomegalovirus clinical isolates that are resistant to ganciclovir and has some in vitro activity against herpes simplex virus, varicella zoster virus (including the TK-deficient aciclovir-resistant strains) and some other viruses.

Adverse effects

- Nephrotoxicity, ameliorated by intravenous hydration.
- Anterior uveitis after intravenous infusion.

Foscarnet

This analogue of inorganic pyrophosphate acts as a non-competitive inhibitor of herpes virus DNA polymerase. It is particularly useful in TK-deficient or mutated invasive HSV isolates resistant to aciclovir. It should only be administered by the intravenous route. It is equally effective against cytomegalovirus. It has very variable CSF penetration.

Adverse effects

- Significant nephrotoxicity (at least 15–20% of cases receiving this treatment). Intravenous fluids ameliorate.
- Hypocalcaemia, hypomagnesaemia and hypokalaemia may induce cardiac arrhythmias.

OTHER ANTIVIRAL AGENTS

Ribavirin

This has in vitro activity against influenza virus, respiratory syncytial virus (RSV), arenaviruses (including Lassa), bunyaviruses, herpes viruses, adenoviruses, poxviruses and retroviruses. Recent clinical studies have shown therapeutic benefit when ribavirin is combined with interferon-α (IFN-α) for the treatment of hepatitis C (p. 968). The drug is well absorbed after oral administration. Ribavirin is administered as an inhaled aerosol in the treatment of RSV pneumonitis or bronchiolitis (p. 689) and orally (in combination with IFN-α) for the treatment of chronic hepatitis C. Inhaled ribavirin is generally well tolerated, although bronchospasm, rash and ocular irritation can occur. Parenteral administration produces a mild haemolytic anaemia which is reversible but may require discontinuation of therapy.

Palivizumab

This monoclonal antibody preparation has recently been licensed in the UK for the management of infants at high risk of RSV infection. The first dose (15 mg/kg i.m., divided between more than one site monthly) should be administered prior to the start of the RSV season each year.

Interferon

The interferons are naturally occurring cytokines that are produced as an early response to viral infection, induce an antiviral state in exposed cells and modulate other immune functions. The addition of a polyethylene glycol (PEG) moiety to the molecule significantly enhances its pharmacokinetics and its efficacy. Currently, IFN-α preparations are used in the treatment of chronic hepatitis B and in combination with ribavirin for the treatment of hepatitis C infections. The drug is only available by injection.

Adverse effects

- Influenza-like syndrome after every dose (modified by premedication with paracetamol).
- Dose-limiting leucopenia, thrombocytopenia and depression.

Conjugation of interferon with polyethylene glycol (pegylated interferon or peginterferon) improves the pharmacokinetics and bioavailability and may be used in therapy of hepatitis C infection.

Amantadine, rimantadine

Amantadine and rimantadine are antiviral agents with some activity against influenza A (but not influenza B). A dose of 100 mg daily of either preparation will prevent 70–80% of symptomatic disease during influenza A epidemics. They are most commonly used either with vaccination to provide short-term prophylaxis, during outbreaks, or to treat early presentation of disease. Treatment must be started within 48 hours of the onset of symptoms and will reduce severity of disease by 1–2 days. Resistance develops very rapidly and both drugs are embryotoxic and teratogenic.

Zanamivir, oseltamivir

Zanamivir (10 mg 12-hourly by inhalation for 5 days) and oseltamivir (75 mg once daily as prophylaxis or 12-hourly for 5 days as treatment) are new agents indicated for the treatment of both influenza A and B (p. 688). UK guidelines are very specific (NICE 2003) and limit use to susceptible patients during known/demonstrable influenza outbreaks. They must be used within 48 hours of the onset of influenza symptoms and have been shown to reduce the duration of fever and illness by 1–2½ days.

3TC (lamivudine)

This drug, currently approved for the treatment of HIV infection (p. 397), has been shown to have excellent activity in animal models against hepatitis B. It is being incorporated into treatment regimens with IFN-α. The drug has significant bone marrow toxicity. The common mode of transmission of both HIV and hepatitis B needs to be recognised. The potential for induction of HIV resistance must be borne in mind should 3TC be selected for hepatitis B therapy.

Adefovir dipivoxil

This drug of the protease inhibitor class was originally developed as an antiretroviral preparation. It is licensed for the treatment of chronic hepatitis B and has some effect in lamivudine-resistant forms of that disease. As with lamivudine, it should be used with caution in dual HIV/HBV infections due to the theoretical development of HIV resistance during its administration.

ANTIPROTOZOAL DRUGS

See pages 342–360.

6

FURTHER INFORMATION

Books and journal articles
Cohen J, Powderly WG. Infectious diseases. 2nd edn. St Louis: Mosby; 2004.
Mandell GL, Bennett JE, Dolin R. Principles and practice of infectious diseases. 6th edn. Edinburgh: Churchill Livingstone; 2005.

Websites
www.dh.gov.uk/PolicyAndGuidance/HealthAndSocialCareTopics/ HealthcareAcquiredInfection/fs/en *Health care-associated infection*.
www.his.org.uk *Hospital Infection Society*.

6

N.R. COLLEDGE

Ageing and disease

COMPREHENSIVE GERIATRIC ASSESSMENT

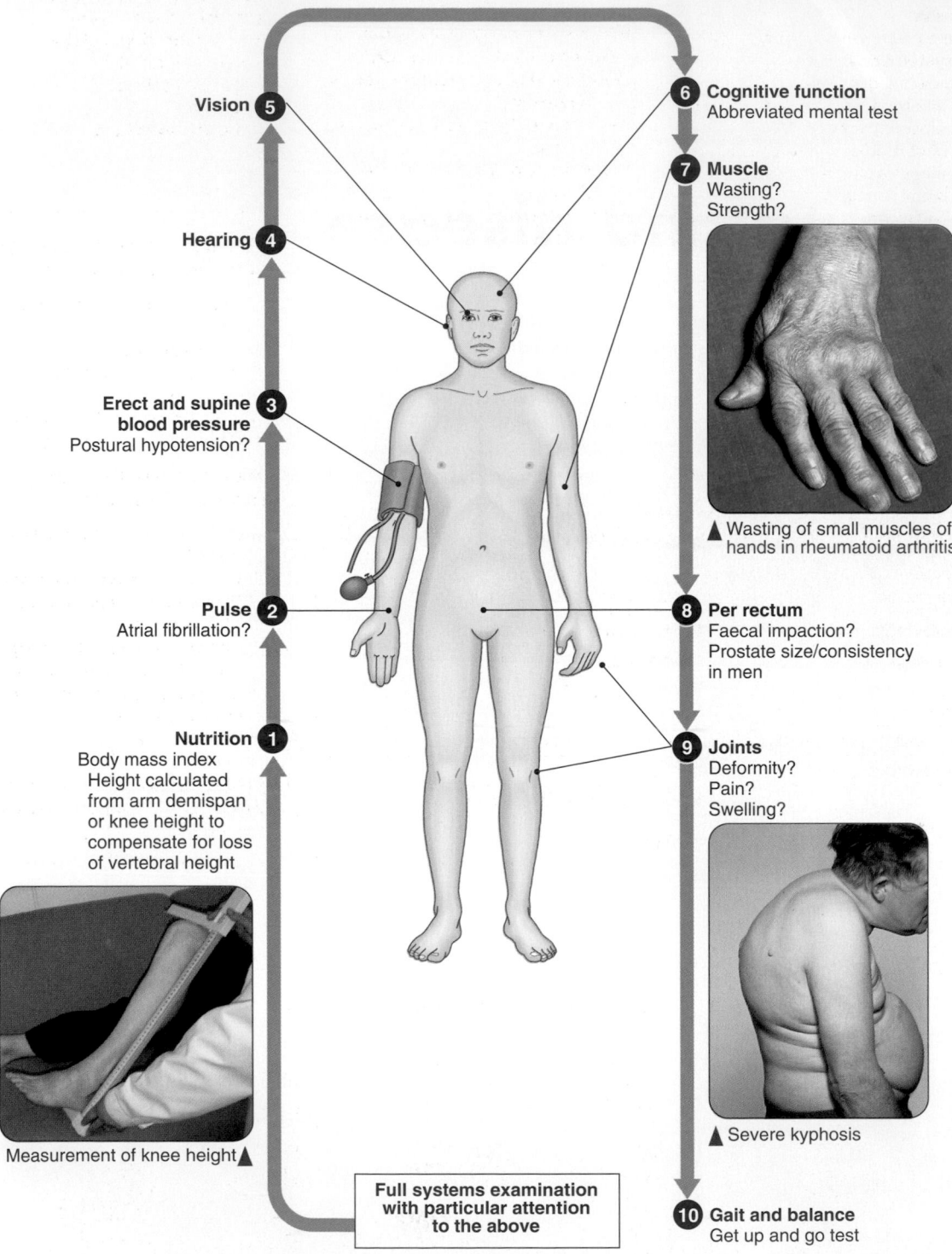

Vision 5

6 Cognitive function
Abbreviated mental test

7 Muscle
Wasting?
Strength?

Hearing 4

▲ Wasting of small muscles of
hands in rheumatoid arthritis

Erect and supine 3
blood pressure
Postural hypotension?

Pulse 2
Atrial fibrillation?

8 Per rectum
Faecal impaction?
Prostate size/consistency
in men

Nutrition 1
Body mass index
Height calculated
from arm demispan
or knee height to
compensate for loss
of vertebral height

9 Joints
Deformity?
Pain?
Swelling?

Measurement of knee height ▲

▲ Severe kyphosis

**Full systems examination
with particular attention
to the above**

10 Gait and balance
Get up and go test

7

HISTORY

- **Slow down** the pace.
- **Ensure the patient can hear**.
- Establish the **speed of onset of the illness**.
- If the presentation is vague, perform a **systematic enquiry**.
- Obtain full details of:
  - **all drugs**, especially any recent prescriptions
  - **past medical history**, even from many years previously
  - **usual function**
    - (a) Can the patient walk normally?
    - (b) Has the patient noticed memory problems?
    - (c) Can the patient perform all household tasks?
- **Corroborative history**: confirm information with a relative or carer and the general practitioner, particularly if the patient is confused or unable to communicate.

SOCIAL ASSESSMENT

Home circumstances

- Living alone or with another.

Activities of daily living (ADL)

- Tasks for which help is needed:
  - domestic ADL: shopping, cooking, housework
  - personal ADL: bathing, dressing, walking
- Informal help: relatives, friends, neighbours
- Formal social services: home help, meals on wheels
- Carer stress.

EXAMINATION

- **Thorough** to identify all comorbidities
- **Tailored to the patient's stamina** and ability to cooperate
- Includes **functional status**:
  - cognitive function
  - gait and balance
  - nutrition
  - hearing and vision.

---

⑥ ABBREVIATED MENTAL TEST

Each correct answer scores 1 mark.

1. What time is it? *(to the nearest hour)*
2. What year is it?
3. What is the name of this place/hospital?
4. How old are you? *(exact year)*
5. What is your date of birth?

Please memorise the following address: 42 West Street.

6. When did the First World War begin?
7. Who is the present monarch?
8. Please count backwards from 20 down to 1.
9. Can you recognise two people? *(e.g. relative or photograph)*
10. Can you tell me the address I asked you to memorise a few minutes ago?

Mini Mental State Examination is used for more detailed assessment (p. 230).

MULTIDISCIPLINARY TEAM (MDT) AND FUNCTIONAL ASSESSMENT	
Team member	**Activity assessed and promoted**
Physiotherapist	Mobility, balance and upper limb function
Occupational therapist	Activities of daily living, e.g. dressing, cooking (Assessment of home environment)
Dietitian	Nutrition
Speech and language therapist	Communication and swallowing
Social worker	Care needs
Nurse	Motivation and initiation of activities Feeding Continence

---

⑩ GET UP AND GO TEST

Ask the patient to stand up from a sitting position, walk 10 m, turn and go back to the chair.

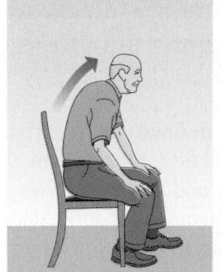
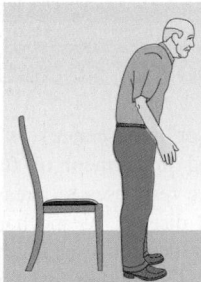
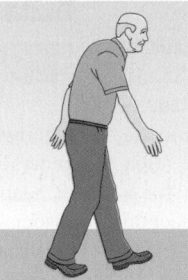
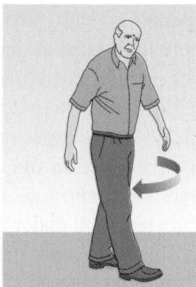
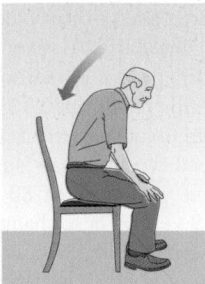

| Difficulty rising? | Unsteady on standing? | Unsteady gait? | Unsteady on turning? | Unsteady on sitting down? |

Geriatric medicine applies the knowledge and clinical skills of the organ-based specialties to a complex group: frail older people. This group is defined by the reduction in physiological capacity that makes them more susceptible to disease and mortality. As a result they frequently have multiple pathology, and illness often presents in atypical ways with confusion, falls, or loss of mobility and day-to-day functioning. Frail older people are also prone to adverse drug reactions, partly because of polypharmacy and partly because of age-related changes in responses to drugs and their elimination (p. 26). Disability is common in old age but patients' function can often be improved by the interventions of the multidisciplinary team, which includes nurses and physiotherapy, occupational and speech therapy, and medical staff.

The older population is extremely diverse. Many older people enjoy an active healthy life into advanced old age. A substantial proportion of 90-year-olds live alone and manage with little support, while some 70-year-olds are severely disabled by chronic disease, often accelerated by cigarette smoking. The terms 'chronological' and 'biological' ageing have been coined to describe these differences, and 'biological' rather than 'chronological' age is generally used as the basis for making decisions about the extent of investigation and intervention that is appropriate to an individual.

Unfortunately, older people have been neglected in research terms and, until recently, were rarely included in randomised clinical trials. There is thus little evidence on which to base practice.

DEMOGRAPHY

There has been a striking change in the demography of developed countries over the past hundred years. In the UK population, the proportion of people aged over 65 years has risen from 5% to 16%, and is projected to increase steadily to 24% in 2061. In contrast, the number of those aged under 16 years in the UK is falling. By 2007, people aged over 65 will outnumber those under 16. Support from younger to older populations may be direct (through living arrangements) or by taxation, so the consequences of this change will be far-reaching. On the other hand, many older people give support to the younger population, through care of children and of other older people.

Over the last 40 years there has been a particularly steep rise in the proportion of people aged over 85. In the UK this rose from 0.7% in 1961 to 1.9% in 2002 and is projected to increase to 3.8% in 2031. Life expectancy in the developed world is now substantial, even in old age (Box 7.1), and women aged 80 years can expect to live for a further 9 years. These changes are having a major impact on health and social services as disability and mental and physical morbidity rise sharply after the age of 75 years. In the UK, the estimated prevalence of severe disability is 2% in those aged 50–64, but 20% in those aged over 85 years.

Although the proportion of the population aged over 65 is greater in developed countries, most older people live in the developing world. Two-thirds of the world population of

7.1 MEAN LIFE EXPECTANCY IN THE DEVELOPED WORLD		
	Males	**Females**
At birth	76 years	81 years
At 60 years	20 years	23 years
At 70 years	13 years	15.5 years
At 80 years	7.5 years	9 years

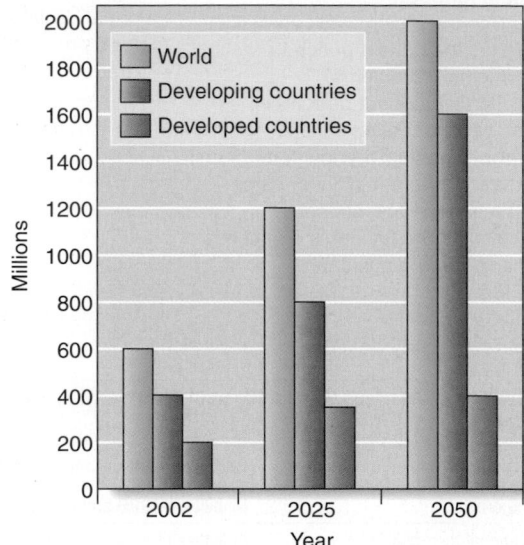

Fig. 7.1 **Number of people aged 60 and over in the world population.**

people aged over 65 live in developing countries at present, and this is projected to rise to 75% in 2025. The pace of population ageing is much faster in developing countries (Fig. 7.1) and so they will have less time to adjust to its impact.

FUNCTIONAL ANATOMY, PHYSIOLOGY AND INVESTIGATIONS

BIOLOGY OF AGEING

Ageing (or senescence) is defined as a progressive generalised impairment of function resulting in the loss of adaptive responses to stress and a growing risk of age-associated disease. Its mechanisms are poorly understood but it is unlikely that ageing has evolved for its own sake. Ageing is not an 'intrinsic' process, as it occurs in the context of an organism's interaction with the environment. Although genes play a part in ageing, a major contributor lies in the build-up of random damage, left unrepaired by inefficient somatic cellular 'housekeeping' mechanisms. Causes of this damage are described below.

Oxidative stress

This occurs when the production of reactive oxygen species (free radicals) exceeds available antioxidant systems. Interaction of these free radicals with DNA in mitochondria and the nucleus leads to mutations and deletions, especially in the mitochondria where DNA repair mechanisms are less efficient. This process continues until oxidative phosphorylation is compromised, adenosine triphosphate (ATP) production declines and cells begin to die.

Protein modification by glycation

Advanced glycosylation end-products are produced by spontaneous reactions between protein and local sugar molecules, a process which is increased by oxidative stress. These products damage the structure and function of the affected protein, which becomes resistant to breakdown. This is the cause of the yellowing of ageing nails and cornea.

Cell senescence

This is a further important phenomenon. Fibroblasts in culture can only undergo a limited number of cell divisions (the Hayflick limit). This suggests a 'biological clock' capable of counting the number of cell divisions, with the possible function of preventing cancer. The site of the 'clock' is thought to be in the telomere end regions of DNA, which shorten with each cell division because polymerase is unable to copy to the end of the 3' strand of linear DNA. This is compounded by poor telomeric DNA repair mechanisms. When telomeres are sufficiently eroded, cells stop dividing. Patients with the premature ageing Werner's syndrome display damaged DNA due to lack of a helicase, which is required for DNA repair and messenger RNA formation, and demonstrate particularly shortened telomeres.

In summary, the process of ageing is multifactorial and we are some way from a complete understanding of its mechanisms.

PHYSIOLOGICAL CHANGES

The physiological features of normal ageing have been identified by examining disease-free populations of older people, in order to separate the effects of pathology from those due to time alone. The principal change that occurs with ageing is a marked increase in inter-individual variation in function; many physiological processes in older people

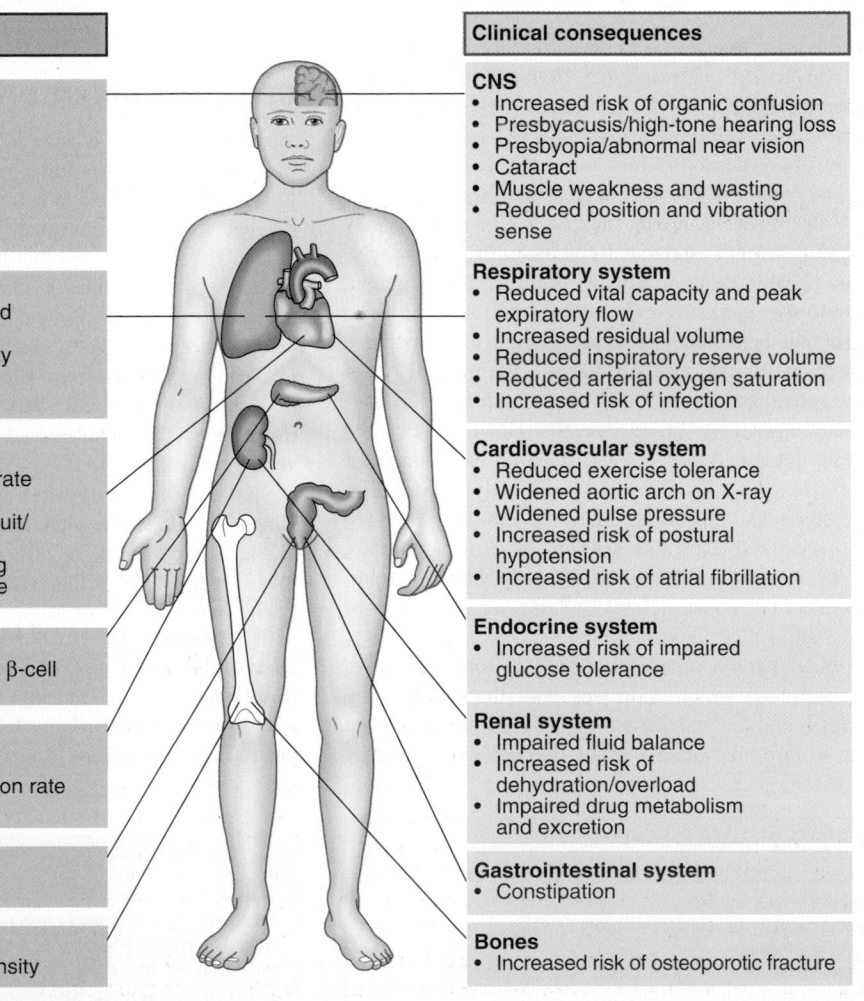

Changes with ageing

CNS
- Neuronal loss
- Cochlear degeneration
- Increased lens rigidity
- Lens opacification
- Anterior horn cell loss
- Dorsal column loss

Respiratory system
- Reduced lung elasticity and alveolar support
- Increased chest wall rigidity
- Increased V̇/Q̇ mismatch
- Reduced immune function

Cardiovascular system
- Reduced maximum heart rate
- Dilatation of aorta
- Reduced elasticity of conduit/capacitance vessels
- Reduced number of pacing myocytes in sinoatrial node

Endocrine system
- Deterioration in pancreatic β-cell function

Renal system
- Loss of nephrons
- Reduced glomerular filtration rate
- Reduced tubular function

Gastrointestinal system
- Reduced motility

Bones
- Reduced bone mineral density

Clinical consequences

CNS
- Increased risk of organic confusion
- Presbyacusis/high-tone hearing loss
- Presbyopia/abnormal near vision
- Cataract
- Muscle weakness and wasting
- Reduced position and vibration sense

Respiratory system
- Reduced vital capacity and peak expiratory flow
- Increased residual volume
- Reduced inspiratory reserve volume
- Reduced arterial oxygen saturation
- Increased risk of infection

Cardiovascular system
- Reduced exercise tolerance
- Widened aortic arch on X-ray
- Widened pulse pressure
- Increased risk of postural hypotension
- Increased risk of atrial fibrillation

Endocrine system
- Increased risk of impaired glucose tolerance

Renal system
- Impaired fluid balance
- Increased risk of dehydration/overload
- Impaired drug metabolism and excretion

Gastrointestinal system
- Constipation

Bones
- Increased risk of osteoporotic fracture

Fig. 7.2 Features and consequences of normal ageing.

deteriorate substantially when measured across populations, but some individuals show little or no change. Environmental factors, such as lack of exercise, poor diet, cigarette smoking and heavy alcohol consumption are thought to play a large part in this, and a healthy lifestyle remains worth encouraging, even when old age has been reached. Genetic factors may also be important in explaining individual variation.

The effects of ageing are usually not enough to interfere with organ function under normal conditions, but reserve capacity is reduced so that organ failure may be precipitated by a relatively minor illness. Some of the changes of ageing are of no clinical significance, such as depigmentation of the hair. Figure 7.2 shows the important changes and their clinical consequences.

FRAILTY

Frailty is defined as the loss of an individual's ability to withstand minor stresses because of reduced reserves in the physiological function of several organ systems. As a consequence, minor illnesses or adverse drug effects result in a disproportionate loss of function and increased risk of death. The same stresses may cause little disturbance in a fit person of the same age.

It is important to understand the difference between 'disability' and 'frailty'; although they frequently coexist, they are separate entities. Disability indicates established loss of function while frailty indicates increased vulnerability to loss of function. Disability may arise from a single pathological event (such as a stroke) in an otherwise healthy individual. After recovery, minor fluctuations in function may occur, but overall it is stable and the patient may otherwise be in good health. When frailty and disability coexist, function deteriorates markedly, even with minor illness, often to the extent that the patient can no longer cope independently.

Unfortunately, the term 'frail' is often used rather vaguely, sometimes to justify a lack of adequate investigation and intervention in older people. However, it can be specifically identified by assessing function in a number of domains (Box 7.2). These are all commonly impaired by disease, illness and indeed age, but their function can often be improved by specific intervention. In clinical practice, frailty per se is rarely measured formally, but a comprehensive assessment (see below) includes an evaluation of each domain.

Frail older people particularly benefit from a comprehensive approach which addresses both the precipitating acute illness and the underlying loss of function. It may be possible to prevent further loss of function through early

intervention; a frail woman with cardiac failure will benefit from specific cardiac investigation and treatment, but even more with an exercise programme to improve her musculoskeletal function, balance and aerobic capacity, and nutritional support to restore lost weight. Establishing a patient's level of frailty also helps inform decisions regarding further investigation and management, and to identify those in need of rehabilitation.

INVESTIGATIONS

COMPREHENSIVE GERIATRIC ASSESSMENT

Although not strictly an investigation, one of the most powerful tools in the management of older people is the Comprehensive Geriatric Assessment, which identifies all the relevant factors contributing to their presentation (pp. 160–161). In frail patients with multiple pathology, there is a tension between this assessment and the need to ensure that they are not exhausted by the process. It may be necessary to perform a comprehensive assessment in stages to take account of the patient's stamina and ability to cooperate. The outcome of the assessment should be a management plan that addresses not only the patient's acute presenting problems, but also improves their overall health and function (Box 7.3).

DECISIONS ABOUT INVESTIGATION

Accurate diagnosis is important at all ages. However, frail older people may not have sufficient stamina or cognitive function to withstand lengthy or invasive procedures, and diagnoses may be revealed which cannot be treated for similar reasons. On the other hand, disability must never be accepted as due to age without adequate investigation. This only leads to inappropriate intervention; for example, the patient no longer able to climb stairs is supplied with a stair lift, when simple tests would have revealed osteoarthritis of a hip and vitamin D deficiency, for which appropriate treatment would have restored the patient's strength to climb stairs once more.

So how is it decided when and how far to investigate? For simple blood tests or plain X-rays, there is no issue in most cases. It becomes more difficult with complex or invasive investigations. The principal factors are described below.

The patient's general health

Does this patient have the physical and mental capacity to tolerate the proposed investigation? Would she be able to manoeuvre on an X-ray table, as required for a barium enema? Does he have the aerobic capacity to undergo

---

7.2 DOMAINS IMPAIRED IN FRAILTY

- Musculoskeletal function
- Aerobic capacity, i.e. cardiorespiratory function
- Cognitive function
- Integrative neurological function (e.g. balance and gait)
- Nutritional status

7.3 COMPREHENSIVE GERIATRIC ASSESSMENT   **EBM**

'Comprehensive Geriatric Assessment programmes linking geriatric evaluation with strong long-term management improve survival and function in old age.'

- Stuck AE, et al. Lancet 1993; 342:1032–1036.

7

bronchoscopy? The more pathologies patients have, the less likely they will be able to withstand an invasive or complex intervention. Information on the outcomes in critically ill older patients is given on page 190.

Will the investigation alter management?

Would the patient be fit for or benefit from the treatment that would be indicated if investigation proved positive? This may be a particular issue if surgery is a possibility. When a patient with severe heart failure and a previous disabling stroke presents with a suspicious mass lesion on chest X-ray, detailed investigation and staging are not appropriate if he or she is not fit for surgery, radical radiotherapy or chemotherapy. On the other hand, if the same patient presented with a pyrexia, investigation for underlying infection would be important, as he or she would be able to tolerate treatment with antibiotics.

The presence of comorbidity is more important than age itself in determining a patient's likely benefit from specific interventions.

The views of the patient and family

Older people often have strong views about their management, and these should be actively sought from the outset when assessing the risks and benefits of investigation and treatment. If the patient wishes, the views of relatives should also be taken into account. If the patient is not able to express a view or lacks capacity because of cognitive impairment or communication difficulties, then relatives' input becomes particularly helpful. They should be asked what they think the patient would have wanted under the circumstances but should never be made to feel responsible for difficult decisions.

Advance directives

Advance directives or 'living wills' are statements made by adults at a time when they have the capacity to decide for themselves about the treatments they would refuse or accept in the future, should they no longer be able to make decisions or communicate them. An advance directive cannot authorise a doctor to do anything that is illegal and doctors are not bound to provide a specific treatment requested, if in their professional opinion it is not clinically appropriate. However, any advance refusal of treatment, made when the patient was able to make decisions based on adequate information about the implications of their decision, is legally binding in the UK. It must be respected where it clearly applies to the patient's present circumstances and where there is no reason to believe that the patient has changed his or her mind.

PRESENTING PROBLEMS IN GERIATRIC MEDICINE

Problem-based practice is integral to geriatric medicine. Most problems are multifactorial and there is rarely a unifying diagnosis. This complexity makes for a rewarding medical challenge. All factors have to be taken into account and attention to detail is paramount. Two patients with the same initial problem are rarely the same in any other way. A wide knowledge of adult medicine is required, as disease in any and often many of the organ systems has to be managed. There are a number of features that are particular to older patients.

Late presentation

Many people (of all ages) accept ill health as a consequence of ageing and may tolerate symptoms for lengthy periods before seeking medical advice. Comorbidities may also contribute to late presentation; in a patient whose mobility is limited by stroke, angina may only present when coronary artery disease is advanced as the patient was unable to exercise sufficiently to cause symptoms at an earlier stage.

Atypical presentation

Infection may present with acute confusion and without clinical pointers to the organ system affected. Stroke may present with falls rather than symptoms of focal weakness. Myocardial infarction may present as weakness and fatigue, without the classical symptoms of chest pain or dyspnoea. The reasons for these atypical presentations are not always easy to explain. Perception of pain is altered in old age, which may explain why myocardial infarction presents in other ways. The pyretic response is blunted in old age so that infection may not be obvious at first. Co-existent dementia may limit the patient's ability to give a history of classical symptoms.

Acute illness and changes in function

It follows from this that 'failure to cope', 'found on floor', 'confusion' and 'off feet' are presentations and *not* diagnoses. When an older patient presents with any of these, the possibility that an acute illness has been the precipitant must always be considered. It can be difficult to know whether this is likely until it is established whether the patient's current status is a change from his or her usual level of function by asking a relative or carer (by telephone if necessary). Investigations aimed at uncovering an acute illness will not be fruitful in a patient whose function has been deteriorating over several months, but if it has suddenly changed, acute illness must be excluded.

Multiple pathology

Presentations in older patients have a more diverse differential diagnosis because multiple pathology is so common. It means that there are usually a number of causes for any single problem, and side-effects from medication may be a contributory factor. A patient may fall because of osteoarthritis of the knees, postural hypotension due to diuretic therapy for hypertension, and poor vision due to cataracts. All these factors have to be addressed to prevent further falls, and this principle holds for most of the common presenting problems in old age.

APPROACH TO PRESENTING PROBLEMS IN OLD AGE

For the sake of clarity the common presenting problems are described individually here, but in real life, older patients

7

often present with several at the same time, particularly confusion, incontinence and falls. These share some underlying causes and may precipitate each other.

The approach to most presenting problems in old age can be summarised as follows:

- *The telephone test*. Find out the patient's usual status (e.g. mobility, cognitive state) from a relative or carer.
- *Check medication*. Have there been any recent changes?
- *Search for and treat any acute illness*. See Box 7.4.
- *Identify and reverse predisposing risk factors*. These depend on the presenting problem.

FALLS

Falls and unsteadiness are very common in older people. Around 30% of those aged 65 and over fall each year, this figure rising to over 40% in those aged over 80 years. Although only 10–15% of falls result in serious injury, they are the principal cause of fractured neck of femur in this age group. Falls also lead to loss of confidence and fear, and are frequently the 'final straw' that makes an older person decide to move to institutional care.

The approach to the patient varies according to the underlying cause of falls, as follows.

Accidental trip

Those who have simply tripped may not require detailed assessment unless they are doing so frequently or have sustained an injury.

Blackouts

A proportion of older people who 'fall' have in fact had a syncopal episode. It is important to ask about loss of consciousness and, if this is a possibility, to perform appropriate investigations (pp. 551 and 1164). Recent research suggests that in small numbers of patients, carotid sinus syndrome (p. 553) may be the cause of otherwise unexplained falls.

Acute illness

Falling is one of the classical atypical presentations of acute illness in the frail. The reduced reserves in older people's integrative neurological function mean that they are less able to maintain their balance when challenged by an acute illness. Suspicion should be especially high when falls have occurred suddenly over a period of a few days. Common underlying illnesses include infection, stroke, metabolic disturbance and heart failure. Thorough examination and

investigation are required to identify these (Box 7.4). It is also important to establish whether any drug has been started recently, as this may precipitate falls. Once an underlying acute illness has been treated, falls may no longer be a problem.

Multiple risk factors

Many patients, especially those with recurrent falls, are frail with multiple medical problems and chronic disabilities. Their tendency to fall is associated with risk factors that have been well established from prospective studies (Box 7.5). The annual risk of falling increases linearly with the number of risk factors present, from 8% with no risk factors to 78% in those with four or more. Obviously, such patients may present with a fall resulting from an acute illness or syncope as above, but they will remain at risk of further falls even when the acute illness has resolved.

It has been shown that an effective way of preventing further falls in this group is multiple risk factor intervention (Box 7.6). Examples of such interventions are shown in Box 7.7 and require a multidisciplinary approach. The most effective is balance and exercise training by physio-

---

7.5 RISK FACTORS FOR FALLS

- Muscle weakness
- History of falls
- Gait or balance abnormality
- Use of a walking aid
- Visual impairment
- Arthritis
- Impaired activities of daily living
- Depression
- Cognitive impairment
- Age over 80 years
- Drugs
  Polypharmacy (four or more drugs)
  Digoxin
  Diuretics
  Drugs associated with sedation: benzodiazepines, phenothiazines, antidepressants
  Type I anti-arrhythmics

EBM

7.6 PREVENTION OF FALLS IN OLDER PEOPLE

'Effective interventions to prevent falls in elderly people include multidisciplinary, multifactorial interventions, muscle strength and balance training, home hazard assessment and modification, withdrawal of psychotropic medication, cardiac pacing in fallers with carotid sinus syndrome and t'ai chi group exercise.'

- Gillespie LD, et al. (Cochrane Review). Cochrane Library, issue 3, 2004. Oxford: Update Software.

For further information: 🖥 www.nice.org.uk

7.4 INVESTIGATIONS TO IDENTIFY ACUTE ILLNESS

- Full blood count
- Urea and electrolytes, liver function tests, calcium and glucose
- Chest X-ray
- Electrocardiogram (ECG)
- Urinalysis for leucocytes and nitrites; if positive, urine culture
- C-reactive protein: useful marker for occult infection
- Blood cultures if pyrexial

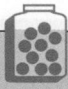

7.7 MULTIFACTORIAL INTERVENTIONS TO PREVENT FALLS

- Balance and exercise training
- Rationalisation of medication, especially sedative drugs
- Correction of visual impairment
- Home environmental hazard assessment and safety education
- Treatment of cardiovascular disorders, including carotid sinus syndrome and postural hypotension

7

7.8 MANAGEMENT OF POSTURAL HYPOTENSION

- Correct dehydration
- Tilt up the head of the bed
- Support stockings (older patients may struggle to get these on)
- Non-steroidal anti-inflammatory drugs (increase circulating volume due to salt and water retention; gastric side-effects limit use)
- Fludrocortisone (causes salt and water retention but poorly tolerated due to cardiac failure)

therapists. An assessment of the patients' home environment for hazards must be delivered by an occupational therapist, who can also provide personal alarms so that patients can summon help, should they fall again. Rationalising medication may help to reduce sedation, although many older patients are reluctant to stop their hypnotic. It will also help reduce postural hypotension, defined as a drop in blood pressure of >20 mmHg systolic or >10 mmHg diastolic pressure on standing from supine. Other measures to reduce postural hypotension are shown in Box 7.8.

The cause of any disability such as loss of strength or gait disturbance should be established, as specific treatment may improve it. For example, a patient's quadriceps muscles may be weak due to osteoarthritis of the hip, which will improve with adequate analgesia and physiotherapy. Gait disturbance due to Parkinson's disease will improve with appropriate drug treatment and physiotherapy. Simple interventions such as providing new glasses or chiropody can have a surprising impact on function.

Bone protection

Osteoporosis prophylaxis should be considered in all older patients who have recurrent falls, particularly if they have already sustained a fracture (p. 1124). In female patients in institutional care, calcium and vitamin D_3 have been shown to reduce fracture rates, and may also reduce falls due to improvements in muscle function. Devices known as hip protectors have also been shown to reduce the risk of hip fracture in those in institutional care, but are poorly tolerated. They consist of polypropylene pads fixed in special underwear to keep them positioned over the greater trochanters. Should patients fall on their hip, the pads disperse the force of the fall away from bone to soft tissues.

ACUTE CONFUSION

The presentation, diagnosis and management of acute confusion are described on page 1187. It is very important to establish the patient's usual cognitive function with a relative or carer, remembering that dementia is a risk factor for acute confusion so they may coexist. Almost any acute illness may present with confusion in old age, and the most common are infection and stroke. The recent addition of a drug is a further common precipitant. Predisposing factors include visual or hearing impairment, alcohol misuse and poor nutrition.

After the telephone test, any acute illness should be sought and treated. Investigation should be performed as in Box 7.4. Computed tomography (CT) of the brain is required in:

- those with focal neurological signs
- those with head injury
- those who fail to improve despite treatment of identified acute illness.

If confused patients become so agitated that their behaviour puts them or others at risk, sedation may be required. Initially, small doses of haloperidol (0.5 mg) or lorazepam (0.5 mg) are the safest drugs to use. Not all patients present with agitation; some become apathetic and withdrawn, and care must be taken to ensure their adequate hydration and nutrition. Acute confusion in old age can be slow to resolve and may not do so completely. It is a marker for the possible subsequent development of dementia.

URINARY INCONTINENCE

Urinary incontinence is defined as the involuntary loss of urine, sufficiently severe to cause a social or hygiene problem. It occurs in all age groups but becomes more prevalent in old age, affecting about 15% of women and 10% of men aged over 65 years. It may lead to skin damage if severe and is very socially restricting. While age-dependent changes in the lower urinary tract predispose older people to incontinence, it is not an inevitable consequence of ageing and always requires investigation. Urinary incontinence is frequently precipitated by acute illness in old age and is commonly multifactorial (Box 7.9).

7.9 CAUSES OF TRANSIENT INCONTINENCE

- Restricted mobility
- Acute confusional state
- Urinary tract infection
- Severe constipation
- Drugs, e.g. diuretics, sedatives
- Hyperglycaemia
- Hypercalcaemia

Initial management is to seek and treat these problems. If incontinence fails to resolve or if the patient has established incontinence, further diagnosis and management should be pursued as described on page 474. The condition can usually be improved with appropriate treatment. Urinary catheterisation should never be viewed as first-line management but may be required as a final resort if the perineal skin is at risk of breakdown or quality of life is impaired by intractable incontinence.

POLYPHARMACY

Polypharmacy is defined as the inappropriate use of multiple drugs, and is common in old age. Older people receive many more prescribed drugs than younger people and this is increasing in the UK (Box 7.10). Even when appropriate—many cardiovascular conditions such as hypertension, myocardial infarction and heart failure dictate the use of

7.10 MEAN NUMBER OF PRESCRIPTION ITEMS DISPENSED BY AGE IN ENGLAND				
Year	0–15 years	15–64 years	65+ years	All ages
2001	4.5	7.2	31.1	11.9
2002	4.4	7.4	33.1	12.4
2003	4.3	7.7	35.0	13.4

7.11 FACTORS LEADING TO POLYPHARMACY

- Multiple pathology
- Poor patient education
- Lack of routine review of all medications
- Patient expectations of prescribing
- Over-use of drug interventions by doctors
- Attendance at multiple specialist clinics
- Poor communication between specialists

several drugs—multiple drugs put older patients at increased risk of adverse drug reactions and interactions, falls and acute confusion. The reasons for this are described on page 26. Adding to the risk is the fact that non-adherence to drug therapy rises with the number of drugs prescribed. Several factors contribute to polypharmacy (Box 7.11).

The clinical presentations of polypharmacy are extremely diverse, so for *any* presenting problem in old age the possibility that the patient's medication is a contributory factor should *always* be considered. Regular review of all medications is the best way of avoiding the problem. Physicians should ask the patient or carer to bring all medication for review rather than relying on previous records. Those drugs that are no longer required or are contraindicated can be discarded.

DIZZINESS

Dizziness is very common, affecting at least 30% of those aged over 65, according to community surveys. It is a good example of the importance of a problem-based rather than an organ-based approach in medicine in old age as it is very commonly multifactorial rather than due to a single condition (pp. 551 and 1164). Acute dizziness is relatively straightforward and common causes include:

- hypotension due to arrhythmia, acute myocardial infarction, gastrointestinal bleed or pulmonary embolism etc.
- acute posterior fossa stroke
- vestibular neuronitis.

However, older people more commonly present with recurrent dizzy spells. They often find it difficult to describe the sensation they experience, so assessment can be very frustrating. Nevertheless the most effective way of establishing the cause(s) of the problem is to determine which of the following is the predominant symptom, even if more than one is often present:

- lightheadedness suggestive of presyncope
- vertigo suggestive of labyrinthine or brain-stem disease
- unsteadiness/poor balance suggestive of joint or neurological disease.

Investigation can then be focused on the specific symptom. For example, a 24-hour ambulatory ECG may be helpful in some patients with presyncope, but not in those with vertigo or unsteadiness. The most common underlying diagnoses in this age group include:

- cerebrovascular disease, either stroke or small vessel disease, which may cause unsteadiness and/or lightheadedness
- degenerative joint disease, especially of weight-bearing joints and cervical spine
- hypotensive medication, which often also exacerbates postural hypotension
- benign paroxysmal positional vertigo (p. 1166).

Most symptoms are provoked by activity. If a patient is experiencing symptoms at rest, arrhythmia should be excluded. Anxiety and poor vision are frequent concomitants of dizziness in old age, but are rarely the only cause. Other causes are described in the algorithms on pages 552 and 1165. If the patient is falling as a result of dizziness, the interventions for falls described above should be applied.

OTHER PROBLEMS

There is a vast range of other possible presenting problems in older people, and they present to many medical specialties. Relevant sections in other chapters are referenced in Box 7.12.

Within each chapter you will find 'In Old Age' panels to highlight the areas in which presentation or management differs in this age group from younger individuals. These are listed at the end of this chapter.

7.12 OTHER PRESENTING PROBLEMS IN OLD AGE

Hypothermia	p. 100
Poor nutrition	p. 118
Infection	pp. 289 and 326
Fluid balance problems	p. 431
Heart failure	p. 542
Hypertension	p. 551
Dizziness and blackouts	pp. 551, 1164
Atrial fibrillation	p. 562
Diabetes mellitus	p. 814
Peptic ulceration	p. 885
Anaemia	p. 1023
Painful joints	p. 1076
Bone disease and fracture	pp. 1121–1130
Immobility	p. 1178
Stroke	p. 1200
Dementia	p. 1217

7

REHABILITATION

Rehabilitation aims to improve the ability of people of all ages to perform day-to-day activities, and to restore their physical, mental and social capabilities as far as possible. Acute illness in older people is often associated with loss of their usual ability to function, and common disabling conditions such as stroke, fractured neck of femur, arthritis and cardio-respiratory disease become increasingly prevalent with advancing age. Figure 7.3 shows the prevalence of the most frequent disabilities in the UK population.

Disability is an interaction between factors intrinsic to the individual and the context in which they live, and interventions at both a medical and a social level are needed in response (Box 7.13). Doctors tend to focus on health conditions and impairments, but patients are more concerned with their effects: the limitation of their activities and restricted participation in everyday life.

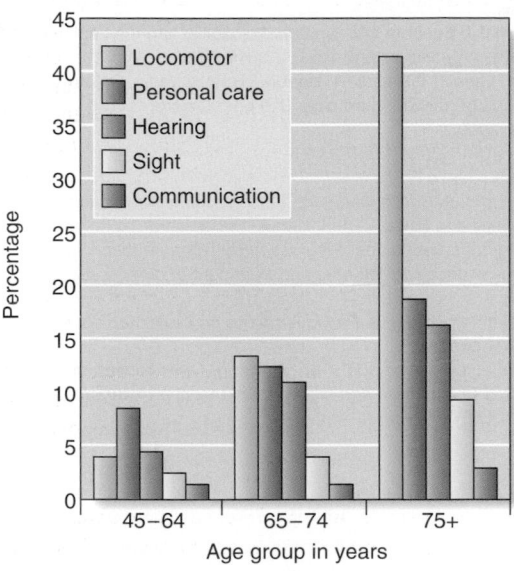

Fig. 7.3 Prevalence of disability in the UK.

The process

Rehabilitation is a problem-solving process focused on improving a patient's function. This includes not only physical function, but also psychological and social functioning. It covers:

- *Assessment.* The nature and extent of the patient's problems are identified from a comprehensive assessment using the framework in Box 7.13. Specific assessment scales such as the Elderly Mobility Scale or Barthel Index of Activities of Daily Living can be used to quantify components of disability but do not determine the underlying causes or the interventions required for individual patients.
- *Goal-setting.* Goals set are specific to the patient's problems, realistic and agreed by the patient with the rehabilitation team.
- *Intervention.* This includes active treatments to achieve the set goals and to maintain the patient's health and quality of life.
- *Reassessment.* There is ongoing re-evaluation of the patient's function and progress towards the set goals, with modification of the interventions if necessary. This requires regular review by all members of the rehabilitation team, the patient and the carer.

Multidisciplinary team working

The core rehabilitation team includes several professional disciplines (Box 7.14), although others may be involved as needed, e.g. audiometry for hearing impairment, podiatry for foot problems and orthotics where prostheses or splinting are required. Good communication and mutual respect are essential. Rehabilitation is *not* where the doctor orders 'Refer to physio' or 'Get a home visit', and takes no further role.

Regular meetings take place to:

- share assessments
- plan and agree rehabilitation goals and interventions
- evaluate progress
- plan discharge.

7

7.13 INTERNATIONAL CLASSIFICATION OF FUNCTIONING AND DISABILITY

Factor	Intervention required
Health condition The underlying disease, e.g. stroke, osteoarthritis	Medical or surgical treatment
Impairment The symptoms or signs of the condition, e.g. hemiparesis, visual loss	Medical or surgical treatment
Activity limitation The resultant loss of function, e.g. walking, dressing	Rehabilitation, assistance, aids
Participation restriction The resultant loss of social function, e.g. cooking, shopping	Adapted accommodation Social services

7.14 THE REHABILITATION TEAM

Team member	Role
Physiotherapist	Promotion of balance, mobility and upper limb function
Occupational therapist	Promotion of activities of daily living, e.g. dressing, cooking Assessment of home environment
Speech and language therapist	Management of speech and swallowing disorders
Dietitian	Management of nutrition
Social worker	Organisation of home support services or institutional care
Nurse	Reinforcement of rehabilitation goals Communication with relatives and other professionals
Doctor	Management of medical problems Coordinator of rehabilitation programme

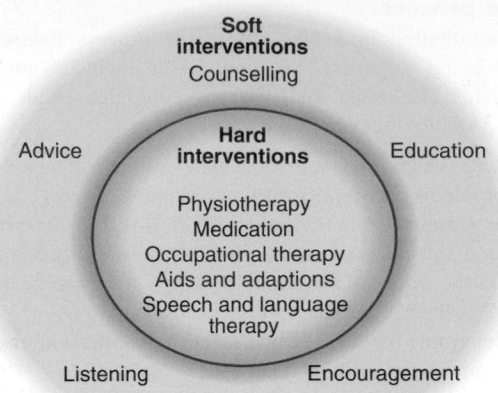

Fig. 7.4 Rehabilitation techniques.

Rehabilitation interventions

The interventions used in rehabilitation can be divided into 'hard', i.e. hands-on treatment by therapists using a functional, task-orientated approach to improve day-to-day activities, and 'soft' interventions such as psychological support and education, often just as important to progress (Fig. 7.4). The emphasis on the type of intervention will be different depending on the patient's disabilities, psychological status and progress. The patient has to be an active participant in the process, working to overcome disability with the encouragement and help of the rehabilitation team.

Rehabilitation outcomes

Effective rehabilitation has a major impact on reducing disability in older patients after acute illness or emergency and elective surgery. There is good evidence that rehabilitation improves functional outcome following stroke and myocardial infarction, and in those with chronic obstructive pulmonary disease. It also reduces mortality after stroke (p. 1207). Rehabilitation obviously involves complex multi-component interventions and it is not clear which has the greatest effect. Is it specific therapy techniques, better delivery and organisation of care, or simply staff enthusiasm? The concept of the 'black box' of rehabilitation has been used to describe this poor understanding of the process, and is the subject of ongoing research.

FURTHER INFORMATION

Books and journal articles
American Geriatrics Society, British Geriatrics Society and American Academy of Orthopedic Surgeons Panel on Falls Prevention. Guideline for the prevention of falls in older persons. Journal of the American Geriatric Society 2001; 49:664–672. *Can be downloaded from the BGS website (below).*

Campbell AJ, Buchner DM. Unstable disability and the fluctuations of frailty. Age and Ageing 1997; 26:315–318.

Grimley Evans J, Williams FT, Beattie LB, et al. (eds). Oxford textbook of geriatric medicine. 2nd edn. Oxford: Oxford University Press; 2000.

Websites
www.bgs.org.uk *British Geriatrics Society: useful publications, guidelines and links.*

www.geriatricsyllabus.com *Provides information on the ageing process and the care and treatment of older people.*

www.helptheaged.org.uk *Provides advice on health and social issues for older patients.*

www.mrc.ac.uk/pdf-ageing_and_health.pdf *Gives causes of age-related disorders and highlights pioneering treatment and prevention.*

7

7.15 INDEX OF 'IN OLD AGE' BOXES

7

Part 2
PRACTICE OF MEDICINE

8

D.F. TREACHER
I.S. GRANT

Critical care and emergency medicine

CLINICAL EXAMINATION OF THE CRITICALLY ILL PATIENT

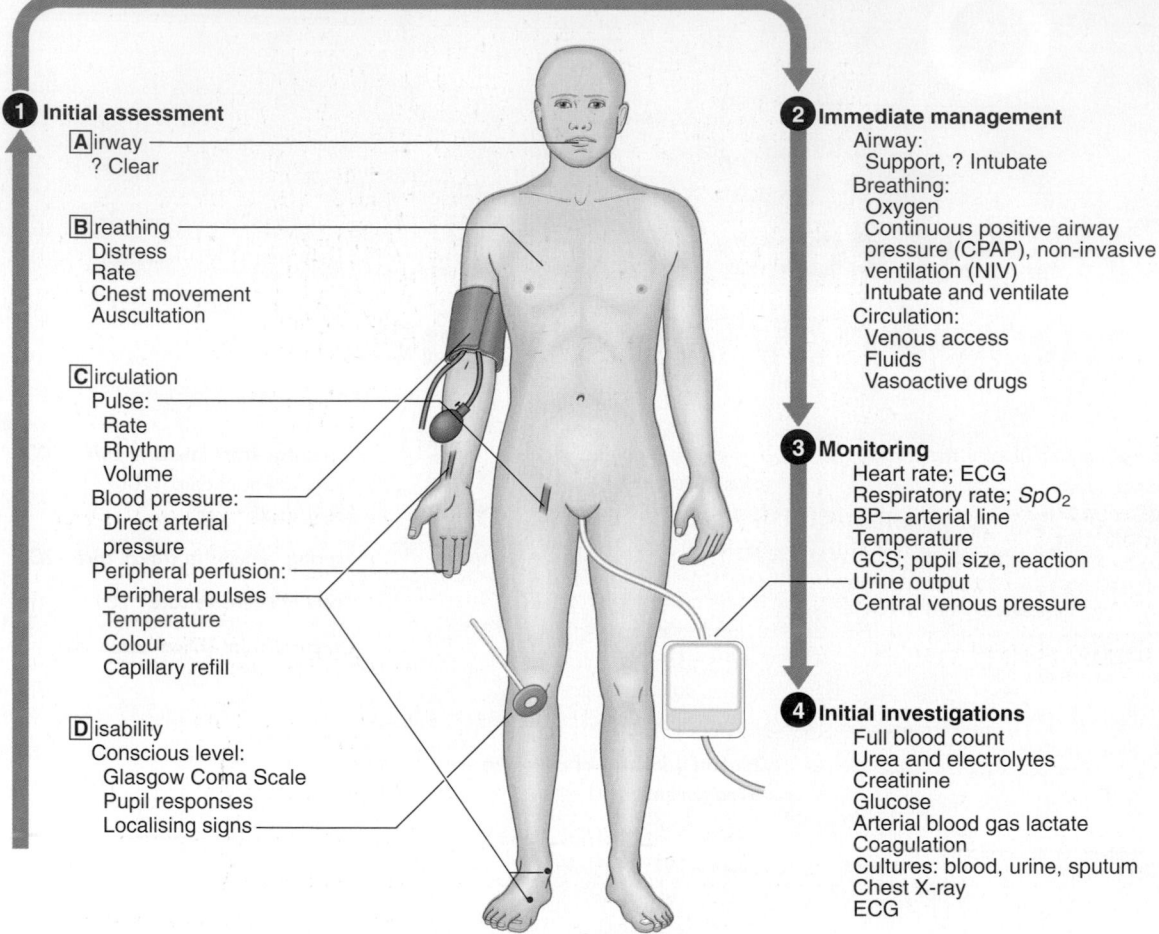

1 Initial assessment

Airway
? Clear

Breathing
Distress
Rate
Chest movement
Auscultation

Circulation
Pulse:
Rate
Rhythm
Volume
Blood pressure:
Direct arterial
pressure
Peripheral perfusion:
Peripheral pulses
Temperature
Colour
Capillary refill

Disability
Conscious level:
Glasgow Coma Scale
Pupil responses
Localising signs

2 Immediate management

Airway:
Support, ? Intubate
Breathing:
Oxygen
Continuous positive airway
pressure (CPAP), non-invasive
ventilation (NIV)
Intubate and ventilate
Circulation:
Venous access
Fluids
Vasoactive drugs

3 Monitoring

Heart rate; ECG
Respiratory rate; SpO_2
BP—arterial line
Temperature
GCS; pupil size, reaction
Urine output
Central venous pressure

4 Initial investigations

Full blood count
Urea and electrolytes
Creatinine
Glucose
Arterial blood gas lactate
Coagulation
Cultures: blood, urine, sputum
Chest X-ray
ECG

Recognising the critically ill patient

Cardiovascular signs
- Cardiac arrest
- Pulse rate <40 or >140 bpm
- Systolic blood pressure (BP) <100 mmHg
- Tissue hypoxia
    Poor peripheral perfusion
    Metabolic acidosis
    Hyperlactataemia
- Poor response to volume resuscitation
- Oliguria: <0.5 ml/kg/hr (check urea, creatinine, K^+)

Respiratory signs
- Threatened or obstructed airway
- Stridor, intercostal recession
- Respiratory arrest
- Respiratory rate < 8 or > 35/min
- Respiratory 'distress': use of accessory muscles; unable to speak in complete sentences
- SpO_2 < 90% on high-flow O_2
- Rising $PaCO_2$ > 8 kPa (> 60 mmHg), or > 2 kPa (> 15 mmHg) above 'normal' with acidosis

Neurological signs
- Threatened or obstructed airway
- Absent gag or cough reflex
- Failure to maintain normal PaO_2 and $PaCO_2$
- Failure to obey commands
- Glasgow Coma Scale (GCS) < 10
- Sudden fall in level of consciousness (GCS fall > 2 points)
- Repeated or prolonged seizures

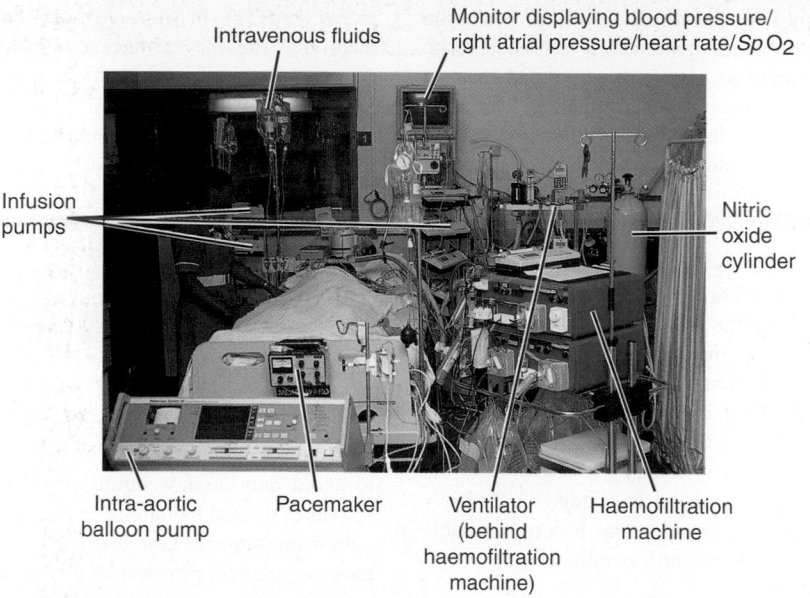

Intravenous fluids

Monitor displaying blood pressure/
right atrial pressure/heart rate/$Sp\,O_2$

Infusion
pumps

Nitric
oxide
cylinder

Intra-aortic
balloon pump

Pacemaker

Ventilator
(behind
haemofiltration
machine)

Haemofiltration
machine

8

A patient with multi-organ failure supported by haemodynamic monitoring, cardiac pacing, a counterpulsation aortic balloon pump, haemofiltration and nitric oxide therapy.

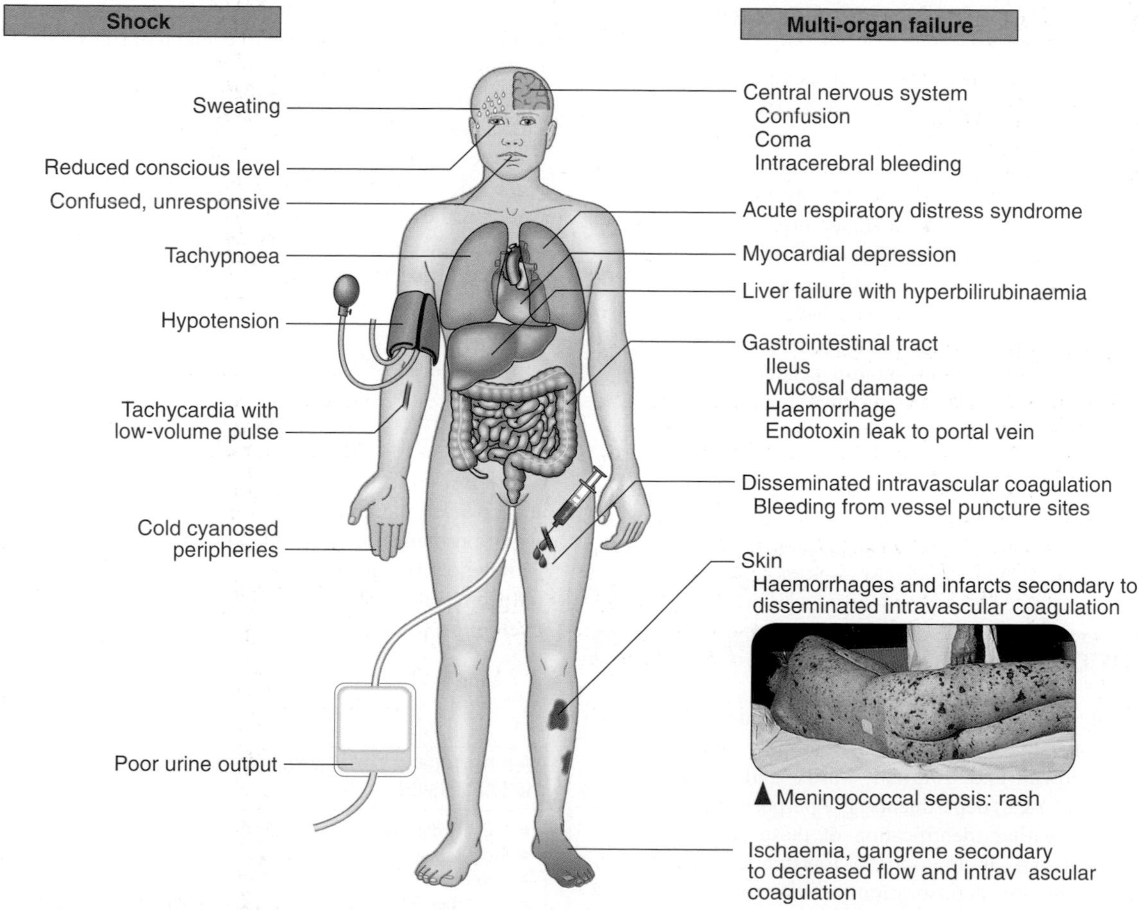

Shock	Multi-organ failure

Sweating

Reduced conscious level

Confused, unresponsive

Tachypnoea

Hypotension

Tachycardia with
low-volume pulse

Cold cyanosed
peripheries

Poor urine output

Central nervous system
  Confusion
  Coma
  Intracerebral bleeding

Acute respiratory distress syndrome

Myocardial depression

Liver failure with hyperbilirubinaemia

Gastrointestinal tract
  Ileus
  Mucosal damage
  Haemorrhage
  Endotoxin leak to portal vein

Disseminated intravascular coagulation
  Bleeding from vessel puncture sites

Skin
  Haemorrhages and infarcts secondary to
  disseminated intravascular coagulation

▲ Meningococcal sepsis: rash

Ischaemia, gangrene secondary
to decreased flow and intrav ascular
coagulation

Some features of shock.

8

A critically ill patient is one at imminent risk of death; the severity of illness must be recognised early and appropriate measures taken promptly to assess, diagnose and manage the illness.

The approach required in managing the critically ill patient differs from that required in less severely ill patients with immediate resuscitation and stabilisation of the patient's condition taking precedence:

Priorities are:

- prompt resuscitation, adhering to advanced life support guidelines (p. 556) and the principles of cardiorespiratory management explained in this chapter
- urgent treatment of life-threatening emergencies such as hypotension, hypoxaemia, hyperkalaemia, hypoglycaemia and dysrhythmias
- analysis of the deranged physiology
- establishing the complete diagnosis in stages as further history and the results of investigations become available
- careful monitoring of the patient's condition and response to treatment.

PROVISION OF CRITICAL CARE

ORGANISATION OF CRITICAL CARE

Critical care embraces both intensive care and high-dependency care. Intensive care units (ICUs) are for the care of very ill patients with potential or established organ failure. Initially established for the provision of mechanical ventilation for patients with respiratory failure, ICUs now monitor and support all the major organ systems. High-dependency care provides an intermediate level of care at a point between intensive care and general ward care; it is appropriate both for patients who have had major surgery and for those with single-organ failure. Ideally the ICU should be adjacent to the high-dependency unit (HDU), allowing the critical care medical team to manage a combined critical care department.

The intensive care specialist (intensivist) should provide a holistic approach that coordinates expert opinions from other specialties (surgeons, physicians, microbiologists) to produce an integrated plan of management that recognises the priorities in the treatment of multiple organ failure.

CRITICAL CARE 'OUTREACH'

Critically ill patients can be found throughout the hospital, in post-operative recovery areas, coronary care units, the acute medical and surgical wards and accident and emergency (A&E) departments. The purpose of 'outreach' is to achieve earlier identification of these patients so that assessment and, if appropriate, transfer to ICU/HDU is arranged before deterioration occurs to the point of imminent or actual cardiorespiratory arrest. Prompt identification and treatment may even avert the need for admission to ICU/HDU. Many hospitals are now setting up medical emergency teams or 'outreach'/'patient at risk'

teams (PARTs). In some hospitals the medical emergency team may be the cardiac arrest team but with a wider remit, while in others this service is provided by the ICU or HDU team.

Criteria that identify deranged physiology (p. 176) are used to alert the ward nursing and junior medical staff to impending problems so that they can summon the outreach team to assess the patient, institute initial resuscitation and supervise transfer to ICU or HDU as appropriate.

ADMISSION GUIDELINES

Rigid rules to determine admission to ICU/HDU are destined to fail because every case must be evaluated on its own merits. Nevertheless, broad guidelines are required to avoid unnecessary suffering and the waste of valuable resources caused by admitting patients who have nothing to gain from intensive care because they either are too well or have no realistic prospect of recovery. The existence of an empty bed does not justify admission. The guiding principle when considering ICU/HDU admission should be the timely use of this resource in patients who have a realistic prospect of recovering to achieve a quality of life that they would value. Patients who do warrant admission should be identified early and admitted without delay since this improves survival and reduces the length of stay on the ICU. The wishes of the patient, if known, should be respected and whatever decision is made should be carefully explained to the patient's family.

If the appropriateness of admission remains uncertain, as may occur in the A&E department when little history is available, the patient should be given the benefit of the doubt and the indication for continued active treatment reviewed as further information becomes available (Box 8.1).

There is now evidence that for patients undergoing high-risk elective or emergency surgery the mortality, morbidity and both ICU and hospital length of stay are reduced by pre-operative admission to ICU/HDU to improve cardiorespiratory status ('pre-optimisation'). Such patients are often elderly with cardiorespiratory disease and poor physiological reserve, and benefit from a protocol of intensive perioperative care. At present many hospitals have major problems in implementing this strategy due to a shortage of critical care beds.

Specific indications for admission to ICU and HDU are given in Box 8.2.

8.1 FACTORS IN THE ASSESSMENT OF A POSSIBLE ICU ADMISSION

- Primary diagnosis and other active medical problems
- Prognosis of underlying condition
- Severity of physiological disturbance—is recovery still possible?
- Life expectancy and anticipated quality of life post-discharge
- Wishes of the patient and/or relatives
- Availability of the required treatment/technology

N.B. Age alone should not be a contraindication to admission.

8

8.2 ADMISSION CRITERIA FOR ICU AND HDU

Admission to ICU

- Patients requiring or likely to require endotracheal intubation and invasive mechanical ventilatory support
- Patients requiring support of two or more organ systems (e.g. inotropes and haemofiltration)
- Patients with chronic impairment of one or more organ systems (e.g. chronic obstructive pulmonary disease (COPD) *or* severe ischaemic heart disease (IHD)) who *also* require support for acute reversible failure of another organ system

Admission to HDU

- Patients who require far more detailed observation or monitoring than can be safely provided on a general ward
    - Direct arterial blood pressure (BP) monitoring
    - Central venous pressure (CVP) monitoring
    - Fluid balance
    - Neurological observations, regular Glasgow Coma Scale (GCS) recording
- Patients requiring support for a single failing organ system but excluding invasive ventilatory support
    - Mask continuous positive airway pressure (CPAP) *or* non-invasive (mask) ventilation (NIPPV)—Box 8.17, page 193
    - Low- to medium-dose inotropic support
    - Renal replacement therapy in an otherwise stable patient
- Patients no longer requiring intensive care but who cannot be safely managed on a general ward

TRANSPORT OF THE CRITICALLY ILL PATIENT

Critically ill patients should be transported to the most appropriate clinical area for their continuing care. Before intra- or inter-hospital transfer is undertaken, the patient's condition must be stabilised. Appropriate monitoring should be set up and if there is clinical evidence of progressive respiratory failure or inability to protect the airway, endotracheal intubation and ventilation are indicated. Intubation, while often essential, may be hazardous in the patient with cardiorespiratory failure, and full monitoring and resuscitation facilities must be available. Hypovolaemia and hypotension should be corrected and this will often require monitoring of the central venous pressure (CVP).

Transfer to another hospital may be necessary for further investigations (such as computed tomography, CT), or to specialist liver failure, neurosurgical or cardiac surgical units. The urgency of providing the specialist treatment has to be balanced against the stability of the patient's condition. It may be more appropriate to admit the patient to the local ICU for initial stabilisation before transfer. All critically ill patients should be accompanied during transfer by an appropriately trained medical escort.

MONITORING

GENERAL PRINCIPLES

On entering an ICU, relatives, students and even clinicians may be intimidated by the numerous tubes and cables attaching each patient to a battery of 'alarming' machines (p. 177). Much of the bedside nurse's time is spent observing, recording and reacting to the information displayed by these monitors, particularly the electrocardiogram (ECG), CVP, arterial blood pressure (BP), temperature and ventilator data. The trends observed over time, interpreted in relation to changes in therapy, are an important guide to the patient's progress.

The critically ill patient should be monitored according to the following principles:

- Regular clinical examination should never be neglected.
- Simple physical signs such as respiratory rate, the appearance of the patient, restlessness, conscious level and indices of poor peripheral perfusion (pale, cold skin, delayed capillary refill in the nail bed) are just as important as a set of blood gases or numbers impressively displayed on expensive monitors.
- If there is conflict between clinical assessment and the information on a monitor, the monitor should be presumed to be wrong until all potential sources of error have been checked and eliminated. For example, CVP measurement may be erroneous because the line is blocked, the system has not been reset to zero after a change in the patient's position, the tip of the cannula is lying in the right ventricle, or another infusion has been attached to the same central line.
- Changes and trends are more important than any single measurement.
- Many monitors have alarms which will activate if certain maximum and minimum values are breached. This is a crucial safety feature and may, for example, help to identify the fact that a patient has become disconnected from the ventilator. Despite the understandable desire to avoid extra noise, the alarm limits should always be set to define physiologically 'safe' limits for the variable being monitored.
- Sophisticated monitoring systems are often invasive and pose certain hazards, particularly infection (Box 8.3). Always ask 'Is it necessary?', and cease monitoring as soon as possible.

MONITORING THE CIRCULATION

Electrocardiogram (ECG)

Standard monitors display a single-lead ECG, record heart rate and identify rhythm changes. More sophisticated machines can print out rhythm strips and monitor ST segment shift, which may be useful in patients with ischaemic heart disease.

Blood pressure

This may be measured intermittently using an automated sphygmomanometer but in critically ill patients continuous intra-arterial monitoring, using a line placed in the radial artery, is preferable. It is important to appreciate that when there is systemic vasoconstriction the mean arterial pressure may be normal or even high although the cardiac output is low. Conversely, if there is peripheral vasodilatation, as in

8.3 COMPLICATIONS AND PITFALLS OF CENTRAL VENOUS AND PULMONARY ARTERY (PA) CANNULATION

At insertion

- Pneumothorax—more likely with subclavian than with internal jugular approach
- Haematoma from accidental arterial puncture
- Air embolism
- Dysrhythmia
- Damage to thoracic duct with left internal jugular or subclavian approach
- Knotting of catheter*
- Pulmonary artery rupture*

In situ

- Sepsis
- Endocarditis
- Thrombosis
- Pulmonary infarct*
- Pulmonary artery rupture*
- Erroneous information
- Inappropriate response to information

* Risk associated specifically with PA catheterisation.

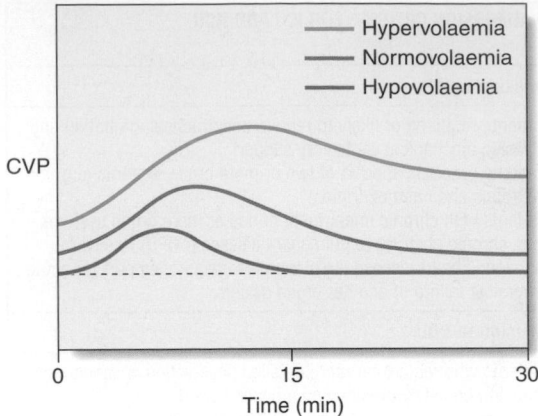

Fig. 8.1 **The different responses observed in central venous pressure (CVP) after a fluid challenge of 250 ml, depending on the intravascular volume status of the patient.**

sepsis, the mean arterial pressure may be low although the cardiac output is high.

Central venous pressure (CVP)

CVP or right atrial pressure (RAP) is monitored using a catheter inserted via either the internal jugular or the subclavian vein with the distal end sited in the upper right atrium. Although on general wards and some HDUs measurements may be made using a saline-filled manometer tube, in ICU the line is transduced as for arterial pressure measurement. The zero reference point used is normally the mid-axillary line (MAL), which approximates to the level of the tricuspid valve or mid-right atrium with the patient lying semi-supine. All intravascular pressures quoted in this chapter are referenced to that point. The classical bedside clinical examination uses the 'sternal angle' as the zero reference point and this lies approximately 6–8 cm (depending on the antero-posterior chest diameter) vertically above MAL. (Values of CVP measured from this reference point will therefore be 6–8 cm lower than values recorded from MAL.)

The CVP is a useful means of assessing the need for intravascular fluid replacement and the rate at which it should be given. If the CVP is low in the presence of a low mean arterial pressure (MAP) or cardiac output, fluid resuscitation is necessary. However, a raised level does not necessarily mean that the patient is adequately volume resuscitated. It must be remembered that right heart function, pulmonary artery pressure, intrathoracic pressure and venous 'tone' also influence CVP and may lead to a raised CVP even when the patient is hypovolaemic. In addition, positive pressure ventilation raises intrathoracic pressure and causes marked swings in atrial pressures and systemic blood pressure in time with respiration. Pressure measurements should be recorded at end-expiration or, if safe, off the ventilator because these values provide the most reliable measure of ventricular end-diastolic transmural pressure.

In severe hypovolaemia the RAP may be sustained by peripheral venoconstriction, and transfusion may initially produce little or no change in the CVP (Fig. 8.1).

Pulmonary artery 'wedge' pressure (PAWP) and PA catheterisation

In most situations the CVP is an adequate guide to the filling pressures of both sides of the heart; however, certain conditions such as pulmonary hypertension or right ventricular dysfunction may lead to raised CVP levels even in the presence of hypovolaemia. If this is suspected, it may be appropriate to insert a pulmonary artery flotation catheter (Fig. 8.2) so that pulmonary artery pressure and PAWP, which approximates to left atrial pressure, can be measured. The mean PAWP normally lies between 8 and 12 mmHg (measured from the mid-axillary line) but in left heart failure it may be grossly elevated and even exceed 30 mmHg. Provided the pulmonary capillary membranes are intact, the optimum PAWP when managing acute circulatory failure in the critically ill patient is generally 12–15 mmHg because this will ensure good left ventricular filling without risking hydrostatic pulmonary oedema.

These catheters may also be used to measure cardiac output, sample blood from the pulmonary artery ('mixed venous' samples) and, by oximetry, provide continuous monitoring of the mixed venous oxygen saturation (SvO_2). Measurement of SvO_2 gives an indication of the adequacy of cardiac output in relation to the body's metabolic requirements and is especially useful in low cardiac output states.

Cardiac output

The most widely used method for cardiac output measurement is the thermodilution technique using a PA catheter. A bolus of cold 5% dextrose is rapidly injected into the right atrium via the CVP line and mixes with the total venous return in the right ventricle, producing a drop in the pulmonary artery temperature that is sensed by a thermistor at the tip of the PA catheter. The cardiac output is derived from the volume and temperature of the injectate and the resulting change in temperature measured in the pulmonary

8

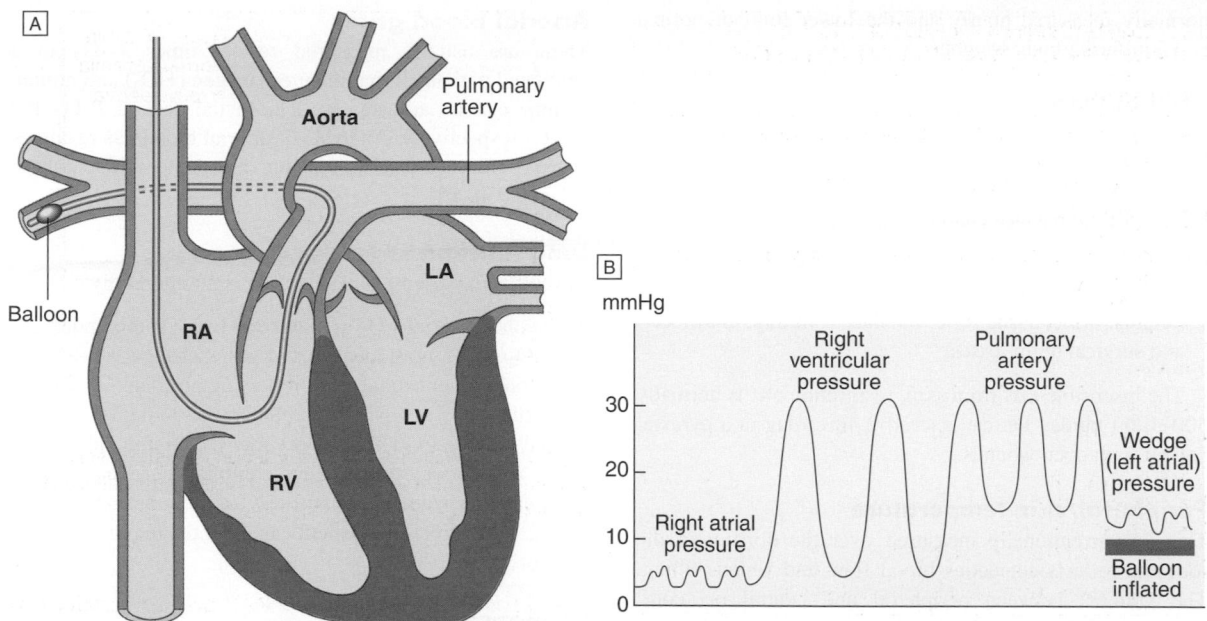

Fig. 8.2 A pulmonary artery catheter. A There is a small balloon at the tip of the catheter and pressure can be measured through the central lumen. The catheter is inserted via an internal jugular, subclavian or femoral vein and advanced through the right heart until its tip lies in the pulmonary artery. When the balloon is deflated the pulmonary artery pressure can be recorded. B Advancing the catheter while inflating the balloon will 'wedge' the catheter in the pulmonary artery. In this position blood cannot flow past the balloon so the tip of the catheter will now record the pressure transmitted from the pulmonary veins and left atrium. This is known as the pulmonary artery wedge pressure and provides an indirect measure of the left atrial pressure.

artery; it is inversely related to the area under the temperature–time curve. Although generally viewed as the 'gold standard' for clinical measurement of cardiac output, the error may be 10–15%.

Thermodilution cardiac output measurement has been refined by the development of PA catheters incorporating a heating element, which raises blood temperature at frequent intervals, with the resultant temperature change also detected by the thermistor. These 'continuous' cardiac output catheters dispense with the need for injections of cold dextrose.

Increasingly less invasive methods for monitoring cardiac output are being used, such as oesophageal Doppler ultrasonography. This involves inserting a 6 mm probe into the distal oesophagus to allow continuous monitoring of the aortic flow signal from the descending aorta (Fig. 8.3). From the stroke distance (area under velocity/time waveform), and using a correction factor that incorporates the patient's age, height and weight, an estimate of left ventricular stroke volume and hence cardiac output can be made. Peak velocity is an indicator of left ventricular performance while flow time is an indicator of left ventricular filling and peripheral resistance. Oesophageal Doppler provides a rapid and clinically useful assessment of volume status and cardiac performance to guide early fluid and vasoactive therapy.

Analysis of arterial pressure waveform is another means of continuously estimating cardiac output, and can be calibrated either by transpulmonary thermodilution (PiCCO) or lithium dilution methods (LidCO).

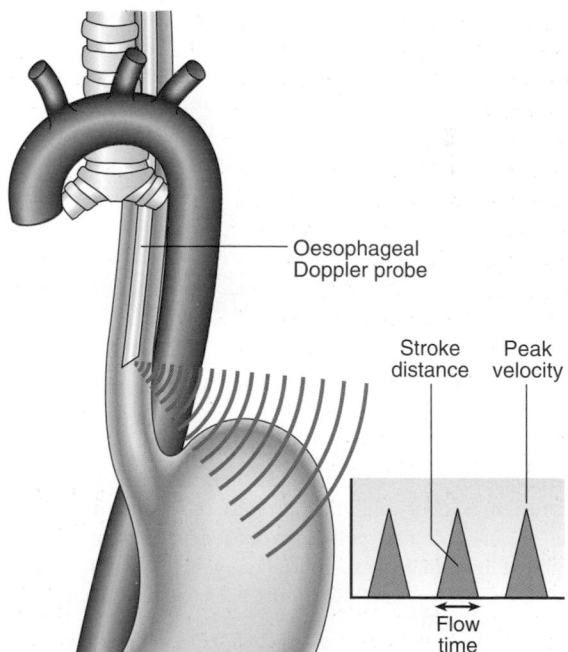

Fig. 8.3 Oesophageal Doppler ultrasonography.

Urine output

This is a sensitive measure of renal perfusion, provided that the kidneys are not damaged (e.g. acute tubular necrosis) or affected by drugs (e.g. diuretics, dopamine), and can be monitored accurately if a urinary catheter is in place. It is normally measured hourly and the lower limit of normal is 0.5 ml/hr/kg body weight.

Fluid balance

Assessing fluid balance in critically ill patients is a difficult but important discipline. Weighing the patient daily can be helpful but is extremely difficult, and assessment is usually based on fluid balance charts which record:

- inputs: oral, nasogastric and intravenous, classified as crystalloid and colloid
- outputs: urine, nasogastric, fistulae, vomiting, diarrhoea and surgical drain losses.

The insensible loss from skin, respiration etc. is normally 500–1000 ml/day but can exceed 2 litres/day in a pyrexial patient with open wounds.

Peripheral/skin temperature

This is conventionally measured over the dorsum of the foot and reflects cutaneous blood flow and venous filling. The gradient between peripheral and central or 'core' temperature (from rectal, oesophageal or tympanic probes) may be used to assess peripheral perfusion; a difference of < 3°C suggests that both intravascular fluid replacement and tissue perfusion are adequate.

Blood lactate, hydrogen ion and base deficit

A metabolic acidosis with base deficit > 5 mmol/l requires explanation (p. 437). It often indicates increased lactic acid production in poorly perfused, hypoxic tissues and impaired lactate metabolism due to poor hepatic perfusion. Serial lactate measurements may therefore be helpful in monitoring tissue perfusion and the response to treatment. Other conditions such as acute renal failure, ketoacidosis and poisoning may be the cause (p. 438). Large volume infusions of fluids containing sodium chloride, e.g. in theatre or during resuscitation, may lead to a hyperchloraemic acidosis.

MONITORING RESPIRATORY FUNCTION

Oxygen saturation (SpO_2)

This is measured by a probe, usually attached to a finger or earlobe. Spectrophotometric analysis is used to determine the relative proportions of saturated and desaturated haemoglobin. The technique is unreliable if peripheral perfusion is poor and may produce erroneous results in the presence of nail polish, excessive movement or high ambient light. In general, arterial oxygenation is satisfactory if SpO_2 is greater than 90%. In the ICU, sudden falls in SpO_2 may be caused by:

- pneumothorax
- displacement of the endotracheal tube
- disconnection from the ventilator
- lung collapse due to thick secretions blocking the proximal bronchial tree
- circulatory collapse causing a poor signal due to impaired peripheral perfusion
- error such as a detached probe.

Arterial blood gases

These are usually measured several times a day in a ventilated patient so that inspired oxygen (FIO_2) and minute volume can be adjusted to achieve the desired PaO_2 and $PaCO_2$ respectively. Analysis of arterial blood gas results is also a useful means of monitoring disturbances of acid–base balance (Ch. 16).

Lung function

In ventilated patients lung function is monitored by:

- alveolar–arterial PO_2 gradient and hypoxaemia index (PaO_2/FIO_2), both measures of gas exchange
- arterial and end-tidal CO_2, reflecting alveolar ventilation
- tidal volume (V_T), respiratory rate (f), minute volume ($V_T \times f$), airway pressure and compliance, reflecting airways resistance, the 'stiffness' of the lungs and the ease with which the patient can meet the required work of breathing.

Capnography

The CO_2 concentration in inspired gas is zero, but during expiration, after clearing the physiological dead space, it rises progressively to reach a plateau which represents the alveolar or end-tidal CO_2 concentration. This cyclical change in CO_2 concentration or capnogram is measured using an infrared sensor inserted between the ventilator tubing and the endotracheal tube. With normal lungs, the end-tidal CO_2 closely mirrors $PaCO_2$, and can be used to assess the adequacy of alveolar ventilation. However, there may be considerable discrepancies if there is lung disease or impaired pulmonary perfusion (for example, due to hypovolaemia). Trends in end-tidal CO_2 are useful in head injury management and during the transport of ventilated patients.

In combination with the gas flow and respiratory cycle data from the ventilator, CO_2 production and hence metabolic rate may be calculated.

PHYSIOLOGY OF THE CRITICALLY ILL PATIENT

OXYGEN TRANSPORT

The major function of the heart, lungs and circulation is the provision of oxygen and other nutrients to the various organs and tissues of the body. During this process carbon dioxide and the other waste products of metabolism are removed. The rate of supply and removal should match the specific metabolic requirements of the individual tissues. This requires adequate oxygen uptake in the lungs, global matching of delivery and consumption, and regional control of the circulation. Failure to supply sufficient oxygen to meet the metabolic requirements of the tissues is the cardinal feature of circulatory failure or 'shock'.

The transport of oxygen from the atmosphere to the mitochondria within individual cells is illustrated in Figure 8.4. The important points to note are that:

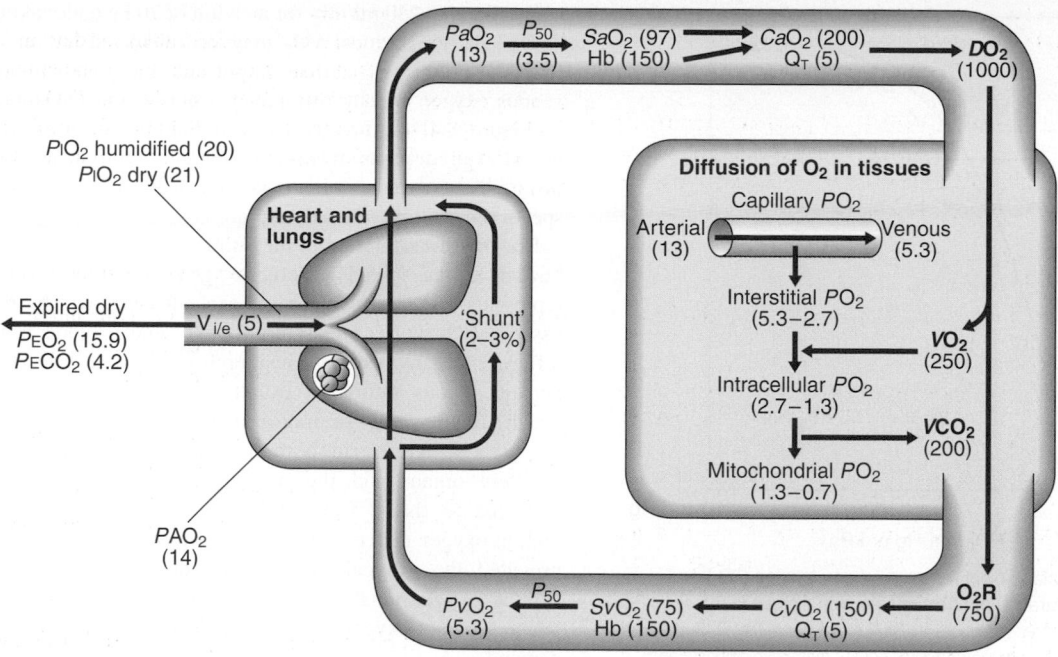

8

Calculations

$CaO_2 = (Hb \times k \times SaO_2/100) + (PaO_2 \times 0.23)$	= 200 ml O_2/l
k = coefficient of haemoglobin oxygen-binding capacity	= 1.36 ml O_2/gram of 100% saturated Hb
$PaO_2 \times 0.23$ = oxygen dissolved in plasma	= 3 ml/l
$DO_2 = Q_T \times CaO_2$	= 1000 ml/min
$VO_2 = Q_T (CaO_2 - CvO_2)$	= 250 ml/min
$OER = VO_2/DO_2 \times 100$	= 25%

Fig. 8.4 Transport of oxygen from inspired gas to the cell, demonstrating the 'oxygen cascade', with equations for calculation of arterial oxygen content, global oxygen delivery, consumption and extraction. Values in parentheses for a normal 70 kg individual (body surface area: 1.67 m²) breathing air (FIO_2: 0.21) at standard atmospheric pressure (P_B: 101 kPa). Partial pressures of O_2, CO_2 in kPa; saturation in %; contents (CaO_2, CvO_2) in ml/litre; Hb in g/l; blood/gas flows (Q_T, $V_{i/e}$) in litre/min; oxygen transport (DO_2, O_2R), VO_2 and VCO_2 in ml/min. To convert kPa to mmHg, multiply by 7.5.

CaO_2 = arterial O_2 content	O_2R = oxygen return	PIO_2 = inspired PO_2	SO_2 = oxygen saturation (%)
CvO_2 = mixed venous O_2 content	PaO_2 = arterial PO_2	PO_2 = oxygen partial pressure (kPa)	SvO_2 = mixed venous SO_2
DO_2 = oxygen delivery	PAO_2 = alveolar PO_2	PvO_2 = venous PO_2	VCO_2 = CO_2 production
Hb = haemoglobin	$PECO_2$ = mixed expired PCO_2	Q_T = cardiac output	$V_{i/e}$ = minute volume: inspired/expired
OER = oxygen extraction ratio	PEO_2 = mixed expired PO_2	SaO_2 = arterial SO_2	VO_2 = oxygen consumption

- The movement of oxygen from pulmonary capillary to systemic tissue capillary, referred to as the global oxygen delivery (DO_2), relies on convection or bulk flow and is the product of cardiac output and arterial oxygen content.
- The regional distribution of oxygen delivery is vital. If skin and muscle receive high blood flows but the splanchnic bed does not, the gut will become hypoxic even if overall oxygen delivery is high.
- The major determinants of the oxygen content of arterial blood (CaO_2) are the arterial oxygen saturation of haemoglobin (SaO_2) and the haemoglobin concentration (over 95% of oxygen carried in the blood is attached to haemoglobin). The shape of the oxyhaemoglobin dissociation curve dictates that increases in PaO_2 beyond the level that ensures SaO_2 is > 90% produce relatively small additional increases in CaO_2 (Fig. 8.5). Consider a

patient who is both anaemic (Hb 60 g/l) and hypoxaemic (SaO_2 75%) when breathing air (FIO_2 0.21). Supplementary oxygen at FIO_2 0.4 will increase SaO_2 to 93%; CaO_2 will increase by 24% but further increases in FIO_2 while increasing PaO_2 cannot produce any further useful increases in SaO_2 or CaO_2. However, increasing Hb to 90 g/l by blood transfusion will result in a further 50% increase in CaO_2.
- The movement of oxygen from tissue capillary to cell occurs by diffusion and depends on the gradient of oxygen partial pressures, diffusion distance and the ability of the cell to take up and use oxygen. Therefore microcirculatory, tissue diffusion and cellular factors, as well as DO_2, influence the oxygen status of the cell.
- Supranormal levels of oxygen delivery cannot compensate for diffusion problems between capillary and cell, nor for metabolic failure within the cell.

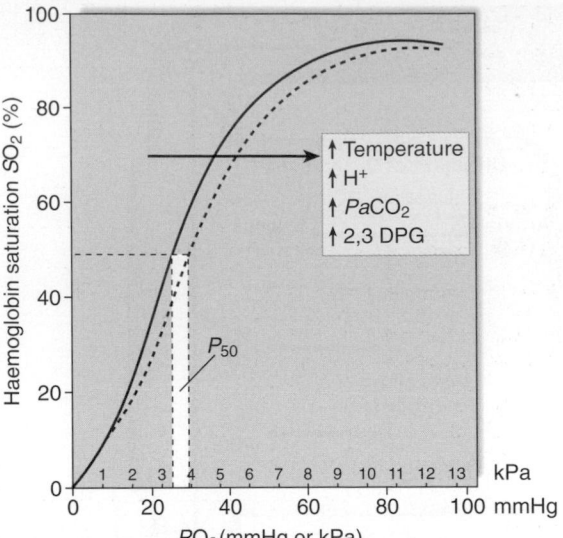

Fig. 8.5   The relationship between oxygen tension (PO_2) and percentage saturation of haemoglobin with oxygen (SO_2). The dotted line illustrates the rightward shift of the curve (i.e. P_{50} increases) caused by increases in temperature, $PaCO_2$, metabolic acidosis and 2,3 diphosphoglycerate (DPG).

OXYHAEMOGLOBIN DISSOCIATION CURVE

The oxyhaemoglobin dissociation curve (Fig. 8.5) describes the relationship between the saturation of haemoglobin (SO_2) and the partial pressure (PO_2) of oxygen in the blood. Due to the shape of the curve, a small drop in PaO_2 below 8 kPa (60 mmHg) will cause a marked fall in SaO_2. Its position and the effect of various physico-chemical factors are defined by the PO_2 at which 50% of the haemoglobin is saturated (P_{50}), which is normally 3.5 kPa (26 mmHg).

A shift in the curve will influence the uptake and release of oxygen by the Hb molecule; for example, if the curve moves to the right, the haemoglobin saturation will be lower for any given oxygen tension and therefore less oxygen will be taken up in the lungs but more will be released to the tissues. As capillary PCO_2 rises, the curve moves to the right, increasing unloading of oxygen in the tissues—a phenomenon known as the Bohr effect.

Traditionally, the optimum haemoglobin concentration for critically ill patients had been considered to be approximately 100 g/l, representing a balance between maximising the oxygen content of the blood and avoiding regional microcirculatory problems due to increased viscosity. However, recent evidence suggests an improved outcome in critically ill patients if the haemoglobin concentration is maintained between 70 and 90 g/l, with the exception of the elderly and patients with coronary artery disease, in whom a level of 100 g/l remains appropriate.

OXYGEN CONSUMPTION

The sum of the oxygen consumed by the various organs represents the global oxygen consumption (VO_2) and is approximately 250 ml/min for an adult of 70 kg undertaking normal daily activities. VO_2 may be calculated indirectly from the product of cardiac output and the arterial mixed venous oxygen content difference (CaO_2–CvO_2), as shown in Figure 8.4, or directly by sampling the inspired and mixed-expired gases from the ventilator and measuring inspired and expired minute volume using either a mass spectrometer or metabolic cart.

The oxygen saturation in the pulmonary artery, otherwise known as the mixed venous oxygen saturation (SvO_2), represents a measure of the oxygen not consumed by the tissues (DO_2–VO_2). The saturation of venous blood from different organs varies considerably; for example, the hepatic venous saturation usually does not exceed 60% but the renal venous saturation may reach 90%, reflecting the great difference in both the metabolic requirements of these organs and the oxygen content of the blood delivered to them. The SvO_2 is influenced by changes both in oxygen delivery (DO_2) and consumption (VO_2) and, provided the microcirculation and the mechanisms for cellular oxygen uptake are intact, can be used to monitor whether global oxygen delivery is adequate to meet overall demand.

The reoxygenation of the blood that returns to the lungs and the resulting arterial saturation (SaO_2) will depend on how closely pulmonary ventilation and perfusion are matched. If part of the pulmonary blood flow perfuses non-ventilated parts of the lung, there will be 'shunting', and the blood entering the left atrium will be desaturated in proportion to the size of this shunt and the level of SvO_2.

RELATIONSHIP BETWEEN OXYGEN CONSUMPTION AND DELIVERY

The tissue oxygen extraction ratio (OER), which is 20–25% in a normal subject at rest, rises as consumption increases or supply diminishes (Fig. 8.6). The maximum OER is approximately 60% for most tissues; at this point no further increase in extraction can occur and any further increase in oxygen consumption or decline in oxygen delivery will cause tissue hypoxia, anaerobic metabolism and increased lactic acid production.

In sepsis the slope of maximum OER decreases, reflecting the reduced ability of tissues to extract oxygen (DE cf. AB on Fig. 8.6), but the curve does not plateau and oxygen consumption continues to increase even at 'supranormal' levels of oxygen delivery. This concept encouraged some physicians to treat septic shock using vigorous intravenous fluid loading and inotropic support, usually with dobutamine, with the aim of achieving very high oxygen deliveries (> 600 ml/min/m²) in the belief that this strategy would increase oxygen consumption, relieve tissue hypoxia, prevent multiple organ failure and improve prognosis. Trials have demonstrated no benefit in ICU patients with established organ failure but suggest that it may be worthwhile if applied before organ failure supervenes (Box 8.4)

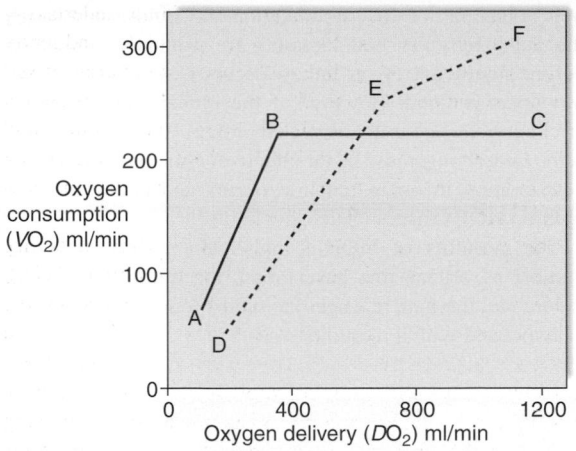

Fig. 8.6 The effects of changing oxygen delivery on consumption.
The solid line (ABC) represents the normal relationship and the dotted line (DEF) the altered relationship believed to exist in sepsis.

8.4 EARLY GOAL-DIRECTED THERAPY IN SEVERE SEPSIS   **EBM**

'In patients with severe sepsis or septic shock managed initially in A&E, early goal-directed therapy (EGT) reduced 60-day mortality from 57% to 44%. Both groups were resuscitated with similar targets for CVP, arterial blood pressure and urine output, but in the EGT group additional goals were central venous oxygen saturation > 70% and haematocrit > 30%, resulting in more rapid fluid resuscitation and higher RBC transfusion rates in the first 6 hours.'

- Rivers E, et al. N Engl J Med 2001; 345:1368–1377.

PATHOPHYSIOLOGY OF THE INFLAMMATORY RESPONSE

The mediators and clinical manifestations of the inflammatory response are described on pages 75–76. In critically ill patients these processes have important consequences (Box 8.5).

Fever, tachycardia with warm peripheries, tachypnoea and a raised white cell count traditionally prompt a diagnosis of sepsis with the implication that the clinical picture is caused by invading microorganisms and their breakdown products. However, other conditions such as pancreatitis, trauma, malignancy, tissue necrosis, aspiration syndromes, liver failure, blood transfusion and drug reactions can all produce the same clinical picture in the absence of infection.

Local inflammation

The body's initial response to a noxious local insult is to produce a local inflammatory response with sequestration and activation of white blood cells and the release of a variety of mediators to deal with the primary 'insult' and prevent further damage either locally or in distant organs.

Normally, a delicate balance is achieved between pro- and anti-inflammatory mediators. However, if the inflammatory response is excessive, local control is lost and a large array of mediators including prostaglandins, leukotrienes, free

---

8.5 TERMINOLOGY USED TO DESCRIBE THE INFLAMMATORY STATE

Infection
- Invasion of normally sterile host tissue by microorganisms

Bacteraemia
- Viable bacteria in the blood

Systemic inflammatory response syndrome (SIRS)
- Encompasses inflammatory response to both infective and non-infective causes such as pancreatitis, trauma, cardiopulmonary bypass, vasculitis etc.
- Defined by presence of two or more of:
  Temperature > 38.0°C or < 36.0°C
  Heart rate > 90/min
  Respiratory rate > 20/min
  $PaCO_2$ < 4.3 kPa (< 32 mmHg) or ventilated
  White blood count > 12×10^9/l or < 4×10^9/l

Sepsis
- Systemic inflammatory response caused by documented infection

Severe sepsis/SIRS
- Sepsis/SIRS with evidence of early organ dysfunction *or* hypotension

Septic/SIRS shock
- Sepsis associated with organ failure *and* hypotension (systolic BP < 90 mmHg or > 40 mmHg fall from baseline) unresponsive to fluid resuscitation

Multiple organ dysfunction syndrome (MODS)
- Development of impaired organ function in critically ill patients with SIRS
- If prompt treatment of underlying cause and suitable organ support are not achieved, then multiple organ failure (MOF) will ensue

---

oxygen radicals and particularly pro-inflammatory cytokines (p. 66) are released into the circulation.

The inflammatory and coagulation cascades are intimately related. The process of blood clotting not only involves platelet activation and fibrin deposition but also causes activation of leucocytes and endothelial cells. Conversely, leucocyte activation induces tissue factor expression and initiates coagulation. Control of the coagulation cascade is achieved through the natural anticoagulants antithrombin (AT) III, activated protein C (APC) and tissue factor pathway inhibitor (TFPI) which not only regulate the initiation and amplification of the coagulation cascade but also inhibit the pro-inflammatory cytokines. Deficiency of ATIII and APC (features of disseminated intravascular coagulation (DIC), see below) facilitates thrombin generation and promotes further endothelial cell dysfunction.

Systemic inflammation

During a severe inflammatory response systemic release of cytokines and other mediators triggers widespread interaction between the coagulation pathways, platelets, endothelial cells and white blood cells, particularly the polymorphonuclear cells (PMNs). These 'activated' PMNs

8

8

express adhesion factors (selectins) causing them initially to adhere to and roll along the endothelium, then to adhere firmly and finally to migrate through the damaged and disrupted endothelium into the extravascular, interstitial space together with fluid and proteins, resulting in tissue oedema and inflammation. A vicious circle of endothelial injury, intravascular coagulation, microvascular occlusion, tissue damage and further release of inflammatory mediators ensues.

All organs may become involved. This manifests in the lungs as the acute respiratory distress syndrome (ARDS) and in the kidneys as acute tubular necrosis (ATN), while widespread disruption of the coagulation system results in the clinical picture of DIC.

The endothelium itself produces mediators that locally control blood vessel tone: endothelin 1, a potent vaso-constrictor, and prostacyclin and nitric oxide (NO, p. 76) which are systemic vasodilators. NO (which is also generated outside the endothelium) is implicated in both the myocardial depression and the profoundly vasodilated circulation (both arterioles and venules) that causes the relative hypovolaemia and systemic hypotension found in septic/SIRS shock.

A major component of the tissue damage in septic/SIRS shock is the inability to take up and use oxygen at mitochondrial level even if global oxygen delivery is supranormal. This effective bypassing of the tissues results in a reduced arteriovenous oxygen difference, a low oxygen extraction ratio, a raised plasma lactate and a paradoxically high mixed venous oxygen saturation (SvO_2).

If both the precipitating cause and accompanying circulatory failure (hypotension and frequently severe hypovolaemia due to venodilatation and fluid loss through the leaky vascular endothelium) are promptly controlled before significant organ failure occurs ('early' shock), the prognosis is good. However, if the global and peripheral circulatory failure is not corrected promptly, and particularly if the underlying cause is not effectively treated, progressive deterioration in organ function occurs and multiple organ failure (MOF) ensues ('late' shock).

The mortality of MOF is high and increases with the number of organs that have failed, the duration of organ failure and the patient's age. Failure of four or more organs is associated with a mortality > 80%.

PRESENTING PROBLEMS IN CRITICAL ILLNESS

CIRCULATORY FAILURE: 'SHOCK'

Circulatory failure or 'shock' exists when the oxygen delivery (DO_2) fails to meet the metabolic requirements of the tissues. In the context of critical illness, 'shock' is often considered to be synonymous with hypotension and to define the state of circulatory failure. While hypotension is a sinister development and requires urgent attention, it is most important to appreciate that hypotension is often a late manifestation of circulatory failure or shock and that the cardiac output and oxygen delivery may be critically low even though the blood pressure remains normal (Box 8.6); the problem should be identified and treatment instituted before the blood pressure falls.

8.6 TYPICAL CIRCULATORY MEASUREMENTS IN A NORMAL ADULT AND IN VARIOUS CARDIORESPIRATORY CONDITIONS THAT MAY CAUSE CIRCULATORY 'SHOCK'

Clinical condition	RAP/CVP (mmHg)	LAP/PAWP (mmHg)	PAP (mmHg)	MAP (mmHg)	Heart rate (/min)	Cardiac output (l/min)	SVR*	PVR*	CaO_2 (ml/l)	DO_2 (ml/min)
Normal	6	11	16	96	70	5	18	1	200	1000
Major haemorrhage	0	4	11	81	120	3	27	2.3	160	480
Left heart failure	8	20	24	96	100	3.7	24	1	180	670
Major pulmonary embolism	12	6	36	81	110	2.5	28	12	160	400
Exacerbation of COPD	11	10	42	82	100	6	12	5	150	900
Septic shock Pre-volume load	3	8	16	55	130	4.5	12	1.3	150	675
Post-volume load	9	15	23	60	120	7.5	7	1.1	140	1050

* Multiply by 80 to give SI units: dyn.sec/cm⁵. To adjust for the size of the patient, the measurements of flow and resistance are frequently indexed by dividing by the patient's body surface area.

(RAP/LAP = right/left atrial pressure; CVP = central venous pressure; PAWP = pulmonary artery wedge pressure; PAP/MAP = pulmonary artery/mean arterial pressure; SVR/PVR = systemic/pulmonary vascular resistance; CaO_2 = arterial oxygen content; DO_2 = global oxygen delivery; COPD = chronic obstructive pulmonary disease)

Note These values are merely examples. The severity of the condition and pre-existing cardiorespiratory disease will affect the precise figures obtained in individual cases. Note that in contrast to other conditions the oxygen delivery is high in septic shock after volume loading. When the circulatory abnormalities have been defined in this way, appropriate management may be planned.

Pressures quoted referenced to zero at mid-axilla as is usual practice in ICU. Subtract vertical distance from mid-axilla to sternal angle (approx. 6–8 mmHg) if sternal angle used as reference point.

The many causes of circulatory failure or 'shock' may broadly be classified into:

- *hypovolaemic*—any condition provoking a major reduction in blood volume, e.g. internal or external haemorrhage, severe burns, dehydration
- *cardiogenic*—any form of severe heart failure, e.g. myocardial infarction, acute mitral regurgitation
- *obstructive*—obstruction to blood flow around the circulation, e.g. major pulmonary embolism, cardiac tamponade, tension pneumothorax
- *neurogenic*—caused by major brain or spinal injury producing disruption of brain stem and neurogenic vasomotor control; may be associated with neurogenic pulmonary oedema
- *anaphylactic*—inappropriate vasodilatation triggered by an allergen (e.g. bee sting)
- *septic/SIRS*—infection or other causes of a systemic inflammatory response that produce widespread endothelial damage with vasodilatation, arteriovenous shunting, microvascular occlusion and tissue oedema, resulting in organ failure.

Clinical assessment and complications

Although dependent to some extent on the underlying cause, a range of clinical features are common to most cases (Box 8.7 and p. 177).

Hypovolaemic, cardiogenic and obstructive causes of circulatory failure produce the 'classical' image of shock, with cold peripheries, weak central pulses and evidence of a low cardiac output. In contrast, neurogenic, anaphylactic and septic shock are usually associated with warm peripheries, bounding pulses and features of a high cardiac

---

8.7 GENERAL FEATURES OF SHOCK

- Hypotension (systolic BP < 100 mmHg)
- Tachycardia (> 100/min)
- Cold, clammy skin
- Rapid, shallow respiration
- Drowsiness, confusion, irritability
- Oliguria (urine output < 30 ml/hr)
- Elevated or reduced central venous pressure (see text)
- Multi-organ failure

---

output. The central venous pressure (jugular venous pressure, JVP) is typically reduced in hypovolaemic and anaphylactic shock but elevated in cardiogenic and obstructive shock, and may be low, normal or high in neurogenic and septic shock. This is an important distinction and direct measurement of the CVP or PAWP (Fig. 8.2, p. 181) may be very helpful if the physical signs are difficult to interpret. Figure 8.7 indicates how the likely diagnosis may be established by careful analysis of the CVP, peripheral perfusion, pulse volume and haematocrit. All forms of shock require early identification and treatment because, if inadequate regional tissue perfusion and cellular dysoxia persist, multiple organ failure will develop.

RESPIRATORY FAILURE INCLUDING ARDS

The majority of patients admitted to ICU/HDU will have respiratory problems either as the primary cause of their admission or secondary to pathology elsewhere. Respiratory failure is formally classified on the basis of blood gas analysis into:

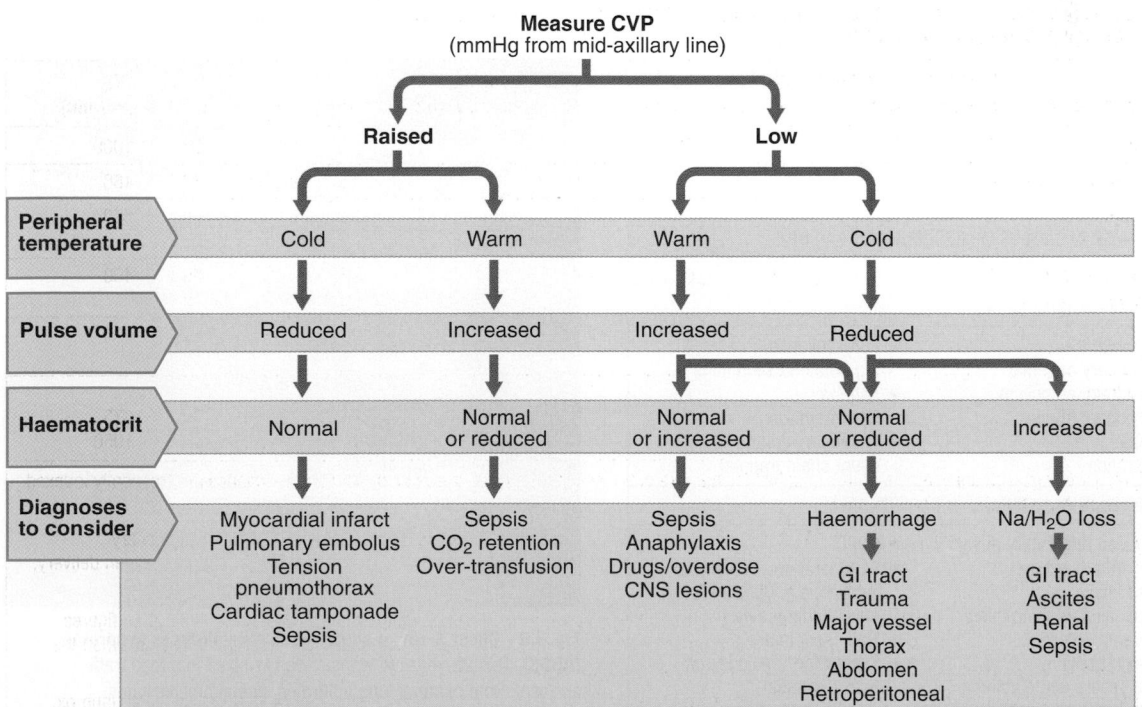

Fig. 8.7 A guide to the initial analysis and diagnosis of circulatory shock.

8

- *type 1*—hypoxaemia ($PaO_2 < 8$ kPa (< 60 mmHg) when breathing air) without hypercapnia caused by a failure of gas exchange due to mismatching of pulmonary ventilation and perfusion
- *type 2*—hypoxaemia with hypercapnia ($PaCO_2 > 6.5$ kPa (> 49 mmHg)) due to alveolar hypoventilation which occurs when the respiratory muscles cannot perform sufficient effective work to clear the carbon dioxide produced by the body.

Although this distinction is conceptually useful, it cannot be applied too rigidly in critically ill patients since they may change from type 1 to 2 as their illness progresses. For example, hypercapnia may develop in pneumonia or pulmonary oedema as the patient tires and can no longer sustain the increased work of breathing.

Pulmonary problems in critically ill patients can also be classified according to the functional residual capacity (FRC, or the lung volume at the end of expiration). Examples of low FRC include lung collapse, pneumonia and pulmonary oedema; examples of a high FRC (i.e. over-distended lungs) include asthma, COPD and bronchiolitis. This allows logical management directed at improving lung compliance and reducing the work of breathing.

The more common causes of acute respiratory failure presenting to ICU/HDU for respiratory support are shown in Box 8.8.

The presentation, differential diagnosis and initial treatment of the primary respiratory conditions causing acute respiratory failure are covered in Chapter 19.

The assessment of respiratory failure in the critically ill patient should be guided by several important principles:

- The patient's appearance (tachypnoea, difficulty speaking in complete sentences, laboured breathing, exhaustion, agitation or increasing obtundation) is more important than measurement of blood gases in deciding when it is appropriate to provide mechanical respiratory support or intubation.

- Adequate supplemental oxygen to maintain $SpO_2 > 94\%$ should be provided. If the inspired oxygen concentration required exceeds 0.6, refer to the critical care team.
- Monitoring of SpO_2 and arterial blood gases is helpful in documenting progress.
- Restless patients dependent on supplementary oxygen or with deteriorating conscious level are at risk. If they remove the mask or vomit, the resulting hypoxaemia or aspiration may be catastrophic.
- An attempt should be made to reduce the work of breathing, e.g. by treating bronchoconstriction or using CPAP (Box 8.17, p. 193).

ACUTE RESPIRATORY DISTRESS SYNDROME (ARDS)

This describes the acute, diffuse pulmonary inflammatory response to either direct (via airway or chest trauma) or indirect blood-borne insults that originate from extra-pulmonary pathology. It is characterised by neutrophil sequestration in pulmonary capillaries, increased capillary permeability, protein-rich pulmonary oedema with hyaline membrane formation, damage to type 2 pneumocytes leading to surfactant depletion, alveolar collapse and reduction in lung compliance. If this early phase does not resolve with treatment of the underlying cause, a fibroproliferative phase ensues and causes progressive pulmonary fibrosis. It is frequently associated with other organ dysfunction (kidney, heart, gut, liver, coagulation) as part of multiple organ failure. The term ARDS is often limited to patients requiring ventilatory support on the ICU, but less severe forms, conventionally referred to as acute lung injury (ALI) and with similar pathology, occur on acute medical and surgical wards. The clinical symptoms and

8.8 COMMON CAUSES OF RESPIRATORY FAILURE IN CRITICALLY ILL PATIENTS
Type 1 respiratory failure

• Pneumonia	• Lung collapse,* e.g. retained secretions
• Pulmonary oedema*	
• Pulmonary embolism	• Asthma
• Pulmonary fibrosis	• Pneumothorax
• ARDS*	• Pulmonary contusion (blunt chest trauma)
• Aspiration	

Type 2 respiratory failure	
• Reduced respiratory drive,* e.g. drug overdose, head injury	• COPD
	• Peripheral neuromuscular disease, e.g. Guillain–Barré, myasthenia gravis
• Upper airway obstruction (oedema, infection, foreign body)	• Flail chest injury
	• Exhaustion* (includes all type 1 causes)
• Late severe acute asthma	

* Secondary complications of other diseases.

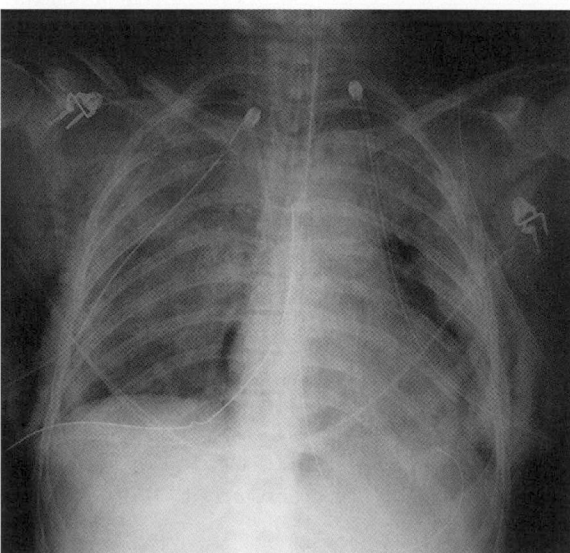

Fig. 8.8 Chest X-ray in acute respiratory distress syndrome (ARDS). This 22-year-old woman was involved in a road traffic accident. Note bilateral lung infiltrates, pneumomediastinum, pneumothoraces with bilateral chest drains, surgical emphysema, and fractures of the ribs, right clavicle and left scapula.

8.9 CONDITIONS PREDISPOSING TO ARDS	
Inhalation (direct)	
• Aspiration of gastric contents	• Blunt chest trauma
• Toxic gases/burn injury	• Near-drowning
• Pneumonia	
Blood-borne (indirect)	
• Sepsis	• Major blood transfusion
• Necrotic tissue	reaction
(particularly bowel)	• Anaphylaxis (wasp, bee,
• Multiple trauma	snake venom)
• Pancreatitis	• Fat embolism
• Cardiopulmonary bypass	• Carcinomatosis
• Severe burns	• Obstetric crises
• Drugs (heroin, barbiturates,	(amniotic fluid embolus,
thiazides)	eclampsia)

8.10 SYSTEMIC CAUSES OF COMA	
Cerebral hypoxia; hypercapnia	
• Respiratory failure	
Cerebral ischaemia	
• Cardiac arrest	• Hypotension
Metabolic disturbance	
• Diabetes mellitus	• Uraemia
Hypoglycaemia	• Hepatic failure
Ketoacidosis	• Hypothermia
Hyperosmolar coma	• Drugs
• Hyponatraemia	• Sepsis

8

signs are not specific, sharing many features with other pulmonary conditions. The criteria defining ARDS are:

- hypoxaemia, defined as $PaO_2/FIO_2 < 26.7$ kPa (< 200 mmHg)
- chest X-ray showing diffuse bilateral infiltrates (Fig. 8.8)
- absence of a raised left atrial pressure: PAWP < 15 mmHg
- impaired lung compliance.

The term ARDS has severe limitations as a diagnostic label since, like jaundice or a raised CVP, it represents a response to a variety of primary conditions (Box 8.9).

RENAL FAILURE

Oliguria is frequently an early sign of systemic problems in critical illness and successful resuscitation is associated with restoration of good urine output, an improving acid–base balance and correction of plasma potassium, urea and creatinine. Acute renal failure (p. 481) in the context of critical illness is usually due to pre-renal factors such as uncorrected hypovolaemia, hypotension or ischaemia causing acute tubular necrosis (ATN). Sepsis is frequently a compounding factor, causing both global hypotension and local ischaemia that is often associated with DIC. In the presence of pre-existing chronic renal impairment or nephrotoxic drugs, acute renal failure may result from relatively minor ischaemic or hypotensive insults. While ATN is by far the most common cause of acute renal failure in the ICU, it is essential not to overlook other causes, such as renal tract obstruction (including a blocked urinary catheter), drug toxicity, acute glomerulonephritis and vasculitis associated with connective tissue diseases such as systemic lupus erythematosus. Appropriate investigations such as urinary microscopy, immunopathological tests and abdominal ultrasound to exclude renal tract obstruction need to be carried out at an early stage.

NEUROLOGICAL FAILURE (COMA)

Impaired consciousness or coma is often an early feature of severe systemic illness (Box 8.10). Prompt assessment of conscious level and management of airway, breathing and circulation are essential to prevent further brain injury, to allow diagnosis and for definitive treatment to be instituted.

Impairment of conscious level is objectively graded according to the Glasgow Coma Scale (GCS, p. 1186), which is also used to monitor progress. Although necessarily limited, careful neurological examination is very important in the unconscious patient. Pupil size and reaction to light, presence or absence of neck stiffness, focal neurological signs and evidence of other organ impairment should be noted. After cardiorespiratory stability is achieved, the cause of the coma must be sought from history (family, witness, general practitioner), examination and investigation, particularly CT. The possibility of drug overdose should always be considered. The direct neurological causes of coma are listed and described in Chapter 26.

SEPSIS

Any or all of the features of SIRS (Box 8.5, p. 185) may be present, together with an obvious focus of infection such as purulent sputum from the chest with shadowing on chest X-ray or erythema around an intravenous line. However, severe sepsis may present as unexplained hypotension (i.e. septic shock) and the speed of onset may simulate a major pulmonary embolus or myocardial infarction. The common sites of infection in critically ill patients and some of the appropriate investigations to consider are listed in Box 8.11.

The patient may be admitted with infection from home ('community-acquired') or may develop it after admission to the unit ('nosocomial'). The likely causative microorganism and the antibiotic sensitivities will depend on this important distinction, which therefore directs the initial choice of antibiotics. Initial investigations should include:

- cultures of blood, sputum, intravascular lines, urine and any wound discharges
- coagulation profile, plasma lactate, arterial blood gases, urinalysis and chest X-ray.

As few as 10% of ICU patients with a clinical diagnosis of 'septic' shock will have positive blood cultures, due to the effects of prior antibiotic treatment and the fact that a patient with an inflammatory state is not necessarily infected.

8

8.11 SITES OF INFECTION IN CRITICALLY ILL PATIENTS

Sites of infection	Investigations and comments
MAJOR	
Intravenous lines (particularly central)	These should always be suspected; if the patient develops evidence of sepsis and the lines have not been changed for > 4 days, they must be replaced
Lungs	The risk of nosocomial pneumonia is high in intubated patients. When the patient has been on the ICU for > 3–4 days, particularly if antibiotics have been administered, the nasopharynx becomes colonised with Gram-negative bacteria which migrate to the lower respiratory tract. Prophylaxis using a combination of parenteral and enteral antibiotics (selective decontamination of the digestive tract) has been shown to reduce incidence of nosocomial pneumonia
Abdomen	Intra-abdominal abscesses or necrotic gut must be considered in patients who have had abdominal surgery. Pancreatitis or acute cholecystitis may develop as a complication of critical illness. Ultrasound, CT, aspiration of collections of fluid/pus and laparotomy are relevant
Urinary tract	A catheter specimen of urine should always be taken in cases of unexplained sepsis but the lower urinary tract is a relatively unusual source of severe sepsis
OTHER	
Heart valves	Transthoracic or transoesophageal echocardiogram
Meninges	Lumbar puncture but check coagulation and platelet count first
Joints and bones	X-ray, gallium or technetium white cell scan
Nasal sinuses, ears, retropharyngeal space	Clinical examination, plain X-ray, CT
Genitourinary tract (particularly post-partum)	Per vaginam examination, ultrasound
Gastrointestinal tract	Per rectum examination, stool culture, *Clostridium difficile* toxin, sigmoidoscopy

8.12 RISK FACTORS FOR NOSOCOMIAL INFECTION

- Mechanical ventilation
- Trauma
- Invasion with catheters—i.v., urinary, nasogastric tubes
- Stress ulcer prophylaxis with H_2-antagonists
- Prolonged length of stay

Specific investigations will be driven by the history and examination. For example, erect/decubitus abdominal X-rays, ultrasound and CT might be considered in cases of suspected intra-abdominal sepsis (Box 8.11).

The most important objective in management is to identify and treat the underlying cause. Nosocomial infections are an increasing problem on critical care units (Box 8.12). Cross-infection is a major concern, particularly with regard to meticillin-resistant *Staphylococcus aureus* (MRSA) and multidrug-resistant Gram-negative organisms, and if this is frequent it should prompt a review of the unit's infection control policies. The most important practice in preventing cross-infection is thorough hand-washing after every patient contact. Limiting the use of antibiotics helps to prevent the emergence of multidrug-resistant bacteria.

DISSEMINATED INTRAVASCULAR COAGULATION (DIC)

This is also known as consumptive coagulopathy and is one of the acquired disorders of haemostasis (p. 1060); it is common in critically ill patients and often heralds the onset of multi-organ failure. The condition is characterised by an increase in prothrombin time, partial thromboplastin time and fibrin degradation products, and a fall in platelets and fibrinogen. The clinically dominant feature may be widespread bleeding from vascular access points, gastrointestinal tract, bronchial tree and surgical wound sites, or widespread microvascular and even macrovascular thrombosis. Management is supportive with infusions of fresh frozen plasma and platelets while the underlying cause is treated.

GENERAL PRINCIPLES OF CRITICAL CARE MANAGEMENT

Critically ill patients should be assessed regularly and at least twice daily on morning and evening ward rounds. Initially, it seems daunting to perform such an assessment,

8.13 THE CRITICALLY ILL OLDER PATIENT

- **ICU demography:** increasing numbers of critically ill older patients are admitted to the ICU; over 50% of patients in many general ICUs are over 65 years old.
- **Outcome:** affected to some extent by age, as reflected in APACHE II, but age should not be used as the sole criterion for withholding or withdrawing ICU support.
- **Cardiopulmonary resuscitation (CPR):** age does affect outcome. Successful hospital discharge following in-hospital CPR is rare in patients over 70 years old in the presence of significant chronic disease.
- **Functional independence:** tends to be lost during an ICU stay.
- **Specific problems:**
  —Skin fragility and ulceration
  —Poor muscle strength: difficulty in weaning from ventilator and in mobilising
  —Confusion/delirium: compounded by sedatives and analgesics
  —High prevalence of underlying nutritional deficiency.

particularly if there is multiple organ failure and no single unifying diagnosis. A systematic approach is required:

- Receive reports of progress from staff; review specialist opinions and medical/social history.
- Review charts.
- Examination: general (rashes, bleeding sites, line sites) and organ-specific.
- Assess information from monitors (check levelling to reference point, zeroing and calibration, determine whether they are still required).
- Fluid balance: note previous 24-hour balances, assess intra- and extravascular state of hydration and set targets for the bedside nurse for the next 24 hours, specifying crystalloid and colloid requirements, the route of administration (enteral or parenteral), and volume and filling pressure limits.
- Nutrition: review calorie intake, route of administration.
- Laboratory results: review haematology including coagulation, biochemistry and bacteriology.
- Review antibiotic therapy: note temperature, white count, line sites etc.
- Review drug chart with ICU pharmacist, consider side-effects and interactions, and identify therapy that can be stopped.
- Review X-rays and other specialist investigations.
- Make an integrated management plan, specifying goals for each organ system.

MANAGEMENT OF MAJOR ORGAN FAILURE

CIRCULATORY SUPPORT

The primary goals (Box 8.14) are to:

- Restore global oxygen delivery (DO_2) by ensuring adequate cardiac output.
- Maintain an MAP that ensures adequate perfusion of vital

organs. The target will be patient-specific depending on pre-morbid factors (e.g. hypertension or coronary artery disease) and may range from 60 to 80 mmHg.

- Avoid levels of left atrial pressure that produce pulmonary oedema and compromise gas exchange. This may limit the degree of volume resuscitation in the presence of acute lung injury/ARDS.

The first objective is to ensure that an 'appropriate' ventricular preload is restored. Vasoactive drugs should *not* be used as a substitute for adequate volume resuscitation.

The key determinants of DO_2 and MAP are cardiac output and arteriolar resistance which are in turn determined by the ventricular 'preload', 'afterload', myocardial contractility and heart rate.

PRELOAD

The atrial filling pressures (RAP or CVP, LAP or PAWP) or preload determine the end-diastolic ventricular volume which, according to Starling's Law and depending on the myocardial contractility, defines the force of the next cardiac contraction (Fig. 18.21, p. 543). The predominant factor influencing preload is venous return, which is determined by the intravascular volume and the venous 'tone' (Box 8.15).

When volume is lost (e.g. major haemorrhage), venous 'tone' increases and this helps to offset the consequent fall in atrial filling pressure and cardiac output. If the equivalent volume is returned gradually, the right atrial pressure will return to normal as the intravascular volume is restored and the reflex increase in venous tone abates. However, if fluid is infused too rapidly there will be insufficient time for the venous and arteriolar tone to fall and pulmonary oedema may occur, even though the intravascular volume has only been restored to the pre-morbid level.

If the preload is low, volume loading with intravenous fluids is the priority and the most appropriate means of improving cardiac output and oxygen delivery. The choice of fluid for volume loading is controversial. No clear advantage of colloid over crystalloid has ever been demonstrated, but adequate filling is achieved with smaller volumes of colloid. Red cells have traditionally been transfused to achieve and maintain an Hb concentration of 100 g/l but, in the absence of significant heart disease, a target of 70–90 g/l may be preferable (Box 24.19, p. 1019). Fluid challenges of 200–250 ml should be titrated against CVP measurements (Fig. 8.1, p. 180).

When the preload is high, due to excessive intravascular volume or impaired myocardial contractility, it is advisable to remove volume from the circulation (diuretics, venesection, haemofiltration) or increase the capacity of the vascular bed using venodilator therapy (glyceryl trinitrate, morphine).

8.14 INITIAL MANAGEMENT OF CIRCULATORY COLLAPSE

- Monitor MAP, CVP
- Correct hypoxaemia
- Correct hypovolaemia
    If CVP < +6 mmHg from mid-axillary line give volume challenge (250 ml normal saline or colloid)
    If CVP > +6 mmHg or poor ventricular function is suspected, use only 100 ml of fluid and consider insertion of PA catheter to direct further treatment with fluids and vasoactive agents
- Achieve target MAP (using vasoactive agents only after hypovolaemia corrected)
- Monitor trend in arterial blood gases, pH, base deficit and lactate
- Consider intubation if
    $PaCO_2$ > 6.5 kPa (> 50 mmHg)
    Respiratory rate > 25/min
    Impaired consciousness: GCS ≤ 7
- Correct acidaemia with i.v. bicarbonate if H^+ > 63 nmol/l (pH < 7.20) and $PaCO_2$ < 6 kPa (< 45 mmHg) (i.e. base excess > −10 mmol/l)

8.15 FACTORS INFLUENCING CENTRAL VENOUS PRESSURE

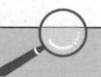

- Intravascular volume
- Venous tone
- Right heart function and 'afterload', i.e. PAP
- Intrathoracic pressure

8

AFTERLOAD

The tension in the ventricular myocardium during systole, or 'afterload', is determined by the resistance to ventricular outflow, which is a function of the peripheral arteriolar resistance. If the considerable assumption is made that flow in the circulation is linear and non-pulsatile, the resistance against which each ventricle works may be calculated as the pressure drop across the resistance bed divided by the flow:

Systemic vascular resistance (SVR) = $(MAP - RAP)/Q_T$

Pulmonary vascular resistance (PVR) = $(PAP - LAP)/Q_T$

If the pressures are measured in mmHg and flow in litres/min, these calculations give the resistances in simple or 'Wood' units; multiplication by 80 converts to SI units. For a normal 70 kg adult:

$SVR = (90 - 0)/5 \times 80 = 1440$ dyn.sec/cm^5

$PVR = (10 - 5)/5 \times 80 = 80$ dyn.sec/cm^5

Understanding the reciprocal relationship between pressure, flow and resistance is crucial for appropriate circulatory management. High resistances produce lower flows at higher pressures for a given amount of ventricular work. Therefore, a systemic vasodilator such as sodium nitroprusside will allow the same cardiac output to be maintained for less ventricular work but with a reduced arterial blood pressure. In hyperdynamic sepsis, the SVR and blood pressure are low but the cardiac output is high; therefore a vasoconstrictor (noradrenaline (norepinephrine), vasopressin) is appropriate to restore BP, albeit with some reduction in cardiac output.

MYOCARDIAL CONTRACTILITY

This determines the work that the ventricle performs under given loading conditions or, put another way, the stroke volume that the ventricle will generate against a given afterload for a particular level of preload.

The relationship between stroke work and filling pressure is shown in Figure 18.21, page 543. The ventricular stroke work is the external work performed by the ventricle with each beat and is calculated from the stroke volume (SV) and the pre- and afterload pressures:

Ventricular stroke work (VSW) = SV × (afterload − preload)

e.g. LVSW = SV × (MAP − LAP) ml.mmHg

Using the data for a normal adult shown in Box 8.6 (p. 186) and multiplying by 0.0136 to convert to SI units of gram.metres, LVSW and RVSW are 80 and 10 g.m respectively.

Consideration of ventricular work is important because it is desirable to maintain satisfactory perfusion and oxygen delivery to all organs at maximum cardiac efficiency and therefore minimise myocardial ischaemia. Myocardial contractility is frequently reduced in critically ill patients due to either pre-existing cardiac disease (usually ischaemic heart disease) or the disease process itself (particularly sepsis).

THERAPEUTIC OPTIONS IN THE MANAGEMENT OF CARDIAC FAILURE

If the cardiac output is inadequate and myocardial contractility is poor, the available treatment options are to:

- *Reduce afterload.* This can be achieved by using an arteriolar dilator (e.g. nitrates, ACE inhibitor), which may be limited by the consequent fall in systemic pressure. A counterpulsation balloon pump offers the ideal physiological treatment because it reduces LV afterload while increasing cardiac output, diastolic pressure and coronary perfusion; it is particularly valuable in treating myocardial ischaemia.

8.16 CIRCULATORY EFFECTS OF COMMONLY USED VASOACTIVE DRUG INFUSIONS

Drug (receptors)	Cardiac contractility	Heart rate	Blood pressure	Cardiac output	Splanchnic blood flow	SVR	PVR
Dopamine (< 5 µg/kg/min) (DA$_1$,β$_1$,α) (> 5 µg/kg/min)) (β$_1$,α,DA$_1$,β$_2$)	↑ ↑↑	→/↑ ↑	→/↑ ↑	↑ ↑↑	→/↑ →	→/↑ ↑	→/↑ ↑
Adrenaline (epinephrine) (β$_1$,α,β$_2$)	↑↑	↑	↑↑	↑↑↑	↓	↑	↑
Noradrenaline (norepinephrine) (α,β$_1$)	→/↑	→/↓	↑↑	→/↓	→/↓	↑↑	↑↑
Isoprenaline (β$_1$,β$_2$)	↑	↑↑	→/↓	↑	→/↑	→/↓	↓
Dobutamine (β$_1$,β$_2$,α)	↑	↑	→/↓	↑↑	→	↓	↓
Dopexamine (β$_2$, DA$_1$, DA$_2$)	↑	↑↑	→/↓	↑	↑	↓	↓
Glyceryl trinitrate (NO)	→	↑	↓	↑	↑	↓	↓
Nitroprusside (NO)	→	↑	↓	↑	↑	↓	↓
Epoprostenol (prostacyclin)	→	↑	↓	↑	↑	↓	↓
Milrinone (PDEI)	→/↑	↑	↓	↑↑	↑	↓	↓

Receptors through which these vasoactive drugs work are given in parentheses and listed in order of the extent of receptor stimulation produced. Note that dopamine acts more like adrenaline at high doses. (α = α-adrenoceptor; β$_1$, β$_2$ = β-adrenoceptors 1 and 2; DA$_1$, DA$_2$ = dopaminergic receptors 1 and 2; NO = acts via local nitric oxide release; PDEI = phosphodiesterase inhibitor.)

The global circulatory effects listed are guidelines only. The magnitude of the response will depend on the circulatory state of the patient when the drug is started, the dose of the drug administered and the receptor distribution and density in specific vascular beds.

- *Increase preload.* However, if there is significant impairment of myocardial contractility, giving intravascular volume to increase filling pressures will only produce a small increase in stroke volume and cardiac output and risks precipitating pulmonary oedema.
- *Improve myocardial contractility.* Box 8.16. lists some characteristics of the commonly used inotropic agents.
- *Control heart rate and rhythm* (pp. 560–575). The optimum heart rate is usually between 90 and 110 per minute. Correction of low serum potassium and magnesium concentrations should be the first stage in treating tachyarrhythmias in the critically ill. Atrial fibrillation is particularly common and troublesome in septic and critically ill patients; amiodarone 300 mg over 30–60 minutes, followed by 900 mg over 24 hours, can be successful in controlling ventricular rate and in restoring and maintaining sinus rhythm.

The management of tamponade and pulmonary embolism is described on pages 645 and 724 respectively and specific aspects of management in sepsis are described later (p. 199).

RESPIRATORY SUPPORT

Respiratory support is indicated to maintain the patency of the airway, correct hypoxaemia and hypercapnia, and reduce the work of breathing. It ranges from oxygen therapy by facemask, through non-invasive techniques such as CPAP (Box 8.17) and non-invasive positive pressure ventilation (NIPPV), to full ventilation via an endotracheal tube or tracheostomy.

OXYGEN THERAPY

Oxygen is given to treat hypoxaemia and ensure adequate arterial oxygenation ($SpO_2 > 90\%$). It should initially be given by facemask or nasal cannulae and the inspired oxygen concentration (FIO_2) can then be adjusted according to the results of pulse oximetry and arterial blood gas analysis. The risk of progressive hypercapnia in certain patients with COPD who are dependent on hypoxic drive has been overstated. If administration of oxygen to ensure $SpO_2 > 90\%$ results in unacceptable hypercapnia, the patient almost certainly requires some form of mechanical respiratory support. The theoretical risks of oxygen toxicity are not relevant if the patient is acutely hypoxaemic. It is vital to maintain cerebral oxygenation even at the risk of pulmonary toxicity because hypoxic cerebral damage is irreversible. More detail on oxygen therapy is given on page 668.

NON-INVASIVE RESPIRATORY SUPPORT

If a patient remains hypoxaemic on high-flow oxygen, other measures are required to improve oxygenation and to reduce the work of breathing. If the patient has respiratory failure associated with decreased lung volume, application of continuous positive airways pressure (CPAP, Box 8.17) will both improve oxygenation by recruitment of under-ventilated alveoli, and reduce the work of breathing by

8.17 MODES AND TERMS USED IN MECHANICAL VENTILATORY SUPPORT

Intermittent positive pressure ventilation (IPPV)

- Generic term for all types of positive pressure ventilation

Controlled mandatory ventilation (CMV)

- Most basic classic form of ventilation
- Pre-set rate and tidal volume
- Does not allow spontaneous breaths
- Appropriate for initial control of patients with little respiratory drive, severe lung injury or circulatory instability

Synchronised intermittent mandatory ventilation (SIMV)

- Pre-set rate of mandatory breaths with pre-set tidal volume
- Allows spontaneous breaths between mandatory breaths
- Spontaneous breaths may be pressure-supported (PS)
- Allows patient to settle on ventilator with less sedation

Pressure controlled ventilation (PCV)

- Pre-set rate; pre-set inspiratory pressure
- Tidal volume depends on pre-set pressure, lung compliance and airways resistance
- Used in management of severe acute respiratory failure to avoid high airway pressure, often with prolonged inspiratory to expiratory ratio (pressure controlled inverse ratio ventilation, PCIRV)

Pressure support ventilation (PSV)

- Breaths are triggered by patient
- Provides positive pressure to augment patient's breaths
- Useful for weaning
- Usually combined with CPAP; may be combined with SIMV
- Pressure support is titrated against tidal volume and respiratory rate

Positive end-expiratory pressure (PEEP)

- Positive airway pressure applied during expiratory phase in patients receiving mechanical ventilation
- Improves oxygenation by recruiting atelectatic or oedematous lung
- May impair venous return and reduce cardiac output

Continuous positive airways pressure (CPAP)

- Positive airway pressure applied throughout the respiratory cycle, via either an endotracheal tube or a tight-fitting facemask
- Fresh gas flow must exceed patient's peak inspiratory flow
- Improves oxygenation by recruitment of atelectatic or oedematous lung
- Mask CPAP discourages coughing and clearance of lung secretions; may increase the risk of aspiration

Bi-level positive airway pressure (BiPAP/BIPAP)

- Describes situation of two levels of positive airway pressure (higher level in inspiration)
- In fully ventilated patients, BiPAP is essentially the same as PCV with PEEP
- In partially ventilated patients, and especially if used non-invasively, BiPAP is essentially PSV with CPAP

Non-invasive intermittent positive pressure ventilation (NIPPV)

- Most modes of ventilation may be applied via a facemask or nasal mask
- Usually PSV/BiPAP (typically 15–20 cmH₂O) often with back-up mandatory rate
- Indications include acute exacerbations of COPD

8

8.18 CLINICAL CONDITIONS REQUIRING MECHANICAL VENTILATION*

Post-operative
- e.g. After major abdominal or cardiac surgery

Respiratory failure
- ARDS
- Pneumonia
- COPD
- Acute severe asthma
- Aspiration
- Smoke inhalation, burns

Circulatory failure
- Following cardiac arrest
- Pulmonary oedema
- Low cardiac output—cardiogenic shock

Neurological disease
- Coma of any cause
- Status epilepticus
- Drug overdose
- Respiratory muscle failure (e.g. Guillain–Barré, poliomyelitis, myasthenia gravis)
- Head injury—to avoid hypoxaemia and hypercapnia, and to reduce intracranial pressure
- Bulbar abnormalities causing risk of aspiration (e.g. cerebrovascular accident, myasthenia gravis)

Multiple trauma

*Additional considerations:
  Metabolic rate (ventilatory requirements rise as metabolic rate increases)
  Nutritional reserve (low potassium or phosphate reduces respiratory muscle power)
  Condition of the abdomen (distension due to surgery or tense ascites causes both discomfort and splinting of the diaphragm, compromising spontaneous respiratory effort and promoting bilateral basal lung collapse)

8.19 INDICATIONS FOR TRACHEAL INTUBATION AND MECHANICAL VENTILATION

- Protection of airway
- Removal of secretions
- Hypoxaemia ($PaO_2 < 8$ kPa (< 60 mmHg); $SpO_2 < 90\%$) despite CPAP with $FiO_2 > 0.6$
- Hypercapnia if conscious level impaired or risk of raised intracranial pressure
- Vital capacity falling below 1.2 litres in patients with neuromuscular disease
- Removing the work of breathing in exhausted patients

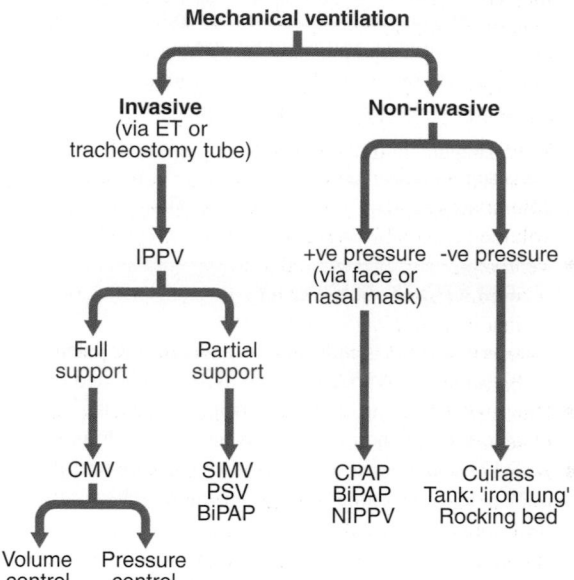

Fig. 8.9   Different types of invasive and non-invasive ventilatory support. (ET = endotracheal; see Box 8.17 for other abbreviations.)

improving lung compliance. CPAP is most successful in clinical situations where alveoli are readily recruited, such as in pulmonary oedema and post-operative collapse/atelectasis. It is also helpful in treating pneumonia, especially in immunocompromised patients. The risk of nosocomial infection is reduced by avoiding endotracheal intubation. A CPAP mask often becomes uncomfortable and gastric distension may occur. Patients must therefore be cooperative, be able to protect their airway and have the strength to breathe spontaneously and cough effectively.

NIPPV refers to ventilatory support by nasal or full facemask. It may avoid the need for endotracheal intubation in patients with type 2 respiratory failure, typically those with exacerbations of COPD, and it may be used during weaning from conventional ventilation. As with mask CPAP, NIPPV requires the patient to be conscious and cooperative.

ENDOTRACHEAL INTUBATION AND MECHANICAL VENTILATION

Over 60% of patients appropriately admitted to ICU require endotracheal intubation and mechanical ventilation, mostly for respiratory failure but also for other reasons (Boxes 8.18 and 8.19).

The final decision to perform tracheal intubation and ventilate a patient should be taken on clinical grounds rather than as a response to the results of particular investigations.

In the conscious patient, intubation requires induction of anaesthesia and muscle relaxation, while in more obtunded patients sedation alone may be adequate. This can be hazardous in the critically ill patient with respiratory and often cardiovascular failure. Continuous monitoring, particularly of heart rate and BP (preferably invasively), is essential, and resuscitation drugs must be immediately available. Hypotension commonly follows sedation or anaesthesia because of direct cardiovascular effects of the drugs and loss of sympathetic drive; positive pressure ventilation may compound this problem by increasing intrathoracic pressure, thereby reducing venous return and hence cardiac output.

The different types of ventilatory support are illustrated in Figure 8.9. Modern ventilators allow considerable flexibility in the level of support from controlled mandatory ventilation to partial ventilatory support modes, and assisted spontaneous breathing which allows the ventilator to respond to patients' demands. Use of partial ventilatory support avoids the requirement for and hazards of paralysis and deep sedation, and allows the patient to be conscious and yet comfortable.

General considerations in the management of the ventilated/intubated patient

- Beware of the restless patient. Try to establish the cause of the problem before simply administering sedation. Possibilities include pneumothorax, hypoxaemia, hypercapnia due to inadequate ventilation, pain, onset of sepsis, cardiac decompensation (pulmonary oedema, dysrhythmia, infarction) and proximal airway obstruction, e.g. secretions.
- Patients who are breathing spontaneously adjust their ventilation to compensate for metabolic derangements; this cannot occur in patients who are ventilated using mandatory modes so the clinician must either correct the underlying metabolic abnormality or make appropriate changes to the ventilator settings. For example, a patient with severe diabetic ketoacidosis will hyperventilate to compensate for the metabolic acidosis; if mechanical ventilation is instituted, there will be a potentially catastrophic fall in pH unless the acidosis is corrected by administering sodium bicarbonate or a high minute volume (artificial hyperventilation) is delivered.
- Ventilator should be set to detect:
  - minimum acceptable minute volume to identify inadvertent disconnection
  - maximum acceptable airway pressure to prevent barotrauma.
- Humidify and warm inspired gas to prevent inspissation of secretions.
- Arrange regular positioning, physiotherapy and suctioning to clear secretions and prevent proximal airway obstruction and distal alveolar collapse. The patient should be in a 30° head-up position to avoid aspiration.
- Obtain a chest X-ray to check the position of the endotracheal tube following intubation (the appropriate position is 4 cm above the carina).
- Bronchoscopy should be readily available to:
  - investigate upper airways obstruction (plugging of the proximal bronchial tree by inspissated mucus is the most common cause)
  - investigate lobar/segmental collapse, and aspirate mucus plug obstructing proximal bronchial tree
  - assist in cases of difficult intubation or tracheostomy tube change
  - obtain bronchoalveolar lavage specimens for microbiology
  - identify the cause of haemoptysis (not always easy)
  - exclude tracheobronchial disruption after thoracic trauma.

Ventilation strategy

The selection of ventilator mode and settings for tidal volume, respiratory rate, positive end-expiratory pressure (PEEP) and inspiratory to expiratory ratio is dependent on the cause of the respiratory failure. The objectives are to:

- improve gas exchange
- minimise damage to the lung by avoiding high lung volumes and FIO_2
- avoid adverse circulatory effects
- make the patient comfortable without heavy sedation or

muscle paralysis by reducing the work of breathing and harmonising interaction between patient and ventilator.

In asthma and conditions with increased lung volumes (high FRC) a prolonged expiratory phase is necessary to prevent progressive lung over-inflation; PEEP and large tidal volumes exacerbate over-distension, produce high alveolar pressures and increase the risk of pneumothorax. High intrathoracic pressures compromise circulatory function, particularly if there is intravascular volume depletion, so that oxygen delivery may actually fall in spite of improved arterial oxygenation.

In patients with alveolar collapse (low FRC), such as those with ARDS, it is appropriate to use a prolonged inspiratory to expiratory ratio and high levels of PEEP (+10 to +15 cmH$_2$O) to recruit alveoli and improve compliance and gas exchange (Boxes 8.20 and 8.21). Recent studies have shown that in ARDS, damage to the lungs can be exacerbated by mechanical ventilation, possibly by over-distension of alveoli and repeated opening and closure of distal airways.

Other management strategies which may be of benefit in severe ARDS include prone ventilation, nitric oxide inhalation and corticosteroids.

Prone ventilation

Prone positioning improves oxygenation significantly in two-thirds of patients with ARDS by reducing thoraco-abdominal compliance and the vertical pleural pressure gradient so that ventilation is more evenly distributed and better matched to perfusion. Multicentre trials using manual pronation have failed to show a survival benefit and trials using an automatic rotating bed are underway.

8.20 PRINCIPLES OF MECHANICAL VENTILATION IN ARDS

- Optimum ventilator settings are:
  Pressure-controlled
  Long inspiratory to expiratory time
  Positive end-expiratory pressure (PEEP)
- Allow $PaCO_2$ to rise (permissive hypercapnia) and tolerate lower oxygen saturations than normal (e.g. 88–90%)
- Avoid:
  Large tidal volumes (ideally 6 ml/kg)
  Airway pressure of more than 35 cmH$_2$O
  FIO_2 of more than 0.8 if possible
- Remember that high intrathoracic pressures compromise circulatory function so oxygen delivery may actually fall in spite of improved oxygenation
- Management must be a balance between improving gas exchange, minimising the risk of subsequent pulmonary fibrosis due to lung injury, and avoiding adverse circulatory effects

---

8.21 OPTIMAL VENTILATION IN ARDS **EBM**

'Ventilation using positive end-expiratory pressure but limiting tidal volumes to 5–7 ml/kg and accepting high $PaCO_2$ levels improves outcome in ARDS.'

- Amato MB, et al. N Engl J Med 1998; 338:347–354.
- Acute Respiratory Distress Syndrome Network. N Engl J Med 2000; 342:1301–1308.

8

Inhaled nitric oxide

Nitric oxide is a very short-acting pulmonary vasodilator. Delivered to the airway in concentrations of between 1 and 20 parts per million, it improves blood flow to ventilated alveoli, thus improving ventilation–perfusion matching. Oxygenation can be improved markedly in some patients but the evidence indicates that the benefit only lasts for 48 hours and outcome is not improved.

Pharmacological therapy

There is now considerable evidence that corticosteroids improve outcome if given in the fibroproliferative stage of ARDS. A trial of corticosteroids is therefore indicated if a patient with ARDS has consistent gas exchange impairment and ventilator dependence at 7–10 days after diagnosis. The recommended dose of methylprednisolone is 2–3 mg/kg/day, decreasing after 7 days and as gas exchange improves. Bronchoscopy and bronchoalveolar lavage should be performed to identify or exclude pulmonary infection before commencing corticosteroid therapy.

Weaning from respiratory support

This is the process of progressively reducing and eventually removing all external ventilatory support and associated apparatus. The majority of patients require mechanical ventilatory support for only a few days and do not need weaning. In these patients simple trials of spontaneous breathing via the endotracheal tube will usually indicate whether the patient can be successfully extubated or not.

In contrast, patients who have required long-term ventilatory support for severe lung disease, e.g. ARDS, may initially be unable to sustain even a modest degree of respiratory work because of residual decreased lung compliance and hence increased work of breathing, compounded by respiratory muscle weakness. These patients therefore require weaning until respiratory muscle strength improves to the point that all support can be discontinued.

Weaning techniques involve the patient breathing spontaneously for increasing periods of the day and a gradual reduction in the level of ventilatory support. This often involves graduation to partial support modes and then non-invasive modes of ventilatory support.

Increasingly, the process of identifying patients able to progress to spontaneous breathing and extubation is done according to a 'weaning protocol'. This entails deciding whether a patient can be safely subjected to a spontaneous breathing trial (Box 8.22). If the patient meets the criteria listed, he or she undergoes the breathing trial for 2–5 minutes. The respiratory rate and tidal volume are noted, and the ratio calculated. If it is less than 105 breaths/min/litre, the patient continues the trial for a further 30 minutes to 2 hours period before extubation.

In the event of failure (increased respiratory rate; decreased tidal volume) gradual weaning of ventilation continues using synchronised intermittent mandatory ventilation (SIMV), pressure support ventilation (PSV) or intermittent periods of spontaneous breathing. Non-invasive ventilation via a facemask can allow earlier extubation in certain groups of patients, e.g. chronic obstructive pulmonary disease, with weaning continuing after removal of the endotracheal tube.

Despite the development of a number of objective tests and indices of the patient's ability to sustain spontaneous ventilation, the decision to extubate and the speed of weaning from mechanical ventilation still rely largely on clinical judgement.

Tracheostomy

Tracheostomy is usually performed electively when endotracheal intubation is likely to be prolonged (over 14 days). Tracheostomies have benefits in terms of patient comfort, aid weaning from ventilation (since sedation can be reduced or stopped), and allow access for tracheal toilet and intermittent respiratory support (Box 8.23).

Tracheostomy is now usually carried out using a percutaneous technique in the ICU, which avoids the need for transfer to the operating theatre. This has led to earlier and more frequent use of tracheostomy. Preliminary evidence indicates that early tracheostomy (at < 3 days) in patients predicted to require prolonged ventilation leads to a reduced length of ICU stay, and decreased morbidity and mortality.

Mini-tracheostomy

The passage of a smaller (4.5 mm internal diameter) tube through the cricothyroid membrane is a useful technique to clear airway secretions in spontaneously breathing patients with a poor cough effort. It can be particularly useful in the HDU and in post-operative patients.

8.22 FACTORS IN DECIDING WHETHER A VENTILATED PATIENT CAN BE WEANED AND SAFELY EXTUBATED
• Has the original indication for mechanical ventilation resolved?
• Is the patient conscious and able to cough and protect his/her airway?
• Is the circulation stable, with a normal or reasonably low left atrial pressure?
• Is gas exchange satisfactory ($PO_2 > 8$ kPa (> 60 mmHg) on $FiO_2 < 0.5$; $PCO_2 < 6$ kPa (< 45 mmHg))?
• Is analgesia adequate?
• Are any metabolic problems well controlled?

8.23 ADVANTAGES AND DISADVANTAGES OF TRACHEOSTOMY
Advantages
• Patient comfort
• Improved oral hygiene
• Reduced sedation requirement
• Enables speech with cuff deflated and a speaking valve attached
• Earlier weaning and ICU discharge
• Access for tracheal toilet
• Reduces vocal cord damage
Disadvantages
• Immediate complications: hypoxia, haemorrhage
• Tracheal damage; late stenosis
• Tracheostomy site infection

8

RENAL SUPPORT

Oliguria (< 0.5 ml/kg/hr for 2–3 hours) requires explanation and early intervention to correct hypoxaemia, hypovolaemia, hypotension and renal hypoperfusion. There is little evidence that specific treatments aimed at inducing a diuresis, such as low-dose dopamine, furosemide or mannitol, have renoprotective action or additional beneficial value in restoring renal function beyond aggressive haemodynamic resuscitation to achieve normovolaemia, normotension and an appropriate cardiac output. Sepsis is frequently implicated in the development of acute renal failure and the focus must be promptly and adequately treated by surgical drainage and antibiotics if renal function is to be restored. Obstruction of the renal tract should always be excluded by abdominal ultrasound and, if present, should be relieved.

If renal function cannot be restored following resuscitation, renal replacement therapy (p. 491) is indicated (Box 8.24).

8.24 INDICATIONS FOR RENAL REPLACEMENT THERAPY

- Fluid overload; pulmonary oedema
- Hyperkalaemia: potassium > 6 mmol/l despite medical management
- Metabolic acidosis: H⁺ > 56 nmol/l (pH < 7.25)
- Uraemia:
  Urea > 30–35 mmol/l (180–210 mg/dl)
  Creatinine > 600 µmol/l (> 6.78 mg/dl)
- Drug removal, in overdose situations
- Sepsis: tentative evidence for mediator removal

The preferred renal replacement therapy in ICU patients is pumped venovenous haemofiltration. This is associated with fewer osmotic fluid shifts and hence greater haemodynamic stability than haemodialysis. It is carried out using a double-lumen central venous catheter placed percutaneously. Haemofiltration should be continuous; higher rates of filtration (preferably > 35 ml/kg/hr) are associated with improved outcome. Intermittent treatment should only be used when the patient is recovering from the primary insult and return of normal renal function is expected. Provided the precipitating cause can be successfully treated, renal failure due to ATN usually recovers between 5 days and several weeks later.

Survival rates from multiple organ failure including acute renal failure have been around 50% for many years but recent evidence suggests that modern haemofiltration techniques are producing better outcomes.

GASTROINTESTINAL AND HEPATIC SUPPORT

The gastrointestinal tract and liver play an important role in the evolution of multiple organ failure, even when the primary diagnosis is not related to the abdomen. Gastrointestinal symptoms such as nausea, vomiting and large nasogastric aspirates may be the earliest signs of regional circulatory failure and, when associated with a tender, distended, silent abdomen, indicate the probable site of the primary pathology. Ischaemic bowel is difficult to diagnose in the critically ill patient but, in the context of an otherwise unexplained lactic acidosis, hyperkalaemia and coagulopathy, urgent laparotomy must be considered (p. 922).

The gut has a very rapid cell turnover rate and fasting alone can produce marked changes in mucosal structure and function. In hypovolaemic and frank shock states, splanchnic vasoconstriction produces gut mucosal ischaemia, damaging the mucosal barrier and allowing toxins to enter the portal circulation and lymphatics. Although equipped to cope with moderate portal toxaemia, the liver may be overwhelmed and will then augment the inflammatory response itself by releasing cytokines into the systemic circulation. For this reason the gut has been described as the 'undrained abscess' or 'motor' of multiple organ failure.

Manifestations of MOF within the gastrointestinal tract include erosive gastritis, stress ulceration, bleeding, ischaemia, pancreatitis and acalculous cholecystitis. Adequacy of gastric mucosal perfusion can be assessed by gastric tonometry, a technique that uses a modified nasogastric tube with a balloon containing either saline or air to measure intramucosal pH (pHi) or PCO_2i. An increased difference between gastric PCO_2 and arterial PCO_2 or an intramucosal acidosis (pHi < 7.32) implies mucosal ischaemia.

Early institution of enteral nutrition is the most effective strategy for protecting the gut mucosa and providing nutritional support. There is evidence suggesting that nasogastric feeds supplemented with arginine, omega 3 fatty acids and nucleotides ('immunonutrition') may improve outcome in critical illness. Glutamine supplementation is logical, although not of proven benefit, since it is a 'conditionally essential' amino acid and the principal energy substrate used by the gut mucosa in critical illness. Total parenteral nutrition (TPN) should only be started if all attempts at implementing enteral feeding, including nasojejunal delivery, have failed; it should be necessary in fewer than 10% of general ICU patients.

Recent evidence from a randomised controlled trial (RCT) demonstrates improved outcomes in the critically ill resulting from tight glycaemic control (Box 8.25). Many patients in ICU will require insulin to maintain a blood sugar between 4.5 and 6.5 mmol/l (~ 80–120 mg/dl), when on either enteral or parenteral feeding.

Ranitidine and sucralfate are both used to reduce the risk of gastrointestinal haemorrhage, although ranitidine is the more effective. Both agents are associated with an increased

8.25 INTENSIVE INSULIN THERAPY IN CRITICALLY ILL PATIENTS

EBM

'Intensive insulin therapy to maintain blood glucose at or below 6.1 mmol/l (110 mg/dl) substantially reduces morbidity and mortality among critically ill patients in a surgical intensive care unit (34% reduction in in-hospital mortality).'

- Van den Berghe G, et al. N Engl J Med 2001; 345:1359–1367

8

incidence of nosocomial pneumonia. Treatment should be stopped when full enteral nutrition has been established and is probably only necessary in patients with a history of peptic ulcer and those who have evidence of MOF, and particularly severe coagulopathy.

The hepatic circulation, 80% of which is derived from the portal venous system, is compromised by the same factors which lead to splanchnic vasoconstriction. Hepatic ischaemia leads to impaired filtering of endotoxin from the portal circulation and, as SIRS develops, inflammatory mediators (e.g. cytokines IL-1, IL-6 and TNF) are released from activated Kupffer cells (hepatic macrophages) into the systemic circulation, increasing the risk of acute renal failure and the other manifestations of MOF developing. Increased metabolic activity in the liver as a result of sepsis and the need for vasoconstricting agents to maintain blood pressure increase hepatic ischaemia. The synthetic inodilator dopexamine with dopaminergic 1 and 2 and β-adrenergic effects may enhance splanchnic blood flow but has not been shown to improve outcome.

Two distinctive hepatic dysfunction syndromes occur in the critically ill:

- *Shock liver or ischaemic hepatitis* results from extreme hepatic tissue hypoxia and is characterised by centrilobular hepatocellular necrosis. Transaminase levels are often massively raised (> 1000–5000 U/l) at an early stage, followed by moderate hyperbilirubinaemia (< 100 μmol/l, < 5.8 mg/dl). There is often associated hypoglycaemia, coagulopathy and lactic acidosis. Following successful resuscitation, hepatic function generally returns to normal.
- *Hyperbilirubinaemia ('ICU jaundice')* frequently develops following trauma or sepsis, particularly if there is inadequate control of the inflammatory process. There is a marked rise in bilirubin levels (predominantly conjugated) but only mild elevation of transaminase and alkaline phosphatase levels. This results from failure of bilirubin transport within the liver and produces the histological appearance of intrahepatic cholestasis. Extrahepatic cholestasis must be excluded by abdominal ultrasound and potentially hepatotoxic drugs should be stopped. Treatment is non-specific and should include early institution of enteral feeding. Therapy that compromises splanchnic blood flow, particularly high doses of vasoconstrictor agents, should be avoided.

NEUROLOGICAL SUPPORT

A diverse range of primary neurological and metabolic conditions require management in the ICU. These include the various causes of coma, spinal cord injury, peripheral neuromuscular disease and prolonged seizures. Intensive care is required to:

- manage acute brain injury with control of raised intracranial pressure
- protect the airway, if necessary by endotracheal intubation
- provide respiratory support to correct hypoxaemia and hypercapnia

- treat circulatory problems, e.g. neurogenic pulmonary oedema in subarachnoid haemorrhage, autonomic disturbances in Guillain–Barré syndrome, spinal shock following high spinal cord injuries
- manage status epilepticus using anaesthetic agents such as thiopental or propofol.

The aim of management in acute brain injury is to optimise cerebral oxygen delivery by maintaining a normal arterial oxygen content and a cerebral perfusion pressure above 70 mmHg. Avoiding secondary insults to the brain such as hypoxaemia and hypotension improves outcome in head injury. Intracranial pressure (ICP) rises in acute brain injury as a result of haematoma, contusions or ischaemic swelling. Raised ICP is damaging both directly to the cerebral cortex and by producing downward pressure on the brain stem, and indirectly by reducing cerebral perfusion pressure, thereby threatening cerebral blood flow and oxygen delivery:

Cerebral perfusion pressure (CPP) = mean BP − ICP

ICP may be measured via pressure transducers inserted directly into the brain tissue or held in place on the dura. The normal upper limit for ICP is 15 mmHg and management should be directed at keeping ICP below 20 mmHg (Box 8.26). Sustained pressures above 30 mmHg are associated with a poor prognosis.

Cerebral perfusion pressure should be maintained above 70 mmHg by ensuring adequate fluid replacement and if necessary by treating hypotension with a vasopressor such as noradrenaline (norepinephrine).

Complex neurological monitoring must be combined with frequent clinical assessment, i.e. GCS, pupil response to light and focal neurological signs. The motor response to pain is a particularly important prognostic sign. No response or extension of the upper limbs is associated with severe injury, and unless there is improvement within a few days prognosis is very poor. A flexor response is encouraging and indicates that a good outcome is still possible.

8.26 STRATEGIES TO CONTROL INTRACRANIAL PRESSURE

- Sedation, analgesia and occasionally paralysis to prevent coughing
- Nurse with 30° head-up tilt and avoid excessive flexion of the head or pressure around the neck that may impair cerebral venous drainage
- Control epileptiform activity with appropriate anticonvulsant therapy; an electroencephalogram (EEG) may be necessary to ensure this is achieved
- Maintain strict glycaemic control with blood glucose between 4 and 8 mmol/l (~ 70–140 mg/dl)
- Aim for a core body temperature of between 36 and 37°C
- Maintain sodium > 140 mmol/l using i.v. normal saline
- Avoid dehydration or fluid overload
- Hyperventilation to reduce the PCO_2 to 4–4.5 kPa (~ 30–34 mmHg) for the first 24 hours
- Osmotic diuretic, mannitol 20% 100–200 ml (0.25–0.5 g/kg), coupled with volume replacement
- Hypnotic infusion, thiopental, titrated to 'burst suppression' on EEG
- Surgery: drainage of haematoma or ventricles; lobectomy, decompressive craniectomy

NEUROLOGICAL COMPLICATIONS IN INTENSIVE CARE

Neurological complications also occur as a result of systemic critical illness. Sepsis may be associated with an encephalopathy characterised by confusion/delirium and associated with cerebral oedema and loss of vasoregulation. Hypotension and coagulopathy may provoke cerebral infarction or haemorrhage. Neurological examination is very difficult if the patient is sedated or paralysed and it is important to stop sedation regularly to reassess the patient's underlying level of consciousness. If there is evidence of a focal neurological deficit or a markedly declining level of consciousness, a CT of the brain should be performed.

Critical illness polyneuropathy is another potential complication in patients with sepsis and MOF. It is due to peripheral nerve axonal loss rather than demyelination and can result in areflexia, gross muscle-wasting and failure to wean from the ventilator, thus prolonging the duration of intensive care. Recovery can take many weeks.

MANAGEMENT OF SEPSIS

Prompt administration of appropriate antibiotics with a spectrum wide enough to cover probable causative organisms, based on an analysis of the likely site of infection, previous antibiotic therapy and the known resistance patterns on the unit, is essential. The haemodynamic changes in septic shock are very variable and are not specific for the Gram status of the infecting organism. The early stages of septic shock are often dominated by hypotension with relative volume depletion due to marked arteriolar and particularly venular dilatation. Sufficient intravenous fluid should be given to ensure that the intravascular volume is not the limiting factor in determining global oxygen delivery. The type of fluid that should be administered and what constitutes 'adequate' volume resuscitation remain controversial. The response to therapy is crucial and frequently unpredictable so it is not appropriate to use rigid protocols. While the patient remains clinically volume-depleted, a continuous crystalloid infusion of at least 1–2 ml/kg/hr should be given, together with full enteral nutrition if tolerated to achieve the planned 24-hour crystalloid balance. Depending on haemoglobin concentration, blood or synthetic colloid should be given as 100–200 ml boluses to assess BP response to volume and to achieve CVP or PAWP targets. A recent meta-analysis has confirmed that albumin should not routinely be used in the resuscitation of critically ill patients (p. 425).

Excessive fluid replacement in pursuit of 'supranormal' goals is not beneficial in patients with established organ failure (p. 184) and may be harmful, producing excessive tissue oedema.

Although ventricular function is frequently impaired, the characteristically low SVR ensures a high cardiac output (once the patient is adequately volume-resuscitated) albeit with low blood pressure.

The choice of the most appropriate vasoactive drug to use should be based on a full analysis of the circulation and

knowledge of the different inotropic, dilating or constricting properties of these drugs (Box 8.16, p. 192). In most cases a vasoconstrictor such as noradrenaline (norepinephrine) is necessary to increase SVR and blood pressure, while an inotrope may be necessary to maintain cardiac output and prevent regional ischaemia. In the later stages of severe sepsis the essential problem is at the level of the micro-circulation. Oxygen uptake and utilisation are impaired due to failure of the regional distribution of flow and direct cellular toxicity despite adequate global oxygen delivery. Tissue oxygenation may be improved and aerobic metabolism sustained by reducing demand, i.e. metabolic rate (Box 8.27).

SPECIFIC THERAPIES

Corticosteroids

Assessment of the pituitary–adrenal axis is difficult in the critically ill but in some series up to 30% of patients have adrenal insufficiency as assessed by baseline cortisol levels and the response to adrenocorticotrophic hormone (ACTH). Corticosteroid replacement therapy is controversial; early studies using short-term, high-dose methylprednisolone showed no benefit but recent studies using lower-dose infusions of hydrocortisone (8 mg/hr) for longer periods (5 days) demonstrated reduced vasoconstrictor requirements in hyperdynamic sepsis and one study has shown an outcome benefit.

Activated protein C

Until recently, numerous large multicentre trials using anti-cytokine and other novel drug therapies to interrupt the inflammatory cascade had all produced disappointing results. However, administration of activated protein C (levels of which frequently fall in critical illness) has recently been shown to produce a substantial reduction in mortality in patients with SIRS (Box 8.28).

8.28 ACTIVATED PROTEIN C IN SEVERE SEPSIS

EBM

'Recombinant human activated protein C reduces 28-day mortality in severe sepsis, even if multiple organ failure has already developed.'

- Taylor FB, et al. J Clin Invest 1987; 79:918–925.
- Bernard GR, et al. N Engl J Med 2001; 344:699–709.

8

SURVIVING SEPSIS CAMPAIGN

The Surviving Sepsis Campaign was launched in 2004 by an international group of critical care and infectious diseases 'experts' representing 11 major organisations with the aim of reducing the worldwide mortality from sepsis by 25% within 5 years. After reviewing and grading the available evidence, the group produced guidelines in the form of packages of care or 'sepsis bundles', each covering an aspect of the care of patients with severe sepsis (Box 8.4, p. 185). The belief is that this approach will eliminate the variable and piecemeal application of new evidence. The guidelines will be updated regularly as new evidence emerges and both the implementation of the guidelines and the outcome from sepsis will be audited to assess the success of the initiative.

DISCHARGE FROM INTENSIVE CARE

Discharge is appropriate when the original indication for admission has resolved and the patient has sufficient physiological reserve to remain safe and continue his or her recovery without the facilities available in intensive care. For long-stay ICU patients who have been ventilator-dependent, 'step-down' to the HDU is appropriate. Discharges from ICU/HDU should preferably take place within normal working hours as there is frequently a lack of skills on the general wards and of suitable junior medical and nursing support out of hours and at weekends.

The shortage of ICU and HDU beds in most hospitals in the UK creates pressure for early discharge but it has been shown that readmission rates and hospital mortality increase if discharge occurs prematurely or out of normal working hours.

The critical care team should give the receiving team a detailed handover, provide a written summary with relevant recent investigations, remain available for advice, and ideally should visit the patient on the ward within the 24 hours after discharge.

WITHDRAWAL OF CARE

Withdrawal of support is appropriate when it is clear that the patient has no realistic prospect of recovery or of surviving with a quality of life that he or she would value. In these situations intensive care will only prolong the dying process and is therefore both futile and an inhumane waste of resources. Nevertheless, when active support is withdrawn, management should remain positive and be directed towards allowing the patient to die with dignity and as free from distress as possible. Patients' wishes in this regard are paramount and increasing use is being made of advance directives or 'living wills'. Communication with the patient, if possible, with the family, with the referring clinicians and between members of the critical care team is crucial (Ch. 1). Failure in this area damages working relations, causes stress and unrealistic expectations, and leads to subsequent unhappiness, anger and litigation.

BRAIN DEATH

The preconditions for considering brain-stem death and the criteria for establishing the diagnosis are listed on page 1187.

When formal criteria for brain-stem death are met it is clearly inappropriate to continue supporting life with mechanical ventilation and, at this stage, the possibility of organ donation should be considered. All intensive care clinicians have a responsibility to approach relatives to seek consent for organ donation, provided there is no contraindication to the use of the organs. This can be a very difficult task but is easier if the patient carried an organ donor card. In the UK each region has a team of transplant coordinators who can help with the process and will provide information and advice about the necessary tests.

SCORING SYSTEMS IN CRITICAL CARE

Admission and discharge criteria vary between units so it is important to define the characteristics of the patients admitted (case mix) in order to assess the effects of the care provided on the outcome achieved (Box 8.29).

Two systems are widely used to measure severity of illness:

- 'APACHE' II—Acute Physiology Assessment and Chronic Health Evaluation
- 'SAPS' 2—Simplified Acute Physiology Score.

These scores include assessment of certain admission characteristics (e.g. age and pre-existing organ dysfunction) and a variety of routine physiological measurements (e.g. temperature, blood pressure, GCS) that reflect the response of the patient to his or her illness. Predicted mortality figures by diagnosis have been calculated from large databases generated from a range of ICUs. These allow a particular unit to evaluate its performance compared to the reference ICUs by calculating standardised mortality ratios (SMRs) for each diagnostic group:

SMR = observed mortality ÷ predicted mortality

A value of unity indicates the same performance as the reference ICUs while a value < 1 indicates a better than predicted outcome. A unit may have a high SMR in a certain diagnostic category and this would prompt investigation into how such patients were managed, with the intention of identifying aspects of care that could be improved.

When combined with the admission diagnosis, scoring systems have been shown to correlate well with the risk of

---

8.29 USES OF CRITICAL CARE SCORING SYSTEMS

- Comparison of the performance of different units
- Assessment of new therapies
- Assessment of changes in unit policies and management guidelines
- Measurement of the cost-effectiveness of care

hospital death. Such outcome predictions can never be 100% accurate and should be viewed as only one of many factors that the clinician considers when deciding whether or not further intervention is appropriate.

COSTS OF INTENSIVE CARE

Measuring the costs of intensive care is complex. The most widely used system is the Therapeutic Intervention Scoring System (TISS), which scores interventions and nursing activities for each day of admission and correlates reasonably well with detailed measurements of staff, equipment and drug costs incurred within the unit. Since it focuses on nurse-based interventions, TISS may also be used as an index of nurse dependency.

Current estimates of the daily cost of intensive care in the UK vary from £1000 to £2000, with high-dependency care accounting for approximately 50% and general ward care 20% of these costs. In the UK, less than 2% of total healthcare expenditure is spent on critical care.

OUTCOME FROM CRITICAL CARE

The most widely used measure to assess outcome from intensive care is mortality. This should be quoted at hospital discharge and at 28 days because mortality at the time of discharge from the unit will be influenced by the unit discharge policy. Mortality is also influenced by case mix, length of stay and organisational aspects of the unit.

The Kings Fund has emphasised the need to demonstrate long-term benefit to justify the increasing costs of critical care provision. Quality of life following discharge should be included in the evaluation of critical care but it is difficult to measure and interpret, not least because no objective premorbid assessment is possible with emergency admissions. However, several units in the UK now run follow-up clinics and have identified that there is a high incidence of physical and psychological problems affecting the patient and his or her family following ICU discharge.

FURTHER INFORMATION

Books and journal articles
Bersten A, Soni N, Oh TE, eds. Oh's intensive care manual. 5th edn. Oxford: Butterworth–Heinemann; 2003.
Davidson AC, Treacher DT, eds. Respiratory intensive care. London: Hodder Arnold; 2002.
Dellinger RP, Carlet JM, Masur H, et al. Surviving Sepsis Campaign guidelines for the management of severe sepsis and septic shock. Critical Care Medicine 2004; 32:858–873.
Fink M, Abraham E, Vincent J-L, et al, eds. Textbook of critical care. 5th edn. London: WB Saunders; 2004.
Hillman K, Bishop G, eds. Clinical intensive care and acute medicine. 2nd edn. Cambridge: Cambridge University Press; 2004.
Hinds CJ, Watson D, eds. Intensive care: a concise textbook. 3rd edn. London: WB Saunders; 2004.
Webb AR, Shapiro MJ, Singer M, et al, eds. Oxford textbook of critical care. Oxford: Oxford University Press; 1999.

Websites
www.esicm.org *Guidelines, recommendations, consensus conference reports.*
www.ics.ac.uk *Clinical guidelines and standards for intensive care.*
www.sicsebm.org.uk *Intensive care evidence-based medicine website. Reviews and critically appraised topics.*
www.survivingsepsis.org *Surviving Sepsis website.*

8

9

A.L. JONES

L. KARALLIEDDE

Poisoning

9

Acute poisoning is one of the most common medical emergencies in the UK, accounting for 10–20% of all acute medical admissions. At least 50% involve more than one drug, with alcohol being the most frequent second agent.

Substances involved in poisoning vary widely between different countries (Box 9.1). In the UK, poisoning with paracetamol accounts for 48% of all overdoses, but only 7% of those in the USA, and in Nepal it is very rare. Poisoning with tricyclic antidepressants, selective serotonin (5-hydroxytryptamine, 5-HT) re-uptake inhibitors and drugs of misuse is very common in the UK and USA. Australia has a similar range of ingested toxins to the UK but envenoming with snakes, spiders and marine creatures is also very common. In South and South-east Asia, pesticide ingestion is endemic, and constitutes the most common cause of death by poisoning. The toxicity of available poisons and the paucity of medical facilities in the developing world mean that the mortality rate for self-poisoning is high at 10–20%, compared with 0.5–1% in most industrialised countries. Reducing deaths from self-harm requires interventions both to lower the incidence of harmful behaviour and to improve the medical management of acute poisoning.

9.1 SUBSTANCES FREQUENTLY INVOLVED IN POISONING

In the United Kingdom

- Analgesics, including paracetamol and non-steroidal anti-inflammatory drugs (NSAIDs)
- Cardiotoxic drugs, especially tricyclic antidepressants
- Drugs of misuse
- Carbon monoxide*
- Alcohol

In South and South-east Asia

- Organophosphorus* and carbamate insecticides
- Aluminium and zinc phosphide
- Snake venoms
- Antimalarial drugs such as chloroquine
- Antidiabetic medication

* Indicates the most common cause of death by poisoning.

GENERAL APPROACH TO THE POISONED PATIENT

TAKING A HISTORY

In most cases, the diagnosis of poisoning is apparent on the basis of the history. However, such information may not always be forthcoming, either because patients do not know what has been taken or because they may have been under the influence of alcohol or the drug itself at the time of ingestion. A few patients deliberately mislead doctors but this is very rare, with the exception of drug misusers.

Full details of the amount and type of substance that has been taken must be recorded, along with the timing of ingestion or exposure. Establishing whether the drugs belonged to the patient, or to a friend or relative, and the source of the drug (i.e. over the counter, prescription, street)

is important in the prevention of future poisoning. The nature of any drug taken should be corroborated or identified from descriptions of the tablets or remaining pills, packets or bottles by the use of drug identification software (e.g. TICTAC®), which can be accessed by many pharmacies and poisons information centres.

Ask the patient why the overdose was taken and take time to listen to the explanation. Reasons often include relationship difficulties, work- or school-related difficulties, drug addiction, psychiatric illness or bereavement. Whilst 'accidental overdose' can occur, in general all patients presenting with poisoning should undergo psychiatric evaluation (pp. 205 and 229).

Details of the past medical history, particularly a history of asthma, jaundice, drug misuse (and by which routes), head injury, epilepsy, cardiovascular problems, previous psychiatric illness and self-harm should be taken. It is important to ask about allergies and alcohol history. Identifying relationship problems and taking a good social history are also important.

CLINICAL FEATURES OF POISONING

First ensure that:

- the Airway is clear
- the patient is Breathing adequately
- the Circulation is not compromised.

If the patient is alert and has a stable circulation, proceed to examination. The only exception is where immediate eye or skin decontamination is required (Fig. 9.2). A standard clinical examination should be carried out on every poisoned patient. Needle marks or previous evidence of self-harm, e.g. razor marks on forearms, should be sought. Examination findings such as pupil size, respiratory rate and heart rate may support the diagnosis in an unconscious patient, but on their own merely help to narrow down the potential list of toxins. Clinical signs that can help identify which toxin has been taken are shown in Figure 9.1. The weight of the patient is important in determining whether toxicity is likely to occur, given the dose ingested, and the dose of any antidote to be calculated (e.g. N-acetylcysteine in paracetamol poisoning).

The Glasgow Coma Scale (GCS, p. 1186) is the method most frequently used to assess the degree of impaired consciousness, though it has never been validated for use in poisoned patients. When patients are unconscious and no history is available, the diagnosis of poisoning depends on the exclusion of other causes of coma (especially meningitis, intracerebral bleeds, hypoglycaemia, diabetic ketoacidosis, uraemia and encephalopathy—p. 1186) and consideration of circumstantial evidence.

ROLE OF THE TOXICOLOGY LABORATORY

In most patients the diagnosis of poisoning is made on the history and clinical signs alone. In some cases, such as poisoning with paracetamol (p. 208), aspirin (p. 209) or iron

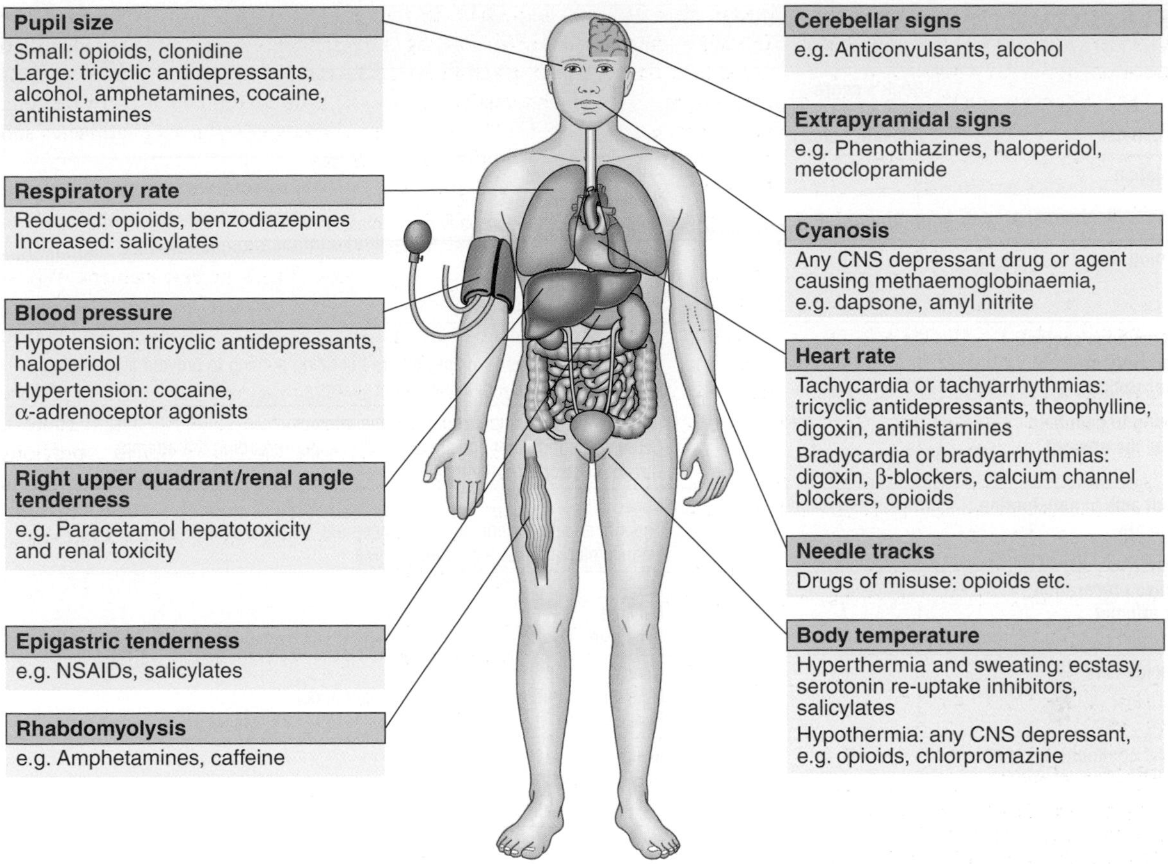

Pupil size

Small: opioids, clonidine
Large: tricyclic antidepressants,
alcohol, amphetamines, cocaine,
antihistamines

Respiratory rate

Reduced: opioids, benzodiazepines
Increased: salicylates

Blood pressure

Hypotension: tricyclic antidepressants,
haloperidol
Hypertension: cocaine,
α-adrenoceptor agonists

**Right upper quadrant/renal angle
tenderness**

e.g. Paracetamol hepatotoxicity
and renal toxicity

Epigastric tenderness

e.g. NSAIDs, salicylates

Rhabdomyolysis

e.g. Amphetamines, caffeine

Cerebellar signs

e.g. Anticonvulsants, alcohol

Extrapyramidal signs

e.g. Phenothiazines, haloperidol,
metoclopramide

Cyanosis

Any CNS depressant drug or agent
causing methaemoglobinaemia,
e.g. dapsone, amyl nitrite

Heart rate

Tachycardia or tachyarrhythmias:
tricyclic antidepressants, theophylline,
digoxin, antihistamines
Bradycardia or bradyarrhythmias:
digoxin, β-blockers, calcium channel
blockers, opioids

Needle tracks

Drugs of misuse: opioids etc.

Body temperature

Hyperthermia and sweating: ecstasy,
serotonin re-uptake inhibitors,
salicylates
Hypothermia: any CNS depressant,
e.g. opioids, chlorpromazine

9

Fig. 9.1   Clinical signs of poisoning by pharmaceutical agents or drugs of misuse.

(Box 9.9, p. 212), subsequent management of the patient depends on measurement of the amount of toxin in the blood.

In unconscious patients, a qualitative screen of the urine (e.g. urine immunofluorescence drugs of misuse screening test) is an effective way to confirm recent use of drugs such as benzodiazepines, cocaine, ecstasy, opioids and cannabis. Routine screens may not, however, detect fentanyl derivatives, tramadol and other synthetic opioids. Occasionally, measuring drugs of misuse and their metabolites in blood by gas chromatography-mass spectroscopy (GC-MS) is required for medico-legal purposes, particularly where there is a fatality, and in such cases urine and serum should be saved for later analysis.

9.2 POISONING IN OLD AGE

- **Renally metabolised drugs** (e.g. metformin, aspirin): accumulate more rapidly and to higher levels due to reduced glomerular filtration rate.
- **CNS depressants:** have a greater sedative action in old age and may precipitate confusion.
- **Suicide rates:** highest in older people in most countries, and attempts are usually by overdose in the UK.
- **Depression and self-harm**: closely associated in old age, so all overdoses in older people should be taken seriously and any underlying depressive illness treated aggressively.

PSYCHIATRIC ASSESSMENT OF THE POISONED PATIENT

To determine the most appropriate placement and supervision for a self-poisoned patient, an initial assessment of suicidal intent must be made. Use of the Beck's depression scale may be helpful (Box 9.3). If the sum of all the scores for each parameter is greater than 4 (e.g. suicide note left and no one likely to find patient after overdose), this indicates significant suicidal intent and that the patient is at risk of further self-harm. A nurse should remain with the patient at all times during the hospital stay.

Suicide attempts were once much more common in women than in men but now the ratios are more equal. There is a higher incidence in lower socio-economic groups, those who lost a parent at an early age, those with alcohol or drug misuse, recipients of child abuse, the unemployed and those with recent broken relationships. A thorough psychiatric and social assessment should be carried out in all patients, once sufficient time has elapsed to allow the toxic effects of any drugs to wear off (p. 229). This can be performed by nurses, physicians or psychiatrists. The interviewer should assess the severity of any symptoms of psychiatric illness and determine what personal or social support is needed. Most patients have depressive and anxiety symptoms, which are reactive to an acute life crisis, superimposed on a

9.3 BECK'S SCORING SYSTEM

Parameter	Beck's score (add up all those relevant below)	Scoring
Isolation	0 1 2	Someone present Someone nearby or in vocal contact No one nearby or in visual/vocal contact
Timing	0 1 2	Intervention probable Intervention not likely Intervention highly unlikely
Precautions against discovery or interruption	0 1 2	None Passive precautions (avoiding others but doing nothing to prevent intervention) Active precautions, e.g. locking door
Acting to gain help after the attempt	0 1 2	Notified potential helper regarding the attempt Contacted but did not specifically notify helper regarding the attempt Did not contact or notify helper
Final acts in anticipation of death	0 1 2	None Thought about or made some arrangement Definite plans made, e.g. changing will
Active preparation for attempt	0 1 2	None Minimal Extensive
Suicide note	0 1 2	None Note written but torn up or note thought about Note present
Overt communication of intent before attempt	0 1 2	None Equivocal communication Unequivocal attempt

background of chronic social and personal difficulties. They need neither psychotropic medication nor specialised psychiatric treatment but do require support, e.g. from a social worker. Admission to a psychiatric ward is necessary for those with major psychiatric illness (p. 234) who remain intent on suicide. In the authors' unit, about 20% of patients make a repeat suicide attempt during the following 12 months and 1% actually kill themselves. Factors associated with an increased risk of suicide include male sex, age over 45, living alone, unemployment, recent bereavement, divorce or separation, chronic ill health, drug or alcohol misuse, violent method used, suicide note written and a history of previous attempts.

Preventing poisoning in the first place is much better than treating it, and a number of important measures have been taken to achieve this (Box 9.4).

GENERAL MANAGEMENT OF THE POISONED PATIENT

The majority of patients who present after poisoning have taken an overdose. Some present with eye or skin contamination and should be treated with appropriate washing or irrigation (Fig. 9.2). Only patients who have ingested significant overdoses need further measures such as gastric

9.4 PREVENTION OF POISONING

Method	Mode of action
Addition of 'Bitrex' and other bittering agents to household products	Prevents significant quantities being ingested as it tastes very bitter
Adding the antidote to the toxin, e.g. combination tablets of methionine and paracetamol	Hepatic-protective glutathione remains replete and hepatocellular injury is prevented
Child-resistant containers	Reduce chance of ingestion by children
Secure location, e.g. locked cupboard	Reduces access
Hazard warning labels	Warn of potential toxicity, routes of exposure and appropriate protective equipment
Education	Warning on safe storage and handling of chemicals and drugs
Supervision	The key to reduced exposure for children
Legislation, e.g. Health and Safety regulations	Safeguards for the use of dangerous chemicals make a safer workplace

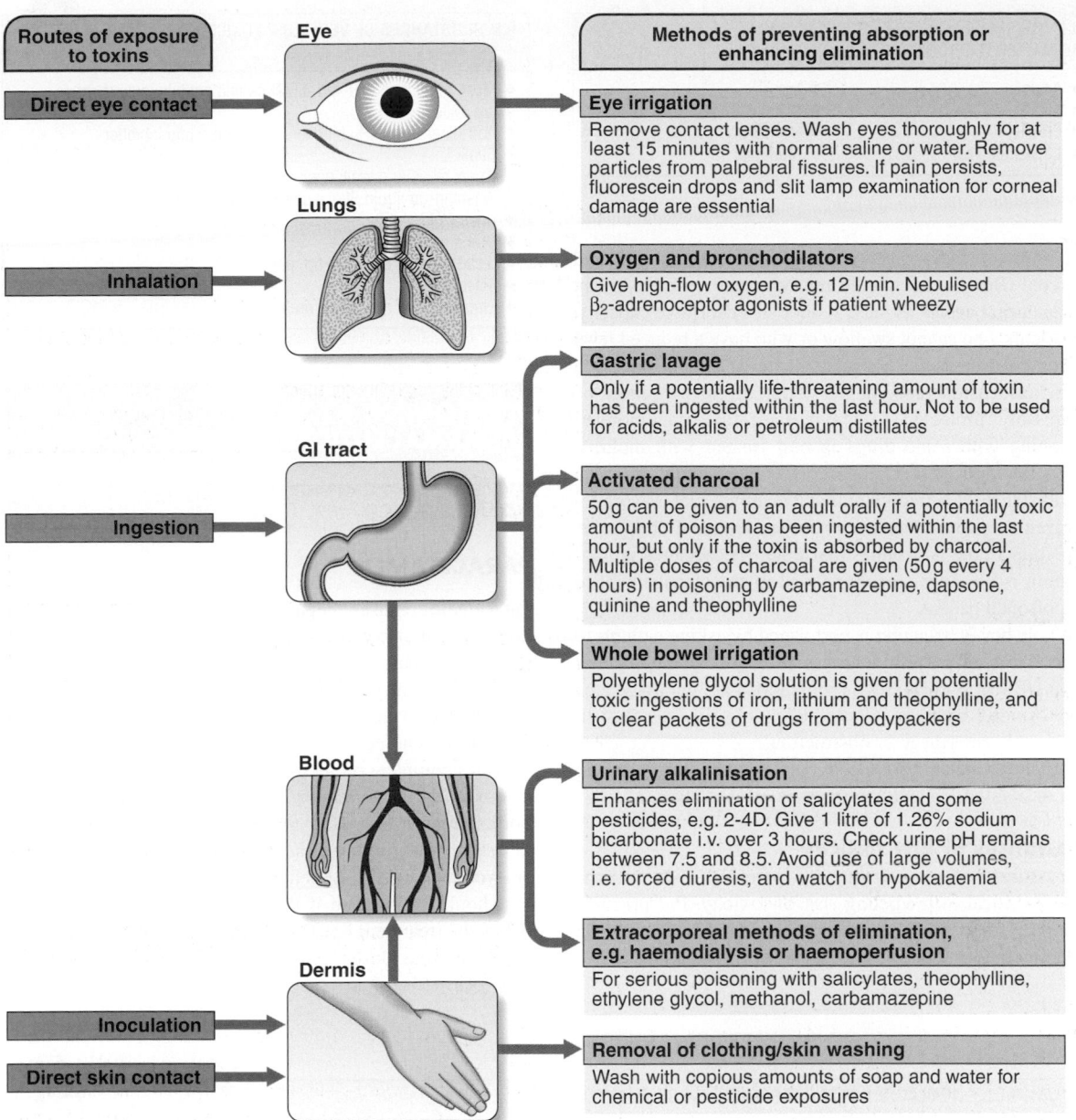

Routes of exposure to toxins		Methods of preventing absorption or enhancing elimination
Direct eye contact	**Eye**	**Eye irrigation** Remove contact lenses. Wash eyes thoroughly for at least 15 minutes with normal saline or water. Remove particles from palpebral fissures. If pain persists, fluorescein drops and slit lamp examination for corneal damage are essential
Inhalation	**Lungs**	**Oxygen and bronchodilators** Give high-flow oxygen, e.g. 12 l/min. Nebulised β_2-adrenoceptor agonists if patient wheezy
Ingestion	**GI tract**	**Gastric lavage** Only if a potentially life-threatening amount of toxin has been ingested within the last hour. Not to be used for acids, alkalis or petroleum distillates
		Activated charcoal 50 g can be given to an adult orally if a potentially toxic amount of poison has been ingested within the last hour, but only if the toxin is absorbed by charcoal. Multiple doses of charcoal are given (50 g every 4 hours) in poisoning by carbamazepine, dapsone, quinine and theophylline
		Whole bowel irrigation Polyethylene glycol solution is given for potentially toxic ingestions of iron, lithium and theophylline, and to clear packets of drugs from bodypackers
	Blood	**Urinary alkalinisation** Enhances elimination of salicylates and some pesticides, e.g. 2-4D. Give 1 litre of 1.26% sodium bicarbonate i.v. over 3 hours. Check urine pH remains between 7.5 and 8.5. Avoid use of large volumes, i.e. forced diuresis, and watch for hypokalaemia
		Extracorporeal methods of elimination, e.g. haemodialysis or haemoperfusion For serious poisoning with salicylates, theophylline, ethylene glycol, methanol, carbamazepine
Inoculation	**Dermis**	**Removal of clothing/skin washing** Wash with copious amounts of soap and water for chemical or pesticide exposures
Direct skin contact		

Fig. 9.2 Routes of exposure to toxins and methods of preventing absorption or enhancing elimination.

decontamination and methods to increase elimination. In the seriously poisoned patient, meticulous supportive care, including the treatment of seizures, coma and cardiovascular complications, is critical to good outcome. Seizures are seen most commonly in poisoning by theophyllines, non-steroidal anti-inflammatory drugs (NSAIDs), anti-convulsants and tricyclic antidepressants, and are best treated by airway management and i.v. diazepam (10 mg for an adult, repeated as necessary; p. 1171). Cardiovascular support measures are discussed on page 191. Ventilatory support may be required until consciousness returns, and complications such as aspiration pneumonia should be treated promptly. Patients must be observed closely for signs of deterioration whilst the effects of the toxin they have

9.5 SINGLE-DOSE ACTIVATED CHARCOAL AFTER POISON INGESTION **EBM**

'Activated charcoal improves outcome when administered within 1 hour of ingestion of a potentially toxic amount of a poison which binds to charcoal.'

- American Academy of Clinical Toxicology; European Association of Poison Control Centres and Clinical Toxicologists. Clin Tox 1997; 35:721–741.

taken wear off. This often approximates to five half-lives of the drug concerned.

Activated charcoal is the most common method used to prevent drug absorption and is given orally as black slurry; owing to its large surface area and porous structure, this is highly effective in adsorbing most toxins (Box 9.5). There

9.6 SUBSTANCES POORLY ADSORBED BY ACTIVATED CHARCOAL	
• Acids	• Iron
• Alkalis	• Lithium
• Ethanol	• Mercury
• Ethylene glycol	• Methanol

9.8 SUBSTANCES OF VERY LOW TOXICITY

- Most antibiotics BUT tetracyclines and antituberculous drugs are toxic
- Anti-ulcer drugs: H$_2$-blockers or proton pump inhibitors
- Chalk
- Paper glues and wallpaper paste
- Washing-up liquid BUT dishwasher tablets are highly corrosive
- Household plants
- Oral contraceptive pills
- 'Lead' pencils and 'felt-tip' pens
- Silica gel
- Emollient and zinc oxide creams

are, however, a few agents that do not bind to activated charcoal (Box 9.6). It should not be mixed with ice cream or flavouring agents as these reduce its adsorptive capacity. In patients who cannot swallow or who have a reduced level of consciousness, the activated charcoal should be given via a nasogastric tube. In all cases, the airway must be adequately protected to avoid aspiration pneumonitis. Poisoning with some drugs is best treated with multiple doses of activated charcoal (Fig. 9.2), and in such circumstances it is important that a laxative, such as sorbitol is given to avoid obstruction due to charcoal 'briquette' formation in the gastrointestinal tract. Ipecacuanha administration is no longer recommended in the management of the poisoned patient.

Whole bowel irrigation is performed by asking patients to drink 1 litre of polyethylene glycol every hour until their rectal effluent is clear. Such preparations are not associated with osmotic changes. Contraindications include gastro-intestinal haemorrhage or obstruction.

Despite popular misconceptions, specific antidotes are only available for a small number of poisons (Box 9.7).

Substances of low toxicity

Every substance, even water, is a potential toxin, but the dose is critical in predicting risk of toxicity. For practical purposes, some substances can be ingested by humans in large amounts without serious sequelae (Box 9.8).

POISONING BY SPECIFIC PHARMACEUTICAL AGENTS

ANALGESICS

PARACETAMOL

Paracetamol causes hepatic damage in overdose. More rarely, it can also cause renal failure. The management of a patient with paracetamol overdose is summarised in Figure 9.3. If a patient presents within 1 hour of the paracetamol overdose, activated charcoal can be given in addition. The antidote of choice is intravenous N-acetylcysteine, which provides complete protection against toxicity if given within 10 hours of the overdose; its efficacy declines thereafter. For this reason, if a patient presents more than 8 hours after ingestion, N-acetylcysteine administration should not be delayed to await a paracetamol blood concentration result, but should be stopped if this is subsequently shown to be below the treatment line. Methionine 12 g orally 4-hourly, to a total of four doses, is a suitable alternative antidote for

9.7 ANTIDOTES AVAILABLE FOR THE TREATMENT OF SPECIFIC POISONINGS	
Poison	**Antidote**
Anticoagulants (e.g. warfarin, rodenticides)	Vitamin K, fresh frozen plasma
β-adrenoceptor antagonists (β-blockers)	I.v. glucagon, adrenaline (epinephrine)
Calcium channel blockers	Calcium gluconate, calcium chloride, glucagon
Cyanide	Oxygen, dicobalt edetate, nitrites, sodium thiosulphate, hydroxocobalamin
Ethylene glycol/methanol	Ethanol, 4-methylpyrazole
Lead	DMSA (2,3-dimercaptosuccinic acid), DMPS (2,3-dimercapto-1-propane sulphonate) Disodium calcium edetate
Mercury	DMPS
Iron salts	Desferrioxamine
Opioids	Naloxone
Organophosphorus insecticides, nerve agents	Atropine, oximes (pralidoxime, obidoxime salts, HI-6, HLo-7)
Paracetamol	N-acetylcysteine, methionine
Cardiac glycosides, e.g. foxglove, digoxin, yellow oleander	Digoxin-specific antibody fragments (F$_{ab}$)

9

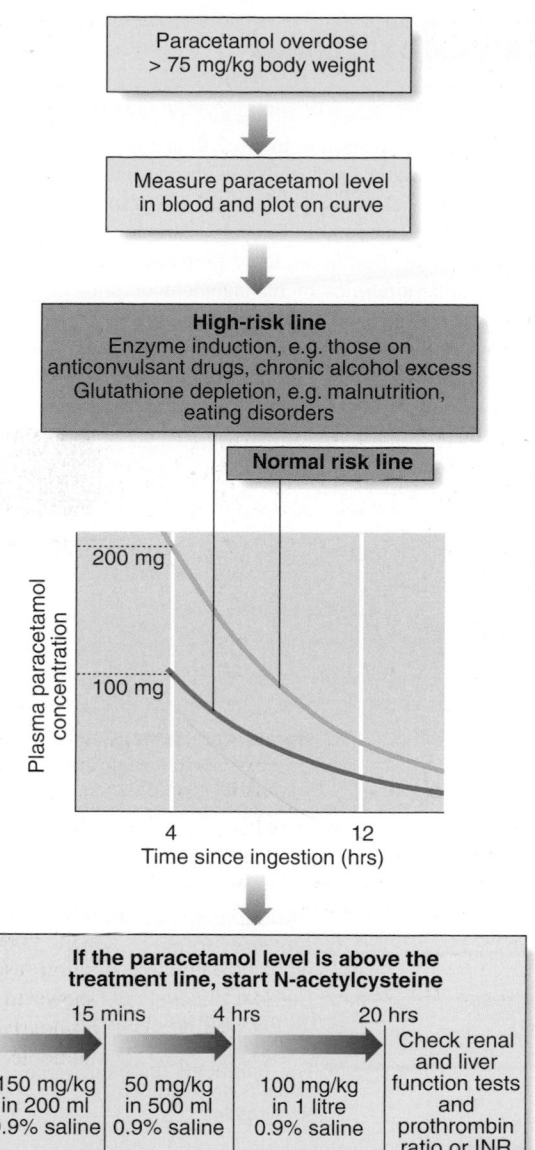

Fig. 9.3 **The management of a paracetamol overdose patient.** Do not check a paracetamol concentration before 4 hours have elapsed; it is uninterpretable. If more than 8 hours have elapsed since ingestion, start the N-acetylcysteine immediately and only stop it if the concentration is below the treatment line. (INR = international normalised ratio)

paracetamol poisoning when N-acetylcysteine is not available. If a patient presents more than 15 hours after ingestion, liver function tests, prothrombin ratio (or international normalised ratio—INR) and renal function tests should be performed, the antidote started, and a poisons information centre or local liver unit contacted for advice. In some cases an arterial blood gas sample will need to be taken. Liver transplantation should be considered in individuals who develop acute liver failure due to paracetamol poisoning (p. 952).

If multiple ingestions of paracetamol have taken place over several hours or days (i.e. a staggered overdose), there is no merit in measuring the plasma paracetamol concen-

tration as it will be uninterpretable. Such patients should be given N-acetylcysteine if the paracetamol dose exceeds 150 mg/kg body weight in any one 24-hour period or 75 mg/kg body weight in 'high-risk groups' (Fig. 9.3).

SALICYLATES (ASPIRIN)

Salicylate ingestion at doses greater than 150, 250 and 500 mg aspirin/kg body weight produces mild, moderate and severe poisoning respectively. Salicylate poisoning can also occur with ingestion of oil of wintergreen or when salicylic ointment (e.g. verruca remover) is applied extensively to skin. Aspirin overdose commonly produces nausea, vomiting, tinnitus and deafness. Direct stimulation of the respiratory centre produces hyperventilation. Peripheral vasodilatation with bounding pulses and profuse sweating occurs in moderately severe poisoning. Petechiae and subconjunctival haemorrhages can occur due to reduced platelet aggregation but this is self-limiting. Signs of serious salicylate poisoning include metabolic acidosis, renal failure and central nervous system (CNS) effects such as agitation, confusion, coma and fits. Rarely, pulmonary and cerebral oedema occur. Death can occur as a consequence of CNS depression and cardiovascular collapse. The development of a metabolic acidosis is a bad prognostic sign, because acidosis results in increased salicylate transfer across the blood–brain barrier.

It is important to measure a plasma salicylate concentration in all but the most trivial overdose. This is best undertaken at 6 hours or later after ingestion because of continued absorption of the drug. The salicylate concentration needs to be interpreted in conjunction with the clinical features and acid–base status of the patient. Any significant metabolic acidosis should be treated with intravenous sodium bicarbonate (8.4%), and the volume given titrated to give an arterial H^+ of 32–40 (pH of 7.4–7.5). Patients are often very dehydrated, and fluid loss from vomiting and sweating must be replaced, although injudicious use of intravenous fluids may precipitate pulmonary oedema. The use of multiple doses of activated charcoal (p. 207) in salicylate poisoning is controversial, but this approach is currently recommended until the salicylate concentration has peaked. Urinary alkalinisation (Fig. 9.2) is indicated for adult patients with salicylate concentrations of 600–800 mg/l. Haemodialysis is very effective at removing salicylate and correcting acid–base and fluid balance abnormalities and should be considered when serum concentrations are above 800 mg/l in adult patients and above 700 mg/l in the elderly. Other indications for haemodialysis in acute salicylate overdose are metabolic acidosis resistant to correction, severe CNS effects such as coma or convulsions, pulmonary oedema and acute renal failure.

NON-STEROIDAL ANTI-INFLAMMATORY DRUGS (NSAIDs)

Overdose of most NSAIDs usually causes little more than minor gastrointestinal upset including mild abdominal pain, vomiting and diarrhoea. However, 10–20% of patients have convulsions; these are usually self-limiting and seldom

9

9

need treatment other than airway protection and oxygen. Those that persist are treated with intravenous diazepam. Serious features include coma, prolonged fits, apnoea and bradycardia but these are very rare. Deaths have been reported after massive overdose of ibuprofen, but not with mefenamic acid. Rarely, renal failure ensues. Features of toxicity tend to occur early and are unlikely to develop later than 6 hours after the overdose. Liver and renal function may be affected, and therefore electrolytes, liver function tests and a full blood count should be checked in all but the most trivial overdoses. The half-lives of most NSAIDs are less than 12 hours, so elimination methods are not needed. Activated charcoal should be given if more than 100 mg/kg body weight of ibuprofen or more than 10 tablets of any other NSAID have been taken in the last hour. Gastrointestinal irritation is treated with oral H_2-blockers (e.g. ranitidine).

CARDIOTOXIC DRUGS

An individual's response to a cardiotoxic drug overdose is highly variable, and those with cardiac disease are more at risk of toxicity, particularly of complications such as pulmonary oedema. Toxicity can be delayed and prolonged with modified-release preparations. The cardiac features and principles of management of poisoning with cardiotoxic drugs are shown in Figure 9.4. In many countries, the more cardiotoxic tricyclic antidepressants are being replaced with the less cardiotoxic selective serotonin re-uptake inhibitors (SSRIs) for the treatment of depression. However, in large doses SSRIs can still cause hypotension and arrhythmias.

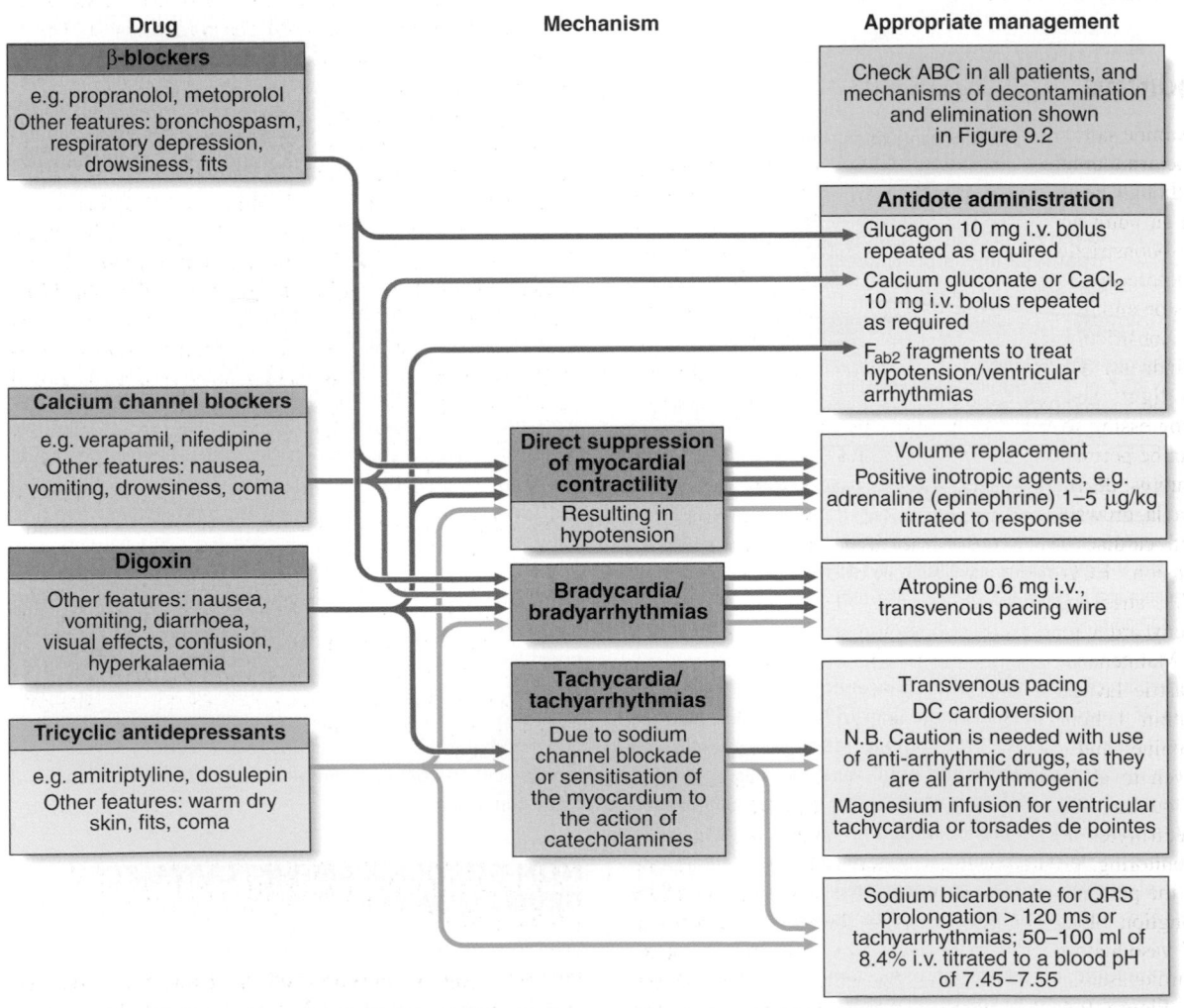

Fig. 9.4 Mechanisms and management of poisoning with cardiotoxic drugs.

ANTIMALARIALS

CHLOROQUINE

Symptoms and signs of chloroquine overdose usually start within 1 hour of ingestion and include nausea, vomiting, agitation, drowsiness, hypokalaemia, headaches and visual disturbances. After large ingestions, coma, convulsions, hypotension (due to the negative inotropic effect), ECG changes (widened QRS and prolonged QT_c interval), and arrhythmias including ventricular tachycardia, torsades de pointes and ventricular fibrillation occur.

Activated charcoal should be given and gastric lavage considered in all patients who present within 1 hour of ingestion of more than 15 mg/kg chloroquine. Cardiovascular complications can be managed as shown in Figure 9.4. The plasma potassium should be monitored, although hypokalaemia may have a protective effect and should not be corrected in the early stages of poisoning. If it persists beyond 8 hours, potassium should be replaced with caution. High-dose diazepam (2 mg/kg body weight i.v. over 30 minutes) may have a protective effect, especially if given in the early stages of severe chloroquine poisoning, but respiratory support should be available.

QUININE

Quinine salts are widely used in the treatment of malaria and nocturnal cramps. The average fatal dose in an adult is 8 g, although deaths have been reported with as little as 1.5 g in an adult and 900 mg in a child. Quinine causes retinal vasoconstriction and has a direct toxic effect on retinal photoreceptor cells. At 6–10 hours after ingestion, blurred vision and impaired colour perception start and can progress to constriction of the visual field, scotoma and complete blindness. The pupils become dilated and unresponsive to light, and fundoscopy shows retinal artery spasm progressing to disc pallor and retinal oedema. Visual loss can be permanent. Other features include nausea, vomiting, tinnitus, deafness, headache and tremor. In large overdoses, ataxia, drowsiness, coma, respiratory depression, haemolysis and cardiac effects can occur. The latter include hypotension, ECG changes (prolongation of the QRS and QT_c, atrioventricular block) and arrhythmias (ventricular tachycardia, torsades de pointes and ventricular fibrillation).

Maintenance of the airway and ventilation is critical. Gastric lavage should be considered if a patient presents within 1 hour of ingestion of more than 15 mg/kg of quinine, and multiple-dose activated charcoal should be given to all patients who have ingested a larger amount of quinine. All patients should have a 12-lead ECG, urea, electrolytes and glucose checked, along with cardiac monitoring. Visual effects of quinine are largely untreatable. In the past many measures were advocated, such as stellate ganglion block and retrobulbar or intravenous injections of vasodilators such as nitrates; these are now obsolete. Cardiovascular complications can be managed as shown in Figure 9.4. Haemodialysis and haemoperfusion are ineffective.

ANTIDIABETIC AGENTS

These include the sulphonylureas (e.g. chlorpropamide, glibenclamide, gliclazide, glipizide, tolbutamide), biguanides (metformin, phenformin) and insulins.

Antidiabetic agents can cause hypoglycaemia when taken in overdose, although insulin is non-toxic if ingested. The onset and duration of hypoglycaemia vary, but can last for several days with the longer-acting agents such as chlorpropamide, and isophane and lente insulins. Hypoglycaemia may manifest as agitation, sweating, confusion, tachycardia, hypothermia, drowsiness, coma or convulsions (p. 823). Permanent neurological damage can occur if the hypoglycaemia is prolonged. Metformin can cause a lactic acidosis in overdose, particularly in elderly patients and those with renal or hepatic impairment, or when co-ingested with ethanol. It is associated with a > 50% mortality. Metformin overdose may also cause nausea and vomiting, diarrhoea, abdominal pain, drowsiness, coma, hypotension and cardiovascular collapse.

Activated charcoal should be given and gastric lavage considered in all patients who present within 1 hour of ingestion of more than the normal therapeutic dose of an oral hypoglycaemic agent. Formal measurement of venous blood glucose (not just visually read strips or meter) and urea and electrolytes should be performed and repeated regularly. For medico-legal purposes (such as when it is suspected that the patient has been poisoned by a third party), a blood sample may be required for subsequent measurement of insulin, pro-insulin and C-peptide levels. Hypoglycaemia should be corrected urgently with 50 ml 50% dextrose, given i.v. if the patient is unconscious or with a sugary drink if the patient is conscious. This should be followed by an infusion of 10% or 20% dextrose titrated to the patient's blood glucose to prevent further hypoglycaemia. Dextrose infusions may be necessary for several days, depending on the agent ingested or injected. Potassium replacement should be guided by frequent measurement of urea and electrolytes. As a general rule, 10–20 mmol potassium chloride should be added to each litre of 5% dextrose i.v. Failure to regain consciousness within a few minutes of normalisation of the blood glucose can indicate that a CNS depressant has also been ingested, that the hypoglycaemia has been prolonged, that there is another cause for the coma (e.g. cerebral haemorrhage) or that the patient has cerebral oedema (p. 825). In cases of severe sulphonylurea overdose resistant to dextrose infusions, use of intravenous octreotide as an antidote may be considered.

DRUGS LESS COMMONLY TAKEN IN OVERDOSE

Box 9.9 gives an overview of the clinical features and management of overdose of other drugs not discussed in detail above.

9

9.9 DRUGS TAKEN LESS COMMONLY IN OVERDOSE

Drug	Features	Management
Anticonvulsants	Cerebellar signs Fits Coma Cardiovascular toxicity	Multiple-dose activated charcoal Cardiovascular support (as Fig. 9.4) I.v. diazepam for fits
Antihistamines	Drowsiness Cardiac arrhythmias	Activated charcoal within 1 hour Cardiovascular support (as Fig. 9.4)
Chlorpromazine/haloperidol	Hypotension Drowsiness Fits	Single-dose activated charcoal Cardiovascular support (as Fig. 9.4) I.v. diazepam for fits
Iron tablets	Vomiting Haematemesis Abdominal pain Coma Convulsions Shock Metabolic acidosis Hepatic failure	Ingestion of < 30 mg elemental iron/kg body weight: No active treatment Ingestion of > 30 mg/kg: Perform gastric lavage/whole bowel irrigation Check a serum iron concentration and if above 90 μmol/l (500 μg/dl) treat with i.v. desferrioxamine, especially if clinical features are present
Isoniazid	Peripheral neuropathy Fits	Activated charcoal I.v. pyridoxine I.v. diazepam for fits
Lithium	Nausea Vomiting Tremors Fits Confusion Coma	Does NOT bind to charcoal Whole bowel irrigation Increased hydration, avoid diuretics In severe cases: haemodialysis
Theophylline	Cardiac arrhythmias Fits Coma	Cardiovascular support (as Fig. 9.4) Multiple-dose activated charcoal I.v. diazepam for fits
Thyroxine	Tremor Tachycardia	Check thyroid function Treat symptomatically with oral propranolol
Zidovudine	Drowsiness Nausea Bone marrow suppression Fits	Activated charcoal Regular full blood count I.v. diazepam for fits

DRUGS OF MISUSE

CANNABIS

The term 'cannabis' refers to all psychoactive substances derived from the dried leaves and flowers of the plant *Cannabis sativa*. Marijuana refers to any part of the plant used to induce effects, and hashish is the dried resin from the flower tops. Cannabis is usually dried and either smoked with tobacco or eaten, and is widely used. Slang terms include grass, pot, ganja, spliff and reefer. When it is smoked, the onset of effect occurs within 10–30 minutes; after ingestion the onset is 1–3 hours. The duration of effect is 4–8 hours. In low doses, cannabis produces euphoria, perceptual alterations and conjunctival injection, followed by relaxation and drowsiness, hypertension, tachycardia, slurred speech and ataxia. High doses produce acute paranoid psychosis, anxiety, confusion, hallucinations, and distortion of time and space. Intravenous misuse of the crude extract of cannabis may cause nausea and vomiting, diarrhoea, abdominal pain, fever, hypotension, pulmonary oedema, acute renal failure, disseminated intravascular coagulation and death. Psychological dependence is common but tolerance and withdrawal symptoms are unusual.

Ingestion or smoking of cannabis rarely results in serious poisoning. For patients with drug-induced psychosis reassurance is usually sufficient but i.v. diazepam may be used for sedation. Hypotension usually responds well to intravenous fluids. All patients who have injected cannabis should be admitted, and fluid and electrolyte balance carefully managed, because of the risks of acute renal failure and pulmonary oedema.

BENZODIAZEPINES

Benzodiazepine dependence tends to result from over-prescription. In general, lone benzodiazepine overdoses are remarkably safe and near-full recovery takes place within 24 hours. Polydrug abusers commonly misuse these drugs and difficulties occur when other CNS depressants, such as tricyclic antidepressants, opioids or alcohol, are taken in

9

addition, or when an overdose occurs in susceptible groups such as older people or those with chronic obstructive pulmonary disease. Drowsiness and mid-position or dilated pupils are common and occur within 3 hours of ingestion. Ataxia, dysarthria, nystagmus and confusion also occur. Coma may follow, but in lone benzodiazepine overdose a GCS grade below 10 (p. 1186) is rare. Minor hypotension and respiratory depression may occur. Respiratory arrest is uncommon but can occur after shorter-acting agents such as midazolam.

Gastric lavage is not advised in pure benzodiazepine overdose. Activated charcoal, if required, can be given within 1 hour of the overdose, particularly in a mixed overdose. Impaired consciousness is treated conventionally, with particular attention to maintenance of the airway. Observation should be for at least 6 hours post-ingestion, or for 24 hours in more serious cases. Oxygen saturation monitoring using a pulse oximeter is useful for ascertaining the adequacy of ventilation. Flumazenil is a specific benzodiazepine antagonist but is not used in the vast majority of cases of poisoning with benzodiazepines. Flumazenil must never be used in patients with a history of convulsions or toxin-induced cardiotoxicity, or in those who have co-ingested tricyclic antidepressants, as seizures and ventricular arrhythmias can be precipitated.

CRACK/COCAINE

Cocaine (hydrochloride) is usually purchased as a white crystalline powder or colourless crystals. It may be sniffed into the nose (or snorted using a tube) from which it is rapidly absorbed, or injected intravenously. 'Crack' is cocaine that has been separated from the hydrochloride base (free-base), melted and smoked in a pipe or mixed with tobacco in a cigarette, to give a rapid onset of effect similar to intravenous use. Crack is usually sold in 'rocks' containing 150 mg of cocaine or as a 'line' of cocaine for snorting that contains 20–30 mg of the drug. While the toxic dose is very variable and depends on individual tolerance, the presence of other drugs and the route of administration, ingestion of any amount over 1 g is potentially fatal.

After intranasal use, effects are experienced within minutes and tend to last 20–90 minutes. With intravenous or oral use the peak 'high' occurs within 10 and 45–90 minutes respectively. Smoking crack causes a peak 'high' within 10 minutes. By these routes the effects begin to resolve in about 20 minutes post-onset. In fatal poisoning, the onset and progression of symptoms are accelerated and death may occur in minutes. Survival beyond 3 hours indicates that the patient is unlikely to die.

Mild to moderate intoxication with cocaine causes euphoria, agitation, aggression, cerebellar signs (p. 1179), dilated pupils, vomiting, pallor, headache, cold sweats, twitching, pyrexia, tachycardia, hallucinations and hypertension. Features of severe intoxication include convulsions, coma, muscular paralysis, severe hypertension and stroke. A toxic psychosis occurs with high levels of consumption, and tactile hallucinations (formication) may be prominent. Coronary artery spasm may result in myocardial ischaemia or infarction, even in patients with normal coronary arteries, and this leads to hypotension, cyanosis and ventricular arrhythmias. Cocaine toxicity should be considered in young healthy adults who present with symptoms of ischaemic heart disease. Hyperthermia associated with rhabdomyolysis, acute renal failure and disseminated intravascular coagulation may also occur.

Activated charcoal should be given in any patient presenting within 1 hour of oral ingestion, irrespective of the amount taken. All patients should be observed with ECG monitoring for a minimum of 2 hours, though ECG changes can be misleading in cocaine toxicity. Troponin T estimations are valuable in assessing the degree of myocardial damage. Blood pressure, heart rate and body temperature should also be monitored and the patient observed carefully for the development of specific complications, which should be managed as shown in Box 9.10.

9.10 COMPLICATIONS AND MANAGEMENT OF ACUTE COCAINE INTOXICATION

Complication	Management
Hypertension	Oral diazepam, nifedipine or doxazosin Avoid β-blockers, which cause hypertension due to unopposed alpha stimulation
Hypertension with encephalopathy, infarction, stroke or proteinuria	I.v. nitrates or sodium nitroprusside Avoid β-blockers
Supraventricular tachycardia	I.v. verapamil; avoid β-blockers
Cocaine-induced angina	I.v. or buccal nitrates are treatment of choice; avoid β-blockers
Cocaine-induced myocardial infarction	Thrombolytic agents usually not necessary because mechanism is spasm rather than thrombosis I.v. nitrates Occasionally angiography may be required
Hyperthermia > 39°C	Cool i.v. fluids, dantrolene; paralyse and ventilate if hyperthermia persists despite these measures
Agitation or psychosis	Oral diazepam; avoid phenothiazines and haloperidol, as they lower the threshold for convulsions
Fits	I.v. diazepam (10 mg initial dose)

ECSTASY/AMPHETAMINES

MDMA (3,4-methylenedioxymethamphetamine, ecstasy) is a 'designer' amphetamine, also known as E, Adam, white dove, white burger, or red and black. It is commonly taken in dance clubs because it produces feelings of euphoria and emotional intimacy, and distorted sensory perceptions. Amphetamines and the newer designer amphetamines are virtually indistinguishable in their clinical effects. There is no evidence they are addictive. Effects occur within 1 hour of ingestion and last 4–6 hours following doses of 75–150 mg but up to 48 hours after the ingestion of 100–300 mg. However, tolerance is common, and most regular users need to take considerably higher doses.

Supraventricular and ventricular arrhythmias are common and may cause death. Agitation or drowsiness is also common. Whilst most patients who have taken ecstasy are profoundly dehydrated, a small proportion develop hyponatraemia, usually through drinking excessive amounts of water in the absence of sufficient exertion to sweat it out. Antidiuretic hormone secretion may also contribute to the development of hyponatraemia. Other features of intoxication include nausea, hyper-reflexia, muscle pain, trismus (jaw-clenching), dilated pupils, blurred vision, sweating, dry mouth, agitation, visual hallucinations, paranoid psychosis and anxiety. Severe intoxication is characterised by coma, convulsions, hypertension and cardiac arrhythmias. A hyperthermic (5-HT-like) syndrome may develop with rigidity, hyper-reflexia and hyperpyrexia (> 39°C) leading to hypotension, rhabdomyolysis, metabolic acidosis, acute renal failure, disseminated intravascular coagulation, hepatocellular necrosis, acute respiratory distress syndrome and cardiovascular collapse. In view of this, urea and electrolytes, creatine kinase, blood glucose, a full blood count and liver function tests must be measured, and a 12-lead ECG performed. All symptomatic cases should have ECG, blood pressure and temperature monitoring for at least 6 hours post-exposure. The complications described above should be treated in the same way as for cocaine (Box 9.10). Selective serotonergic antagonists (e.g. cyproheptadine/ketanserin) may become available for use in patients with a 5-HT-like syndrome to reduce temperature and rigidity via central mechanisms.

GAMMAHYDROXYBUTYRATE (GHB)

GHB is marketed illegally for body-building and weight loss and as a replacement for L-tryptophan. Slang terms include liquid X, cherry meth, easy lay, scoop and GBH. It is commonly dissolved in water to produce a clear, colourless liquid that tastes of seaweed. Many misusers simply 'guzzle' it until they reach an adequate high, which is often achieved shortly before becoming unconscious. Owing to the drowsiness that may occur, it is sometimes mixed with amphetamines to prolong the 'high' for several hours. The severity and duration of effects seem to be dose-dependent. Doses of 10–30 mg/kg cause mild effects such as nausea, diarrhoea, confusion, vertigo, tremor, extra-

pyramidal signs, agitation and euphoria, whereas higher doses (30–50 mg/kg) cause drowsiness, coma, bradycardia, hypotension and respiratory depression. More than 50 mg/kg causes decreased cardiac output and increasingly severe respiratory depression, fits and coma. The effects are potentiated by other CNS depressants (e.g. alcohol, benzodiazepines, opioids and neuroleptic drugs). Bizarrely, patients often recover quickly (within 1–2 hours), and self-extubation and rapid reversal of coma are seen. Coma usually resolves spontaneously within 2–4 hours, but may persist as long as 96 hours.

Urea, electrolytes and glucose should be measured in all but the most trivial of cases. Activated charcoal treatment is recommended within 1 hour for ingestion of more than 20 mg/kg. All patients should be observed for a minimum of 2 hours, with monitoring of blood pressure, heart rate, respiratory rate and oxygenation. Patients who remain symptomatic thereafter should be admitted and observed until symptoms resolve, but require supportive care only.

LSD

d-Lysergic acid diethylamide (LSD) is a synthetic hallucinogen. Common slang terms are acid, trips, dots, paper mushrooms or 'L'. LSD is usually ingested as small squares of impregnated absorbent paper, which are often printed with a distinctive design, or as 'microdots'. Perceptual changes occur within 40 minutes of oral ingestion. Vision is affected most often with heightened visual awareness of objects, especially colours. Images may be distorted in shape or size and true hallucinations occur. These may be pleasurable but are sometimes terrifying, the experience then being referred to as a 'bad trip'.

Patients presenting to hospital usually do so because of a 'bad trip', panic reaction, vivid visual hallucinations or aggression, or after a suicide attempt. The individual may be found wandering in a confused, agitated state. Dilated pupils are common. Peak effects are seen within 30–60 minutes of an oral dose. LSD itself is of low acute toxicity; fatalities are a result of the behavioural changes it induces, which lead to accidents such as drowning. Flashbacks can occur within hours or months after acute or chronic misuse and may be precipitated by physical or emotional stress. During these flashbacks, the psychotic effects of LSD are experienced again with their original intensity.

Patients with psychotic reactions or CNS depression should be observed in hospital, in a quiet, dimly lit room to minimise external stimulation. Where sedation is required, diazepam is the drug of choice; haloperidol is used if diazepam is ineffective. The use of chlorpromazine in LSD intoxication has been associated with cardiovascular collapse.

OPIOIDS

These include heroin, morphine, methadone, codeine, pethidine, dihydrocodeine and dextropropoxyphene. They give a rapid, intensely pleasurable experience, often accompanied by heightened sexual arousal. Physical dependence occurs within a few weeks of regular high-dose injection; as a result, the dose is escalated and the addict's life becomes increasingly centred around obtaining and taking the drug. The withdrawal syndrome, which can start within 12 hours, presents with intense craving, rhinorrhoea, lacrimation, yawning, perspiration, shivering, piloerection, vomiting, diarrhoea and abdominal cramps. Examination reveals tachycardia, hypertension, mydriasis and facial flushing.

Accidental overdose is common. The hallmarks of opioid analgesic poisoning are:

- depressed respiration
- pinpoint or small pupils
- depressed conscious level
- signs of intravenous drug misuse (e.g. needle track marks).

Severe poisoning is indicated by respiratory depression, hypotension, non-cardiogenic pulmonary oedema and hypothermia. Death occurs by respiratory arrest or from aspiration of gastric contents. Poisoning with dextropropoxyphene (the opioid component of co-proxamol) may also result in cardiac conduction effects, particularly QRS prolongation, ventricular arrhythmias and heart block. Co-proxamol has been withdrawn in the UK because of an associated excess of deaths due to the dextropropoxyphene moiety in the elderly population and those with chronic obstructive pulmonary disease. Unconscious patients should always have their paracetamol concentration checked because of the wide use of combination opioid/paracetamol drugs. Symptoms of opioid poisoning can be prolonged for up to 48 hours, particularly after ingestion of methadone, which has a long half-life.

The airway should be cleared and, if necessary, respiratory support provided. Supplementary high-flow oxygen should be administered. The need for endotracheal intubation can often be avoided by prompt administration of adequate doses of the opioid antagonist naloxone (see below). Oxygen saturation monitoring and arterial blood gases indicate the adequacy of ventilation in those whose respiration has been compromised. The management of coma (p. 1186), fits (p. 1167) and hypotension (Fig. 9.4, p. 210) is detailed elsewhere. Non-cardiogenic pulmonary oedema in severe cases does not usually respond to diuretic therapy, and continuous positive airways pressure (CPAP) or positive end-expiratory pressure (PEEP) ventilatory support (p. 193) may be required.

Naloxone is a specific opioid antagonist that reverses the above features of opioid toxicity. It should be used as a bolus dose (0.8–2 mg i.v.) in adults, repeated every 2 minutes as necessary until the level of consciousness and respiratory rate increase and the pupils dilate. A total dose of as much as 10–20 mg may be required in some cases. Administration of too much naloxone should be avoided as it can precipitate a withdrawal reaction, characterised by gastrointestinal effects, sweating and fits. It is best to titrate repeat bolus doses, aiming for a GCS of 13–14 (not 15). After the initial i.v. bolus, an infusion of naloxone may be needed because its half-life is much shorter than the half-lives of most opioids. As a guide, two-thirds of the bolus dose initially required to wake the patient should be infused each hour. Patients must be carefully observed for recurrence of coma and respiratory depression, usually for at least 18–24 hours. It is particularly important that patients are observed for recurrence of CNS depression for at least 4–6 hours after the last dose of naloxone is given. Naloxone has been reported to cause pulmonary oedema and ventricular arrhythmias, but these are too infrequent to justify avoiding its use.

MANAGEMENT OF BODYPACKERS

Bodypackers ingest drugs of misuse (particularly cocaine and heroin) wrapped in cling film or packed into condoms for the purpose of drug smuggling. It is important to ask exactly what is in the packets and how they are wrapped, and to obtain an abdominal X-ray to help establish where the packets are located and how many are present (Fig. 9.5). If they are in the stomach, they can be removed endoscopically, taking extreme care not to rupture the packages. Alternatively, they can be allowed to pass through with the help of a laxative such as lactulose. Paraffin-based laxatives should not be used, as these may corrode the packaging material and increase the risk of packet rupture. If packages are in the small or large bowel, either laxatives can be given, or whole bowel irrigation can be performed to aid their speedy excretion (p. 208). Patients should be admitted and observed closely until all packets are recovered. Rupture of the packets can be rapidly fatal because of the large doses carried. Packets carried in the vagina or rectum should be removed manually.

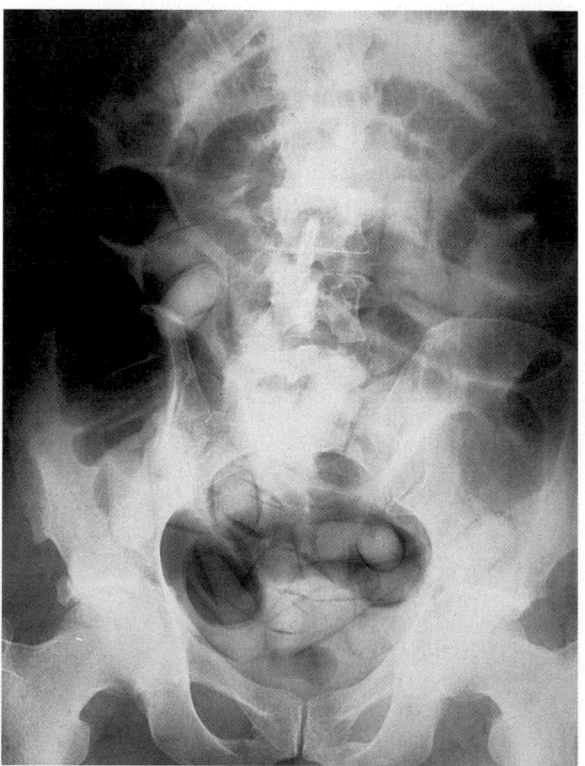

Fig. 9.5 Abdominal X-ray of a bodypacker showing multiple drug-filled condoms.

9

CHEMICALS AND PESTICIDES

CARBON MONOXIDE AND SMOKE

Carbon monoxide (CO) is a major cause of death by poisoning, and is particularly dangerous because it is colourless, non-irritant and odourless. It is produced by the incomplete combustion of organic substances particularly in homes by gas cookers and certain types of heating system which burn natural gas, wood, coal or paraffin, and in vehicle exhaust fumes. The risk of poisoning is greatest where ventilation is poor. CO binds to haemoglobin to form carboxyhaemoglobin (COHb), reducing the oxygen-carrying capacity of the blood. It also acts as a chemical asphyxiant as it impairs the function of cytochrome oxidases and thus utilisation of oxygen by tissues.

The early clinical features of acute severe carbon monoxide poisoning are headache, nausea and vomiting, ataxia and nystagmus, drowsiness, hyperventilation, hyper-reflexia and shivering. Later features incude lethargy, coma, convulsions, hypotension, respiratory depression, cardio-vascular collapse and death. Some patients are disinhibited, agitated or aggressive rather than drowsy. ECG abnormalities (ST segment depression, T-wave abnormalities, ventricular tachycardia or ventricular fibrillation) are often seen. Cerebral oedema is common and cerebellar signs, hyper-reflexia or extensor plantars can be present. CO-induced rhabdomyolysis leading to myoglobinuria and renal failure has been reported. Low-level CO poisoning may exacerbate angina and produce subtle neurobehavioural deficits, with the ability to sustain attention or performance most sensitive to disruption. Poisoning during pregnancy is likely to cause miscarriage or premature labour due to fetal hypoxia.

Patients recovering from CO poisoning may suffer neurological sequelae including tremor, personality changes, memory impairment, loss of visual acuity, inability to concentrate and Parkinsonian features. Chronic 'low-level' CO poisoning causes symptoms difficult to distinguish from influenza, such as nausea, vomiting, headache, lethargy, and aches and pains.

The COHb concentration is of value in confirming exposure to CO, although it may not be elevated sufficiently to be diagnostic in chronic cases. Normal values are up to 3–5% and can be as high as 6–10% in smokers. However, the COHb concentration measured in hospital does not correlate well with the severity of poisoning, even acutely, because blood COHb concentrations fall rapidly on cessation of exposure and following oxygen therapy during ambulance transfer to hospital. An ECG should be performed in all those with acute poisoning, especially in patients with pre-existing heart disease. Arterial blood gas analysis should be performed in all those with serious poisoning. Oxygen saturation readings by pulse oximetry are misleading, as this measures both COHb and oxyhaemoglobin.

The first step in treating CO poisoning is to remove the patient from the source of exposure. The airway, breathing and circulation must be adequately maintained and oxygen

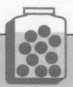

9.11 INDICATIONS FOR CONSIDERING HYPERBARIC OXYGEN THERAPY IN CARBON MONOXIDE POISONING

- Focal neurological signs, especially cerebellar ones
- COHb concentration > 40% at any time
- Patient is pregnant
- Patient is unconscious at any time

given as soon as possible. The half-life of COHb whilst breathing air ranges from 4 to 6 hours. On 100% oxygen at ambient pressure, the half-life of COHb is reduced to approximately 40 minutes. Thus, high-flow oxygen should be given, e.g. 12 litres per minute, ideally through a tightly fitting facemask such as those used for CPAP. It should be continued until the COHb is less than 5% and for at least 6 hours after exposure. Sometimes this takes 12–20 hours. Intravenous $NaHCO_3$ should be avoided, as it impairs oxygen release to tissues. Excessive intravenous fluid administration should also be avoided, particularly in the elderly, because of the risk of pulmonary oedema. Convulsions are controlled with diazepam. Most deaths occur in those who have arrested at the scene or who are unconscious on arrival in hospital.

The use of hyperbaric oxygen is controversial; Box 9.11 lists the current indications for its consideration. In theory, at 2.5 atmospheres, it reduces the half-life of COHb to 20 minutes and increases the amount of dissolved oxygen by a factor of 10. The logistical difficulties of transporting sick patients to hyperbaric chambers should not be under-estimated.

ORGANOPHOSPHORUS INSECTICIDES/ NERVE AGENTS

Organophosphorus (OP) compounds are widely used as pesticides in agriculture, for eradication of vectors of malaria and filariasis, and as chemical warfare agents (Box 9.12). OP pesticide intoxications are estimated at 3 million per year worldwide with approximately 300 000 deaths. The fatality rate following deliberate ingestion of OP pesticides in developing countries in Asia is approximately 20% and may reach 70% during certain seasons and at rural hospitals.

OP nerve agents are used in chemical warfare. G agents are absorbed by inhalation or percutaneously; they are volatile and disappear rapidly after use. V agents are contact

9.12 ORGANOPHOSPHORUS COMPOUNDS

Nerve agents	
• G agents: sarin, tabun, soman	• V agents: VX, VE

Insecticides	
Dimethyl compounds	**Diethyl compounds**
• Dichlorvos	• Chlorpyrifos
• Fenthion	• Diazinon
• Malathion	• Parathion-ethyl
• Methamidophos	• Quinalphos

poisons unless aerosolised, and contaminate ground for weeks or months. They are related to OP pesticides but have much higher acute toxicity, particularly percutaneously. The toxicology and management of nerve agent and pesticide poisoning are similar.

Mechanism of toxicity

OPs inactivate acetylcholinesterase (AChE) by phosphorylation leading to the accumulation of acetylcholine (ACh) at cholinergic synapses (Fig. 9.6). Recovery follows the reappearance of active AChE following synthesis or spontaneous hydrolysis of phosphorylated AChE. The phosphorylated AChE may lose a chemical group so that its inactivation becomes irreversible; this is known as 'ageing'. The rate of ageing differs and is more rapid with dimethyl compounds (3.7 hours) than diethyl compounds (31 hours) (Box 9.12). Nerve agents (especially soman) cause ageing within minutes.

Sequential triphasic illness follows OP intoxication (Fig. 9.6):

- acute cholinergic phase
- intermediate syndrome (IMS)
- organophosphate-induced delayed polyneuropathy (OPIDN).

Several disorders reported following OP poisoning cannot be attributed to inhibition of AChE alone. The consequences of inhibition of other enzyme systems by OPs are as yet uncertain.

Clinical features

The onset, severity and duration of poisoning depend on the route of exposure and agent involved.

Acute cholinergic syndrome

The acute cholinergic syndrome may occur within minutes of exposure, usually within one hour. Sulphurated OPs have a characteristic pungent garlic-like odour which can be detected in the breath, vomit and/or clothing. The pathognomonic features are miosis and muscle fasciculation, but these may not be obvious in children. Other muscarinic and nicotinic features are shown in Figure 9.7. Bradycardia would be predicted from the mechanism of action, but tachycardia occurs in 20% of cases. Central nervous dysfunction is often the presenting feature in the very young.

Flaccid paralysis of limb, respiratory and sometimes extra-ocular muscles may follow. Central depression of the respiratory centre, copious secretions, bronchoconstriction and muscle paralysis contribute to respiratory failure. Unconsciousness and convulsions may occur early. The acute cholinergic phase usually lasts 48–72 hours, with most patients requiring intensive cardiorespiratory support and monitoring.

Nerve agents cause eye pain and conjunctival injection, and the eyes may take on a glassy 'marble' appearance. A relative absence of lacrimation has been reported. The onset of miosis is rapid. A transient tachycardia occurs in the majority. Sublethal doses can markedly degrade performance of complex tasks and this may be prolonged.

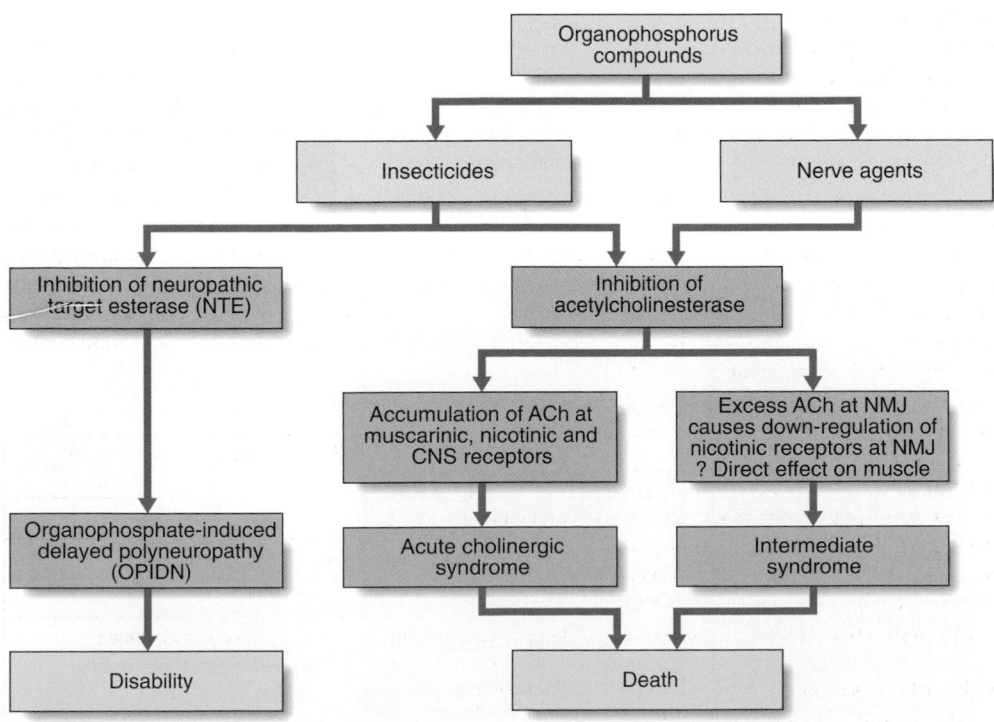

Fig. 9.6 **Mechanism of action of organophosphorus compounds.** (ACh = acetycholine; NMJ = neuromuscular junction)

Parkinsonian features, pancreatitis, transient hepatic dysfunction, vocal cord paralysis and pyrexia may occur before the onset or during treatment of IMS (see below). A profuse offensive diarrhoea follows oral ingestion and may lead to fluid and electrolyte imbalance. There have been isolated reports of myocardial sequelae (arrhythmias and cardiomyopathy), alterations of the immune system and neuropsychological disturbances, but these are extremely rare. Early deaths from OP pesticide self-poisoning result from respiratory failure and cardiovascular collapse.

The intermediate syndrome (IMS)

This begins 48 hours after poisoning in approximately 20% of patients, but may be delayed for 72–96 hours. It follows the resolution of the acute phase, although in some instances it occurs whilst some of the symptoms of the acute phase are still present. Muscle weakness causing respiratory distress and failure (without accompanying muscarinic signs such as salivation) are the cardinal features, attributed to receptor dysfunction at the neuromuscular junction.

The onset of the IMS is often rapid, with progression of muscle weakness from the ocular muscles to the neck (the patient cannot raise their head from the pillow) and proximal limbs, to the respiratory muscles (intercostals and diaphragm) over the course of 24 hours. Increasing respiratory difficulty causes anxiety, sweating and use of accessory muscles of respiration. If endotracheal intubation and ventilation are not instituted early, cyanosis, coma and death follow rapidly. Paralysis may continue for 2–18 days. Unless OPIDN develops, recovery from IMS is complete with adequate ventilatory care.

Organophosphate-induced delayed polyneuropathy (OPIDN)

This occurs about 1–3 weeks after acute exposure and an uncertain period following chronic exposure, due to degeneration of long myelinated nerve fibres. A distinct acute or intermediate phase may not always precede its development. Cramping muscle pains in the legs are followed by numbness and paraesthesiae in the distal upper and lower limbs. Acute weakness of the lower limbs follows and spreads to the hands, causing a shuffling gait, and foot- and wrist-drop. Muscle wasting and deformity, such as clawing of the hands, follow. Sensory loss is variable and is often mild and inconspicuous. Physical examination reveals symmetrical flaccid weakness of the distal muscles, especially in the legs. The dominant hand may be more affected. Tendon reflexes are reduced or lost, absent ankle reflexes being a constant feature. Later, mild pyramidal tract signs (spasticity, hypertonicity, hyper-reflexia and clonus) may develop.

Recovery from OPIDN is incomplete and may be limited to the hands and feet, although substantial functional recovery after 1–2 years may occur in younger patients. Dichlorvos and nerve agents are not associated with OPIDN.

Management (Fig. 9.7)

Cholinesterase (ChE) estimations (plasma butyryl cholinesterase and red cell AChE) are the only useful biochemical tool for confirming exposure to OPs, but are a poor guide to management and prognosis. There is approximate correlation between ChE activity and clinical effects: ~50%

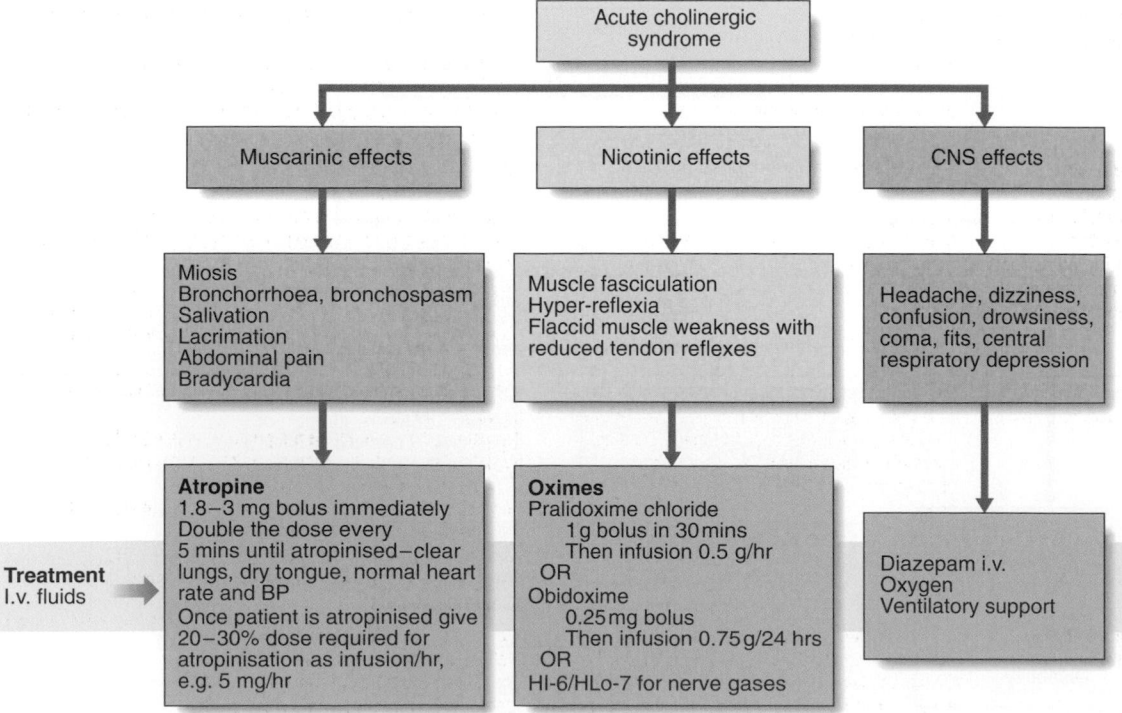

Fig. 9.7 Management of poisoning with organophosphorus compounds.

activity in subclinical poisoning, 20–50% in mild poisoning and less than 10% in severe poisoning. In occupational exposure, pre-exposure values are important to protect workers from toxicity, but are obviously not available in cases of deliberate self-poisoning.

Acute cholinergic syndrome

Further contamination is prevented by removal from the site of exposure and of contaminated clothing and contact lenses. The airway is cleared and high-flow oxygen administered. Direct mouth-to-mouth/nose resuscitation must be avoided. Contaminated clothing and contact lenses should be double-bagged, the skin washed with soap and water, and the eyes irrigated. Following ingestion, gastric lavage may be undertaken within an hour of intake, followed by activated charcoal via nasogastric tube, after establishing

intravenous access and airway protection. Convulsions are controlled with intravenous diazepam. Monitoring of ECG, blood gases, temperature, urea and electrolytes, amylase and glucose is mandatory. Severe cases should be managed in an intensive care unit, and may require supported ventilation.

Complete and early atropinisation is essential in early management. Speed of administration is as important as use of sufficient doses (Fig. 9.7). Atropine reverses ACh-induced bronchospasm, bronchorrhoea, bradycardia and hypotension and, as it crosses the blood–brain barrier, may also have therapeutic effects within the CNS. Excess atropine causes agitation, confusion, urinary retention, ileus, hyperthermia and tachycardia. Hyperthermia is a serious complication in hot wards but may be controlled by restricting the amount of atropine given to a minimum, active cooling, and sedation to reduce muscle activity.

9

9.13 CHEMICALS TAKEN LESS COMMONLY IN OVERDOSE		
Toxin	**Clinical features**	**Management**
Acids and alkalis, i.e. corrosives	Acid injures stomach but alkali injures oesophagus; aspiration causes pneumonitis Serious GI injury can result Later, strictures or malignant transformation can occur	Gastric lavage contraindicated Do not give neutralising chemicals Chest X-ray needed to exclude perforation Early endoscopy or Gastrografin studies to assess extent of damage and need for surgery
Button batteries containing lithium or mercury	Obstruction, corrosion of GI tract Heavy metal toxicity	Abdominal X-ray will locate position Remove endoscopically if battery not passed from stomach into small bowel within 24 hours
Bleach	Irritation around mouth Serious GI corrosion if deliberate ingestion of a large amount	Milk if small amounts ingested, e.g. accidental mouthful by a child Endoscopy for adults as per acid (see above)
Essential oils, e.g. clove oil	Fits and hepatotoxicity	Gastric lavage if even a few ml have been taken by a child
Ethanol, e.g. alcoholic drinks, mouthwashes, antiseptics, perfumes	Fatal dose of absolute ethanol is 6–10 ml/kg body weight in adults Blood alcohol concentrations of > 5 g/l associated with coma Convulsions, hypotension, respiratory depression and/or circulatory failure	Check blood alcohol concentration Protect airway to prevent aspiration; intubation and ventilation may be required Ensure adequate hydration; in a chronic alcoholic, give i.v. thiamine (Pabrinex) before dextrose Consider haemodialysis if blood ethanol concentration is > 5 g/l or arterial H^+ > 100 (pH < 7)
Lead, e.g. chronic occupational exposure, leaded paint, water contaminated by lead pipes, use of kohl cosmetics	Gastrointestinal: colicky abdominal pain Haematological: microcytic anaemia, basophilic stippling Neurological: encephalopathy, headache, motor neuropathy Nephrotoxicity Hypertension Hypocalcaemia	Check blood lead concentration Full blood count and blood film Urea and electrolytes, liver function tests, calcium Abdominal X-ray for children to detect pica; long bone X-ray for children for 'lead lines' Remove the patient from the source of lead poisoning Chelation therapy for blood lead concentrations > 450 µg/l: DMSA (2,3 dimercaptosuccinic acid). Seek poisons centre advice
Methanol or ethylene glycol, e.g. antifreeze	Methanol metabolised to formate, causing profound metabolic acidosis and ocular toxicity Ethylene glycol metabolised to acids, causing metabolic acidosis; oxalate causes renal damage due to calcium oxalate crystals in urine	Ethylene glycol and methanol assays not widely available as an urgent assay Diagnosed by presence of a high anion gap, osmolal gap (> 10 mOsm) and presence of oxalate crystals in urine (in 50% of cases ethylene glycol) Antidotes oral ethanol, i.v. ethanol or i.v. 4-methylpyrazole (non-sedating): inhibit alcohol dehydrogenase Haemodialysis should be considered in severe cases, especially if methanol or ethylene glycol concentration in blood is > 500 mg/l
Petroleum distillates, white spirit, kerosene	Vomiting common; aspiration results in severe pulmonary complications (cough, choking, wheeze, dyspnoea); peak in 24 hrs and settle 3–4 days later In more severe cases chemical pneumonitis or lipoid pneumonia can develop; deaths have occurred	Gastric lavage contraindicated Activated charcoal ineffective Oxygen and nebulised bronchodilators Chest X-ray to assess pulmonary effects

9.14 PESTICIDES TAKEN LESS COMMONLY IN OVERDOSE		
Toxin	**Clinical features**	**Management**
Paraquat	Buccal ulceration Progressive respiratory fibrosis Respiratory failure Renal failure	Multiple doses of activated charcoal if urine screen test is positive Check blood paraquat concentration; if above survival curve, patient will probably die, as no measures are effective
Organochlorines	Clinical effects begin within minutes to hours Nausea, vomiting, agitation, fasciculations, paraesthesiae of the face and extremities Severe: seizures, coma, respiratory depression and death; ventricular irritability or dysrhythmias Complications include hyperthermia, rhabdomyolysis, pulmonary oedema, disseminated intravascular coagulation	Nasogastric aspiration may be useful if a liquid preparation has been taken Activated charcoal is given within 1 hour of ingestion Seizures should be treated with benzodiazepines Patients should be kept on a cardiac monitor
Pyrethroid insecticides	Contact dermatitis, skin paraesthesiae or a stinging or burning sensation—may last for 12–18 hours Spills on the face and eyes cause pain, lacrimation, photophobia and oedema of the eyelids Allergic reactions documented Inhalation causes dyspnoea, nausea, headaches Ingestion causes epigastric pain, nausea, vomiting, headache, coma, convulsions, pulmonary oedema	Symptomatic and supportive care Washing the skin makes irritation worse
Superwarfarins (warfarin-like rodenticides), e.g. brodifacoum, bromodialone	Increased risk of bleeding, e.g. haemoptysis, haematuria, epistaxis, GI haemorrhage—may be delayed, even weeks after ingestion	Monitor INR/prothrombin ratio If greater than twice normal give vitamin K1 (0.25 g/kg) by slow i.v. injection In severe bleeding, a transfusion of fresh frozen plasma or specific clotting factors may be necessary

Urinary retention should be excluded in those who become agitated and confused.

When the diagnosis of OP poisoning is uncertain, administration of a 'test dose' of atropine 1 mg i.v. is helpful. A marked increase in heart rate (> 20–25 bpm) and skin flushing eliminates the possibility of significant cholinergic poisoning.

The role of the oximes, which reactivate phosphorylated AChE, is contentious and dosage and duration of therapy are uncertain. Oximes are of more benefit with OPs which age slowly. Their benefit in excess of 24–48 hours after nerve agent poisoning is uncertain. Regimes for pralidoxime and obidoxime are shown in Figure 9.7. If administered too rapidly, severe hypotension may occur. A response should be seen within 30 minutes, with resolution of fasciculation, convulsions, muscle weakness and coma.

Cost and lack of availability restrict the use of oximes in developing countries, and there is an urgent need for realistic guidelines and more reliable antidotes.

IMS

Ventilatory support should be instituted before a patient develops respiratory failure to maintain a PaO_2 > 13 kPa (97 mmHg), $PaCO_2$ of 4–6 kPa (30–45 mmHg) and H^+ < 50 (pH > 7.3) (p. 191). Diazepam or midazolam may be used for sedation during ventilation. Weaning from respiratory support should be initiated by changing to pressure support, starting with approximately 20 cm water and a positive end-expiratory pressure of 10 cm water. Parenteral nutrition is often required.

OPIDN

There are no specific therapeutic measures. Regular physiotherapy may reduce deformity caused by muscle-wasting.

CARBAMATE INSECTICIDES

Carbamate insecticides (e.g. aldicarb, carbofuran, methomyl) inhibit a number of tissue esterases, especially AChE. The mechanism of action, clinical features and management are similar to those of OP compounds. However, clinical features are less severe and duration of toxicity is shorter, as the carbamate/ChE complex dissociates quickly with a half-life of 30–40 minutes and does not undergo ageing. Deaths have, however, occurred and pancreatitis has been reported as a sequel.

Atropine may be given intravenously in frequent small doses (0.5–1.0 mg i.v. for an adult) until signs of atropinisation develop. Diazepam may be used to relieve anxiety. The use of oximes is unnecessary and may be detrimental.

ALUMINIUM AND ZINC PHOSPHIDE

These rat poisons have recently become a common means of self-poisoning in northern India, with a mortality rate of 60%. When ingested, both compounds react with water in the stomach to yield phosphine—a potent pulmonary toxicant which causes severe burning retrosternal pain and

9

vomiting followed by profound hypotension. Subjects become restless, tachypnoeic, hypotensive and oliguric or anuric. Even a few tablets can be fatal. Both hypomagnesaemia and hypermagnesaemia have been reported, as have hepatic toxicity and myocarditis. Detecting phosphine in the exhaled air or stomach aspirate using either a silver nitrate-impregnated strip or specific phosphine detector tube is diagnostic, but gas chromatography provides the most sensitive indicator. Supportive therapy remains the only available form of management as there is no specific antidote. Many physicians undertake gastric lavage with vegetable oil to reduce the release of toxic phosphine. If hypomagnesaemia is present, magnesium sulphate (10 mmol i.v. bolus) has been reported to decrease the incidence of cardiac arrhythmias. Most patients die despite optimal supportive care.

CHEMICALS AND PESTICIDES LESS COMMONLY TAKEN IN OVERDOSE

Boxes 9.13 and 9.14 give an overview of the clinical features and management for other chemicals and pesticides.

ENVENOMING

SNAKE BITES

Snake bite is a common life-threatening condition in many tropical countries; farmers, hunters and rice-pickers are at particular risk and prompt medical treatment is vital. The virtually global presence of venomous snakes explains the worldwide estimates of 3–5 million victims per year, with nearly 50 000 deaths and a staggering 400 000 amputations. As many as 40% of bites inflicted by venomous snakes do not produce signs of envenoming. As it is difficult to predict which bites will produce symptoms or the clinical outcome, all victims of snake bite should be brought under medical care as quickly as possible.

Poisonous species of snake fall into the families shown in Box 9.15.

Snake venoms are complex mixtures of proteins and small polypeptides with enzymatic activity (Fig. 9.8). The classification of snake venoms into neurotoxins, haematotoxins (haemorrhagic or coagulopathic) or cardiotoxins is toxicologically misleading, as these effects often occur in combination, and pure neurotoxicity, coagulopathy or myotoxicity is rare. A snake venom is capable of producing changes concomitantly in one or more systems of the body. Further, within a snake family, qualitative or quantitative differences in the chemistry of venoms occur at species level. Such differences may also occur within a species, depending on geographic area. For example, the venom composition and clinical manifestations of a Russell's viper (*Daboia russellii*) bite in eastern parts of India differ significantly from those in western parts of India.

Clinical features and assessment

Key questions to ask a victim are:

- Where on the body were you bitten?
- How long ago?
- By what sort of snake?

Friends and relatives will frequently bring the snake with the patient; it should be handled as little as possible since it may only be injured rather than dead. The amount of venom

9.15 VENOMOUS SNAKES AND ANTIVENINS		
Snake family	**Location**	**Antivenin**
Atractaspididae e.g. Burrowing asps, stiletto snakes, Natal black snake	Africa (from South Africa to Israel)	No specific antivenin. Treat symptomatically, e.g. coronary vasoconstriction, atrioventricular conduction abnormalities
Colubridae e.g. Boomslang, Australian brown tree snake	Africa, Australia	Brown snake antivenin (CSL Australia)
Viperidae e.g. Russell's viper, European adder Subfamily: **Crotalidae** e.g. Pit vipers, rattlesnakes, moccasins	South and South-east Asia, Europe (Old World) Absent in America and Australia North and South America, South Asia Absent in Australia and Africa	Vipera Tab (European viper antivenom) Polyvalent Haffkine antivenin (India) Vins polyvalent antivenin (Sri Lanka) Crotalidae polyvalent antivenin—Wyeth antivenin (equine) CroFab-Protherics Crotalidae polyvalent immune Fab (ovine)
Elapidae e.g. Cobras, coral snakes, krait (*Bungarus*), mambas, Australian snakes	Australia, South and South-east Asia, United States, Africa	Multivalent coral snake antivenin (Costa Rica) SAMIR polyvalent antivenin (South Africa) Polyvalent (CSL) elapid antivenin (Australia) Polyvalent Haffkine antivenin (India, Sri Lanka) Thai Red Cross cobra antivenin (Thailand)
Hydrophiidae e.g. Sea snakes—*Enhydrina schistosa*	Indo-Pacific region, Australia, South-east Asia All warmer seas except the Atlantic	CSL sea snake antivenin CSL tiger snake antivenin

9

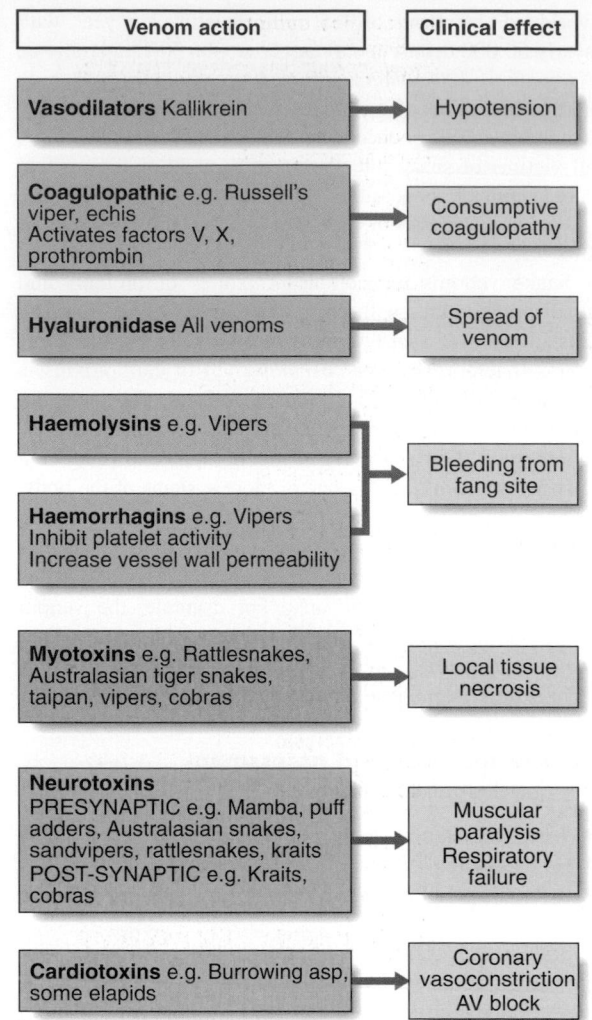

Venom action	Clinical effect
Vasodilators Kallikrein	Hypotension
Coagulopathic e.g. Russell's viper, echis Activates factors V, X, prothrombin	Consumptive coagulopathy
Hyaluronidase All venoms	Spread of venom
Haemolysins e.g. Vipers	Bleeding from fang site
Haemorrhagins e.g. Vipers Inhibit platelet activity Increase vessel wall permeability	
Myotoxins e.g. Rattlesnakes, Australasian tiger snakes, taipan, vipers, cobras	Local tissue necrosis
Neurotoxins PRESYNAPTIC e.g. Mamba, puff adders, Australasian snakes, sandvipers, rattlesnakes, kraits POST-SYNAPTIC e.g. Kraits, cobras	Muscular paralysis Respiratory failure
Cardiotoxins e.g. Burrowing asp, some elapids	Coronary vasoconstriction AV block

Fig. 9.8 Snake venoms and mechanisms of toxicity. Blue boxes indicate enzymatic proteins, while red boxes indicate non-enzymatic proteins. Myotoxins may be either.

injected via a bite is highly variable, depending on the length of time since the snake last ate and on its aggression. The pattern of clinical features is shown in Figure 9.9.

Snake venom detection kits are available in some countries. The venom is detected from a dry swab of the bite site using monoclonal antibody techniques. The 20-minute whole blood-clotting test is a useful bedside tool in remote areas; a 2–3 ml sample of venous blood from the victim is left undisturbed at ambient temperature for at least 20 minutes. The vessel containing the blood is then tipped once and may be compared with a normal control. If it has not clotted, there is haemostatic disturbance from systemic envenoming. All patients should have a full blood count, urea and electrolytes, liver function tests, creatine kinase, troponins and an ECG performed.

Management

First-aid measures include reassuring the patient, immobilising the bitten area to minimise venom spread, and identifying the snake. Application of a firm bandage to occlude lymphatic drainage is appropriate, but tourniquets are unhelpful since they do not prevent the spread of venom and are frequently applied incorrectly. Incisions at the bite site and attempts to suck out the venom by mouth should not be made. A large-bore intravenous cannula should be inserted on an unaffected limb. Blood pressure, coagulation, and renal, neurological and cardiorespiratory status must be monitored, as hypotension, anaphylactic shock, renal failure and respiratory distress may all develop rapidly. All patients with suspected envenoming should be observed for 12–24 hours, as the initial manifestations may be delayed, especially with elapid bites. Pain and vomiting should be managed symptomatically. Aspirin should not be used for analgesia since this may aggravate bleeding. In severe coagulopathy with thrombocytopenia causing disseminated intravascular coagulation, large quantities of fresh frozen plasma, cryoprecipitate and platelets are required if the response to antivenin is poor.

The most appropriate therapy for envenoming is timely administration of the species-appropriate antivenin (Box 9.15); indications are given in Box 9.16. Before starting antivenin therapy, enquiry must be made as to any history of allergy and an intradermal sensitivity test performed by injecting 0.02 ml of saline-diluted antiserum at a site distant from the bite. The injection site is then observed for at least 10 minutes for the development of redness, hives, pruritus or other adverse effects. In general, the shorter the interval between injection and reaction, the greater the degree of sensitivity. A syringe containing 0.5 ml 1:1000 adrenaline (epinephrine) must be available whenever antivenin is administered. Unfortunately, a negative skin test does not rule out a reaction following administration of the full antivenin dose. The rate of administration of antivenin should be based on the severity of the case and the patient's tolerance to the antivenin. The entire initial dose should be given as soon as possible and preferably within 4 hours of the bite. In severe envenoming, however, antivenin given up to 24 hours after the bite has been shown to reverse coagulation deficits.

There are three types of antivenin reaction: early anaphylactoid, pyrogenic or late (Ch. 4). If an immediate anaphylactoid reaction occurs, administration of antivenin should be immediately discontinued and the patient given an oral antihistamine or intramuscular adrenaline (epinephrine; 0.5 ml of 1:1000) as appropriate. Infusion of the antivenin can be restarted, but at a slower rate. Corticosteroids are commonly given to treat serum sickness, although their value remains to be established. Bites by large snakes may

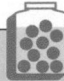

9.16 INDICATIONS FOR ANTIVENIN ADMINISTRATION IN SNAKE BITES

- Cardiogenic shock
- Spontaneous systemic bleeding
- Incoagulable blood
- Neurotoxicity
- Haematuria
- Other evidence of haemolysis/rhabdomyolysis
- Rapidly progressive extensive local swelling
- Bites on digits by snakes with known necrotic venoms

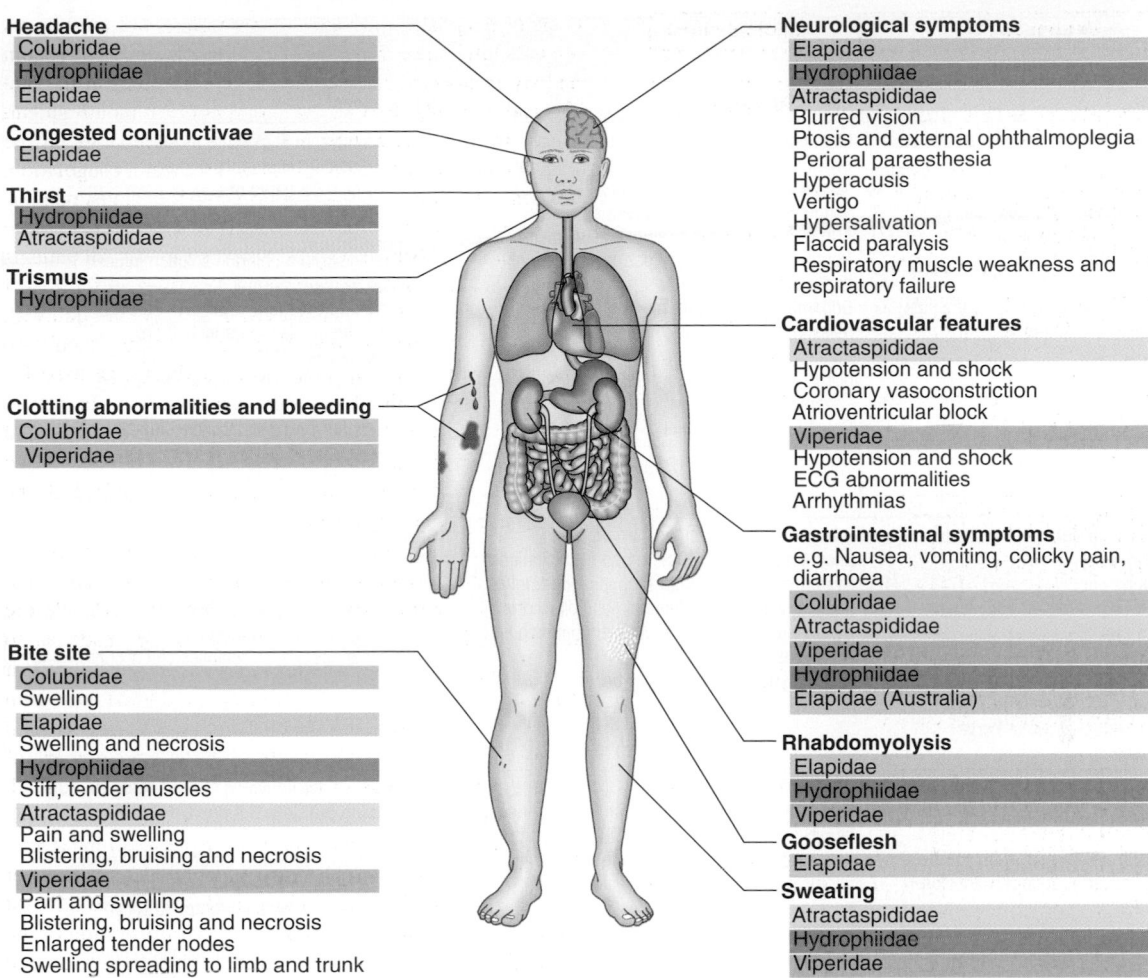

Headache
Colubridae
Hydrophiidae
Elapidae

Congested conjunctivae
Elapidae

Thirst
Hydrophiidae
Atractaspididae

Trismus
Hydrophiidae

Clotting abnormalities and bleeding
Colubridae
Viperidae

Bite site
Colubridae
Swelling
Elapidae
Swelling and necrosis
Hydrophiidae
Stiff, tender muscles
Atractaspididae
Pain and swelling
Blistering, bruising and necrosis
Viperidae
Pain and swelling
Blistering, bruising and necrosis
Enlarged tender nodes
Swelling spreading to limb and trunk

Neurological symptoms
Elapidae
Hydrophiidae
Atractaspididae
Blurred vision
Ptosis and external ophthalmoplegia
Perioral paraesthesia
Hyperacusis
Vertigo
Hypersalivation
Flaccid paralysis
Respiratory muscle weakness and
respiratory failure

Cardiovascular features
Atractaspididae
Hypotension and shock
Coronary vasoconstriction
Atrioventricular block
Viperidae
Hypotension and shock
ECG abnormalities
Arrhythmias

Gastrointestinal symptoms
e.g. Nausea, vomiting, colicky pain,
diarrhoea
Colubridae
Atractaspididae
Viperidae
Hydrophiidae
Elapidae (Australia)

Rhabdomyolysis
Elapidae
Hydrophiidae
Viperidae

Gooseflesh
Elapidae

Sweating
Atractaspididae
Hydrophiidae
Viperidae

Fig. 9.9 Clinical features of snake bite.

need relatively high antivenin doses, particularly in children or small adults. Additional antivenin (e.g. the contents of 1–5 vials) should be administered if swelling progresses or if systemic features of envenoming increase in severity and new manifestations such as hypotension or reduced haematocrit appear. The use of ancillary drugs, such as anticholinesterases for neurotoxic envenoming, remains contentious.

If pulses are lost in a bitten limb, compartment syndrome should be suspected and surgical assessment requested. Wound débridement and later skin grafting are occasionally required, especially in cobra and viper bites, but should never be carried out until the coagulation profile is normal. Awareness and avoidance of the habitat of snakes are the major means of preventing snakebite.

SPIDER BITES

Approximately 35 000 species of spider, ranging in size from 1 mm to over 10 cm, are found world-wide and in all habitats. Although nearly all spiders are venomous and bite, most species are not associated with severe envenoming. Factors affecting the clinical features of a spider bite include the species, size, maturity and sex of the spider, the quantity of venom injected, the bacterial flora on the mouthparts, and the number and duration of bites. For the victim, the severity of envenoming depends on age and pre-existing health, and on the size and site of the bite.

Most spiders associated with significant envenoming belong to the *Atrax*, *Hadronyche*, *Latrodectus*, *Loxosceles* and *Phoneutria* species. The important features of these spiders and management of envenoming are presented in Box 9.17.

The majority of spider bites cause only minor effects, but any spider bite may cause local swelling, pain, erythema and pruritus. There may be a local tissue reaction varying from formation of a weal to a vesicle, which may ulcerate. The tarantulas or 'bird-eating spiders' (*Theraphosid*) usually cause only local pain. Local lymphadenopathy may occur. Occasionally spider hairs, spider secretions or even their webs may produce allergic reactions in sensitised individuals. Some species possess irritating hairs which may be a particular problem in the eye. The term 'necrotic arachnidism' refers to any tissue injury which occurs following a spider bite. For local pain, opioids may be used along with local measures such as ice packs. Local anaesthetic infiltration or regional local anaesthetic blocks

9.17 SPIDER BITES

Spider	Clinical reaction	Management
Black widow spider (Lactrodectus mactans) USA and Australia Jet-black body with red hour-glass mark on underside of abdomen Venom (alpha-latrotoxin): opens ion channels with release of ACh, noradrenaline, dopamine, glutamate; destabilises membranes	Most bites painless with little or no local reaction Onset of symptoms in 15 mins–1 hr: generalised severe pain in back or abdomen, with rigid abdominal muscles and severe cramps ACh excess: salivation, sweating, vomiting Noradrenaline excess: hypertension, tachycardia, arrhythmias Dopamine and glutamate excess: hallucinations, delirium, hysteria Periorbital oedema, skin rash and pyrexia may occur, as may respiratory muscle paralysis and cardiovascular collapse Coma in severe poisoning	Specific antivenin is given to those who have heart disease or respiratory distress, are pregnant, are < 16 or > 65 years of age, or have signs of envenoming or serious poisoning 1 vial of antivenin added to 15–100 ml of 0.9% (w/v) sodium chloride solution infused over 20–30 mins; normal dose is 1–2 vials. Dramatic improvement within 10–20 mins; most symptoms disappear in 1–2 hrs. May also be given i.m. to good effect Oxygen, i.v. access and cardiac monitoring indicated in symptomatic patients Oral diazepam may help muscle cramps Calcium gluconate (10%, 10 ml i.v.) has been recommended for pain relief Monitor patients with severe pain for at least 24 hrs
Funnel-web spider (Atrax and Hadronyche) Australia Dark brown to black; body length 15–45 mm Venom (robustoxin): neurotoxin that causes 'autonomic storm'— widespread release of ACh and noradrenaline at motor nerve synapses	Bite very painful with local erythema, piloerection, local sweating and fasciculations Systemic reactions: salivation, perioral tingling, nausea, vomiting, abdominal pain, diarrhoea, dyspnoea and signs of pulmonary oedema, hypertension and coma Acute myocardial injury may occur	Specific antivenin: minimum dose is 2 ampoules (diluted in 0.9% saline) i.v. but 4 or more ampoules may be required Patients should be closely observed for at least 12 hrs in minor envenoming and longer if antivenin is needed, as relapses can occur
Brown recluse spider (Loxosceles reclusa) USA Yellow to dark brown, with dark, violin-shaped markings immediately behind eye Venom induces injury to arteries and veins, which become occluded with thrombus and capillary stasis; tissue infarction results. Local necrosis has been attributed to sphingomyelinase D (also known as phospholipase D)	Painless bite, often missed Pain may develop in 6 hrs, with local erythema: bluish-grey or purple macule surrounded by pale halo, haemorrhagic bleb followed by necrosis which dries in 7 days. Ulcerating wound heals very slowly Systemic reactions (rare but particularly in children; may be delayed for 72–96 hrs): nausea, vomiting, pyrexia, weakness, chills, headache, joint pains. Severe intravascular haemolysis associated with thrombocytopenia, haemoglobinuria and haematuria may lead to renal failure in 24–72 hrs Deaths are due to circulatory or renal failure	Polyvalent spider antivenin is used in severe envenoming but does not prevent development of skin lesions Dapsone used early may be effective at reducing necrosis. Hyperbaric oxygen is still under investigation as possible therapy to speed healing of bite wound Monitoring of renal function, full blood count Maintenance of hydration to prevent haemoglobinuria. Renal failure is treated by haemodialysis Haemolysis is treated with blood transfusion
Redback spider (Lactrodectus hasselti) Urban habitats in Australia Black/brown with orange/red stripe on upper abdomen Venom: neurotoxin causing release and subsequent depletion of neurotransmitters	Painful bites so spider is recognised at the time. Local erythema, sweating and swelling Pain progresses to entire limb and may become generalised Nausea, vomiting, hypertension, headache, fever, arthralgia	Ice pack for local pain relief CSL redback spider antivenin: indicated in those with more than mild to moderate pain, systemic symptoms or signs of envenoming; 1 ampoule is efficacious in > 90%
Banana spider (Phoneutria fera) South America Grey/brown, up to 5 cm in size Venom: activates sodium channels of excitable membranes with release of ACh and catecholamines	Immediate onset of local burning pain that can affect whole limb, swelling, redness, sweating at site of bite Tachycardia, agitation, vomiting, salivation, hypertension, priapism in children, diarrhoea Highest-risk groups in Brazil are children < 10 years and adults > 70 years	Pain relief: opioids, ice packs, local anaesthetic infiltration or regional anaesthetic blocks Supportive care: children may develop pulmonary oedema Antivenin in severe or moderate envenoming and in high-risk groups

may be useful following *Phoneutria* bites. Calcium gluconate (10 ml of 10% solution i.v.) may be useful after *Latrodectus* bites. Corticosteroids and blood transfusions may be required for the subsequent generalised haemolysis and haemoglobinuria that can follow *Loxosceles* bites.

Most bites require no first aid measures but in the case of the Australian funnel-web spider, compression bandaging and funnel-web antivenin are required. The efficacy of the antivenin for systemic reactions is such that there have been no published deaths since its introduction.

SCORPION STINGS

In many tropical regions of the world, scorpions are the most important venomous animals after snakes. Most scorpion species produce a venom which causes only minor local reactions in humans, but in Mexico, Tunisia, Algeria, Morocco and Libya scorpion stings are a serious health hazard.

Scorpions do not attack humans and try to escape when disturbed. Stings occur after a person accidentally steps on or involuntarily presses the scorpion (when it is trapped inside shoes or clothes) or when reaching under dead wood or stones. Clothes and shoes need to be inspected closely and shaken, and sitting or sleeping places checked when camping in rural districts where scorpions are common (southern USA, Mexico, North Africa, parts of India and South Africa).

Two types of scorpion venom exist:

- The venom of the genera *Hadrurus, Vejovis* and *Uroctonus* has local effects only, including sharp burning, swelling and discoloration at the bite site. Very rarely, anaphylaxis occurs. However, in envenoming by the more poisonous species, *Leiurus*, which is common in the Middle East, more protracted surveillance is necessary and if systematic manifestations develop, transfer to an area with intensive care facilities is required.
- The second type of venom, produced by the genera of the poisonous varieties of *Centruroides* and *Mesobuthus*, contains neurotoxins which block sodium channels. This leads to spontaneous depolarisation of parasympathetic and sympathetic nerves which results in tachycardia, hypertension, sweating, piloerection, hyperglycaemia and ultimately pulmonary oedema (especially with *Mesobuthus* species) and seizures. The sharp pain after a sting is quickly followed by paraesthesiae and numbness in the area due to peripheral nerve effects, muscle fasciculation and finally drowsiness. With *Centruroides* and *Mesobuthus* there is no swelling at the sting site.

Local pain and paraesthesiae are best treated with local compresses and oral analgesics. Patients with significant envenoming should be hospitalised for at least 12 hours and observed for cardiovascular and neurological sequelae. More severe symptoms may require airway support and 1–2 vials of intravenous antivenin. The effectiveness of antivenin is controversial, but it is beneficial in the very young, the elderly or those with severe hypertension. True anaphylaxis to antivenin occurs rarely. Serum sickness is common after antivenin administration but is usually self-limiting and easily controlled with corticosteroids and histamines. Tachyarrhythmias can be treated with intravenous metoprolol or esmolol. Prazosin, an α-adrenoceptor antagonist, is indicated if hypertension or pulmonary oedema develops. Prazosin also stimulates the secretion of insulin (which often falls during envenoming) and thus prevents hyperglycaemia. Other treatments, such as calcium or sympathomimetic drugs, are of little value.

MARINE ENVENOMING AND POISONING

There is an enormous diversity and complexity of venoms and poisons in marine animals. Illness and even death may be caused by stings and bites, by ingestion of the poisonous flesh (e.g. puffer fish), and by skin contact (Box 9.18). The mechanism the animal uses to administer the toxin is important as the venom may be deposited at one site (as following blue-ringed octopus bites) or over an area (as with jellyfish stings). When single-celled organisms (dinoflagellates) are ingested by molluscs, crabs or fish, the toxins present can cause serious illness subsequently if these are eaten by humans (p. 331). Mussels and oysters may contain neurotoxic poisons.

9

9.18 SIGNIFICANTLY TOXIC MARINE ANIMALS AND THEIR ENVENOMING

Source	Symptoms/signs	Management
Venomous sponges	Delayed onset of burning, stinging and itching of skin Oedema can compromise circulation	Remove spicules Wash affected area with soap and water Aspirin/paracetamol for pain Parenteral corticosteroids, or local application if not available
Jellyfish toxins	Immediate localised pain Myocardial toxicity Haemolysis Necrosis of skin Vascular spasm	Effective antivenin available for box jellyfish (*Chironex fleckeri*)
Sea anemone	Severe burning pain at site of sting (may be delayed) Blanching, wheal formation, erythema, oedema, vesicles, possible necrosis	Analgesics Systemic antihistamine and hydrocortisone Antibiotics for sting site infection
Ciguatera poisoning	Diarrhoea, abdominal pain, nausea, vomiting Burning sensation of skin on contact with cold water, pruritus, paraesthesia Myalgia, arthralgia Progressive flaccid paralysis	Intravenous rehydration Respiratory and cardiovascular support
Blue-ringed octopus	Painless bite Intense chemical venom causes bulbar and respiratory paralysis within 4–10 hours	Monitor respiratory function Prompt mechanical ventilatory support

Of the marine poisonings, ciguatera (caused by the consumption of fish contaminated with lipid-soluble toxins called ciguatoxins) is a major public health problem in the tropical and subtropical Pacific region (p. 331). Some of the commoner marine poisonings are described in Box 9.18.

Prevention of marine envenoming includes wearing protective clothing when wading, swimming, snorkelling or scuba diving. Knowledge of risk areas and risk seasons (e.g. summertime in the tropics for jellyfish) is a necessity prior to underwater activities and diving, and instructions given by beach patrols and lifeguards should be followed. Strange-looking objects or unfamiliar marine structures should not be handled, nor should attempts be made to capture unfamiliar live marine animals.

ENVIRONMENTAL POISONING AND ILLNESS

ARSENISM

Chronic arsenic exposure from drinking water has been reported in many countries of the world, especially India, Bangladesh, Nepal, Thailand, Taiwan, China, Mexico and South America. A large proportion of the drinking water (ground water) has a high arsenic content placing large population groups (70 million in Bangladesh and 45 million in West Bengal) at risk. The World Health Organisation guideline value for arsenic content in tube well water is 10 μg/l.

Health effects associated with chronic exposure to arsenic in drinking water are shown in Box 9.19. In exposed individuals, high concentrations of arsenic are present in bone, hair and nails. Chronic arsenic exposure has been associated with an increased risk of skin cancer and possibly cancers of the lung, liver, bladder, kidney and colon. Specific treatments are of no benefit in chronic arsenic toxicity and recovery from the peripheral neuropathy may never be complete. The emphasis should be on the prevention of exposure to arsenic in drinking water. Iron oxide-coated sand has been found to be a promising medium for arsenic removal from household drinking water supplies in China.

FLUOROSIS

Though water-borne fluorides at levels of 1 part per million are associated with significant immunity to dental caries, the presence of excessive quantities of fluoride in drinking water leads to a characteristic sequence of pathological changes in teeth, bone and periarticular tissues (p. 127). A yellowish-brown mottling of teeth (permanent teeth being particularly affected) is an early and easily recognisable feature of chronic toxicity. This is important, as skeletal involvement may not be clinically obvious until advanced changes have taken place in bone. Radiological changes, however, are seen in the skeleton at an early stage and provide the only means of early diagnosis of relatively asymptomatic fluorosis. Such early cases are usually young adults who complain of vague pains in the small joints of the hands and feet and sometimes in the knees and spine. Subjects may be misdiagnosed as suffering from rheumatoid arthritis or osteoarthritis. The changes in bone and periarticular tissues limit movement of the limbs and may cause back pain. Lesions may progress to cause serious disability, particularly kyphosis, due to progressive joint ankylosis. Changes in the bones of the thoracic cage may lead to rigidity that causes dyspnoea on exertion. In calcium-deficient children, the toxic effects of fluoride manifest even at marginally high exposures to fluoride.

In endemic areas, such as Jordan, Turkey, Chile, India, Bangladesh, China and Tibet, fluorosis is a major public health problem. The maximum impact is seen in communities engaged in physically strenuous agricultural or industrial activities. Dental fluorosis is endemic in East Africa and some West African countries.

FURTHER INFORMATION

Books and journal articles
Dart RC. Medical toxicology. 3rd edn. Philadelphia: Lippincott, Williams & Wilkins; 2004.

Websites
www.atsdr.cdc.gov *Agency for Toxic Substances and Disease Registry (ATSDR) home page: includes information on toxicological profiles, chemical-specific fact sheets, HazDat (database of hazardous substance release and health effects) and ToxFAQs, frequently asked questions about contaminants found at hazardous waste sites.*
www.spib.axl.co.uk *Toxbase, the clinical toxicology database of the UK National Poisons Information Service.*
www.toxinology.com *The website of the Women's and Children's Hospital Adelaide Toxinology Department.*
www.toxnet.nlm.nih.gov *National Library of Medicine's Toxnet: a hazardous substances databank, including Toxline for references to literature on drugs and other chemicals.*

Telephone numbers
Australian Poison Centre Network 131126 (from anywhere within Australia).
UK National Poisons Information Service 0870 243 2241.

9.19 CLINICAL FEATURES OF CHRONIC ARSENIC POISONING

- Anorexia, nausea, vomiting and weight loss
- Increased salivation and metallic taste in the mouth
- Low-grade fever
- Skin lesions
    Hyperpigmentation and 'raindrop' pigmentation
    Palmar and plantar keratosis
    Multiple epitheliomas
- Mee's lines (transverse white lines on finger nails)
- Neuropathy
    Predominantly sensory
    Motor involvement may mimic Guillain–Barré syndrome (p. 1249)
- Vasospasm and peripheral vascular disorders resulting in gangrene (black foot disease)
- Splenomegaly and hypersplenism
- Hepatic portal fibrosis
- Bone marrow depression

M.C. SHARPE

S.G. POTTS

10

Medical psychiatry

Psychiatric disorders have traditionally been considered as mental rather than physical illnesses. This is because they manifest with disordered psychological functioning in the areas of emotion, perception, thinking and memory, and/or have no established biological basis. However, recent research has challenged this assumption; mental disorders are now known to be associated with abnormalities of the brain, and some physical illnesses to be profoundly affected by psychological factors. In practice, both physical and mental aspects of all illness have to be considered to achieve optimal patient care.

Psychiatric terminology is confusing. Psychiatric illnesses are referred to as 'disorders'. As they are diagnosed predominantly by recognising patterns of symptoms, they should really be considered 'syndromes' but since much is known about their natural history, response to treatment and aetiology, the term 'disorder' reflects a status intermediate between syndrome and established disease. Many psychiatric disorders represent extremes of normality and are therefore defined by a specified level of subjective distress and/or impairment. For example, anxiety or depression may refer to a normal state, a symptom or a disorder. Other terms include 'psychosis' which is used to describe an illness in which the person has an altered perception of reality as evidenced by delusions and/or hallucinations, and 'neurosis' when the person has excessive worry or distress but no change in their perception of reality.

10.1 CLASSIFICATION OF PSYCHIATRIC DISORDERS

Stress-related disorders
- Acute stress disorder
- Adjustment disorder
- Post-traumatic stress disorder

Anxiety disorders
- Generalised anxiety
- Phobic anxiety
- Panic disorder
- Obsessive-compulsive disorder

Affective (mood) disorders
- Depressive disorder
- Mania and bipolar disorder

Schizophrenia and delusional disorders

Substance misuse
- Alcohol
- Drugs

Organic
- Acute, e.g. delirium
- Chronic, e.g. dementia

Disorders of adult personality and behaviour
- Personality disorder
- Factitious disorder

Eating disorders
- Anorexia nervosa
- Bulimia nervosa

Somatoform disorders
- Somatisation disorder
- Dissociative (conversion) disorder
- Pain disorder
- Hypochondriasis
- Body dysmorphic disorder
- Somatoform autonomic dysfunction

Neurasthenia

Puerperal mental disorders

CLASSIFICATION OF PSYCHIATRIC DISORDERS

There are two main psychiatric classifications in current use: the American Psychiatric Association's Diagnostic and Statistical Manual (4th edition), or DSM-IV, and the World Health Organization's International Classification of Disease (10th edition), ICD-10. The two systems are very similar but ICD-10 is more widely used outside the United States. The classification of clinical syndromes in this chapter is based on ICD-10 (Box 10.1).

EPIDEMIOLOGY OF PSYCHIATRIC DISORDERS

Psychiatric disorders are amongst the most common of human illnesses. Their relative frequency depends on the setting (Box 10.2). In the general population, depression, anxiety disorders and adjustment disorders are common (10%) and psychosis is rare (less than 1%); in general hospitals, organic disorders such as delirium (10% in the elderly) are especially common; in specialist psychiatric services, however, psychoses are amongst the most common disorders seen.

10.2 PREVALENCE OF PSYCHIATRIC DISORDERS BY MEDICAL SETTING

	General practice	Medical/surgical		Psychiatric services
		Outpatients	Inpatients	
Adjustment disorders	++	++	+++	++
Depression/anxiety	++	++	+++	+++
Alcohol abuse	++	++	+++	+++
Personality disorders	++	++	++	+++
Somatoform disorders	+	+++	++	+
Delirium	−	−	+++	−
Psychosis	−	−	−	+++
(− rare; + uncommon; ++ common; +++ very common)				

AETIOLOGY OF PSYCHIATRIC DISORDERS

The aetiology of psychiatric disorders is multifactorial, with a combination of biological, psychological and social causes. Each of these factors may predispose, precipitate or perpetuate the illness (Box 10.3).

BIOLOGICAL FACTORS

Genetic

Genes are a causal factor in several psychiatric disorders, including schizophrenia and bipolar affective disorder. Whilst some disorders such as Huntington's disease are due to a single gene, in most disorders multiple genes are involved.

Brain structure and function

Brain structure usually appears normal in psychiatric disorders, although there may be generalised atrophy in Alzheimer's disease and enlarged ventricles in schizophrenia. On the other hand, brain function is commonly altered. There may be changes in the level of neurotransmitters, such as dopamine, noradrenaline (norepinephrine) and 5-hydroxytryptamine (5-HT, serotonin), and differences in regional activity, as shown on single photon emission tomography (SPECT) or magnetic resonance imaging (MRI) scans. Damage to the brain, as in head injury or stroke, may precipitate psychiatric illness.

PSYCHOLOGICAL AND BEHAVIOURAL FACTORS

Perceived stress and trauma

Early childhood experiences, such as emotional deprivation or abuse, increase the risk of developing psychiatric illnesses such as depression and eating disorders as an adult. Events in adult life perceived as stressful may trigger a psychiatric illness: for example, post-traumatic stress disorder.

Personality

The relationship between personality and psychiatric illness can be difficult to assess because the development of psychiatric illness can change a patient's personality. However, some personality types do predispose to illness. For example, a neurotic personality increases the risk of depression. Abnormal personality may also perpetuate psychiatric illness once it is established, leading to a poorer prognosis.

Behaviour

A person's behaviour may predispose to the development of a disorder (e.g. excess alcohol intake leading to dependence) or perpetuate it, as in persistent avoidance of the feared situation in phobia.

SOCIAL AND ENVIRONMENTAL FACTORS

Social isolation

The lack of a close, confiding relationship predisposes to psychiatric illnesses such as depression. The reduced social support resulting from illness may also perpetuate it.

Stressors

Social and environmental stressors can precipitate illness in vulnerable people. Their effect is modified by how they are perceived by the individual, although some may be so severe that they precipitate illness in most people. Events perceived as losses (such as bereavement) commonly precede the onset of depression, and events perceived as threats commonly precipitate anxiety.

10

DIAGNOSING PSYCHIATRIC DISORDERS

The differences between a psychiatric and a medical assessment are:

- a greater emphasis on the history
- the systematic examination of the patient's mental state
- the routine interviewing of an informant (usually a relative or friend who knows the patient), especially when the illness affects the patient's ability to give an accurate history.

A full psychiatric history and detailed mental state examination (MSE) may take an hour or more, but a briefer psychiatric examination should be part of the assessment of *all* patients.

PSYCHIATRIC INTERVIEW

The aims of the interview are:

- to establish a positive relationship with the patient
- to elicit the symptoms, their history and background information (Box 10.4)
- to examine the mental state
- to provide information, reassurance and advice.

Some aspects of the patient's mental state may be observed whilst the history is being taken, but specific enquiry must be made for important features.

10.3 CLASSIFICATION OF AETIOLOGICAL FACTORS IN PSYCHIATRIC DISORDERS

Predisposing

- Increase susceptibility to psychiatric disorder
- Established in utero or in childhood
- Operate throughout patient's lifetime (e.g. genetic factors, congenital defects, chronic physical illness, disturbed family background)

Precipitating

- Trigger an episode of illness
- Determine its time of onset (e.g. stressful life events, acute physical illness)

Perpetuating

- Delay recovery from illness (e.g. lack of social support, chronic physical illness)

10.4 TOPICS COVERED DURING INTERVIEW

Presenting problem

Reason for referral
- Why the patient has been referred and by whom

Presenting complaints
- The patient should be asked to describe the symptoms for which help is requested

History of present illness
- The patient should be asked to describe the course of the illness from the time when symptoms were first noticed. The interviewer asks direct questions to determine the nature, duration and severity of symptoms and any associated factors

Background

Family history
- Description of parents and siblings, and a record of mental illness in relatives

Personal history
- Birth history, major events in childhood, schooling, higher education, occupational history, relationship, marriage, children, current social circumstances

Previous medical and psychiatric history
- Previous health, accidents and operations; use of alcohol, tobacco and other drugs. Direct questions may be needed concerning previous psychiatric history since this may not be volunteered: 'Have you ever been treated for depression or nerves?' or 'Have you ever suffered a nervous breakdown?'

Previous personality
- The characteristic patterns of behaviour and thinking which determine a person's adjustment to the environment—including attitudes, moral values, interests, quality of relationships with other people and reactions to stress. The most useful information may be obtained from an informant who has known the patient well for many years

MENTAL STATE EXAMINATION

General appearance and behaviour

Any unusual features are noted, including abnormalities of alertness and motor behaviour such as restlessness or retardation. The level of consciousness should be noted, especially in the assessment of possible delirium.

Speech

Speed and fluency should be observed, including slow (retarded) speech and word-finding difficulty. 'Pressure of speech' describes rapid speech that is difficult to interrupt.

Mood

This can be judged by facial expression, posture and movements. Patients should also be asked if they feel sad or depressed, or lack ability to experience pleasure (anhedonia). Are they anxious, worried or tense? Is mood elevated with elation, excess energy and a reduced need for sleep?

Thoughts

The content of thought is elicited by asking 'What are your main concerns?' Is thinking negative, guilty or hopeless, suggesting depression? Are there thoughts of self-harm? If so, enquiry should be made about plans. Does the patient think that he or she is especially powerful, important or gifted (grandiose thoughts), suggesting mania or is he/she excessively worried about many things, suggesting anxiety?

The form of thinking may also be abnormal. For example, in schizophrenia, patients may display loosened associations, making it difficult to follow their train of thought. There may also be abnormalities of thought possession, when patients experience the intrusion of alien thoughts or the broadcasting of their own (p. 242).

Abnormal beliefs

A delusion is a false belief, out of keeping with a patient's cultural background, which is held with unshakable conviction despite evidence to the contrary (p. 232).

10.5 MINI-MENTAL STATE EXAMINATION (MMSE)

Patient name _____

Date of birth _____ Date of test _____

Max. points	Patient score	
		Orientation
5	( )	What is the (year) (season) (date) (day) (month)?
5	( )	Where are we (country) (county) (town/city) (building) (floor)?
		Registration
3	( )	Name three common objects (e.g. 'apple', 'table', 'penny'). Take 1 second to say each. Then ask the patient to repeat all three after you have said them. Give 1 point for each correct answer. Then repeat them until he/she learns all three. Count trials and record. Trials ( )
		Attention
5	( )	Spell 'world' backwards. The score is the number of letters in the correct order. (D_L_R_O_W_)
		Recall
3	( )	Ask for the three objects repeated above. Give 1 point for each correct answer. (Note: recall cannot be tested if all three objects were not remembered during registration)
		Language
2	( )	Name a 'pencil' and a 'watch'. (2 points)
1	( )	Repeat the following: 'No ifs, ands or buts.' (1 point)
3	( )	Follow a three-stage command: 'Take this paper in your right hand, fold it in half, and put it on the floor.' (3 points)
1	( )	Read and obey the following: (1 point) CLOSE YOUR EYES
1	( )	Write a sentence. (1 point)
1	( )	Copy the following design. Give 1 point if no construction problem
30	( )	**Total**

Examiner _____

Abnormal perceptions

Illusions are abnormal perceptions of real stimuli. Hallucinations are sensory perceptions which occur in the absence of external stimuli: for example, hearing voices when no one is present (p. 232).

Cognitive function

The Mini-Mental State Examination (MMSE) is a useful screening questionnaire to detect cognitive impairment (Box 10.5). A score of less than 24 out of 30 indicates cognitive impairment. The degree of cognitive impairment in delirium typically fluctuates and may be missed by a single assessment.

- *Concentration.* Serial 7s is a test in which the patient is asked to subtract 7 from 100 and then 7 from the answer, down to zero.
- *Orientation.* This is assessed by asking the patient about place—his or her exact location; time—what day, date, month and year it is now; and person—details of personal identity such as name, date of birth, marital status and address.
- *Intellectual abilities.* These can be gauged from the history of the patient's educational background and attainments but can also be assessed during the interview from the patient's fluency, vocabulary and grasp of the interviewer's questions.
- *Memory.* Registration of memories is tested by asking the patient to repeat immediately simple new information such as a name and address. Short-term memory is assessed by asking him/her to repeat it after an interval of 5 minutes, during which time the patient's attention should be diverted elsewhere. Long-term memory is checked by assessing the recall of events of the previous day, month and year.

Patients' understanding of illness ('insight')

Patients should be asked what they think their symptoms are due to, and what they fear might happen in the future. Lack of insight is a failure to accept that one is ill, and is characteristic of acute psychosis.

PRESENTING PROBLEMS IN PSYCHIATRIC ILLNESS

ANXIETY SYMPTOMS

Anxiety may be transient, persistent, episodic or limited to specific situations. The symptoms of anxiety are both psychological and somatic (Box 10.6). The differential diagnosis of anxiety is shown in Box 10.7. Most commonly it is transient, as an adjustment disorder (p. 239), and subsides without treatment. Other more persistent forms of anxiety are described in detail on pages 239–240. Anxiety may occasionally be a manifestation of a medical condition such as thyrotoxicosis (Box 10.7).

DEPRESSED MOOD

Depressive disorder is common, occurring in a quarter to a half of medical inpatients. The symptoms of depression are

---

10.6 SYMPTOMS OF ANXIETY DISORDER

Psychological

● Apprehension	● Fear of impending disaster
● Irritability	● Poor concentration
● Worry	● Depersonalisation

Somatic

● Palpitations	● Frequent desire to pass urine
● Fatigue	● Chest pain
● Tremor	● Initial insomnia
● Dizziness	● Breathlessness
● Sweating	● Headache
● Diarrhoea	

10.7 DIFFERENTIAL DIAGNOSIS OF ANXIETY

● Normal response to threat	● Organic (medical) cause
● Adjustment disorder	Hyperthyroidism
● Generalised anxiety disorder	Paroxysmal arrhythmias
● Panic disorder	Phaeochromocytoma
● Phobic disorder	Alcohol and benzodiazepine
	withdrawal
	Hypoglycaemia
	Temporal lobe epilepsy

---

both mental and physical (Box 10.8). In the physically ill patient, diagnosis of comorbid depression is based mainly on careful assessment of the core psychological symptoms: namely, persistently lowered mood and anhedonia.

Differential diagnosis

Depressive disorder must be differentiated from depressive adjustment disorder (p. 239). Adjustment disorders are self-limiting reactions to adversity, including physical illness. They are common, transient and do not require treatment beyond general support. On the other hand, depressive disorders (p. 240) are characterised by more severe and persistent mood disturbance and do require specific treatment. In some cases, depression may occur as a result of a direct effect of a medical condition or its treatment on neurotransmitter function or neural pathways in the brain, when it is referred to as an organic mood disorder (Box 10.9).

10.8 SYMPTOMS OF DEPRESSIVE DISORDERS

Psychological

● Depressed mood	● Loss of interest
● Reduced self-esteem	● Loss of enjoyment (anhedonia)
● Pessimism	● Suicidal thinking
● Guilt	

Somatic

● Reduced appetite	● Loss of libido
● Weight change	● Bowel disturbance
● Disturbed sleep	● Motor retardation (slowing of
● Fatigue	activity)

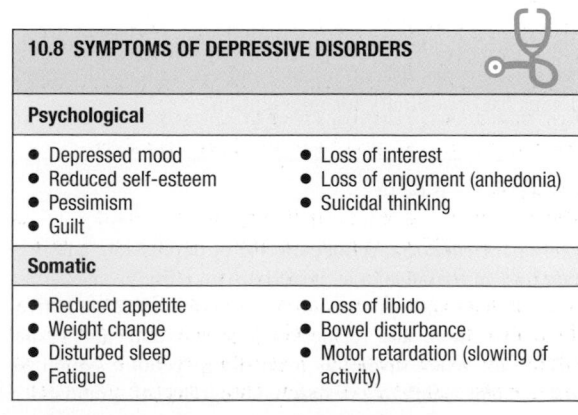

10.9 ORGANIC AFFECTIVE DISORDERS*

Neurological

- Cerebrovascular disease
- Cerebral tumour
- Multiple sclerosis
- Parkinson's disease
- Huntington's disease
- Alzheimer's disease
- Epilepsy

Endocrine

- Hypothyroidism
- Hyperthyroidism
- Cushing's syndrome
- Addison's disease
- Hyperparathyroidism

Infections

- Infectious mononucleosis
- Herpes simplex
- Brucellosis
- Typhoid
- Toxoplasmosis

Connective tissue disease

- Systemic lupus erythematosus

Malignant disease

Drugs

- Reserpine, methyldopa
- Phenothiazines
- Phenylbutazone
- Corticosteroids, oral contraceptives
- Interferon

*Diseases that may cause organic affective disorders by direct action on the brain.

10.10 RISK FACTORS FOR SUICIDE

- Psychiatric illness (depressive illness, schizophrenia)
- Age over 45
- Male sex
- Living alone
- Unemployed
- Recently bereaved, divorced or separated
- Chronic physical ill health
- Drug or alcohol misuse
- Suicide note written
- History of previous attempts (especially if a violent method was used)

Suicide

Depression is the major risk factor for suicide, especially when it co-occurs with a medical condition or substance misuse. Other risk factors are shown in Box 10.10. When depression is suspected, tactful enquiry should always be made into suicidal thoughts, plans and impulses. This does not increase the risk of suicide; indeed, failure to enquire denies the opportunity for intervention.

ELATED MOOD

Elation, or euphoria, is the converse of depression, and may manifest in hypomania as infectious joviality, over-activity, lack of sleep and appetite, undue optimism, over-talkativeness, irritability, and recklessness in spending and sexual behaviour. When severe, as in mania, psychotic symptoms are evident, such as delusional degrees of grandiosity.

Elevated mood is much less common than depression, and where it arises in medical settings it may be secondary to drug or alcohol misuse, an organic disorder or medical treatment. Where none of these applies, the patient may have a bipolar mood disorder (p. 242) and specialist treatment is indicated.

DELUSIONS AND HALLUCINATIONS

Delusions

Various types of delusion are identified on the basis of their content. They may be persecutory, e.g. a conviction that one is being tracked by hostile intelligence agencies; hypochondriacal, as in the unfounded conviction that one has cancer; or grandiose, such as the belief that one has special powers or status. The most extreme form of delusion is nihilistic, e.g. 'My head is missing,' 'I have no body,' 'I am dead.' Delusions should be differentiated from overvalued ideas: beliefs which are strongly held but which fall short of delusions.

Hallucinations

These are perceptions without external stimuli. They can occur in any sensory modality, most commonly visual or auditory. Typical examples are hearing voices when no one else is present, or seeing demonic faces on a blank white wall. Hallucinations have the character and quality of ordinary perceptions and are perceived as originating in the external world, not the patient's own mind (when they are termed pseudo-hallucinations). Those occurring at the edges of sleep are normal; they are called hypnogogic when falling asleep and hypnopompic on waking. Hallucinations should be distinguished from illusions, which are misperceptions of real external stimuli such as mistaking a shrub for a person in poor light.

Differential diagnosis

Agitation, terror or the fear of being thought 'mad' may make patients unable or unwilling to volunteer their abnormal beliefs or to describe their experiences. Careful enquiry is therefore required. The nature of hallucinations can be important diagnostically; 'running commentary' voices which discuss the patient in the third person are strongly associated with schizophrenia, for example. In general, auditory hallucinations suggest a functional psychosis such as schizophrenia, while hallucinations in other sensory modalities, especially vision but also taste and smell, suggest an organic cause such as delirium or temporal lobe epilepsy.

Hallucinations and delusions often co-occur, and if their content is appropriate to coexisting emotional symptoms, they are described as mood-congruent. Thus a patient with a severe depressive illness may feel desolate, believe themselves responsible for all the evils in the world, and hear voices saying 'You're worthless. Go and kill yourself.' In this case the diagnosis is made on the basis of the concurrence of symptoms in different areas (belief, mood, perception, impulse). Incongruence between hallucinations, delusions and mood suggests schizophrenia.

10

Where hallucinations and delusions arise with disturbed consciousness and impaired cognition, the cause is probably an organic disorder, most commonly delirium and/or dementia (p. 247). The diagnosis is made by assessing the nature, extent and time course of any cognitive disturbances, and by investigating for underlying causes.

DISTURBED AND AGGRESSIVE BEHAVIOUR

Disturbed and aggressive behaviour is common in hospitals, especially in emergency departments. Most behavioural disturbance arises not from medical or psychiatric illness, but from alcohol intoxication and personality. The key principles of management are to establish control of the situation and thereby ensure the safety of the patient and others, and simultaneously to assess the cause of the disturbance in order to remedy it. Establishing control requires the presence of an adequate number of trained staff, an appropriate physical environment and sedation, as set out in Figure 10.1. Hospital security staff and the police may also need to be involved. In all cases staff responses to the patient are important; a calm, non-threatening approach by a doctor or nurse who can understand and address the patient's fears often may be all that is required.

The most widely used sedating agents are antipsychotic drugs such as haloperidol and/or benzodiazepines such as diazepam. The choice of drug, dose, route and rate of administration will depend on the patient's age, sex and physical health, as well as the likely cause of the disturbed behaviour. The benefits of sedation must be balanced against the risks. Haloperidol can cause acute dystonias and oculogyric crises, while the benzodiazepines can precipitate respiratory depression in patients with lung disease, and encephalopathy in those with liver disease. Thus appropriate sedation for a frail elderly woman with emphysema and delirium may be a low dose (0.5 mg) of oral haloperidol, while a threatening young man having an acute psychotic episode may need at least 10 mg of intravenous diazepam and a similar dose of haloperidol. A parenterally administered anticholinergic agent such as procyclidine should be available to treat extrapyramidal effects arising from haloperidol. When benzodiazepines are used, flumazenil (p. 212) should be on hand to reverse respiratory depression. When benzodiazepines are used in large doses, oxygen and ventilation should be available.

Differential diagnosis

Many factors may contribute to disturbed behaviour, although little may be learned from an attempted interview with an uncooperative patient. Other sources of information about the patient are therefore crucial and include medical and psychiatric records, and discussion with nursing staff, family members and other informants, including the patient's general practitioner. Key information is psychiatric, medical (especially neurological) or criminal history; current psychiatric and medical treatment; current or previous alcohol and drug misuse; recent stressors; and the

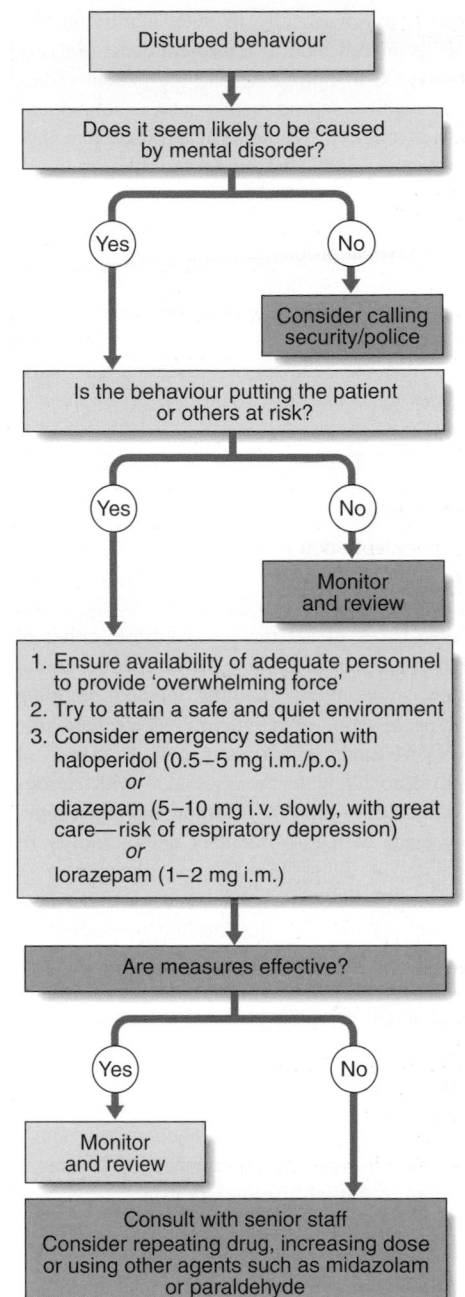

Fig. 10.1   Acute management of disturbed behaviour.

time course and accompaniments of the current episode in terms of mood, belief and behaviour.

Simple observation of patients' behaviour may yield useful clues. Do they appear to be responding to hallucinations? Are they alert or variably drowsy and confused? Are there physical features suggesting drug or alcohol misuse or withdrawal? Are there new injuries or old scars, especially on the head? Do they smell of alcohol or solvents? Do they bear marks of drug injection? Are they grubby and unkempt, suggesting a gradual development of their condition?

10

If the person is psychiatrically ill, then admission to a psychiatric facility is indicated. If a medical cause is likely, psychiatric transfer is inappropriate and the patient should be managed in a medical setting, with whatever nursing and security support is required. Where it is clear that there is no medical or psychiatric illness, the person should be removed from the hospital, to police custody if necessary.

Measures such as restraint, sedation, the investigation and treatment of medical problems, and psychiatric transfer all raise legal as well as medical issues (p. 251). In most countries, including the UK, the law confers upon doctors the right and indeed the duty to intervene against a patient's wishes in cases of acute behavioural disturbance if this is urgently necessary to protect the patient or other people.

SELF-HARM

Self-harm (SH) is a common reason for medical presentation. The term 'attempted suicide' is potentially misleading as most such patients are not unequivocally trying to kill themselves. Most cases of SH involve overdose, either of prescribed or non-prescribed drugs (Ch. 9). Less common methods include asphyxiation, drowning, hanging, jumping from a height or in front of a moving vehicle, and the use of firearms. Methods which carry a high chance of being fatal are more likely to be associated with serious psychiatric illness. Self-cutting is common and often repetitive, but only leads to medical contact on a minority of occasions.

The incidence of SH has changed over time and varies between countries. In the UK, the lifetime prevalence of suicidal ideation is 15% and that of SH is 4%. SH is more common in women than in men and in young adults than in the elderly. In contrast, completed suicide is more common in men and in the elderly (Box 10.10). There is a higher incidence among lower socioeconomic groups, particularly those living in crowded, socially deprived urban areas. Patients often have a deprived family background. There is also an association with alcohol misuse, child abuse, unemployment and recently broken relationships.

Differential diagnosis

The main differential diagnosis is from accidental poisoning and from so-called 'recreational' overdose in drug users. SH is not a diagnosis but a presentation, and may be associated with any psychiatric disorder; the most common are adjustment disorders, substance and alcohol misuse, depressive disorders and personality disorders. In many cases there is no psychiatric diagnosis.

Initial management

A thorough psychiatric and social assessment should be carried out in all cases (Fig. 10.2), although some patients will discharge themselves before this can take place. In most UK hospitals, assessment is undertaken by psychiatrists, although other doctors, physicians, nurses and social workers can also be trained to do this. Psychiatric assessment should not delay urgent medical or surgical treatment, and may need to be deferred until the patient is

well enough for interview, and the sedating or intoxicating effect of the drugs and any alcohol taken have worn off. The purpose of the psychiatric assessment is to:

- establish the short-term risk of suicide
- identify potentially treatable problems, whether medical, psychiatric or social.

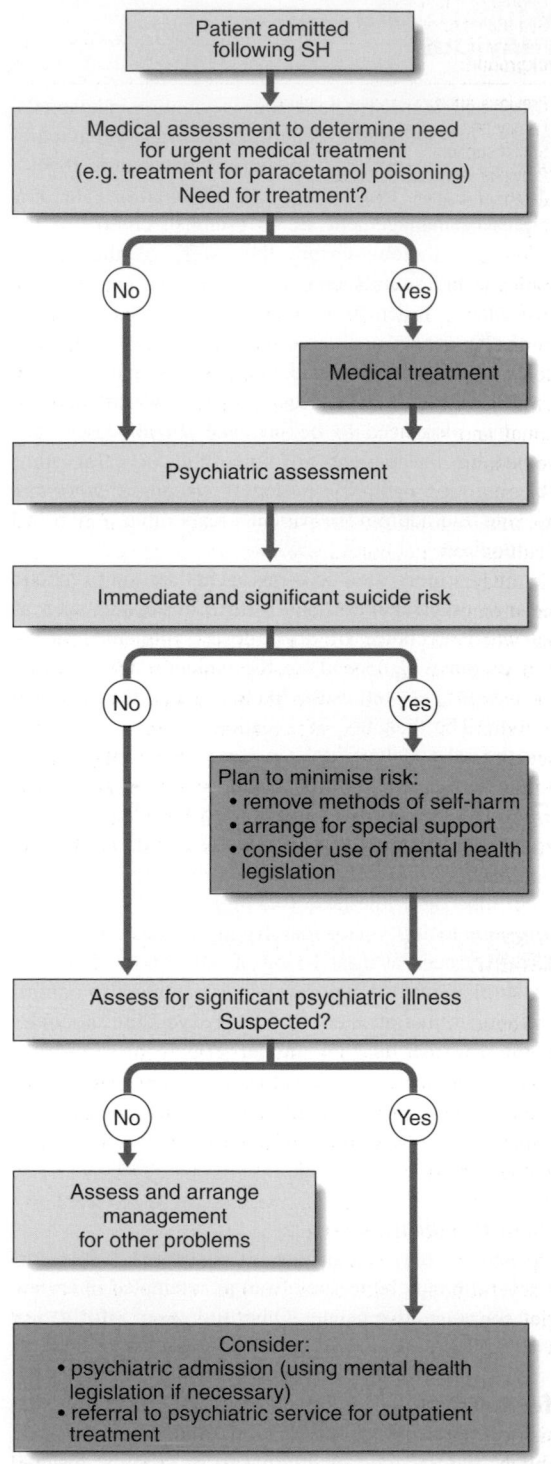

Fig. 10.2 Assessment of patients admitted following self-harm (SH).

10.11 ASSESSMENT OF PATIENTS AFTER SELF-HARM

Current attempt

- Patient's account
- Degree of intent at the time: preparations, plans, precautions against discovery, note
- Method used, particularly whether violent
- Degree of intent now
- Symptoms of psychiatric illness

Background

- Previous attempts and their outcome
- Family and personal history
- Social support
- Previous response to stress
- Extent of drug and alcohol misuse

10.12 MEDICAL PSYCHIATRY IN OLD AGE

- **Organic psychiatric disorders**: especially common so cognitive function should always be assessed and, if impaired, an associated medical condition or adverse drug effect suspected.
- **Disturbed behaviour**: delirium is the most common cause.
- **Depression**: common. Just because a person is old and frail does not mean that depression is 'to be expected' and that it should not be treated.
- **Self-harm**: associated with an increased risk of completed suicide.
- **Medically unexplained symptoms**: common and often associated with depressive disorder.
- **Loneliness, poverty and lack of social support**: must be taken into consideration in management decisions.

Topics to be covered when assessing a patient are listed in Box 10.11. The history should cover events occurring immediately before and after the act and especially any evidence of planning. The nature and severity of any current psychiatric symptoms must be assessed, along with the personal and social supports available if the patient is to leave hospital.

The majority of patients have depressive and anxiety symptoms on a background of chronic social and personal difficulties and alcohol misuse, and do not require psychotropic medication or specialised psychiatric treatment. They do need emotional support and practical advice from a GP, social worker or community psychiatric nurse. Admission to a psychiatric ward is necessary only for those with a major psychiatric illness who remain intent on suicide or who require temporary respite from intolerable circumstances, or when further assessment of the mental state is essential. Approximately 20% of SH patients make a repeat attempt during the following year and 1–2% kill themselves. Factors associated with an increased risk of suicide after SH are listed in Box 10.10.

CONFUSION

This vague term covers a range of primarily cognitive problems but also includes disturbances in mood, perception, belief and behaviour. 'Confusion' usually presents as a problem when patients cannot comply with medical care; they may repeatedly wander off the ward, pull out essential cannulae and catheters, and hit out at nurses. The apparently confused patient may have deficits in any or all cognitive domains. Cognitive assessments range from simple screening questions to detailed psychometric testing which can take several hours. All doctors should be able to undertake a brief cognitive assessment as outlined above (p. 230 and Box 10.5).

Differential diagnosis

A history from the patient and informants is essential to establish the time course, variability and functional consequences of any cognitive deficit. Mental state examination is necessary to seek evidence of associated mood

disorder, hallucinations, delusions or behavioural abnormalities, and physical examination to identify medical illness. A clinical assessment should distinguish between organic disorders such as delirium, dementia, and focal deficits secondary to brain lesions; psychiatric disorders such as pseudo-dementia and dissociative disorder; and malingering (p. 251). Further investigation will usually be needed to identify the specific causes of any delirium (Chs 9 and 26).

ALCOHOL MISUSE

Misuse of alcohol is a world-wide problem, and is growing in the UK. It can present in medical settings in a multitude of ways, which are discussed further on page 244 and in Box 10.30. In many cases, the link to alcohol will be all too obvious but in others it may not. Denial and concealment of alcohol intake is common and a high index of suspicion is essential. The patient should be asked to describe a typical week's drinking, quantified in terms of units of alcohol (1 unit contains approximately 9 g alcohol and is the equivalent of half a pint of beer, a single measure of spirits or a small glass of table wine). Drinking becomes hazardous at levels above 21 units weekly for men and 14 units weekly for women. The history from the patient may need corroboration by the GP, earlier medical records and family members. The mean cell volume (MCV) and γ-glutamyl transferase (GGT) may be raised, but are abnormal in only half of problem drinkers, so normal results do not exclude an alcohol problem. When abnormal, they may be helpful in challenging denial and monitoring treatment response. The prevention and management of alcohol-related problems is discussed on pages 245–246.

SUBSTANCE MISUSE

The misuse of drugs of all kinds is widespread in the UK and many other countries, despite being illegal. As well as the general headings listed for alcohol problems in Box 10.30 (p. 245), there are two additional sets of problems associated with drug misuse: those linked with the route of administration rather than the substance taken, and problems arising from pressure applied to doctors by the patient to

10

10.13 SUBSTANCE MISUSE: ADDITIONAL PRESENTING PROBLEMS

Complications arising from the route of use

Intravenous
- Local: abscesses, cellulitis, thrombosis
- Systemic
  Bacterial: endocarditis
  Viral: hepatitis, human immunodeficiency virus (HIV)

Nasal
- Erosion of nasal septum, epistaxis

Smoking
- Oral, laryngeal and lung cancer

Inhalation
- Burns, chemical pneumonitis, rashes

Pressure to prescribe misused substance

- Manipulation, deceit and threats
- Factitious description of illness
- Malingering

---

prescribe the misused substances (Box 10.13). Assessment and management are described on page 247.

PSYCHOLOGICAL FACTORS AFFECTING MEDICAL CONDITIONS

Psychological factors influence the presentation, management and outcome of medical conditions. Risk factors are shown in Box 10.14. The most common psychological problems in the medically ill are adjustment, anxiety and depressive disorders. However understandable these diagnoses appear, if they are severe and persistent, active management should be considered. Anxiety may present as an increase in somatic symptoms such as breathlessness, tremor or palpitations, or as the avoidance of treatment. It is most common in those facing difficult or painful treatment, deterioration of their illness or death. Depressive disorders may also manifest as increased symptoms such as pain or fatigue, and disability. These are most common in patients who have suffered actual or anticipated loss such as a terminal diagnosis or disfiguring surgery.

Treatment is by psychological and/or pharmacological therapies, as described below. Care is required when prescribing psychotropic drugs in the medically ill, in order to avoid exacerbating the medical condition or causing interactions with other prescribed drugs.

10.14 RISK FACTORS FOR PSYCHOLOGICAL PROBLEMS ASSOCIATED WITH MEDICAL CONDITIONS

- Previous history of depression or anxiety
- Lack of social support
- New diagnosis of a serious medical condition
- Deterioration of or failure of treatment for medical condition
- Unpleasant, disabling or disfiguring treatment
- Change in medical care, e.g. discharge from hospital
- Impending death

MEDICALLY UNEXPLAINED SOMATIC SYMPTOMS

Patients commonly present to doctors with somatic symptoms. These may be clearly associated with a medical condition. When they are disproportionate to, or occur in the absence of a physical disease, they are termed medically unexplained symptoms. These occur in a quarter to a half of patients attending general medical clinics. Almost any symptom can be medically unexplained. Common examples include:

- pain (including back, chest, abdominal and headache)
- fatigue
- dizziness
- fits, 'funny turns' and feelings of weakness.

These patients may receive a diagnosis of a functional somatic syndrome such as irritable bowel syndrome (Box 10.15) but may also merit a psychiatric diagnosis such as a somatoform disorder, on the basis of the same symptoms. This double diagnosis reflects different perspectives on the same problem rather than two conditions. The psychiatric classification is based on the number of somatic symptoms and associated psychological symptoms (Box 10.16).

Differential diagnosis

The main medical differential diagnosis is from symptoms of a medical disease. Diagnostic difficulties are most likely with unusual presentations of common diseases and with rare diseases. A medical and psychiatric assessment should be completed in all cases (Fig. 10.3). The most common psychiatric diagnoses are anxiety or depressive disorders. The remainder have somatoform disorders (p. 249).

10.15 FUNCTIONAL SOMATIC SYNDROMES

• **Gastroenterology**	Irritable bowel syndrome, non-ulcer dyspepsia
• **Gynaecology**	Premenstrual syndrome, chronic pelvic pain
• **Rheumatology**	Fibromyalgia
• **Cardiology**	Atypical or non-cardiac chest pain
• **Respiratory medicine**	Hyperventilation syndrome
• **Infectious diseases**	Chronic (post-viral) fatigue syndrome
• **Neurology**	Tension headache, non-epileptic attacks
• **Dentistry**	Temporomandibular joint dysfunction, atypical facial pain
• **Ear, nose and throat**	Globus syndrome
• **Allergy**	Multiple chemical sensitivity

10.16 PSYCHIATRIC DIAGNOSES FOR MEDICALLY UNEXPLAINED SOMATIC SYMPTOMS

- **Hypochondriasis**: predominant worry about disease
- **Somatisation**: predominant concern about symptoms
  Somatic presentation of depression and anxiety
  Simple somatoform disorders: small number of symptoms
  Somatisation disorder (Briquet's syndrome): chronic multiple symptoms
- **Conversion disorder**: Loss of function
- **Body dysmorphic disorder**: Dislike of body parts

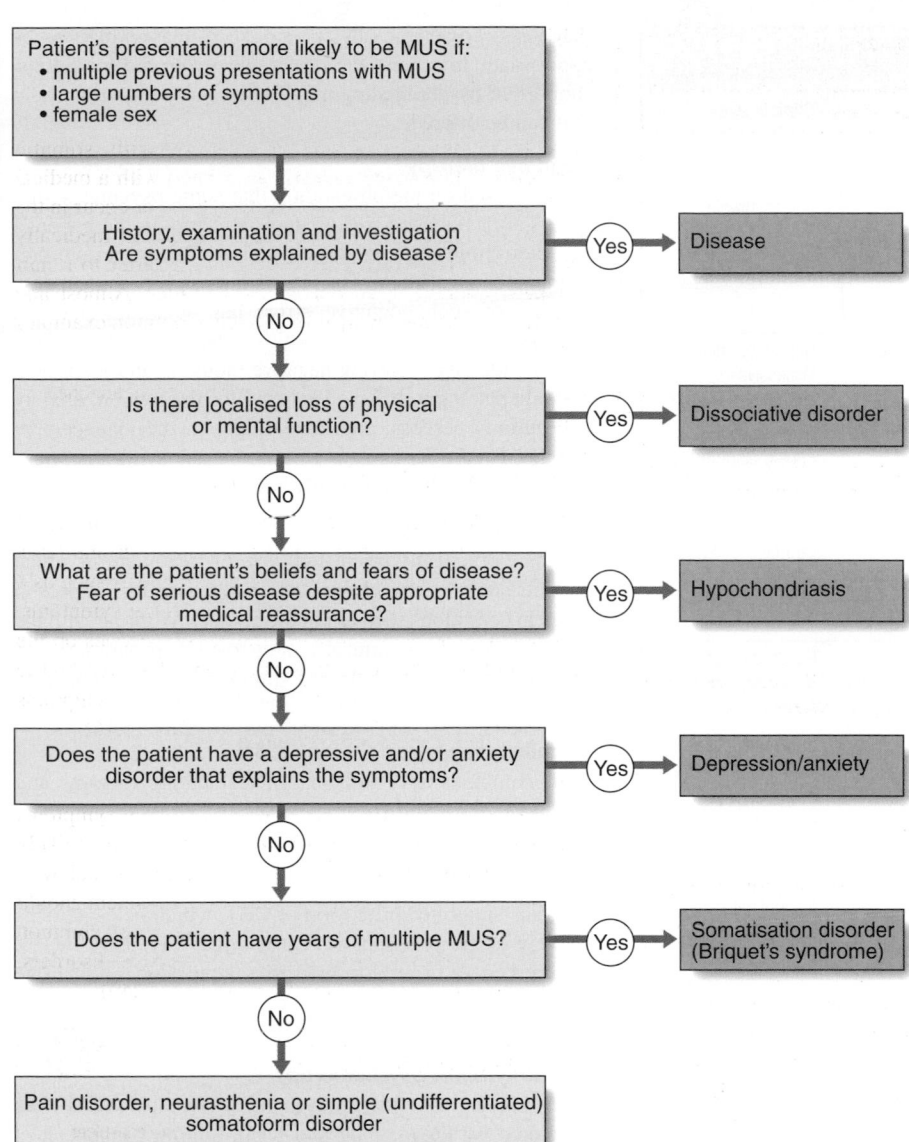

Patient's presentation more likely to be MUS if:
• multiple previous presentations with MUS
• large numbers of symptoms
• female sex

History, examination and investigation
Are symptoms explained by disease? — Yes → Disease

No

Is there localised loss of physical
or mental function? — Yes → Dissociative disorder

No

What are the patient's beliefs and fears of disease?
Fear of serious disease despite appropriate
medical reassurance? — Yes → Hypochondriasis

No

Does the patient have a depressive and/or anxiety
disorder that explains the symptoms? — Yes → Depression/anxiety

No

Does the patient have years of multiple MUS? — Yes → Somatisation disorder
(Briquet's syndrome)

No

Pain disorder, neurasthenia or simple (undifferentiated)
somatoform disorder

**Fig. 10.3   Diagnosis of medically
unexplained symptoms (MUS).**

10

TREATING PSYCHIATRIC DISORDERS

The multifactorial origin of most psychiatric disorders means that there may be multiple targets for treatment.

SOCIAL INTERVENTIONS

Factors such as unemployment may not be readily amenable to intervention but others, such as access to benefits and poor housing, are. Patients can be helped to take an active problem-solving approach to such issues. In the UK, befrienders and day centres can reduce social isolation, benefits advisers can ensure appropriate financial assistance, and medical recommendations can be made to local Housing Departments to move patients to more appropriate accommodation.

BIOLOGICAL TREATMENTS

These aim to modify brain function. Psychotropic drugs are widely used for various purposes, and a pragmatic classification is set out in Box 10.17. It should be noted that some drugs have applications in more than one condition; for example, antidepressants are widely used in the treatment of anxiety *and* chronic pain. Specific subgroups of psychotropic drugs are discussed more fully in the sections on the appropriate disorders.

Electroconvulsive therapy (ECT) entails producing a convulsion by the administration of high-voltage, brief direct current impulses to the head while the patient is anaesthetised and paralysed by muscle relaxants. It is now remarkably safe, has few side-effects, and is of proven efficacy for severe depressive illness. There may be amnesia for events occurring a few hours before ECT (retrograde)

10.17 CLASSIFICATION OF PSYCHOTROPIC DRUGS

Action	Main groups	Clinical use
Antipsychotic	Phenothiazines Butyrophenones Thioxanthenes Diphenylbutylpiperidines Substituted benzamides Dibenzodiazepine* Benzisoxazole* Thienobenzodiazepines*	Schizophrenia Mania Acute confusion
Antidepressant	Tricyclics and related drugs	Depressive illness Obsessive-compulsive disorder
	Monoamine oxidase inhibitors	Depressive illness Phobic disorders
	Amine precursors	Depressive illness (in combination)
	Noradrenergic re-uptake inhibitors and SSRIs (selective serotonin re-uptake inhibitors)	Depressive illness
Mood-stabilising	Lithium	Prophylaxis of manic depression Acute mania
	Carbamazepine	Prophylaxis of manic depression
	Sodium valproate	Prophylaxis of manic depression
Anti-anxiety	Benzodiazepines	Anxiety disorders Insomnia Alcohol withdrawal
	β-adrenoceptor antagonists	Anxiety (somatic symptoms)
	Buspirone	Anxiety disorders

*Atypical antipsychotics.

and after it (anterograde). Permanent anterograde amnesia has been claimed to occur but is infrequent. Although ECT, and to a lesser extent psychosurgery, still have a place, drugs are the most commonly used biological interventions.

PSYCHOLOGICAL TREATMENTS

These treatments are used in many psychiatric disorders and also in the management of non-psychiatric conditions. They are based on talking with patients, either individually or in groups. Sometimes discussion is supplemented by 'homework' or tasks to complete between sessions. Psychological treatments take a number of forms based on the duration and frequency of contact, the specific techniques applied and their underlying theory.

General or supportive psychotherapy

This should form part of all medical treatment. It involves empathic listening, in which the doctor encourages the patient to describe symptoms, express feelings and reflect on associated problems. The doctor should offer an explanation of the symptoms (and where possible a diagnosis), practical advice and such reassurance as is appropriate. In patients with incurable or chronic conditions, supportive psychotherapy may be the most important help that can be offered.

Cognitive therapy

This is based on the observation that some psychiatric disorders are associated with systematic errors in the patient's conscious thinking: for example, a tendency to interpret events in a negative way or see them as unduly threatening. A triad of such cognitive errors has been described in depression (Box 10.18). Cognitive therapy aims to help patients identify recurring negative thoughts and learn how to challenge them. It is widely used for depression, anxiety and bulimia nervosa, and increasingly in the management of other conditions such as chronic fatigue syndrome, non-cardiac chest pain and irritable bowel syndrome.

Behaviour therapy

This is a practically orientated form of treatment, in which patients are helped to change their behaviour. It is of proven value in conditions such as phobic anxiety. Working with the patient through a carefully constructed programme of graded exposure to the feared stimulus can be remarkably effective.

Cognitive behaviour therapy (CBT)

This combines the methods of behaviour therapy and cognitive therapy. It is the most widely available and most extensively researched psychological treatment.

Problem-solving therapy

This is a simplified brief form of CBT, which helps patients actively tackle problems in a structured way (Box 10.19). It is of benefit in mild to moderate depression, and can be delivered by non-psychiatric doctors and nurses after brief training.

Psychodynamic psychotherapy

Also known as 'interpretive psychotherapy', this was pioneered by Freud, Jung and Klein amongst others. It is based upon the theory that early life experience generates

10.18 THE NEGATIVE COGNITIVE TRIAD ASSOCIATED WITH DEPRESSION

- Negative view of self, e.g. 'I am no good'
- Negative view of current life experiences, e.g. 'The world is an awful place'
- Negative view of the future, e.g. 'The future is hopeless'

10.19 STAGES OF PROBLEM-SOLVING THERAPY

- Define and list problems
- Choose one to work on
- List possible solutions
- Evaluate these and choose the best
- Try it out
- Evaluate the result

Repeat until problems are resolved.

10

powerful motivating forces, of which the patient is unconscious. Psychotherapy aims to help the patient to become aware of these unconscious factors on the assumption that, once identified, they have less effect. It uses the relationship between the therapist and the patient as a therapeutic tool; the patients' relationships with others, particularly parents, may be replicated or transferred to their relationship with the therapist. Explicit discussion of this transference is the basis for the treatment, which traditionally requires frequent sessions over a period of months or even years.

Interpersonal therapy (IPT) is a specific form of brief psychotherapy which focuses on patients' current interpersonal relationships and is an effective treatment for mild to moderate depression.

PSYCHIATRIC DISORDERS

STRESS-RELATED DISORDERS

ACUTE STRESS REACTION

Following a stressful event such as a diagnosis of AIDS or cancer, or a major accident, some people develop a characteristic pattern of symptoms. These include a sense of bewilderment, anxiety, anger, depression, increased activity or under-activity, and withdrawal. The symptoms are transient; they start to subside within a few hours and usually resolve completely within 3 days of their onset.

ADJUSTMENT DISORDER

A more common psychological response to physical illness is a less severe but more prolonged emotional reaction. The predominant symptom is usually depression and/or anxiety, which is insufficiently persistent or intense for a diagnosis of depressive or anxiety disorder. There may also be anger, aggressive behaviour and excessive alcohol use. Symptoms develop within a month of the onset of the stress, and their duration and severity reflect the course of the underlying physical condition, resolution tending to occur with physical recovery.

Grief reactions following bereavement are a particular type of adjustment disorder, which manifest as a brief period of emotional numbing, followed by a period of distress lasting several weeks, during which sorrow, tearfulness, sleep disturbance, loss of interest and a sense of futility are common. Perceptual distortions may occur, including misinterpreting sounds as the dead person's voice. 'Pathological grief' describes a grief reaction that is abnormally intense or persistent.

Management and prognosis

Ongoing contact with and support from a doctor or other who can listen, reassure, explain and advise are helpful. Most patients do not require psychotropic medication, although benzodiazepines reduce arousal in acute stress reactions and can aid sleep in adjustment disorders. Psychotherapy is required for some patients with abnormal grief reactions. These conditions usually resolve with time but

a minority of patients may develop depressive or anxiety disorders.

POST-TRAUMATIC STRESS DISORDER (PTSD)

This is a delayed and protracted response to a stressful event of an exceptionally threatening or catastrophic nature, defined as being outside the range of everyday human experience and which would cause distress in almost everyone. Examples include natural disasters, terrorist activity, serious accidents and witnessing violent deaths. PTSD may also occur after distressing medical treatments. There is usually a delay ranging from a few days to several months between the traumatic event and the onset of symptoms. Typical symptoms are recurrent intrusive memories (flashbacks) of the traumatic event, as well as sleep disturbance, nightmares (usually of the traumatic event) from which the patient awakes in a state of anxiety, symptoms of autonomic arousal, emotional blunting and avoidance of situations which evoke memories of the trauma. Anxiety and depression are associated features and excessive use of alcohol or drugs frequently complicates the clinical picture.

Management and prognosis

Immediate counselling for those who have survived a major catastrophe is unhelpful and even potentially harmful if forced on people (Box 10.20). It should therefore only be given to those who request it. The main aims are to provide support, direct advice and the opportunity for catharsis by reliving the trauma. In established PTSD, structured psychological approaches (particularly cognitive therapy) and antidepressant medication are effective. There is some evidence that a novel therapy called eye movement desensitisation and reprocessing (EMDR) is effective. The condition runs a fluctuating course, with most patients recovering within 2 years. In a small proportion the symptoms become chronic.

EBM
10.20 EARLY DEBRIEFING FOR POST-TRAUMATIC STRESS DISORDER (PTSD)
'At present the routine use of individual debriefing in the aftermath of individual trauma cannot be recommended. Early counselling has been found to be unhelpful and possibly even harmful.'
● Rose S, et al. (Cochrane Review). Cochrane Library, issue 2, 2005. Oxford: Update Software.
For further information: 🖥 www.cochrane.org

ANXIETY DISORDERS

These are characterised by the emotion of anxiety, anxious thoughts, avoidance behaviour and the somatic symptoms of sympathetic arousal. Anxiety disorders are divided into three main subtypes: phobic, paroxysmal (panic) and generalised (Box 10.21). The nature and prominence of the somatic symptoms often lead the patient to present initially to medical services. Anxiety may be stress-related and phobic anxiety may follow an unpleasant incident. Patients often also have depression.

10

10.21 CLASSIFICATION OF ANXIETY DISORDERS

	Phobic anxiety disorder	Panic disorder	Generalised anxiety disorder
Occurrence of anxiety	Situational	Paroxysmal	Persistent
Associated behaviour	Avoidance	Escape	Agitation
Associated cognitions	Fear of situation	Fear of symptoms	Worry
Somatic symptoms	On exposure	Episodic	Persistent

PHOBIC ANXIETY DISORDER

A phobia is an abnormal or excessive fear of an object or situation, which leads to avoidance of it. A generalised phobia of going out alone or being in crowded places is called agoraphobia. Phobic responses can develop to medical interventions such as venepuncture.

PANIC DISORDER

Panic disorder entails attacks of severe anxiety, which are not restricted to any particular situation or circumstances and are therefore unpredictable. Somatic symptoms such as chest pain and palpitations are common. The symptoms are in part due to involuntary over-breathing (hyperventilation). Patients often fear they are suffering from a serious illness such as a heart attack or stroke, and may therefore seek emergency medical attention. Panic disorder is often associated with agoraphobia.

GENERALISED ANXIETY DISORDER

This is chronic anxiety associated with uncontrollable worry. Somatic symptoms of muscle tension and bowel disturbance often lead to a medical presentation.

Management of anxiety disorders

Psychological treatment
Explanation and reassurance are essential, especially when patients fear they have a serious medical condition. Psychological treatments may be needed for those who do not respond, including relaxation, graded exposure (desensitisation) to feared situations for phobic disorders, and CBT for panic.

Drug treatment
Antidepressants are the drugs of choice. Benzodiazepines are useful in the short term but long-term use can lead to dependence. A β-blocker such as propranolol can help when peripheral somatic symptoms are prominent. Phobic disorders usually require graded exposure treatment as well as drug therapy.

OBSESSIVE-COMPULSIVE DISORDER

Obsessive-compulsive disorder (OCD) is characterised by obsessive thoughts which are recurrent, unwanted and usually anxiety-provoking, and by compulsions which are repeated acts that relieve feelings of tension. An example is repeated hand-washing because of thoughts of contamination. The differential diagnosis is from normal checking and from delusional beliefs. OCD is equally common in men and women.

Management and prognosis
OCD usually responds to antidepressant drugs such as clomipramine, and to CBT which helps patients expose themselves to the feared thought or situation without performing the anxiety-relieving compulsions. Relapses are common and the condition often becomes chronic.

MOOD DISORDERS

Mood or affective disorders include:

- *unipolar depression*: the patient suffers one or more episodes of lowered mood
- *bipolar disorder*: the patient also experiences episodes of elevated mood, usually but not always interspersed with episodes of depression
- *dysthymia*: describes a particularly chronic low-grade depression.

Clinically significant depression is referred to as major depressive disorder.

DEPRESSION

Major depressive disorder has a prevalence of 5–10% in the general population and up to 20% in medical patients. It is a major cause of disability and of suicide. If comorbid with a medical condition, depression magnifies disability, diminishes adherence to medical treatment and rehabilitation, and may even shorten life expectancy.

Aetiology
There is a genetic predisposition to depression, especially when of early onset, although the number and identity of the specific genes are unknown. Adverse experiences and emotional deprivation early in life also predispose to depression. Depressive episodes are often but not always triggered by adverse life events (especially those that involve loss), including medical illnesses. Associated biological factors include hypofunction of monoamine neurotransmitter systems (5-HT and noradrenaline (norepinephrine)) and abnormal hypothalamo-pituitary-adrenal axis (HPA) regulation, which results in elevated cortisol levels that do not suppress with dexamethasone. Exclusion of Cushing's syndrome is described on page 779.

10.22 POINTERS TO AN ORGANIC CAUSE FOR PSYCHIATRIC DISORDER

- Late age of onset of psychiatric illness
- No previous history of psychiatric illness
- No family history of psychiatric illness
- No apparent psychological precipitant

Diagnosis

The symptoms are listed in Box 10.8 (p. 231). It may be mild, moderate or severe, and episodic, recurrent or chronic. It can be both a complication of a medical condition, and a cause of MUS (see below), so physical examination is essential; and an associated medical condition should always be considered (Box 10.22).

Management and prognosis

There is good evidence for the efficacy of both drug and psychological treatments for depression, and in practice the choice is determined by patient preference and local availability. Severe depression complicated by psychosis, risk of starvation or intractable suicide risk may require ECT.

Drug treatment

Antidepressant drugs are effective in patients whose depression is a complication of medical illness as well as in those where it is the primary problem (Box 10.23). These agents are all effective in moderate and severe degrees of depression. Commonly used antidepressants are shown in Box 10.24.

- *Tricyclic antidepressants (TCAs).* These have well-established efficacy and are the most effective antidepressants for treating chronic pain. They inhibit the re-uptake of the amines noradrenaline (norepinephrine) and 5-HT at synaptic clefts. There is a delay of 2–3 weeks between the start of treatment and the onset of therapeutic effect. Side-effects can be particularly troublesome during this period; they include anticholinergic effects, postural hypotension, lowering of the seizure threshold and cardiotoxicity. TCAs may be dangerous in overdose and in people who have coexisting medical conditions, such as heart disease, glaucoma and prostatism.
- *Selective serotonin re-uptake inhibitors (SSRIs).* Less cardiotoxic, less sedative and with fewer anticholinergic effects than tricyclics, these can still cause headache, nausea, anorexia and sexual dysfunction.
- *Newer antidepressants.* A variety are available, including venlafaxine, mirtazapine, reboxetine and duloxetine. They have different profiles of action and adverse effects but none has been shown to be more effective than the more established agents listed above.
- *Monoamine oxidase inhibitors (MAOIs).* These increase the availability of neurotransmitters at synaptic clefts by inhibiting metabolism of noradrenaline (norepinephrine) and 5-HT. They are now rarely prescribed in the UK, but it is still important to know of their dangerous interactions with drugs such as amphetamines, and foods rich in tyramine such as cheese and red wine. Amines

10.23 ANTIDEPRESSANTS IN THE MEDICALLY ILL

EBM

'Limited trial data support the use of antidepressants in depressed patients who are also physically ill.'

- Gill D, Hatcher S. (Cochrane Review). Cochrane Library, issue 2, 2001. Oxford: Update Software.
- van Heeringen K, Zivkov M. Br J Psychiatry 1996; 169:440–443.

For further information: 💻 www.cochrane.org

10.24 ANTIDEPRESSANT DRUGS

Group	Drug	Usual dose
Tricyclics	Amitriptyline	75–150 mg daily
	Imipramine	75–150 mg daily
	Dosulepin	75–150 mg daily
	Clomipramine	75–150 mg daily
SSRIs	Citalopram	20–40 mg daily
	Escitalopram	10–20 mg daily
	Fluoxetine	20 mg daily
	Fluvoxamine	100–300 mg daily
	Sertraline	50–100 mg daily
	Paroxetine	20–50 mg daily
Monoamine oxidase inhibitors (MAOIs)	Phenelzine	45–90 mg daily
	Tranylcypromine	20–40 mg daily
	Moclobemide	300–600 mg daily
Noradrenergic re-uptake inhibitors and SSRIs	Venlafaxine	75–375 mg daily
Selective noradrenaline (norepinephrine) re-uptake inhibitor	Reboxetine	8–12 mg daily
Noradrenergic and specific serotonergic inhibitor	Mirtazapine	15–45 mg daily

accumulate in the systemic circulation causing a potentially fatal hypertensive crisis.

- *Moclobemide.* This is a reversible and selective inhibitor of monoamine oxidase subtype A, which causes minimal potentiation of the pressor response to dietary tyramine.

The various antidepressant agents are equally effective and about three-quarters of patients will respond to treatment. Successful treatment requires the patient to take an appropriate dose of an effective drug for an adequate period. Improvement may take 2–4 weeks. The patient's progress must be monitored and, after recovery, treatment should be continued for at least 6 months to reduce the high risk of relapse; the dose should then be tapered off over several weeks to avoid discontinuation symptoms. In England and Wales, NICE guidelines help with the choice of an antidepressant regimen (www.nice.org.uk).

Psychological treatments

Both CBT and interpersonal therapy are as effective as antidepressants for mild to moderately severe depression. Antidepressant drugs are, however, preferred for more severe depression. Drug and psychological treatments can be used in combination.

Over 50% of people who have had one depressive episode and over 90% of people who have had three or more

10

episodes will have another. The risk of suicide in an individual who has had a depressive disorder is ten times greater than in the general population.

BIPOLAR DISORDER (MANIC DEPRESSION)

Bipolar disorder is a relapsing mood disturbance with periods of both depressed and elevated mood, known as hypomania, or mania when severe. The typical age of onset and lifetime risk of 1% are similar to those of schizophrenia.

Aetiology

The aetiology is largely genetic and bipolar disorder is strongly heritable (80%). Relatives of someone with bipolar disorder have an increased incidence of both bipolar and unipolar depressive disorder. Life events, physical illness and prescribed drugs may play a role in triggering episodes.

Diagnosis

Isolated episodes of mania/hypomania do occur but they are usually followed by an episode of depression. Psychosis may occur in both the depressive and the manic phases, with delusions and hallucinations that are usually in keeping with the mood disturbance. This is described as an affective psychosis. Patients who present with symptoms of both bipolar disorder and schizophrenia may be given a diagnosis of schizoaffective disorder.

Management and prognosis

Depression is treated as described above. Manic episodes usually respond well to antipsychotic drugs (Box 10.27). Prophylaxis to prevent recurrent episodes is important. The main drugs used are lithium, carbamazepine and sodium valproate. Caution must be exercised when stopping these as a relapse may follow.

- *Lithium carbonate* is the drug of choice. It is also used for acute mania, and in combination with a tricyclic as an adjuvant treatment for resistant depression. It has a narrow therapeutic range so regular blood monitoring is required to maintain a serum level of 0.5–1.0 mmol/l. Toxic effects include nausea, vomiting, tremor and convulsions. With long-term treatment, weight gain, hypothyroidism, nephrogenic diabetes insipidus (p. 796) and renal failure can occur. Thyroid and renal function should be checked before treatment is started and every 6 months thereafter. Lithium has a significant teratogenic effect and should never be prescribed during the first trimester of pregnancy.
- *Carbamazepine* and *sodium valproate* are established anticonvulsant drugs that have been used successfully as prophylaxis in bipolar disorder, usually as second-line alternatives to lithium. Common side-effects with carbamazepine are drowsiness, ataxia, headache, rashes and nausea; with valproate, nausea, ataxia and tremor.

The relapse rate is very high, although patients may be perfectly well between episodes. After one episode the annual average risk of relapse is about 10–15%, and after more than three episodes the annual average risk of relapse is about 20–30%. There is a substantially increased life-time risk of suicide.

SCHIZOPHRENIA

Schizophrenia is a psychosis characterised by delusions, hallucinations and lack of insight. Acute schizophrenia may present with disturbed behaviour, marked delusions, hallucinations and disordered thinking, or with insidious social withdrawal and less obvious delusions and hallucinations. The prevalence is similar world-wide at about 1% and the disorder is equally common in men and women. The children of one affected parent have approximately a 10% risk of developing the illness, but this rises to 50% if both parents are affected. Schizophrenia can present at any age but does so most commonly in young adults.

Aetiology

Schizophrenia was traditionally described as a 'functional' as opposed to 'organic' psychosis, because examination of the brain indicated no apparent pathology. However, modern forms of brain imaging have identified minor structural abnormalities, including an enlargement of the lateral ventricles and an overall decrease in brain size with relatively greater reduction in temporal lobe volume. There is evidence of a genetic contribution, probably involving many susceptibility genes, each of small effect. These interact with environmental influences such as urban birth, low social class, obstetric complications and other insults to the brain in early life. Episodes of acute schizophrenia may be precipitated by social stressors. Consequently, schizophrenia is now viewed as a neuro-developmental disorder, caused by abnormalities of brain development associated with genetic predisposition and early environmental influences, and triggered by stress.

Diagnosis

Schizophrenia usually presents with an acute episode and may progress to a chronic state. Acute schizophrenia should be suspected in any individual with bizarre behaviour accompanied by delusions and hallucinations, that is not due to organic brain disease or substance misuse. The diagnosis is made on clinical grounds with investigations used principally to rule out organic brain disease. The characteristic clinical features include symptoms described originally by Schneider as of the 'first rank' in importance when making the diagnosis (Box 10.25). Hallucinations are typically auditory, although they can occur in any sensory modality. They are commonly of voices heard outside the head that talk to or about the person. Sometimes the voices repeat the person's thoughts. Patients may also describe 'passivity of thought'; this is experienced as disturbances of the normal private boundary of thinking, and expressed in the belief that their thoughts are being broadcast to others and thoughts that are not their own are being 'inserted' into or 'withdrawn' from their mind. Other first-rank symptoms are delusions of control, and believing that one's emotions, impulses or acts are controlled by others. Another characteristic phenomenon is delusional perception, a delusional belief which arises suddenly in association with a perception (e.g. 'I saw the moon and I immediately knew

10.25 SYMPTOMS OF SCHIZOPHRENIA

First-rank symptoms of acute schizophrenia

- A = Auditory hallucinations—second or third person/écho de la pensée
- B = Broadcasting, insertion/withdrawal of thoughts
- C = Controlled feelings, impulses or acts ('passivity' experiences/ phenomena)
- D = Delusional perception (a particular experience is bizarrely interpreted)

Symptoms of chronic schizophrenia (negative symptoms)

- Flattened (blunted) affect
- Apathy and loss of drive (avolition)
- Social isolation
- Poverty of speech
- Poor self-care

10.26 DIFFERENTIAL DIAGNOSIS OF SCHIZOPHRENIA

Alternative diagnosis	Distinguishing features
Other functional psychoses	
Delusional disorders	Absence of specific features of schizophrenia
Psychotic depression	Prominent depressive symptoms
Manic episode	Prominent manic symptoms
Schizoaffective disorder	Mood and schizophrenia symptoms both prominent
Puerperal psychosis	Acute onset after childbirth
Organic disorders	
Drug-induced psychosis	Evidence of drug or alcohol misuse
Side-effects of prescribed drugs	Levodopa, methyldopa, corticosteroids, anti-malarial drugs
Temporal lobe epilepsy	Other evidence of seizures
Delirium	Visual hallucinations; impaired consciousness
Dementia	Age; established cognitive impairment
Huntington's disease	Family history; choreiform movements; dementia

10.27 ANTIPSYCHOTIC DRUGS

Group	Drug	Usual dose
Phenothiazines	Chlorpromazine	100–1500 mg daily
	Trifluoperazine	5–30 mg daily
	Fluphenazine	20–100 mg fortnightly
Butyrophenones	Haloperidol	5–30 mg daily
Thioxanthenes	Flupentixol	40–200 mg fortnightly
Diphenylbutylpiperidines	Pimozide	4–30 mg daily
Substituted benzamides	Sulpiride	600–1800 mg daily
Dibenzodiazepine*	Clozapine	25–900 mg daily
Benzisoxazole*	Risperidone	2–16 mg daily
Thienobenzodiazepines*	Olanzapine	5–20 mg daily

*Atypical antipsychotics.

he was evil'). In addition to these so-called 'first-rank' symptoms, many others may occur. These include thought disorder manifest by incomprehensible speech, and abnormalities of movement in which the patient can become immobile or adopt awkward postures for prolonged periods (catatonia).

The main differential diagnosis of schizophrenia is from:

- Other functional psychoses, particularly psychotic depression and mania, in which delusions and hallucinations are congruent with a marked mood disturbance (negative in depression and grandiose in mania). If it is impossible to differentiate schizophrenia from affective disorder, the diagnosis of schizoaffective disorder is made. Schizophrenia must also be differentiated from specific delusional disorders that are not associated with the other typical features of schizophrenia (Box 10.26).
- Organic psychoses including delirium, in which there is impairment of consciousness and loss of orientation with typically visual hallucinations and drug misuse, the latter particularly in young people. Schizophrenia must also be differentiated from more specific organic psychoses such as temporal lobe epilepsy, in which olfactory hallucinations and distortion of visual perception may occur (Box 10.26).

Some of those who develop acute schizophrenia go on to develop a chronic state. The acute so-called positive symptoms resolve, or at least do not dominate the clinical picture, leaving so-called negative symptoms which include blunted mood, apathy, social isolation, poverty of speech and poor self-care. Patients with chronic schizophrenia may also manifest positive symptoms, particularly when under stress, and it can be difficult for those who do not know the patient to judge whether or not these are signs of an acute relapse.

Management

Acute schizophrenia usually requires admission to hospital because patients lack insight that they are ill and are unwilling to accept drug treatment. In some cases, they may be at risk of harming themselves or others. Chronic schizophrenia is commonly managed in the community.

Drug treatment

Antipsychotic agents (also called neuroleptics or major tranquillisers) are effective against the positive symptoms of schizophrenia in the majority of cases. They take 2–3 weeks to be maximally effective, but have some beneficial effects shortly after administration. Once symptoms have been controlled, treatment with antipsychotic medication is usually continued to prevent relapse. In a patient with a first episode of schizophrenia, this will usually be for 1–2 years, but in patients with multiple psychotic episodes, treatment may be required for many years. The benefits of prolonged treatment must be weighed against the adverse effects, which include tardive dyskinesia (abnormal movements commonly of the face, over which the patient has no voluntary control). For long-term use, antipsychotic agents are often given in slow-release (depot) injected form to improve patient adherence.

There are a number of antipsychotic agents available (Box 10.27). These may be divided into conventional

10

(typical, first-generation) drugs such as chlorpromazine and haloperidol, and newer or atypical (also so-called novel or second-generation) drugs such as clozapine. All are believed to work by blocking D_2 dopamine receptors in the brain. Patients who have not responded to conventional drugs may respond to newer agents, which are also less likely to produce unwanted extrapyramidal side-effects but do tend to cause greater weight gain. Clozapine can also cause an agranulocytosis and consequently requires regular monitoring of the white blood cell count, initially on a weekly basis. Details of the side-effects of antipsychotic drugs are listed in Box 10.28.

Serious adverse effects of antipsychotic drugs include:

- *Neuroleptic malignant syndrome*, which is uncommon but serious. It is characterised by fever, tremor and rigidity, and confusion. Characteristic laboratory findings are an elevated creatinine phosphokinase and leucocytosis. Antipsychotic medication must be immediately stopped and supportive therapy provided, often in an intensive care unit. Treatment includes ensuring hydration and reducing hyperthermia. Dantrolene sodium and bromocriptine may be helpful. Mortality is 20% untreated and 5% with treatment.
- *Prolongation of the QT_c interval*, which may be associated with ventricular tachycardia, torsades de pointes and sudden death. Treatment is by stopping the drug, monitoring the ECG and treating serious arrhythmias (p. 560).

Psychological treatment

Psychological treatment, including general support for the patient and his or her family, is now seen as an essential component of the therapeutic plan. CBT may help patients to cope with their symptoms and also to adhere to treatment with antipsychotic drugs. There is good evidence that family education reduces the rate of relapse while family therapy may help a patient to live with other members of the family.

Social treatment

After an acute episode of schizophrenia has been controlled by drug therapy, social and occupational rehabilitation is required. The illness is likely to have caused major disruption to patients' relationships and their ability to manage their previous accommodation and occupation. They will consequently need help to obtain housing and employment and to re-establish a social network. A graded return to employment and sometimes a period of sheltered accommodation are required.

Patients with chronic or recurrent schizophrenia have particular difficulties. They may need long-term sheltered accommodation. This was previously provided in mental hospitals but now tends to be in supervised accommodation in the community. They may also require sheltered employment if they are unable to participate effectively in the labour market. Ongoing contact with a health worker allows monitoring for signs of relapse so that treatment can be administered early. This is sometimes called 'assertive outreach', with multidisciplinary teams working to agreed plans (a 'care programme approach'). Partly because of a tendency to inactivity, smoking and a poor diet, patients with chronic schizophrenia are at increased risk of cardiovascular disease, diabetes and tuberculosis, and require medical as well as psychiatric care.

Prognosis

About a quarter of those who develop an acute schizophrenic episode have a good outcome. A third deteriorate to chronic schizophrenia, and the remainder recover after each episode but suffer relapses. Prophylactic treatment with antipsychotic drugs reduces the rate of relapse in the first 2 years after an episode of schizophrenia from 70% to 40%. Schizophrenia is associated with suicide, 1 in 10 patients taking their own lives.

ALCOHOL MISUSE AND DEPENDENCE

Alcohol consumption associated with social, psychological and physical problems constitutes harmful use. The criteria for alcohol dependence, a more restricted term, are shown in Box 10.29. Approximately one-quarter of male patients in general hospital medical wards in the UK have a current or previous alcohol problem.

Aetiology

Availability of alcohol and social patterns of use appear to be the most important factors. Genetic factors may play

---

10.28 SIDE-EFFECTS OF ANTIPSYCHOTIC DRUGS

Weight gain due to increased appetite

Effects due to dopamine blockade*
- Parkinsonism
- Akathisia (motor restlessness)
- Acute dystonia
- Tardive dyskinesia
- Gynaecomastia
- Galactorrhoea

Effects due to cholinergic blockade
- Dry mouth
- Blurred vision
- Constipation
- Urinary retention
- Impotence

Hypersensitivity reactions
- Cholestatic jaundice
- Photosensitive dermatitis
- Blood dyscrasias (neutropenia with clozapine)

Ocular complications (long-term use)
- Corneal and lens opacities

* Less severe with clozapine, risperidone and olanzapine because of strong 5-HT-blocking effect and relatively weak dopamine blockade.

10.29 CRITERIA FOR ALCOHOL DEPENDENCE

- Narrowing of the drinking repertoire (restriction to one type of alcohol, e.g. spirits)
- Priority of drinking over other activities (salience)
- Tolerance of effects of alcohol
- Repeated withdrawal symptoms
- Relief of withdrawal symptoms by further drinking
- Subjective compulsion to drink
- Reinstatement of drinking behaviour after abstinence

some part in predisposition to dependence. The majority of alcoholics do not have an associated psychiatric illness, but a few drink heavily in an attempt to relieve anxiety or depression.

Diagnosis

Alcohol misuse may emerge during the patient's history, although patients may minimise their intake. It may also present via its effects on one or more aspects of the patient's life, listed below. Alcohol dependence commonly presents with withdrawal in those admitted to hospital, as they can no longer maintain their high alcohol intake in this setting.

Complications of chronic alcohol misuse

Social problems include absenteeism from work, unemployment, marital tensions, child abuse, financial difficulties and problems with the law, such as violence and traffic offences.

Psychological problems

- *Depression* is common and is usually reactive to the numerous social problems which heavy drinking creates. Alcohol also has a direct depressant effect. Attempted suicide and completed suicide are often associated with alcohol misuse.
- *Anxiety* is relieved by alcohol. People who are socially anxious may consequently use alcohol in this way and may develop dependence. Conversely, alcohol withdrawal increases anxiety.
- *Alcoholic hallucinosis* is a rare condition in which alcoholic individuals experience auditory hallucination in clear consciousness.
- *Alcohol withdrawal* is described in Box 10.30. Symptoms usually become maximal about 2 days after the last drink, and can include seizures ('rum fits').
- *Delirium tremens* is a form of delirium associated with severe alcohol withdrawal. It has a significant mortality and morbidity (Box 10.30).

Effects on the brain

The familiar features of drunkenness are ataxia, slurred speech, emotional incontinence and aggression. Very heavy drinkers may experience periods of amnesia for events which occurred during bouts of intoxication, termed 'alcoholic blackouts'. Established alcoholism may lead to alcoholic dementia, a global cognitive impairment resembling Alzheimer's disease, but which does not progress if the patient becomes abstinent. Indirect effects on behaviour can result from head injury, hypoglycaemia and portosystemic encephalopathy (p. 950).

A rare but important effect of chronic alcohol misuse is the Wernicke–Korsakoff syndrome. This organic brain disorder results from damage to the mamillary bodies, dorsomedial nuclei of the thalamus and adjacent areas of grey matter. It is caused by a deficiency of thiamin (vitamin B_1), which is most commonly caused by long-standing heavy drinking and an inadequate diet. Without prompt treatment (see below), the acute presentation of Wernicke's encephalopathy (nystagmus, ophthalmoplegia, ataxia and confusion) can progress to the irreversible deficits of Korsakoff's syndrome (severe short-term memory deficits and confabulation). In those who die in the acute stage,

---

10.30 CONSEQUENCES OF CHRONIC ALCOHOL MISUSE

Acute intoxication

- Emotional and behavioural disturbance
- Medical problems: hypoglycaemia, aspiration of vomit, respiratory depression
- Complicating other medical problems
- Accidents, and injuries sustained in fights

Withdrawal phenomena

- Psychological symptoms: restlessness, anxiety, panic attacks
- Autonomic symptoms: tachycardia, sweating, pupil dilation, nausea, vomiting
- Delirium tremens: agitation, hallucinations, illusions, delusions
- Seizures

Harmful use

MEDICAL CONSEQUENCES

Neurological
- Peripheral neuropathy
- Cerebellar degeneration
- Cerebral haemorrhage
- Dementia

Hepatic
- Fatty change and cirrhosis
- Liver cancer

Gastrointestinal
- Oesophagitis, gastritis
- Pancreatitis
- Oesophageal cancer
- Mallory–Weiss syndrome
- Malabsorption
- Oesophageal varices

Respiratory
- Pulmonary TB
- Pneumonia

Skin
- Spider naevi
- Palmar erythema
- Duypuytren's contractures
- Telangiectasiae

Cardiac
- Cardiomyopathy
- Hypertension

Musculoskeletal
- Myopathy
- Fractures

Endocrine and metabolic
- Pseudo-Cushing's syndrome
- Hypoglycaemia
- Gout

Reproductive
- Hypogonadism
- Fetal alcohol syndrome
- Infertility

PSYCHIATRIC AND CEREBRAL CONSEQUENCES
- Depression
- Alcoholic hallucinosis
- Alcoholic 'blackouts'
- Wernicke's encephalopathy: nystagmus, opthalmoplegia, ataxia, confusion
- Korsakoff's syndrome: short-term memory deficits, confabulation

---

microscopic examination of the brain shows hyperaemia, petechial haemorrhages and astrocytic proliferation.

Effects on other organs

These are protean and virtually any organ (Box 10.30) can be involved; alcohol has replaced syphilis as the great mimic of disease. These effects are discussed in detail in the relevant chapters.

Management and prognosis

Advice about the harmful effects of alcohol and safe levels of consumption is often all that is needed. In more

10

serious cases, patients may have to be advised to alter leisure activities or change jobs if these are contributing to the problem. Supportive psychotherapy is often crucial in helping the patient make the necessary changes in lifestyle. Psychological treatment is used for patients who have recurrent relapses and is usually available at specialised centres. Support is also provided by voluntary organisations such as Alcoholics Anonymous (AA) in the UK.

If alcohol dependence is suspected, withdrawal syndromes can be prevented, or treated once established, with benzodiazepines. Large doses may be required (e.g. diazepam 20 mg 6-hourly), tailed off over a period of 5–7 days as symptoms subside. Prevention of the Wernicke–Korsakoff complex requires the immediate use of high doses of thiamin, which may be given parenterally in the form of Pabrinex (p. 1218). There is no treatment for Korsakoff's syndrome once it has arisen. The risk of side-effects, such as respiratory depression with benzodiazepines and anaphylaxis with Pabrinex, is small when weighed against the risks of no treatment.

Disulfiram (200–400 mg daily) can be given as a deterrent to patients who have difficulty resisting the impulse to drink after becoming abstinent. It blocks the metabolism of alcohol, causing acetaldehyde to accumulate. When alcohol is consumed, an unpleasant reaction follows with headache, flushing and nausea. Disulfiram is always an adjunct to other treatments, especially supportive psychotherapy. Acamprosate (666 mg 8-hourly) has recently been introduced to maintain abstinence by reducing the craving for alcohol. Only rarely are antidepressants required; depressive symptoms, if present, usually resolve with abstinence. Antipsychotics (e.g. chlorpromazine 100 mg 8-hourly) are required for alcoholic hallucinosis.

Many but not all who become dependent on alcohol relapse after treatment. Chronic alcohol misuse greatly increases the risk of death from accidents, disease and suicide.

SUBSTANCE MISUSE DISORDER

Dependence on and misuse of both illegal and prescribed drugs is a major problem world-wide. Drugs of misuse are described in detail in Chapter 9. They can be grouped as follows.

Sedatives
These commonly give rise to physical dependence, the manifestations being tolerance and a withdrawal syndrome. They include benzodiazepines, opiates (including morphine, heroin, methadone and dihydrocodeine) and barbiturates (now rarely prescribed). Overdosage can be dangerous with the opiates and benzodiazepines, primarily as a result of respiratory depression (Ch. 9). Withdrawal from opiates is notoriously unpleasant, and withdrawal from benzodiazepines (Box 10.31) and barbiturates may be dangerous because of seizures.

Intravenous opiate users are prone to bacterial infections, hepatitis B, hepatitis C (pp. 963–968) and HIV infection (Ch. 14) through needle contamination. Accidental overdose

10.31 BENZODIAZEPINE WITHDRAWAL SYMPTOMS

- Anxiety
- Heightened sensory perception
- Hallucinations
- Epileptic seizures
- Ataxia
- Paranoid delusions

is common, mainly because of the varied and uncertain potency of illicit supplies of the drug. The withdrawal syndrome, which can start within 12 hours of the drug's last use, presents with intense craving, rhinorrhoea, lacrimation, yawning, perspiration, shivering, piloerection, vomiting, diarrhoea and abdominal cramps. Examination reveals tachycardia, hypertension, mydriasis and facial flushing.

Stimulants
These include amphetamines and cocaine. They are less dangerous than the sedatives in overdose, although they can cause cardiac and cerebrovascular problems through their pressor effects. With prolonged heavy use, psychiatric disturbance can be prominent. Physical dependence syndromes do not arise, but withdrawal causes a rebound lowering in mood and can give rise to an intense craving for further use, especially in any form of drug with a rapid onset and offset of effect such as crack cocaine. Chronic amphetamine ingestion can cause a syndrome identical to paranoid schizophrenia. A toxic psychosis occurs with high levels of cocaine consumption, and tactile hallucinations (formication) may be prominent.

Hallucinogens
The hallucinogens are a disparate group of drugs that cause changes in mood and prominent sensory experiences. They include cannabis, ecstasy, lysergic acid diethylamide (LSD) and *Psilocybin* (magic mushrooms).

A toxic confusional state can occur after heavy cannabis consumption. Acute psychotic episodes are well recognised, especially in those with a family or personal history of psychotic illness, and there is evidence that prolonged heavy use increases the risk of developing schizophrenia. Paranoid psychoses have been reported in association with ecstasy. Flashback experiences can occur several months after the last dose of LSD, when the psychotic experiences are relived with their original intensity. A chronic psychotic illness has also been reported after regular LSD use.

Organic solvents
Solvent inhalation (glue sniffing) is popular in some adolescent groups. Solvents produce acute intoxication characterised by euphoria, excitement, dizziness and a floating sensation. Further inhalation leads to loss of consciousness; death can occur from the direct toxic effect of the solvent, or from asphyxiation if the substance is inhaled from a plastic bag.

Aetiology
Many of the aetiological factors for alcohol misuse also apply to drug dependence. The main factors are cultural pressures, particularly within a peer group, and availability of a drug. In the case of some drugs, medical over-

prescribing has increased their availability, but there has also been a relative decline in the price of illegal drugs. Many drug users take a range of drugs—so-called polydrug misuse.

Diagnosis

As with alcohol, the diagnosis either may be apparent from the history, or may only be made once the patient presents with a complication. Drug screening of samples of urine or blood can be very valuable in confirming the diagnosis, especially if the patient persists in denial.

Management and prognosis

The first step is to determine whether patients wish to stop using the drug. If not, they need advice about harm minimisation: for example, advice to use clean needles for those who inject. For those who are physically dependent on sedative drugs, substitute prescribing (using methadone, for example, in opiate dependence) may help stabilise the chaos in their lives sufficiently to allow a gradual reduction in dosage until they reach abstinence. Some specialist units offer inpatient detoxification. For details on the medical management of overdose, see Chapter 9.

The drug lofexidine, a centrally acting α-agonist, can be useful in treating the autonomic symptoms of opiate withdrawal, as can clonidine, although this carries a risk of hypotension and is best used by specialists. Long-acting opiate antagonists such as naltrexone may also have a place, again in specialist hands, in blocking the euphoriant effects of the opiate, which may aid in breaking patterns of addiction.

In some cases complete opiate withdrawal is not successful and the patient functions better if maintained on regular doses of oral methadone as an outpatient. This decision should only be taken by a specialist, and long-term supervision requires the patient to attend a specialist drug treatment centre.

Substitute prescribing is neither necessary nor possible for the hallucinogens and stimulants, so the principles of management are the same as those that should accompany prescribing for the sedatives. These include identifying problems associated with the drug misuse which may serve to maintain it, and intervening where possible. Intervention may be directed at physical ill health, psychiatric comorbidity, social problems or family disharmony.

Relapsing patients and those with complications should be referred to specialist drug misuse services. Support can also be provided by self-help groups and voluntary bodies such as Narcotics Anonymous in the UK.

DELIRIUM, DEMENTIA AND ORGANIC DISORDERS

Delirium, dementia and other organic problems are primarily medical conditions rather than psychiatric disorders. Nevertheless they are included in psychiatric classifications and sometimes misdiagnosed as mental illnesses.

DELIRIUM (ACUTE CONFUSIONAL STATE, ACUTE ORGANIC BRAIN SYNDROME OR ENCEPHALOPATHY)

Delirium is common in acute medical settings, affecting more than half of patients in high-dependency and intensive care units. Aetiology, assessment and management are described in Chapters 26 and 7.

DEMENTIA (CHRONIC ORGANIC BRAIN SYNDROME)

Dementia affects 5% of those over 65 and 20% of those over 85. It is defined as a global impairment of cognitive function, and although memory is most affected in the early stages, deficits in visuo-spatial function, language ability, concentration and attention gradually become apparent. Aetiology and investigation are described in Chapter 26. Management is essentially symptomatic and supportive. The anticholinesterase inhibitors such as donepezil may arrest progression for a time in Alzheimer-type dementia, while addressing the underlying vascular risk factors may slow deterioration in vascular dementia, but neither can be reversed. Psychotropic drugs may help where there is associated disturbance of sleep, perception or mood, but should be used with care, especially since emerging evidence shows increased mortality when the atypical antipsychotics are used. Sedation is not a substitute for good community support for patients and carers or, in the later stages, attentive residential nursing care. In the UK incapacity and mental health legislation may be required to manage patients' financial and domestic affairs, as well as to determine safe placement. Most dementias have a progressive course, which may be gradual (as in Alzheimer's disease) or step-wise (as in vascular dementia).

PERSONALITY DISORDERS

Personality is the set of behavioural traits which best describes any given individual and their patterns of interaction with the world. Behavioural traits are enduring tendencies to behave in particular ways. The intensity of particular traits varies from person to person, although many, such as shyness or irritability, are displayed to some degree by most people.

A personality disorder is diagnosed when an individual's personality causes persistent and severe problems for the person themselves, those around them or society in general. For example, shyness may be so pronounced that the individual never ventures into any situation where he/she fears scrutiny, so that his/her life becomes narrow and empty. Psychopathic or antisocial personality disorder describes a persistent pattern of behaviour characterised by a lack of concern for others. This may manifest as repeatedly breaking the law, disregard for safety and a lack of guilt concerning the adverse effects of one's actions on others.

Personality disorder is classified into 8–10 types (such as emotionally unstable, antisocial or schizotypal), depending on the particular behavioural traits in question. There are differences between ICD-10 and DSM-IV classifications, and there have been repeated changes to these. A patient who meets diagnostic criteria for one subtype commonly meets criteria for two or three others. As allocation to one particular subtype gives little guidance to management or prognosis, classification is of limited value. Personality disorder commonly accompanies other psychiatric conditions, making treatment of those conditions more difficult and therefore affecting their prognosis.

Aetiology

Some personality disorders are inherited to a degree but most are more clearly related to an unsatisfactory upbringing and childhood abuse.

Management and prognosis

Personality disorder is largely untreatable. There is little evidence of benefit from psychotropics, and limited evidence for the value of psychotherapy. Any such treatment has to be intensive and/or long-term if it is to effect any substantial change, which means it is unlikely to be available or acceptable to the large numbers of patients to whom the diagnosis may apply. By definition, personality disorders tend to persist throughout life, although they may become less extreme with age.

EATING DISORDERS

There are two well-defined eating disorders, anorexia nervosa (AN) and bulimia nervosa (BN), which share some overlapping features. Ninety per cent of cases are female. There is a much higher prevalence of abnormal eating behaviour in the population which does not meet diagnostic criteria for AN or BN, and a higher prevalence still of obesity, which is usually considered to be more a disorder of lifestyle or physiology than psychology.

ANOREXIA NERVOSA

There is marked weight loss, arising from food avoidance, often in combination with bingeing, purging, excessive exercise, or the use of diuretics and laxatives. Occasionally more extreme measures such as blood-letting are encountered. There is profound body image disturbance so that, despite their emaciation, patients still feel overweight and are terrified of weight gain. These preoccupations are intense and pervasive, and the false beliefs at times held with a conviction approaching the delusional. Anxiety and depressive symptoms are common accompaniments. Downy hair (lanugo) may develop on the back, forearms and cheeks. Extreme starvation is associated with a wide range of physiological and pathological bodily changes. All organ systems may be affected, although the most serious problems are cardiac and skeletal (Box 10.32).

Aetiology

This is unknown but probably includes genetic and environmental factors, including social pressure on women to be thin.

10.32 PHYSICAL CONSEQUENCES OF EATING DISORDERS

Cardiac

- ECG abnormalities: T wave inversion, ST depression and prolonged QTc interval
- Arrhythmias, including profound sinus bradycardia and ventricular tachycardia

Haematological

- Anaemia, thrombocytopenia and leucopenia

Endocrine

- Pubertal delay or arrest
- Growth retardation and short stature
- Amenorrhoea
- Sick euthyroid state

Metabolic

- Uraemia
- Renal calculi
- Impaired bone mineralisation with osteoporosis

Gastrointestinal

- Constipation
- Abnormal liver function tests

10.33 DIAGNOSTIC CRITERIA FOR EATING DISORDERS

Anorexia nervosa

- Weight loss of at least 15% of total body weight (or body mass index ≤17.5)
- Avoidance of high-calorie foods
- Distortion of body image so that patients regard themselves as fat even when grossly underweight
- Amenorrhoea for at least 3 months

Bulimia nervosa

- Recurrent bouts of binge eating
- Lack of self-control over eating during binges
- Self-induced vomiting, purgation or dieting after binges
- Weight maintained within normal limits

Diagnosis

The condition usually emerges in adolescence, with a marked female preponderance. Diagnostic criteria are shown in Box 10.33. Differential diagnosis includes other causes of weight loss including psychiatric disorders such as depression, and medical conditions such as inflammatory bowel disease, malabsorption, hypopituitarism and cancer. The diagnosis is made on the presence of a pronounced fear of fatness despite being thin, and on the absence of alternative causes of weight loss.

Management and prognosis

The aims of management are to ensure the patient's physical well-being, whilst helping her to increase her weight to the normal range by addressing abnormal beliefs and behaviour. This requires a good therapeutic relationship. Treatment is usually given on an outpatient basis, inpatient treatment being indicated only if weight loss is intractable

10

and severe (for example, less than 65% of normal), or if there is a risk of death from medical complications or from suicide. There is a limited evidence base for treatment, although individual psychological treatments, particularly CBT and family therapy, are used. Psychotropic drugs are of little benefit except in those with clear-cut comorbid depressive disorder.

Weight gain is best managed in a collaborative fashion. Compulsory admission and re-feeding (including tube feeding) are very occasionally resorted to when patients are at risk of death and other measures have failed. Whilst this may produce a short-term improvement in weight, it probably does not change long-term prognosis. About 20% of patients with anorexia nervosa have a good outcome, a further 20% develop a chronic intractable disorder and the rest have an intermediate outcome. There is a long-term mortality rate of 10–20%, either due to the complications of starvation or from suicide.

BULIMIA NERVOSA

In bulimia nervosa, patients are usually at or near normal weight (unlike in AN), but display a morbid fear of fatness. Despite this they recurrently embark on eating binges, often followed by corrective measures such as self-induced vomiting. The prevalence is similar to or slightly greater than that of AN, but only a small proportion of sufferers reach treatment services.

Diagnosis
BN usually begins later in adolescence than AN, and is even more predominantly a female malady. Diagnostic criteria are shown in Box 10.33. Physical signs of repeated self-induced vomiting include pitted teeth (from gastric acid), calluses on knuckles and parotid gland enlargement. There are many associated physical complications including the dental and oesophageal consequences of repeated vomiting, as well as electrolyte abnormalities, cardiac arrhythmias and renal problems (Box 10.32).

Management and prognosis
CBT achieves short- and long-term improvements. Guided self-help and interpersonal psychotherapy may also be of value. There is also evidence for benefit from the SSRI fluoxetine, although high doses (60 mg daily) and long courses (1 year) are required; this appears to be independent of the antidepressant effect.

Bulimia does not carry the mortality associated with AN, and few sufferers 'cross over' to anorexia. At 10 years, approximately 10% are still unwell, 20% have a subclinical degree of BN, and the remainder have recovered.

SOMATOFORM DISORDERS

The essential feature of these disorders is somatic symptoms which are not explained by a medical condition and not better diagnosed as part of a depressive or anxiety disorder. Several syndromes are described within this category; there is considerable overlap between them in both aetiology and clinical presentation.

Aetiology
The cause of somatoform disorders is incompletely understood but contributory factors include depression or anxiety, the erroneous interpretation of somatic symptoms as evidence of disease, and preoccupation with physical illness. A family history or previous history of a particular condition may have shaped concerns about illness. Patients may selectively emphasise somatic symptoms to doctors because they do not want to accept their problems as psychiatric. A doctor who either dismisses the complaints as non-existent or over-emphasises the possibility of disease may unwittingly reinforce the patient's concerns about illness.

SOMATISATION DISORDER (BRIQUET'S SYNDROME)

This syndrome runs a chronic and fluctuating course over many years. Symptoms start in early adult life and may be referred to any part of the body. It is much more common in women. Common complaints include pain, vomiting, nausea, headache, dizziness, menstrual irregularities and sexual dysfunction. Patients may undergo a multitude of negative investigations and unhelpful operations, particularly hysterectomy and cholecystectomy. There is no proven treatment but minimisation of iatrogenic harm is important.

HYPOCHONDRIACAL DISORDER

Patients with hypochondriasis have a fear or belief that they have a serious, often fatal, disease that persists despite appropriate medical reassurance. They characteristically seek many medical opinions and investigations in a futile attempt to gain reassurance. CBT may be helpful. The condition may become chronic.

In a small proportion of cases, the conviction that disease is present reaches delusional intensity, the best-known example being that of parasitic infestation ('delusional parasitosis'), which leads patients to consult dermatologists. Antipsychotic medication may be effective.

BODY DYSMORPHIC DISORDER

This describes a preoccupation with bodily shape or appearance, with the belief that one is disfigured in some way (previously known as dysmorphophobia). People with this condition may make inappropriate requests for cosmetic surgery. CBT may be helpful. The belief in disfigurement may sometimes be delusional and in such cases treatment with antipsychotic drugs may help.

SOMATOFORM AUTONOMIC DYSFUNCTION

This describes somatic symptoms referable to bodily organs which are largely under the control of the autonomic nervous system. The most common examples involve the cardiovascular system (cardiac neurosis), respiratory system (psychogenic hyperventilation) and gut (psychogenic

10

vomiting and irritable bowel syndrome). Antidepressant drugs and CBT may be helpful.

SOMATOFORM PAIN DISORDER

This describes severe, persistent pain which cannot be explained by a medical condition. Antidepressant drugs (especially tricyclics and dual action drugs such as duloxetine and mirtazapine) are helpful, as are some of the anticonvulsant drugs, particularly carbamazepine and gabapentin. CBT and multidisciplinary pain management teams are also useful.

NEURASTHENIA (CHRONIC FATIGUE SYNDROME)

Neurasthenia is characterised by excessive fatigue after minimal physical or mental exertion, poor concentration, dizziness, muscular aches and sleep disturbance. This pattern of symptoms may follow a viral infection such as infectious mononucleosis, influenza or hepatitis. Symptoms overlap considerably with those of depression and anxiety. There is evidence that many patients improve with carefully graded exercise and CBT.

DISSOCIATIVE (CONVERSION) DISORDER

This has replaced the term 'hysteria' in the ICD-10 classification. It is characterised by a loss or distortion of neurological function not fully explained by organic disease. The most common symptoms mimic lesions in the motor or sensory nervous system (Box 10.34). Dissociative disorder can also involve psychological functions, especially memory and general intelligence. The aetiology of dissociation is unknown. It has been considered to be the result of unconscious psychological processes and there is an association with adverse childhood experiences including physical and sexual abuse. Organic disease may facilitate dissociative mechanisms and provide a model for symptoms; thus, for example, non-epileptic seizures may occur in those with epilepsy. Coexisting depression should be treated with CBT or antidepressant drugs.

10.34 COMMON PRESENTATIONS OF DISSOCIATIVE (CONVERSION) DISORDER

- Gait disturbance
- Loss of function in limbs
- Aphonia
- Non-epileptic seizures
- Sensory loss
- Blindness

GENERAL MANAGEMENT OF PATIENTS WITH MEDICALLY UNEXPLAINED COMPLAINTS

The management of the various syndromes of medically unexplained complaints described above is based on general principles (Box 10.35) and specific measures for individual syndromes.

Reassurance

Patients should be asked what they are most worried about. Clearly it may be unwise to state categorically that the patient has no disease but it can be emphasised that the probability of having disease is low. If patients repeatedly ask for reassurance about the same issue, they may have hypochondriasis.

Explanation

Patients need a positive explanation for their symptoms. It is unhelpful to say that symptoms are psychological or 'all in the mind', but useful to describe a plausible physiological mechanism for the symptom that emphasises the link with psychological factors such as stress and which demonstrates that the symptoms are reversible. For example, in irritable bowel syndrome, psychological stress results in increased activation of the autonomic nervous system which leads to constriction of smooth muscle in the gut wall, which in turn causes pain.

Advice

This should focus on how to overcome probable perpetuating factors: for example, by resolving stressful social problems or by practising relaxation. The doctor can offer to review progress, to prescribe (for example) an antidepressant drug and, if appropriate, to refer for physiotherapy or psychological treatments. The attitudes of relatives may need to be addressed if they have adopted an over-protective role, unwittingly reinforcing the patient's disability.

Drug treatment

Antidepressant drugs are helpful even if the patient is not depressed (Box 10.36).

Psychological treatment

There is moderate evidence for the effectiveness of CBT (Box 10.37). Other psychological treatments may also have a role.

10.35 GENERAL MANAGEMENT PRINCIPLES FOR MEDICALLY UNEXPLAINED SYMPTOMS

- Take a full, sympathetic history
- Exclude disease but avoid unnecessary investigation or referral
- Seek specific treatable psychiatric syndromes
- Demonstrate to patients that you believe their complaints
- Establish a collaborative relationship
- Give the patient a positive explanation including but not over-emphasising psychological factors
- Encourage a return to normal functioning

EBM

10.36 ANTIDEPRESSANTS FOR MEDICALLY UNEXPLAINED SOMATIC SYMPTOMS

'Antidepressant drugs are moderately effective for medically unexplained symptoms; the odds ratio for improvement with antidepressant treatment compared with placebo was 3.4.'

- O'Malley PG, et al. J Fam Pract 1999; 48:980–990.
- van Heeringen K, Zivkov M. Br J Psychiatry 1996; 169:440–443.

EBM

10.37 CBT FOR MEDICALLY UNEXPLAINED SOMATIC SYMPTOMS

'CBT for medically unexplained symptoms is superior to non-specific treatment.'

- Kroenke K, Swindle R. Psychother Psychosom 2000; 69:205–215.
- Speckens AE, et al. BMJ 1995; 311:1328–1332.

Rehabilitation

Where there is chronic disability, particularly in dissociative disorder, conventional physical rehabilitation may be the best approach.

Shared care with the GP

Ongoing care is required for patients with chronic intractable symptoms, especially somatisation disorder. Review by the same specialist, interspersed with visits to the GP, is the best way to avoid unnecessary re-referral for investigation, to ensure that treatable aspects of the patient's problems such as depression are actively managed, and also to prevent the GP from becoming demoralised by feelings of helplessness.

FACTITIOUS DISORDERS AND MALINGERING

It is important to distinguish somatoform disorders from factitious disorder and malingering.

FACTITIOUS DISORDER

This describes the repeated and deliberate production of the signs or symptoms of disease, apparently to obtain medical care. It is uncommon and typically presents in young women who work in paramedical professions. Examples include the dipping of thermometers into hot drinks to fake a fever, or patients with diabetes who deliberately induce hypo- and hyperglycaemic episodes. The factitious disorder is usually medical but may relate to a psychiatric illness with reports of hallucinations or depressive illness.

Münchausen's syndrome

This refers to a severe form of factitious disorder. Patients are usually older and male with a solitary, peripatetic lifestyle in which they travel widely, sometimes visiting several hospitals in one day. Although the condition is rare, such patients are memorable because they present so frequently and so dramatically. The history can be convincing enough to persuade doctors to undertake investigations or initiate treatment, including exploratory surgery. It may be possible to trace the patient's history, and show that he has presented similarly elsewhere, often changing name several times. Some emergency departments hold lists of such patients.

Management is by gentle but firm confrontation with clear evidence of the fabrication of illness, together with an offer of psychological support. Treatment is usually declined but recognition of the condition may help to avoid further iatrogenic harm.

MALINGERING

Malingering is a description of behaviour, not a psychiatric diagnosis. It refers to the conscious simulation of signs of disease and disability. Patients have motives which are clear to them but which they conceal from doctors. Examples include the avoidance of burdensome responsibilities (such as work or court appearances) or the pursuit of financial gain (fraudulent claims for benefits or compensation). Malingering can be hard to detect at clinical assessment, but is suggested by evasion or inconsistency in the history.

PUERPERAL DISORDERS

There are three common psychiatric complications of childbirth. When managing these conditions, it is important to consider both the mother and the baby, and also their relationship.

POST-PARTUM BLUES

These are characterised by irritability, labile mood and tearfulness. Most women are affected to some degree. Symptoms begin soon after childbirth, peak on about the fourth day and then resolve. They may be related to hormonal or psychological changes associated with childbirth. No treatment is required other than to reassure the mother.

POST-PARTUM DEPRESSION

This occurs in 10–15% of women. Women with a previous history of depression are at risk. Explanation and reassurance are important. The usual psychological and drug treatments for depression should be considered as well as practical help with childcare. If hospital admission is required, it should ideally be to a mother and baby unit. Further episodes of depression, both after childbirth and in response to other stressors, are likely.

PUERPERAL PSYCHOSIS

This has its onset in the first 2 weeks after childbirth. It is a rare but serious complication affecting about 1 in 500 women and usually takes the form of a manic or depressive psychosis, although a schizophrenic psychosis can also occur. Delirium is rare with modern obstetric management but should still be considered in the differential diagnosis. Management depends on the type of psychosis which presents. In addition it is important to consider the baby, and especially so to establish whether the mother has ideas of harming it. If so, the risk to the baby must be assessed and, if necessary, the baby temporarily removed. Most women recover but are at a 25% increased risk of puerperal psychosis with the next pregnancy, and a 50% lifetime risk. Admission to a psychiatric mother and baby unit may be required.

PSYCHIATRY AND THE LAW

Medicine takes place in a legal framework, made up of legislation (statute law) drafted by parliament or other governing bodies, and common law (case law) built up from court judgements over time. Psychiatry differs from other branches of medicine in that patients can be subject to

10

legislative requirements to remain in hospital or to undergo treatments they refuse, such as the administration of antipsychotic drugs to a patient with acute schizophrenia who lacks insight, and whose symptoms pose risks to himself or to others.

The UK has three different Mental Health Acts, covering England and Wales, Scotland, and Northern Ireland, and all of these are undergoing revision. Other countries may have very different provisions. It is important for practitioners to be familiar with the relevant provisions that apply in their jurisdictions, and are likely to arise in the clinical settings in which they work.

Scotland has an Incapacity Act, with detailed provisions covering medical treatments for patients incapable of consenting, whether this incapacity arises from physical or mental illness. Similar legislation is being introduced elsewhere in the UK. In general, the guiding principle in British law is that people should be free to make their own decisions about medical treatment, except where their ability to decide is impaired by mental illness or physical incapacity, and where there are clear risks to the health and safety of themselves or others. Any restrictions or compulsions applied should be the minimum necessary, and they should only be applied for as long as is necessary; there should also be provisions for appeals and oversight.

FURTHER INFORMATION

Books and journal articles

Harrison P, Geddes J, Sharpe M. Lecture notes on psychiatry. 9th edn. Oxford: Blackwell Science; 2005.

Johnstone EC, Freeman C, Zealley A (eds). Companion to psychiatric studies. 7th edn. Edinburgh: Churchill Livingstone; 2004.

Levenson JL (ed). American Psychiatric Publishing textbook of psychosomatic medicine. Washington DC: American Psychiatric Publishing; 2005.

Mayou R, Sharpe M, Carson A (eds). ABC of psychological medicine. London: BMJ Books; 2003.

Websites

http://cebmh.warne.ox.ac.uk/cebmh/ *Website of Centre for Evidence-based Mental health.*

www.depressionalliance.org *Information on depression.*

www.mja.com.au/public/mentalhealth/articles/singh/sinbox5.html/ *Managing chronic somatisation disorder.*

www.niaaa.nih.gov/ *Information on alcoholism.*

www.nimh.nih.gov/practitioners/ *General information on depression, anxiety etc.*

www.nimh.nih.gov/publicat/schizoph.htm *Information on schizophrenia.*

www.rcpsych.ac.uk/info/index.htm *Royal College of Psychiatrists: mental health information.*

www.who.int/mental_health/ *WHO website on mental health and brain disorders.*

10

D.A. CAMERON
G.C.W. HOWARD

Oncology

Oncology derives in part from the Greek *onkos* (mass, tumour), and describes the study of malignant disease. There are a number of common synonyms for malignant disease such as cancer, but this term technically only applies to tumours of epithelial origin (Box 11.1). The oldest treatment for malignancy is surgery, but there is now an increasing range of non-surgical treatments, encompassing both radiotherapy (clinical oncology) and drug treatments (medical oncology).

Malignancy is common, developing at some time in the life of more than one-third of the population (Fig. 11.1). It is the second most common cause of death in the Western world, after cardiovascular disease. However, there is significant variation with age, sex and geography in the incidence of the various malignancies, as well as in the resources available for detection and treatment. Amongst the more common solid tumours such as lung and breast cancer,

the incidence is often higher in developed countries. The incidence of lung cancer is four times higher in the UK than in India, although it is becoming increasingly common throughout the world. Breast cancer accounts for around 20–25% of all female cancers in both India and the UK, but the incidence in the UK per 100 000 women is three times higher than in Mumbai. In contrast, carcinoma of the cervix is the second most common cause of cancer death in women in the Caribbean, with an incidence almost four times higher than in the UK.

EPIDEMIOLOGY

Epidemiology can help us understand the causes of cancer by examining patterns of distribution of cases by age, sex, other illnesses, social class, geography and so on. Sometimes these give strong pointers to the molecular or cellular causes of the disease, such as the association between aflatoxin production within contaminated food supplies and certain *p53* gene mutations in hepatocellular carcinomas. However, for many solid cancers such as breast and colorectal, there is evidence of a multi-factorial pathogenesis, even when there is a principal environmental cause (Box 11.2). Smoking is now established beyond all doubt as a major cause of lung cancer, but there must be additional modifying influences since not all smokers develop cancer; these may be based in the individual's genotype. Similarly, most carcinomas of the cervix are related to infection with particular strains of the human papillomavirus (HPV 16 and 18), although other factors such as early age at first sexual intercourse contribute. For carcinomas of the bowel or

11.1 SYNONYMS FOR MALIGNANT DISEASE

Synonym	Definition
Neoplasia	New growth: includes benign disease
Tumour	Swelling: includes benign/inflammatory disease
Cancer, carcinoma	Malignancy of epithelial cell origin
Sarcoma	Malignancy of mesothelial cell origin
Lymphoma	Malignancy of lymphoid organs (usually glands)
Leukaemia	Malignancy of white blood cells

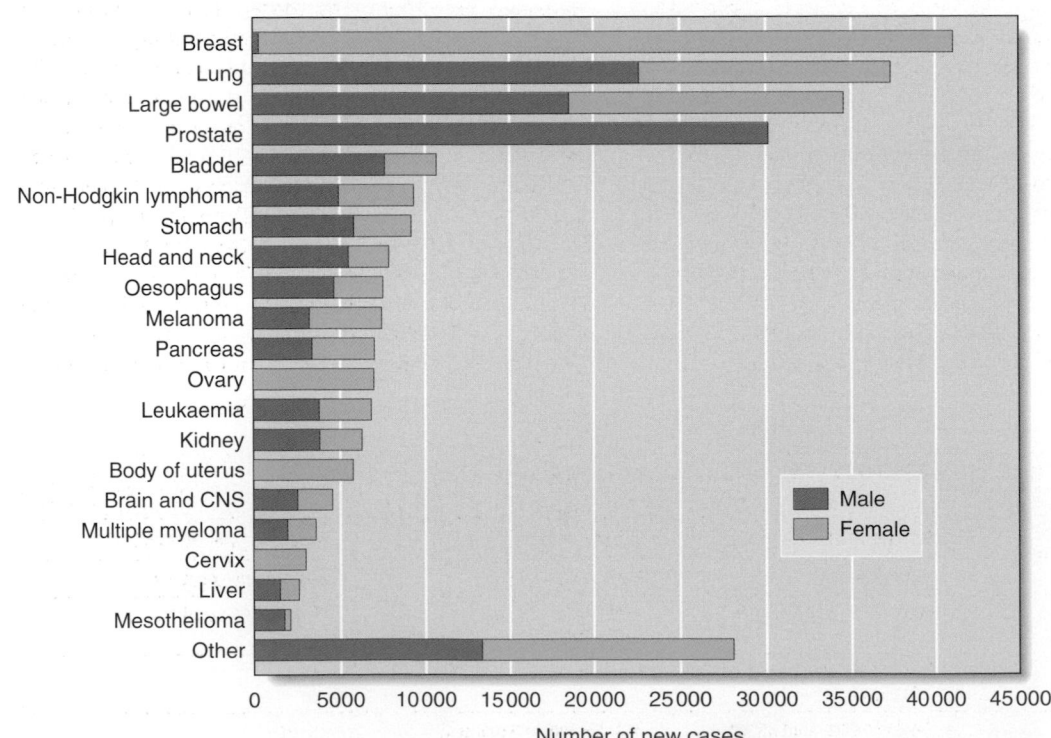

Fig. 11.1 The 20 most commonly diagnosed cancers, UK 2001.

11.2 EPIDEMIOLOGICAL CAUSES OF CANCER	
Drugs	
• Cytotoxics	→ Leukaemia
Infection	
• Schistosomiasis	→ Squamous bladder cancer
• Human papillomavirus 16 and 18	→ Cervical cancer
Genetics	
• Breast cancer gene 1/2	→ Breast and ovarian cancer
• Hereditary non-polyposis colorectal cancer gene	→ Colon and endometrial cancer
• Adenopolyposis coli gene	→ Colorectal cancer
Lifestyle	
• Western (specific cause still unclear)	→ Breast and colorectal cancer
• Tobacco	→ Lung, bladder, head and neck cancer
• Alcohol	→ Oesophageal cancer
• Aflatoxin	→ Liver cancer
Occupational	
• Asbestos	→ Mesothelioma
• Aniline dyes	→ Bladder cancer
• Ultraviolet (UV) light	→ Skin cancers

breast, the strongest aetiological factors appear to be environmental and genetic. For example, the risk of breast cancer in women of Far Eastern origin remains relatively low when they first migrate to a country with a Western lifestyle, but rises in subsequent generations to approach that of the resident population of the host country. The precise environmental factor that causes this change is unclear, but may include diet (higher intake of saturated fat and/or dairy products), reproductive patterns (later onset of first pregnancy) and lifestyle (increased use of artificial light and shift in diurnal rhythm). Additionally, a small number of genes have been identified that significantly increase the risk of developing breast cancer (*BRCA1*, *BRCA2*, *AT* (ataxia telangiectasia)). None of these has 100% penetrance so that there must be additional modulating factors, as yet undefined. For most patients, the precise cause of a cancer is less important than the diagnosis itself, although some may be concerned that there is an increased risk for their offspring, which means that exploration of a possible genetic contribution is a key part of management.

PREVENTION AND SCREENING

Knowledge of the cause of cancer seems an obvious route to prevention, but although we know that smoking is the cause of most lung cancer in the world, prevention has proved much more difficult. Modification of a population's lifestyle involves not only education but also political change. It is clear from many studies that the risk of breast cancer is related to a woman's lifetime oestrogen exposure, and this has given some possibilities for therapeutic intervention. Premature menopause, iatrogenic or otherwise, reduces the risk of developing breast cancer but is associated with a number of other unwanted consequences such as osteoporosis. Therapeutic intervention using, for example, tamoxifen (see below) has been shown to reduce the incidence of breast cancer but not mortality, and is not without toxicity. An alternative is prophylactic surgery, such as mastectomy or colectomy, in those at high risk of developing cancers in these tissues, but this is clearly not an option for a whole population.

Even if the key to reducing the death rate from cancer is preventing it in the first place, earlier diagnosis creates the potential to cure more patients. When patients are diagnosed with a cancer on the basis of symptoms, the cancer may have already spread in a significant proportion, so that loco-regional treatment (usually surgical) may be insufficient for a cure. Earlier identification of a cancer in an asymptomatic population could therefore 'catch' more cancers before they spread, rendering more patients curable by loco-regional treatment alone. This is the concept behind screening for malignancy, which has now been successfully applied to two major cancers in many developed countries (Box 11.3). Population-based mammographic screening for women between 50 and 65 years old has been shown, with some controversy, to reduce the mortality from breast cancer. Patients cannot be 'forced' to be screened, so the screening method has to be acceptable to a high enough proportion of the candidate population to be effective (Box 11.4).

Screening is not without its pitfalls. Only a tiny minority of most populations will have the disease, and screening requires considerable organisation, resources, and diagnosticians able to identify the occasional abnormal sample

11.3 CANCERS WITH POTENTIAL FOR SCREENING			
Malignancy	**Method of screening**	**Benefits**	**National programmes?**
Breast cancer	Mammography	Reduced mortality	Yes—many countries
Cervical cancer	Cervical smear cytology	?Reduced mortality (indirectly inferred)	Yes—many countries
Prostate cancer	Serum prostate-specific antigen (PSA) level	Possible reduced mortality	No
Colorectal cancer	Single flexible sigmoidoscopy Faecal occult blood test	Possible reduced mortality None	Some No

11

11.4 KEY REQUIREMENTS OF A SCREENING PROGRAMME

- Acceptable to the majority of the target population
- A high enough detection rate of early tumours to be effective
- Low false-positive rate (reducing unnecessary interventions)
- Affordable by the health-care system
- An effective intervention
- Deliverable

11.5 ONCOLOGY IN OLD AGE

- **Incidence:** around 50% of cancers occur in the 15% of the population aged over 65 years.
- **Screening:** women aged over 65 in the UK are not invited to breast cancer screening but can request it. Uptake is low despite increasing incidence with age.
- **Presentation:** may be later for some cancers. When symptoms are non-specific, patients (and their doctors) may initially attribute them to age alone.
- **Life expectancy:** an 80-year-old woman can expect to live 8 years, so cancer may still shorten life and an active approach remains appropriate.
- **Prognosis:** histology, stage at presentation and observation for a brief period are better guides to outcome than age alone.
- **Rate of progression:** malignancy may have a more indolent course. This is poorly understood but may be due to reduced effectiveness of angiogenesis with age, inhibiting the development of metastases.
- **Response to treatment:** equivalent to that in younger people. This is well documented for a range of cancers and for surgery, radiotherapy, chemotherapy and hormonal therapy.
- **Treatment selection:** chronological age is of minor importance compared to comorbid illness and patient choice. Although older patients can be treated effectively and safely, aggressive intervention is not appropriate for all individuals. Symptom control may be all that is possible or desired by the patient.

or X-ray amongst hundreds of normal ones, as missing these would invalidate the whole process. Similarly, a positive result must have a reasonably high chance of indicating malignancy to avoid generating unnecessary anxiety and further investigation. It must be clear that the earlier diagnosis of a cancer improves the cure rate, as otherwise the individual is simply subjected to more years as a 'cancer patient'. If it is not possible to cure more patients it may be better to delay diagnosis until there are symptoms, rather than screening the population.

PHYSIOLOGY, CLINICAL ASSESSMENT AND INVESTIGATIONS

The key to understanding the clinical behaviour of cancers lies in their biology. Malignancies generally arise because of mutations in the DNA of at least one cell which then no longer behaves normally. Most commonly, mutations give malignant cells a growth advantage, so that these take up an increasing proportion of the tissue of origin. Most malignant cells acquire the ability to invade, causing both local spread beyond normal tissue boundaries and distant dissemination (or metastases). These properties of growth and invasion give rise to the common presentations of cancers. However,

almost all malignant cells retain some phenotypic properties of their original tissue, which is why lymphoma, sarcoma and breast cancer do not present or behave in the same manner. Full details of the molecular biology of the cancer cell are given on page 48; this forms the key to understanding how treatments for cancer work.

Successful 'medical' (i.e. drug or radiotherapy) treatment of malignancy depends in part on the tumour biology. Proliferating tumour cells have an increased propensity to die, usually in a controlled or programmed manner known as apoptosis. Most of the current treatments for malignancy rely on this interplay between life and death and, by inducing DNA damage or interfering with growth factor pathways, trigger cell death (Fig. 11.2). Mutations or altered expression of key proteins in this pathway, such as *p53* and the *BCL*-2 family, may however prevent cells from undergoing apoptosis, and thus in part explain the limited sensitivity of cancer cells to DNA-damaging therapies. Normal human cells also undergo apoptosis and therefore many anticancer treatments cause loss of normal cells which manifests as toxicity, particularly in tissues with a high cell turnover. This inherent non-specificity of cancer treatments often results in a narrow margin between efficacy and toxicity or a 'narrow therapeutic index'. The apparent failure of medical treatments to cure some cancers is probably because of the dose-limiting effects of potential injury to healthy tissues. Much research has focused on methods of escalating treatment doses by preventing or reducing normal tissue damage, such as autologous bone marrow support for myelo-ablative chemotherapy. This has not become an established treatment for solid tumours, but has a role in haematological malignancies (p. 1039). There is now a shift in emphasis as our increased understanding of the molecular biology of cancers can help design more targeted therapies, such as antibodies to proteins encoded for by key oncogenes such as Her-2 neu, thereby avoiding toxicity.

CLINICAL ASSESSMENT

In order to plan the management of a patient with malignancy, the following information is required:

- the nature of the primary malignancy (site, type, pathology)
- the extent of the disease (stage)
- the patient's general condition and comorbidity
- the available treatment options.

The presentation of a malignancy can involve both local and systemic features (Boxes 11.6 and 11.7). The local signs or symptoms are usually due to mass effect or invasion of local tissues. In contrast, systemic features may be the result of metastases or the non-metastatic manifestations of malignant disease.

From the history, details of the tumour-related problem should be established along with potential risk factors. In breast cancer, family history, early menarche, late menopause and benign breast disease are associated with increased risk, while early full-term pregnancy reduces risk. An impression of the rate of development of the disease may

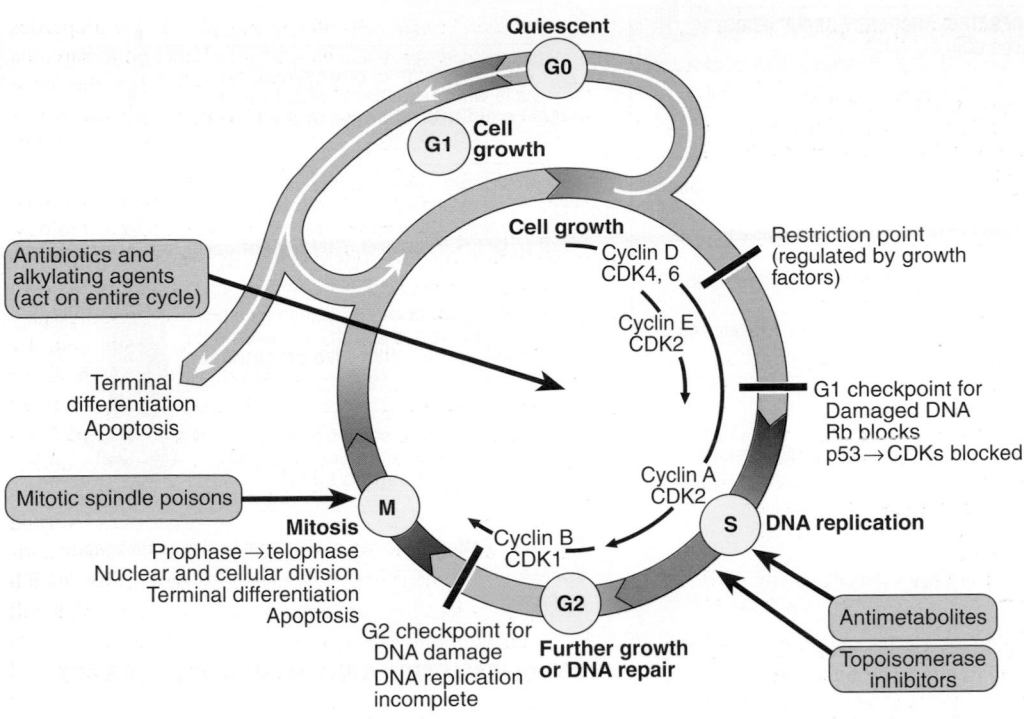

Fig. 11.2 **The cell cycle and sites of action of chemotherapeutic agents.** See page 43 for a full explanation of the cell cycle. Some groups of agents (Box 11.18, p. 266) act on the cell cycle in its entirety, others at specific points in the cycle. (Rb = retinoblastoma (gene); CDK = cyclin-dependent kinase).

11

11.6 LOCAL FEATURES OF MALIGNANT DESEASE

Symptom	Site/tumour
Haemorrhage	Stomach, colon, bronchus, endometrium, bladder, kidney
Lump	Breast, lymph node (any site), testicle
Pain	Bone (primary sarcoma, secondary)
Skin abnormality	Melanoma, basal cell carcinoma (rodent ulcer)
Ulcer	Oesophagus, stomach, anus, skin
Obstruction Pain, cough, recurrent infection Odynophagia, dysphagia, early satiety, vomiting Altered bowel habit, pain, distension	Bronchus Gastro-oesophageal Colon, rectum
Abdominal swelling (ascites)	Ovary, gastric cancer
Fracture	Metastatic cancer (breast, prostate, kidney, bronchus, thyroid)

11.7 NON-METASTATIC MANIFESTATIONS OF MALIGNANT DISEASE

Feature	Common associations
Weight loss and anorexia	Gastrointestinal tumours
Fatigue	Any
Hypercalcaemia	Myeloma, breast, renal tumours
Prothrombotic tendency	Pancreas and other gastrointestinal tumours
Hormonal effects Syndrome of inappropriate antidiuretic hormone secretion (SIADH) Ectopic adrenocorticotrophic hormone (ACTH)	Small-cell lung cancer
Neuropathies and myopathies Eaton–Lambert myasthenia-like syndrome Subacute cerebellar degeneration	Small-cell lung cancer
Skin abnormalities Acanthosis nigricans Dermatomyositis/polymyositis	Gastro-oesophageal tumours Gastric, lung tumours

help determine prognosis and treatment. A thorough clinical examination is essential to identify sites of metastases, and to identify any other conditions that may have a bearing on the management plan.

The overall fitness of a patient can be evaluated using a variety of scales. One of the most common is the Eastern Cooperative Oncology Group (ECOG) performance scale (Box 11.8). The outcome for patients with a performance status of 3 or 4 is worse in almost all malignancies than for those with a status of 0 to 2. Treatment decisions must take such assessments into account.

INVESTIGATIONS

Tumour imaging and sampling are required. Sampling may be achieved under direct vision as at endoscopy, bronchoscopy or colonoscopy, or with ultrasound or computed tomography (CT) guidance. Superficial masses or lesions may be biopsied or fine needle aspirates may be taken. In cases where treatment is initially or largely non-surgical, precise measurement of initial tumour size helps to assess subsequent response to therapy.

11.8 EASTERN COOPERATIVE ONCOLOGY GROUP (ECOG) PERFORMANCE STATUS SCALE

- **0** Fully active, able to carry on all usual activities without restriction and without the aid of analgesics
- **1** Restricted in strenuous activity but ambulatory and able to carry out light work or pursue a sedentary occupation. This group also contains patients who are fully active, as in grade 0, but only with the aid of analgesics
- **2** Ambulatory and capable of all self-care but unable to work. Up and about more than 50% of waking hours
- **3** Capable of only limited self-care, confined to bed or chair more than 50% of waking hours
- **4** Completely disabled, unable to carry out any self-care and confined totally to bed or chair

Special investigations such as serum tumour marker tests and a series of standard radiological tests to 'stage' the disease may follow (see below).

PATHOLOGY

The pathologist studies the tissue sample for evidence of cellular abnormalities which reflect mutations:

- greater numbers of cells than in normal tissue
- increased size
- a higher nuclear to cytoplasmic ratio
- a higher proliferation rate (evidenced by visible mitotic figures).

In addition, the cells may be in an abnormal location; they may have penetrated (invaded) the basement membrane or moved (metastasised) from their tissue of origin, e.g. to lymph nodes/liver. There is, however, a continuum from benign to malignant (Fig. 11.3).

Immunohistochemistry

Highly specific monoclonal antibodies, associated with a coloured stain, are used to detect various intracellular and cell-surface proteins to achieve a specific diagnosis (Box 11.9). This technique can be used to determine the tissue of origin of a very undifferentiated tumour, identify important subtypes of common cancers (small-cell, neuro-endocrine) which have different prognoses or require different therapies, and establish the presence of oestrogen receptors in breast cancers, which assists therapeutic planning (Fig. 11.4).

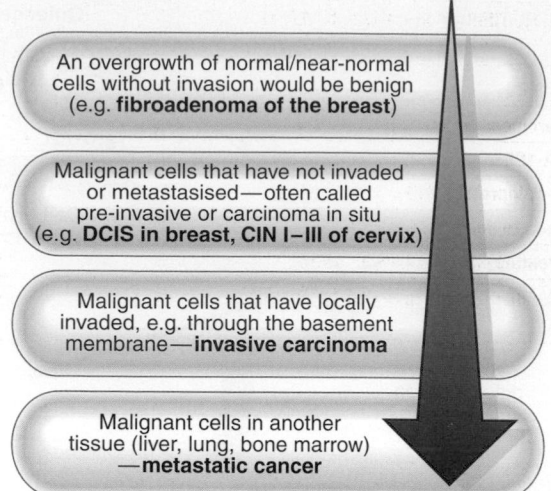

An overgrowth of normal/near-normal cells without invasion would be benign (e.g. **fibroadenoma of the breast**)

Malignant cells that have not invaded or metastasised—often called pre-invasive or carcinoma in situ (e.g. **DCIS in breast, CIN I—III of cervix**)

Malignant cells that have locally invaded, e.g. through the basement membrane—**invasive carcinoma**

Malignant cells in another tissue (liver, lung, bone marrow) —**metastatic cancer**

Fig. 11.3 Pathological expression from benign to malignant disease. (DCIS = ductal carcinoma in situ; CIN = cervical intra-epithelial neoplasia)

BIOCHEMISTRY AND TUMOUR MARKERS

In addition to classical pathological features, many tumours are associated with abnormalities in peripheral blood. This may be due to the tumour secreting proteins into the circulation, which are detectable on routine testing (Box 11.10). Many of these so-called tumour markers can be used for diagnosis, and in some types of cancer levels reflect the extent (stage) of the disease. Commonly, markers are antigens that are usually only expressed in the fetus, but they may be produced by a tumour in an adult, causing levels that are much higher than normal. Hormone levels can also be used as tumour markers—for example, oestrogen may be produced by ovarian granulosa cell tumours, and human chorionic gonadotrophin (HCG) by choriocarcinomas and teratomas. Few markers are uniquely associated with the tumour, so that the currently available serum tumour markers are not completely specific. Their main use is to assess a cancer's response to treatment and to monitor for recurrence rather than as a diagnostic test.

STAGING

Staging is the determination of the extent of the malignancy. It entails clinical examination and imaging to establish

11.9 IMMUNOHISTOCHEMISTRY MARKERS			
Name	**Oncogene?**	**Routine use?**	**Tumour type**
S-100	No	Yes	Neural crest origin (e.g. melanoma)
Cam 5.2	No	Yes	Small-cell cancer (e.g. lung)
Carcinoembryonic antigen (CEA)	No	Yes	Colon and other gastrointestinal tumours
CA-125	No	Yes	Ovary
Oestrogen receptor (ER)	No	Yes	Breast cancer (present in other tumours, e.g. ovary)
Her-2	Yes	No	Breast cancer (present in other tumours, e.g. lung, ovary, gastric)

11.10 TUMOUR MARKERS IN BLOOD

Name	Fetal antigen?	Normally detected?	Tumours
Carcinoembryonic antigen (CEA)	Yes	Yes	Gastrointestinal tract, lung, breast
CA-125	Yes	Yes	Ovary
α-Fetoprotein (AFP)	Yes	Yes (very low)	Hepatocellular carcinoma and malignant teratoma
Lactate dehydrogenase (LDH)	No	Yes	Most, reflecting tumour burden or necrosis
Prostate-specific antigen (PSA)	No	Yes	Prostate, some breast cancers
Human chorionic gonadotrophin (HCG)	No	Only in pregnancy	Malignant teratoma, seminoma, choriocarcinoma, gastrointestinal tumours

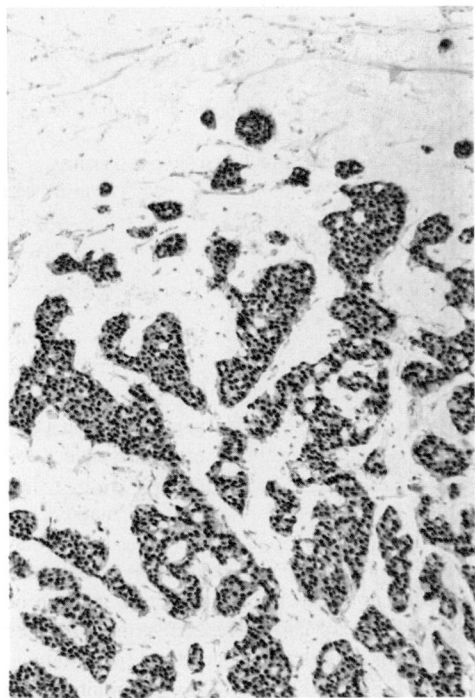

Fig. 11.4 Breast cancer specimen stained for the expression of oestrogen receptors using a monoclonal antibody. Note the heterogeneity of staining.

possible sites or extent of disease involvement (Fig. 11.5 and Box 11.11). The tests used depend on the likely patterns of spread. The outcome is recorded using a standard staging system to enable comparison between different groups of patients. Therapeutic decisions and prognostic predictions can then be made using the evidence base for the disease. One of the most commonly used systems is the T (tumour), N (regional lymph nodes) and M (metastatic sites) approach of the Union Internationale contre le Cancer (UICC) (Box 11.12). For some tumours the most widely used system is not the UICC; colorectal cancer, for example, is often staged using the Dukes system (p. 928).

PRESENTING PROBLEMS IN ONCOLOGY

With the advent of screening and public awareness campaigns, the vast majority of patients with cancer in developed countries present with local symptoms to organ-based specialties. Therefore the details of the clinical presentation and management of most of the common solid tumours are discussed in the relevant organ-based chapters. A small number of patients present as an emergency. In addition, most cancer treatments used are given close to their tolerance, which may result in complications that can be life-threatening and require urgent intervention.

11

11.11 STAGING TESTS

Primary	Common	Less common/ geographical variation
Breast	Chest X-ray, bone scan	Bone marrow, CT of abdomen/thorax
Lymphoma	CT abdomen and thorax, bone marrow	Bone scan
Prostate	Bone scan, CT pelvis	
Colon	Ultrasound, CT liver	
Lung	Chest X-ray, CT chest and upper abdomen	Bone marrow, bone scan

11.12 TNM CLASSIFICATION

T*	Extent of primary tumour
N*	Extent of regional lymph node involvement
M	Presence or absence of metastases

Extent of disease

T0	Excised tumour
T1	
T2	Increases in primary tumour size
T3	

Increased involvement of nodes

N1	
N2	Increases in involvement
N3	

Presence of metastases

M0	Not present
M1	Present

* Exact criteria for size and region of nodal involvement have been defined for each anatomical site.

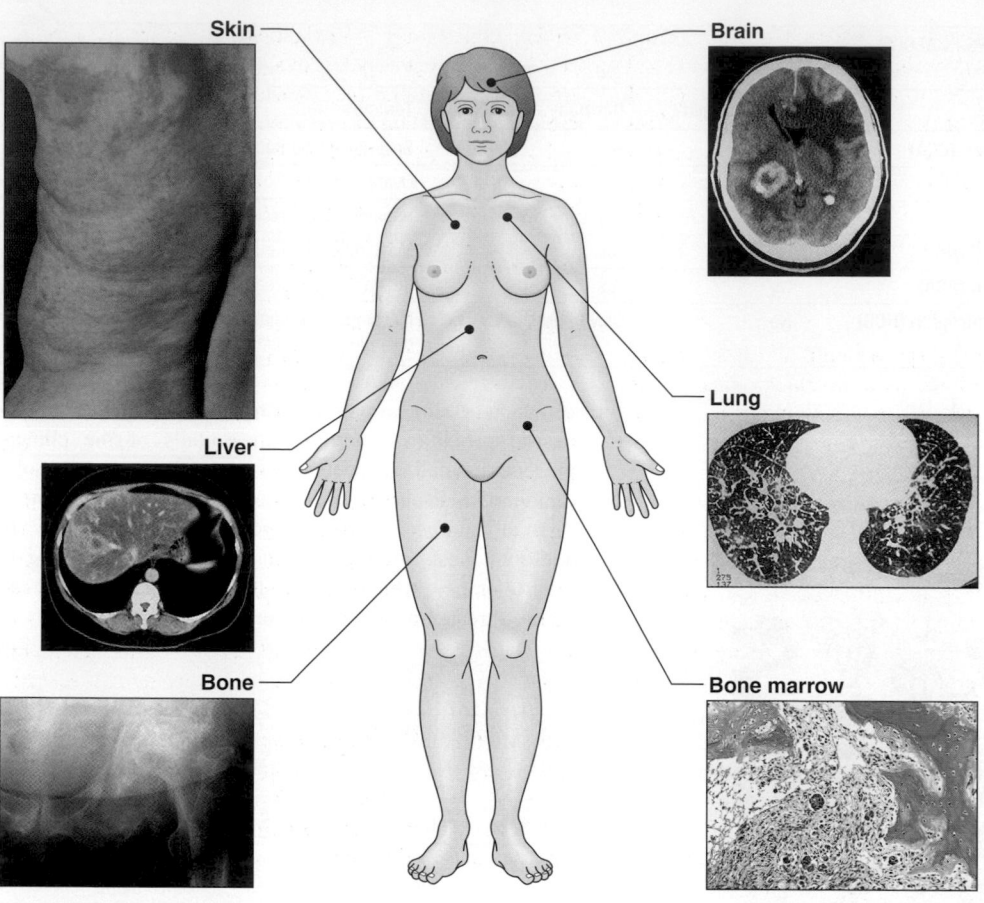

Fig. 11.5 Common sites of metastasis for breast and other cancers.

ONCOLOGICAL EMERGENCIES

As these are described in detail in the specific system-based chapters, only a brief outline is given here.

NEUTROPENIC SEPSIS/FEVER

Fever of 38°C for over 1 hour in a patient with a neutrophil count $< 1.0 \times 10^9/l$ indicates possible septicaemia (p. 1014). This is most commonly a complication of myelosuppressive chemotherapy but can be a complication of the underlying disease, particularly in leukaemias or very occasionally in metastatic solid tumours with extensive bone marrow replacement. It is life-threatening and requires urgent assessment and therapy. Presenting symptoms include obvious infection (fever, chills, influenza-like myalgia, headache), non-specific malaise and profound shock (p. 186). Those with shock and multi-organ failure should be managed in a specialist or intensive care unit, using agreed protocols for antibiotics that reflect local sensitivity patterns. A detailed description of the management of neutropenic sepsis is given on pages 189–190.

SPINAL CORD COMPRESSION

This is an emergency that is difficult to treat effectively. The spinal cord resides within a confined bony framework, so that tumour tissue quickly expands to damage nerve tissue directly by pressure or indirectly by interfering with blood supply. Pain, sensorimotor and sphincter symptoms vary according to the level of the cord compressed (p. 1243).

Immediate diagnosis and therapy are essential as the neurological deficit following treatment is closely related to the severity prior to treatment. Plain X-rays may show bony destruction, but magnetic resonance imaging (MRI) is essential to demonstrate tumour detail. Needle biopsy may be appropriate to establish histology. Treatment should be commenced with dexamethasone 16 mg i.v. then 4 mg 6-hourly. Urgent radiotherapy is the mainstay of therapy, but surgical decompression may be appropriate in some patients (p. 1245). Useful function can be regained if treatment starts within 24 hours of the development of weakness or sphincter disturbance. Tragically, warning signs of a band-like pain just below the lesion, or early evidence of neurological damage distal to the lesion, are often missed by patients and clinicians alike.

HYPERCALCAEMIA

As a consequence of direct bone involvement with metastatic disease or ectopic tumour production of a hormone (almost always parathormone-related peptide, PTHrP), increased osteoclast activity produces a rise in serum calcium, which cannot be compensated for by the normal homeostatic mechanisms. The clinical manifestations are essentially the same as for any other cause of elevated serum calcium (p. 773), except that the duration is usually shorter and renal stone formation consequently rare. The basic physiological problem is dehydration, consequent upon the diuretic effect of the elevated urinary calcium, and so the key to successful management is fluid replacement as well as prevention of further calcium release with bisphosphonate therapy. Details of this are given on page 774.

CARDIAC TAMPONADE

Occlusion of the pericardial space with fluid causes cardiac compression, which results in a dramatic reduction in cardiac output (p. 542). Patients present with breathlessness, collapse, tachycardia and hypotension. Clinical signs are described on page 542. Chest X-ray may reveal an enlarged and globular heart, and echocardiography confirms the presence of a significant pericardial effusion. Treatment involves aspiration of the pericardial fluid through a catheter placed under echocardiographic guidance, and a sample of fluid should be sent for cytological examination (p. 645). Recurrent pericardial tamponade is fortunately uncommon. If it occurs, surgical intervention with drainage into the left pleural cavity or peritoneal cavity may be necessary.

SUPERIOR VENA CAVAL OBSTRUCTION

Obstruction of the superior vena cava (SVCO) in the mediastinum reduces the filling of the right atrium and ventricle and causes venous engorgement and later oedema in the head, neck, arms and upper thorax. The symptoms are breathlessness, blackouts, and headaches which are worse on leaning forwards. Clinically, the venous engorgement is usually obvious, with fixed dilated external jugular veins (p. 712).

The majority of cases (> 85% in the UK) are due to malignancy, but there are benign causes such as mediastinal fibrosis, so unless the patient is already known to have cancer, a tissue diagnosis is necessary before treatment begins. The mainstay of treatment for SVCO due to malignant disease is radiotherapy, and two of the more common causes, small-cell lung cancer and lymphoma, are often exquisitely radiosensitive. In many patients, secondary thrombosis within the SVC occurs and therefore, particularly in recurrent SVCO, percutaneous insertion of a stent within the SVC may be necessary.

ADENOCARCINOMA OF UNKNOWN ORIGIN

Some patients develop evidence of metastatic cancer without a prior or concurrent diagnosis of a primary site. Management will depend on the individual's circumstances as well as the site(s) involved and the likely primary sites. The overriding principle, however, is to ensure that a curable diagnosis has not been overlooked. For example, lung metastases from a testicular teratoma do not preclude cure, nor do one or two liver metastases from a colorectal cancer. Early discussion with an oncologist is essential and also

avoids unnecessary investigation: for example, a single HCG-based pregnancy test in a young man with lung metastases might confirm the presence of a teratoma and allow rapid administration of potentially curative chemotherapy.

For most patients, histological examination of an accessible site of metastasis is required. It is better to perform a biopsy rather than aspiration as the tissue architecture can help the pathologist to determine likely primary sites, and the greater amount of tissue in a biopsy specimen permits the use of immunohistochemistry. For example, the expression of oestrogen receptors suggests breast cancer; significant levels of CA-125 suggest a diagnosis of epithelial ovarian carcinoma. Review of specimens by a panel of experienced pathologists may help secure a diagnosis. Extensive imaging to search for the primary is rarely indicated: a careful history to identify symptoms and risk factors (including familial) will often permit a judicious choice of imaging. Treatment should not necessarily wait for a definitive diagnosis; appropriate analgesia, radiotherapy or surgical palliation can all be helpful. Some patients remain free of cancer for some years after resection of a single metastasis of an adenocarcinoma of unknown primary, justifying this approach in selected patients.

In those with no obvious primary, systemic chemotherapy may achieve some reduction in tumour burden and alleviation of symptoms. In these circumstances, a regimen based on platinum and/or 5-fluorouracil may be used, but long-term survival is rare.

BONE METASTASES OF UNKNOWN PRIMARY

Some patients present with symptoms from bone metastases such as pain, fracture, nerve root or spinal cord compression (Fig. 11.5). As well as treatment for the symptoms, investigation to identify the primary is indicated. It is not necessary to look for all possible primary sites (e.g. bronchus, thyroid) as cure is highly unlikely in this situation. It is, however, necessary to screen for a primary which may respond to treatment once metastases have developed e.g. myeloma and breast cancer. The X-ray appearances may be helpful. Large well-defined lytic lesions may suggest a renal primary; widespread sclerotic disease in an elderly man suggests prostate cancer. Although these are the common causes of bone metastases, all cancers can spread to bone and a careful history may point to further investigations that may prove fruitful.

BRAIN METASTASES OF UNKNOWN PRIMARY

Metastasis to the brain (Fig. 11.6) may be the first presentation of some cancers. The prognosis in the majority is poor. The clinical features of headache, local effects and seizures are described in detail on page 1236. The diagnosis should also be considered when a patient with cancer develops persistent nausea and vomiting. The diagnosis is

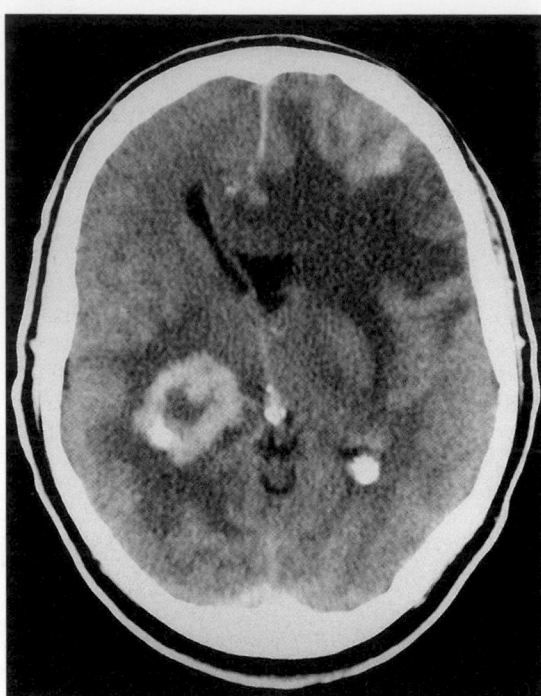

Fig. 11.6 **CT showing multiple cerebral metastases and significant oedema and midline shift.**

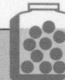

11.13 GOALS OF NON-SURGICAL TREATMENT

Curative

- Choriocarcinoma
- Teratoma
- Seminoma
- High-grade lymphoma
- Cervical cancer
- Head and neck cancer

Radical, occasionally curative

- Small-cell lung cancer
- Stage III ovarian cancer

Adjuvant (with surgery)

- Breast cancer
- Stage I–II ovarian cancer
- Colorectal cancer
- Osteogenic sarcoma

Palliative

- Metastatic breast cancer
- Stage IV ovarian cancer
- Advanced gastrointestinal cancers
- Metastatic sarcoma
- Metastatic prostate cancer
- Advanced lung cancer

11.14 CHEMOTHERAPY IN TESTICULAR TERATOMA `EBM`

'Adjuvant chemotherapy following orchidectomy reduces relapse rates from 50% to 1% in stage 1 teratoma and where there is lymphovascular invasion.'

- Management of adult testicular germ cell tumours. SIGN publication no. 28; 1998.

For further information: 💻 www.sign.ac.uk

made by CT or MRI. Multiple lesions often represent secondaries but solitary lesions can also be metastatic. Biopsy should be considered as a tissue diagnosis may be important for management and prognosis; testicular cancer may be treatable and surgical intervention in renal cancer may result in long-term survival.

The mainstay of treatment is dexamethasone to reduce cerebral oedema, and it may possibly protect the brain during radiotherapy. Most patients are treated with palliative radiotherapy, although there is little definitive evidence for this approach (p. 1237). For some, especially those with single lesions and/or low-volume or indolent extracranial metastases, a neurosurgical opinion should be sought as to whether surgical resection would be appropriate.

GENERAL MANAGEMENT PRINCIPLES

Patients must be informed of the diagnosis and the stage and prognosis for the disease, to allow an informed discussion about treatment options. The initial consultation must be unhurried and empathetic so that the patient's history, fears and concerns can be fully ascertained. The doctor needs to establish good communication and a rapport with the patient. Patients' responses to the diagnosis of cancer vary from shock to denial, anxiety, depression or inappropriate fatalism. Oncologists have to remain sensitive to patients' needs and fears, yet still be able to discuss the appropriateness of starting and stopping treatment. The future cannot be foreseen with certainty, so discussions with patients and relatives must take account of the variability in outcome and response to treatment, but in a way that does

not undermine their confidence. It is not helpful to give patients '6 months to live', or to describe a treatment as having been 'successful' when residual disease may be present. Integral to treatment planning is a decision about the aims of therapy (Box 11.13) and these should be clear to the doctor, to the patient and to the patient's family.

Treatment for cancer can be divided into:

- *Curative treatment*
- *Palliative treatment*—given to alleviate symptoms, with an emphasis on quality rather than quantity of life (Ch. 12). However, sometimes the best way of achieving symptomatic control is to reduce the amount of cancer with systemic anti-cancer treatment.
- *Adjuvant treatments*—given after primary therapy such as surgery, when there is no known residual disease but a defined risk of recurrence which can be reduced by another treatment (Box 11.14). For example, radiotherapy, chemotherapy and hormonal therapy each incrementally reduce the risk of recurrent breast cancer.

Not all treatments fall neatly into these categories. For example, chemotherapy for metastatic ovarian, breast and colorectal cancer prolongs life but cannot be considered curative (Box 11.15).

Many treatments for cancer are associated with significant morbidity and sometimes mortality. It is therefore of paramount importance to the patient and clinician to define the goal of a treatment strategy at the outset, accepting that this may need to be revised in the light of subsequent assessment. If the goal of therapy is cure then clearly a greater degree of toxicity will be acceptable than if it is palliative.

TREATMENT PLANNING

Increasingly, multiple treatments are being used to obtain optimal results, particularly where the aim of treatment is cure. Usually, a strategy is designed by a multidisciplinary team which includes representatives from all the specialties that may be involved in the management of the patient (e.g. medical and clinical oncologists and specialist surgeons).

ASSESSMENT OF RESPONSE

For treatments where there is measurable disease (such as the primary cancer or metastatic disease), it is important to formally assess response, usually at defined times such as after radiotherapy or a certain number of courses of chemotherapy. Where possible, marker lesions such as clinically measurable lymph nodes or radiologically imageable lung or liver metastases should be assessed, and response defined as either complete or partial, static or progressive disease. If the primary cancer has been excised and the treatment is adjuvant, this is not possible, so a course of therapy is defined and completed, as long as toxicity is acceptable. With palliative therapy, assessment of response is more subjective and may focus on an improvement in general well-being, pain control or performance status. Whether objectively or subjectively, it is important to assess response to therapy accurately, so that ineffective treatment is stopped as soon as possible.

SANCTUARY SITES

Systemic therapies have poor penetration of the brain and testes, as a consequence of which potentially radical drug treatment can fail. For leukaemias (p. 1039) this poses a major problem and requires additional therapy. In solid tumour oncology, limited small-cell lung carcinoma has a subsequent high incidence of symptomatic and life-threatening brain metastases, which can be reduced by additional therapy with prophylactic cranial irradiation (PCI, Box 11.16). Patients with breast cancer that over-

expresses the Her-2 oncogene also have a high risk of developing brain metastases (up to one-third of patients with metastatic disease) and the benefit of PCI in small-cell lung cancer is leading to studies to determine whether a similar approach might be justified in this aggressive subtype of breast cancer.

THERAPIES

SURGERY

Surgery has a pivotal role in the management of cancer. There are three main situations where it is necessary.

Biopsy
In the vast majority of cases, a histological or cytological diagnosis of cancer is necessary, and tissue will also provide important information such as tumour type and differentiation, to assist subsequent management. Although newer techniques such as fine needle aspiration under radiological control have a role, surgical biopsy is still the mainstay.

Excision
The main curative management of most solid cancers is surgical excision. In early localised cases of colorectal, breast and lung cancer, cure rates are high with surgery. There is increasing evidence that outcome is related to surgical expertise, and most multidisciplinary teams include surgeons experienced in the management of a particular cancer. There are some cancers where surgery is one of two or more options for primary management, and the role of the multidisciplinary team is to recommend appropriate treatment for a specific patient. Examples include prostate and transitional cell carcinoma of the bladder where both radiotherapy and surgery may be equally effective.

Palliation
Surgical procedures are often the quickest and most effective way of palliating crippling symptoms such as faecal incontinence with a defunctioning colostomy and urinary frequency with a bypass; fungating skin lesions may benefit from 'toilet' surgery. Other specific indications for surgical intervention are fixation of pathological fractures and decompression of spinal cord compression.

A more specialist role for surgery is resection of residual masses after chemotherapy and, in very selected cases, resection of metastases.

11

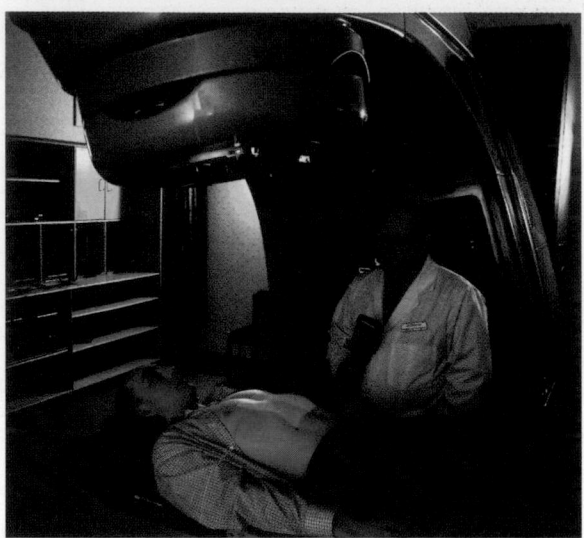

Fig. 11.7 **Linear accelerator.** The light beam identifies the entry point of the X-ray beam. The red laser lights help to reproduce the patient's position for each daily treatment.

RADIOTHERAPY

Radiotherapy means the treatment of cancer with ionising radiation, and for certain localised cancers it may be curative. Ionising radiation can be delivered by radiation emitted from the decay of a radioactive isotope or by high-energy radiation beams, usually X-rays. These can be delivered by three methods:

- *Teletherapy*—from a distance by a linear accelerator
- *Brachytherapy*—direct application of a radioactive source on to or into a tumour. This allows the delivery of a very high localised dose of radiation because the dose falls off rapidly with distance from the source. It is integral to the management of localised cancers of the head and neck and cancer of the cervix and endometrium.
- *Intravenous injection of a radioisotope*—such as ^{131}-iodine for cancer of the thyroid and ^{89}-strontium for the treatment of bone metastases from prostate cancer.

The majority of treatments are now delivered by linear accelerators (Fig. 11.7). These machines use wave guides to accelerate electrons to high energies to produce electron or X-ray beams that are used for treatment. Whatever the method of delivery, the biological effect of ionising radiation is to cause lethal and sublethal damage to DNA. Given a high enough dose, any cancer can be sterilised in this way, but normal tissues are also radio-sensitive to varying degrees and radiotherapy delivery has to be designed to obtain a therapeutic gain. The ideal way to achieve this would be to treat the tumour and no normal tissue at all. This is impossible because, to cover microscopic spread and to allow for organ and patient movement, it is necessary for some normal tissue to be within the irradiated volume. However, modern sophisticated planning techniques using CT and MRI allow much better

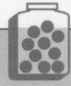

- Bone pain
- Haemoptysis
- Haematuria
- Ulceration of superficial lesions
- Spinal cord compression
- Superior vena caval obstruction
- Brain metastases

visualisation of normal and tumour tissue. In addition, techniques such as conformal radiotherapy, where shaped rather than conventional square or rectangular beams are used, allow much closer matching of the high dose volume to the tumour, reducing the volume of normal tissue irradiated by up to 40% compared to non-conformal techniques.

Radiobiological differences between normal and tumour tissues are also used to obtain therapeutic gain. Fundamental to this is fractionation, which entails delivering the radiation as a number of small, usually daily, doses. This allows normal cells to recover from some sublethal and potentially lethal irradiation damage, but recovery occurs to a lesser degree in malignant cells. Fractionation regimens vary from centre to centre but radical treatments given with curative intent are often delivered in 20–30 fractions given daily, 5 days a week over 4–6 weeks.

As well as having a significant role in the curative management of some cancers, radiotherapy can be extremely useful for the alleviation of symptoms (Box 11.17). For palliative treatments such as these, a smaller number of fractions, such as 1–5, is usually adequate.

Both normal and malignant tissues have a range of radiosensitivities. Germ cell tumours and lymphomas are extremely radiosensitive and relatively low doses are adequate to sterilise and often to cure them. However, most cancers require doses close to or beyond that which can be tolerated by adjacent normal structures. Normal tissue also varies in its radiosensitivity, the central nervous system, small bowel and lung being amongst the most sensitive.

The side-effects of radiotherapy (Fig. 11.8) depend on the normal tissues treated, their radiosensitivity and the dose delivered.

Acute side-effects

An acute inflammatory radiation reaction occurs towards the end of most radical treatments. It is localised to the area treated, such as a skin reaction (Fig. 11.8) with breast or chest wall radiotherapy, and proctitis and cystitis with treatment to the bladder or prostate. These acute reactions settle over a period of a few weeks after treatment, assuming normal tissue tolerance has not been exceeded.

Late reactions

These persist or develop 6 weeks or more (some may take years) after treatment and should only occur in 5–10% of patients. Severity will vary but the damage is permanent. This highlights the care needed when changing a radio-therapy technique or dose as the side-effects may not be apparent for many years. Examples of late effects are brachial plexopathy and subcutaneous fibrosis after breast cancer treatment, and shrinkage and fibrosis of the bladder

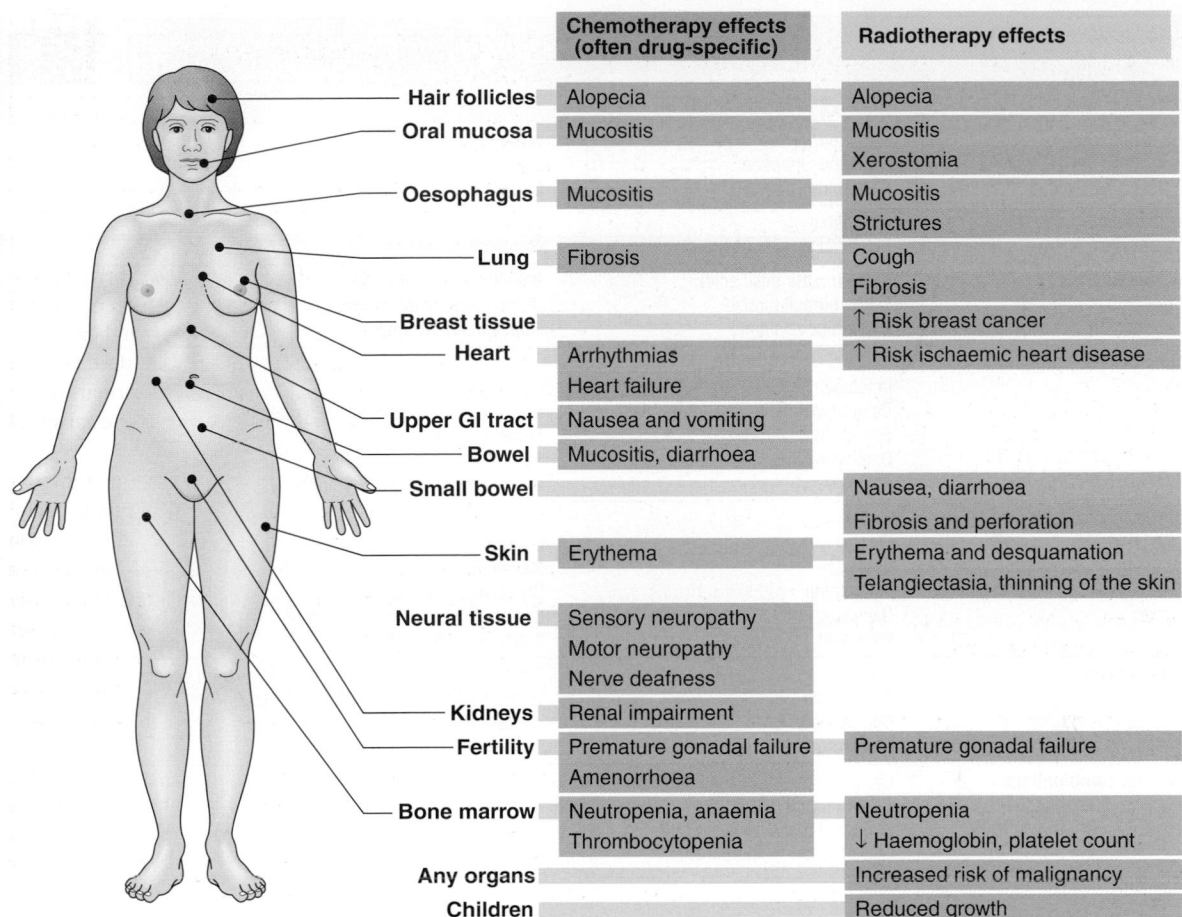

	Chemotherapy effects (often drug-specific)	Radiotherapy effects
Hair follicles	Alopecia	Alopecia
Oral mucosa	Mucositis	Mucositis Xerostomia
Oesophagus	Mucositis	Mucositis Strictures
Lung	Fibrosis	Cough Fibrosis
Breast tissue		↑ Risk breast cancer
Heart	Arrhythmias Heart failure	↑ Risk ischaemic heart disease
Upper GI tract	Nausea and vomiting	
Bowel	Mucositis, diarrhoea	
Small bowel		Nausea, diarrhoea Fibrosis and perforation
Skin	Erythema	Erythema and desquamation Telangiectasia, thinning of the skin
Neural tissue	Sensory neuropathy Motor neuropathy Nerve deafness	
Kidneys	Renal impairment	
Fertility	Premature gonadal failure Amenorrhoea	Premature gonadal failure
Bone marrow	Neutropenia, anaemia Thrombocytopenia	Neutropenia ↓ Haemoglobin, platelet count
Any organs		Increased risk of malignancy
Children		Reduced growth

Fig. 11.8 Acute (in red) and late (in blue) side-effects of chemotherapy and radiotherapy.

11

after treatment for bladder cancer. There is a risk of cancer induction after therapeutic doses of radiotherapy, which varies depending on the site treated and whether the patient has had other treatment such as chemotherapy.

CHEMOTHERAPY

The potential for nitrogen mustard to destroy proliferating bone marrow and lymphoid cells was recognised in the 1940s, and rapidly led to the first use of alkylating cytotoxic agents. The second class of cytotoxics arose from research on folic acid metabolism in leukaemic cells, leading to the discovery of methotrexate, the first antimetabolite. In general, cytotoxic agents have a broader range of intra-cellular effects than radiotherapy, although they also damage DNA. Chemotherapeutic drugs are classified by their mode of action, with most only being active in proliferating tissues (Box 11.18). They are not specifically designed to target malignant cells and therefore their common side-effects relate to these anti-proliferative actions.

Combination therapy

In order to overcome drug resistance and to limit the side-effects of different drugs, chemotherapy is most commonly given as a combination of agents. Combinations usually include drugs from different classes, each of which may be independently active and the combination of which should not have additive deleterious effects. Drugs are conventionally given by intravenous injection every 3–4 weeks, allowing enough time for the patient to recover from short-term toxic effects (Fig. 11.8) before the next dose. Between four and eight such cycles of treatment are usually given in total. More recently, a number of other strategies have been developed. For example, 5-fluorouracil (5-FU), which has a very short half-life, has increased efficacy when given by continuous intravenous infusion, using a semi-permanent in-dwelling intravenous catheter. However, the use of such catheters is not without risk, and the potential of oral 5-FU is now being explored, using precursors such as capecitabine. Other oral chemotherapeutic agents have been developed over the past 30 years, although not many have replaced their intravenous counterparts. Schedules of administration at weekly or 2-weekly intervals have also found their place in the management of both solid and haematological malignancies.

Each tumour type has specific regimens that are used at various stages of the disease, and some examples are given in the section on treatment of common solid tumours (p. 269).

11.18 COMMONLY USED CYTOTOXICS		
Mode of action	**Drug**	**Uses**
Alkylating agents	Melphalan	Myeloma
	Cyclophosphamide	Breast cancer, lymphoma
	Ifosfamide	Sarcomas
Antibiotics	Bleomycin	Teratoma
	Mitomycin	GI cancer, breast cancer
Antimetabolites (target in parentheses)	Methotrexate (folic acid)	Breast cancer, osteosarcoma, intrathecal chemotherapy
	5-fluorouracil (uracil)	GI cancers, breast cancer
	Cytarabine (cytidine)	Leukaemias, lymphoma
Topoisomerase inhibitors Topo-I	Irinotecan	Colorectal cancer
Topo-II	Doxorubicin (has other effects too)	Breast cancer, sarcoma and lymphoma
	Epirubicin	Breast cancer
	Daunorubicin	Sarcoma
	Etoposide	Lung cancer, sarcoma, lymphoma
Mitotic spindle poisons Vinca alkaloids	Vincristine	Lymphoma
	Vindesine	Melanoma
	Vinorelbine	Breast and lung cancer
Taxanes	Docetaxel	Breast, lung and prostate cancer
	Paclitaxel	Breast, lung and ovarian cancer
Miscellaneous	Cisplatin	Teratoma, lung cancer, cervical and ovarian cancer
	Carboplatin	Teratoma, lung cancer, ovarian cancer
	Dacarbazine	Lymphoma, melanoma
	Procarbazine	Lymphoma
Common combinations	Cyclophosphamide, methotrexate, 5-fluorouracil (CMF)	
	Carboplatin and paclitaxel	
	Cisplatin and 5-fluorouracil	

Supportive care

Most cytotoxics have a narrow therapeutic window or index. Unfortunately, even at minimally effective doses, they have significant side-effects, as shown in Figure 11.8. Considerable supportive therapy is required to enable patients to tolerate sufficient therapy to achieve its potential benefit.

Administration

Most drugs have to be given intravenously, and many are vesicant or locally irritant if there is an extravasation (Fig. 11.9). Chemotherapy should therefore never be given

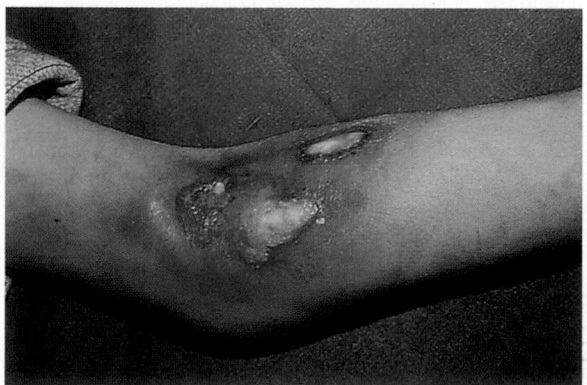

Fig. 11.9 Extravasation. Skin necrosis due to extravasation of anthracycline chemotherapy (e.g. doxorubicin, daunorubicin).

into an antecubital fossa vein, and so some patients receive their chemotherapy using indwelling central venous catheters (such as a Hickman line or Port-a-Cath) to minimise the risk of damage. Otherwise the patient must be carefully observed, and the chemotherapy stopped at the first sign of any extravasation. Equally, these drugs are potentially dangerous to the person giving the therapy, because cytotoxics are potentially carcinogenic to them, and also potentially teratogenic. There must be policies for the use of gloves and aprons and safe disposal of syringes containing cytotoxics.

Adverse effects

Nausea and vomiting are common, and used to be greatly feared. However, with modern anti-emetics, such as the combination of dexamethasone and highly selective 5-hydroxytryptamine (5-HT, serotonin) receptor antagonists (e.g. ondansetron), most patients now receive chemotherapy without any significant problems. Myelosuppression is common to almost all cytotoxics. This not only limits the dose of drug, but also can cause life-threatening complications. The risk of neutropenia can be reduced with the use of specific growth factors that accelerate the repopulation of myeloid precursor cells. The most commonly used is granulocyte colony-stimulating factor (G–CSF), which is widely used in conjunction with chemotherapy regimens that induce a high rate of neutropenia (p. 1014). More recently it has also been used to 'accelerate' the administration of chemotherapy, enabling

11.19 TOXICITY OF CHEMOTHERAPEUTIC AGENTS

Cytotoxic	Toxicity	Antidote/precaution
Almost all	Bone marrow suppression	Delay next cycle until recovery Use of colony-stimulating factors (G–CSF)
Most drugs	Gonadal failure and teratogenicity	For patient, relatives and staff Careful handling of syringes as well as patient body fluids Prior preservation of ovarian tissue, sperm
	Risk of extravasation	Careful monitoring during administration Use of semi-permanent catheters for administration
	Actual extravasation	Rapid application of local policies and antidotes (drug-specific)
Anthracyclines	Cardiac muscle damage	Do not use if pre-existing damage Regular monitoring of ejection fraction, and maximal total dose Dexrazoxane (not widely used)
Cisplatin, ifosfamide	Renal damage	Do not use if low creatinine clearance Maintain high fluid loading during/after chemotherapy
Ifosfamide, cyclophosphamide	Haemorrhagic cystitis	Maintain high fluid throughput Co-administration of mesna
Docetaxel	Peripheral oedema	Pre-treatment with dexamethasone
Vinca alkaloids	Peripheral neuropathy	Maximal dose of 2 mg vincristine/administration Careful monitoring during therapy
Paclitaxel, cisplatin	Peripheral neuropathy	None: careful monitoring during therapy

11

11.20 HORMONAL TREATMENTS

Drug/approach	Therapeutic target	Hormone	Disease
Luteinising hormone-releasing hormone (LHRH) agonists	Pituitary	LH, follicle-stimulating hormone (FSH) → Secondary oestrogen → Secondary androgens	Breast cancer Prostate cancer
Ovarian ablation	Ovarian function	Oestrogen synthesis	Breast cancer
Testicular ablation	Testicular function	Androgen synthesis	Prostate cancer
Anti-oestrogens (e.g. tamoxifen)	Oestrogen receptor	Oestrogen function	Breast cancer
Aromatase inhibitors	Aromatase enzyme	Oestrogen synthesis	Breast cancer
Progestogens	Unclear	Oestrogen synthesis Direct on endometrium	Breast cancer Endometrial cancer

standard doses to be given at shorter intervals where the rate-limiting factor has been the time taken for the peripheral neutrophil count to recover. Such accelerated chemotherapy regimens have now been demonstrated to offer therapeutic advantages in small-cell lung cancer, lymphoma and possibly breast cancer. Other side-effects may be specific to a drug or to a class of drugs, and there may not always be a specific antidote, so that careful attention to detail is required during the administration of any chemotherapy (Box 11.19).

HORMONAL TREATMENTS

Since breast cancers arise from the epithelium of breast ducts which are sensitive to oestrogen and progesterone, it is not surprising that they sometimes retain hormonal sensitivity. The best predictor for the sensitivity of breast cancer to hormonal therapy is the presence of detectable levels of the intracellular protein oestrogen receptor (ER-α), and assessment of this is now standard in the pathological diagnosis of breast cancer. Dramatically reducing circulating oestrogen can reduce the proliferation of cancer cells and increase their loss through apoptosis leading to tumour shrinkage (Fig. 11.10). Oestrogen synthesis can be inhibited by various means at different levels, including intratumoral production. In the correctly chosen patient, adjuvant hormonal therapy reduces the risk of relapse and death at least as much as chemotherapy, and in advanced disease can induce stable disease and remissions that may last months to years, with acceptable toxicity (see below). Hormonal manipulation may be effective in other cancers (Box 11.20). In prostate cancer, reductions in the level of the growth-promoting androgens can provide good long-term control of advanced disease, but there is no convincing evidence that it is an effective therapy following potentially curative surgery. Progestogens are active in the treatment of breast cancer and endometrial cancer.

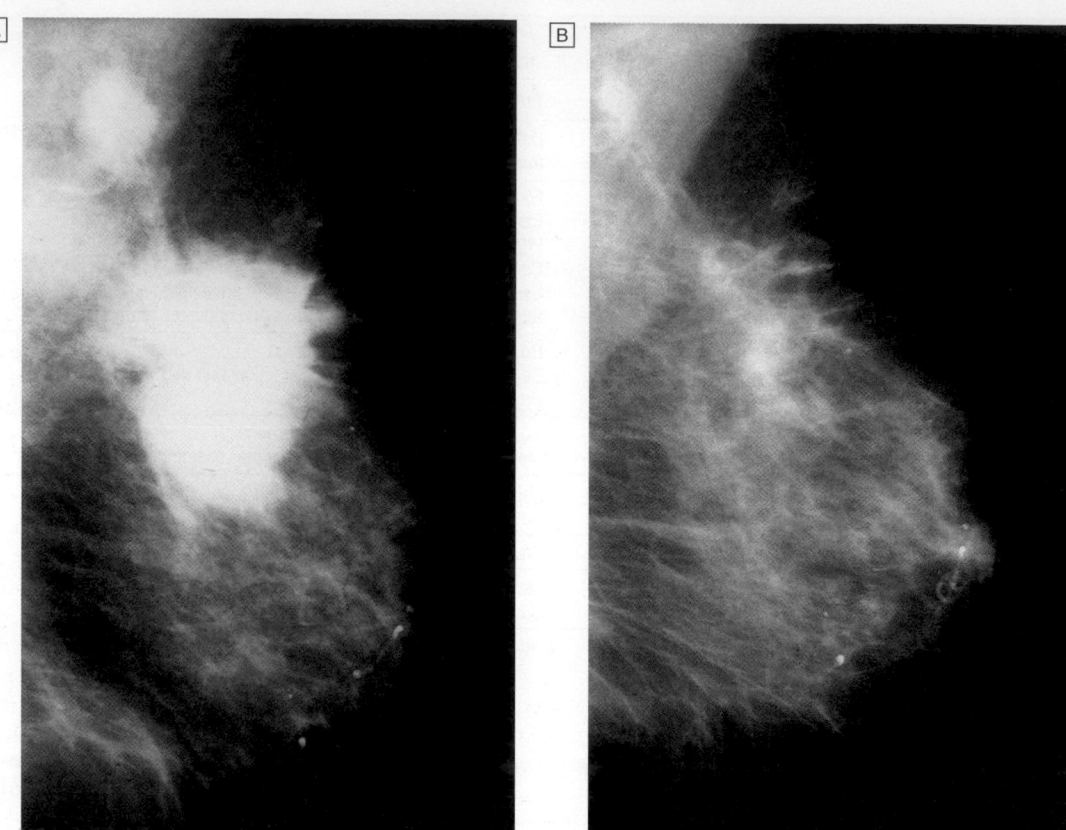

Fig. 11.10   Serial mammograms showing a breast cancer responding to hormone therapy. [A] Large tumour with involved axillary nodes before treatment. [B] After 3 months of hormone therapy alone, the tumour has shrunk significantly.

BIOLOGICAL TREATMENTS

Immunological treatments

A profound stimulus to the patient's immune system can sometimes alter the natural history of a malignancy, and the discovery of interferons stimulated much research. Although solid tumours show little benefit, interferons are active in melanoma and lymphoma, and there is evidence that they are beneficial as adjuvants (after surgery and chemotherapy respectively) to delay recurrence. Whether interferon-induced stimulation of the immune system is capable of eradicating microscopic disease remains unproven. More powerful immune responses can be achieved with potent agents like interleukin-2 (IL-2), but the accompanying systemic toxicity is a problem still to be overcome.

The immune system is now being harnessed by the use of monoclonal antibodies directed against specific antigens carried by tumour cells. To date only a few such antigens have been successfully targeted with antibodies that are licensed for clinical use. Rituximab is an antibody against the common B-cell antigen CD20. It increases complete response rates and improves survival in diffuse large-cell non-Hodgkin lymphoma when combined with chemo-therapy, and is also effective in palliating advanced follicular non-Hodgkin lymphoma (p. 1049). In addition, the onco-gene *Her-2* is over-expressed in around one-third of breast cancers, and in a number of other solid tumours. The monoclonal antibody trastuzumab is an effective single-agent therapy, and also improves survival in patients with advanced breast cancer when it is given in conjunction with chemotherapy. Unfortunately, trastuzumab can induce cardiac failure by an unknown biological mechanism, especially in combination with the potentially cardiotoxic cytotoxic drug, doxorubicin.

Bisphosphonates

Administration of bisphosphonates can inhibit osteoclast function (p. 1068), reducing bone turnover, bone pain and the risk of skeletal events, and there is some evidence to suggest that prophylactic use of these compounds may prevent skeletal complications in advanced (and potentially even early stage) breast cancer and myeloma. There is evidence that they are also effective for treatment of bone metastases in most tumour types, including prostate and renal cancer, although their use in these other solid tumours is not yet routine.

NOVEL AND TARGETED THERAPIES

Molecular biology has allowed the development of drugs to block the particular pathways responsible for the growth of a cancer. This creates the potential to target cancer cells more selectively, with reduced toxicity to normal tissues. However, although some effective treatments have been produced, understanding why a therapy might *not* work is itself revealing more complex patterns of tumour biology!

Some novel anti-cancer therapies developed using molecular biological insights have reached the clinic. For example, gefitinib and imatinib are both based on inhibiting a cell surface tyrosine kinase receptor. The former was designed to inhibit the activity of the epidermal growth factor receptor, which is over-expressed in many solid tumours, such as lung and breast cancer. However, the drug's activity does not depend on the amount of over-expression (unlike trastuzumab which targets a closely related receptor, Her-2), but on whether or not the gene coding for the receptor has a mutation in the hinge region of the receptor, presumably making it permanently active. Imatinib was developed to inhibit the *BCR-ABL* gene product tyrosine kinase that is responsible for chronic myeloid leukaemia (p. 1044), which it does extremely effectively. It is also active in a type of sarcoma (GIST, see below) which has over-expression of another cell surface tyrosine kinase, c-kit. As with any new drug, there are sometimes unexpected side-effects, but both of these agents have a good tolerability profile and this makes them more acceptable than conventional chemotherapy, which in the case of GIST is also less effective. Over the next few years many more such agents will come into clinical use, with the potential to revolutionise our approach to some cancers.

TREATMENT OF COMMON SOLID TUMOURS

The treatments of most common solid tumors are described in the relevant chapters (lung, p. 705; gastrointestinal, pp. 891, 903, 909 and 923; liver, p. 983; haematological, p. 1039; kidney and genitourinary tract, p. 512; skin, p. 1301; brain, p. 1236). Other important cancers are discussed briefly here.

BREAST CANCER

The treatment of a patient with breast cancer rests with diagnosis, multidisciplinary assessment and a combination of local and systemic therapy. Whether a patient is diagnosed as a result of symptoms or through screening, the approach is the same. The assessment of clinical, radiological and pathological findings is required:

- *Clinical examination* may help distinguish cyst from solid lump.
- *Mammography* may identify malignant calcification or other features of concern, or the presence of a cyst. This may be complemented by ultrasound, and MRI may help if the findings are equivocal.
- *Cytology* from fine needle aspirate (FNA) and/or histopathology from a core biopsy including measurement of tumour grade, oestrogen receptor status (ER) and in some cases progesterone receptor (PR)

and/or Her-2 status. These can be performed (probably more accurately) on a definitive resection specimen (wide local excision or mastectomy).

Once a diagnosis of invasive cancer is made, further staging is performed (Box 11.11, p. 259).

Local disease

Patients are treated with a combination of radical local therapy and systemic anti-cancer therapy. If breast conservation is possible and desired by the patient, surgical excision is performed if it is likely to remove all known disease. In other cases, particularly when there is extensive pre-invasive cancer, mastectomy may be needed. If the relative size of a tumour to the breast is too big for breast conservation, an alternative approach is to give systemic anti-cancer therapy before surgery, which has been shown to reduce the need for mastectomy with no effect on overall survival. Successful breast conservation is followed by locoregional radiotherapy, although in older women with low-risk cancers the added benefit may not outweigh the disadvantages. All women should be considered for adjuvant systemic therapy, either hormonal or chemotherapy or both (Box 11.21). For women with *very* low-risk tumours, the benefit of this may be too small to justify it in all cases.

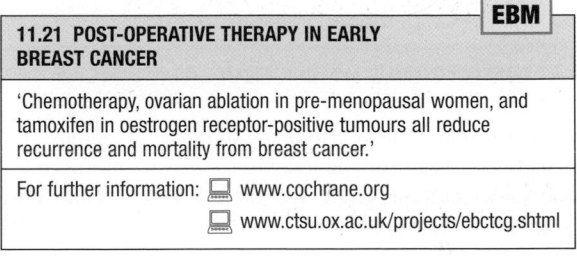

11.21 POST-OPERATIVE THERAPY IN EARLY BREAST CANCER **EBM**

'Chemotherapy, ovarian ablation in pre-menopausal women, and tamoxifen in oestrogen receptor-positive tumours all reduce recurrence and mortality from breast cancer.'

For further information: 🖥 www.cochrane.org
🖥 www.ctsu.ox.ac.uk/projects/ebctcg.shtml

The exact choice of systemic therapy is beyond the scope of this chapter, but where chemotherapy is indicated it most commonly consists of an anthracycline, either in combination or in sequence with either an alkylator such as cyclophosphamide or a taxane. When the likelihood of benefit is small, treatments should not be offered except as a last resort. Patients with breast cancers that do not express any hormonal receptors (ER- and PR-negative cancers) should not be offered adjuvant endocrine therapy such as tamoxifen or an aromatase inhibitor, as it will only increase the risk of toxicity. Similar predictors of response to chemotherapy are not at present defined, but may be in the future.

Metastatic disease

The treatment is primarily systemic with chemotherapy and/or hormonal therapy; there is little role for surgery. Local treatment to an ulcerating primary may be given (such as radiotherapy or 'toilet' mastectomy), but most will improve with effective systemic therapy. However, when previous hormonal therapies have failed to work, or if the patient's disease is rapidly growing and involving vital organs such as liver or lung, effective control is more likely with chemotherapy.

11

OVARIAN CANCER

This is commonly diagnosed with evidence of metastases at presentation, although in many patients these are confined to the peritoneal cavity. Most types of ovarian cancer are among the most chemosensitive of solid tumours, and chemotherapy therefore has an equal role to surgery. Patients usually first have the tumour excised by a surgeon with a specialist interest. The best long-term outcomes are seen when the largest residual lesions are around 1–2 cm^3 or less. Several cycles of platinum-based chemotherapy are then given, following which it may be appropriate to carry out further surgery. Even for patients with disease that has spread within the peritoneal cavity, long-term survival is possible. The distinction between a radical and a palliative approach is therefore not one that is made at first diagnosis, unless it is clear that the patient is too ill for surgery or chemotherapy. Unfortunately, the disease relapses in the majority of patients, despite effective initial therapy. Further treatments with both surgery and chemotherapy are usually offered, but cure is rarely possible and the focus switches to a palliative approach.

For patients presenting with localised disease (whether confined to one or both ovaries), surgical resection is usually followed by adjuvant chemotherapy except in low-grade cases.

ENDOMETRIAL AND CERVICAL CANCER

For many years, a large part of the workload of radiotherapy departments has been the treatment of cancer of the cervix and endometrium. These are the sites most commonly treated with intra-cavitary radioactive isotopes, usually caesium. Applicators may be inserted into the vagina and/or the uterus under a general anaesthetic to guide placement and maintain the position of the isotope. For reasons of radioprotection, an afterloading technique is usually used whereby the radioactive sources are inserted into the preplaced applicators automatically using a system such as a Selectron (Fig. 11.11).

CARCINOMA OF THE CERVIX

The most common is squamous cell carcinoma. The disease is usually staged using the FIGO (Fédération Internationale de Gynécologie et d'Obstétrique) staging system. Investigations include an examination under anaesthetic and cystoscopy to assess local extent, as well as staging by intravenous urography (IVU), chest X-ray and blood tests.

Treatment depends on the stage:

- *Pre-malignant disease* (cervical intra-epithelial neoplasia, CIN): local ablation with laser therapy or diathermy.
- *Microinvasive disease*: cone biopsy or a simple hysterectomy in older patients past child-bearing age will be curative in the majority of cases.

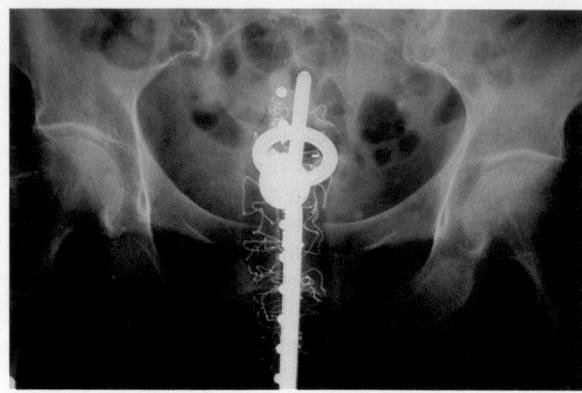

Fig. 11.11 Selectron treatment of cervical cancer. An X-ray taken after the insertion of metal applicators into the vaginal vault and endometrium. Radioactive sources will be inserted into the applicators remotely (afterloading technique). The fine lines are in gauze packing, to keep the applicators in place.

- *Invasive but localised disease*: radical surgery with a Wertheim's hysterectomy or radical radiotherapy offers potential cure. There are advantages and disadvantages associated with both of these treatments and patient preference is an important consideration. Often radiotherapy is offered to older patients and those not fit for surgery.

In selected cases where there is a high risk of recurrence, there may be a role for post-operative radiotherapy. Where there is incurable disease, chemotherapy with a combination such as methotrexate and cisplatin may be beneficial.

CARCINOMA OF THE CORPUS UTERI

The mainstay of treatment is surgery. An examination under anaesthetic and dilatation and curettage are essential as part of the staging investigations. The FIGO staging system is used. The extent of surgery will depend on the stage of the disease, but will include an abdominal hysterectomy and bilateral salphingoophorectomy with a lymphadenectomy in those at high risk of nodal spread. Post-operative radiotherapy may be necessary depending on the risk of loco-regional recurrence and may include intra-cavitary treatment to the vaginal vault as well as external beam treatment to the pelvis.

For inoperable, recurrent and metastatic disease, medroxy-progesterone produces an objective response in 30% of cases.

HEAD AND NECK CANCER

The head and neck cancers incorporate an important group of diseases whose management is complex and demanding, both radiotherapeutically and surgically. The more common sites of malignancy include the nasopharynx, hypopharynx, maxillary antrum, larynx and salivary glands. The management of each individual cancer cannot be described here in detail but fundamental principles are relevant to all

11

sites. Close collaboration of a multidisciplinary team including a clinical oncologist, ENT surgeon, maxillofacial and plastic surgeon is crucial to the optimal management of these patients.

Many head and neck cancers are curable if diagnosed at an early stage but cure often comes at the cost of treatment that is associated with very significant morbidity. For most sites, the results of primary radiotherapy and primary surgery are similar and decisions regarding the most appropriate management are based on the functional result and patient preference. Both treatment modalities may be associated with very significant toxicity and, in the case of surgery, there is considerable mutilation with a cosmetic result that may be far from optimal. In general, radiotherapy may be best in the treatment of early cancers where cure rates are relatively high and the functional results better than surgery. For more extensive local disease, surgery usually forms the mainstay of treatment with post-operative radiation reserved for cases where there is a high risk of local recurrence.

Surgery and radiotherapy are demanding on both patient and clinician. Because of the complex anatomy and the close apposition of radiosensitive structures to the volume requiring to be irradiated, the planning and delivery of radiotherapy requires the most sophisticated of techniques. CT planning and shaped radiation beams are required for safe delivery of a tumoricidal dose without compromising local adjacent radiosensitive structures such as brain stem, spinal cord and optic chiasma.

SARCOMA

There are many different types of sarcoma, but the fundamental distinction is between osteosarcomas (bone tumours) and the remainder of soft-tissue origin. When the diagnosis of a soft-tissue sarcoma is suspected, the patient should be referred to a centre with a multidisciplinary team with a major interest in these uncommon tumours. Extensive imaging of the suspected lesion helps determine the optimal method of both diagnosis and primary surgical treatment; diagnostic resection is not usually the best way to proceed. In the absence of definite metastases (the lung is the most common site for most types), surgical resection is the primary therapeutic modality. Peripheral lesions may require amputation, but where that can be avoided, resection, particularly of high-grade sarcomas, should be followed by radiotherapy. The role of systemic therapy in adult soft-tissue sarcoma is controversial, with improvements in recurrence but not in overall survival, except in some subgroups. This is in contrast to the paediatric

tumours, which also arise in young adults, where chemotherapy has significantly contributed to the improved cure rate. However, many centres would offer adjuvant chemotherapy to fit adult patients with large high-grade sarcomas of most histological subtypes.

Similarly, high-quality surgery, together with adjuvant chemotherapy, is key to the successful treatment of osteosarcomas. There is evidence that amputations may be needed less often following primary chemotherapy, and this is almost always given first (an approach that can also be applied to some soft-tissue sarcomas). Radiotherapy has little role to play, whereas the use of systemic chemotherapy significantly improves the chance of cure. Patients with less than 5% of the primary tumour still viable after chemotherapy have the highest chance of cure.

Following successful treatment of the primary sarcoma, follow-up of patients should include regular radiological examination of both the primary site and the lungs. Recurrent disease at either site can sometimes be successfully cured surgically (with or without further chemotherapy).

There is one type of soft tissue sarcoma, gastrointestinal stromal tumour (GIST), which is the paradigm of molecular targeted therapy. Extraordinarily resistant to conventional chemotherapy or radiotherapy, almost every case of this tumour has a mutation in the c-kit cell surface receptor tyrosine kinase. Imatinib (p. 269) inhibits tyrosine kinase and can shrink the majority of cases of advanced tumours. It has not yet been demonstrated to improve survival if given after surgical resection of a primary tumour, although many expect that current trials will find it effective in the adjuvant setting as well.

FURTHER INFORMATION

Books and journal articles

De Vita VT, Hellman S, Rosenburg SA, eds. Cancer: principles and practice of oncology. 7th edn. Philadelphia: Lippincott Williams & Wilkins; 2005.

Franks LM, Teich NM. Introduction to the cellular and molecular biology of cancer. 3rd edn. Oxford: Oxford University Press; 1997.

Tannock IF, Hill RP, Bristow RG, et al. The basic science of oncology. 4th edn. New York: McGraw-Hill; 2004.

Websites

http://info.cancerresearchuk.org/cancerstats/ *Information on UK cancer statistics and what they mean.*

www.cancer.org *Website of the American Cancer Society; aimed at patients and relatives but gives some basic data on cancer and its treatment.*

www.sign.ac.uk/guidelines/index.html *Evidence-based SIGN guidelines for cancer (and other diseases).*

11

12

D. OXENHAM

Palliative care and pain management

Palliative care is the active total care of patients with far advanced, rapidly progressive and ultimately fatal disease. The focus is quality of life rather than cure. It encompasses a distinct body of knowledge and skills that all good physicians must possess to allow them to care effectively for patients at the end of life. In palliative care there is a fundamental change of emphasis in decision-making: investigations and treatments are kept appropriate to the stage of the patient's disease and the prognosis. The principles of palliative care may be applied to any chronic disease state in addition to the terminal phase.

Because of its focus on symptoms, palliative medicine specialists are expert in cancer pain management. In this chapter, cancer pain control and non-malignant pain control are described, including the similarities and differences in their management.

PAIN

The International Association for the Study of Pain (IASP) has defined pain as 'an unpleasant sensory and emotional experience associated with actual or potential tissue damage or described in terms of such damage'. Pain perception does not therefore correlate with the degree of tissue damage, and each patient's experience and expression of pain are different. Effective pain treatment facilitates recovery from injury or surgery, aids rapid recovery of function, and may minimise chronic pain and disability. Unfortunately, there may be obstacles to the delivery of good pain relief, such as poor assessment and concerns about the use of opioid analgesia.

PAIN CLASSIFICATION AND MECHANISMS

Pain can be classified into two main types:

- *nociceptive*: due to direct stimulation of peripheral nerve endings (e.g. wounds, fractures, burns, angina)
- *neuropathic*: due to dysfunction of the pain perception system within the peripheral or central nervous system as a result of injury, disease or surgical damage (e.g. continuing pain experienced from a limb which has been amputated—'phantom limb pain'). It is important to identify this early (Box 12.1) because it is more difficult to treat once established.

12.1 FEATURES OF NEUROPATHIC PAIN

- Burning, stabbing or pulsing pain
- Spontaneous pain, without ongoing tissue damage
- Pain in an area of sensory loss
- The presence of a major neurological deficit (e.g. spinal cord trauma)
- Pain in response to non-painful stimuli—'allodynia'
- Increased pain in response to painful stimuli—'hyperalgesia'
- Unpleasant abnormal sensations—'dysaesthesias'
- Poor relief with opioids alone

The pain perception system is described in detail on page 1185. There is considerable plasticity (changeability) in all the peripheral and central components of the pain pathway, with several areas of modulation within the system. The 'pain pathway' cannot therefore be viewed as a simple hard-wired circuit of nerves connecting tissue pain receptors to the brain, but should be seen as a dynamic system where a continuing pain stimulus can cause central changes leading to increased pain perception in the pain centres of the brain. Early and appropriate treatment of pain is important as it reduces the potential for the development of these changes.

ASSESSMENT AND MEASUREMENT OF PAIN

Accurate assessment of the patient is the first step in providing good analgesia.

History and measurement of pain

A history of the patient's general health status should be taken with a full pain history, to establish its causes and underlying diagnoses. Patients may have more than one pain, e.g. bone and neuropathic pain from skeletal metastases (Box 12.2). A diagram of the body on which the patient can mark the pain site can be helpful. If patients are asked to score pain, they consistently rate it higher than their physicians and nurses, and patient-rated pain measurement is therefore an essential part of overall assessment and assessment of the effect of treatment. Methods include:

- *verbal rating scale*: different verbal descriptions used to rate pain—'no pain', 'mild pain', 'moderate pain' and 'severe pain'
- *11 point scale*: a question such as 'Over the past 24 hours, how would you rate your pain if 0 is no pain and 10 is the worst pain you could imagine?'

Psychological aspects of chronic pain

Perception of pain is influenced by many factors other than the painful stimulus, and pain cannot therefore be easily classified as wholly physical or psychogenic in any individual (Fig. 12.1). Patients who suffer chronic pain will be affected emotionally, and conversely emotional stress can exacerbate physical pain (p. 236). Full assessment for symptoms of anxiety and depression is fundamental to effective pain management.

Examination

This should include careful assessment of the painful area, looking for signs of neuropathic pain (Box 12.1) or bony tenderness, suggestive of bone metastases. In patients with cancer, do not assume that all pains are due to the cancer or its metastases.

Appropriate investigations

Investigations should be directed towards diagnosis of an underlying cause, remembering possible reversible causes even in patients with terminal cancer. Imaging may be

12.2 TYPES OF PAIN

Type of pain	Features	Management options
Bone pain	Tender area over bone Possible pain on movement	NSAIDs Bisphosphonates Radiotherapy
Increased intracranial pressure	Headache, worse in the morning, associated with vomiting and occasionally confusion	Corticosteroids Radiotherapy Codeine
Abdominal colic	Intermittent severe spasmodic, associated with nausea or vomiting	Antispasmodics
Liver capsule pain	Right upper quadrant abdominal pain, often associated with tender enlarged liver	Corticosteroids (Poor relief with opioids and NSAIDs)
Neuropathic pain	Box 12.1	Anticonvulsants, e.g. gabapentin, pregabalin Antidepressants, e.g. amitriptyline Ketamine
Ischaemic pain	Diffuse severe aching pain associated with evidence of poor perfusion	Poorly responsive to opioids NSAIDs Ketamine
Incident pain	Episodic pain usually related to movement or bowel spasm	Intermittent short-acting opioids Nerve block

12

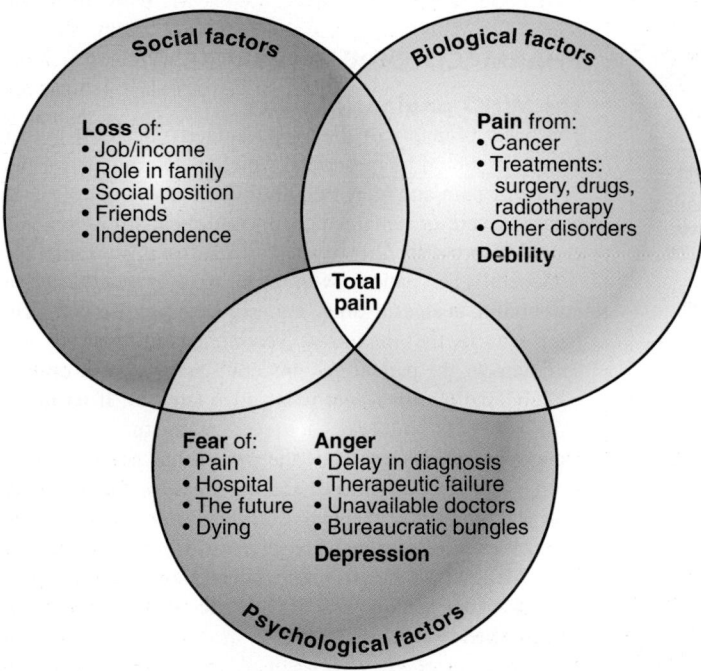

Fig. 12.1 Components of pain.

indicated, such as plain X-ray for fracture or MRI for spinal cord compression.

MANAGEMENT OF PAIN

Many of the principles of pain management apply to any painful condition. However, some interventions, such as strong opioids, either have, or are perceived to have, a greater chance of harm in patients with a good prognosis. Acute pain post-surgery or following trauma should be controlled with medication without causing unnecessary side-effects or risk to the patient (Fig. 12.2). Chronic, non-malignant pain is more difficult. It may be impossible to relieve pain completely and there is a greater emphasis on non-pharmacological treatments and enabling the patient to cope with pain.

Two-thirds of patients with cancer experience moderate or severe pain. One-quarter will have three or more different pains. Many of these pains are of a mixed aetiology and 50% of pain from cancer has a neuropathic element. Specific features of different pains and treatments are listed in

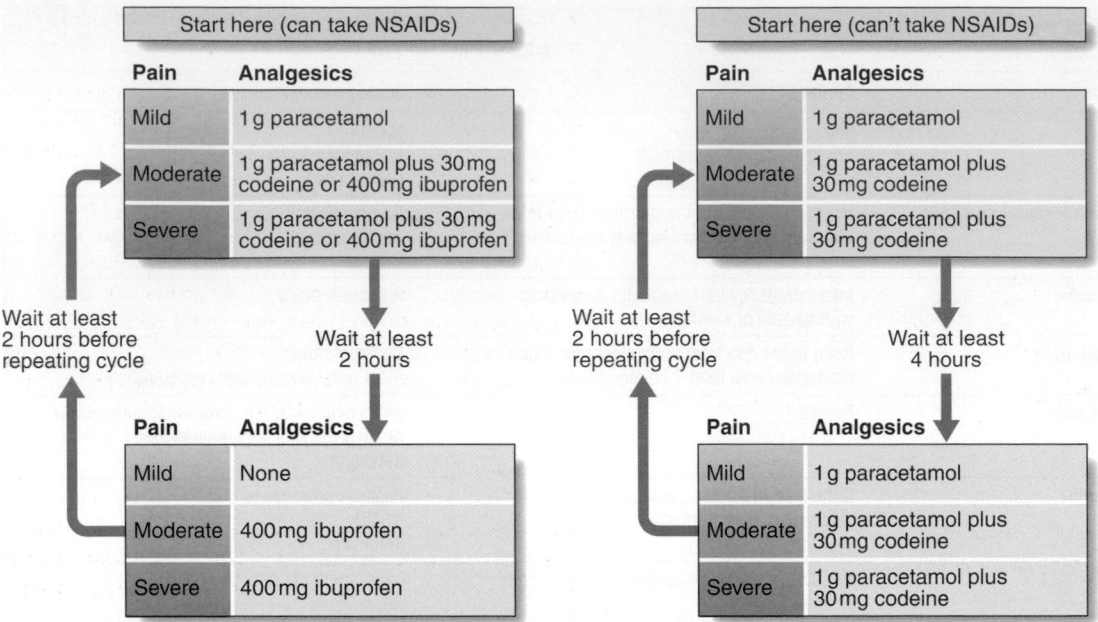

Fig. 12.2 Acute pain management.

12.3 OPIOID MYTHS

Myth	Fact
Pain is inevitable in cancer and many other diseases	**Pain can usually be controlled**
Opioids should be avoided because of dangerous side-effects	**Opioids can cause side-effects and sometimes the therapeutic window is narrow. However, side-effects are treatable and reversible**
The use of opioids commonly leads to addiction	**Addiction is very rare in patients who have pain and no previous history of addiction**
Taking opioids leads to more rapid decline and earlier death	**Opioids do not cause organ damage or serious harm. NSAIDs and paracetamol are more likely to cause irreversible damage**

Box 12.2. Careful evaluation will identify the likely pain mechanism and appropriate treatment.

Treatment is classified as pharmacological, non-pharmacological and complementary. It is fundamental to cancer pain management that a patient's fears about opioids are explored, and reassurance given that when used for cancer pain, psychological dependence and tolerance are not a concern (Box 12.3).

Nearly all types of pain respond to morphine to some degree. Some are completely opioid-responsive but some are relatively unresponsive. Neuropathic and ischaemic pains are often relatively unresponsive, as is severe pain on movement ('incident' pain). If a patient has an opioid-unresponsive or poorly responsive pain, it will only be relieved by opioids at a dose which causes significant side-effects. In this situation, pain relief is better achieved with the correct use of adjuvant analgesics (see below).

PHARMACOLOGICAL TREATMENTS

The WHO analgesic ladder

The basic principle of the WHO ladder (Fig. 12.3) is that analgesia should be prescribed which is appropriate for the degree of pain and increased until the pain is controlled. If pain is severe or remains poorly controlled, strong opioids should be prescribed.

Generally, a patient with mild pain is started on a non-opioid analgesic drug, e.g. paracetamol 1 g 6-hourly (step 1). If the maximum recommended dose is not sufficient or the patient has moderate pain, a weak opioid, e.g. codeine 60 mg 6-hourly, is added (step 2). If adequate pain relief is still not achieved with the maximum recommended dosages or if the patient has severe pain, a strong opioid is substituted for the weak opioid (step 3). It is important not to move 'sideways' (change from one drug to another of equal potency) on a particular step of the ladder. All patients with severe pain should receive a full trial of strong opioids with appropriate adjuvant analgesia, as described below.

Non-opioids

Paracetamol. This is effective when taken alone or in combination with opioids for mild to moderate pain. For severe pain it is inadequate alone, but remains a useful and well-tolerated adjunct.

Non-steroidal anti-inflammatory drugs (NSAIDs). These are effective in the treatment of mild to moderate pain, and are also useful adjuncts in the treatment of severe pain. Adverse effects (p. 1090) may be serious, especially in the elderly.

Weak opioids

Codeine and dihydrocodeine are weak opioids. They have lower analgesic efficacy than strong opioids and a ceiling dose. They are effective for mild to moderate pain.

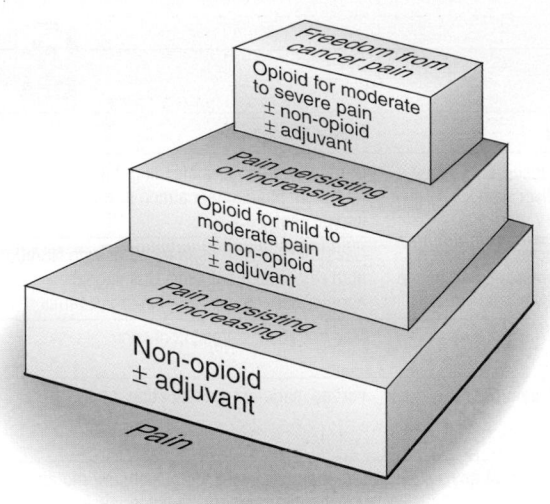

Fig. 12.3   The WHO analgesic ladder.

Strong opioids

Immediate-release (IR) oral morphine takes about 20 minutes to take effect and usually provides pain relief for 4 hours. Most patients with continuous pain should initially be prescribed IR oral morphine every 4 hours (i.e. six times daily), which will provide continuing pain relief over the whole 24-hour period. Controlled-release (CR) morphine lasts for 12 or 24 hours but takes much longer to take effect. It should only be used once the correct dose has been found by a process of dose titration with IR morphine until adequate pain relief is achieved.

In addition to the regular dose, an extra dose of IR morphine should be prescribed 'as required' for when the patient has any pain not controlled by the regular prescription ('breakthrough' pain). The dose should be the same as the regular 4-hourly dose. The frequency of breakthrough doses should be dictated by their efficacy and any side-effects, rather than by a fixed time interval. A patient may require hourly doses if pain is severe, but this should lead to early review. The patient and/or carer should note the timing of any breakthrough doses and the reason for them. This should be reviewed daily and the regular 4-hourly dose increased for the next 24 hours on the basis of:

- frequency of and reasons for breakthrough analgesia
- degree and acceptability of side-effects.

The regular 24-hour dose should then be increased by the sum of the breakthrough doses over the previous 24 hours, unless there are significant problems with unacceptable side-effects. When the correct dose has been established, a CR preparation can be prescribed, usually twice daily.

Worldwide, the most effective and appropriate route of administration is oral, though transdermal preparations of strong opioids (usually fentanyl) are extremely useful in certain situations (e.g. patients with dysphagia, or reluctant to take regular tablets). Diamorphine is a highly soluble strong opioid used for subcutaneous infusions, particularly in the last few days of life, but is only available in certain countries.

Common side-effects of opioids are shown in Box 12.4. Nausea and vomiting occur initially but usually settle after a few days. Opioids can cause confusion and drowsiness which are dose-related and reversible. In acute dosing, respiratory depression can occur but this is rare in a patient on regular opioids.

Opioid toxicity

All patients will develop dose-related side-effects such as nausea, drowsiness, confusion or myoclonus at some point; the dose at which this occurs varies from 10 to 5000 mg of morphine depending on the patient and the type of pain. This is termed morphine toxicity and is managed by reducing the dose and returning to IR morphine so that dose adjustments can be made more rapidly. Parenteral rehydration may be necessary and the pain should be reassessed to ensure appropriate adjuvants are being used. Switching to an alternative strong opioid may be helpful.

Alternatives to morphine include oxycodone, transdermal fentanyl, hydromorphone and occasionally methadone, which may produce a better balance of benefit against side-effects. Oxycodone and fentanyl have no renally excreted active metabolites and may be particularly useful in patients with renal failure. Pethidine is used in acute pain management but should not be used to manage chronic pain because of its short half-life and ceiling dose.

Adjuvant analgesics

An adjuvant analgesic is a drug with a primary indication other than pain but which is analgesic in some painful

12.4 OPIOID SIDE-EFFECTS	
Side-effect	**Management**
Constipation	Regular laxative, e.g. co-danthramer or co-danthrusate (starting dose 2 capsules o.d.; titrate laxative)
Dry mouth	Frequent sips of iced water, soft white paraffin to lips, chlorhexidine mouthwashes 12-hourly, sugar-free gum, water or saliva sprays
Nausea/vomiting	Haloperidol 1.5–3 mg nocte or metoclopramide/domperidone 10 mg 8-hourly In cases of constant nausea a parenteral antiemetic is necessary to break the nausea cycle
Sedation	Explanation very important Expect to settle in about 2–3 days Avoid other sedating medication where possible Ensure appropriate use of adjuvant analgesics which can have an opioid-sparing effect

12

12.5 ADJUVANT ANALGESICS

Drug	Dosage	Indications	Side-effects*
NSAIDs e.g. diclofenac	50 mg oral 8-hourly (SR 75 mg 12-hourly) 100 mg per rectum once a day	Bone metastases, soft tissue infiltration, liver pain, inflammatory pain	Gastric irritation and bleeding, fluid retention, headache; caution in renal impairment
Corticosteroids e.g. dexamethasone	8–16 mg per day; use morning (titrate down to lowest dose which controls pain)	Raised intracranial pressure, nerve compression, soft tissue infiltration, liver pain	Gastric irritation if used together with NSAID, fluid retention, confusion, Cushingoid appearance, candidiasis, hyperglycaemia
Gabapentin	100–300 mg nocte (starting dose) (titrate to 600 mg 8-hourly)	Neuropathic pain of any aetiology	Mild sedation, tremor, confusion
Carbamazepine (evidence for all anticonvulsants)	100–200 mg nocte (starting dose)	Neuropathic pain of any aetiology	Vertigo, sedation, constipation, rash
Amitriptyline (evidence for all tricyclics)	25 mg nocte (starting dose) 10 mg (elderly)	Neuropathic pain of any aetiology	Sedation, dizziness, confusion, dry mouth, constipation, urinary retention; avoid in cardiac disease

*In the elderly all drugs can cause confusion.

12

12.6 TREATMENT OF NEUROPATHIC PAIN | EBM

'Tricyclic antidepressants, a variety of anticonvulsants, and gabapentin are effective treatments for neuropathic pain.'

- Guideline 44. Control of pain in patients with cancer. Edinburgh: Scottish Intercollegiate Guidelines Network; 2000.

For further information: 🖥 www.sign.ac.uk

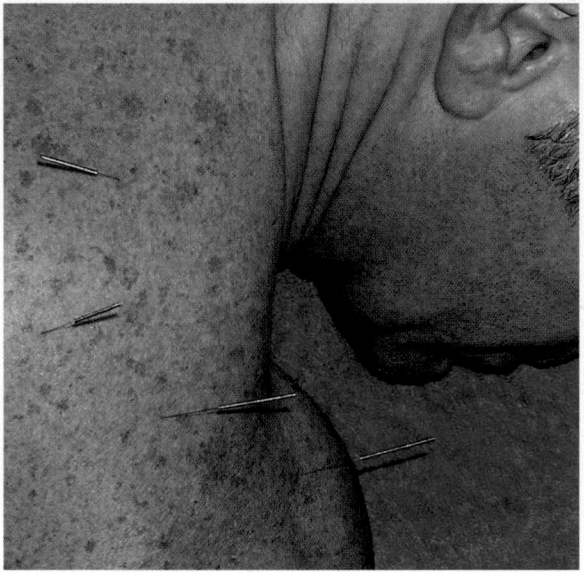

Fig. 12.4   Acupuncture.

conditions and may enhance the effect of primary analgesia. At each step of the WHO analgesic ladder, an adjuvant analgesic should be considered, the choice depending on the type of pain (Boxes 12.5 and 12.6).

NON-PHARMACOLOGICAL AND COMPLEMENTARY TREATMENTS

Radiotherapy
Radiotherapy has a place in the management of bone metastases (Box 12.2, p. 275).

Physiotherapy
One of the key aims of pain management is to alleviate suffering and restore function, so physiotherapy and active mobilisation must be considered early. Pain may respond to spinal manipulation, massage, application of heat or cold, and exercise. Immediate cold application (e.g. ice packs) reduces subsequent swelling and inflammation after sports injury.

Psychological techniques
Psychological techniques include simple relaxation, hypnosis, cognitive behavioural therapies and biofeedback (p. 238). These train the patient in coping strategies and behavioural techniques. This is clearly more relevant in chronic non-malignant pain than in cancer pain.

Stimulation therapies
Acupuncture (Fig. 12.4) has been used successfully in Eastern medicine for centuries. It causes release of endogenous analgesics (endorphins) within the spinal cord. Transcutaneous electrical nerve stimulation (TENS) may have a similar mechanism of action to acupuncture and can be used in both acute and chronic pain.

Herbal medicine and homeopathy
These are widely used for pain, but often with little evidence for efficacy (p. 15). Safety regulations for these treatments are limited compared with conventional drugs, and the doctor should be wary of unrecognised side-effects which may result.

PRESENTING PROBLEMS IN PALLIATIVE CARE

COUGH

Intractable cough is a difficult symptom to manage. There are many causes (p. 657) in cancer and patients with other intractable illnesses (motor neurone disease, cardiac failure, chronic obstructive pulmonary disease). Antitussives such as codeine linctus are sometimes effective, particularly to aid sleep at night. Specific treatments for the underlying condition should also be given.

BREATHLESSNESS

The sensation of breathlessness is the result of a complex interaction between different factors at the levels of production (the pathophysiological cause), perception (the severity of breathlessness perceived by the patient) and expression (the symptoms expressed by an individual patient). Assessment and treatment should therefore be targeted at modifying perception, particularly when there is no reversible pathophysiology. Perception and expression of breathlessness can be significantly improved even if there is no reversible 'cause' (Box 12.7).

Clearly reversible causes of breathlessness (p. 658) should be sought and managed, remembering that investigation and treatment should be appropriate to the prognosis and stage of disease. A therapeutic trial of corticosteroids (dexamethasone 6 mg for 5 days) and/or nebulised salbutamol is helpful in many patients.

Perception of breathlessness may be affected by specific anxieties and beliefs about breathlessness, and these should be explored. The most common fear is that the patient will die during an attack of breathlessness; although this is understandable, reassurance can be given that it is unlikely. Another frequently expressed fear is that breathlessness will continue to worsen until it is continuous and unbearable, leading to a distressing and undignified death. The patient can again be reassured that this is uncommon and can be effectively managed with benzodiazepines and other drugs.

Some patients have specific panic–breathlessness cycles where breathlessness leads to panic which leads to worsening breathlessness and worsening panic. These should be identified and explained to the patient. A rapidly acting benzodiazepine such as sublingual lorazepam or non-drug measures such as relaxation techniques may help.

Discussion with a physiotherapist about energy conservation and pacing of activity may also be useful.

Perception of breathlessness may also be altered by night-time or regular morphine, or by regular benzodiazepines. Oxygen may be no more effective than a fan or piped air for non-hypoxic breathlessness and again the patient's perception of the need for oxygen can be gently explored and modified.

NAUSEA AND VOMITING

Different causes (p. 866) of nausea and vomiting are associated with different clinical presentations. Large-volume vomiting with little nausea is common in intestinal obstruction, whereas constant nausea with little or no vomiting is often due to metabolic abnormalities or drugs. Vomiting related to raised intracranial pressure is worse in the morning.

Different receptors are activated depending on the cause or causes of the nausea (Fig. 12.5). For example, dopamine receptors in the chemotactic trigger zone in the fourth ventricle are stimulated by metabolic and drug causes of nausea, whereas gastric irritation stimulates histamine receptors in the vomiting centre via the vagus nerve.

12

EBM

12.7 PALLIATIVE TREATMENT OF BREATHLESSNESS

'Interventions based on psychosocial support, breathing control and coping strategies can help patients to cope with the symptom of breathlessness and reduce physical and emotional distress.'

• Bredin M, et al. BMJ 1999; 318:901.

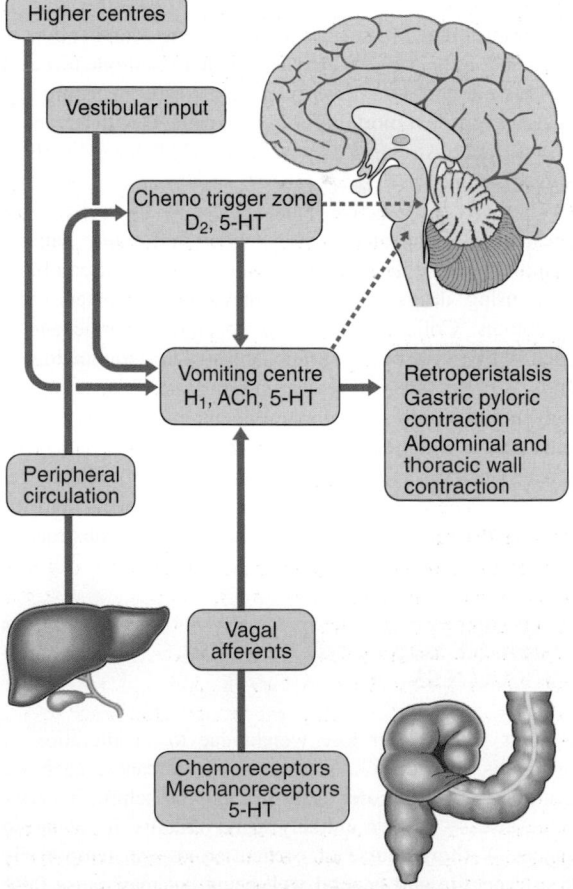

Fig. 12.5 Mechanisms of nausea. (ACh = acetylcholine; 5-HT = serotonin, 5-hydroxytryptamine; H_1 = histamine; D_2 = dopamine)

12.8 RECEPTOR SITE ACTIVITY OF ANTIEMETIC DRUGS

Area	Receptors	Drugs
Chemo trigger zone	Dopamine$_2$ 5-HT	Haloperidol Metoclopramide
Vomiting centre	Histamine$_1$ Acetylcholine	Cyclizine Levomepromazine Hyoscine
Gut (gastric stasis)		Metoclopramide
Gut distension (vagal stimulation)	Histamine$_1$	Cyclizine
Gut (chemoreceptors)	5-HT	Levomepromazine

Reversible causes (e.g. hypercalcaemia, constipation) should be treated appropriately. Potential drug causes should be considered and medication rationalised if possible. As different classes of antiemetic drug act at different receptors, antiemetic therapy should be based on a careful assessment of the probable causes and a rational decision to use a particular class of drug (Box 12.8). The subcutaneous route is often required initially to overcome gastric stasis and poor absorption of oral medicines.

GASTROINTESTINAL OBSTRUCTION

Gastrointestinal obstruction is a frequent complication of intra-abdominal cancer. Patients may have multiple levels of obstruction and symptoms may vary greatly in nature and severity. Surgical mortality is high in patients with advanced disease and obstruction may be effectively managed without surgery in any case.

The key to effective management is to address the presenting symptoms—colic, abdominal pain, nausea, vomiting, intestinal secretions, individually or in combination, using drugs which do not cause or worsen other symptoms. Colic responds well to anticholinergic agents such as hyoscine butylbromide, and somatostatin analogues such as octreotide will reduce intestinal secretions. Nausea will improve with metoclopramide although this is contraindicated in the presence of colic because of its prokinetic effect. Cyclizine will improve nausea but may reduce gut motility. There is some evidence that corticosteroids (dexamethasone 8 mg) shorten the length of obstructive episodes.

WEIGHT LOSS AND GENERAL WEAKNESS

Patients with cancer lose weight due to an alteration of metabolism by the tumour known as the cancer cachexia syndrome. NSAIDs and megestrol may be helpful in early-stage disease but are unlikely to be effective in advanced cancer. A short course of corticosteroids can temporarily boost appetite and general well-being but may cause false weight gain by promoting fluid retention. While they can improve appetite and elevate mood, corticosteroids must be carefully used as they can cause neuropsychiatric disturbances in addition to physical side-effects.

ANXIETY AND DEPRESSION

It is important to identify depression even in patients with far advanced disease as this may still respond to treatment (p. 231). Sometimes appropriate management of physical symptoms alone will resolve anxiety and/or depression; however, in some cases concomitant treatment of depression and/or anxiety with a combination of drugs and psychotherapeutic approaches may be necessary. It is important not to assume that depression is 'understandable' because of an unpleasant physical symptom and therefore has no solution other than removing the symptom. Anxiety and depression may still be amenable to therapy even if the underlying physical problem remains.

DELIRIUM AND TERMINAL AGITATION

Many patients become confused or agitated in the last days of life. Opioid toxicity is a common cause. It is important to identify other causes (pp. 235 and 1187) which may be reversible, although at this stage it may be difficult or inappropriate to do so. Effective management of any distressing confusion remains extremely important. Opioids are not a good option and patients should be prescribed a neuroleptic agent (haloperidol) for confusion and adequate doses of benzodiazepines (diazepam or midazolam) to relieve distress. Some patients become profoundly distressed and require large doses of benzodiazepines.

THE DYING PHASE

TALKING ABOUT DYING

Talking about dying is difficult for health professionals, as it brings with it feelings of failure, loss of hope and fear of causing distress. Some patients have a great fear of death and never wish to discuss the possibility; others welcome the chance to talk about death and the dying process, express their wishes and gain reassurance that these will be respected; in general, their wish is for a dignified and peaceful death. Families also are grateful for the chance to prepare themselves for the death of a patient, by timely and gentle discussion with their doctor or other health professionals.

DIAGNOSING DYING

For many patients there comes a time when death is predictable and inevitable, when further active intervention will be futile and will cause distress rather than produce benefit. At least two-thirds of patients dying in hospital have a death that is predictable and measures should be taken to plan good care for the patient and family.

When patients with cancer become bed-bound, semi-comatose, no longer able to take tablets and only able to take sips of water, they are likely to be dying and many will have died within 2 days. Patients with other conditions also reach a stage where death is predictable and close. Doctors are sometimes poor at recognising that a patient is dying, and should listen to the views of other members of the multidisciplinary team.

MANAGEMENT

Once a decision has been reached that a patient has entered the dying phase, there is a significant and important change in management. Symptom control, relief of distress and care for the family are the most important facets of care (Box 12.9). Medication and investigation are only justifiable if they contribute to these ends. When patients can no longer drink because they are dying, intravenous fluids are not necessary and may cause worsening of bronchial secretions. Medicines should always be available for the relief of pain (e.g. morphine or diamorphine), nausea (e.g. levomepromazine), confusion (e.g. haloperidol), distress (e.g. diazepam or midazolam) and respiratory secretions (e.g. hyoscine hydrobromide). If these cause drowsiness or even worsening renal failure, it is reasonable to continue them if the principal aim of relieving distress is achieved.

12.9 CHECKLIST FOR THE DYING PHASE

- Stop non-essential medication
- Stop routine observations
- Ensure availability of parenteral medication for symptom relief
- Assess patient and family's awareness of condition
- Assess religious and spiritual needs
- Ensure family understands plan of care
- Ensure continued assessment and management of symptoms
- Arrange appropriate care after death

ETHICAL ISSUES AT THE END OF LIFE

In Europe between 25 and 50% of all deaths are associated with some form of decision which may affect the length of a patient's life. The most common form of decision involves withdrawing or withholding further treatment (for example, not treating a chest infection in a patient who is clearly dying). Less commonly, medicines are given which shorten a patient's life utilising the principle of double effect (see below). It is important to have a framework for considering such decisions; one of the most helpful employs four ethical principles which balance degrees of importance where they conflict (p. 11). These include: respecting a patient's wishes (autonomy); benefiting the patient and not causing harm (beneficence and non-maleficence); and being fair and legal (justice). Difficulties arise when these principles conflict: for example, when a patient wishes treatment which a doctor judges to be harmful or which is illegal. A decision has to be taken as to which principle is most

important. Is it better to respect a patient's wishes even if it causes harm, or to prevent harm by not respecting the patient's wishes?

A futile treatment is one which has no chance of achieving worthwhile benefit, i.e. it cannot achieve a result that the patient would consider, now or in the future, as worthwhile. Doctors are not required to institute a futile treatment and may choose not to discuss this with a patient where the discussion would cause distress.

INCAPACITY AND ADVANCE DIRECTIVES

Patients' wishes are very important in Western countries, although this is not true in all cultures. If a patient is unable to express their view because of communication or cognitive impairment, they lack 'capacity'. In order to decide what the patient would have wished had they been able, it is important to gain as much information as possible about the patient's previously expressed wishes and views from relatives and other health professionals. An advance directive is a previously recorded, written document of a patient's wishes (p. 165). It should carry the same weight in decision-making as a patient's contemporaneously expressed wishes, but may not be sufficiently specific to be used in a particular clinical situation.

REHYDRATION

Deciding whether to give intravenous fluids can be difficult when a patient is very unwell and the prognosis is uncertain. If a patient is clearly dying and has a prognosis of a few days (e.g. with disseminated malignancy), rehydration may cause harm by increasing bronchial secretions, and will not benefit the patient by prolonging life or relieving symptoms. A patient with a major stroke, who is unable to swallow but who is expected to live more than a few days, will develop renal impairment and thirst if not given fluids, and should be hydrated unless this treatment is considered futile.

DOUBLE EFFECT

At the end of life, the principle of double effect allows symptom control to be given to patients even though it may shorten their life, providing the 'good' effect (control of symptoms) outweighs the 'bad' effect (shortening of life) and there is no other means to achieve the same result. The intention must be to control symptoms rather than shorten life and no more medication should be given than achieves symptom control.

EUTHANASIA

In Britain and Europe between 3 and 6% of dying patients ask a doctor to end their lives. Many of these requests are temporary; some are associated with poor control of physical symptoms or a depressive illness. All expressions of a wish to die are an opportunity to help the patient discuss unresolved issues and problems, and these should be addressed.

Reversible causes, such as pain or depression, should be treated. Sometimes patients who are taking life-prolonging treatments, such as ACE inhibitors or anticoagulation, may choose to discontinue these following discussion and the provision of adequate alternative symptom control. There remain, however, a small number of patients who have a sustained, competent wish to end their lives despite good control of physical symptoms. Public ethical and legal debate over this issue is likely to continue.

PALLIATIVE CARE IN NON-MALIGNANT CONDITIONS

There is a growing recognition that the principles and some of the specific interventions developed in the palliative care of patients with cancer are equally applicable to other conditions. As oncological treatments advance, some cancers have become more like chronic illnesses and have better prognoses than advanced cardiac failure or diabetes mellitus. Studies have also demonstrated that these non-malignant diseases have an equally high burden of symptoms, and psychological and family distress. Clearly many of the principles of palliative care can be directly transferred to such disease states. Breathlessness from any cause can be alleviated even when there is no reversible 'cause', nausea can be evaluated and appropriate drugs chosen, and any predicted death can be managed effectively and compassionately. Access to specialist palliative care services should be on the basis of need rather than diagnosis and these services may need to consider expanding or focusing on those in most need of specialist help.

FURTHER INFORMATION

Books and journal articles

Ellershaw J, Wilkinson S. Care of the dying: a pathway to excellence. Oxford: Oxford University Press; 2003.

Kaye P. AZ pocketbook of symptom control. Northampton: EPL; 1994.

Twycross R. Introducing palliative care. Oxford: Radcliffe Medical; 2003.

Websites

www.pallcare.info General information about palliative care and end-of-life issues.

www.palliativedrugs.co.uk Information for health professionals about the use of drugs in palliative care. It highlights drugs given for unlicensed indications or by unlicensed routes and the administration of multiple drugs by continuous subcutaneous infusion.

12

13

W.T.A. TODD

D.N.J. LOCKWOOD

S. SUNDAR

Infectious diseases

CLINICAL EXAMINATION OF THE FEBRILE PATIENT

13

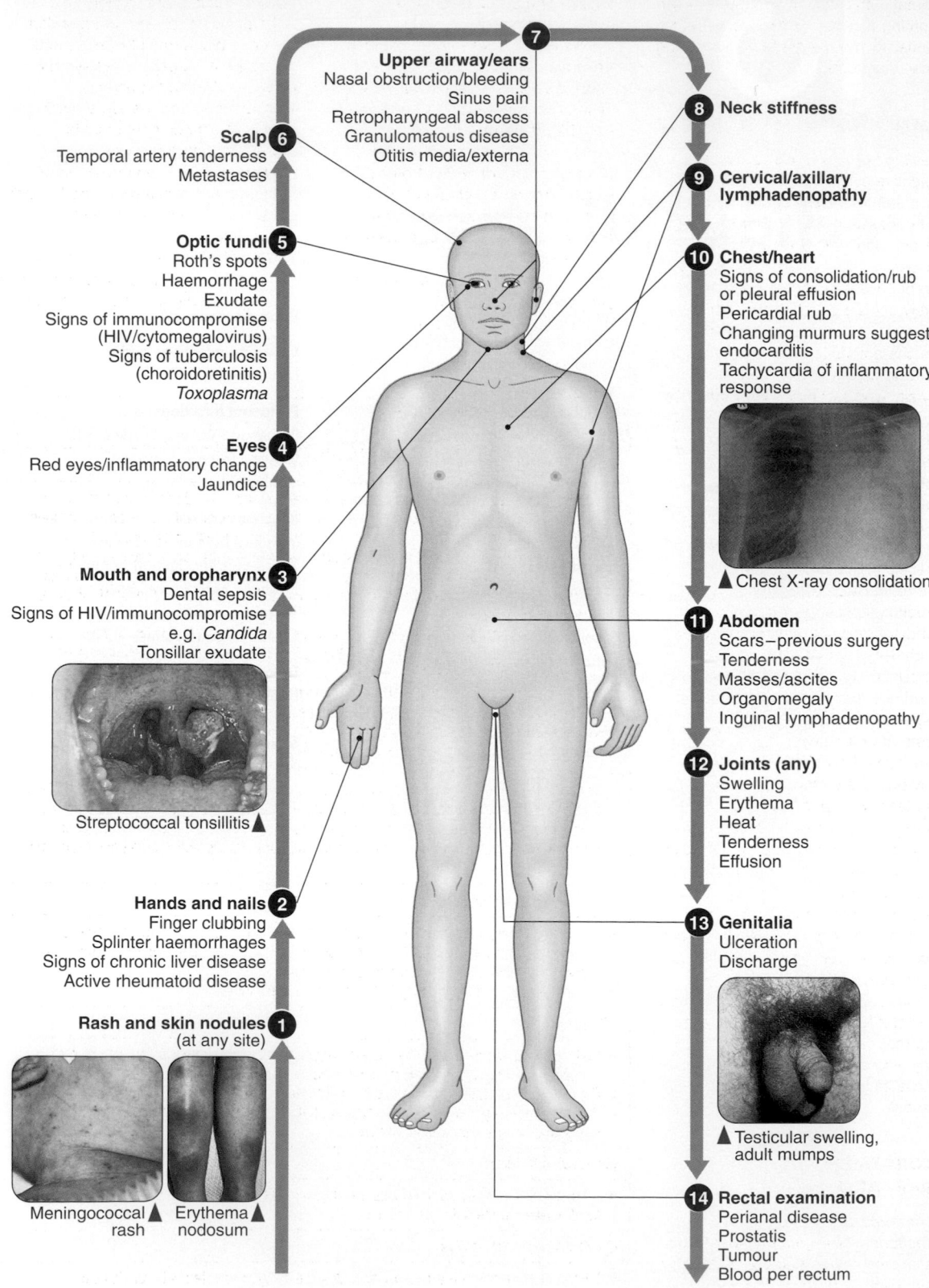

7 Upper airway/ears
Nasal obstruction/bleeding
Sinus pain
Retropharyngeal abscess
Granulomatous disease
Otitis media/externa

6 Scalp
Temporal artery tenderness
Metastases

5 Optic fundi
Roth's spots
Haemorrhage
Exudate
Signs of immunocompromise
(HIV/cytomegalovirus)
Signs of tuberculosis
(choroidoretinitis)
Toxoplasma

4 Eyes
Red eyes/inflammatory change
Jaundice

3 Mouth and oropharynx
Dental sepsis
Signs of HIV/immunocompromise
e.g. *Candida*
Tonsillar exudate

Streptococcal tonsillitis ▲

2 Hands and nails
Finger clubbing
Splinter haemorrhages
Signs of chronic liver disease
Active rheumatoid disease

1 Rash and skin nodules
(at any site)

Meningococcal ▲   Erythema ▲
rash   nodosum

8 Neck stiffness

**9 Cervical/axillary
lymphadenopathy**

10 Chest/heart
Signs of consolidation/rub
or pleural effusion
Pericardial rub
Changing murmurs suggesting
endocarditis
Tachycardia of inflammatory
response

▲ Chest X-ray consolidation

11 Abdomen
Scars–previous surgery
Tenderness
Masses/ascites
Organomegaly
Inguinal lymphadenopathy

12 Joints (any)
Swelling
Erythema
Heat
Tenderness
Effusion

13 Genitalia
Ulceration
Discharge

▲ Testicular swelling,
adult mumps

14 Rectal examination
Perianal disease
Prostatis
Tumour
Blood per rectum

Of all the manifestations of infection in the human host, fever is the most common and most constant (p. 136). A systematic and logical approach to the presenting features of fever is therefore essential to the elements of infectious disease diagnosis.

PRESENTATION OF FEVER

- *'Feeling hot'*. It is wise to obtain objective evidence of raised body temperature. A feeling of heat does not necessarily imply fever (p. 136).
- *Rigors*. Shivering (followed by excessive heat or sweating) implies a rapid rise in body temperature but rarely gives a clue to aetiology.
- *Excessive sweating*. Night sweats are characteristic of tuberculosis, but sweating from any cause is usually worse at night. Non-infective causes of sweating include alcohol misuse, anxiety, thyrotoxicosis, diabetes mellitus, lymphoma and excessive heating of the environment.
- *Recurrent fever*. There are various causes of recurrent fever, some specific (p. 320), but the source is often a focus of bacterial infection (abscess), frequently subdiaphragmatic: cholecystitis or cholangitis, intra-abdominal, retroperitoneal or psoas abscess, or urinary tract infection (especially associated with obstruction or calculi).
- *Headache*. Fever from any cause may provoke headache. Severe headache and photophobia, although characteristic of meningitis, may accompany any septic process, e.g. pyelonephritis, pneumonia and bacterial enteritis.
- *Delirium*. Mental confusion during fever is well described and relatively more common in young children and in old age.
- *Muscle pain*. Myalgia is characteristic of viral infections such as influenza and that caused by enterovirus, but may also accompany septicaemic illness including meningococcal disease.

HISTORY-TAKING IN FEBRILE PATIENTS

- *Symptoms of common respiratory infections*. These include sore throat, nasal discharge, sneezing and sinus pain. Elicit symptoms of lower respiratory tract infection (cough, sputum, wheeze or breathlessness).
- *Genitourinary symptoms*. Ask specifically about frequency of micturition, dysuria, loin pain, and vaginal or urethral discharge (urinary tract infection, pelvic inflammatory disease and sexually transmitted infection (STI)). Also enquire about sexual contacts with or without protective contraception (STI, blood-borne viruses).
- *Abdominal symptoms*. Ask about diarrhoea, with or without blood, weight loss and abdominal pain (gastroenteritis, intra-abdominal sepsis, inflammatory bowel disease, malignancy).
- *Joint symptoms*. Active arthritis is suggested by joint pain, swelling or limitation of movement.
- *Rash*. Enquire about appearance and distribution.
- *Travel history* (pp. 288 and 296). Always ask about foreign travel. If the patient has been in an endemic area, malaria must be excluded, whatever the presenting symptoms.
- *Drug history*. Drug fever is uncommon and therefore easily missed. The culprits include penicillins and cephalosporins, sulphonamides, antituberculous agents, anticonvulsants (particularly phenytoin), methyldopa and quinidine.
- *Alcohol consumption*. Alcoholic hepatitis, cirrhosis and hepatocellular carcinoma are all recognised causes of fever.

EXAMINATION OF THE FEBRILE PATIENT

❶ Rash

- Erythematous rashes (irregular erythematous patches that pale on pressure and may be papular) may be non-infective, e.g. as a reaction to medication. Infectious causes include human erythrovirus 19 infection which produces a characteristic 'slapped cheek' appearance (Fig. 13.8, p. 302). Measles, now uncommon in the UK, is often accompanied by upper respiratory tract symptoms, conjunctivitis and photophobia. The widespread toxic erythema of streptococcal infection (scarlet fever) or the punctate erythema of rubella are also characteristic.
- A purpuric or petechial rash does not pale on pressure. It should alert the physician to meningococcal disease but in this case the rash may be erythematous (blanching on pressure) or absent (10–20%). The differential diagnosis includes petechiae induced by vomiting (superior vena cava distribution), vasculitic lesions and thrombocytopenia or disseminated intravascular coagulopathy and sepsis from any cause.
- Vesicular rashes may be caused by chickenpox, shingles, herpes simplex infection, Coxsackie A virus infection (hand, foot and mouth disease) and erythema multiforme.
- Nodular skin lesions are caused by disseminated fungal infection and malignancy. Erythematous painful lesions on extensor surfaces of the limbs suggest erythema nodosum related to tuberculosis, sarcoid or drug reactions. Cancers of the colon, bladder and ovary often metastasise to the abdominal wall; nodules on the scalp or chest wall suggest a breast or bronchial primary. Leukaemia and lymphoma may produce skin papules, nodules or plaques.

❸ Mouth and oropharynx

- Vesicular lesions, tonsillar exudates and palatal petechiae suggest possible infectious aetiologies (viral, e.g. Coxsackie, streptococcal pharyngitis or infectious mononucleosis).
- Hairy leucoplakia of the tongue suggests HIV disease.
- Oropharyngeal candidiasis may indicate immune deficiency.

❹ Eyes

- Red eye suggests conjunctivitis, scleritis or uveitis. Consider immune complex disorders, connective tissue disease, Reiter's syndrome, reactive arthritis etc.
- Conjunctival petechiae may be due to endocarditis.
- Proptosis may suggest thyroid eye disease. If it is unilateral, consider orbital infiltration by malignancy or granulomatous disease.

❽ Neck stiffness

- Stiffness on forward flexion implies meningeal irritation; stiffness in all directions suggests local disease of the spine or soft tissues.

❾ Cervical lymph nodes

- Enlargement of anterior and tonsillar nodes is usually associated with tonsillitis or pharyngitis; posterior lymphadenopathy may suggest a glandular fever syndrome or HIV infection.

13

Infectious agents, the epidemiology of infection, micro-organism–host interactions and general aspects of the investigation and management of infectious diseases have all been discussed in Chapter 6, Principles of infectious disease.

To summarise, disease due to infection differs from other diseases in a number of ways:

- Most importantly, it is caused by living microorganisms that can usually be identified, thus establishing the aetiology early in the illness. Many such organisms are sensitive to antimicrobial agents and most infections are potentially curable, unlike many non-infectious degenerative and chronic diseases.
- Communicability is another factor which differentiates infections from non-infectious diseases. Transmission of pathogenic organisms to other people, directly or indirectly, may lead to an outbreak requiring specific expertise in its management.
- Many infections are preventable by hygienic measures, by vaccines or by the judicious use of drugs (chemoprophylaxis).

This present chapter discusses the clinical management of those patients with infectious diseases that are not covered in the system-based chapters. Where appropriate, relevant cross-references to these system-based chapters are given and every effort has been made to avoid repetition.

PRESENTING PROBLEMS IN INFECTIOUS DISEASES

PYREXIA OF UNKNOWN ORIGIN

Pyrexia of unknown origin (PUO) is a common presenting problem and may be defined as a consistently elevated body temperature of more than 37.5°C persisting for more than 2 weeks with no diagnosis after initial investigation. Many causes of PUO are listed in Box 13.1. Causes of fever are not necessarily mutually exclusive; however, some characteristic presentations are discussed in the following sections.

The following account applies to immunocompetent individuals in developed countries with community-acquired PUO. Inevitably, infection will account for a higher percentage of PUO in developing countries. Fever in old age merits special attention (Box 13.8, p. 289).

History
- *Travel abroad and countries of origin.* A careful history of any countries the patient has visited or lived in is important. Malaria, respiratory infections, viral hepatitis and dengue are the most common causes of imported fever in the United Kingdom. For other causes see pages 288–296.
- *Personal and social history.* A sexual history is revealing. Possible recent exposure to sexually transmitted infections should be established, and an assessment made of the lifetime risk of sexually acquired HIV

13.1 AETIOLOGY OF PYREXIA OF UNKNOWN ORIGIN IN DEVELOPED COUNTRIES
Infections (30%)

• Sepsis
    Abscess at any site; cholecystitis/cholangitis
    Urinary tract infection: prostatitis
    Dental and sinus infections
    Bone and joint infections
• Imported infections, e.g. malaria, dengue, brucellosis
• Enteric fevers
• Infective endocarditis
• Tuberculosis (particularly extrapulmonary)
• Viral infections (cytomegalovirus—CMV, Epstein–Barr virus—EBV, human immunodeficiency virus—HIV) and toxoplasmosis
• Fungal infections

Malignancy (20%)
• Lymphoma and myeloma • Leukaemia • Solid tumours (renal, liver, colon, stomach, pancreas)
Connective tissue disorders (15%)
• Vasculitic disorders (including polyarteritis nodosa and rheumatoid disease with vasculitis) • Temporal arteritis/polymyalgia rheumatica • Systemic lupus erythematosus (SLE) • Still's disease • Polymyositis • Rheumatic fever
Miscellaneous (20%)
• Inflammatory bowel disease • Liver disease: cirrhosis and granulomatous hepatitis • Sarcoidosis • Drug reactions • Atrial myxoma • Thyrotoxicosis • Hypothalamic lesions • Familial Mediterranean fever
No diagnosis or resolves spontaneously (15%)

infection. Illicit drug usage, particularly by injection, is important (HIV, hepatitis B and C, infective endocarditis and disseminated staphylococcal infection).
- *Occupational or recreational history.* Check on exposure to birds (psittacosis) or animals (toxoplasmosis, Q fever, brucellosis, leptospirosis) and on consumption of unpasteurised milk or milk products (brucellosis, tuberculosis and Q fever).

Investigations and management
First, confirm that the temperature is genuine and measure it 4-hourly. It is essential to reassess the patient clinically at regular intervals while investigations are under way. History-taking should be repeated and expanded, and physical examination performed every few days to recognise emerging physical signs, such as the appearance of enlarged lymph nodes, a heart murmur or missing pulses (embolisation, vasculitis).

PUO should be investigated in a stepwise fashion in order of increasing complexity and invasiveness. The differential diagnosis will depend on geographical location and HIV status. Pursue diagnostic clues immediately, but otherwise

13

proceed in a progressive manner, starting with blood tests and moving to imaging techniques and, finally, more invasive procedures such as 'blind' biopsies. A suggested scheme of investigation based on this principle is summarised in Boxes 13.2–13.4.

Serology

Serological tests should be utilised for both infectious aetiologies and autoimmune causes of fever (Box 13.3).

13.2 EARLY TESTS IN THE INVESTIGATION OF PUO IN DEVELOPED COUNTRIES

- Full blood count (FBC) and differential
- Erythrocyte sedimentation rate (ESR) and C-reactive protein (CRP)
- Serum ferritin
- Urea, creatinine and electrolytes
- Liver function tests (LFTs) and γ-glutamyl transferase
- Blood glucose
- Bone biochemistry
- Creatine phosphokinase
- Malaria blood films (if travel history)
- Urinalysis
- Midstream urine (MSU) for microscopy and culture
- Faeces culture
- Sputum for routine microscopy and culture, and microscopy and culture for mycobacteria
- Blood cultures × 3
- Chest X-ray
- Ultrasound examination of abdomen
- Electrocardiogram (ECG)

13.3 USEFUL SEROLOGICAL INVESTIGATIONS IN THE MANAGEMENT OF PUO IN DEVELOPED COUNTRIES

Viral

- CMV infection
- Infectious mononucleosis
- HIV infection
- Hepatitis A, B and C infection
- Erythrovirus infection

If travel history:
- Arbovirus infection

Bacterial

- Chlamydial infection
- Q fever
- Brucellosis
- *Mycoplasma* infection
- Syphilis
- Leptospirosis
- Lyme disease
- *Yersinia* infection
- Streptococcal infection

If travel history:
- Rickettsial infection
- Melioidosis
- Relapsing fever
- Bartonellosis

Fungal

- Cryptococcosis (antigen detection)

If travel history:
- Histoplasmosis
- Coccidioidomycosis

Protozoal and parasitic

- Toxoplasmosis

If travel history:
- Schistosomiasis
- Amoebiasis
- Leishmaniasis
- Trypanosomiasis

Imaging

Appropriate imaging (Box 13.4) in a sequential manner is invaluable in the investigation of PUO. Chest and abdominal X-rays may show lymphadenopathy or the absence of a psoas shadow. Ultrasound is rapid and non-invasive but often requires to be augmented by computed tomography (CT) or magnetic resonance imaging (MRI) or specialised nuclear medical scans such as labelled white cell imaging.

The role of biopsies in investigation

Liver biopsy

Liver biopsy is a low-yield investigation which carries an estimated mortality of approximately 0.01%. The procedure may occasionally be required to diagnose tuberculosis, lymphoma, or granulomatous disease including sarcoidosis. Biopsy material should always be sent for culture, including that for tuberculosis. It is unlikely to be helpful in patients with normal LFTs and normal liver parenchyma on imaging.

Many cases of PUO involving the liver may be elucidated without biopsy. Raised transaminases should prompt serological screening for viral hepatitis, while elevations of

13

13.4 FURTHER NON-INVASIVE INVESTIGATIONS IN THE MANAGEMENT OF PUO

Nucleic acid detection (polymerase chain reaction, PCR)

- Increasingly used, e.g. for tuberculosis, herpes simplex virus (HSV), CMV, HIV, erythrovirus, dengue, *Toxoplasma,* Whipple's disease

Immunology

- Autoantibody screen, including anti-double-stranded DNA, anti-neutrophil cytoplasmic antibody (ANCA)
- Immunoglobulins
- Complement (C3 and C4) levels
- Cryoglobulins

Tuberculosis screening tests

- Tuberculin (Mantoux) test
- Early morning specimen of urine (EMSU) × 3 for mycobacterial microscopy and culture

Imaging techniques

Ultrasound of abdomen
- Liver tumour or metastases, liver abscess
- Dilated intrahepatic bile ducts
- Renal tumour, abscess or hydronephrosis
- Ascites

Echocardiogram
- Vegetations
- Atrial myxoma
- Intracardiac thrombus

CT/MRI of thorax and abdomen
- Enlarged lymph nodes
- Organomegaly
- Tumours and abscesses
- Lung and liver metastases/ primary tumours

Limited skeletal survey
- Multiple myeloma
- Bone metastases

Isotope bone scan
- Malignancy
- Osteomyelitis/septic arthritis

Labelled white cell scan
- Abscesses/local sepsis
- Inflammatory bowel disease

γ-glutamyl transferase (GT) and liver alkaline phosphatase may point to metastases or biliary disease (infection or obstruction). Glandular fever syndromes, Q fever and syphilis frequently involve the liver as part of a wider systemic process, and are usually best diagnosed serologically.

Bone marrow biopsy

Overall, the diagnostic yield of a bone marrow biopsy in PUO is about 15%, a figure that is likely to be lower if there are no abnormalities in the peripheral blood. A biopsy is most useful in revealing haematological malignancy, myelodysplasia and tuberculosis. It may also lead to a diagnosis of brucellosis, enteric fever or visceral leishmaniasis. Bone marrow should always be sent for culture as well as microscopy.

Temporal artery biopsy

Temporal artery biopsy should be considered in patients over the age of 50, even if the ESR is not significantly elevated. Since arteritis is patchy, diagnostic yield is increased if a 5 cm section of artery is removed for examination.

Prognosis in PUO

The overall mortality of PUO is 30–40% (5% in patients aged under 55 years, 40% in those age over 55 years). Older patients are more likely to have a malignancy. If no cause is found on exhaustive investigation, the long-term mortality is low. On long-term follow-up of these patients no single disease features strongly and in most cases the fever settles spontaneously.

Factitious fever

This is defined as fever, or the appearance of fever, that is engineered by the patient (p. 251). The desired effect is usually accomplished by manipulating the thermometer and/or temperature chart, or by inducing infection by the self-injection of contaminated materials. This practice tends to be relatively more common in female patients and those with a medical or nursing background. The condition may be part of the behaviour pattern characteristic of Munchausen's syndrome; in an individual case 'secondary gain', i.e. psychological motivation, may or may not be apparent. Factitious fever must be excluded as soon as possible; diagnostic clues are summarised in Box 13.5.

13.5 CLUES TO THE DIAGNOSIS OF FACTITIOUS FEVER	

- A patient who looks well
- Bizarre temperature chart with absence of diurnal variation and/or temperature-related changes in pulse rate
- Temperature > 41°C
- Absence of sweating during defervescence
- Normal ESR and CRP despite high fever
- Evidence of self-injection or self-harm
- Useful methods for the detection of factitious fever include supervised (observed) temperature measurement and measuring the temperature of freshly voided urine

FEVER IN THE RETURNING TRAVELLER/ TROPICAL RESIDENT

Presentation of illness as fever is common both in patients returning from the tropics and in tropical residents. Infections that could be acquired in the tropics or during a tropical residence should be considered. Non-tropical infection may also present after tropical travel and it is important to enquire about all systems, as discussed in the investigation of PUO (see above). The most common final diagnoses in febrile patients returning from the tropics are malaria, typhoid fever, viral hepatitis and dengue fever. Malaria should always be excluded by performing three blood films (p. 345).

History

Vital questions to ask anyone returning from the tropics are listed in Box 13.6.

13.6 KEY QUESTIONS FOR DIAGNOSING A FEVER IN THE TROPICS	

- Where have you been?
- What have you done?
- How long where you there?
- Did you have insect bites or contact with animals?
- Did you take precautions/prophylaxis against malaria?

13.7 SPECIFIC EXPOSURES THAT ASSIST IN DIAGNOSIS OF FEVER FROM THE TROPICS	
Exposure	**Infection or disease**
Mosquito bite	Malaria, dengue fever, filariasis
Tsetse fly bite	African trypanosomiasis
Tick bite	Typhus, Lyme disease, Crimean–Congo haemorrhagic fever, babesiosis, Kyasanur forest disease
Louse bite	Typhus
Flea bite	Plague, tularaemia
Sandfly bite	Leishmaniasis, arbovirus infection
Infected person contact	Viral haemorrhagic fevers (Lassa, Ebola, Marburg, Crimean–Congo), viral hepatitis, typhoid fevers, meningococcal disease, HIV infection, hepatitis B
Animal contact	Q fever, brucellosis, anthrax, viral haemorrhagic fevers, histoplasmosis, rabies, plague
Raw or uncooked foods	Enteric bacterial infections, viral hepatitis
Untreated water	Enteric bacterial infections, viral hepatitis
Unpasteurised milk	Brucellosis, salmonellosis, abdominal tuberculosis
Fresh-water swimming	Schistosomiasis, leptospirosis
Unprotected sexual contact	HIV infection, viral hepatitis B, syphilis, gonococcal bacteraemia

Geography and exposures

It is important to establish which countries were visited and the arrival and departure dates. Most tropical infections are transmitted more easily in rural than in urban centres.

The potential infections acquired by an aid worker who has been located in a rural African community are different from those of a business traveller who has stayed in five-star hotels. A detailed living history should be taken, covering living and sleeping conditions, whether bed nets were used, what type of food and water was consumed, and whether there was any contact with animals, hospitals or fresh water. Sometimes particular exposures (Box 13.7) point to a specific diagnosis, e.g. unprotected intercourse with a commercial sex worker.

A sexual history should always be taken. It is also useful to ask about local remedies which patients may have used, either conventional modern medicine or traditional medical preparations. Remember that locally manufactured medications may have low amounts of bio-available drugs.

Vaccinations and prophylaxis

Ask about vaccinations and their validity; those against yellow fever and against hepatitis A and B virtually rule out these infections. Oral and injectable typhoid vaccinations are 70–90% effective. Enquire about malaria prophylaxis and establish precisely which tablets, if any, were being taken. Consult appropriate literature about possible resistance to antimalarial drugs in the country in question.

Examination

A careful examination is vital and must be repeated regularly. Particular attention should be paid to the skin, throat, eyes, nail beds, lymph nodes, abdomen and heart. Patients may be unaware of tick bites or eschars (Fig. 13.1). The temperature should be measured at least twice daily.

13.8 FEVER IN OLD AGE

- **Temperature measurement:** fever may be missed because oral temperatures are unreliable in older people. Rectal measurement may be needed but core temperature is increasingly measured using eardrum reflectance.
- **Associated acute confusion:** frequent with fever, especially in those with underlying cerebrovascular disease or other causes of dementia.
- **Prominent causes of PUO:** include endocarditis, tuberculosis and intra-abdominal sepsis. Non-infective causes include polmyalgia rheumatica and temporal arteritis.
- **Common infective causes in the very frail** (e.g. nursing home residents): include pneumonia, urinary infection, soft tissue infection and gastroenteritis.

13

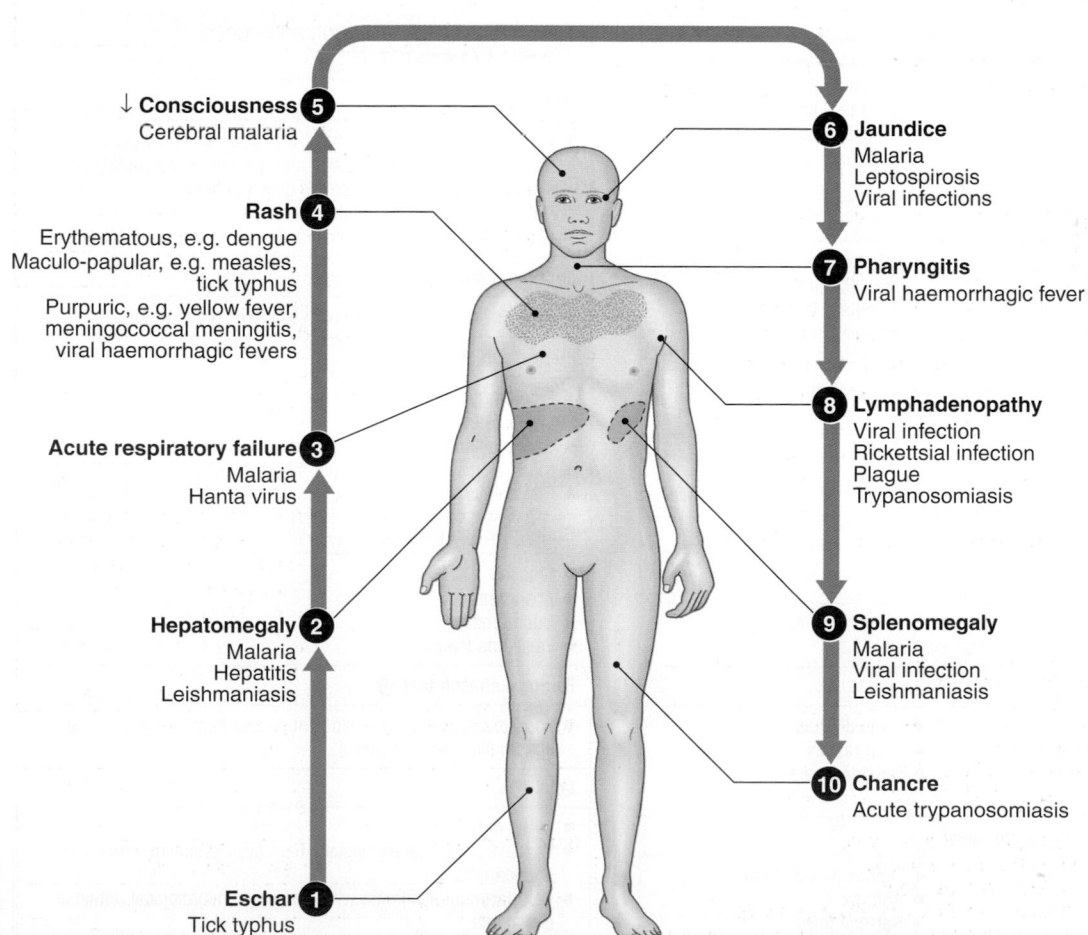

5 ↓ Consciousness
Cerebral malaria

4 Rash
Erythematous, e.g. dengue
Maculo-papular, e.g. measles, tick typhus
Purpuric, e.g. yellow fever, meningococcal meningitis, viral haemorrhagic fevers

3 Acute respiratory failure
Malaria
Hanta virus

2 Hepatomegaly
Malaria
Hepatitis
Leishmaniasis

1 Eschar
Tick typhus

6 Jaundice
Malaria
Leptospirosis
Viral infections

7 Pharyngitis
Viral haemorrhagic fever

8 Lymphadenopathy
Viral infection
Rickettsial infection
Plague
Trypanosomiasis

9 Splenomegaly
Malaria
Viral infection
Leishmaniasis

10 Chancre
Acute trypanosomiasis

Fig. 13.1 Acute fever in/from the tropics: clinical examination.

13.9 DIFFERENTIAL WHITE CELL COUNTS (WCC): ACUTE FEVER IN THE ABSENCE OF LOCALISING SIGNS

WCC differential	Potential diagnoses	Futher investigations
Neutrophil leucocytosis	Bacterial sepsis *Leptospira* and *Borrelia* infections	Blood culture
	Leptospirosis	Culture of blood and urine, serology
	Tick-borne relapsing fever	Blood film
	Louse-borne relapsing fever	Blood film
	Amoebic liver abscess	Ultrasound
Normal WCC and differential	Typhoid fever	Blood, stool and urine culture
	Typhus	Serology
	Arboviral infection	Serology (PCR and viral culture)
Lymphocytosis	Viral fevers	Serology
	Infectious mononucleosis	Monospot test
	Rickettsial fevers	Serology

13.10 PATTERNS OF RASH ASSOCIATED WITH INFECTION

Macular or maculo-papular

- Measles*
- Rubella
- Enteroviral infections
- Herpes virus type 6 infections
- Infectious mononucleosis
- Toxoplasmosis
- Drug rashes
- CMV infections
- HIV seroconversion illness
- Typhoid and paratyphoid fevers
- Rickettsial infections
- Dengue fever
- Secondary syphilis

Haemorrhagic

- Meningococcal infection
- Viral haemorrhagic fevers
- Leptospirosis
- Septicaemia with disseminated intravascular coagulation
- Rickettsial infections

Urticarial

- Toxocariasis
- Fascioliasis
- Strongyloidiasis
- Schistosomiasis

Vesicular/pustular

- Chickenpox*
- Shingles*
- Herpes simplex infections*
- Hand, foot and mouth disease
- Herpangina (mouth)
- Poxviruses (monkey pox)

Nodular

- Erythema nodosum (primary tuberculosis and leprosy, streptococcal infection, *Mycoplasma*)

Erythematous

- Scarlet fever*
- Toxic shock syndrome*
- Human erythrovirus 19 infection*
- Lyme disease
- Drug rashes
- Dengue fever

Chancres (ulcerating nodules)

- Syphilis (p. 411)
- Trypanosomiasis
- Typhus (tick and mite)
- Anthrax
- Rat-bite fever

* Rash is illustrated later in this chapter.

Investigations

Initial investigations in all settings should start with thick and thin blood films for malaria parasites, FBC, urinalysis and chest X-ray if indicated. Box 13.9 gives the diagnoses that should be considered in acute fever with no localising signs.

FEVER ASSOCIATED WITH A RASH

Many infective processes produce skin manifestations as part of the disease, either as a result of infection or a toxin or as part of an immune reaction. Different patterns of rash associated with fever (Box 13.10) may provide helpful clues to the diagnosis. It is therefore important to ask about and examine carefully for a rash that may be transient or minimal or may have characteristic features that aid in diagnosis (e.g. the non-blanching purpuric rash of meningococcal septicaemia, p. 177). Recognition of typical patterns of rash often helps to narrow down and focus subsequent investigations.

Although the combination of fever and rash frequently indicates infection in the mind of the patient, there are many non-infectious causes of this combination (Ch. 27).

13.11 FEVER IN THE INJECTION DRUG-USER: CLINICAL EXAMINATION*

Mouth ❺

- Many injection drug-users have very poor dental hygiene as a result of self-neglect, poor diet and the use of oral methadone syrup. Dental sepsis may be the cause of fever. Look for signs of HIV infection, such as oropharyngeal candidiasis or oral hairy leucoplakia. Kaposi's sarcoma is rare in heterosexual drug-users

Jugular venous pulse ❻

- Systolic 'V' waves may occur in tricuspid endocarditis

Pleural rub or effusion ❽

- Pulmonary infarction as a result of deep venous thrombosis (DVT) and pulmonary embolus
- Septic pulmonary emboli from infected DVT
- Small septic emboli from right-sided endocarditis
- Pneumonia causing pleurisy

Groin injection sites ❿

- Sinuses
- Abscesses
- Haematomas
- False aneurysm

Femoral stretch test ⓫

- Passive extension of the hip joint causes pain and reflex muscle spasm (ilio-psoas abscess)

Legs ⓬

- Signs of DVT
- Vasculitic or ischaemic lesions from arterial spasm, emboli or endocarditis
- Compartment syndrome with associated neurological deficit or ischaemia

* Numbers refer to Figure 13.3.

13

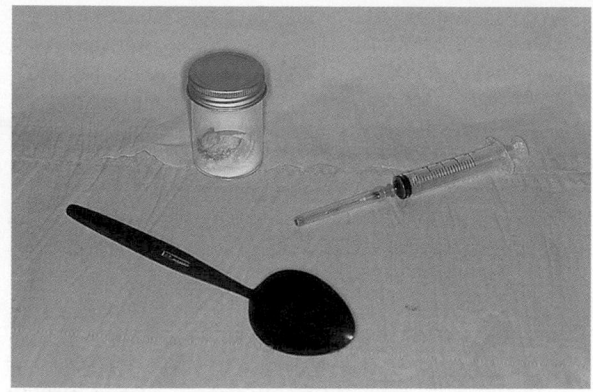

Fig. 13.2 Sharing any injecting equipment may transmit blood-borne viruses.

FEVER IN THE INJECTION DRUG-USER

History

Duration

The duration of injecting drug usage is important as the risk of blood-borne virus infections (hepatitis B and C, and HIV) increases with each year of injecting behaviour.

Site

The site of drug injection is also important. Femoral vein injecting may be associated with vascular complications such as deep venous thrombosis (50% of which are septic) and accidental arterial injection with false aneurysm formation and the compartment syndrome. Septic complications include local or ilio-psoas abscess, and septic arthritis

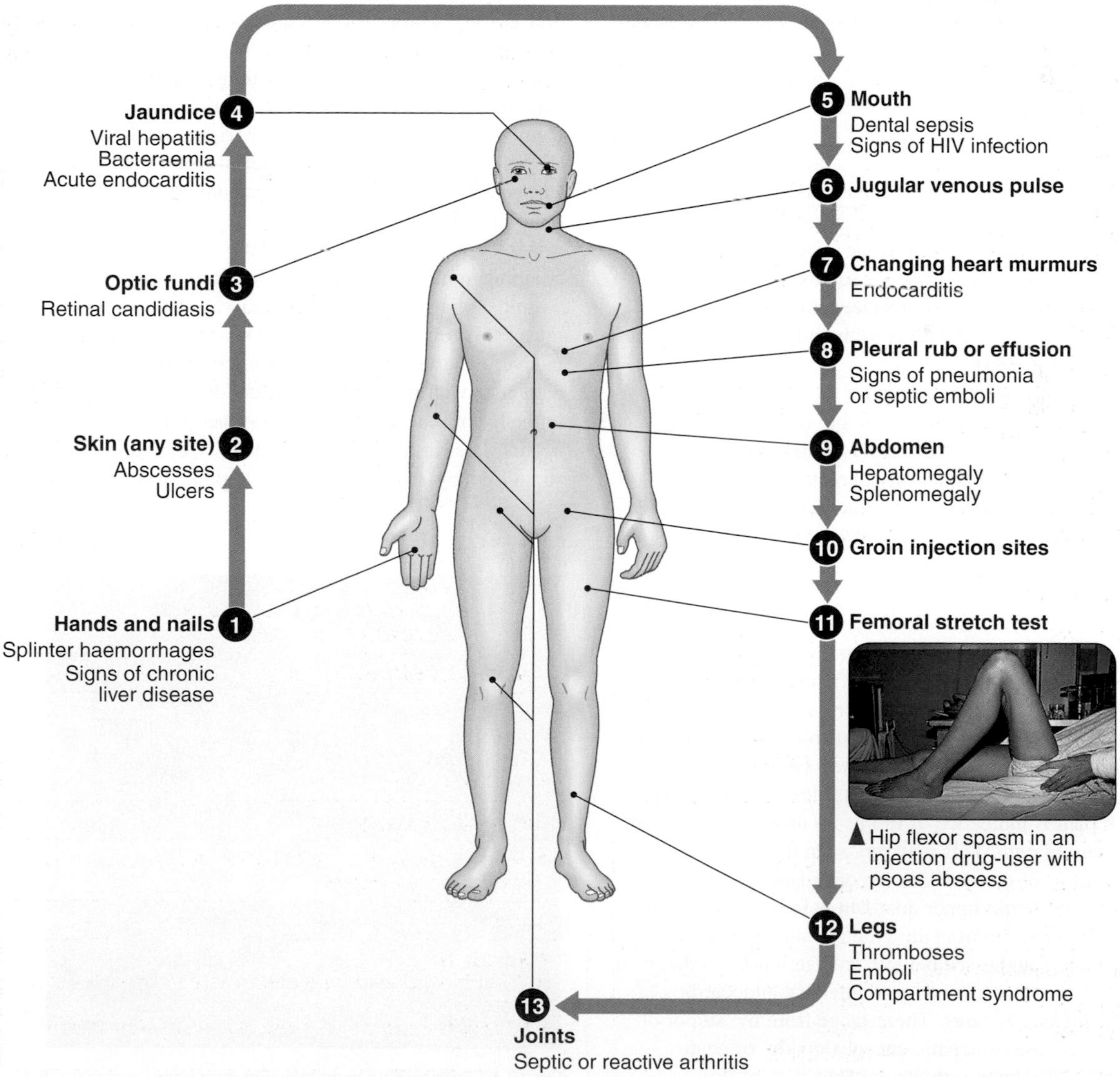

13

Jaundice ④
Viral hepatitis
Bacteraemia
Acute endocarditis

⑤ Mouth
Dental sepsis
Signs of HIV infection

Optic fundi ③
Retinal candidiasis

⑥ Jugular venous pulse

⑦ Changing heart murmurs
Endocarditis

⑧ Pleural rub or effusion
Signs of pneumonia
or septic emboli

Skin (any site) ②
Abscesses
Ulcers

⑨ Abdomen
Hepatomegaly
Splenomegaly

⑩ Groin injection sites

Hands and nails ①
Splinter haemorrhages
Signs of chronic
liver disease

⑪ Femoral stretch test

▲ Hip flexor spasm in an
injection drug-user with
psoas abscess

⑫ Legs
Thromboses
Emboli
Compartment syndrome

⑬
Joints
Septic or reactive arthritis

Fig. 13.3 Fever in the injection drug-user: clinical examination.

of the hip joint or sacro-iliac joint. In the UK subcutaneous and intramuscular injection has been associated with infection by clostridial species, the spores of which contaminate the heroin. *Clostridium novyi* causes a local septic lesion with significant toxin production. The resulting toxaemia produces shock and multi-organ failure, often associated with a marked leukaemoid neutrophil response in the peripheral blood. There is a high mortality. Tetanus, wound botulism and gas gangrene are other anaerobic clostridial infections which may also result from injection into soft tissues.

Technical details

The technical details of injection drug usage are also important. Sharing of needles and other injecting paraphernalia (including spoons and filters) greatly increases the risk of blood-borne virus infection (Fig. 13.2). Some users lubricate their needles by licking them prior to injection, thus introducing mouth organisms such as anaerobic streptococci and *Bacteroides* species. Contamination of commercially available lemon juice, used to dissolve heroin before injection, has been associated with blood-stream infection with *Candida* species.

Clinical assessment

See Figure 13.3 and Box 13.11.

- *Skin.* Recent injection sites may indicate deep infection or abscess formation. They may also be the site of a necrotising skin infection. If the injection sites are over joints, then septic arthritis due to direct inoculation may have occurred. Skin manifestations of immunosuppression with or without HIV disease should be sought (p. 384).
- *Joints.* Pain and redness suggest seeding from bacteraemia or direct injection into the joint space. Frequently there is associated osteomyelitis.
- *Breathlessness.* Gradual-onset breathlessness may represent opportunistic infection secondary to HIV/immunosuppression (p. 389). Acute onset with or without pleuritic pain may indicate septic emboli from a distant injection site or from a right-sided (tricuspid or pulmonary valve) endocarditis.
- *New murmurs or evidence of cardiac decompensation.* These suggest either right- or left-sided endocarditis, or the cardiomyopathy of generalised sepsis.
- *Myalgia and muscle pains.* Apart from non-specific features of bacteraemia, associated swellings represent intramuscular abscess formation. Flexion at the hip plus back pain is indicative of ilio-psoas abscess (Fig. 13.3).
- *Abdominal pain.* This may represent the non-specific discomfort of opiate-induced constipation. More specifically, right upper quadrant pain may indicate the capsular swelling of acute viral hepatitis (jaundice should be sought; see below), and similar left-sided pain a splenic infarct secondary to infective endocarditis.
- *Neurological features.* These range from the stupor of drug overdose or hepatic encephalopathy of acute hepatitis B infection to the agitated state of drug withdrawal (excitement, tachycardia, sweating, marked myalgia, confusion) which is often mistaken for a manifestation of infection. Focal neurological signs may point to septic emboli with cerebral abscess formation. Headache and drowsiness may signal meningitis or encephalitis. Frank psychosis may be a manifestation of both acute drug intoxication and withdrawal, but may also indicate an infective encephalitis due, for example, to herpes simplex virus or an enteroviral infection. Local paralysis or spasms, especially of cranial nerves, should alert the physician to tetanus or botulism.

Diagnosis and management

Acute viral hepatitis (p. 962) may present with fever and immunologically mediated manifestations such as reactive arthritis. Jaundice may be delayed for a few days, or occasionally may be so mild as to be overlooked. Serological tests may reveal evidence of recent infection with hepatitis A or B; in acute hepatitis C antibody is not usually detectable until several weeks after onset of illness. Other causes of jaundice in this situation include bacteraemia, acute bacterial endocarditis and acute drug toxicity, e.g. from oral ecstasy usage. Blood cultures and urinary toxicology are important diagnostic tools.

Chest signs and radiological lung abnormalities may be caused by pneumonia, or by septic pulmonary emboli from peripheral thromboses or right-sided endocarditis (Fig. 13.4). Blood-borne bacterial infection should be suspected if lung abscesses or pneumatoceles are detected radiologically.

An acute compartment syndrome is an occasional complication of groin injection. Rapid rise in pressure within fascial compartments leads to acute ischaemia and muscle necrosis. The syndrome may follow massive DVT or inadvertent arterial injection; characteristic signs include leg pain and swelling and neurological deficit, e.g. sensory loss in the leg or foot. Disappearance of peripheral arterial pulses occurs late in the natural history. Clinical diagnosis is supported by the finding of myoglobinuria and/or raised

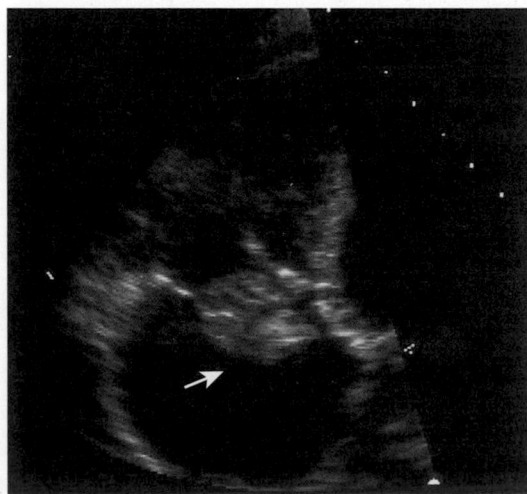

Fig. 13.4 Endocarditis in an injecting drug user. Large vegetation on the tricuspid valve (arrow).

13.12 ORAL ANTIBIOTICS IN STAPHYLOCOCCAL ENDOCARDITIS IN INJECTION DRUG-USERS

'If i.v. drug administration is impractical in patients with right-sided staphylococcal endocarditis, oral ciprofloxacin plus rifampicin is effective and is associated with less drug toxicity than intravenous therapy.'

- Helman AW, et al. Am J Med 1996; 101:68–76.

---

serum creatine kinase levels. Once compartment syndrome is diagnosed, urgent surgical decompression by fasciotomy is essential to preserve function and avoid the need for amputation.

Diagnosis and treatment of endocarditis are discussed on page 629. In drug-users right-sided endocarditis caused by *Staphylococcus aureus* is customarily treated with high-dose intravenous flucloxacillin. Additional gentamicin is probably unnecessary. A 28-day course of oral ciprofloxacin and rifampicin gives results comparable to intravenous therapy and is a useful alternative in this group of patients (Box 13.12).

Local sepsis in drug-users is usually caused by skin organisms (staphylococci and streptococci) and occasionally by anaerobes. Clindamycin and co-amoxiclav are therefore appropriate antibiotics for oral therapy.

FEVER IN THE NEUTROPENIC PATIENT

Neutropenia is defined as a neutrophil count of less than $1.5 \times 10^9/l$. Patients with neutropenia, particularly less than $1.0 \times 10^9/l$, from either drug toxicity (including deliberate chemotherapy for cancer treatment), marrow invasion or failure, are particularly prone to bacterial infections. Gram-positive organisms have now superseded Gram-negative infections as the most common pathogens in this condition, particularly where any line infection or in-dwelling catheter is present.

It is both appropriate and potentially life-saving to start empirical broad-spectrum antibiotic therapy in these cases as soon as neutropenia is recognised and relevant specimens (blood culture, line removal and culture, urine or other body fluid culture) have been taken.

The most common regimen for neutropenic sepsis is a broad-spectrum penicillin such as piperacillin (or tazobactam) plus gentamicin i.v., with the addition of parenteral antifungal therapy, e.g. amphotericin B, if fever has not resolved in 48 hours (p. 1014).

ACUTE DIARRHOEA

Acute diarrhoea (p. 869) is an extremely common presenting problem. It is usually due to faecal–oral transmission of bacterial toxins, viruses, bacteria or protozoal organisms (Box 13.13). Acute diarrhoea is the predominant symptom in acute infective gastroenteritis. A frequent accompaniment of the diarrhoea is the passage of blood per rectum; there are a number of causes (Box 13.14).

13.13 CAUSES OF ACUTE DIARRHOEA

Infectious

Toxin-mediated
- *Bacillus cereus* (p. 326)
- Staphylococcal enterotoxin (p. 325)
- Clostridial spp. enterotoxin (p. 326)
- Scombrotoxic (p. 331)

Infective food poisoning
- Rotavirus gastroenteritis (p. 311)
- *Campylobacter* (p. 326)
- *Salmonella* (p. 328)
- Verocytotoxigenic *E. coli* (p. 328)
- Other *E. coli*, e.g. travellers' diarrhoea (p. 328)
- *Shigella* (p. 330)
- *Clostridium difficile* (p. 329)
- Norovirus (p. 311)
- Cholera (p. 330)

Protozoal
- Giardiasis (p. 359)
- Amoebic dysentery (p. 358)
- *Cryptosporidium* (pp. 360 and 387)
- Isosporiasis (p. 388)
- Microsporidiosis (p. 388)

Systemic illness
- Sepsis (+ sepsis syndrome, p. 317)
- Meningococcal sepsis (p. 189)
- Pneumonia (especially 'atypical disease', p. 687)
- Malaria (p. 342)

Non-infectious

Gastrointestinal
- Acute diverticulitis (p. 929)
- Inflammatory bowel disease
  Ulcerative colitis (p. 910)
  Crohn's disease (p. 910)
- Bowel malignancy (p. 923)
- Pelvic inflammatory disease (p. 410)
- Overflow from constipation (p. 930)

Metabolic upset
- Ketosis (e.g. diabetic decompensation)
- Vasoactive intestinal peptide release (p. 858)
- Carcinoid syndrome (p. 903)
- Uraemia (p. 485)

Drugs and toxins
- NSAIDs
- Cytotoxic agents
- Antibiotics
- Ciguatera fish poisoning (p. 331)
- Dinoflagellates (p. 331)
- Plant toxins (p. 331)
- Heavy metals (p. 331)

13.14 CAUSES OF BLOODY DIARRHOEA

Infectious

- *Campylobacter* spp. (p. 326)
- *Shigella* dysentery (p. 330)
- Non-typhoidal salmonellae (p. 328)
- Enterohaemorrhagic *E. coli* (EHEC, p. 328)
- Entero-invasive *E. coli* (EIEC, p. 328)
- *Clostridium difficile* (p. 329)
- *Vibro parahaemolyticus* (p. 330)
- *Entamoeba histolytica* (amoebic dysentery, p. 358)

Non-infectious

- Diverticular disease (p. 929)
- Rectal or colonic malignancy (p. 923)
- Inflammatory bowel disease (p. 910)
- Bleeding haemorrhoids (p. 933)
- Anal fissure (p. 933)
- Ischaemic colitis (p. 923)
- Intussusception

13

13

Diarrhoea may also be a symptom of systemic upset in addition to being a specific indicator of gastroenteritic infection or disease. Stress, whether psychological or physical, will produce loose stools in susceptible individuals without overt gastrointestinal disease. Sepsis from a non-gastrointestinal site frequently results in diarrhoea; for example, up to 30% of patients with lobar pneumonia have diarrhoea as a presenting symptom.

FOOD POISONING AND GASTROENTERITIS

Acute gastroenteritis is a major cause of morbidity and mortality. Infants and young children are particularly at risk. The World Health Organization (WHO) estimates that there are more than 1000 million cases of acute diarrhoea annually in developing countries, with 3–4 million deaths. Even in developed countries diarrhoea remains an important problem, with 38 million cases annually in the US. Although other causes are important (Box 13.13), the majority of episodes may be directly linked to infection or infectious agents spread by the faecal–oral route and transmitted either on fomites, on contaminated hands, or in food or water. Measures such as the provision of clean potable water, appropriate disposal of human and animal sewage with separation from water supplies, and simple principles of food hygiene are all very effective means of halting the spread of these infections. Fluid replacement, ideally oral, is vital in the management of these cases.

The clinical features of food-borne disease all involve gastrointestinal upset but the pattern of symptomatology is dependent on the pathogenic mechanisms involved. Some organisms (*Bacillus cereus*, *Staph. aureus* and *Vibrio cholerae*) elute exotoxins which exert their major effects on the stomach and small bowel, where they cause mucosal inflammation. They frequently produce vomiting and/or a so-called 'secretory' diarrhoea. This is watery without blood and faecal leucocytosis. In general, the 'incubation period' of these intoxications, i.e. the time from ingestion to the onset of symptoms, is short and, other than dehydration, little systemic upset occurs. Other organisms, such as *Shigella*, *Salmonella*, *Campylobacter* and enterohaemorrhagic *E. coli*, may directly invade the mucosa of the small bowel or produce cytotoxins that damage and ulcerate the mucosa with inflammation, typically affecting the terminal small bowel and colon. Here the incubation period is longer and more systemic upset occurs with prolonged diarrhoea. If the colon is inflamed, blood and leucocytes may be present in the stool.

ASSESSMENT OF THE PATIENT WITH ACUTE DIARRHOEA

History

This should include questioning about appropriate suspect foods, the duration and frequency of diarrhoea, the presence of blood, abdominal pain and tenesmus, and whether family or community members have been affected. Fever and bloody diarrhoea suggest an invasive, dysenteric process. Incubation periods of less than 18 hours suggest toxin-mediated food poisoning; a period longer than 5 days suggests diarrhoea caused by protozoa or helminths.

Examination

The degree of dehydration can be assessed by skin turgor and blood pressure measurement. The urine output and ongoing stool losses should be measured carefully.

Investigations

These should include stool inspection for blood and microscopy for leucocytes. Stool culture should be performed where possible but often the results will come too late to influence immediate management. An FBC and serum electrolytes will also indicate the degree of inflammation and dehydration. In a malarious area a blood film for malaria parasites should be obtained.

MANAGEMENT OF ACUTE DIARRHOEA

All patients with acute, potentially infective diarrhoea should be appropriately isolated to minimise person-to-person spread of infection. Regardless of the cause of diarrhoea, significant fluid loss will occur if it continues without adequate fluid replacement.

There are three elements to the management of acute diarrhoea in individual cases:

- fluid replacement
- antibiotics/antimicrobial therapy
- adjunctive antidiarrhoeal therapy.

Fluid replacement

By far the most important aspect of the management of acute gastroenteritis is replacement of fluid losses; occasionally, this is life-saving. Most clinicians significantly underestimate the potential for serious dehydration produced by relatively mild gastroenteritis, particularly in a tropical/subtropical setting.

Although normal daily fluid intake in an adult is 1–2 litres with approximately 8 litres entering the upper small bowel, there is considerable fluid movement, particularly across the small bowel (Fig. 22.7, p. 856). Infective and toxic processes in the gut disturb or reverse the resorptive power of the colon/small intestine, resulting in marked dehydration. Cholera is the archetype of this process, where 10–20 litres of fluid may be lost in 24 hours.

The fluid lost in diarrhoea is isotonic, so a source of electrolytes, in either continued food intake or replacement fluid, is required. The absorption of electrolytes from the gut is an active process requiring energy. Infected mucosa is capable of very rapid fluid and electrolyte transport if an energy source is available. During gastroenteritis a source of carbohydrate, either starch or sugar, is required; otherwise fluids, even with electrolyte content, will not be absorbed. This is the basis of oral rehydration solution (ORS). Many commercial equivalents are available. Those in developed countries often have relatively high sucrose levels (for supposed palatability) and reduced sodium levels (Box 13.15).

ORS can be just as effective as intravenous replacement fluid even in the management of cholera. If intravenous fluid is used, it adds to the cost and to the potential danger from infection if hygiene is suboptimal.

13.15 COMPOSITION OF ORAL REHYDRATION SOLUTION AND OTHER REPLACEMENT FLUIDS				
Fluid	Na	K	Cl	KCalories/l
WHO	90	20	80	54
Dioralyte	60	20	60	71
Pepsi	6.5	0.8	–	400
7-up	7.5	0.2	–	320
Apple juice	0.4	26	–	480
Orange juice	0.2	49	–	400
Breast milk	22	36	28	670

Regardless of the type of fluid replacement used, there are three elements to the calculation of appropriate volumes:

- replacement of established losses
- replacement of ongoing losses
- replacement of normal daily requirement.

The most common mistake in the management of gastroenteritis of any cause is inadequate fluid replacement.

Replacement of established losses
The average adult with 48 hours of moderate diarrhoea (6–10 stools per 24 hours) will be 1–2 litres depleted from diarrhoea alone. Any associated vomiting will compound this. Adults with this symptomatology should therefore be given rapid replacement of 1–1.5 litres, either orally (ORS) or by intravenous infusion (normal saline) within the first 2–4 hours of their presentation. Careful calculation of fluid requirements is needed for children.

Longer symptomatology or more persistent/severe diarrhoea rapidly produces fluid losses comparable to diabetic ketoacidosis and is a metabolic emergency requiring active intervention.

Replacement of ongoing losses
The average adult's diarrhoeal stool accounts for a loss of 200 ml of isotonic fluid. Stool losses should be carefully charted and an estimate of ongoing replacement fluid calculated. Currently, commercially available rehydration sachets are conveniently produced to provide 200 ml of ORS. One sachet per diarrhoea stool is an appropriate and effective means of ongoing rehydration.

Replacement of normal daily requirement
The average adult has a minimal daily requirement of 1–1.5 litres of fluid in addition to the calculations above. In mild to moderate gastroenteritis adults should be encouraged to drink normally and infants should continue to breastfeed. Additional fluids should be given to replace established and ongoing losses, including insensible losses. Wherever possible, continue normal dietary intake.

Antimicrobial agents
Antibiotics in non-specific gastroenteritis have been shown to shorten symptoms by only 1 day in an illness usually lasting 1–3 days. The benefit of this, when related to the potential for the development of antimicrobial resistance (10–30% of *Salmonella* and *Campylobacter* are now resistant to ciprofloxacin), does not support this treatment.

13.16 SEVERITY MARKERS IN ACUTE GASTROENTERITIS
Chronic conditions
<ul><li>Age > 65</li><li>Diabetes mellitus</li><li>Rheumatoid or other autoimmune disease</li><li>Chronic renal disease</li><li>Valvular heart disease (especially with valve replacements)</li><li>Acquired or secondary immunodeficiency</li><li>Any internal prostheses</li></ul>
Current drug therapy
<ul><li>Diuretic therapy</li><li>Angiotensin-converting enzyme (ACE) inhibitor therapy</li><li>Corticosteroid therapy</li><li>Cytotoxic therapy</li><li>Proton pump or H_2-receptor blockers</li></ul>
Current illness
<ul><li>Number of stools per 24 hours</li><li>Presence of blood per rectum</li><li>Abdominal pain</li><li>Associated systemic toxicity</li></ul>

Antimicrobials in *Salmonella* illness increase the stool carriage time (Box 13.43, p. 328). Recent evidence has suggested that in EHEC (VTEC) infections the use of antibiotics may make the complication of haemolytic uraemic syndrome (HUS, p. 498) more likely due to increased toxin release from organisms. Antibiotics should therefore not be used routinely in bloody diarrhoea in childhood.

Dysentery produced by *Sh. dysenteriae* is a clear indication for antibiotic therapy, and the use of antimicrobials may be advantageous in cholera epidemics for reducing infectivity and controlling the spread of infection. Generally, in mild to moderate cases of gastroenteritis there should be a very high threshold for antibiotic use. However, severe disease or certain clinical conditions (Box 13.16) will lower this threshold far enough to make a decision to administer antimicrobials appropriate.

Antidiarrhoeal, antimotility and antisecretory agents
In general these agents are not recommended and their use may even be contraindicated in the management of infective or potentially infective gastroenteritis.

Although widely used, antimotility agents such as loperamide, diphenoxylate or opiates are potentially dangerous in dysentery in childhood (causing intussusception). Their use should be avoided in any case with bloody stool. Antisecretory agents such as bismuth and chlorpromazine may be effective but can cause significant sedation. They do not reduce stool fluid losses, although the stools may appear more bulky. Adsorbents such as kaolin or charcoal have little effect.

CHRONIC DIARRHOEA

This is defined as diarrhoea persisting for more than 14 days. The differential diagnosis can be wide, and parasitic

13

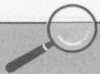

13.17 CAUSES OF CHRONIC DIARRHOEA IN THE TROPICS

- *Giardia intestinalis*
- Strongyloidiasis
- Hypolactasia (primary and secondary)
- Enteropathic *E. coli*
- Tropical sprue
- Chronic calcific pancreatitis
- HIV enteropathy
- Intestinal flukes
- Chronic intestinal schistosomiasis

and bacterial causes, tropical malabsorption, inflammatory bowel disease and neoplasia should all be considered (Box 22.18, p. 870). Box 13.17 gives the causes of chronic diarrhoea in the tropics; most are considered later in this chapter. Tropical sprue is defined as clinical malabsorption with no defined aetiology. It was typically associated with a long period of residence in the tropics or with overland travel but is now rarely seen. *Giardia* infection may progress to a malabsorption syndrome that mimics tropical sprue (p. 870).

Clinical assessment

The key signs and symptoms are diarrhoea with pale, bulky stools, abdominal symptoms with distension and flatulence, nutritional deficiencies and general ill health.

Investigations

Malabsorption should be investigated systematically (p. 871). Appropriate tests should be carried out to establish a parasitic cause of chronic diarrhoea.

Management

Specific causes of chronic diarrhoea should be treated appropriately. If no cause is found, empirical treatment for *Giardia lamblia* infection with metronidazole is often helpful.

SPLENOMEGALY IN THE RETURNING TRAVELLER/TROPICAL RESIDENT

Splenomegaly (p. 1015) is occasionally the presenting feature of a tropically acquired infection (Box 13.18). If it is moderate or massive, then endocarditis, splenic abscess, visceral leishmaniasis and hyper-reactive malarial splenomegaly should be considered.

Investigations

These will be guided by the context of the splenomegaly, particularly the travel and exposure history. Every patient should have several thick and thin blood films examined for malaria parasites, blood cultures, an FBC and film examination. Serologies where appropriate can help diagnose a viral infection. Imaging can detect a splenic abscess and indicate whether portal hypertension is present. The diagnosis of visceral leishmaniasis will require a bone marrow or splenic aspirate.

Hyper-reactive malarial splenomegaly (tropical splenomegaly syndrome)

In some malarious areas gross splenomegaly is associated with an exaggerated immune response to malaria in adults

13.18 CAUSES OF TROPICAL SPLENOMEGALY

Mild

Parasite infection
- Malaria
- Katayama fever
- Toxoplasmosis
- Trypanosomiasis

Viral
- EBV
- Hepatitis
- Dengue
- CMV
- HIV

Bacterial
- Typhoid
- Brucellosis

Spirochaetal
- Leptospirosis

Fungal
- Histoplamosis

Moderate
- Subacute bacterial endocarditis
- Splenic abscess
- Portal hypertension due to schistosomiasis
- Disseminated tuberculosis

Massive
- Visceral leishmaniasis
- Hyper-reactive malarial splenomegaly

who have high antibody titres to malaria (immunofluorescent antibody titre < 1 in 128) and low or negative parasitaemias.

Splenomegaly and anaemia usually resolve over a period of months of continuous treatment with proguanil 100 mg daily and chloroquine 600 mg weekly. Long-term treatment may be needed to prevent relapse. Complicating folate deficiency is treated with folic acid 5 mg daily.

EOSINOPHILIA

Eosinophilia is associated with parasite infections, particularly those with a tissue migration phase during their life cycle. Eosinophils have an important role in mediating antibody-dependent damage to helminths, phagocytosing immune complexes and modulating type 1 hypersensitivity reactions (p. 83). Anybody with an eosinophil count of $> 0.4 \times 10^9$ should be investigated for both parasitic and non-parasitic causes of eosinophilia. Box 13.19 gives the main causes of eosinophilia, Box 13.20 the main parasitic causes and Box 13.21 the tropical diseases that are *not* associated with eosinophilia.

The response to parasite infections is often different when travellers to and residents of endemic areas are compared.

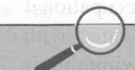

13.19 CAUSES OF EOSINOPHILIA

- Metazoan parasite infections
- Atopy and allergic drug reactions
- Skin diseases
- Pulmonary eosinophilia
- HIV, human T-cell lymphotropic virus 1 (HTLV 1)
- Lymphomas
- Leukaemias
- Polyarteritis nodosa
- Sarcoidosis
- Hypereosinophilic syndrome

13

13.20 PARASITE INFECTIONS THAT CAUSE EOSINOPHILIA

Infestation	Pathogen	Clinical syndrome associated with eosinophilia
Strongyloidiasis	Strongyloides stercoralis	
Soil-transmitted helminthiases		
Hookworm	Necator americanus Ancylostoma duodenale	
Ascariasis	Ascaris lumbricoides	Löffler's syndrome
Toxocariasis	Toxocara canis	Visceral larva migrans
Schistosomiasis	Schistosoma haematobium S. mansoni S. japonicum	Katayama fever Chronic infection
Filariases		
Loiasis	Loa loa	
Wuchereria bancrofti	W. bancrofti	
Brugia malayi	B. malayi	
Mansonella perstans	M. perstans	
Onchocerciasis	Onchocerca volvulus	
Cysticercosis	Taenia saginata T. solium	Migratory phase
Hydatid disease	Echinococcus granulosus	Leakage from cyst
Liver flukes	Fasciola hepatica Clonorchis sinensis Opisthorchis felineus	Migratory phase

13.21 TROPICAL INFECTONS NOT ASSOCIATED WITH EOSINOPHILIA

- Amoebiasis
- Arboviral infections
- Brucellosis
- Enteric fever
- Giardiasis
- Leishmaniasis
- Leprosy
- Malaria
- Trypanosomiasis
- Tuberculosis
- Tapeworms other than cysticercosis

Travellers will often have recent and light infections associated with eosinophilia. Residents have often been infected for a long time, have evidence of chronic pathology and no longer have an eosinophilia.

History

A careful geographical history of where the patient has travelled and the known endemic areas for diseases such as schistosomiasis, onchocerciasis and the filariases will indicate possible causes for the eosinophilia. Establish how long patients spent in endemic areas and ask about any occupational and behavioural risks (Box 13.7, p. 288). Contact with fresh water in sub-Saharan Africa, particularly swimming in Lake Malawi, is an important risk factor for schistosomiasis. Walking barefoot is a risk factor for acquiring any of the soil-transmitted helminthiases.

Symptoms that would suggest a parasitic cause for eosinophilia include transient rashes (schistosomiasis, strongyloidiasis), fever (Katayama syndrome—p. 368), itching (onchocerciasis), haematuria, haematospermia

(schistosomiasis) or migrating subcutaneous swellings (loiasis, gnathostomiasis) (Box 13.22).

Investigations

To establish a parasitic infestation, direct visualisation of adult worms, larvae or ova is the best evidence. Serological evidence may be helpful but a serological response may not distinguish between an active and an old infection. Radiological investigations may also provide circumstantial

13.22 CLINICAL FEATURES ASSOCIATED WITH HELMINTHIC INFECTIONS AND EOSINOPHILIA

Urticarial rashes
- Strongyloidiasis, onchocerciasis, fascioliasis, hydatid disease, trichinosis

Cutaneous larva migrans
- Ancylostoma braziliense

Dermatitis
- Onchocerciasis

Migratory subcutaneous swellings
- Loiasis, gnathostomiasis

Lymphangitis, orchitis
- Lymphatic filariasis

Myositis
- Trichinosis, cysticercosis

Febrile hepatosplenomegaly
- Schistosomiasis, toxocariasis

Pneumonitis
- Migratory stage of larval helminths (Löffler's syndrome), lymphatic filariasis (tropical pulmonary eosinophilia), systemic strongyloidiasis

Enteritis and colitis
- Strongyloidiasis, capillariasis, trichinosis, rarely other intestinal worms

Meningitis
- Angiostrongyliasis, strongyloidiasis

13.23 INITIAL INVESTIGATION OF EOSINOPHILIA

Investigation	Pathogens sought
Stool microscopy	Ova, cysts and parasites
Terminal urine	Ova of Schistosoma haematobium
Duodenal aspirate	Filariform larvae of Strongyloides, liver fluke ova
Day bloods	Microfilariae Brugia malayi, Loa loa
Night bloods	Microfilariae Wuchereria bancrofti
Skin snips	Onchocerca volvulus
Serology	Schistosomiasis, filariasis, strongyloidiasis, hydatid, trichinosis etc.

13

evidence of parasite infestation. Box 13.23 gives the initial investigations for eosinophilia.

SKIN CONDITIONS IN THE RETURNING TRAVELLER/TROPICAL RESIDENT

Community-based studies in the tropics consistently show that skin infections (bacterial and fungal), scabies and eczema are the most common skin problems there. These are dealt with in Chapter 27, except for necrotising, clostridial and *Bacteroides* soft tissue infections, which are described later in this chapter. Cutaneous leishmaniasis and onchocerciasis have defined geographical distributions (pp. 352 and 365). In travellers, secondarily infected insect bites, pyoderma, cutaneous larva migrans and non-specific dermatitis are common skin lesions. Enquire about habitation, work and travel when investigating these lesions (Box 13.6, p. 288). A number of other skin and subcutaneous conditions (Box 13.24) are not considered elsewhere but are common enough in the tropics, or in returning travellers, to warrant consideration on their own merit here.

Investigation of skin lesions

Skin swabs should be taken for bacterial and fungal culture. Skin biopsies are helpful in diagnosing parasitic infections and persistent reactions to insect bites. Culture of biopsy material may be needed to diagnose fungal and mycobacterial infections.

CUTANEOUS LARVA MIGRANS

Cutaneous larva migrans (CLM) is the most common linear lesion seen in travellers. Intensely pruritic, linear, serpiginous lesions result from the larval migration of the dog hookworm *(Ancylostoma caninum)*. The track moves across the skin at a rate of 2–3 cm/day. This contrasts with the rash of *Strongyloides* (p. 361), which is fast-moving and evanescent. Dog hookworms rarely establish infection in humans. The most common site for CLM is the foot but elbows, breasts and buttocks may be affected. Most patients with CLM have recently visited a beach where the affected part was exposed. The diagnosis is clinical. Treatment may be local with 12-hourly application of 15% tiabendazole cream, or systemic with a single dose of albendazole (400 mg) or ivermectin (150–200 µg/kg).

TROPICAL ULCER

Tropical ulcer is due to a synergistic bacterial infection caused by a fusobacterium *(F. ulcerans*, an anaerobe), and *Treponema vincenti*. It is common in hot humid regions. The

13.24 COMMON CAUSES OF SKIN LESIONS IN THE TROPICS

Lesion type	Aetiology	Clinical features
Papules		
Scabies (p. 1297)	*Sarcoptes scabiei*	Nocturnal pruritus, excoriated papules and raised linear burrows (sides of fingers and finger webs)
Insect bites	Mosquito	Pruritic weal, flare or papule
	Flea	Discrete pruritic papule with central haemorrhagic punctum
	Tick	Painful swelling with central necrosis and erythematous margin
	Bedbug	Pruritic papules in a linear configuration
Prickly heat	Heat with humidity	Erythematous, papular and vesicular eruption around sweat glands
Ringworm (p. 1297)	*Tinea corporis*	Circular, raised, sharply marginated scaly lesions
Onchocerciasis (p. 365)	*Onchocerca volvulus*	Widespread pruritic, papular rash
Linear lesions		
Cutaneous larva migrans	*Ancylostoma caninum*	Severely pruritic serpiginous track
Larva currens	*Strongyloides stercoralis*	Pruritic, fast-moving linear urticaria
Ulcers		
Ecthyma (p. 1293)	*Staphylococcus aureus*, β-haemolytic streptococcus	Crusted ulcer
Oriental sore, Delhi boil, chiclero ulcer etc.	*Leishmania*	Indolent, slow-healing ulcer
Anthrax (p. 332)	*Bacillus anthracis*	Single black, oedematous, painless lesion
Rickettsial eschar	*Rickettsia conorii* and *R. tsutsugamushi*	Small ulcer with black centre, systemic illness
Buruli ulcer	*Mycobacterium ulcerans*	Nodule and ulceration
Tropical ulcer	*Fusobacterium ulcerans* and *Treponema vincenti*	Sharply defined painful ulcer, usually on lower leg
Vesicles		
Insect bites	Spanish fly (*Lytta vesicatoria*) Rove beetle	Blister produced from contact with insect toxins
Subcutaneous swellings		
Myiasis	*Dermatobia hominis* larva, *Cordylobia anthropophaga* larva	Larva protruding from subcutaneous cavity
Tungiasis (jiggers)	*Tunga penetrans*	Small black dot, developing into an inflammatory nodule
Fungal infections	*Sporothrix schenckii*	Hard, non-tender subcutaneous nodules, which later ulcerate
Dracunculiasis	*Dracunculus medinensis*	Erythema, ulceration and induration; worm may protrude

13

ulcer is most common on the lower legs and develops as a papule that rapidly breaks down to a sharply defined, painful ulcer. The base of the ulcer has a foul slough. Penicillin and metronidazole are useful in the early stages but rest, elevation and dressings are the mainstays of treatment.

JIGGERS (TUNGIASIS)

This is widespread in tropical America and Africa and is caused by the sand flea *Tunga penetrans*. The pregnant flea burrows into the skin around toes and produces large numbers of eggs. The burrows are intensely irritating and the whole inflammatory nodule should be removed with a sterile needle. Secondary infection of tunga lesions is common.

MYIASIS

Myiasis is due to skin infestation with larvae of the South American botfly, *Dermatobia hominis*, and the African Tumbu fly, *Cordylobia anthropophaga*. The larvae develop in a subcutaneous space with a central sinus. This orifice is the air source for the larvae, and periodically the larval respiratory spiracles protrude through the sinus. Patients with myiasis feel movement within the larval burrow and experience intermittent sharp, lancinating pains. Myiasis is diagnosed clinically and should be suspected with any furuncular lesion accompanied by pain and a crawling sensation in the skin. The larva may be extruded by squeezing gently on the burrow and catching it with tweezers. Alternatively, it may be suffocated by blocking the respiratory orifice with petroleum jelly. Secondary infection of myiasis is remarkably infrequent and rapid healing follows removal of intact larvae.

VIRAL INFECTIONS

Viruses are simple infectious agents consisting of a portion of genetic material, RNA or DNA, enclosed in a protein coat which is antigenically unique for that species. They are essentially inert and cannot exist in a free-living state, needing to infect host cells to survive. Once in the intracellular environment, they utilise host material for protein synthesis and genetic reproduction. All viral infections must therefore originate from an infected source by either direct or vector-mediated spread.

CLASSIFICATION OF VIRAL INFECTIONS

The taxonomy of viral infections in humans is shown in Box 13.25.

COMMON VIRAL INFECTIONS AND CHILDHOOD EXANTHEMS

An exanthem describes the rash that characterises an eruptive fever. World-wide the common childhood exanthemas

---

13.25 VIRUSES INVOLVED IN HUMAN DISEASE

Classification/viruses involved	Clinical syndromes
DNA VIRUSES	
Adenoviruses	Upper respiratory tract infection/pharyngitis
	Acute diarrhoea
Herpes viruses	
Herpes simplex types 1 and 2	Acute/recurrent vesicular rash
Varicella zoster	Chickenpox/shingles
Cytomegalovirus	Acute/recurrent hepatorenal infection
Human herpes virus 6 and 7	Roseola infantum
Epstein–Barr virus	Infectious mononucleosis
	Burkitt's lymphoma
Human herpes virus 8	Nasopharyngeal carcinoma
	Kaposi's sarcoma
Papovaviruses	
Human papillomavirus	Common wart
Polyoma (human BK and JC)	Progressive multifocal leucoencephalopathy
Human erythrovirus 19	Erythema infectiosum
Poxviruses	
Variola	Smallpox
Monkey pox	
Cowpox	
Vaccinia	Smallpox vaccination
Orf virus	
Molluscum contagiosum	
RNA VIRUSES	
Picornaviruses	
Poliovirus	
Coxsackie viruses	Gut/neurological illness
Echoviruses	
Enteroviruses 68–72	
Hepatitis A	
Rhinoviruses	Upper respiratory tract infection
Rheoviruses	
Rheovirus	Mild upper respiratory tract infection/gut disease
Rotavirus	Gastroenteritis
Togaviruses	
Rubella	German measles
Alphaviruses	Mosquito-borne encephalitides
Flaviviruses	
Yellow fever	Yellow/haemorrhagic fever
Dengue	
Other arboviruses	Haemorrhagic fevers
Hepatitis C	Chronic hepatitis
Bunyaviruses	
Congo–Crimean fever	Acute hepatitis
Hantavirus	Gastroenteritis
Calicivirus	
Hepatitis E	Acute gastroenteritis
Norvovirus	
Astrovirus	Acute epidemic lower respiratory tract infection
Orthomyxoviruses	
Influenza A, B	
Paramyxoviruses	
Measles	
Mumps	
Respiratory syncytial virus	
Rhabdoviruses	Rabies
Retroviruses	
HIV-1 and 2	HIV infection syndrome/AIDS
Arenaviruses	
Lassa	Lassa fever
Lymphocytic choriomeningitis	
Filoviruses	
Marburg and Ebola viruses	
Hepadnavirus	
Hepatitis B	

13

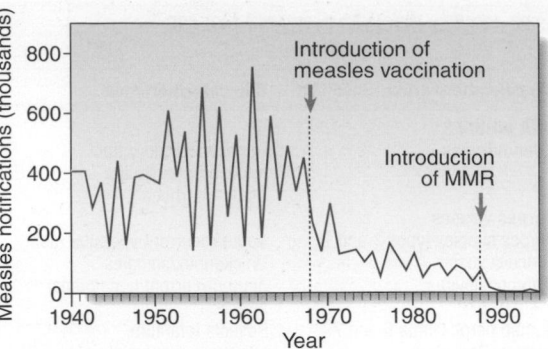

Fig. 13.5 Effectiveness of measles vaccination in England and Wales. (MMR = measles/mumps/rubella vaccine)

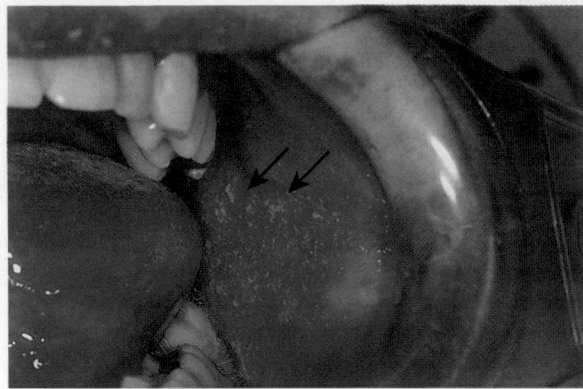

Fig. 13.6 Koplik's spots (arrows) seen on buccal mucosa in the early stages of clinical measles.

still represent a significant cause of morbidity and mortality. Comprehensive immunisation programmes, where consistently maintained, have eradicated many of these conditions from developed countries. Lapses in vaccine coverage and reintroduction of the wild virus often result in adults contracting these conditions, usually with much more severe consequences.

MEASLES

This paramyxovirus infection is endemic world-wide. It is probably the most infectious of all microbial agents. Before immunisation campaigns, measles occurred in almost 100% of children. Maternal antibody gives protection for the first 6 months of life. In temperate areas there is a natural epidemic cycle every 2–3 years, less obvious in the tropics. With live attenuated vaccine, the condition is potentially completely controllable by immunisation (Fig. 13.5). The WHO has set the objective of eradicating measles by the year 2010 as part of its expanded programme of immunisation. Incomplete vaccination of only 70–80% of the population may lead to outbreaks in older children and adults, in whom complications are more frequent. This necessitates repeat mass immunisation campaigns or second dosing of vaccine in an older age group. Natural illness produces life-long immunity.

Clinical features

Infection is by droplet spread with an incubation period of 14 days to onset of rash. A prodromal illness 1–3 days before the rash appears heralds the most infectious, 'catarrhal' stage with upper respiratory symptoms, conjunctivitis and the presence of Koplik's spots on the internal buccal mucosa (Fig. 13.6). These small white spots surrounded by erythema are pathognomonic of measles. At this stage the patient is miserable, irritable and photophobic, corresponding to the peak of a second viraemia. As natural antibody develops, the rash appears (Fig. 13.7), lasting 5–6 days and gradually fading with 'staining' in the pale-skinned. Generalised lymphadenopathy and diarrhoea are common, with bacterial pneumonia in approximately 4% of cases. Convulsions occur in approximately 1% and long-term damage can result in the rare occurrence of subacute sclerosing panencephalitis (SSPE) up to 7 years

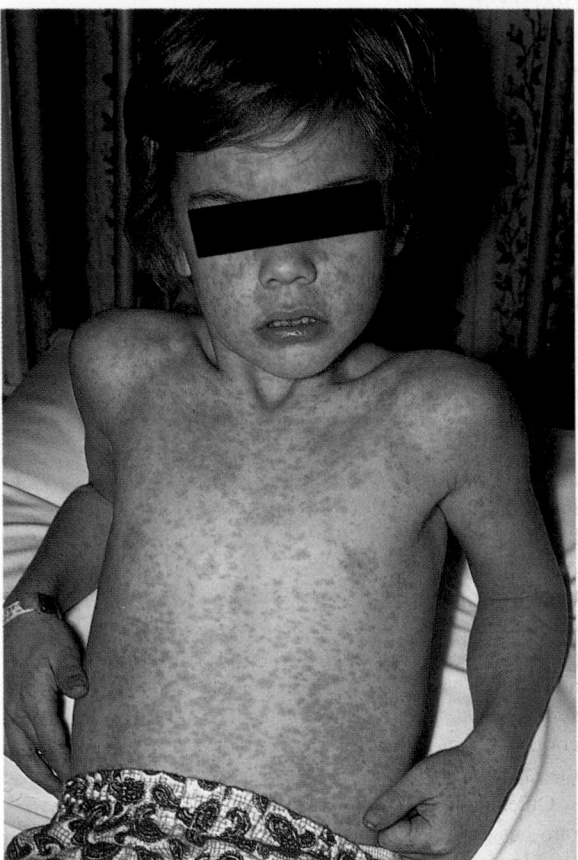

Fig. 13.7 Typical measles rash.

after infection. The typical rash may be missing in the immunocompromised and persistent infection with a giant cell pneumonitis or rapidly progressive encephalitis may occur. As with many childhood exanthemas, disease is more severe and prolonged in adults.

Measles is a serious disease in the malnourished, vitamin-deficient or immunocompromised. Mortality clustering at the extremes of age is 1:1000 in developed countries, compared to up to 1:4 in developing countries. Death usually results from bacterial superinfection such as pneumonia, diarrhoeal disease or cancrum oris.

13.26 ANTIBIOTICS TO PREVENT PNEUMONIA AFTER MEASLES

'Antibiotics should be given only if a child has clinical signs of pneumonia or other evidence of sepsis.'

- Shann F, et al. (Cochrane Review). Cochrane Library, issue 4, 2000. Oxford: Update Software.

For further information: 💻 www.cochrane.org

13.27 RUBELLA INFECTION: RISK OF CONGENITAL MALFORMATION

Stage of gestation	Likelihood of malformations
1–2 months	65–85% chance of illness, multiple defects/spontaneous abortion
3 months	30–35% chance of illness, usually a single defect, deafness or congenital heart disease
4 months	10% risk of congenital defects, most commonly deafness
> 20 weeks	Occasional deafness

Management

Normal immunoglobulin attenuates the disease in the immunocompromised or in non-immune pregnant women. Vaccination can be used in outbreaks and vitamin A may improve the outlook in uncomplicated disease. Antibiotic therapy is only effective where signs of superinfection already exist and should not be used empirically (Box 13.26).

RUBELLA (GERMAN MEASLES)

Rubella is endemic in countries without universal vaccination policies. Outbreaks occur in spring and early summer, with epidemics every 7–10 years. The virus is transmitted by aerosol, with infectivity from up to 1 week before and 1 week after the onset of the rash. In non-immunised communities 80–85% of young adults have evidence of past infection. In childhood most cases are subclinical. In 1941 Sir Norman Gregg recognised the association between rubella infection in early pregnancy and significant congenital abnormalities.

Initial infection via the upper respiratory tract and local lymph nodes is followed by viraemia to target organs such as skin, joints and placenta. If placental infection takes place in the first trimester, persistence of the virus is likely and has the potential for severe congenital disease (Box 13.27). Adenopathy lasting several weeks occurs, usually with the involvement of post-auricular, post-cervical and sub-occipital nodes and occasional splenomegaly. A maculo-papular non-confluent rash starts simultaneously on the face and moves to the trunk. Petechial lesions ('Forchheimer spots') appear on the soft palate, associated with a mild coryza/conjunctivitis. Fever occurs only on the first day of the rash.

Other than with congenital infection, complications are rare but are more common in adult females. An immune-mediated arthritis/arthralgia affects 30% of women and involves the fingers, wrists and knees; it takes 1–2 months to resolve. Encephalitis occurs in approximately 1 in every 5000 cases, with a 20–50% mortality. Recovery is complete in survivors. A mild hepatitis is frequently seen and haemorrhagic manifestations occur in 1:3000 cases.

Diagnosis

Laboratory confirmation of the diagnosis of rubella is required, particularly if there has been contact with a pregnant woman. Detection of rubella-specific IgG with absent IgM indicates previous infection. Specific IgM or rising IgM is indicative of recent infection. However, this may persist for 1–3 months and occur as a reaction in other common rashes such as human erythrovirus 19 and EBV infections. The most important investigation in early pregnancy is the detection of maternal rubella-specific IgG which indicates established immunity and allows the patient to be reassured that there is no serious risk of congenital disease.

Prevention

Rubella vaccine should be given to all children at the age of 12–15 months and again at about 4 years.

HUMAN ERYTHROVIRUS 19 (PARVOVIRUS B19)

This virus (previously known as parvovirus B19) occurs world-wide and produces a mild or subclinical infection in normal hosts. Clinical manifestations are summarised in Box 13.28. A biphasic illness occurs with symptoms during viraemia and at a later immune complex stage of the disease. Transmission is air-borne, although blood-borne, infection has been described in haemophiliacs. A week after infection non-specific symptoms occur and a few days later the immune response commences, accompanied by bone marrow depression. Reduction of erythroid precursors progresses to thrombocytopenia, lymphopenia and neutro-penia. This is transient and rarely clinically significant. The disease is relevant in individuals with a short red cell life, such as those with sickle-cell disease or spherocytosis where significant anaemia may progress to life-threatening levels. Haematopoiesis usually recovers spontaneously after 10–14 days. Two to three weeks after infection, the immune-mediated, classic red 'slapped cheek' rash with circumoral pallor (Fig. 13.8) and arthralgia appears. A second-stage erythematous maculo-papular rash may occur on the trunk and limbs. Apart from rare cases in the immuno-compromised, there is spontaneous recovery. Infection during the first two trimesters of pregnancy can result in intra-uterine infection and impact on fetal bone marrow; it causes 10–15% of non-immune (non-Rhesus-related) hydrops fetalis. This is rare, occurring in only 1:30 000 infected pregnancies.

Diagnosis

Erythrovirus 19 DNA may be detected in the serum and a PCR test will remain positive from then until some 4 months after infection. IgM responses, although commonly used for diagnostic purposes, may persist for months. During the

13

13.28 CLINICAL FEATURES OF HUMAN ERYTHROVIRUS 19 INFECTION

Disease caused by erythrovirus 19	Affected age group	Clinical manifestations
Fifth disease (erythema infectiosum)	Small children	Three clinical stages: a 'slapped cheek' appearance, followed by a reticulate eruption on the body and limbs, then a stage of resolution. Often the child is quite well throughout
Gloves and socks syndrome	Young adults	Fever and an acral purpuric eruption with a clear margin at the wrists and ankles. Mucosal involvement also occurs
Arthropathies	Adults and occasionally children	Polyarthropathy affecting small joints. In children it tends to involve the larger joints in an asymmetrical distribution
Red cell aplasia	Adults, those with haematological disease, the immunosuppressed	Can cause a mild anaemia but in an individual with an underlying haematological abnormality can precipitate an aplastic crisis
Hydrops fetalis	Transplacental fetal infection	Asymptomatic or symptomatic maternal infection can cause fetal anaemia with an aplastic crisis leading to non-immune hydrops fetalis and spontaneous abortion. Human erythrovirus 19 is the most common identifiable cause of hydrops fetalis

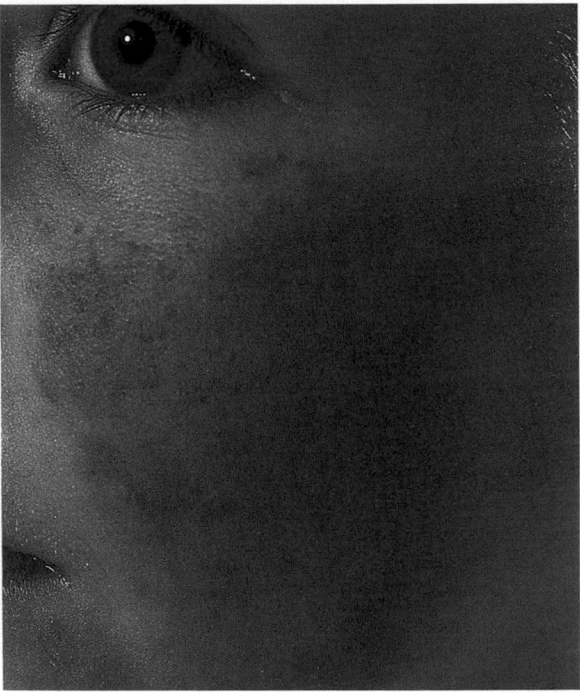

Fig. 13.8   Slapped cheek syndrome. The typical facial rash of human erythrovirus 19 infection.

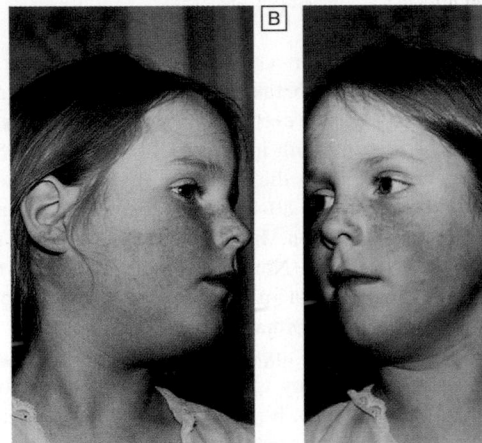

Fig. 13.9   Typical unilateral mumps. [A] Note the loss of angle of the jaw on the affected (right) side. [B] Comparison showing normal (left) side.

early stages of erythropoietic disturbance, haemophago-cytosis may be demonstrable in the bone marrow and occasionally in peripheral blood.

Management
In the normal individual, this infection is self-limiting and symptomatic relief for arthritic symptoms should be given. Passive prophylaxis with normal immunoglobulin has been suggested for non-immune pregnant women exposed to infection. The pregnancy should be closely monitored by ultrasound scanning, and any suggestion of hydrops should result in consideration of fetal transfusion.

MUMPS

This paramyxovirus is endemic world-wide. In non-vaccinated populations, it occurs in epidemics every 2–3 years, primarily infecting 5–9-year-old children. If vaccination has been employed without complete eradication of the disease, there is increased susceptibility in older teenagers. Infection is by droplets or direct salivary spread and initial infection is through the upper respiratory tract. A primary viraemia seeds the virus to target organs: parotid glands, other exocrine glands, meninges and sites of gametogenesis. The incubation period of 16–18 days ends with 2–3 days of infectivity and a second viraemia. Infectivity lasts for 5–7 days.

Classical tender parotid enlargement, which is bilateral in 75%, follows a prodrome of pyrexia and malaise (Fig. 13.9). Other salivary glands are involved in approximately 10% of cases.

Complications commonly occur. Oophoritis and orchitis only occur post-pubertally. Oophoritis causing abdominal pain is present in 5% of post-pubertal mumps in women.

Around 35% of post-pubertal males with mumps develop orchitis; 33% of these cases are bilateral. Some degree of testicular atrophy does result but sterility is most unlikely. Meningitis occurs in approximately 50% of cases. In non-vaccinated communities mumps is the most common cause of sporadic viral meningitis. The cerebrospinal fluid (CSF) pleocytosis is lymphocytic, often $0.2–0.4 \times 10^9$/l. A raised protein and reduced glucose level mimicking early bacterial meningitis may be present. Mumps meningitis is three times more common in males than females. Encephalitis is found in two forms: acute and post-infectious. It occurs in 1:6000 cases and has a mortality of 1.4%.

Transient hearing loss and labyrinthitis are recognised but uncommon. However, 1:20 000 cases will have persisting measurable deafness.

There appears to be no apparent added danger to the immunocompromised and natural infection results in life-long immunity. Abortion may occur if infection takes place in the first trimester of pregnancy but in the later trimesters infection appears to carry no added risk.

Management
Symptomatic relief is important. Prednisolone up to 40 mg orally for 4 days may be used to relieve the discomfort of orchitis.

Prevention
Mumps vaccine is given, usually as part of the MMR combined vaccine, after the first birthday and at a pre-school visit. If used widely, this will markedly reduce the incidence of natural infection and abolish the epidemic pattern of disease (Fig. 13.10).

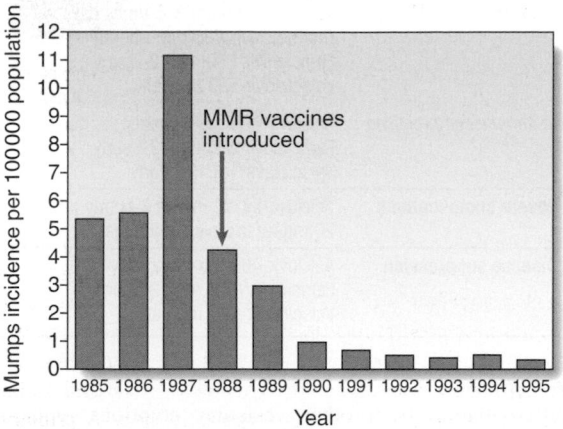

Fig. 13.10   Effect of mumps vaccination on incidence of disease.

HUMAN HERPES VIRUS 6 AND 7 (HHV-6 AND HHV-7)

These viruses (Box 13.25) were only identified in the 1990s. They are associated with a benign febrile illness of children with a maculo-papular erythematous rash: 'roseola infantum'/'exanthem subitum'. In the immunocompromised they cause lymphadenopathy.

13.29 HERPES VIRUS INFECTIONS	
Virus	**Infection**
Herpesvirus hominis (herpes simplex, HSV) Type 1	Herpes labialis ('cold sores') Keratoconjunctivitis Finger infections ('whitlows') Encephalitis Primary stomatitis Genital infections
Type 2	Genital infections Neonatal infection (acquired during vaginal delivery)
Varicella zoster virus (VZV) (p. 305)	Chickenpox Shingles (herpes zoster)
Cytomegalovirus (CMV) (p. 308)	Congenital infection Disease in immunocompromised patients Pneumonitis Retinitis Enteritis Generalised infection
Epstein–Barr virus (EBV) (p. 307)	Infectious mononucleosis Burkitt's lymphoma Nasopharyngeal carcinoma Oral hairy leucoplakia (AIDS patients)
Human herpes virus 6 (HHV-6) and 7 (HHV-7)	Exanthem subitum ? Disease in immunocompromised patients
Human herpes virus 8 (HHV-8) (p. 306)	Associated with Kaposi's sarcoma

13

VIRAL INFECTIONS OF THE SKIN

A number of viral infections produce manifestations predominantly in the skin. The herpes virus group consists of at least eight organisms (Box 13.29), all with particular tropism for specific body tissues and the potential for latency after primary infection. Recurrent disease occurs due to changes in immune surveillance or immune deficiency. Skin disease is particularly related to infection with herpes simplex and varicella zoster viruses.

HERPES SIMPLEX VIRUS (HSV)

Types 1 and 2 of this common virus affect humans. Type 1 HSV produces mucocutaneous lesions, predominantly of the head and neck (Fig. 13.11), whilst type 2 disease is a sexually transmitted anogenital infection (pp. 384 and 415). By puberty 30–100% of UK adults will have antibodies to HSV, depending on socioeconomic status. The source of infection is a case of primary or active recurrent disease. Primary infection normally occurs as a gingivostomatitis in infancy and may be subclinical or mistaken for 'teething'. It may present as a keratitis (dendritic ulcer), viral paronychia ('whitlow'—Fig. 13.12), vulvovaginitis, cervicitis (often unrecognised), balanitis or rarely as encephalitis.

Recurrent disease, involving reactivation of HSV from latency in the dorsal root ganglion, produces the classical

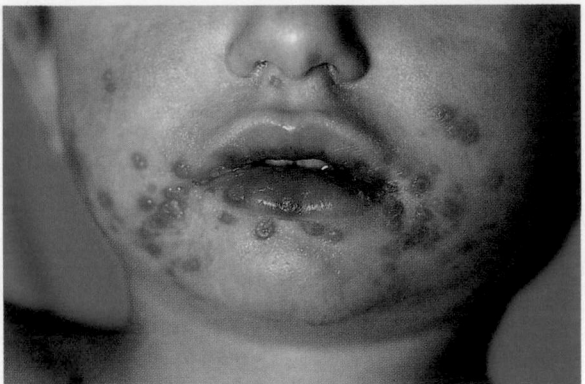

Fig. 13.11   Acute herpes simplex (HSV-1). There were also vesicles in the mouth—herpetic stomatitis.

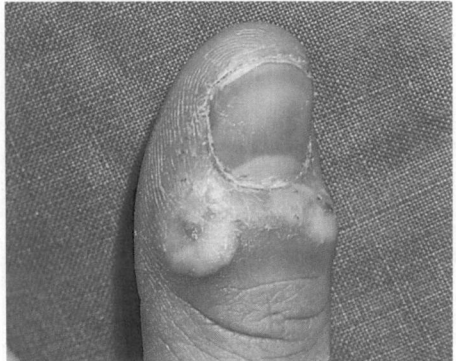

Fig. 13.12   Herpetic whitlow.

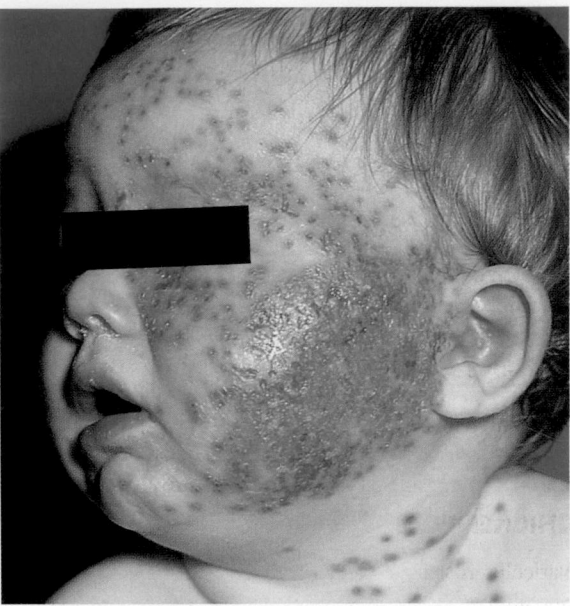

Fig. 13.13   Eczema herpeticum. HSV-1 infection spreads rapidly in eczematous skin.

13.30 THERAPY FOR HERPES SIMPLEX VIRUS INFECTION	
Disease state	**Treatment**
Primary HSV	Famciclovir 250 mg 8-hourly Valaciclovir 500 mg 12-hourly Aciclovir 200 mg 5 times daily
Severe and preventing oral intake	Aciclovir 5 mg/kg 8-hourly i.v.
Recurrent HSV-1 or 2	Aciclovir ointment 3–5 times daily Oral aciclovir 200 mg 6-hourly Famciclovir 250 mg 12-hourly Valaciclovir 500 mg daily
In immunocompromised	Aciclovir 400 mg 6-hourly Famciclovir 500 mg 12-hourly Valaciclovir 1 g 12-hourly
Severe complications	Aciclovir i.v. 10 mg/kg 8-hourly (up to 20 mg/kg in severe encephalitis)
Disease suppression	Aciclovir 400 mg 12-hourly Famciclovir 250 mg 12-hourly Valaciclovir 500 mg daily

'cold sore' or 'herpes labialis'. Prodromal hyperaesthesia is followed by rapid vesiculation, pustulation and crusting. Recurrences can be precipitated by disturbance of local skin integrity by ultraviolet light or systemic upset from menstruation or fever of any cause. Type 2 (genital) disease is a common cause of recurrent painful genital ulceration (p. 415).

Complications

Neonatal HSV disease, contracted from the birth canal, may be disseminated and is potentially fatal. Active HSV in a pre-term mother is an indication for either elective caesarean section or antiviral therapy. Active antiviral therapy should also be administered in the immunocompromised (lymphoma, leukaemia or HIV/AIDS, Box 13.30.

HSV infection in patients with eczema can result in a spreading and potentially serious infection, eczema herpeticum (Fig. 13.13). Dendritic ulcers may produce corneal scarring and permanently damage eyesight. These require aggressive antiviral therapy.

Encephalitis, the most serious complication of HSV disease, may occur following either primary or secondary disease. A haemorrhagic necrotising temporal lobe cerebritis produces temporal lobe epilepsy and decreasing conscious level/coma. Without treatment, mortality is 80%. Any suggestion of HSV encephalitis is an indication for immediate empirical systemic antiviral therapy.

Diagnosis

Differentiation from other vesicular eruptions requires demonstration of virus by PCR, electron microscopy or culture from vesicular fluid. CSF PCR is very useful in HSV encephalitis. Serology is of limited value, only confirming primary infection.

Management

The acyclic antivirals are the treatment of choice for HSV infection. Therapy must commence in the first 48 hours of clinical disease (primary or recurrent); thereafter it is unlikely to influence clinical outcome or modify the disease process. Severe manifestations should be treated regardless of the time of presentation (Box 13.30).

13

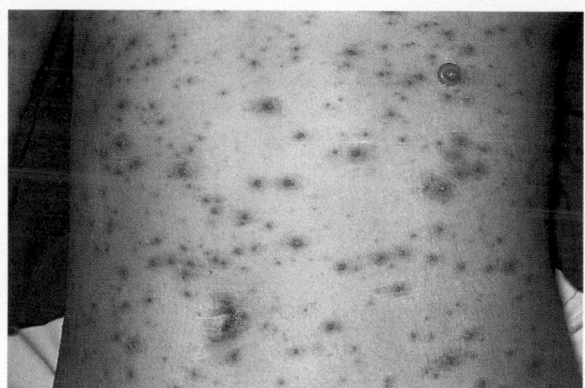

Fig. 13.14   Chickenpox.

13.31 ACICLOVIR FOR CHICKENPOX/SHINGLES   **EBM**

'Aciclovir shortens symptoms in chickenpox by an average of 1 day. In shingles aciclovir reduces pain by 10 days and the risk of post-herpetic neuralgia by 8%. Aciclovir is therefore cost-effective in shingles but not chickenpox.'

- Nathwani D, et al. Infect Dis Clin Prac 1995; 4:138–145.
- Trying SK. Arch Fam Med; 2000; 9:863–869.

CHICKENPOX

Varicella zoster virus (VZV) is dermo- and neurotropic. Spread by the aerosol route, it is highly infectious to susceptible individuals. Disease in children is usually well tolerated. It is more severe in adults, pregnant women and the immunocompromised. Pneumonitis can be fatal and is more likely in smokers, pregnant women and the immunocompromised. The incubation period is 14–21 days, after which a vesicular eruption begins (Fig. 13.14), often on mucosal surfaces first, followed by rapid dissemination in a centripetal distribution (most dense on trunk and sparse on limbs). New lesions occur every 2–4 days, each crop associated with fever. The rash progresses from small pink macules to vesicles and pustules within 24 hours. These then crust. Infectivity lasts until crusts separate. Due to intense itch secondary bacterial infection from scratching is the most common complication of primary chickenpox. Self-limiting cerebellar ataxia may rarely occur 7–10 days after recovery from the rash. Maternal infection in early pregnancy carries a 3% risk of neonatal damage, and disease within 5 days of delivery can lead to severe neonatal varicella.

Diagnosis

Usually this is clinically obvious from the classical appearance of the rash (Fig. 13.14). Aspiration of vesicular fluid and PCR or tissue culture will confirm the diagnosis. Electron microscopy cannot distinguish HSV from VZV. Serological examination for rising titres of antibody is only useful in primary infection. Chickenpox can recur as a subclinical infection following primary disease.

Management

Aciclovir, valaciclovir and famciclovir, although effective if commenced within 48 hours of rash appearance, do not have a licence in the UK for uncomplicated primary VZV infection. They are required in the management of the immunocompromised or any case of pneumonitis (Box 13.31).

Human VZV immunoglobulin may be used to attenuate infection in highly susceptible contacts of chickenpox such as:

- bone marrow recipients
- patients with debilitating disease
- HIV-positive contacts without VZV immunity
- pregnant women with no known VZV antibody (screen for antibody if in doubt)
- immunosuppressed contacts who have received high-dose corticosteroids in the previous 3 months
- neonates whose mothers develop chickenpox between 1 week before and 4 weeks after delivery
- neonates in contact with chickenpox/shingles whose mothers have no history of chickenpox or any demonstrable antibody
- premature infants of less than 30 weeks' gestation, or weighing less than 1 kg at birth who contact chickenpox or shingles.

VZV vaccine, now in use in the USA, offers effective protection.

SHINGLES (HERPES ZOSTER)

This is produced by reactivation of latent VZV from the dorsal root ganglion of sensory nerves. Commonly seen in the elderly, it may present in younger patients with immune deficiency or after intra-uterine infection.

Although thoracic dermatomes are most commonly involved (Fig. 13.15), the ophthalmic division of the trigeminal nerve is frequently implicated; vesicles may appear on the cornea and lead to ulceration. Geniculate ganglion involvement causes the Ramsay Hunt syndrome of facial palsy, ipsilateral loss of taste and buccal ulceration, plus a rash in the external auditory canal. This may be mistaken for Bell's palsy (p. 1249). Bowel and bladder

13

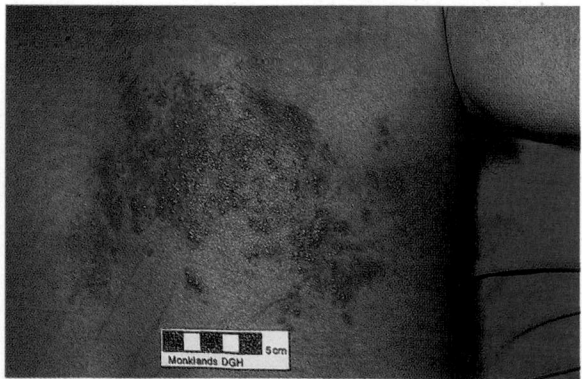

Fig. 13.15   Typical 'shingles' varicella zoster virus infection reactivating in a thoracic dermatome: 'a band of roses from Hell'.

dysfunction occurs with sacral nerve root involvement. The virus occasionally causes myelitis or encephalitis.

Clinical features

Burning discomfort in the affected dermatome progresses to frank neuralgia. Discrete vesicles appear in the dermatome 3–4 days later and often coalesce. This is associated with a brief viraemia and influenza-like features, and potentially produces distant satellite 'chickenpox' lesions elsewhere.

Severe disease, multiple dermatomal involvement or recurrence suggests underlying immune deficiency. Chickenpox may be contracted from a case of shingles but not the reverse.

Complications

The most common and troublesome complication is post-herpetic neuralgia: persistence of pain for 1–6 months or more following healing of the rash.

Management

Early therapy with aciclovir 800 mg 5 times daily or valaciclovir 1 g 8-hourly, or aciclovir 10 mg/kg i.v. 8-hourly in severe infection and in the immunocompromised has been shown to reduce both early- and late-onset pain, especially in patients over 65 (Box 13.31). Post-herpetic neuralgia requires aggressive analgesia and the use of transcutaneous nerve stimulation (a 'TENS' machine), along with neurotransmitter modification with agents such as amitriptyline 25–100 mg daily or gabapentin (commencing at 300 mg daily and building slowly to 300 mg 12-hourly or more.

HUMAN HERPES VIRUS 8 (HHV-8)

This virus (Box 13.25) has been linked to Kaposi's sarcoma tumour cells in both AIDS-related and endemic non-AIDS-related forms. There is some sero-epidemiological evidence that the infection may be transmitted via the sexual route, explaining the increased incidence of Kaposi's sarcoma among men who have sex with men (MSM) who are HIV sufferers. Contradictory evidence in children from endemic areas has thrown some doubt on this theory.

HAND, FOOT AND MOUTH DISEASE

This systemic infection is usually caused by Coxsackie virus A16. Mostly affecting children and occasionally adults, it often causes local or household outbreaks. A relatively mild illness of fever and lymphadenopathy develops after an incubation period of approximately 10 days; 2–3 days later a vesicular rash appears on palmoplantar surfaces of hands and feet, with associated mouth lesions that ulcerate rapidly. A papular erythematous rash may appear on buttocks and thighs.

The disease is self-limiting, lasting a maximum of 2 weeks, but the lesions are painful and may require analgesia.

HERPANGINA

This infection, caused by Coxsackie viruses (A1–10, 16 and 22, B1–5), primarily affects children and teenagers. It is characterised by discrete vesicles at the soft/hard palate junction, often associated with high fever, an extremely sore throat and headache.

The lesions are short-lived, rupturing after 2–3 days and rarely persisting for more than 1 week. Treatment is symptomatic. Culture or PCR of the lesions differentiates herpangina from HSV.

POXVIRUS INFECTIONS

These DNA viruses are potentially important pathogens but nowadays rarely cause significant human disease.

Smallpox (variola)

This severe disease, with a 30% mortality in the unvaccinated and no current effective therapy, was eradicated world-wide in 1980 by a successful international vaccination campaign coordinated by the WHO. The classical form is characterised by a typical deep-seated centrifugal vesicular/pustular rash, worst on the face and extremities, with no cropping (i.e. unlike chickenpox); the rash is accompanied by fever, severe myalgia and odynophagia. Interest in the disease has re-emerged due to its potential as a bioterrorist weapon (p. 342). In view of this threat some developed countries have reintroduced vaccination for key health-care personnel and re-evaluated national plans for the containment of disease.

Monkey pox

Despite the name, the animal reservoirs for this virus are probably small squirrels and rodents. It causes a rare zoonotic infection in primitive communities in the rainforest belt of central Africa, producing a vesicular rash indistinguishable from smallpox. Little to no person-to-person transmission occurs.

Cowpox

Humans in contact with infected cows develop large vesicles, usually on the hands or arms and associated with fever and regional lymphadenitis. The reservoir is thought to be wild rodents, and the virus also produces symptomatic disease in cats and a range of other animals.

Vaccinia virus

This poxvirus, derived in the laboratory, is the basis of the existing vaccine to prevent smallpox. Widespread vaccination is no longer recommended due to the likelihood of local spread from the vaccination site (potentially life-threatening in those with eczema (eczema vaccinatum) or immune deficiency) and of encephalitis (1:10–30 000 doses).

Orf

See page 1297.

Molluscum contagiosum

See page 1296.

SYSTEMIC VIRAL INFECTIONS

INFLUENZA

See page 688.

INFECTIOUS MONONUCLEOSIS (IM)

Virology and epidemiology

The disease is caused by the Epstein–Barr virus (EBV), a gamma herpes virus. In developing countries and poorer societies in developed nations subclinical infection in childhood is virtually universal. In richer communities, particularly among upper socioeconomic groups, primary infection may be delayed until adolescence or early adult life. Under these circumstances about 50% of infections result in typical IM. The virus is usually acquired from asymptomatic excreters. Saliva is the main means of spread, either by droplet infection or environmental contamination in childhood, or by kissing among adolescents and adults. There is a good correlation between sexual maturity and IM, and the age/sex distribution of the disease resembles that of gonorrhoea. IM is not highly contagious, isolation is unnecessary and documented outbreaks seldom occur.

Clinical features

A presumptive diagnosis of IM must include one or more of the following clinical features: lymphadenopathy, especially posterior cervical, pharyngeal inflammation or exudates, fever, splenomegaly, palatal petechiae, periorbital oedema, clinical or biochemical evidence of hepatitis, and a non-specific rash.

The diagnosis of IM outside the usual age range is difficult. In children under 10 years the illness is mild and short-lived, but in adults over 30 years of age it can be severe and prolonged. In both groups pharyngeal symptoms are often absent. IM may present with jaundice, as a PUO or with an unusual complication (Box 13.32).

Investigations

To establish the diagnosis, 20% or more of peripheral lymphocytes must have an atypical morphology (Fig. 13.16)

13.32 COMPLICATIONS OF INFECTIOUS MONONUCLEOSIS	
Common	
• Severe pharyngeal oedema	• Chronic fatigue syndrome (10%)
• Antibiotic-induced rash	
Uncommon	
Neurological	
• Cranial nerve palsies	• Transverse myelitis
• Polyneuritis	• Meningoencephalitis
Haematological	
• Haemolytic anaemia	• Thrombocytopenia
Renal	
• Glomerulonephritis	• Interstitial nephritis
Cardiac	
• Myocarditis	• Pericarditis
Pulmonary	
• Interstitial pneumonitis	
Rare	
• Ruptured spleen	• Agranulocytosis
• Respiratory obstruction	• Agammaglobulinaemia
• Arthritis	

and the serum must contain the characteristic heterophile antibody. This antibody, present during the acute illness and convalescence, agglutinates erythrocytes of other species, e.g. sheep and horse. It has a specific absorption pattern, detected by the classical Paul–Bunnell titration or by a more convenient slide test such as the 'Monospot'. Sometimes antibody production is delayed, so an initially negative test should be repeated. However, many children and 10% of adolescents with IM do not produce heterophile antibody at any stage.

Specific EBV serology (immunofluorescence) can be used to confirm the diagnosis if necessary. Acute infection is characterised by:

- antiviral capsid (VCA) antibodies in the IgM class
- antibodies to EBV early antigen (EA)
- absent antibodies to EBV nuclear antigen (anti-EBNA).

Management

Treatment is largely symptomatic: for example, aspirin gargles to relieve a sore throat. If a throat culture yields a β-haemolytic streptococcus, a course of erythromycin should be prescribed. Amoxicillin and similar semi-synthetic penicillins should be avoided because they commonly induce a maculo-papular rash in patients with IM (Fig. 13.17).

13

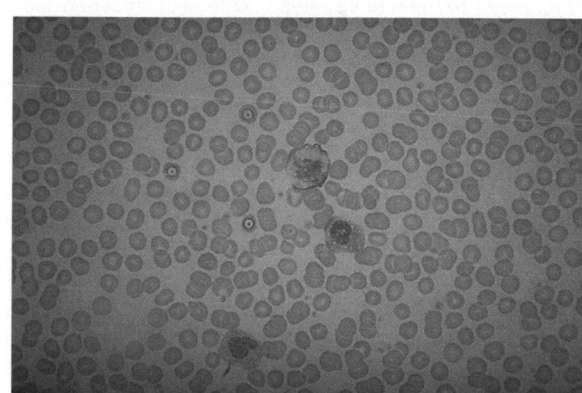

Fig. 13.16   Infectious mononucleosis: atypical lymphocytes in peripheral blood.

Fig. 13.17   Skin reactions to ampicillin and amoxicillin are common in infectious mononucleosis.

When pharyngeal oedema is severe a short course of corticosteroids, e.g. prednisolone 30 mg daily for 5 days, may help to relieve the swelling.

Return to work or school is governed by the patient's physical fitness rather than laboratory tests. However, contact sports should be avoided until splenomegaly has completely resolved because of the danger of splenic rupture. Unfortunately, about 10% of patients with IM suffer a chronic relapsing syndrome.

ACQUIRED CYTOMEGALOVIRUS INFECTION

Virology and epidemiology

Cytomegalovirus (CMV) is a beta herpes virus. Like EBV, it circulates readily among children, especially in crowded communities. Although most primary infections are asymptomatic, many children continue to excrete virus for months or years.

A second peak in virus acquisition occurs among teenagers and young adults. CMV infection is persistent, and is characterised by subclinical cycles of active virus replication and by persistent low-level virus shedding. Most post-childhood infections are therefore acquired from asymptomatic excreters who shed virus in saliva, urine, semen and genital secretions. Sexual transmission and oral spread are common among adults, but infection may also be acquired by women caring for children with asymptomatic infections. The peak incidence occurs between the ages of 25 and 35, rather later than with EBV-related mononucleosis.

Clinical features

Most post-childhood CMV infections are subclinical, although some young adults develop a mononucleosis-like syndrome which accounts for 20–50% of heterophile antibody-negative IM. Some patients have a prolonged influenza-like illness lasting 2 weeks or more. Physical signs such as a palpable liver and spleen resemble those of IM, but in CMV mononucleosis hepatomegaly is relatively more common, while lymphadenopathy, pharyngitis and tonsillitis are found less often. Jaundice is uncommon and usually mild. Unusual complications include neurological involvement, autoimmune haemolytic anaemia, pericarditis, pneumonitis and arthropathy.

Investigations

Atypical lymphocytosis is not as prominent as in IM and heterophile antibody tests are negative. LFTs are often abnormal, with an alkaline phosphatase level raised out of proportion to transaminases. Serological diagnosis depends on the detection of CMV-specific IgM antibody.

Management

Only symptomatic treatment is available. Amoxicillin and similar antibiotics should not be prescribed because of the risk of a skin reaction. Since CMV infection in immunocompetent subjects is self-limiting, the use of potentially toxic antiviral agents is usually inappropriate.

Gestational CMV infection

Most CMV infections in pregnancy are subclinical. However, heterophile antibody-negative 'glandular fever' in pregnancy requires full investigation, as CMV can cause congenital infection and disease at any stage of gestation. The risk of spread to the fetus is around 40%, and 10% of infected infants will have long-term central nervous system sequelae.

DENGUE

The dengue flavivirus is a common cause of fever in and from the tropics. It is endemic in South-east Asia and India and is also seen in Africa; there have been recent large epidemics in the Caribbean and Americas (Fig. 13.18). The principal vector is *Aedes aegypti*, which breeds in standing water; collections of water in containers and tyre dumps are a particular risk in large cities. *Aedes albopictus* is a vector in some South-east Asian countries. There are four serotypes of dengue virus, all producing a similar clinical syndrome; homotypic immunity is life-long but heterotypic immunity between serotypes lasts only a few months. The incubation period from being bitten by an infected mosquito is usually 2–7 days.

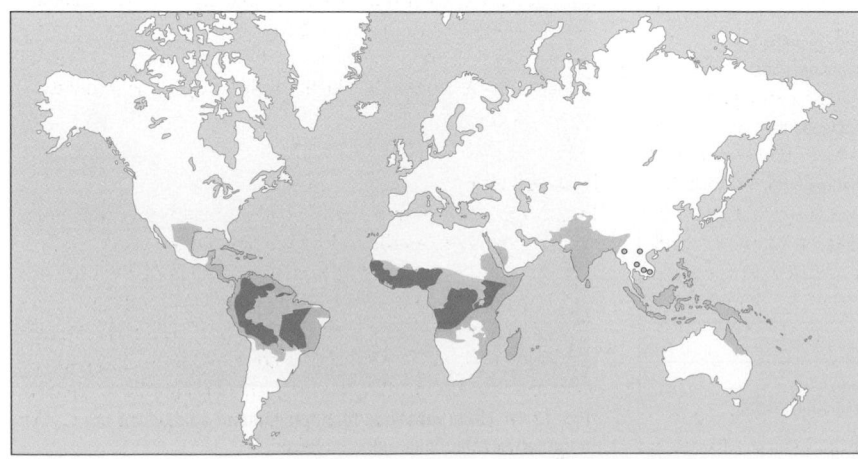

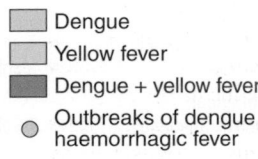
Dengue
Yellow fever
Dengue + yellow fever
Outbreaks of dengue haemorrhagic fever

Fig. 13.18 Endemic zones of yellow fever and dengue.

13.33 CLINICAL FEATURES OF DENGUE FEVER	

Prodrome

- 2 days of malaise and headache

Acute onset

- Fever, backache, arthralgias, headache, generalised pains ('breakbone fever'), pain on eye movement, lacrimation, anorexia, nausea, vomiting, relative bradycardia, prostration, depression, lymphadenopathy, scleral injection

Fever

- Continuous or 'saddle-back', with break on fourth or fifth day; usually lasts 7–8 days

Rash

- Transient macular in first 1–2 days. Maculo-papular, scarlet morbilliform from days 3–5 on trunk, spreading centrifugally and sparing palms and soles. May desquamate on resolution

Convalescence

- Slow

Clinical features

The disease varies in severity. The clinical features are listed in Box 13.33. Asymptomatic infections are common. The morbilliform rash characteristically blanches under pressure.

Dengue haemorrhagic fever or dengue shock syndrome

This occurs mainly in children in south-east Asia (Fig. 13.18 and Box 13.35). In mild forms there is thrombocytopenia and haemoconcentration. In the most severe form, after 3–4 days of fever, hypotension and circulatory failure develop with features of a capillary leak syndrome. Minor (petechiae, ecchymoses, epistaxis) or major (gastrointestinal bleeding) haemorrhagic signs may occur. The pathogenesis is unclear but pre-existing immunity to a dengue virus serotype, heterotypic to the one causing the current infection, predisposes to the syndrome. In vitro such heterotypic antibody causes enhanced virus entry and replication in monocytes; it is believed that enhancing antibody from previous dengue infection with a different serotype, or from acquired maternal antibody in infants, facilitates development of a very heavy viral load. Disseminated intravascular coagulation, complement activation and release of vasoactive mediators may contribute to the pathogenesis of the syndrome, possibly triggered by immunopathological mechanisms. Cytokine release is thought to be the cause of vascular damage at the site of post-capillary endothelial junctions. Even with good treatment the case fatality may be up to 10%. Adults rarely have classical dengue shock syndrome but may have a stormy and fatal course characterised by elevated liver enzymes, haemostatic abnormalities and gastrointestinal bleeding.

Investigations

Diagnosis of dengue is easier in an endemic area when a patient has the characteristic symptoms and signs. However, mild cases may have a similar presentation to other viral infections. Leucopenia is usual and thrombocytopenia common. The diagnosis is confirmed by either a fourfold rise in IgG antibody titres, isolation of dengue virus from blood or detection of dengue virus genomic sequences by real-time PCR (p. 142). Serological tests may detect cross-reacting antibodies from other flaviviruses, including yellow fever vaccine.

Management and prevention

There is no specific treatment. The severe pains can be relieved by paracetamol. Aspirin should be avoided. Volume replacement, blood transfusions and management of shock are indicated in the capillary leak syndrome. Corticosteroids have not been shown to help. No existing antivirals are effective.

Breeding places of *Aedes* mosquitoes should be abolished and the adults destroyed by insecticides. There is as yet no vaccine and in any case a tetravalent vaccine would be needed to cover all four serotypes. Until the *Aedes* mosquito can be controlled or a cost-effective vaccine developed, the incidence of dengue can be expected to continue to escalate.

YELLOW FEVER

Yellow fever, caused by a flavivirus, is normally a zoonosis of monkeys that inhabit tropical rainforests in West and Central Africa and South and Central America, where it may cause devastating epidemics (Fig. 13.18). It is transmitted by mosquitoes living in tree-tops. *Aedes africanus* in Africa and the *Haemagogus* species in America are the vectors. The infection is brought down to humans either by infected mosquitoes when trees are felled, or by monkeys raiding human settlements. In towns yellow fever may be transmitted between humans by *Aedes aegypti*, which breeds efficiently in small collections of water. The distribution of this mosquito is far wider than that of yellow fever and poses a continual risk of spread. It is surprising that there is no yellow fever in Asia; this may be because there are strain differences between the Asian and African *Aedes* mosquitoes or there may be unrecognised demographic obstacles to transmission.

Yellow fever causes between 200 000 and 300 000 deaths each year, mainly in sub-Saharan Africa, where it remains a major public health problem. Humans are infectious during the viraemic phase, which starts 3–6 days after the bite of the infected mosquito and lasts for 4–5 days. The incubation period is 3–6 days.

Pathology

In the liver, acute mid-zonal necrosis leads to deposits of hyalin called Councilman bodies, and intranuclear eosinophilic inclusions called Torres bodies. Another characteristic feature is the absence of inflammatory infiltrate. The kidneys show tubular degeneration, which may partly be due to reduced blood flow. Widespread petechial haemorrhages are most marked in the stomach and duodenum. Haemorrhage is due to liver damage and disseminated intravascular coagulation.

13

13.34 DIAGNOSIS OF YELLOW FEVER

- Clinical features in endemic area
- Virus isolation from blood in first 24 days
- Fourfold rise in antibody titre
- Post-mortem liver biopsy
- Differentiation from malaria, typhoid, viral hepatitis, leptospirosis, haemorrhagic fevers, aflatoxin poisoning

Clinical features

Yellow fever is often a mild febrile illness lasting less than 1 week. In severe cases the disease starts suddenly with rigors and high fever. Backache, headache and bone pains are severe. Nausea and vomiting then develop. The face is flushed and the conjunctivae are injected. Bradycardia and leucopenia are characteristic of this phase of the illness, which lasts 3 days and is followed by a period of remission lasting a few hours or days. The fever then returns with acute hepatic and renal failure. There is jaundice and a haemorrhagic diathesis with petechiae, haemorrhages into the mucosa and gastrointestinal bleeding plus oliguria. Patients commonly die in the third stage, often after a period of coma.

Investigations

Diagnostic procedures are listed in Box 13.34.

Management

Treatment is supportive, with meticulous attention to fluid and electrolyte balance, urine output and blood pressure. Blood transfusions, plasma expanders and peritoneal dialysis may be necessary. Patients should be isolated as their blood and body products may contain viral particles.

Prevention

A single vaccination with the 17D non-pathogenic strain of virus gives full protection for at least 10 years. The vaccine does not produce appreciable side-effects, unless there is allergy to egg protein. Vaccination is not recommended in people who are immunosuppressed, whether this is the result of immunosuppressive therapy or of underlying disease.

VIRAL HAEMORRHAGIC FEVERS

The viral haemorrhagic fevers are zoonoses caused by several different viruses (Box 13.35). They are endemic world-wide, each virus having its own niche. They are mainly rural and transmission is associated with poverty and poor medical facilities. Serological surveys have shown that Lassa fever is widespread in West Africa, where it accounts for 15% of adult hospital admissions and 50% of adults have antibodies. Although Lassa fever remains very rare in Britain, with about 1 case arriving in the country every 2 years, experience of managing this infection is greater than managing others in the group. Ebola and Marburg viruses cause small epidemics but have high fatality rates. The most recent Ebola outbreak was in Angola in 2005. Kyasanur forest disease is a tick-borne viral haemorrhagic fever currently confined to a small focus in Karnataka, India; there are about 500 cases annually. Monkeys are the principal hosts but with forest felling there are fears that this disease will increase. All of these viral illnesses except Ebola have mild self-healing forms.

Pathogenesis

These viruses cause endothelial dysfunction with the development of leaky capillary syndrome. Bleeding is due to this and associated platelet dysfunction. Hypovolaemic shock and acute respiratory distress syndrome develop (p. 187).

13.35 COMMON VIRAL HAEMORRHAGIC FEVERS

Disease	Reservoir	Transmission	Geography	Mortality rate	Clinical features[1]
Lassa fever	Multimammate rats (*Mastomys natalensis*) Patient	Urine Body fluids	West Africa	Up to 50%	Encephalopathy ARDS (Responds to ribavirin)
Marburg/Ebola virus	? Monkeys	Body fluids	Central Africa	25–90%	Thrombocytopenia Blood oozing
Yellow fever	Monkeys	Mosquitoes	Tropical Africa, South and Central America	10–60%	Hepatic failure Blood oozing
Dengue	Humans	*Aedes aegypti*	Tropical and subtropical coasts	Nil–10%[2]	Joint and bone pain Petechiae
Crimean–Congo	*Ixodes* tick	*Ixodes* tick	Africa, Asia, Eastern Europe	15–70%	Thrombocytopenia Blood oozing Petechiae
Bolivian and Argentinian	Rodents (*Calomys* spp.)	Urine	South America	?	Thrombocytopenia Petechiae
Haemorrhagic fever with renal syndrome (Hantan fever)	Rodents	Faeces	Northern Asia, northern Europe	30%	Petechiae Renal failure ARDS

[1] All potentially have circulatory failure.
[2] Mortality of uncomplicated and haemorrhagic dengue fever, respectively.

Clinical features

All viral haemorrhagic fevers have similar non-specific presentations with fever, malaise, body pains, sore throat and headache. On examination conjunctivitis, throat injection, an erythematous or petechial rash, haemorrhage, lymphadenopathy and bradycardia may be noted.

In Lassa fever joint and abdominal pain are prominent. A macular blanching rash may be present but bleeding is unusual, occurring in only 20% of hospitalised patients. Haemorrhage is a late feature of established severe disease and most patients will present with earlier symptoms. Bradycardia and ECG abnormalities are common. Encephalopathy may develop. Deafness affects 30% of survivors.

Investigations

There is leucopenia, thrombocytopenia and proteinuria. In Lassa fever an aspartate amino transferase (AST) > 150 U/l is associated with a 50% mortality.

Diagnosis

The clue to the viral aetiology will come from the travel and exposure history, so it is important to be aware of the incubation periods for these illnesses. For example, Lassa fever will not present more than 21 days after the patient leaves an endemic area. In Lassa fever retrosternal pain, pharyngitis and proteinuria have a positive predictive value of 80% in West Africa. Enquiry should be made about insect bites, particularly mosquitoes and ticks, hospital visits and attendance at ritual funerals (Ebola virus infection). The causative virus may be isolated, or antigen detected, in maximum security laboratories from serum, pharynx, pleural exudate and urine. The diagnosis of Lassa fever should be considered in non-endemic areas in patients presenting with fever within 21 days of leaving West Africa, particularly if they have organ failure or haemorrhagic features; most patients suspected of having a viral haemorrhagic fever in the UK turn out to have malaria.

Management

It is important to exclude other causes of fever, especially malaria, typhoid and respiratory tract infections. Particular care must be taken with body fluids. Patients returning from rural Africa with a fever should be managed in isolation until a diagnosis is made. General supportive measures, preferably in a special unit, are required. Ribavirin is given intravenously (100 mg/kg, then 25 mg/kg daily for 3 days and 12.5 mg/kg daily for 4 days). Once haemorrhagic fever is confirmed, full pressure isolation is mandatory and good infection control practices will prevent further transmission.

Prevention

Ribavirin has been used as prophylaxis in close contacts in Lassa fever but there are no formal trials of its efficacy.

GASTROINTESTINAL VIRAL INFECTIONS

NOROVIRUS (NORWALK AGENT)

Norovirus has been identified both in outbreaks related to infected food handlers and in endemic person-to-person gastroenteritis. Seroprevalence surveys suggest that many adults are susceptible to this infection.

These viruses spread by faeco–oral transmission, or by aerosol spread if susceptible individuals are in the vicinity of a sufferer actively vomiting.

After a 48-hour incubation period there is a brisk 2–3-day illness with marked nausea, predominant vomiting and little diarrhoea. Stepwise transmission of illness through nurseries and families remains very common. Norovirus outbreaks in health-care facilities are becoming a major problem.

CALICIVIRUS

This virus may produce seasonal symptoms. Seroprevalence surveys suggest that the infection is more common than its rate of identification in cases of gastroenteritis would suggest.

ROTAVIRUS

Rotaviruses are the major cause of diarrhoeal illness in young children, accounting for 30–50% of cases admitted to hospital in developed countries, and 10–20% of deaths due to gastroenteritis in developing countries. Infection is endemic in developing countries and there are winter epidemics in developed countries. These viruses are easily transmitted and resist alcohol denaturation; person-to-person spread, especially by health-care workers in hospitals, is well documented. The virus infects enterocytes, causing decreased surface absorption and loss of enzymes on the brush border. The incubation period is 48 hours and patients present with watery diarrhoea, vomiting, fever and abdominal pain. Diagnosis is aided by commercially available enzyme immunoassay kits which simply require fresh or refrigerated stool for effective demonstration of the pathogens.

The disease is self-limiting but dehydration needs appropriate management (p. 294). Immunity develops to natural infection. Rotavirus vaccines have been developed and gave good protection to children in Venezuela but were associated with intussusception; this has hampered vaccine uptake.

ASTROVIRUSES

Astroviruses are less frequently identified as a cause of infection/diarrhoea than rotaviruses (accounting for some 10% of the incidence of the latter). Seroprevalence in the community mimics rotavirus and they are therefore probably under-diagnosed.

HEPATITUS VIRUSES (A, B, C)

See Chapter 23.

OTHER VIRUSES

Adenoviruses are frequently identified from stool culture and implicated as a cause of diarrhoea. Two serotypes (40

13

13

and 41) appear to be more frequently found in association with diarrhoea rather than the more common upper respiratory types 1–7.

RESPIRATORY VIRAL INFECTIONS

These infections are described in Chapter 19; see also Box 13.25 (p. 299).

Adenoviruses, rhinoviruses and enteroviruses (Coxsackie viruses and echoviruses) (Box 19.42, p. 689) often produce non-specific symptoms. The individual infections each produce lasting specific immunity but the number of different serotypes in each class accounts for the apparent recurrence of common upper respiratory symptoms.

VIRAL INFECTIONS WITH NEUROLOGICAL INVOLVEMENT

A number of viral infections show neurotropism with disease manifestations predominantly in the central or peripheral nervous systems (Box 13.25, p. 299). These are described in Chapter 26.

JAPANESE B ENCEPHALITIS

This flavivirus is an important cause of encephalitis in Japan, China, South-east Asia and India. These regions are endemic for Japanese B encephalitis and epidemics also occur. In China, despite 70 million children being immunised, there are still 10 000 cases annually. Swine and birds are the virus reservoirs; transmission is by mosquitoes.

Clinical features
There is an initial systemic illness with fever, malaise and anorexia, followed by photophobia, vomiting, headache and changes in brain-stem function. Most children die from respiratory failure and frequently have evidence of cardiac and respiratory instability, reflecting viraemic spread via the vertebral vessels and infection of brain-stem nuclei. Other patients have evidence of multifocal CNS disease that involves the basal ganglia, thalamus and lower cortex, and develop tremors, dystonia and parkinsonian symptoms. Asymptomatic infection is common; of symptomatic infections there is a case fatality rate of 25%, and 50% of survivors are left with neurological sequelae.

Diagnosis
Other infectious causes of encephalitis should be excluded (p. 1228). Serological testing can be carried out. There is a CSF antigen test.

Management
Treatment should be supportive, anticipating and treating complications. Vaccination for travellers to endemic areas during the wet monsoon period is effective prophylaxis. Some endemic countries include this vaccination in their childhood regimens.

NIPAH VIRUS ENCEPHALITIS

In 1999 a newly discovered paramyxovirus in the Hendra group, the Nipah virus, caused an epidemic of encephalitis amongst Malaysian pig farmers. Infection is through direct contact with pig secretions. Mortality is around 30%. Antibodies to the Hendra virus are present in 76% of cases.

BACTERIAL INFECTIONS

BACTERIAL INFECTIONS OF THE SKIN AND SOFT TISSUES

Staphylococci are perhaps one of the most successful human pathogens. They normally colonise skin and mucous membranes but readily enter breaches in these natural barriers, especially if foreign material – e.g. soil, plastic cannulae, prosthetics – is present.

STAPHYLOCOCCAL INFECTIONS

Bacteria are prokaryotic, with a defined cell wall and cellular organelles but no defined nucleus. They are capable of free living but many organisms have a long-standing association with the human body, colonising skin, body cavities and the gut lumen in a normal commensal relationship. The differentiation between colonisation and infection can be difficult, requiring a combination of clinical acumen and microbiological expertise.

They are particularly dangerous if they gain access to the blood stream, having the potential to cause disease in many different situations (Fig. 13.19). Any evidence of

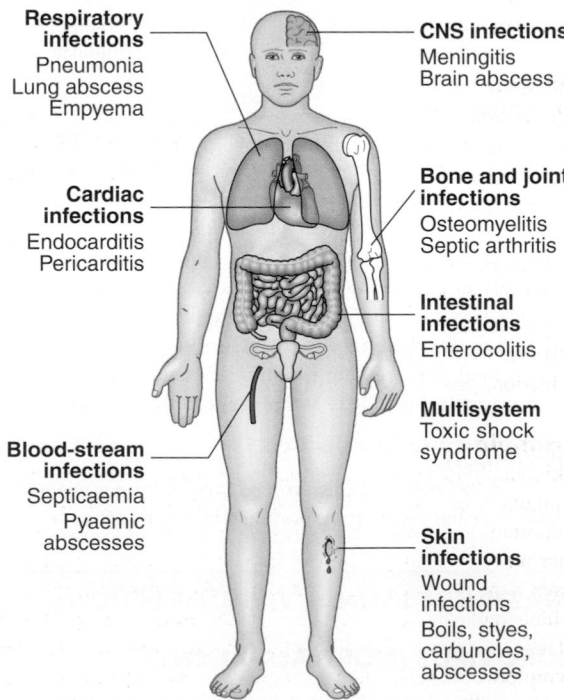

Respiratory infections
Pneumonia
Lung abscess
Empyema

Cardiac infections
Endocarditis
Pericarditis

Blood-stream infections
Septicaemia
Pyaemic abscesses

CNS infections
Meningitis
Brain abscess

Bone and joint infections
Osteomyelitis
Septic arthritis

Intestinal infections
Enterocolitis

Multisystem
Toxic shock syndrome

Skin infections
Wound infections
Boils, styes, carbuncles, abscesses

Fig. 13.19 Infections caused by *Staphylococcus aureus*.

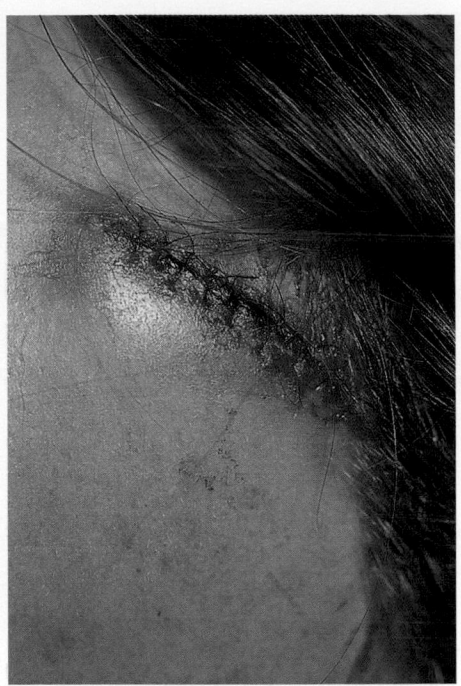

Fig. 13.20 Typical staphylococcal wound infection.

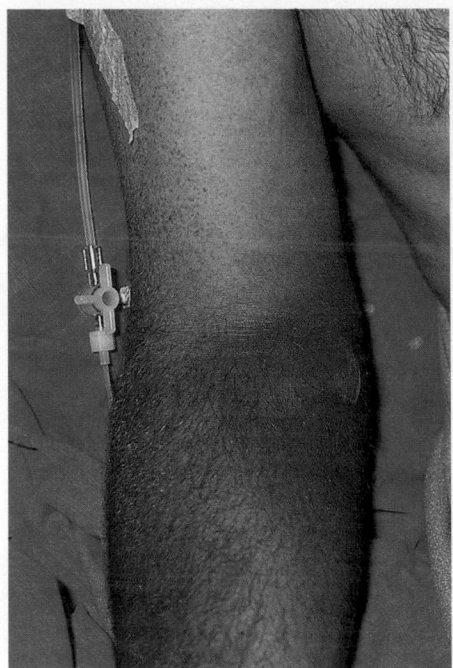

Fig. 13.21 Cannula-related infection.

spreading cellulitis or its occurrence in the mid-facial region indicates the need for urgent antistaphylococcal antibiotics such as flucloxacillin to prevent secondary sepsis.

Ecthyma, folliculitis, furuncles and carbuncles

These lesions are invariably caused by *Staphylococcus aureus*. They are described and illustrated on pages 1293–1294. They represent superficial skin infection with this ubiquitous organism.

Wound infections

Many wound infections are caused by staphylococci and may significantly prolong hospital stays in otherwise uncomplicated surgery (Fig. 13.20). Infection control and aseptic surgical technique are the best means of prevention. Antibiotic prophylaxis in clean surgery is also well established as a method of reducing wound infection.

Treatment is by drainage of any abscesses plus adequate dosage of antistaphylococcal antibiotics. These should be instituted early in the course of any post-operative wound infection, particularly where implants have been inserted.

Cannula-related infection

Skin staphylococci, e.g. *Staph. epidermidis* associated with cannula sepsis (Fig. 13.21) and thrombophlebitis, are an important and, unfortunately, extremely common reason for morbidity following hospital admission. These organisms have a predilection for plastic, rapidly forming a biofilm which remains as a source of bacteraemia as long as the plastic is in situ. Local poultice application may relieve symptoms but antibiotic treatment with benzylpenicillin and flucloxacillin is necessary if there is any suggestion of spreading infection.

Meticillin-resistant *Staph. aureus* (MRSA)

Staph. aureus has, perhaps more than any other organism, shown the ability to develop resistance to antibiotic therapy (p. 144). In the 1960s the so-called 'hospital staphylococcus', resistant to penicillin, caused severe problems in 'clean' orthopaedic and other prosthetic surgery. The introduction of meticillin and flucloxacillin re-established effective treatment for these infections. Resistance to meticillin due to the production of an additional penicillin-binding protein has been recognised in *Staph. aureus* for more than 30 years. Hospitals world-wide now experience MRSA as a major health care-acquired pathogen, and the recent recognition of resistance to vancomycin/teicoplanin (glycopeptides) in either glycopeptide intermediate *Staph. aureus* (GISA) or, rarely, vancomycin-resistant (VRSA) strains threatens our ability to manage serious infections produced by such organisms. MRSA now accounts for up to 40% of staphylococcal bacteraemia in developed countries, requiring care in both infection control and specific therapy of these infections. Clinicians must be aware of the potential danger of these infections and be prepared to take whatever appropriate infection control measures are locally advised (Box 6.17, p. 140).

Injection site infection in injection drug-users

Poor hygiene and injection techniques in injection drug-users, along with sharing unsterile equipment, often lead to skin and subcutaneous tissue sepsis. Mixed infections including staphylococci are involved in such cases (Fig. 13.22). A diagnostic aspiration of skin lesions with appropriate microbiological investigation should be undertaken.

Broad-spectrum antibiotics should be started and modified according to microbiological results.

13

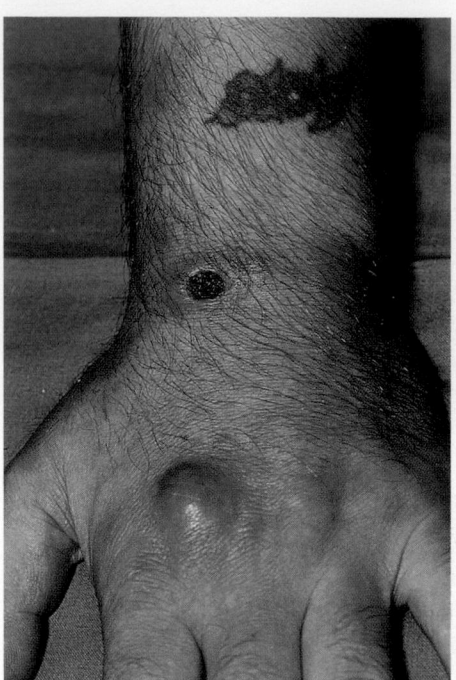

Fig. 13.22   Skin abscesses in an injection drug-user.

Secondary spread

In any patient with superficial staphylococcal infections, especially injection drug-users, the possibility of endocarditis must always be considered (p. 629).

Staphylococcal scalded skin syndrome and bullous impetigo

See pages 1293 and 1294.

Staphylococcal toxic shock syndrome (TSS)

This serious and life-threatening disease is associated with infection by *Staph. aureus* which is producing toxic shock syndrome toxin 1 (TSST1). It is most commonly seen in young women during, or immediately after, menstruation and is associated with the use of highly absorbent intra-vaginal tampons. *Staph. aureus* has been shown to grow in and around the tampon with the liberation of TSST1. TSS has also been described in both sexes in any age group associated with toxin-producing staphylococcal infections. The toxin acts as a 'super-antigen', triggering significant T-helper cell activation and very high peripheral polymorphonuclear leucocyte numbers.

TSS has an abrupt onset with high fever, generalised systemic upset (myalgia, headache, sore throat and vomiting), a generalised erythematous blanching rash resembling scarlet fever, and hypotension. It rapidly progresses over a matter of hours to multisystem involvement with cardiac, renal and hepatic compromise, leading to death in 10–20%. Recovery is accompanied at 7–10 days by desquamation (Fig. 13.23).

Diagnosis

The diagnosis is clinical (fever, rash, hypotension plus systemic upset in any person with distant staphylococcal

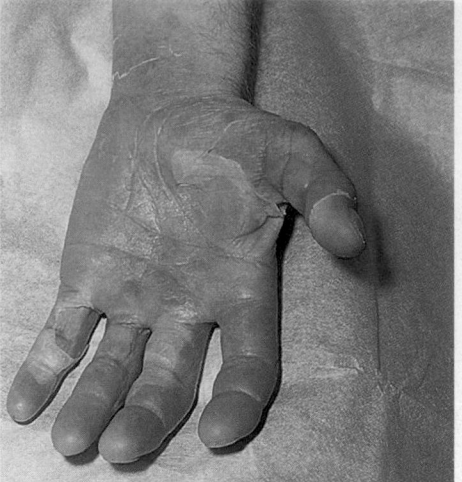

Fig. 13.23   Full-thickness desquamation after toxic shock syndrome.

infection). It may be confirmed in menstrual cases by vaginal examination, the finding of a retained tampon and microbiological examination by Gram stain demonstrating typical staphylococci. Subsequent culture and demonstration of toxin production are confirmatory.

Management

Immediate and aggressive fluid resuscitation with an intravenous antistaphylococcal antibiotic (flucloxacillin or vancomycin) is required. The rapid progression of symptoms and signs may require intensive care. Women who recover should be advised not to use tampons for at least 1 year and should also be warned that, due to an inadequate antibody response to TSST1, the condition can recur.

STREPTOCOCCAL INFECTIONS

Streptococcal scarlet fever

Group A and occasionally group C and G streptococci are implicated. A diffuse erythematous rash occurs, which blanches on pressure (Fig. 13.24), classically with circumoral pallor. The tongue, initially coated, becomes red and swollen ('strawberry tongue'—Fig. 13.25). The source is often a relatively uncomplicated streptococcal pharyngitis or tonsillitis. Common in school-age children, scarlet fever can occur in young adults who have contact with young children. The disease lasts about 7 days, the rash disappearing in 7–10 days followed by a fine desquamation. Residual petechial lesions in the antecubital fossa may be seen ('Pastia's sign'—Fig. 13.26).

Treatment involves active therapy for the underlying infection (benzylpenicillin or orally available penicillin) plus symptomatic measures.

Streptococcal toxic shock syndrome

This is associated with severe group A streptococcal skin infections producing pyogenic exotoxin A. Initially, an influenza-like illness occurs with, in 50% of cases, signs of necrotising fasciitis. A faint erythematous rash, mainly on

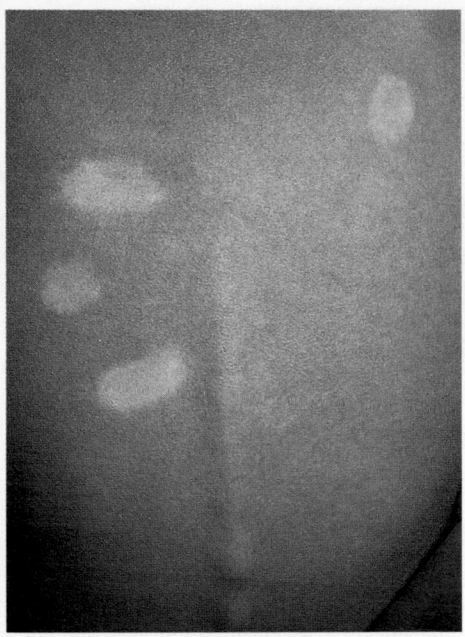

Fig. 13.24   Scarlet fever. Note blanching on pressure.

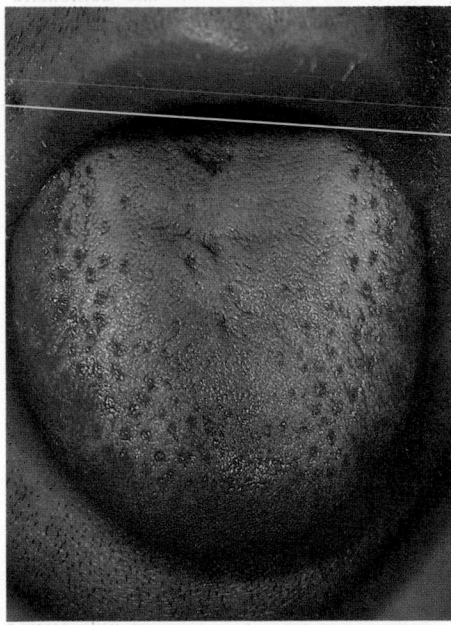

Fig. 13.25   The 'strawberry tongue' of acute streptococcal disease.

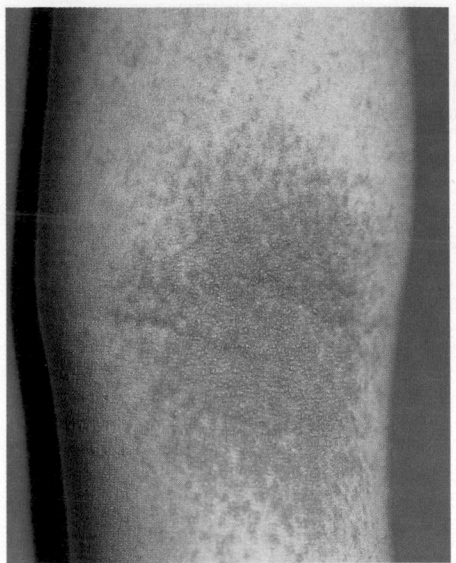

Fig. 13.26   Pastia's sign. Petechial rash in the cubital fossa.

13.36 STREPTOCOCCAL AND RELATED INFECTIONS

Strep. pyogenes	
• Skin and soft tissue infection (including erysipelas, impetigo, necrotising fasciitis)	• Tonsillitis
	• Puerperal sepsis
	• Scarlet fever
• Streptococcal toxic shock syndrome	• Glomerulonephritis
	• Rheumatic fever
• Bone and joint infection	

Alpha-haemolytic streptococci (Strep. mitis, sanguis, mutans, salivarius)	
• Endocarditis	• Septicaemia in immunosuppressed

Group B streptococci	
• Neonatal infections including meningitis	• Female pelvic infections

Enterococcus faecalis	
• Endocarditis	• Urinary tract infection

Anaerobic streptococci (Peptostreptococcus spp.)	
• Peritonitis	• Liver abscess
• Dental infections	• Pelvic inflammatory disease

N.B. All streptococci can cause septicaemia.

13

the chest, rapidly progresses to a toxic multisystem shock-like state. Without aggressive management, multi-organ failure will develop.

If necrotising fasciitis is present, it should be treated as described on page 316. Fluid resuscitation must be undertaken, linked to parenteral antistreptococcal antibiotic therapy, usually with benzylpenicillin with or without clindamycin.

Other streptococcal infections are shown in Box 13.36.

Cellulitis, erysipelas and impetigo
See pages 1293 and 1295.

SEVERE NECROTISING SOFT TISSUE INFECTIONS

Cellulitis may rapidly progress to extensive necrosis of subcutaneous tissue and overlying skin. Several different clinical presentations are recognised, depending upon the causative organism, the structure and anatomical level

13.37 SEVERE NECROTISING SOFT TISSUE INFECTIONS

- Necrotising fasciitis
- Clostridial anaerobic cellulitis (confined to skin and subcutaneous tissue)
- Non-clostridial anaerobic cellulitis
- Progressive bacterial synergistic gangrene (*Staph. aureus* + microaerophilic streptococcus)
- Pyomyositis (discrete abscesses within individual muscle groups)
- Clostridial myonecrosis (gas gangrene)
- Anaerobic streptococcal myonecrosis (non-clostridial infection mimicking gas gangrene)
- Group A streptococcal necrotising myositis (streptococcal myositis without abscess formation)

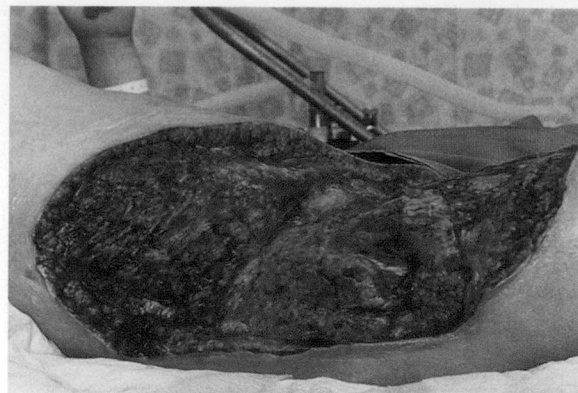

Fig. 13.27   Excision following necrotising fasciitis in an injection drug-user.

involved, and the predisposing conditions in the patient (Box 13.37).

Aggressive intravenous antibiotic therapy against anaerobic, Gram-negative and Gram-positive organisms is required. Urgent surgical débridement should be considered if the lesion is not rapidly controlled.

Necrotising fasciitis

There are two major categories of necrotising fasciitis:

- *Type 1* is a polymicrobial infection with Enterobacteriaceae and anaerobic organisms. It often occurs following surgery or in diabetic or immunocompromised patients.
- *Type 2* (sometimes known as streptococcal gangrene) is caused by pure growth of *Strep. pyogenes* Lancefield group A.

Both types produce a severe, rapidly progressive and destructive inflammation of the dermis, subcutaneous tissues, subcutaneous fat and tissue planes including the deep fascia. Necrotising fasciitis is associated with profound toxaemia and multisystem failure. The whole process is hyperacute, often arising from an apparently minor breach in skin integrity. The affected area is erythematous, hot, shiny and exquisitely tender.

The skin rapidly changes and frank, full-thickness gangrene resembling a thermal burn ensues. The central area of skin involvement becomes anaesthetic due to cutaneous nerve damage. Central anaesthesia surrounded by exquisitely tender erythematous skin is pathognomonic of necrotising fasciitis. Systemic toxicity develops with high fever, marked leucocytosis and often hypocalcaemia due to subcutaneous fat necrosis. Subcutaneous gas may be present in type 1 necrotising fasciitis. Recently, a form of this condition has been recognised which occurs in tropical regions after contact with shellfish. It is due to *Vibrio fulnificus* and is associated with liver disease.

Management

Necrotising fasciitis requires urgent and extensive surgical débridement (Fig. 13.27) and appropriate antibiotic therapy against Gram-positive, anaerobic and Gram-negative organisms. Usually intravenous benzylpenicillin and a quinolone, plus either clindamycin or metronidazole, are used. Despite this, mortality is between 30% and 80% and up to 50% may require amputation of affected limbs and/or plastic surgical management. Culture of débrided tissue plus Gram staining of exudate from lesions help to delineate and confirm the infecting organism. Empirical antibiotic therapy (p. 145) should be started prior to microbiological confirmation.

Clostridial soft tissue infections

Although *Clostridia* may colonise or contaminate wounds, no action is required unless evidence of spreading infection is present. In anaerobic cellulitis, usually due to *Cl. perfringens* or other strains infecting devitalised tissue following a wound, gas forms locally and extends along tissue planes, but bacteraemia and invasion of healthy tissue are not found. Prompt surgical débridement of devitalised tissue with penicillin or clindamycin therapy usually results in an excellent outcome.

Gas gangrene or myonecrosis is defined as acute invasion of healthy living muscle undamaged by previous trauma. It usually (70% of cases) develops following deep penetrating injury sufficient to create an anaerobic (ischaemic) environment and allow clostridial introduction and proliferation. *Cl. perfringens* accounts for the majority of these infections. Severe pain at the site of the injury progresses rapidly over 18–24 hours. Skin colour changes from pallor to bronze/purple discoloration and the skin is tense and exquisitely tender. Gas in tissues may be obvious with crepitus on clinical examination or visible on X-ray, CT or ultrasound. Signs of systemic toxicity develop rapidly with high leucocytosis, multi-organ dysfunction, raised creatine kinase and evidence of disseminated intravascular haemolysis. *Cl. tetani* and *Cl. botulinum* contaminating imported heroin can cause 'wound tetanus' and 'wound botulism' in injection drug-users. Antibiotic therapy with high-dose intravenous penicillin, clindamycin, cephalosporins and metronidazole is very effective, and should be coupled with aggressive surgical débridement of the affected tissues. Use of hyperbaric oxygen is controversial.

Bacteroides infection

Bacteria of the *Bacteroides fragilis* group are commonly found in the gastrointestinal tract and cause both skin and soft tissue infections and bacteraemia. They are often associated with mixed infections in compromised hosts such as diabetics and are frequently linked to rectal or colonic pathology, surgery or pelvic disease. Antimicrobial resistance is widespread in this group which are nevertheless usually sensitive to β-lactam–β-lactamase inhibitor combinations, metronidazole or carbapenems.

TREPONEMATOSES

Syphilis

This disease is described on page 411.

Endemic treponematoses

Yaws

Yaws is a granulomatous disease, mainly involving the skin and bones, which is caused by *Treponema pertenue*, morphologically indistinguishable from the causative organisms of syphilis and pinta. The three infections induce similar serological changes and possibly some degree of cross-immunity. Organisms are transmitted by bodily contact from a patient with infectious yaws through minor abrasions of the skin of another patient, usually a child. The mass WHO campaigns between 1950 and 1960 treated over 60 million people and eradicated yaws from many areas, but the disease has persisted patchily throughout the tropics; there was a resurgence in the 1980s and 1990s in West and Central Africa and the South Pacific.

Pathology. A proliferative granuloma containing numerous treponemes develops at the site of the inoculation. This primary lesion is followed by secondary eruptions. In addition, there may be hypertrophic periosteal lesions of many bones, with underlying cortical rarefaction. Lesions of late yaws are characterised by destructive changes which closely resemble the osteitis and gummas of tertiary syphilis and which heal with much scarring and deformity. The incubation period is 3–4 weeks.

Clinical features. In early yaws the primary lesion or 'mother yaw' is usually on the leg or buttocks. The secondary eruption usually follows a few weeks or months later, as crops of papillomas covered with a whitish-yellow exudate, especially in the flexures and around the mouth. Sometimes a lesion erupts through the palm or sole, and walking becomes painful ('wet crab yaws'). Phalanges, nasal bones and tibiae swell and become distorted. Most of the lesions of early yaws will eventually subside, even if untreated.

In the 'latent yaws' stage, following the spontaneous resolution of 'early yaws', serological changes may persist, to be followed by further manifestations of 'early yaws' or, after an interval of as much as 5–10 years, by the tertiary lesions of 'late yaws'.

In late yaws, solitary or multiple lesions appear as nodules or ulcers in the skin, hyperkeratotic lesions of palms or soles ('dry crab yaws') and gummatous lesions of bone. They heal with scarring. Lesions of the facial and palatal bones cause terrible disfigurement (gangosa).

Investigations and management. See Box 13.38.

Prevention. The disease disappears with improved housing and cleanliness. In few fields of medicine have

13.38 DIAGNOSIS AND TREATMENT OF YAWS, PINTA AND BEJEL	

Diagnosis of early stages

- Detection of spirochaetes in exudate of lesions by dark ground microscopy

Diagnosis of latent and early stages

- Positive serological tests, as for syphilis (p. 412)

Treatment of all stages

- Single intramuscular injection of 1.2 g long-acting (e.g. benzathine) benzylpenicillin

chemotherapy and improved hygiene achieved such dramatic success as in the control of yaws.

Pinta and bejel

These two treponemal infections occur in poor rural populations with low standards of domestic hygiene, but are found in separate parts of the world. They have features in common, notably that they are transmitted by contact, usually within the family and not sexually, and in the case of bejel, through common eating and drinking utensils. Their diagnosis and management are as for yaws (Box 13.38).

Pinta. Pinta is probably the oldest of the human treponemal infections and *T. carateum* the parent of the organism that came to Europe with the return of Christopher Columbus's sailors in 1493, starting the epidemic of venereal syphilis known as the 'Great Pox'. It is found only in South and Central America, where its incidence is declining. The early lesions are scaly papules or dyschromic patches on the skin. The late lesions are often depigmented and disfiguring. The infection is confined to the skin.

Bejel. Bejel is the Middle Eastern name for non-venereal syphilis, which has a patchy distribution across sub-Saharan Africa, the Middle East, Central Asia and Australia. It has been eradicated from Eastern Europe. Transmission is most commonly from the mouth of the mother or child and the primary mucosal lesion is seldom seen. The early and late lesions resemble those of secondary and tertiary syphilis (pp. 411–412) but cardiovascular and neurological disease are rare.

SYSTEMIC BACTERIAL INFECTIONS

SEPSIS SYNDROME

Sepsis syndrome is systemic invasion of microbes and their toxins, which results in a disease state characterised by high fever, rigors and tachypnoea, with or without localising signs and the development of shock. Although bacteria can be recovered from the blood following minor surgical procedures, catheterisation and so on, these are easily eliminated by host defences (bacteraemia). However, some organisms, like *Staphylococcus aureus* (p. 312), *Neisseria meningitides* (p. 1225), *Escherichia coli* (p. 328) and other Gram-negative organisms, may escape defence mechanisms, especially in the presence of conditions compromising the immune system (e.g. diabetes mellitus, cirrhosis of

13

the liver, invasive procedures or devices, injection drug use etc.).

Clinical features

In severe sepsis, hypotension unresponsive to fluids, along with organ dysfunction (septic shock), may develop (p. 189). If is often difficult to implicate a causative organism in the absence of attributable clinical features. However, certain features such as generalised erythroderma (toxic shock syndrome, *Staph. aureus, Strep. pyogenes*) and petechial or haemorrhagic rash (*N. meningitides*) may provide certain clues. In elderly or unvaccinated splenectom-ised individuals, *Strep. pneumoniae* may cause septicaemia without localising features. The incidence of polymicrobial infection has progressively increased in recent years.

Progression of the disease results in damage to different organs (multi-organ failure). Confusion, delirium and coma suggest encephalopathy, especially in the elderly. Increasing alveolar–capillary permeability leads to ventilation/perfusion mismatch, and acute respiratory distress syn-drome (ARDS) may ensue. Acute renal failure may occur due to prolonged hypotension and/or toxic injury, leading to acute tubular necrosis. Hepatic dysfunction, indicated by hyperbilirubinaemia and elevated enzyme levels, is a common occurrence in sepsis. Disseminated intravascular coagulation (DIC) is a frequent complication of severe septicaemia.

Investigations

A polymorphonuclear leucocytosis is frequently found. As organ involvement develops, elevated urea, serum creatinine, bilirubin and hepatic enzymes are seen. Progressive thrombocytopenia and other coagulation abnormalities indicate the presence of DIC. Arterial blood gas analysis may show alkalosis due to hyperventilation, but a metabolic acidosis may follow and indicates a poor prognosis. The chest X-ray may show features of ARDS. Blood culture is the most valuable tool in detecting the causative organism; multiple cultures are often needed. Culture of material from septic foci, if present, should always be performed.

Management

Prompt antimicrobial therapy should be started after blood and other specimens have been sent for culture. Broad cover including both Gram-negative and Gram-positive organisms is desirable, and once culture and sensitivity reports are available, specific antibiotics can be chosen. Correction of metabolic imbalance, ventilatory support and vasopressor agents in hypotension are important measures in severe sepsis. Corticosteroids (200–300 mg of hydrocortisone daily for 5 days) may improve survival in patients with septic shock. Administration of drotrecogin alfa (activated protein C) has been shown to improve survival in patients with severe sepsis and septic shock.

OSTEOMYELITIS

In addition to the conditions described above, osteomyelitis (p. 1118), with or without discitis (inflammation of the intervertebral disc), may sometimes present with fever without localising signs. In acute osteomyelitis, especially with haematogenous spread, fever antedates any localising feature. Common in children, the disease more frequently affects growing bones. In a minority of patients, acute osteomyelitis becomes chronic despite treatment. Fever is not a feature of the chronic disease. Discitis is almost always associated with vertebral osteomyelitis. Infection occurs via the haematogenous route and the elderly are more likely to be affected. The disease is usually insidious in onset, with pain in the neck or other areas, and with or without low-grade fever. In addition to pyogenic causes, tuberculosis is an important cause.

ENDOCARDITIS

In a significant number of patients fever is the only presenting symptom of infective endocarditis (p. 629) and there is no indication of cardiac involvement. A careful cardiac examination may provide the clue, although the presence of typical vegetations on two-dimensional or transoesophageal echocardiography eventually confirms the diagnosis.

BRUCELLOSIS

Microbiology and epidemiology

Brucellosis is an enzootic infection (i.e. endemic in animals). Although six species of *Brucella* are known, only four are important to humans: *B. melitensis* (goats, sheep and camels), *B. abortus* (cattle), *B. suis* (pigs) and *B. canis* (dogs).

B. melitensis is enzootic in the Middle East, Africa, India, Central Asia and South America. *B. abortus* is found in Africa, Asia and South America, and *B. suis* in South Asia. *B. melitensis* causes the most severe disease; *B. suis* is often associated with abscess formation.

Infected animals may excrete brucellae in their milk for long periods of time and human infection is acquired by ingesting contaminated milk, cheese, yoghurt and butter. Uncooked meat and offal may also spread infection. Animal urine, faeces, vaginal discharge and uterine products may act as sources of infection through abraded skin or via splashes and aerosols to the respiratory tract and conjunctiva.

Clinical features

Brucellae are intracellular organisms that can survive for long periods within the reticulo-endothelial system. This explains many of the features of clinical brucellosis, including the chronicity of the disease and the tendency to relapse even after adequate antimicrobial therapy.

Acute illness is characterised by a high swinging temperature, rigors, sweating, lethargy, headache, and joint and muscle pains. Occasionally, there is delirium, abdominal pain and constipation. Physical signs are non-specific: for example, a palpable spleen or enlarged lymph nodes. Enlargement of the spleen may lead to hypersplenism and thrombocytopenia.

Localisation of infection, which occurs in about 30% of patients, is more likely if diagnosis and treatment are

13

13.39 FOCAL MANIFESTATIONS OF BRUCELLOSIS

Musculoskeletal

- Suppurative arthritis; synovitis, bursitis
- Osteomyelitis
- Spinal spondylitis
- Paravertebral or psoas abscess

Central nervous system

- Meningitis
- Cranial nerve palsies
- Intracranial or subarachnoid haemorrhage
- Stroke
- Myelopathy
- Radiculopathy

Ocular

- Uveitis
- Retinal thrombophlebitis

Cardiac

- Myocarditis
- Endocarditis

delayed. Focal manifestations of infection are summarised in Box 13.39.

Diagnosis

Definitive diagnosis of brucellosis depends on the isolation of the organism. Blood cultures are positive in 75–80% of infections caused by *B. melitensis* and 50% of those caused by *B. abortus*. The non-radiometric 'Bactec' system gives a good isolation rate, but if brucellosis is suspected, prolonged incubation and blind subcultures are recommended. Bone marrow culture should not be used routinely but may increase the diagnostic yield, particularly if antibiotics have been given before specimens are taken. CSF culture in neurobrucellosis is positive in about 30% of cases.

World-wide, the serum agglutination test is the serological technique most commonly employed to detect brucellosis. The test has many pitfalls and good quality control is essential. Agglutination should be carried out to a high dilution (at least 1/640) to avoid the prozone phenomenon whereby non-agglutinating IgG and IgA molecules completely block the agglutinating reaction. Significant agglutination titres may persist for months or years after recovery and in endemic areas a single titre of 1/320 or a fourfold rise in titre is needed to support a diagnosis of acute infection. The test usually takes several weeks to become positive but should eventually detect 95% of acute infections. The pre-treatment of serum with 2-mercaptoethanol helps to distinguish between IgG and IgM responses. The enzyme-linked immunosorbent assay (ELISA) also identifies IgM and IgG antibodies; IgM decreases rapidly within the first few months of illness.

Specialist laboratory techniques including the use of the anti-human globulin (Coombs) test may be necessary to distinguish chronic disease from past inactive infection.

Management

Aminoglycosides show synergistic activity with tetracyclines when used against brucellae. Standard therapy therefore consists of doxycycline 100 mg 12-hourly for 6 weeks, with streptomycin 1 g i.m. daily for the first 2 weeks. The relapse rate with this treatment is about 5%. An alternative oral regimen consists of doxycycline 100 mg 12-hourly plus rifampicin 900 mg (15 mg/kg) daily for 6 weeks, but failure and relapse rates are higher, particularly with spondylitis. Rifampicin may antagonise doxycycline activity by reducing serum levels through enzyme induction.

Chronic illness should be treated for a minimum of 3 months and many authorities would extend this to 6 months, depending upon the condition of the patient and the result of sequential serological tests. The optimum therapy for neurobrucellosis is unknown, and there is no current agreement on the combination or number of drugs to use. Treatment should continue for at least 3 months, and longer if CSF pleocytosis persists.

LYME BORRELIOSIS

Microbiology and epidemiology

The causative agent of Lyme disease (named after the town of Old Lyme in Connecticut, USA) is a flagellated spirochaetal bacterium of the genus *Borrelia*. *B. burgdorferi* is the type species found in the northern hemisphere. In Europe two additional genospecies are also encountered, *B. afzelii* and *B. garinii*. The reservoir of infection is maintained in ixodid (hard) ticks that feed on a variety of large mammals, particularly deer. Birds may spread ticks over a wide area. The organism is transmitted to humans, who are incidental hosts, via the bite of infected ticks; larval, nymphal and adult forms are all capable of spreading infection.

Lyme disease is found in the USA, Europe, Russia, China, Japan and Australia. Incidence parallels the burden of infection among tick vectors and peaks in the summer.

Clinical features

Clinical features can be classified into three stages: early localised, early disseminated and late disease. Progression may be arrested at any stage.

Early localised disease

The characteristic feature is a skin reaction around the site of the tick bite, known as erythema migrans. Initially, a red macule or papule appears 2–30 days after the bite. It then enlarges peripherally with central clearing, and may persist for months. Atypical forms of erythema migrans are fairly common. Other acute manifestations such as fever, headache and regional lymphadenopathy may develop with or without the rash.

Early disseminated disease

During this stage the organism seeds to other organs via the blood stream and lymphatics. There may be a pronounced systemic reaction with malaise, arthralgia, and occasionally metastatic areas of erythema migrans. Neurological involvement may follow weeks or months after infection. Common features include lymphocytic meningitis, cranial nerve palsies (especially unilateral or bilateral facial palsy) and peripheral neuropathy. Radiculopathy, often painful, may present a year or more after initial infection. Carditis, sometimes accompanied by atrioventricular conduction defects, is not uncommon in the USA but appears to be rare in Europe.

13

13

Late disease

Late manifestations include arthritis, polyneuritis and encephalopathy. Prolonged arthritis particularly affecting large joints is a well-described feature but is rare in the UK. Brain parenchymal involvement causing neuropsychiatric abnormalities may also be encountered, but is again very rare in the UK. Acrodermatitis chronica atrophicans is an uncommon late complication seen more frequently in Europe than North America. Doughy, patchy discoloration occurs on the peripheries, eventually leading to shiny atrophic skin. The lesions are easily mistaken for those of peripheral vascular disease.

Diagnosis

The diagnosis of Lyme borreliosis is primarily clinical. Culture from biopsy material is not generally available, has a low yield, and may take longer than 6 weeks. Antibody detection is therefore the best means of confirming the diagnosis. This lacks specificity and is frequently negative early in the course of the disease, although sensitivity increases to 90–100% in disseminated or late disease. Immunofluorescence or ELISA can give false positive reactions in a number of conditions including other spirochaetal infections, infectious mononucleosis, rheumatoid arthritis and SLE. Immunoblot (Western blot) techniques are more specific but technically demanding. Antibody responses may not become detectable until several weeks after the onset of infection, and may be suppressed by antibiotic therapy. True positive results may reflect past rather than active infection. DNA detection by PCR has been applied to blood, urine, and biopsies of skin and synovium. PCR positivity in CSF is useful in confirming the diagnosis of neuroborreliosis but has low sensitivity.

Management

It is questionable whether asymptomatic patients with positive antibody tests should be treated. However, erythema migrans always requires therapy because of the risk of progressive disease; in untreated patients organisms can be recovered from skin biopsies long after the skin eruption has resolved. Standard therapy consists of a 14-day course of doxycycline (200 mg daily) or amoxicillin (500 mg 8-hourly). Some 15% of patients with early disease will develop a mild Jarisch–Herxheimer reaction during the first 24 hours of therapy. In pregnant women, small children or those allergic to amoxicillin, 14-day treatment with cefuroxime axetil (500 mg 12-hourly) or erythromycin (250 mg 6-hourly) is equally effective.

Disseminated disease and arthritis require prolonged therapy; a minimum of 30 days' treatment with either doxycycline or amoxicillin plus probenecid is required. Arthritis may respond poorly, and prolonged or repeated courses may be necessary. Neuroborreliosis is treated with parenteral β-lactam antibiotics for 3–4 weeks. Ceftriaxone (2 g daily), cefotaxime (2 g 8-hourly) or benzylpenicillin (3 g 6-hourly) have all been used successfully. The cephalosporins may be superior to penicillin in this situation.

Prevention

Protective clothing and insect repellents should be used in tick-infested areas. Since the risk of borrelial transmission is lower in the first few hours of a blood feed, prompt removal of ticks is advisable. Unfortunately, larval and nymphal ticks are tiny and may not be noticed. The value of prophylactic antibiotics is difficult to evaluate. Where risk of transmission is high, a single 200 mg dose of doxycycline, given within 72 hours of exposure, has been shown to prevent erythema migrans. A recombinant vaccine OspA in adjuvant (three injections of 30 μg at 0, 1, and 2 or 12 months) offers up to 76% protection, and is now commercially available.

RELAPSING FEVER

This term applies to two distinct types of relapsing fever due to systemic infection by borrelial spirochaetes: louse-borne relapsing fever and tick-borne relapsing fever, both characterised by recurrent febrile illnesses following an initial amelioration of symptoms.

Louse-borne relapsing fever

The human body louse, *Pediculus humanus*, causes itching. Borreliae *(B. recurrentis)* are liberated from the infected lice when they are crushed during scratching, which also inoculates the borreliae into the skin.

Pathology

The borreliae multiply in the blood, where they are abundant in the febrile phases, and invade most tissues, especially the liver, spleen and meninges. Hepatitis causing jaundice is frequent in severe infections and there may be petechial haemorrhages in the skin, mucous membranes and serous surfaces of internal organs. Thrombocytopenia is marked.

Clinical features

Onset is sudden with fever. The temperature rises to 39.5–40.5°C accompanied by a tachycardia, headache, generalised aching, injected conjunctivae (Fig. 13.28) and, frequently, a petechial rash, epistaxis and herpes labialis. As the disease progresses, the liver and spleen frequently become tender and palpable, and jaundice is common. There may be severe serosal and intestinal haemorrhage. Mental confusion and meningism may occur. The fever ends in crisis between the fourth and tenth days, often associated with profuse sweating, hypotension, and circulatory and cardiac failure. There may be no further fever but in a

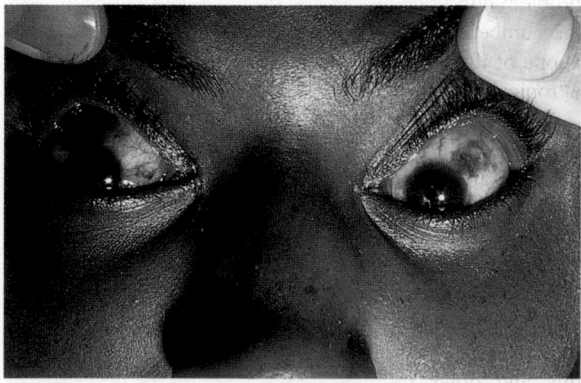

Fig. 13.28 Louse-borne relapsing fever. Injected conjunctivae.

proportion of patients, after an afebrile period of about 7 days, there may be one or more relapses which are usually milder and less prolonged. In the absence of specific treatment the mortality rate may be as high as 40%, especially among the elderly and malnourished.

Investigations
The organisms are demonstrated in the blood during fever either by dark ground illumination of a wet film or by staining thick and thin films.

Management
The problems of treatment are to eradicate the organism, to minimise the severe Jarisch–Herxheimer reaction (JHR— p. 413) which inevitably follows successful chemotherapy, and to prevent relapses. The safest treatment is procaine penicillin 300 mg i.m., followed the next day by 0.5 g tetracycline. Tetracycline alone is effective and prevents relapse, but may give rise to a worse reaction. Doxycycline 200 mg once by mouth, as an alternative to tetracycline, has the advantage of also being curative for typhus, which often accompanies epidemics of relapsing fever. JHR is best managed in a high-dependency unit with expert nursing and medical care.

Prevention
The patient, clothing and all contacts must be freed from lice as in epidemic typhus.

Tick-borne relapsing fever
Soft ticks (*Ornithodoros* spp.) transmit *B. duttoni* (and several other borrelia species) through saliva while feeding on their host. Those sleeping in mud houses are at risk, as the tick hides in crevices during the day and feeds on human beings during the night. Rodents are the reservoir in all parts of the world, except in East Africa where humans are the reservoir. Clinical manifestations are similar to the louse-borne disease but spirochaetes are detected in fewer patients on dark field microscopy. A 7-day course of treatment with either tetracycline (500 mg 6-hourly) or erythromycin (500 mg 6-hourly) is needed.

LEPTOSPIROSIS

Microbiology and epidemiology
Leptospirosis has emerged as an important public health problem during the last few years due to sudden upsurge in the number of reported cases and outbreaks world-wide. It is one of the most common zoonotic diseases, favoured by a tropical climate and flooding during the monsoon.

Leptospires are tightly coiled, thread-like organisms about 5–7 microns in length which are actively motile by rotating and bending; each end is bent into a hook. *Leptospira interrogans* is pathogenic for humans. The genus can be separated into more than 200 serovars belonging to 23 serogroups.

Leptospirosis appears to be ubiquitous in wildlife and in many domestic animals. The most frequent hosts are rodents, especially the common rat (*Rattus norvegicus*). In this and other reservoir species the organisms persist indefinitely in the convoluted tubules of the kidney without causing apparent disease, and are shed into the urine in massive numbers. Particular leptospiral serogroups are associated with characteristic animal hosts; *L. ictero-haemorrhagiae* is the classical parasite of rats, *L. canicola* of dogs, *L. hebdomadis* of cattle, and *L. pomona* of pigs. There is nevertheless considerable overlap in host–serogroup associations.

Leptospires can enter their human hosts through intact skin or mucous membranes, but entry is facilitated by cuts and abrasions. Prolonged immersion in contaminated water will also favour invasion as the spirochaete can survive in water for months. After a relatively brief bacteraemia, invading leptospires are distributed throughout the body; in humans the main organs affected are the kidneys, liver, meninges and brain. The mechanism of tissue damage is uncertain since it is often associated with the lysis of the organisms rather than their multiplication. Leptospirosis is common in the tropics and also in freshwater sports enthusiasts.

Clinical features
The incubation period averages 1–2 weeks. Four main clinical syndromes can be discerned.

Bacteraemic leptospirosis
This can occur with any serogroup. It produces a non-specific illness in which there is high fever accompanied by weakness, muscle pain and tenderness (especially of the calf and back), intense headache and photophobia, and sometimes diarrhoea and vomiting. Conjunctival congestion is the only notable physical sign. The illness comes to an end after about 1 week, or else merges into one of the other forms of infection.

Aseptic meningitis
Classically associated with *L. canicola* infection, this illness is very difficult to distinguish from viral meningitis. The conjunctivae may be congested but there are no other differentiating signs. Laboratory clues to the correct diagnosis include a neutrophil leucocytosis, abnormal LFTs, and the occasional presence of albumin and casts in the urine.

Icteric leptospirosis (Weil's disease)
Less than 10% of symptomatic infections result in severe icteric illness. Weil's disease is a dramatic life-threatening event, characterised by fever, haemorrhages, jaundice and renal impairment. Conjunctival hyperaemia is a frequent feature. The patient may have a transient macular erythematous rash, but the characteristic skin changes are those of purpura, with large areas of bruising. In severe cases there may be epistaxis, haematemesis and melaena, or bleeding into the pleural, pericardial or subarachnoid spaces. Thrombocytopenia, probably related to activation of endothelial cells with platelet adhesion and aggregation, is present in 50% of cases. Jaundice is deep and the liver is enlarged, but there is usually little evidence of hepatic failure or encephalopathy. Renal failure, primarily caused by impaired renal perfusion and acute tubular necrosis, becomes manifest as oliguria or anuria, with the presence of albumin, blood and casts in the urine.

13

Weil's disease may also be associated with myocarditis, encephalitis and aseptic meningitis. Uveitis and iritis may appear months after apparent clinical recovery.

Pulmonary syndrome

A pulmonary syndrome has long been recognised in the Far East, and has recently been described during an outbreak of leptospirosis in Nicaragua. This syndrome is characterised by haemoptysis, patchy lung infiltrates on chest X-ray, and respiratory failure. Total bilateral lung consolidation and ARDS (p. 187) develop in fatal cases. Severe disease with a pulmonary syndrome or with multi-organ dysfunction can be associated with very high mortality (> 50%).

Diagnosis

Results of routine laboratory tests are non-specific but may nevertheless be helpful. The characteristic change in the peripheral blood is a polymorphonuclear leucocytosis. Severe infections are often accompanied by thrombocytopenia and elevated blood levels of creatine phosphokinase. In jaundiced patients LFTs are mildly hepatitic in pattern with moderately raised transaminases; the prothrombin time may be a little prolonged. The CSF in leptospiral meningitis shows a variable cellular response, a moderately elevated protein level and a normal glucose content.

In the tropics dengue, malaria, typhoid fever, scrub typhus and hantavirus infection are important differential diagnoses.

Definitive diagnosis of leptospirosis depends upon isolation of the organism, serological tests or the detection of specific DNA.

- Blood cultures are most likely to be positive if taken before the tenth day of illness. Special media are required and cultures may have to be incubated for several weeks.
- Leptospires appear in the urine during the second week of illness and in untreated patients may be recovered on culture for several months.
- At present the serological investigation of choice is the microscopic agglutination test (MAT); seroconversion or a fourfold rise in titre between acute and convalescent sera is confirmatory. However, serology becomes positive only by the end of the first week. Less cumbersome assays including IgM ELISA and immunofluorescent techniques, while several rapid immunochromatographic tests have become commercially available. Their sensitivity remains low (~50%) in the first week but rise (~86%) during weeks 2–4. Their specificity, however, remains high and the results are comparable with ELISA.
- PCR shows great promise as a rapid and specific means of diagnosis. The technique can detect leptospiral DNA in blood in early symptomatic disease, and is positive in urine from the eighth day and for many months afterwards. Highly sensitive real-time PCR, capable of differentiating between pathogenic and non-pathogenic species with a detection limit of 2 leptospires (in serum) to 10 leptospires (in urine) has been developed.

Management and prevention

Antibiotic regimens for the treatment of leptospirosis are a form of care for which the evidence is insufficient to provide clear guidelines for practice. Therapy with either doxycycline or intravenous penicillin has been reported to be effective but may not prevent the development of renal failure. Doxycycline is given in oral doses of 100 mg 12-hourly for 1 week. Intravenous benzylpenicillin is administered as 1.5 mega-units 6-hourly for 1 week. Parenteral ceftriaxone 1 g daily is equally effective as penicillin. A Jarisch–Herxheimer reaction (p. 413) may occur during treatment but is usually mild. Uveitis is treated with a combination of systemic antibiotics and local corticosteroids.

The general care of the patient is critically important. Blood should be taken early for grouping and cross-matching, and haemorrhage treated by prompt blood transfusion. Renal failure demands very careful management since it is the usual cause of death. The renal damage is, however, essentially reversible, and peritoneal dialysis or haemodialysis may be life-saving.

Trials in military personnel have shown that infection with *L. interrogans* can be prevented by taking prophylactic doxycycline 200 mg weekly.

PLAGUE

Epidemics of plague, such as the 'Black Death', have attacked humans since ancient times. The disease continues to have a rat reservoir. Plague foci are widely distributed throughout the world and human cases are reported from about ten countries per year. An outbreak of plague in India in 1994 centred on Surat (Fig. 13.29). The causative organism, *Yersinia pestis*, is a small Gram-negative bacillus that is spread between rodents by their fleas. If domestic rats become infected, infected fleas may bite humans. In the late stages of human plague, *Y. pestis* may be expectorated and spread between humans by droplets. 'Pneumonic plague' may follow. Hunters and trappers can contract plague from handling rodents. *Y. pestis* can be used in biological warfare because of its capacity for mass production and aerosol transmission, and the high fatality rate associated with pneumonic plague.

Pathology

Organisms inoculated through the skin are taken rapidly to the draining lymph nodes where they elicit a severe inflammatory response that may be haemorrhagic. If the infection is not contained, septicaemia ensues and necrotic, purulent or haemorrhagic lesions develop in many organs. Oliguria and shock follow, and disseminated intravascular coagulation may result in widespread haemorrhage. Inhalation of *Y. pestis* causes alveolitis. The incubation period is 3–6 days, shorter in pneumonic plague.

Bubonic plague

In this, the most common form of the disease, the onset is usually sudden with a rigor, high fever, dry skin and severe headache. Soon, aching and swelling at the site of the affected lymph nodes begin. The groin is the most common

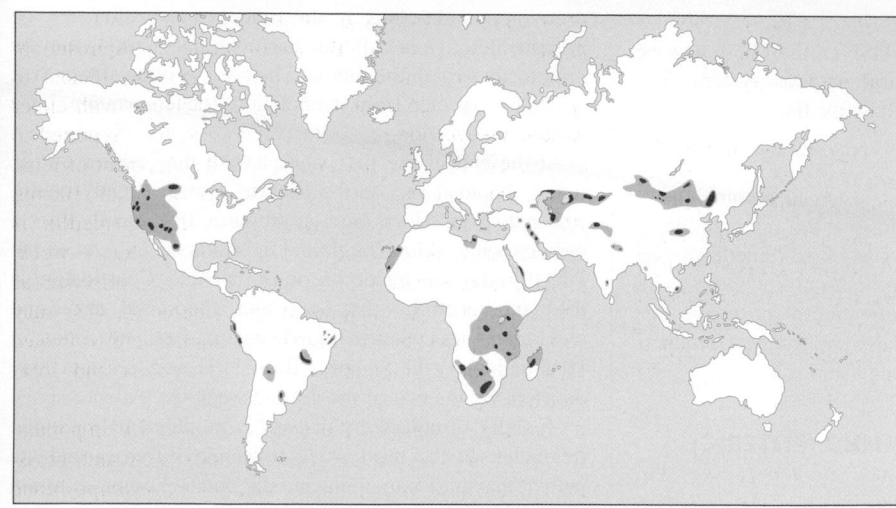

Frequent transmission

Infrequent or suspected transmission

Fig. 13.29 Foci of the transmission of plague.

13

site of the bubo, made up of the swollen lymph nodes and surrounding tissue. Some infections are relatively mild but in the majority of patients toxaemia quickly increases with a rapid pulse, hypotension and mental confusion. The spleen is usually palpable.

Septicaemic plague

Those not exhibiting a bubo usually deteriorate rapidly. The elderly are more prone to develop this form of illness. The patient is toxic and may have gastrointestinal symptoms such as nausea, vomiting, abdominal pain and diarrhoea. DIC may occur, manifested by bleeding from various orifices or puncture sites, along with ecchymoses. Hypotension, shock, renal failure and ARDS may lead to further deterioration. Meningitis, pneumonia and expectoration of blood-stained sputum containing *Y. pestis* may complicate septicaemic or occasionally bubonic plague. The septicaemic form carries a high mortality.

Pneumonic plague

The onset is very sudden with cough and dyspnoea. The patient soon expectorates copious blood-stained, frothy, highly infective sputum, becomes cyanosed and dies. X-rays of the lung show a lobar opacity.

Investigations

Early diagnosis is urgent and requires a high index of clinical suspicion. Delayed diagnosis is associated with a high case fatality rate. An aspirate from a bubo, sputum or the buffy coat (leucocyte fraction) of blood is used to show the characteristic bipolar staining organisms by staining with methylene blue or by immunofluorescence. Blood, sputum and aspirate should be cultured. DNA diagnosis through PCR and rapid diagnostic tests (RDTs) have been developed to improve on the sensitivity of the existing methods. Plague is notifiable under the international health regulations.

Management

If the diagnosis is suspected on clinical and epidemiological grounds, treatment must be started as soon as, or even before, samples have been collected for laboratory diag-

nosis. Streptomycin (1 g 12-hourly) or gentamicin (1 mg/ kg 8-hourly) is the drug of choice. Tetracycline (500 mg 6-hourly) and chloramphenicol (12.5 mg/kg 6-hourly) are alternatives. Fluoroquinolones (ciprofloxacin and levofloxacin) appear to be as effective as the drugs listed above. Treatment may also be needed for acute circulatory failure, DIC and hypoxia.

Prevention and infection control

Rats and fleas should be controlled. In endemic areas people should avoid handling and skinning wild animals. The patient should be isolated for the first 48 hours or until clinical improvement begins. Attendants must wear gowns, masks and gloves. Exposed symptomatic or asymptomatic people who have been in close contact with a patient with pneumonic plague should receive post-exposure antibiotic prophylaxis (doxycycline 100 mg or ciprofloxacin 500 mg 12-hourly) for 7 days.

A formalin-killed vaccine is available for those at occupational risk but offers little protection against pneumonic plague. A recombinant subunit vaccine (protein antigens F1 + V) is in development.

LISTERIOSIS

Listeria monocytogenes is an environmental bacterium which can contaminate food, including poultry and cheese. Outbreaks have been associated with soft cheeses, undercooked chicken, fish or meat and pâtés. Although food-borne outbreaks of gastroenteritis have been reported in immunocompetent individuals, *Listeria* causes invasive infection especially in pregnancy, the immunosuppressed due to drugs or AIDS, those with diabetes mellitus, those who misuse alcohol and those at extremes of age. In pregnant females, in addition to systemic symptoms like fever and myalgia, listeriosis causes chorioamnionitis, fetal deaths, abortions and neonatal infection. In other susceptible individuals, it causes systemic illness due to bacteraemia without focal symptoms. Meningitis similar to other bacterial meningitis but with normal CSF sugar is the next most common presentation.

Diagnosis

Diagnosis is made by blood and CSF culture; both may be positive in disease of the central nervous system. The organism grows readily in the culture media.

Management

The most effective regimen still consists of a combination of intravenous penicillin or aminopenicillin (amoxicillin or ampicillin) plus an aminoglycoside. A sulfamethoxazole/trimethoprim combination can be used in those with penicillin sensitivity. Cephalosporins are of no use in this infection. Proper treatment of dairy/poultry/meat products before eating is the key to reducing listeriosis.

TYPHOID AND PARATYPHOID (ENTERIC) FEVERS

In developing countries typhoid and paratyphoid fevers, which are transmitted by the faecal–oral route, are important causes of fever. Elsewhere they are relatively rare.

Aetiology

The enteric fevers are caused by infection with *Salmonella typhi* and *S. paratyphi* A and B (see also p. 328). High levels of transmission continue in India, sub-Saharan Africa and Latin America. The bacilli may live in the gallbladder of carriers for months or years after clinical recovery and pass intermittently in the stool and less commonly in the urine. The incubation period of typhoid fever is about 10–14 days; that of paratyphoid is somewhat shorter.

Pathology

After a few days of bacteraemia, the bacilli localise mainly in the lymphoid tissue of the small intestine. The typical lesion is in the Peyer's patches and follicles. These swell at first, then ulcerate and ultimately heal, but during this sequence they may perforate or bleed.

Clinical features

Typhoid fever

Clinical features are outlined in Box 13.40. The onset may be insidious. The temperature rises in a stepladder fashion for 4 or 5 days. There is malaise, with increasing headache, drowsiness and aching in the limbs. Constipation may be present, although in children diarrhoea and vomiting may be prominent early in the illness. The pulse is often slower than would be expected from the height of the temperature, i.e. a relative bradycardia.

At the end of the first week a rash may appear on the upper abdomen and on the back as sparse, slightly raised, rose-red spots, which fade on pressure. It is usually visible only on white skin. Cough and epistaxis occur. Around the 7th–10th day the spleen becomes palpable. Constipation is then succeeded by diarrhoea and abdominal distension with tenderness. Severe diarrhoea has been described in HIV patients with typhoid. Bronchitis and delirium may develop. By the end of the second week the patient may be profoundly ill unless the disease is modified by antibiotic treatment. In the third week toxaemia increases and the patient may pass into coma and die. Such extreme cases are rare in countries with developed health services.

Following recovery, up to 5% of patients become chronic carriers of *S. typhi* and classically such patients have gallbladder disease.

Paratyphoid fever

The course tends to be shorter and milder than that of typhoid fever and the onset is often more abrupt with acute enteritis. The rash may be more abundant and the intestinal complications less frequent.

Complications

These are given in Box 13.41. Haemorrhage from, or a perforation of, the ulcerated Peyer's patches may occur at the end of the second week or during the third week of the illness. A drop in temperature to normal or subnormal levels may occur in those with intestinal haemorrhage. This can be falsely reassuring as it occurs even before there is clinical evidence of bleeding such as melaena. Additional complications may involve almost any viscus or system because of the septicaemia present during the first week; these include cholecystitis, pneumonia, myocarditis, arthritis, osteomyelitis and meningitis. Bone and joint infection is seen, especially in children with sickle-cell disease.

Investigations

In the first week the diagnosis may be difficult because in this invasive stage with bacteraemia the symptoms are those of a generalised infection without localising features. A white blood count may be helpful as there is typically a

13.40 CLINICAL FEATURES OF TYPHOID FEVER	
First week	
• Fever	• Relative bradycardia
• Headache	• Constipation
• Myalgia	• Diarrhoea and vomiting in children
End of first week	
• Rose spots on trunk	• Abdominal distension
• Splenomegaly	• Diarrhoea
• Cough	
End of second week	
• Delirium, complications, then coma and death (if untreated)	

13.41 COMPLICATIONS OF TYPHOID FEVER	
Bowel	
• Perforation	• Haemorrhage
Septicaemic foci	
• Bone and joint infection	• Cholecystitis
• Meningitis	
Toxic phenomena	
• Myocarditis	• Nephritis

leucopenia. Blood culture is the most important diagnostic method in a suspected case. The faeces will contain the organism more frequently during the second and third weeks. The Widal reaction detects antibodies to the causative organisms. However, it is not a reliable diagnostic test and should be interpreted with caution, particularly in typhoid-vaccinated patients.

Management

Several antibiotics are effective in enteric fever. Chloramphenicol (500 mg 6-hourly), ampicillin (750 mg 6-hourly) and co-trimoxazole (2 tablets or i.v. equivalent 12-hourly) are important therapies but are losing their effect due to resistance in many areas of the world, especially India and South-east Asia. The fluoroquinolones remain the drugs of choice (e.g. ciprofloxacin 500 mg 12-hourly). Extended-spectrum cephalosporins, ceftriaxone and cefotaxime, are useful alternatives but have a slightly increased treatment failure rate. Azithromycin (500 mg once daily) has been shown to be an alternative where fluoroquinoline resistance is present but has not been validated in severe disease. Treatment should be continued for 14 days. Pyrexia may persist for up to 5 days after the start of specific therapy. Even with effective chemotherapy there is still a danger of complications, recrudescence of the disease and the development of a carrier state. The chronic carrier should be treated for 4 weeks with ciprofloxacin; cholecystectomy may be necessary in some cases.

Prevention

Improved sanitation and living conditions reduce the incidence of typhoid. Travellers to countries where enteric infections are endemic should be inoculated with one of the three available typhoid vaccines (two inactivated injectable and one oral live attenuated).

TULARAEMIA

Tularaemia is primarily a zoonotic disease of the northern hemisphere. It is caused by a highly infectious Gram-negative bacillus, *Francisella tularensis*. *F. tularensis* can survive for months in nature, and thus is a potential weapon for bioterrorism. Wild rabbits, domestic dogs or cats are the reservoirs and ticks are the vectors. Infection is introduced either through the bite of ticks, or from animals through skin, abrasions resulting in the most common 'ulceroglandular' variety of the disease (70–80%), characterised by skin, ulceration with regional lymphadenopathy. There is a purely 'glandular' form of the disease. Inhalation of the infected aerosols may result in pulmonary tularaemia, presenting as pneumonia. Rarely, the portal of entry of infection may be the conjuctiva, leading to a nodular, ulcerated conjunctivitis with regional lymphadenopathy (an 'oculoglandular' form).

Diagnosis

Demonstration of a single high titre ($\geq$ 1:160) or a fourfold rise in 2–3 weeks in the tularaemia tube agglutination test confirms the diagnosis. Bacterial yield from the lesions is extremely poor. PCR and real-time PCR (p. 142) have been developed for reliable and rapid diagnosis.

Management

Treatment consists of a 7–10-day course of parenteral aminoglycosides, streptomycin (7.5–10 mg/kg 12-hourly) or gentamicin (5 mg/kg in three divided doses). *F. tularensis* is not susceptible to most other antibiotics.

MELIOIDOSIS

Melioidosis is caused by *Burkholderia (Pseudomonas) pseudomallei*, a saprophyte found in soil and water (paddy fields). Infection is by inoculation and inhalation. Patients with diabetes or severe burns are susceptible. The disease is most common in South India, East Asia and northern Australia.

Pathology

A bacteraemia is followed by the formation of abscesses in the lungs, liver and spleen.

Clinical features

There is high fever, prostration and sometimes diarrhoea, with signs of pneumonia and enlargement of the liver and spleen. The chest X-ray resembles that of acute caseous tuberculosis. In more chronic forms multiple abscesses recur in subcutaneous tissue and bone.

Investigations

Culture of blood, sputum or pus may yield *B. pseudomallei*. Except in fulminating infections, antibodies may be detected by indirect haemagglutination, direct agglutination and complement-fixation tests.

Management

In the acute illness prompt treatment, without waiting for confirmation by culture, may be life-saving. Ceftazidime 100 mg/kg (2 g 8-hourly), imipenem 50 mg/kg (1 g 6-hourly) or meropenem (0.5–1 g 8-hourly) is given for about 2–3 weeks. This is followed by maintenance therapy of doxycycline 200 mg daily, plus co-trimoxazole (sulfamethoxazole 1600 mg plus trimethoprim 320 mg 12-hourly) for a minimum of 12 weeks, and chloramphenicol (500 mg 6-hourly) for the first 4 weeks. In patients with severe melioidosis in septic shock, granulocyte–colony stimulating factor (G–CSF) significantly reduces mortality. Abscesses should be drained surgically. In chronic cases profound wasting is a major clinical problem. In the absence of intensive care, the disease carries a significant mortality.

GASTROINTESTINAL BACTERIAL INFECTIONS

FOOD POISONING (see also p. 294)

Bacterial causes of acute gastroenteritis
See Box 13.13, page 293.

STAPHYLOCOCCAL FOOD POISONING

Staph. aureus is a common commensal of the anterior nares. With poor hygiene, transmission takes place via the hands of

13

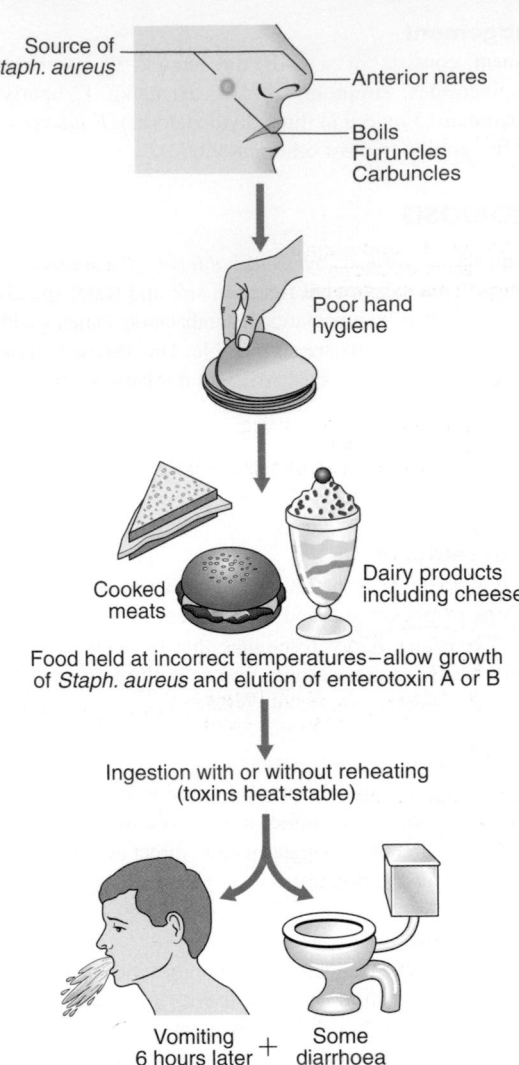

Fig. 13.30   Staphylococcal food poisoning.

13

13.42 INFECTIOUS DIARRHOEA IN OLD AGE

- **Incidence:** is not increased, but the impact of these illnesses is greater.
- **Mortality:** the majority of deaths due to gastroenteritis in the developed world are in adults aged over 70 years. Most are presumed to be caused by dehydration leading to organ infarction and failure.
- **Increased risk:** due to age-associated achlorhydria, diminished intestinal motility and frequent antibiotic use.
- *Cl. difficile* **diarrhoea:** age is associated with its development in the community, hospital and nursing home settings, partly due to antibiotic exposure.

BACILLUS CEREUS

Rapid onset of vomiting within hours of food consumption is caused by the ingestion of the pre-formed toxins of *B. cereus*. Fried rice or freshly made vanilla sauces are frequent sources. The organism grows and produces enterotoxin during storage; 1–4 hours after ingestion, brisk vomiting and some diarrhoea occur, with rapid resolution within 24 hours.

A form with longer incubation occurs if viable bacteria are ingested and toxin formation takes place within the gut lumen. The incubation period is 12–24 hours and watery diarrhoea and cramps are the predominant symptoms. The disease is self-limiting but can be quite severe (Fig. 13.31).

Management

Rapid and judicious fluid replacement and appropriate notification of the public health authorities are all that is required.

CLOSTRIDIUM PERFRINGENS

Spores of *Cl. perfringens* are widespread in the guts of large animals and in soil. If contaminated meat products are incompletely cooked and stored in anaerobic conditions, *Cl. perfringens* spores germinate and viable organisms multiply to give large numbers. Subsequent reheating of the food causes heat-shock sporulation of the organisms during which they elute an enterotoxin. Symptoms (diarrhoea and cramps) occur some 6–12 hours following ingestion (Fig. 13.32).

'Point source' outbreaks, in which a number of cases all become symptomatic following ingestion, classically occur after school or canteen lunches where meat stews are served. Clostridial enterotoxins are potent and most people who ingest them will be symptomatic. The illness is usually self-limiting.

CAMPYLOBACTER JEJUNI

This infection is essentially a zoonosis, the organisms originating in the gut of cattle and poultry. The most common source of the infection is meat, such as chicken, or contaminated milk products. There has been an association with pet puppies. *Campylobacter* infection is now the most common cause of bacterial gastroenteritis in the UK, accounting for some 100 000 cases per annum, most of which are sporadic.

food handlers to foodstuffs such as dairy products, including cheese, and cooked meats. Inappropriate storage of these foods allows growth of the organism and production of one or more heat-stable enterotoxins (Fig. 13.30).

Clinical features

Following ingestion, symptoms of nausea and profuse vomiting develop within 1–6 hours. Diarrhoea may not be marked. These toxins act as super-antigens, stimulating a non-specific T-cell activation and a significant neutrophil leucocytosis. This may be clinically misleading. Most cases settle rapidly but severe dehydration and rare fatalities have occurred due to acute fluid loss and shock.

Management

Antiemetics and appropriate fluid replacement are the mainstays of treatment. Suspect food should be cultured for staphylococci and demonstration of toxin production. The public health authorities should be notified if food vending is involved.

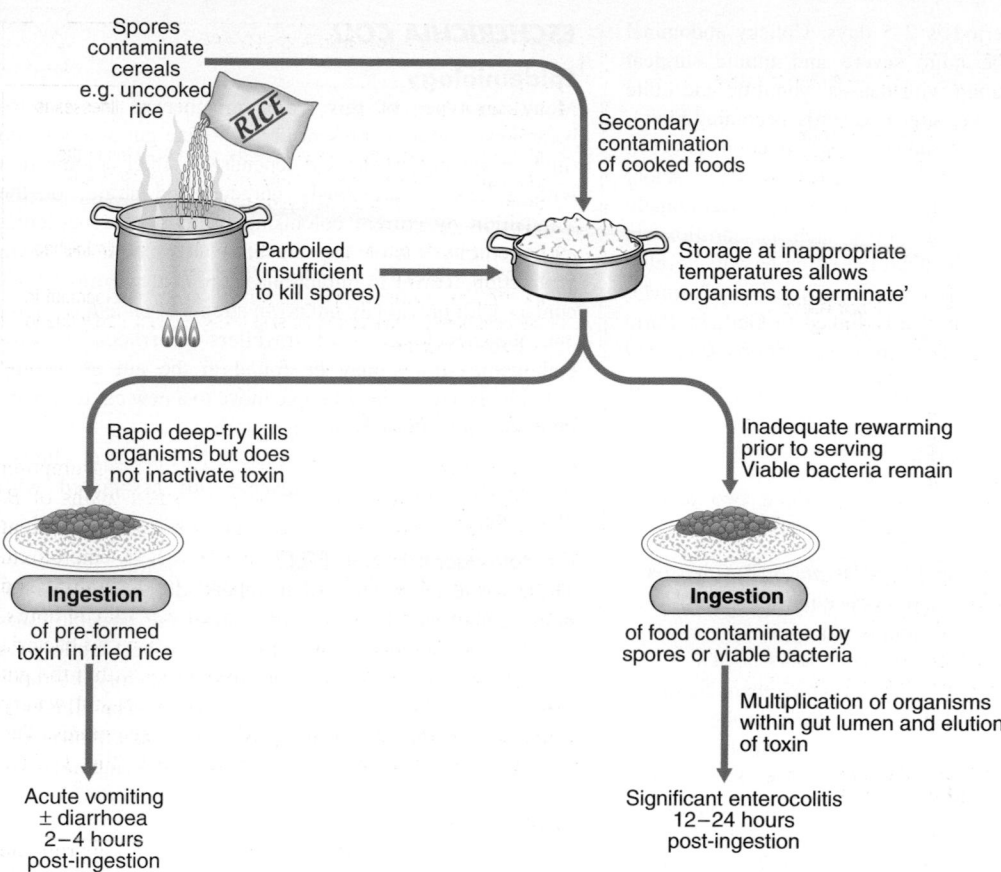

Fig. 13.31 *Bacillus cereus* food poisoning.

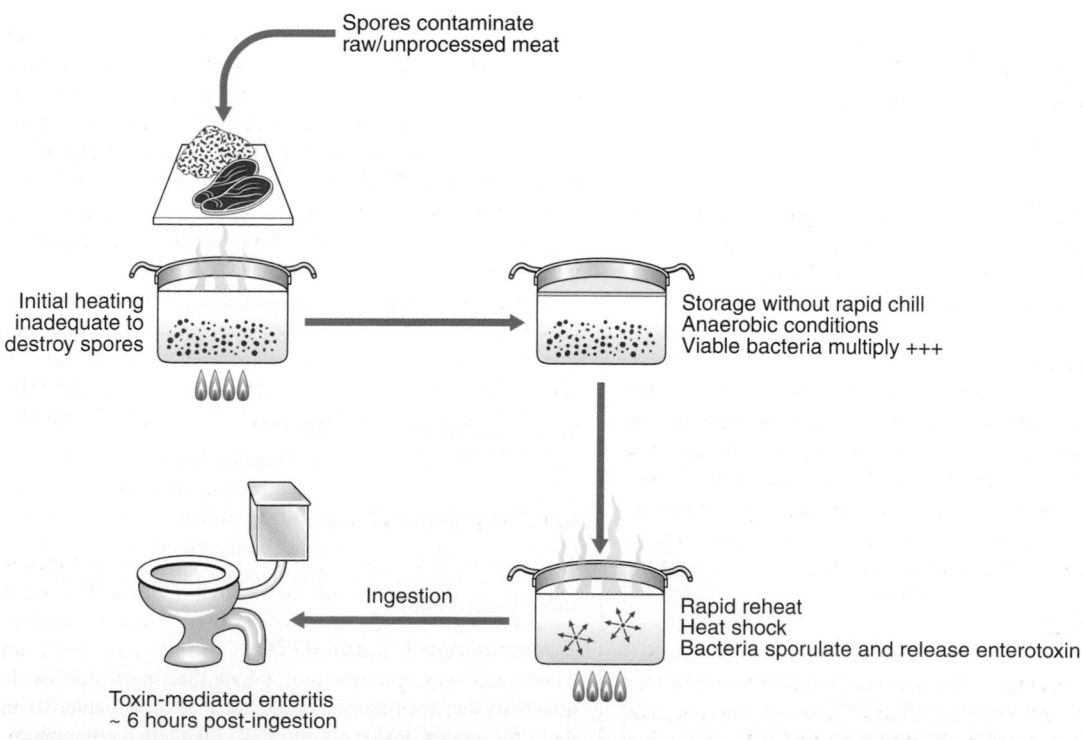

Fig. 13.32 *Clostridium perfringens* food poisoning.

13

The incubation period is 2–5 days. Colicky abdominal pain, which may be quite severe and mimic surgical pathology, ensues, along with nausea, vomiting and quite significant diarrhoea, the latter frequently becoming blood-stained. The majority of *Campylobacter* infections affect fit young adults and are self-limiting after 5–7 days. About 10–20% will have prolonged symptomatology, occasionally meriting treatment with antibiotics such as ciprofloxacin or a macrolide. Approximately 1% of cases will develop bacteraemia and possible distant foci of infection. *Campylobacter* species have been clearly linked to Guillain–Barré syndrome and post-infectious reactive arthritis (pp. 1249 and 1108).

SALMONELLA SPECIES

These Gram-negative organisms produce two distinct clinical entities:

- The serotypes *S. typhi* and *S. paratyphi* A, B, C have a purely human reservoir and produce the septicaemic illness 'enteric fever' (typhoid or paratyphoid fever—p. 324).
- All other *Salmonella* serotypes, of which there are more than 2000, are subdivided into five distinct subgroups which produce gastroenteritis. They are widely distributed throughout the animal kingdom. Some strains have a clear relationship to particular animal species, e.g. *S. arizonae* and pet reptiles. Transmission is by contaminated water or food, particularly poultry, egg products and related fast foods, direct person-to-person spread or the handling of exotic pets such as salamanders, lizards or turtles. The incidence of *Salmonella* enteritis is falling in the UK due to an aggressive culling policy in broiler chicken stocks coupled with vaccination. Two serotypes remain important in the UK: *S. enteritidis* phage type 4 and *S. typhimurium* dt.104. The latter may be significantly resistant to commonly used antibiotics such as ciprofloxacin.

The incubation period of *Salmonella* gastroenteritis is 12–72 hours and the predominant feature is diarrhoea. Vomiting may be present at the outset and blood is quite frequently noted in the stool. Approximately 5% of cases will be bacteraemic. Reactive (post-infective) arthritis occurs in approximately 2% of cases. Evidence of bacteraemia is a clear indication for antibiotic therapy, as salmonellae are notorious for persistent infection and often colonise endothelial surfaces such as an atherosclerotic aorta or a major blood vessel. Antibiotics are not indicated for uncomplicated *Salmonella* gastroenteritis (Box 13.43).

13.43 ANTIBIOTICS IN *SALMONELLA* GASTROENTERITIS   **EBM**

'In otherwise healthy adults or children with non-severe *Salmonella* diarrhoea, antibiotics have no clinical benefit over placebo, increase side-effects and prolong *Salmonella* detection.'

- Sirinavin S, Garner P (Cochrane Review). Cochrane Library, issue 1, 2001. Oxford: Update Software.

ESCHERICHIA COLI

Epidemiology

Many serotypes of this major member of the Enterobacteriaceae may be present in the human gut at any given time. Production of disease depends on either colonisation with a new or previously unrecognised strain, or the acquisition by current colonising bacteria of a particular pathogenicity factor for mucosal attachment or toxin production. Travel to unfamiliar areas of the world allows contact with previously unknown strains of endemic *E. coli* and the development of travellers' diarrhoea. Enteropathogenic strains may be found in the gut of healthy individuals and, if these people move to a new environment, close contacts may develop symptoms.

The genus *Escherichia* can cause five different clinico-pathological patterns of disease, all associated with diarrhoea.

Enterotoxigenic E. coli (ETEC)

These cause most cases of travellers' diarrhoea in developing countries, although other causes are possible (Box 13.44). The organisms produce either a heat-labile or a heat-stable enterotoxin, causing marked secretory diarrhoea and vomiting after 1–2 days' incubation. The illness is usually mild and self-limiting after 3–4 days. Antibiotics have been used to limit the duration of symptoms and prophylaxis may help to prevent this disease (Box 13.45).

13.44 MOST COMMON CAUSES OF TRAVELLERS' DIARRHOEA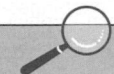

- Enterotoxigenic *E. coli* (ETEC)
- *Shigella* spp.
- *Campylobacter jejuni*
- *Salmonella* spp.
- *Pleisomonas shigelloides*
- Non-cholera *Vibrio* spp.
- *Aeromonas* spp.

13.45 ANTIBIOTICS IN TRAVELLERS' DIARRHOEA   **EBM**

'Antibiotics reduce the duration of acute non-bloody diarrhoea in patients over 5 years old, but with a risk of side-effects.'

For further information: 💻 www.cochrane.org

Entero-invasive E. coli (EIEC)

This illness is very similar to *Shigella* dysentery (p. 330) and is caused by invasion and destruction of colonic mucosal cells. No enterotoxin is produced. Acute watery diarrhoea, abdominal cramps and some scanty blood-staining of the stool are common. The symptoms are rarely severe and are usually self-limiting.

Enteropathogenic E. coli (EPEC)

These are very important in infant diarrhoea. Ability to attach to the gut mucosa, inducing a specific 'attachment and effacement' lesion, is the basis of their pathogenicity. This causes destruction of microvilli and disruption of normal absorptive capacity. The symptoms vary from mild non-bloody diarrhoea to quite severe illness. Bacteraemia/septicaemia is virtually unheard of.

Entero-aggregative E. coli (EAEC)

These strains have the genetic codes for adherence to the mucosa but also produce a locally active enterotoxin and demonstrate a particular 'stacked brick' aggregation in the small bowel. They have been associated with prolonged diarrhoea in children in South America, South-east Asia and India.

Enterohaemorrhagic E. coli (EHEC)

A number of distinct 'O' serotypes of E. coli possess both the genetic codes for attachment and effacement (see 'EPEC' above) and plasmids encoding for two distinct enterotoxins (verocytotoxin) which are identical to toxins produced by Shigella ('shiga-toxins 1 and 2'). E. coli O157:H7 is perhaps the best known of these verocyto-toxigenic E. coli (VTEC), but others, including types O126 and O11, are also implicated. Although the incidence is considerably lower than Campylobacter and Salmonella, it is increasing in the developing world.

The reservoir of infection is in the gut of herbivores. Contaminated meat products, such as hamburgers, have long been recognised as a source of this infection. The organism has an extremely low infecting dose (10–100 organisms). Run off water from pasture lands where cattle have grazed which is used to irrigate vegetable crops, as well as contaminated milk, lettuce, radish shoots and apple juice, have all been implicated as sources (Fig. 13.33).

The incubation period is between 1 and 7 days. Initial watery diarrhoea becomes frankly and uniformly blood-stained in 70% of cases and is associated with severe and often constant abdominal pain. There is little systemic upset, vomiting or fever. Enterotoxins, if produced, have both a local effect on the bowel and a distant effect on particular body tissues such as glomerular apparatus, heart and brain. The potentially life-threatening haemolytic uraemic syndrome (HUS—p. 498) occurs in 10–15% of sufferers from this infection, arising 5–7 days after the onset of symptoms. It is most likely at the extremes of age, is heralded by a high peripheral leucocyte count and may be induced, particularly in children, by antibiotic therapy.

Management

HUS is treated by dialysis if necessary and may be averted by active intervention with processes such as plasma exchange.

ANTIBIOTIC-ASSOCIATED DIARRHOEA (CL. DIFFICILE INFECTION)

A history of any antibiotic therapy in the 6 weeks prior to the onset of diarrhoea can be related to the finding of Cl. difficile or its toxins in the stool. This is a potent cause of diarrhoea (Box 13.42) and can produce life-threatening pseudomembranous colitis. This diagnosis (p. 931) should be actively considered in the elderly and treated with metronidazole 400 mg 8-hourly for 10 days. If there is no response, then vancomycin may be used (125 mg orally 6-hourly for 1 week).

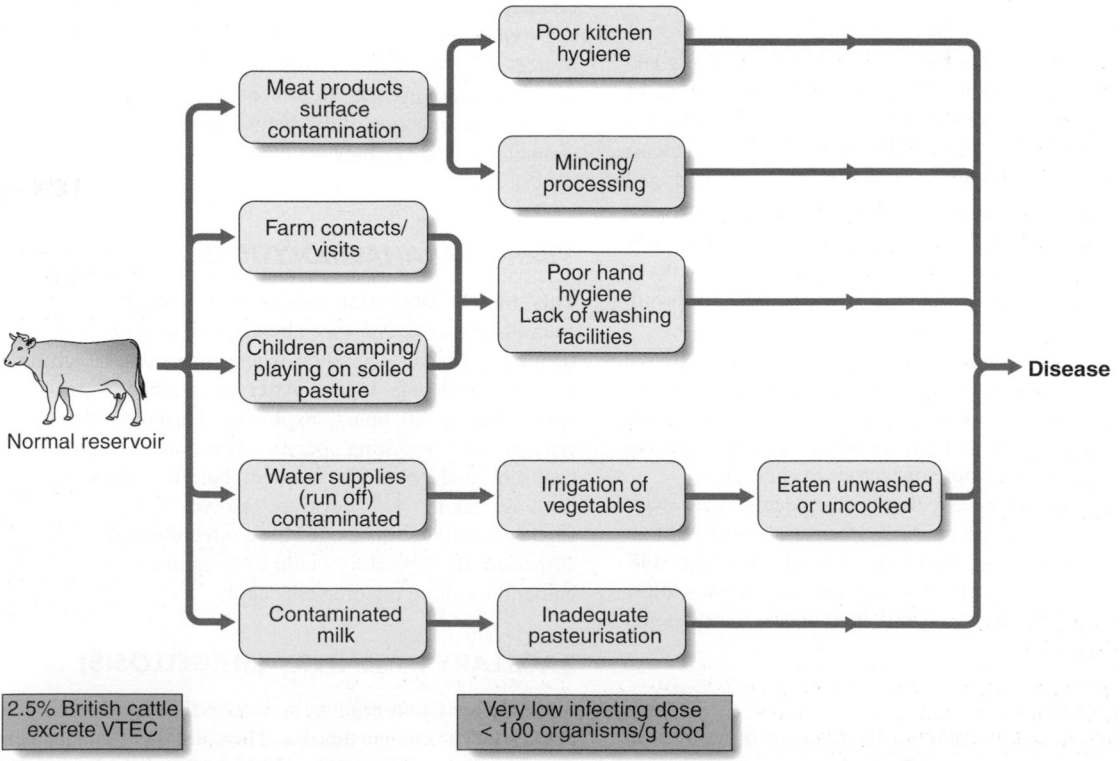

Fig. 13.33 Verocytotoxigenic E. coli infections.

YERSINIA ENTEROCOLITICA

This organism, commonly found in pork, causes mild to moderate gastroenteritis and can produce significant mesenteric adenitis after an incubation period of 3–7 days. It predominantly causes disease in children but adults may also be affected. The illness resolves slowly, with 10–30% of cases complicated by persistent arthritis or Reiter's syndrome (p. 1108).

VIBRIO CHOLERAE

Cholera, caused by *Vibrio cholerae* serotype 01, is the archetype bacterial cause of acute watery diarrhoea. Following its origin in the Ganges valley, devastating epidemics have occurred, often in association with large religious festivals, and pandemics have spread world-wide. The seventh pandemic, due to the El Tor biotype, began in 1961 and spread via the Middle East to become endemic in Africa. In 1990 it reached Peru and spread throughout South and Central America. Since August 2000 there has been a massive outbreak in South Africa. El Tor is more resistant than classical *Vibrio*, and causes prolonged carriage in 5% of infections. A new classical toxigenic strain, serotype 0139, established itself in Bangladesh in 1992 and started a new pandemic.

Infection spreads via the stools or vomit of symptomatic patients or of the much larger number of subclinical cases. It survives for up to 2 weeks in fresh water and 8 weeks in salt water. Transmission is normally through infected drinking water, shellfish and food contaminated by flies, or on the hands of carriers.

Clinical features

Severe diarrhoea without pain or colic begins suddenly and is succeeded by vomiting. Following the evacuation of normal gut faecal contents, typical 'rice-water' material is passed consisting of clear fluid with flecks of mucus. Classical cholera produces enormous loss of fluid and electrolytes, leading to intense dehydration with muscular cramps. Shock and oliguria develop but mental clarity remains. Death from acute circulatory failure may occur rapidly unless fluid and electrolytes are replaced. Improvement is rapid with proper treatment.

The majority of infections, however, cause mild illness with slight diarrhoea. Occasionally, a very intense illness, 'cholera sicca', occurs, with loss of fluid into dilated bowel, killing the patient before typical gastrointestinal symptoms appear. The disease is more dangerous in children.

Clinical diagnosis is easy during an epidemic. Otherwise the diagnosis should be confirmed bacteriologically. Stool dark field microscopy shows the typical 'shooting star' motility of *V. cholerae*. Rectal swab or stool cultures allow identification. Cholera is notifiable under international health regulations.

Management

Maintenance of circulation by replacement of water and electrolytes is paramount. Early intervention improves prognosis. A clinical assessment of dehydration is made from the appearance of the patient. Oral rehydration solution (ORS, p. 294) is effective and safe for all but the most severely dehydrated patients. The addition of resistant starch to ORS reduces faecal fluid loss and shortens the duration of diarrhoea in adolescents and adults with cholera. The effect is caused by enhanced sodium absorption in the colon due to short-chain fatty acids produced in the colon from non-absorbed carbohydrates. Ringer-Lactate is the best fluid for intravenous replacement. Vomiting usually stops once the patient is rehydrated, and fluid should then be given orally up to 500 ml hourly. The fluid required is calculated every 8 hours from the urine volume, stool and vomit output, and estimated insensible loss (as much as 5 litres/24 hours in a hot humid climate). Total fluid requirements may exceed 50 litres over a period of 2–5 days. Accurate records are greatly facilitated by the use of a 'cholera cot' which has a reinforced hole under the patient's buttocks beneath which a graded bucket is placed.

In children careful attention to fluid balance is required; they are prone to hypoglycaemia.

Three days' treatment with tetracycline 250 mg 6-hourly, a single dose of doxycycline 300 mg or ciprofloxacin 1 g in adults all reduce the duration of excretion of *Vibrio* and the total volume of fluid needed for replacement.

Prevention

Strict personal hygiene is vital and drinking water should come from a clean piped supply or be boiled. Flies must be denied access to food. Parenteral vaccination with a killed suspension of *V. cholerae* may provide limited protection. Oral vaccines containing killed *V. cholerae* and the B subunit of cholera toxin are available but are of limited efficacy.

In epidemics public education, and control of water sources and population movement are vital. Mass single-dose vaccination and treatment with tetracycline are valuable. Disinfection of discharges and soiled clothing, and scrupulous hand-washing by medical attendants reduce the danger of spread.

VIBRIO PARAHAEMOLYTICUS

This marine organism produces a disease similar to enterotoxigenic *E. coli* (see above). It is acquired from raw seafood and is very common where ingestion of such food is widespread (e.g. Japan). After an incubation period of approximately 20 hours, explosive diarrhoea, abdominal cramps and vomiting occur. Systemic symptoms of headache and fever are frequent but the illness is self-limiting, taking 4–7 days to resolve. Rarely, a severe septicaemic illness arises. If *Vibrio* infection of this nature is suspected, the laboratory ought to be notified since specific halophilic culture requirements apply.

BACILLARY DYSENTERY (SHIGELLOSIS)

Shigellae are Gram-negative rods, closely related to *E. coli*, that invade the colonic mucosa. There are four main groups: *Sh. dysenteriae*, *flexneri*, *boydii* and *sonnei*. In the tropics bacillary dysentery is usually caused by *Sh. flexneri*, whilst

13

in the UK most cases are caused by *Sh. sonnei*. Shigellae are often multi-resistant to antibiotics, especially in tropical countries. Such organisms have been responsible for epidemics of bacillary dysentery in Bangladesh and other tropical countries. The organism only infects humans and its spread is facilitated by its low infecting dose of around 10 organisms.

Epidemiology

Spread may occur via contaminated food or flies, but transmission by unwashed hands after defaecation is by far the most important factor. Outbreaks occur in mental hospitals, residential schools and other closed institutions, and dysentery is a constant accompaniment of wars and natural catastrophes which bring crowding and poor sanitation in their wake.

Clinical features

Disease severity varies from mild *Sh. sonnei* infections that may escape detection to more severe *Sh. flexneri* infections, while those due to *Sh. dysenteriae* may be fulminating and cause death within 48 hours.

In a moderately severe illness, the patient complains of diarrhoea, colicky abdominal pain and tenesmus. Stools are small, and after a few evacuations contain blood and purulent exudate with little faecal material. Fever, dehydration and weakness with tenderness over the colon occur. Arthritis or iritis may occasionally complicate bacillary dysentery (Reiter's syndrome, p. 1108), and may be associated with HLA–B27. *Shigella* infection may spread rapidly amongst promiscuous MSM.

Management

Oral rehydration therapy or, if diarrhoea is severe, intravenous replacement of water and electrolyte loss will be necessary. Antibiotic therapy with ciprofloxacin 500 mg 12-hourly for 3 days is effective in known shigellosis and appropriate in epidemics. The use of antidiarrhoeal medication should be avoided in all but the mildest cases.

Prevention

The prevention of faecal contamination of food and milk and the isolation of cases may be difficult except in limited outbreaks. Hand-washing is very important.

NON-INFECTIOUS CAUSES OF FOOD POISONING

Whilst acute food poisoning and gastroenteritis are frequently caused by bacteria or their toxins, a number of non-infectious causes must be considered in the differential diagnosis.

Plant toxins

Legumes and beans produce oxidants which are toxic to people with glucose-6-phosphate dehydrogenase (G6PD) deficiency (p. 1032). Consumption produces headache, nausea and fever progressing to potentially severe haemolysis, haemoglobinuria and jaundice (favism). Red kidney beans, if incompletely cooked, cause acute

abdominal pain and diarrhoea from their lectin content. Adequate cooking abolishes this.

Alkaloids develop in potato tubers exposed to light causing green discoloration. Ingestion induces acute vomiting and anticholinesterase-like activity.

Fungi and mushrooms of the *Psilocybe* spp. produce hallucinogens. Many fungal species induce a combination of gastroenteritis and cholinergic symptoms of blurred vision, salivation, sweating and diarrhoea. *Amanita phalloides* (death head mushroom) causes acute abdominal cramps and diarrhoea followed by inexorable hepatorenal failure, often fatal.

Chemical toxins

Paralytic shellfish toxin

Saxitoxin from dinoflagellates, responsible for 'red tides', is concentrated in bivalve molluscs, e.g. mussels, clams, oysters, cockles and scallops. Consumption produces gastrointestinal symptoms within 30 minutes, followed by respiratory paralysis. The UK water authorities ban the harvesting of molluscs at certain times of the year associated with excessive dinoflagellate numbers.

Ciguatera fish poisoning

Warm-water coral reef fish derive ciguatoxin from dinoflagellates in their food chain. Consumption produces gastrointestinal symptoms 1–6 hours later with associated paraesthesiae of the lips and extremities, distorted temperature sensation, myalgia and progressive flaccid paralysis. In the South Pacific and Caribbean there are 50 000 cases per year with a case fatality of 0.1%. Exotic fish imports are a major source in the UK. The gastrointestinal symptoms resolve rapidly but the neuropathic features may persist for months.

Scombrotoxic fish poisoning

Under poor storage conditions histidine in scombroid fish—tuna, mackerel, bonito, skipjack and the canned dark meat of sardines—may be converted by bacteria to histamine and other chemicals. Consumption produces symptoms within minutes with flushing, burning, sweating, urticaria, pruritus, headache, colic, nausea and vomiting, diarrhoea, bronchospasm and hypotension. Management is with salbutamol and antihistamines. Occasionally, intravenous fluid replacement is required.

Heavy metals

Thallium and cadmium can cause acute vomiting and diarrhoea resembling staphylococcal enterotoxin poisoning.

RESPIRATORY BACTERIAL INFECTIONS

Most of these infections are described in Chapter 19.

DIPHTHERIA

In many parts of the developing world diphtheria remains an important cause of illness. It was eradicated from much of the developed world by mass vaccination in the mid-20th century. Recent outbreaks have occurred in the former

13

Soviet Union and continue to occur in South-east Asia. The disease is notifiable in all countries of Europe and North America and international guidelines have been issued by the WHO for the management of infection.

Infection with *Corynebacterium diphtheriae* occurs most commonly in the upper respiratory tract, and sore throat is frequently the presenting feature. The disease is usually spread by droplet infection from cases or carriers. The organisms remain localised at the site of infection and serious consequences result from the absorption of a soluble exotoxin which damages the heart muscle and the nervous system. Infection may occur rarely on the conjunctiva or in the genital tract, or may complicate wounds, abrasions or diseases of the skin, especially in chronic lesions and those who misuse alcohol.

The average incubation period is 2–4 days. Cases must be isolated until cultures from three daily nose and throat swabs are negative.

Clinical features (Box 13.46)

The disease begins insidiously. Fever is seldom significant although tachycardia is usually marked. The diagnostic feature is the 'wash-leather' elevated greyish-green membrane on the tonsils. It has a well-defined edge, is firm and adherent, and is surrounded by a zone of inflammation. There may be swelling of the neck ('bull-neck') and tender enlargement of the lymph nodes. In the mildest infections, especially in the presence of a high degree of immunity, a membrane may never appear and the throat is merely slightly injected.

With anterior nasal infection there is nasal discharge, frequently blood-stained. In laryngeal diphtheria a husky voice and high-pitched cough signal potential respiratory obstruction requiring urgent tracheostomy. If infection spreads to the uvula, fauces and nasopharynx, the patient is gravely ill. Death from acute circulatory failure may occur within the first 10 days.

Late complications occur as a result of toxin action on the heart or nervous system. About 25% of survivors of the early toxaemia may later develop myocarditis with arrhythmias or cardiac failure. These are usually reversible with no permanent damage other than heart block in survivors.

Neurological involvement occurs in 75% of cases. After tonsillar or pharyngeal diphtheria it usually starts after 10 days with palatal palsy. Paralysis of accommodation often follows, manifest by difficulty in reading small print.

13.46 CLINICAL FEATURES OF DIPHTHERIA	
Acute infection	
• Membranous tonsillitis • *or* Nasal infection • *or* Laryngeal infection • *or* Skin/wound/conjunctival infection (rare)	
Complications	
• Laryngeal obstruction or paralysis • Myocarditis • Peripheral neuropathy	

Generalised polyneuritis with weakness and paraesthesia may follow in the next 10–14 days. Recovery from such neuritis is always ultimately complete.

Management

A clinical diagnosis of diphtheria must be notified to the public health authorities and the patient sent urgently to a hospital for infectious diseases. Treatment should begin once appropriate swabs have been taken before waiting for microbiological confirmation. Three main areas of management are:

- administration of diphtheria antitoxin
- administration of antibiotics
- strict isolation procedures.

Antitoxin has no neutralising effect on toxin already fixed to tissues so must be injected intramuscularly without awaiting the result of a throat swab. However, since the antitoxin is hyperimmune horse serum, undesirable reactions to this foreign protein may occur. A potentially lethal immediate anaphylactic reaction (p. 86) with dyspnoea, pallor and collapse is recognised. 'Serum sickness' with fever, urticaria and joint pains may occur 7–12 days after injection. A careful history of previous horse serum injections or allergic reactions should alert the physician. A small test injection of serum should be given half an hour before the full dose in every patient. Adrenaline (epinephrine) solution must be available to deal with any immediate type of reaction (0.5–1.0 ml of 1/1000 solution i.m.). An antihistamine is also given.

In a severely ill patient the risk of anaphylactic shock is outweighed by the mortal danger of diphtheritic toxaemia and up to 100 000 units of antitoxin are injected intravenously if the test dose has not given rise to symptoms. For disease of moderate severity, 16 000–40 000 units i.m. will suffice, and for mild cases 4000–8000 units.

Penicillin 1200 mg 6-hourly i.v. or amoxicillin 500 mg 8-hourly should be administered for 2 weeks to eliminate *C. diphtheriae*. Patients allergic to penicillin can be given erythromycin. Due to poor immunogenicity all sufferers should be immunised with diphtheria toxoid following recovery. Patients must be managed in strict isolation attended by staff with a clearly documented immunisation history until three swabs 24 hours apart are culture-negative.

Prevention

Active immunisation should be given to all children (Box 6.15, p. 139). If diphtheria occurs in a closed community, contacts should be given erythromycin, which is more effective than penicillin in eradicating the organism in carriers. All contacts should also be immunised or given a booster dose of toxoid. Booster doses are required every 10 years to maintain immunity. Low-dose toxoid should be given to prevent severe reactions.

ANTHRAX

There are three recognised forms of infection with *Bacillus anthracis*:

13

- cutaneous anthrax
- gastrointestinal anthrax
- inhalational (pulmonary) anthrax.

The ease of production of *B. anthracis* spores makes this infection a candidate for biological warfare or bioterrorism (p. 341).

Cutaneous anthrax

This skin lesion is associated with occupational exposure to anthrax spores during processing of hides and bone products, or with bioterrorism. It accounts for the vast majority of clinical cases. Animal infection is a serious problem in Africa, India, Pakistan and the Middle East.

Spores are inoculated into exposed skin. A single lesion develops as an irritable papule on an oedematous haemorrhagic base. This progresses to a depressed black eschar. Despite extensive oedema, pain is infrequent.

Gastrointestinal anthrax

This is associated with the ingestion of meat products that have been contaminated or incompletely cooked. The caecum is the seat of the infection, which produces nausea, vomiting, anorexia and fever, followed in 2–3 days by severe abdominal pain and bloody diarrhoea. Toxaemia and death can develop rapidly thereafter.

Inhalational anthrax

This form of the disease is extremely rare unless associated with bioterrorism. Without rapid and aggressive therapy at the onset of symptoms, the mortality is greater than 90%. Fever, dyspnoea, cough, headache and symptoms of septicaemia develop 3–14 days following exposure. Typically, there is little on the chest X-ray other than widening of the mediastinum and pleural effusions.

Management

B. anthracis can be cultured from lesional skin swabs. Skin lesions are readily curable with early antibiotic therapy. Treatment is with ciprofloxacin 500 mg daily until penicillin susceptibility is confirmed; the regimen can then be changed to benzylpenicillin 600 000 units i.m. 6-hourly or phenoxymethylpenicillin 500 mg 6-hourly. Aggressive fluid resuscitation and the addition of an aminoglycoside may improve the outlook. Ventilatory assistance will be required in inhalational disease. Prophylaxis with ciprofloxacin (500 mg 12-hourly) is recommended for anyone at high risk of exposure to biological warfare.

BACTERIAL INFECTIONS WITH NEUROLOGICAL INVOLVEMENT

BACTERIAL MENINGITIS

See page 1225.

BOTULISM

Botulism is a syndrome of paralysis and neurological dysfunction produced by the neurotoxins of *Cl. botulinum*. This organism may contaminate many different foodstuffs, from canned meat and salmon to home produced and preserved vegetables. Contaminated honey has been implicated in outbreaks involving neonates. Wound botulism is a growing problem in injection drug-users. Anaerobic conditions are necessary for the organism's growth. Ingestion of this extremely potent neurotoxin in even picogram amounts causes predominately bulbar and ocular palsies (difficulty in swallowing, blurred or double vision, ptosis), progressing to limb weakness and respiratory paralysis.

Management includes assisted ventilation and general supportive measures until the toxin eventually dissociates from nerve endings at 6–8 weeks following ingestion.

TETANUS

See page 1232.

MYCOBACTERIAL INFECTIONS

EXTRAPULMONARY TUBERCULOSIS

See page 697.

LEPROSY

Leprosy (Hansen's disease) is a chronic granulomatous disease affecting skin and nerve; it is caused by *Mycobacterium leprae*. The clinical form of the disease is determined by the degree of cell-mediated immunity (CMI) (p. 69) expressed by that individual towards *M. leprae* (Fig. 13.34). High levels of CMI with elimination of leprosy bacilli produce tuberculoid leprosy, whereas absent CMI

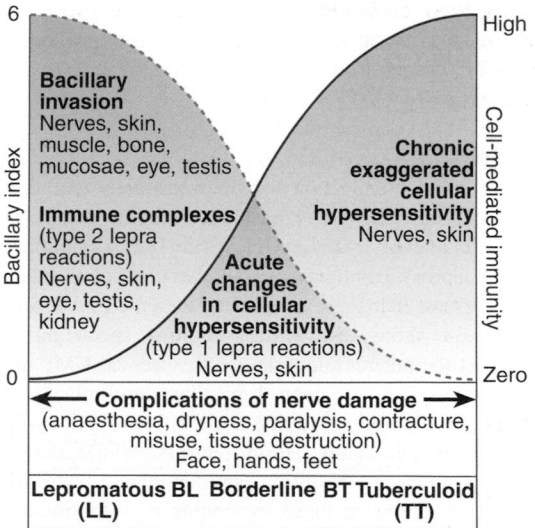

Fig. 13.34 Leprosy: mechanisms of damage and tissue affected. Mechanisms under the broken line are characteristic of disease near the lepromatous end of the spectrum, and those under the solid line characteristic of the tuberculoid end. They overlap in the centre where, in addition, instability predisposes to type 1 lepra reactions. At the peak in the centre neither bacillary growth nor cell-mediated immunity has the upper hand. (BL = borderline lepromatous; BT = borderline tuberculoid)

results in lepromatous leprosy. The medical complications of leprosy are due to nerve damage, immunological reactions and bacillary infiltration. Nerve damage accompanying leprosy is a serious complication causing considerable morbidity. Leprosy patients are frequently stigmatised and using the word 'leper' is inappropriate.

Organism

M. leprae still cannot be grown in vitro. It has a doubling time of 12 days and is a hardy organism which withstands drying for up to 5 months. The genome of *M. leprae* has undergone massive gene decay and differs from *M. tuberculosis* by only 29 functional genes. Analysis of these proteins will be critical for understanding the survival and pathogenesis of *M. leprae*.

Epidemiology

Some 4 million people have or are disabled by leprosy. World-wide active transmission continues, with around 750 000 new cases detected annually, many of them children. About 70% of the world's leprosy patients live in India, with Brazil, Indonesia, Mozambique, Madagascar, Tanzania and Nepal being the next most endemic countries. All new cases seen in the UK have acquired their infection abroad. Age, sex and household contact are important determinants of leprosy risk; leprosy incidence reaches a peak at 10–14 years, and an excess of male cases has regularly been found. HIV infection is not a risk factor for leprosy. HIV/leprosy co-infected patients have typical skin lesions and typical leprosy histology and granuloma formation, even with low circulating CD4 counts.

Transmission

Untreated lepromatous patients discharge bacilli from the nose. Infection occurs through the nose, followed by haematogenous spread to skin and nerve. The incubation period is 2–5 years for tuberculoid cases and 8–12 years for lepromatous cases.

Pathogenesis

M. leprae has a predilection for Schwann cells and skin macrophages, and the host response is critical in determining the outcome of infection. There are three important aspects of leprosy pathogenesis: the spectrum of immune responses, nerve damage and immune-mediated reactions. Figure 13.34 shows the Ridley–Jopling spectrum of response. At the tuberculoid pole, well-expressed CMI and delayed hypersensitivity control bacillary multiplication; organised epithelioid granulomas are seen in tissue biopsies. In the lepromatous form, there is cellular anergy towards *M. leprae*, resulting in abundant bacillary multiplication. Between these two poles is a continuum, varying from patients with moderate CMI (borderline tuberculoid) to patients with little cellular response (borderline lepromatous). The polar groups are stable but the central groups are immunologically unstable.

Both T cells and macrophages are important in the response to *M. leprae* antigens. Tuberculoid patients have a Th1-type response to *M. leprae*, producing interleukin-2 (IL-2) and interferon-γ (IFN-γ), and positive lepromin (a soluble *M. leprae* preparation) skin tests. This strong cell-mediated response clears antigen, but with local tissue destruction. Lepromatous patients have a specific cell-mediated T-cell and macrophage anergy to *M. leprae* and poor lymphocyte responses to *M. leprae* antigens in vitro. They are negative on lepromin skin testing. They produce Th2-type cytokines.

Nerve damage occurs across the spectrum in skin lesions and peripheral nerves. In tuberculoid disease epithelioid granulomas are found. In lepromatous leprosy bacilli are found in Schwann cells and the perineurium. Immune-mediated events are responsible for leprosy reactions (see below).

Clinical features

Patients commonly present with skin lesions or the effects of a peripheral nerve lesion, weakness or an ulcer in an anaesthetic hand or foot. Borderline patients may present with a reaction (see below), nerve pain, sudden palsy and multiple new skin lesions. Box 13.47 gives the cardinal signs of leprosy.

- *Skin.* The most common skin lesions are macules or plaques. In lepromatous leprosy, papules, nodules or diffuse infiltration of the skin occur. Tuberculoid patients have few, hypopigmented lesions whilst lepromatous patients have numerous, sometimes confluent lesions.
- *Anaesthesia.* Anaesthesia occurs in skin lesions when dermal nerves are involved or in the distribution of a large peripheral nerve. In skin lesions the small dermal sensory and autonomic nerve fibres are damaged, causing local sensory loss and loss of sweating within that area.
- *Peripheral neuropathy.* Peripheral nerve trunks are affected at 'sites of predilection'. These are the ulnar (elbow), median (wrist), radial (humerus) causing wrist drop, radial cutaneous (wrist), common peroneal (knee), posterior tibial and sural nerves at the ankle, facial nerve as it crosses the zygomatic arch, and great auricular in the posterior triangle of the neck. Damage to peripheral nerve trunks produces characteristic signs with regional sensory loss and dysfunction of muscles supplied by that peripheral nerve. All these nerves should be examined for enlargement and tenderness and tested for motor and sensory function. The central nervous system is not affected.
- *Eye involvement.* Blindness due to leprosy is a devastating complication for a patient with anaesthetic hands and feet. Eyelid closure is impaired when the facial (7th) nerve is affected. Damage to the trigeminal (5th) nerve causes anaesthesia of the cornea and conjunctiva. The cornea is then susceptible to trauma and ulceration.

13.47 CARDINAL FEATURES OF LEPROSY

- Skin lesions, typically anaesthetic at tuberculoid end of spectrum
- Thickened peripheral nerves
- Acid-fast bacilli on skin smears or biopsy

13

Tuberculoid leprosy (TT)

Tuberculoid leprosy (Fig. 13.35) has a good prognosis; it may self-heal and peripheral nerve damage is limited.

Borderline tuberculoid (BT)

The skin lesions (Fig. 13.36) are similar to those in tuberculoid leprosy but are more numerous. Damage to peripheral nerves may be widespread and severe. These patients are prone to type 1 reactions with consequent nerve damage.

Borderline leprosy (BB)

Borderline leprosy is unstable and patients have numerous skin lesions varying in size, shape and distribution. Annular lesions with a broad, irregular edge and a sharply defined, punched-out centre are characteristic. Nerve damage is variable.

Borderline lepromatous leprosy (BL)

Borderline lepromatous leprosy is characterised by widespread small macules. They may experience both type 1 and type 2 reactions. Peripheral nerve involvement is widespread.

Lepromatous leprosy (LL)

The earliest lesions are ill defined; gradually, the skin becomes infiltrated and thickened. Facial skin thickening leads to the characteristic leonine facies (Fig. 13.37). Dermal nerves are destroyed, sweating is lost, and a 'glove and stocking' neuropathy is common. Nerve damage to large peripheral nerves occurs late in the disease. Nasal collapse occurs secondary to bacillary destruction of the bony nasal spine. Testicular atrophy is caused by diffuse infiltration and the acute orchitis that occurs with type 2 reactions. This results in azoospermia and gynaecomastia (Box 13.48).

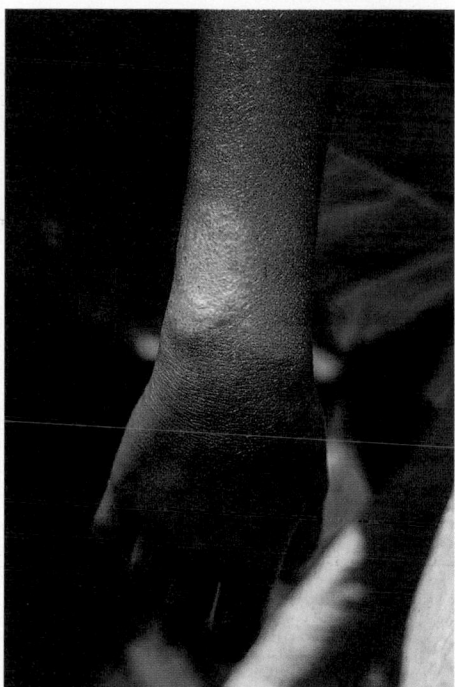

Fig. 13.35   Tuberculoid leprosy. Single lesion with a well-defined active edge and anaesthesia within the lesion.

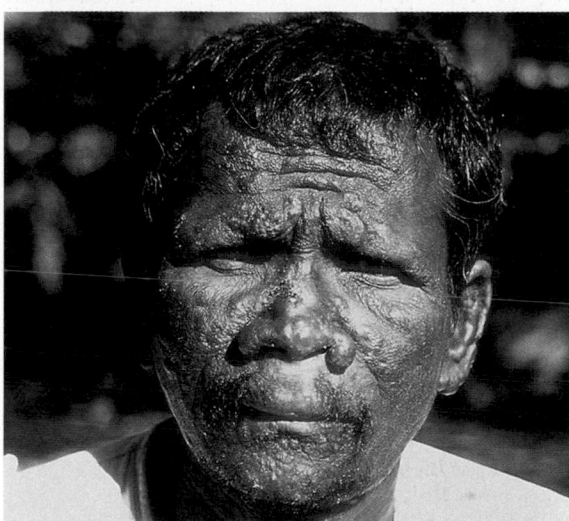

Fig. 13.37   Lepromatous leprosy. Widespread nodules and infiltration with loss of the eyebrows. This man also has early collapse of the nose.

Pure neural leprosy

This occurs principally in India and accounts for 10% of patients. There is asymmetrical involvement of peripheral nerve trunks and no visible skin lesions. On nerve biopsy all types of leprosy have been found.

Leprosy reactions

Leprosy reactions (Box 13.49) are events superimposed on the cardinal features shown in Box 13.47.

Type 1 (reversal) reactions

These occur in 30% of borderline patients (BT, BB, BL) and are delayed hypersensitivity reactions caused by increased recognition of *M. leprae* antigens in skin and nerve sites. Skin lesions become erythematous (Fig. 13.38); peripheral nerves become tender and painful. Loss of nerve function can be sudden, with foot drop occurring overnight. Reversal reactions may occur spontaneously, after starting treatment and also after completion of multidrug therapy.

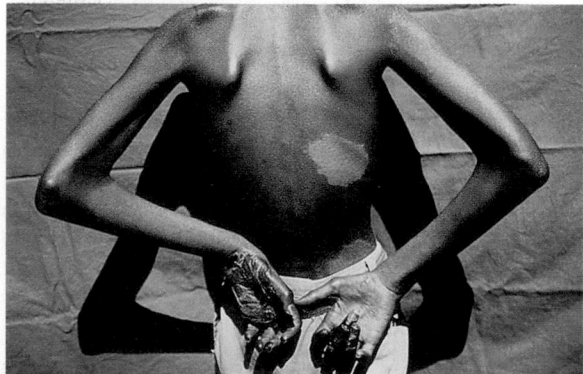

Fig. 13.36   Borderline tuberculoid leprosy with severe nerve damage. This boy has several well-defined, hypopigmented, macular, anaesthetic lesions. He has severe nerve damage affecting both ulnar and median nerves bilaterally and has sustained severe burns to his hands.

13.48 CLINICAL CHARACTERISTICS OF THE POLAR FORMS OF LEPROSY

Clinical and tissue-specific features	Lepromatous	Tuberculoid
Skin and nerves		
Number and distribution	Widely disseminated	One or a few sites, asymmetrical
Skin lesions		
Definition		
Clarity of margin	Poor	Good
Elevation of margin	Never	Common
Colour		
Dark skin	Slight hypopigmentation	Marked hypopigmentation
Light skin	Slight erythema	Coppery or red
Surface	Smooth, shiny	Dry, scaly
Central healing	None	Common
Sweat and hair growth	Impaired late	Impaired early
Loss of sensation	Late	Early and marked
Nerve enlargement and damage	Late	Early and marked
Bacilli (bacterial index)	Many (5 or 6+)	Absent (0)
Natural outcome	Progression	Healing
Other tissues	Upper respiratory mucosa, eye, testes, bones, muscle	None
Reactions	Immune complexes	Cell-mediated

13.49 REACTIONS IN LEPROSY

	Lepra reaction type 1 (reversal)	Lepra rection type 2 (erythema nodosum leprosum)
Mechanism	Cell-mediated hypersensitivity	Immune complexes
Clinical features	Painful tender nerves, loss of function Swollen skin lesions` New skin lesions	Tender papules and nodules; may ulcerate Painful tender nerves, loss of function Iritis, orchitis, myositis, lymphadenitis Fever, oedema
Management	Prednisolone 40 mg, reducing over 3–6 months[1]	Moderate: prednisolone 40 mg daily Severe: thalidomide[2] or prednisolone 40–80 mg, reducing over 1–6 months; local if eye involved[3]

[1]Indicated for any new impairment of nerve or eye function.
[2]See text for details.
[3]1% hydrocortisone drops or ointment and 1% atropine drops.

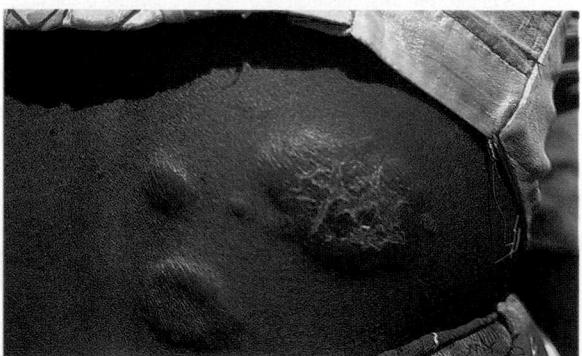

Fig. 13.38 Reversal reactions. Erythematous, oedematous lesions.

Type 2 (erythema nodosum leprosum—ENL) reactions
These are partly due to immune complex deposition and occur in BL and LL patients who produce antibodies and have a high antigen load. They manifest with malaise, fever and crops of small pink nodules on the face and limbs.

Iritis and episcleritis are common. Other signs are acute neuritis, lymphadenitis, orchitis, bone pain, dactylitis, arthritis and proteinuria. ENL may continue intermittently for several years.

Investigations
The diagnosis is clinical, made by finding a cardinal sign of leprosy and supported by finding acid-fast bacilli in slit skin smears or typical histology in a skin biopsy. Skin lesions should be tested for anaesthesia. The peripheral nerves should be palpated for thickening and tenderness. Neither serology nor PCR testing for *M. leprae* DNA is sensitive or specific enough for diagnosis.

Slit skin smears
The bacterial load is assessed by scraping dermal material on to a glass slide. The smears are then stained and acid-fast bacilli are scored on a logarithmic scale: the bacterial index (BI). Smears are useful for confirming the diagnosis and monitoring response to treatment.

Differential diagnosis

Skin

The anaesthesia of tuberculoid and borderline tuberculoid lesions differentiates them from fungal pityriasis versicolor, vitiligo, post-inflammatory depigmentation, psoriasis and eczema. The presence of acid-fast bacilli in smears differentiates lepromatous nodules from onchocerciasis, Kaposi's sarcoma and post-kala-azar dermal leishmaniasis.

Nerves

Leprosy is the most common cause of peripheral nerve thickening. Uncommon conditions such as Charcot–Marie–Tooth disease and amyloid are differentiated from leprosy by the absence of skin lesions and acid-fast bacilli. Comparison should always be made with nerves on the other side. The causes of other polyneuropathies such as HIV infection, diabetes, alcoholism, vasculitides and heavy metal poisoning should all be considered where appropriate.

Outside leprosy-endemic areas doctors often fail to diagnose leprosy. Of new patients seen between 1995 and 1999 at the Hospital for Tropical Diseases, London, diagnosis had been delayed in over 80% of cases. Patients had been misdiagnosed by dermatologists, neurologists, orthopaedic surgeons and rheumatologists. These delays had serious consequences for patients, with over half of them having nerve damage and disability. Leprosy should always be considered as a possible cause of peripheral neuropathy or neuropathic ulcers in patients of Indian or African origin.

Management

Effective treatment (Box 13.50) can only be achieved with the patient's cooperation and confidence. All leprosy patients should be given an appropriate multidrug combination. Patients can be classified into paucibacillary (skin smear-negative tuberculoid and BT) and multibacillary (skin smear-positive BT, all BB, BL and LL). The first-line anti-leprosy drugs are rifampicin, clofazimine and dapsone. Box 13.51 gives the drug combinations, doses and duration of treatment. Studies from India have shown that multibacillary patients with an initial BI > 4 need longer treatment, for at least 24 months.

Rifampicin is a potent bactericidal for *M. leprae* but should always be given in combination with other anti-leprotics since a single-step mutation can confer resistance to rifampicin. Dapsone is bacteriostatic. It commonly causes mild haemolysis but rarely anaemia. Clofazimine is a red, fat-soluble crystalline dye, weakly bactericidal for *M. leprae*. Skin discoloration (red to purple-black) and ichthyosis are troublesome side-effects, particularly on pale skins. New drugs bactericidal for *M. leprae* have been identified, notably the fluoroquinolones pefloxacin and ofloxacin, minocycline and clarithromycin. These agents are now established second-line drugs. Minocycline causes a grey pigmentation of skin lesions.

More than 12 million patients have been treated successfully with multidrug treatment (MDT). Clinical improvement has been rapid and toxicity rare. The treatment duration has been shortened. Monthly supervision of the rifampicin component has been crucial to success. At the end of 6 months' treatment for borderline disease there may still be signs of inflammation which should not be mistaken for active infection. The distinction between relapse and reaction may be difficult. WHO studies have reported a cumulative relapse rate of 1.07% for paucibacillary leprosy and 0.77% for multibacillary leprosy at 9 years after completion of MDT. *M. leprae* is such a slow-growing organism that relapse only occurs after many years. A single-dose triple drug combination (rifampicin, ofloxacin and minocycline) has been tested in India for patients with single skin lesions. Although single-dose treatment is clinically less effective than the conventional 6-month treatment for paucibacillary leprosy, it is an operationally attractive field regimen and has been recommended for use by the WHO.

13

13.50 PRINCIPLES OF LEPROSY TREATMENT

- Stop the infection with chemotherapy
- Treat reactions
- Educate the patient about leprosy
- Prevent disability
- Support the patient socially and psychologically

13.51 MODIFIED WHO-RECOMMENDED MULTIDRUG THERAPY REGIMENS IN LEPROSY

Type of leprosy*	Monthly supervised drug treatment	Daily self-administered drug treatment	Duration of treatment
Paucibacillary	Rifampicin 600 mg	Dapsone 100 mg	6 months
Multibacillary	Rifampicin 600 mg Clofazimine 300 mg	Clofazimine 50 mg Dapsone 100 mg	12 months
Paucibacillary single-lesion	Ofloxacin 400 mg Rifampicin 600 mg Minocycline 100 mg		Single dose

*WHO classification for field use when slit skin smears are not available:
- paucibacillary single-lesion leprosy (one skin lesion)
- paucibacillary (2–5 skin lesions)
- multibacillary (more than 5 skin lesions).
In this field classification WHO recommends treatment of multibacillary patients for 12 months only.

Treatment of reactions

The principles of treating immune-mediated reactions are:

- Control the acute inflammation and ease the pain.
- Treat the neuritis.
- Halt eye damage.

Type 1 reactions should be treated with oral prednisolone starting at 40 mg daily, and reduced by 5 mg/day each month. ENL is difficult to treat and requires high-dose corticosteroids (40–80 mg daily, tapered down rapidly) or thalidomide. The chronicity of ENL reactions makes corticosteroid dependency a problem in these patients. Thalidomide is effective at controlling ENL but its teratogenic side-effects in early pregnancy limit its use in women of child-bearing age. Chloroquine can also be used.

Patient education

Educating leprosy patients about their disease is vital for successful management. Patients should be reassured that after 3 days of chemotherapy they are not infectious and can lead a normal social life. It should be emphasised that gross deformities are not inevitable, and that care of anaesthetic limbs is as important as chemotherapy.

Prevention of disability

The morbidity and disability associated with leprosy are secondary to nerve damage. Nerve damage produces anaesthesia, dryness and muscle weakness. These three factors lead to misuse of the affected limb, with resultant ulceration, infection and, ultimately, severe deformity. Monitoring sensation and muscle power in hands, feet and eyes should be part of the routine follow-up so that new nerve damage is detected early. The patient with an anaesthetic hand or foot needs to develop daily self-care and protection when performing dangerous tasks. Soaking dry hands and feet followed by rubbing with oil keeps the skin moist and supple. Physiotherapy can prevent contractures, muscle atrophy and over-stretching of paralysed muscles.

Anaesthetic feet need protective footwear. For anaesthesia alone, a well-fitting 'trainer' with firm soles and shock-absorbing inners provides adequate protection. Once there is deformity, then special footwear is needed to protect pressure points and ensure even weight distribution.

Patients should be taught to work out the causation of any injury so that recurrence can be avoided. Plantar ulceration occurs secondary to increased pressure over bony prominences and is treated by rest. Unlike ulcers in diabetic feet, ulcers in leprosy heal if they are protected from weight-bearing. No weight-bearing is permitted until the ulcer has healed. Appropriate footwear should be provided to prevent recurrence.

Social, psychological and economic rehabilitation

The social and cultural background of the patient determines many of the problems that may be encountered. The patient may have difficulty in coming to terms with leprosy. The community may reject the patient. Education, employment, support from family, friends and doctor, and plastic surgery to correct stigmatising deformity all have a role to play.

Leprosy in women

Women with leprosy are in double jeopardy; not only may they develop post-partum nerve damage but they are also at particular risk of social ostracisation with rejection by spouse and family.

Prognosis

The majority of patients, especially those who have no nerve damage at the time of diagnosis, do well on MDT, with resolution of skin lesions. Borderline patients are at risk of developing type 1 reactions which may result in devastating nerve damage.

Prevention and control

The previous strategy of vertical leprosy campaigns has now been superseded by integrated programmes with primary health-care workers in many countries now responsible for case detection and providing MDT. It is not yet clear how successful this will be, especially in the time-consuming area of disability prevention.

BCG vaccination has been shown to give good but variable protection against leprosy; adding killed *M. leprae* to BCG does not give enhanced protection.

BURULI ULCER

This ulcer is caused by *Mycobacterium ulcerans* and occurs world-wide in tropical rainforests. In 1999 a survey in Ghana found 6500 cases; there are an estimated 10 000 cases in West Africa as a whole.

Pathogenesis

The ulcer starts with acute necrosis. Clumps of acid-fast bacilli are present on the ulcer floor. Later, healing occurs with granuloma formation.

Clinical features

The initial lesion is a small subcutaneous nodule on the arm or leg. This breaks down to form a shallow, necrotic ulcer with deeply undermined edges which extends rapidly. Healing may occur after 6 months but the accompanying fibrosis causes contractures and deformity.

Management

A combination of rifampicin and streptomycin can cure the infection. Infected tissue should be removed surgically.

Prevention

Health campaigns in Ghana have successfully focused on early removal of the small, pre-ulcerative nodules.

RICKETTSIAL INFECTIONS

RICKETTSIAL FEVERS

The rickettsial fevers are the most common tick-borne infections. Patients present acutely with headache, rash and sometimes neurological disturbance. It is important to ask about exposures that would put patients at risk of bites

13.52 ESSENTIAL FEATURES OF RICKETTSIAL INFECTIONS

Disease	Reservoir	Vector	Primary complex[1]	Rash	Gangrene	Target organs	Mortality
SPOTTED FEVER GROUP							
Rocky Mountain spotted fever	Rodents, dogs, ticks	*Ixodes* tick	Often	Morbilliform Haemorrhagic	Often	Bronchi, myocardium, brain, skin	2–12%[2]
Other tick-borne typhus	Rodents, dogs, ticks	*Ixodes* tick	Usual	Maculo-papular	–	Skin, meninges	Rare[3]
TYPHUS GROUP							
Scrub typhus	Rodents	*Trombicula* mite	Often	Maculo-papular	Unusual	Bronchi, myocardium, brain, skin	Rare[3]
Epidemic typhus	Humans	Louse	–	Morbilliform Haemorrhagic	Often	Brain, skin, bronchi, myocardium	Up to 40%
Endemic typhus	Rats	Flea	–	Slight	–	–	Rare[3]

[1] Eschar at bite site and local lymphadenopathy.
[2] Highest in adult males.
[3] Except in infants, older people and the debilitated.

or contact with ticks, lice or fleas. There are two main groups of rickettsial fevers; these are compared in Box 13.52.

Pathogenesis

The rickettsiae are intracellular Gram-negative organisms which parasitise the intestinal canal of arthropods. Infection is usually conveyed to humans through the skin from the excreta of arthropods, but the saliva of some biting vectors is infected. The organisms multiply in capillary endothelial cells, producing lesions in the skin, central nervous system, heart, lungs, kidneys and skeletal muscles. Endothelial proliferation, associated with a perivascular reaction, may cause thrombosis and purpura. In epidemic typhus the brain is the target organ; in scrub typhus the cardiovascular system and lungs in particular are attacked. An eschar is often found in tick- and mite-borne typhus. This often crusted necrotic sore at the site of the bite is due to vasculitis following immunological recognition of the inoculated organism. Regional lymph nodes often enlarge.

Spotted fever group

Rocky Mountain spotted fever

Rickettsia rickettsii is transmitted by tick bites. It is widely distributed and increasing in western and south-eastern states of the USA and also in South America. The incubation period is about 7 days. The rash appears on about the third or fourth day, looking at first like measles, but in a few hours the typical maculo-papular eruption develops. The rash spreads in 24–48 hours from wrists, forearms and ankles to the back, limbs and chest, and then to the abdomen where it is least pronounced. Larger cutaneous and subcutaneous haemorrhages may appear in severe cases. The liver and spleen become palpable. At the extremes of life the mortality is 5–10%.

Tick-borne South African typhus

R. conorii causes Mediterranean and African tick typhus, which also occurs on the Indian subcontinent. Infected

ticks may be picked up by walking on grasslands or dogs may bring ticks into the house. Careful examination might reveal a diagnostic eschar, and the maculo-papular rash on the trunk, limbs, palms and soles. There may be delirium and meningeal signs in severe infections but recovery is usual.

Typhus group

Scrub typhus fever

Scrub typhus is caused by *R. tsutsugamushi*, transmitted by mites. It occurs in the Far East, Myanmar, Pakistan, Bangladesh, India, Indonesia, the South Pacific islands and Queensland, particularly where patches of forest cleared for plantations have attracted rats and mites.

In many patients one eschar or more develops, surrounded by an area of cellulitis and enlargement of regional lymph nodes. The incubation period is about 9 days.

Mild or subclinical cases are common. The onset of symptoms is usually sudden with headache, often retro-orbital, fever, malaise, weakness and cough. In severe illness the general symptoms increase, with apathy and prostration. An erythematous maculo-papular rash often appears on about the 5th–7th day and spreads to the trunk, face and limbs including the palms and soles, with generalised painless lymphadenopathy. The rash fades by the 14th day. The temperature rises rapidly and continues as a remittent fever with sweating until it falls by lysis on about the 12th–18th day. In severe infection the patient is prostrate with cough, pneumonia, confusion and deafness. Cardiac failure, renal failure and haemorrhage may develop. Convalescence is often slow and tachycardia may persist for some weeks.

Epidemic (louse-borne) typhus

Epidemic typhus is caused by *R. prowazekii* and is transmitted by infected faeces of the human body louse, usually through scratching the skin. Patients suffering from epidemic typhus infect the lice, which leave when the patient is febrile. In conditions of overcrowding the disease spreads rapidly. It is prevalent in parts of Africa, especially Ethiopia and Rwanda, and in the South American Andes and Afghanistan. Large epidemics have occurred in Europe, usually as a sequel to war. The incubation period is usually 12–14 days.

There may be a few days of malaise but the onset is more often sudden with rigors, fever, frontal headaches, pains in the back and limbs, constipation and bronchitis. The face is flushed and cyanotic, the eyes are congested and the patient becomes dull and confused.

The rash appears on the 4th–6th day. In its early stages it disappears on pressure but soon becomes petechial with subcutaneous mottling. It appears first on the anterior folds of the axillae, sides of the abdomen or backs of hands, then on the trunk and forearms. The neck and face are seldom affected. During the second week symptoms increase in severity. Sores develop on the lips. The tongue becomes dry, brown, shrunken and tremulous. The spleen is palpable, the pulse feeble and the patient stuporous and delirious. The temperature falls rapidly at the end of the second week and the patient recovers gradually. In fatal cases the patient usually dies in the second week from toxaemia, cardiac or renal failure, or pneumonia.

Endemic (flea-borne) typhus
Flea-borne or 'endemic' typhus caused by *R. mooseri* is endemic world-wide. Humans are infected when the faeces or contents of a crushed flea which has fed on an infected rat are introduced into the skin. The incubation period is 8–14 days. The symptoms resemble those of a mild louse-borne typhus. The rash may be scanty and transient.

Investigation of rickettsial infection
Routine blood investigations are unhelpful. Diagnosis is made on clinical grounds and response to treatment. Differential diagnoses include malaria, typhoid, meningococcal sepsis and leptospirosis.

The Weil–Felix reaction is the agglutination of the somatic antigens of non-motile *Proteus* species by the patient's serum. It is now seldom used due to its lack of specificity and sensitivity.

Species-specific antibodies may be detected by complement fixation, microagglutination and fluorescence in specialised laboratories.

Management of the rickettsial diseases
The different rickettsial fevers vary greatly in severity but all respond to tetracycline or chloramphenicol 500 mg 6-hourly for 7 days. Louse-borne typhus and scrub typhus can be treated with a single dose of 200 mg doxycycline, repeated for 2–3 days to prevent relapse. Chloramphenicol- and doxycycline-resistant strains of *R. tsutsugamushi* have been reported from Thailand and patients here may need treatment with rifampicin.

Nursing care is important, especially in epidemic typhus. Sedation may be required for delirium and blood transfusion for haemorrhage. Relapsing fever and typhoid are common intercurrent infections in epidemic typhus, and pneumonia in scrub typhus. They must be sought and treated. Convalescence is usually protracted, especially in older people.

Prevention of rickettsial infections

Vector and reservoir control
Lice, fleas, ticks and mites need to be controlled with insecticides.

Q FEVER

Q fever occurs world-wide and is caused by the rickettsia-like organism *Coxiella burnetii*, an obligate intracellular organism that can survive in the extracellular environment. Cattle, sheep and goats are important reservoirs and the organism is transmitted by inhalation of aerosolised particles.

Clinical features
The incubation period is 3–4 weeks. The initial symptoms are non-specific with fever, headache and chills; in 20% of cases a maculo-papular rash occurs. Other presentations include pneumonia and hepatitis. Chronic Q fever may present with osteomyelitis, encephalitis and endocarditis.

Investigations
Diagnosis is usually serological and the stage of the infection can be distinguished by isotype tests and phase-specific antigens. Phase I and II IgM titres peak at 4–6 weeks. In chronic infections IgG titres to phase I and II antigens may be raised.

Management
Prompt treatment of acute Q fever with doxycycline reduces fever duration. Treatment of Q fever endocarditis is problematic, requiring prolonged therapy with doxycycline and rifampicin; even then, organisms are not always eradicated.

BARTONELLOSIS

This group of diseases is caused by intracellular Gram-negative rods closely related to the rickettsia. The principal human pathogens are *Bartonella quintana* and *B. henselae*. Bartonella infections are associated with the following clinical conditions:

- *Trench fever*. This is a relapsing fever with severe leg pain. The disease is not fatal but is very debilitating.
- *Bacteraemia and endocarditis in the homeless*. The endocarditis is associated with severe damage to the heart valves.
- *Cat scratch disease*. *B. henselae* causes this common benign lymphadenopathy in children and young adults. A vesicle or papule develops on the head, neck or arms after a cat scratch. The lesion resolves spontaneously but there may be regional lymphadenopathy that persists for up to 4 months before also resolving spontaneously.
- *Bacillary angiomatosis*. This is an HIV-associated disease.

Investigations
Bartonellae can be grown from the blood but this requires prolonged incubation using enriched media. Serological

diagnosis can be made by haemagglutination, immuno-fluorescent antibody (IFA) testing and ELISA.

Management

Bartonella isolates are susceptible to β-lactams, rifampicin, erythromycin and tetracyclines. Antibiotic use is guided by clinical need. Cat scratch disease usually resolves spontaneously but *Bartonella* endocarditis requires valve replacement and combination antibiotic therapy.

CHLAMYDIAL INFECTIONS

- *Chlamydia trachomatis* (Box 13.53) causes trachoma (see below), lymphogranuloma venereum and sexually transmitted genital infections (p. 415).
- *Chlamydia psittaci* causes psittacosis (p. 690).
- *Chlamydia pneumoniae* is a cause of atypical pneumonia (p. 690).

13.53 CHLAMYDIAL INFECTIONS

Organism	Disease caused
Chlamydia trachomatis	Trachoma Lymphogranuloma venereum Cervicitis, urethritis, proctitis
Chlamydia psittaci	Psittacosis
Chlamydia pneumoniae	Atypical pneumonia Acute/chronic sinusitis

TRACHOMA

Trachoma is a chronic keratoconjunctivitis caused by *Chlamydia trachomatis*, and is the most common cause of avoidable blindness. The classic trachoma environment is described as dry and dirty; children have eye and nose discharges. Transmission occurs through flies, on fingers and within families. In endemic areas the disease is most common in children.

Pathology

The infection lasts for years, may be latent over long periods and may recrudesce. The conjunctiva of the upper lid is first affected with vascularisation and cellular infiltration. Scarring causes inversion of the lids (entropion) so that the lashes rub against the cornea (trichiasis). The cornea becomes vascularised and opaque.

Clinical features

The onset is usually insidious and infection may not be apparent to the patient. Early symptoms include conjunctival irritation and blepharospasm, but the problem may not be detected until vision begins to fail. The early follicles of trachoma are characteristic (Fig. 13.39), but clinical differentiation from conjunctivitis due to other viruses may be difficult.

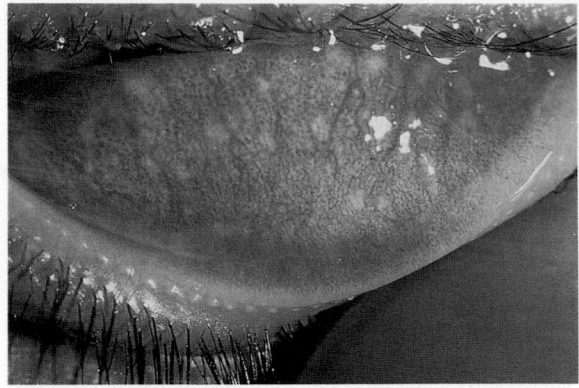

Fig. 13.39 Trachoma. Trachoma is characterised by hyperaemia and numerous pale follicles.

Investigations

Intracellular inclusions may be demonstrated in conjunctival scrapings by staining with iodine or immunofluorescence. Chlamydia may be isolated in chick embryo or cell culture.

Management

A single dose of azithromycin (20 mg/kg) has been shown to be superior to 6 weeks of 12-hourly tetracycline eye ointment for individuals and in mass treatment programmes. Deformity and scarring of the lids, and corneal opacities, ulceration and scarring require surgical treatment after control of local infection.

Prevention

Personal and family cleanliness should be improved. Proper care of the eyes of newborn and young children is essential. Family contacts should be examined. Population surveys identify communities with severe blinding disease. The WHO is promoting the SAFE strategy for trachoma control (**S**urgery, **A**ntibiotics, **F**acial cleanliness and **E**nvironmental improvement).

PRION DISEASES

Prions are defined on page 130. They cause the transmissible spongiform encephalopathies, including Creutzfeldt–Jakob disease, described on page 1234.

EMERGING INFECTIONS AND BIOTERRORISM

SEVERE ACUTE RESPIRATORY SYNDROME (SARS)

SARS (p. 695) is a highly infectious atypical pneumonia caused by a coronavirus now named SARS-CoV. In a significant proportion of infected patients, it causes severe disease and may be fatal. It appears to have originated in Guangdong Province in China in November 2002, although the first reports of the disease came from Vietnam and Hong

Kong in early 2003. Since then it has been reported from all parts of the world.

AVIAN FLU/INFLUENZA

Influenza virus subtypes A, B and C can infect humans; however, only subtype A commonly does so, causing influenza pandemics (p. 688). Wild birds are naturally infected by subtype A (avian flu) and do not become ill. However, when poultry birds are infected, due to species-jumping, they develop severe and often fatal disease. People handling infected birds may contract avian flu, which can occasionally be fatal. In recent years, several epidemics of avian flu, with subsequent human infection, have been reported, especially from South-east Asian countries and, in 2005, Eastern Europe.

WEST NILE FEVER

This infection is a zoonosis caused by West Nile virus, a flavivirus transmitted from birds and animals by *Culex* mosquitoes. Originally confined to Israel and the Nile region, it has recently spread, probably via infected birds, to a large area over the eastern seaboard of the USA and to parts of Europe (e.g. Portugal). After 3–14 days' incubation, the majority of cases present with a 'flu-like syndrome with relatively mild meningitic or encephalitic symptoms. A small proportion of elderly or very young sufferers (< 1%) present with a severe encephalitic illness with cranial nerve signs, ataxia and extrapyramidal features; these may evolve to the Guillain-Barré syndrome (p. 1249). If there is a history of travel to relevant areas the diagnosis should be sought by IgM serology or demonstration of the virus from CSF samples. Supportive therapy is all that can be offered and the disease carries a significant mortality.

BIOTERRORISM

Bioterrorism describes the intimidation of civilians, military forces and their governments through the release of harmful organisms or toxins. In recent years there has been an increase in the incidence of terrorism through biological agents. These agents can be disseminated in innumerable ways—through contamination of food and water, dispersal through aerosols, and even detonators filled with harmful material. Potential organisms that can be used in bioterrorism are listed in Box 13.54.

Outbreaks of an uncommon infectious disease in clusters, febrile illness associated with sepsis, pneumonia, respiratory failure or a rash, or a botulism-like syndrome with flaccid muscle paralysis, especially if occurring in otherwise healthy persons, should suggest a possible act of bioterrorism. Weapons-grade anthrax in the US postal system in 2001 resulted in 22 anthrax cases with five deaths. A rapid response to contain the threat is key to minimising morbidity, mortality and terror. Steps such as rapid identification of the organism, prompt isolation and treatment of the victims, protection of care providers and post-exposure chemoprophylaxis are important. Heightened surveillance, use of information technology to alert and educate the population, and strategic vaccination can successfully minimise and contain the threat.

13.54 ORGANISMS WITH THE POTENTIAL FOR USE IN BIOTERRORISM
Bacteria
• Anthrax (*Bacillus anthracis*)*   • Plague (*Yersinia pestis*)*   • Tularaemia (*Francisella tularensis*)*   • Brucellosis (*Brucella* spp.)   • Food safety threats (e.g. *Salmonella* spp., *Escherichia coli* 0157:H7, *Shigella*)   • Glanders (*Burkholderia mallei*)   • Melioidosis (*Burkholderia pseudomallei*)   • Psittacosis (*Chlamydia psittaci*)   • Q fever (*Coxiella burnetii*)   • Typhus fever (*Rickettsia prowazekii*)   • Water safety threats (e.g. *Vibrio cholerae*)
Viruses
• Smallpox (*Variola major*)   • Viral haemorrhagic fevers (filoviruses, e.g. Ebola, Marburg; arenaviruses, e.g. Lassa, Machupo)*   • Viral encephalitis (alphaviruses, e.g. Venezuelan equine encephalitis, Eastern equine encephalitis, Western equine encephalitis)   • Emerging infectious diseases such as Nipah virus and hantavirus
Toxins
• Botulism (*Clostridium botulinum* toxin)   • Epsilon toxin of *Clostridium perfringens*   • Ricin toxin from *Ricinus communis* (castor beans)   • Staphylococcal enterotoxin B
* Agents with highest potential.

Anthrax

Due to its use in recent years as a bioterrorist weapon, anthrax has assumed considerable significance. *Bacillus anthracis* is a Gram-positive spore-forming bacillus; the extremely resistant spores can survive for decades. The inhalational (pulmonary) form of anthrax is the most lethal (p. 333).

Smallpox

The aetiological agent for smallpox is variola virus; it belongs to the family Poxviridae. The world was declared free of smallpox in 1980 after a concerted vaccination programme. However, 76 laboratories world-wide retain the virus. Potential for the use of smallpox as a bioterrorist weapon is great, as deliberate release of this virus could result in major epidemics in the currently unvaccinated majority of the population (p. 306).

PROTOZOAL INFECTIONS (Box 13.55)

BLOOD AND TISSUE PARASITES

MALARIA

Malaria is caused by *Plasmodium falciparum*, *P. vivax*, *P. ovale* and *P. malariae*. It is transmitted by the bite of female anopheline mosquitoes and occurs throughout the tropics and subtropics at altitudes below 1500 metres (Fig. 13.40). There are up to 250 million clinical cases per

13

13.55 PROTOZOAL INFECTIONS

Site of infection	Disease	Organisms involved
Blood stream/ systemic	Malaria	Plasmodium falciparum Plasmodium vivax Plasmodium malariae Plasmodium ovale
	Babesiosis	Babesia bovis Babesia divergens Babesia microti
	Leishmaniasis	Leishmania donovani Leishmania tropica Leishmania major Leishmania aethiopica, infantum, mexicana, amazonensis, brasiliensis etc.
	Trypanosomiasis African	Trypanosoma brucei gambiense Trypanosoma rhodesiense
	South American	Trypanosoma cruzi
	Toxoplasmosis	Toxoplasma gondii
Gastrointestinal/ mucosal	Amoebiasis Giardiasis Cryptosporidiosis Cyclosporiasis Trichomoniasis (pp. 406 and 409)	Entamoeba histolytica Giardia lamblia Cryptosporidium parvum Cyclospora cayetanensis Trichomona hominis

near airports in Europe have acquired malaria from accidentally imported mosquitoes.

Pathogenesis

Life cycle of the malarial parasite

The female anopheline mosquito becomes infected when it feeds on human blood containing gametocytes, the sexual forms of the malarial parasite (Figs 13.41 and 13.42). Development in the mosquito takes from 7–20 days. Sporozoites inoculated by an infected mosquito disappear from human blood within half an hour and enter the liver. After some days merozoites leave the liver and invade red blood cells, where further asexual cycles of multiplication take place, producing schizonts. Rupture of the schizont releases more merozoites into the blood and causes fever, the periodicity of which depends on the species of parasite.

P. vivax and *P. ovale* may persist in liver cells as dormant forms, hypnozoites, capable of developing into merozoites months or years later. Thus the first attack of clinical malaria may occur long after the patient has left the endemic area, and the disease may relapse after treatment with drugs that kill only the erythrocytic stage of the parasite.

P. falciparum and *P. malariae* have no persistent exo-erythrocytic phase but recrudescences of fever may result

year and over 1 million die, mainly children. Following WHO-sponsored campaigns focusing on prevention and effective treatment, the incidence of malaria was greatly reduced between 1950 and 1960, but since 1970 there has been a resurgence. Furthermore, *P. falciparum* has now become resistant to chloroquine, notably in Asia and Africa. Due to increased travel and neglect of chemoprophylaxis, over 2000 cases are imported annually into Britain. Most are due to *P. falciparum*, usually from Africa, and of these 1% die because of late diagnosis. Immigrants returning home after a long residence in the UK are particularly at risk. They have lost their partial immunity and do not realise that they should be taking malaria prophylaxis. A few people living

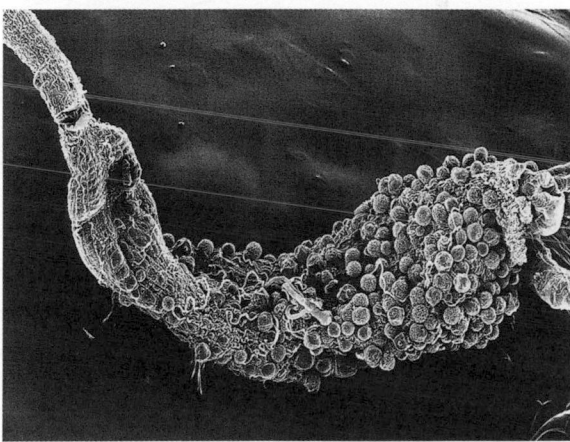

Fig. 13.41 Scanning electron micrograph of *P. falciparum* oöcysts lining the anopheline mosquito's stomach.

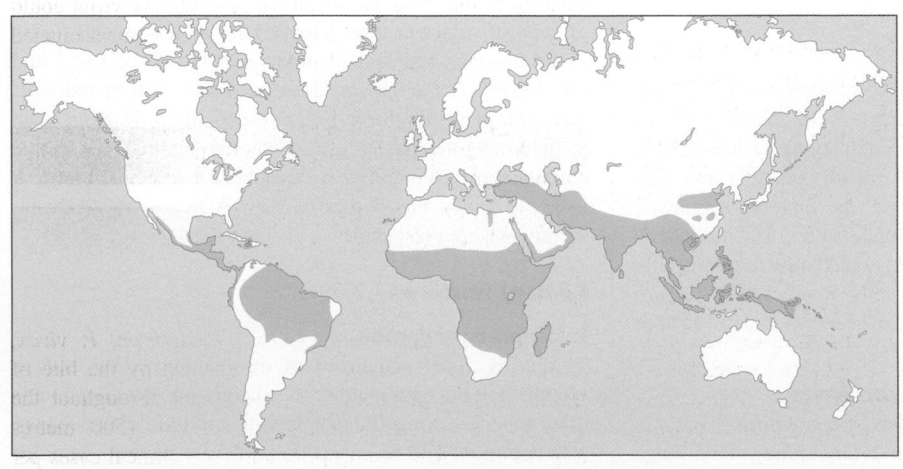

Fig. 13.40 Distribution of malaria.

13

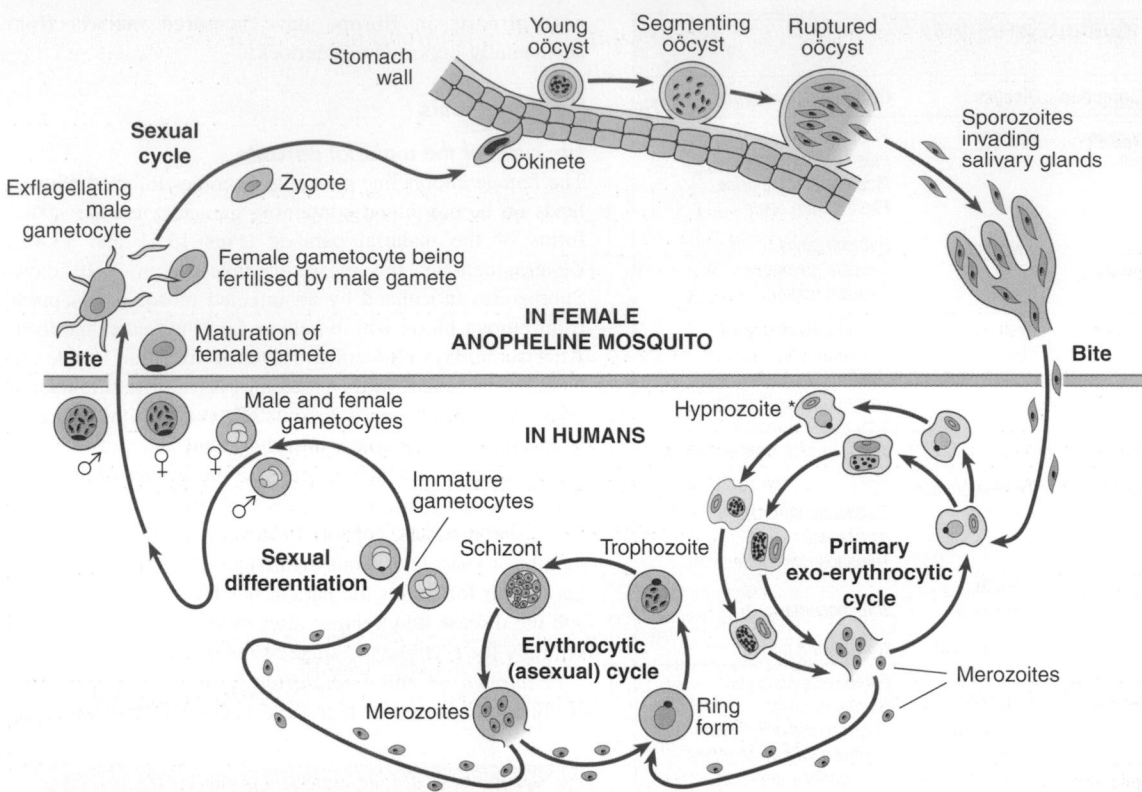

Fig. 13.42 **Malarial parasites: life cycle.** Hypnozoites(*) are present only in *P. vivax* and *P. ovale* infections.

Cycle/feature	*P. vivax, P. ovale*	*P. malariae*	*P. falciparum*
13.56 RELATIONSHIPS BETWEEN LIFE CYCLE OF PARASITE AND CLINICAL FEATURES OF MALARIA			
Pre-patent period (minimum incubation)	8–25 days	15–30 days	8–25 days
Asexual cycle	48 hrs synchronous	72 hrs synchronous	< 48 hrs asynchronous
Periodicity of fever	'Tertian'	'Quartan'	Aperiodic
Exo-erythrocytic cycle	Persistent as hypnozoites	Pre-erythrocytic only	Pre-erythrocytic only
Delayed onset	Common	Rare	Rare
Relapses	Common up to 2 years	Recrudescence many years later	Recrudescence up to 1 year

from multiplication in the red cells of parasites which have not been eliminated by treatment and immune processes (Box 13.56).

Pathology

The pathology in malaria is due to haemolysis of infected red cells and adherence of infected red blood cells to capillaries. Malaria is always accompanied by haemolysis and in a severe or prolonged attack anaemia may be profound. Anaemia is worsened by dyserythropoiesis, splenomegaly and depletion of folate stores. Haemolysis is most severe with *P. falciparum*, which invades red cells of all ages but especially young cells. *P. vivax* and *P. ovale* invade reticulocytes, and *P. malariae* normoblasts, so that infections remain lighter.

Effects on red blood cells and capillaries

In *P. falciparum* malaria, red cells containing schizonts adhere to capillary endothelium in brain, kidney, liver, lungs

and gut. The vessels become congested and the organs anoxic. Rupture of schizonts liberates toxic and antigenic substances that may cause further damage. Thus the main effects of malaria are haemolytic anaemia and, with *P. falciparum*, widespread organ damage (Box 13.57 and Fig. 13.43). *P. falciparum* does not grow well in red cells that contain haemoglobin F, C or especially S. Haemoglobin S heterozygotes (AS) are protected against the lethal complications of malaria. *P. vivax* cannot enter red cells that lack the Duffy blood group. West Africans and African-Americans are protected.

Clinical features

P. falciparum *infection*

This is the most dangerous of the malarias. The onset is often insidious, with malaise, headache and vomiting, and is often mistaken for influenza. Cough and mild diarrhoea are also common. The fever has no particular pattern. Jaundice

13.57 SEVERE MANIFESTATIONS AND COMPLICATIONS OF *FALCIPARUM* MALARIA AND THEIR IMMEDIATE MANAGEMENT

Manifestation/complication	Immediate management
Coma (cerebral malaria)	Maintain airway Nurse on side Exclude other treatable causes of coma (e.g. hypoglycaemia, bacterial meningitis) Avoid harmful ancillary treatments such as corticosteroids, heparin and adrenaline (epinephrine) Intubate if necessary
Hyperpyrexia	Tepid sponging, fanning, cooling blanket Antipyretic drug
Convulsions	Maintain airway Treat promptly with diazepam or paraldehyde injection
Hypoglycaemia	Measure blood glucose Give 50% dextrose injection followed by 10% dextrose infusion (glucagon may be ineffective)
Severe anaemia (packed cell volume < 15%)	Transfuse fresh whole blood or packed cells if pathogen screening is available
Acute pulmonary oedema	Nurse at 45°, give oxygen, venesect 250 ml of blood into donor bag, give diuretic, stop intravenous fluids Intubate and add PEEP/CPAP (p. 193) in life-threatening hypoxaemia Haemofilter
Acute renal failure	Exclude pre-renal causes Check fluid balance, urinary sodium If urine output is inadequate despite fluid replacement, give diuretic/dopamine Peritoneal dialysis (haemofiltration or haemodialysis if available)
Spontaneous bleeding and coagulopathy	Transfuse screened fresh whole blood (cryoprecipitate/fresh frozen plasma and platelets if available) Vitamin K injection
Metabolic acidosis	Exclude or treat hypoglycaemia, hypovolaemia and Gram-negative septicaemia Give oxygen
Shock ('algid malaria')	Suspect Gram-negative septicaemia Make blood cultures Give parenteral antimicrobials Correct haemodynamic disturbances
Aspiration pneumonia	Give parenteral antimicrobial drugs Change position Physiotherapy Give oxygen
Hyperparasitaemia (e.g. > 10% of circulating erythrocytes parasitised in non-immune patient with severe disease)	Consider exchange or partial exchange transfusion, manual or haemophoresis

13

is common due to haemolysis and hepatic dysfunction. The liver and spleen enlarge and become tender. Anaemia develops rapidly.

A patient with *falciparum* malaria, apparently not seriously ill, may develop dangerous complications (Box 13.57). Cerebral malaria is the most grave complication and is manifested by either confusion or coma, usually without localising signs. Children die rapidly without any special symptoms other than fever. Immunity is impaired in pregnancy, and abortion from parasitisation of the maternal side of the placenta is frequent. Splenectomy increases the risk of severe malaria.

P. vivax *and* P. ovale *infection*
In many cases the illness starts with several days of continued fever before the development of classical bouts of fever on alternate days. Fever starts with a rigor. The patient feels cold and the temperature rises to about 40°C. After half an hour to an hour the hot or flush phase begins.

It lasts several hours and gives way to profuse perspiration and a gradual fall in temperature. The cycle is repeated 48 hours later. Gradually the spleen and liver enlarge and may become tender. Anaemia develops slowly. Herpes simplex is common. Relapses are frequent in the first 2 years after leaving the malarious area.

P. malariae *infection*
This is usually associated with mild symptoms and bouts of fever every third day. Parasitaemia may persist for many years with the occasiolnal recrudescence of fever, or without producing any symptoms. *P. malariae* causes glomerulonephritis and the nephrotic syndrome in children.

Diagnosis
Thick and thin blood films should be taken whenever malaria is suspected. In the thick film erythrocytes are lysed, releasing all blood stages of the parasite. This, as well as the

13

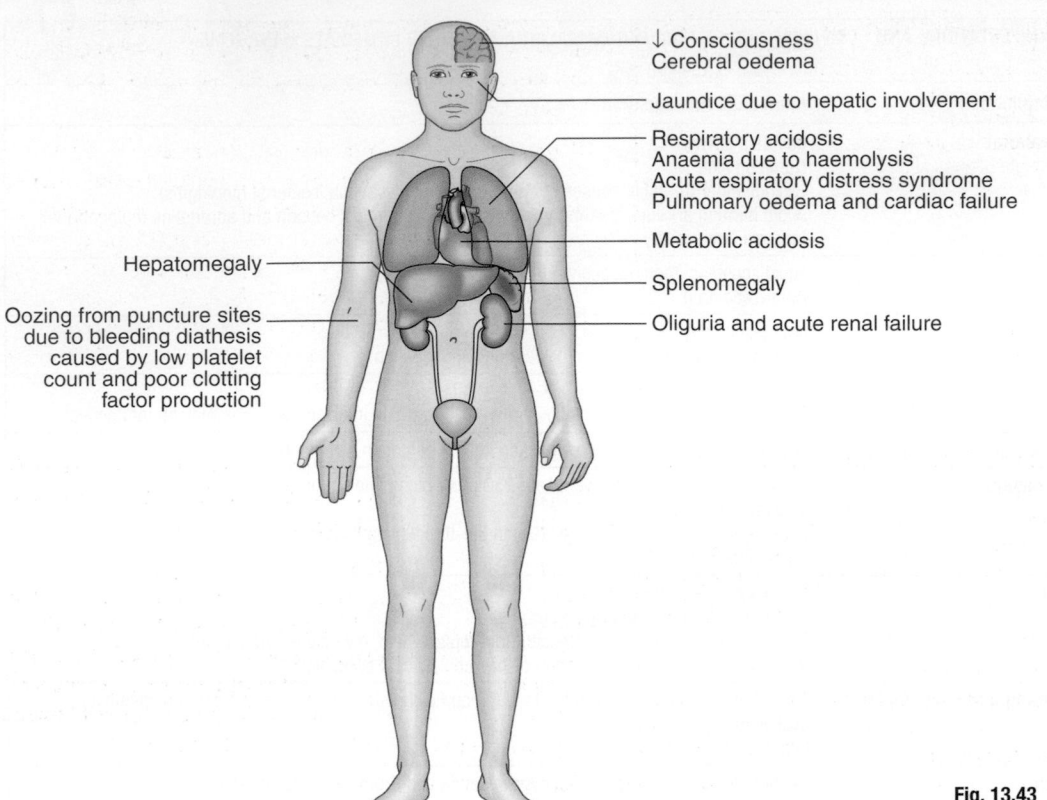

↓ Consciousness
Cerebral oedema

Jaundice due to hepatic involvement

Respiratory acidosis
Anaemia due to haemolysis
Acute respiratory distress syndrome
Pulmonary oedema and cardiac failure

Metabolic acidosis

Splenomegaly

Oliguria and acute renal failure

Hepatomegaly

Oozing from puncture sites
due to bleeding diathesis
caused by low platelet
count and poor clotting
factor production

Fig. 13.43   Organ involvement in severe malaria.

fact that more blood is used in thick films, facilitates the diagnosis of low-level parasitaemias. A thin film is essential to confirm the diagnosis, to identify the species of parasite and, in *P. falciparum* infections, to quantify the parasite load (by counting the percentage of infected erythrocytes). *P. falciparum* parasites may be very scanty, especially in patients who have been partially treated. With *P. falciparum*, only ring forms are normally seen in the early stages. With the other species all stages of the erythrocytic cycle may be found. Gametocytes appear after about 2 weeks. They persist after treatment and are harmless, but are the source for infecting mosquitoes. Immunochromatographic 'dipstick' tests for *P. falciparum* antigen are now marketed and provide a useful non-microscopic means of diagnosing this infection. They should be used in parallel with blood film examination but are about 100 times less sensitive than a carefully examined blood film.

Management

Chemotherapy of mild P. falciparum *malaria*

P. falciparum is now resistant to chloroquine almost world-wide, so quinine is the drug of choice. Quinine dihydrochloride or sulphate 600 mg *salt* (10 mg/kg) 8-hourly by mouth is given until the patient is clinically better and the blood is free of parasites (usually 3–5 days). The dose should be reduced to 12-hourly intervals if quinine toxicity develops. This regimen should be followed by a single dose of sulfadoxine 1.5 g combined with pyrimethamine 75 mg, i.e. 3 tablets of Fansidar. In pregnancy a 7-day course of quinine alone should be given. If sulphonamide

sensitivity is suspected, quinine may be followed by doxycycline 100 mg daily for 7 days. Decreased efficacy of quinine has been reported in some areas, notably the Thailand/Myanmar border. Alternatives to quinine plus Fansidar are atovaquone 250 mg plus proguanil 100 mg (Malarone) 4 tablets once daily for 3 days, or artemether 200 mg/day orally for 5 days then mefloquine 500 mg in 2 doses 2 hours apart. Mefloquine may occasionally cause alarming neuropsychiatric side-effects which can persist for several days due to its plasma half-life of 14 days. Policy in Africa is moving towards artemisinin combination therapy. This combines an astemisinin drug (artemether or artesunate) with another drug. Currently co-artemether (artemether-lumefantrine) and artesunate+amodiaquine are the most widely used.

Management of complicated P. falciparum *malaria*

Severe malaria is a medical emergency and cerebral malaria is the most common presentation and cause of death in adults with malaria. Cerebral malaria is assumed when asexual parasites are present in the blood film and the patient has impaired consciousness and other encephalopathies have been excluded, particularly bacterial meningitis and locally occurring viral encephalitides. Complications of severe malaria include hypoglycaemia, severe anaemia, renal failure and metabolic acidosis (Box 13.57). Severe malaria should be considered in any non-immune patient with a parasite count greater than 2%.

The management of severe malaria should include early and appropriate antimalarial chemotherapy, active treatment of complications, correction of fluid, electrolyte

13.58 INEFFECTIVE ANCILLARY TREATMENTS IN MALARIA

- Corticosteroids (dexamethasone)
- Other anti-inflammatory agents
- Other anti-cerebral oedema agents (urea, mannitol, invert sugar)
- Low molecular weight dextran
- Adrenaline (epinephrine)
- Heparin
- Epoprostenol
- Pentoxifylline
- Hyperbaric oxygen
- Ciclosporin A
- Hyperimmune serum
- Iron-chelating agents (desferrioxamine B)
- Anti-tumour necrosis factor antibodies

and acid–base balance, and avoidance of harmful ancillary treatments (Box 13.58).

Quinine is indicated if a chloroquine-resistant infection is at all likely. Although quinine resistance has increased in South-east Asia and South America, there is still no high-grade resistance that precludes its use in severe malaria. Quinine is given as an intravenous infusion over 4 hours. Treatment should be started with a loading dose infusion of 20 mg/kg quinine *salt*. Up to a maximum of 1.4 g quinine can be given over 4 hours, then after 8–12 hours maintenance dosage at 10 mg/kg quinine *salt* up to a maximum of 700 mg. The dose should be repeated at intervals of 8–12 hours until the patient can take drugs orally. The loading dose should *not* be given if the patient has received quinine, quinidine or mefloquine during the previous 24 hours. Quinine may instead be given intramuscularly but may cause muscle necrosis; the hydrochloride is less irritant than the dihydrochloride. Those with cardiac disease should be monitored by ECG, with special attention to QRS duration and QT_c. Artemisinin derivatives may also be used as antimalarial chemotherapy. Four recently published randomised controlled trials have compared parenteral quinine and intramuscular artemether and none has shown a clear and unequivocal benefit for either drug in outcome measures as either mortality or incidence of neurological sequelae. Artesunate should be given as a loading dose 2.4 mg/kg then 1.2 mg/kg i.v. 12-hourly to a total dose of 600 mg. It can be given intramuscularly in children. Artemether is given as a loading dose 3.2 mg/kg i.m., then 1.6 mg/kg i.m. daily to a total of 640 mg. This should be changed to an oral formulation as soon as possible. Mefloquine should not be used for severe malaria since no parenteral form is available.

The management of severe malaria involves careful attention to all the major organ systems (Box 13.57). Numerous ancillary treatments have been tested but none has proven beneficial (Box 13.58).

Exchange transfusion has not been tested in randomised controlled trials but may be beneficial for non-immune patients with persisting high parasitaemias (> 10% circulating erythrocytes).

Cheap and affordable drugs are urgently needed for the treatment of severe malaria. A combination of chlorproguanil and dapsone (Lapdap) is in third-stage research trials in uncomplicated malaria in sub-Saharan African children.

P. vivax, *P. ovale* and *P. malariae* infections should be treated with chloroquine: 600 mg chloroquine *base* followed by 300 mg *base* in 6 hours, then 150 mg *base* 12-hourly for 2 more days.

Radical cure of malaria due to P. vivax and P. ovale

Relapses can be prevented by taking one of the antimalarial drugs in suppressive doses. Radical cure is achieved in most patients with a course of primaquine (15 mg daily for 14 days), which destroys the hypnozoite phase in the liver. Haemolysis may develop in those who are glucose-6-phosphate dehydrogenase (G6PD)-deficient. Cyanosis due to the formation of methaemoglobin in the red cells is more common but not dangerous.

Prevention

Every person going to a malarious area should receive anti-malaria advice. This comprises avoiding bites and taking appropriate chemoprophylaxis.

Avoiding mosquito bites

Long sleeves and trousers should be worn outside the house, especially at night when the anopheline mosquitoes bite. Repellent creams and sprays can be used. Screened windows, the use of a mosquito net and burning repellent coils or tablets also reduce the risk. Impregnation of bed nets with permethrin also reduces mosquito biting.

Chemoprophylaxis

Clinical attacks of malaria may be preventable with drugs such as proguanil which attack the pre-erythrocytic form, and also by drugs such as atovaquone 250 mg plus proguanil 100 mg (Malarone), doxycycline, chloroquine or mefloquine after the parasite has entered the erythrocyte ('suppression'). Box 13.59 gives the recommended doses for protection of the non-immune. It is important to determine the degree of risk of malaria in the area to be visited and the degree of chloroquine resistance. These factors will guide the recommendations for prophylaxis and are summarised in the *British National Formulary* (BNF) in the UK and similar publications in other countries. Expert advice is required for individuals unable to tolerate the first-line agents listed, or in whom they are contraindicated. Doses for children vary, depending on age and body weight. Reference should be made to standard dosage recommendations (BNF). Chemoprophylaxis is begun 1 week before entering the malarious area and is continued for 4 weeks after leaving it. Resistance to the cheap and well-tolerated drug proguanil is increasing, and frequently coincides with the much more serious spread of chloroquine resistance. Chloroquine should not be taken continuously as a prophylactic for more than 5 years without regular ophthalmic examination, as it may cause irreversible retinopathy. Pregnant and lactating women may take proguanil or chloroquine safely. Mefloquine is contraindicated in the first trimester of pregnancy. Fansidar should not be used for chemoprophylaxis, as deaths have occurred from agranulocytosis or Stevens–Johnson syndrome (p. 1308). Mefloquine is useful in areas of multiple drug resistance, such as East and Central Africa and Papua New Guinea. Experience shows it to be safe for at least 2 years. There are several contraindications to its use (Box 13.59).

13

13.59 CHEMOPROPHYLAXIS OF MALARIA

Area	Antimalaria tablets	Adult prophylactic dose	Regimen
Chloroquine resistance high[1]	Mefloquine[2] *or* Doxycycline *or* Malarone	250 mg 100 mg 1 tablet from 1–2 days before travelling to 1 week after return	One tablet weekly Daily Daily
Chloroquine resistance moderate	Chloroquine[3] *plus* Proguanil	150 mg base 100 mg	Two tablets weekly Two tablets daily
Chloroquine resistance absent	Chloroquine *or* Proguanil	150 mg base 100 mg	Two tablets weekly One or two tablets daily

[1] Choice of regimen is determined by area to be visited, length of stay, level of malaria transmission, level of drug resistance, presence of underlying disease in the traveller and concomitant medication taken.
[2] Contraindicated in the first trimester of pregnancy, lactation, cardiac conduction disorders, epilepsy, psychiatric disorders; may cause neuropsychiatric disorders.
[3] British preparations of chloroquine usually contain 150 mg base, French preparations 100 mg base and American preparations 300 mg base.

Malaria control in endemic areas

There are major initiatives under way to reduce malaria in endemic areas. The provision of permethrin-impregnated bed nets has been shown to reduce mortality in African children. The WHO now has a 'Roll back malaria' programme. New combination drugs such as artemether-lumefatrine and pyronaridine are being assessed in trials. In developing new drugs known targets can be better exploited by new 4-aminoquinolones, and new targets can be identified such as phospholipid biosynthesis. Inhibitors of this are at an early stage of development. Trial vaccines are being evaluated in Thailand and Africa.

BABESIOSIS

This is caused by a tick-borne intra-erythrocytic protozoon parasite. Patients present with fever 1–4 weeks after a tick bite. Severe illness is seen in splenectomised patients. The diagnosis is made by blood film examination. Treatment is with quinine and clindamycin.

LEISHMANIASIS

Leishmaniasis is caused by unicellular flagellate intracellular protozoa belonging to the genus *Leishmania* (order Kinetoplastidae). It comprises several diverse clinical syndromes which can be placed into three broad groups of disorders:

- visceral leishmaniasis (VL, kala-azar)
- cutaneous leishmaniasis (CL)
- mucosal leishmaniasis (ML).

Although most clinical syndromes are caused by zoonotic transmission (Fig. 13.44) of parasites from animals (chiefly canine and rodent reservoirs) to humans through phlebotomine sandfly vectors, humans are the only known reservoir (anthroponotic) in major VL foci in India and Sudan (Fig. 13.45). There are 21 leishmanial species responsible for these disorders. The disease occurs in 88 countries around the world, with an estimated annual incidence of 2 million new cases (500 000 for VL, and 1.5 million for CL; Figs 13.47 and 13.51).

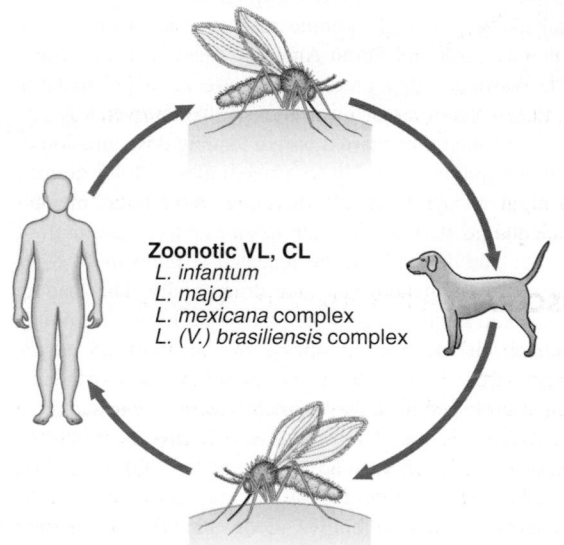

Zoonotic VL, CL
L. infantum
L. major
L. mexicana complex
L. (V.) brasiliensis complex

Fig. 13.44 Zoonotic transmission of leishmaniasis.

Life cycle (Fig. 13.46)

Flagellar promastigotes (10–20 μm) are introduced by the feeding female sandfly. Sandfly saliva helps *Leishmania* evade immunity. The promastigotes are taken up by macrophages where they lose their flagellae and transform into amastigotes (2–4 μm). These multiply, ultimately causing lysis of the macrophages and infection of another cell. Sandflies pick up amastigotes when feeding on infected patients or animal reservoirs. In the sandfly, the parasite transforms into a flagellar promastigote which multiplies by binary fission in the gut of the vector and migrates to the proboscis to infect a new host.

Vector

Different species of sandfly vector (*Phlebotomus* in the eastern hemisphere, *Lutzomyia* and *Psyodopygus* in the western hemisphere) are responsible for transmission of leishmaniasis. Sandflies live in hot and humid climates in the cracks and crevices of mud or straw houses and lay eggs in organic matter. People living in such conditions are more prone to acquire the disease. Female sandflies bite during

13

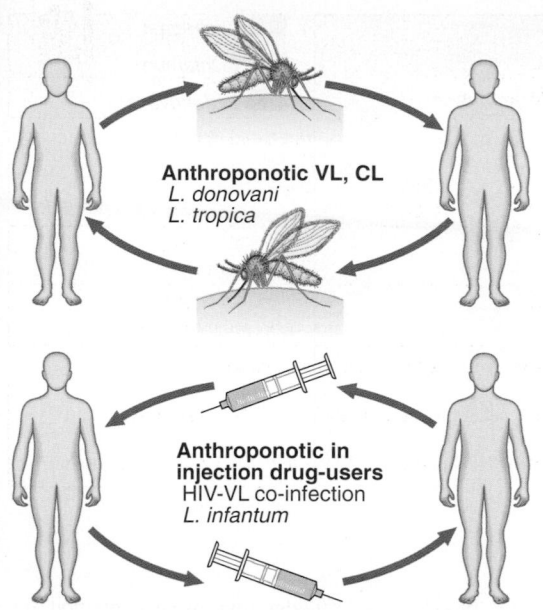

Fig. 13.45 Anthroponotic transmission of leishmaniasis.

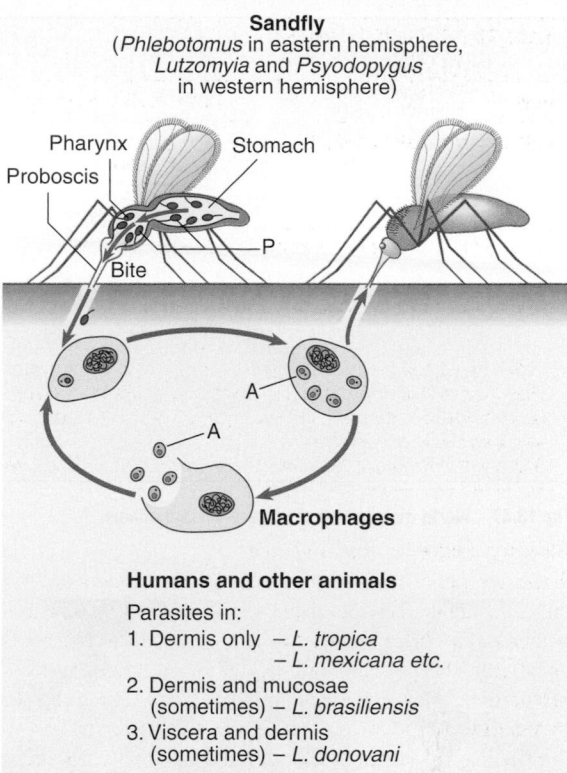

Fig. 13.46 Life cycle of *Leishmania.* (A = amastigote (Leishman–Donovan body); P = promastigote

the night and preferentially feed on animals; humans are incidental hosts.

VISCERAL LEISHMANIASIS (KALA-AZAR)

Visceral leishmaniasis is caused by the protozoon *Leishmania donovani* complex and transmitted by the phlebotomine sandfly (Fig. 13.46). Rarely, a dermatotropic species (e.g. *Leishmania tropica*) may cause visceral disease. India, Sudan, Bangladesh and Brazil account for 90% of cases of VL, while other affected regions include the Mediterranean, East Africa, China, Arabia, Israel and other South American countries (Fig. 13.47). Transmission has also been reported to follow blood transfusion in northern Europe. The disease can present unexpectedly in immunosuppressed patients—for example, after renal transplantation and in AIDS.

Pathogenesis

The great majority of people infected with flagellar promastigotes remain asymptomatic and control the infection. Those unable to do so develop clinical disease. In visceral diseases the spleen, liver, bone marrow and lymph nodes are primarily involved.

Clinical features

On the Indian subcontinent both adults and children are equally affected; on other continents it is predominantly a disease of small children and infants, except in HIV co-infection (adult disease). Malnutrition increases susceptibility to the visceral disease. The incubation period ranges from weeks to months (occasionally several years).

The first sign of infection is high fever, usually accompanied by rigor and chills. Fever intensity decreases over time and patients may become afebrile for intervening periods ranging from weeks to months. This is followed by a relapse of fever, often of lesser intensity. Splenomegaly

develops quickly in the first few weeks and becomes massive as the disease progresses. Hepatomegaly occurs later, to a lesser degree than splenomegaly. Lymphadenopathy is seen in the majority of cases in Africa, the Mediterranean and South America but is rare on the Indian subcontinent. Blackish discoloration of the skin, from which the disease derived its name, kala-azar (the Hindi word for 'black fever'), is a feature of advanced illness, and is now rarely seen. Pancytopenia with its consequent clinical manifestations is a common feature. Moderate to severe anemia develops rapidly, and can result in congestive cardiac failure and associated clinical features. Thrombocytopenia, often compounded by hepatic dysfunction, may result in bleeding from retina, gastrointestinal tract and nose. In progressive disease, hypoalbuminaemia may manifest as pedal oedema, ascites and anasarca.

As the disease advances, there is profound immunosuppression and secondary infections are very common. These include tuberculosis, pneumonia, severe amoebic or bacillary dysentery, gastroenteritis, herpes zoster and chickenpox. Skin infections, boils, cellulitis and scabies are common occurrences. Without adequate treatment most patients with clinical VL are likely to die.

Investigations

Pancytopenia is the most dominant feature, with granulocytopenia and monocytosis. Polyclonal hypergammaglobulinaemia, chiefly IgG followed by IgM, and hypoalbuminaemia are seen later on in the course of the

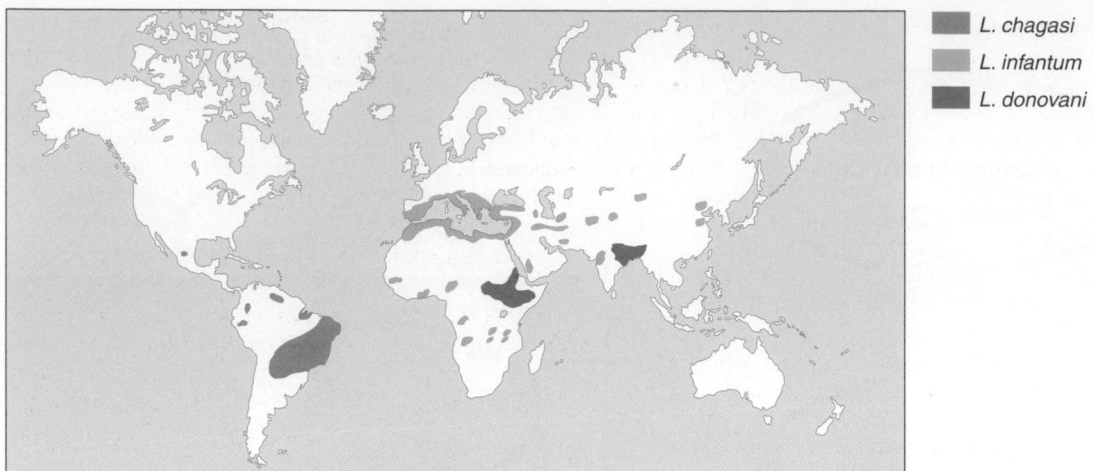

Fig. 13.47 World distribution of visceral leishmaniasis.

- L. chagasi
- L. infantum
- L. donovani

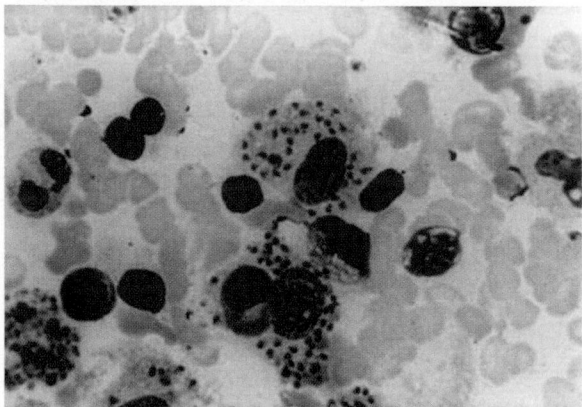

Fig. 13.48 Splenic smear showing numerous intracellular, and a few extracellular, amastigotes.

disease. Patients are anergic to the leishmanin antigen skin test (LST), and there is antigen-specific immunosuppression when peripheral blood mononuclear cells are challenged with *Leishmania* antigen ex vivo. After successful chemotherapy there is recovery of immunity and the LST becomes positive. Immunological parameters measuring T-helper lymphocyte activity suggest absence of a polarised response as both the pro-inflammatory Th1 cytokine, interferon-γ, and the anti-inflammatory Th2 cytokine, interleukin-10, are detected in lesions.

Diagnosis

Demonstration of amastigotes (Leishman–Donovan bodies) in splenic smears is the most efficient means of diagnosis, with 98% sensitivity (Fig. 13.48); however, it carries a risk of serious haemorrhage in inexperienced hands. Safer methods like bone marrow or lymph node smears are not as sensitive. Parasites may be demonstrated in buffy coat smears, especially in immunosuppressed patients. Sensitivity can be improved by culturing the aspirate material. However, this is an expensive process only available in well-equipped laboratories. PCR for DNA detection from the

peripheral blood is an efficient non-invasive method for diagnosis, but is only performed in specialised laboratories. PCR is also used for species identification. Serodiagnosis, by ELISA or immunofluorescence antibody test, is employed in developed countries. In endemic regions, a highly sensitive and specific direct agglutination test of stained promastigotes and an equally efficient rapid immunochromatographic k39 strip test have become popular. These tests remain positive for several months after cure has been achieved, so do not predict response to treatment or relapse. A significant proportion of the healthy population in an endemic region will be positive for these tests due to past exposure. Formal gel (aldehyde) or other similar tests based on the detection of raised globulin have limited value and should not be employed for the diagnosis of VL.

Differential diagnosis

This includes malaria, typhoid, tuberculosis, schistosomiasis and many other infectious and neoplastic conditions, some of which may coexist with VL. Fever, splenomegaly, pancytopenia and non-response to antimalarial therapy may provide the clue before specific laboratory diagnosis is made.

Management

Pentavalent antimonials

Antimony (Sb) compounds were the first drugs to be used for the treatment of leishmaniasis and remain the mainstay of treatment in most parts of the world. The exception is the Indian subcontinent, especially Bihar state, where almost two-thirds of cases are refractory to Sb treatment. Traditionally, pentavalent antimony is available as sodium stibogluconate (100 mg/ml) in English-speaking countries and meglumine antimoniate (85 mg/ml) in French ones. The daily dose is 20 mg/kg body weight, given either intravenously or intramuscularly for 28–30 days. Side-effects are common and include arthralgias, myalgias, raised hepatic transaminases, pancreatitis, especially in patients co-infected with HIV, and ECG changes (T wave inversion and reduced amplitude). Severe cardiotoxicity, manifested by concave ST segment elevation, prolongation of QT_c > 0.5 msec, ventricular ectopics, runs of ventricular tachycardia, torsades de pointes, ventricular fibrillation and sudden death, is not uncommon. The incidence of cardiotoxicity and death can be very high with improperly manufactured Sb.

Amphotericin B

The antifungal drug, amphotericin B deoxycholate given once daily or on alternate days at a dose of 0.75–1.00 mg/kg for 15–20 doses, is used in patients with Sb failure or as a first-line drug in regions with a significant level of Sb unresponsiveness. It has a cure rate of nearly 100%. Infusion-related side-effects, e.g. high fever with rigor, thrombophlebitis, diarrhoea and vomiting, are extremely common. Serious adverse events, such as renal or hepatic toxicity, hypokalaemia, thrombocytopenia, myocarditis and occasional death, are not uncommon.

Lipid formulations (amphotericin B lipid complex—Abelcet) and liposomal amphotericin B (AmBisome) are less toxic and have been tested widely for the treatment of VL. AmBisome is approved by the US Food and Drug Administration for this purpose. Drug doses vary according to geographical location. On the Indian subcontinent a total dose of 10–15 mg/kg is considered adequate, whereas in Africa 14–18 mg, and in South America and Europe 21–24 mg is needed for immunocompetent patients. High daily doses (5–7.5 mg/kg) of the lipid formulations are well tolerated, thus reducing hospital stay and cost. The high price of lipid formulations precludes their use in endemic regions, although in Europe and other developed countries liposomal amphotericin B remains the drug of choice.

Miltefosine

This oral drug, an alkyl phospholipid, has been approved in India, Germany and Colombia for the treatment of VL. A daily dose of 50 mg (patient's body weight < 25 kg) to 100 mg (≥ 25 kg), or 2.5 mg/kg body weight for children, for 28 days cures over 90% of patients. Side-effects include mild to moderate vomiting and diarrhoea, and rarely skin allergy or nephrotoxicity. Since it is a teratogenic drug, it cannot be used in pregnancy; female patients are advised not to become pregnant for the duration of treatment and another 2 months, because of its half-life of nearly 1 week.

Paromomycin

An aminoglycoside, this has undergone trials in India and Africa, and is highly effective if given intramuscularly at 15 mg/kg body weight daily for 3 weeks. No significant auditory or renal toxicity is seen.

Pentamidine isetionate

This was used to treat Sb-refractory patients with VL. However, declining efficacy and serious side-effects such as type 1 diabetes mellitus, hypoglycaemia and hypotension have led to it being abandoned.

Response to treatment

A good response results in abatement of fever, a feeling of well-being, gradual decrease in splenic size, weight gain and recovery of blood counts. Patients should be followed regularly for a period of 6–12 months, as a small minority may experience a relapse of the disease during this period irrespective of the treatment regimen. Relapse is indicated by enlargement of the spleen, return of fever, weight loss and decline in blood counts. Depending upon the geographical location, patients can be retreated either with Sb or conventional or lipid amphotericin B.

HIV-visceral leishmaniasis co-infection
(Fig. 13.45)

HIV-induced immunosuppression (Ch. 14) increases the risk of contracting VL 100–1000 times. Most cases of HIV-VL co-infection have been reported from Spain, France, Italy and Portugal, although the numbers are increasing in Africa (mainly Ethiopia) and Brazil and on the Indian subcontinent.

Atypical clinical presentations of VL in patients co-infected with HIV pose a diagnostic challenge. The clinical triad of fever, splenomegaly and hepatomegaly is found in less than half the patients with a CD4 count under 50 cells/ mm³. VL may present with gastrointestinal involvement (stomach, duodenum or colon), ascites, pleural or peri-cardial effusion, or involvement of lungs, tonsil, oral mucosa or skin. Diagnostic principles remain the same as those in non-HIV patients. Parasites are numerous and easily demonstrable, even in buffy coat preparations. Sometimes amastigotes are found in unusual sites such as bronchoalveolar lavage fluid, pleural fluid or biopsies of the gastrointestinal tract. Immunofluorescence, Western blot, ELISA and other serological tests used singly have low sensitivity. PCR of the blood or its buffy coat are ≥ 95% sensitive, and accurately track recovery and relapse.

Treatment of VL in a setting of HIV co-infection remains essentially the same as in immunocompetent patients but there are some differences in outcome. Conventional amphotericin B (0.7 mg/kg/day for 28 days) may be more effective in achieving initial cure than Sb^v (20 mg/kg/day for 28 days), although in some studies similar results have been reported. Using high-dose AmBisome (4 mg/kg on days 1–5, 10, 17, 24, 31 and 38), a high cure rate is possible. However, these co-infected patients have a tendency to relapse within 1 year. For prevention of relapse, the role of maintenance chemotherapy is debatable. Highly active antiretroviral therapy (HAART) has led to a remarkable decline in the incidence of VL co-infection.

Post-kala-azar dermal leishmaniasis (PKDL)

After treatment and recovery from the visceral disease in India and Sudan some patients develop dermatological manifestations. In India dermatological changes occur in a small minority of patients 6 months to ≥ 3 years after the initial infection. They are seen as macules, papules, nodules (most frequently) and plaques which have a predilection for the face, especially the area around the chin. The face often appears erythematous (Fig. 13.49). Hypopigmented macules can occur over all parts of the body and are highly variable in extent and location. There are no systemic symptoms and no spontaneous healing.

The diagnosis is clinical, supported by demonstration of scanty parasites in lesions by slit skin smear and culture.

13

13

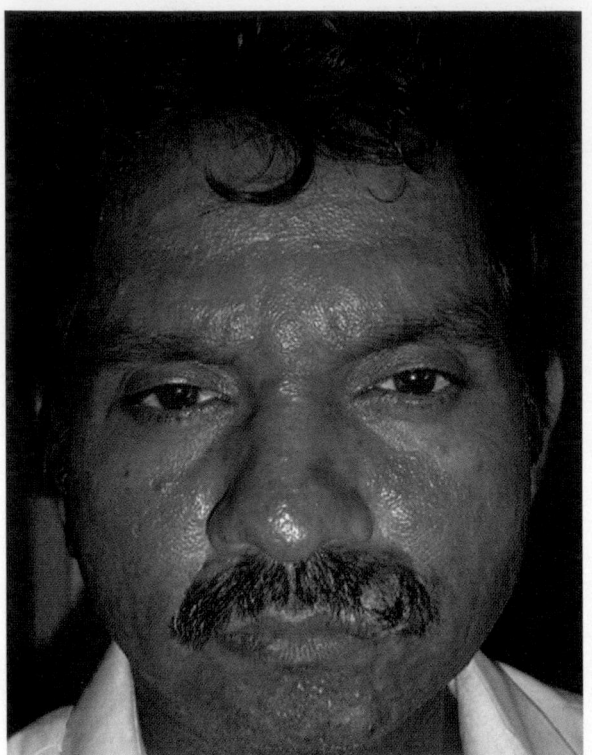

Fig. 13.49   Indian post-kala-azar dermal leishmaniasis.

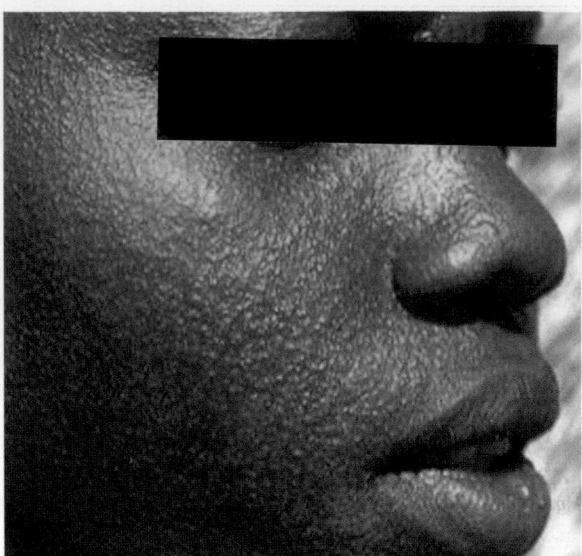

Fig. 13.50   Micronodular rash of Sudanese post-kala-azar dermal leishmaniasis.

Immunofluorescence and immunohistochemistry are other methods for demonstration of the parasite in skin tissues. In the majority of patients serological tests (direct agglutination test or k39 strip tests) are positive.

Treatment of PKDL is difficult. Sb for 120 days or several courses of amphotericin B infusions are required. In the absence of a physical handicap, most patients are reluctant to complete the treatment.

PKDL patients are a human reservoir, and focal outbreaks have been linked to patients with PKDL in areas previously free of VL. In Sudan 50% of patients with VL develop PKDL, experiencing skin manifestations concurrently with VL or shortly afterwards (within 6 months). In addition to the dermatological features described above, a measles-like micropapular rash (Fig. 13.50) may be seen all over the body. In Sudan, children are more frequently affected than in India, where PKDL is a disease of adults. Spontaneous healing occurs in about three-quarters of cases within 1 year. In patients with persistent PKDL treatment with Sb for 2 months is considered adequate.

Prevention and control

A multipronged approach is needed. Sandflies are extremely sensitive to insecticides and vector control through insecticide spray is very important. Mosquito nets or curtains treated with insecticides will keep out the tiny sandflies. In endemic areas with zoonotic transmission, infected or stray dogs should be destroyed.

In areas with anthroponotic transmission, early diagnosis and treatment of human infections, to reduce the reservoir and control epidemics of VL, is extremely important.

Serology is useful for screening of suspected cases in the field. No vaccine is currently available.

CUTANEOUS AND MUCOSAL LEISHMANIASIS

Cutaneous leishmaniasis

CL (oriental sore) occurs in both the Old World and the New World. In the Old World, it is found around the Mediterranean basin, throughout the Middle East and Central Asia as far as Pakistan, and in sub-Saharan West Africa and Sudan (Fig. 13.51). Anthroponotic CL is caused by *L. tropica*, and is confined to urban or suburban areas of the Old World. Afghanistan is currently the biggest focus, but Pakistan, western deserts of India, Iran, Iraq, Syria and other areas of the Middle East are also highly endemic. The causative organisms for Old World zoonotic CL are *L. major*, *L. tropica* and *L. aethiopica* (Box 13.60). In recent years there has been an increase in the incidence of zoonotic CL in both the Old and the New World due to urbanisation and deforestation which have led to domestication of transmission cycles; the building of dams and new irrigation schemes have also caused an increase in the population of animal reservoirs. New World CL is caused by the *L. mexicana* complex, composed of *L. mexicana*, *L. amazonensis* and *L. venezuelensis*, and by the *Viannia* subgenus *L. (V.) brasiliensis* complex constituted by *L. (V.) guyanensis*, *L. (V.) panamensis*, *L. (V.) brasiliensis* and *L. (V.) peruviana*.

The geographical origin of the parasite is critical. In the Old World cutaneous disease is mild, while in the Americas the disease may involve the nose and mouth. CL is commonly imported into Britain and should be considered in the differential diagnosis of an ulcerating skin lesion, especially in travellers who have visited endemic areas of the Old World or forests in Central and South America.

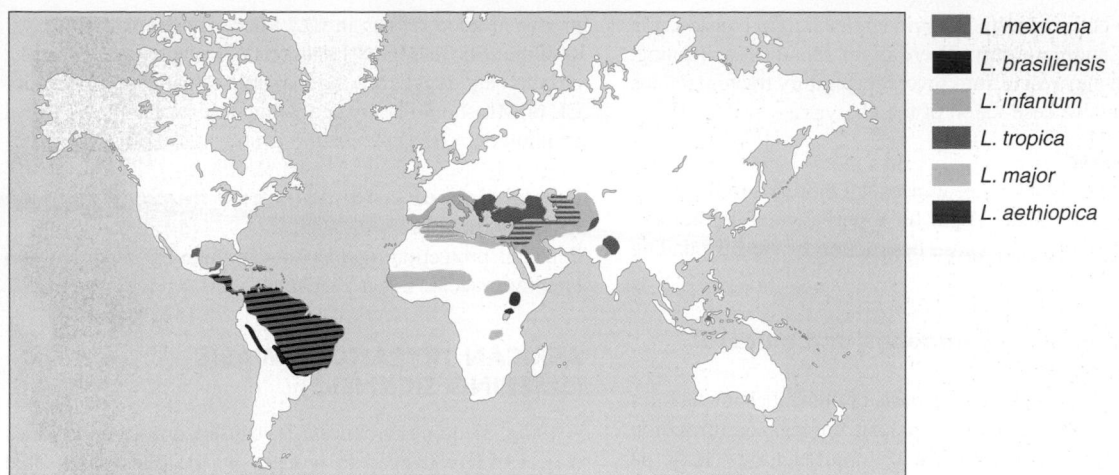

Fig. 13.51 World distribution of cutaneous leishmaniasis.

Legend:
- L. mexicana
- L. brasiliensis
- L. infantum
- L. tropica
- L. major
- L. aethiopica

13.60 TYPES OF OLD WORLD *LEISHMANIA*

Leishmania species	Host	Clinical features
L. tropica	Dogs	Slow evolution, less severe
L. major	Gerbils, desert rodents	Rapid necrosis, wet sores
L. aethiopica	Hyraxes	Solitary facial lesions with satellites

Pathogenesis

Inoculated parasites are taken up by dermal macrophages where they multiply and form a focus for lymphocytes, epithelioid cells and plasma cells. Self-healing may occur with necrosis of infected macrophages, or the lesion may become chronic with ulceration of the overlying epidermis, depending upon the aetiological pathogen.

Clinical features

The incubation period is 2–3 months (range 2 weeks to 5 years). In all types of CL, the common feature is development of a papule followed by ulceration of the skin with raised borders, usually at the site of the bite of the vector. Lesions, single or multiple, start as small red papules that increase gradually in size, reaching 2–10 cm in diameter. A crust forms, overlying an ulcer with a granular base (Fig. 13.52). These ulcers develop a few weeks to months after the bite. There can be satellite lesions, especially in *L. major* and occasionally in *L. tropica* infections. Regional lymphadenopathy, pain, pruritus and secondary bacterial infections may occur. Clinically, lesions of *L. mexicana* and *L. peruviana* closely resemble those seen in the Old World, but lesions on the pinna of the ear are common, and are chronic and destructive. *L. mexicana* is responsible for chiclero ulcers, the self-healing sores of Mexico. If immunity is good, there is usually spontaneous healing in *L. tropica*, *L. major* and *L. mexicana* lesions. In some patients with anergy to *Leishmania*, the skin lesions of *L. aethiopica*, *L. mexicana* and *L. amazonensis* infections

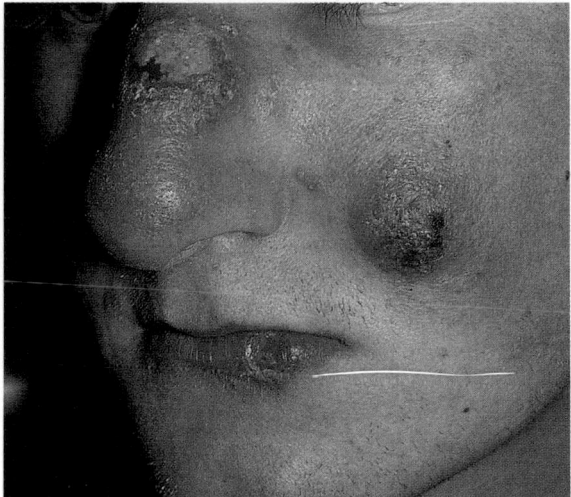

Fig. 13.52 Cutaneous leishmaniasis.

progress to the development of diffuse CL; this is characterised by spread of the infection from the initial ulcer, usually on the face, to involve the whole body in the form of non-ulcerative nodules. Occasionally, in *L. tropica* infections, sores that have apparently healed relapse persistently (recidivans or lupoid leishmaniasis).

Mucosal leishmaniasis

The *Viannia* subgenus extends widely from the Amazon basin as far as Paraguay and Costa Rica and is responsible for deep sores and mucosal leishmaniasis. In *L. (V.) brasiliensis* complex infections, cutaneous lesions may be followed by mucosal spread of the disease simultaneously or even years later. Young men with chronic lesions are particularly at risk, and between 2% and 40% of infected persons develop 'espundia', metastatic lesions in the mucosa of the nose or mouth. This is characterised by thickening and erythema of the nasal mucosa, typically starting at the junction of the nose and upper lip. Later, ulceration develops. The lips, soft palate, fauces and larynx may also be invaded and destroyed, leading to considerable suffering and deformity. There is no spontaneous healing, and death may result from severe respiratory tract infections due to massive destruction of the pharynx.

Pathogenesis

Microscopically, the appearances are similar to Old World CL. Mucosal lesions begin as a perivascular infiltration; later, endarteritis may cause destruction of the surrounding tissues.

Investigations in cutaneous and mucosal leishmaniasis

CL is often diagnosed on the basis of clinical characteristics of the lesions. However, parasitological confirmation is important because clinical manifestations may be mimicked by other infections and granulomatous diseases. Amastigotes can be demonstrated by making a slit skin smear and staining the material obtained with Giemsa stain; alternatively, they can be cultured from the sores early during the infection. Parasites seem to be particularly difficult to isolate from sores caused by *L. brasiliensis*, responsible for the vast majority of cases in Brazil. Touch preparations from biopsies and histopathology usually have a low sensitivity. Culture of fine needle aspiration material has been reported to be the most sensitive method. ML is more difficult to diagnose parasitologically. The leishmanin skin test is positive except in diffuse CL. PCR is used increasingly for diagnosis and speciation, greatly improving the diagnostic rates for both CL and ML. Speciation may be important for therapeutic reasons.

Management of cutaneous and mucosal leishmaniasis

There are few good randomised controlled trials of treatment for CL or ML. Small lesions may self-heal. There is no ideal therapy. Treatment should be individualised on the basis of the causative organism, severity of the lesions, availability of drugs, tolerance of the patient for toxicity, and local resistance patterns. Small lesions may be treated by freezing with liquid nitrogen or curettage. Topical application of paromomycin 15% plus methylbenzethonium chloride 12% is beneficial in both Old and New World CL. When the lesions are multiple or in a disfiguring site, it is better to treat with parenteral Sb in a dose of 20 mg/kg for 20 days. The same Sb regimen is indicated to prevent the development of mucosal disease, if there is any chance that a lesion acquired in South America is due to an *L. brasiliensis* strain. Intralesional Sb has also been used with encouraging results in both Old and New World CL. Intralesional antimony (0.2–0.8 ml/lesion) up to 2 g seems to be rapidly effective in suitable cases, well tolerated and economic, and is safe in patients with cardiac, liver or renal diseases. Two to four doses (2–4 mg/kg) of alternate-day administration of pentamidine is effective in New World CL. Ketoconazole 600 mg daily for 4 weeks has shown some potential against *L. mexicana* infection. In Saudi Arabia, fluconazole 200 mg daily for 6 weeks reduced healing times and cured 79% of patients with CL due to *L. major.* In India itraconazole 200 mg daily for 6 weeks

produced good results in CL. ML is treated with 28 days' systemic Sb. In ML, 8 injections of pentamidine (4 mg/kg on alternate days) cure the majority of patients. Refractory CL or ML should be treated with conventional or liposomal amphotericin B.

Prevention of cutaneous and mucosal leishmaniasis

Personal protection against sandfly bites is important. No effective vaccine is yet available.

AFRICAN TRYPANOSOMIASIS (SLEEPING SICKNESS)

African sleeping sickness is caused by trypanosomes (Fig. 13.53) conveyed to humans by the bites of infected tsetse flies, and is unique to sub-Saharan Africa. Two trypanosomes affect humans in Africa: *Trypanosoma brucei gambiense* and *T. rhodesiense. Gambiense* trypanosomiasis has a wide distribution in West and Central Africa; *rhodesiense* trypanosomiasis is found in parts of East and Central Africa, where it is currently on the increase (Fig. 13.54). In West Africa transmission is mainly at the riverside, where the fly rests in the shade of trees. The rural populations earning their livelihood from agriculture, fishing and animal husbandry are susceptible. Local people

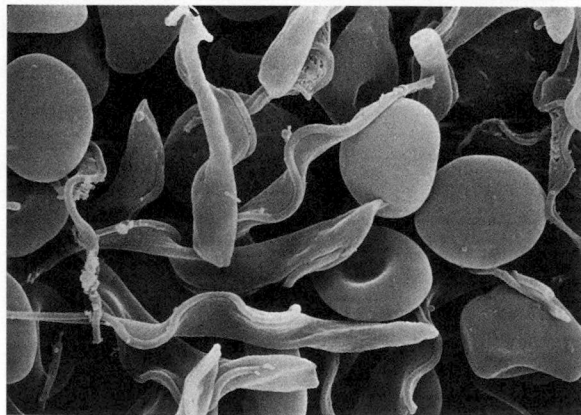

Fig. 13.53   Trypanosomiasis. Scanning electron micrograph showing trypanosomes swimming among erythrocytes.

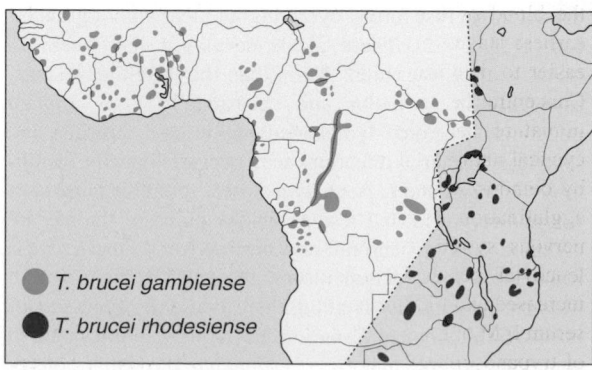

T. brucei gambiense

T. brucei rhodesiense

Fig. 13.54   Geographical distribution of African trypanosomiasis.

and tourists visiting forests infested with tsetse flies and animal reservoirs may become infected. Animal reservoirs of *T. gambiense* have not been identified. *T. rhodesiense* has a large reservoir in numerous wild animals and transmission takes place in the shade of woods bordering grasslands.

Clinical features

A bite by a tsetse fly is painful and commonly becomes inflamed, but if trypanosomes are introduced, the site may again become painful and swollen about 10 days later ('trypanosomal chancre') and the regional lymph nodes enlarge ('Winterbottom's sign'). Within 2–3 weeks of infection the trypanosomes invade the blood stream. The disease is characterised by an early haematolymphatic stage and a late encephalitic stage in which the parasite crosses the blood–brain barrier and chronic encephalopathy develops.

Rhodesiense *infections*

In these infections the disease is more acute and severe than in *gambiense* infections, so that within days or a few weeks the patient is usually severely ill and may have developed pleural effusions and signs of myocarditis or hepatitis. There may be a petechial rash. The patient may die before there are signs of involvement of the central nervous system. If the illness is less acute, drowsiness, tremors and coma develop.

Gambiense *infections*

The distinction between early and late stages may not be apparent in *gambiense* infections. The disease usually runs a slow course over months or years, with irregular bouts of fever and enlargement of lymph nodes. These are characteristically firm, discrete, rubbery and painless, and are particularly prominent in the posterior triangle of the neck. The spleen and liver may become palpable. After some months, in the absence of treatment, the central nervous system is invaded. This is shown clinically by headache and changed behaviour, blunting of higher mental functions, insomnia by night and sleepiness by day, mental confusion and eventually tremors, pareses, wasting, coma and death.

Investigations

Trypanosomiasis should be considered in any febrile patient from an endemic area. In *rhodesiense* infections thick and thin blood films, stained as for the detection of malaria, will reveal trypanosomes. The trypanosomes may be seen in the blood or from puncture of the primary lesion in the earliest stages of *gambiense* infections, but it is usually easier to demonstrate them by puncture of a lymph node. Concentration methods include buffy coat microscopy and miniature anion exchange chromatography. Due to the cyclical nature of parasitaemia, the diagnosis is often made by demonstration of antibodies using a simple, rapid card agglutination trypanosomiasis test (CATT). If the central nervous system is affected, the cell count ($> 20 \times 10^9$ leucoytes per litre) and protein content of the CSF are increased and the glucose is diminished. Very high levels of serum IgM or the presence of IgM in the CSF are suggestive of trypanosomiasis. Recognition of central nervous system involvement is critical as failure to treat it might be fatal.

13.61 DRUGS USED TO TREAT HUMAN AFRICAN TRYPANOSOMIASIS
***Gambiense* trypanosomiasis**
Stage 1 ● First-line: pentamidine ● Second-line: eflornithine or melarsoprol
Stage 2 ● First-line: melarsoprol ● Second-line: eflornithine
***Rhodesiense* trypanosomiasis**
Stage 1 ● First-line: suramin ● Second-line: melarsoprol
Stage 2 ● First-line: melarsoprol ● Second-line: nifurtimox combined with melarsoprol

Management

Unfortunately, therapeutic options for African trypanosomiasis are limited and most of the antitrypanosomal drugs are toxic and expensive. The prognosis is good if treatment is begun early before the brain has been invaded. At this stage intravenous suramin, after a test dose of 100–200 mg, should be given, 1 g on days 1, 3, 7, 14 and 21 for *rhodesiense* infections. For *gambiense* infections, intramuscular or intravenous pentamidine 4 mg/kg for 10 days is given (Box 13.61). Once the nervous system is affected, treatment with melarsoprol (an arsenical) is effective for both East and West African diseases. It is used in a dose of 2–3.6 mg/kg/day i.v. for the first course and 3.6 mg/kg thereafter. Two 3-day treatment courses are given at an interval of 7 days, and the 3-day cycle is repeated 10–21 days later. Treatment-related mortality with melarsoprol is 4–12% due to reactive encephalopathy. For central nervous system infections due to *gambiense*, eflornithine (DFMO), an irreversible inhibitor of ornithine decarboxylase, 100 mg/kg i.v. 6-hourly for 14 days, is considered to be a safer option.

Prevention

In endemic *gambiense* areas various measures may be taken against tsetse flies, and field teams help to detect and treat early human infection. In *rhodesiense* areas control is difficult.

AMERICAN TRYPANOSOMIASIS (CHAGAS DISEASE)

Chagas disease occurs widely in South and Central America. The cause is *Trypanosoma cruzi*, transmitted to humans from the faeces of a reduviid (triatomine) bug in which the trypanosomes have a cycle of development before becoming infective to humans. Bugs live in the wild (forests) in crevices, burrows and palm trees. *Triatoma infestans* has become domesticated in the Southern Cone countries (Argentina, Brazil, Chile, Paraguay and Uruguay). It lives in the mud and wattle walls and thatch roofs of simple rural

13

houses, and emerges at night to feed and defecate on the sleeping occupants. Infected faeces are rubbed in through the conjunctiva, mucosa of mouth or nose, or abrasions of the skin. Over 100 species of mammal, domestic, peridomestic and wild, may serve as reservoirs of infection. In some areas blood transfusion accounts for about 5% of cases. Congenital transmission occasionally occurs.

Pathology

The trypanosomes migrate via the blood stream, develop into amastigote forms in the tissues and multiply intracellularly by binary fission. In the acute phase (primarily cell-mediated) inflammation of parasitised as well as non-parasitised cardiac muscles and capillaries occurs, resulting in acute myocarditis. In the chronic phase focal myocardial atrophy, signs of chronic passive congestion and thrombo-embolic phenomena, cardiomegaly and apical cardiac aneurysm are salient findings in the cardiac form. Focal myositis and discontinuous lesions of the intramural myenteric plexus, predominantly in the oesophagus and colon, are seen in the digestive form.

Clinical features

Acute phase

The acute phase is seen in only 1–2% of infected individuals before the age of 15 years. Young children (1–5 years) are most commonly affected. The entrance of *T. cruzi* through an abrasion produces a dusky-red firm swelling and enlargement of regional lymph nodes. A conjunctival lesion, although less common, is more characteristic; the unilateral firm reddish swelling of the lids may close the eye and constitutes 'Romaña's sign'. In a few patients an acute generalised infection soon appears, with a transient morbilliform or urticarial rash, fever, lymphadenopathy and enlargement of the spleen and liver. In a small minority of patients acute myocarditis and heart failure or neurological features, including personality changes and signs of meningoencephalitis, may be seen. The acute infection may be fatal to infants.

Chronic phase

About 50–70% of infected patients become seropositive and develop an indeterminate form when no parasitaemia is detectable. They have a normal lifespan with no symptoms but are a natural reservoir for the disease and maintain the life cycle of parasites. After a latent period of several years, 10–30% of chronic cases develop low-grade myocarditis, and damage to conducting fibres causes a cardiomyopathy characterised by cardiac dilatation, arrhythmias, partial or complete heart block and sudden death. In nearly 10% of patients damage to Auerbach's plexus results in dilatation of various parts of the alimentary canal, especially the colon and oesophagus, so-called 'mega' disease. Dilatation of the bile ducts and bronchi is also a recognised sequela. Autoimmune processes may be responsible for much of the damage. There are geographical variations of the basic pattern of disease. Reactivation of Chagas disease can occur in patients with AIDS if the CD4 count falls lower than 200 cells/mm^3 (p. 381).

Investigations

T. cruzi is easily detectable in a blood film in the acute illness. In chronic disease it may be recovered in up to 50% of cases by xenodiagnosis in which infection-free, laboratory-bred reduviid bugs are allowed to feed on the patient; subsequently, the hind gut or faeces of the bug are examined for parasites. Parasite DNA detection by PCR is a highly sensitive method for documentation of infection. ELISA and indirect immunofluorescence are the two highly sensitive (99%) methods used for serodiagnosis, followed by an indirect haemagglutination test.

Management

The acute phase, congenital disease and indeterminate form of the chronic phase (within 10 years of infection) should be treated with parasiticidal drugs. Nifurtimox is given orally. The dose, which has to be carefully supervised to minimise toxicity while preserving parasiticidal activity, is 10 mg/kg divided into three equal doses, daily by mouth for 60–90 days. The paediatric dose is 15 mg/kg daily. Cure rates of 80% in acute disease are obtained. Benznidazole is an alternative drug given at a dose of 5–10 mg/kg daily by mouth, in two divided doses for 60 days; children receive 10 mg/kg daily. Both nifurtimox and benznidazole are toxic, with adverse reaction rates of 30–55%. Specific drug treatment of the cardiac or digestive form is not usually undertaken and does not reverse established tissue damage. Surgery may be needed for 'mega' disease.

Prevention

Preventative measures include improving housing and destruction of reduviid bugs by spraying of houses with insecticides. Blood donors should be screened.

ACQUIRED TOXOPLASMOSIS

Parasitology and epidemiology

Toxoplasma gondii is a coccidian intracellular parasite found in all species of warm-blooded animal. The sexual phase of the parasite's life cycle (Fig. 13.55) occurs in the small intestinal epithelium of the domestic cat. Oöcysts are shed in cat faeces and are spread to intermediate hosts (pork, lamb), including humans, through widespread contamination of soil. Oöcysts may survive in moist conditions for weeks or months. Once they are ingested by the intermediate host the parasite undergoes transformation, inside the intestinal epithelium, into rapidly dividing tachyzoites through cycles of asexual multiplication, and then infects other tissues. This leads to the formation of microscopic tissue cysts containing bradyzoites which persist for the lifetime of the host. Cats become infected or reinfected by ingesting tissue cysts in prey such as rodents and birds.

Human acquisition of infection occurs via oöcyst-contaminated soil, salads and vegetables, or by the ingestion or tasting of raw or undercooked meats containing tissue cysts. Sheep, pigs and rabbits are the most important food sources. Outbreaks of toxoplasmosis have been linked to the consumption of unfiltered water. In developed countries toxoplasmosis is the most common protozoal infection; around 22% of adults in the UK are seropositive. Most

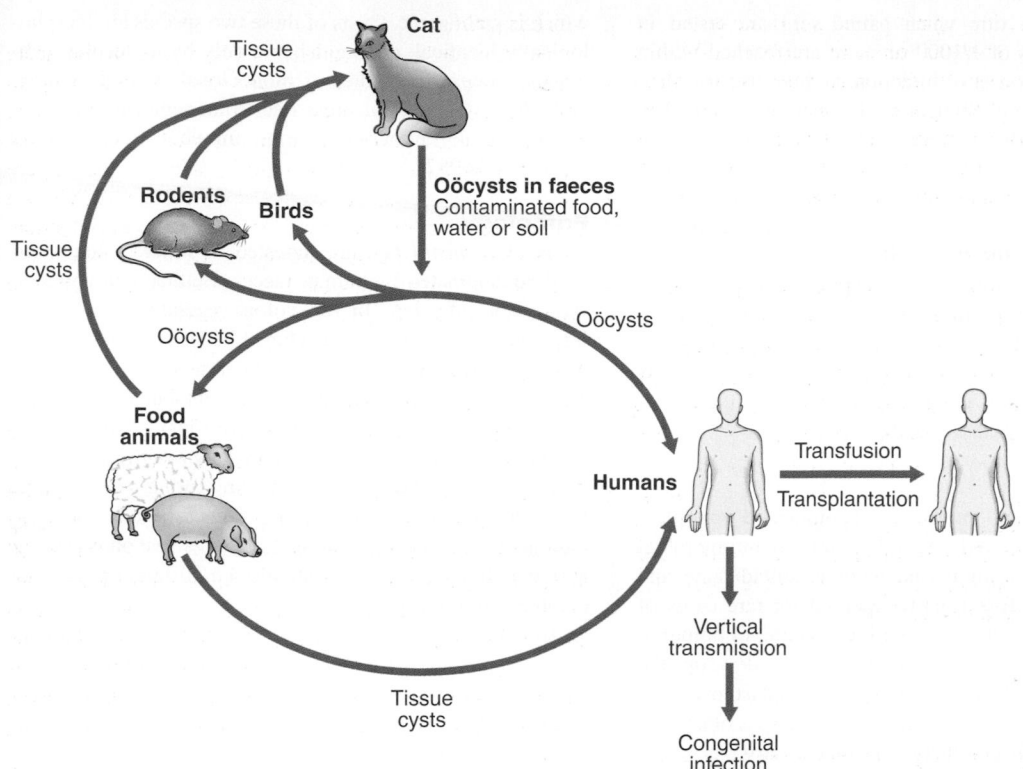

Fig. 13.55 Life cycle of *Toxoplasma gondii*.

13

primary infections are subclinical; however, toxoplasmosis is thought to account for about 15% of heterophile antibody-negative glandular fever. In countries like India or Brazil 42–60% of pregnant females are seropositive for *Toxoplasma*. In AIDS (p. 392), toxoplasmosis is an important opportunistic infection with considerable morbidity and mortality.

Clinical features

In most immunocompetent individuals, including children and pregnant women, the infection goes unnoticed. In about 10% of patients it causes a self-limiting illness. The peak incidence of clinical illness is in adults aged 25–35 years. The most common presenting feature is painless enlargement of lymph nodes. In particular, the cervical nodes are involved, but lymphadenopathy can be local or generalised and may involve the mediastinal, mesenteric or retroperitoneal groups. The spleen is seldom palpable. Most patients have no systemic symptoms, but some complain of malaise, fever, fatigue, muscle pain, sore throat and headache. Complete resolution usually occurs within a few months, although symptoms and lymphadenopathy tend to fluctuate unpredictably and some patients do not recover completely for a year or more. Sites other than lymph nodes are seldom involved clinically but, very infrequently, some patients may develop encephalitis, myocarditis, polymyositis, pneumonitis or hepatitis. Retinochoroiditis (Fig. 13.56) is nearly always the result of remote or congenital infection but has also been reported to arise de novo in the acquired form of the disease. Generalised toxoplasmosis has been described after accidental laboratory infection with highly virulent strains.

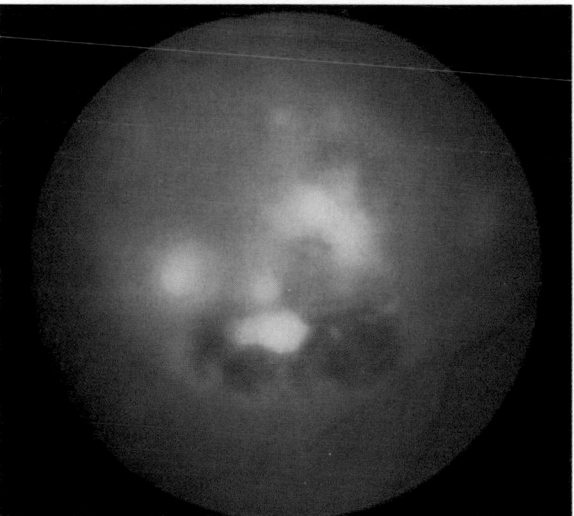

Fig. 13.56 Retinochoroiditis due to toxoplasmosis.

Investigations

In contrast to the immunocompromised patients in whom the diagnosis often requires direct detection of parasites, indirect serology is often used in immunocompetent individuals. During pregnancy it is critical to differentiate between recent and past infection. Avidity tests for IgG are reliable and the presence of high-avidity antibodies excludes infection acquired in the preceding 3–4 months. Other tests for serological diagnosis include the Sabin–Feldman dye test (indirect fluorescent antibody test), which detects IgG antibody. Recent infection is indicated by a fourfold or greater increase in titre when paired sera are tested in parallel. Peak titres of 1/1000 or more are reached within 1–2 months of the onset of infection, and the dye test then becomes an unreliable indicator of recent infection. The detection of significant levels of *Toxoplasma*-specific IgM antibody using double sandwich IgM ELISA and IgM immunosorbent agglutination assay (ISAGA) may be useful in confirming acute infection. False positives or persistence of IgM antibodies for years after infection make interpretation difficult; however, negative IgM antibodies virtually rule out acute infection.

If necessary, the presence of *Toxoplasma* organisms in a lymph node biopsy can be sought by staining sections histochemically with *T. gondii* antiserum, or by the use of PCR to detect *Toxoplasma*-specific DNA.

Management

In immunocompetent subjects uncomplicated toxoplasmosis is self-limiting and responds poorly to antimicrobial therapy. Treatment with pyrimethamine, sulfadiazine and folinic acid is therefore usually reserved for rare cases of severe or progressive disease, and for infection in immunocompromised patients. A few individuals develop the chronic fatigue syndrome after acute toxoplasmosis, but there is no evidence that their immune response is other than normal and antimicrobial therapy is unnecessary.

CONGENITAL TOXOPLASMOSIS

Acute toxoplasmosis, mostly subclinical, affects 0.3–1% of pregnancies with a 60% transmission rate to the fetus. The chance of transmission is lowest in early pregnancy and greatest in the third trimester. However, the overall incidence and severity of congenital disease (40% of infected fetuses) are greatest in the first trimester, but extend into the third trimester of pregnancy. Many fetal infections are subclinical at birth but long-term sequelae occur in almost all cases. The main features are retinochoroiditis, microcephaly and hydrocephalus. In a pregnancy with an established recent infection, spiramycin (3 g daily in divided doses) should be given until term. Once fetal infection is established, treatment with sulfadiazine, pyrimethamine plus calcium folinate is recommended (spiramycin does not cross the placental barrier). The cost/benefit of routine *Toxoplasma* screening and treatment in pregnancy is being debated in many countries. There is insufficient evidence to determine the effects on mother or baby of current antiparasitic treatment for women who seroconvert in pregnancy.

GASTROINTESTINAL PROTOZOAL INFECTIONS

AMOEBIASIS

Amoebiasis is caused by *Entamoeba histolytica*, which is spread between humans by its cysts. It is common throughout the tropics and occasionally acquired in the UK. The parasite is now known to consist of two separate species: *E. dispar* (non-pathogenic) and *E. histolytica*, which is pathogenic. Cysts of these two species are morphologically identical, distinguishable only by molecular techniques, isoenzyme studies or monoclonal antibody typing. Only *E. histolytica* can give rise to amoebic dysentery or extraintestinal amoebiasis, e.g. amoebic liver abscess (pp. 359 and 987).

Pathology

Cysts of *E. histolytica* are ingested in water or uncooked food contaminated by human faeces. Lettuce is a common vehicle of infection. In the colon vegetative trophozoite forms emerge from the cysts (Fig. 13.57). The parasite may invade the mucous membrane of the large bowel, producing lesions that are maximal in the caecum but found as far down as the anal canal. These are flask-shaped ulcers varying greatly in size and surrounded by healthy mucosa. A localised granuloma (amoeboma), presenting as a palpable mass in the rectum or a filling defect in the colon on radiography, is a rare complication. This responds well to anti-amoebic treatment so should be differentiated from colonic carcinoma.

Amoebic ulcers may cause severe haemorrhage but rarely perforate the bowel wall. Cutaneous amoebiasis causes progressive genital, perianal or peri-abdominal surgical wound ulceration.

Clinical features

Intestinal amoebiasis or amoebic dysentery

The incubation period of amoebiasis ranges from 2 weeks to many years, followed by a chronic course with grumbling abdominal pains and two or more unformed stools a day. Diarrhoea alternating with constipation is common, as is mucus, sometimes with streaks of blood; the stools often have an offensive odour. There may be tenderness along the line of the colon, especially over the caecum (which may simulate acute appendicitis) and pelvic colon. Acute bowel symptoms, with very frequent motions and the passage of much blood and mucus, simulating bacillary dysentery or ulcerative colitis, occur particularly in older people, in the puerperium and with superadded pyogenic infection of the ulcers.

Diagnosis

Any exudate should be examined at once under the microscope for motile trophozoites containing red blood cells. Movements cease rapidly as the stool preparation cools. Sigmoidoscopy may reveal typical flask-shaped ulcers, which should be scraped and examined immediately for *E. histolytica*. Several stools may need to be examined in chronic amoebiasis before cysts are found. In endemic areas one-third of the population are symptomless passers of amoebic cysts.

Antibodies are detectable by immunofluorescence in over 95% of patients with hepatic amoebiasis and intestinal amoeboma but in only about 60% of dysenteric amoebiasis.

Management

Intestinal amoebiasis responds quickly to oral metronidazole (800 mg 8-hourly for 5 days) or tinidazole (2 g daily for 3 days). Diloxanide furoate 500 mg should be given orally

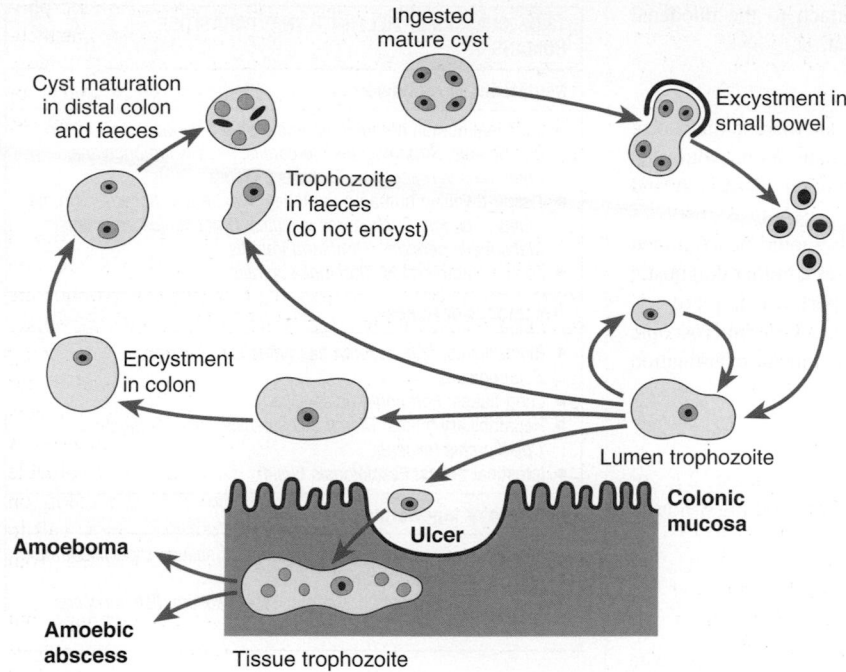

Fig. 13.57 **Amoebiasis.** The life cycle of *Entamoeba histolytica*.

13

8-hourly for 10 days after treatment to eliminate luminal cysts. Hepatic amoebiasis is dealt with on page 987.

Prevention

Personal precautions against contracting amoebiasis consist of not eating fresh uncooked vegetables or drinking unboiled water.

AMOEBIC LIVER ABSCESS

This often occurs without a history of recent diarrhoea. It is common in the tropics and an important cause of imported fever in Britain. The life cycle of the amoeba is shown in Figure 13.57.

Pathogenesis

Amoebic trophozoites emerge from the vegetative cyst form in the colon and may invade the bowel mucosa. They may enter a portal venous radicle and be carried to the liver where they multiply rapidly and destroy the parenchyma, causing an amoebic abscess. The liquid contents at first have a characteristic pinkish colour which may later change to chocolate brown.

Clinical features

The abscess is usually found in the right hepatic lobe. Early symptoms may be local discomfort only and malaise; later, a swinging temperature and sweating may develop. An enlarged, tender liver, cough and pain in the right shoulder are characteristic, but symptoms may remain vague and signs minimal (p. 987). The absence of toxicity in the presence of a high swinging fever is noticeable. The less common abscess in the left lobe is difficult to diagnose. There is usually neutrophil leucocytosis and a raised diaphragm, with diminished movement on the right side. A large abscess may penetrate the diaphragm and rupture into the lung, from where its contents may be coughed up. Rupture into the pleural cavity, the peritoneal cavity or pericardial sac is less common but more serious.

Investigations

An amoebic abscess of the liver is suspected from the clinical and radiographic appearances and confirmed by ultrasonic scanning. Aspirated pus from an amoebic abscess has the characteristic appearance described above but only rarely contains free amoebae.

Antibodies are detectable by immunofluorescence in over 95% of patients with hepatic amoebiasis.

Management

Early hepatic amoebiasis responds promptly to treatment with metronidazole (800 mg 8-hourly for 5 days) or tinidazole (2 g daily for 3 days) as above. The luminal amoebicide diloxanide furoate (500 mg 8-hourly for 10 days) is given to eliminate the intestinal infection. If the abscess is large or threatens to burst, or if the response to chemotherapy is not prompt, aspiration is required and repeated if necessary. Rupture of an abscess into the pleural cavity, pericardial sac or peritoneal cavity necessitates immediate aspiration or surgical drainage. Small serous effusions resolve without drainage.

GIARDIASIS

Infection with *Giardia intestinalis*, also known as *G. lamblia*, is found world-wide and is common in the tropics. It particularly affects children, tourists and immuno-suppressed individuals, and is the parasite most commonly imported into the UK. The cysts remain viable in water for up to 3 months and infection usually occurs by ingesting contaminated water. The parasites attach to the duodenal and jejunal mucosa, causing inflammation.

Clinical features

After an incubation period of 1–3 weeks, there is diarrhoea, abdominal pain, weakness, anorexia, nausea and vomiting. On examination there may be abdominal distension and tenderness.

Stools obtained at 2–3-day intervals should be examined for cysts. Duodenal or jejunal fluid gives a higher diagnostic yield. Thus if endoscopy is being performed, giardiasis should be considered and juice aspirated for microscopic examination. On jejunal biopsy fresh mucus examination may show *Giardia* on the epithelial surface.

Management

Treatment is with a single dose of tinidazole 2 g, or metronidazole 2 g once daily for 3 days or 400 mg 8-hourly for 10 days.

CRYPTOSPORIDIOSIS

Cryptosporidium parvum is a coccidian protozoal parasite of humans and domestic animals. Infection is acquired by the faecal–oral route through contaminated water supplies. The incubation period is approximately 7–10 days, and is followed by watery diarrhoea and abdominal cramps. The illness is usually self-limiting, but in immunocompromised patients, especially those with AIDS, the illness can be devastating, with persistent severe diarrhoea and substantial weight loss (p. 387).

CYCLOSPORIASIS

Cyclospora cayetanensis is a newly recognised coccidian protozoal parasite of humans. It has been reported from Nepal, the Indian subcontinent and South America. Infection is acquired by ingestion of contaminated water. The incubation period is approximately 2–11 days, and is followed by acute onset of diarrhoea with abdominal cramps. The disease can remit and relapse. Although usually self-limiting, the illness may last as long as 6 weeks with significant associated weight loss and malabsorption. The disease is more severe in immunocompromised individuals. Diagnosis is by detection of oöcysts on faecal microscopy. Treatment may be necessary in a few cases, and the agent of choice is co-trimoxazole 960 mg 12-hourly for 7 days.

INFECTIONS CAUSED BY HELMINTHS

Helminths (from the Greek *Helmins*, meaning worm) include several classes of parasitic worm (Box 13.62), large multicellular organisms with complex tissues and organs.

Three groups of helminths parasitise humans:

- annelids (segmented worms), which include leeches
- nematodes (roundworms)
- platyhelminths (flatworms), which include trematodes (flukes) and cestodes (tapeworms).

13.62 CLASSES OF HELMINTH THAT PARASITISE HUMANS

Nematodes or roundworms

- Intestinal human nematodes: *Ancylostoma duodenale, Necator americanus, Strongyloides stercoralis, Ascaris lumbricoides, Enterobius vermicularis, Trichuris trichiura*
- Tissue-dwelling human nematodes: *Wuchereria bancrofti, Brugia malayi, Loa loa, Onchocerca volvulus, Dracunculus medinensis, Mansonella perstans, Dirofilaria immitis*
- Zoonotic nematodes: *Trichinella spiralis*

Trematodes or flukes

- Blood flukes: *Schistosoma haematobium, S. mansoni, S. japonicum*
- Lung flukes: *Paragonimus* species
- Hepatobiliary flukes: *Clonorchis sinensis, Fasciola hepatica, Opisthorchis felineus*
- Intestinal flukes: *Fasciolopsis buski*

Cestodes or tapeworms

- Intestinal tapeworms: *Taenia saginata, T. solium, Diphyllobothrium latum, Hymenolepis nana*
- Tissue-dwelling cysts or worms: *Taenia solium, Echinococcus granulosus*

INTESTINAL HUMAN NEMATODES

Disease is caused by adult nematodes living in the human gut. There are two types: the hookworms which have a soil stage and develop into larvae which then penetrate the host, and a group of nematodes which survive in the soil merely as eggs that have to be ingested for the cycle to continue. The geographical distribution of hookworms is limited by the larval requirement for warmth and humidity.

ANCYLOSTOMIASIS (HOOKWORM)

Ancylostomiasis is caused by parasitisation of the small intestine with *Ancylostoma duodenale* or *Necator americanus*. It is one of the main causes of anaemia in the tropics. In the early stages of infection eosinophilia is common. The adult hookworm is 1 cm long and lives in the duodenum and upper jejunum. Eggs are passed in the faeces. In warm, moist, shady soil the larvae develop into the filariform infective stage; they then penetrate human skin and are carried to the lungs (Fig. 13.58). After entering the alveoli they ascend the bronchi, are swallowed and mature in the small intestine, reaching maturity 4–7 weeks after infection.

Hookworm infection is widespread in the tropics and subtropics. *A. duodenale* is endemic in the Far East and Mediterranean coastal regions and is also present in Africa, while *N. americanus* is endemic in West, East and Central Africa and Central and South America, as well as in the Far East.

Pathology

The larvae may cause allergic inflammation at the site of entry through the skin. When infection is heavy, the passage through the lungs may cause pulmonary eosinophilia. The

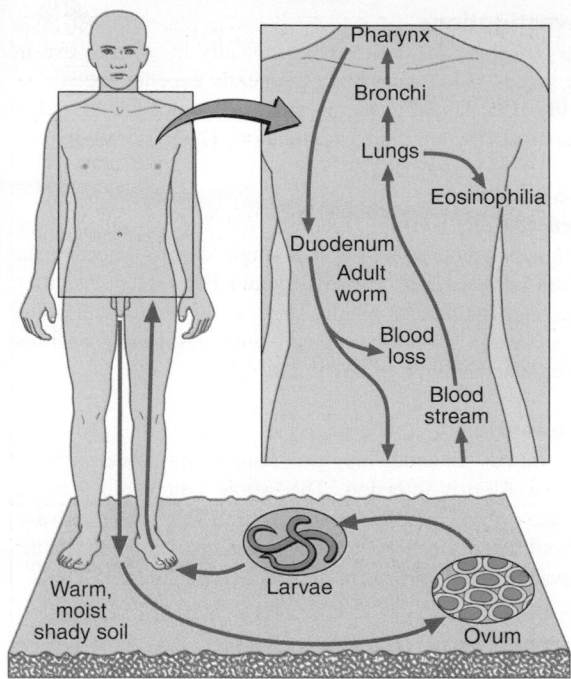

Fig. 13.58 **Ancylostomiasis.** Life cycle of *Ancylostoma*.

(Labels in figure: Pharynx, Bronchi, Lungs, Eosinophilia, Duodenum, Adult worm, Blood loss, Blood stream, Warm, moist shady soil, Larvae, Ovum)

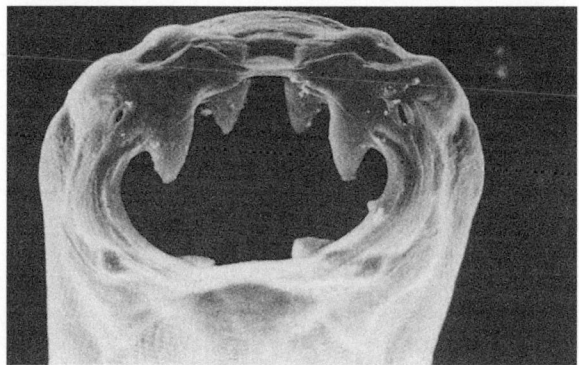

Fig. 13.59 *Ancylostoma duodenale.* Electron micrograph showing the ventral teeth.

worms attach themselves to the mucosa of the small intestine by their buccal capsule (Fig. 13.59) and withdraw blood. The mean daily loss of blood from one *A. duodenale* is 0.15 ml and from *N. americanus* 0.03 ml. The degree of iron and protein deficiency which develops depends not only on the load of worms but also on the nutrition of the patient and especially on the iron stores. In a light infection there may be no anaemia.

Clinical features

Dermatitis, usually on the feet (ground itch), may be experienced at the time of infection. The passage of the larvae through the lungs in a heavy infection causes a paroxysmal cough with blood-stained sputum, associated with patchy pulmonary consolidation. When the worms have reached the small intestine, vomiting and epigastric pain resembling peptic ulcer disease may occur. Sometimes frequent loose stools are passed. Iron deficiency anaemia,

protein-losing enteropathy and hypoproteinaemia may develop in the undernourished. High-output cardiac failure may result from the chronic iron deficiency anaemia. The mental and physical development of children may be retarded. A well-nourished person with a light infection may be asymptomatic.

Investigations

There is eosinophilia. The characteristic ovum can be recognised in the stool. If hookworms are present in numbers sufficient to cause anaemia, faecal occult blood testing will be positive and many ova will be present.

Management

Mebendazole 100 mg 12-hourly for 3 days is preferred, but for single-dose treatment albendazole (400 mg) is the best choice. Anaemia associated with hookworm infection responds well to oral iron. The management of anaemic heart disease is best accomplished by treatment with anthelmintics and iron. Blood transfusion should only be used with great care in very severely anaemic patients (< 40 g/l).

STRONGYLOIDIASIS

Strongyloides stercoralis is a very small nematode (2 mm × 0.4 mm) which parasitises the mucosa of the upper part of the small intestine, often in large numbers, causing persistent eosinophilia. The eggs hatch in the bowel but only larvae are passed in the faeces. In moist soil they moult and become the infective filariform larvae. After penetrating human skin they undergo a development cycle similar to that of hookworms but the female worms burrow into the intestinal mucosa and submucosa. Some larvae in the intestine may develop into filariform larvae which may then penetrate the mucosa or the perianal skin and lead to autoinfection and persistent infection. Patients with *Strongyloides* infection persisting for more than 35 years have been described. Strongyloidiasis occurs in the tropics and subtropics and is especially prevalent in the Far East.

Pathology

Worms burrow into the intestinal mucosa, inducing an inflammatory reaction. Eosinophilia commonly persists. Actively motile larvae are passed in the faeces.

Clinical features

These are shown in Box 13.63. The classic triad of symptoms consists of abdominal pain, diarrhoea and urticaria. Cutaneous manifestations, either urticaria or larva currens, are characteristic and occur in 66% of patients. Systemic strongyloidiasis (the *Strongyloides* hyperinfestation syndrome), with dissemination of larvae throughout the body, occurs in association with immune suppression (intercurrent disease, HTLV 1 infection, corticosteroid treatment). Patients present with severe, generalised abdominal pain, abdominal distension and shock. Massive larval invasion of the lungs causes cough, wheeze and dyspnoea; cerebral involvement has manifestations ranging from subtle neurological signs to coma. Gram-negative sepsis frequently complicates the picture.

13

13.63 CLINICAL FEATURES OF STRONGYLOIDIASIS

Penetration of skin by infective larvae

- Itchy rash

Presence of worms in gut

- Abdominal pain, diarrhoea, steatorrhoea, weight loss

Allergic phenomena

- Urticarial plaques and papules, wheezing, arthralgia

Autoinfection

- Transient itchy linear urticarial weals across abdomen and buttocks (larva currens)

Systemic (super)infection

- Diarrhoea, pneumonia, meningoencephalitis, death

Investigations

There is eosinophilia. The faeces should be examined microscopically for motile larvae. Excretion is intermittent so repeated examinations may be necessary. Larvae can also be found in jejunal aspirate or detected using the string test. Serology (ELISA) is helpful, but definitive diagnosis depends upon finding the larvae. Larvae may also be cultured from faeces.

Management

Ivermectin 200 µg/kg as a single dose, or two doses of 200 µg/kg on successive days, is effective. Albendazole is given orally in a dose of 15 mg/kg body weight 12-hourly for 3 days. A second course may be required. For the *Strongyloides* hyperinfestation syndrome, ivermectin is given at 200 µg/kg on days 1, 2, 15 and 16.

ASCARIS LUMBRICOIDES (ROUNDWORM)

This pale yellow nematode is 20–35 cm long. Humans are infected by eating food contaminated with mature ova. *Ascaris* larvae hatch in the duodenum, migrate through the lungs, ascend the bronchial tree, are swallowed and mature in the small intestine. This tissue migration can provoke both local and general hypersensitivity reactions with pneumonitis, eosinophilic granulomas, bronchial asthma and urticaria.

Clinical features

Intestinal ascariasis causes symptoms ranging from occasional vague abdominal pain through to malnutrition. The large size of the adult worm and its tendency to aggregate and migrate can result in severe obstructive complications. In endemic areas ascariasis causes up to 35% of all intestinal obstructions, most commonly in the terminal ileum. Obstruction can be complicated further by intussusception, volvulus, haemorrhagic infarction and perforation. Other complications include blockage of the bile or pancreatic duct and obstruction of the appendix by adult worms.

Investigations

The diagnosis is made microscopically by finding ova in the faeces. Adult worms are frequently expelled rectally or orally. Occasionally, the worms are demonstrated radiographically by a barium examination. There is eosinophilia.

Management

Mebendazole 100 mg 12-hourly for 3 days, albendazole 400 mg or piperazine 4 g as a single dose is effective for intestinal ascariasis. Patients should be warned that they may expel numerous whole, large worms. Obstruction due to ascariasis should be treated with nasogastric suction, piperazine and intravenous fluids.

Prevention

Community chemotherapy programmes have been used to reduce *Ascaris* infection. The whole community can be treated every 3 months and over several years. Alternatively, schoolchildren can be targeted; treating them lowers the prevalence of ascariasis in the whole community.

ENTEROBIUS VERMICULARIS (THREADWORM)

This helminth is common throughout the world. It affects children especially. After the ova are swallowed, development takes place in the small intestine, but the adult worms are found chiefly in the colon.

Clinical features

The gravid female worm lays ova around the anus, causing intense itching, especially at night. The ova are often carried to the mouth on the fingers and so reinfection takes place (Fig. 13.60). In females the genitalia may be involved. The adult worms may be seen moving on the buttocks or in the stool.

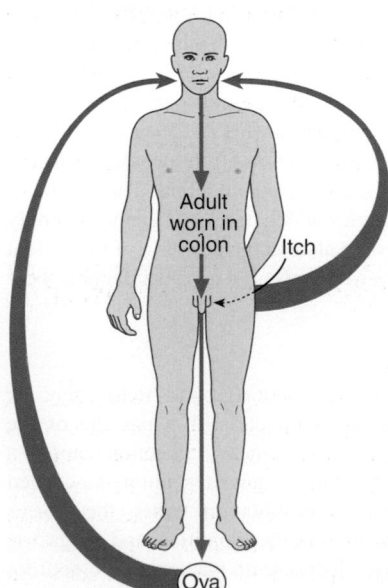

Fig. 13.60 Threadworm. Life cycle of *Enterobius vermicularis*.

13

Investigations

Ova are detected by applying the adhesive surface of cellophane tape to the perianal skin in the morning. This is then examined on a glass slide under the microscope. A perianal swab, moistened with saline, is an alternative method for diagnosis.

Management

A single dose of mebendazole 100 mg, albendazole 400 mg or piperazine 4 g is given and may be repeated after 2 weeks to control auto-reinfection. Where infection constantly recurs in a family, each member should be treated as above. During this period all nightclothes and bed linen are laundered. Fingernails must be kept short and hands washed carefully before meals. Subsequent therapy is reserved for those family members who develop recurrent infection.

TRICHURIS TRICHIURA (WHIPWORM)

Infections with whipworm are common all over the world under unhygienic conditions. Infection is contracted by the ingestion of earth or food contaminated with ova which have become infective after lying for 3 weeks or more in moist soil. The adult worm is 3–5 cm long and has a coiled anterior end resembling a whip. Whipworms inhabit the caecum, lower ileum, appendix, colon and anal canal. There are usually no symptoms, but intense infections in children may cause persistent diarrhoea or rectal prolapse, and stunting. The diagnosis is readily made by identifying ova in faeces. Treatment is with mebendazole in doses of 100 mg 12-hourly for 3–5 days or a single dose of albendazole 400 mg.

PREVENTION OF SOIL-TRANSMITTED HELMINTHIASES

This is achieved by preventing contact with faecally contaminated soil; the provision of adequate sewerage disposal could eliminate hookworm infestation. The use of footwear also reduces hookworm infection. Transmission of intestinal nematodes is through contaminated soil or unwashed hands. Safe disposal of faeces, the provision of clean drinking water and strict personal hygiene form the basis of control.

TISSUE-DWELLING HUMAN NEMATODES

FILARIASES

Filarial worms are tissue-dwelling nematodes. The larval stages are inoculated by biting mosquitoes or flies, each specific to a particular filarial species. The larvae develop into adult worms (2–50 cm long) which, after mating, produce millions of microfilariae (170–320 microns long) that migrate in blood or skin. The life cycle is completed when the vector takes up microfilariae while feeding on humans, normally the only host.

13.64 PATHOGENICITY OF FILARIAL INFECTIONS DEPENDING ON SITE AND STAGE OF WORMS

Worm species	Adult worm	Microfilariae
Wuchereria bancrofti and *Brugia malayi*	Lymphatic vessels[+++]	Blood[−] Pulmonary capillaries[++]
Loa loa	Subcutaneous[+]	Blood[+]
Onchocerca volvulus	Subcutaneous[+]	Skin[+++] Eye[+++]
Mansonella perstans	Retroperitoneal[−]	Blood[−]
Mansonella streptocerca	Skin[+]	Skin[++]

(+++ severe; ++ moderate; + mild; − rarely pathogenic)

Disease is due to the host's immune response to the worms (both adult and microfilariae), particularly dying worms, and its pattern and severity vary with the site and stage of each species (Box 13.64). The worms are long-lived; microfilariae survive 2–3 years and adult worms 10–15 years. The infections are chronic and worst in individuals constantly exposed to reinfection.

LYMPHATIC FILARIASIS

Infection with the filarial worms *Wuchereria bancrofti* and *Brugia malayi* is associated with clinical outcomes ranging from subclinical infection to hydrocele and elephantiasis. *W. bancrofti* is transmitted by night-biting *Culex quinquefasciatus* mosquitoes. The adult worms, 4–10 cm in length, live in the lymphatics, and the females produce microfilariae which at night circulate in large numbers in the peripheral blood. In the mosquito, ingested microfilariae develop into infective larvae. The infection is widespread in tropical Africa, the North African coast, coastal areas of Asia, Indonesia and northern Australia, the South Pacific islands, the West Indies and also in North and South America. *B. malayi* is similar to *W. bancrofti* and is found in Indonesia, Borneo, Malaysia, Vietnam, South China, South India and Sri Lanka.

Pathology

Four factors are central to the pathogenesis of lymphatic filariasis: the living adult worm, the inflammatory response caused by the death of the worm, microfilariae and secondary infections. Toxins released by the adult worm cause lymphangiectasia. Dilatation of the lymphatic vessel leads to lymphatic dysfunction and the chronic clinical manifestations of lymphatic filariasis, lymphoedema and hydrocele. Death of the adult worm results in acute filarial lymphangitis. Lymphatic obstruction persists after death of the adult worm. Secondary bacterial infections cause tissue destruction. Microfilariae are central to the pathogenesis of tropical pulmonary eosinophilia (Fig. 13.61).

Clinical features

Acute filarial lymphangitis presents with fever, pain, tenderness and erythema along the course of inflamed lymphatic vessels. Inflammation of the spermatic cord,

13

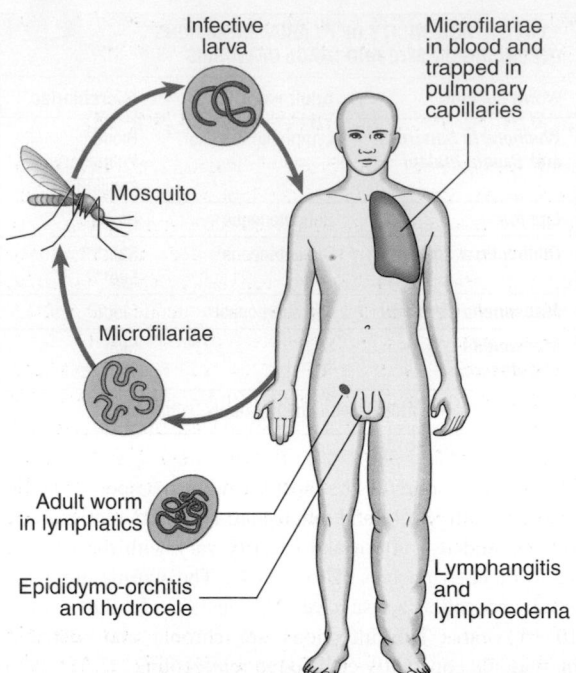

Fig. 13.61 *Wuchereria bancrofti* and *Brugia malayi*. Life cycle of organisms and pathogenesis of lymphatic filariasis.

epididymitis and orchitis are common. The whole episode lasts a few days but may recur several times a year. Temporary oedema becomes more persistent and regional lymph nodes enlarge. Progressive enlargement, coarsening, corrugation and fissuring of the skin and subcutaneous tissue develop gradually, causing irreversible 'elephantiasis'. The scrotum may reach an enormous size. Chyluria and chylous effusions are milky and opalescent; on standing, fat globules rise to the top. Elephantiasis develops only in association with repeated skin sepsis.

The acute lymphatic manifestations of filariasis must be differentiated from thrombophlebitis and infection. The oedema and lymphatic obstructive changes must be distinguished from congestive cardiac failure, malignancy, trauma and idiopathic abnormalities of the lymphatic system.

Tropical pulmonary eosinophilia

This condition is seen mainly in India and is likely to be due to microfilariae trapped in the pulmonary capillaries and destroyed by allergic inflammation. Patients present with paroxysmal cough, wheeze and fever. The chest X-ray shows miliary changes or mottled opacities. LFTs show a restrictive picture. If untreated, this progresses to debilitating chronic interstitial lung disease.

There is no specific therapy for this condition but the lymphatic damage can be managed actively as outlined for filarial elephantiasis.

Investigations

In the earliest stages of lymphangitis the diagnosis is made on clinical grounds, supported by eosinophilia and sometimes by positive filarial serology. Filarial infections cause the highest eosinophilia of all helminthic infections.

Microfilariae are found in the peripheral blood at night and can be seen moving in a wet blood film or by microfiltration of a sample of lysed blood. They are usually present in hydrocele fluid which may occasionally yield an adult filaria. By the time elephantiasis develops, microfilariae become difficult to find. Calcified filariae may sometimes be demonstrable by radiography. Movement of adult worms can be seen on scrotal ultrasound. Indirect fluorescence and ELISA detect antibodies in over 95% of active cases and 70% of established elephantiasis. The test becomes negative 1–2 years after cure. Serological tests cannot distinguish the different filarial infections. In tropical pulmonary eosinophilia, serology is strongly positive and IgE levels are massively elevated but circulating microfilariae are not found.

Management

Treatment of the individual is aimed at reversing and halting disease progression. Diethylcarbamazine (DEC) kills microfilariae and adult worms. The dose is 6 mg/kg daily orally in three divided doses for 12 days. The full dose must be reached slowly, starting with 50 mg and doubling daily unless serious allergic reactions ensue. Most adverse effects seen with DEC treatment are due to the host response to dying microfilariae, and the reaction intensity is directly proportional to the microfilarial load. The main symptoms are fever, headache, nausea, vomiting, arthralgia and prostration. These usually occur within 24–36 hours of the first dose of DEC. Antihistamines or corticosteroids may be required to control these allergic phenomena. Both the 12-day course and a single dose of DEC reduce microfilaria levels by about 90% 6–12 months after treatment. No carefully controlled trials have evaluated the effects of DEC treatment alone on the chronic manifestations of lymphatic filariasis. Ivermectin may also be used.

Chronic lymphatic pathology

Experience in India and Brazil shows that active management of chronic lymphatic pathology can alleviate symptoms. Patients should be taught meticulous local care of their lymphoedematous limbs with assiduous skin care to prevent secondary bacterial and fungal infections. Tight bandaging, massage and bed rest with elevation of the affected limb may help to control the lymphoedema. Prompt diagnosis and antibiotic therapy of bacterial cellulitis are important in preventing further lymphatic damage and worsening of existing elephantiasis. Patient education is a critical feature of lymphoedema treatment, both to alter fatalistic beliefs about inevitable progression of disease and to foster motivation. Plastic surgery may be indicated in established elephantiasis. Great relief can be obtained by removal of excess tissue but recurrences are probable unless new lymphatic drainage is established. Hydroceles can be repaired surgically; chyluria can also be corrected surgically.

Prevention

Treatment of the whole population in endemic areas with annual single-dose DEC, 100 mg for adults (50 mg for children), has reduced but not eliminated the infection. Ivermectin, alone or in combination with albendazole, is

13

under evaluation as an alternative to DEC. This mass treatment should be combined with mosquito control programmes.

NON-FILARIAL ELEPHANTIASIS

This occurs in certain filaria-free geographical areas and affects one or both legs. It is due to lymphatic damage by silicates absorbed from volcanic soil. There is no specific therapy for this condition but the lymphatic damage can be managed actively as outlined above for filarial elephantiasis.

LOIASIS

Loiasis is caused by infection with the filaria *Loa loa*. The adults, 3–7 cm × 4 mm, chiefly parasitise the subcutaneous tissue of humans. The larval microfilariae circulate harmlessly in the peripheral blood in the daytime. The vector is *Chrysops*, a forest-dwelling, day-biting fly.

Pathology

The adult worms move harmlessly about in the subcutaneous tissues and other interstitial planes. From time to time a short-lived, inflammatory, oedematous swelling (a Calabar swelling) is produced around an adult worm. Heavy infections, especially when treated, may cause encephalitis. The incubation period is commonly over a year but may be just 3 months.

Clinical features

The infection is often symptomless. The first sign is usually a Calabar swelling, an irritating, tense, localised swelling that may be painful, especially if it is near a joint. The swelling is generally on a limb; it measures a few centimetres in diameter but sometimes is more diffuse and extensive. It usually disappears after a few days but may persist for 2 or 3 weeks. A succession of such swellings may appear at irregular intervals, often in adjacent sites. Sometimes there is urticaria and pruritus elsewhere. Occasionally, a worm may be seen wriggling under the skin, especially that of an eyelid, and may cross the eye under the conjunctiva, taking many minutes to do so.

Investigations

Diagnosis is by demonstrating microfilariae in blood taken during the day, but they may not always be found in patients with Calabar swellings. Antifilarial antibodies are positive in 95% of patients; there is massive eosinophilia. Occasionally, a calcified worm may be seen on X-ray.

Management

DEC (see above) is curative, gradually increased to a dose of 9–12 mg/kg daily which is continued for 21 days. Treatment may precipitate a severe reaction in patients with a heavy microfilaraemia characterised by fever, joint and muscle pain, and encephalitis; microfilaraemic patients should be given corticosteroid cover.

Prevention

Protection is afforded by building houses away from trees and by having dwellings wire-screened. Protective clothing and repellents are also useful. DEC in a dose of 5 mg/kg daily for 3 days each month is partially protective.

ONCHOCERCIASIS (RIVER BLINDNESS)

Onchocerciasis is the result of infection by the filarial *Onchocerca volvulus*. The infection is conveyed by flies of the genus *Simulium* which inflict a painful bite. The flies breed in rapidly flowing, well-aerated water, the larvae being attached to submerged vegetation, rocks or crabs. Adult flies bite during the day both inside and outside houses. Humans are the only known definitive hosts.

Onchocerciasis is endemic in sub-Saharan Africa, Yemen, and a few foci in Central and South America. It is currently estimated that 17.7 million people are infected, with 500 000 being visually impaired and 270 000 blind. Due to onchocerciasis huge tracts of fertile land lie virtually untilled, and individuals and communities are impoverished.

Pathology

Infective larvae of *O. volvulus* are introduced into the skin by the bite of an infected *Simulium* fly (Fig. 13.62). The worms mature in 2–4 months and live for up to 17 years in subcutaneous and connective tissues. At sites of trauma, over bony prominences and around joints, fibrosis may form nodules around adult worms which otherwise cause no direct damage. Innumerable microfilariae, discharged by the female *O. volvulus*, move actively in these nodules and in the adjacent tissues, are widely distributed in the skin, and may invade the eye. Live microfilariae elicit little tissue reaction, but dead ones may cause severe allergic inflammation leading to hyaline necrosis and loss of collagen and elastin. Death of microfilariae in the eye causes conjunc-

13

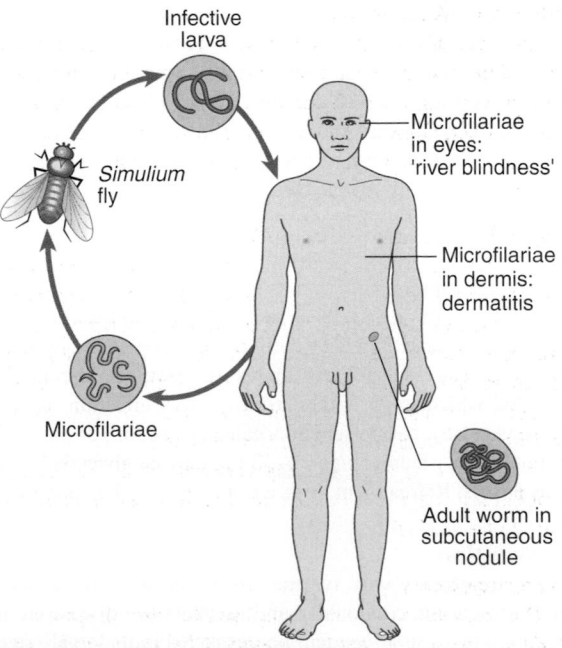

Fig. 13.62 *Onchocerca volvulus.* Life cycle of organism and pathogenesis of onchocerciasis.

tivitis, sclerosing keratitis with pannus formation, uveitis which may lead to glaucoma and cataract and, less commonly, choroidoretinitis and optic neuritis.

Clinical features

The infection may remain symptomless for months or years. The first symptom is usually itching, localised to one quadrant of the body and later becoming generalised and involving the eyes. Evanescent oedema of part or all of a limb is an early sign, followed by papular urticaria spreading gradually from the site of infection. This is difficult to see on dark skins, in which the most common signs are papules excoriated by scratching, spotty hyperpigmentation from resolving inflammation, and more chronic changes of a rough, thickened or inelastic, wrinkled skin. Superficial lymph nodes enlarge and may hang down in folds of loose skin at the groins. Hydrocele, femoral hernias and scrotal elephantiasis occur. Firm subcutaneous nodules (onchocercomas) occur in chronic infection, and are palpable and 1 cm or more in diameter.

Eye disease is most common in highly endemic areas and is associated with chronic heavy infections and nodules on the head. Early manifestations include itching, lacrimation, conjunctival injection and evidence of the features listed under 'Pathology'. Classically, 'snowflake' deposits are seen in the edges of the cornea.

Investigations

The finding of nodules or characteristic lesions of the skin or eyes in a patient from an endemic area, associated with eosinophilia, is suggestive. Skin snips or shavings, taken with a corneoscleral punch or scalpel blade from calf, buttock and shoulder, are placed in saline under a cover slip on a microscope slide and examined after 4 hours. Microfilariae are seen wriggling free in all but the lightest infections. If the test is negative, a test dose of DEC is given to see whether it aggravates the rash. Slit-lamp examination may reveal microfilariae moving in the anterior chamber of the eye or trapped in the cornea. A nodule may be removed and incised, showing the coiled, thread-like adult worm. Filarial antibodies may be detected in up to 95% of patients, but antibody positivity can be much lower in lightly infected expatriates.

Management

Ivermectin, in a single dose of 100–200 µg/kg, kills microfilariae and prevents their return for 9 months. It is non-toxic and does not trigger severe reactions, in contrast to DEC which is no longer used for this infection. In the rare event of a severe reaction causing oedema or postural hypotension, prednisolone 20–30 mg may be given daily for 2 or 3 days. Retreatment with ivermectin may be necessary.

Prevention

Mass treatment with ivermectin is in use. It reduces morbidity in the community and prevents eye disease from getting worse. *Simulium* can be destroyed in its larval stage by the application of insecticide to streams. Long trousers, skirts and sleeves discourage the fly from biting.

DRACUNCULIASIS (GUINEA WORM)

Another tissue-dwelling nematode is the Guinea worm (*Dracunculus medinensis*). Infestation manifests when the female worm, over a metre long, emerges from the skin. Humans are infected by ingesting a small crustacean, *Cyclops*, which inhabits wells and ponds and contains the infective larval stage of the worm. The worm was widely distributed across Africa and the Middle East but after a successful eradication programme is now seen only in sub-Saharan Africa.

Management

Traditionally, the protruding worm is extracted by winding it out gently over several days on a matchstick. The worm must never be broken. Antibiotics for secondary infection and prophylaxis of tetanus are also required.

Prevention

The global elimination campaign is based on the provision of clean drinking water and eradication of water fleas from drinking water. The latter is being achieved by simple filtration of water through a plastic mesh filter and chemical treatment of water supplies.

OTHER FILARIASES

Mansonella perstans

This filarial worm is transmitted by the midges *Culicoides austeni* and *C. grahami*. It is common throughout equatorial Africa as far south as Zambia, and also in Trinidad and parts of northern and eastern South America.

M. perstans has never been shown to cause disease but it may be responsible for a persistent eosinophilia and occasional allergic manifestations. *M. perstans* is resistant to ivermectin and DEC and the infection may persist for many years.

Dirofilaria immitis

This dog heart worm infects humans with skin and lung lesions. It is not uncommon in the US, Japan and Australia.

ZOONOTIC NEMATODES

TRICHINOSIS (TRICHINELLOSIS)

Trichinella spiralis is a nematode that parasitises rats and pigs and is only transmitted to humans if they eat partially cooked infected pork, usually as sausage or ham. Bear meat is another source. Symptoms result from invasion of intestinal submucosa by ingested larvae, which develop into adult worms, and the secondary invasion of tissues by fresh larvae produced by these adult worms. The main tissue invaded is striated muscle, in which the larvae encyst. Outbreaks have occurred in the UK as well as in other countries where pork is eaten.

Clinical features

The clinical features of trichinosis are determined by the larval numbers. A light infection with a few worms may be asymptomatic; a heavy infection causes nausea and diarrhoea 24–48 hours after the infected meal. A few days later, the symptoms associated with larval invasion predominate: fever and oedema of the face, eyelids and conjunctivae. Invasion of the diaphragm may cause pain, cough and dyspnoea; involvement of the muscles of the limbs, chest and mouth causes stiffness, pain and tenderness in affected muscles. Larval migration may cause acute myocarditis and encephalitis. An eosinophilia is usually found after the second week. An intense infection may prove fatal but those who survive recover completely.

Investigations

Commonly, a group of people who have eaten infected pork from a common source develop symptoms at about the same time. Biopsy from the deltoid or gastrocnemius after the third week of symptoms in suspected cases may reveal encysted larvae. Serological tests are also helpful.

Management

Treatment is with albendazole 20 mg/kg daily for 7 days. Given early in the infection this may kill newly formed adult worms in the submucosa and thus reduce the number of larvae reaching the muscles. Corticosteroids are necessary to control the serious effects of acute inflammation.

CUTANEOUS LARVA MIGRANS (p. 298)

This is caused by the larvae of the zoonotic nematodes, *Ancylostoma braziliense* and *A. caninum*.

TREMATODES (FLUKES)

These leaf-shaped worms are parasitic to humans and animals. Their complex life cycles may involve one or more intermediate hosts, often freshwater molluscs.

SCHISTOSOMIASIS

Schistosomiasis (bilharziasis) is one of the most important causes of morbidity in the tropics and is being spread by irrigation schemes. Schistosome eggs have been found in Egyptian mummies dated 1250 BC. Recent travellers, especially those overlanding through Africa, may present with eosinophilia; residents of schistosomiasis-endemic areas are more likely to present with chronic urinary tract pathology or portal hypertension.

There are three species of the genus *Schistosoma* which commonly cause disease in humans: *S. haematobium*, *S. mansoni* and *S. japonicum*. *S. haematobium* was discovered by Theodor Bilharz in Cairo in 1861 and the disease is sometimes called bilharziasis. The ovum is passed in the urine or faeces of infected individuals and gains access to fresh water where the ciliated miracidium inside it is liberated; it enters its intermediate host, a species of freshwater snail, in which it multiplies (Fig. 13.63A). Large numbers of fork-tailed cercariae are then liberated into the water, where they may survive for 2–3 days. Cercariae can penetrate the skin or the mucous membrane of the mouth of their definitive host, humans. They transform into

13

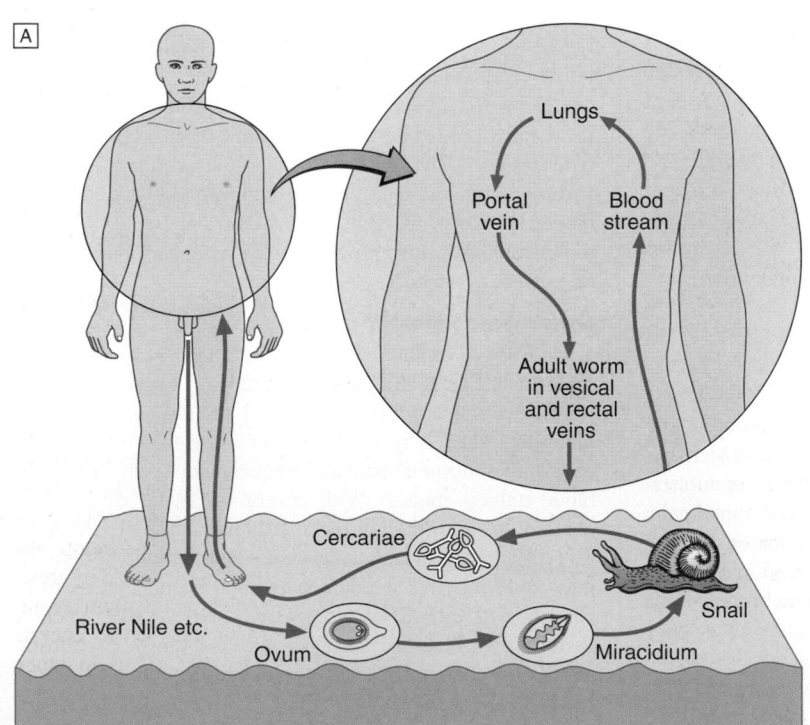

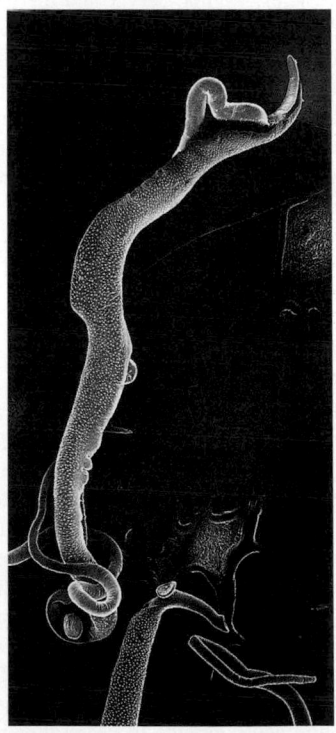

Fig. 13.63 *Schistosoma.* [A] Life cycle. [B] Scanning electron micrograph of adult schistosome worms showing the larger male worm embracing the thinner female.

13.65 PATHOGENESIS OF SCHISTOSOMIASIS

Stage	Time	S. haemotobium	S. mansoni and S. japonicum
Cercarial penetration	Days	Papular dermatitis at site of penetration	As for S. haematobium
Larval migration and maturation	Weeks	Pneumonitis, myositis, hepatitis, fever, 'serum sickness', eosinophilia, seroconversion	As for S. haematobium
Early egg deposition	Months	Cystitis, haematuria Ectopic granulomatous lesions: skin, CNS etc. Immune complex glomerulonephritis	Colitis, granulomatous hepatitis, acute portal hypertension As for S. haematobium
Late egg deposition	Years	Fibrosis and calcification of ureters, bladder: bacterial infection, calculi, hydronephrosis, carcinoma Pulmonary granulomas and pulmonary hypertension	Colonic polyposis and strictures, periportal fibrosis, portal hypertension As for S. haematobium

schistosomulae and moult as they pass through the lungs and are carried by the blood stream to the liver and so to the portal vein where they mature. The male worm is up to 20 mm in length and the more slender cylindrical female, usually enfolded longitudinally by the male, is rather longer (Fig. 13.63B). Within 4–6 weeks of infection they migrate to the venules draining the pelvic viscera, where the females deposit ova.

Pathology

The pathological changes and symptoms depend on species and stage of infection (Box 13.65). Most of the disease is due to the passage of eggs through mucosa and to the granulomatous reaction to eggs deposited in tissues. The eggs of *S. haematobium* pass mainly through the wall of the bladder, but may also involve rectum, seminal vesicles, vagina, cervix and uterine tubes. *S. mansoni* and *S. japonicum* eggs pass mainly through the wall of the lower bowel or are carried to the liver. The most serious, although rare, consequences of the ectopic deposition of eggs are transverse myelitis and paraplegia. Granulomas are composed of macrophages, eosinophils, epithelioid and giant cells around an ovum. Later there is fibrosis and eggs calcify, often in sufficient numbers to become radiologically visible. Eggs of *S. haematobium*, and of the other two species after the development of portal hypertension, may reach the lungs.

Clinical features

During the early stages of infection there may be itching lasting 1–2 days at the site of cercarial penetration. After a symptom-free period of 3–5 weeks acute schistosomiasis (Katayama syndrome) may present with allergic manifestations such as urticaria, fever, muscle aches, abdominal pain, headaches, cough and sweating. On examination hepatomegaly, splenomegaly, lymphadenopathy and pneumonia may be present. There is eosinophilia and schistosomiasis serology may be positive. These allergic phenomena may be severe in infections with *S. mansoni* and *S. japonicum* but are rare with *S. haematobium*. The features subside after 1–2 weeks. Chronic schistosomiasis is due to egg deposition and occurs months to years after infection. The symptoms and signs depend upon the intensity of infection and the species of infecting schistosome.

Schistosoma haematobium

Humans are the only natural hosts of *S. haematobium*, which is highly endemic in Egypt and East Africa, and occurs throughout Africa and the Middle East (Fig. 13.64). Infection can be acquired after a brief exposure such as swimming in freshwater lakes in Africa.

Painless terminal haematuria is usually the first and most common symptom. Frequency of micturition follows, due to bladder neck obstruction. Later the disease may be complicated by frequent urinary tract infections, bladder or ureteric stone formation, hydronephrosis, renal functional abnormalities and ultimately renal failure with a contracted calcified bladder. Pain is often felt in the iliac fossa or in the loin and radiates to the groin. In several endemic areas there is a strong epidemiological association of *S. haematobium* infection with squamous cell carcinoma of the bladder. Disease of the seminal vesicles may lead to haemospermia. Females may develop schistosomal papillomas of the vulva, and schistosomal lesions of the cervix may be mistaken for cancer. Intestinal symptoms may follow involvement of the bowel wall. Ectopic worms cause skin or cord lesions. The severity of *S. haematobium* infection varies greatly, and many with a light infection are asymptomatic. However, as adult worms can live for 20 years or more and lesions may progress, these patients should always be treated.

Schistosoma mansoni

S. mansoni is endemic throughout Africa, the Middle East, Venezuela, Brazil and the Caribbean (Fig. 13.64).

Characteristic symptoms begin 2 months or more after infection. They may be slight, no more than malaise, or consist of abdominal pain and frequent stools which contain blood-stained mucus. With severe advanced disease increased discomfort from rectal polyps may be experienced. The early hepatomegaly is reversible but portal hypertension may cause massive splenomegaly, fatal haematemesis from oesophageal varices, or progressive ascites. Liver function is initially preserved because the pathology is fibrotic rather than cirrhotic. *S. mansoni* infections predispose to the carriage of *Salmonella*.

Schistosoma japonicum

In addition to humans the adult worm infects the dog, rat, fieldmouse, water buffalo, ox, cat, pig, horse and sheep.

13

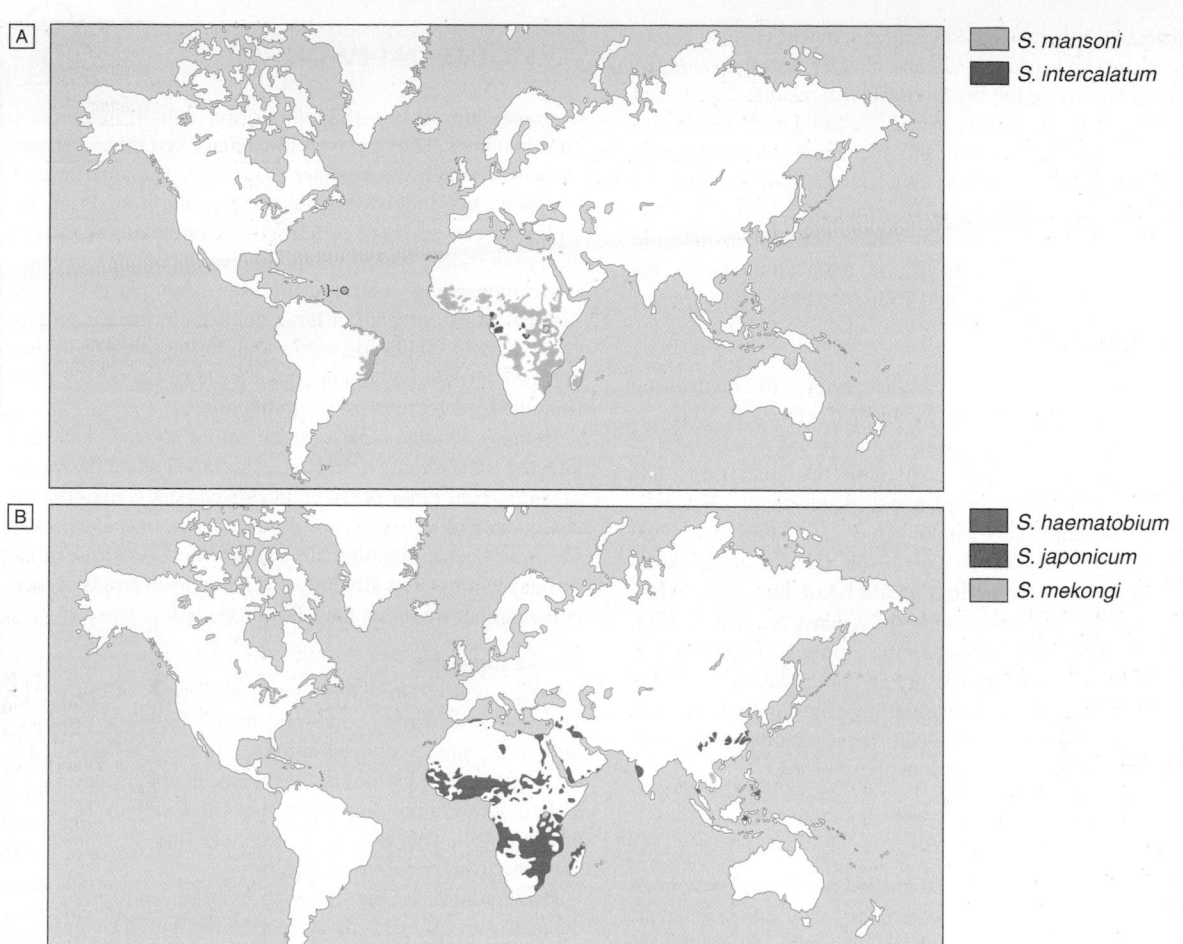

Fig. 13.64 Geographical distribution of schistosomiasis.

S. japonicum is prevalent in the Yellow River and Yangtze–Jiang basins in China, where the infection is a major public health problem. It also has a focal distribution in the Philippines, Indonesia and Thailand. There is now no human transmission of this parasite in Japan. A related parasite, *S. mekongi*, occurs in Laos, Thailand and Myanmar. The pathology of *S. japonicum* is similar to that of *S. mansoni*, but as this worm produces more eggs, the lesions tend to be more extensive and widespread. The clinical features resemble those of severe infection with *S. mansoni*, with added neurological features. The small bowel as well as the large may be affected, and hepatic fibrosis with splenic enlargement is usual. Deposition of eggs or worms in the central nervous system, especially in the brain, causes symptoms in about 5% of infections, notably epilepsy, hemiplegia, blindness and paraplegia.

Investigations

Diagnosis depends on demonstrating eggs or serological evidence of infection. In *S. haematobium* infection, dipstick urine testing shows blood and albumin. The terminal spined eggs can be found by microscopic examination of the centrifuged deposit of terminal stream urine. Ultrasound is useful for assessing the urinary tract and can be performed easily in the field. Bladder wall thickening, hydronephrosis and bladder calcification can be detected. Cystoscopy reveals 'sandy' patches, bleeding mucosa and later distortion.

In a heavy infection with *S. mansoni* or *S. japonicum* the characteristic egg with its lateral spine can usually be found in the stool. When the infection is light, or of long duration, a rectal biopsy can be examined. Sigmoidoscopy may show inflammation or bleeding. Biopsies should be examined for ova. There is eosinophilia. Serological tests (ELISA) are useful as screening tests but remain positive after chemotherapeutic cure.

Management

The object of specific treatment is to kill the adult schistosomes and so stop egg-laying. It may not be possible to kill all adult worms by mass treatment campaigns in communities where reinfection is likely, but a reduction in egg output of around 90% is often achieved and this significantly reduces morbidity and possibly transmission.

Praziquantel is the drug of choice for all forms of schistosomiasis. The drug produces parasitological cure in 80% of treated individuals and over 90% reduction in egg counts in the remaining individuals. Side-effects are uncommon but include nausea and abdominal pain.

Praziquantel therapy in early infection will reverse pathologies such as hepatomegaly and bladder wall thickening.

Surgery may be required to deal with residual lesions but large vesical granulomas usually respond well to chemotherapy. Ureteric stricture and the small fibrotic urinary bladder may require plastic procedures. Removal of rectal papillomas by diathermy or by other means may provide relief. Granulomatous masses in the brain or spinal cord may require neurosurgery if the manifestations do not respond to chemotherapy and corticosteroids.

Prevention

So far no satisfactory single means of controlling schistosomiasis has been established. The life cycle is terminated if the ova in urine or faeces are not allowed to contaminate fresh water containing the snail host. The provision of latrines and of a safe water supply, however, remains a major problem in rural areas throughout the tropics. Furthermore, *S. japonicum* has so many hosts besides humans that latrines would be of little avail. Mass treatment of the population helps against *S. haematobium* and *S. mansoni* but this method has so far had little success with *S. japonicum*. Attack on the intermediate host, the snail, presents many difficulties and has not on its own proved successful on any scale. For personal protection, contact with infected water must be avoided.

LIVER FLUKES

Liver flukes infect at least 20 million people and remain an important public health problem in many endemic areas. They are associated with abdominal pain, hepatomegaly and relapsing cholangitis. *Clonorchis sinensis* is a major aetiological agent of bile duct cancer. The three major flukes have similar life cycles and pathologies, as outlined in Box 13.66.

CESTODES (TAPEWORMS)

Cestodes are ribbon-shaped worms which inhabit the intestinal tract. They have no alimentary system and absorb nutrients through the tegumental surface. The anterior end, or scolex, has suckers for attaching to the host. From the scolex arises a series of progressively developing segments, the proglottides, which when shed may continue to show active movements. Cross-fertilisation takes place between segments. Ova, present in large numbers in mature proglottides, remain viable for weeks and during this period they may be consumed by the intermediate host. Larvae liberated from the ingested ova pass into the tissues.

Humans acquire tapeworm by eating undercooked beef infected with *Cysticercus bovis*, the larval stage of *Taenia saginata* (beef tapeworm), undercooked pork containing the larval stage of *T. solium* (pork tapeworm), or undercooked freshwater fish containing larvae of *Diphyllobothrium latum* (fish tapeworm). Usually only one adult tapeworm is present in the gut but up to ten have been reported.

Taenia saginata

Infection with *T. saginata* occurs in all parts of the world. The adult worm may be several metres long and produces little or no intestinal upset in human beings, but knowledge of its presence, by noting segments in the faeces or on underclothing, may distress the patient. Ova may be found in the stool. The ova of *T. saginata* and *T. solium* are indistinguishable microscopically.

Praziquantel is the drug of choice, and prevention depends on efficient meat inspection and the thorough cooking of beef. Niclosamide is an alternative (see below).

Taenia solium

T. solium, the pork tapeworm, is common in central Europe, South Africa, South America and parts of Asia. It is not

13.66 DISEASES CAUSED BY FLUKES IN THE BILE DUCT

	Clonorchiasis	Opisthorchiasis	Fascioliasis
Parasite	*Clonorchis sinensis*	*Opisthorchis felineus*	*Fasciola hepatica*
Other mammalian hosts	Dogs, cats, pigs	Dogs, cats, foxes, pigs	Sheep, cattle
Mode of spread	Ova in faeces, water	As for *C. sinensis*	Ova in faeces on to wet pasture
1st intermediate host	Snails	Snails	Snails
2nd intermediate host	Freshwater fish	Freshwater fish	Encysts on vegetation
Geographical distribution	Far East, especially South China	Far East, especially North-east Thailand	Cosmopolitan, including UK
Pathology	*E. coli* cholangitis, abscesses, biliary carcinoma	As for *C. sinensis*	Toxaemia, cholangitis, eosinophilia
Symptoms	Often symptom-free, recurrent jaundice	As for *C. sinensis*	Unexplained fever, tender liver, may be ectopic, e.g. subcutaneous fluke
Diagnosis	Ova in stool or duodenal aspirate	As for *C. sinensis*	As for *C. sinensis*, also serology
Prevention	Cook fish	Cook fish	Avoid contaminated watercress
Treatment	Praziquantel 25 mg/kg 8-hourly for 2 days	As for *C. sinensis* but for 1 day only	Triclabendazole 10 mg/kg single dose; repeat treatment may be required*

*In UK available from the Hospital for Tropical Diseases, London.

as large as *T. saginata*. The adult worm is found only in humans following the eating of undercooked pork containing cysticerci.

CYSTICERCOSIS

Human cysticercosis is acquired by ingesting tapeworm ova, either by ingesting ova from contaminated fingers or by eating contaminated food (Fig. 13.65). The larvae are liberated from eggs in the stomach, penetrate the intestinal mucosa and are carried to many parts of the body where they develop and form cysticerci, 0.5–1 cm cysts that contain the head of a young worm. They do not grow further or migrate. Common locations are the subcutaneous tissue, skeletal muscles and brain.

Clinical features

When superficially placed, cysts can be palpated under the skin or mucosa as pea-like ovoid bodies. Here they cause few or no symptoms, and will eventually die and become calcified.

Heavy brain infections, especially in children, may cause features of encephalitis. More commonly, however, cerebral signs do not occur until the larvae die, 5–20 years later. Epilepsy, personality changes, staggering gait or signs of internal hydrocephalus are the most common features.

Investigations

Calcified cysts in muscles can be recognised radiologically. In the brain, however, less calcification takes place and

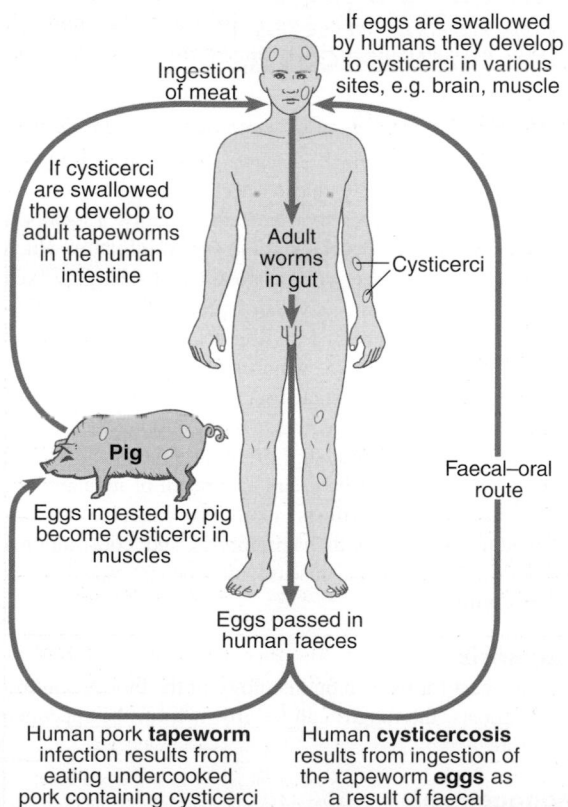

Human pork **tapeworm** infection results from eating undercooked pork containing cysticerci

Human **cysticercosis** results from ingestion of the tapeworm **eggs** as a result of faecal contamination of food

If eggs are swallowed by humans they develop to cysticerci in various sites, e.g. brain, muscle

Ingestion of meat

If cysticerci are swallowed they develop to adult tapeworms in the human intestine

Adult worms in gut — Cysticerci

Pig

Eggs ingested by pig become cysticerci in muscles

Faecal–oral route

Eggs passed in human faeces

Fig. 13.65 Cysticercosis. Life cycle of *Taenia solium*.

larvae are only occasionally demonstrated radiologically; usually CT or MRI will show them. Epileptic fits starting in adult life should suggest the possibility of cysticercosis if the patient has lived in or travelled to an endemic area. The subcutaneous tissue should be palpated and any nodule excised for histology. Radiological examination of the skeletal muscles may be helpful. Antibody detection by fluorescent antibody test, ELISA or immunoblotting is available for serodiagnosis.

Management and prevention

Niclosamide, followed by a mild laxative (after 1–2 hours) to prevent retrograde intestinal autoinfection, is useful only for the intestinal infection. Praziquantel improves the prognosis of cerebral cysticercosis; the dose is 50 mg/kg in three divided doses daily for 10 days. Albendazole, 15 mg/kg daily for a minimum of 8 days, has now become the drug of choice for parenchymal neurocysticercosis. Prednisolone, 10 mg 8-hourly, is also given for 14 days, starting 1 day before the albendazole or praziquantel. In addition, anti-epileptic drugs should be given until the reaction in the brain has subsided. Operative intervention is indicated for hydrocephalus. Studies from India and Peru suggest that most small solitary cerebral cysts will resolve without treatment.

Cooking pork well will prevent infection with *T. solium*. Cysticercosis is avoided if food is not contaminated by ova or segments. Great care must be taken by nurses and other adults while attending a patient harbouring an adult worm.

ECHINOCOCCUS GRANULOSUS (TAENIA ECHINOCOCCUS) AND HYDATID DISEASE

Dogs are the definitive hosts of the tiny tapeworm *E. granulosus*. The larval stage, a hydatid cyst, normally occurs in sheep, cattle, camels and other animals that are infected from contaminated pastures or water. By handling a dog or drinking contaminated water, humans may ingest eggs (Fig. 13.66). The embryo is liberated from the ovum in the small intestine and gains access to the blood stream and thus to the liver. The resultant cyst grows very slowly, sometimes intermittently, and may outlive the patient. It may calcify or rupture, giving rise to multiple cysts. The disease is common in the Middle East, North and East Africa, Australia and Argentina. Foci of infection persist in rural Wales and Scotland. *E. multilocularis*, which has a cycle between foxes and voles, causes a similar but more severe infection, 'alveolar hydatid disease', which invades the liver like cancer.

Clinical features

A hydatid cyst is typically acquired in childhood and it may, after growing for some years, cause pressure symptoms. These vary, depending on the organ or tissue involved. In nearly 75% of patients with hydatid disease the right lobe of the liver is invaded and contains a single cyst. In others a cyst may be found in lung, bone, brain or elsewhere.

Investigations

The diagnosis depends on the clinical, radiological and ultrasound findings in a patient who has lived in close

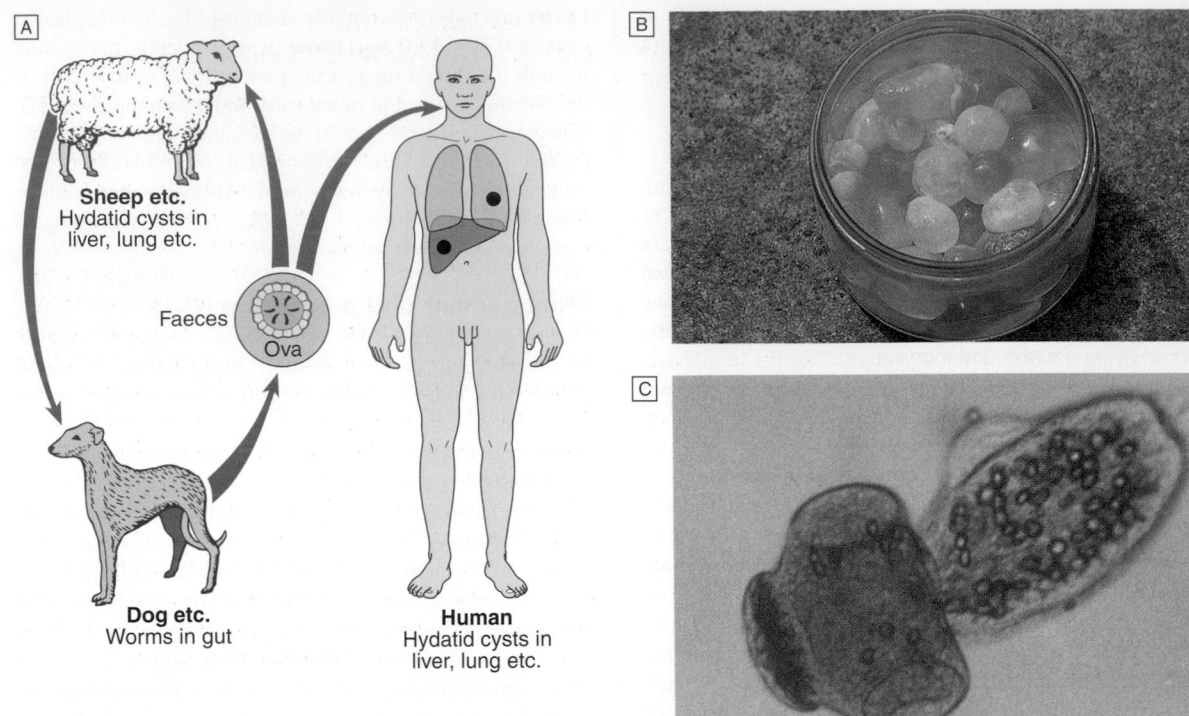

Fig. 13.66 **Hydatid disease.** [A] Life cycle of *Echinococcus granulosus*. [B] Daughter cysts removed at surgery. [C] Within the daughter cysts are the protoscolices.

13

contact with dogs in an endemic area. Complement fixation and ELISA are positive in 70–90% of patients.

Management and prevention

Hydatid cysts should be excised wherever possible. Great care is taken to avoid spillage and cavities are sterilised with 0.5% silver nitrate or 2.7% sodium chloride. Albendazole (400 mg 12-hourly for 3 months) is used for inoperable disease, and to reduce the infectivity of cysts pre-operatively. Praziquantel 20 mg/kg 12-hourly for 14 days kills protoscolices perioperatively.

Prevention is difficult in situations where there is a close association with dogs and sheep. Personal hygiene, satisfactory disposal of carcasses, meat inspection and deworming of dogs can greatly reduce the prevalence of disease.

OTHER TAPEWORMS

There are many other cestodes whose adult or larval stages may infect humans. Sparganosis is a condition in which an immature worm develops in humans, usually subcutaneously, as a result of eating or applying to the skin the secondary or tertiary intermediate host.

FUNGAL INFECTIONS

Superficial fungal infections of the skin (ringworm, dermatophytosis) are described in Chapter 27.

DEEP FUNGAL INFECTIONS OF THE SKIN AND SUBCUTANEOUS TISSUES

SPOROTRICHOSIS

Sporotrichosis is a fungal disease caused by *Sporothrix schenckii* and is usually due to accidental inoculation of the fungus growing on a thorny plant. Usually, a localised subcutaneous nodule develops at the site of infection which subsequently ulcerates with a pustular discharge (fixed cutaneous). The disease may then spread along the cutaneous lymphatic channels, resulting in multiple cutaneous nodules along their route, which ulcerate and produce a pustular discharge (lymphocutaneous). Other rarer forms of sporotrichosis include patients with cutaneous disease presenting with arthritis; later, draining sinuses may form. Pulmonary sporotrichosis occurs as a result of inhalation of the conidia and manifests itself as chronic cavitary fibronodular disease with haemoptysis and constitutional symptoms. Disseminated disease may occur, especially in patients with AIDS.

Diagnosis

Typical yeast forms seen on histology of the biopsy confirm the diagnosis; the fungus can be grown from the specimen in culture.

Management

Oral itraconazole (200–400 mg daily for 3–6 months) is the treatment of choice for cutaneous and lymphocutaneous disease. Alternative agents include a saturated solution of potassium iodide (SSKI), initiated with 5 drops and increased to 40–50 drops 8-hourly for 3–6 months, and terbinafine (500 mg daily for 24 weeks). Amphotericin B should be used for systemic life-threatening illness.

MYCETOMA

Mycetoma, in this restricted sense, is a chronic suppurative infection of the deep soft tissues and bones, most commonly of the limbs but also of the abdominal or chest wall or head. It is caused either by anaerobic filamentous bacteria, *Actinomycetes* (60%—actinomycetoma), or by true fungi, *Eumycetes* (40%—eumycetoma). Both groups produce characteristically coloured grains, the colour depending on the organism. The disease occurs mostly in the tropics and subtropics.

Pathology
The histology is that of a chronic granuloma with a fibrous stroma and cyst-like spaces in which lie the characteristic grains.

Clinical features
The causative organism is usually introduced by a thorn and the infection is most common on the foot (Madura foot). The mycetoma begins as a painless swelling at the site of implantation, which grows and spreads steadily within the soft tissues, causing further swelling and eventually penetrating bones. Nodules develop under the epidermis and these rupture, revealing sinuses through which grains (fungal colonies) are discharged. Some sinuses may heal with scarring while fresh sinuses appear elsewhere. Deeper tissue invasion and involvement of bone are rapid and greater in actinomycetoma than eumycetoma.

There is little pain and usually no fever or lymphadenopathy, but there is progressive disability. When the lesion is in the scalp, the skull may be affected but the dura mater appears to be an effective barrier. *Nocardia brasiliensis* often affects the skin of the back. It is seldom localised and may spread widely.

Investigations
Diagnosis is confirmed by demonstration of fungal grains in aspiration cytology, pus or tissue biopsy. Culture is usually necessary for species identification. Serology may be helpful.

Management
Localised lesions that can be excised without residual disability are best so treated. Medical treatment of fungal mycetomas is unsatisfactory. Drug treatment for eumycetoma is either with ketoconazole or itraconazole 200–400 mg in two divided doses for 6–12 months. *Madurella mycetomatis* is the most sensitive to therapy, responding to ketoconazole in about 60% of cases. Amputation should be considered carefully as it may deprive patients of their livelihood.

Actinomycetes may be susceptible to treatment with combinations of either streptomycin or amikacin and dapsone or co-trimoxazole for several months. *Nocardia* infection may respond to dapsone alone.

CHROMOMYCOSIS (CHROMOBLASTOMYCOSIS)

Chromomycosis is a fungal disease most commonly occurring in the tropics and subtropics. Of the several fungi implicated in this disease, the most common is *Fonsecaea pedrosoi*, but others include *F. compacta*, *Cladophialophora carrionii* and *Phialophora verrucosa*. Chromomycosis is a disease of cutaneous and subcutaneous tissue caused by inoculation of the fungus in the body through trauma. People walking barefoot are commonly affected, and lesions of the feet are most common. Lesions may start several months after the injury in the form of a papule which later turns into a painless, itchy, scaly nodule or plaque. Later there may be hypertrophy of the tissue leading to a verrucous and cauliflower-like appearance. Diagnosis is by demonstration of dematiaceous (brown-pigmented), rounded thick-walled sclerotic bodies in the biopsy. Culture is necessary to confirm the aetiological agent. Oral itraconazole (200 mg daily) or terbinafine (250 mg daily) for 6–12 months may be needed. Cryosurgery with liquid nitrogen has been employed to good effect in some patients, either alone or in combination with these drugs.

13

SYSTEMIC FUNGAL INFECTIONS

CANDIDIASIS

Approximately 10% of the known 200 species of *Candida* are involved in human disease. Most infections and 50% of systemic infections are caused by *C. albicans*. Other species increasingly implicated are *C. tropicalis*, *C. glabrata* and *C. krusei*. The latter two are inherently resistant to fluconazole and, because of the drug's regular use as a prophylactic in oncology and haematology units, are becoming common. The majority of *Candida* infections originate from the patient's endogenous flora in the oropharyngeal or genitourinary regions. The most common infections are oropharyngeal or vaginal candidiasis or 'thrush'. These conditions frequently arise when, broad-spectrum antibiotic therapy has disrupted normal commensal bacterial flora or when CD4 T lymphocyte numbers are depleted as in HIV/AIDS (p. 386).

Neutrophils form the main defence against systemic infection with *Candida* spp. Hence systemic candidiasis is most common in neutropenic patients, whatever the cause. Immunosuppression and debility, especially in organ transplant recipients, injection drug-users, and patients with leukaemia, diabetes, cirrhosis, uraemia, cancer or auto-immune disease (such as systemic lupus erythematosus), significantly increase the risk of *Candida* infection. The condition is often occult and so should be suspected in these cases.

Clinical features
These are not constant but three typical manifestations occur:

- Between 5% and 50% of cases will have ophthalmic involvement, with characteristic 'cotton wool' exudates on the retina progressing to a vitreous haze. If left untreated, this may progress to frank ophthalmitis and permanent loss of sight.

- Characteristic skin lesions occur in approximately 10% of cases. These often occur on the extremities in the form of non-tender pink/red nodules that occasionally coalesce as infection progresses.
- In leukaemic patients chronic disseminated hepatosplenic candidiasis occurs, typically manifested as persistent fever in neutropenia despite antibacterial therapy. The fever persists despite resolution of the neutropenia and is associated with a raised alkaline phosphatase and multiple lesions in liver and spleen on imaging. This infection may last for months despite therapy.

A particular constellation of skin lesions, ophthalmitis and osteoarthritis, due to systemic candidiasis in injection drug-users, is recognised and thought to be due to candidal contamination of citric acid or lemon juice used to dissolve heroin.

Bone and joint involvement, peritonitis and abdominal organ involvement, meningitis and endocarditis are well recognised and require specialist advice.

Management

Positive blood cultures for *Candida* spp. must never be ignored and require aggressive therapy with systemic antifungals.

Amphotericin B (p. 154) remains the mainstay of therapy and use of the lipid formulations helps to reduce renal side-effects. Fluconazole is useful, provided the organism has been confirmed as *C. albicans*. The newer antifungals, voriconazole and caspofungin (p. 155), are alternatives.

HISTOPLASMOSIS

Histoplasmosis is caused by *Histoplasma capsulatum*; this is a yeast in its parasitic phase but a filamentous fungus of soil at other times. A variant, *H. duboisii*, is found in parts of tropical Africa.

H. capsulatum multiplies in soil enriched by the droppings of birds and bats, and the spores remain viable for years. Natural infections are found in several species of small mammal, including bats. Infection is by inhalation of infected dust. The infection is an especial hazard for explorers of caves and people who clear out bird (including chicken) roosts.

H. capsulatum is found in all parts of the USA, especially in the east central states, and less commonly in Latin America from Mexico to Argentina, Europe, North, South and East Africa, Nigeria, Malaysia, Indonesia and Australia. Disseminated histoplasmosis is also seen in immunocompromised patients, such as those who have contracted AIDS (p. 385).

Pathology

The parasite in its yeast phase multiplies mainly in monocytes and macrophages, and produces areas of necrosis in which the parasites may abound. From these foci the blood stream may be invaded, producing metastatic lesions in the liver, spleen and lymph nodes. Pulmonary histoplasmosis may cause pathological changes similar to those of tuberculosis, including the production of a primary complex with enlarged regional lymph nodes, multiple small discrete lesions and occasionally cavitation. Healed lesions may calcify.

Clinical features

Histoplasma infection is usually asymptomatic or self-limiting. Pulmonary symptoms are the most common disease presentation, with non-productive cough, pleuritic pain and an influenza-like illness. On examination lymphadenopathy, rashes and pulmonary crackles may be found. Patients with pre-existing lung disease, such as emphysema or fibrosis, may develop chronic histoplasmosis with fever, cough, dyspnoea and weight loss. Disseminated *Histoplasma* infection occurs when there is progressive disease with extrapulmonary involvement. The reticulo-endothelial system is usually involved causing fever, anorexia and weight loss. Cutaneous and mucosal lesions, lymphadenopathy, hepatosplenomegaly and meningitis may develop. Disseminated disease with central nervous system involvement is seen in AIDS patients.

Investigations

In an area where the disease occurs, histoplasmosis should be suspected in every obscure infection in which there are pulmonary signs or where there are enlarged lymph nodes or hepatosplenomegaly. Tissue is obtained by biopsy for an impression smear, histology and culture. Radiological examination in long-standing cases may show calcified lesions in the lungs, spleen or other organs. In the more acute phases of the disease single or multiple soft pulmonary shadows with enlarged tracheobronchial nodes are seen.

Delayed hypersensitivity to the intradermal injection of histoplasmin develops in patients with either active or healed infections but is usually negative in acute disseminated disease. Complement-fixing antibodies are detected within 3 weeks of the onset of an acute primary infection and increase in titre as the disease progresses. Precipitating antibodies may also be detected.

Management

Specific treatment with amphotericin B is indicated only in severe infections; the dosage (0.5 mg/kg in 500 ml of 5% glucose) is given intravenously over a 6-hour period, gradually increasing to a maximum of 1 mg/kg. Treatment is given on alternate days to a total adult dose of 2 g. If badly tolerated, the dose may have to be reduced. Side-effects (anorexia, nausea, fever, headache and venous thrombosis) may be controlled by the addition of 10 mg prednisolone to the intravenous solution. Plasma urea rises and haemoglobin falls during treatment but later return to normal. Amphotericin may have to be continued for up to 3 months or longer, depending on the clinical response. Severe dyspnoea in histoplasmosis should be treated with prednisolone 20–40 mg daily for a few days. Itraconazole 200–400 mg daily can be used in patients with chronic

13

pulmonary histoplasmosis and chronic disseminated histoplasmosis.

HISTOPLASMA DUBOISII

H. duboisii, the fungus of African histoplasmosis, is larger than the classical *H. capsulatum*. It is found throughout East, Central and West Africa.

The disease differs in several ways from *H. capsulatum* infection. The bones, skin, lymph nodes and liver develop granulomatous lesions or cold abscesses resembling tuberculosis, but the lungs are seldom involved. The visceral form with liver and splenic invasion is often fatal, while ulcerative skin lesions and bone abscesses follow a more benign course.

Radiological examination may show rounded foci of bone destruction, sometimes associated with abscess formation. Multiple lesions of the ribs are common and the bones of the limbs may be involved. Systemic disease is treated in the same way as *H. capsulatum* infections. A solitary lesion in bone may require only local surgical treatment.

ASPERGILLOSIS

This is the most common respiratory mycosis in the UK and is discussed on page 703.

COCCIDIOIDOMYCOSIS

This is caused by *Coccidioides immitis* and is found in the southern USA, and Central and South America. The disease is acquired by inhalation. The infection behaves like tuberculosis or histoplasmosis. In 60% of cases it is asymptomatic, but in 40% of cases it affects the lungs, lymph nodes and skin. Rarely, it may be carried by the blood stream to the bones, adrenals, meninges and other organs. Pulmonary coccidioidomycosis has two forms: primary and progressive. Primary coccidioidomycosis behaves like primary tuberculosis or histoplasmosis and is often asymptomatic. The progressive form of the disease is associated with marked systemic upset and features of lobar pneumonia. When it develops slowly it may resemble chronic tuberculosis. Infections, including subclinical attacks, are followed by immunity.

The fungi grow readily on culture media but as they are highly infective, diagnostic investigations are limited to intradermal, complement fixation and precipitin tests.

Amphotericin B (as for histoplasmosis), itraconazole, ketoconazole or fluconazole may be helpful but relapse is common. Some localised pulmonary lesions can be treated by surgery.

PARACOCCIDIOIDOMYCOSIS

This is caused by *Paracoccidioides brasiliensis* and occurs in South America. Mucocutaneous lesions occur early. Involvement of lymphatic nodes and the lungs is prominent and the gastrointestinal tract may also be attacked. Most patients respond to ketoconazole 200 mg/day for at least 6 months; itraconazole 100–200 mg daily is an alternative.

Liver function must be monitored for either agent. For those who do not respond, amphotericin B (as for histoplasmosis) may be used.

BLASTOMYCOSIS

North American blastomycosis is caused by *Blastomyces dermatitidis*. It also occurs in Africa. Systemic infection begins in the lungs and mediastinal lymph nodes and resembles pulmonary tuberculosis. Bones, skin and the genitourinary tract may also be affected. Treatment is with itraconazole 200–400 mg daily, ketoconazole 200–400 mg daily or amphotericin B (see above).

CRYPTOCOCCOSIS

This is caused by *Cryptococcus neoformans*. Its distribution is world-wide. It causes local gumma-like tumours and granulomatous lesions of the lung, bones, brain and meninges. The CSF, which shows a lymphocytic pleocytosis, is often at high pressure and management may require regular removal of 10–15 ml CSF to prevent features of raised intracranial pressure. It often contains the fungus when the nervous system is affected. Immunocompromised individuals are at special risk, including those with HIV infection (p. 394).

The diagnosis is made by culture or recognition of spores in the CSF, biopsy and serological detection of antigen.

Amphotericin B is the treatment of choice and should be given intravenously (p. 154) with flucytosine orally. The azoles, particularly second-generation agents such as voriconazole, are emerging as important in the long-term management of this condition. Surgical removal of local pulmonary lesions may be necessary. Recovery may be monitored by the fall in antigen titre. Cryptococcal meningitis is particularly important in HIV infection (p. 394).

FURTHER INFORMATION

Books and journal articles

Abrutyn E, Goldmann D, Scheckler W. Saunders Infection Control Reference Service with CD-ROM: The expert's guide to the guidelines. 2nd edn. Philadelphia: WB Saunders; 2001.

Ahmed AO, van Leeuwen W, Fahal A, et al. Mycetoma caused by *Madurella mycetomatis*: a neglected infectious burden. Lancet Infect Dis 2004; 4(9):566–574.

British Medical Association/Royal Pharmaceutical Society of Great Britain. British national formulary (BNF). London: Pharmaceutical Press/BMJ Books; 2005.

Britton WJ, Lockwood DN. Leprosy. Lancet 2004; 363:1209–1219.

Cohen J, Powderly W. Infectious diseases. 2nd edn. St Louis: Mosby; 2004.

Cook GC, Zumla AI (eds). Manson's tropical diseases. 21st edn. Philadelphia: WB Saunders; 2002.

Davies CR, Kaye P, Croft SL, Sundar S. Leishmaniasis: new approaches to disease control. BMJ 2003; 326:377–382.

Gibbons RV, Vaughn DW. Dengue: an escalating problem. BMJ 2002; 324(7353):1563–1566.

Greenwood BM, Bojang K, Whitty CJ, Targett GA. Malaria. Lancet 2005; 365:1487–1498.

Mabey DC, Solomon AW, Foster A. Trachoma. Lancet 2003; 362(9379):223–229.

Stich A, Abel PM, Krishna S. Human African trypanosomiasis. BMJ 2002; 325(7357):203–206.

Mandell G, Bennett J, Dolin R. Principles and practice of infectious diseases. 6th edn. Edinburgh: Churchill Livingstone; 2005.

Richter J, Hatz C, Haussinger D. Ultrasound in tropical and parasitic diseases. Lancet 2003; 362(9387):900–902.

Websites

www.cdc.gov *Centers for Disease Control and Prevention, USA. Emerging infections are at* www.cdc.gov/ncidod/eid.

www.hpa.org.uk *Aspects of infection and its control.*

www.paho.org *Pan American Health Organization.*

www.who.int/en/ *World Health Organization.*

13

E.G.L. WILKINS

Human immunodeficiency virus infection and the human acquired immunodeficiency syndrome

CLINICAL EXAMINATION IN HIV INFECTION

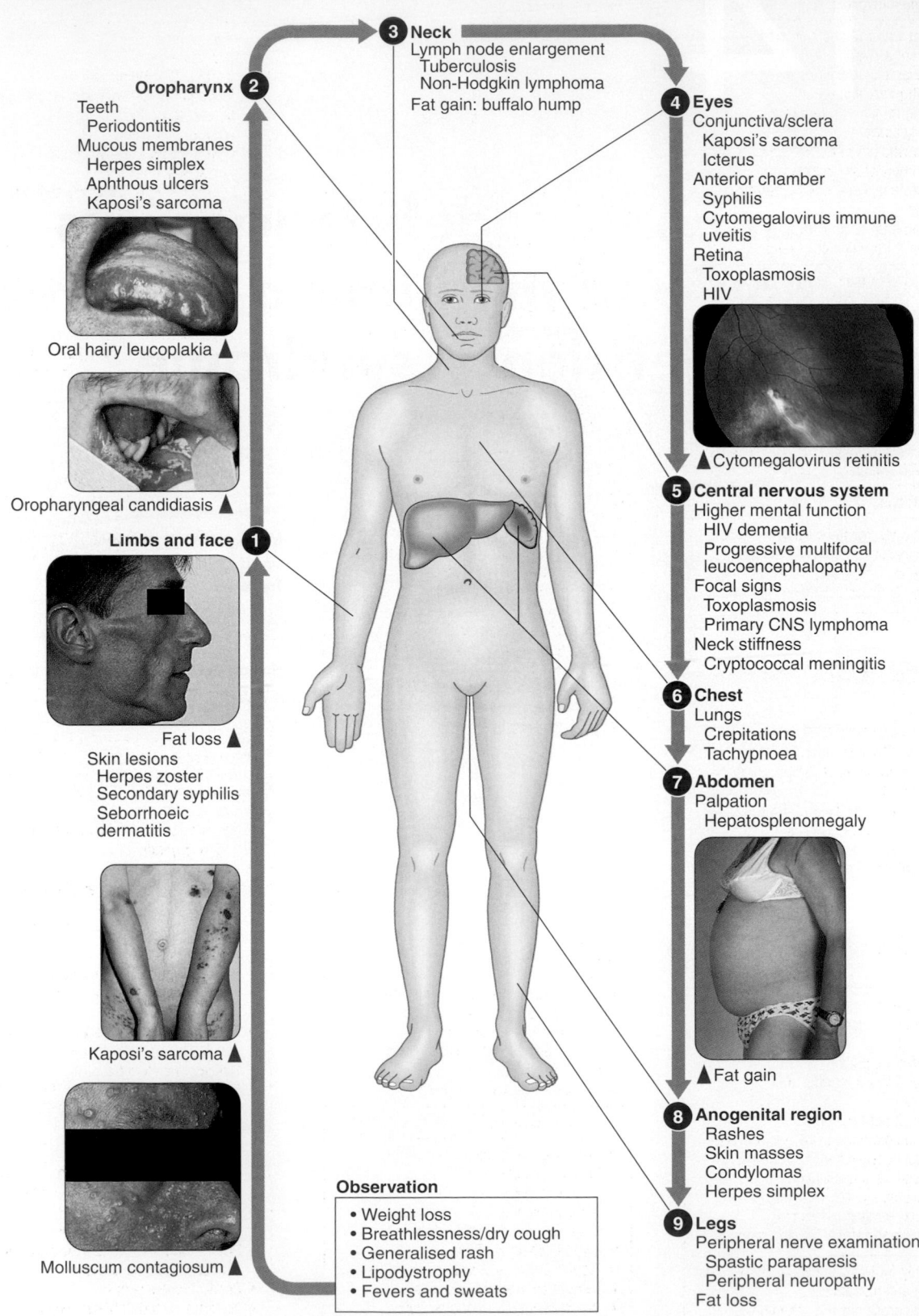

2 Oropharynx
Teeth
  Periodontitis
Mucous membranes
  Herpes simplex
  Aphthous ulcers
  Kaposi's sarcoma

Oral hairy leucoplakia ▲

Oropharyngeal candidiasis ▲

1 Limbs and face

Fat loss ▲
Skin lesions
  Herpes zoster
  Secondary syphilis
  Seborrhoeic
  dermatitis

Kaposi's sarcoma ▲

Molluscum contagiosum ▲

3 Neck
Lymph node enlargement
  Tuberculosis
  Non-Hodgkin lymphoma
Fat gain: buffalo hump

4 Eyes
Conjunctiva/sclera
  Kaposi's sarcoma
  Icterus
Anterior chamber
  Syphilis
  Cytomegalovirus immune
  uveitis
Retina
  Toxoplasmosis
  HIV

▲ Cytomegalovirus retinitis

5 Central nervous system
Higher mental function
  HIV dementia
  Progressive multifocal
  leucoencephalopathy
Focal signs
  Toxoplasmosis
  Primary CNS lymphoma
Neck stiffness
  Cryptococcal meningitis

6 Chest
Lungs
  Crepitations
  Tachypnoea

7 Abdomen
Palpation
  Hepatosplenomegaly

▲ Fat gain

8 Anogenital region
  Rashes
  Skin masses
  Condylomas
  Herpes simplex

9 Legs
Peripheral nerve examination
  Spastic paraparesis
  Peripheral neuropathy
Fat loss

Observation
• Weight loss
• Breathlessness/dry cough
• Generalised rash
• Lipodystrophy
• Fevers and sweats

14

CLINICAL POINTERS

Risk behaviour/group

- Contact with HIV-endemic area
  Recent arrival
  Sexual tourist/expatriate
  Health-care worker
  Blood transfusion recipient
- Sexually active
  Men who have sex with men
  Commercial sex worker
  Unprotected sex with numerous
  partners
- Injection drug user
- Partner of HIV-infected person

Confirmed diagnosis in risk group

- Herpes zoster
- Active tuberculosis
- Recurrent pneumococcal pneumonia
- Dementia
- B-cell lymphoma
- Paul–Bunnell-negative glandular fever
- Necrotising gingivitis
- Other HIV symptomatic disease (Box 14.5)
- Other AIDS-defining disease (Box 14.6)

Investigations

- Thrombocytopenia/atypical lymphocytosis
- Lymphopenia
- Positive markers for hepatitis B,
  hepatitis C or syphilis

PRE-TEST COUNSELLING

- Discuss purpose of test
- Carry out risk assessment
- Explore knowledge and explain natural
  history of HIV
- Discuss transmission and risk reduction
- Assess likely coping strategy
- Explain test procedure
- Obtain informed consent

LABORATORY CONFIRMATION

- Serology using commercial enzyme-
  linked immunosorbent assay (ELISA)
  screening test[1]
- Test result negative:
  Second test 3 months after last
  exposure
- Test result positive
  Result confirmed using two different
  immunoassays and/or Western blot
  Second sample checked
- Nucleic acid amplification test[2] if:
  Seroconversion suspected
  Confirming vertical transmission

[1] Commonly for HIV-1 antibody, HIV-2
antibody and p24 antigen.
[2] E.g. polymerase chain reaction (PCR) or
branched-chain DNA assay.

CLINICAL EXAMINATION

- See opposite.

KEY HISTORY POINTS

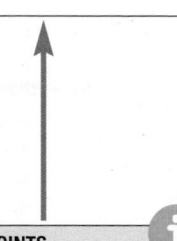

HIV (assessing time of HIV acquisition/likelihood of resistance)

- Previous negative HIV test
- History consistent with seroconversion
  (p. 400)
- Known HIV-infected ex-/current partner
  ? On medication
- Episodes of 'unsafe' sex in high-risk
  situations (e.g. saunas)
- Previous antenatal screening
- History of herpes zoster

General

- Birthplace, residence, occupation
- Tuberculosis: past history or contact
- Travel history/animal contacts
- Immunisation history (BCG, hepatitis A
  and B)
- Recreational drug use
- Past sexually transmitted infections
- Partner and children
- Others' knowledge of status (to contact
  if needed)
- GP awareness and permission to inform

POST-TEST COUNSELLING

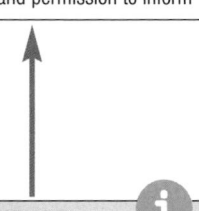

Test result negative

- Discuss transmission and need for
  behaviour modification
  Safer sex, needle exchange
- Advise second test 3 months after
  last exposure
- Support if uninfected partner

Test result positive

- Explain significance and
  implications of result
  Fear of disclosure
  Discrimination/social rejection
- Organise urgent medical follow-up
- Assess coping strategy
- Provide verbal and written information
- Discuss confidentiality issues
- Organise emotional and practical
  support (names/numbers)

BASELINE INVESTIGATIONS

All

- CD4 count
- Viral load (VL)
- Hepatitis B (HBV) status
- Hepatitis C (HCV) antibody
- HIV resistance test
- Cervical smear in women
- Hepatitis A (HAV) IgG antibody
- *Toxoplasma* antibody
- Cytomegalovirus (CMV) IgG antibody
- *Treponema* serology
- Genitourinary medicine screen

CD4 < 200 cells/mm^3

- Chest X-ray
- HCV-RNA
- Cryptococcal antigen
- Stool for ova, cysts and parasites

CD4 < 100 cells/mm^3

- CMV-PCR
- Dilated fundoscopy
- Electroencephalogram (ECG)
- Mycobacterial blood cultures

FURTHER ISSUES

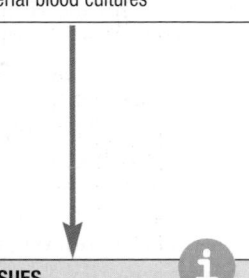

Immunisations

- Hepatitis A and hepatitis B if
  non-immune
- Pneumovax (at initial diagnosis and
  then 3–5-yearly)
- Influenza (yearly)
- Consider tetanus booster (if injection
  drug user)

Counselling

- Safe sex/behaviour modification
- Cryptosporidial risk and need to
  boil water
- *Toxoplasma* risk and safe handling of
  cats/litter; undercooked meat
- Live vaccines and travel
- Over-the-counter medicines if on highly
  active antiretroviral therapy (HAART)
- Plans for pregnancy

Repeat tests

- Treponemal antibody 3–4 times/year
- HBV markers every 1–2 years
- HCV antibody every 1–2 years
- HBVs antibody in immunised persons
  to assess need for booster
- Cervical smear yearly
- *Toxoplasma* and CMV serology if
  negative initially, yearly

14

EPIDEMIOLOGY AND BIOLOGY OF HIV

The acquired immunodeficiency syndrome (AIDS) was first recognised in 1981. It is caused by the human immunodeficiency virus (HIV-1). HIV-2 causes a similar illness to HIV-1 but is less aggressive and restricted mainly to western Africa. The viruses almost certainly originated from closely related African primate viruses, simian immunodeficiency viruses (SIVs). Sequence analysis has led to the estimate that HIV-1 was introduced into humans in the early 1930s. Since 1981 AIDS has grown to be the second leading cause of disease burden world-wide and the leading cause of death in Africa, where it accounts for over 20% of deaths. Immune deficiency is a consequence of continuous high-level HIV replication leading to virus and immune-mediated destruction of the key immune effector cell, the CD4 lymphocyte.

GLOBAL EPIDEMIC AND REGIONAL PATTERNS

In 2004, the World Health Organization (WHO) estimated that there were 39.4 million people living with HIV/AIDS, 4.9 million new infections and 3.1 million deaths. The cumulative death toll since the epidemic began is over 20 million, the vast majority of cases occurring in sub-Saharan Africa where over 13 million children have been orphaned. In Botswana, South Africa, Swaziland and Zimbabwe, 25–40% of adults are infected, with rates of 5–15% in most other sub-Saharan African countries. A total of 64% of all persons with HIV live in sub-Saharan Africa, with South Africa accounting for one-third of AIDS deaths globally. Since 2002, the steepest increases have been seen in East Asia (50%), attributable largely to the epidemic occurring in China, and in Eastern Europe and Central Asia (40%), where alarming increases have been seen in the Ukraine, Latvia and Russia. In Vietnam, Thailand, Cambodia, Nepal and Myanmar, HIV is now well established. In India, it is estimated that 5.1 million persons are currently infected; in Tamil Nadu district 50% of sex-workers are infected, and in Manipur over 5% of pregnant women are positive. In northern India, HIV is well established in injection drug-users, of whom 25–50% are infected. Given that Asia is home to 60% of the world's population, these changes have huge implications.

Many different cultural, social and behavioural aspects determine the regional characteristics of HIV disease. In the USA and northern Europe, the epidemic has predominantly been in men who have sex with men, whereas in southern and Eastern Europe, Vietnam, Malaysia, North-east India and China the incidence has been greatest in injection drug-users. In Africa, the Caribbean and much of South-east Asia the dominant routes of transmission are heterosexual and from mother to child (vertical). The economic and demographic impact of HIV infection in developing countries is profound as it affects the most economically productive and fertile ages and is also eroding the health and economic advances made in the last few decades. Unlike the situation in developed nations, fewer than 5% of patients in resource-poor countries are able to access antiretroviral drugs.

The epidemic in industrialised nations is changing. Heterosexual transmission has become the dominant route, with racial and ethnic minorities representing an increasing fraction. Around 58% of infections in the UK in 2003 were acquired heterosexually and 75% of these were acquired abroad in a country with a high prevalence of HIV, mainly sub-Saharan Africa. High-risk sexual behaviour is also increasing in many developed countries, including in persons aware of their HIV-positive status.

MODES OF TRANSMISSION

HIV is present in blood, semen and other body fluids such as breast milk and saliva. Exposure to infected fluid leads to a risk of contracting infection, which is dependent on the integrity of the exposed site, the type and volume of body fluid, and the viral load. HIV can enter either as free virus or within cells. The modes of spread are sexual (man to man, heterosexual and oral), parenteral (blood or blood product recipients, injection drug-users and those experiencing occupational injury) and vertical. The transmission risk after exposure is over 90% for blood or blood products,

14.1 FACTORS INCREASING THE RISK OF ACQUISITION OF HIV	
Common to all transmission categories	
• High viral load	• AIDS
• Lower CD4 cell count	• Seroconversion
Vertical transmission	
• Older gestational age	• Vaginal vs elective
• Prolonged rupture of membranes	caesarean delivery
• Chorioamnionitis	• No peripartum
• Fetal trauma (e.g. scalp electrodes)	prophylaxis
• Lower birth weight	• First-born twin
Breastfeeding	
• Longer duration feeding	• Younger age
• Lower parity	• Mastitis
Sexual transmission	
• Sexually transmitted infections (STIs), especially genital ulcers	• Male–male vs heterosexual sex
• Cervical ectopy	• Non-circumcised
• Receptive vs insertive anal sex	• Increased number of
• Rectal or vaginal trauma	partners
• Menstruation	
Injection drug use transmission	
• Sharing equipment	• Intravenous use
• Frequency of use	• Cocaine use
• Linked commercial sex	• Incarceration
• Lower income	
Occupational transmission	
• Deep injury	• Previous arterial or
• Visible blood on device	venous device siting

14

14

14.2 PREVENTION MEASURES FOR HIV TRANSMISSION

Sexual

- Comprehensive sex education programmes in schools
- Public awareness campaigns for HIV
- Easily accessible/discreet testing centres
- Safe sex practices (avoiding penetrative intercourse, delaying sexual debut, condom use, fewer sexual partners)
- Targeting safe sex methods to high-risk groups
- Control of STIs
- Effective treatment of HIV-infected persons
- Post-sexual exposure prophylaxis

Parenteral

- Blood product transmission (donor questionnaire, routine screening of donated blood, blood substitute use)
- Injection drug use (education, needle/syringe exchange, avoidance of 'shooting galleries', sharing and support for methadone maintenance programmes)

Perinatal

- Routine 'opt-out' antenatal HIV antibody testing
- Counselling about planning/risks of pregnancy if HIV-seropositive
- Measures to reduce vertical transmission (p. 400)

Occupational

- Education/training (universal precautions, needlestick avoidance)
- Post-exposure prophylaxis

15–40% for the vertical route, 0.5–1.0% for injection drug use, 0.2–0.5% for genital mucous membrane spread and under 0.1% for non-genital mucous membrane spread. Important factors increasing the risk of acquisition and measures available to reduce it are outlined in Boxes 14.1 and 14.2.

World-wide, the major route of transmission (> 75%) is heterosexual. About 5–10% of new HIV infections are in children and more than 90% of these are infected during pregnancy, birth or breastfeeding. The rate of mother-to-child transmission is higher in developing countries (25–44%) than in industrialised nations (13–25%); postnatal transmission via breast milk may account for some of this increased risk. Of those infected vertically, 80% are infected close to the time of delivery and 20% in utero. Around 70% of patients with haemophilia A and 30% of those with haemophilia B had been infected through contaminated blood products by the time HIV antibody screening was adopted in the USA and Europe in 1985. In developed nations, because of routine antibody screening, the likelihood of acquiring HIV from blood products is now less than 1:500 000 and arises from donors in the seroconverting phase of infection. However, the WHO estimates that because of the lack of adequate screening facilities in resource-poor countries, 5–10% of blood transfusions globally are with HIV-infected blood. There have been approximately 100 definite and 200 possible cases of HIV acquired occupationally in health-care workers. Infection related to health-care settings is substantially higher in developing nations, where it is estimated that 40% of syringes/needles used in injections are reused without sterilisation.

VIROLOGY AND IMMUNOLOGY

HIV is a single-stranded RNA retrovirus from the Lentivirus family. After mucosal exposure, HIV is transported to the lymph nodes via dendritic, CD4 or Langerhans cells, where infection becomes established. Dendritic cells express various receptors (e.g. DC–SIGN) that facilitate capture and transport of HIV-1. Free or cell-associated virus is then disseminated widely through the blood with seeding of 'sanctuary' sites (e.g. central nervous system) and latent CD4 cell reservoirs. With time, there is gradual attrition of the CD4 cell population, resulting in increasing impairment of cell-mediated immunity and susceptibility to opportunistic infections.

Each mature virion is spherical and has a lipid membrane lined by a matrix protein that is studded with glycoprotein (gp)120 and gp41 spikes surrounding a cone-shaped protein core. This core houses two copies of the single-stranded RNA genome and viral enzymes. The virus infects the CD4 cell in a complicated sequence of events beginning with engagement of the viral gp120 and the CD4 cell receptor (stage 1, Fig. 14.1), which results in a conformational change in gp120. This permits interaction with one of two chemokine co-receptors (CXCR4 or CCR5: stage 2) which is followed by membrane fusion and cellular entry involving gp41 (stage 3). Other cells expressing the CD4 cell receptor and permissive to infection are monocyte–macrophages, follicular dendritic cells and microglial cells in the central nervous system.

After penetrating the cell and uncoating, a DNA copy is transcribed from the RNA genome by the reverse transcriptase (RT) enzyme (stage 4) that is carried by the infecting virion. Reverse transcription is an error-prone process, and multiple mutations arise with ongoing replication (hence the rapid generation of viral resistance to drugs). This DNA is transported into the nucleus and integrated randomly within the host cell genome via integrase enzyme (stage 5). Integrated virus is known as proviral DNA. On host-cell activation, this DNA copy is used as a template to transcribe new RNA copies (stage 6), which are processed and exported from the nucleus, viral mRNA then being translated into viral peptide chains (stage 7). The precursor polyproteins are then cleaved by the viral protease enzyme to form new viral structural proteins and viral enzymes such as the reverse transcriptase and protease. These then migrate to the cell surface and are assembled using the host cellular apparatus to produce infectious viral particles. These bud from the cell surface, incorporating the host cell membrane as their own lipid bilayer coat, and cell lysis occurs (stage 9). Once maturation is complete, the new infectious virus (virion) is then available to infect uninfected cells and repeat the process. All of these processes are enabled by three viral genes (*GAG*, *POL* and *ENV*), as well as the products of six regulatory genes (*VIF, VPR, VPU, NEF, TAT* and *REV*). It has been calculated that each day more than 10^{10} virions are produced and 10^9 CD4 cells destroyed. This represents a daily turnover of 30% of the total viral burden and 6–7% of the total body CD4 cells. A small percentage of T cells (< 0.01%) either produce small

Stage	Steps in replication	Drug targets
1	Attachment to CD4 receptor	
2	Binding to co-receptor CCR5 or CXCR4	CCR5/CXCR4 receptor inhibitors
3	Fusion	Fusion inhibitors
4	Reverse transcription	Nucleoside and non-nucleoside reverse transcription inhibitors
5	Integration	Integrase inhibitors
6	Transcription	
7	Translation	
8	Cleavage of polypeptides and assembly	Protease inhibitors
9	Viral release	

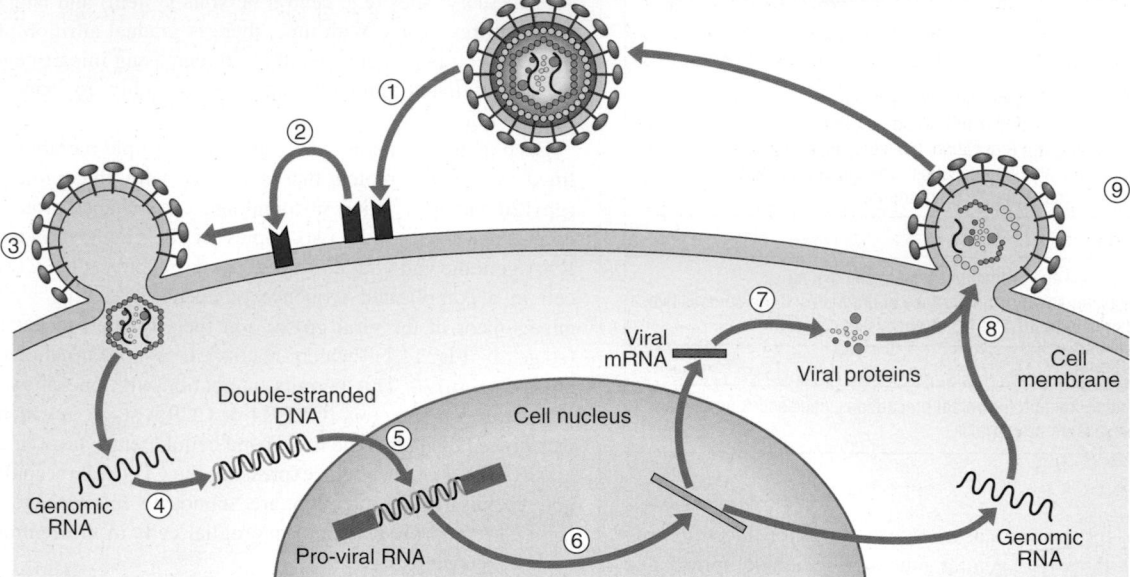

Fig. 14.1   Life cycle of HIV.

quantities of virus or enter a post-integration latent phase and represent the main reservoir of HIV. Together with virion-associated immune complexes bound to follicular dendritic cells, they can refuel infection if host defences fail or highly active antiretroviral therapy (HAART, p. 397) is discontinued. Within these cells there is ongoing low-level replication even when plasma levels of HIV are below the level of detection as a result of antiretroviral treatment. They are important as sanctuary sites from antiviral therapy, as continuing sources of virus (including the generation of drug-resistant strains) and as eventual targets for eradication strategies. The half-life of the virus is 1–2 hours in plasma, 1.5 days in productively infected CD4 cells and over 12 months in latently infected CD4 cells.

On the basis of DNA sequencing, HIV-1 can be sub-divided into group M ('major', world-wide distribution), group O ('outlier', divergent from group M) and group N (rare, highly divergent) types. Groups O and N are restricted to West Africa and may screen weakly positive or negative on routine antibody testing. Groups M and O can be sub-divided further into subtypes. There are 11 subtypes for group M, lettered A–K (Box 14.3), and these are responsible for the global epidemic of HIV. Many countries host several group M subtypes (e.g. in Africa) and genetic recombinants have been identified (e.g. AE) which now predominate in West Africa and Thailand. Increased HIV diversity has

14.3 HIV AND GENETIC VARIANTS

Virus Group	Subtype	Predominant area	Association
HIV-1 M	A	Africa	Heterosexual
		Eastern Europe	IDU
	B	Europe, North America	MSM, IDU
		Australia	MSM
		Thailand	IDU
	C	Southern Africa, India	Heterosexual
	D	East and Central Africa	Heterosexual
	AE	Thailand	Heterosexual
O/N		West Africa	Heterosexual
HIV-2		West Africa	Heterosexual

(MSM = men who have sex with men; IDU = injection drug-users)

implications for diagnostic tests, treatments and vaccine development. In Europe, the prevalence of non-B subtypes has increased dramatically and accounts for 10–25% of new infections. HIV-2 is an important but separate retrovirus which has at least five subtypes. The virus differs from HIV-1 in that patients have lower viral loads, slower CD4 decline, lower rates of vertical transmission, and slower progression to AIDS (12-fold lower).

As CD4 cells are pivotal in orchestrating the immune response, any depletion in numbers renders the body susceptible to opportunistic infections and oncogenic virus-related tumours. The predominant opportunist infections seen in HIV disease are intracellular parasites (e.g. *Mycobacterium tuberculosis*) or pathogens susceptible to cell-mediated rather than antibody-mediated immune responses. The reduction in the number of CD4 cells circulating in peripheral blood is tightly correlated with the amount of plasma viral load. (The exact mechanisms underlying the decline are not fully understood but it is not restricted to virus-infected cells.) Both are monitored closely in patients and are used as measures of disease progression. Virus-specific CD8 cytotoxic T-cell lymphocytes develop rapidly after infection and are the most important element in recognising, binding and lysing infected CD4 cells. They play a crucial role in controlling HIV replication after infection and determine the viral 'set-point' and subsequent rate of disease progression.

14.4 CLINICAL FEATURES OF PRIMARY INFECTION	

- Fever with rash
- Pharyngitis with cervical lymphadenopathy
- Myalgia/arthralgia
- Headache
- Mucosal ulceration

NATURAL HISTORY AND CLASSIFICATION OF HIV

Primary infection

Primary infection is symptomatic in 70–80% of cases and usually occurs 2–6 weeks after exposure. The major clinical manifestations are listed in Box 14.4. Rarely, presentation may be neurological (aseptic meningitis, encephalitis, myelitis, polyneuritis). This coincides with a surge in plasma HIV-RNA levels to > 1 million copies/ml (peak between 4 and 8 weeks), and a fall in the CD4 count to 300–400 cells/mm³, but occasionally to below 200 when opportunistic infections (e.g. oropharyngeal candidiasis, *Pneumocystis carinii* (*jirovecii*) pneumonia) may rarely occur (Fig. 14.2). Symptomatic recovery occurs after 1–2 weeks but occasionally may take up to 10 weeks and parallels the return of the CD4 count and fall in the viral load. In many patients the illness is mild and only identified by retrospective enquiry at later presentation. However, the CD4 count rarely recovers to its previous value.

Diagnosis is made by detecting HIV-RNA in the serum or by immunoblot assay (which shows antibodies developing to early proteins). The appearance of specific anti-HIV antibodies in serum (seroconversion) takes place later at 3–12 weeks (median 8 weeks), although very rarely seroconversion may take place after 3 months. Factors likely to indicate a faster progression of HIV are the presence and duration of symptoms, evidence of candidiasis, and neurological involvement. The level of the viral load post-seroconversion strongly correlates with subsequent progression of disease. The differential diagnosis of primary HIV includes acute Epstein–Barr virus (EBV), cytomegalovirus (CMV), streptococcal pharyngitis, toxoplasmosis and secondary syphilis.

Asymptomatic infection

Asymptomatic infection (category A disease in the Centers for Disease Control (CDC) classification) follows and lasts for a variable period, during which the infected individual remains well with no evidence of disease except for the possible presence of persistent generalised lymphadenopathy (PGL, defined as enlarged glands at ≥ 2 extra-inguinal sites). At this stage the bulk of virus replication takes place within lymphoid tissue (e.g. follicular dendritic cells). There is sustained viraemia with a decline in CD4 count dependent on the height of the viral load but usually between 50 and 150 cells/year (Fig. 14.2).

14

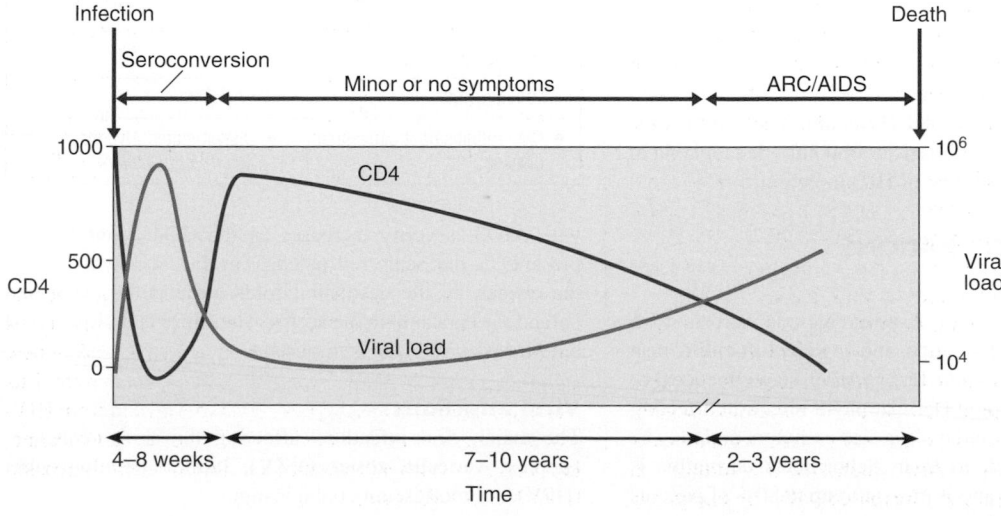

Fig. 14.2 Virological and immunological progression of HIV infection. (ARC = AIDS-related complex)

14.5 HIV SYMPTOMATIC DISEASES

- Oral hairy leucoplakia
- Recurrent oropharyngeal candidiasis
- Recurrent vaginal candidiasis
- Severe pelvic inflammatory disease
- Bacillary angiomatosis
- Cervical dysplasia
- Idiopathic thrombocytopenic purpura
- Weight loss*
- Chronic diarrhoea*
- Herpes zoster
- Peripheral neuropathy
- Low-grade fever/night sweats*

* But not AIDS-defining.

14.6 AIDS-DEFINING DISEASES

- Oesophageal candidiasis
- Cryptococcal meningitis
- Chronic cryptosporidial diarrhoea
- CMV retinitis or colitis
- Chronic mucocutaneous herpes simplex
- Disseminated *Mycobacterium avium intracellulare*
- Pulmonary or extrapulmonary tuberculosis
- *Pneumocystis carinii* (*jirovecii*) pneumonia
- Progressive multifocal leucoencephalopathy
- Recurrent non-typhi *Salmonella* septicaemia
- Cerebral toxoplasmosis
- Extrapulmonary coccidioidomycosis
- Invasive cervical cancer
- Extrapulmonary histoplasmosis
- Kaposi's sarcoma
- Non-Hodgkin lymphoma
- Primary cerebral lymphoma
- HIV-associated wasting
- HIV-associated dementia

Mildly symptomatic disease

Mildly symptomatic disease (CDC Classification category B disease) then develops in the majority, indicating some impairment of the cellular immune system. These diseases correspond to AIDS-related complex (ARC) conditions but by definition are not AIDS-defining (Box 14.5). The median interval from infection to the development of symptoms is around 7–10 years, although subgroups of patients exhibit 'fast' or 'slow' rates of progression.

Acquired immunodeficiency syndrome (AIDS)

AIDS (CDC Classification category C disease) is defined by the development of specified opportunistic infections, tumours etc. (Box 14.6). The correlation between CD4 count and HIV-related diseases is presented in Box 14.7.

14.7 CORRELATIONS BETWEEN CD4 COUNT AND HIV-ASSOCIATED DISEASES

> 500 cells/mm³

- Acute primary infection
- Recurrent vaginal candidiasis
- Persistent generalised lymphadenopathy

< 500 cells/mm³

- Pulmonary tuberculosis
- Pneumococcal pneumonia
- Herpes zoster
- Oropharyngeal candidiasis
- Oral hairy leucoplakia
- Extra-intestinal salmonellosis
- Kaposi's sarcoma
- HIV-associated idiopathic thrombocytopenic purpura
- Cervical intra-epithelial neoplasia II–III
- Lymphoid interstitial pneumonitis

< 200 cells/mm³

- *Pneumocystis carinii* (*jirovecii*) pneumonia
- Mucocutaneous herpes simplex
- *Cryptosporidium*
- *Microsporidium*
- Oesophageal candidiasis
- Miliary/extrapulmonary tuberculosis
- HIV-associated wasting
- Peripheral neuropathy

< 100 cells/mm³

- Cerebral toxoplasmosis
- Cryptococcal meningitis
- Primary CNS lymphoma
- Non-Hodgkin lymphoma
- HIV-associated dementia
- Progressive multifocal leucoencephalopathy

< 50 cells/mm³

- CMV retinitis/gastrointestinal disease
- Disseminated *Mycobacterium avium intracellulare*

PRESENTING PROBLEMS IN HIV INFECTION

MUCOCUTANEOUS DISEASE

Mucocutaneous manifestations are common in HIV and range from the trivial to markers of significant systemic infection (Boxes 14.8 and 14.9). Most patients are affected at some time and for many it is a major problem. Dermatological problems may present atypically, coexist with other pathologies and be harder to manage than in an HIV-negative person. Type and severity of rash are often dependent upon the level of CD4 count. The presence of either oropharyngeal candidiasis or oral hairy leucoplakia in a young person is suggestive of HIV infection.

SPECIFIC SKIN CONDITIONS

Fungal infections

Early HIV-associated skin diseases include xerosis with pruritus, seborrhoeic dermatitis, and an itchy folliculitic rash which may be fungal *(Malassezia furfur)*, staphylococcal or eosinophilic in aetiology. Dermatophyte infection affecting skin (feet, body, face) and nails is also common, and may be extensive and difficult to treat. Seborrhoeic dermatitis is very common in HIV and is present in up to 80% of patients

with AIDS; severity increases as the CD4 count falls. It presents as dry scaly red patches on the face (typically on the cheeks, in the nasolabial folds, around the eyebrows, behind the ears and on the scalp). The cause is multifactorial but *Malassezia furfur* is important.

Viral infections

The major viral infections affecting the skin are herpes simplex, varicella zoster (VZV), human papillomavirus (HPV) and molluscum contagiosum.

14

14.8 DIFFERENTIAL DIAGNOSIS OF HIV-RELATED SKIN DISEASE

Early HIV

Infection
- Herpes simplex
- Varicella zoster
- Human papillomavirus (HPV)
- Impetigo
- Dermatophytosis
- Scabies
- Syphilis
- HIV seroconversion

Other
- Xeroderma
- Pruritus
- Seborrhoeic dermatitis
- Drug reaction (co-trimoxazole/nevirapine)
- Itchy folliculitis
- Psoriasis
- Acne

Late HIV

Common
- Kaposi's sarcoma
- Molluscum contagiosum
- Chronic mucocutaneous herpes simplex

Rare
- Bacillary angiomatosis
- CMV
- Non-Hodgkin lymphoma
- *Cryptococcus*
- Histoplasmosis
- Mycobacterial (tuberculosis/atypical)

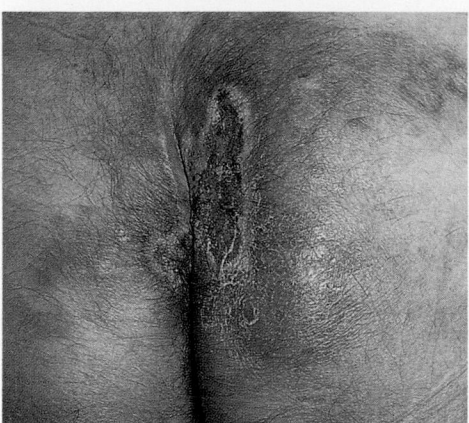

Fig. 14.3 Severe mucocutaneous herpes simplex. Perianal or perioral infection is not uncommon in later-stage HIV infection.

14.9 DIFFERENTIAL DIAGNOSIS OF HIV-RELATED ORAL DISEASE

Early HIV

- Oral hairy leucoplakia
- Herpes simplex
- Oropharyngeal candidiasis
- Aphthous ulcers
- Periodontitis
- Syphilis
- HPV
- Herpes zoster

Late HIV

- Kaposi's sarcoma
- Drug reaction
- Lymphoma
- CMV

ophthalmic or very dense, or when the CD4 count is < 200 cells/mm^3, parenteral aciclovir must be used.

Human papillomavirus infection is frequent amongst HIV patients and is usually anogenital (p. 417); disease may be extensive and very difficult to manage. Lesions on the hands and feet (especially periungual) are also common and may attain considerable size, requiring surgery. Occasionally, myriads of flat-topped papules occur over the body and face. Both oncogenic (16, 18, 31, 33) and non-oncogenic (6, 11) genotypes are found. There is often improvement on HAART.

Molluscum contagiosum is an epidermal poxvirus infection. It is found in approximately 10% of AIDS patients (pp. 378 and 1296). The lesions are usually 2–5 mm diameter papules with a central umbilicus and most frequently affect the face, neck, scalp and genital region. Lesions may become widespread and attain a large size (giant mollusca). With improvement in CD4 counts, lesions usually disappear.

Bacterial and parasitic infections

Bacterial infections include *Staphylococcus aureus* (folliculitis, cellulitis and abscesses), bacillary angiomatosis and syphilis (primary and secondary, pp. 411–412). Bacillary angiomatosis is a bacterial infection due to the cat-scratch bacillus, *Bartonella henselae*. Skin lesions range from solitary superficial reddish-purple lesions resembling Kaposi's sarcoma or pyogenic granuloma, to multiple subcutaneous nodules or even hyperpigmented plaques. Lesions are painful and may bleed or ulcerate. The infection may become disseminated with fevers, lymphadenopathy and hepatosplenomegaly. Diagnosis is made by Warthin–Starry silver staining which reveals aggregates of bacilli.

In HIV, scabies (due to the mite *Sarcoptes scabiei*—p. 1297) may cause intensely pruritic, encrusted papules affecting most areas. Classically, the interdigital web spaces, wrists, periumbilical area, buttock and sides of the feet are involved. Commonly in HIV the infestation may be heavy, the rash hyperkeratotic (Norwegian scabies) and the patient highly infectious. Uniquely, the face and neck are often affected. Rarely, cutaneous disease may be a manifestation of mycobacterial infection (tuberculosis or an atypical mycobacterium) or disseminated fungal infection.

Herpes simplex (type 1 or 2) may affect the lips, mouth, skin or anogenital area and is seen in 20% of cases. In later-stage HIV, the lesions are usually chronic, extensive, harder to treat and recurrent (Fig. 14.3). Persistent and severe anogenital ulceration is usually herpetic and a marker for underlying HIV.

Varicella zoster usually presents with a dermatomal vesicular rash on an erythematous base and may be the first clue to a diagnosis of HIV infection. It can occur at any stage but is more frequent with failing immunity. In patients with a low CD4 count (< 100 cells/mm^3) the rash may be more severe, multidermatomal, persistent or recurrent, or may become disseminated. Involvement of the trigeminal nerve, scarring on recovery and associated motor defects are probably also more common. Diagnosis of herpetic infection can be confirmed by culture, smear preparations showing characteristic inclusion bodies, electron microscopy or biopsy. Treatment should be given for all cases of active disease, irrespective of the time since onset of rash. In patients with severe mucocutaneous herpes simplex or herpes zoster which is disseminated, multidermatomal,

14

SPECIFIC ORAL CONDITIONS

Candidiasis

Candida infection in HIV is almost exclusively mucosal, affects nearly all patients with CD4 counts that drop below 200 cells/mm^3 and in early disease is nearly always caused by *C. albicans* (p. 378). Pseudomembranous candidiasis describes white patches on the buccal mucosa that can be scraped off to reveal a red raw surface. The tongue, palate and pharynx may also be involved. Less common is erythematous candidiasis; patients present with a sore mouth, reddened mucosa and a smooth shiny tongue. Hypertrophic candidiasis (leucoplakia-like lesions which do not scrape off but respond to antifungal treatment) and angular cheilitis may also be present.

Diagnosis is clinical but it is important to perform a mouth swill for culture, speciation and sensitivities in patients unresponsive to fluconazole or other azole drugs. The cause is usually *C. albicans*, although occasionally non-*albicans Candida* may be responsible (e.g. *C. glabrata*, *C. krusei*), in which case azole resistance is more likely. Prophylaxis is not recommended and therapeutic courses of azoles should be given with each attack.

Oesophageal infection may coexist, although in up to 30% no oropharyngeal candidiasis is visible. Up to 80% of patients with pain on swallowing have *Candida* oesophagitis (see p. 881 for differential diagnosis) with pseudomembranous plaques visible on barium swallow and endoscopy (Fig. 14.4). The pain is usually associated with dysphagia and, when untreated, leads to weight loss. Treatment is with an oral azole drug. Where azole-resistant candida is present, caspofungin or amphotericin can be used.

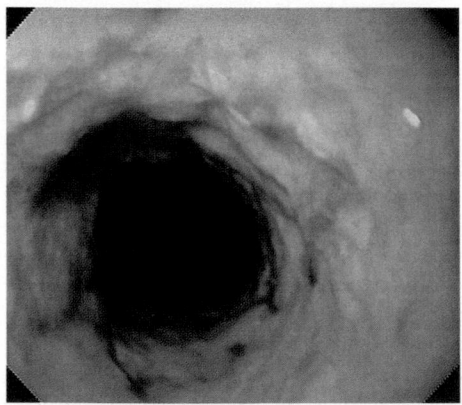

Fig. 14.4 Oesophageal candidiasis. Endoscopy may show pseudomembranous plaques or extensive confluent infection.

Oral hairy leucoplakia

Oral hairy leucoplakia has the appearance of corrugated white plaques running vertically on the side of the tongue and is virtually pathognomonic of HIV disease in the context of HIV risk factors (p. 378). It is usually asymptomatic and does not require treatment. The aetiology is closely associated with EBV. High-dose aciclovir is sometimes effective in eradicating the infection but relapse often follows cessation of treatment.

14.10 FIRST-LINE TREATMENTS IN HIV-RELATED MUCOCUTANEOUS DISEASE	
Condition	**Treatment**
Seborrhoeic dermatitis/ capitis	Topical antifungal/hydrocortisone cream Ketoconazole shampoo
Herpes infections	Aciclovir or valaciclovir
Bacillary angiomatosis	Doxycycline or azithromycin
Molluscum contagiosum	Curettage or cryotherapy
Oral candidiasis	Fluconazole or another azole compound
Severe oral hairy leucoplakia	Aciclovir or valaciclovir
Anogenital HPV	Podophyllin, imiquimod or cryotherapy
Scabies	Permethrin, malathion or benzyl benzoate
Kaposi's sarcoma	HAART, radiotherapy Liposomal doxorubicin or daunorubicin
Syphilis	Penicillin (procaine or benzathine) or doxycycline

Kaposi's sarcoma

This is discussed in more detail on page 396.

INVESTIGATIONS AND MANAGEMENT

Diagnosis of mucocutaneous conditions in HIV, including Kaposi's sarcoma, is usually clinical. Rarely, bacterial, viral or fungal cultures are necessary. Any person with an unusual rash, especially one persistent and unresponsive to topical antifungal/corticosteroid combinations, or in the presence of severe immune compromise (CD4 < 50 cells/mm^3), merits a skin biopsy for histology and culture. First-line treatment is outlined in Box 14.10.

GASTROINTESTINAL DISEASE

Pain on swallowing, weight loss and chronic diarrhoea are common presenting features of later-stage HIV and indicate disease at different sites in the gastrointestinal tract. A range of opportunistic organisms and HIV-related tumours may be responsible (Fig. 14.5).

SPECIFIC CONDITIONS

Cytomegalovirus (CMV)

Gastrointestinal CMV occurs in up to one-third of patients with AIDS and is only seen if the CD4 count is < 100 cells/mm^3 (usually < 50). It may cause disease throughout the entire gastrointestinal tract, including the liver and biliary tree, but most commonly affects the oesophagus and colon.

Oesophageal CMV accounts for 10–20% of oesophageal disease and presents with gradual onset of localised pain on swallowing, retrosternal pain, dysphagia, fever and weight loss. The diagnosis is suspected when there is failure to respond to an empirical course of fluconazole (oesophageal

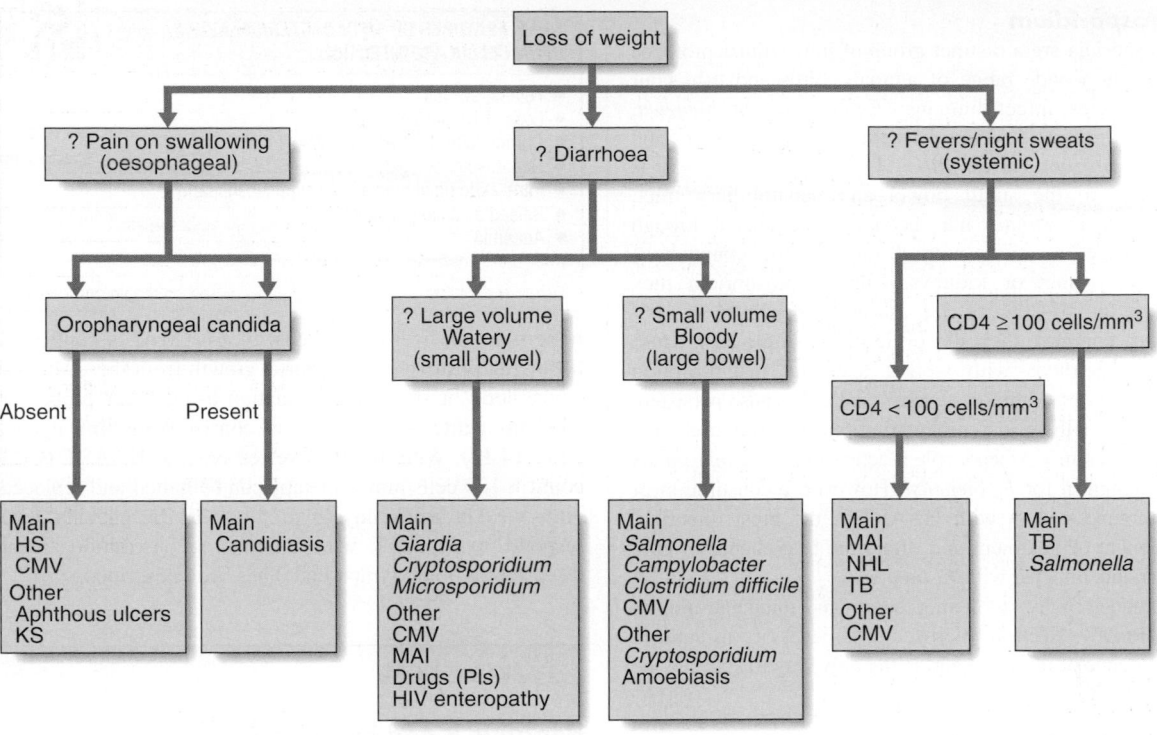

Fig. 14.5 Presentation and differential diagnosis of HIV-related gastrointestinal disorders. (HS = herpes simplex; CMV = cytomegalovirus; KS = Kaposi's sarcoma; MAI = *Mycobacterium avium intracellulare*; PI = protease inhibitor; NHL = non-Hodgkin lymphoma; TB = tuberculosis)

14

candidiasis accounts for up to 80% of patients with pain on swallowing), distal focal disease on barium swallow, or inflammation with erosions/ulcers on endoscopy. Confirmation is by biopsy showing classical intracellular 'owl's-eye' inclusion bodies or by immunofluorescence. Rarely, strictures may complicate long-standing disease.

CMV colitis may occur in up to 5% of patients. Presentation is usually with watery diarrhoea, often accompanied by blood, colicky abdominal pain, weight loss and fever. It should be suspected in patients with pathogen-negative diarrhoea or with thickened and dilated large bowel on abdominal X-ray. Endoscopy may show a range of abnormalities from generalised hyperaemia to segmental or confluent shallow or deep ulcers. Again diagnosis depends on biopsy. As up to 20% of cases have disease proximal to the splenic flexure, colonoscopy should be performed where possible. Toxic megacolon (p. 914), haemorrhage and perforation may complicate infection.

Cryptosporidium

Cryptosporidium is a highly contagious zoonotic protozoal enteric pathogen that infects a wide range of animals. It accounts for 15–20% of the causes of diarrhoea, characteristically producing large-volume watery stools and abdominal pain. If the CD4 count is over 200 cells/mm^3, infection is usually self-limiting (> 80%). Below this level, a cholera-like illness or severe chronic watery diarrhoea with malabsorption and weight loss may occur. Prior to the advent of HAART, the majority of these patients would die from their infection.

Diagnosis is confirmed by stool microscopy in 90% using acid-fast or immunofluorescence stains. Cryptosporidia are also readily identifiable on duodenal biopsy, which may be necessary as stainable oöcysts are intermittently or never seen in the stool of some patients (10%) (Fig. 14.6). Treatment is rarely successful unless the CD4 count can be increased above 200 cells/mm^3 with HAART. *Cryptosporidium* can rarely cause acalculous cholecystitis (p. 993), sclerosing cholangitis (p. 980) and pneumonitis when the CD4 is < 50 cells/mm^3. All HIV patients with CD4 counts below 200 cells/mm^3 should be advised to boil drinking water as cysts are chlorine-resistant, and to minimise contact with animals (especially young).

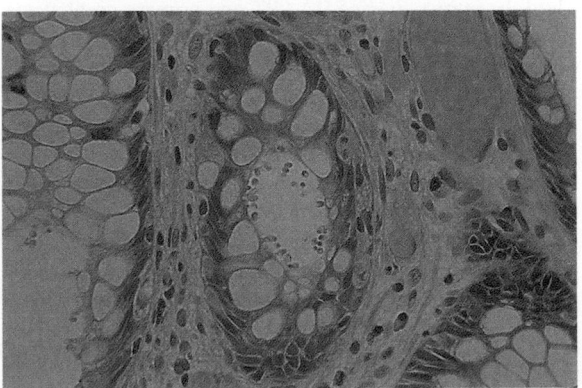

Fig. 14.6 Cryptosporidial infection. Duodenal biopsy may be necessary to confirm cryptosporidiosis or microsporidiosis.

Microsporidium

Microsporidia are a distinct group of intracellular protozoa carried by a wide range of animals, birds and fish. Four main species infect humans: *Enterocytozoon bieneusi*, *Encephalitozoon hellem, Encephalitozoon cuniculi,* and *Encephalitozoon intestinalis*. In HIV, *E. bieneusi* is restricted to the small bowel and hepatobiliary tract, whereas *E. intestinalis* may become disseminated through macrophage infection, with disease in the conjunctiva, respiratory tract or kidneys. Like cryptosporidia they account for 10–20% of the causes of diarrhoea in HIV patients, complete their life cycle in the single host, cause chronic diarrhoea with weight loss and malabsorption (although not as rapid or severe), and only cause persistent disease when there is significant immune compromise (CD4 < 100 cells/mm³). Albendazole is active against *E. intestinalis* and fumagillin for *E. bieneusi*. However, reconstitution of the immune system with HAART is the most important component of treatment and offers the best chance of cure for patients infected with *E. bieneusi*.

Diagnosis is by stool microscopy and duodenal biopsy. Occasionally, electron microscopy is necessary to confirm the presence of infection and is the only way to speciate the microsporidia.

Other infections

Isospora (Africa and Latin America) and *Cyclospora* (Asia) are common to their localities and cause watery diarrhoea, weight loss and malabsorption akin to *Cryptosporidium*, accounting overall for 2–4% of cases in the UK. Diagnosis is by stool microscopy and treatment for both is co-trimoxazole.

Giardia, Entamoeba histolytica, adenovirus and bacterial overgrowth also occur more frequently in HIV patients.

HIV enteropathy is a term given to a complex of chronic diarrhoea and partial villous atrophy for which no other cause can be found (10–20% of cases).

Of the standard enteric pathogens, *Salmonella* is important because of the increased probability of bacteraemia and recurrent disease, and *Clostridium difficile* toxin-associated colitis because of the frequent use of antimicrobials.

Mycobacterium avium intracellulare (MAI)

Until the introduction of HAART and primary prophylaxis, disseminated MAI occurred in up to 35% of all patients with a median CD4 count of 13 cells/mm³ at presentation. Like other opportunistic infections, the incidence has now fallen by 90% but it remains a problem in late-stage AIDS, especially those cases that are newly diagnosed.

The organism is an environmental mycobacterium commonly found in water and food. Acquisition of infection is probably from the respiratory and gastrointestinal tracts, where colonisation precedes disseminated infection in two-thirds of patients. All organs are affected, with heavy infiltration of organisms and little inflammatory response; the reticulo-endothelial system bears the major burden of infection (Box 14.11).

Mycobacterial disease is confirmed by identifying acid-fast bacilli on Ziehl–Neelsen staining of induced sputum,

> **14.11 FEATURES OF *MYCOBACTERIUM AVIUM INTRACELLULARE* INFECTION**
>
> - Fevers, sweats
> - Loss of weight/appetite
> - Chronic diarrhoea and abdominal pain
> - Hepatosplenomegaly
> - Intra-abdominal/mediastinal lymphadenopathy
> - Raised alkaline phosphatase
> - Anaemia

bone marrow, liver or duodenal biopsy. MAI is confirmed following positive mycobacterial growth from these sites or from blood or stool, and speciation using DNA probes or conventional tests. Therapy must consist of multiple agents (Box 14.12). With an effective response to HAART (CD4 count > 100 cells/mm³), therapy can be halted and replaced with weekly azithromycin prophylaxis. In patients who respond to HAART with immune reconstitution, focal disease (e.g. joint, lymph node) has been described.

LIVER DISEASE

Hepatitis B and hepatitis C

The contribution of hepatitis B and C co-infection is becoming increasingly recognised. The majority of persons with HIV have evidence of hepatitis B virus exposure. Carriage rate depends on the mode of acquisition (highest for injection drug-users), place of birth and ethnic group (reflecting vertical transmission), immunisation history (although response rates are lower in HIV patients) and the likelihood of immune clearance after infection. This is determined by whether infection preceded HIV infection (carriage rate 5–10%) or came after (rate increased and dependent on CD4 count when infected).

Hepatitis C (HCV)

Only 15–20% of patients ever clear their initial infection and the major determinant of co-infection rate is the mode of acquisition (> 80% for haemophiliacs, 70–80% for injection drug-users, 10–15% for MSM and 3–5% for heterosexuals). Co-infected patients have a higher HCV viral load, accelerated natural progression to cirrhosis (5–8 years after infection) and an increased risk of complications. Response to 12 months' combination therapy with pegylated α-interferon and ribavirin is dependent on the genotype (~65% with genotypes 2 or 3 as opposed to ~27% with other genotypes). The presence of cirrhosis also reduces the likelihood of cure.

Hepatitis B (HBV)

Co-infected patients have higher DNA levels and the disease is more aggressive, although the immunosuppression seen in more advanced disease affords some protection because hepatic damage is immune-mediated. Treatment should be considered for all patients who have active viral replication (HBVeAg-positive or high levels of HBV-DNA) and biopsy evidence of active disease. The choice of treatment depends on whether therapy is also required for HIV.

14.12 FIRST-LINE TREATMENTS IN HIV-RELATED GASTROINTESTINAL DISORDERS

Condition	Treatment
Candida	Fluconazole or another azole compound Amphotericin or caspofungin (if azole-resistant)
Herpes simplex	Aciclovir or valaciclovir
Cytomegalovirus	Ganciclovir, valganciclovir, cidofovir or foscarnet
Cryptosporidium	Paramomycin and azithromycin
Microsporidium[1]	Albendazole or fumagillin
Mycobacterium avium intracellulare	Rifabutin, ethambutol, azithromycin, ciprofloxacin
Isospora and *Cyclospora*	Co-trimoxazole
Hepatitis B[2]	Pegylated α-interferon or adefovir (no HIV treatment required) Tenofovir and 3TC or FTC (HIV treatment required)
Hepatitis C	Pegylated α-interferon and ribavirin
Kaposi's sarcoma	Liposomal doxorubicin or daunorubicin Paclitaxel (refractory disease)
Non-Hodgkin lymphoma	Chemotherapy

[1] See text.
[2] Tenofovir and 3TC or FTC should only be given in the context of HAART.

14.13 DIFFERENTIAL DIAGNOSIS OF HIV-RELATED PULMONARY DISEASE: CHEST X-RAY FINDINGS

Appearance	Major causes
Diffuse infiltrate	*Pneumocystis carinii* pneumonia, tuberculosis, Kaposi's sarcoma, non-Hodgkin lymphoma, atypical bacterial pneumonia, lymphoid interstitial pneumonitis
Nodules/focal consolidation	Kaposi's sarcoma, tuberculosis, non-Hodgkin lymphoma, *Cryptococcus*, pyogenic bacterial pneumonia
Hilar lymphadenopathy	Tuberculosis, Kaposi's sarcoma, non-Hodgkin lymphoma, *Cryptococcus*, *Histoplasma*
Pleural effusion	Kaposi's sarcoma, tuberculosis, pyogenic bacterial pneumonia, cavity-based lymphoma

14

For both HBV and HCV, therapy may be associated with a flare of hepatitis because of improved immune responsiveness. When the CD4 count is < 200 cells/mm³ at initial diagnosis, HCV-RNA should be assessed because HCV antibody may be absent. All patients should be screened for HBV and HAV and immunised if not protected. Hepatitis is described on pages 962–969.

RESPIRATORY DISEASE

More than half of patients with AIDS will develop pulmonary disease at some time. Several factors influence the likely cause, including CD4 count, ethnicity, age, risk group, prophylactic history and geographical location. The history is vital in discriminating acute bacterial pneumonia (rapid onset, pleuritic chest pain, rigors) from *Pneumocystis carinii* pneumonia (subacute onset, breathlessness, dry cough), a common differential in later-stage disease. The chest X-ray is also important in distinguishing presenting syndromes (Box 14.13).

SPECIFIC CONDITIONS

Pneumocystis carinii

Pneumocystis carinii (now renamed *jirovecii*) pneumonia (PCP) was the first major indicator disease for HIV at the beginning of the epidemic and is still the most common AIDS-defining illness. The organism is a fungus on genetic analysis but has a life cycle (cyst, sporozoite and tropho-

zoite), morphology and drug susceptibility pattern characteristic of a protozoan. It cannot be cultured, but the cyst and trophozoite are easily stained (Giemsa, methenamine-silver or immunofluorescence). PCP represents reactivation of latent infection acquired in childhood in the majority of patients but re-infection probably also occurs. Transmission is likely to be air-borne and the source other infected humans.

The incidence of PCP has fallen dramatically with the advent of HAART and routine primary prophylaxis in those persons with CD4 counts less than 200 cells/mm³. The risk of developing PCP is inversely correlated with the CD4 count. Cases rarely occur when the CD4 count is > 200 cells/mm³, whereas 40% of patients with a CD4 count of < 100 cells/mm³ and not taking primary prophylaxis will develop the disease annually. In those taking prophylaxis, PCP may still occur but at a lower CD4 count and with a better prognosis.

Co-trimoxazole also provides prophylaxis for *Toxoplasma gondii* and bacterial respiratory tract infections; it is inexpensive. Side-effects (typically a rash but occasionally Stevens–Johnson syndrome (p. 1308), leucopenia, thrombocytopenia and hepatitis) occur in approximately 20–25% of patients.

Dapsone, atovaquone or aerosolised pentamidine inhaled every 2–4 weeks are effective alternatives.

Typical presenting features are described in Box 14.14. There may also be other markers of HIV (e.g. oropharyngeal candidiasis or mucocutaneous herpes simplex). Non-specific diagnostic tests include a chest X-ray, and there is raised lactate dehydrogenase (from lung damage), exercise-induced O₂ desaturation, hypoxaemia on arterial blood gases and impaired carbon monoxide transfer factor. The chest X-ray appearances may be normal in early disease (15–20%) but classically demonstrate perihilar ground-glass changes (Fig. 14.7); later, an acute respiratory distress syndrome (ARDS) picture is common. Atypical appearances (20%) include unilateral infiltration, upper lobe disease (often when on inhaled pentamidine prophylaxis), focal consolidation, cavitation or nodular shadows. Complications

14.14 CLINICAL FEATURES OF *PNEUMOCYSTIS CARINII* PNEUMONIA

- 2–3-week history
- Fever with dry cough
- Disproportionate breathlessness
- No response to standard antibiotics
- Few signs on auscultation
- Exercise-related desaturation

14.15 FIRST-LINE TREATMENTS IN HIV-RELATED PULMONARY DISEASE

Condition	Treatment
Pneumocystis carinii (moderate to severe)	Co-trimoxazole, pentamidine, or clindamycin and primaquine Adjunctive corticosteroid therapy reduces mortality
P. carinii (mild)	Co-trimoxazole,[1] atovaquone, pentamidine[2]
Mycobacterium tuberculosis	Rifampicin, isoniazid, ethambutol, pyrazinamide
M. avium intracellulare	Rifabutin, ethambutol, azithromycin, ciprofloxacin
Pulmonary Kaposi's sarcoma	Liposomal doxorubicin or daunorubicin Paclitaxel (refractory disease)
Community-acquired pneumonia	Cefotaxime and clarithromycin
Cryptococcus neoformans	Amphotericin B or fluconazole

[1] Oral.
[2] Inhaled.

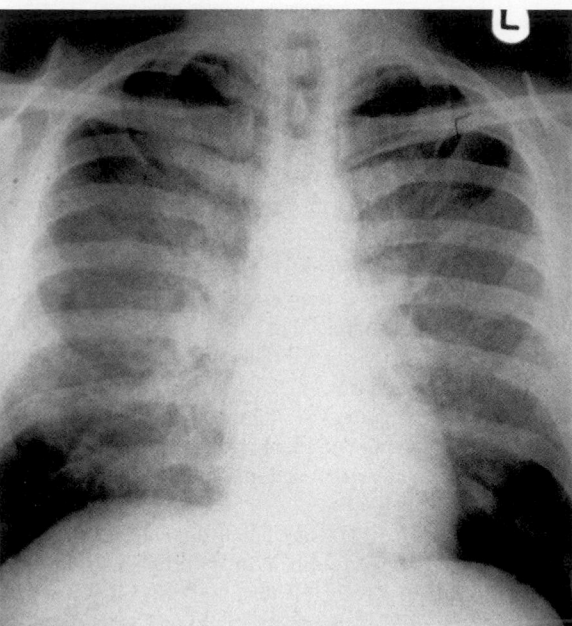

Fig. 14.7 *Pneumocystis* pneumonia. Typical chest X-ray appearance. Note the sparing at the apex and base of both lungs.

Mycobacterium tuberculosis

Approximately one-third of the 40 million HIV-infected persons in the world are co-infected with *M. tuberculosis*; 75% of these people reside in sub-Saharan Africa, where in some countries up to 30% of patients with tuberculosis (TB) are co-infected with HIV. Patients with HIV are at greater risk of:

- reactivating latent infection (7–10% annual risk compared to 5–10% lifetime risk in a non-HIV-infected individual)
- acquiring TB from an open contact (10–20% compared to 5–10%)
- developing progressive primary disease (30–40% compared to 5–10%)
- developing disseminated, miliary or extrapulmonary disease (> 60% compared to < 25%)
- developing second episodes of TB from exogenous infection.

Escalating TB case rates in sub-Saharan Africa are largely attributable to the explosive HIV epidemic. The present estimated annual new case and death rates (8 million and 2 million respectively) are expected to continue to rise inexorably. *M. tuberculosis* also affects HIV adversely with enhanced replication and acceleration of the disease process.

The clinical presentation depends mainly on immune function. When the CD4 count is > 200 cells/mm³, disease is more likely to be reactivated upper-lobe open cavitatory disease (Fig. 14.8); as immunosuppression increases, miliary, atypical pulmonary and extrapulmonary (especially pericardial, abdominal and meningeal) TB become progressively more common, as does mycobacteraemia (identified in up to half of those with CD4 < 200 cells/mm³). Constitutional symptoms of fever and night sweats are usually present. Approximately 5% of patients with smear-positive pulmonary TB have normal chest X-rays. Confirmation of the clinical diagnosis when the immune

include pneumothorax, bacterial superinfection, respiratory failure, corticosteroid-induced candidiasis and extra-pulmonary disease.

The differential diagnosis includes *M. tuberculosis* (p. 695), lymphoma, unusual fungi (*Histoplasma, Penicillium, Cryptococcus, Coccidioides*), pulmonary Kaposi's sarcoma, atypical pneumonia (*Mycoplasma* etc.) and *Nocardia* (Box 14.13). Specific diagnostic tests are cytology of nebulised hypertonic saline-induced sputum (30–80% sensitivity), bronchoscopy with lavage (90%) or together with transbronchial biopsy (95%). PCR of bronchoalveolar lavage fluid, induced sputum or saliva is sensitive and specific but does not distinguish active from treated infection or colonisation.

Treatment is outlined in Box 14.15. Clinical and radio-logical deterioration within the first 48 hours of treatment is not uncommon. Poor prognostic factors include delayed diagnosis, not being on prophylaxis, low CD4 count, extensive chest X-ray changes, low hypoxaemia ratio, high lactate dehydrogenase, hypoalbuminaemia, pneumothorax and additional pulmonary infection. There is some evidence that prolonged co-trimoxazole use may result in drug resistance with an increased risk of treatment failure.

14

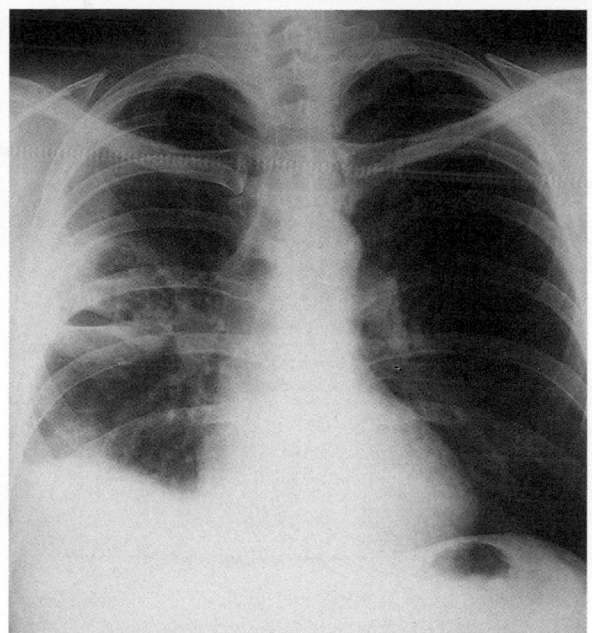

Fig. 14.8 Chest X-ray of pulmonary tuberculosis in HIV infection. Appearances are often atypical but in this case there is a typical large cavity accompanied by a pleural effusion.

system is relatively preserved is by sputum microscopy (Ziehl–Neelsen and auramine stains) and radiometric culture. Rapid diagnostic tests involving nucleic acid amplification are being employed more frequently for sputum analysis in smear-negative pulmonary cases and are also important in rapid speciation and determining rifampicin resistance. In patients with late-stage HIV and low CD4 counts, diagnosis is usually made by mycobacterial culture of blood, bone marrow or tissue.

Response to quadruple anti-TB combination therapy is good, although mortality is increased because of other disseminated bacterial infections (e.g. *Salmonella* and pneumococcal). Rifampicin-induced P450 CYP3A4 activity makes the choice of HAART complicated; efavirenz combined with two NRTIs is recommended if rifampicin is being used. Drug reactions are more common in HIV-infected persons (especially rashes and hepatitis), and may be life-threatening with thiacetazone and streptomycin which must be avoided. If compliance is likely to be a problem, daily or thrice-weekly directly observed therapy (DOT) should be considered (p. 701). A syndrome resulting from HAART-induced immune reconstitution occurs in up to 10% of patients. This usually occurs 4–6 weeks after initiation of TB therapy and is most common in those with a nadir CD4 < 50 cells/mm^3 and a brisk CD4 response to HAART. It may present as focal disease away from the original site. It reflects immune activation to dead or dying mycobacteria, or previously unrecognised TB. Treatment is with non-steroidal anti-inflammatory drugs (NSAIDs) or corticosteroids.

In the early 1990s, nosocomially acquired multidrug-resistant TB (MDRTB) presented a serious public health problem, initially in the USA but soon followed by southern European countries. By definition resistance is present to rifampicin and isoniazid but also usually to the remaining first-line and often many of the second-line agents; treatment often entails 6–7 drug combinations. Case fatality rates were initially > 80%. Strengthened infection control procedures have meant that such outbreaks are now infrequent in developed countries. Prophylaxis with isoniazid (with or without rifampicin) reduces the risk of TB by 70% in patients with positive tuberculin skin tests (and no history of BCG). However, this protection is lost on discontinuing the drugs. Its place in HIV infection is uncertain.

Bacterial infections

Bacterial pneumonia (p. 687) is a common cause of morbidity and mortality in HIV. The incidence, severity, likelihood of bacteraemia and recurrent pneumonia, and mortality rate are all increased compared to non-HIV-infected persons. Susceptibility to particular respiratory pathogens is influenced by risk group, the level of immune depletion, age and the presence of neutropenia. *Streptococcus pneumoniae* (150-fold greater risk in advanced HIV) is the cause of 40% of all pneumonias where a pathogen is identified, and 70% of those with bacteraemia. *Haemophilus influenzae* (10–15%) and *Staph. aureus* (5%) can occur at any CD4 count, whereas *Pseudomonas* (5%) and *Nocardia* infections are more likely in later-stage disease. *Legionella* is also found more frequently. Chest X-ray appearances may be atypical. The infection usually responds to standard antibiotic therapy.

Kaposi's sarcoma and non-Hodgkin lymphoma are discussed in more detail on pages 396–397. Initial first-line treatments are detailed in Box 14.10.

NERVOUS SYSTEM AND EYE DISEASE

Disease of the central and peripheral nervous system is common in HIV. It may be a direct consequence of HIV infection or an indirect result of CD4 cell depletion. Presentation may be as a space-occupying lesion, encephalitis, meningitis, myelitis, spinal root disease or neuropathy (Fig.14.9 and Box 14.16).

14.16 PRESENTATION AND DIFFERENTIAL DIAGNOSIS OF HIV-RELATED DISORDERS OF THE NERVOUS SYSTEM	
Presentation	**Main causes**
Focal brain disease	Toxoplasmosis, PCNSL, PMFL, TB, syphilis, CMV
Diffuse brain disease	HIV, VZV, herpes simplex, syphilis
Headache, meningitis	HIV seroconversion, *Cryptococcus*, TB, syphilis
Spastic paraparesis	HIV-vacuolar myelopathy, transverse myelitis from VZV, herpes simplex, human T-cell lymphotropic virus 1 or syphilis
Weakness/numbness in legs, incontinence	CMV, non-Hodgkin lymphoma
Pain, numbness in legs	HIV, drugs (ddC, d4T, ddl)
Floaters, flashing lights, field defects	CMV, HIV, toxoplasmosis, retinal necrosis, syphilis

14

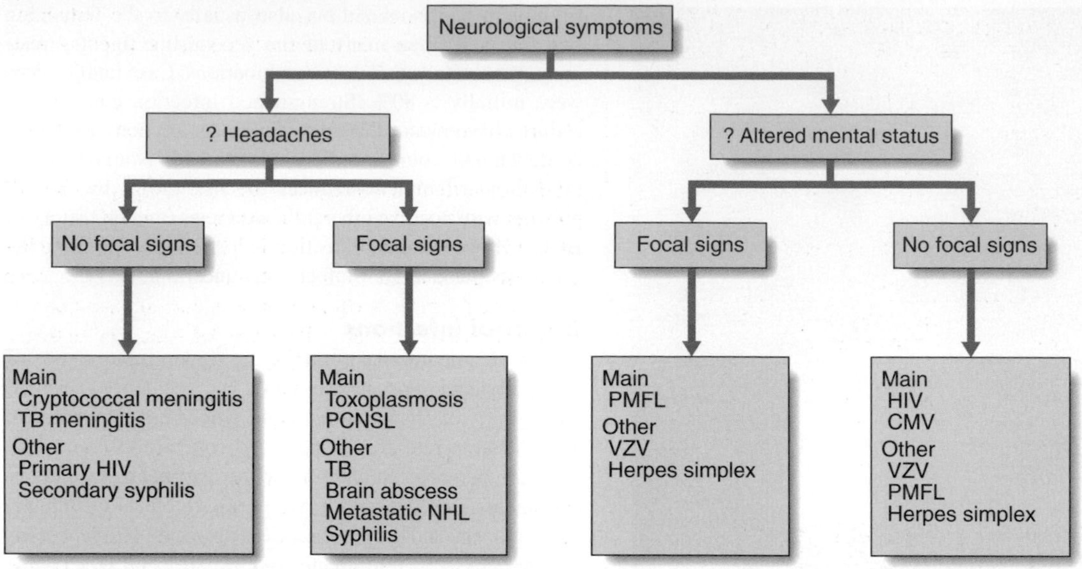

Neurological symptoms

? Headaches → No focal signs / Focal signs

? Altered mental status → Focal signs / No focal signs

No focal signs

Main
Cryptococcal meningitis
TB meningitis
Other
Primary HIV
Secondary syphilis

Focal signs

Main
Toxoplasmosis
PCNSL
Other
TB
Brain abscess
Metastatic NHL
Syphilis

Focal signs

Main
PMFL
Other
VZV
Herpes simplex

No focal signs

Main
HIV
CMV
Other
VZV
PMFL
Herpes simplex

Fig. 14.9 Presentation and differential diagnosis of HIV-related neurological disorders. (PCNSL = primary CNS lymphoma; TB = tuberculosis; NHL = non-Hodgkin lymphoma; PMFL = progressive multifocal leucoencephalopathy; VZV = varicella zoster virus; CMV = cytomegalovirus)

14

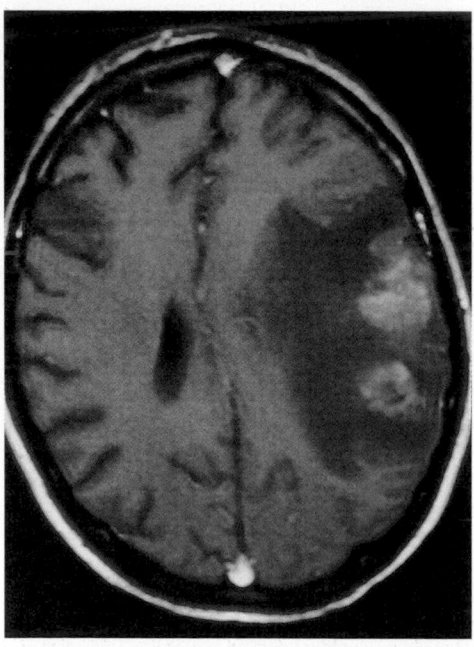

Fig. 14.10 Cerebral toxoplasmosis. Multiple cortical ring-enhancing lesions with surrounding oedema are characteristic.

Toxoplasma gondii

Toxoplasma infection results in a mild or subclinical illness in immunocompetent individuals, with the formation of latent tissue cysts that persist for life and have a predilection for brain tissue. The prevalence of latent infection varies between regions and increases with age. The infection rate, as judged by seroconversion, is 0.5–1% per year. In the presence of advanced HIV-induced immunosuppression, there is a > 30% chance that a seropositive patient will

reactivate these dormant cysts and develop clinical cerebral toxoplasmosis (Fig. 14.10). Patients usually present with a short history of headache, fever and drowsiness, which are soon followed by confusion, seizures and focal signs. The localising neurology reflects the tendency for lesions to occur in the cortex, basal ganglia and brain stem. Imaging using contrast-enhanced computed tomography (CT) or magnetic resonance imaging (MRI) typically shows multiple ring-enhancing lesions with marked surrounding oedema and mass effect. *Toxoplasma* DNA may be detectable in the cerebrospinal fluid (CSF) if lumbar puncture is not contraindicated because of raised intracranial pressure. Despite the characteristic imaging, it is often impossible to distinguish *Toxoplasma* encephalitis from primary CNS lymphoma with confidence. However, the response to a trial of anti-*Toxoplasma* therapy (Box 14.17) is usually diagnostic, with clinical improvement within 1 week and significant shrinkage of lesions within 2 weeks in over 90%. Despite the excellent response, there remains a significant neurological morbidity (up to 15%) and occasional mortality. Dexamethasone should be given if there is significant mass effect.

Primary CNS lymphoma (PCNSL)

PCNSL usually complicates late-stage HIV (CD4 < 50 cells/ mm^3), occurring in approximately 5% of AIDS patients and accounting for 20% of all focal CNS lesions. Tumours are nearly always high-grade, diffuse, B-cell neoplasms and are closely associated with EBV (found in over 90%). The time course of the disease is weeks to months, with features of raised intracranial pressure developing early and focal signs later; seizures occur in 15%. Characteristically, imaging demonstrates a large, single, homogeneously enhancing periventricular lesion with mild to moderate surrounding oedema and mass effect (Fig. 14.11). Ring enhancement may be present if central necrosis develops; periventricular

14.17 FIRST-LINE TREATMENTS FOR HIV-RELATED DISORDERS OF THE NERVOUS SYSTEM

Diagnosis	Treatment
Cerebral toxoplasmosis	Pyrimethamine* and sulfadiazine or clindamycin
Primary multifocal leucoencephalopathy	Cidofovir and HAART
Primary CNS lymphoma	Radiotherapy, HAART, methotrexate
HIV dementia	HAART
CMV encephalitis/ radiculitis/retinitis	Ganciclovir, cidofovir, foscarnet, or valganciclovir (oral)
Cryptococcal meningitis	Amphotericin B and 5-flucytosine, or fluconazole

* Folinic acid should be given with pyrimethamine.

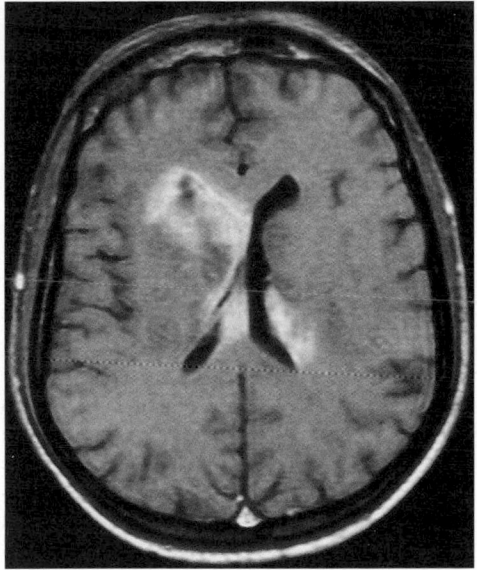

Fig. 14.11 Primary CNS lymphoma. A single enhancing periventricular lesion with moderate oedema is typical.

spread is typical. Multiple lesions are found in half of patients but rarely number more than 2–3. However, a solitary lesion is four times more likely to be PCNSL than *Toxoplasma*. CSF abnormalities are detectable in the majority but cytology is positive in only 25%. The presence of EBV-DNA in the CSF has a high sensitivity and specificity for PCNSL. Functional neuroimaging studies such as positron emission tomography (PET) may distinguish lymphoma (which results in a 'hot spot') from other mass lesions. Biopsy is definitive but carries a significant risk of morbidity, may be non-diagnostic in up to one-third, and may be misleading because of the presence of dual pathology. Distinction from cerebral toxoplasmosis may be impossible although, in the absence of *Toxoplasma* antibodies, this diagnosis is very unlikely. Failure to improve clinically on a trial of anti-*Toxoplasma* therapy or on scanning after 2 weeks is consistent with PCNSL.

Treatment is usually palliative with dexamethasone and symptomatic relief. Occasional responses to HAART and high-dose methotrexate have been reported. Whole-brain irradiation may provide temporary respite. Life expectancy is measured in months.

Progressive multifocal leucoencephalopathy (PMFL)

PMFL is a fatal demyelinating disease caused by the JC papovavirus that occurs in approximately 2–3% of AIDS patients at very low CD4 counts. Seroprevalence studies demonstrate that up to 90% of young adults have been exposed to JC virus, most infections occurring in childhood. It is assumed that with advancing HIV-induced immune depletion, reactivation of latent JC virus occurs. Patients usually present with focal deficits (80%), slow-onset visual field defects (25%) and ataxia; seizures are uncommon. MRI is the investigation of choice and shows high-intensity, bilateral (80%), occipitoparietal white matter signals on T2-weighted images (Fig. 14.12). There is never any mass effect and contrast enhancement is seen in < 10%. The presence of JC-DNA in CSF is diagnostic. Treatment with HAART and/or cidofovir can occasionally induce prolonged clinical remission with resolution of the MRI changes but most patients progress to death over 3–12 months.

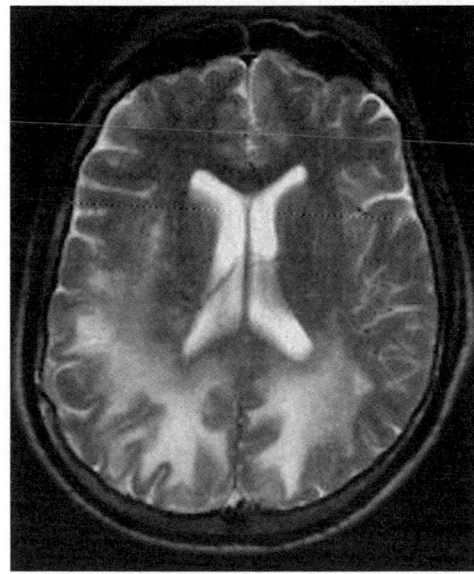

Fig. 14.12 Progressive multifocal leucoencephalopathy. Non-enhancing white matter lesions without surrounding oedema are seen.

Other focal brain disease

A less frequent cause of focal disease is CMV, which presents with headache, neck stiffness, confusion, a lymphocytic CSF and periventricular changes on MRI. Retinitis is present in over half of patients. CMV-DNA can usually be detected in CSF. *M. tuberculosis*, *Cryptococcus neoformans* and *Treponema pallidum* predominantly affect the meninges but can produce mass lesions with focal neurology.

HIV-associated dementia

HIV is a neurotropic virus and infects the CNS early during infection. Aseptic meningitis or encephalitis may

14

occur at seroconversion, and minor cognitive defects such as mental slowness and poor memory may develop as the disease progresses. Dementia occurs in late disease and is characterised by global deterioration of cognitive function, severe psychomotor retardation, paraparesis, ataxia, and urinary and faecal incontinence. Changes in affect are common and depression or psychosis may be the predominant feature. Higher plasma and CSF viral load, lower CD4 count and age are predictors for HIV-associated dementia. The incidence has fallen dramatically as a result of HAART. Investigations show diffuse cerebral atrophy with widened sulci and enlarged ventricles on imaging, and a raised protein in the CSF. An electroencephalogram (EEG) may show features consistent with encephalopathy.

Combination therapy using agents providing optimal CNS penetration improves minor cognitive defects in early disease, and may slow or even reverse the progression of HIV-associated dementia. Appropriate psychotropic medication may also be necessary.

Cryptococcosis

Cryptococcus neoformans is a budding encapsulated yeast; it is the most common cause of meningitis associated with late-stage HIV (CD4 < 50 cells/mm³) and occurs in 5% of AIDS patients. Rarely, non-meningeal (lung, prostate or skin) and disseminated disease may occur. Patients usually present with a 2–3-week history of headache, fever, vomiting and mild confusion; neck stiffness is often absent (< 25%). Less common are seizures, photophobia and blurred vision; papilloedema is found in 10% but focal features are rare. Around 10% of patients are asymptomatic. Protein, cell counts and glucose may be normal in the CSF, although numerous organisms are present on India ink stain (60–80%), cultures are usually positive (> 95%), and the CSF and serum cryptococcal antigen are strongly positive (95%). Although clinically disseminated infection is rare, the organism may be cultured from blood, urine, gut or bone marrow. The antigen titre, the number of organisms, the CSF white cell count and opening pressure, and the admission level of consciousness, as well as the delay before commencing treatment, are all prognostically significant. Deafness and blindness are the most common complications and result from prolonged raised intracranial pressure, arachnoiditis and direct cryptococcal nerve infiltration.

Between 10% and 20% of patients require treatment for raised intracranial pressure with repeated lumbar punctures, a lumbar drain, acetazolamide or shunting. Around 5–10% of patients die within the first 2 weeks of therapy, death being mainly related to raised intracranial pressure.

Spinal cord, nerve root and peripheral nerve disease

A variety of neuropathies occur in HIV infection. At seroconversion, Guillain–Barré syndrome, transverse myelitis, facial palsy, brachial neuritis, polyradiculitis and peripheral neuropathy have all rarely been described.

Vacuolar myelopathy is a slowly progressive myelitis resulting in paraparesis with no sensory level. Ataxia and incontinence occur in advanced cases. The CSF may show a raised protein but is frequently normal; MRI of the spine is normal. Diagnosis is by exclusion.

A predominantly distal HIV-related sensory neuropathy of the lower limbs affects up to 30% of patients. It is associated with a lower CD4 (usually < 200 cells/mm³), higher viral load, older age and wasting. It results from axonal degeneration, unmyelinated nerve fibres bearing the brunt. Hyperaesthesia, pain in the soles of the feet and paraesthesia are common. Diminished pin-prick, light touch and vibration sensation, accompanied by loss of ankle reflexes, is found in 75% and is typical. The nucleoside reverse transcriptase inhibitor (NRTI) drugs, especially ddC, d4T and ddI, can produce an identical picture but with remission if the offending agent is withdrawn early on. Treatment is often difficult, although amitriptyline, lamotrigine and recombinant nerve growth factor are beneficial. HAART has minimal effect on halting or reversing the process. Treatment is supportive.

Polyradiculitis occurs in late-stage HIV (CD4 count < 50 cells/mm³) and is nearly always a result of CMV. It causes rapidly progressive flaccid paraparesis, saddle anaesthesia, loss of lower limb reflexes and sphincter dysfunction. Pain in the legs and back is an early symptom. A neutrophil CSF pleocytosis, nerve root involvement on nerve conduction studies, and the presence of CMV-DNA demonstrated by PCR confirm the diagnosis. Despite treatment, functional recovery may not occur.

Lastly, proximal myopathy can result from HIV (when it may occur at any stage) or zidovudine (ZDV) (< 1% of patients). Presentation is with pain, slowly progressive weakness involving the major muscle groups, tender muscles and raised creatine kinase. Distinction can usually be made by muscle biopsy, when typical 'red-ragged' fibres indicating mitochondrial damage are seen with ZDV myopthy.

CMV is discussed in more detail on page 308.

Psychiatric disease

Significant psychiatric morbidity is not uncommon (Box 14.18). Mild cognitive dysfunction is a common occurrence in later-stage disease and usually improves with HAART

14.18 ISSUES IN MENTAL HEALTH
Pre-test
• Fear of being infected
Positive result
• Confidentiality • Stigmatisation • Discrimination
Early-stage disease
• Life expectancy • Drug side-effects
Late-stage disease
• Facing up to death • Living wills

(see above). Disorders of mental state may also result from drugs directly (e.g. efavirenz) or indirectly (e.g. those affecting sexual dysfunction). Psychiatric morbidity is a major risk factor for poor compliance to drugs, which is a critical component of HAART management. Psychiatric disease is described in Chapter 10.

Retinitis

CMV co-infection is very common in HIV-infected adults, with over 95% of MSM and 50% of other risk groups being seropositive. Prior to HAART, approximately one-quarter of patients with CD4 counts $< 100/mm^3$ would proceed to develop active CMV retinitis within 24 months (through either reactivation or re-infection). Since the advent of HAART, there has been a 90% fall in the incidence of CMV infections. Clinical features and differential diagnosis are listed in Box 14.19. A few asymptomatic patients with a CD4 < 50 cells/mm^3 are diagnosed on screening dilated fundoscopy. Macular disease is rare but is the most sight-threatening. If it is left untreated, the leading edge will progressively advance. No recovery of vision occurs in affected areas and there is always a risk of retinal detachment because of necrosis. High-dose (induction) treatment must commence immediately, followed by a reduced maintenance dose. Patients who respond to HAART, with an increase in the CD4 count to > 200 cells/mm^3, HIV and CMV viral suppression and inactive retinal disease can probably discontinue maintenance therapy safely but must be monitored closely for relapse. If the CD4 count falls, maintenance treatment should be reintroduced. Some patients with quiescent disease may develop immune recovery uveitis in response to HAART, with intraocular inflammation, macular oedema and cataract formation. Treatment involves oral and intraocular corticosteroids; visual loss may occur if treatment is not promptly instigated. Toxoplasmosis is discussed on page 356 and syphilis on page 411.

Depending on the neurological presentation, appropriate investigations include blood for *Toxoplasma* antibody and CMV antigen/PCR, as well as CSF to detect JC virus, EBV, herpes simplex, VZV, CMV, *Toxoplasma* and *M. tuberculosis* using PCR. Cryptococcal antigen and treponemal antibody testing should also be performed on blood and CSF. Initial first-line treatments are detailed in Box 14.17.

MISCELLANEOUS CONDITIONS

HAEMATOLOGICAL CONDITIONS

Disorders of all three major cell lines may occur in HIV, being most frequent in later-stage disease (anaemia 70%, leucopenia 50% and thrombocytopenia 40%), when pancy-topenia may also be seen. Numerous causes for anaemia exist, including marrow infiltration with opportunistic infections (MAI, TB, CMV) or neoplasms (non-Hodgkin lymphoma); bone marrow suppression from drugs (ZDV) or as a direct effect of HIV; and chronic blood loss (Kaposi's sarcoma) or malabsorption (chronic protozoal infections) in gastrointestinal tract disease. Haemolytic anaemia is uncommon but is seen with lymphoma. Leucopenia is usually seen in the context of marrow replacement as above or drug toxicity (e.g. ZDV, co-trimoxazole, ganciclovir, chemotherapy agents). Lymphopenia ($< 1.0 \times 10^9$/l) is a good marker of HIV. Thrombocytopenia may appear early (5–10%) and be the first indicator of HIV, or in later-stage disease. The disease is very similar to idiopathic thrombo-cytopenic purpura, with detectable platelet antibodies and short-lived response to intravenous immunoglobulin. However, the treatment of choice is HAART.

RENAL, CARDIAC AND ENDOCRINE CONDITIONS

HIV-associated nephropathy (HIVAN) is the most important renal condition and is seen most frequently in patients of African descent and those with low CD4 counts. Several drugs used in HIV management are also associated with renal disease, including indinavir (renal stones), tenofovir, pentamidine, cidofovir and co-trimoxazole. HIVAN usually presents with nephrotic syndrome, chronic renal disease or a combination of both. HAART may have some effect in slowing progression of renal disease. Doses of NRTIs must be adjusted according to creatinine clearance.

With increasing life expectancy and drug-related toxicity, cardiac disease will become a more and more important issue. HIV-related dilated cardiomyopathy can be detected in 25–40% of AIDS patients but symptomatic heart disease is rare (3–6%). Cardiomyopathy may very rarely be a result of ZDV through drug-induced mitochondrial dysfunction. Patients with HIV are also at increased risk of coronary artery disease, due partly to HAART-induced hyperlipidaemia.

Hypoadrenalism may be seen in up to one-quarter of AIDS patients and patients complaining of fatigue should be screened for it (p. 776). Postural hypotension and characteristic biochemistry (hyperkalaemia, hyponatraemia) may be absent. Hypopituitarism has also been described (p. 794).

14.19 CYTOMEGALOVIRUS RETINITIS

Clinical presentation

- Subacute history
- Floaters, flashing lights
- Field defects/reduced visual acuity
- Haemorrhagic exudates
    - Along retinal vessels
    - Well-demarcated peripheral disease
- 10% bilateral

Differential diagnosis

- Toxoplasmosis
- Syphilis
- Acute retinal necrosis
- Progressive outer retinal necrosis
- HIV retinopathy

NEOPLASMS

Kaposi's sarcoma (1000-fold higher rate than in non-HIV-infected) and non-Hodgkin lymphoma (100-fold greater) are the most common opportunistic malignancies associated with HIV and are AIDS-defining diagnoses. Increased incidence rates are also seen with Hodgkin lymphoma (five-fold higher) and anogenital cancers (five-fold higher).

SPECIFIC CONDITIONS

Kaposi's sarcoma (KS)

Prior to the HIV epidemic, KS was a rare tumour restricted to elderly males of Mediterranean or Jewish descent, immunosuppressed transplant recipients, and children and young adults in sub-Saharan Africa. Together with PCP, it has become a hallmark of AIDS and is particularly seen in MSM, bisexuals and patients from sub-Saharan Africa; haemophiliacs, injection drug-users and non-African heterosexuals rarely develop KS. Epidemiologically, the disease was strongly suspected of being a sexually transmissible agent and the identification of a novel herpes virus (HHV8) confirmed this link. In HHV8-co-infected MSM, there is a 10-year cumulative risk of 30–50% for developing KS with a median time to development of 3–5 years. Although HHV8 represents a predominantly sexually transmitted infection in the developed countries (exposure of the virus to rectal mucosa presenting the greatest risk), non-sexual and non-parenteral horizontal routes of transmission (possibly salivary) are more important in sub-Saharan Africa.

Histologically, the tumour consists of spindle cells, endothelial cells, fibroblasts and inflammatory cells. Clinical features are listed in Box 14.20. As the disease progresses, the skin lesions become more numerous and larger. Disease may be very indolent or fulminant, with rapid visceral involvement and clinical deterioration. This is more likely with lower CD4 counts. Hepatosplenomegaly usually indicates disease of these organs. Pulmonary KS occurs in 10–15% of patients and presents with breathlessness, cough, haemoptysis, chest pain and fever. Typically,

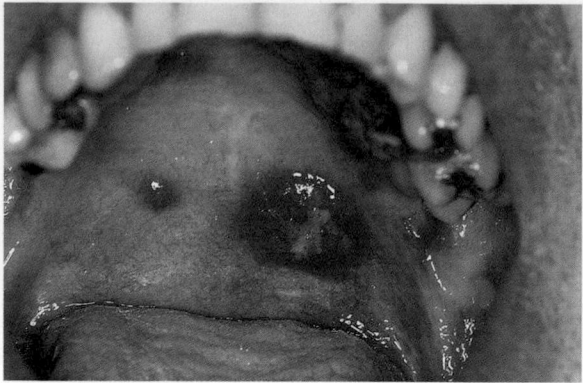
Fig. 14.13 Oral Kaposi's sarcoma. A full examination is important to detect disease that may affect the palate, gums, fauces or tongue.

disease affects middle and lower zones with patchy coarse reticulonodular shadowing and mediastinal lymphadenopathy; a pleural effusion is present in approximately 25%.

Prognosis in KS depends upon the CD4 count and the extent of disease. For limited and localised disease, therapeutic options include surgical excision, intralesional chemotherapy, liquid nitrogen or laser therapy, radiation or retinoic acid gel. Radiotherapy is also valuable for localised disease where lymphoedema is prominent or where symptoms relate to mass effects (e.g. oral lesions). For widespread mucocutaneous or visceral KS, chemotherapy should be used. First-line agents are cyclical liposomal doxorubicin or daunorubicin (response rate 60%). For refractory or relapsed disease, paclitaxel gives a response rate of 70%. With the widespread use of HAART, there has been a 68% fall in the incidence of KS. It is also apparent that combination therapy alone can result in regression of mucocutaneous lesions and even visceral disease, as well as maintaining remission. It is therefore a vital component of management. Cavity-based lymphoma (< 2% of cases of non-Hodgkin lymphoma) and Castleman's disease are other HHV8-associated conditions seen rarely with HIV.

HIV-associated lymphoma

In the majority of patients, lymphoma (p. 1047) represents a late manifestation of HIV, with risk increasing as immunocompromise worsens (median CD4 count at diagnosis is 50 cells/mm^3). It is the initial AIDS-defining illness in 2–3% of patients. The risk is increased 100-fold over non-infected persons for non-Hodgkin lymphoma (NHL) and fivefold for Hodgkin lymphoma, with a lifetime risk of developing NHL of 5–10%. It is seen in all groups at risk for HIV. HAART has reduced the incidence of NHL by 40%, with an effect dependent on the histological type (most noticeable with PCNSL—p. 392—whereas there is no effect with Burkitt's lymphoma), the time on combination treatment and the CD4 count (greatest effect where < 50 cells/mm^3). However, this is a modest effect compared to the decreases seen in opportunistic infections. Histological subtypes have distinct associations with herpes viruses and underlying genetic mutations. Over 95% of AIDS-associated lymphomas are of B-cell lineage and comprise several histological types (Box 14.21).

14.20 FEATURES OF KAPOSI'S SARCOMA	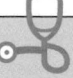

Cutaneous

- Purple non-tender, non-pruritic papules
- May ulcerate on feet
- Often associated with oedema and lymphadenopathy
- Crease line arrangements
- Favoured sites: nose, genitals, lower limbs

Oral

- Favoured sites: palate, gum margins, fauces (Fig. 14.13)
- Predictor of gastrointestinal and respiratory tract disease

Visceral

- Pulmonary, pleural effusion
- Gastrointestinal tract
- Hepatosplenomegaly
- Ocular

14.21 FEATURES OF HIV-ASSOCIATED NON-HODGKIN LYMPHOMA
Histological types
• Diffuse large cell • Large cell immunoblastic • Burkitt's • Small cleaved cell • Primary effusion (HHV8)
Clinical features
• Stage IVB • Lymphadenopathy • Extranodal involvement • Disseminated disease
Poor prognostic factors
• Previous AIDS diagnosis • Disseminated disease • Age >35 years • Not being on HAART • Injection drug-user risk group

After diagnosis of NHL or Hodgkin lymphoma, a staging evaluation is required (Ann Arbor classification—p. 1048). This requires CT of the thorax, abdomen and pelvis, bone marrow aspirate and biopsy, and lumbar puncture for cytology. HAART therapy is associated with significant improvement in predicting response to chemotherapy, event-free remission and overall survival. Management includes chemotherapy, support of bone marrow reserves, prevention of infection and control of HIV. Multi-agent chemotherapy is used (e.g. EPOCH), although lower doses are often employed because there appears to be no advantage in higher-dose regimens and HIV patients are more susceptible to side-effects. Rituximab may improve responses when added to standard chemotherapy. Intrathecal chemotherapy should be used for patients with meningeal involvement. The remission rate in persons with less than two poor prognosis risk factors is over 50%, with prolonged remission over 24 months seen in 20–30%. Use of HAART with chemotherapy is safe, although certain agents, in particular ZDV (marrow suppression) and d4T/ddC/ddI (peripheral neuropathy), may aggravate the side-effects of chemotherapy agents. Following chemotherapy, it may take up to 1 year for the CD4 count to return to pre-treatment levels. Where possible, its introduction should not be delayed. For primary CNS lymphoma, see page 392.

Genital cancer

HIV-infected persons have a fivefold greater risk of developing anogenital (vulval/vaginal, anal, penile) and in situ cervical (cervical intra-epithelial neoplasia III) cancer. This is closely associated with HPV co-infection, which is more frequently observed in HIV (60% of females; 90% of males), including the most oncogenic genotypes (HPV-16, 18, 31, 33, 35). Patients are more likely to have multiple genotypes, which persist with time, and to demonstrate a more rapid progression from dysplasia to in situ cancer. Both a higher viral load and a lower CD4 count are associated with higher co-infection rates. Invasive cervical cancer is an AIDS-defining diagnosis. Disease tends to

present late and is more aggressive. Annual cervical smears should be taken from all HIV-infected women and regular anal smears considered for MSM. Anal cancer is rare but is being increasingly diagnosed in HIV patients.

MANAGEMENT OF HIV

Management of HIV involves both treatment of the virus and prevention of opportunistic infections. The aims of HIV treatment are to:

• reduce the viral load to an undetectable level (< 50 copies/ml) for as long as possible
• improve the CD4 count (above 200 cells/mm³ significant HIV-related events rarely occur)
• increase the quantity and improve the quality of life without unacceptable drug-related side-effects or lifestyle alteration
• reduce transmission (mother-to-child and person-to-person).

The drugs that are currently used, their side-effects and a glossary of terms and abbreviations are given in Boxes 14.22, 14.23 and 14.24.

14

DRUGS

NUCLEOSIDE REVERSE TRANSCRIPTASE INHIBITORS (NRTIs)

The drugs in this class are zidovudine (ZDV), didanosine (ddI), zalcitabine (ddC), lamivudine (3TC), stavudine (d4T), abacavir and emtricitabine (FTC), which have appeared sequentially. The NRTIs act through intracellular phosphorylation to the triphosphate form and incorporation into

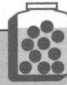

14.22 ANTIRETROVIRAL DRUGS	
Nucleoside reverse transcriptase inhibitors (NRTIs)	
• Zalcitabine (ddC) • Didanosine (ddI) • Lamivudine (3TC)	• Zidovudine (ZDV) • Stavudine (d4T) • Abacavir • Emitricitabine (FTC)
Non-nucleoside reverse transcriptase inhibitors (NNRTIs)	
• Nevirapine • Efavirenz	• Delavirdine[1]
Protease inhibitors (PIs)	
• Indinavir[2] • Ritonavir • Nelfinavir • Lopinavir[3] • Atazanavir[2]	• Fosamprenavir[2] • Saquinavir[2] • Amprenavir[1,2] • Tipranavir[1,2]
Others	
• Tenofovir	• Enfuvirtide (T-20)

[1] Restricted use.
[2] Usually given with boosting low-dose ritonavir.
[3] Co-formulated with low-dose ritonavir.

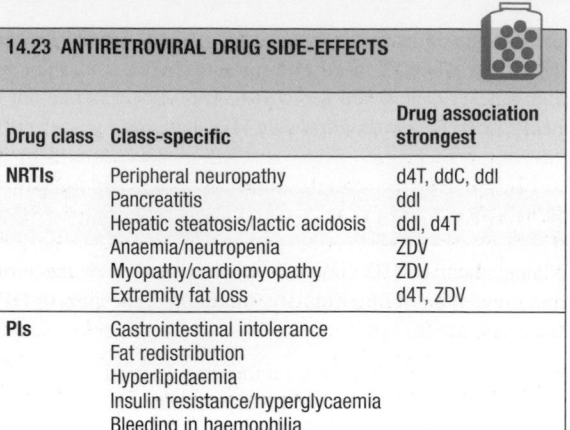

14.23 ANTIRETROVIRAL DRUG SIDE-EFFECTS

Drug class	Class-specific	Drug association strongest
NRTIs	Peripheral neuropathy	d4T, ddC, ddI
	Pancreatitis	ddI
	Hepatic steatosis/lactic acidosis	ddI, d4T
	Anaemia/neutropenia	ZDV
	Myopathy/cardiomyopathy	ZDV
	Extremity fat loss	d4T, ZDV
PIs	Gastrointestinal intolerance	
	Fat redistribution	
	Hyperlipidaemia	
	Insulin resistance/hyperglycaemia	
	Bleeding in haemophilia	
	Liver enzyme derangement	
NNRTIs	Rash/Stevens–Johnson syndrome	Nevirapine
	Hepatitis	Nevirapine

14.24 TREATMENT GLOSSARY

Term	Explanation
CD4 cells	In the context of this chapter, refers to CD4 lymphocytes
Class	Type of drug defined by mode of action (e.g. NRTI)
HAART	Highly active antiretroviral therapy (combination treatment)
Immune therapy	Drugs designed to improve CD4 or CD8 responses
NNRTI	Non-nucleoside reverse transcriptase inhibitor
NRTI	Nucleoside reverse transcriptase inhibitor
PI	Protease inhibitor
Resistance test	In vitro assessment of drug susceptibility
Undetectable VL	Plasma VL below detection (< 50 copies/ml)
Viral load (VL)	Quantitative level of plasma RNA virus
Virological failure	Detectable VL despite treatment

the DNA where they inhibit further lengthening of the complementary strand to the viral RNA template. Each drug specifically competes with a natural nucleoside (e.g. ZDV with thymidine, 3TC with cytidine). CNS penetration is good with all NRTIs, and both ZDV and abacavir have been demonstrated to be of benefit in AIDS dementia. Tenofovir is a nucleotide drug which only requires two phosphorylation steps to the triphosphate form. Its activity and characteristics are identical to the NRTIs. The inclusion of two NRTIs, or one NRTI and tenofovir, remains the cornerstone of HAART.

Resistance occurs to all NRTIs unless they are part of a maximally suppressive HAART regimen; resistance to 3TC and FTC is rapid and high-level. Occasionally, certain single mutations in the viral reverse transcriptase may result in broad resistance to several or all of the NRTIs and tenofovir. These can be selected by combining drugs that have overlapping resistance profiles and a low genetic barrier to resistance. Many of the major and longer-term side-effects

probably have a common pathway through inhibition of mitochondrial DNA synthesis, although displaying some organ specificity (Box 14.23). Once-daily administration (ddI, 3TC, FTC, tenofovir and abacavir) and NRTI co-formulations (ZDV/3TC, abacavir/3TC, FTC/tenofovir and ZDV/3TC/abacavir) improve adherence. Hypersensitivity (rash, fever, influenza-like illness) to abacavir occurs in 5–8% in the first 6 weeks and can be life-threatening if not recognised early or if the patient is rechallenged with the drug.

PROTEASE INHIBITORS (PIs)

The first PI was saquinavir (hard gel formulation), followed by indinavir, ritonavir, nelfinavir, saquinavir (soft gel), amprenavir and lopinavir/ritonavir. More recently, two PIs (atazanavir and fosamprenavir) have become available; they allow for once-daily administration with fewer tablets. The subsequent fall in morbidity and mortality can be directly linked to the introduction of these drugs and their use in HAART. PIs prevent post-translational cleavage of polypeptides into functional virus proteins. When they are given with two NRTIs the combination controls viral replication in plasma and tissues, and allows reconstitution of the immune system.

Short- and long-term side-effects are not infrequent. Fat redistribution occurred in 20–30% of patients treated with HAART including a PI after 2 years (p. 378). The syndrome is characterised by peripheral fat-wasting (cheeks, temples, limbs and buttocks), localised collections (buffalo hump, peripheral lipomatosis, and breast enlargement in women) and central adiposity. One-quarter of patients have a pattern of predominant peripheral fat loss, one-quarter central fat gain, and half a mixed pattern. Thymidine NRTIs are probably the main cause of fat loss. PI use may also be associated with insulin resistance (60%), abnormal glucose tolerance (35%) and frank diabetes (8%). Increases in total cholesterol, low-density lipoprotein (LDL) and/or triglycerides, and decreases in high-density lipoprotein (HDL) occur in 30–50% of patients. The major exception is atazanavir. Coronary artery disease appears to be more common in HIV. This is a result partly of the metabolic risk factors and partly of the greater frequency of other recognised risk factors in those with HIV such as smoking. Although the frequency of these clinical and metabolic complications may vary between different PIs, all have been implicated except atazanavir. Individual PI side-effects include renal stones (indinavir), hyperbilirubinaemia (atazanavir), and rash (amprenavir).

PIs are metabolised by the P450 cytochrome system (mainly the CYP3A4 isoenzyme), giving rise to the potential for multiple drug interactions. Common drugs that interact with PIs (in particular ritonavir) are rifampicin, midazolam, simvastatin and certain antihistamines. The potent enzyme inhibition produced by ritonavir can be used to raise the trough level of co-administered PIs such as lopinavir (where the combination has been formulated as a single tablet). Ritonavir-boosting significantly reduces the likelihood of drug failure from viral resistance and allows the number of pills to be reduced, as well as dietary restrictions to be relaxed. Adequate plasma levels are necessary for, and predictive of, successful treatment. Monitoring the levels (therapeutic drug monitoring) and adjusting the dose accordingly may be necessary to optimise the antiviral effect and reduce toxicity.

NON-NUCLEOSIDE REVERSE TRANSCRIPTASE INHIBITORS (NNRTIs)

There are two main NNRTIs: nevirapine and efavirenz. Activity is through inhibiting reverse transcriptase by binding near to the active enzyme site. NNRTIs do not require intracellular activation and are not active against HIV-2. Efavirenz and nevirapine have similar potency to PIs when combined with two NRTIs, a half-life over 24 hours allowing for once-daily dosing (although nevirapine is normally given twice daily), good bioavailability, low tablet number and apparent freedom from long-term side-effects. The major disadvantage is the potential for development of cross-resistance to all current drugs in this class through a single mutational change.

Rash is the major class-specific side-effect (Box 14.23). CNS side-effects, including dizziness, vivid dreams, insomnia, depression and poor concentration, are described in half the patients treated with efavirenz. These usually resolve by 4 weeks and are only sufficiently severe to require discontinuation in 2–5%. A hypersensitivity hepatitis occurs in 1–2% of patients commencing nevirapine and these patients need to have their liver function tests monitored regularly on starting treatment. It is seen more frequently at CD4 counts > 250 cells/mm^3 and in females. No association with fat redistribution has been identified for the NNRTIs.

The CYP3A4 isoenzyme is induced by nevirapine, and both inhibited and induced by efavirenz. As a result, both efavirenz and nevirapine induce the metabolism of certain PIs, requiring dose increases if given concurrently. They also reduce methadone levels by approximately 50% and may precipitate opiate withdrawal.

NEW DRUGS

Enfuvirtide (T-20) is a new class of antiretroviral drug which prevents viral entry into cells by targeting the gp41 and preventing fusion. It is highly active but has to be injected subcutaneously 12-hourly and therefore is reserved for patients with more advanced disease and fewer options. Other entry inhibitors target the chemokine receptors CCR5 and CXCR4; these have the benefit of oral administration. Other drugs in current clinical trials show activity against resistant virus (tipranavir, TMC-114, TMC-125). For many patients, these new drugs represent their only realistic chance of achieving virological control.

TREATMENT

THE NAÏVE PATIENT

The decision to start therapy is a major one and is influenced by the patient's symptom status, CD4 count and wishes. The

risk of HIV-related opportunistic infection increases and treatment is less effective when the CD4 count is < 200 cells/mm^3. Also, the higher the viral load (VL), the faster the CD4 count falls. In general, treatment should be commenced when the CD4 count falls below 250 cells/mm^3 or the patient is symptomatic. A potent combination (HAART) should always be used (Boxes 14.25 and 14.26). When treatment is started, certain factors need to be considered (Boxes 14.27 and 14.28). Commencing antiretroviral therapy is not a medical emergency and there is always time to decide on the optimum regimen for a particular patient. All patients should have a viral resistance test performed before commencing therapy as there is a 5–10% incidence of primary viral resistance.

With careful and appropriate choice of HAART, the chance of a VL of < 50 copies/ml at 24 weeks is over 80%. The factors that reduce the probability of achieving prolonged viral suppression are:

14.25 INDICATIONS TO START HAART	
CD4 count (cells/mm^3)	Decision
Seroconversion	Consider[1]
> 350	Monitor 2–3 monthly
200–350	Monitor/recommend based on symptoms and VL[2]
< 200	Recommend

[1] If severely symptomatic.
[2] Symptomatic patients should commence treatment. The higher the VL, the earlier treatment should be recommended.

14.26 RECOMMENDED COMBINATION TREATMENTS FOR THE NAÏVE PATIENT[1]			
Regimen	A	B	C
Preferred	Efavirenz Lopinavir/ritonavir	ZDV Abacavir Tenofovir ddI	3TC FTC
Alternative	Fosamprenavir/ritonavir Saquinavir/ritonavir Nevirapine[2]		

[1] One drug from columns A, B and C.
[2] Only when CD4 <250 cells/mm^3 in females or <400 cells/mm^3 in males.

14.27 FACTORS TO CONSIDER WHEN CHOOSING HAART

- Ease of compliance
- Fit of the drug regimen around the patient's lifestyle
- Wishes of the patient
- Stage of disease
- Coexisting/past medical history
- Possibility of additive side-effects (e.g. ddI and neuropathy)
- Potential for drug interactions with non-HIV medications
- Antagonistic NRTI combinations (ZDV/d4T and ddC/3TC)
- CNS penetration
- Possibility of acquisition of resistant virus

14.28 COMBINATION THERAPY IN HIV INFECTION | EBM

'In antiretroviral-naïve patients, PI-based HAART reduces progression to AIDS and death compared to dual NRTI regimens. Triple combinations based on an NNRTI or a ritonavir-boosted PI have antiviral and immunological efficacy.'

- Yazdanpanah Y, et al. BMJ 2004; 328:249.
- Gallant JE, et al. JAMA 2004; 292:191.

- suboptimal potency of the regimen
- a high baseline VL
- a slow VL fall or failure to achieve an undetectable level
- poor adherence
- prior exposure to antiretroviral drugs
- drug interaction or toxicity
- primary acquisition or development of resistant virus.

THE 'TREATMENT-EXPERIENCED' PATIENT

A change in antiretroviral therapy may be necessary because of drug side-effects (early or late), difficulties in adherence or virological failure. In a patient with a previously undetectable VL, virus rebound is usually the first evidence of treatment failure.

With increasing time on a failing regimen, the VL rises towards baseline levels, resistance mounts, the CD4 count falls and clinical progression occurs. In essence, most early failures are related to adherence difficulties and most late failures are a result of virological resistance. A resistance test should be obtained before switching the failing regimen; any change should be guided by this result and also take into account prior drug exposure. In certain situations, therapeutic drug monitoring may be helpful in confirming that virological failure is not related to inadequate PI or NNRTI levels. As a rule, as many new agents as possible should be used, including expanded access drugs. In the absence of alternative options, continuing a failing regimen may be worthwhile if the drugs used are disabling the replicative capacity of the virus. Occasionally, HAART must be stopped because of life-threatening drug toxicity or overriding medical problems where predicted drug interactions will occur. In this situation, the prolonged half-life of the NNRTIs must be covered by substitution of a PI or continuation of the other components of HAART for 2 weeks. Discontinuing treatment is also necessary when the patient requests it and in terminal care.

ENHANCING THE IMMUNE SYSTEM

In the knowledge that HAART alone will not cure a patient of HIV because of the long-lived cellular latency of the virus, focus has turned towards the possibility of bolstering the immune system with the hope that virological control without drugs may be achievable. Theoretically, this can be achieved by allowing wild virus stimulation of the immune system through interrupting therapy in a controlled and safe setting (structured therapeutic interruption, STI) or by direct anti-HIV cytotoxic T-cell stimulation through immunisation with viral proteins. Whether either approach will prove to be

beneficial in the long term is uncertain but STI studies to date suggest not. Interleukin-2 is a cytokine that mobilises CD4 cells and increases production, leading to a significant rise in circulating CD4 cell numbers. It is the subject of large-scale trials to define its value and place in treatment.

SPECIAL SITUATIONS

SEROCONVERSION

Seroconversion (primary infection) occurs 2–6 weeks after exposure (p. 383). Very little published data exist as to the merits or potential dangers of antiretroviral treatment at this time. Nevertheless, there is a body of opinion that seroconversion may represent a therapeutic window of opportunity associated with long-term benefit. In patients with severe and prolonged seroconversion illness, HAART is indicated. Otherwise, potential benefits from early treatment include retaining any anti-HIV CD8 cell function, reducing latent and sanctuary site infection, altering viral load set-point to a lower level, and possibly reducing risk of transmission. However, the potential for long-term drug side-effects, adherence difficulties, and the fact that it may be many years before clinical problems supervene argue against treatment at this stage.

CHILDREN

The general principles for the drug management of HIV in children are the same as those for adults. The CD4 percentage is a better marker of immunological health until 6 years of age, and of the need to initiate HAART. Treatment should be commenced in all infants presenting with an AIDS-defining illness, a CD4% < 20, a rapidly falling CD4 percentage and/or a viral load persistently > 10^6 copies/ml. Treatment should also be commenced in children > 12 months of age with an AIDS-defining illness or a CD4% < 15, and considered if the CD4% is < 20 or viral load > 10^6 copies/ml. Not all antiretroviral drugs are available in a suitable formulation for children (suspension, powder, crushable tablet or a capsule that can be opened). Co-ordinated, comprehensive family-centred systems of care are necessary to support the child and parents in order to optimise compliance with medications.

PERINATAL TRANSMISSION

There is now clear evidence that reduction in perinatal transmission of HIV can be achieved with short-course perinatal prophylaxis using single-drug regimens of ZDV or nevirapine. The likelihood of transmission is decreased to the order of 8.3–18% for ZDV alone, 2.6–10.2% for ZDV and 3TC, 8.2% for nevirapine, and 0.8–1.8% for ZDV and caesarean section. Higher rates of reduction are observed in industrialised countries, when drugs are started at 16 weeks, when they are continued in the neonate for 4–6 weeks, and when HAART is used. The risk of transmission is < 1% when the maternal VL is < 1000 copies/mm³. All patients should be treated in an effort to prevent transmission. Nevirapine is not now advised for pregnant women with

CD4 counts > 250 cells/mm^3 because of a 6–7% risk of hypersensitivity hepatitis. Ritonavir-boosted saquinavir or lopinavir is now recommended. ZDV should be commenced as an intravenous infusion at the onset of labour and the neonate should be treated for 4–6 weeks. Unfortunately, single-dose nevirapine in the absence of other drugs is associated with a 30–50% chance of NNRTI resistance in mother and infected child. Screening for HIV in the baby (RNA or pro-viral DNA) should be performed at birth (not on cord blood), 6 weeks and 4–6 months. If negative, vertical transmission has not occurred.

POST-EXPOSURE PROPHYLAXIS

Combination therapy is now recommended for occupational post-exposure prophylaxis (PEP) where the risk is deemed to be significant, although there is no evidence for this practice. The first dose should be given as soon as possible. However, protection is not absolute and health-care workers have been reported to seroconvert despite taking a full course of three drugs started within hours of exposure. PEP is also being used in non-occupational settings such as condom breakage in HIV-serodiscordant partners, victims of rape, relapses in injection drug-users, and sharps-related home exposures in families of HIV patients. As for occupational PEP, a careful risk assessment should be made. Benefits are greatest in those presenting early, where the risk of transmission is high and where adherence is likely. Approximately 77% of persons receiving PEP experience side-effects and only 40% complete therapy. Recommended PEP is ZDV, 3TC and indinavir or nelfinavir for 28 days.

PREVENTION OF INFECTION

Patients should be immunised with hepatitis A and hepatitis B vaccines if there is no evidence of naturally acquired infection. HBV surface antibody levels need to be monitored and boosters given when < 100 U/ml. Pneumococcal vaccine (every 3–5 years) and influenza vaccine (every year) should be given to all patients. Response to all immunisations is lower when the CD4 count is < 200 cells/mm^3, although some protection is afforded. Live attenuated vaccines should be avoided (BCG, oral polio) or restricted to those with high CD4 counts (yellow fever). Nevertheless, MMR (measles/mumps/rubella) vaccine is safe and can be given.

Prophylaxis against infection is another vital aspect of management. Primary prophylaxis (Box 14.29) is to prevent the initial disease occurring and secondary prophylaxis is to prevent recurrence of infection. Primary prophylaxis is introduced at certain CD4 count levels when there is a risk of infection occurring (Box 14.30). Secondary prophylaxis is started after successful treatment of the opportunistic infection, usually with the same drugs used to treat the infection but at lower doses. There is now firm evidence that when HAART has been successful, drugs for the primary prophylaxis of *P. carinii* (*jirovecii*) pneumonia and *Toxoplasma* can be stopped when the CD4 threshold at which they were introduced is reached.

14.29 PRIMARY PROPHYLAXIS IN HIV	EBM

'The incidence of several opportunistic infections is reduced by primary prophylaxis: for PCP, by 68% with either co-trimoxazole or pentamidine; for toxoplasmosis, to 3% with co-trimoxazole; and for MAI, by 56% with weekly azithromycin and 73% with daily clarithromycin.'

- Bucher HC, et al. J Acquir Immune Defic Syndr Hum Retrovirol 1997; 15:104–114.
- Oldfield EC, et al. Clin Infect Dis 1998; 26:611–619.

14.30 PROPHYLAXIS OF OPPORTUNISTIC INFECTIONS

Organism/infection	Indication	First-line
Pneumocystis	CD4 < 200 cells/mm^3	Co-trimoxazole
Toxoplasmosis	CD4 < 100 cells/mm^3	Co-trimoxazole
Cryptococcus[1]	CD4 < 100 cells/mm^3	Itraconazole
Penicillium[1]	CD4 < 100 cells/mm^3	Itraconazole
Tuberculosis[2]	Positive tuberculin skin test	Rifampicin and isoniazid
MAI	CD4 < 50 cells/mm^3	Azithromycin

[1] In areas of the world where these infections are common.
[2] Place in primary prophylaxis uncertain.

14

Vaccine development is slow. An effective, safe and cheap vaccine would radically alter the future global epidemic of HIV. Subunit and synthetic peptide vaccines (e.g. gp120 with an adjuvant) are safe but elicit inadequate cell-mediated immunity. Construct vaccines with a live viral vector (e.g. canary pox or adenovirus) with HIV genes inserted stimulate good CD8 responses and are on trial. However, the massive viral turnover and the frequent generation of antigenically distinct variants provide a significant challenge.

HUMAN T-CELL LYMPHOTROPIC VIRUS (HTLV) INFECTIONS

There are two other retroviruses, HTLV 1 and HTLV 2, that are associated with disease in humans.

HTLV 1 is endemic in Japan, the Caribbean and certain areas of West Africa. It is transmitted by blood transfusion, by drug users sharing needles and from mother to child, principally through breastfeeding. It can also be transmitted by sexual intercourse, especially from male to female. HTLV 1 is associated with adult T-cell leukaemia/lymphoma and with a degenerative neurological disease characterised by demyelination of the long motor neurons in the spinal cord; this is known as tropical spastic paraparesis in the Caribbean and HTLV 1-associated myelopathy in Japan. These diseases also occur in Europe and North America in immigrants from areas of the world where HTLV 1 infection is endemic.

HTLV 2, a much more rarely isolated virus than HTLV 1, has been found in Native Americans and in Africa, and also injection drug-users in the USA. Its role in human disease is uncertain. Although it was first isolated from a case of hairy cell leukaemia, it is infrequently associated with this disease.

FURTHER INFORMATION

Books and journal articles
Bartlett JG. Medical management of HIV infection. *Updated regularly on the Web at www.hopkins-aids.edu.*

Gazzard B, ed. AIDS care handbook. 2nd edn. London: Mediscript; 2002.

Websites
www.bhiva.org
www.i-base.org.uk
www.hivandhepatitis.com
www.medscape.com

15

G.R. SCOTT

Sexually transmitted infections

CLINICAL EXAMINATION IN MEN

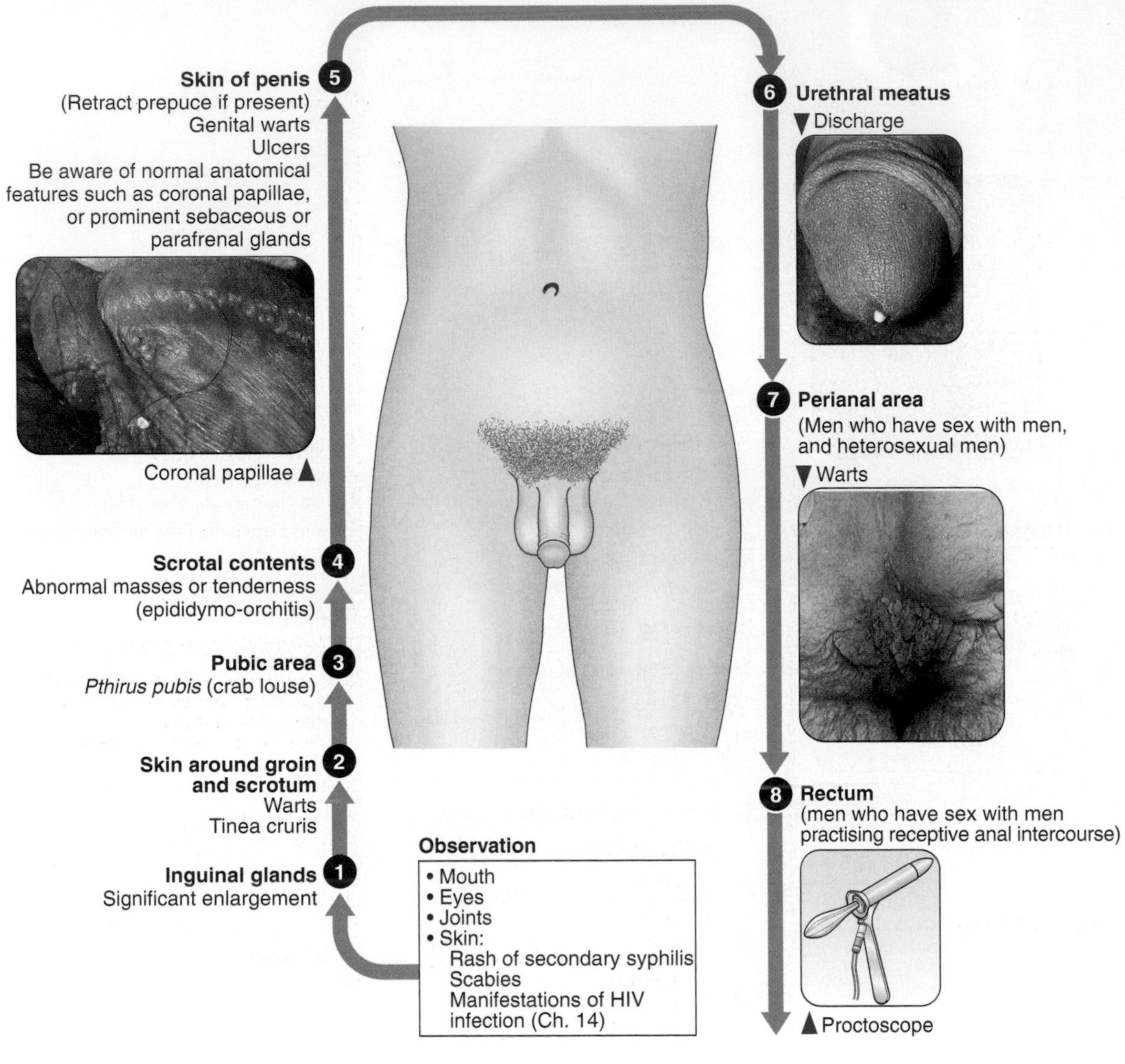

15

Skin of penis ⑤
(Retract prepuce if present)
Genital warts
Ulcers
Be aware of normal anatomical
features such as coronal papillae,
or prominent sebaceous or
parafrenal glands

Coronal papillae ▲

Scrotal contents ④
Abnormal masses or tenderness
(epididymo-orchitis)

Pubic area ③
Pthirus pubis (crab louse)

Skin around groin ②
and scrotum
Warts
Tinea cruris

Inguinal glands ①
Significant enlargement

⑥ **Urethral meatus**
▼ Discharge

⑦ **Perianal area**
(Men who have sex with men,
and heterosexual men)
▼ Warts

⑧ **Rectum**
(men who have sex with men
practising receptive anal intercourse)

▲ Proctoscope

Observation

- Mouth
- Eyes
- Joints
- Skin:
  Rash of secondary syphilis
  Scabies
  Manifestations of HIV
  infection (Ch. 14)

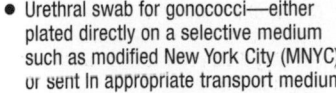

INVESTIGATIONS FOR SEXUALLY TRANSMITTED INFECTIONS IN HETEROSEXUAL MALES

- Urethral swab for gonococci—either plated directly on a selective medium such as modified New York City (MNYC) or sent in appropriate transport medium
- Urethral swab or first void urine (FVU) for chlamydia
- Serological test for syphilis (STS), e.g. enzyme immunoassay (EIA) for anti-treponemal IgG antibody
- HIV test (see note)

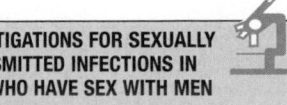

INVESTIGATIONS FOR SEXUALLY TRANSMITTED INFECTIONS IN MEN WHO HAVE SEX WITH MEN

- Pharyngeal, urethral and rectal swabs for gonococci
- Urethral swab or FVU, and rectal swab for chlamydia
- STS (repeat testing may be necessary because of negative results in the first few weeks following exposure)
- Serological tests for hepatitis A/B (with a view to vaccination if seronegative)
- HIV test (see note)

HIV TESTING

It should be standard practice to offer HIV testing as part of STI screening because the benefits of early diagnosis outweigh other considerations. Extensive pre-test counselling is not required in most instances, but it is important to establish efficient pathways for referral of patients at high risk in whom the clinician wishes specialist support, and for those diagnosed HIV-positive.

CLINICAL EXAMINATION IN WOMEN

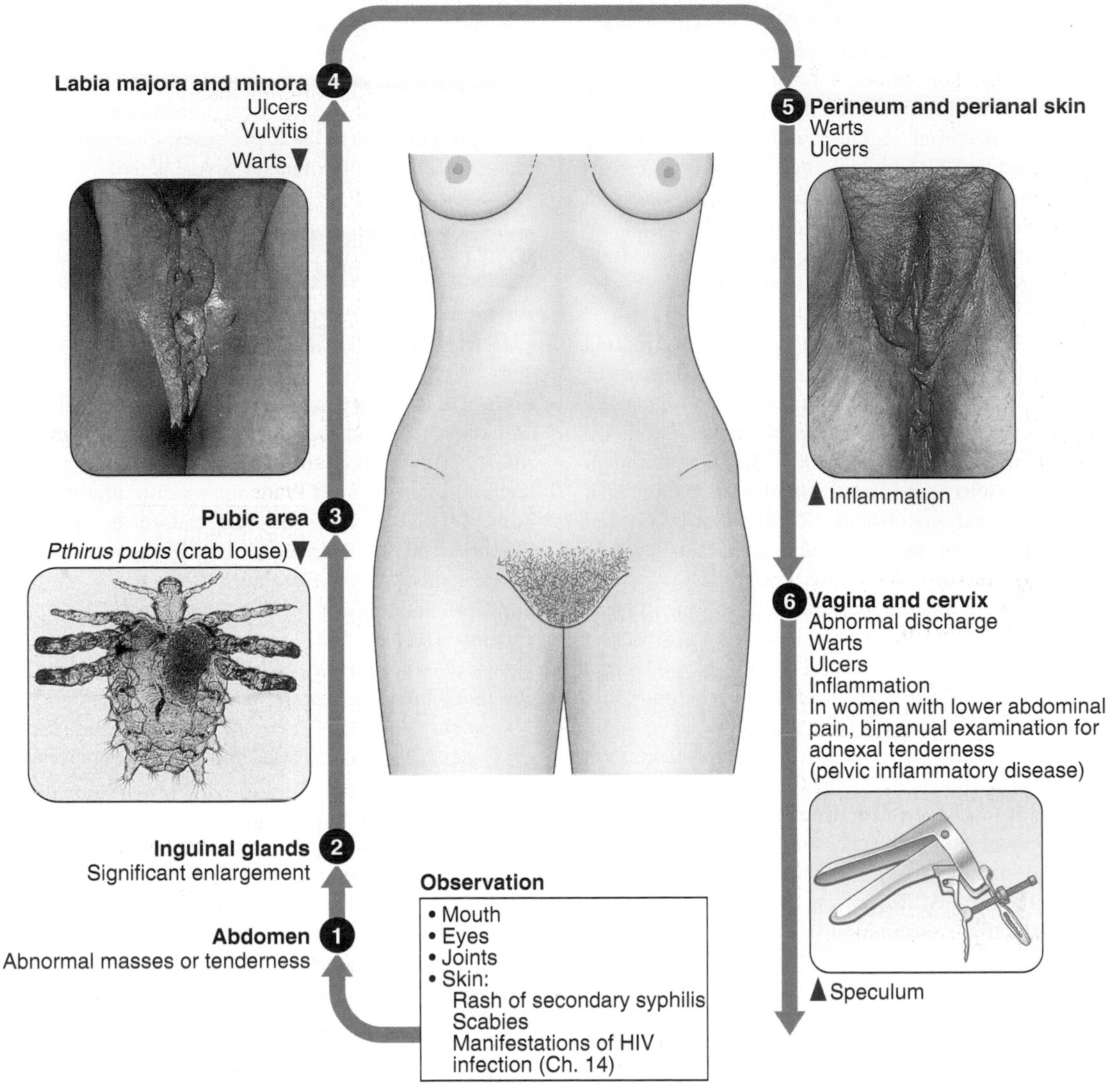

Labia majora and minora ④
Ulcers
Vulvitis
Warts ▼

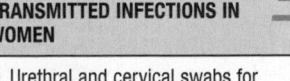

Pubic area ③
Pthirus pubis (crab louse) ▼

Inguinal glands ②
Significant enlargement

Abdomen ①
Abnormal masses or tenderness

⑤ **Perineum and perianal skin**
Warts
Ulcers

▲ Inflammation

⑥ **Vagina and cervix**
Abnormal discharge
Warts
Ulcers
Inflammation
In women with lower abdominal
pain, bimanual examination for
adnexal tenderness
(pelvic inflammatory disease)

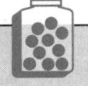

▲ Speculum

Observation
- Mouth
- Eyes
- Joints
- Skin:
  Rash of secondary syphilis
  Scabies
  Manifestations of HIV
  infection (Ch. 14)

15

INVESTIGATIONS FOR SEXUALLY TRANSMITTED INFECTIONS IN WOMEN

- Urethral and cervical swabs for gonococci
- Cervical swab for chlamydia
- Wet mount for microscopy or high vaginal swab (HVS) for culture of *Trichomonas*
- Serological test for syphilis (STS)
- HIV test (see note)

MANAGEMENT GOALS IN SUSPECTED STI

- Relief of any symptoms
- Screening for treatable STI that may not be causing symptoms
- Tracing and treatment of sexual contacts who may also be infected
- Advice to reduce risk of infection in the future

THOSE AT PARTICULAR RISK FROM STIs*

- Sex workers, male and female
- Clients of sex workers
- Men who have sex with men
- Injecting drug users (sex for money or drugs) and their partners
- Frequent travellers

* Adapted from WHO/UNAIDS, 1997.

Sexually transmitted infections (STIs) are a group of contagious conditions whose principal mode of transmission is by intimate sexual activity involving the moist mucous membranes of the penis, vulva, vagina, cervix, anus, rectum, mouth and pharynx, along with their adjacent skin surfaces. A wide range of infections may be sexually transmitted, including syphilis, gonorrhoea, human immunodeficiency virus (HIV), genital herpes, genital warts, chlamydia and trichomoniasis. Bacterial vaginosis and genital candidiasis are not regarded as STIs although they are common causes of vaginal discharge in sexually active women. Chancroid, lymphogranuloma venereum and granuloma inguinale are usually seen in tropical countries. Hepatitis viruses A, B, C and D (pp. 926–968) may be acquired sexually, as well as by other routes.

The World Health Organization estimates that 340 million curable STIs occur each year, including 170 million cases of *Trichomonas vaginalis,* 92 million cases of *Chlamydia trachomatis,* 62 million cases of gonorrhoea and 12 millon cases of syphilis. In the UK in 2004, the most common treatable STIs diagnosed were chlamydia (more than 100 000 cases) and gonorrhoea (22 000 cases). Genital warts are the second most common complaint seen in genitourinary medicine (GUM) departments.

As coincident infection with more than one STI is frequently seen, GUM clinics routinely offer a full set of investigations at the patient's first visit (pp. 404–405), regardless of the reason for attendance. In other settings, less comprehensive investigation may be appropriate.

The extent of the examination largely reflects the likelihood of HIV infection or syphilis. Most heterosexuals in the UK are at such low risk of these infections that routine extragenital examination is unnecessary. This is not the case in parts of the world where HIV is endemic, or for men who have sex with men (MSM) in the UK. In other words, the extent of the examination is determined by the sexual history.

APPROACH TO PATIENTS WITH A SUSPECTED STI

Patients concerned about the possible acquisition of an STI are often anxious. Staff must be friendly, sympathetic and reassuring; they should have the ability to put patients at ease, whilst emphasising that clinic attendance is confidential. The history focuses on genital symptoms, with reference to genital ulceration, rash, irritation, pain, swelling and urinary symptoms, especially dysuria. In men, the clinician should ask about urethral discharge, and in women, vaginal discharge, pelvic pain or dyspareunia. Enquiry about general health should include menstrual and obstetric history, cervical cytology, recent medication, especially with antimicrobial or antiviral agents, previous STI and allergy. Immunisation status for hepatitis A and B should be noted, as should information about recreational drug use.

A detailed sexual history is imperative, as this informs the clinician of the degree of risk for certain infections as well as specific sites that should be sampled; for example, rectal samples should be taken from men who have had unpro-tected anal sex with other men. Sexual partners, whether male or female, and casual or regular, should be recorded. Sexual practices—insertive or receptive vaginal, anal, oro-genital or oroanal—should be noted. Choice of contraception should be recorded for women, together with condom use for both sexes.

The presence of an STI in a child may be indicative of sexual abuse, although vertical transmission may explain some presentations in the first 2 years. In an older child, STI may be the result of voluntary sexual activity.

PRESENTING PROBLEMS IN MEN

URETHRAL DISCHARGE

In the UK the most important causes of urethral discharge are gonorrhoea and chlamydia. In a significant minority of cases, tests for both of these infections are negative, a scenario often referred to as non-specific urethritis (NSU). Some of these cases may be caused by *Trichomonas vaginalis,* herpes simplex virus (HSV), mycoplasmas or ureaplasmas. A small minority seem not to have an infectious aetiology.

Gonococcal urethritis usually causes symptoms within 7 days of exposure. The discharge is typically profuse and purulent. Chlamydial urethritis has an incubation period of 1–4 weeks, and tends to result in milder symptoms than gonorrhoea; there is overlap, however, and microbiological confirmation should always be sought.

Investigations

A presumptive diagnosis of urethritis can be made from a Gram-stained smear of the urethral exudate (Fig. 15.1), which will demonstrate significant numbers of poly-morphonuclear leucocytes (≥ 5 per high-power field). A working diagnosis of gonococcal urethritis is made if Gram-negative intracellular diplococci (GNDC) are seen; if no GNDC are seen, a label of non-specific urethritis is applied.

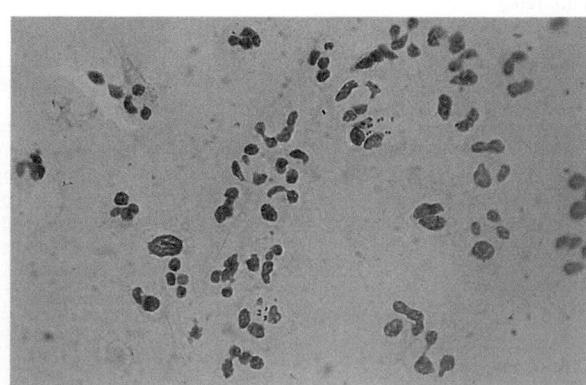

Fig. 15.1 A Gram-stained urethral smear from a man with gonococcal urethritis. Gram-negative diplococci are seen within polymorphonuclear leucocytes.

15

If microscopy is not available, swabs and/or urine samples should be taken and empirical antimicrobials prescribed.

A urethral swab should always be sent for culture of *Neisseria gonorrhoeae*; in addition, a first void urine (FVU) sample or a specific urethral swab should be sent for detection of chlamydial DNA by a nucleic acid amplification test (NAAT) such as polymerase chain reaction (PCR). NAATs are likely to replace the need for routine culture for gonorrhoea. Tests for other potential causes of urethritis are not performed routinely.

A swab should also be taken from the pharynx because gonococcal infection at this site is not reliably eradicated by single-dose therapy. In MSM swabs for gonorrhoea and chlamydia should be taken from the rectum.

Management

This depends upon local epidemiology and the availability of diagnostic resources. Treatment is often presumptive, with prescription of multiple antimicrobials to cover the possibility of gonorrhoea and/or chlamydia. This is likely to include a single-dose treatment for gonorrhoea, which is desirable because it eliminates the risk of non-adherence. The recommended agents for treating gonorrhoea vary according to local antimicrobial resistance patterns (p. 414). Appropriate treatment for chlamydia (p. 415) should also be prescribed because concurrent infection is present in up to 50% of men with gonorrhoea. Non-gonococcal, non-chlamydial urethritis is treated as for chlamydia.

Patients should be advised to avoid sexual contact until it is confirmed that any infection has resolved, and whenever possible, recent sexual contacts should be traced. The task of contact tracing—also called partner notification—is best performed by trained nurses based in GUM clinics; it is standard practice in the UK to treat current sexual partners of men with gonococcal or non-specific urethritis without waiting for microbiological confirmation.

If symptoms clear, a routine test of cure is not necessary, but patients should be re-interviewed to confirm that there was no immediate vomiting or diarrhoea after treatment, that there has been no risk of re-infection, and that traceable partners have sought medical advice.

GENITAL ITCH AND/OR RASH

Patients may present with many combinations of penile/genital symptoms that may be acute or chronic, and infectious or non-infectious. Box 15.1 provides a guide to diagnosis.

Balanitis refers to inflammation of the glans penis, often extending to the under-surface of the prepuce when it is called balanoposthitis. Tight prepuce and poor hygiene may be aggravating factors. Candidiasis is sometimes associated

15

15.1 DIFFERENTIAL DIAGNOSIS OF GENITAL ITCH AND/OR RASH IN MEN							
Likely diagnosis	Acute or chronic	Itch	Pain	Discharge (non-urethral)	Specific characteristics	Diagnostic test	Treatment
Subclinical urethritis	Either	±	−	±	Often intermittent	Gram stain and urethral swabs	As for urethral discharge
Candida	Acute	✓	−	White	Postcoital	Microscopy	Antifungal cream, e.g. clotrimazole
Anaerobic (erosive) balanitis	Acute	±	−	Yellow	Offensive	Microscopy	Saline bathing ± metronidazole
Pthirus pubis ('crab lice')	Either	✓	−	−	Lice and nits seen attached to pubic hairs	Can be by microscopy, but usually visual	According to local policy —often permethrin
Lichen planus (p. 1292)	Either	±	−	−	Violaceous papules ± Wickham's striae	Clinical	None or mild topical corticosteroid, e.g. hydrocortisone
Lichen sclerosus (p. 1281)	Chronic	±	−	−	Ivory white plaques, scarring	Clinical or biopsy	Strong topical corticosteroid, e.g. clobetasol
Plasma cell balanitis of Zoon	Chronic	−	−	±	Shiny, inflamed circumscribed areas	Clinical or biopsy	Strong topical corticosteroid, e.g. clobetasol
Dermatoses, e.g. eczema or psoriasis	Either	✓	−	−	Similar to lesions elsewhere on skin	Clinical	Mild topical corticosteroid, e.g. hydrocortisone
Genital herpes	Acute	±	✓	−	Atypical ulcers are not uncommon	Swab for HSV PCR	Oral antiviral, e.g. aciclovir
Circinate balanitis	Either	−	−	−	Painless erosions with raised edges; usually as part of Reiter's syndrome (p. 1108)	Clinical	Mild topical steroid, e.g. hydrocortisone

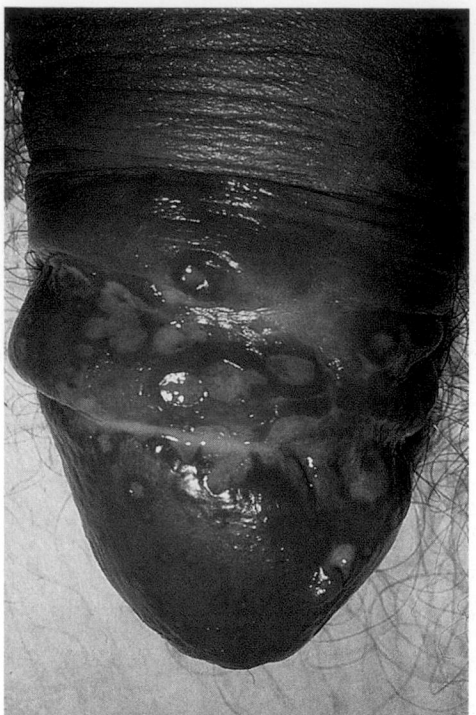

Fig. 15.2   Penile herpes simplex (HSV-2) infection.

15

with immune deficiency, diabetes mellitus, and the use of broad-spectrum antimicrobials, corticosteroids or anti-mitotic drugs. Local saline bathing is usually helpful, especially when no cause is found.

GENITAL ULCERATION

The most common cause of ulceration is genital herpes. Classically, multiple painful ulcers affect the glans, coronal sulcus or shaft of penis (Fig. 15.2), but solitary lesions occur rarely. Perianal ulcers may be seen in MSM. Diagnosis is made by gently scraping material from lesions and sending this in an appropriate transport medium for culture or detection of HSV DNA by PCR.

In the UK, the possibility of any other ulcerating STI is remote unless the patient is an MSM and/or has had a sexual partner from a region where tropical STIs are more common. The classic lesion of primary syphilis (chancre) is single, painless and indurated; however, multiple lesions are seen rarely and anal chancres are often painful. Diagnosis is made in GUM clinics by dark-ground microscopy, but in other settings by serological tests for syphilis (p. 412). Other rare infective causes seen in the UK include varicella zoster virus (pp. 305–306) and trauma with secondary infection. Tropical STI such as chancroid, lymphogranuloma venereum (LGV) and granuloma inguinale are described in Box 15.10 (p. 416). Inflammatory causes include Stevens–Johnson syndrome (p. 1308), Behçet's syndrome (p. 1142) and fixed drug reactions. In older patients, malignant and pre-malignant conditions such as squamous cell carcinoma and erythroplasia of Queyrat (intra-epidermal carcinoma) should be considered.

GENITAL LUMPS

The most common cause of genital 'lumps' is warts (p. 417). These are classically found in areas of friction during sex such as the parafrenal skin and prepuce of the penis. Warts may also be seen in the urethral meatus, and less commonly on the shaft or around the base of the penis. Perianal warts are surprisingly common in men who do not have anal sex.

The differential diagnosis includes molluscum contagiosum and skin tags. Adolescent boys may confuse normal anatomical features such as coronal papillae (p. 404), parafrenal glands or sebaceous glands (Fordyce spots) with warts.

PROCTITIS IN MEN WHO HAVE SEX WITH MEN

STIs that may cause proctitis in MSM include gonorrhoea, chlamydia, herpes and syphilis. The serovars of *Chlamydia trachomatis* that cause LGV (L1–3) have been associated with outbreaks of severe proctitis in the Netherlands and the UK. Symptoms include mucopurulent anal discharge, rectal bleeding, pain and tenesmus.

Examination may show mucopus and erythema with contact bleeding (Fig. 15.3). A PCR test for HSV and a request for identification of LGV serovars should be arranged in addition to the diagnostic tests on page 404 if chlamydial infection is detected. Treatment is directed at the individual infections (see below).

MSM may also present with gastrointestinal symptoms from infection with organisms such as *Entamoeba histolytica* (p. 358), *Shigella* spp (p. 330), *Campylobacter* spp (p. 326) and *Cryptosporidium* spp (p. 360).

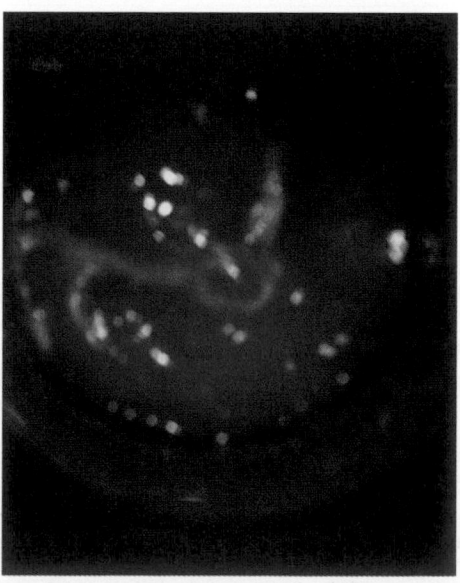

Fig. 15.3   Proctitis showing mucopus in the lumen of the rectum.

PRESENTING PROBLEMS IN WOMEN

VAGINAL DISCHARGE

The natural vaginal discharge may vary considerably, especially under differing hormonal influences such as puberty, pregnancy or prescribed contraception. A sudden or recent change in discharge, especially if associated with alteration of colour and/or smell, or vulval itch/irritation is more likely to indicate an infective cause than a gradual or long-standing change.

Local epidemiology is particularly important when assessing possible causes. In the UK, most cases of vaginal discharge are not sexually transmitted, being due to either candidal infection or bacterial vaginosis (BV). World-wide, the most common treatable STI causing vaginal discharge is trichomoniasis; other possibilities include gonorrhoea and chlamydia. HSV may cause increased discharge, although vulval pain and dysuria are usually the predominant symptoms. Non-infective causes include retained tampons, malignancy and/or fistulae.

Speculum examination often allows a relatively accurate diagnosis to be made. In BV, the discharge is characteristically homogeneous and off-white in colour. Vaginal pH is greater than 4.5, and Gram stain microscopy reveals scanty or absent lactobacilli with significant numbers of Gram-variable organisms, some of which may be coating vaginal squames (so-called Clue cells, Fig. 15.4). In candidiasis, there may be vulval and vaginal erythema, and the discharge is typically curdy in nature. Vaginal pH is usually less than 4.5, and Gram stain microscopy reveals fungal spores and pseudohyphae. Trichomoniasis tends to cause a profuse yellow or green discharge and is usually associated with significant vulvovaginal inflammation. Diagnosis is made by observing motile flagellate protozoa on a wet-mount microscopy slide of vaginal material.

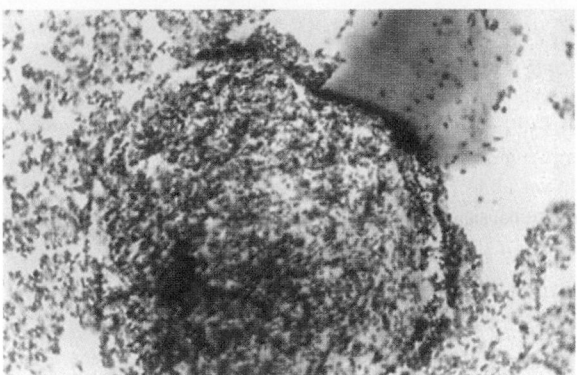

Fig. 15.4 Gram stain of a Clue cell from a patient with bacterial vaginosis. The margin of this vaginal epithelial cell is obscured by a coating of anaerobic organisms.

If examination reveals the discharge to be cervical in origin, the possibility of chlamydial or gonococcal infection is increased and appropriate cervical swabs should be taken (p. 405). In addition, Gram stain of cervical and urethral material may reveal GNDC, allowing presumptive treatment for gonorrhoea to be given. If gonococcal cervicitis is suspected, swabs should also be taken from the pharynx and rectum; infections at these sites are not reliably eradicated by single-dose therapy and a test of cure will therefore be required.

GUM clinics in the UK routinely offer sexually active women presenting with vaginal discharge an STI screen (p. 405). In other settings such as primary care or gynaecology, testing for chlamydia and gonorrhoea should be strongly considered in young women (< 25 years old), those who have changed partner recently, and those not using a barrier method of contraception, even if a non-STI cause of discharge is suspected clinically.

Treatment of infections causing vaginal discharge is shown in Box 15.2.

15

15.2 INFECTIONS THAT CAUSE VAGINAL DISCHARGE		
Cause	**Clinical features**	**Treatment (in pregnancy seek specialist advice)**
Candidiasis	Vulval and vaginal inflammation Curdy white discharge adherent to walls of vagina Low vaginal pH	Clotrimazole[1] 500 mg pessary once at night and clotrimazole cream 12-hourly *or* Econazole[1] pessary 150 mg for 3 nights and econazole cream 12-hourly (topical creams for 7 days) *or* Fluconazole[2] 150 mg orally stat
Trichomoniasis	Vulval and vaginal inflammation Frothy yellow/green discharge	Metronidazole[3] 400 mg 12-hourly orally for 5–7 days *or* Metronidazole[3] 2 g orally as a single dose
Bacterial vaginosis	No inflammation White homogeneous discharge High vaginal pH	Metronidazole[3] 2 g stat or 400 mg 12-hourly orally for 5–7 days Metronidazole[3] vaginal gel 0.75% daily for 5 days Clindamycin[1,4] vaginal cream 2% daily for 7 days
Streptococcal/ staphylococcal infection	Purulent vaginal discharge	Choice of antibiotic depends on sensitivity tests

[1]Clotrimazole, econazole and clindamycin damage latex condoms and diaphragms.
[2]Avoid in pregnancy and breastfeeding.
[3]Avoid alcoholic drinks until 48 hours after finishing treatment. Avoid high-dose regimens in pregnancy or breastfeeding.
[4]Pseudomembranous colitis has been reported with the use of clindamycin cream.

LOWER ABDOMINAL PAIN

Pelvic inflammatory disease (PID, infection or inflammation of the Fallopian tubes and surrounding structures) is part of the extensive differential diagnosis of lower abdominal pain in women, especially those who are sexually active. The possibility of PID is increased if, in addition to acute/subacute pain, there is dyspareunia, abnormal vaginal discharge and/or bleeding. There may also be systemic features such as fever and malaise. On examination, lower abdominal pain is usually bilateral, and vaginal examination reveals adnexal tenderness with or without cervical excitation. Unfortunately, a definitive diagnosis can only be made by laparoscopy. A pregnancy test should be performed (in addition to the diagnostic tests listed on page 405) because the differential diagnosis includes ectopic pregnancy.

Broad-spectrum antibiotics, including those active against gonorrhoea and chlamydia such as ofloxacin and metronidazole, should be prescribed if PID is suspected, along with appropriate analgesia. Delaying treatment increases the likelihood of adverse sequelae such as abscess formation, and tubal scarring that may lead to ectopic pregnancy or infertility. Hospital admission may be indicated in women with severe symptoms.

GENITAL ULCERATION

The most common cause of ulceration is genital herpes. Classically, multiple painful ulcers affect the introitus, labia and perineum, but solitary lesions occur rarely. Inguinal lymphadenopathy and systemic features such as fever and malaise are more common than in men. Diagnosis is made by gently scraping material from lesions and sending this in an appropriate transport medium for culture or detection of HSV DNA by PCR. In the UK, the possibility of any other ulcerating STI is remote unless the patient has had a sexual partner from a region where tropical STIs are more common (Box 15.10, p. 416).

Inflammatory causes include lichen sclerosus (p. 1281),

Stevens–Johnson syndrome (p. 1308), Behçet's syndrome (p. 1142) and fixed drug reactions. In older patients, malignant and pre-malignant conditions such as squamous cell carcinoma should be considered.

GENITAL LUMPS

The most common cause of genital 'lumps' is warts. These are classically found in areas of friction during sex, such as the fourchette and perineum. Perianal warts are surprisingly common in women who do not have anal sex.

The differential diagnosis includes molluscum contagiosum, skin tags and normal papillae or sebaceous glands.

CHRONIC VULVAL PAIN AND/OR ITCH

Women may present with a range of chronic symptoms that may be intermittent or continuous (Box 15.3).

Recurrent candidiasis may lead to hypersensitivity to candidal antigens, with itch and erythema becoming more prominent than increased discharge. Effective treatment may require regular oral antifungals, e.g. fluconazole 150 g once every 2–4 weeks plus a combined antifungal/corticosteroid cream such as Daktacort or Canesten HC.

PREVENTION OF STI

CASE-FINDING

Early diagnosis and treatment facilitated by active case-finding will help to reduce the spread of infection by limiting the period of infectivity; tracing and treating sexual partners will also reduce the risk of re-infection. Unfortunately, the majority of individuals with an STI are asymptomatic and therefore unlikely to seek medical attention. Improving access to diagnosis in primary care or non-medical settings, especially through opportunistic testing, may help. However, the impact of medical intervention through improved access alone is likely to be small.

15.3 CHRONIC VULVAL PAIN AND/OR ITCH					
Likely diagnosis	Itch	Pain	Specific characteristics	Diagnostic test	Treatment
Candida	✓	±	Usually cyclical	Microscopy	Oral antifungal, e.g. fluconazole 150 mg
Lichen planus	±	–	Violaceous papules ± Wickham's striae	Clinical	No treatment, or mild topical corticosteroid, e.g. hydrocortisone
Lichen sclerosus	±	–	Ivory white plaques, scarring ± labial resorption	Clinical or biopsy	Strong topical corticosteroid, e.g. clobetasol
Vestibulitis	–	✓	Dyspareunia common, pain on touching erythematous area	Clinical	Refer to specialist vulva clinic
Vulvodynia	–	✓	Pain usually neuropathic in nature	Clinical	Refer to specialist vulva clinic
Dermatoses, e.g. eczema or psoriasis	✓	–	Similar to lesions elsewhere on skin	Clinical	Mild topical corticosteroid, e.g. hydrocortisone
Genital herpes	±	✓	Atypical ulcers are not uncommon	Swab for HSV PCR	Oral antiviral, e.g. aciclovir

CHANGING BEHAVIOUR

The prevalence of STIs is driven largely by sexual behaviour. Primary prevention encompasses efforts to delay the onset of sexual activity and limit the number of sexual partners thereafter. Encouraging the use of barrier methods of contraception will also help to reduce the risk of transmitting or acquiring STIs. This is especially important in the setting of 'sexual concurrency', i.e. where sexual relationships overlap.

Unfortunately, there is contradictory evidence as to which (if any) interventions can reduce sexual activity. Knowledge alone does not translate into behaviour change, and broader issues such as poor parental role modelling, low self-esteem, peer group pressure in the context of the increased sexualisation of our societies, gender power imbalance and homophobia all need to be addressed. Throughout the world there is a critical need to enable women to protect themselves from indisciplined and coercive male sexual activity. Economic collapse and the turmoil of war regularly lead to situations where women must turn to prostitution to feed themselves and their children, and an inability to negotiate safe sex increases their risk of acquiring STI including HIV.

SEXUALLY TRANSMITTED BACTERIAL INFECTIONS

SYPHILIS

Syphilis is caused by infection, through abrasions in the skin or mucous membranes, with the spirochaete *Treponema pallidum*. In adults the infection is usually sexually acquired; however, transmission by kissing, blood transfusion and percutaneous injury has been reported. Transplacental infection of the fetus can occur.

The natural history of untreated syphilis is variable. Infection may remain latent throughout, or clinical features may develop at any time. The classification of syphilis is shown in Box 15.4. All infected patients should be treated. Penicillin remains the drug of choice for all stages of infection.

ACQUIRED SYPHILIS

Early syphilis

Primary syphilis

The incubation period is usually between 14 and 28 days with a range of 9–90 days. The primary lesion or chancre (Fig. 15.5) develops at the site of infection, usually in the genital area. A dull red macule develops, becomes papular and then erodes to form an indurated ulcer (chancre). The draining inguinal lymph nodes may become moderately enlarged, mobile, discrete and rubbery. The chancre and the lymph nodes are both painless and non-tender, unless there is concurrent or secondary infection. Without treatment, the chancre will resolve within 2–6 weeks to leave a thin atrophic scar.

Chancres may develop on the vaginal wall and on the cervix. Extragenital chancres are found in about 10% of patients, affecting sites such as the finger, lip, tongue, tonsil, nipple, anus or rectum. Anal chancres often resemble fissures and may be painful.

Secondary syphilis

This occurs 6–8 weeks after the development of the chancre when treponemes disseminate to produce a multisystem disease. Constitutional features such as mild fever, malaise and headache are common. Over 75% of patients present with a rash on the trunk and limbs that may later involve the palms and soles; this is initially macular but evolves to maculo-papular or papular forms, which are generalised, symmetrical and non-irritable. Scales may form on the papules later. Without treatment, the rash may last for up to 12 weeks. Condylomata lata (papules coalescing to plaques) may develop in warm, moist sites such as the vulva or perianal area. Generalised non-tender lymphadenopathy is present in over 50% of patients. Mucosal lesions, known as mucous patches, may affect the genitalia, mouth, pharynx or larynx and are essentially modified papules, which become eroded. Rarely, confluence produces characteristic 'snail track ulcers' in the mouth.

Other features such as meningitis, cranial nerve palsies, anterior or posterior uveitis, hepatitis, gastritis, glomerulonephritis or periostitis are sometimes seen.

The differential diagnosis of secondary syphilis can be extensive, but in the context of a suspected STI, primary HIV infection is the most important alternative condition to consider (Ch. 14).

The clinical manifestations of secondary syphilis will resolve without treatment but relapse may occur, usually

15

15.4 CLASSIFICATION OF SYPHILIS		
Stage	**Acquired**	**Congenital**
Early	Primary Secondary Latent	Clinical and latent
Late	Latent Benign tertiary Cardiovascular Neurosyphilis	Clinical and latent

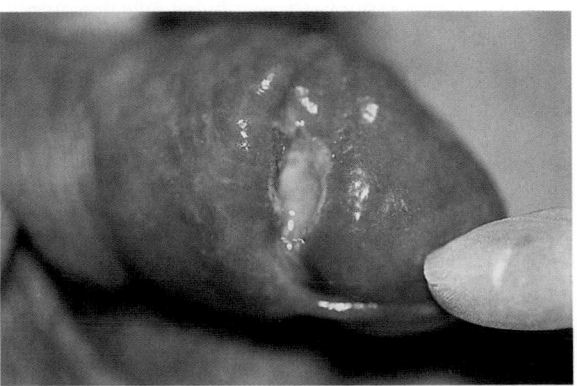

Fig. 15.5 Primary syphilis. A painless ulcer (chancre) is shown in the coronal sulcus of the penis. This is usually associated with inguinal lymphadenopathy.

within the first year of infection. Thereafter, the disease enters the phase of latency.

Latent syphilis

This phase is characterised by the presence of positive syphilis serology or the diagnostic cerebrospinal fluid (CSF) abnormalities of neurosyphilis in an untreated patient with no evidence of clinical disease. It is divided into early latency (within 2 years of infection), when syphilis may be transmitted sexually, and late latency, when the patient is no longer sexually infectious. Transmission of syphilis from a pregnant woman to her fetus, and rarely by blood transfusion, is possible for several years following infection.

Late syphilis

Late latent syphilis

This may persist for many years or for life. Without treatment over 60% of patients might be expected to suffer little or no ill health. Coincidental prescription of antibiotics for other illnesses such as respiratory tract or skin infections may treat latent syphilis serendipitously.

Benign tertiary syphilis

This may develop between 3 and 10 years after infection but is now rarely seen in the UK. Skin, mucous membranes, bone, muscle or viscera can be involved. The characteristic feature is a chronic granulomatous lesion called a gumma, which may be single or multiple. Healing with scar formation may impair the function of the structure affected. Skin lesions may take the form of nodules or ulcers whilst subcutaneous lesions may ulcerate with a gummy discharge. Healing occurs slowly with the formation of characteristic tissue paper scars. Mucosal lesions may occur in the mouth, pharynx, larynx or nasal septum, appearing as punched-out ulcers. Of particular importance is gummatous involvement of the tongue, healing of which may lead to leucoplakia with the attendant risk of malignant change. Gummas of the tibia, skull, clavicle and sternum have been described, as has involvement of the brain, spinal cord, liver, testis and, rarely, other organs. Resolution of active disease should follow treatment, though some tissue damage may be permanent. Paroxysmal cold haemoglobinuria (p. 1034) may be seen.

Cardiovascular syphilis

This may present many years after initial infection. Aortitis which may involve the aortic valve and/or the coronary ostia is the key feature. Clinical features include aortic incompetence, angina and aortic aneurysm (p. 605). The condition typically affects the ascending aorta and sometimes the aortic arch; aneurysm of the descending aorta is rare. Treatment with penicillin will not correct anatomical damage and surgical intervention may be required.

Neurosyphilis

This may also take years to develop. Asymptomatic infection is associated with CSF abnormalities in the absence of clinical signs. Meningovascular disease, tabes dorsalis or general paralysis of the insane characterises the symptomatic forms (p. 1233). Neurosyphilis and cardiovascular syphilis may coexist and are sometimes referred to as quaternary syphilis.

15.5 CLINICAL FEATURES OF CONGENITAL SYPHILIS

Early congenital syphilis (neonatal period)

- Maculo-papular rash
- Condylomata lata
- Mucous patches
- Fissures around mouth, nose and anus
- Rhinitis with nasal discharge (snuffles)
- Hepatosplenomegaly
- Osteochondritis/periostitis
- Generalised lymphadenopathy
- Choroiditis
- Meningitis
- Anaemia/thrombocytopenia

Late congenital syphilis

- Benign tertiary syphilis
- Periostitis
- Paroxysmal cold haemoglobinuria
- Neurosyphilis
- 8th nerve deafness
- Interstitial keratitis
- Clutton's joints (painless effusion into knee joints)

Stigmata

- Hutchinson's incisors (anterior–posterior thickening with notch on narrowed cutting edge)
- Mulberry molars (imperfectly formed cusps/deficient dental enamel)
- High arched palate
- Maxillary hypoplasia
- Saddle nose (following snuffles)
- Rhagades (radiating scars around mouth, nose and anus following rash)
- Salt and pepper scars on retina (from choroiditis)
- Corneal scars (from interstitial keratitis)
- Sabre tibia (from periostitis)
- Bossing of frontal and parietal bones (healed periosteal nodes)

CONGENITAL SYPHILIS

Congenital syphilis is rare where antenatal serological screening is practised. Antisyphilitic treatment in pregnancy treats the fetus, if infected, as well as the mother.

Treponemal infection may give rise to a variety of outcomes after 4 months of gestation when the fetus becomes immunocompetent:

- miscarriage or stillbirth, premature or at term
- birth of a syphilitic baby (a very sick baby with hepatosplenomegaly, bullous rash and perhaps pneumonia)
- birth of a baby who develops signs of early congenital syphilis during the first few weeks of life (Box 15.5)
- birth of a baby with latent infection who either remains well or develops congenital syphilis/stigmata later in life (Box 15.5).

Investigations in adult cases

T. pallidum may be identified in serum collected from chancres, or from moist or eroded lesions in secondary syphilis using a dark-field microscope, a direct fluorescent antibody test or PCR.

The serological tests for syphilis are listed in Box 15.6. Many centres use treponemal enzyme immunoassays (EIAs) for IgG and IgM antibodies to screen for syphilis. EIA for antitreponemal IgM becomes positive at approximately 2 weeks, whilst non-treponemal tests become positive

15

15.6 SEROLOGICAL TESTS FOR SYPHILIS

Non-treponemal (non-specific) tests

- Venereal Diseases Research Laboratory (VDRL) test
- Rapid plasma reagin (RPR) test

Treponemal (specific) antibody tests

- Treponemal antigen-based enzyme immunoassay (EIA) for IgG and IgM
- *T. pallidum* haemagglutination assay (TPHA)
- *T. pallidum* particle agglutination assay (TPPA)
- Fluorescent treponemal antibody-absorbed (FTA-ABS) Test

about 4 weeks after primary syphilis. All positive results in asymptomatic patients must be confirmed by repeat tests.

Biological false positive reactions occur occasionally; these are most commonly seen with Venereal Diseases Research Laboratory (VDRL) or rapid plasma reagin (RPR) tests (when treponemal tests will be negative). Acute false positive reactions may be associated with infections such as infectious mononucleosis, chickenpox and malaria, and may also occur in pregnancy. Chronic false positive reactions may be associated with autoimmune diseases. False negative results for non-treponemal tests may be found in secondary syphilis because extremely high antibody levels can prevent the formation of the antibody–antigen lattice necessary for the visualisation of the flocculation reaction (the prozone phenomenon).

In benign tertiary and cardiovascular syphilis, examination of CSF should be considered because asymptomatic neurological disease may coexist. The CSF should also be examined in patients with clinical signs of neurosyphilis (p. 1233) and in both early and late congenital syphilis. Chest X-ray, ECG and echocardiogram are useful in the investigation of cardiovascular syphilis. Biopsy may be required to diagnose gumma.

Endemic treponematoses such as yaws, endemic (non-venereal) syphilis (bejel) and pinta (p. 317) are caused by treponemes morphologically indistinguishable from *T. pallidum* that cannot be differentiated by serological tests. A VDRL or RPR test may help to elucidate the correct diagnosis because adults with late yaws usually have low titres.

Investigations in suspected congenital syphilis

Passively transferred maternal antibodies from an adequately treated mother may give rise to positive serological tests in her baby. In this situation, non-treponemal tests should become negative within 3–6 months of birth. A positive EIA test for antitreponemal IgM suggests early congenital syphilis. A diagnosis of congenital syphilis mandates investigation of the mother, her partner and any siblings.

Management

Penicillin is the drug of choice. Specific regimens depend on the stage of infection. Longer courses are required in late syphilis and in HIV co-infection. Doxycycline is indicated for patients allergic to penicillin, except in pregnancy (see below). Azithromycin has also been advocated, but recent outbreaks in UK cities have been associated with strains of

T. pallidum such as Street 14 that are resistant to macrolides. All patients must be followed up to ensure cure, and partner notification is of particular importance. Resolution of clinical signs in early syphilis with declining titres for non-treponemal tests, usually to undetectable levels within 6 months for primary syphilis and 12–18 months for secondary syphilis, are indicators of successful treatment. Specific treponemal antibody tests may remain positive for life. In patients who have had syphilis for many years there may be little serological response following treatment.

Pregnancy

Penicillin is the treatment of choice in pregnancy. Erythromycin stearate can be given if there is penicillin hypersensitivity, but crosses the placenta poorly; the newborn baby must therefore be treated with a course of penicillin and consideration given to retreating the mother. Some specialists recommend penicillin desensitisation for pregnant mothers so that penicillin can be given during temporary tolerance. The author has successfully prescribed ceftriaxone 250 mg i.m. for 10 days in this situation. Babies should be treated in hospital with the help of a pediatrician.

Treatment reactions

Anaphylaxis. Penicillin is a common cause; on-site facilities should be available for management (p. 86).

Jarisch–Herxheimer reaction. This is an acute febrile reaction that follows treatment and is characterised by headache, malaise and myalgia; it resolves within 24 hours. It is common in early syphilis and rare in late syphilis. Fetal distress or premature labour can occur in pregnancy. The reaction may also cause worsening of neurological (cerebral artery occlusion) or ophthalmic (uveitis, optic neuritis) disease, myocardial ischaemia (inflammation of the coronary ostia) and laryngeal stenosis (swelling of a gumma). Prednisolone 10–20 mg orally 8-hourly for 3 days is recommended to prevent the reaction in patients with these forms of the disease; antisyphilitic treatment can be started 24 hours after introducing corticosteroids. In high-risk situations it is usually wise to initiate therapy in hospital.

Procaine reaction. Fear of impending death occurs immediately after the accidental intravenous injection of procaine penicillin and may be associated with hallucinations or fits. Symptoms are short-lived, but verbal assurance and sometimes physical restraint are needed. The reaction can be prevented by aspiration before intramuscular injection to ensure the needle is not in a blood vessel.

GONORRHOEA

Gonorrhoea is caused by infection with *Neisseria gonorrhoeae* and may involve columnar epithelium in the lower genital tract, rectum, pharynx and eyes. Transmission is usually the result of vaginal, anal or oral sex. Gonococcal conjunctivitis may be the result of accidental infection from contaminated fingers. Untreated mothers may infect their babies during delivery, resulting in ophthalmia neonatorum (Fig. 15.6). Infection of children beyond the neonatal period is usually indicative of sexual abuse.

15

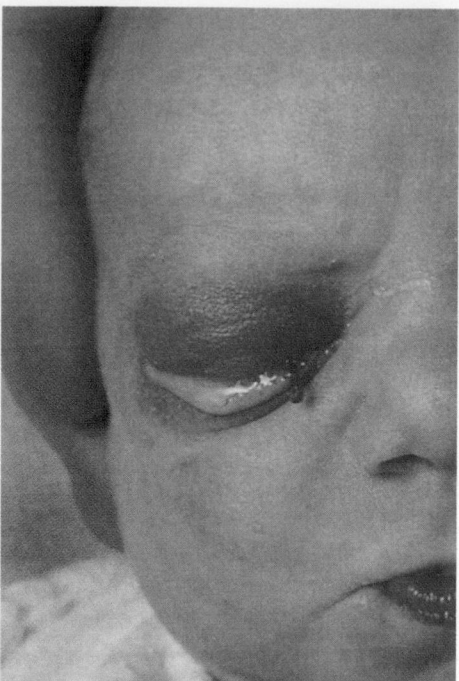

Fig. 15.6 Gonococcal ophthalmia neonatorum.

15.7 TREATMENT OF UNCOMPLICATED ANOGENITAL GONORRHOEA

Uncomplicated infection

- Cefixime 400 mg stat *or*
- Ciprofloxacin 500 mg orally stat[1,2] *or*
- Ofloxacin 400 mg orally stat[1,2] *or*
- Amoxicillin 3 g *plus* probenecid 1 g orally stat[3]

Quinolone resistance

- Ceftriaxone 250 mg i.m. stat *or*
- Spectinomycin 2 g i.m. stat[4]

Pregnancy and breastfeeding

- Cefixime 400 mg stat *or*
- Ceftriaxone 250 mg i.m. stat *or*
- Amoxicillin 3 g *plus* probenecid 1 g orally stat[3] *or*
- Spectinomycin 2 g i.m. stat[4]

Pharyngeal gonorrhoea

- Cefixime 400 mg stat *or*
- Ceftriaxone 250 mg i.m. stat *or*
- Ciprofloxacin 500 mg[1,2] orally stat *or*
- Ofloxacin 400 mg[1,2] orally stat

[1] Contraindicated in pregnancy and breastfeeding.
[2] If prevalence of quinolone resistance for *N. gonorrhoeae* < 5%.
[3] If prevalence of penicillin resistance for *N. gonorrhoeae* < 5%.
[4] May only be available in specialist clinics.

Clinical features

The incubation period is usually 2–10 days. In men the anterior urethra is commonly infected, causing urethral discharge and dysuria, but symptoms are absent in about 10% of cases. Examination will usually show a mucopurulent or purulent urethral discharge. Rectal infection in MSM is usually asymptomatic but may present with anal discomfort, discharge or rectal bleeding. Proctoscopy may reveal either no abnormality, or clinical evidence of proctitis (Fig. 15.3, p. 408) such as inflamed rectal mucosa and mucopus.

In women, the urethra, paraurethral glands/ducts, Bartholin's glands/ducts or endocervical canal may be infected. The rectum may also be involved either due to contamination from a urogenital site or as a result of anal sex. Occasionally, the rectum is the only site infected. About 80% of women who have gonorrhoea are asymptomatic. There may be vaginal discharge or dysuria but these symptoms are often due to additional infections such as chlamydia (see below), trichomoniasis or candidiasis, making full investigation essential (p. 405). Lower abdominal pain, dyspareunia and intermenstrual bleeding may be indicative of PID. Clinical examination may show no abnormality or pus may be expressed from urethra, paraurethral ducts or Bartholin's ducts. The cervix may be inflamed, with mucopurulent discharge and contact bleeding.

Pharyngeal gonorrhoea is the result of receptive orogenital sex and is usually symptomless. Gonococcal conjunctivitis is an uncommon complication, presenting with purulent discharge from the eye(s), severe inflammation of the conjunctivae and oedema of the eyelids, pain and photophobia. Gonococcal ophthalmia neonatorum presents similarly with purulent conjunctivitis and oedema of the eyelids. Conjunctivitis must be treated urgently to prevent corneal damage.

Disseminated gonococcal infection (DGI) is seen rarely, and typically affects women with asymptomatic genital infection. Symptoms include arthritis of one or more joints, pustular skin lesions and fever. Gonococcal endocarditis has been described.

Investigations

Gram-negative intracellular diplococci may be seen on microscopy of smears from infected sites (Fig. 15.1, p. 406). Pharyngeal smears are difficult to analyse due to the presence of other diplococci so the diagnosis must be confirmed by culture.

Management of adults

Uncomplicated gonorrhoea responds to a single adequate dose of a suitable antimicrobial (many UK centres currently use oral cefixime 400 mg, Box 15.7); cure rates should exceed 95%. Longer courses of antibiotics are required for complicated infection. Partner(s) of patients with gonorrhoea should be seen as soon as possible.

Delay in treatment may lead to complications (Box 15.8).

15.8 COMPLICATIONS OF DELAYED THERAPY IN GONORRHOEA

- Acute prostatitis
- Epididymo-orchitis
- Bartholin's gland abscess
- PID (may lead to infertility or ectopic pregnancy)
- Disseminated gonococcal infection

CHLAMYDIAL INFECTION

CHLAMYDIAL INFECTION IN MEN

Chlamydia is transmitted and presents in a similar way to gonorrhoea; however, urethral symptoms are usually milder and may be absent in over 50% of cases. Conjunctivitis is also milder than in gonorrhoea; pharyngitis does not occur. The incubation period varies from 1 week to a few months. Without treatment, symptoms may resolve but the patient remains infectious for several months. Complications such as epididymo-orchitis and Reiter's syndrome, or sexually acquired reactive arthropathy (SARA, p. 1108) are rare. Sexually transmitted pathogens such as chlamydia or gonococci are usually responsible for epididymo-orchitis in men aged less than 35 years, whereas bacteria such as Gram-negative enteric organisms are more commonly implicated in older men.

Treatments for chlamydia are listed in Box 15.9. Non-specific urethritis is treated identically. The partner(s) of men with chlamydia should be treated even if laboratory tests for chlamydia are negative. Investigation is not mandatory, but serves a useful epidemiological purpose; moreover, positive results encourage further attempts at contact-tracing.

CHLAMYDIAL INFECTION IN WOMEN

The cervix and urethra are commonly involved. Infection is asymptomatic in about 80% of patients but may cause vaginal discharge, dysuria, intermenstrual and/or postcoital bleeding. Lower abdominal pain, dyspareunia and intermenstrual bleeding are features of PID. Examination may reveal mucopurulent cervicitis, contact bleeding from cervix, evidence of PID or no obvious clinical signs. Treatment options are listed in Box 15.9. The patient's male partner(s) should be investigated and treated.

Some infections may clear spontaneously but others persist. PID, with the risk of tubal damage and subsequent infertility or ectopic pregnancy, is an important long-term complication. Other complications include perihepatitis, chronic pelvic pain, conjunctivitis and Reiter's syndrome or SARA. Perinatal transmission may lead to ophthalmia neonatorum and/or pneumonia in the neonate.

15.9 TREATMENT OF CHLAMYDIAL INFECTION	

Standard regimens

- Azithromycin 1 g orally as a single dose[1] *or*
- Doxycycline 100 mg 12-hourly orally for 7 days[2]

Alternative regimens

- Erythromycin 500 mg 6-hourly orally for 7 days *or* 500 mg 12-hourly for 2 weeks *or*
- Ofloxacin 200 mg 12-hourly orally for 7 days[2]

[1]Safety in pregnancy and breastfeeding has not been fully assessed.
[2]Contraindicated in pregnancy and breastfeeding.
[3]Avoid alcoholic drinks during and for 48 hours after therapy.

OTHER SEXUALLY TRANSMITTED BACTERIAL INFECTIONS

Chancroid, granuloma inguinale and LGV as causes of genital ulcers in the tropics are described in Box 15.10 overleaf. LGV is also a cause of proctitis in MSM (p. 408).

SEXUALLY TRANSMITTED VIRAL INFECTIONS

GENITAL HERPES SIMPLEX

Infection with herpes simplex virus type 1 (HSV-1) or type 2 (HSV-2) produces a wide spectrum of clinical problems (p. 303). Transmission is usually sexual (vaginal, anal, orogenital or oroanal), but perinatal infection of the neonate may also occur. Primary infection at the site of HSV entry, which may be symptomatic or asymptomatic, establishes latency in local sensory ganglia. Recurrences, either symptomatic or asymptomatic viral shedding, are a consequence of HSV reactivation. The first symptomatic episode is usually the most severe. Although HSV-1 is classically associated with orolabial herpes and HSV-2 with anogenital herpes, HSV-1 now accounts for more than 50% of anogenital infections in the UK.

Clinical features

The first symptomatic episode presents with irritable vesicles that soon rupture to form small, tender ulcers on the external genitalia (Figs 15.2, p. 408, and 15.7). Lesions

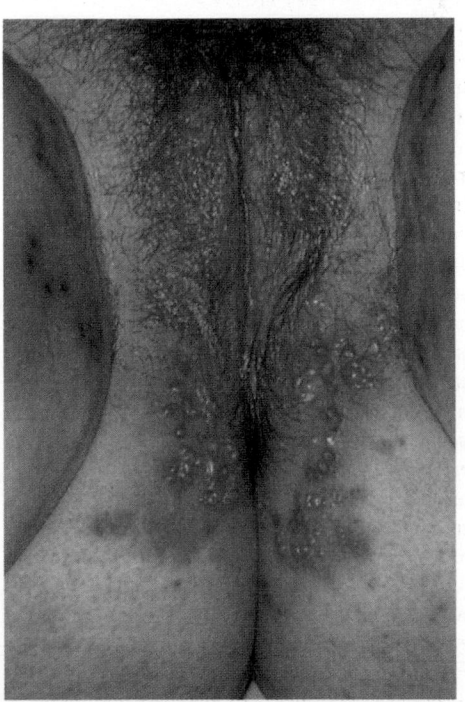

Fig. 15.7 Herpetic ulceration of the vulva.

15

15.10 SALIENT FEATURES OF LYMPHOGRANULOMA VENEREUM, CHANCROID AND GRANULOMA INGUINALE (DONOVANOSIS)

Infection and distribution	Organism	Incubation period	Genital lesion	Lymph nodes	Diagnosis	Management
Lymphogranuloma venereum (LGV) East/West Africa, India, South-east Asia, South America, Caribbean	*Chlamydia trachomatis* types L1, 2, 3	3–30 days	Small, transient, painless ulcer, vesicle, papule; often unnoticed	Tender, usually unilateral, matted, adherent, multilocular, suppurative bubo; inguinal/femoral nodes involved; there may be late sequelae[1]	Serological tests for L1–3 serotypes; swab from ulcer or bubo pus for *Chlamydia*	Doxycycline[2] 12-hourly orally for 21 days *or* Erythromycin 500 mg 6-hourly orally
Chancroid Africa, Asia, Central and South America	*Haemophilus ducreyi* (short Gram-negative bacillus)	3–10 days	Single or multiple painful ulcers with ragged undermined edges	As above but unilocular, suppurative bubo; inguinal nodes involved in ~50%	Microscopy and culture of scrapings from ulcer or pus from bubo	Azithromycin[3] 1 g orally once *or* Ceftriaxone 250 mg i.m. once *or* Ciprofloxacin[2] 500 mg 12-hourly orally for 3 days *or* Erythromycin 500 mg 6-hourly orally for 7 days
Granuloma inguinale Australia, Caribbean, India, South Africa, South America, Papua New Guinea	*Klebsiella granulomatis* (Donovan bodies)	3–40 days	Ulcers or hypertrophic granulomatous lesions; usually painless[4]	Initial swelling of inguinal nodes, then spread of infection to form abscess or ulceration through adjacent skin	Microscopy of cellular material for intracellular bipolar-staining Donovan bodies	Azithromycin[3] 1 g weekly orally *or* 500 mg daily orally *or* Doxycycline[2] 100 mg 12-hourly orally *or* Ceftriaxone 1 g i.m. daily *or* Erythromycin 500 mg 6-hourly orally Treatment for at least 3 weeks and until lesions have healed

[1] The genito-ano-rectal syndrome is a late manifestation of LGV.
[2] Doxycycline and ciprofloxacin are contraindicated in pregnancy and breastfeeding.
[3] The safety of azithromycin in pregnancy and breastfeeding has not been fully assessed.
[4] Mother-to-baby transmission of granuloma inguinale may rarely occur.

Partners of patients with LGV, chancroid and granuloma inguinale should be investigated and treated, even if asymptomatic.

at other sites (e.g. urethra, vagina, cervix, perianal area, anus or rectum) may cause dysuria, urethral or vaginal discharge, or anal, perianal or rectal pain. Constitutional symptoms such as fever, headache and malaise are common. Inguinal lymph nodes become enlarged and tender, and there may be nerve root pain in the 2nd and 3rd sacral dermatomes.

Extragenital lesions may develop at other sites such as the buttock, finger or eye due to auto-inoculation. Oropharyngeal infection may result from orogenital sex. Complications such as urinary retention due to autonomic neuropathy, and aseptic meningitis are occasionally seen.

First episodes usually heal within 2–4 weeks without treatment; recurrences are usually milder and of shorter duration than the initial attack. They occur more often in HSV-2 infection and their frequency tends to decrease with time. Prodromal symptoms such as irritation or burning at the subsequent site of recurrence, or neuralgic pains affecting buttocks, legs or hips are seen commonly. The first symptomatic episode may be a recurrence of a previously undiagnosed primary infection. Recurrent episodes of asymptomatic viral shedding are important in the transmission of HSV.

Diagnosis
Swabs are taken from vesicular fluid or ulcers for detection of DNA by PCR or tissue culture and typing. Electron microscopy of such material will only give a presumptive diagnosis, as herpes group viruses appear similar. Type-specific antibody tests are available but are not sufficiently accurate for general use.

Management
First episode
The following 5-day oral regimens are all recommended and should be started within 5 days of the beginning of the episode, or whilst lesions are still forming:

- aciclovir 200 mg five times daily
- famciclovir 250 mg 8-hourly
- valaciclovir 500 mg 12-hourly.

Analgesia may be required and saline bathing can be soothing. Treatment may be continued for longer than 5 days if new lesions develop. Occasionally intravenous therapy may be indicated if oral therapy is poorly tolerated or aseptic meningitis occurs.

Catheterisation via the suprapubic route is advisable for urinary retention due to autonomic neuropathy because the transurethral route may introduce HSV into the bladder.

Recurrent genital herpes

Symptomatic recurrences are usually mild and may require no specific treatment other than saline bathing. For more severe episodes patient-initiated treatment at onset, with one of the following 5-day oral regimens, should reduce the duration of the recurrence:

- aciclovir 200 mg five times daily
- famciclovir 125–150 mg 12-hourly
- valaciclovir 500 mg 12-hourly.

In a few patients, treatment started at the onset of prodromal symptoms may abort recurrence.

Suppressive therapy may be required for patients with frequent recurrences, especially if these occur at intervals of less than 4 weeks. Treatment should be given for a minimum of 1 year before stopping to assess recurrence rate. About 20% of patients will experience reduced attack rates thereafter, but for those whose recurrences remain unchanged, resumption of suppressive therapy is justified. Aciclovir 400 mg 12-hourly is most commonly prescribed.

Management in pregnancy

If her partner is known to be infected with HSV, a pregnant woman with no previous anogenital herpes should be advised to protect herself during sexual intercourse because the risk of disseminated infection is increased in pregnancy. Consistent condom use during pregnancy may reduce transmission of HSV. Genital herpes acquired during the first or second trimester of pregnancy is treated with aciclovir as clinically indicated. Although aciclovir is not licensed for use in pregnancy in the UK, there is considerable clinical evidence to support its safety. Third-trimester acquisition has been associated with life-threatening haematogenous dissemination and should be treated with aciclovir.

Vaginal delivery should be routine in women who are symptomless in late pregnancy. Caesarean section (CS) is sometimes considered if there is a recurrence at the beginning of labour, although the risk of neonatal herpes through vaginal transmission is very low. CS is often recommended if primary infection occurs after 34 weeks because the risk of viral shedding is very high in labour.

HUMAN PAPILLOMAVIRUS (HPV) AND ANOGENITAL WARTS

HPV DNA typing has demonstrated over 90 genotypes (p. 1295), of which HPV-6, HPV-11, HPV-16 and HPV-18 most commonly infect the genital tract through sexual transmission. It is important to differentiate between the benign genotypes (HPV-6 and 11) that cause anogenital warts, and genotypes such as 16 and 18 that are associated with dysplastic conditions and cancers of the genital tract but are not a cause of benign warts. All genotypes usually result initially in subclinical infection of the genital tract rather than clinically obvious lesions affecting penis, vulva, vagina, cervix, perineum or anus.

Anogenital warts are the result of HPV-driven hyperplasia and usually develop after an incubation period of between 3 months and 2 years. They may be single or multiple, exophytic, papular or flat. Perianal warts (p. 404), whilst being more commonly found in MSM, are also found in heterosexual men and in women. Rarely, a giant condyloma (Buschke–Lewenstein tumour) develops with local tissue destruction. Atypical warts should be biopsied. In pregnancy warts may dramatically increase in size and number, making treatment difficult. Rarely, they are large enough to obstruct labour and in this case delivery by CS will be required. Perinatal transmission of HPV rarely leads to anogenital warts, or possibly laryngeal papillomas, in the neonate.

A variety of treatments are available including the following:

- *Podophyllotoxin, 0.5% solution or 0.15% cream* (contraindicated in pregnancy) applied 12-hourly for 3 days, followed by 4 days' rest, for up to 4 weeks is suitable for home treatment of external warts.
- *Imiquimod* cream (contraindicated in pregnancy) applied 3 times weekly (and washed off after 6–10 hours) for up to 16 weeks is also suitable for home treatment of external warts.
- *Cryotherapy* using liquid nitrogen to freeze warty tissue is suitable for external and internal warts but often requires repeated clinic visits.
- *Hyfrecation*—electrofulguration that causes superficial charring—is suitable for external and internal warts. Hyfrecation results in smoke plume which contains HPV DNA and the potential to cause respiratory infection in the operator/patient. Masks should be worn during the procedure and adequate extraction of fumes should be provided.
- *Surgical removal.*

The use of condoms to prevent the transmission of HPV to non-infected partners should be encouraged. However, HPV may affect parts of the genital area not protected by condoms. HPV vaccines are under development.

MOLLUSCUM CONTAGIOSUM

Infection by molluscum contagiosum virus, both sexual and non-sexual, produces flesh-coloured umbilicated hemispherical papules usually up to 5 mm in diameter after an incubation period of 3–12 weeks (Fig. 15.8). Larger lesions may be seen in HIV infection (p. 385). Lesions are often multiple and, once established in an individual, may spread by auto-inoculation. They are found on the genitalia, lower abdomen and upper thighs when sexually acquired. Facial lesions are highly suggestive of underlying HIV infection. Diagnosis is made on clinical grounds and by expression of the central core, in which the typical pox-like viral particles can be seen on electron microscopy (differentiating molluscum contagiosum from genital warts). Typically, lesions persist for an average of 2 years before spontaneous resolution occurs. Treatment regimens are therefore cosmetic; they include cryotherapy, hyfrecation, topical

15

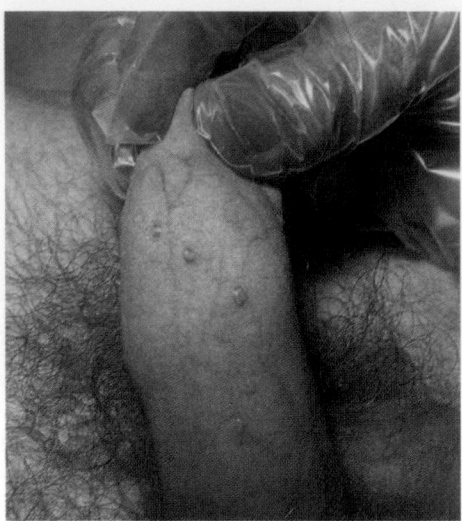

Fig. 15.8 Molluscum contagiosum of the shaft of the penis.

applications of 0.15% podophyllotoxin cream (contraindicated in pregnancy) or expression of the central core.

VIRAL HEPATITIS

The hepatitis viruses A–D (pp. 962–968) may be sexually transmitted:

- *Hepatitis A (HAV).* Insertive oroanal sex, insertive digital sex, insertive anal sex and multiple sexual partners have been linked with HAV transmission in MSM. HAV transmission in heterosexual men and women is also possible through oroanal sex.
- *Hepatitis B (HBV).* Insertive oroanal sex, anal sex and multiple sexual partners are linked with HBV infection in MSM. Heterosexual transmission of HBV is well documented and commercial sex workers are at particular risk. Hepatitis D (HDV) may also be sexually transmitted.
- *Hepatitis C.* Sexual transmission of HCV is well documented in MSM, and less so in heterosexuals. Sexual transmission is less efficient than for HBV.

The sexual partner(s) of patients with HAV and HBV should be seen as soon as possible and offered immunisation (pp. 137–139) where appropriate. Patients with HAV should abstain from all forms of unprotected sex until non-infectious. Those with HBV should likewise abstain from unprotected sex until they are non-infectious or until their partners have been vaccinated successfully. No active or passive immunisation is available for protection against HCV but the consistent use of condoms is likely to protect susceptible partners. Active immunisation against HAV and HBV should be offered to susceptible people at risk of infection. Many STI clinics offer HAV immunisation to MSM along with routine HBV immunisation; a combined HAV and HBV vaccine is available.

FURTHER INFORMATION

Books and journal articles
Adler M, Cowan F, French P, et al. ABC of sexually transmitted infections. London: BMJ Books; 2004.
Clutterbuck D. Specialist training in sexually transmitted infections and HIV. London: Mosby; 2004.
McMillan A, Young H, Ogilvie MM, Scott GR. Clinical practice in sexually transmissible infections. London: Saunders; 2002.
Mayaud P, Mabey D. Approaches to the control of sexually transmitted infections in developing countries: old problems and modern challenges. Sexually Transmitted Infections 2004; 80:174–182.

Websites
www.bashh.org/guidelines/ceguidelines.htm *Updates on treatment of all STIs.*

15

16

M.J. FIELD
L. BURNETT
D.R. SULLIVAN
P. STEWART

Clinical biochemistry and metabolism

There is a world-wide trend towards increased use of laboratory-based diagnostic investigations, and biochemical investigations in particular. It has been estimated that 60–70% of all critical decisions taken in regard to patients in health-care systems in developed countries involve a laboratory service or result.

This chapter considers a diverse group of disorders not considered elsewhere, whose primary manifestation is in abnormalities of biochemistry laboratory results, or whose underlying pathophysiology involves disturbance in specific biochemical pathways. It describes the more common metabolic diseases which affect adults. Note that discussion of diabetes mellitus and other endocrine disorders is to be found in Chapters 20 and 21.

BIOCHEMICAL INVESTIGATIONS

There are three broad reasons why a clinician may request a biochemical laboratory investigation:

- to screen an asymptomatic subject for the presence of disease
- to assist in diagnosis of a patient's presenting complaint, when an abnormal result confirms the presence of a disease, or a normal result rules it out
- to monitor changes in test results, as a marker of disease progression or of effects of treatment.

Contemporary medical practice has become increasingly reliant on laboratory investigation, and in particular, on biochemical laboratory investigation. This has both been limited by, and has driven, extraordinary improvements in the analytical capacity and speed of response of laboratory instrumentation.

Three operational themes can be seen in modern clinical biochemistry laboratories:

- Large central biochemistry laboratories feature extensive utilisation of automation and information technology. Specimens are transported from clinical areas to the laboratory using high-speed transport systems (such as pneumatic transport tubes), and identified with machine-readable labels (such as barcodes). Laboratory instruments have been miniaturised and tightly integrated with robot transport systems to enable multiple common analyses to be performed rapidly on a single sample. Statistical process control techniques are used to assure the quality of analytical results, and are also increasingly being used to monitor other aspects of the laboratory, such as the time taken to complete the analysis ('turn-around time').
- Point-of-care testing (POCT) involves bringing selected laboratory analytical systems into clinical areas, to the patient's bedside, or even connected to an individual patient. These systems allow the clinician to receive the results of analysis almost instantaneously, although often at greater cost than using a central laboratory.
- The range and diversity of analyses that can now be performed has widened considerably with the introduction into the clinical laboratory of many techniques borrowed from the chemical or other industries (Box 16.1). This has enabled testing for what were previously regarded as esoteric substances and conditions.

Good medical practice involves appropriate ordering of laboratory investigations and correct interpretation of test results. The key principles, including the concepts of sensitivity and specificity, are described in Chapter 1 (pp. 6–8).

16.1 RANGE OF ANALYTICAL MODALITIES USED IN THE CLINICAL BIOCHEMISTRY LABORATORY

Analytical modality	Analyte	Typical applications
Ion-selective electrodes	Blood gases, electrolytes (e.g. Na, K, Cl)	Point-of-care testing (POCT) High-throughput analysers
Colorimetric chemical reaction, or coupled enzymatic reaction	Simple mass or concentration measurement (e.g. creatinine, phosphate) Simple enzyme activity	High-throughput analysers
Ligand assay (usually immunoassay)	Specific proteins Hormones Drugs	Increasingly available as POCT or high-throughput analysers
Chromatography: gas chromatography (GC), high-pressure liquid chromatography (HPLC), thin-layer chromatography (TLC) Mass spectroscopy (MS)	Organic compounds	Therapeutic drug monitoring (TDM) Drug screening (e.g. drugs of misuse) Vitamins Biochemical metabolites
Spectrophotometry, turbidimetry, nephelometry, fluorimetry	Haemoglobin derivatives Specific proteins Immunoglobulins	Xanthochromia Lipoproteins Paraproteins
Electrophoresis	Proteins Some enzymes	Paraproteins Isoenzyme analysis
Atomic absorption (AA) Inductively coupled plasma/mass spectroscopy (ICP-MS)	Trace elements and metals	Quantitation of heavy metals

INTEGRATED WATER AND ELECTROLYTE BALANCE

One of the most common uses of the clinical biochemistry laboratory is to monitor electrolyte and acid–base status. The diverse clinical consequences of these biochemical disorders are illustrated in Box 16.2. Some whole-body electrolyte disturbances (notably of sodium) result in major clinical problems with minimal disturbance in measured biochemical parameters. However, these will also be considered for convenience in this section.

Before considering individual electrolytes and acid–base balance in turn, it is important to review the relationships between them.

16.2 MANIFESTATIONS OF DISORDERED WATER, ELECTROLYTE AND ACID–BASE STATUS		
Primary disturbance	Altered physiology	Clinical effect
Sodium	ECF volume	Circulatory changes
Water	ECF osmolality	Cerebral changes
Potassium	Action potential in excitable tissues	Neuromuscular weakness, cardiac effects
Hydrogen ion	Acid–base balance (pH)	Altered tissue function, respiratory compensation
Magnesium	Cell membrane stability	Neuromuscular, vascular and cardiac effects
Phosphate	Cellular energetics	Widespread tissue effects

(ECF = extracellular fluid)

WATER AND ELECTROLYTE DISTRIBUTION

In a typical adult male, the total body water (TBW) is approximately 60% of the body weight (somewhat more for infants and somewhat less for women). Of a TBW of 40 litres, more than half is located inside cells (the intracellular fluid or ICF) while the remainder, some 15 litres, is in the extracellular fluid (ECF) compartment (Fig. 16.1). Of the ECF, the plasma is itself a small fraction (some 3 litres) while the remainder is interstitial fluid within the tissues but outside the cells.

Figure 16.1 also illustrates some of the major differences in composition between the main body fluid compartments. The dominant cation in the ICF is potassium, while the dominant cation in the ECF is sodium. Phosphates and negatively charged proteins constitute the major intracellular anions, while chloride and, to a lesser extent, bicarbonate dominate the ECF anions. An important difference between the plasma and interstitial compartments of the ECF is that only plasma contains significant concentrations of protein.

The major force maintaining the difference in cation concentration between the ICF and ECF is the activity of the sodium–potassium pump (Na,K-activated ATPase) integral

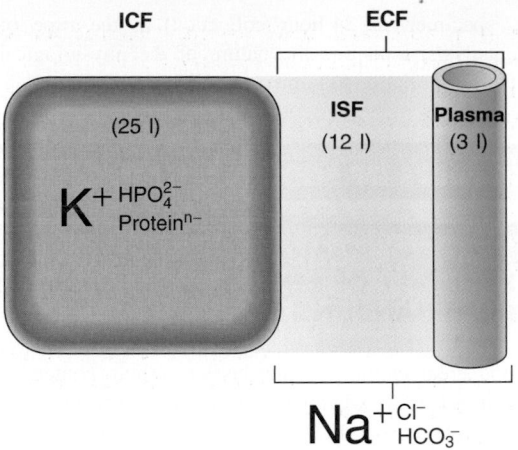

Fig. 16.1 Normal distribution of body water and electrolytes. Schematic representation of volume (l = litres) and composition (dominant ionic species only shown) of the intracellular fluid (ICF) and extracellular fluid (ECF) in a 70 kg male. The main difference in composition between the plasma and interstitial fluid (ISF) is the presence of appreciable concentrations of protein in the plasma (not shown) but not the ISF.

to all cell membranes. Maintenance of the cation gradients across cell membranes is essential for many cell processes, including the excitability of conducting tissues such as nerve and muscle. The difference in protein content between the plasma and the interstitial fluid compartment is maintained by the protein permeability barrier at the capillary wall. This protein concentration gradient contributes to the balance of forces across the capillary wall favouring fluid retention within the capillaries (the colloid osmotic, or oncotic, pressure of the plasma), thus maintaining an adequate circulating plasma volume.

These basic concepts are relevant to understanding the origin and consequences of many of the fluid and electrolyte disturbances to be discussed in this chapter. They also provide a background to the principles of management of these disorders, particularly intravenous fluid therapy (p. 425).

INVESTIGATION OF WATER AND ELECTROLYTES

A number of practical matters should be considered in sampling body fluids for electrolyte tests. Because the blood consists of both intracellular (red cell) and extracellular (plasma) components, it is important to avoid haemolysis during or after collection of the sample, which causes contamination of the plasma compartment by intracellular elements, particularly potassium. Blood should not be drawn from an arm into which an intravenous infusion is being given, to avoid contamination by the infused fluid. Repeat or serial measurements of plasma electrolytes are frequently necessary when a marked abnormality has been detected and corrective therapy has been instituted.

Since the kidney acts to maintain the constancy of the body fluids by adjusting urine volume and composition, it is frequently helpful to obtain a simultaneous sample of urine

16

('spot' specimen or 24-hour collection) at the time of blood analysis, to define the nature of the physiological disturbance in relation to homeostatic balance.

DISORDERS OF SODIUM BALANCE

FUNCTIONAL ANATOMY AND PHYSIOLOGY OF RENAL SODIUM HANDLING

Since the great majority of the body's sodium content is located in the ECF, where it is by far the most abundant cation, total body sodium is a principal determinant of ECF volume. Thus the regulation of sodium excretion by the kidney is crucially important in maintaining normal ECF and hence plasma volume, in the face of wide variations in sodium intake, typically in the range 50–250 mmol/day.

The functional unit involved in renal excretory function is the nephron (Fig. 16.2). The glomerulus is the site of ultrafiltration of the blood, resulting in the generation of a cell- and protein-free fluid, resembling plasma in electrolyte composition, being delivered into the initial part of the tubular system (more detail on the structure and function of the glomerulus is given in Ch. 17). The glomerular filtra-

tion rate (GFR) is approximately 125 ml/min (equivalent to 180 litres/day) in a typical adult. Over 99% of this filtered fluid is reabsorbed into the blood in the peritubular capillaries during its passage through successive segments of the nephron, largely as a result of tubular reabsorption of sodium. The processes mediating this sodium reabsorption, and the factors which regulate it, are key to understanding clinical disturbances and pharmacological interventions.

Nephron segments

At least four different functional segments of the nephron can be defined in terms of their mechanism for sodium reabsorption (Fig. 16.3).

Proximal tubule

This is responsible for the reabsorption of some 65% of the filtered sodium load. The cellular mechanism is complex but some of the key features are shown in Figure 16.3A. The basolateral membrane contains a high density of Na,K-ATPase pump units which remove sodium from the cell into the blood. The filtered sodium in the luminal fluid enters the cell via a number of apical membrane processes. One of these involves the cotransport of sodium with glucose, and there are other species of cotransporters coupling sodium to the entry of amino acid, phosphate and other organic molecules. A quantitatively more significant mechanism is the entry of sodium by countertransport with H^+ ions, using the sodium–hydrogen exchanger (NHE-3). Intracellular H^+ ions are generated by the breakdown of carbonic acid, produced in the cell through the hydration of carbon dioxide, catalysed by the enzyme carbonic anhydrase. A large component of the transepithelial flux of sodium, water and other dissolved solutes occurs *between* the cells, through the 'shunt' pathway. Overall, fluid and electrolyte reabsorption is almost isotonic in this segment, as water reabsorption is matched very closely to sodium fluxes. A component of this water flow also passes *through* the cells, via aquaporin-1 (AQP-1) water channels, which are not sensitive to hormonal regulation.

The loop of Henle

The thick ascending limb of the loop of Henle (Fig. 16.3B) reabsorbs a further 25% of the filtered sodium but is impermeable to water, resulting in dilution of the luminal fluid. Again, the primary driving force for sodium reabsorption is the Na,K-ATPase on the basolateral cell membrane, but in this segment sodium enters the cell from the lumen via a specific carrier molecule, the Na,K,2Cl cotransporter ('triple cotransporter', or NKCC2) which allows electroneutral entry of these ion species driven by the 'downhill' electrochemical gradient acting on sodium. Some of the potassium accumulated inside the cell recirculates across the apical membrane back into the lumen through a specific potassium channel (ROMK), providing a continuing supply of potassium to match the high concentrations of sodium and chloride available in the lumen to bind to the cotransporter. A small positive transepithelial potential difference exists in the lumen of this segment relative to the interstitium, and this serves to drive cations such as sodium, potassium, calcium and magnesium between the cells, forming a reabsorptive shunt pathway.

16

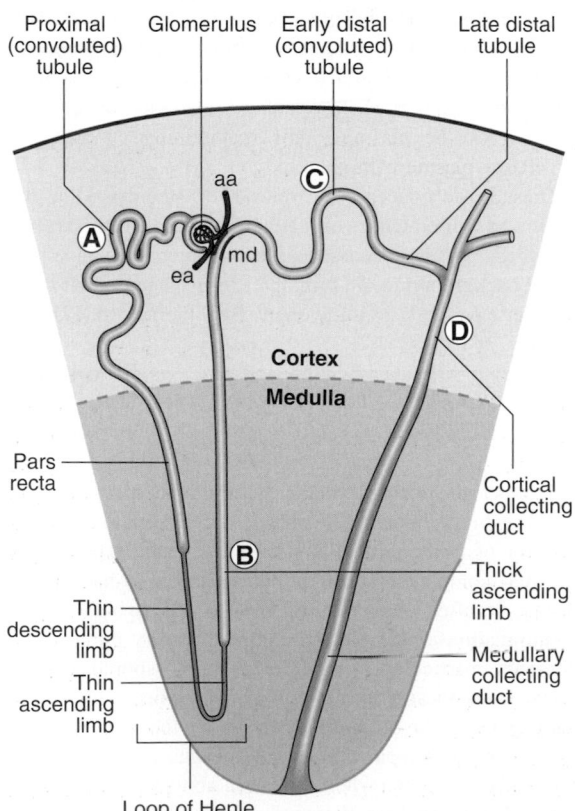

Fig. 16.2 The nephron. Letters A–D refer to tubular segments shown in more detail in Figure 16.3. (aa = afferent arteriole; ea = efferent arteriole; md = macula densa)

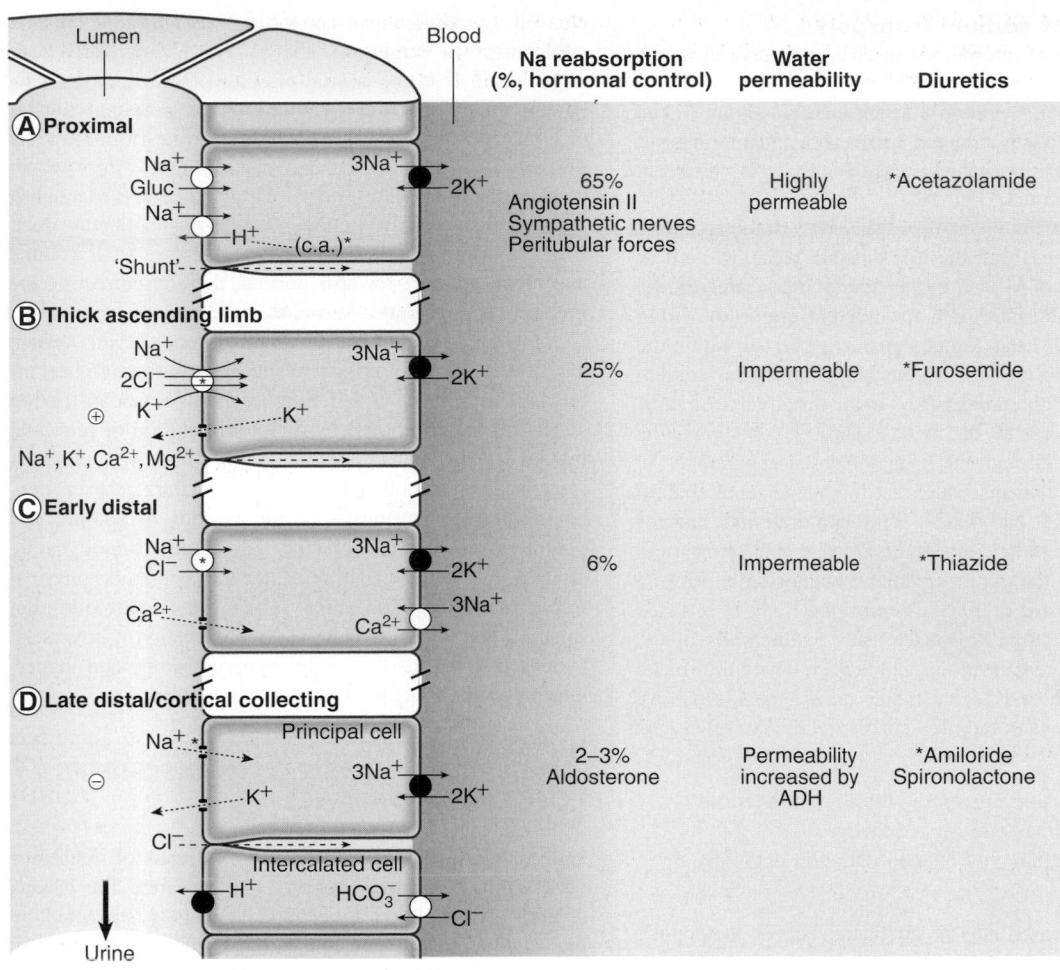

Fig. 16.3   Principal transport mechanisms in segments of the nephron. See text for further details. Asterisk indicates site of diuretic action in each segment. Black circles indicate primary active transport pumps; open circles are carrier molecules without direct linkage to ATP hydrolysis. (c.a. = carbonic anhydrase)

16

Early distal tubule

Some 6% of filtered sodium is reabsorbed in the early distal (also called distal convoluted) tubule (Fig. 16.3C), again driven by the activity of the basolateral Na,K-ATPase. In this segment, entry of sodium into the cell from the luminal fluid is via a sodium–chloride cotransport carrier (NCCT). This segment is also impermeable to water, resulting in further dilution of the luminal fluid. There is no significant transepithelial flux of potassium in this segment, but calcium is reabsorbed through the mechanism shown in Figure 16.3C; a basolateral sodium–calcium exchanger leads to low intracellular concentrations of calcium, promoting calcium entry from the luminal fluid through a calcium channel.

Late distal tubule and collecting ducts

The late distal tubule and cortical collecting duct are anatomically and functionally continuous (Fig. 16.3D). Here sodium entry from the luminal fluid is via the epithelial sodium channel (ENaC) through which sodium passes alone, generating a substantial lumen-negative transepithelial potential difference. Potassium is accumulated in

the cell by the basolateral Na,K-ATPase, and passes into the luminal fluid down its electrochemical gradient, through an apical potassium channel (ROMK). Only a fraction of the sodium reabsorptive flux is balanced by potassium secretion. A further component of this flux is accompanied by chloride ions, passing largely between cells, and by hydrogen ion secretion mediated by an H^+-ATPase located on the luminal membrane of the intercalated cells, which constitute approximately one-third of the epithelial cells in this nephron segment. This part of the nephron has a variable permeability to water, depending on the availability of antidiuretic hormone (ADH, or vasopressin) in the circulation. All ion transport processes in this segment are stimulated by the steroid hormone aldosterone. This can increase the sodium reabsorption in this segment over the range 2–3% of the filtered sodium load.

A further small component of sodium reabsorption occurs in the medullary collecting duct. This segment reabsorbs less than 1% of the filtered load, and is a site of action of atrial natriuretic peptide (ANP) which inhibits this reabsorptive mechanism.

Regulation of sodium transport

A large number of interrelated mechanisms serve to match urinary sodium excretion to sodium intake closely. These mechanisms operate via an afferent (sensor) signal linked to the ECF volume and related parameters, and a number of efferent (effector) mechanisms capable of altering the renal sodium excretion rate (Fig. 16.4).

Important sensing mechanisms include volume receptors in the cardiac atria and the intrathoracic veins, as well as pressure receptors located in the central arterial tree (aortic arch and carotid sinus) and the afferent arterioles within the kidney. A further afferent signal is generated within the kidney itself; during low volume conditions, the sodium concentration of the tubular fluid in the distal nephron falls, and this is detected by the macula densa which signals the release of renin through the juxtaglomerular apparatus.

Efferent mechanisms which act to change renal sodium excretion are of two kinds, neurohumoral and haemodynamic. The most important of the neurohormonal mechanisms is the renin–angiotensin–aldosterone (RAA) system (Fig. 20.18, p. 777). The enzyme renin is released from specialised smooth muscle cells in the walls of the afferent and efferent arterioles, at the point where they make contact with the early distal tubule (at the macula densa), forming the juxtaglomerular apparatus. Renin release is stimulated by:

- reduced perfusion pressure in the afferent arteriole
- increased sympathetic nerve activity
- decreased sodium chloride concentration in the distal tubular fluid.

The renin released into the circulation acts on the peptide substrate angiotensinogen (manufactured in the liver), producing angiotensin I in the circulation. This in turn is cleaved by angiotensin-converting enzyme (ACE) into angiotensin II, largely in the pulmonary capillary bed. Angiotensin II is the central effector of the RAA system, having multiple actions: stimulation of proximal tubular sodium reabsorption, release of aldosterone from the zona glomerulosa of the adrenal cortex, and direct vasoconstriction of small arterioles. Aldosterone acts to amplify sodium retention by its action in the cortical collecting duct. The net effect of these actions is to restore ECF volume and blood pressure towards normal, thereby correcting the initiating hypovolaemic stimulus.

As shown in Figure 16.4, the sympathetic nervous system also acts to enhance sodium retention, both through haemodynamic mechanisms (afferent arteriolar vasoconstriction and GFR reduction) and by direct stimulation of proximal tubular sodium reabsorption. The other humoral mediators illustrated, on the other hand, inhibit sodium reabsorption, contributing to natriuresis during periods of sodium and volume excess. Hypovolaemia also has haemodynamic effects which reduce GFR and alter the peritubular physical forces around the proximal tubule, increasing filtration fraction, thereby decreasing sodium excretion. Conversely, increased renal perfusion in hypervolaemia and hypertension results in increased sodium excretion.

PRESENTING PROBLEMS IN DISORDERS OF SODIUM BALANCE

When sodium balance is disturbed, as a result of imbalance between intake and excretion, any tendency for plasma sodium concentration to change is usually corrected by the osmotic mechanisms controlling water balance (p. 428). As a result, disorders in sodium balance present chiefly as altered ECF volume rather than altered sodium concentration. Clinical manifestations of altered volume are illustrated in Box 16.3.

SODIUM DEPLETION (USUALLY ASSOCIATED WITH HYPOVOLAEMIA)

Aetiology and clinical assessment

Sodium depletion can occur occasionally under extreme environmental conditions as a result of inadequate intake of

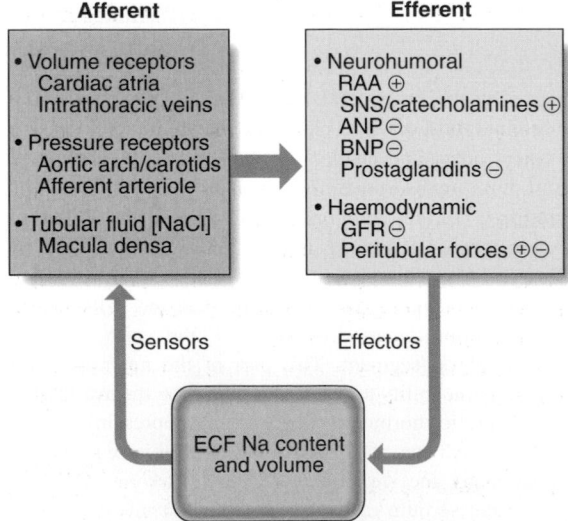

Fig. 16.4 Mechanisms involved in the regulation of sodium transport. (ANP = atrial natriuretic peptide; BNP = brain natriuretic peptide; ECF = extracellular fluid; GFR = glomerular filtration rate; RAA = renin–angiotensin–aldosterone system; SNS = sympathetic nervous system. ⊕ indicates an effect to reduce Na excretion, while ⊖ indicates an effect to increase Na excretion)

16.3 CLINICAL FEATURES OF HYPOVOLAEMIA AND HYPERVOLAEMIA		
	Hypovolaemia	**Hypervolaemia**
Symptoms	Thirst Dizziness on standing Weakness	Ankle swelling Abdominal swelling Breathlessness
Signs	Low JVP Postural hypotension Tachycardia Dry mouth Reduced skin turgor Reduced urine output Weight loss Confusion, stupor	Peripheral oedema Raised JVP Pulmonary crepitations Pleural effusion Ascites Weight gain Hypertension (sometimes)
(JVP = jugular venous pressure)		

16

16.4 CAUSES OF SODIUM AND WATER DEPLETION

Mechanism	Examples
Inadequate intake	Environmental deprivation, inadequate therapeutic replacement
Gastrointestinal sodium loss	Vomiting, diarrhoea, nasogastric suction, external fistula
Skin sodium loss	Excessive sweating, burns
Renal sodium loss	Diuretic therapy, mineralocorticoid deficiency, tubulointerstitial disease (sometimes)
Internal sequestration*	Bowel obstruction, peritonitis, pancreatitis, crush injury

* A cause of circulatory volume depletion, although total body sodium and water may be normal or increased.

16.5 BASIC DAILY WATER AND ELECTROLYTE REQUIREMENTS

	Requirement per kg	Typical 70 kg adult
Water	35–45 ml/kg	2.5–3.0 l/day
Sodium	1.5–2 mmol/kg	100–140 mmol/day
Potassium	1.0–1.5 mmol/kg	70–100 mmol/day

16.6 COMPOSITION OF SOME ISOTONIC INTRAVENOUS FLUIDS (1 LITRE)*

Fluid	D-glucose	Calories	Na^+	Cl^-	Other
5% dextrose	50 g	200	0	0	0
Normal saline	0	0	154	154	0
Hartmann's solution	0	0	131	111	K^+ 5 Ca^{2+} 2 $Lactate^-$ 29

* Electrolytes shown in mmol.

salt, but it is much more commonly due to pathological losses of sodium-containing fluids, as shown in Box 16.4. Loss of whole blood, as in acute haemorrhage, is also an obvious cause of hypovolaemia, and elicits the same mechanisms for the conservation of sodium and water as do the other conditions listed above.

Diagnosis of hypovolaemia is based on clinical evaluation, seeking the characteristic symptoms and signs (Box 16.3) in the context of a relevant precipitating illness. Supportive evidence may be obtained from the clinical biochemistry laboratory, but it is important to note that plasma sodium concentration may be within the normal range if losses of salt and water proceed in parallel. On the other hand, abnormalities may be expected in a number of other parameters reflecting appropriate renal, hormonal and haemodynamic responses. Typically, the plasma urea concentration rises, as urea excretion is affected by both glomerular filtration and urine flow rate. Thus while the plasma creatinine may be relatively well preserved early in hypovolaemic states, reflecting maintenance of near-normal GFR, the plasma urea will rise as urinary flow rate is reduced as a consequence of activation of sodium- and water-retaining mechanisms in the nephron. Plasma uric acid may also rise, reflecting activation of compensatory proximal tubular reabsorption, and the urine osmolality increases as urine concentrating mechanisms are activated. Urine sodium concentration, on the other hand, falls as a result of activation of sodium-retaining mechanisms. Under these circumstances, sodium excretion may fall to less than 0.1% of the filtered sodium load.

Management

Management of sodium and water depletion has two main components:

- treatment of the cause where possible, to stop ongoing salt and water losses
- replacement of salt and water deficits, and provision of ongoing maintenance requirements, usually through the intravenous route when depletion is severe.

Intravenous fluid therapy

Box 16.5 shows the daily maintenance requirements for water and electrolytes in a typical adult, and Box 16.6 summarises the composition of some widely available intravenous fluids. The choice of fluid and the rate of administration will depend on the clinical circumstances, as assessed at the bedside and from laboratory data.

In the absence of normal oral intake (as in a fasting or post-operative patient in hospital), maintenance quantities of fluid, sodium and potassium should be provided. If any deficits or continuing pathological losses are identified, additional fluid and electrolytes will be required. In prolonged periods of fasting (greater than a few days), attention needs also to be given to providing sufficient caloric and nutritional intake to prevent catabolism of body energy stores (p. 117).

The choice of intravenous fluid therapy relates to the concepts in Figure 16.1 (p. 421). If fluid containing neither sodium nor protein is given, it will distribute in the body fluid compartments in proportion to the normal distribution of total body water. Thus, giving 1 litre of 5% dextrose will contribute relatively little (approximately 3/25 of the infused volume) towards expansion of the plasma volume. This makes 5% dextrose ineffective at restoring the circulation and perfusion of vital organs. Intravenous infusion of an isotonic (normal) saline solution, on the other hand, results in more effective expansion of the extracellular fluid, although again a minority of the infused volume (some 3/15) will contribute to plasma volume.

Carrying this reasoning further, it might be expected that a solution containing plasma proteins would be largely

16.7 ALBUMIN INFUSIONS IN HYPOVOLAEMIA   EBM

'For patients with hypovolaemia there is no evidence that albumin reduces mortality when compared with cheaper alternatives such as saline.'

- The Albumin Reviewers. Cochrane Library, issue 4, 2000.

For further information: 🖳 www.cochrane.org

retained within the plasma, thus maximally expanding the circulating fluid volume and improving tissue perfusion. Recent clinical studies have not verified any overall advantage of such infusions, however, and a special role for albumin solutions can no longer be supported (Box 16.7). On the other hand, resuscitation fluids containing synthetic colloids (based on carbohydrate polymers or gelatin) may be more effective in the short-term resuscitation of volume-depleted patients than solutions containing sodium chloride alone.

SODIUM EXCESS (USUALLY ASSOCIATED WITH HYPERVOLAEMIA)

Aetiology and clinical assessment

In the presence of normal function of the heart and kidneys, an excessive intake of salt and water is compensated for by increased excretion and so is unlikely to lead to clinically obvious features of hypervolaemia. However, diseases affecting the kidney, heart or liver frequently set in train a sequence of events leading to the clinical features of hypervolaemia shown in Box 16.3. Important causes of sodium excess are given in Box 16.8.

Peripheral oedema is the most common physical sign associated with these conditions (p. 480). The volume expansion seen in the three most common systemic dis-

16.8 CAUSES OF SODIUM AND WATER EXCESS	
Mechanism	**Examples**
Impaired renal function (Ch. 17)	Primary renal disease
Primary hyperaldosteronism* (p. 786)	Conn's syndrome

Secondary hyperaldosteronism (Fig 16.5)	Congestive cardiac failure
	Cirrhotic liver disease
	Nephrotic syndrome
	Other hypoalbuminaemic states
	  Protein-losing enteropathy
	  Malnutrition
	Idiopathic/cyclical oedema
	Renal artery stenosis*

* Conditions in this table *other than* primary hyperaldosteronism and renal artery stenosis are typically associated with generalised oedema.

orders associated with sodium and fluid overload (cardiac failure, cirrhosis and nephrotic syndrome) is largely due to secondary responses to the circulatory insufficiency associated with the primary disorder. These concepts are illustrated in Figure 16.5. Note that in renal failure (not shown), the prime cause of volume expansion is the profound reduction in GFR impairing sodium and water

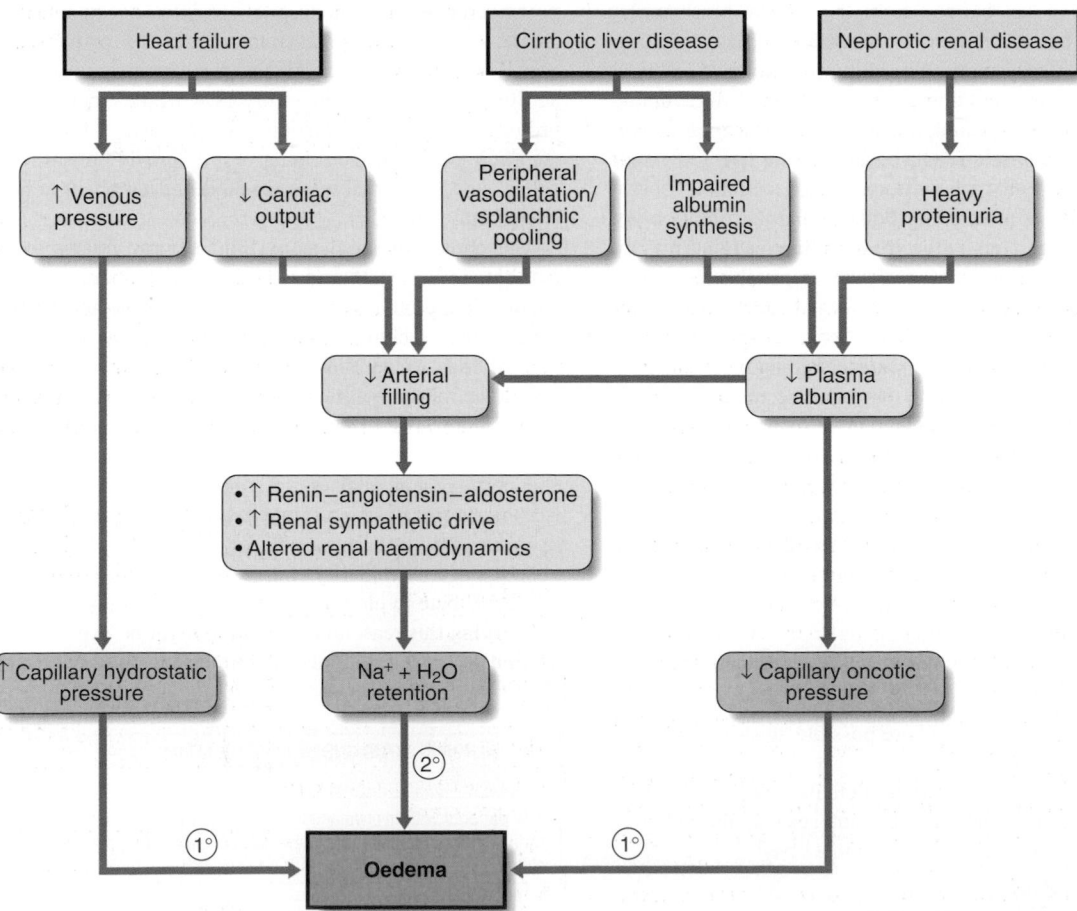

Fig. 16.5 **Pathophysiology of sodium excess and oedema in cardiac failure, cirrhosis and nephrotic syndrome.** (ECF = extracellular fluid)

excretion, and secondary tubular mechanisms are of less importance. Further detail on each of the conditions referred to here is given in other chapters of this book.

Management

The management of ECF volume overload involves a number of components:

- specific treatment (where available) directed at the cause, e.g. ACE inhibitors in heart failure, corticosteroids in minimal change nephropathy
- restriction of dietary sodium to more nearly match the diminished excretory capacity, e.g. 50–80 mmol/day
- treatment with diuretic drugs.

DIURETIC THERAPY

Diuretics are important in the treatment of conditions of ECF expansion due to salt and water retention. They act by inhibiting sodium reabsorption at various locations along the nephron (Fig. 16.3, p. 423). Their potency and adverse effects relate to their mechanism and site of action.

Mechanisms of action

In the proximal tubule, carbonic anhydrase inhibitors (e.g. acetazolamide) inhibit the intracellular production of H^+ ions, thereby reducing the fraction of sodium reabsorption which is exchanged for H^+ by the apical membrane sodium–hydrogen exchanger. These drugs have limited usefulness, however, since only a limited fraction of proximal sodium reabsorption uses this mechanism, and much of the unreabsorbed sodium can be reabsorbed by downstream segments of the nephron.

In the thick ascending limb of the loop of Henle, loop diuretics (e.g. furosemide) inhibit sodium reabsorption by blocking the action of the apical membrane Na,K,2Cl cotransporter. Because this segment reabsorbs a significant fraction of the filtered sodium, these drugs are potent diuretics, in common use in serious oedematous disorders.

In the early distal (distal convoluted) tubule, thiazide drugs inhibit sodium reabsorption by blocking the sodium–chloride cotransporter in the apical membrane. Since this segment reabsorbs a much smaller fraction of the filtered sodium, the thiazide drugs are less potent than the loop diuretics, but are widely used as part of the treatment of hypertension and in less severe oedema disorders.

All diuretic drugs acting in the proximal, loop and early distal segments cause excretion not only of sodium (and with it water), but also of potassium. This occurs largely as a result of delivery of increased amounts of sodium to the late distal/cortical collecting duct site, where sodium reabsorption is associated with secretion of potassium into the lumen. Thus drugs acting before this site cause a degree of potassium depletion, which can be amplified if circulating aldosterone levels are high. By contrast, drugs acting to inhibit sodium reabsorption in the late distal/cortical collecting duct segment are associated with reduced potassium secretion, and are described as 'potassium-sparing'. One target of drug action in this segment is the apical sodium channel in the principal cells, which is blocked by drugs such as amiloride and triamterene. Another is the cytoplasmic receptor for aldosterone, which is blocked by spironolactone and eplerenone.

An important feature of the most commonly used diuretic drugs (furosemide, thiazides and amiloride) is that they act on their target transport molecules from the luminal side of the tubular epithelium. Since they are highly protein-bound in the plasma, very little reaches the urinary fluid by glomerular filtration, but there are active transport mechanisms for secreting organic acids and bases, including these drugs, across the proximal tubular wall, resulting in adequate drug concentrations being delivered to later tubular segments. This secretory process may be impaired by certain other drugs, and also by accumulated organic anions as occurs in chronic renal failure and chronic liver failure.

Osmotic diuretics are a further class of drug which act independent of any specific transport mechanism. These substances are freely filtered but are not reabsorbed by any part of the tubular system. They thus entrain fluid osmotically within the tubular lumen and therefore limit the extent of sodium reabsorption in multiple segments. Mannitol is the most commonly used such drug, and must be given by intravenous infusion to achieve short-term diuresis in conditions associated with cell swelling, such as cerebral oedema.

Clinical use of diuretics

In the selection of a diuretic drug for use in the treatment of hypertension or oedema disorders, the following principles should be observed:

- Use the minimum effective dose.
- Use for as short a period of time as necessary.
- Monitor regularly for adverse effects.

The choice of diuretic drug class will be determined by the required potency of action, the presence of coexistent conditions, and the anticipated side-effect profile.

The adverse effects encountered with the most commonly used classes of diuretic (loop drugs and thiazide drugs) are summarised in Box 16.9. Volume depletion and electrolyte disorders can be largely predicted from their mechanism of action. The metabolic side-effects listed are rarely of clinical

16.9 ADVERSE EFFECTS OF DIURETIC THERAPY (LOOP-ACTING AND THIAZIDE CLASSES)	
Renal side-effects	
• Hypovolaemia	• Hyperuricaemia
• Hyponatraemia	• Hypomagnesaemia
• Hypokalaemia	• Hypercalciuria (loop)
• Metabolic alkalosis	• Hypocalciuria (thiazide)
Metabolic side-effects	
• Glucose intolerance/hyperglycaemia	
• Hyperlipidaemia	
Miscellaneous side-effects	
• Hypersensitivity reactions	
• Acute pancreatitis/cholecystitis (thiazides)	
• Erectile dysfunction	

significance and may reflect effects on K^+ channels, which influence insulin secretion (p. 808). Since most drugs from these classes are sulphonamides, there is a relatively high incidence of hypersensitivity reactions, and some idiosyncratic side-effects in a variety of organ systems are occasionally seen. An important difference between the loop and thiazide classes of drug is that calcium excretion is enhanced by loop drugs, but inhibited by the thiazides. This can be deduced from the transport mechanisms in the respective nephron segments (Fig. 16.3, p. 423).

The side-effect profile of the potassium-sparing diuretics differs in a number of important respects from other diuretics. Specifically, the disturbances in potassium, magnesium and acid–base balance are in the opposite direction, so that normal or increased levels of potassium and magnesium are found in the blood, and there is a tendency to metabolic acidosis, especially when renal function is impaired.

Diuretic resistance can be encountered under a variety of circumstances, including impaired renal function, activation of sodium-retaining mechanisms, impaired oral bioavailability (e.g. due to gastrointestinal disease), and decreased renal blood flow. In these circumstances short-term use of intravenous therapy with a loop-acting agent such as furosemide may be useful. However, rational use can also be made of combinations of diuretic drugs taken by the oral route. Either a loop or thiazide drug can be combined with a potassium-sparing drug, and all three classes can be used together for short periods, with carefully supervised clinical and laboratory monitoring.

DISORDERS OF WATER BALANCE

Daily water intake can vary over a wide range, from 500 ml to several litres a day. While a certain amount of water is lost through the stool, sweat and the respiratory tract, the kidneys are chiefly responsible for adjusting water excretion to maintain constancy of body water content and body fluid osmolality (normal range 280–300 mmol/kg).

FUNCTIONAL ANATOMY AND PHYSIOLOGY OF RENAL WATER HANDLING

While regulation of total ECF volume is largely achieved through the kidneys' control of sodium excretion, there must also be mechanisms to allow for the excretion of a 'pure' water load when free water intake is high, and for the avid retention of water by the kidneys when access to water is restricted.

These functions are largely achieved by the properties of the loop of Henle and the collecting ducts. The counter-current configuration of flow in adjacent limbs of the loop sets up a gradient of tissue osmolality from plasma-like in the renal cortex through to hypertonic levels (around 1200 mmol/kg) in the inner part of the medulla. At the same time, the fluid emerging from the thick ascending limb is hypotonic compared to plasma, because it has been diluted by the reabsorption of sodium, but not water, from the thick ascending limb and early distal tubule. As this dilute fluid passes from the cortex through the collecting duct system to the renal pelvis, it traverses the medullary interstitial gradient of osmolality set up by the operation of the loop of Henle.

Further changes in the urine osmolality on passage through the collecting ducts depend on the level in the plasma of the peptide antidiuretic hormone (ADH, or vasopressin), which is released by the posterior pituitary gland under conditions of increased plasma osmolality or other stimuli such as hypovolaemia (Ch. 20).

- When ADH levels are minimal, such as during adequate water intake and low–normal plasma osmolality, the collecting ducts remain impermeable to water, and the luminal fluid osmolality remains low, resulting in the excretion of a dilute urine (minimum osmolality 50 mmol/kg in a healthy young person).
- When ADH levels are elevated (during water restriction and high plasma osmolality, or severe volume depletion), the water permeability of the collecting ducts is greatly increased through the action of ADH, through its V2 receptor, to enhance collecting duct water permeability via the insertion of aquaporin AQP2 channels into the luminal cell membrane. This results in osmotic reabsorption of water along the entire length of the collecting duct, with maximum urine osmolality approaching that in the medullary tip (1200 mmol/kg).

Parallel to these changes in ADH release are changes in water-seeking behaviour triggered by the sensation of thirst, which also becomes activated as plasma osmolality rises from normal to above-normal levels.

In summary for adequate dilution of the urine, there must be:

- adequate solute delivery to the loop of Henle and early distal tubule
- normal function of the loop of Henle and early distal tubule
- no ADH in the circulation.

If any of these processes are faulty, water retention and hyponatraemia may result.

Conversely, to achieve concentration of the urine there must be:

- adequate solute delivery to the loop of Henle
- normal function of the loop of Henle
- ADH release into the circulation
- ADH action on the collecting ducts.

Failure of any of these steps may be expected to result in inappropriate water loss, with resultant hypernatraemia.

PRESENTING PROBLEMS IN DISORDERS OF WATER BALANCE

Disturbances in body water metabolism, in the absence of changes in sodium balance, manifest principally as abnormalities of plasma sodium concentration, and hence of plasma osmolality. The main consequence of changes in plasma osmolality, especially when rapid, is altered cerebral function. This is because when extracellular osmolality changes abruptly, water flows rapidly across cell membranes with resultant cell swelling (during hypo-osmolality) or shrinkage (during hyperosmolality). Cerebral cell function is very sensitive to such volume changes, particularly during cell swelling where an increase in intracerebral pressure occurs due to the constraints posed by the bony skull, resulting in impairment of cerebral perfusion.

HYPONATRAEMIA

Aetiology and clinical assessment

Hyponatraemia (plasma Na < 135 mmol/l) is a common electrolyte abnormality, often detected asymptomatically, but it may also be associated with profound disturbances of cerebral function, manifesting as anorexia, nausea, vomiting, confusion, lethargy, seizures and coma. The degree of cerebral symptomatology depends more on the rate of development of the electrolyte abnormality than on its severity. This is because when the plasma osmolality falls rapidly, water flows into cerebral cells which become swollen and ischaemic. However, when hyponatraemia develops more gradually, cerebral neurons have time to respond by reducing the intracellular osmolality, through reduction in cell potassium and by reduced synthesis of intracellular organic osmolytes (Fig. 16.6). The osmotic gradient favouring water movement into the cells is thus reduced, and patients may present with minimal symptomatology.

The causes of hyponatraemia are best organised according to any associated change in ECF volume status, i.e. the total body sodium (Box 16.10). In all cases, there is a retention of water relative to sodium, and it is the clinical examination rather than the electrolyte test results which gives clues to the underlying problem.

One artefactual cause of apparent hyponatraemia should be remembered. This can occur in the presence of severe hyperlipidaemia or hyperproteinaemia, where the aqueous fraction of the plasma specimen is reduced because of the

16.10 CAUSES OF HYPONATRAEMIA	
Volume status	**Examples**
Hypovolaemic (sodium deficit with a relatively smaller water deficit)	Renal Na losses Diuretic therapy (especially thiazides) Adrenocortical failure Gastrointestinal Na losses Vomiting Diarrhoea
Euvolaemic (water retention alone)	Primary polydipsia Excessive electrolyte-free water infusion SIADH* Hypothyroidism
Hypervolaemic (sodium retention with relatively greater water retention)	Congestive cardiac failure Cirrhosis Nephrotic syndrome Chronic renal failure (during free water intake)
* SIADH = syndrome of inappropriate antidiuretic hormone secretion, Box 16.11.	

volume occupied by the macromolecules (although this artefact is dependent on the assay technology). Transient hyponatraemia may also occur due to osmotic shifts of water out of cells during hyperosmolar states caused by acute hyperglycaemia or by mannitol infusion.

Hyponatraemia with hypovolaemia

Hyponatraemia in association with a sodium deficit ('depletional hyponatraemia') can arise as a result of renal salt losses during diuretic therapy, or aldosterone deficiency such as in Addison's disease. A similar pattern can arise due to gastrointestinal losses of sodium, especially following vomiting, and also through skin losses in burns. Patients in this category have clinical features of hypovolaemia (Box 16.3, p. 424). Laboratory findings supportive of this assessment include low urinary sodium concentration and elevated plasma renin activity.

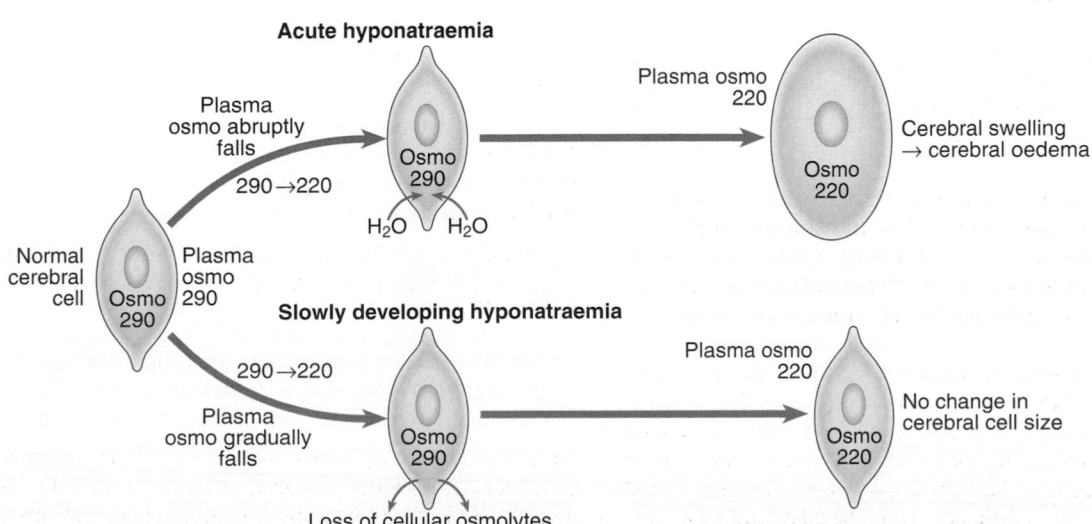

Fig. 16.6 Hyponatraemia and the brain. Numbers represent osmolality in mmol/kg. (Osmo = osmolality)

16

16.11 SYNDROME OF INAPPROPRIATE ANTIDIURETIC HORMONE SECRETION (SIADH): CAUSES AND DIAGNOSIS

Causes

- Tumours, especially small-cell lung cancer
- CNS disorders: stroke, trauma, infection, psychosis
- Pulmonary disorders: pneumonia, tuberculosis
- Drugs
    - Anticonvulsants, e.g. carbamazepine
    - Psychotropics, e.g. haloperidol
    - Antidepressants, e.g. amitriptyline, fluoxetine
    - Cytotoxics, e.g. cyclophosphamide, vincristine
    - Hypoglycaemics, e.g. chlorpropamide
    - Opiates, e.g. morphine
- Sustained pain, stress, nausea, e.g. post-operative state, acute porphyria
- Idiopathic

Diagnosis

- Low plasma sodium concentration (typically < 130 mmol/l)
- Low plasma osmolality (< 270 mmol/kg)
- Urine osmolality not minimally low (> 150 mmol/kg)
- Urine sodium concentration not minimally low (> 30 mmol/l)
- Low–normal plasma urea, creatinine, uric acid
- Exclusion of other causes of hyponatraemia (Box 16.10)
- Appropriate clinical context (above)

16.12 URINE Na AND OSMOLALITY IN THE DIFFERENTIAL DIAGNOSIS OF HYPONATRAEMIA*

Urine Na (mmol/l)	Urine osmolality (mmol/kg)	Possible diagnoses
Low (< 30)	Low (< 100)	Primary polydipsia Malnutrition Beer excess
Low	High (> 150)	Salt depletion Hypovolaemia
High (> 40)	Low	Diuretic action (acute phase)
High	High	SIADH Cerebral salt-wasting Adrenal insufficiency

* Note that intermediate urine results are of indeterminate significance, and diagnosis depends on a comprehensive clinical assessment.

Hyponatraemia with euvolaemia

Patients in the second group ('dilutional hyponatraemia') have no major disturbance of body sodium content, and are clinically euvolaemic. Excess body water may be the result of abnormally high intake, either orally (primary polydipsia) or as a result of medically infused fluids (as intravenous dextrose solutions, or by absorption of sodium-free bladder irrigation fluid after prostatectomy).

Water retention may also occur in the syndrome of inappropriate secretion of ADH (SIADH). In this condition an endogenous source of ADH (either cerebral or tumour-derived) promotes renal water retention in the absence of an appropriate physiological stimulus (Box 16.11). The clinical diagnosis requires the patient to be euvolaemic, with no evidence of organ system disease potentially associated with hyponatraemia (heart, liver, kidney). Supportive laboratory findings are shown in Box 16.11. The plasma has low concentrations of sodium, chloride, urea and uric acid, with a correspondingly low osmolality. The urine, which should physiologically be maximally dilute in the face of low plasma osmolality, is typically greater than the plasma osmolality. However, the diagnosis can still be sustained with urine osmolalities as low as 100–150 mmol/kg, since the urine ought to be maximally dilute (~50 mmol/kg) in the presence of water overload. The urine sodium concentration is typically high (above 30 mmol/l) suggesting that there is no force promoting sodium retention (although diuretic use and mineralocorticoid deficiency can also produce high urine sodium).

Hyponatraemia with hypervolaemia

The third pattern of hyponatraemia is where excess water retention is associated with sodium retention and volume expansion, as in heart failure and other oedematous disorders.

Investigations

Plasma and urine electrolytes and osmolality (Box 16.12) are usually the only tests required to classify the hyponatraemia. Doubt about clinical signs of ECF volume may be resolved with measurement of plasma renin activity.

Note that assay of plasma ADH is not generally helpful in distinguishing between these categories of hyponatraemic states. This is because ADH is activated both in hypovolaemic states and in most chronic hypervolaemic states, as the impaired circulation in those disorders activates ADH release through non-osmotic mechanisms. Indeed, these disorders may have higher circulating ADH levels than patients with SIADH. The only disorders listed in Box 16.10 in which ADH is not normal or elevated are primary polydipsia and iatrogenic water intoxication, in which the hypo-osmolar plasma suppresses ADH release.

Management

The treatment for hyponatraemia is critically dependent on the rate of development and severity, and on the underlying cause. In general, if hyponatraemia has developed rapidly (over hours to days), morbidity will be high due to cerebral oedema, and it is generally safe to correct the plasma sodium relatively rapidly. This can include infusion of hypertonic (3%) sodium chloride solutions, especially when the patient is obtunded or convulsing.

On the other hand, rapid correction of hyponatraemia which has developed slowly (over weeks to months) can itself be hazardous to the brain. This is because cerebral cells adapt to slowly developing hypo-osmolality by reducing the intracellular osmolality, thus maintaining normal cell volume (Fig. 16.6). Under these conditions, an abrupt increase in extracellular osmolality can lead to water shifting out of the cerebral neurons, abruptly reducing their volume and risking detachment from their myelin sheaths. The resulting 'myelinolysis' can produce permanent structural and functional damage to midbrain structures, and is generally fatal. The rate of correction of the plasma Na concentration in chronic asymptomatic hyponatraemia should not exceed 10 mmol/l/day, and an even slower rate would generally be safer.

Specific treatment measures should be related to the underlying cause. For hypovolaemic patients, this will involve controlling the source of sodium loss, and administering intravenous saline if clinically warranted. Patients with dilutional hyponatraemia will generally respond to fluid restriction in the range 600–1000 ml/day, accompanied where possible by withdrawal of the precipitating stimulus (e.g. a drug causing SIADH). Where an inadequate rise in plasma Na results, treatment with demeclocycline (600–900 mg/day) may enhance water excretion, by interfering with collecting duct responsiveness to ADH. An effective alternative for subjects with persistent hyponatraemia due to prolonged SIADH is oral urea therapy (30–45 g/day), which provides a solute load to promote water excretion. Hypervolaemic patients need optimal treatment of the underlying condition, accompanied by cautious use of diuretics in conjunction with strict fluid restriction. Potassium-sparing diuretics may be particularly useful in this context where there is significant secondary hyperaldosteronism.

HYPERNATRAEMIA

Aetiology and clinical assessment

Just as hyponatraemia represents a failure of the mechanisms for diluting the urine during free access to water, so hypernatraemia (plasma Na > 150 mmol/l) reflects an inadequacy of the kidney in concentrating the urine in the face of relatively restricted water intake. This can be due to failure to generate an adequate medullary concentration gradient (low GFR states, loop diuretic therapy), but more commonly it is due to failure of the ADH system, either because no ADH is released from the pituitary (central or 'cranial' diabetes insipidus, p. 796) or because the collecting duct cells are unable to respond to circulating ADH (nephrogenic diabetes insipidus, either inherited or acquired).

Patients with hypernatraemia generally have reduced cerebral function, either as a primary problem or as a consequence of the hypernatraemia itself, which results in dehydration of cerebral neurons and brain shrinkage. In the presence of an intact thirst mechanism and preserved capacity to obtain water, hypernatraemia may not progress very far as water intake proceeds. Where adequate water is not obtained, dizziness, confusion, weakness and ultimately coma and death can result.

As for hyponatraemia, the causes of hypernatraemia are best grouped according to the simultaneous disturbance, if any, in total body sodium content (Box 16.13). It is important to note the risk of iatrogenic induction of hypernatraemia, and to reiterate that whatever the underlying cause, sustained or severe hypernatraemia must reflect an impaired thirst mechanism or responsiveness to thirst, which would otherwise lead to sufficient water being ingested to prevent this disorder progressing.

Management

Treatment of hypernatraemia depends on both the rate of development and the underlying cause. If there is reason to think that the condition has developed rapidly, cerebral

16.13 CAUSES OF HYPERNATRAEMIA

Volume status	Examples

Hypovolaemic (sodium deficit with a relatively greater water deficit)	Renal Na losses
	  Diuretic therapy (especially osmotic diuretic, or loop diuretic during water restriction)
	  Glycosuria (HONK, p. 815)
	Gastrointestinal Na losses
	  Colonic diarrhoea
	Skin Na losses
	  Excessive sweating

Euvolaemic (water deficit alone)	Diabetes insipidus (central or nephrogenic)
Hypervolaemic (sodium retention with relatively less water retention)	Enteral or parenteral alimentation I.v. or oral salt administration Chronic renal failure (during water restriction)

16.14 HYPONATRAEMIA AND HYPERNATRAEMIA IN OLD AGE

- **Decline in GFR:** older patients are predisposed to both hyponatraemia and hypernatraemia, mainly because as GFR declines with age, the capacity of the kidney to dilute or concentrate the urine is impaired.
- **Hyponatraemia:** occurs when free water intake continues in the presence of a low dietary salt intake and/or diuretic drugs (particularly thiazides).
- **ADH release:** water retention is aggravated by any condition which stimulates ADH release, especially heart failure. Moreover, the ADH response to non-osmotic stimuli may be brisker in older subjects. Appropriate water restriction is a key part of the management.
- **Hypernatraemia:** occurs when water intake is inadequate, due to physical restrictions preventing access to drinks and/or blunted thirst. Both are frequently present in patients with advanced dementia or following a severe stroke.
- **Dietary salt:** hypernatraemia is aggravated if dietary supplements or medications with a high sodium content (especially effervescent preparations) are administered. Appropriate prescription of fluids is a key part of the management.

shrinkage may be acute, and correction with appropriate volumes of intravenous hypotonic fluid may be attempted relatively rapidly. However, in older, institutionalised patients it is more likely that the disorder has developed slowly, and extreme caution should be exhibited in lowering the plasma sodium rapidly, to avoid the risk of cerebral oedema in the osmotically adapted cerebral neurons. Where possible, the underlying cause should also be addressed, especially where this involves the simple cessation of salt administration to patients with blunted thirst.

Elderly patients are predisposed, in different circumstances, to both hyponatraemia and hypernatraemia, and a high index of suspicion of these electrolyte disturbances is appropriate in aged patients with recent alterations in behaviour (Box 16.14).

DISORDERS OF POTASSIUM BALANCE

Potassium is the major intracellular cation (Fig. 16.1, p. 421), and the steep concentration gradient for potassium across

16

the cell membrane of excitable cells plays an important part in generating the resting membrane potential and allowing the propagation of the action potential which is crucial to normal functioning of nerve, muscle and cardiac tissues.

Factors influencing the distribution of potassium between the intracellular and extracellular fluid compartments can alter plasma potassium concentration, without any overall change in total body potassium content. Potassium is driven into the cells from the plasma by extracellular alkalosis and by a number of hormones, including insulin, catecholamines (through the β_2 receptor) and aldosterone. These influences alone can produce hypokalaemia, while the contrary changes (extracellular acidosis, insulin lack, insufficiency or blockade of catecholamines or aldosterone) can contribute to hyperkalaemia due to redistribution of potassium outside the cells.

FUNCTIONAL ANATOMY AND PHYSIOLOGY OF RENAL POTASSIUM HANDLING

In the steady state, the kidney is responsible for the excretion of some 90% of the daily intake of potassium, typically 80–100 mmol/day. Potassium is freely filtered at the glomerulus; around 65% is reabsorbed in the proximal tubule and a further 25% in the thick ascending limb of the loop of Henle, reflecting the pattern of sodium reabsorption in these two sites. However, in the early distal tubule little potassium is transported, while in the late distal/cortical collecting duct tubule a significant secretory flux of potassium into the urine ensures that this cation is removed from the blood in proportion to the ingested load.

The mechanism whereby potassium secretion occurs in the distal parts of the nephron is shown in Figure 16.3D (p. 423). The movement of potassium from blood to lumen is dependent on active uptake across the basal cell membrane by the Na,K-ATPase, followed by diffusion of potassium through a luminal membrane potassium channel (ROMK) into the tubular fluid. The electrochemical gradient for potassium movement into the lumen is contributed to both by the high cell potassium and by the negative luminal potential difference relative to the blood.

A number of factors influence the rate of potassium secretion. Luminal influences include the rate of sodium delivery and fluid flow past the late distal/cortical collecting duct site, and this is a major factor in the increased potassium loss during therapy with diuretics acting earlier in the nephron. Agents interfering with the generation of the negative luminal potential impair potassium secretion, and this is the basis of reduced potassium secretion during therapy with potassium-sparing diuretics such as amiloride. Factors acting from the blood side of this tubule segment include plasma potassium and pH, such that hyperkalaemia and alkalosis stimulate potassium secretion directly. However, the most important factor in the acute and chronic adjustment of potassium secretion to match metabolic potassium load is the corticosteroid hormone aldosterone.

As shown in Figure 16.7, a negative feedback relationship exists between the plasma potassium and aldosterone. In

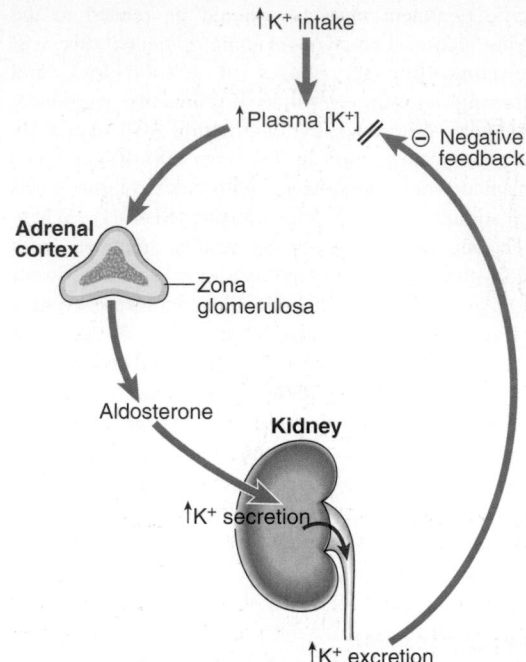

Fig. 16.7 Feedback control of plasma potassium concentration.

addition to its regulation by the renin–angiotensin system, aldosterone is released from the adrenal cortex in direct response to an elevated plasma potassium, and aldosterone acts on the kidney to stimulate potassium secretion, as well as hydrogen secretion and sodium reabsorption, in the late distal/cortical collecting duct segment. The resulting increased potassium excretion serves to dampen the accumulation of potassium in the plasma, keeping plasma concentrations tightly controlled in the narrow normal range (3.5–5.0 mmol/l). Since the plasma aldosterone concentration is the net effect of two different stimuli, factors reducing angiotension II levels may indirectly impair potassium balance by blunting the rise in aldosterone which would otherwise be provoked by hyperkalaemia. This is the basis for the potential for hyperkalaemia developing during therapy with ACE inhibitors and related drugs.

PRESENTING PROBLEMS IN DISORDERS OF POTASSIUM BALANCE

HYPOKALAEMIA

Aetiology and clinical assessment

Patients with hypokalaemia (plasma K < 3.5 mmol/l) typically present with muscular weakness and associated tiredness. Cardiac effects include ventricular ectopics or more serious arrhythmias, and potentiation of the adverse effects of digoxin. Typical ECG changes occur, affecting particularly the T wave (Fig. 16.8). Functional bowel obstruction may occur due to paralytic ileus. Long-standing hypokalaemia damages renal tubular structures (hypokalaemic nephropathy) and interferes with the tubular response to ADH (acquired nephrogenic diabetes insipidus) resulting in polyuria and polydipsia.

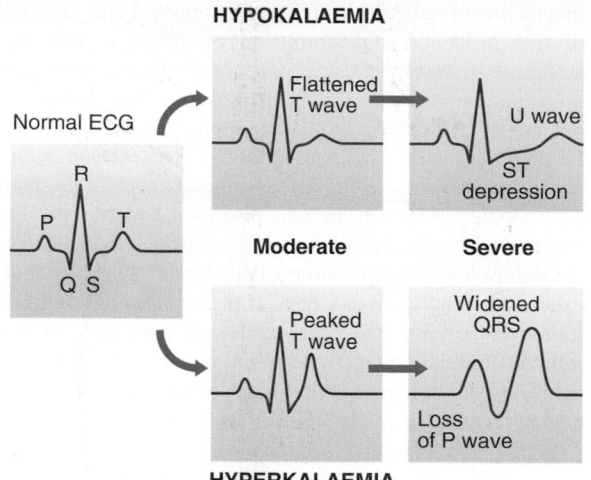

HYPOKALAEMIA

Normal ECG

Flattened
T wave

U wave

ST
depression

Moderate   Severe

Peaked
T wave

Widened
QRS

Loss
of P wave

HYPERKALAEMIA

Fig. 16.8 **The ECG in hypokalaemia and hyperkalaemia.**

concentration. An inadequate intake of potassium can be a factor contributing to hypokalaemia, but only in extreme cases is it likely to be a sufficient explanation. Generally, hypokalaemia implies abnormal potassium loss from the body, either through the kidney or the gastrointestinal tract. Where there is no obvious clinical clue to which pathway is involved, measurement of urinary potassium may be helpful; if the kidney is the route of potassium loss, the urine potassium is relatively high (more than 30 mmol/day), whereas potassium loss through the gastrointestinal tract is usually associated with renal potassium retention, resulting in a lower urinary potassium (generally less than 20 mmol/day, although paradoxically, if gastrointestinal fluid loss is also associated with hypovolaemia, activation of the renin–angiotensin–aldosterone system may cause loss of potassium through the kidney as well).

The renal causes can be divided into those with or without hypertension. Hypertensive disorders with hypokalaemia may be due to excess mineralocorticoid activity such as aldosterone oversecretion in Conn's syndrome. Apparent mineralocorticoid excess can be produced by excess liquorice intake, or treatment with carbenoxolone which inhibit the renal enzyme which normally inactivates cortisol and prevents inappropriate activation of mineralocorticoid receptors. Liddle's syndrome produces a similar phenotype,

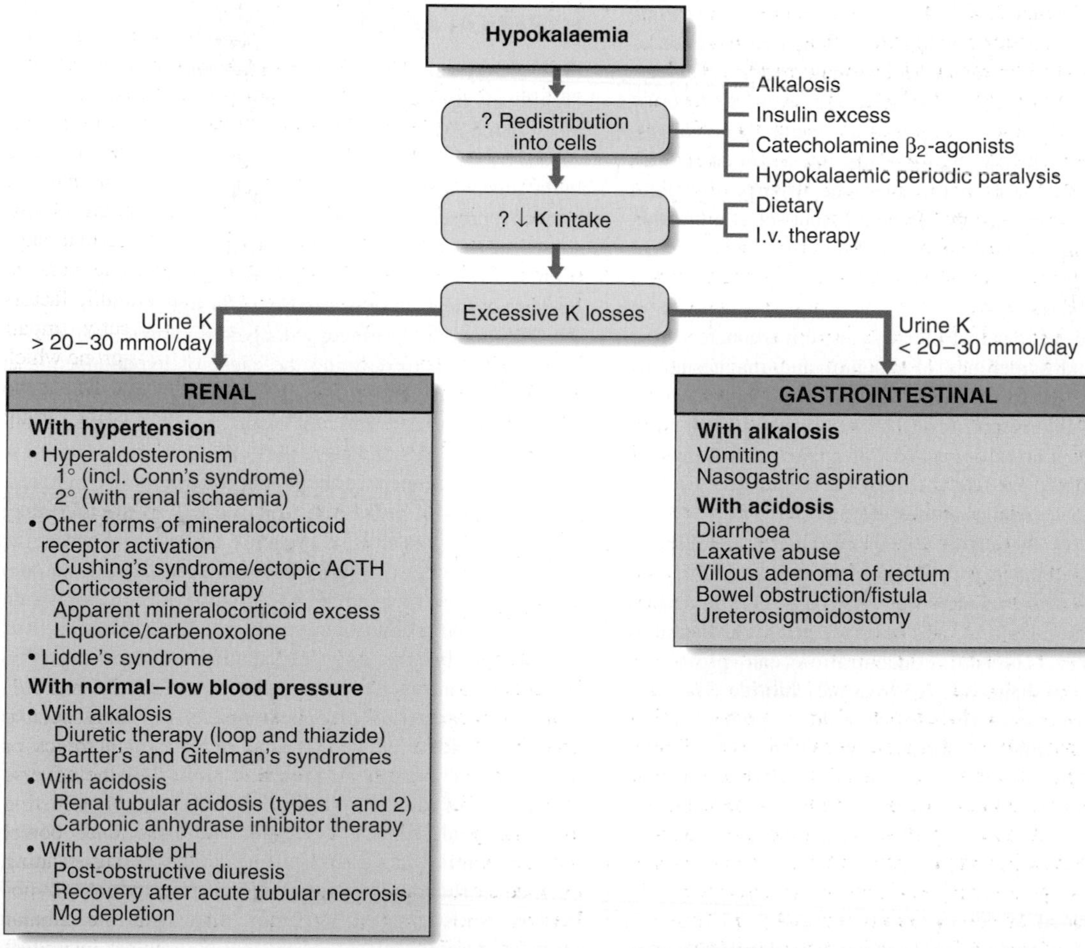

The main causes of hypokalaemia, and an approach to the differential diagnosis, are shown in Figure 16.9. A first consideration is to exclude redistribution of potassium into cells as the prime cause, since correction of the factors involved (see above) may be sufficient to correct the plasma

16

Hypokalaemia

? Redistribution
into cells

— Alkalosis
— Insulin excess
— Catecholamine β_2-agonists
— Hypokalaemic periodic paralysis

? ↓ K intake

— Dietary
— I.v. therapy

Excessive K losses

Urine K
> 20−30 mmol/day

Urine K
< 20−30 mmol/day

RENAL

With hypertension
- Hyperaldosteronism
  1° (incl. Conn's syndrome)
  2° (with renal ischaemia)
- Other forms of mineralocorticoid
  receptor activation
  Cushing's syndrome/ectopic ACTH
  Corticosteroid therapy
  Apparent mineralocorticoid excess
  Liquorice/carbenoxolone
- Liddle's syndrome

With normal−low blood pressure
- With alkalosis
  Diuretic therapy (loop and thiazide)
  Bartter's and Gitelman's syndromes
- With acidosis
  Renal tubular acidosis (types 1 and 2)
  Carbonic anhydrase inhibitor therapy
- With variable pH
  Post-obstructive diuresis
  Recovery after acute tubular necrosis
  Mg depletion

GASTROINTESTINAL

With alkalosis
Vomiting
Nasogastric aspiration

With acidosis
Diarrhoea
Laxative abuse
Villous adenoma of rectum
Bowel obstruction/fistula
Ureterosigmoidostomy

Fig. 16.9 **Diagnostic decision tree for hypokalaemia.** (ACTH = adrenocorticotrophic hormone)

due to a genetic defect causing overactivity of epithelial sodium channels in the distal nephron.

If blood pressure is normal or low, renal potassium loss can be classified according to the associated acid–base change. If hypokalaemia is associated with alkalosis, and diuretic use has been excluded, an inherited tubular transport defect may be suspected. In Bartter's syndrome there is a defect in the mechanism for sodium reabsorption in the thick ascending limb of Henle, due to a mutation causing malfunction of the NKCC2 carrier or other transporters involved in reabsorption in this segment. The clinical and biochemical features are similar to chronic treatment with furosemide. In Gitelman's syndrome there is a mutation causing malfunction of the NCCT carrier in the early distal tubule. The clinical and biochemical features are similar to chronic thiazide treatment.

Note that while both Bartter's and Gitelman's syndromes are characterised by hypokalaemia and hypomagnesaemia, urinary calcium excretion is increased in Bartter's syndrome but decreased in Gitelman's syndrome, analogous to the effects of the loop and thiazide diuretics, respectively, on calcium transport (p. 428).

If hypokalaemia is associated with a normal blood pressure but with metabolic acidosis, renal tubular acidosis (proximal or 'classical' distal) should be suspected (p. 438).

When hypokalaemia is due to potassium wasting through the gastrointestinal tract, the cause is usually obvious clinically. In some cases, where there is occult induction of vomiting or surreptitious use of aperients, a useful generalisation is that upper gastrointestinal losses (above the pylorus) are characteristically associated with metabolic alkalosis, whereas losses below the pylorus are associated with metabolic acidosis. In both cases, the urinary potassium excretion would be expected to be low (but see qualification mentioned above regarding high aldosterone states).

Investigations

Measurement of plasma electrolytes, bicarbonate, urine potassium and sometimes of calcium and magnesium is usually sufficient to establish the diagnosis. Plasma renin activity and aldosterone levels will identify patients with primary hyperaldosteronism (p. 786) and other forms of mineralocorticoid excess, when renin is suppressed; in other causes of hypokalaemia renin is elevated.

Occasionally the cause of hypokalaemia is obscure, especially when the history is incomplete or unreliable, and the urine K is indeterminate. Many such cases are associated with metabolic alkalosis, and in this setting the measurement of urine chloride concentration can provide a helpful guide to diagnosis. A low urine chloride (less than 30 mmol/l) is characteristic of vomiting (spontaneous or self-induced), while a chloride above 40 mmol/l suggests diuretic therapy (acute phase) or a tubular disorder such as Bartter's or Gitelman's syndrome. Differentiation between these latter possibilities can be assisted by performing a screen of urine for diuretic drugs.

Management

Treatment of hypokalaemia involves first determining the cause and correcting this where possible. If the problem is mainly one of redistribution of potassium into cells, reversal of this influence (e.g. correction of alkalosis) may be sufficient to restore plasma potassium without providing potassium supplements. In most cases, however, a form of potassium replacement will be required. This can generally be achieved with slow-release KCl tablets, but in more acute circumstances intravenous potassium chloride will be necessary. The rate of administration depends on the severity of hypokalaemia and the presence of cardiac or neuromuscular complications, but should generally not exceed 10 mmol of K per hour. If higher rates of administration are needed, the concentration of potassium in the infused fluid may be increased to 40 mmol/l if a peripheral vein is used, but higher concentrations must be infused into a large 'central' vein with continuous cardiac monitoring.

In the less common situation of hypokalaemia being associated with systemic acidosis, alkaline salts of potassium such as potassium bicarbonate can be given by mouth. Where magnesium depletion is also present, replacement of magnesium may be necessary to allow correction of hypokalaemia to occur. In appropriate circumstances, use of a potassium-sparing diuretic such as amiloride can assist in the correction of hypokalaemia, hypomagnesaemia and metabolic alkalosis, especially when these are due to use of a loop or thiazide diuretic.

HYPERKALAEMIA

Aetiology and clinical assessment

Significant hyperkalaemia can be a dangerous electrolyte disturbance, because of the risk of diastolic cardiac arrest caused by the marked slowing of action potential conduction in the presence of potassium levels above 7 mmol/l. Patients typically present with progressive muscular weakness, but sometimes there are no symptoms until cardiac arrest occurs. Typical ECG changes are shown in Figure 16.8. Peaking of the T wave is an early ECG sign, but widening of the QRS complex presages a dangerous cardiac arrhythmia.

An approach to defining the cause of hyperkalaemia is shown in Figure 16.10. It is important to exclude artefacts due to in vitro haemolysis of blood specimens, but if there is doubt about this and there are consistent changes present in the ECG, treatment for hyperkalaemia should be initiated. Redistribution of potassium from the ICF to the ECF may occur in the presence of systemic acidosis, or when the relevant hormones (insulin, catecholamines and aldosterone) are reduced or blocked (p. 432). While a high potassium intake may be a contributory cause of hyperkalaemia, it is unlikely to be the only explanation if renal excretion mechanisms are intact.

Impaired excretion of potassium into the urine may be associated with a reduced GFR, as in acute or chronic renal failure. In the presence of preserved GFR, the problem may be a failure of tubular potassium secretory mechanisms.

Acute renal failure is associated with particularly severe hyperkalaemia when there is a concomitant potassium load, such as in rhabdomyolysis or in sepsis, particularly when acidosis is also present. In chronic renal failure, adaptation to a moderately elevated plasma potassium commonly develops, but a further rise can occur during intercurrent

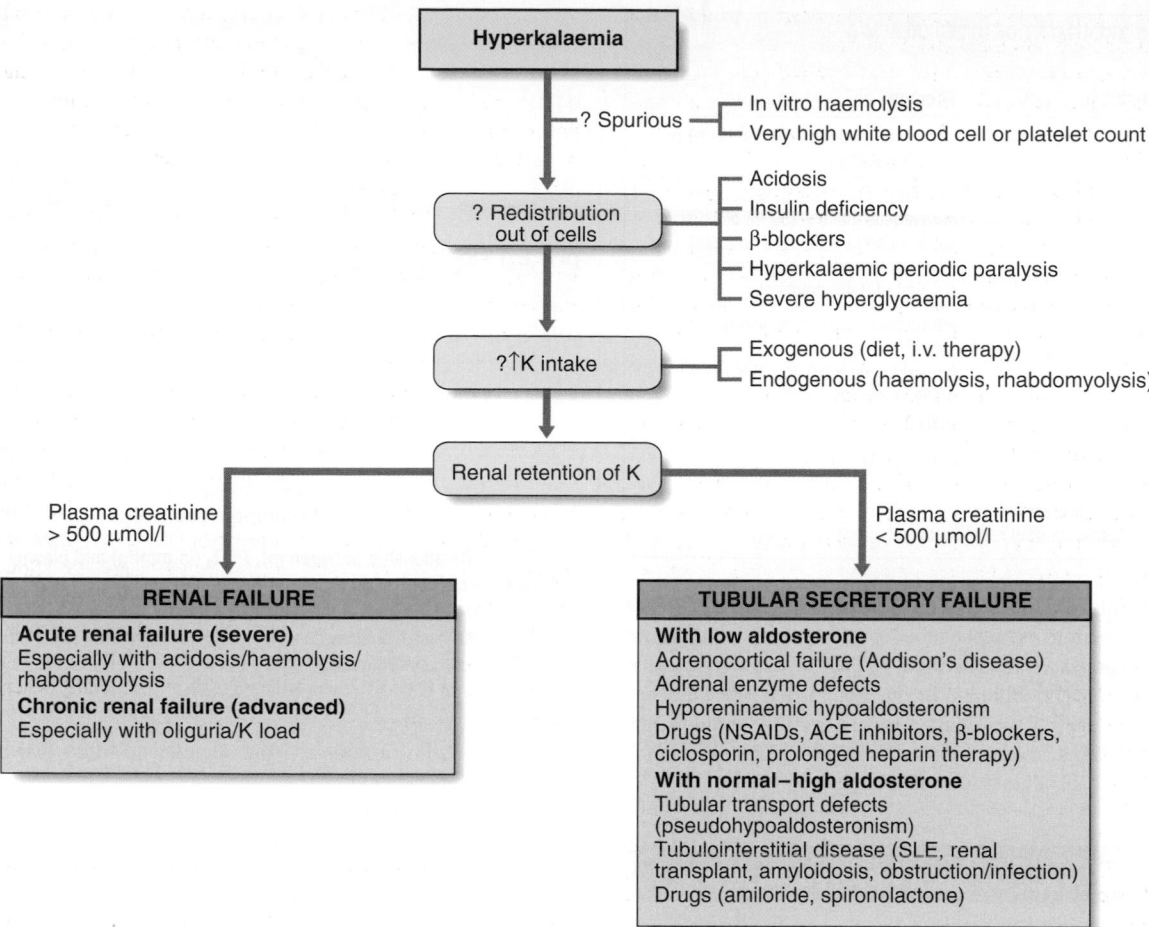

Fig. 16.10 Diagnostic decision tree for hyperkalaemia. Creatinine of 500 μmol/l = 5.67 mg/dl.

events which destabilise the new steady-state, e.g. a dietary load of potassium, hypovolaemia or drugs (see below).

Hyperkalaemia can also develop when tubular potassium secretory processes are impaired, even if the GFR is well maintained. In some cases, this is due to inadequate circulating aldosterone, as in Addison's disease, ACE inhibitor therapy, or other situations where the renin–angiotensin–aldosterone system is inactivated (e.g. hyporeninaemic hypoaldosteronism which typically occurs in association with neuropathy in diabetes and is thought to reflect impaired β-adrenergic stimulation of renin release, or therapy with angiotensin receptor antagonists, non-steroidal anti-inflammatory drugs (NSAIDs) or β-blocking drugs). In another group of conditions, tubular potassium secretion is impaired, even in the presence of high aldosterone levels. Such aldosterone resistance can occur in a variety of diseases involving inflammation in the tubulointerstitium (e.g. systemic lupus erythematosus (SLE), renal transplant), during therapy with potassium-sparing diuretics, and in a number of inherited disorders of tubular transport.

In all conditions of aldosterone deficiency or aldosterone resistance, hyperkalaemia may be associated with acid retention, giving rise to the pattern of hyperkalaemic distal ('type 4') renal tubular acidosis (p. 438).

Investigations

Results for plasma electrolytes, creatinine and bicarbonate, together with consideration of the clinical scenario, will usually provide the explanation for hyperkalaemia. In aldosterone deficiency, plasma sodium concentration is characteristically low, although this can occur in many causes of hyperkalaemia. Addison's disease should be excluded unless there is an obvious alternative diagnosis, as described on pages 782–784.

Management

Treatment of hyperkalaemia depends on the severity and the rate of development. In the absence of neuromuscular symptoms or ECG changes, reduction of potassium intake and correction of underlying abnormalities may be sufficient. However, in acute and/or severe hyperkalaemia more urgent measures must be taken (Box 16.15).

If ECG changes are present, the first step should be infusion of calcium gluconate to stabilise conductive tissue membranes (calcium has the opposite effect of potassium on conduction of an action potential). Measures to shift potassium from the ECF to the ICF should be taken, as they generally act rapidly and may avert arrhythmic complications of hyperkalaemia. Ultimately, a means of removing

16.15 TREATMENT OF HYPERKALAEMIA

Mechanism	Therapy
Stabilise cell membrane potential[1]	Intravenous calcium gluconate (10 ml of 10% solution)
Shift K into cells	Inhaled β_2 agonist, e.g. salbutamol Intravenous glucose (50 ml of 50% solution) and insulin (5 U Actrapid) Intravenous sodium bicarbonate[2] (100 ml of 8.4% solution)
Remove K from body	Intravenous furosemide and normal saline[3] Ion-exchange resin (e.g. Resonium) orally or rectally Dialysis

[1] If ECG changes suggestive of hyperkalaemia (K typically > 7 mmol/l).
[2] If acidosis present.
[3] If adequate residual renal function.

potassium from the body will generally be necessary. When renal function is reasonably preserved, loop diuretics (accompanied by intravenous saline if hypovolaemia is present) may be effective in this regard, but in established renal failure, ion-exchange resins acting through the gastrointestinal tract may need to be used. In this situation urgent dialysis should also be arranged.

16 DISORDERS OF ACID–BASE BALANCE

The pH of the arterial plasma is normally 7.40, corresponding to a H^+ concentration of 40 nmol/l. An increase in H^+ concentration corresponds to a decrease in pH. To preserve function of many pH-sensitive enzymes, this parameter is under tight homeostatic regulation, such that the H^+ concentration does not vary outside the range 36–44 nmol/l (pH 7.44–7.36) under normal circumstances. Abnormal acid–base balance occurs in a wide range of diseases.

FUNCTIONAL ANATOMY AND PHYSIOLOGY OF ACID–BASE HOMEOSTASIS

A variety of physiological mechanisms act to prevent wide swings in the pH of the ECF. The first is the action of blood and tissue buffers, of which the most important is the carbonic acid/bicarbonate buffer system. This involves the reaction of H^+ ions with bicarbonate to form carbonic acid, which, under the influence of the enzyme carbonic anhydrase (c.a.), dissociates to form CO_2 and water, as follows:

$$CO_2 + H_2O \overset{c.a.}{\rightleftharpoons} H_2CO_3 \rightleftharpoons H^+ + HCO_3^-$$

This buffer system is important because bicarbonate is present in relatively high concentration in the ECF (21–28 mmol/l), and two of its key components are under physiological control: the CO_2 by the lungs, and the bicarbonate, by the kidneys. These relationships are illustrated

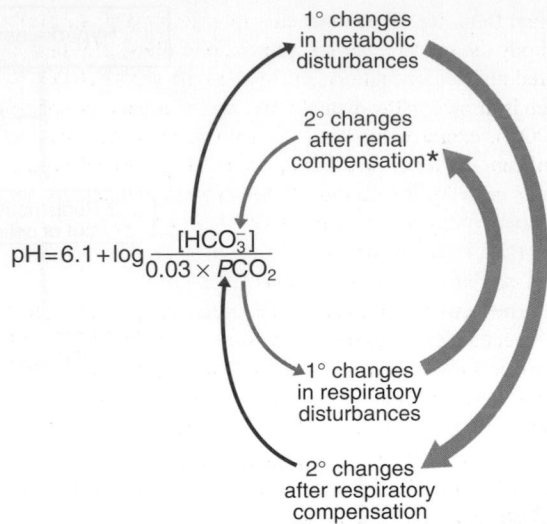

$$pH = 6.1 + \log \frac{[HCO_3^-]}{0.03 \times PCO_2}$$

Fig. 16.11   Relationship between pH, PCO_2 (in mmHg) and plasma bicarbonate concentration (in mmol/l). * Note that changes in HCO_3^- concentration are also part of the renal correction for sustained metabolic acid–base disturbances as long as the kidney itself is not the cause of the primary disturbance.

in Figure 16.11 (a form of the Henderson–Hasselbalch equation).

Respiratory compensation for acid–base disturbances can occur quickly, due to alterations in ventilatory drive mediated through pH changes in the brain stem. In response to acid accumulation, ventilation is increased, serving to reduce the PCO_2 and hence drive up the pH (p. 657). Conversely, systemic alkalosis leads to inhibition of ventilation (although this is limited by the development of hypoxia).

The kidney provides a third line of defence against disturbances of arterial pH. When acid accumulates due to chronic respiratory or metabolic (non-renal) causes, the kidney has the long-term capacity to enhance urinary excretion of acid, effectively increasing the plasma bicarbonate.

Renal control of acid–base balance

There are several components to the kidneys' contribution to maintaining acid–base balance. First, the proximal tubule reabsorbs some 85% of the filtered bicarbonate ions, through the mechanism for H^+ secretion illustrated in Figure 16.3A (p. 423). This is dependent on the enzyme carbonic anhydrase both in the cytoplasm of the proximal tubular cells and on the luminal surface of the brush border membranes. The system has a high capacity but does not lead to significant acidification of the luminal fluid.

Distal nephron segments have an important role in determining net acid excretion by the kidney. In the intercalated cells of the cortical collecting duct and the outer medullary collecting duct cells, acid is secreted into the lumen by an H^+-ATPase. This excreted acid is generated in the tubular cell from the hydration of CO_2 to form carbonic acid, which dissociates into an H^+ ion secreted luminally, and a bicarbonate ion which passes across the basolateral membrane into the blood. The secreted H^+ ions contribute to the reabsorption of any residual bicarbonate present in the luminal fluid, but also contribute net acid for removal from the body, bound to a variety of urinary buffers. The first is filtered non-bicarbonate buffer, such as phosphate (HPO_4^{2-}) which is titrated in the distal lumen to dihydrogen phosphate ($H_2PO_4^-$), excreted in the urine with sodium. The second significant buffer is ammonia, which is generated within tubular cells by the action of the enzyme glutaminase on glutamine. NH_3 reacts with secreted acid to form ammonium (NH_4^+) which becomes trapped in the luminal fluid and is excreted with chloride ions.

The net removal of acid by the kidney, using these latter two mechanisms, amounts to some 1 mmol/kg/day of hydrogen ions, which equals the non-volatile acid load arising from the metabolism of dietary protein. Thus a slightly alkaline plasma pH of 7.4 (H^+ 40 nmol/l) is maintained by the kidney's capacity to generate an acidic urine (pH typically 5–6) in which the net daily excess of metabolic acid can be excreted.

PRESENTING PROBLEMS IN DISORDERS OF ACID–BASE BALANCE

Patients with disturbances of acid–base balance may present clinically either with the effects of tissue malfunction due to disturbed pH (such as altered cardiac and CNS function), or with secondary changes in respiration as a response to the underlying metabolic change (e.g. Kussmaul respiration during metabolic acidosis). The clinical picture is often dominated by the cause of the acid–base change, such as uncontrolled diabetes or primary lung disease. Frequently the acid–base disturbance only becomes evident when the venous plasma bicarbonate concentration is noted to be abnormal, or when a full arterial blood gas analysis shows abnormalities in the pH, PCO_2 or bicarbonate (the 'base excess' may also be provided with these data; this is the difference between the patient's bicarbonate level and the normal bicarbonate, measured in vitro with the PCO_2 adjusted to 5.33 kPa (40 mmHg)).

The common patterns of abnormality in the blood gas parameters in acid–base disturbances are shown in Box 16.16. (Note that the terms acidosis and alkalosis strictly refer to the underlying direction of the acid–base change, while acidaemia and alkalaemia more correctly refer to the net change present in the blood.) Interpretation of arterial blood gases is also described on page 657.

In metabolic disturbances, respiratory compensation is almost immediate, so that the predicted compensatory change in PCO_2 is achieved soon after the onset of the metabolic disturbance. In respiratory disorders, on the other hand, a small initial change in bicarbonate occurs as a result of chemical buffering of CO_2, largely within red blood cells, but the kidney achieves further compensatory changes in bicarbonate concentration as a result of long-term adjustments in acid secretory capacity, requiring days to weeks. When clinically obtained acid–base parameters do not accord with the predicted compensation shown, a mixed acid–base disturbance should be suspected (p. 440).

METABOLIC ACIDOSIS

Aetiology and clinical assessment

Metabolic acidosis occurs when an acid other than carbonic acid (due to CO_2 retention) accumulates in the body, resulting in a fall in the plasma bicarbonate. The pH fall which would otherwise occur is blunted by hyperventilation, resulting in a reduced PCO_2. If the kidneys are intact (i.e. not the cause of the initial disturbance), renal excretion of acid can be gradually increased over days to weeks, raising the plasma bicarbonate and hence the pH towards normal in the new steady state.

Two patterns of metabolic acidosis can be defined (Box 16.17), depending on the nature of the accumulating acid:

- In pattern A, where a mineral acid (HCl) accumulates, or where there is a primary loss of bicarbonate buffer from the ECF, there is no addition to the plasma of a new acidic anion. In this case, the 'anion gap', calculated as the difference between the main measured cations ($Na^+ + K^+$) and the anions ($Cl^- + HCO_3^-$), is unchanged from normal, since the plasma chloride increases to replace the depleted bicarbonate levels. This 'gap', normally around 15 mmol/l, is made up of anions such as phosphate, sulphate and multiple negative charges on plasma protein molecules.
- In pattern B, an accumulating acid is accompanied by its corresponding anion, which adds to the unmeasured anion gap, while the chloride concentration remains normal.

16

16.16 PRINCIPAL PATTERNS OF ACID–BASE DISTURBANCE

Disturbance	Blood H^+	Primary change	Compensatory response	Predicted compensation
Metabolic acidosis	> 40[1]	HCO_3 < 24 mmol/l	PCO_2 < 5.33 kPa[2]	PCO_2 fall in kPa = 0.16 × HCO_3 fall in mmol/l
Metabolic alkalosis	< 40[1]	HCO_3 > 24 mmol/l	PCO_2 > 5.33 kPa[2,3]	PCO_2 rise in kPa = 0.08 × HCO_3 rise in mmol/l
Respiratory acidosis	> 40[1]	PCO_2 > 5.33 kPa[2]	HCO_3 > 24 mmol/l	Acute: HCO_3 rise in mmol/l = 0.75 × PCO_2 rise in kPa Chronic: HCO_3 rise in mmol/l = 2.62 × PCO_2 rise in kPa
Respiratory alkalosis	< 40[1]	PCO_2 < 5.33 kPa[2]	HCO_3 < 24 mmol/l	Acute: HCO_3 fall in mmol/l = 1.50 × PCO_2 fall in kPa Chronic: HCO_3 fall in mmol/l = 3.75 × PCO_2 fall in kPa

[1] H^+ of 40 nmol/l ≡ pH of 7.40.
[2] PCO_2 of 5.33 kPa ≡ 40 mmHg.
[3] PCO_2 does not rise above 7.33 kPa (55 mmHg); further hypoventilation prevents adequate oxygenation.

16.17 CAUSES OF METABOLIC ACIDOSIS	
Disorder	**Mechanism**
A. NORMAL ANION GAP	
Inorganic acid addition	Therapeutic infusion or poisoning with of NH_4Cl, HCl
Gastrointestinal base loss	Loss of HCO_3 in diarrhoea, small bowel fistula, urinary diversion procedure
Renal tubular acidosis (RTA)	Urinary loss of HCO_3 in proximal RTA; impaired tubular acid secretion in distal RTA
B. INCREASED ANION GAP	
Endogenous acid load	
Diabetic ketoacidosis	Accumulation of ketones[1] with hyperglycaemia
Starvation ketosis	Accumulation of ketones without hyperglycaemia
Lactic acidosis	Tissue hypoxia (e.g. shock) or liver disease
Renal failure	Accumulation of organic acids
Exogenous acid load	
Aspirin poisoning	Accumulation of salicylate[2]
Methanol poisoning	Accumulation of formate
Ethylene glycol poisoning	Accumulation of glycolate, oxalate

[1] Ketones include the acid anions acetoacetate and β-hydroxybutyrate (p. 809).
[2] Salicylate poisoning is also associated with respiratory alkalosis due to direct ventilatory stimulation.

16.18 CAUSES OF RENAL TUBULAR ACIDOSIS (RTA)	
Type	**Examples**
Proximal RTA ('type 2')	Congenital, e.g. Fanconi's syndrome, cystinosis, Wilson's disease Paraproteinaemia, e.g. myeloma Amyloidosis Hyperparathyroidism Heavy metal toxicity, e.g. Pb, Cd, Hg Drugs, e.g. carbonic anhydrase inhibitors, ifosfamide
Classical distal RTA ('type 1')	Congenital Hyperglobulinaemia Autoimmune connective tissue diseases, e.g. SLE Toxins and drugs, e.g. toluene, lithium, amphotericin
Hyperkalaemic distal RTA ('type 4')	Hypoaldosteronism (primary or secondary) Obstructive nephropathy Drugs, e.g. amiloride, spironolactone Renal transplant rejection

Box 16.17 summarises the main causes of metabolic acidosis, in terms of the anion gap.

When the anion gap is increased (pattern B), the cause is usually apparent from associated clinical features such as uncontrolled diabetes, renal failure or shock, or may be suggested by associated symptoms, such as visual complaints in methanol poisoning (p. 219). It is noteworthy that a number of causes of increased anion gap acidosis are associated with alcoholism, including starvation ketosis, lactic acidosis and intoxication by methanol or ethylene glycol.

Lactic acidosis may be confirmed by the measurement of plasma lactate, which will be increased over the normal maximal level of 2 mmol/l by as much as tenfold. Two types of lactic acidosis have been defined:

- Type 1, due to tissue hypoxia and peripheral generation of lactate, as in patients with circulatory failure and shock.
- Type 2, due to impaired metabolism of lactate as in liver disease. A number of drugs and toxins also impair lactate metabolism, including metformin.

Other organic anions can be measured when specifically suspected.

Normal anion gap metabolic acidosis (pattern A) is usually due either to diarrhoea, where the clinical diagnosis is generally obvious, or to renal tubular acidosis.

Renal tubular acidosis (RTA)

This condition should be suspected where there is a hyperchloraemic (normal anion gap) acidosis with no evidence of gastrointestinal disturbance, and the urine pH is inappropriately high (i.e. greater than 5.5 in the presence of systemic acidosis). The defect can affect one of three tubular processes: reabsorption of bicarbonate in the proximal tubule (proximal RTA), acid secretion in the late distal/cortical collecting duct intercalated cells (classical distal RTA), or sodium reabsorption in the principal cells of this nephron segment, with secondary effects to reduce secretion of both potassium and acid (hyperkalaemic distal RTA).

Typical causes of each type of RTA are shown in Box 16.18. Inherited causes are due to defects in the molecular mechanisms mediating acid or bicarbonate transport in the respective tubular segments (Fig. 16.3, p. 423). However, many causes are acquired, and the metabolic acidosis may serve as an early clue to the diagnosis of those conditions.

Sometimes the distal type of RTA is 'incomplete' and the plasma bicarbonate concentration is normal under resting conditions. In this context the diagnosis can be revealed by performing an acid challenge test, involving the ingestion of ammonium chloride sufficient to lower the plasma bicarbonate. In incomplete distal RTA the urine pH remains above 5.3.

A number of features allow differentiation of proximal from distal RTA. The proximal form is frequently associated with urinary wasting of amino acids, phosphate and glucose (Fanconi's syndrome) as well as bicarbonate and potassium. In severe acidosis, patients with proximal RTA can lower the urine pH once the plasma bicarbonate has fallen below 16 mmol/l and leakage of bicarbonate has subsided, since distal H^+ secretion mechanisms are intact. In classical distal RTA, by contrast, acid accumulation is relentless and progressive, resulting in mobilisation of calcium from bone and consequent osteomalacia with hypercalciuria, stone formation and nephrocalcinosis. Potassium is also lost in classical distal RTA, while it is retained in hyperkalaemic distal RTA.

Management

The first step in management of metabolic acidosis is identifying and correcting the cause when possible (Box

16.17). This may involve control of diarrhoea, treatment of diabetes, correction of shock, cessation of drug administration, or dialysis to remove toxins. Since metabolic acidosis is frequently associated with sodium and water depletion, resuscitation with appropriate intravenous fluids will often be needed. Use of intravenous bicarbonate in this setting is controversial. Because rapid correction of acidosis has some inherent risks (e.g. induction of hypokalaemia or reduced plasma ionised calcium), use of bicarbonate infusions is best reserved for situations where the underlying disorder cannot be readily corrected and where the acidosis is severe ($H^+ > 70$ nmol/l, pH < 7.15) and associated with evidence of tissue dysfunction.

The acidosis associated with RTA can sometimes be controlled by treating the underlying cause (Box 16.18). Usually, however, supplements of sodium and potassium bicarbonate are necessary to achieve the target of a plasma bicarbonate level above 18 mmol/l with normokalaemia in types 1 and 2 RTA, while diuretics or corticosteroids (as appropriate) may be effective in reversing the underlying disturbance in type 4 RTA.

METABOLIC ALKALOSIS

Aetiology and clinical assessment
Metabolic alkalosis is characterised by an increase in the plasma bicarbonate concentration and the plasma pH (Box 16.16). There is a compensatory rise in PCO_2 due to hypoventilation, but this is limited by the need to avoid hypoxia. The causes are best classified by the accompanying disturbance of ECF volume.

Hypovolaemic metabolic alkalosis is the most common pattern, typified by disorders such as sustained vomiting where acid-rich fluid is lost directly from the body. This pattern also occurs during treatment with most diuretic drugs (other than carbonic anhydrase inhibitors and potassium-sparing drugs), since the diuretic action involves increased acid loss into the urine.

Normovolaemic (or hypervolaemic) metabolic alkalosis occurs in settings where both bicarbonate retention and volume expansion occur simultaneously. Classical causes include corticosteroid excess states such as primary hyperaldosteronism (Conn's syndrome, p. 786), Cushing's syndrome (p. 779) and corticosteroid therapy (p. 784). Occasionally, overuse of antacid salts for treatment of dyspepsia can produce a similar pattern.

Several factors act to sustain or amplify metabolic alkalosis, particularly that developing in the context of volume depletion. In the case of sustained vomiting (Fig. 16.12), the loss of acid is the immediate trigger for generating metabolic alkalosis, but it is maintained by other physiological responses; the loss of sodium and fluid leads to hypovolaemia, triggering both proximal sodium bicarbonate reabsorption and further distal acid secretion, via the stimulus of aldosterone. Hypokalaemia, due to potassium loss in the vomitus as well as through the kidney under the influence of aldosterone, itself stimulates distal acid excretion. Additionally, the compensatory rise in PCO_2 enhances tubular acid secretion. The net result is an inappropriately acid urine and a failure of the kidney to effect

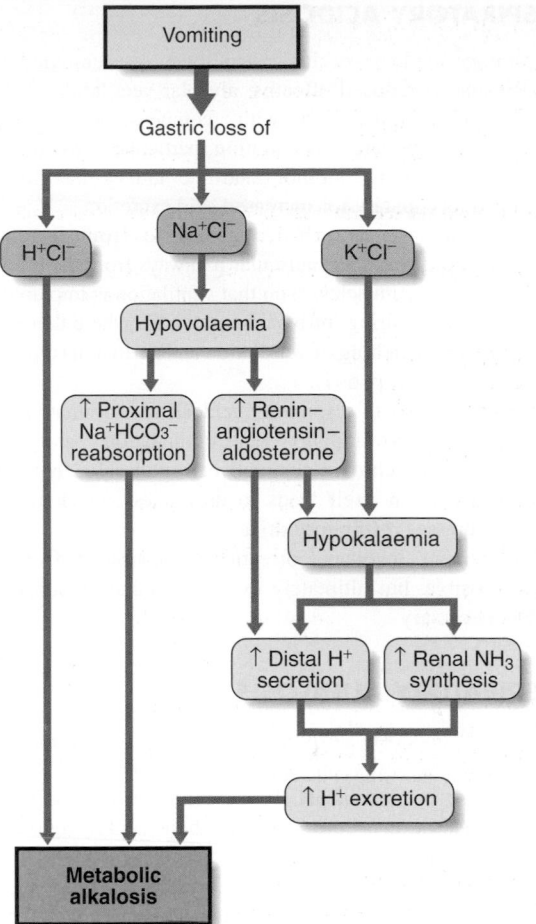

Fig. 16.12 Generation and maintenance of metabolic alkalosis during prolonged vomiting. Loss of $H^+ Cl^-$ generates metabolic alkalosis which is maintained by renal changes.

long-term correction of the systemic pH disturbance, at least until adequate replenishment of the circulating volume and hence reversal of secondary hyperaldosteronism.

Clinically, apart from manifestations of the underlying cause, there may be few symptoms or signs related to alkalosis itself. When the rise in systemic pH is abrupt, plasma ionised calcium falls and signs of increased neuromuscular irritability such as tetany may develop (p. 774).

Management
In metabolic alkalosis associated with hypovolaemia, treatment involves provision of adequate intravenous fluid, specifically isotonic sodium chloride, which interrupts the volume-conserving mechanisms and allows the kidney to excrete the excess alkali in the urine. Replacement of potassium helps correct the hypokalaemia and its consequences in the kidney.

In metabolic alkalosis associated with normal or increased volume, treatment should focus on correcting the underlying cause, specifically the removal or blockade of excess mineralocorticoid activity. The approach depends on the underlying endocrinological diagnosis (Ch. 20).

RESPIRATORY ACIDOSIS

Respiratory acidosis occurs when there is accumulation of CO_2 due to reduced effective alveolar ventilation. This results in a rise in the PCO_2, with a compensatory increase in plasma bicarbonate concentration, particularly when the disorder is of long duration and the kidney has fully developed its capacity for increased acid excretion.

This acid–base disturbance can arise from lesions anywhere along the neuromuscular pathways from the brain to the respiratory muscles, such that ventilation is impaired. It can also arise during intrinsic lung disease where there is significant mismatching of ventilation and perfusion (type II respiratory failure, p. 667).

Clinical features of respiratory acidosis are dominated by the cause of hypoventilation (e.g. obtundation, paralysis, chest wall injury, chronic obstructive lung disease), but the CO_2 accumulation itself leads to drowsiness which itself further depresses respiratory drive.

Management involves correction of causative factors where possible, but ultimately external ventilatory support may be necessary.

RESPIRATORY ALKALOSIS

Respiratory alkalosis develops when there is a period of sustained hyperventilation resulting in a reduction of PCO_2 and increase in plasma pH. If the condition is sustained, renal compensation occurs such that tubular acid secretion is reduced and the plasma bicarbonate falls.

This acid–base disturbance is frequently of short duration, as in anxiety states or over-vigorous assisted ventilation. It can be prolonged in the context of pregnancy, pulmonary embolism, chronic liver disease, and ingestion of certain drugs which stimulate the brain stem respiratory centre (e.g. salicylates).

Clinical features are those associated with the cause, but there is frequently also agitation associated with perioral and digital tingling, due to a reduction in ionised calcium caused by increased binding of calcium to albumin in the alkalotic ECF. In severe cases, Trousseau's sign and Chvostek's sign may be positive, and tetany or seizures may develop (p. 775).

Management involves correction of identifiable causes, reduction of anxiety, and sometimes a period of rebreathing into a closed bag to allow CO_2 levels to rise.

MIXED ACID–BASE DISORDERS

In patients with complex illnesses, it is not uncommon for more than one independent disturbance of acid–base metabolism to be present at the same time. In these situations, the arterial pH will represent the net effect of all primary and compensatory changes. Indeed, the pH may be normal, but the presence of underlying acid–base disturbances can be gauged from concomitant abnormalities in the PCO_2 and bicarbonate concentration.

In assessing these disorders, all clinical influences on the patient's acid–base status should be identified, and reference should be made to the table of predicted compensation given in Box 16.16 (p. 437). Where the compensatory change is discrepant from the rules of thumb provided, the presence of more than one disturbance of acid–base metabolism may be suspected.

DISORDERS OF DIVALENT ION METABOLISM

The present section excludes discussion of calcium disorders, which are considered in Chapters 20 (pp. 772–775) and 25 (p. 1127).

FUNCTIONAL ANATOMY AND PHYSIOLOGY OF MAGNESIUM METABOLISM

Like potassium, magnesium is mainly an intracellular cation. It is important to the function of many enzymes, including the Na,K-ATPase, and can regulate both potassium and calcium channels. Its overall effect is to stabilise excitable cell membranes.

Renal handling of magnesium involves filtration of free plasma magnesium (about 70% of the total) with extensive reabsorption (50–70%) in the loop of Henle, although significant reabsorption also occurs in the proximal and distal tubules. Reabsorption is enhanced by parathyroid hormone (PTH).

PRESENTING PROBLEMS IN DISORDERS OF MAGNESIUM METABOLISM

HYPOMAGNESAEMIA

Aetiology and clinical assessment

A plasma magnesium concentration below the normal range (0.8–1.0 mmol/l) is usually a reflection of magnesium depletion (Box 16.19). Reduced intake is rarely sufficient alone to cause magnesium depletion, and generally there is excessive loss from either the gastrointestinal tract (notably in chronic diarrhoea) or the kidney (during prolonged use of loop diuretics). Excessive alcohol ingestion can cause magnesium depletion through both gut and renal losses. Some inherited tubular transport disorders result in urinary magnesium wasting, notably Gitelman's syndrome (p. 434).

Hypomagnesaemia is frequently associated with hypocalcaemia, probably because magnesium is required for the normal secretion of PTH in response to a fall in serum calcium, and because hypomagnesaemia induces resistance to PTH in bone. Clinical features of hypomagnesaemia and hypocalcaemia are similar; there may be tetany, cardiac arrhythmias (notably torsades de pointes, p. 568), central nervous excitation and seizures, as well as vasoconstriction and hypertension. Magnesium depletion is also associated (through uncertain mechanisms) with hyponatraemia and hypokalaemia, which may mediate some of the clinical manifestations.

16.19 CAUSES OF HYPOMAGNESAEMIA

Mechanism	Examples
Inadequate intake	Starvation, malnutrition (esp. alcoholism), parenteral alimentation
Excessive losses Gastrointestinal	Prolonged vomiting/nasogastric aspiration, chronic diarrhoea/laxative abuse, malabsorption, small bowel bypass surgery, fistulae
Urinary	Diuretic therapy (loop, thiazide), alcohol, tubulotoxic drugs (gentamicin, cisplatin), volume expansion (e.g. primary hyperaldosteronism), diabetic ketoacidosis, post-obstructive diuresis, recovery from acute tubular necrosis, inherited tubular transport defect (Bartter's syndrome, Gitelman's syndrome, primary renal magnesium wasting)
Complex formation	Acute pancreatitis, foscarnet therapy, hungry bone syndrome

Management

Treatment involves identification and correction of the cause where possible. Oral magnesium salts have limited effectiveness due to poor absorption and may cause diarrhoea. Where symptoms are present, treatment should be with intravenous magnesium chloride, at a rate not exceeding 0.5 mmol/kg in the first 24 hours. When intravenous access is not available, magnesium sulphate can be given intramuscularly. If hypomagnesaemia is due to diuretic treatment, adjunctive use of a potassium-sparing agent will also reduce magnesium loss into the urine.

HYPERMAGNESAEMIA

Aetiology and clinical assessment

This is a much less common abnormality than hypomagnesaemia. The cause nearly always involves acute or chronic renal failure, but adrenocortical insufficiency also predisposes to magnesium retention. Any cause of increased intake, either through medications containing magnesium (antacids, laxatives, enemas) or through iatrogenic parenteral therapy, will greatly increase the risk when renal impairment is present.

Clinical features include bradycardia, hypotension, reduced consciousness and respiratory depression.

Management

Management of hypermagnesaemia involves ceasing all magnesium intake, improving renal function if possible, and promoting urinary magnesium excretion using a loop diuretic with intravenous hydration, if residual renal function allows. Calcium gluconate may be given intravenously to reverse overt cardiac effects. Ultimately, if renal function is minimal, dialysis may be necessary to remove the magnesium load.

FUNCTIONAL ANATOMY AND PHYSIOLOGY OF PHOSPHATE METABOLISM

Inorganic phosphate (mainly present as HPO_4^{2-}) is intimately involved in cell energy metabolism, intracellular signalling and bone and mineral balance (Ch. 25). The normal plasma concentration is 0.7–1.4 mmol/l. It is freely filtered at the glomerulus and approximately 65% is reabsorbed by the proximal tubule, via an apical sodium–phosphate cotransport carrier. A further 10–20% is reabsorbed in the distal tubules, leaving a fractional excretion of some 10% to pass into the urine, usually as $H_2PO_4^-$. Proximal reabsorption is decreased by parathyroid hormone, volume expansion and glucose infusion.

PRESENTING PROBLEMS IN DISORDERS OF PHOSPHATE METABOLISM

HYPOPHOSPHATAEMIA

Aetiology and clinical assessment

The causes of a reduced plasma phosphate concentration are shown in Box 16.20. Phosphate may redistribute into cells during periods of increased energy utilisation (as in refeeding after a period of starvation) and during systemic alkalosis. However, an overall body deficit is likely to be present in severe hypophosphataemia, on the basis of inadequate intake or absorption through the gut, or due to excessive renal losses, notably during primary hyperparathyroidism (p. 775) or diuretic states. An inherited defect of proximal sodium–phosphate cotransport is the basis of familial hypophosphataemic rickets.

Clinical manifestations of phosphate depletion reflect the widespread involvement of phosphate in tissue metabolism. Defects appear in the blood (impaired function and survival of all cell lines), skeletal muscle (weakness, respiratory failure), cardiac muscle (congestive cardiac failure), smooth muscle (ileus), the central nervous system (decreased consciousness, seizures and coma) and bone, where severe prolonged hypophosphataemia leads to osteomalacia (p. 1126).

16.20 CAUSES OF HYPOPHOSPHATAEMIA

Mechanism	Examples
Redistribution into cells	Refeeding after starvation, respiratory alkalosis, treatment for diabetic ketoacidosis
Inadequate intake or absorption	Malnutrition, malabsorption, chronic diarrhoea, phosphate binders (antacids), vitamin D deficiency or resistance
Increased renal excretion	Hyperparathyroidism, ECF volume expansion with diuresis, osmotic diuresis, proximal tubular transport defect (Fanconi's syndrome, familial hypophosphataemic rickets, cancer-induced hypophosphataemia)

Management

Management involves administering oral phosphate supplements and high-protein/high-dairy dietary supplements which are rich in naturally occurring phosphate. Intravenous treatment with sodium or potassium phosphate salts can be used in critical situations, but there is a risk of precipitating hypocalcaemia and metastatic calcification.

HYPERPHOSPHATAEMIA

Aetiology and clinical assessment

Phosphate accumulation is usually the result of decreased renal function, in acute or chronic renal failure. Phosphate excretion is also reduced in hypoparathyroidism (and pseudohypoparathyroidism) (p. 773). Redistribution of phosphate from cells into the plasma can be a contributing factor to hyperphosphataemia in the tumour lysis syndrome and in catabolic states. Phosphate accumulation will be aggravated in any of these conditions when the patient is taking phosphate-containing preparations or inappropriate vitamin D therapy.

The clinical features relate to hypocalcaemia and metastatic calcification, particularly in chronic renal failure and tertiary hyperparathyroidism where a high calcium–phosphate product occurs.

Management

Management involves volume expansion with normal saline which promotes phosphate excretion if renal function is normal. In the presence of renal failure, dietary phosphate restriction and the use of oral phosphate binders (such as calcium carbonate) are important, as discussed on page 489).

DISORDERS OF AMINO ACID METABOLISM

Congenital disorders of amino acid metabolism usually present in the neonatal period and may involve life-long treatment regimens. However, some disorders, particularly those involved in amino acid transport, may not present until later in life.

PHENYLKETONURIA

Phenylketonuria (PKU) is caused by a deficiency of enzymatic activity of phenylalanine hydroxylase. It is inherited as an autosomal recessive disorder. As a result of this enzyme deficiency, phenylalanine accumulates to high levels in the neonate's blood, causing mental retardation.

Diagnosis of PKU is almost always made by routine neonatal screening. Treatment involves life-long adherence to a low-phenylalanine diet. Early and adequate dietary treatment will prevent major mental retardation, although there may still be a slight reduction in IQ.

HOMOCYSTINURIA

Homocystinuria is caused by cystathionine β-synthase deficiency and inherited as an autosomal recessive trait. This results in increased urinary excretion of homocystine and methionine. Many cases of homocystinuria are diagnosed through newborn screening programmes.

There is a wide spectrum of clinical manifestations, involving the eyes (ectopia lentis—displacement of the lens), central nervous system (mental retardation, delayed developmental milestones, seizures, psychiatric disturbances), skeleton (resembling Marfan syndrome, and also with generalised osteoporosis), vascular system (thrombotic lesions of arteries and veins) and skin (hypopigmentation).

Treatment is dietary, involving a methionine-restricted, cystine-supplemented diet, as well as large doses of pyridoxine.

DISORDERS OF CARBOHYDRATE METABOLISM

The most common disorder of carbohydrate metabolism is diabetes mellitus, which is discussed in Chapter 21. There are also some rare inherited defects.

GALACTOSAEMIA

Galactosaemia is caused by a mutation in the galactose-1-phosphate uridylyltransferase gene (GALT) and is usually inherited as an autosomal recessive disorder. The neonate is unable to metabolise galactose, one of the hexose sugars contained in lactose.

Vomiting or diarrhoea usually begins within a few days of ingestion of milk, and the neonate may become jaundiced. Failure to thrive is the most common clinical presentation. The classic form of the disease results in hepatomegaly, cataracts and mental retardation, and fulminant infection with *Escherichia coli* is a frequent complication. Treatment involves life-long avoidance of galactose- and lactose-containing foods.

The widespread inclusion of galactosaemia in newborn screening programmes has resulted in the identification of a number of milder variants (e.g. 'Duarte' variant).

GLYCOGEN STORAGE DISEASES

Glycogen represents a rapidly mobilisable storage form of glucose, enabling glucose to be released as needed during exercise or between meals. Glycogen storage diseases (GSD, or glycogenoses) result from an inherited defect in one of the many enzymes responsible for the formation or breakdown of glycogen.

There are about eleven major types of GSD which are classified by a number, by the name of the defective enzyme or eponymously after the physician who first described the condition (Box 16.21). Most forms of GSD are inherited as autosomal recessive disorders.

A diagnosis of GSD is made on the basis of the patient's symptoms, a physical examination and the results of biochemical tests. Occasionally, a muscle or liver biopsy is required to confirm the enzyme defect.

16.21 GLYCOGEN STORAGE DISEASES (GSD)

GSD	Eponym	Enzyme defect	Clinical features and complications
I	Von Gierke	Glucose-6-phosphatase deficiency	Childhood presentation, hypoglycaemia, hepatomegaly
II	Pompe	α-glucosidase (acid maltase) deficiency	Classical presentation in infancy, muscle weakness (may be severe)
III	Cori	Debrancher enzyme deficiency	Childhood presentation, hepatomegaly, mild hypoglycaemia
IV	Andersen	Brancher enzyme deficiency	Presentation in infancy, severe muscle weakness (may affect heart), cirrhosis
V	McArdle	Muscle glycogen phosphorylase deficiency	Exercise-induced fatigue and myalgia
VI	Hers	Liver phosphorylase deficiency	Mild hepatomegaly
VII	Tarui	Muscle phosphofructokinase deficiency	Exercise-induced fatigue and myalgia
VIII		Liver phosphorylase kinase deficiency	Very mild disease; hepatomegaly, growth retardation, elevated hepatic enzymes, hyperlipidaemia, fasting hyperketosis
IX		Liver glycogen phosphorylase kinase deficiency	Mild hepatomegaly. Inheritance can be autosomal or X-linked recessive
0		Hepatic glycogen synthase deficiency	Fasting hypoglycaemia, post-prandial hyperglycaemia

DISORDERS OF COMPLEX LIPID METABOLISM

Complex lipids are key components of the cell membrane (p. 40). Their synthesis and metabolism are coordinated in organelles called lysosomes. The lysosomal storage diseases are a heterogeneous group of disorders in which there is a missing enzyme in the lysosomes (Box 16.22). Lack of this enzyme results in an inability to break down complex glycolipids or other intracellular macromolecules. These disorders have diverse clinical manifestations, typically including mental retardation. Some of these disorders are becoming treatable using human enzyme replacement therapy (Box 16.22), while others (such as Tay–Sachs disease) can be prevented through community participation in genetic carrier screening programmes.

DISORDERS OF BLOOD LIPIDS AND LIPOPROTEINS

The term 'lipid' refers to substances with poor water solubility. These include biologically important materials such as sterols, including cholesterol, that are composed of hydrocarbon rings, and glycerides, such as triglyceride (TG) and phospholipid, that are chiefly composed of hydrocarbon chains. Despite their poor water solubility, these materials

16.22 LYSOSOMAL STORAGE DISEASES

Lysosomal storage disease	Clinical features	Enzyme/deficiency	Human enzyme replacement therapy
Fabry's disease	Variable age of onset. Neurological (pain in extremities). Dermatological (hypohidrosis, angiokeratomas) Cerebrovascular (renal, cardiac, CNS)	α-galactosidase A	In clinical practice
Gaucher's disease (various types)	Splenic and liver enlargement, with variable severity of disease. Some types also have neurological involvement	Glucocerebrosidase	In clinical practice for some types
Mucopolysaccharidosis (MPS) (various types, including Hurler's, Hunter's, Sanfilippo's, Morquio's syndromes)	Vary with syndrome. Can cause mental retardation, skeletal and joint abnormalities, abnormal facies, obstructive respiratory diseases and recurrrent respiratory infections	Each MPS type has a different enzyme deficiency	In clinical practice for some types, clinical trials underway for other types
Niemann–Pick disease	Most common presentation is as a progressive neurological disorder, accompanied by organomegaly. Some variants do not have neurological symptoms	Acid sphingomyelinase	Clinical trials planned for some types
GM2-gangliosidosis (various types, including Tay–Sachs, Sandhoff's diseases)	Severe progressive neurological disorder. Sandhoff's disease also characterised by organomegaly	Hexosaminidase A, B	

16

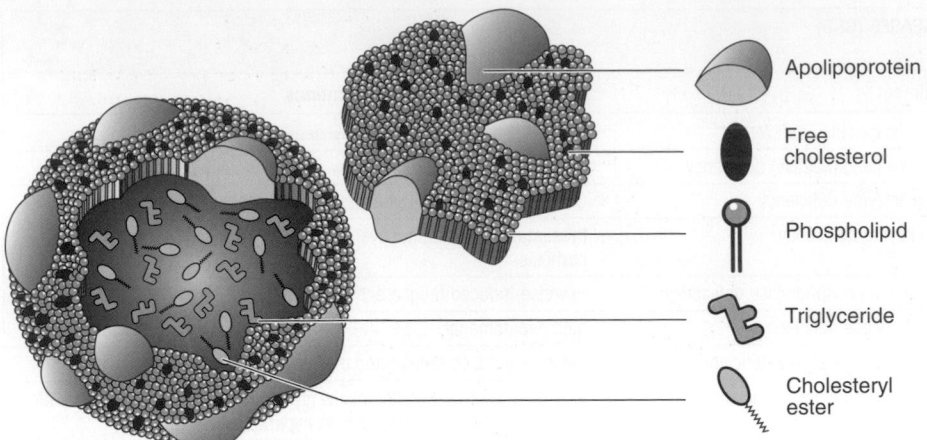

Apolipoprotein

Free
cholesterol

Phospholipid

Triglyceride

Cholesteryl
ester

Fig. 16.13   Structure of
lipoproteins.

16

must be assimilated from the diet and transported within the body; this is achieved by incorporating lipids within lipoproteins. Plasma cholesterol and TG are clinically important because they are major treatable risk factors for cardiovascular disease, whilst severe hypertriglyceridaemia also predisposes to acute pancreatitis.

FUNCTIONAL ANATOMY, PHYSIOLOGY AND INVESTIGATION OF LIPID METABOLISM

Lipids can be transported and metabolised in vivo by virtue of the detergent-like properties of apolipoproteins. The laws of physical chemistry dictate that in the aqueous in vivo environment of the blood and tissue fluids, apolipoproteins combine with lipids to form spherical or disc-shaped lipoproteins, which consist of a hydrophobic core and a less hydrophobic coat (Fig. 16.13). The structure of some apolipoproteins also enables them to act as enzyme co-factors or cell receptor ligands. Thus, variation in lipid and apolipoprotein composition results in the formation of distinct classes of lipoprotein that perform specific metabolic functions.

Dietary lipid

The intestinal absorption of dietary lipid is described on page 854 (see also Fig. 16.14). Enterocytes lining the gut extract monoglyceride and free fatty acids from micelles and re-esterify them into TG. TG is combined with a truncated form of apolipoprotein B (Apo B48) as it is synthesised. This process produces chylomicrons that are secreted basolaterally into lymphatic lacteals. These newly secreted chylomicrons enter the circulation via the thoracic duct where they are remodelled by the transfer of additional apolipoproteins. Chylomicrons are then acted on by lipoprotein lipase located on the endothelium of tissue capillary beds to release fatty acids that may be used locally for energy or storage in tissues such as muscle or adipose tissue. The residual 'remnant' chylomicron particle is avidly cleared by receptors in the liver. Complete absorption of dietary lipids takes about 6–10 hours, so chylomicrons should not be detectable in the plasma after a 12-hour fast.

Intestinal cholesterol derived from the diet and biliary excretion is also absorbed in chylomicrons.

The effect of dietary cholesterol on plasma cholesterol level is less than might be expected, because intestinal cholesterol transport is limited beyond low to moderate intakes. Nevertheless, inhibition of intestinal cholesterol absorption can reduce plasma levels.

The main dietary determinant of plasma cholesterol is intake of saturated (and trans-unsaturated) fatty acids, which reduce the expression of receptors that remove cholesterol from the circulation (see below). Dietary determinants of plasma TG are complex. Excessive intakes of carbohydrate, fat or alcohol may each contribute to increased plasma TG by different mechanisms.

Endogenous lipid

In the fasting state, the liver is the major source of plasma lipids (Fig. 16.14). The liver may acquire lipids by uptake, synthesis or conversion from other macronutrients. These lipids are transported to other tissues by secretion of TG-rich very low-density lipoproteins (VLDL), which differ from chylomicrons in that they contain full-length apolipoprotein B100. Following secretion into the circulation, VLDL undergo a metabolic process similar to that of chylomicrons. Hydrolysis of VLDL TG releases fatty acids into tissues and converts VLDL into 'remnant' particles, referred to as intermediate-density lipoproteins (IDL). Most IDL are rapidly cleared by receptors in the liver, but some are processed by hepatic lipase. Materials other than apolipoprotein B100, free and esterified cholesterol are removed with the result that the particle is converted to a low-density lipoprotein (LDL).

LDL is a source of cholesterol for maintenance of cell and tissue homeostasis (Fig. 16.14). LDL cholesterol is internalised by receptor-mediated endocytosis via the LDL receptor. Delivery of cholesterol via this pathway down-regulates further expression of the LDL receptor gene and reduces the synthesis and activity of the rate-limiting enzyme for cholesterol synthesis, HMGCoA reductase. These negative feedback pathways, together with the modulation of cholesterol esterification, control the intra-cellular free cholesterol level within a narrow range.

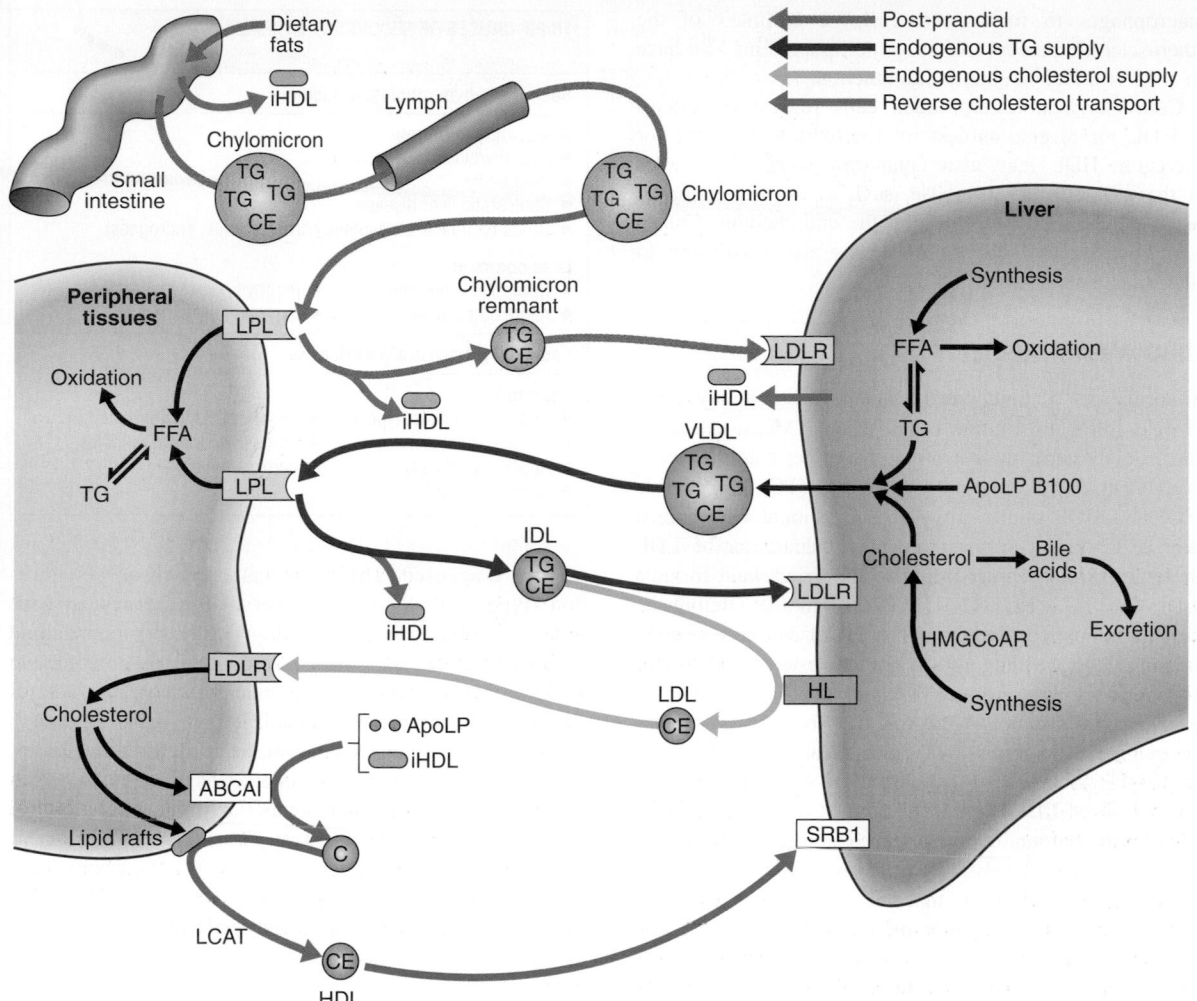

Fig. 16.14 Absorption, transport and storage of lipids. Pathways of lipid transport are shown; in addition cholesterol ester transfer protein exchanges triglyceride and cholesterol ester between VLDL/chylomicrons and iHDL/HDL. (ABCA1 = ATP-binding cassette A1; CE = cholesterol ester; FFA = free fatty acids; HDL = mature high-density lipoprotein; iHDL = immature high-density lipoprotein; HL = hepatic lipase; HMGCoAR = hydroxy-methyl-glutaryl-coenzyme A reductase; IDL= intermediate-density lipoprotein; LCAT = lecithin cholesterol acyl transferase; LDL = low-density lipoprotein; LDLR = low-density lipoprotein receptor (Apo B100 receptor); LPL = lipoprotein lipase; SRB1 = scavenger receptor B1; TG = triglyceride; VLDL = very low-density lipoprotein)

Reverse cholesterol transport

Peripheral tissues are further guarded against excessive cholesterol accumulation by high-density lipoproteins (HDL, Fig. 16.14). Lipid-poor apolipoprotein A1, which has been derived from the liver, intestine and the outer layer of chylomicrons and VLDL, accepts cellular cholesterol and phospholipid from a specific membrane transporter known as ATP-binding cassette A1 transporter. This produces small HDLs that are able to accept more free cholesterol from cholesterol-rich regions of the cell membrane that are known as 'rafts'. The esterification of cholesterol by lecithin cholesterol acyl transferase maintains an uptake gradient. HDLs release their cholesterol to the liver and other cholesterol-requiring tissues via the scavenger receptor B1.

HDL may transfer cholesterol to VLDL or chylomicrons in exchange for TG by the action of cholesterol ester transfer protein. When TG is elevated, this may reduce HDL-cholesterol. It may also affect LDL, resulting in 'small,

dense' LDL particles that are more atherogenic in the blood vessel wall. Animal species that lack cholesterol ester transfer protein are resistant to atherosclerosis, suggesting that this process may have a detrimental effect on progression of cardiovascular disease.

LIPIDS AND CARDIOVASCULAR DISEASE

Plasma lipoprotein levels are major modifiable risk factors for cardiovascular disease. Increased levels of atherogenic lipoproteins, especially LDL, but also IDL and possibly chylomicron remnants, contribute to the development of atherosclerosis (p. 578). Increased plasma concentration and reduced diameter favour subendothelial accumulation of these lipoproteins. Following chemical modifications such as oxidation, the lipoproteins are no longer cleared by normal mechanisms. They trigger a self-perpetuating inflammatory response during which they are taken up by macrophages to form foam cells—a hallmark of the atherosclerotic process. Atherogenic lipoproteins also have an adverse effect on endothelial function.

Conversely, cholesterol-laden cells release cholesterol to HDL for reverse cholesterol transport to the liver for excretion. HDL may also counteract some components of the inflammatory response, such as the expression of vascular adhesion molecules by the endothelium. Consequently, low HDL cholesterol levels also predispose to atherosclerosis.

LIPID MEASUREMENT

Abnormalities of lipid metabolism most commonly come to light following routine blood testing. Measurement of plasma cholesterol alone is not sufficient for comprehensive assessment. Levels of total cholesterol (TC), triglyceride (TG) and HDL cholesterol (HDL-C) should be obtained after a 12-hour fast to permit the calculation of LDL cholesterol (LDL-C) according to the Friedewald formula (LDL-C = TC – HDL-C – (TG/2.2) mmol/l). (Before the formula is applied, lipid levels in mg/dl can be converted to mmol/l by dividing by 38 for cholesterol and 88 for triglycerides.) The formula becomes unreliable when TG levels exceed 4 mmol/l (350 mg/dl). Non-fasting samples are unaffected in terms of TC and measured LDL-C, but they differ in terms of TG and HDL-C, and hence the calculation of LDL-C is invalidated. Consideration must be given to confounding factors such as recent illness, after which cholesterol levels temporarily decrease in proportion to severity. Measurements that will affect major decisions, such as initiation of drug therapy, should be confirmed with a repeat measurement.

Elevated TG, which is common in obesity, diabetes and insulin resistance (Chs 5 and 21), is frequently associated with low HDL and increased 'small, dense' LDL. Under these circumstances, LDL-C may underestimate risk. This is one situation in which measurement of apolipoprotein B may provide additional useful information.

PRESENTING PROBLEMS IN DISORDERS OF LIPIDS

Lipid measurements are usually performed for the following reasons: screening for primary or secondary prevention of cardiovascular disease; investigation of patients with clinical features of lipid disorders (Fig. 16.15); and testing relatives of patients with one of the single gene defects causing dyslipidaemia.

AETIOLOGY AND CLINICAL ASSESSMENT

The first step is to consider the effect of other diseases and drugs that may cause secondary lipid disturbances (Box 16.23). Overt or subclinical hypothyroidism (p. 750) may cause hypercholesterolaemia, so measurement of thyroid stimulating hormone is warranted in most cases, even in the absence of typical symptoms and signs. Following exclusion of secondary causes, primary lipid abnormalities

16.23 CAUSES OF SECONDARY HYPERLIPIDAEMIA
Secondary hypercholesterolaemia
Moderately common
• Hypothyroidism
• Pregnancy
• Cholestatic liver disease
• Drugs (diuretics, ciclosporin, corticosteroids, androgens)
Less common
• Nephrotic syndrome   • Porphyria
• Anorexia nervosa   • Hyperparathyroidism
Secondary hypertriglyceridaemia
Common
• Diabetes mellitus (type 2)   • Hepatocellular disease
• Chronic renal disease   • Drugs (β-blockers, retinoids,
• Abdominal obesity   corticosteroids)
• Excess alcohol

may be diagnosed. The numerical Fredrickson classification (types I to V) is no longer in use because it adds little to clinical decision-making. Instead, primary lipid abnormalities are classified according to the predominant lipid problem: hypercholesterolaemia, hypertriglyceridaemia or mixed hyperlipidaemia (Box 16.24). Although single gene disorders are encountered in all three categories, the most common cause is an interaction between numerous genetic and environmental factors (i.e. 'polygenic'). Clinical features (Fig. 16.15) of dyslipidaemia may occur in association with these categories.

Predominant hypercholesterolaemia

Polygenic hypercholesterolaemia is the most common cause of mild to moderate increase in LDL-C (Box 16.24). Physical signs such as corneal arcus and xanthelasma may be found in this as well as other forms of lipid disturbance (Fig. 16.15). Risk of cardiovascular disease is proportional to the degree of LDL-C elevation, together with other major risk factors, particularly HDL-C.

Familial hypercholesterolaemia (FH) causes moderate to severe hypercholesterolaemia with a prevalence of at least 0.2% in most populations. It is usually due to an autosomal dominantly inherited mutation of the LDL receptor gene, but a similar syndrome can arise with defects in the ligand-binding domain of apolipoprotein B100 or a sterol-sensitive protease known as NARC-1. Most patients with these abnormalities exhibit LDL levels that are approximately twice as high as in unaffected subjects of the same age and gender. Family history reveals that approximately 50% of each generation suffers hypercholesterolaemia, often with very premature cardiovascular disease. FH may be accompanied by xanthomas of the Achilles or extensor digitorum tendons (Fig. 16.15), which are strongly suggestive (but not pathognomonic) for FH. The onset of corneal arcus before age 40 is also suggestive of this condition.

In populations in which there is a 'founder gene' effect or consanguineous marriage, homozygous FH occasionally occurs, resulting in more extensive xanthomas and precocious cardiovascular disease in childhood. A recessive form of this condition has also been described recently.

16

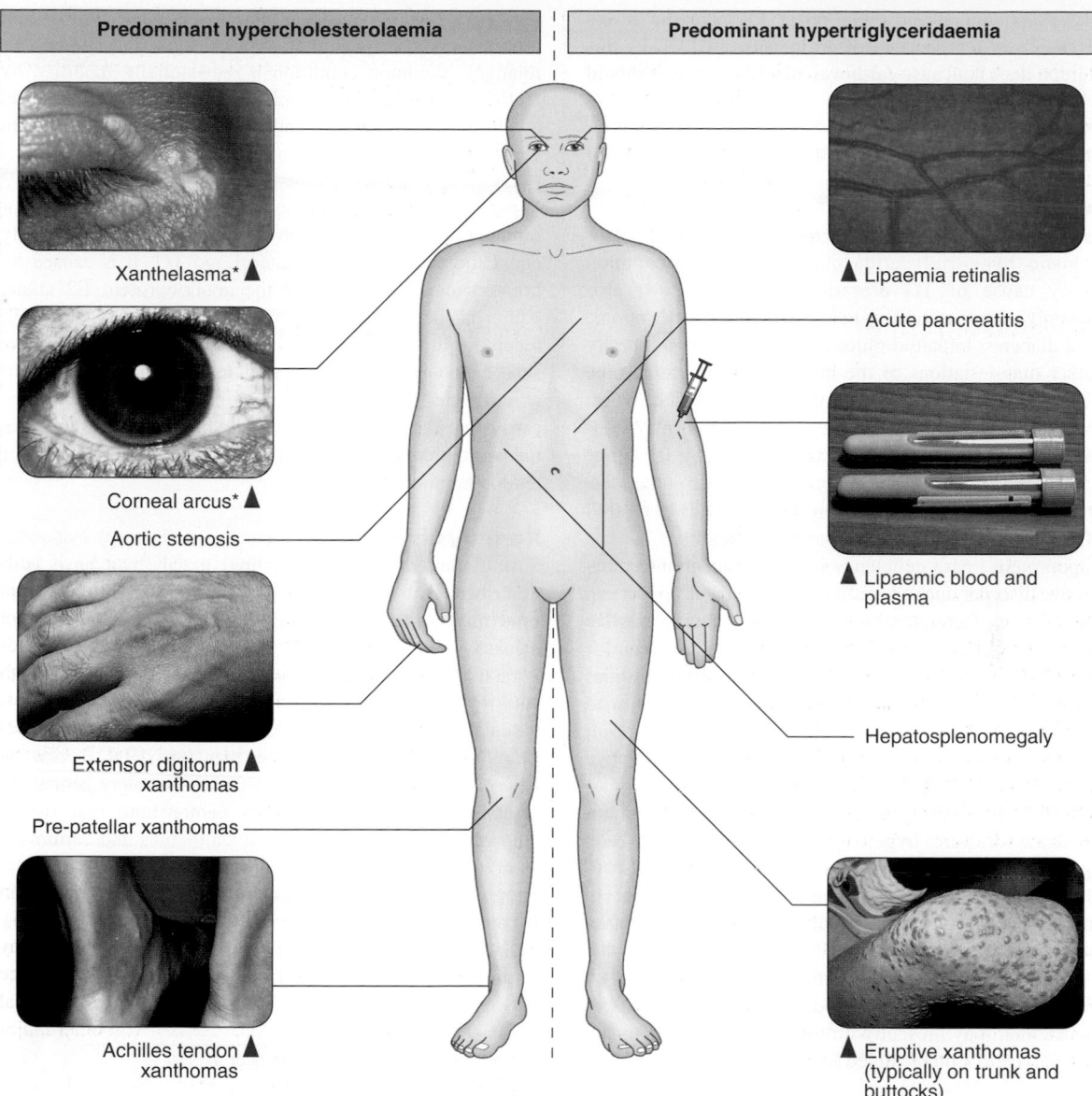

Fig. 16.15 **Clinical manifestations of hyperlipidaemia.** *Note that xanthelasma and corneal arcus may be non-specific, especially in later life.

16.24 CLASSIFICATION OF HYPERLIPIDAEMIA

Disease	Elevated lipid results	Elevated lipoprotein	CHD risk	Pancreatitis risk
Predominant hypercholesterolaemia (mostly polygenic)	TC ± TG	LDL ± VLDL	+	−
Familial hypercholesterolaemia (LDL receptor defect, defective Apo B100, defective NARC-1 protease)	TC ± TG	LDL ± VLDL	+++	−
Hyperalphalipoproteinaemia	TC	HDL	− −	−
Predominant hypertriglyceridaemia (mostly polygenic)	TG	VLDL ± LDL	Variable	+
Lipoprotein lipase deficiency	TG > TC	Chylo	?	+++
Familial hypertriglyceridaemia	TG + TC	VLDL + Chylo	?	++
Mixed hyperlipidaemia (mostly polygenic)	TC + TG	VLDL + LDL	Variable	+
Familial combined hyperlipidaemia*	TC and/or TG	LDL and VLDL	++	+
Dysbetalipoproteinaemia*	TC and/or TG	IDL	+++	+

* Familial combined hyperlipidaemia and dysbetalipoproteinaemia may also present as predominant hypercholesterolaemia or predominant hypertriglyceridaemia. (Chylo = chylomicrons; CHD = coronary heart disease; TC = total cholesterol; TG = triglycerides)

16

Hyperalphalipoproteinaemia refers to increased levels of HDL-C. In the absence of an increase in LDL-C, this condition does not cause cardiovascular disease, so it should not be regarded as pathological.

Familial combined hyperlipidaemia, and dysbetalipoproteinaemia, may present with the pattern of predominant hypercholesterolaemia ('mixed hyperlipidaemia' below).

Predominant hypertriglyceridaemia

Polygenic hypertriglyceridaemia is the most common primary cause of TG elevation (Box 16.24). It also commonly occurs secondary to excess alcohol, medications, type 2 diabetes, impaired glucose tolerance, central obesity or other manifestations of the insulin resistance syndrome (p. 813). It is often accompanied by post-prandial hyperlipidaemia and reduced HDL-C, both of which may contribute to cardiovascular risk. Excessive dietary fat intake or other exacerbating factors may precipitate a massive increase in TG levels, which, if they exceed 10 mmol/l (880 mg/dl), may pose a risk of acute pancreatitis.

Lipoprotein lipase deficiency is an infrequent autosomal recessive disorder due to hereditary deficiency of lipoprotein lipase or its co-factor, apolipoprotein C2. It causes massive hypertriglyceridaemia that is resistant to drug treatment. It may commence in childhood and is associated with episodes of acute abdominal pain and pancreatitis. In common with other causes of severe hypertriglyceridaemia, it may result in hepatosplenomegaly, lipaemia retinalis and eruptive xanthomas (Fig. 16.15).

Familial hypertriglyceridaemia refers to dominant inheritance of pure hypertriglyceridaemia. It has been suggested that it may represent a secondary response to impaired bile acid resorption and that it seems not to increase the risk of cardiovascular disease. On the other hand, it predisposes to levels of hypertriglyceridaemia that are sufficient to pose a risk of pancreatitis.

Familial combined hyperlipidaemia, and dysbetalipoproteinaemia, may present with the pattern of predominant hypertriglyceridaemia ('mixed hyperlipidaemia', below).

Mixed hyperlipidaemia

It is difficult to define the distinction between predominant hyperlipidaemias and mixed hyperlipidaemia quantitatively. The term 'mixed' usually implies the presence of hypertriglyceridaemia as well as an increase in LDL or IDL. Treatment of massive hypertriglyceridaemia may improve TG faster than cholesterol, thus mimicking mixed hyperlipidaemia.

Primary mixed hyperlipidaemia is usually polygenic and, like predominant hypertriglyceridaemia, often occurs in association with type 2 diabetes, impaired glucose tolerance, central obesity or other manifestations of the insulin resistance syndrome (p. 813). Both components of mixed hyperlipidaemia may contribute to the risk of cardiovascular disease.

Familial combined hyperlipidaemia is a dominantly inherited disorder caused by overproduction of atherogenic apolipoprotein B-containing lipoproteins. It results in elevation of cholesterol, TG or both in different family members at different times. It is associated with an increased risk of cardiovascular disease but it does not produce any pathognomonic physical signs. In practice, this relatively common condition is substantially modified by factors such as age and weight. It may not be a monogenic condition, but rather one end of a heterogeneous spectrum that overlaps with the insulin resistance syndrome.

Dysbetalipoproteinaemia (also referred to as type 3 hyperlipidaemia, broad-beta dyslipoproteinaemia or remnant hyperlipidaemia) involves accumulation of roughly equal molar levels of cholesterol and TG. It is caused by homozygous inheritance of the apolipoprotein E2 allele, which is the isoform least avidly recognised by the LDL receptor. In conjunction with other exacerbating factors such as obesity and diabetes, it leads to accumulation of atherogenic IDL and chylomicron remnants. Premature cardiovascular disease is common and it may also result in the formation of palmar xanthomas, tuberous xanthomas or tendon xanthomas.

Rare dyslipidaemias

Several rare disturbances of lipid metabolism have been described (Box 16.25). They provide important insights into lipid metabolism and its impact on risk of cardiovascular disease.

Fish eye disease and Apo A1 Milano demonstrate that very low HDL levels do not necessarily cause cardiovascular disease, but Apo A1 deficiency, Tangier disease and LCAT deficiency demonstrate that low HDL-C can be atherogenic under some circumstances. Sitosterolaemia and cerebrotendinous xanthomatosis demonstrate that sterols other than cholesterol can cause xanthomas and cardiovascular disease, while abetalipoproteinaemia and hypobetalipoproteinaemia suggest that low levels of apolipoprotein B-containing lipoproteins reduce the risk of cardiovascular disease at the expense of fat-soluble vitamin deficiency, leading to retinal lesions and peripheral neuropathy.

16.25 MISCELLANEOUS AND RARE FORMS OF HYPERLIPIDAEMIA		
Condition	Lipoprotein pattern	CVD risk
Tangier disease	Very low HDL, low TC	+
Apo AI deficiency	Very low HDL	+
Apo AI Milano	Very low HDL	−
Fish eye disease	Very low HDL, high TG	−
LCAT deficiency	Very low HDL, high TG	?
Sitosterolaemia	High plant sterols including sitosterol	+
Cerebrotendinous xanthomatosis	Bile acid defect (cholestanol)	+
(HDL = high-density lipoprotein; LCAT = lecithin cholesterolacyl transferase; TC = total cholesterol; TG = triglycerides)		

MANAGEMENT OF DYSLIPIDAEMIA

Lipid-lowering therapies have a key role in the secondary and primary prevention of cardiovascular diseases (p. 580). Assessment of absolute risk, treatment of all modifiable

16

risk factors and optimisation of lifestyle factors, especially diet and exercise, are central to management in all cases.

Patients with the greatest absolute risk of cardiovascular disease derive the greatest benefit from treatment. Public health organisations recommend thresholds for the introduction of lipid-lowering therapy based on the identification of patients in very high-risk categories or those calculated to be at high absolute risk according to algorithms or tables such as the Joint British Societies Coronary Risk Prediction Chart (see Appendix). These tables, which are based on large epidemiological studies, should be re-calibrated for the local population, if possible. In general, patients who already have cardiovascular disease, diabetes mellitus or an absolute risk of cardiovascular disease of greater than 20% in the ensuing 10 years, are arbitrarily regarded as having sufficient risk to justify drug treatment.

Public health organisations also recommend target levels for patients receiving drug treatment. High-risk patients should aim for HDL-C > 1 mmol/l (38 mg/dl) and fasting TG < 2 mmol/l (~180 mg/dl), whilst target levels for LDL-C have been reduced from 2.5 to 2.0 mmol/l (76 mg/dl) or less. In general, total cholesterol should be < 5 mmol/l (190 mg/dl) during treatment, and < 4 mmol/l (~150 mg/dl) in high-risk patients and in secondary prevention of cardiovascular disease.

Non-pharmacological treatment
Patients with lipid abnormalities should receive medical advice and, if necessary, dietary counselling to:

- reduce intake of saturated and trans-unsaturated fat to less than 7–10% of total energy
- reduce the intake of cholesterol to less than 250 mg/day
- replace sources of saturated fat and cholesterol with alternative foods such as lean meat, low-fat dairy products, polyunsaturated spreads and low glycaemic index carbohydrates
- reduce energy-dense foods such as fats and soft drinks, whilst increasing activity and exercise to achieve stable or negative energy balance (i.e. weight maintenance or weight loss)
- increase consumption of cardioprotective and nutrient-dense foods such as vegetables, unrefined carbohydrates, fish, pulses, legumes, fruit etc.
- adjust alcohol consumption, reducing intake if excessive or if associated with hypertension, hypertriglyceridaemia or central obesity
- achieve additional benefits with supplementary intake of foods containing lipid-lowering nutrients such as n-3 fatty acids, dietary fibre and plant sterols.

Response to diet is usually apparent within 3–4 weeks but dietary adjustment may need to be introduced gradually. Hyperlipidaemia in general, and hypertriglyceridaemia in particular, can be very responsive to these measures. Explanation, encouragement and other measures should be undertaken to reinforce patient compliance. Even minor weight loss can substantially reduce cardiovascular risk, especially in centrally obese patients (p. 113).

All other modifiable cardiovascular risk factors should be assessed and treated. Where possible, intercurrent drug treatments that adversely affect the lipid profile should be replaced.

Pharmacological management
The main diagnostic categories provide a useful framework for management and the selection of first-line pharmacological treatment (Fig. 16.16).

Predominant hypercholesterolaemia
Predominant hypercholesterolaemia is treated with one or more of the cholesterol-lowering drugs.

16

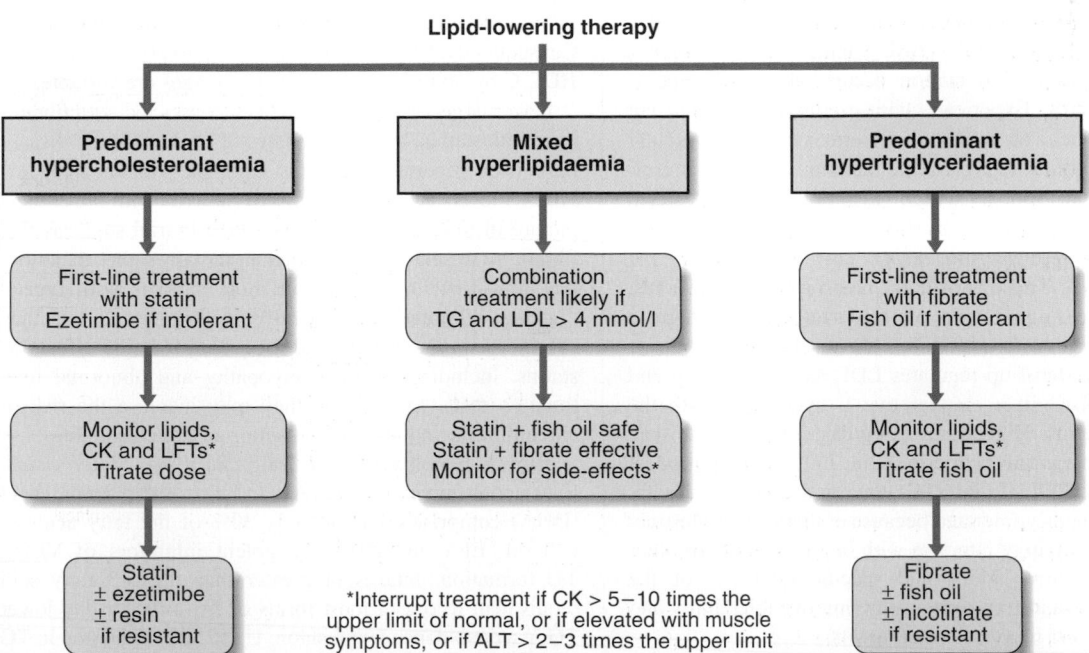

Fig. 16.16 Flow chart for the drug treatment of hyperlipidaemia. To convert TG in mmol/l to mg/dl, multiply by 88. To convert LDL-cholesterol in mmol/l to mg/dl, multiply by 38. (CK = creatinine kinase; LDL = low-density lipoprotein; LFTs = liver function tests; TG = triglyceride)

HMGCoA reductase inhibitors (statins). Statins inhibit cholesterol synthesis, thereby up-regulating activity of the LDL receptor. This increases clearance of LDL and its precursor, IDL, thereby causing a secondary reduction in LDL synthesis. As a result, statins reduce LDL-C by up to 60%, reduce TG by up to 40% and increase HDL-C by up to 10%. They also reduce the concentration of intermediate metabolites such as isoprenes, which may lead to other effects such as suppression of the inflammatory response. There is clear evidence of protection against stroke, and total and coronary mortality, as well as a reduction in cardiovascular events in high-risk patients (Box 16.26).

Statins are generally well tolerated and serious side-effects are rare (well below 2%). Myalgia, asymptomatic increase in creatine kinase (CK), myositis and, infrequently, rhabdomyolysis are the most important category, along with liver function test abnormalities. Side-effects are more likely in patients who are elderly, debilitated or receiving other drugs that interfere with statin degradation, which usually involves cytochrome P450 3A4.

16.26 BENEFITS OF TREATING PATIENTS WITH HYPERCHOLESTEROLAEMIA WITH STATINS **EBM**

'Meta-analysis of major RCTs involving over 90 000 subjects receiving statins for an average of 5 years showed reduced coronary mortality of 19% (95% confidence interval 15–24%), stroke 17% (12–22%) and total mortality 12% (9–16%) per 1 mmol/l reduction in LDL-C.'

- Baigent C, et al. Lancet 2005; 366:1267–1278.

Cholesterol absorption inhibitors, such as ezetimibe. These inhibit the intestinal mucosal transporter NPC1L1 that absorbs dietary and biliary cholesterol. Depletion of hepatic cholesterol up-regulates hepatic LDL receptor activity. This mechanism of action is synergistic with the effect of statins. Monotherapy with the standard 10 mg/day dose reduces LDL-C by 15–20%. Slightly greater (17–25%) incremental LDL-C reduction occurs when ezetimibe is added to statins. Experience with ezetimibe is limited but it seems to be well tolerated. Its effect on cardiovascular disease endpoints is yet to be determined. Plant sterol-supplemented foods, which also reduce cholesterol absorption, lower LDL-C by 7–15%.

Bile acid sequestering resins, such as colestyramine and colestipol. These prevent the reabsorption of bile acids, thereby increasing de novo bile acid synthesis from hepatic cholesterol. As with ezetimibe, the resultant depletion of hepatic cholesterol up-regulates LDL receptor activity and reduces LDL-C in a manner that is synergistic with the action of statins. High doses (24 g/day colestyramine) can achieve substantial reductions in LDL-C and modest increases in HDL-C, but TG may rise. Resins are safe, but they are poorly tolerated because of their gastrointestinal effects and they may interfere with bio-availability of other drugs. New formulations and specific inhibitors of the intestinal bile acid transporter may improve tolerability and rekindle interest in this class of agents.

Nicotinic acid (vitamin B₃). In pharmacological doses, this reduces peripheral fatty acid release with the result that cholesterol and TG decline whilst HDL-C increases.

Flushing occurs universally, and other side-effects include gastric irritation, liver function disturbances and exacerbation of gout and hyperglycaemia. Slow-release formulations and low-dose aspirin may reduce flushing. Trials suggest a beneficial effect on atherosclerosis and cardiovascular events.

Routine treatment of predominant hypercholesterolaemia generally requires continuation of diet plus the use of a statin in sufficient doses to achieve target LDL-C levels. Therapy may have to be interrupted or ceased if there are clear-cut muscle side-effects, CK elevation beyond 10 times the upper limit of normal, or sustained ALT elevation beyond 2–3 times the upper limit of normal (and not accounted for by fatty liver, p. 971). Patients who do not reach LDL targets on the highest tolerated statin dose may receive ezetimibe, plant sterols, nicotinic acid or resins, and these agents may also be added when patients are intolerant of statins. Nicotinic acid may also be used as an alternative in statin intolerance. It is also very effective in combination with a statin, but caution is required because the risk of side-effects is increased. Post-menopausal oestrogen replacement therapy, which may reduce LDL-C and increase HDL-C and TG, is no longer recommended for cardiovascular disease prevention (p. 766).

Predominant hypertriglyceridaemia

Predominant hypertriglyceridaemia is treated with one of the triglyceride-lowering drugs (Fig. 16.16).

Fibrates. These stimulate peroxisome proliferator activated receptor (PPAR)-alpha, which controls the expression of gene products that mediate the metabolism of triglyceride and HDL. As a result, synthesis of fatty acids, triglyceride and VLDL is reduced whilst that of lipoprotein lipase, which catabolises TG, is enhanced. In addition, the promotor regions of genes such as apolipoprotein A1 and ATP binding cassette A1 are up-regulated, leading to increased reverse cholesterol transport via HDL. Consequently, fibrates reduce TG by up to 50% and increase HDL-C by up to 20%, but LDL-C changes are variable.

Fewer large-scale trials have been conducted with fibrates than with statins, but reduced rates of cardiovascular disease have been reported in studies amongst patients with low HDL-C levels and in subgroups of patients with the clinical picture of insulin resistance. The FIELD trial suggests that fibrates represent selective adjuvant therapy rather than first-line lipid-lowering therapy in most patients with type 2 diabetes. Fibrates are generally well tolerated but they exhibit a similar profile and frequency of side-effects as statins, including myalgia, myopathy and abnormal liver function tests. In addition, they may increase the risk of cholelithiasis and prolong the action of anticoagulants.

Highly polyunsaturated long-chain n-3 fatty acids. Eicosapentaenoic acid (EPA) and docosahexaenoic acid (DHA) comprise approximately 30% of the fatty acids in fish oil. EPA and DHA are potent inhibitors of VLDL TG formation. Intakes of greater than 2 g n-3 fatty acid (equivalent to 6 g of most forms of fish oil) per day lower TG in a dose-dependent fashion. Up to 50% reduction in TG may be achieved with 15 g fish oil per day or fish oil concentrates. Changes in LDL-C and HDL-C are variable. Fish oil fatty acids have also been shown to inhibit platelet

16

16.27 MANAGEMENT OF HYPERLIPIDAEMIA IN THE ELDERLY

- **Prevalence of atherosclerotic cardiovascular disease:** greatest in old age.
- **Associated cardiovascular risk:** lipid levels become less predictive, as do other risk factors apart from age itself.
- **Benefit of statin therapy:** maintained up to the age of 80 years but evidence is lacking beyond this.
- **Life expectancy and statin therapy:** lives saved by intervention are associated with shorter life expectancy than in younger patients, and so the impact of statins on quality-adjusted life years is smaller in old age.

aggregation and improve models of ventricular arrhythmia. Dietary and pharmacological trials indicate that n-3 fatty acids reduce mortality from coronary heart disease. Fish oils appear to be safe and well tolerated.

Patients with predominant hypertriglyceridaemia who do not respond to lifestyle intervention can be treated with either fibrates, fish oil or nicotinic acid, depending on individual response and tolerance. If target levels are not achieved, the fibrates or nicotinic acid and fish oil can be combined. Massive hypertriglyceridaemia may require more aggressive limitation of dietary fat intake (< 10–20% energy as fat). Any degree of insulin deficiency should be corrected because insulin is required for optimal activity of lipoprotein lipase. The initial target for patients with massive hypertriglyceridaemia is TG < 10 mmol/l (880 mg/dl), to reduce the risk of acute pancreatitis.

Mixed hyperlipidaemia

Mixed hyperlipidaemia can be difficult to treat. Statins alone are less effective first-line therapy once fasting TG exceeds approximately 4 mmol/l (~350 mg/dl). Fibrates alone are first-line therapy for dysbetalipoproteinaemia, but they may not control the cholesterol component in other forms of mixed hyperlipidaemia. Combination therapy is often required. Statin plus fish oil is relatively safe and effective when TG is not too high and in future fibrate plus ezetimibe may be effective. Statin plus nicotinic acid or statin plus fibrate is effective, but the risk of myopathy is greater.

Monitoring of therapy

The effect of drug therapy can be assessed after 6 weeks (12 weeks for fibrates), and it is prudent to review side-effects, lipid response, CK and liver function tests at this stage. Follow-up should encourage continued compliance (especially diet and exercise), monitoring for side-effects and cardiovascular symptoms or signs, measurement of weight, blood pressure and lipids as well as review of absolute cardiovascular disease risk status.

Some special issues relevant to treating hyperlipidaemia in the elderly are given in Box 16.27.

DISORDERS OF HAEM METABOLISM—THE PORPHYRIAS

The porphyrias are rare disorders of the haem biosynthetic pathway (Fig. 16.17). Most of the described forms are due to partial enzyme deficiencies with a dominant mode of inheritance, and all have been associated with specific mutations. They are commonly categorised as either hepatic or erythropoietic, depending on whether the major site of excess porphyrin production is in the liver or the red cell.

The porphyrias are characterised by a low penetrance in the order of 25%. Environmental factors are important in modifying disease expression in some forms of porphyria. In the most common of these conditions, porphyria cutanea tarda (PCT), these include alcohol, excess iron, exogenous oestrogens and exposure to various chemicals, while many cases are associated with hepatitis C infection.

Clinical features

The clinical features of porphyria fall into two broad categories. Photosensitive skin manifestations, attributable to excess production and accumulation of porphyrins in the skin, occur in PCT, congenital erythropoietic porphyria (CEP), hereditary coproporphyria (HCP), variegate porphyria (VP) and erythrohepatic protoporphyria (EHP). Pain, erythema, bullae, erosions, hirsutism and hyperpigmentation are characteristic, and occur predominantly on areas of the skin that are exposed to sunlight (Fig. 27.6, p. 1272). The skin also becomes especially sensitive to damage from mild trauma.

The other pattern of presentation is with an acute relapsing and remitting neurological syndrome, characteristic of acute intermittent porphyria (AIP), HCP, VP and ALA dehydratase deficiency (plumboporphyria). This presents invariably with acute abdominal pain together with features of autonomic dysfunction such as tachycardia, hypertension and constipation. Other frequent associations include neuropsychiatric manifestations, hyponatraemia due to inappropriate ADH release (p. 430), and acute neuropathy (p. 1246), which is usually motor, and can result in some cases in respiratory failure. The forms HCP and VP can present with either symptom pattern or with a mixed picture.

There is no proven explanation for the episodic pattern of these attacks. However, they are often provoked by drugs such as anticonvulsants, sulphonamides, oestrogen and progesterone, especially the oral contraceptive pill, or by alcohol and even fasting. In a significant number of cases, no precipitant can be identified.

Diagnosis

The diagnosis of porphyria and categorisation into various forms has traditionally relied on the pattern of the porphyrins and porphyrin precursors found in blood, urine and faeces (Box 16.28). This is straightforward when the metabolites are significantly elevated, but this is not always the case.

More recently, measurement of the enzymes that are deficient in the various porphyrias has provided further important diagnostic information. However, there is often considerable overlap between enzyme activities in normal and abnormal populations. Furthermore, some of the specific enzymes occur in the cell mitochondria, for which it is difficult to obtain suitable specimens for analysis.

The genes of the haem biosynthetic pathway have now been characterised. This has made it possible to identify all affected individuals in families with known mutations, a

16

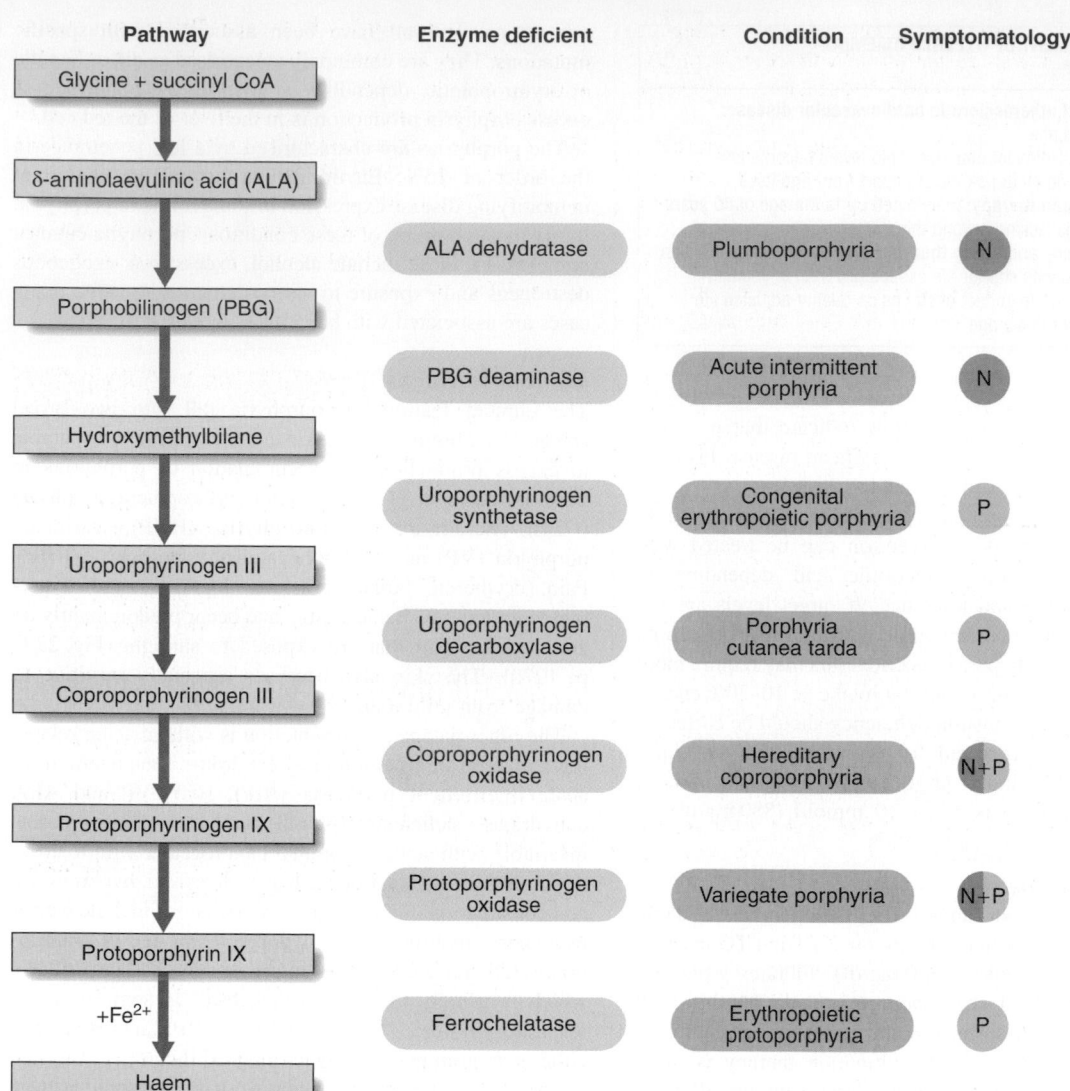

Fig. 16.17 Haem biosynthetic pathway and enzyme defects responsible for the porphyrias. (N = neurovisceral; P = photosensitive)

16

16.28 DIAGNOSTIC BIOCHEMICAL FINDINGS IN THE PORPHYRIAS

Condition	Elevated porphyrins and precursors		
	Blood	Urine	Faeces
ALA dehydratase deficiency (plumboporphyria)	Proto IX*	ALA, Copro III*	
Acute intermittent porphyria (AIP)		ALA, PBG	
Congenital erythropoietic porphyria (CEP)	Uro I	Uro I	Copro I
Porphyria cutanea tarda (PCT)		Uro I	Isocopro
Hereditary coproporphyria (HCP)		ALA, PBG, Copro III	Copro III
Variegate porphyria (VP)		ALA, PBG, Copro III	Proto IX
Erythrohepatic protoporphyria (EHP)	Proto IX		Proto IX

* The paradoxical rise in coproporphyrin III (Copro III) and protoporphyrin (Proto) in this very rare condition is poorly understood.
Refer to Fig. 16.17 above for metabolic pathways. Uro I (uroporphyrin I) and Copro I (coproporphyrin I) are metabolites of hydroxymethylbilane.
Isocopro (isocoproporphyrin) is a metabolite of uroporphyrinogen III. Copro III (coproporphyrin III) is a metabolite of coproporphyrinogen III.

significant advance considering that penetrance of porphyria is low and most attacks do not occur without an identified precipitant. At this time, well over 100 mutations have been found to cause AIP alone.

In the clinical situation where there are active cutaneous manifestations of porphyria, or where a subject presents in an acute attack, metabolite excretory patterns are always grossly abnormal and diagnostic of the particular porphyria. Finding normal metabolites in this circumstance effectively excludes porphyria. Furthermore, metabolites usually remain abnormal for long periods after an acute attack, and in some individuals never return to normal.

The diagnosis may not be so straightforward in patients in remission, and investigation can be very difficult in patients with a positive family history but no clinical or metabolite manifestations. Porphyria rarely manifests before puberty, nor can it be readily diagnosed from metabolite patterns after menopause. In those circumstances, measurement of enzyme activities related to the possible porphyria, and especially finding a disease-specific mutation, can now clarify the situation.

Management

For patients predisposed to neurovisceral attacks, general management includes avoidance of any agents that are known to precipitate acute porphyria. Specific management includes intravenous glucose, as provision of 5000 kilojoules per day can terminate acute attacks through a reduction in ALA synthetase activity. More recently, administration of haem (in various forms such as haematin or haem arginate) has been shown to reduce metabolite excretory rates, relieve pain and lead to accelerated recovery. Cyclical acute attacks in women sometimes respond to suppression of the menstrual cycle using gonadotrophin-releasing hormone analogues.

There are few specific or effective measures to treat the photosensitive manifestations. The primary goal is to avoid sun exposure and skin trauma. Barrier sun creams containing zinc or titanium oxide are the most effective products. New colourless zinc creams have improved patient acceptance. Beta-carotene is used in some patients with EHP with some efficacy. In PCT, a course of venesections to remove iron can result in long-lasting clinical and biochemical remission, especially if exposure to identified precipitants such as alcohol or oestrogens is reduced. Alternatively, a prolonged course of chloroquine therapy may be effective.

FURTHER INFORMATION

Books and journal articles

Anderson KE, Sassa S, Bishop D, et al. Disorders of heme biosynthesis: X-linked sideroblastic anemia and the porphyrias. In: Scriver CR, Beaudet AL, Sly WS, eds. The metabolic and molecular basis of inherited disease. 8th edn. New York: McGraw Hill; 2000, pp 2961–3062.

Burtis CA, Ashwood ER, Bruns D, eds. Tietz textbook of clinical chemistry and molecular diagnostics. 4th edn. Philadelphia: WB Saunders; 2005.

Davidson MH, Toth PP. Combination therapy in the management of complex dyslipidemias. Current Opinion in Lipidology 2004; 15:423–431.

Field MJ, Pollock CA, Harris DC. The renal system. Edinburgh: Churchill Livingstone; 2001.

Gotto AM, Pownall HJ. Manual of lipid disorders: reducing the risk for coronary heart disease. 3rd edn. Baltimore: Lippincott Williams & Wilkins; 2002.

Rose BD, Post TW. Clinical physiology of acid–base and electrolyte disorders. 5th edn. New York: McGraw-Hill; 2001.

Websites

www.kidneyatlas.org *Atlas of Diseases of Kidney (see especially Volume 1, Section 1: Disorders of water, electrolytes and acid–base).*

www.lipidsonline.org

www.ncbi.nlm.nih.gov/entrez/query.fcgi?db=OMIM *Online Mendelian inheritance in man (OMIM).*

16

J. GODDARD
A.N. TURNER
A.D. CUMMING
L.H. STEWART

Kidney and urinary tract disease

CLINICAL EXAMINATION OF THE KIDNEY AND URINARY TRACT

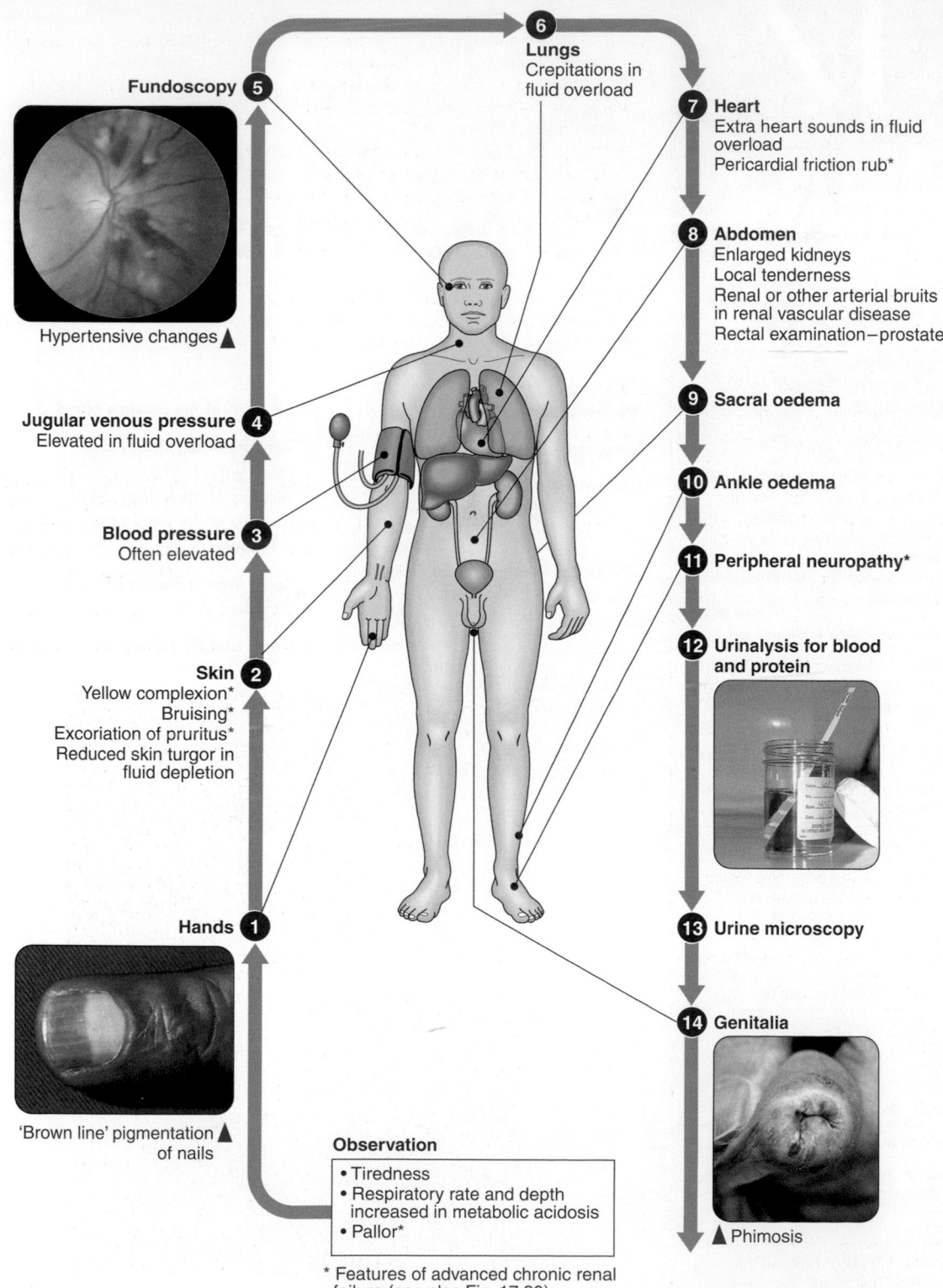

6 Lungs
Creptations in
fluid overload

Fundoscopy 5

Hypertensive changes ▲

7 Heart
Extra heart sounds in fluid
overload
Pericardial friction rub*

8 Abdomen
Enlarged kidneys
Local tenderness
Renal or other arterial bruits
in renal vascular disease
Rectal examination—prostate

Jugular venous pressure 4
Elevated in fluid overload

9 Sacral oedema

10 Ankle oedema

Blood pressure 3
Often elevated

11 Peripheral neuropathy*

**12 Urinalysis for blood
and protein**

Skin 2
Yellow complexion*
Bruising*
Excoriation of pruritus*
Reduced skin turgor in
fluid depletion

13 Urine microscopy

Hands 1

14 Genitalia

'Brown line' pigmentation ▲
of nails

Observation
- Tiredness
- Respiratory rate and depth
  increased in metabolic acidosis
- Pallor*

▲ Phimosis

* Features of advanced chronic renal
  failure (see also Fig. 17.20)

17

Diseases of the kidneys and urinary tract are often clinically 'silent'. Detection then depends on biochemical testing, e.g. measurement of plasma creatinine or testing of urine for abnormal constituents. Severe renal disease may present with non-specific symptoms, e.g. tiredness or breathlessness due to renal failure and associated anaemia, or oedema due to fluid retention. In end-stage renal failure, a wide range of physical signs may be present, including some iatrogenic features, as seen opposite. In less severe disease, physical findings may be few.

CARDINAL SYMPTOMS OF DISEASE OF THE KIDNEYS AND URINARY TRACT

Lower urinary tract symptoms

- Dysuria, frequency, urgency —lower urinary tract infection
- Impaired urinary flow, hesitancy, dribbling of urine, incomplete emptying of bladder—bladder outflow obstruction
- Urinary retention, incontinence/enuresis —sphincter or bladder wall dysfunction

Upper urinary tract symptoms

- Loin pain/tenderness—renal infection, renal infarction or rarely obstruction and glomerulonephritis
- Renal or ureteric colic—severe loin pain due to acute obstruction of the renal pelvis and ureter by calculus or blood clot; may radiate to the iliac fossa, groin and genitalia

Abnormal urine volume

- Anuria or oliguria—acute renal failure or obstruction to the flow of urine
- Polyuria or nocturia—failure of the kidneys to concentrate urine (e.g. diabetes insipidus, chronic renal failure)

Abnormal urinary constituents

- Proteinuria—suggests glomerular disease; massive proteinuria causes oedema
- Haematuria—disease anywhere in the urinary tract

Hypertension

- Acute or chronic parenchymal disease or renovascular disease

Uraemia

- A group of symptoms and signs of advanced renal failure

Diseases of the testes and epididymis

- Local swelling, pain and tenderness sometimes causing abdominal pain, inflammation and torsion

⑧ ABDOMEN

Technique for palpating the kidneys

- Lie the patient flat with the abdominal muscles relaxed.
- Use both hands—place one hand posteriorly just below the lower ribs and the other anteriorly over the upper quadrant.
- Push the two hands towards each other as the patient breathes out.
- Then feel for the lower pole of the kidney moving down between the hands as the patient breathes in.
- If palpable, push the kidney backwards and forwards between the two hands ('ballotting'). This helps to confirm that it is the kidney.
- Assess the size, surface and consistency of a palpable kidney; e.g. polycystic kidneys are often massively enlarged with an irregular, nodular surface.

The right kidney, and occasionally the lower pole of the left kidney, may be palpable in normal slim adults. Kidneys may be palpably enlarged in: polycystic kidney disease, hydronephrosis/pyonephrosis, solitary cyst, compensatory hypertrophy in a single kidney, renal tumours and renal amyloid. Local tenderness may reflect infection or inflammation.

Possible findings

- Transplanted kidney—palpable in the iliac fossa, with an overlying scar.
- Distension of the bladder—smooth midline mass arising from the pelvis, dull to percussion.
- Arterial bruits—heard on either side of the epigastrium. May arise from renal artery stenosis; there is usually also evidence of vascular disease elsewhere.
- Inspection of the male genitalia—looking particularly for testicular masses.
- Rectal examination—assesses extent and nature of prostatic enlargement. Benign enlargement is characteristically smooth and regular; an enlarged, hard, irregular prostate suggests prostatic cancer.

⑬ URINE MICROSCOPY

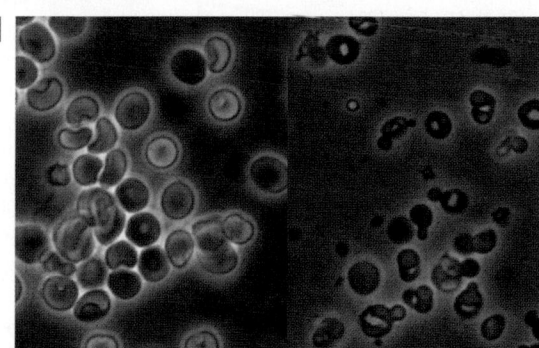

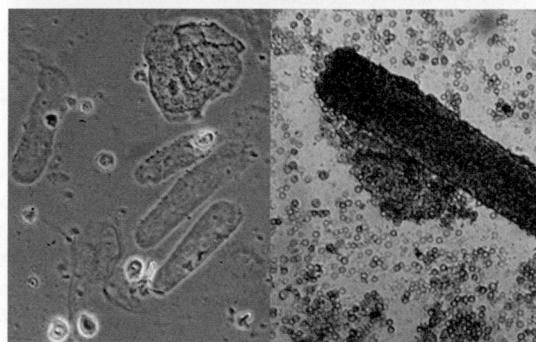

Urine microscopy. A Phase contrast images of red blood cells (× 400) showing on the right glomerular bleeding with many dysmorphic forms including acanthocytes (teardrop forms), and on the left bleeding from lower in the urinary tract. B On the left, phase contrast images show hyaline casts, a normal feature of urine (× 160). On the right, numerous red cells and a large red cell cast in acute glomerular inflammation (× 100, not phase contrast).

17

Renal medicine ranges from the management of common conditions (e.g. urinary tract infection) to the use of complex technology to replace renal function (e.g. dialysis and transplantation). There are close links with the surgical specialties of urology and transplantation. This chapter describes the common disorders of the kidneys and urinary tract which are encountered in everyday practice, as well as giving an overview of the highly specialised field of renal replacement therapy. Selective disorders of renal tubular function, which manifest themselves by alterations in electrolyte and acid–base balance, are described in Chapter 16.

FUNCTIONAL ANATOMY, PHYSIOLOGY AND INVESTIGATIONS

RENAL AND URINARY TRACT ANATOMY AND FUNCTION

THE KIDNEYS

Functions of the kidneys

In health, the volume and composition of body fluids are tightly regulated and the kidneys are largely responsible. This is achieved by making large volumes of an ultrafiltrate of plasma (120 ml/min, 170 litres/day) at the glomerulus, and selectively reabsorbing components of this ultrafiltrate at points along the nephron. The rates of filtration and reabsorption are under the control of many hormonal and haemodynamic signals.

Some metabolites either are not reabsorbed from the filtrate, or are actively secreted into it. The kidney is primarily responsible for excretion of many metabolic breakdown products (including ammonia, urea and creatinine from protein, and uric acid from nucleic acids), drugs and toxins.

In addition, the kidney has a number of hormonal functions. Three of these are particularly important:

- The kidney is the main source of erythropoietin, which is produced by interstitial peritubular cells in response to hypoxia. Replacement of erythropoietin reverses the anaemia of chronic renal failure (p. 488).
- The kidney is essential for vitamin D metabolism; it hydroxylates 25-hydroxycholecalciferol to the active form, 1,25-dihydroxycholecalciferol. Failure of this process contributes to the hypocalcaemia and bone disease of chronic renal failure (p. 490).
- Renin is secreted from the juxtaglomerular apparatus in response to reduced afferent arteriolar pressure, stimulation of sympathetic nerves, and changes in sodium content of fluid in the distal convoluted tubule at the macula densa. Renin generates angiotensin II (Fig. 18.26, p. 549), which causes aldosterone release from the adrenal cortex, constricts the efferent arteriole of the glomerulus and thereby increases glomerular filtration pressure (Fig. 17.1D). Angiotensin II also induces systemic vasoconstriction. By these mechanisms, the kidneys 'defend' circulating blood volume, blood pressure and glomerular filtration during circulatory shock. However, the same mechanisms lead to systemic hypertension in renal ischaemia.

Anatomy of the kidneys

Adult kidneys are 11–14 cm (three lumbar vertebral bodies) in length, and are located retroperitoneally on either side of the aorta and inferior vena cava. The right kidney is usually a few centimetres lower because the liver lies above it. Both kidneys rise and descend several centimetres with respiration.

Each kidney contains ~1 million functional units, or 'nephrons'. These consist of the glomerulus (where filtration of plasma occurs), proximal convoluted tubule, loop of Henle and distal convoluted tubule (where selective reabsorption of fluid and solutes from the filtrate occurs), and the collecting duct (Fig. 16.2, p. 422). The collecting ducts of multiple nephrons drain into the renal pelvis and ureter (Fig. 17.1B). There is a rich blood supply (20–25% of cardiac output), although there is considerable physiological variation in renal blood flow. Intralobular branches of the renal artery give rise to the glomerular afferent arterioles which supply the capillaries within the glomerulus. The efferent arteriole, leading from the glomerulus, supplies the distal nephron and medulla in a 'portal' circulation.

Glomeruli

The glomerulus contains three main cell types: endothelial cells lining the glomerular capillaries, epithelial cells and mesangial cells (Fig. 17.1D). Mesangial cells lie in the central region of the glomerulus. They have similarities to vascular smooth muscle cells (e.g. contractility), but also some macrophage-like properties.

Filtration occurs across the glomerular basement membrane (GBM), produced by fusion of the basement membranes of epithelial and endothelial cells. The glomerular capillary endothelial cells contain pores (fenestrae) which allow access of circulating molecules to the underlying GBM. On the outer side of the GBM, glomerular epithelial cells (podocytes) put out multiple long foot processes which interdigitate with those of adjacent epithelial cells (Fig. 17.1E). As well as maintaining the filtration barrier, podocytes are involved in the regulation of filtration and of GBM turnover.

The filtration barrier at the glomerulus is normally almost absolute to proteins the size of albumin (67 kDa) or larger, while proteins of 20 kDa or smaller are able to filter freely. Between these sizes the ability of individual molecules to cross the GBM is influenced by their shape and charge. Anionic (negatively charged) proteins are relatively less freely filtered than cationic proteins. Little lipid is filtered.

Filtration pressure at the GBM is controlled by afferent and efferent arteriolar tone. Autoregulation maintains a constant glomerular filtration rate (GFR) by altering this arteriolar tone over a wide range of systemic blood pressure and renal perfusion pressure. In response to a reduction in perfusion pressure, angiotensin II mediates constriction of the efferent arteriole, which restores filtration pressure (see above).

Tubules and interstitium

Tubular cells are polarised, with a brush border (proximal tubular cells) and specialised functions at both basal and apical surfaces. As described on pages 422–423, different

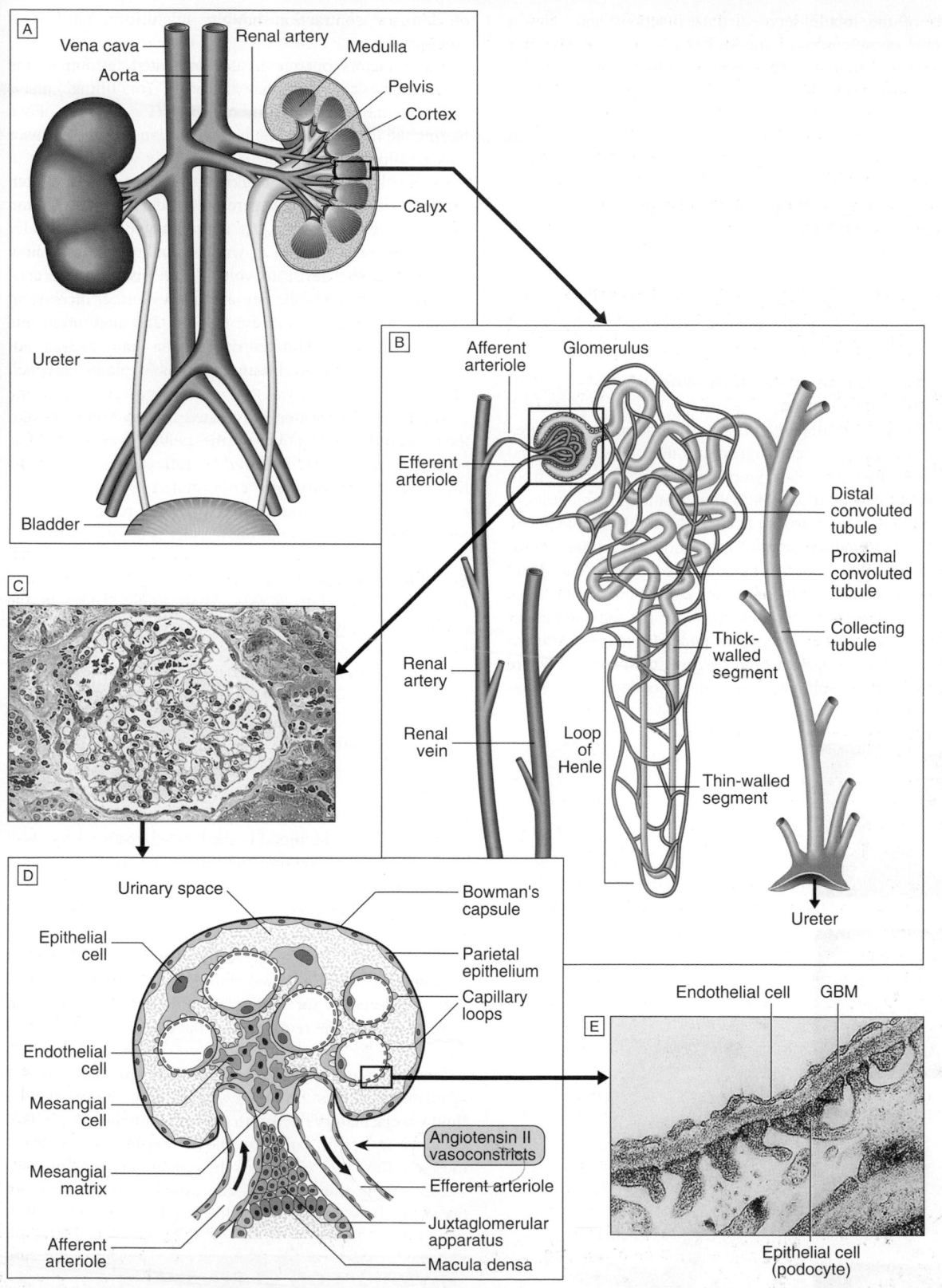

Fig. 17.1 Functional anatomy of the kidney. Ⓐ Anatomical relationships of the kidney. Ⓑ A single nephron. For the functions of different segments, see Figures 16.2 and 16.3, pages 422–423. Ⓒ Histology of a normal glomerulus. Ⓓ Schematic cross-section of a glomerulus showing five capillary loops, to illustrate structure and show cell types. Ⓔ Electron micrograph of the filtration barrier. (GBM = glomerular basement membrane)

17

parts of the tubule serve distinct functions and carry a specific complement of transporter, channel and receptor molecules. Interstitial cells between tubules are less well understood. Fibroblast-like cells in the cortex produce erythropoietin in response to hypoxia. In the medulla, lipid-laden interstitial cells are believed to be important in prostaglandin production.

COLLECTING SYSTEM AND LOWER URINARY TRACT

The key functions of this part of the urinary system (Fig. 17.2) are to allow free passage of urine to the bladder, and to store urine in the bladder for controlled voiding (i.e. to maintain urinary 'continence').

Mechanisms of micturition and urinary continence

Continence is dependent on anatomical structures (Fig. 17.2), and on neurological and muscle (sphincter and detrusor) function. Parasympathetic nerves arising from S2–4 stimulate detrusor contraction, resulting in micturition. Sympathetic nerves arising from T10–L2 relay in the pelvic ganglia and produce detrusor relaxation and contraction of the bladder neck (both via α-adrenoceptors). The distal sphincter mechanism is innervated by somatic motor fibres from sacral segments S2–4 which reach the sphincter either by the pelvic plexus or via the pudendal nerves. Afferent sensory impulses pass to the cerebral cortex, from where reflex-increased sphincter tone and associated suppression

of detrusor contraction inhibits micturition until it is appropriate.

These factors operate in a coordinated fashion in the micturition cycle, which has a 'storage' (or 'filling') phase and a 'voiding' (or 'micturition') phase (Fig. 17.14, p. 474). During the filling phase, the high compliance of the detrusor muscle allows the bladder to fill steadily without a rise in intravesical pressure. As bladder volume increases, stretch receptors in its wall cause reflex bladder relaxation and increased sphincter tone. At approximately 75% bladder capacity there is a desire to void. Voluntary control is now exerted over the desire to void, which disappears temporarily. Compliance of the detrusor allows further increase in capacity until the next desire to void. Just how often this desire needs to be inhibited depends on many factors, not the least of which is finding a suitable place in which to void.

The act of micturition is initiated first by voluntary and then by reflex relaxation of the pelvic floor and distal sphincter mechanism, followed by reflex detrusor contraction. These actions are coordinated by the pontine micturition centre. Intravesical pressure remains greater than urethral pressure until the bladder is empty.

Erectile function

Blood inflow into the corpus cavernosum of the penis is under tonic sympathetic control via nerves from the thoraco-lumbar plexus which maintain smooth muscle contraction. In response to afferent input from the glans penis and from higher centres, pelvic splanchnic parasympathetic nerves actively relax the cavernosal smooth muscle via neurotransmitters such as nitric oxide, acetylcholine, vasoactive intestinal polypeptide (VIP) and prostacyclin, with consequent dilatation of the lacunar space. At the same time, draining venules are compressed, and possibly actively constricted, trapping blood in the lacunar space with consequent elevation of pressure and tumescence of the penis.

Prostate function

Exocrine glands within the prostate produce fluid which comprises about 20% of the volume of ejaculated seminal fluid and is rich in lipids and phospholipids. Seminal vesicle secretions account for about 60% and contain fructose and prostaglandins. The remainder of the ejaculate is formed in the testes.

Smooth muscle fibres within the prostate, under sympathetic control, contract at orgasm to move seminal fluid via ejaculatory ducts into the bulbar urethra (emission). Contraction of the bulbocavernosus muscle (via a spinal muscle reflex) then ejaculates the semen out of the urethra. These smooth muscle fibres can also effect some control over urine flow through the bulbar urethra.

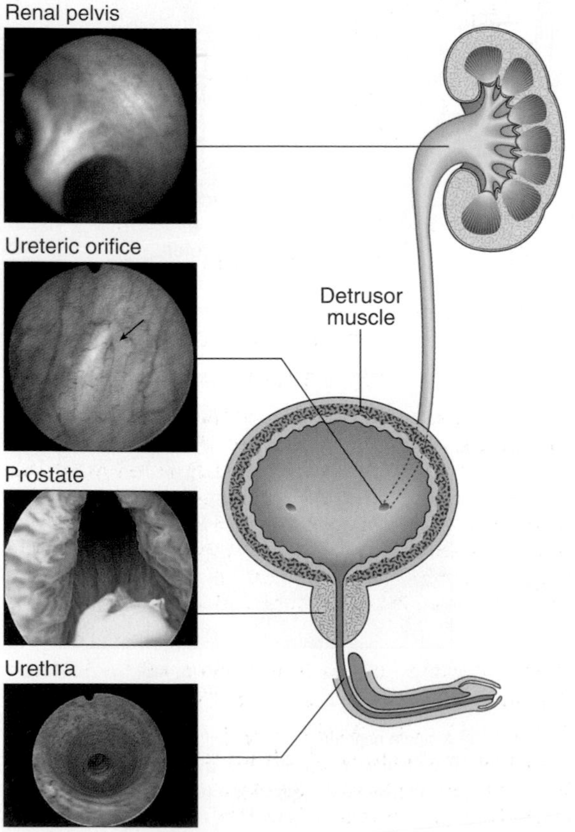

INVESTIGATION OF RENAL AND URINARY TRACT DISEASE

TESTS OF FUNCTION

Renal excretory function can be assessed by measuring serum levels of compounds excreted by the kidney,

Renal pelvis

Ureteric orifice

Detrusor muscle

Prostate

Urethra

Fig. 17.2 Endoscopic views of the male urinary tract.

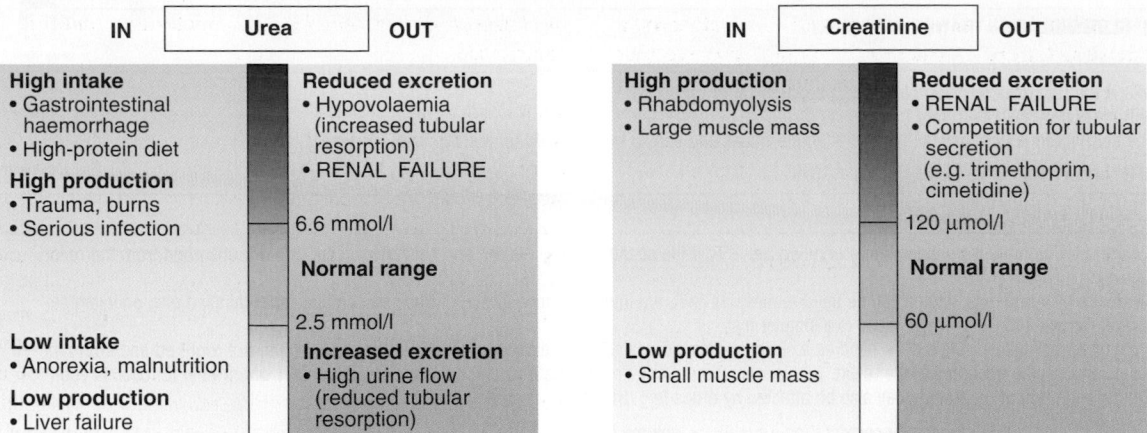

Fig. 17.3 Factors affecting blood levels of urea and creatinine. Factors affecting intake and production are shown to the left ('in'); those affecting excretion are shown to the right ('out'). Creatinine intake is omitted as dietary creatinine (from meat) only rarely influences blood levels. (Urea 2.5–6.6 mmol/l ≈ 15–40 mg/dl. Creatinine 60–120 µmol/l ≈ 0.68–1.36 mg/dl.)

commonly the products of protein catabolism (urea and creatinine). Blood urea is a poor guide to renal excretory function as it varies with protein intake, liver metabolic capacity and renal perfusion (Fig. 17.3). Serum creatinine is more reliable as it is produced from muscle at a constant rate and almost completely filtered at the glomerulus. If muscle mass remains constant, changes in creatinine concentration reflect changes in GFR. However, an increase outside the normal range is typically not seen until GFR is reduced by about 50% (Fig. 17.4), and isolated measurements of serum creatinine may give a misleading impression of renal function, particularly if muscle mass is unusually small (or large).

Urine measurements to derive creatinine clearance provide a reasonable approximation of the GFR (Box. 17.1). More accurate measurement of GFR is now most easily undertaken by ascertaining the clearance of ^{51}Cr-labelled ethylenediamine–tetraacetic acid (EDTA).

Tests of tubular function, including concentrating ability, ability to excrete a water load and ability to excrete acid (p. 420), are valuable in some circumstances.

Urinalysis

Examination of an aliquot of urine provides important information on kidney function. Dipsticks may be used to screen for blood and protein semi-quantitatively (p. 456). Urine microscopy (p. 457) can detect red cells of glomerular origin and red cell casts, indicative of intrinsic renal disease, and is routinely used to screen for white blood cells and bacteria seen in urine infections. Crystals (e.g. of calcium oxalate, cysteine or urate) may be seen in renal calculus disease, although calcium oxalate and urate crystals are also sometimes found in normal urine that has been left to stand. Urine pH can provide diagnostic information in the assessment of renal tubular acidosis (p. 438), and a persistently low specific gravity will be found in diabetes insipidus (p. 796).

Timed urine collections (Box 17.1) can be used to measure creatinine clearance as a surrogate for GFR and can provide a quantitative measure of urinary protein loss. Timed urine collections are also used to measure the urinary excretion rates (and thus, if in dietary equilibrium, the

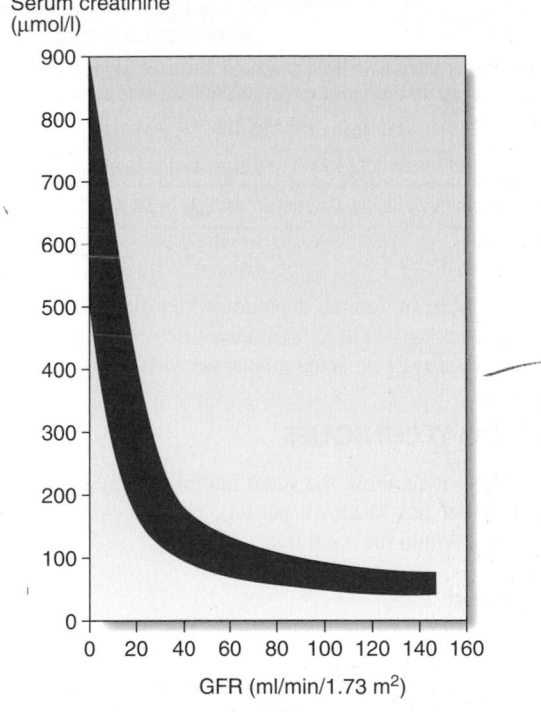

Fig. 17.4 Serum creatinine and the glomerular filtration rate (GFR). The inverse reciprocal relationship between GFR and serum creatinine is shown for a group of patients with renal disease. The red band indicates the range of values obtained. Note that some individuals have a GFR as low as 30–40 ml/min without serum creatinine rising out of the normal range. A normal GFR is 120 ± 25 ml/min/1.73 m². A normal creatinine varies between laboratories but is typically ≤ 120 µmol/l. (To convert creatinine from µmol/l to mg/dl, divide by 88.4.)

intake) of compounds such as calcium, oxalate and urate that can form renal calculi (p. 471). However, it is notoriously difficult to obtain accurately timed samples.

Simple measurement of tubular excretory function can be made by comparison of blood and urine ratios of electrolytes to creatinine. Fractional excretion of sodium (= urinary Na/plasma Na × plasma creatinine/urine creati-

17

17.1 GLOMERULAR FILTRATION RATE (GFR)

- GFR is the rate at which fluid passes into nephrons after filtration
- GFR measures renal excretory function
- The normal range depends on the size of an individual, and should be corrected for surface area—typically 1.73 m^2

GFR normal range = 120 ± 25 ml/min/1.73 m^2

Measuring clearance to estimate GFR

- Clearance of a solute from plasma into urine equals GFR, if the solute is freely filtered and neither secreted into nor absorbed from the renal tubules
- Clearance of exogenous solutes can be used to measure GFR, e.g inulin. Disappearance of trace amounts of radio-labelled ethylenediamine-tetraacetic acid (EDTA) from the blood is a simpler test
- Creatinine clearance (CrCl) is often used as a surrogate measure of GFR. Timed urine collections (typically 24 hrs) are required and errors in collection limit the accuracy of the result. Tubular secretion of creatinine (small) causes CrCl to exaggerate GFR when renal function is poor. Tubular secretion of creatinine may also be affected by drugs (e.g. trimethoprim, cimetidine)

$$\text{CrCl (ml/min)} = \frac{\text{urine creatinine concentration (μmol/l)} \times \text{volume (ml)}}{\text{plasma creatinine concentration (μmol/l)} \times \text{time (min)}}$$

Estimating GFR from plasma measurements

- Equations can be used to estimate GFR from serum creatinine alone. The Cockcroft and Gault (C&G) equation is reasonably accurate at normal to moderately impaired renal function. However, it was designed to estimate CrCl, not GFR

$$\text{CrCl (C\&G)} = \frac{(140 - \text{age}) \times \text{lean body weight (kg)} \times (1.22 \text{ males or } 1.04 \text{ females})}{\text{serum creatinine (μmol/l)}}$$

- Complex equations have been developed which are better at poorer levels of renal function, e.g. the Modification of Diet in Renal Disease (MDRD) study equation (online eGFR (MDRD) available at www.renal.org/eGFR)

$$\text{CrCl} = 186 \times (\text{creatinine in μmol/l/88.4})^{-1.154} \times (\text{Age in yrs})^{-0.203} \times (0.742 \text{ if female}) \times (1.210 \text{ if black})$$

- These equations do not perform well in unusual circumstances, such as extremes of body (and muscle) mass

To convert creatinine in mg/dl to μmol/l, multiply by 88.4.

---

nine) is reduced in volume depletion when the tubules are avidly conserving sodium, and increased in the tubular damage associated with acute tubular necrosis.

IMAGING TECHNIQUES

Plain X-rays may show the renal outlines (if perinephric fat and bowel gas shadows permit), opaque calculi and calcification within the renal tract.

Ultrasound

This quick, non-invasive technique is the first and often the only method required for renal imaging. It can show renal size and position, detect dilatation of the collecting system (suggesting obstruction, Fig. 17.5), distinguish tumours and cysts, and show other abdominal, pelvic and retroperitoneal pathology. In addition, it can image the prostate and bladder, and estimate completeness of emptying in suspected bladder outflow obstruction. Images are often less clear in obese individuals. In chronic renal disease ultrasonographic density of the renal cortex is increased and corticomedullary differentiation is lost.

Doppler techniques are used to show blood flow in extrarenal and larger intrarenal vessels. The resistivity index is the ratio of peak systolic and diastolic velocities, and is influenced by the resistance to flow through small intrarenal arteries. It may be elevated in various diseases, including acute glomerulonephritis and rejection of a renal transplant. Severe renal artery stenosis causes damping of flow in intrarenal vessels with high peak velocities.

17.2 RENAL COMPLICATIONS OF RADIOLOGICAL INVESTIGATIONS

Contrast nephrotoxicity

- An acute deterioration in renal function, sometimes life-threatening, commencing < 48 hrs after administration of i.v. radiographic contrast media

Risk factors
- Pre-existing renal impairment
- Use of high-osmolality, ionic contrast media and repetitive dosing in short time periods
- Diabetes mellitus
- Myeloma

Prevention
- Hydration—e.g. free oral fluids plus i.v. isotonic saline 500 ml then 250 ml/hr during procedure
- Avoid nephrotoxic drugs; withhold non-steroidal anti-inflammatory drugs (NSAIDs); omit metformin for 48 hrs after procedure
- N-acetyl cysteine may provide protection (Box 17.3)
- If the risks are high, consider alternative methods of imaging

Cholesterol atheroembolism

- Typically follows days to weeks after intra-arterial investigations (p. 499)

EBM

17.3 N-ACETYL CYSTEINE AND RADIOCONTRAST-INDUCED NEPHROPATHY

'N-Acetyl cysteine reduces the incidence of contrast nephropathy. However, this finding is not consistent across all trials.'

- Nallamathu BK. Am J Med 2004; 117(12):938–947.

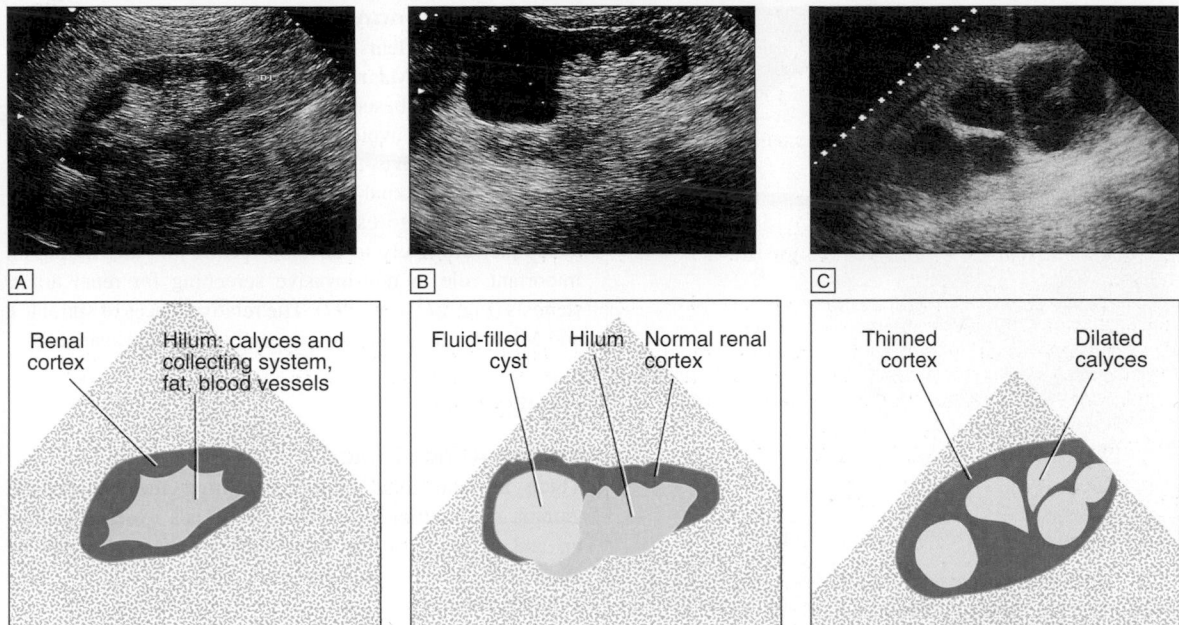

Fig. 17.5 Renal ultrasound. [A] Normal kidney. The normal cortex is less echo-dense (blacker) than the adjacent liver. [B] A simple cyst occupies the upper pole of an otherwise normal kidney. [C] The renal pelvis and calyces are dilated by a chronic obstruction to urinary outflow. The thinness and increased density of the remaining renal cortex indicate chronicity.

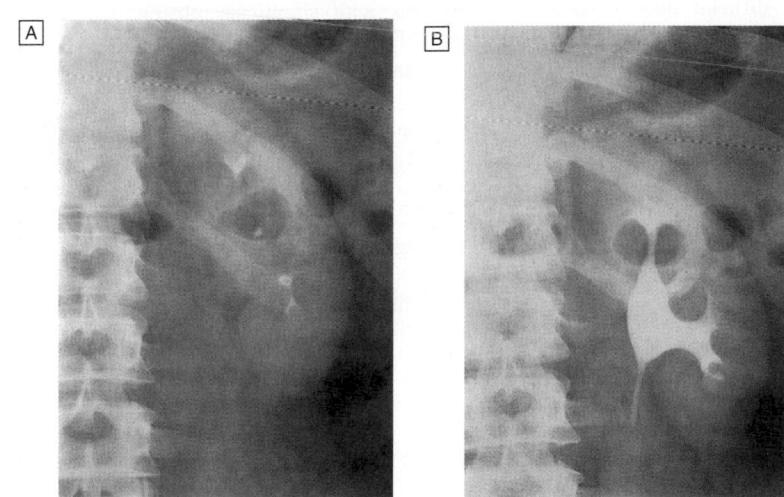

Fig. 17.6 Intravenous urography (IVU).
[A] Nephrogram phase at 1 minute. [B] Collecting system at 5 minutes.

The disadvantages of renal ultrasound are that it is operator-dependent and that the printed images convey only a fraction of the information gained by performing the investigation in real time.

Intravenous urography (IVU)

While intravenous urography has been largely replaced by ultrasound for routine renal imaging, the technique provides excellent definition of the collecting system and ureters, and remains superior to ultrasound for examining renal papillae, stones and urothelial malignancy (Fig. 17.6). X-rays are taken at intervals following administration of an intravenous bolus of an iodine-containing compound that is excreted by the kidney. An early image (1 minute after injection) will demonstrate the nephrogram phase of renal perfusion in patients with an adequate renal arterial supply. This is followed by contrast filling the collecting system, ureters and bladder. The disadvantages of this technique are the need for an injection, time requirement, dependence on adequate renal function for good images, and risk of exposure to contrast medium (Box 17.2) and irradiation.

Pyelography

Pyelography (direct injection of contrast medium into the collecting system from above or below) offers the best views of the collecting system and upper tract, and is commonly used to identify the cause of urinary tract obstruction (p. 476). Antegrade pyelography requires the insertion of a fine needle into the pelvicalyceal system under ultrasound or radiographic control. Contrast is injected to outline the

463

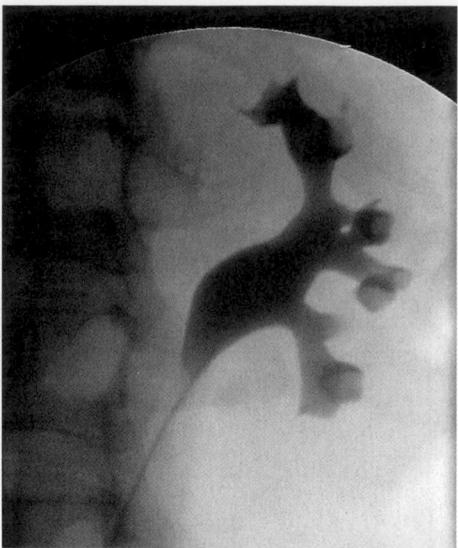

Fig. 17.7   Retrograde pyelography. The best views of the normal collecting system are shown by pyelography. A catheter has been passed into the left renal pelvis at cystoscopy. The anemone-like calyces are sharp-edged and normal. (Compare with the obstructed system shown in Fig. 17.10.)

collecting system, and particularly to localise the site of obstruction. This approach is much more difficult and hazardous in a non-obstructed kidney. In the presence of obstruction, percutaneous nephrostomy drainage can be established, and often stents can be passed through any obstruction. Retrograde pyelography can be performed by inserting catheters into the ureteric orifices at cystoscopy (Fig. 17.7).

Renal arteriography and venography

The main indication for renal arteriography is to investigate suspected renal artery stenosis (p. 496) or haemorrhage. Therapeutic balloon dilatation and stenting of the renal artery may be undertaken, and bleeding vessels or arterio-venous fistulae occluded.

Computed tomography (CT)

CT is particularly useful for characterising mass lesions within the kidney (Fig. 17.40A, p. 513), or combinations of cysts with masses. It gives clear definition of retroperitoneal anatomy regardless of obesity.

Spiral CT is a rapid-sequence technique, with images obtained immediately following a large bolus injection of intravenous contrast media to outline vascular structures. New developments in spiral CT enable three-dimensional arteriograms to be obtained. This produces high-quality images of the main renal vessels and is of value in trauma, renal haemorrhage and the investigation of possible renal artery stenosis. The speed of image acquisition also enables functional assessment and enhancement of vascular structures, e.g. angiomyolipomas.

CT is also useful for demonstrating renal stones, and in many centres CT urography is replacing IVU as the first radiological investigation for renal colic. However, there are risks of exposure to contrast medium (Box 17.2).

Magnetic resonance imaging (MRI)

MRI offers excellent resolution and distinction between different tissues. Magnetic resonance angiography (MRA) uses gadolinium-based contrast media which are non-nephrotoxic, and avoids the risk of atheroemboli which accompany invasive angiography. It can produce good images of main renal vessels, although the resolution is not yet sufficient to exclude branch artery stenosis. These techniques are likely to develop further and are finding an important role in non-invasive screening for renal artery stenosis (Fig. 17.27, p. 497). The relative places of spiral CT and MRA for this condition depend upon local availability.

OTHER TESTS

Radionuclide studies

These are functional studies requiring the injection of gamma ray-emitting radiopharmaceuticals which are taken up and excreted by the kidney, a process which can be monitored by an external gamma camera.

Diethylenetriamine–pentaacetic acid labelled with technetium (^{99m}Tc-DTPA) is excreted by glomerular filtration. DTPA injection and analysis of uptake and excretion provides information regarding the arterial perfusion of each kidney. A typical pattern of prolonged transit time, delayed peak activity and reduced excretion is seen in renal artery stenosis. In patients with significant obstruction of the outflow tract, persistence of the nuclide in the renal pelvis is seen (Fig. 17.10), and a loop diuretic fails to accelerate its disappearance.

Dimercaptosuccinic acid labelled with technetium (^{99m}Tc-DMSA) is filtered by glomeruli and partially bound to proximal tubular cells. Following intravenous injection, images of the renal cortex show the shape, size and function of each kidney (Fig. 17.8). This is a sensitive method of demonstrating early cortical scarring that is of particular value in children with vesico-ureteric reflux and pyelonephritis. It is also possible to assess the relative contribution of each kidney to total function.

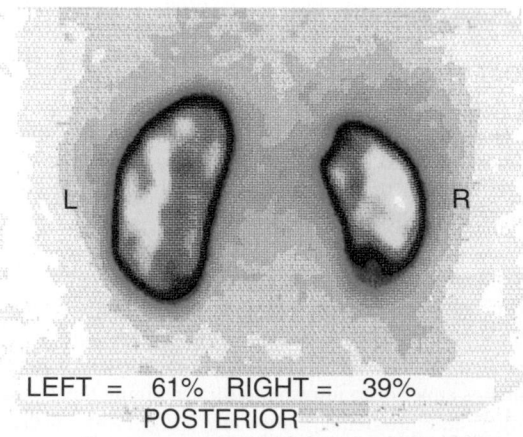

LEFT = 61%   RIGHT = 39%
POSTERIOR

Fig. 17.8   DMSA isotope renogram. A posterior view is shown of a normal left kidney and a small right kidney (with evidence of cortical scarring at upper and lower poles) which contributes only 39% of total renal function.

17

17.4 RENAL BIOPSY

Indications

- Acute renal failure that is not adequately explained
- Chronic renal failure with normal-sized kidneys
- Nephrotic syndrome or glomerular proteinuria in adults
- Nephrotic syndrome in children that has atypical features or is not responding to treatment
- Isolated haematuria or proteinuria with renal characteristics or associated abnormalities

Contraindications

- Disordered coagulation or thrombocytopenia. Aspirin and other agents causing platelet dysfunction should be omitted for elective biopsies
- Uncontrolled hypertension
- Kidneys < 60% predicted size
- Solitary kidney (except transplants) (relative contraindication)

Complications

- Pain, usually mild
- Bleeding into urine, usually minor but may produce clot colic and obstruction
- Bleeding around the kidney, occasionally massive and requiring angiography with intervention, or surgery
- Arteriovenous fistula, rarely significant clinically

Renal biopsy

Renal biopsy is used to establish the nature and extent of renal disease in order to judge the prognosis and need for treatment (Box 17.4). The procedure is performed transcutaneously with ultrasound guidance to ensure accurate needle placement into a renal pole. Radiographic screening after contrast administration or other methods may also be used. Light microscopy, electron microscopy and immuno-histological assessment of the specimen may all be required.

PRESENTING PROBLEMS IN RENAL AND URINARY TRACT DISEASE

PATTERNS OF PRESENTATION

The broad categories of renal and urinary tract disease, and their typical manifestations, are shown in Figure 17.9.

Symptoms from the lower urinary tract are an extremely common group of presenting complaints. Less commonly, urinary tract disorders lead to obstruction to urinary flow (Fig. 17.10), which may present with pain or with loss of renal function.

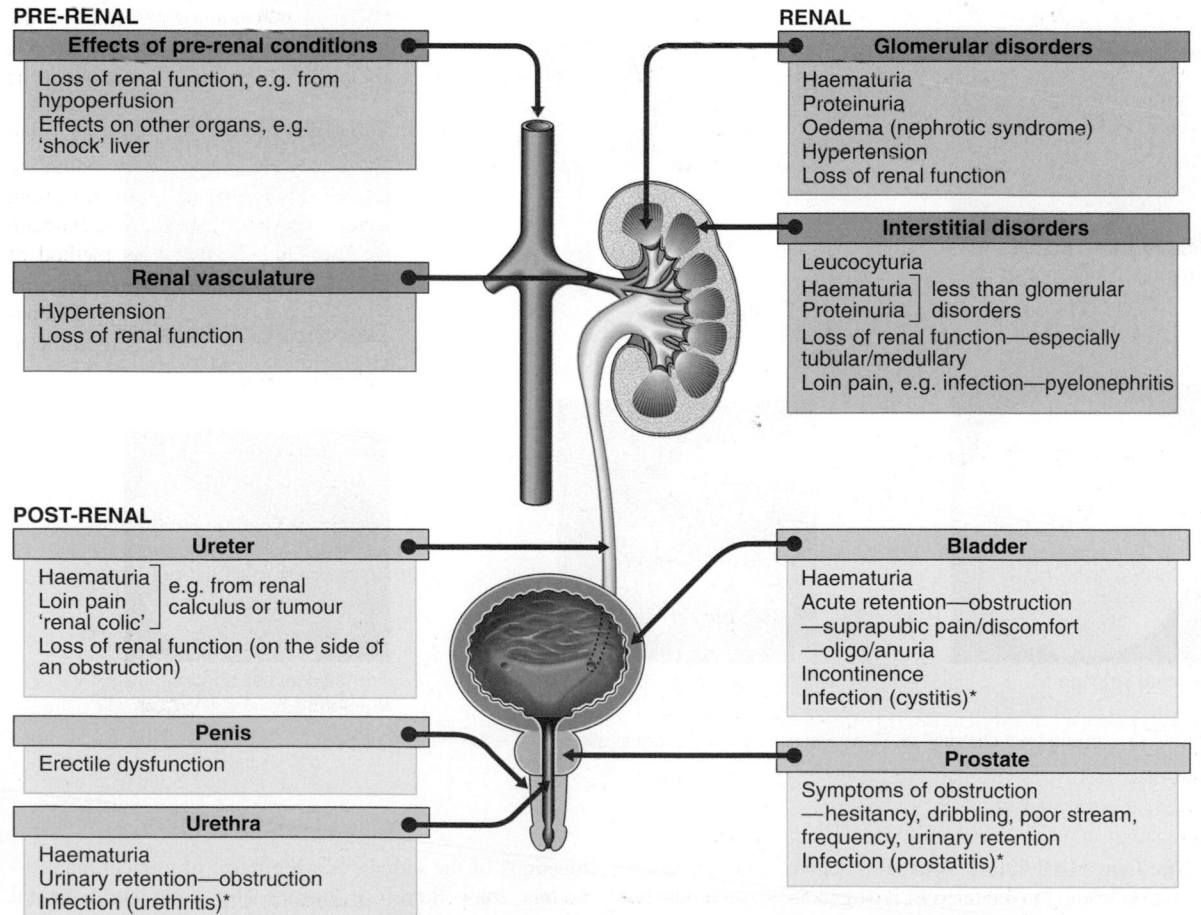

Fig. 17.9 Classification and manifestations of renal and urinary tract disease. Consequences of loss of renal function and effects on other organs are described on pages 481–491. (* Lower urinary tract infection: haematuria, dysuria, frequency, urgency, cloudy and smelly urine.)

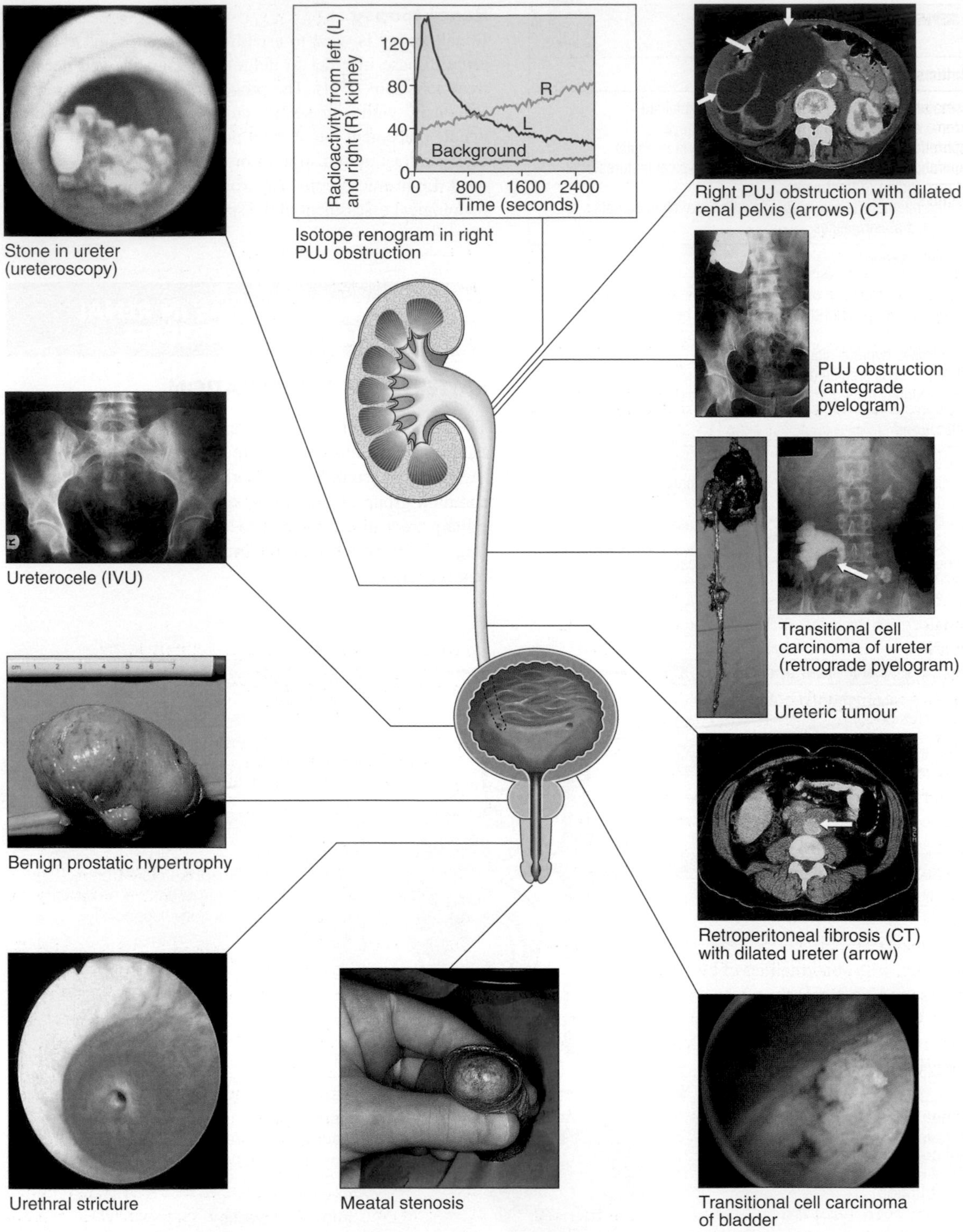
Stone in ureter (ureteroscopy)
Radioactivity from left (L) and right (R) kidney
120
80
40
0
R
L
Background
0
800
1600
2400
Time (seconds)
Isotope renogram in right PUJ obstruction
Right PUJ obstruction with dilated renal pelvis (arrows) (CT)
PUJ obstruction (antegrade pyelogram)
Ureterocele (IVU)
Transitional cell carcinoma of ureter (retrograde pyelogram)
Ureteric tumour
Benign prostatic hypertrophy
Retroperitoneal fibrosis (CT) with dilated ureter (arrow)
Urethral stricture
Meatal stenosis
Transitional cell carcinoma of bladder

Fig. 17.10 Urinary tract obstruction. Some common causes and their locations. (PUJ = pelviureteric junction)

The term 'renal failure' is used to denote failure of renal excretion leading to retention of nitrogenous waste products of metabolism including creatinine and urea. Other aspects of renal function may fail at the same time, including the regulation of fluid and electrolyte status and the endocrine functions of the kidney. A wide range of clinical manifestations may therefore occur. The most fundamental categorisation of renal failure is into acute or chronic types, and this is aided by knowledge of previous renal function for comparison.

17.5 NEPHRITIC AND NEPHROTIC SYNDROMES
Nephritic syndrome[1]
• Haematuria (brown urine) • Oedema and generalised fluid retention • Hypertension • Oliguria
Nephrotic syndrome[2]
• Overt proteinuria—usually > 3.5 g/24 hrs (urine may be frothy) • Hypoalbuminaemia (< 30 g/l) • Oedema and generalised fluid retention • Intravascular volume depletion with hypotension, or expansion with hypertension, may occur
[1] The complete form is classically seen in post-infectious glomerulo-nephritis, may occur in acute IgA nephropathy, and occasionally occurs in other types of glomerulonephritis. The presence of one or more features is common to many types of glomerular disease. [2] Classically seen in non-inflammatory and subacute inflammatory/proliferative glomerular disorders.

17.6 RISK FACTORS FOR URINARY TRACT INFECTION
Incomplete bladder emptying
• Bladder outflow obstruction • Neurological problems (e.g. multiple sclerosis, diabetic neuropathy) • Gynaecological abnormalities (e.g. uterine prolapse) • Vesico-ureteric reflux (p. 509)
Foreign bodies
• Urethral catheter or ureteric stent
Loss of host defences
• Atrophic urethritis and vaginitis in post-menopausal women • Diabetes mellitus

Non-inflammatory and subacute inflammatory/proliferative glomerular disorders may present with substantial proteinuria resulting in nephrotic syndrome (p. 479). Inflammatory glomerular disorders more typically cause haematuria in association with early signs of disturbed renal function, such as hypertension. If progressive, obvious signs of impaired excretion of water and solutes develop. The onset of these features in close succession has been described as the nephritic syndrome (Box 17.5), but in pure form this condition is rarely seen, except in countries where post-infectious glomerulonephritis is common. Mixed inflammatory and nephrotic features are more common. It is important to recognise such disease, especially if renal impairment is progressing, as the inflammatory group includes some renal disorders which are amenable to treatment.

Many patients do not present acutely and are essentially asymptomatic, with abnormalities of blood or urine detected on routine screening. Recently, a new classification of stages of chronic kidney disease has been proposed; most patients requiring renal replacement therapy have a progressive course through these stages (Box 17.28, p. 486).

CYSTITIS AND URINARY TRACT INFECTION

Urinary tract infection (UTI) is the most common bacterial infection managed in general medical practice and accounts for 1–3% of consultations. Up to 50% of women have a UTI at some time. The prevalence of UTI in women is about 3% at the age of 20, increasing by about 1% in each subsequent decade. In males UTI is uncommon, except in the first year of life and in men over 60, in whom urinary tract obstruction due to prostatic hypertrophy may occur. UTI causes morbidity and, in a small minority of cases, renal damage and chronic renal failure.

When the urinary tract is anatomically and physiolo-gically normal and local and systemic defence mechanisms are intact, bacteria are confined to the lower end of the urethra. UTI is defined as multiplication of organisms in the urinary tract. It is usually associated with the presence of neutrophils and > 10^5 organisms/ml in a midstream sample of urine (MSU).

Aetiology

Organisms causing UTI in the community include:

• *Escherichia coli* derived from the gastrointestinal tract (about 75% of infections)
• *Proteus*
• *Pseudomonas* species
• streptococci
• *Staphylococcus epidermidis*.

In hospital, *E. coli* still predominates, but *Klebsiella* or streptococci are more common than in the community. Certain strains of *E. coli* have a particular propensity to invade the urinary tract.

The first stage in the development of UTI is colonisation of the periurethral zone with pathogenic organisms. Urine is an excellent culture medium for bacteria; in addition, the urothelium of susceptible persons may have more receptors to which virulent strains of *E. coli* become adherent. In women, the ascent of organisms into the bladder is easier than in men because of the relatively short urethra and absence of bactericidal prostatic secretions. Sexual inter-course may cause minor urethral trauma and transfer bacteria from the perineum into the bladder. Instrumen-tation of the bladder may also introduce organisms. Multi-plication of organisms then depends on a number of factors, including the size of the inoculum and virulence of the bacteria. Conditions which predispose to UTI are shown in Box 17.6.

Some patients, usually female, have symptoms suggestive of urethritis and cystitis but no bacteria are cultured from the urine (the 'urethral syndrome'). Possible explanations include infection with organisms not readily cultured by ordinary methods (e.g. *Chlamydia*, certain anaerobes), intermittent or very low-count bacteriuria, reaction to toilet preparations or disinfectants, symptoms related to sexual

17

17.7 THE SPECTRUM OF PRESENTATIONS OF URINARY TRACT INFECTION

- Asymptomatic bacteriuria
- Symptomatic acute urethritis and cystitis
- Acute pyelonephritis (p. 470)
- Acute prostatitis (p. 512)
- Septicaemia (usually Gram-negative bacteria)

intercourse, or post-menopausal atrophic vaginitis. Antibiotics are not indicated.

Clinical assessment

Typical features of cystitis and urethritis include:

- abrupt onset of frequency of micturition
- scalding pain in the urethra during micturition (dysuria)
- suprapubic pain during and after voiding
- intense desire to pass more urine after micturition, due to spasm of the inflamed bladder wall (urgency)
- urine that may appear cloudy and have an unpleasant odour
- microscopic or visible haematuria.

Systemic symptoms are usually slight or absent. However, infection in the lower urinary tract can spread (Box 17.7); prominent systemic symptoms with fever and loin pain suggest the presence of acute pyelonephritis (p. 470) and may be an indication for hospitalisation. Prostatis (p. 512) is suggested by systemic symptoms and prostatic tenderness.

The differential diagnosis includes urethritis due to sexually transmitted disease (p. 406) or Reiter's syndrome.

Investigations

An approach to investigation is shown in Box 17.8.

In an otherwise healthy woman with a single lower urinary tract infection and no indications of a complicated infection, urine culture prior to treatment is not mandatory. It is necessary, however, in patients with recurrent infection or after failure of initial treatment, during pregnancy, or in patients susceptible to serious infection (e.g. older people, those with diabetes, the immunocompromised or those with an indwelling catheter).

Definitive diagnosis rests on the combination of typical clinical features with findings in the urine. Neutrophils are usually present in the urine in symptomatic infections. Interpretation of bacterial counts in the urine, and of what is a 'significant' culture, is based on probabilities. Urine taken by suprapubic aspiration should be sterile, so the presence of any organisms is significant. If the patient has symptoms and there are neutrophils in the urine, a small number of organisms is significant. In asymptomatic patients, $> 10^5$/ml organisms is usually regarded as significant (asymptomatic bacteriuria, see below).

Urine dipstick tests can be used to test for UTI. One tests for nitrite—most urinary pathogens can reduce nitrate to nitrite. Another tests for leucocyte esterase, suggesting the presence of neutrophils. If either test is positive, UTI is probable; if they are both negative, UTI is unlikely.

Investigations to detect underlying predisposing factors for UTI are used more selectively, most commonly in patients with recurrent infections (Box 17.8).

Management

Antibiotics are recommended in all cases of proven UTI (Box 17.9). If urine culture has been performed, treatment

17

17.8 INVESTIGATION OF PATIENTS WITH URINARY TRACT INFECTION

Investigation	Indications
Culture of MSU, or urine obtained by suprapubic aspiration	All patients
Microscopic examination or cytometry of urine for white and red cells	All patients
Dipstick examination of urine for nitrite and leucocyte esterase*	All patients
Dipstick examination of urine for blood, protein and glucose	All patients
Full blood count	Infants; children; adults with acute pyelonephritis or prostatitis
Plasma urea, electrolytes, creatinine	Infants; children; acute pyelonephritis; recurrent UTI
Blood culture	Fever, rigors or evidence of septic shock
Pelvic examination	Women with recurrent UTI
Rectal examination	Men (to examine prostate)
Renal ultrasound or CT	To identify obstruction, cysts, calculi Infants, children, men after single UTI Women who have (1) acute pyelonephritis; (2) recurrent UTI after antibiotic treatment; (3) UTI or asymptomatic bacteriuria in pregnancy
Intravenous urogram (IVU)	Alternative to ultrasound, particularly to image the collecting system after voiding
Micturating cysto-urethrogram (MCU) or radioisotope study to identify and assess severity of vesico-ureteric reflux or impaired bladder emptying	Selected infants and children; to look for reflux and renal scars
Cystoscopy	Patients with haematuria or a suspected bladder lesion

* May substitute for microscopy and culture in uncomplicated infection.

17.9 ANTIBIOTIC REGIMENS FOR TREATMENT OF URINARY TRACT INFECTIONS IN ADULTS

Drug	Treatment of urinary tract infection		Treatment of acute pyelonephritis		Treatment of bacterial prostatitis		Prophylactic or suppressive therapy
	Dose	Duration of course	Dose	Duration of course	Dose	Duration of course	Dose
Trimethoprim	200 mg daily	3 days	200 mg daily	7–14 days	200 mg 12-hourly	4–6 weeks	100 mg/night
Nitrofurantoin	50 mg 6-hourly	3 days	50 mg 6-hourly	7-14 days			
Co-amoxiclav	250/125 mg 8-hourly	3 days	250/125 mg 8-hourly	7–14 days			250/125 mg/night
Ciprofloxacin[1]	100 mg 12-hourly	3 days	250–500 mg 12-hourly oral *or* 100 mg 12-hourly i.v.	7–14 days	250 mg 12-hourly	4–6 weeks	
Norfloxacin[1]	400 mg 12-hourly	3 days	400 mg 12-hourly	7–14 days	400 mg 12-hourly	4–6 weeks	
Cefuroxime[1]			250 mg 12-hourly oral *or* 750 mg 6–8-hourly i.v.	7–14 days Start treatment. i.v in seriously ill patient			
Gentamicin			3–5 mg/kg i.v. daily[2]	7–14 days			
Cefalexin	500 mg 12-hourly	3 days	500 mg 12-hourly	3 days			250 mg/night

[1] Modification of dosage is necessary when renal function is impaired.
[2] Dose determined by plasma [creatinine] and [gentamicin].

may be started while awaiting the result. Treatment for 3 days is the norm and is less likely to induce antibiotic resistance than more prolonged therapy. Trimethoprim is the usual choice for initial treatment. Between 10% and 40% of organisms causing UTI are resistant to trimethoprim, the lower rates being seen in community-based practice. Nitrofurantoin, quinolone antibiotics such as ciprofloxacin and norfloxacin, and cefalexin are also generally effective. Co-amoxiclav or amoxicillin should only be used when the organism is known to be sensitive. Penicillins and cephalosporins are safe to use in pregnancy but trimethoprim, sulphonamides, quinolones and tetracyclines should be avoided.

A fluid intake of at least 2 litres/day is usually recommended, although this is not based on evidence and may make matters worse for patients with severe dysuria. Urinary alkalinising agents such as potassium citrate may help symptomatically but are not of proven efficacy.

Modifications of treatment for patients with acute pyelonephritis or prostatitis are shown in Box 17.9 and discussed on pages 470 and 512, respectively.

PERSISTENT OR RECURRENT UTI

Treatment failure, with persistence of the causative organism on repeat culture, suggests that an underlying cause is present (Box 17.6), which should be investigated (Box 17.8) and treated, if possible. Reinfection with a different organism, or with the same organism after an interval, may also occur. In women, recurrent infections are common and further investigation is only justified if infections are frequent (three or more per year) or unusually

17.10 PROPHYLACTIC MEASURES TO BE ADOPTED BY WOMEN WITH RECURRENT URINARY INFECTIONS

- Fluid intake of at least 2 litres/day
- Regular complete emptying of bladder
- If vesico-ureteric reflux is present, practise double micturition (empty the bladder then attempt micturition 10–15 minutes later)
- Good personal hygiene
- Emptying of the bladder before and after sexual intercourse
- Cranberry juice may be effective

17

severe. Men and children with recurrent infections, and patients with signs of pyelonephritis or systemic infection should also be investigated.

If the underlying cause cannot be removed, suppressive antibiotic therapy (Box 17.9) can be used to prevent recurrence and reduce the risk of septicaemia and renal damage. Urine is cultured at regular intervals; a regime of two or three antibiotics in sequence, rotating every 6 months, is often used in an attempt to reduce the emergence of resistant organisms. Other simple measures may help to prevent recurrence (Box 17.10).

Recurrent UTI, particularly in the presence of an underlying cause, may result in permanent renal damage, whereas uncomplicated infections rarely (if ever) do so. (See chronic pyelonephritis on page 509.)

ASYMPTOMATIC BACTERIURIA

This is defined as $> 10^5$/ml organisms in the urine of apparently healthy asymptomatic patients. Approximately 1% of children under the age of 1, 1% of schoolgirls, 0.03% of schoolboys and men, 3% of non-pregnant adult

17.11 URINARY INFECTION IN OLD AGE

- **Prevalence of asymptomatic bacteriuria:** rises with age. Amongst the frailest in institutional care it rises to ~40% in women and 30% in men.
- **Contributory factors:** include an increased prevalence of underlying structural abnormalities, post-menopausal oestrogen deficiency and increased residual urine in women, and prostatic hypertrophy with reduced bactericidal activity of prostatic secretions in men.
- **Decision to treat:** there is little evidence for the benefit of treating asymptomatic bacteriuria in old age. It does not improve chronic incontinence or decrease mortality or morbidity from symptomatic urinary infection. It risks adverse effects from the antibiotic and promoting the emergence of resistant organisms.
- **Source of infection:** the urinary tract is the most frequent source of bacteraemia in older patients admitted to hospital.
- **Incontinence:** new or increased incontinence is a common presentation of UTI in older women.
- **Treatment:** post-menopausal women with acute lower urinary tract symptoms may require longer than 3 days' therapy.

women and 5% of pregnant women have asymptomatic bacteriuria. It is increasingly common in those aged over 65. There is no evidence that this condition causes renal scarring in adults who are not pregnant and have a normal urinary tract, and in general, treatment is not indicated. Up to 30% of patients will develop symptomatic infection within 1 year. In infants and pregnant women, treatment is required and investigation is indicated. Where the urinary tract is abnormal, asymptomatic bacteriuria is also more significant and may require intervention.

CATHETER-RELATED BACTERIURIA

In patients with a urethral catheter, bacteriuria increases the risk of Gram-negative bacteraemia fivefold. However, bacteriuria is common, and almost universal during long-term catheterisation. Treatment is usually avoided in asymptomatic patients as this may promote antibiotic resistance. Careful sterile insertion technique is important, and the catheter should be removed as soon as it is not required.

LOIN PAIN

Dull ache in the loin is rarely due to renal disease but may be due to renal stone, renal tumour, acute pyelonephritis or obstruction of the renal pelvis. This is most commonly caused by a congenital abnormality of the pelvi-ureteric junction (PUJ, p. 508), where typically the pain is precipitated by a large fluid intake. More rarely, upper urinary tract obstruction is caused by retroperitoneal fibrosis (p. 509), a sloughed renal papilla, tumour or blood clot.

ACUTE PYELONEPHRITIS

The kidneys are infected in a minority of patients with lower urinary tract infection or bacteriuria, although the exact proportion is unknown. Acute renal infection (pyelonephritis) presents as a classic triad of loin pain, fever and tenderness over the kidneys. The renal pelvis is inflamed and small abscesses are often evident in the renal parenchyma

(Fig. 17.35C, p. 505). Histological examination shows focal infiltration by neutrophils, which can often be seen within the tubules.

Pathogenesis

Renal infection is almost always caused by organisms ascending from the bladder, and the bacterial profile is the same as for lower urinary tract infection (p. 467). Rarely, bacteraemia may give rise to renal or perinephric abscesses, most commonly due to staphylococci. One or more complicating factors are often present; pre-existing renal damage, such as cyst formation or scarring, facilitates infection. The renal medulla may be particularly susceptible to infection because of the low oxygen tension, high osmolality and high concentrations of H^+ and ammonia, which impair leucocyte function. The high osmolality favours conversion of bacteria to antibiotic-resistant L-forms.

Clinical assessment

There is usually acute onset of pain in one or both loins, which may radiate to the iliac fossae and suprapubic area and is associated with tenderness and guarding in the lumbar region. About 30% of patients have dysuria due to associated cystitis. Fever is usually present and may be associated with rigors, vomiting and hypotension. Examination of urine reveals neutrophils, organisms, red cells and tubular epithelial cells.

Rarely, acute pyelonephritis is associated with papillary necrosis. Fragments of renal papillary tissue are passed per urethra and can be identified histologically. They may cause ureteric obstruction, and if this occurs bilaterally or in a single kidney, may cause acute renal failure. Predisposing factors include diabetes mellitus, chronic urinary obstruction, analgesic nephropathy and sickle-cell disease.

The differential diagnosis of acute pyelonephritis includes acute appendicitis, diverticulitis, cholecystitis and salpingitis. In perinephric abscess, there is marked pain and tenderness and often bulging of the loin on the affected side. Patients are extremely ill, with fever, leucocytosis and positive blood cultures. Urinary symptoms are absent, and urine contains neither pus cells nor organisms.

Investigations and management

Appropriate investigations are shown in Box 17.8. Bacteria and neutrophils in the urine of a patient with typical clinical features confirm the diagnosis.

Renal tract ultrasound should be performed as soon as possible, to exclude a perinephric collection and obstruction as a predisposing factor. If obstruction is present, drainage by a percutaneous nephrostomy should be considered.

Adequate fluid intake must be ensured, if necessary by the intravenous route.

Antibiotics are continued for 7–14 days. Severe cases require intravenous therapy, with a cephalosporin, quinolone or gentamicin (Box 17.9), later switching to an oral agent. In less severe cases, oral antibiotics can be used throughout. Penicillins and cephalosporins are safe in pregnancy; other antibiotics should usually be avoided.

Urine should be cultured during and after treatment.

17

RENAL COLIC

Aetiology

Acute loin pain radiating to the groin ('renal colic'), together with haematuria, is typical of ureteric obstruction most commonly due to calculi, although a sloughed renal papilla, tumour or blood clot may be responsible.

Urinary calculi

Urinary calculi consist of aggregates of crystals containing small amounts of proteins and glycoprotein. Different types vary in frequency around the world, probably as a consequence of dietary and environmental factors, but genetic factors may also contribute. In Europe, 80% of renal stones contain crystals of calcium (most commonly as oxalate, but also as phosphate). About 15% contain magnesium ammonium phosphate (struvite; these are often associated with infection), and small numbers of pure cystine or uric acid stones are found. Rarely, drugs may form stones (e.g. indinavir, ephedrine).

In developing countries, bladder stones are common, particularly in children. In developed countries, the incidence of childhood bladder stones is low; renal stones in adults are more common. In a North American survey, 12% of men and 5% of women had experienced a renal stone by the age of 70 years. It is surprising that stones and nephrocalcinosis are not more common, since some of the constituents are present in urine in concentrations which exceed their maximum solubility in water. However, urine contains proteins, glycosaminoglycans, pyrophosphate and citrate which help to keep otherwise insoluble salts in solution.

Urinary concretions vary greatly in size. There may be particles like sand anywhere in the urinary tract, or large round stones in the bladder. Staghorn calculi fill the whole renal pelvis and branch into the calyces (Fig. 17.11); they are usually associated with infection and composed largely of struvite. Deposits of calcium may be present throughout the renal parenchyma, giving rise to nephrocalcinosis, especially in patients with renal tubular acidosis, hyperparathyroidism, vitamin D intoxication and healed renal tuberculosis.

A number of risk factors are known for renal stone formation (Box 17.12). However, in developed countries, most calculi occur in healthy young men in whom investigations reveal no clear predisposing cause.

Clinical assessment

When a stone becomes impacted in the ureter, an attack of renal colic develops. The patient is suddenly aware of pain in the loin, which radiates round the flank to the groin and often into the testis or labium, in the sensory distribution of the first lumbar nerve. The pain steadily increases in intensity to reach a peak in a few minutes. The patient is restless, and generally tries unsuccessfully to obtain relief by changing position or pacing the room. There is pallor, sweating and often vomiting, and the patient may groan in agony. Frequency, dysuria and haematuria may occur. The intense pain usually subsides within 2 hours, but may continue unabated for hours or days. It is usually constant during attacks, although slight fluctuations in severity may

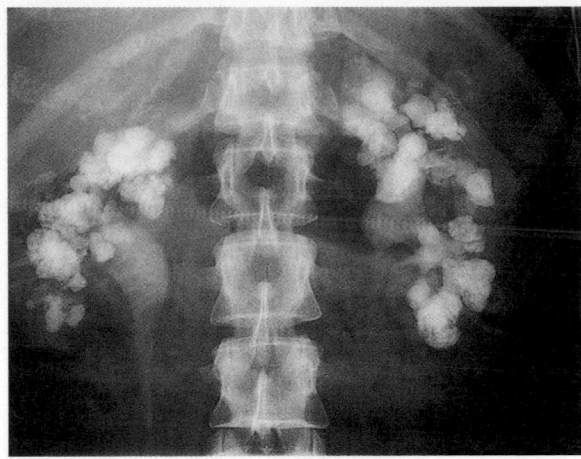

Fig. 17.11 Bilateral staghorn calculi. The intravenous pyelogram demonstrates that, while some dye is being excreted by the right kidney, there is little function on the left.

17.12 PREDISPOSING FACTORS FOR KIDNEY STONES

Environmental and dietary

- Low urine volumes: high ambient temperatures, low fluid intake
- Diet: high protein intake, high sodium, low calcium
- High sodium excretion
- High oxalate excretion
- High urate excretion
- Low citrate excretion

Acquired causes

- Hypercalcaemia of any cause (p. 772)
- Ileal disease or resection (leads to increased oxalate absorption and urinary excretion)
- Renal tubular acidosis type I (distal, p. 438)

Congenital and inherited causes

- Familial hypercalciuria
- Medullary sponge kidney
- Cystinuria
- Renal tubular acidosis type I (distal)
- Primary hyperoxaluria

occur. Contrary to general belief, attacks rarely consist of intermittent severe pains coming and going every few minutes. Subsequent to an attack of renal colic there may be intermittent dull pain in the loin or back.

Investigations

The diagnosis of renal colic is usually made easily from the history and by finding red cells in the urine. Investigations are required to confirm the presence of a stone, and to identify the site of the stone and degree of obstruction. About 90% of stones are seen on a plain abdominal X-ray. When the stone is in the ureter an IVU shows delayed excretion of contrast from the kidney and a dilated ureter down to the stone (Fig. 17.12). IVU remains the most commonly used investigation world-wide, but spiral CT gives the most accurate assessment and will identify non-opaque stones (e.g. uric acid). Ultrasound may show dilatation of the ureter if the stone is obstructing urine flow. The stone may also cast an acoustic shadow.

Patients with a first renal stone should have a minimum set of investigations (Box 17.13); the yield of more detailed

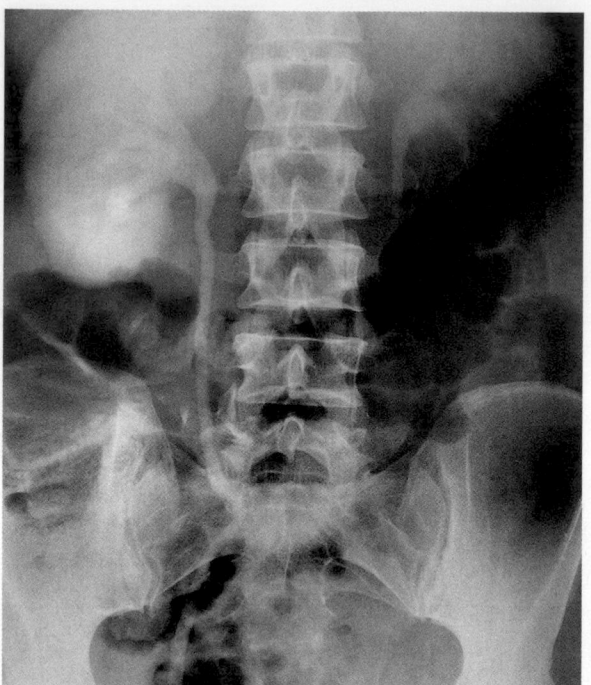

Fig. 17.12 Unilateral obstruction. Intravenous urogram of a patient with a stone (not visible) at the lower end of the right ureter. This film, taken 2 hours post-contrast injection, demonstrates persistence of contrast medium in the right kidney, pelvicalyceal system and ureter, whereas only a small amount remains visible in the normal left pelvicalyceal system.

17.13 INVESTIGATIONS FOR RENAL STONES

Sample	Test	First stone	Recurrent stones
Stone	Chemical composition—most valuable when possible	✓	✓
Blood	Calcium	✓	✓
	Phosphate	✓	✓
	Uric acid	✓	✓
	Urea and electrolytes	✓	✓
	Parathyroid hormone—only if calcium or calcium excretion high		(✓)
Urine	Dipstick test for protein, blood, glucose	✓	✓
	Amino acids		✓
24-hour urine	Urea		✓
	Creatinine clearance		✓
	Sodium		✓
	Calcium		✓
	Oxalate		✓
	Uric acid		✓

17.14 MEASURES TO PREVENT CALCIUM STONE FORMATION

Diet

Fluid
- At least 2 litres output per day (intake 3–4 litres)—check with 24-hr urine collections
- Intake distributed throughout the day (especially before bed)

Sodium
- Restrict intake

Protein
- Moderate; not high

Calcium
- Plenty in diet (because calcium forms an insoluble salt with dietary oxalate, lowering oxalate absorption and excretion)
- Avoid supplements away from meals (increase calcium excretion without reducing oxalate excretion)

Oxalate
- Avoid foods that are rich in oxalate (e.g. rhubarb)

N.B. Citrate supplementation of unproven value.

Drugs

Thiazide diuretics
- Reduce calcium excretion
- Valuable in recurrent stone-formers and patients with hypercalciuria

Allopurinol
- If urate excretion high

Avoid
- Vitamin D supplements as they increase calcium absorption and excretion

investigation is low, and hence usually reserved for those with recurrent or multiple stones, or those with complicated or unexpected presentations (e.g. in the very young). Chemical analysis of stones is helpful. Since most stones pass spontaneously through the urinary tract, urine should be sieved for a few days after an episode of colic in order to collect the calculus for analysis.

Management

The immediate treatment of renal pain or renal colic is bed rest and application of warmth to the site of pain. Renal colic is often unbearably painful and demands powerful analgesia, e.g. morphine (10–20 mg), pethidine (100 mg) intramuscularly or diclofenac as a suppository (100 mg). Patients are advised to drink 2 litres per day. Around 90% of stones less than 4 mm in diameter will pass spontaneously, but only 10% of stones of more than 6 mm will pass and these may require active intervention. Immediate action is required if there is anuria or if severe infection occurs in the stagnant urine proximal to the stone (pyonephrosis).

Attempts to develop drugs that dissolve stones have so far been unsuccessful. However, most stones can now be fragmented by extracorporeal shock wave lithotripsy (ESWL; Fig. 17.13), in which shock waves generated outside the body are focused to the stone, breaking it into small pieces which can pass easily down the ureter. This requires free drainage of the distal urinary tract.

Endoscopic surgery is often required for stones, but open surgery is now almost never needed except for large bladder stones. All stones are potentially infected and surgery should be covered with appropriate antibiotics.

Management to prevent further stone formation should be guided by the results of the investigations in Box 17.13, but some general principles apply to almost every patient with calcium-containing stones (Box 17.14). More specific measures apply to some stone types. Urate stones can be

17

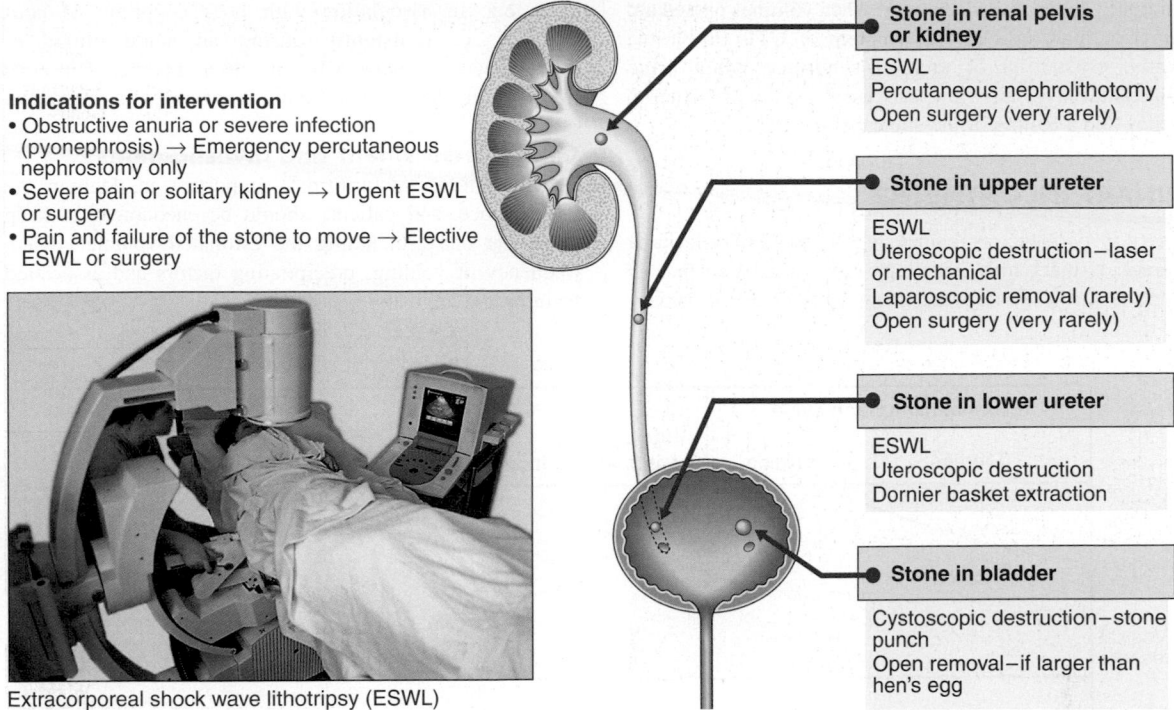

Indications for intervention
- Obstructive anuria or severe infection (pyonephrosis) → Emergency percutaneous nephrostomy only
- Severe pain or solitary kidney → Urgent ESWL or surgery
- Pain and failure of the stone to move → Elective ESWL or surgery

Extracorporeal shock wave lithotripsy (ESWL)

Stone in renal pelvis or kidney

ESWL
Percutaneous nephrolithotomy
Open surgery (very rarely)

Stone in upper ureter

ESWL
Uteroscopic destruction–laser or mechanical
Laparoscopic removal (rarely)
Open surgery (very rarely)

Stone in lower ureter

ESWL
Uteroscopic destruction
Dornier basket extraction

Stone in bladder

Cystoscopic destruction–stone punch
Open removal–if larger than hen's egg

Fig. 17.13 Surgical options for urinary stones.

prevented by allopurinol, and this may also reduce calcium stone formation in patients with a high urate excretion. Stones formed in cystinuria can be reduced by penicillamine therapy. It may be helpful to attempt to alter urine pH with ammonium chloride (low pH discourages phosphate stone formation) or sodium bicarbonate (high pH discourages urate and cystine stone formation).

EXCESSIVE MICTURITION

POLYURIA

An inappropriately high urine volume (> 3 litres/day) may result from increased urinary solute excretion (osmotic diuresis) or may represent pure water diuresis (Box 17.15). In the assessment of polyuria accurate documentation of intake is essential. In primary or psychogenic polydipsia, the increased urine output is an appropriate response to increased water intake. Typically, plasma sodium concentration will be low to normal in such patients. Polyuria with increased free water clearance (i.e. water free of solute) in the absence of an excessive intake is indicative of impaired urinary concentrating ability, as seen in diabetes insipidus. Plasma sodium will be high to normal in such patients; an increased thirst will usually prevent abnormally high plasma sodium concentrations, but restricted access to water may result in hypernatraemia. Free water clearance is calculated by measuring osmotic clearance:

$$\text{Osmotic clearance} = \text{urine volume} \times \frac{\text{urine osmolality}}{\text{plasma osmolality}}$$

Free water clearance = urine volume − osmotic clearance

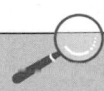

17.15 CAUSES OF POLYURIA

- Excess fluid intake
- Osmotic, e.g. hyperglycaemia, hypercalcaemia
- Cranial diabetes insipidus (reduced antidiuretic hormone (ADH) secretion)
    Idiopathic (50%), mass lesion, trauma, infection
- Nephrogenic diabetes insipidus (tubular dysfunction)
    Genetic tubular defects
    Drugs/toxins, e.g. lithium, diuretics
    Interstitial renal disease
    Hypokalaemia, hypercalcaemia

Investigation of polyuria includes measurement of plasma electrolytes, glucose and calcium. Investigation of suspected diabetes insipidus is described on page 797.

NOCTURIA

Waking up at night to void urine may be a consequence of polyuria but may also result from fluid intake or diuretic use in the late evening. Nocturia also occurs in chronic kidney disease, and in prostatic enlargement where it is associated with poor stream, hesitancy, incomplete bladder emptying, terminal dribbling and urinary frequency due to partial urethral obstruction (p. 510 and Fig. 17.14). Nocturia may also occur in sleep disturbance without functional abnormalities of the urinary tract.

FREQUENCY

Frequency describes micturition more often than a patient's expectations. It may be a consequence of polyuria, most

17

commonly due to diuretic therapy, when volumes passed are normal or high. It is also a symptom of UTIs (urethritis, cystitis, prostatitis) or urethral syndrome when urine volumes are typically low and associated with dysuria, urgency and a feeling of incomplete emptying.

URINARY INCONTINENCE

Urinary incontinence is defined as any involuntary leakage of urine. Urinary tract pathology causing incontinence is described below. It may also occur with a normal urinary tract, e.g. in association with poor cognition or poor mobility, or transiently during an acute illness or hospitalisation, especially in older people. Diuretics (medication, alcohol or caffeine) may worsen incontinence.

Clinical assessment and investigations

The pattern of micturition is important in defining the incontinence, and patients should be encouraged to keep a voiding diary, including the estimated volume voided, frequency of voiding, precipitating factors and associated features, e.g. urgency.

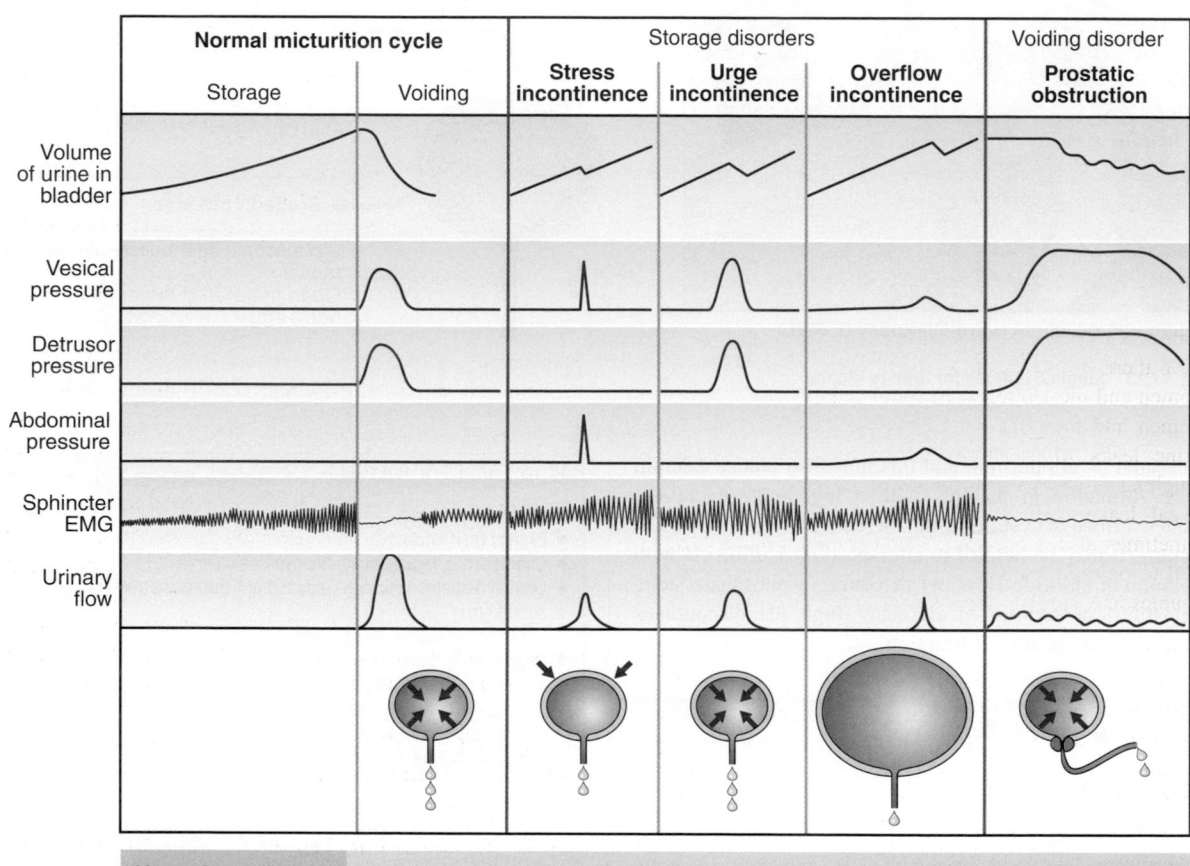

Normal micturition cycle		Storage disorders			Voiding disorder
Storage	Voiding	Stress incontinence	Urge incontinence	Overflow incontinence	Prostatic obstruction

Normal micturition cycle	Storage	Minimal pressure rise in bladder as it fills. No detrusor activity, sphincter muscle tone increased during filling
	Voiding	Sphincter relaxes, detrusor contracts and vesical pressure increases. Good urine flow until bladder empty
Stress incontinence		As for normal but during cough there is passive increase in the vesical pressure (no active detrusor contraction). This vesical pressure is greater than urethral pressure transiently with resultant urine leakage
Urge incontinence		As for normal but during filling there is abnormal detrusor contraction; this results in a raised vesical pressure, and if this is greater than the urethral pressure, leakage occurs
Overflow incontinence		Bladder is very full. No detrusor contractions but minimal increases in abdominal and vesical pressure result in urine leakage (as in stress incontinence)
Prostatic obstruction		This shows only the voiding phase; the storage phase is the same as the normal. During voiding there is a strong detrusor contraction resulting in high vesical pressure. Despite this high pressure there is poor flow because of the obstruction in the prostatic urethra. Flow is typically wavy as the prostatic obstruction is somewhat elastic and varies throughout the void

Fig. 17.14 Urodynamic abnormalities in patients with urinary incontinence. (EMG = electromyogram)

Examination includes an assessment of cognitive function and mobility, and of perineal sensation and anal sphincter tone since the innervation is from the same sacral nerve roots that supply the bladder and urethral sphincter. A general neurological assessment is required to detect disorders such as multiple sclerosis that may affect the nervous supply of the bladder, and the lumbar spine should be inspected for features of spina bifida occulta. Rectal examination is needed to assess the prostate in men and to exclude faecal impaction as a cause of incontinence. Genital examination should identify phimosis and paraphimosis in men, and vaginal mucosal atrophy, cystoceles or rectoceles in women.

Urinalysis and culture should be performed in all patients. An assessment of post-micturition volume should be made, either by post-micturition ultrasound or catheterisation. Urine flow rates and full urodynamic assessment may also be helpful in selected cases (Fig. 17.14).

Incontinence syndromes

Stress incontinence

In stress incontinence leakage occurs because passive bladder pressure exceeds the urethral pressure, due to either poor pelvic floor support or a weak urethral sphincter. Most often there is an element of both. This is very common in women and most often seen following childbirth. It is rare in men and then usually follows surgery to the prostate. Urine leaks when abdominal pressure rises, e.g. when coughing or sneezing. In women, perineal inspection may reveal leakage of urine when the patient coughs, and sometimes also a prolapse. Females in particular respond well to physiotherapy but if incontinence is persistent and troublesome, surgical treatment is indicated.

Urge incontinence

In urge incontinence leakage usually occurs because of detrusor over-activity producing an increased bladder pressure which overcomes the urethral sphincter (motor urgency). Urgency with or without incontinence may also be driven by a hypersensitive bladder (sensory urgency) resulting from UTI or bladder stone. The incidence of urge incontinence increases with age, occurring in 17% of the population aged over 65 years and around 50% of those requiring nursing home care. It is also seen in men with lower urinary tract obstruction and most often remits after the obstruction is relieved (p. 510).

The diagnosis is often made simply on the basis of symptoms and the exclusion of urinary retention by bladder ultrasound; confirmation requires urodynamic testing (Fig. 17.14). The mainstay of treatment is bladder retraining, teaching patients to hold more urine voluntarily in their bladder, assisted by anticholinergic medication. Surgery is restricted to patients who have severe day-time incontinence despite such treatment.

Continual incontinence

This suggests the presence of a fistula, usually between the bladder and vagina (vesicovaginal) or the ureter and vagina (ureterovaginal). This is most common following gynaecological surgery but is also seen in patients with

17.16 INCONTINENCE IN OLD AGE

- **Prevalence:** urinary incontinence affects 15% of women and 10% of men aged over 65 years.
- **Cause:** incontinence may be transient due to an acute confusional state, urinary infection, medication (such as diuretics), faecal impaction or restricted mobility, and these should be treated before embarking on further specific investigation.
- **Detrusor over-activity:** established incontinence in old age is most commonly due to detrusor over-activity which may be caused by damage to central inhibitory centres or local detrusor muscle abnormalities.
- **Catheterisation:** poor manual dexterity or cognitive impairment may necessitate the help of a carer to assist with intermittent catheterisation.

gynaecological malignancy or following radiotherapy. In parts of the world where obstetric services are scarce, prolonged obstructed labour can be a common cause of vesicovaginal fistulae. Continual incontinence may also be seen in infants with congenital ectopic ureters. Occasionally, stress incontinence is so severe that the patient leaks continuously. Diagnosis is confirmed by inspection of the perineum and by IVU. Treatment is surgical.

Overflow incontinence

This occurs when the bladder becomes chronically over-distended. It is most commonly seen in men with benign prostatic hyperplasia or bladder neck obstruction (p. 510), but may occur in either sex as a result of failure of the detrusor muscle (atonic bladder). The latter state may be idiopathic but more commonly is the result of damage to the pelvic nerves, either from surgery (commonly, hysterectomy or rectal excision), trauma or infection, or from compression of the cauda equina from disc prolapse, trauma or tumour. Incomplete bladder emptying can be identified by ultrasound, which reveals a significant post-micturition volume (> 100 ml). Obstructed bladders should be treated surgically. Unobstructed bladders will need to be drained, preferably by intermittent self-catheterisation. Urodynamic testing may help clarify the aetiology.

Post-micturition dribble

This is very common in men, even in the relatively young. It is due to a small amount of urine becoming trapped in the U-bend of the bulbar urethra, which leaks out when the patient moves. It is more pronounced if associated with a urethral diverticulum or urethral stricture. It may occur in females with a urethral diverticulum and may mimic stress incontinence.

Neurological causes

Neurological disease resulting in abnormal bladder function is almost always associated with obvious neurological signs; these are described on page 1199.

REDUCED MICTURITION

OLIGURIA/ANURIA

On a normal diet, between 300 and 500 ml/day of urine is required to excrete the solute load at maximum concen-

17

tration. Volumes below this are termed oliguria. Anuria is the (almost) total absence of urine (< 50 ml/day). A low measured urine volume is an important finding and is a consequence of reduced production, obstruction to urine flow or both.

Reduced urine production

The volume of urine produced by the kidney is the result of the difference between glomerular filtration and tubular reabsorption. Urine volumes are variable in renal failure. When GFR is very low, urine volumes may still be normal if tubular reabsorption is correspondingly low; hence urine volume is a poor indicator of chronic kidney disease. Oligo/anuria may be caused by a reduction in urine production, as typically seen in pre-renal acute renal failure, when GFR is reduced but intact tubular homeostatic mechanisms increase reabsorption to conserve salt and water. A high solute load or associated tubular dysfunction may, however, produce normal or high urine volumes in such cases until the pre-renal insult becomes severe and GFR minimal, e.g. in diabetic ketoacidosis with marked glycosuria. Urine volumes are variable in acute renal failure due to intrinsic renal disease. Typically, renal infarction is associated with a sudden cessation of urine production (if bilateral or in a single functioning kidney). Rapidly progressive glomerulonephritis is often associated with a rapid onset of oligo/anuria.

Urinary tract obstruction

A reduced urine volume may also be caused by obstruction to urine flow. The most common causes of urinary tract obstruction are urinary calculi (p. 471) and prostatic enlargement (benign or malignant, p. 510), or pelvic and retroperitoneal tumours in an older age group. Acute urinary retention is seen after general anaesthesia in about 50% of cases, particularly in conjunction with pre-existing prostatic enlargement. In young men, bladder neck dyssynergia may also cause obstruction. Urethral strictures (more likely if there is a history of instrumentation), trauma or urethral infection, urethral valves, phimosis or meatal stenosis are other common causes (Fig. 17.10, p. 466). Poor flow and post-micturition residual bladder volume are also seen in atonic bladders (e.g. in neurological disorders such as multiple sclerosis and spina bifida) when there is reduced/absent detrusor muscle activity and a failure of the distal sphincter to relax.

Obstruction may be acute or chronic, and partial or complete. Acute obstruction is often associated with pain due to distension of the urinary tract that may be exacerbated by a fluid load. The site of the pain can indicate the site of the obstruction. Obstruction at the bladder neck (acute urinary retention) is associated with lower midline abdominal discomfort due to bladder dilatation. Ureteric obstruction, e.g. from a renal calculus, typically presents as loin pain radiating to the groin. Higher obstructions, e.g. at the level of the renal pelvis, may present as flank pain. Chronic obstruction rarely produces pain but may produce a dull ache.

To produce oligo/anuria, the obstruction must be complete and distal to the bladder neck, bilateral, or unilateral on the side of a single functioning kidney. If an obstruction is not relieved, the pressure transmitted back to the nephrons will result in cessation of glomerular filtration. Hence, in the assessment of oligo/anuria, it is important to diagnose and relieve urinary tract obstruction rapidly. All patients presenting with acutely reduced urinary volumes should be palpated/percussed for a full bladder and catheterised. Radiological assessment, typically by ultrasound, should be undertaken promptly to identify obstruction. It is important to note that, if there is failure of urine production because of concomitant acute renal failure, urinary tracts may not be particularly dilated. Relief of an acute obstruction is usually accompanied by a rapid return of renal function, although tubular function may be impaired, resulting in polyuria and failure to conserve electrolytes (e.g. phosphate).

Partial obstruction can be associated with normal or even high urine volumes due to chronic tubular injury, with a loss of tubular concentrating ability. This chronic tubular injury can also produce a type 1 renal tubular acidosis (p. 438). Over time, even partial obstruction will cause tubular atrophy and irreversible renal failure.

ERECTILE DYSFUNCTION

Causes of erectile failure are shown in Box 17.17. Vascular, neuropathic and psychological causes are most common. With the exception of diabetes mellitus, endocrine causes are relatively uncommon and are characterised by loss of libido as well as erectile dysfunction. Erectile dysfunction and reduced libido occur in over 50% of men with advanced chronic kidney disease or on dialysis. From experience gained in diabetes clinics, erectile dysfunction is a markedly under-diagnosed problem. It is important to be able to discuss matters frankly with the patient, and to establish whether there are associated features of hypogonadism (p. 766), and whether erections occur at any other time (e.g. if the patient has erections on wakening in the morning, vascular and neuropathic causes are much less likely).

Investigations

Blood should be taken for glucose, glycated haemoglobin, prolactin, testosterone, luteinising hormone (LH) and follicle-stimulating hormone (FSH). A number of further tests are available but are rarely employed because they do

17.17 CAUSES OF ERECTILE DYSFUNCTION	

With reduced libido

- Hypogonadism
- Depression

With intact libido

- Psychological problems, including anxiety
- Vascular insufficiency (atheroma)
- Neuropathic causes (e.g. diabetes mellitus, alcohol excess, multiple sclerosis)
- Drugs (e.g. β-blockers, thiazide diuretics)

not usually influence management. These include nocturnal tumescence monitoring (using a plethysmograph placed around the shaft of the penis overnight) to establish whether blood supply and nerve function are sufficient to allow erections to occur during sleep; intracavernosal injection of papaverine or prostaglandin E1 to test the adequacy of blood supply; internal pudendal artery angiography; and tests of autonomic and peripheral sensory nerve conduction.

Management

Psychotherapy which includes the sexual partner is most useful for psychological problems. Neuropathy and vascular disease are unlikely to improve, but several treatments are available. First-line therapy is usually with oral phosphodiesterase inhibitors (e.g. sildenafil) which potentiate the vasodilator action of nitric oxide on cyclic guanosine monophosphate (cGMP). Coadministration of phosphodiesterase inhibitors with nitric oxide donors ('nitrate' drugs) is contraindicated because of the risk of severe hypotension. Caution should also be exercised in patients with chronic disease including ischaemic heart disease, principally because the unaccustomed stress of sexual activity may precipitate cardiac ischaemia or dysrhythmia. Other treatments for impotence include self-administered intracavernosal injection or urethral gel administration of prostaglandin E1; vacuum devices which achieve an erection which is maintained by a tourniquet around the base of the penis; and prosthetic implants, either of a fixed rod or inflatable reservoir. Hypogonadism should be treated as described on page 767.

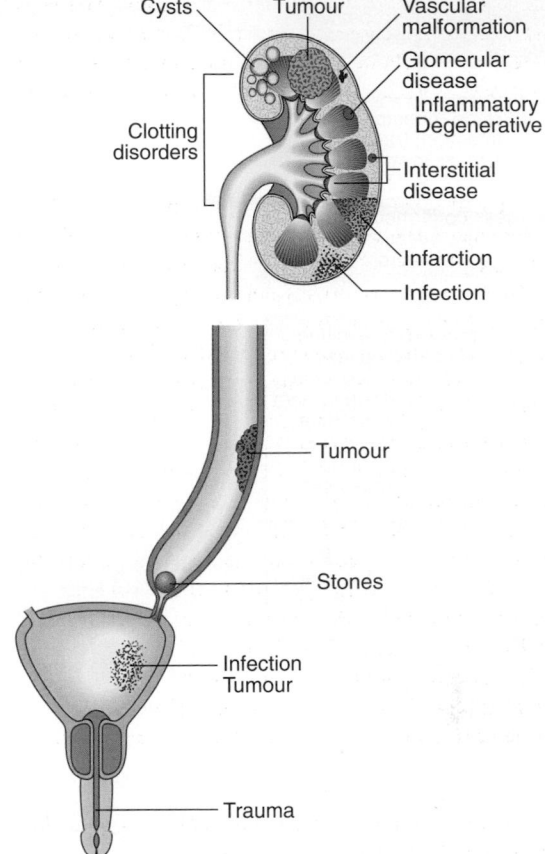

Fig. 17.15 Causes of haematuria.

HAEMATURIA

Haematuria may be visible and reported by the patient (macroscopic haematuria), or invisible and detected on dipstick testing of urine (microscopic haematuria). It indicates bleeding from anywhere in the renal tract (Fig. 17.15).

Microscopy shows that normal individuals have occasional red blood cells in the urine (up to 12 500 rbc/ml). The detection limit for dipstick testing is 15–20 000 rbc/ml, which is sufficiently sensitive to detect all significant bleeding. However, dipstick tests are also positive in the presence of free haemoglobin or myoglobin. Urine microscopy (p. 457) can be valuable in confirming haematuria and

in establishing the cause of bleeding (Box 17.18). Other causes of red or dark urine may sometimes be confused with haematuria but produce negative dipstick tests and microscopy (Box 17.19). True positive tests may occur during menstruation, infection or strenuous exercise, but persistent haematuria requires further investigation to exclude malignancy.

Macroscopic (visible) haematuria is more likely to be caused by tumours (p. 512 and Box 17.20). Severe infections or renal infarction can also cause macroscopic haematuria, usually accompanied by pain. Recurrent episodes of

17

17.18 INTERPRETATION OF DIPSTICK-POSITIVE HAEMATURIA		
Dipstick test positive	**Urine microscopy**	**Suggested cause**
Haematuria	White blood cells	Infection
	Abnormal epithelial cells	Tumour
	Red cell casts	
	Dysmorphic erythrocytes (phase contrast microscopy)	Glomerular bleeding*
Haemoglobinuria	No red cells	Intravascular haemolysis
Myoglobinuria	No red cells	Rhabdomyolysis

* Glomerular bleeding implies that the GBM is fractured. It can occur physiologically following very strenuous exertion but usually indicates intrinsic renal disease and is an important feature of the nephritic syndrome (Box 17.5, p. 467).

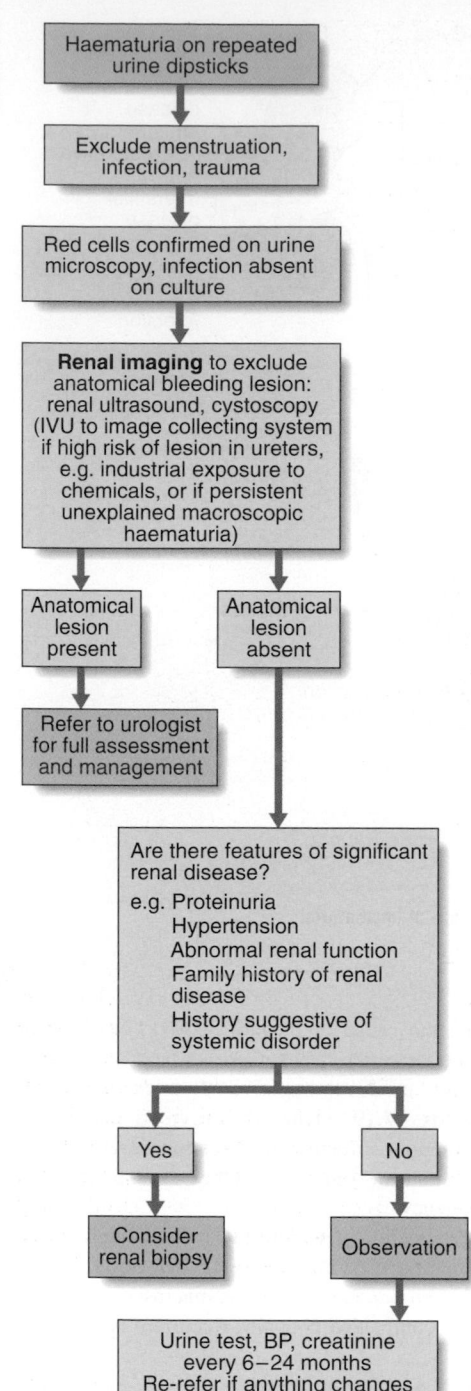

Fig. 17.16   Investigation of haematuria.

painless gross haematuria in association with respiratory infections are characteristic of IgA nephropathy (p. 500).

Investigations and management

Investigation of haematuria (Fig. 17.16), whether microscopic or macroscopic, should be directed first at the exclusion of an anatomical bleeding lesion, particularly in older patients or others at risk of carcinoma of the bladder or other malignancy. If haematuria occurs with proteinuria or

17.19 DIPSTICK-NEGATIVE DARK URINE	
Cause	**Urine colour**
Food dyes e.g. Acanthocyanins (beetroot)	Red
Drugs e.g. Phenolphthalein	Pink when alkaline
Senna/other anthaquinones	Orange
Rifampicin	Orange
Levodopa	Darkens on standing
Porphyria	Darkens on standing
Alkaptonuria	
Bilirubinuria e.g. Obstructive jaundice	Dark Dipstick-positive for bilirubin, negative for haemoglobin

EBM

17.20   HAEMATURIA AND UROTHELIAL MALIGNANCY

'Macroscopic haematuria has a positive predictive value of 83% for bladder cancer and 22% for all urothelial tumours, rising to 41% in patients over the age of 40.'

● Buntinx F, et al. Fam Pract 1997; 14(1):63–68.

clinical features of renal disease (Box 17.5, p. 467), inflammatory renal disease (pp. 465 and 499) should be considered and a renal biopsy may be indicated. Where there are no features of significant renal disease and malignancy has been excluded, patients with isolated microscopic haematuria may be managed by observation alone and biopsy is rarely warranted. Although this scenario occasionally precedes significant renal disease (e.g. Alport's syndrome, IgA nephropathy), it is commonly caused by the usually benign condition of thin basement membrane disease (p. 504), insignificant vascular malformations, renal cysts or renal stones. In 'loin pain–haematuria' syndrome, benign glomerular bleeding is associated with loin pain.

Management of haematuria depends upon the cause.

PROTEINURIA

Moderate amounts of low molecular weight protein do pass through the GBM. These proteins are normally reabsorbed by tubular cells so that less than 150 mg/day appears in urine. As shown in Box 17.21, larger amounts indicate renal damage; any renal disease or injury may cause proteinuria. Proteinuria is usually asymptomatic, although large amounts may make urine froth easily.

Relatively minor leakage of albumin into the urine may occur transiently after vigorous exercise, during fever or UTI and in heart failure. Such proteinuria does not reach nephrotic levels and tests should be repeated once the stimulus is no longer present. Occasionally, proteinuria occurs only during the day, and the first morning sample is negative. In the absence of other signs of renal disease, such 'orthostatic proteinuria' is usually regarded as benign.

17.21 QUANTIFYING PROTEINURIA

24-hr urine protein	Protein/creatinine ratio[1] (random sample)	Significance
< 0.03 g	< 3.5 (female)[2] < 2.5 (male)[2]	Normal
0.03–0.3 g	~3.5–15[2,4]	Microalbuminuria
0.3–0.5 g	~15–50[3]	Dipsticks positive
0.5–2.5 g	~50–250[3]	Source equivocal
> 2.5 g	> 250[3]	Glomerular disease likely
> 4.0 g	> 400[3]	Nephrotic range—always glomerular

[1] Urine protein (mg/l)/urine creatinine (mmol/l).
[2] Usually measured as albumin/creatinine ratio.
[3] Usually measured as total protein/creatinine ratio.
[4] Not detectable with standard dipsticks but can be detected with specific 'albustix'.

Low molecular weight proteins may also appear in the urine in larger quantities than 150 mg/day, indicating failure of reabsorption by damaged tubular cells, i.e. 'tubular proteinuria'. This can be demonstrated by analysis of the size of excreted proteins or by specific assays for such proteins (e.g. β_2-microglobulin, molecular weight 12 kDa). The amounts of such protein rarely exceed 1.5–2 g/24 hours, and proteinuria greater than this almost always indicates significant glomerular disease.

The amount of protein in urine should be quantified to guide further investigations (Fig. 17.17). Quantification in a 24-hour urine collection is the gold standard, but these collections are arduous and often inaccurate. Use of the protein/creatinine (mg/mmol) ratio in single samples makes allowance for the variable degree of urinary dilution and can allow extrapolation of 24-hour values (Box 17.21). Changes in this ratio give valuable information about the progression of renal disease.

In many types of renal disease, the severity of proteinuria is a marker for an increased risk of progressive loss of renal function. There is circumstantial evidence that protein in the glomerular filtrate is toxic to the kidneys, and treatments that are effective at lowering the risk of progression of renal failure (e.g. angiotensin-converting enzyme (ACE) inhibitors in diabetic nephropathy) also reduce proteinuria.

MICROALBUMINURIA

Microalbuminuria describes the urinary excretion of small amounts of normal albumin protein. The presence of albumin in the urine is a clear sign of glomerular abnormality and can identify the very early stages of progressive glomerular disease, e.g. in diabetic nephropathy (p. 841). Because significant renal damage will have occurred before dipstick tests become positive, patients with diabetes mellitus should be screened regularly for microalbuminuria. Persistent microalbuminuria has also been associated with an increased risk of atherosclerosis and cardiovascular mortality; neither the mechanism of proteinuria nor an explanation of these associations has yet been found.

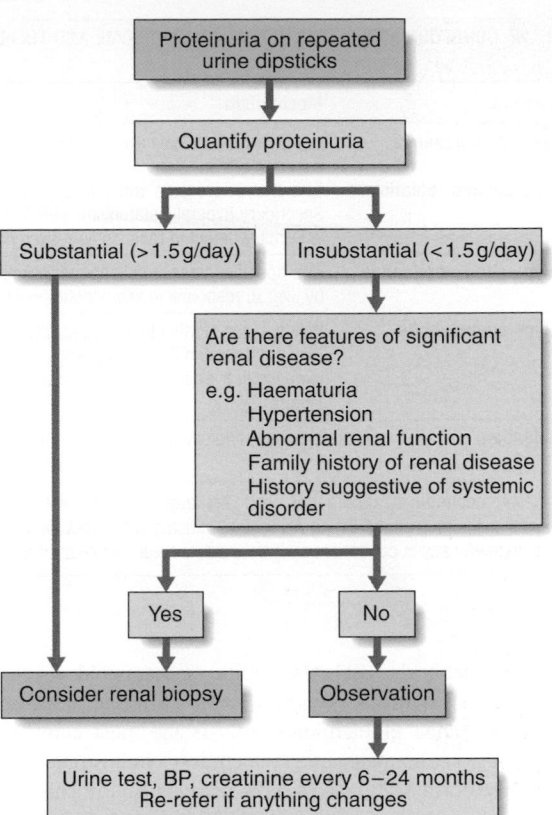

Fig. 17.17 Investigation of proteinuria.

BENCE JONES PROTEINURIA

Patients with a clone of B lymphocytes secreting free immunoglobulin light chains (molecular weight 25 kDa) filter these freely into the urine, and Bence Jones protein can then be identified in fresh urine samples. This may occur in amyloidosis (p. 79) and plasma cell dyscrasias, but is particularly important as a marker for myeloma (p. 1052). Bence Jones protein is poorly identified by dipstick tests, and the sulphosalicylic acid precipitation test is insufficiently sensitive. Therefore, immunodetection methods should be performed when Bence Jones proteinuria is suspected.

NEPHROTIC SYNDROME

Nephrotic syndrome refers to the secondary phenomena that occur when substantial amounts of protein are lost in the urine (Box 17.5, p. 467). The consequences are shown in Box 17.22. Dependent oedema accumulates predominantly in the lower limbs in adults, extending to the genitalia and lower abdomen as it becomes more severe. In the morning, the upper limbs and face may be more affected. In children, ascites occurs early and oedema is often seen only in the face. Blood volume may be normal, reduced or increased. Avid renal sodium retention is an early and universal feature; the mechanisms are shown in Figure 16.5, p. 426.

The diseases that cause nephrotic syndrome always affect the glomerulus (Fig. 17.30, p. 499) and tend to be non-inflammatory, or subacute examples of inflammatory

17

17.22 CONSEQUENCES OF THE NEPHROTIC SYNDROME AND THEIR MANAGEMENT

Feature	Mechanism	Consequence	Management
Hypoalbuminaemia	Urinary protein losses exceed synthetic capacity of liver	Reduced oncotic pressure Oedema	Diuretics and a low-sodium diet*
Avid sodium retention	Low oncotic pressure and intravascular volume Secondary hyperaldosteronism ± Primary defect in renal sodium excretion	Oedema	
Hypercholesterolaemia	Non-specific increase in lipoprotein synthesis by liver in response to low oncotic pressure	High rate of atherosclerosis	Lipid-lowering drugs (e.g. HMG CoA reductase inhibitors, p. 450)
Hypercoagulability	Relative loss of inhibitors of coagulation (e.g. antithrombin II, protein C and S) and increase in liver synthesis of procoagulant factors	Venous thromboembolism	Case for routine anticoagulation in all patients with chronic or severe nephrotic syndrome
Infection	Hypogammaglobulinaemia (urinary losses)	Pneumococcal infection	Consider vaccination, particularly in children

* Severe nephrotic syndrome may need very large doses of combinations of diuretics acting on different parts of the nephron (e.g. loop diuretic plus thiazide plus amiloride). In occasional patients with hypovolaemia, intravenous salt-poor albumin infusions may help to establish a diuresis, although efficacy is controversial. Over-diuresis risks secondary impairment of renal function through hypovolaemia.

glomerulonephritis. Diabetes mellitus and amyloidosis can also cause nephrotic syndrome. In children, because minimal change glomerulonephritis is the most common diagnosis, initial management includes administration of high-dose corticosteroids. In older patients, and in children where this therapy is unsuccessful, a renal biopsy is required unless there is strong evidence for a specific aetiology (e.g. a long history of diabetes with other microvascular complications and a demonstrated progression from microalbuminuria, and with hypertension but no haematuria). Supportive management in patients with nephrotic syndrome is described in Box 17.22.

OEDEMA

Aetiology

'Pitting' oedema reflects increased interstitial fluid, which can result from disruption of the 'Starling forces' which dictate fluid transit across capillary basement membranes (Box 17.23). It is usually influenced by the effect of gravity on venous hydrostatic pressure and so accumulates in the ankles during the day and improves overnight ('dependent' oedema). Non-pitting oedema may reflect protein deposition: for example, in myxoedema associated with hypothyroidism (p. 750). In developed countries the most common causes of oedema are local venous problems and heart failure (p. 542), but it is important to identify other causes.

Lower limb oedema is common in morbid obesity. Although venous obstruction often contributes, the oedema may be multifactorial: for example, being exacerbated by right heart failure caused by sleep apnoea.

'Idiopathic oedema' occurs most commonly in women, typically varies with the menstrual cycle, and is characterised by marked diurnal variation in weight (more than 1.5 kg over 12 hours). This probably reflects variation in capillary permeability rather than extracellular fluid volume.

Clinical assessment

A substantial volume (litres) of extracellular fluid may accumulate without any clinical signs. In adults dependent regions or immobile limbs are usually the first site of oedema formation, where it is easy to mistake the first signs of generalised oedema for a local problem. Ankle swelling is characteristic, but oedema develops over the sacrum in bed-bound patients. It rises higher up the lower limbs with increasing severity, to affect the genitalia and abdomen. Ascites is common and often an earlier feature in children or

17.23 CAUSES OF OEDEMA

Low plasma oncotic pressure

Low serum albumin due to
• Increased loss—nephrotic syndrome
• Decreased synthesis—liver failure
• Malnutrition/malabsorption

Increased capillary permeability

Leakage of proteins into the interstitium, reducing the osmotic pressure gradient which draws fluid into the lymphatics and blood
• Local—infection/inflammation
• Systemic—severe sepsis
• Drug-related, e.g. calcium channel blockers

Increased hydrostatic pressure

High venous pressure/obstruction
• Deep venous thrombosis or venous insufficiency—local oedema
• Pregnancy
• Pelvic tumour
• Congestive heart failure
• Intravascular volume expansion (iatrogenic, renal failure, Conn's syndrome)

Lymphatic obstruction
• Infection—filariasis, lymphogranuloma venereum (pp. 416 and 363)
• Malignancy
• Radiation injury
• Congenital abnormality

17

young adults, and in liver disease. Pleural effusions are common and can be a feature of any cause of generalised oedema. Facial oedema on waking is common in adults with low oncotic pressure oedema and in young patients. Features of intravascular volume depletion (tachycardia, postural hypotension) may occur when oedema is due to decreased oncotic pressure or increased capillary permeability. If oedema is localised—for example, to one ankle but not the other—then features of venous thrombosis, inflammation and lymphatic disease should be sought.

Investigations

The cause of oedema is usually apparent from the history and examination of the cardiovascular system and abdomen, combined with testing the urine for protein and measuring the serum albumin level. Where ascites or pleural effusions in isolation are causing diagnostic difficulty, aspiration of fluid with measurement of protein and glucose, and microscopy for cells, will usually clarify the diagnosis (p. 665).

Management

Specific causes (e.g. venous thrombosis) should be treated. Diuretics are commonly used for oedema, but are also commonly abused. Where there is sodium retention and generalised oedema, restriction of sodium (and sometimes fluid) intake is rational, along with diuretic treatment. Mild fluid retention will respond to a thiazide or to a low dose of a loop diuretic such as furosemide or bumetanide. However, in oedema caused by venous or lymphatic obstruction or by increased capillary permeability, diuretics are likely to be hazardous, as they will cause hypovolaemia with secondary hyperaldosteronism and rebound exaggeration of oedema. Local treatments, such as the use of compression either continuously (e.g. compression stockings) or intermittently (with a mechanical device), can be useful in these circumstances.

In nephrotic syndrome, renal failure and severe cardiac failure, very large doses of diuretics, sometimes in combination, may be required to achieve a negative sodium and fluid balance.

HYPERTENSION

Hypertension is a very common feature of renal parenchymal and vascular disease and is an early feature of glomerular disorders. Renal mechanisms are also likely to be important in essential hypertension, and most inherited disorders of blood pressure have been attributed to altered salt- and water-handling by the kidney. In renal interstitial disorders, increased sodium loss (through reduced reabsorption from glomerular filtrate) may lead to hypotension. However, as GFR declines, hypertension becomes an increasingly common feature, regardless of the aetiology of the renal disease. When renal function is replaced by dialysis, control of hypertension often becomes easier as salt and volume balance are controlled. Obsessional attention to fluid balance in haemodialysis patients may reduce or remove the need for hypotensive drugs. Control of hypertension is very important in patients with renal impairment because of its close relationship with further decline of renal function (p. 488) and with the adverse cardiovascular risk in renal disease.

ACUTE RENAL FAILURE

Acute renal failure (ARF) refers to a sudden and usually reversible loss of renal function, which develops over a period of days or weeks and is usually accompanied by a reduction in urine volume. There are many possible causes (Fig. 17.18) and it is frequently multifactorial. The clinical picture is often dominated by the underlying condition (e.g.

17

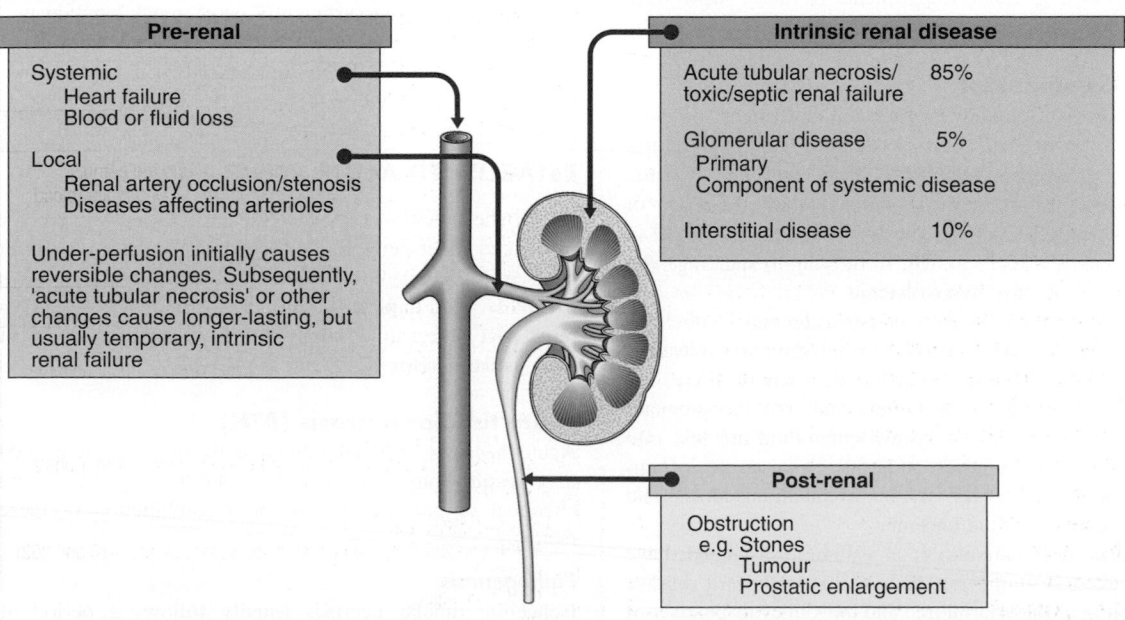

Fig. 17.18 Causes of acute renal failure.

septic shock, trauma). If the cause cannot be rapidly corrected and renal function restored, temporary renal replacement therapy may be required (p. 491).

REVERSIBLE PRE-RENAL ACUTE RENAL FAILURE

Because haemodynamic disturbances can initially produce acute renal dysfunction that has the potential to be rapidly reversed, prompt recognition and treatment are important. These topics are considered separately from established acute renal failure.

Pathogenesis

The kidney can regulate its own blood flow and GFR over a wide range of perfusion pressures. When the perfusion pressure falls—as in hypovolaemia, shock, heart failure or narrowing of the renal arteries—the resistance vessels in the kidney dilate to facilitate flow. Vasodilator prostaglandins are important, and this mechanism is markedly impaired by NSAIDs (p. 517). If autoregulation of blood flow fails, the GFR can still be maintained by selective constriction of the post-glomerular (efferent) arteriole. This is mediated through the release of renin and generation of angiotensin II, which preferentially constricts this vessel. ACE inhibitors interfere with this response (p. 517).

More severe or prolonged under-perfusion of the kidneys may lead to failure of these compensatory mechanisms and hence an acute decline in GFR. The renal tubules are intact and become hyperfunctional; that is, tubular reabsorption of sodium and water is increased, partly through physical factors associated with changes in blood and urine flow and partly through the influence of angiotensins, aldosterone and vasopressin. This leads to the formation of a low volume of urine which is concentrated (osmolality > 600 mOsm/kg) but low in sodium (< 20 mmol/l). These urinary changes may be absent in patients with impaired tubular function, e.g. pre-existing renal impairment, or those who have received loop diuretics.

Clinical assessment

There may be marked hypotension and signs of poor peripheral perfusion, such as delayed capillary return. However, pre-renal ARF may occur without systemic hypotension, particularly in patients taking NSAIDs or ACE inhibitors (see above). Postural hypotension (a fall in blood pressure > 20/10 mmHg from lying to standing) is a valuable sign of early hypovolaemia.

The cause of the reduced renal perfusion may be obvious, but concealed blood loss can occur into the gastrointestinal tract, following trauma (particularly where there are fractures of the pelvis or femur) and into the pregnant uterus. Large volumes of intravascular fluid are lost into tissues after crush injuries or burns, or in severe inflammatory skin diseases or sepsis. Metabolic acidosis and hyperkalaemia are often present.

In sepsis most patients, once volume-resuscitated, have a vasodilated systemic circulation; this leads to a relative under-filling of the arterial tree and the kidney responds as it would to absolute hypovolaemia. When it is severe or

---

17.24 LOW-DOSE DOPAMINE IN ACUTE RENAL FAILURE | EBM

'Dopamine at low, 'renal' doses has been used in the belief that it may increase renal blood flow in critically ill patients (as it does in normal individuals) and prevent ARF. However, evidence from clinical trials does not support its use.'

● ANZICS Clinical Trials Group. Lancet 2000; 356:2139–2143.
● O'Leary MJ, et al. BMJ 2001; 322:1437–1438.

---

prolonged, sepsis is an important cause of established ARF with acute tubular necrosis. The combination of sepsis and NSAIDs is a potent cause of ARF.

Management

● Establish and correct the underlying cause of the ARF.
● If hypovolaemia is present, restore blood volume as rapidly as possible (with blood, plasma or isotonic saline (0.9%), depending on what has been lost).
● Optimise systemic haemodynamics. Monitoring of the central venous pressure or pulmonary wedge pressure as an adjunct to clinical examination may aid in determining the rate of administration of fluid. Critically ill patients may require invasive haemodynamic monitoring to assess cardiac output and systemic vascular resistance, and the use of inotropic drugs to restore an effective blood pressure (p. 197).
● Correct metabolic acidosis.
  — Restoration of blood volume will correct acidosis by restoring kidney function.
  — Isotonic sodium bicarbonate (e.g. 500 ml of 1.26%) may be used.
● Recent trials do not support the use of low-dose dopamine in severely ill patients at risk of ARF (Box 17.24).

Prognosis

If treatment is given sufficiently early, renal function will usually improve rapidly; in such circumstances residual renal impairment is unlikely. In some cases, however, treatment is ineffective and renal failure becomes established.

ESTABLISHED ACUTE RENAL FAILURE

Established ARF may develop following severe or prolonged under-perfusion of the kidney (pre-renal ARF). In such cases, the histological pattern of acute tubular necrosis is usually seen. In patients without an obvious cause of pre-renal ARF, alternative 'renal' and 'post-renal' causes must be considered (Box 17.25 and Fig. 17.18).

Acute tubular necrosis (ATN)

Acute necrosis of renal tubular cells (Fig. 17.35, p. 505) may result from ischaemia or nephrotoxicity, caused by chemical or bacterial toxins, or a combination of these factors.

Pathogenesis

Ischaemic tubular necrosis usually follows a period of shock, during which renal blood flow is greatly reduced.

17

17.25 DIFFERENTIAL DIAGNOSIS OF ACUTE RENAL FAILURE IN A HAEMODYNAMICALLY STABLE, NON-SEPTIC PATIENT

Urinary tract obstruction (Fig. 17.10, p. 466)

- Suggested by a history of loin pain, haematuria, renal colic or difficulty in micturition but often clinically silent
- Can usually be excluded by renal ultrasound—essential in any patient with unexplained ARF
- Prompt relief of the obstruction restores renal function

Vascular event

- Due to major vascular occlusion or small-vessel diseases (pp. 496–499), notably malignant hypertension and haemolytic uraemic syndrome/thrombotic thrombocytopenic purpura
- May be precipitated by ACE inhibitors in critical renal artery stenosis (p. 496)
- Urine usually shows minimal abnormalities but there may be haematuria in renal infarction

Rapidly progressive glomerulonephritis (RPGN) (p. 503)

- Typically, significant (dipsticks 3+) haematuria and proteinuria (often with red cell casts or 'glomerular' red cells)
- Sometimes associated with systemic features (e.g. systemic vasculitis, systemic lupus erythematosus (SLE), Goodpasture's (anti-GBM) disease)
- Useful blood tests include: antineutrophil cytoplasmic antibodies (ANCA), antinuclear antibodies (ANA), anti-GBM antibodies, complement, immunoglobulins
- Renal biopsy shows aggressive glomerular inflammation, usually with crescent formation

Acute interstitial nephritis (p. 504)

- Usually caused by an adverse drug reaction
- Characterised by small amounts of blood and protein in urine, often with leucocyturia
- Kidneys are normal size
- Requires cessation of drug and often prednisolone treatment

Drugs

For example:
- Haemodynamic effects (e.g. NSAIDs, ACE inhibitors)
- Acute allergic interstitial nephritis (see above and p. 504)
- Direct toxicity to the tubule (e.g. aminoglycosides)

Even when systemic haemodynamics are restored, renal blood flow can remain as low as 20% of normal, due to swelling of the endothelial cells of the glomeruli and peritubular capillaries, and oedema of the interstitium. Blood flow is further reduced by vasoconstrictors such as thromboxane, vasopressin, noradrenaline (norepinephrine) and angiotensin II, partly counterbalanced by the release of intrarenal vasodilator prostaglandins. Thus, in ischaemic ATN there is reduced oxygen delivery to the tubular cells. These cells are vulnerable to ischaemia because they have high oxygen consumption in order to generate energy for solute reabsorption, particularly in the thick ascending limb of the loop of Henle.

The ischaemic insult ultimately causes death of tubular cells (Fig. 17.35B, p. 505), which may shed into the tubular lumen causing tubular obstruction. Focal breaks in the tubular basement membrane develop, allowing tubular contents to leak into the interstitial tissue and cause interstitial oedema.

In nephrotoxic ATN a similar sequence occurs, but it is initiated by direct toxicity of the causative agent to tubular cells. Examples include the aminoglycoside antibiotics, such as gentamicin, the cytotoxic agent cisplatin, and the antifungal drug amphotericin B.

Recovery from ATN

Fortunately, tubular cells can regenerate and re-form the basement membrane. If the patient is supported during the regeneration phase, kidney function usually returns. During recovery there is often a diuretic phase in which urine output increases rapidly and remains excessive for several days before returning to normal. This is due in part to loss of the medullary concentration gradient, which normally allows concentration of the urine in the collecting duct, and which depends on continued delivery of filtrate to the ascending limb of the loop of Henle and active tubular transport. The medullary concentration gradient is gradually 'washed out' in ATN, and is not re-established until glomerular filtration and tubular function are restored. Not all patients have a diuretic phase, depending on the severity of the renal damage and the rate of recovery.

Features of established ARF

These reflect the causal condition, such as trauma, septicaemia or systemic disease, together with features of renal failure. The rate of rise in plasma urea and creatinine is determined by the rate of protein catabolism (tissue breakdown). In ARF associated with catabolic states, such as severe infections, major surgery or trauma, the daily rise in plasma urea often exceeds 5 mmol/l (30 mg/dl). At first the patient may feel well but, unless dialysis is instituted, the clinical features described below eventually appear.

Alterations in urine volume

Patients are usually oliguric (urine volume < 500 ml daily). Anuria (complete absence of urine) is rare and usually indicates acute urinary tract obstruction or vascular occlusion. In about 20% of cases, the urine volume is normal or increased, but with a low GFR and a reduction of tubular reabsorption (non-oliguric ARF). Excretion is inadequate despite good urine output, and the plasma urea and creatinine increase.

Disturbances of water, electrolyte and acid–base balance

Hyperkalaemia is common, particularly with massive tissue breakdown, haemolysis or metabolic acidosis (p. 437). Dilutional hyponatraemia occurs if the patient has continued to drink freely despite oliguria or has received inappropriate amounts of intravenous dextrose. Metabolic acidosis develops unless prevented by loss of hydrogen ions through vomiting or aspiration of gastric contents. Hypocalcaemia, due to reduced renal production of 1,25-dihydroxycholecalciferol, is common.

Other features

- 'Uraemic' features include initial anorexia, nausea and vomiting followed by drowsiness, apathy, confusion, muscle-twitching, hiccoughs, fits and coma.

17

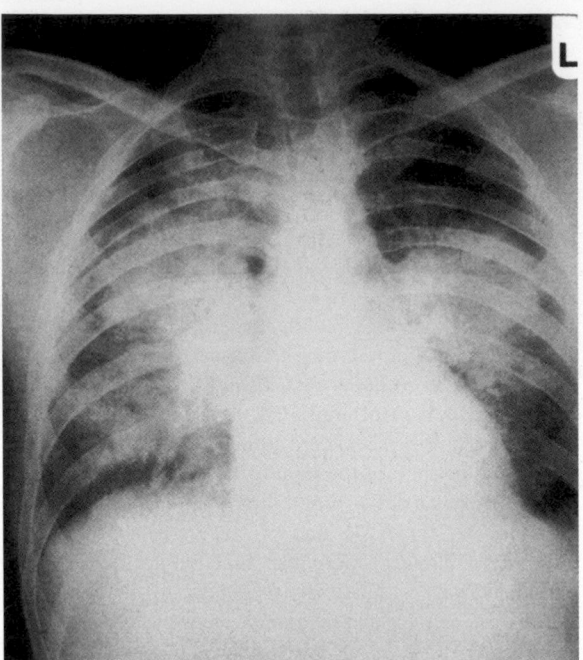

Fig. 17.19 Pulmonary oedema in acute renal failure. The appearances are indistinguishable from left ventricular failure but the heart size is usually normal. Blood pressure is often high.

- Respiratory rate may be increased due to acidosis, pulmonary oedema or respiratory infection. Pulmonary oedema (Fig. 17.19) may result from the administration of excessive amounts of fluids relative to urine output and because of increased pulmonary capillary permeability.
- Anaemia is common, due to excessive blood loss, haemolysis or decreased erythropoiesis. Bleeding is more likely because of disordered platelet function and disturbances of the coagulation cascade. Spontaneous gastrointestinal haemorrhage may occur, often late in the illness, although this is less common with effective dialysis and the use of agents that reduce gastric acid production.
- Severe infections may complicate ARF because humoral and cellular immune mechanisms are depressed.

Management

Emergency resuscitation
Hyperkalaemia (a plasma K^+ concentration > 6 mmol/l) must be treated immediately, as described in Box 16.15 (p. 436), to prevent the development of life-threatening cardiac arrhythmias.

Circulating blood volume should be optimised to ensure adequate renal perfusion. Hypovolaemia must be treated as for reversible pre-renal ARF (p. 482), with monitoring of central venous or pulmonary wedge pressure as required. Patients with pulmonary oedema usually require dialysis to remove sodium and water.

Severe acidosis can be ameliorated with isotonic sodium bicarbonate (e.g. 500 ml of 1.26%) if volume status allows. In an anuric or volume-overloaded patient, renal replacement therapy may be required.

17.26 SUGGESTED SCREENING TESTS IN ACUTE RENAL FAILURE

Haematology

- Full blood count
- Blood film: in case of fragmentation of RBC
- Clotting screen, including fibrinogen
- Group and save: in case blood products or procedures that carry the risk of bleeding (e.g. renal biopsy) are required

Biochemistry

- Urea, electrolytes and creatinine
- Calcium
- Urinalysis: for qualitative assessment of haematuria and proteinuria
- Urine microscopy: for identification of dysmorphic RBC or casts
- Quantitative urinary protein measurement

Microbiology

- Blood cultures
- C-reactive protein (ESR is misleading in ARF)
- Mid-stream urine
- Other cultures, e.g. wound, sputum, catheters
- Hepatitis and HIV serology: urgent if dialysis is needed (isolation of dialysis machine if positive)

Imaging etc.

- Renal ultrasound: usually required urgently to confirm/refute two equal-sized, unobstructed kidneys
- Chest X-ray
- ECG: if > 40 years or there are risk factors for cardiac disease

If diagnosis is not known

Consider:
- Immunoglobulins and protein electrophoresis
- Urinary Bence Jones protein
- Complement
- ANA and dsDNA if ANA is positive
- Extractable nuclear antigen (ENA): if a connective tissue disorder is suspected
- Rheumatoid factor
- ANCA and anti-GBM: in all possible inflammatory renal disease
- Cryoglobulins: if cryoglobulinaemia is clinically suspected
- Myoglobin/creatine kinase: if rhabdomyolysis is possible
- Anti-streptolysin O titre: if post-streptococcal glomerulonephritis is possible
- Other serology: if clinically suspected, e.g. leptospirosis, syphilis, Hantavirus
- Pulmonary function: in systemic disease
- Carbon monoxide transfer coefficient: if lung haemorrhage is suspected

Addressing the underlying cause of the ARF
This may be obvious or revealed by simple initial investigations (e.g. ultrasound showing urinary tract obstruction). If not, a range of investigations, including renal biopsy, may be necessary (Box 17.26). In many cases, more than one factor contributes to the renal dysfunction.

There is no specific treatment for ATN, other than restoring renal perfusion. Intrinsic renal disease may require specific therapy; for example, immunosuppressive drugs are of value in some causes of rapidly progressive glomerulonephritis (p. 503), and plasma infusion and plasma exchange may be indicated in microangiopathic diseases (p. 498).

'Post-renal' obstruction should be relieved urgently. If pelvic or ureteric dilatation is found and not explained by bladder outlet obstruction, percutaneous nephrostomy is undertaken to decompress the urinary system (p. 464). With rapid intervention, dialysis can usually be avoided. Injection of dye through the nephrostomy tube (antegrade pyelography) reveals the site of the obstruction. Once obstruction has been relieved and blood chemistry is returning to normal, the underlying cause is treated whenever possible. Sometimes obstruction is caused by pelvic malignancies, such as carcinoma of the cervix, uterus or colon, which are so advanced that intervention is inadvisable.

Fluid and electrolyte balance

After initial resuscitation, daily fluid intake should equal urine output, plus an additional 500 ml to cover insensible losses; such losses are higher in febrile patients and in tropical climates. If abnormal losses occur, as in diarrhoea, additional fluid and electrolyte replacement is required. Measurement of fluid intake and urine output is subject to error so the patient should be weighed daily. Large changes in body weight, the development of oedema or signs of fluid depletion indicate that fluid intake should be reassessed.

Since sodium and potassium are retained, intake of these substances should be restricted.

Protein and energy intake

In patients in whom dialysis is likely to be avoided, accumulation of urea is slowed by dietary protein restriction (to about 40 g/day) and by suppression of protein catabolism by giving as much energy as possible in the form of fat and carbohydrate. Patients treated by dialysis may have more dietary protein (70 g protein daily, 10–12 g nitrogen).

It is important to give adequate energy and nitrogen to hypercatabolic patients (e.g. sepsis, burns). In some patients, feeding via a nasogastric tube may be helpful. Parenteral nutrition (p. 119) may be required, especially in critically ill patients, because of vomiting or diarrhoea, or if the bowel is not intact.

Infection control

Patients with ARF are at risk of intercurrent infection. Regular clinical examination and microbiological investigation, as clinically indicated, are required to diagnose and treat this complication promptly.

Drugs

Vasoactive drugs such as NSAIDs and ACE inhibitors may prolong ARF and temporary withdrawal should be considered. Many drugs are excreted renally and dose adjustment may be required in ARF to avoid accumulation.

Renal replacement therapy (p. 491)

This may be required as supportive management in ARF.

Recovery from ARF

This is usually indicated by a gradual return of urine output, and subsequently a steady improvement in plasma biochemistry. Some patients, primarily those with ATN or after relief of chronic urinary obstruction, develop a 'diuretic phase'. Fluid should be given to replace the urine output as appropriate. Supplements of sodium chloride, sodium bicarbonate and potassium chloride, and sometimes calcium, phosphate and magnesium, may be needed to com-

17.27 ACUTE RENAL FAILURE IN OLD AGE

- **Physiological change:** nephrons decline in number from the age of 30; creatinine clearance declines at a rate of about 10 ml/min per decade after the age of 50 years.
- **Creatinine:** as muscle mass falls with age, less creatinine is produced each day. Serum creatinine can be a misleading guide to renal function in poorly nourished older people.
- **Renal tubular function:** declines with age, leading to loss of urinary concentration, acidification and toxin excretion.
- **Drugs:** increased drug prescription in older people (e.g. diuretics, ACE inhibitors and NSAIDs) may contribute to loss of renal function.
- **Acute renal failure:** due to reduction in function, older people are susceptible to acute renal failure. Infection, renal vascular disease, prostatic obstruction, hypovolaemia and severe cardiac dysfunction are common causes.
- **Mortality from acute renal failure:** rises with age, primarily because of comorbid conditions.

pensate for increased urinary losses. After a few days urine volume falls to normal as the concentrating mechanism and tubular reabsorption are restored.

Prognosis

In uncomplicated ARF, such as that due to simple haemorrhage or drugs, mortality is low even when renal replacement therapy is required. In ARF associated with serious infection and multiple organ failure, mortality is 50–70%. Outcome is usually determined by the severity of the underlying disorder and other complications, rather than by renal failure itself.

CHRONIC RENAL FAILURE

Chronic renal failure (CRF) refers to an irreversible deterioration in renal function which classically develops over a period of years (Box 17.28). Initially, it is manifest only as a biochemical abnormality. Eventually, loss of the excretory, metabolic and endocrine functions of the kidney leads to the development of the clinical symptoms and signs of renal failure, which are referred to as uraemia. When death is likely without renal replacement therapy, it is called end-stage renal failure (ESRF). The social and economic consequences of CRF are considerable. In the UK, over 37 000 patients (632 per million) are kept alive by renal replacement therapy and approaching 110 new patients per million of the adult population are accepted for long-term dialysis treatment each year. Of these, 50% are aged over 65. The incidence of CRF is much higher in some countries due to differences in regional and racial incidences of disease, as well as differences in medical practice. For example, in the USA, incident rates are over 300 per million population, with nearly half of these patients having a primary diagnosis of diabetes mellitus.

Aetiology

CRF may be caused by any condition which destroys the normal structure and function of the kidney. Common

17

17.28 STAGES OF CHRONIC RENAL DISEASE[1]

Stage	Description	GFR (ml/min/1.73m²)	Action
1	Kidney damage[2] with normal or high GFR	≥ 90	Investigate, e.g. haematuria and proteinuria (see below)
2 3	Kidney damage with slightly low GFR Moderately low GFR	60–89 30–59	Renoprotection—blood pressure control, dietary modifications
4 5	Severe low GFR Kidney failure	15–29 < 15 or dialysis	Prepare for renal replacement therapy (if appropriate)

[1]US National Kidney Foundation Kidney Disease Quality Outcomes Initiative classification of stages of chronic kidney disease (Am J Kidney Dis 2002; 39(suppl 1):S1–266).
[2]Kidney damage means pathological abnormalities or markers of damage, including abnormalities in blood or urine tests or imaging studies or GFR < 60 ml/min/1.73 m² for 3 months. Symptoms unusual until $\geq$ stage 3.

17.29 COMMON CAUSES OF CHRONIC RENAL FAILURE

Disease	Proportion of end-stage renal failure	Comments
Congenital and inherited	5%	e.g. Polycystic kidney disease, Alport's syndrome
Renal artery stenosis	5%	
Hypertension	5–25%	It is uncertain whether such variation is due to true racial differences or to differences in diagnostic labelling
Glomerular diseases	10–20%	IgA nephropathy is most common
Interstitial diseases	5–15%	
Systemic inflammatory diseases	5%	e.g. SLE, vasculitis
Diabetes mellitus	20–40%	Large racial and national differences exist—higher rate is from USA
Unknown	5–20%	

17

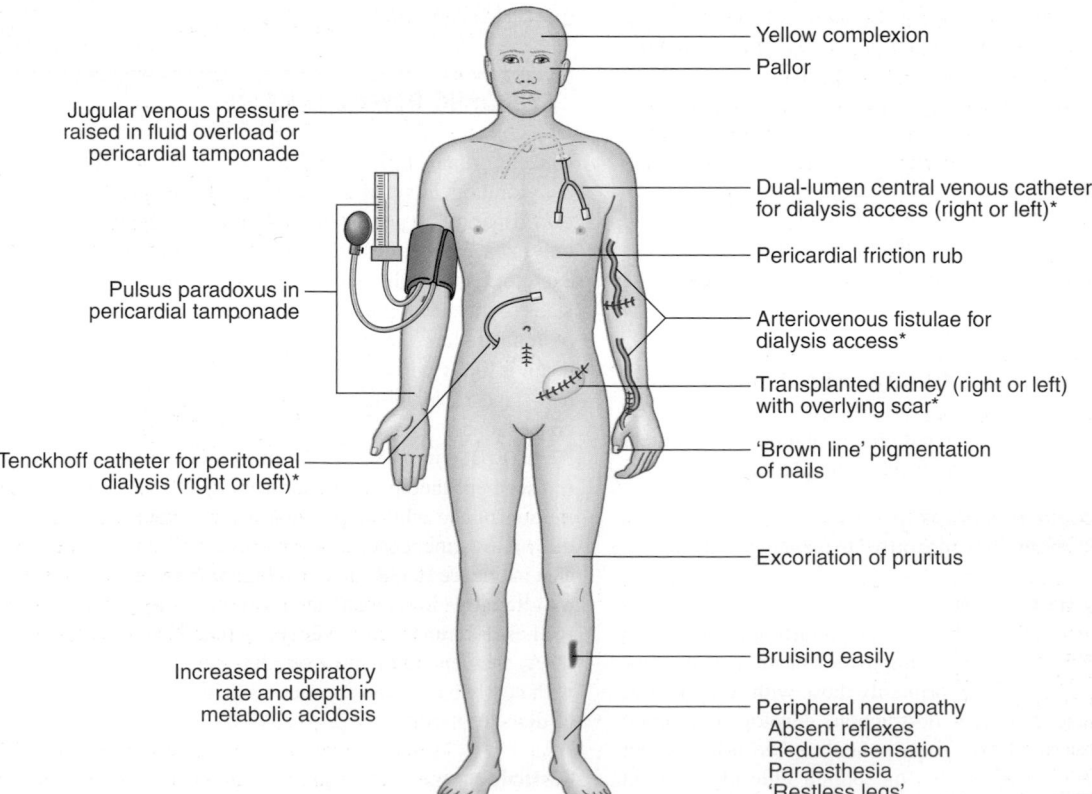

Yellow complexion
Pallor
Jugular venous pressure raised in fluid overload or pericardial tamponade
Dual-lumen central venous catheter for dialysis access (right or left)*
Pericardial friction rub
Pulsus paradoxus in pericardial tamponade
Arteriovenous fistulae for dialysis access*
Transplanted kidney (right or left) with overlying scar*
'Brown line' pigmentation of nails
Tenckhoff catheter for peritoneal dialysis (right or left)*
Excoriation of pruritus
Bruising easily
Increased respiratory rate and depth in metabolic acidosis
Peripheral neuropathy
  Absent reflexes
  Reduced sensation
  Paraesthesia
  'Restless legs'

Fig. 17.20   Physical signs in chronic renal failure. (* Features of renal replacement therapy)

causes are shown in Box 17.29. A precise diagnosis is not always established. Patients often have bilateral small kidneys at presentation, and in such a situation renal biopsy is usually inadvisable because of the difficulty in making a histological diagnosis in severely damaged kidneys and the fact that treatment is unlikely to improve renal function significantly.

Pathogenesis

Disturbances in water, electrolyte and acid–base balance contribute to the clinical picture in patients with CRF, but the exact pathogenesis of the clinical syndrome of uraemia is unknown. Many substances present in abnormal concentration in the plasma have been suspected as being 'uraemic toxins', and uraemia is probably caused by the accumulation of various intermediary products of metabolism.

Clinical assessment

Renal failure may present as a raised blood urea and creatinine found during routine examination, often accompanied by hypertension, proteinuria or anaemia. When renal function deteriorates slowly, patients may remain asymptomatic until GFR falls below 30 ml/minute (stage 4 or 5, Box 17.28). Nocturia, due to the loss of concentrating ability and increased osmotic load per nephron, is often an early symptom. Thereafter, due to the widespread effects of renal failure, symptoms and signs may develop that are related to almost every body system (Fig. 17.20). Patients may present with complaints which are not obviously renal in origin, such as tiredness or breathlessness.

In ESRF (stage 5, Box 17.28) patients appear ill and anaemic. They do not necessarily retain fluid, and may show signs of sodium and water depletion. There may be unusually deep respiration related to metabolic acidosis (Kussmaul's respiration), anorexia and nausea. Later, hiccoughs, pruritus, vomiting, muscular twitching, fits, drowsiness and coma ensue.

Investigations and management

There are several aspects to the management of CRF:

- Identify the underlying renal disease.
- Look for reversible factors which are making renal function worse (Box 17.30).
- Attempt to prevent further renal damage.

17.30 REVERSIBLE FACTORS IN CHRONIC RENAL FAILURE

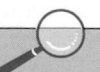

- Hypertension
- Reduced renal perfusion
    - Renal artery stenosis
    - Hypotension due to drug treatment
    - Sodium and water depletion
    - Poor cardiac function
- Urinary tract obstruction
- Urinary tract infection
- Other infections: increased catabolism and urea production
- Nephrotoxic medications

17.31 SUGGESTED SCREENING TESTS IN CHRONIC RENAL FAILURE

Haematology

- Full blood count: institution of erythropoietin treatment if anaemic
- Haematinics: supplementation if deficient to optimise response to erythropoietin

Biochemistry

- Urea, electrolytes and creatinine: dietary restriction of potassium
- Calcium, phosphate and albumin: dietary restriction of phosphate, calorie maintenance in advanced renal impairment
- Parathyroid hormone: treatment of secondary hyperparathyroidism with 1-α-hydroxylated vitamin D
- Lipids, glucose ± HbA$_{1c}$: aggressive metabolic control

Microbiology

- Hepatitis and HIV serology: if dialysis is needed (vaccination against hepatitis B if no previous infection; isolation of dialysis machine if positive)

Imaging etc.

- Renal ultrasound: to confirm/refute two equal-sized unobstructed kidneys
- Chest X-ray: heart size, pulmonary oedema
- ECG: if > 40 years or there are risk factors for cardiac disease
- Renal artery imaging: if renovascular disease is suspected

Immunology

- Group and save
- Tissue typing — if transplantation
- Cytomegalovirus, Epstein–Barr virus, varicella zoster virus — is considered

If diagnosis is not known

Consider:
- Immunoglobulins and protein electrophoresis
- Urinary Bence Jones protein
- Complement
- ANA: and dsDNA if ANA is positive
- ENA: if a connective tissue disorder is suspected
- Rheumatoid factor
- ANCA: in all possible inflammatory renal disease
- Anti-GBM: in all possible inflammatory renal disease
- Cryoglobulins: if cryoglobulinaemia is clinically suspected

---

- Attempt to limit the adverse effects of the loss of renal function.
- Institute renal replacement therapy (dialysis, transplantation, pp. 491 and 494) when appropriate.

At presentation the nature of the underlying disease should be determined, if possible, by history, examination, testing of biochemistry, immunology, radiology and biopsy (Box 17.31). The degree of renal failure is assessed and complications are documented. In some cases the cause may be amenable to specific therapy, e.g. immunosuppression in some types of glomerulonephritis.

Retarding the progression of CRF

Once the plasma creatinine exceeds about 300 μmol/l (3.4 mg/dl), there is usually progressive deterioration in renal function, irrespective of aetiology. The rate of deterioration is very variable between patients but is relatively

17

constant for an individual patient. A plot of the reciprocal of the plasma creatinine concentration against time predicts when dialysis will be required and detects any unexpected worsening of renal failure (Fig. 17.21). Changes in the slope may reflect changes in treatment: for example, blood pressure control or other interventions.

Control of blood pressure

In many types of renal disease, but particularly in diseases affecting glomeruli, control of blood pressure may retard deterioration of GFR. This has been proven for diabetic nephropathy, but is probably true for other diseases as well, particularly those associated with heavy proteinuria. No threshold for this effect has been found; reduction of any level of blood pressure is beneficial. Various target blood pressures have been suggested: for example, 130/85 mmHg for CRF alone, lowered to 125/75 mmHg for those with proteinuria > 1 g/day. Achieving these targets often requires multiple drugs and may be limited by toxicity or non-compliance. The very high incidence of left ventricular hypertrophy, heart failure and occlusive vascular disease in patients with long-standing renal disease also justifies vigorous efforts to control blood pressure.

ACE inhibitors have been shown to be more effective at retarding the progression of renal failure than other therapies which lower systemic blood pressure to a similar degree (Box 17.32). This may be because they reduce glomerular perfusion pressure by dilating the efferent arteriole, although this causes an immediate reduction in GFR when therapy is initiated. Reduction in proteinuria is a good prognostic sign, but it is not clear whether this is causally related to prognosis. ACE inhibitors should be used, where tolerated (check creatinine and potassium), in all patients with incipient or overt diabetic nephropathy or protein-uria > 1 g/day (protein/creatinine ratio > 100 mg/mmol) independent of the presence of hypertension. Angiotensin II receptor antagonists also reduce glomerular perfusion pressure, and the same effect may be achieved by certain non-dihydropyridine calcium antagonists.

Diet

In animals, progressive renal disease can be retarded by various manipulations of diet, most notably by restricting dietary protein. In humans results are less clear-cut; low-protein diets are difficult to adhere to and carry a risk of inducing malnutrition. This remains a controversial area but, for most patients living in areas where renal replacement therapy is available, severe protein restriction is not recommended. Moderate restriction (to 60 g protein per day, Box 17.33) should be accompanied by an adequate intake of calories to prevent malnutrition. Anorexia and muscle loss may indicate a need to commence dialysis treatment.

Limiting the adverse effects of CRF

Anaemia

Anaemia is common; it usually correlates with the severity of renal failure and contributes to many of the non-specific symptoms of CRF. Several mechanisms are implicated, including:

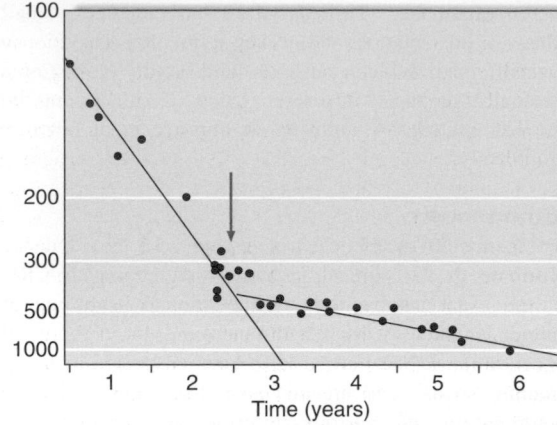

Serum creatinine (μmol/l)

Fig. 17.21 Plot of the reciprocal of serum creatinine concentration against time over a 6-year period in a patient with progressive renal failure caused by membranous nephropathy. Serial plasma creatinine estimations permit prediction of the time to end-stage renal disease. The 'break point' (arrow) at which the gradient of the line is dramatically reduced was associated with a 6-month course of treatment with chlorambucil and prednisolone.

EBM

17.32 ANGIOTENSIN-CONVERTING ENZYME (ACE) INHIBITORS IN NON-DIABETIC CHRONIC RENAL FAILURE (CRF)

'ACE inhibitors reduce proteinuria and slow the decline in GFR in non-diabetic patients with hypertension, CRF and proteinuria, independently of the extent of blood pressure reduction.'
  See Boxes 21.52 and 21.54 (p. 842), on the role of ACE inhibitors in diabetic subjects with renal disease.

● Lewis EJ, et al. N Engl J Med 1993; 329:1456–1462.

For further information: 🖳 www.cochrane.org

EBM

17.33 DIETARY PROTEIN RESTRICTION IN CHRONIC RENAL FAILURE

'Restriction of dietary protein intake delays the progression of chronic renal failure.'

● Klahr S, et al. N Engl J Med 1994; 330:877–884.

For further information: 🖳 www.cochrane.org

● relative deficiency of erythropoietin
● diminished erythropoiesis due to toxic effects of uraemia on marrow precursor cells
● reduced red cell survival
● increased blood loss due to capillary fragility and poor platelet function
● reduced dietary intake and absorption of iron and other haematinics.

Plasma erythropoietin is usually within the normal range and thus inappropriately low for the degree of anaemia. In patients with polycystic kidneys, anaemia is often less severe or absent, while in some interstitial disorders it appears disproportionately severe for the degree of renal failure. This is probably because of the effects of these disorders on the interstitial fibroblasts that secrete erythropoietin.

Recombinant human erythropoietin is effective in correcting the anaemia of CRF. The target haemoglobin is usually between 100 and 120 g/l. Complications of treatment include increased blood pressure, and adjustment of antihypertensive medication is often necessary. There is also an increase in blood coagulability and an increased incidence of thrombosis of the arteriovenous fistulae used for haemodialysis. If anaemia is corrected slowly, these effects are less common. Erythropoietin is less effective in the presence of iron deficiency, active inflammation or malignancy, or in patients with aluminium overload which may occur in dialysis. These factors should be sought and, if possible, corrected before treatment. Iron supplementation should be used to keep ferritin > 100 µg/l and transferrin saturation > 20%.

Fluid and electrolyte balance

Due to the reduced ability of the failing kidney to concentrate the urine, a relatively high urine volume is needed to excrete products of metabolism and a fluid intake of around 3 litres/day is desirable. Some patients with so-called 'salt-wasting' disease may require a high sodium and water intake, including supplements of sodium salts, to prevent fluid depletion and worsening of renal function. This is most often seen in patients with renal cystic disease, obstructive uropathy, reflux nephropathy or other tubulo-interstitial diseases, and is not seen in patients with glomerular disease. These patients benefit from taking 5–10 g/day (85–170 mmol/day) of sodium chloride by mouth. It is usual to start with 2–3 g/day and increase the dose as required. The limit for additional salt is set by the development of peripheral or pulmonary oedema, or aggravation of hypertension. Sodium bicarbonate may be substituted in part for sodium chloride when acidosis requires correction.

Limitation of potassium intake (e.g. 70 mmol/day) and sodium intake (e.g. 100 mmol/day) may be required in late CRF if there is evidence of accumulation. Disproportionate fluid retention in milder renal failure, sometimes leading to episodic pulmonary oedema, is particularly associated with renal artery stenosis.

Acidosis

Declining renal function is associated with metabolic acidosis (p. 437), which is often asymptomatic. Sustained acidosis results in protons being buffered in bone in place of calcium, thus aggravating metabolic bone disease. Acidosis may also contribute to reduced renal function and increased tissue catabolism.

The plasma bicarbonate should be maintained above 22 mmol/l by giving sodium bicarbonate supplements (starting dose of 1 g 8-hourly, increasing as required). The increased sodium intake may induce hypertension or oedema; calcium carbonate (up to 3 g daily) is an alternative that is also used to bind dietary phosphate.

Cardiovascular disease and lipids

CRF is an independent risk factor for occlusive cardio-vascular disease. Atherosclerosis is common and may be accelerated by hypertension. Vascular calcification, accel-erated by a high calcium × phosphate product, may develop and be sufficiently severe to cause limb ischaemia. Pericarditis is common in untreated or inadequately treated ESRF. It may lead to pericardial tamponade and, later, constrictive pericarditis.

Hypertension develops in approximately 80% of patients with CRF. In part, this is caused by sodium retention. Chronically diseased kidneys also tend to hypersecrete renin, leading to high circulating concentrations of renin, angiotensin II and aldosterone. This is exaggerated if there is renal under-perfusion related to renal vascular disease. Hypertension must be controlled, as it causes further vascular and glomerular damage and worsening of renal failure.

Hypercholesterolaemia is almost universal in patients with significant proteinuria, and increased triglyceride levels are also common in patients with CRF. It has been suggested that as well as influencing the development of vascular disease, this may accelerate the progression of chronic renal disease. HMG-CoA reductase inhibitors (p. 450) achieve substantial reductions in lipids in chronic renal disease, and long-term studies are under way in this group of patients. However, many believe that the high incidence of vascular disease in CRF justifies the treatment of these abnormalities in advance of proof from controlled trials.

Infection

Cellular and humoral immunity are impaired, with increased susceptibility to infection. Infections are the second most common cause of death in dialysis patients, after cardio-vascular disease; they must be recognised and treated promptly.

Bleeding

There is an increased bleeding tendency in renal failure which manifests in patients with advanced disease as cutan-eous ecchymoses and mucosal bleeds. Platelet function is impaired and bleeding time prolonged. Adequate dialysis treatment partially corrects the bleeding tendency.

Renal osteodystrophy

This metabolic bone disease which accompanies CRF con-sists of a mixture of osteomalacia, hyperparathyroid bone disease (osteitis fibrosa), osteoporosis and osteosclerosis (Fig. 17.22). Osteomalacia (p. 1126) results from diminished activity of the renal 1α-hydroxylase enzyme, with failure to convert cholecalciferol to its active metabolite, 1,25-dihydroxycholecalciferol. A deficiency of the latter leads to diminished intestinal absorption of calcium, hypo-calcaemia and reduction in the calcification of osteoid in bone. The parathyroid glands are stimulated by the low plasma calcium, and also by hyperphosphataemia, consequent upon reduced urinary phosphate excretion in CRF. Osteitis fibrosa results from this secondary hyperparathyroidism in the presence of hyperphosphataemia (in osteomalacia, phosphate levels are normally low; p. 1127). In some patients tertiary or autonomous hyperparathyroidism with hypercalcaemia develops. Osteosclerosis is seen mainly in the sacral area, at the base of the skull and in the vertebrae; the cause of this unusual reaction is not known.

17

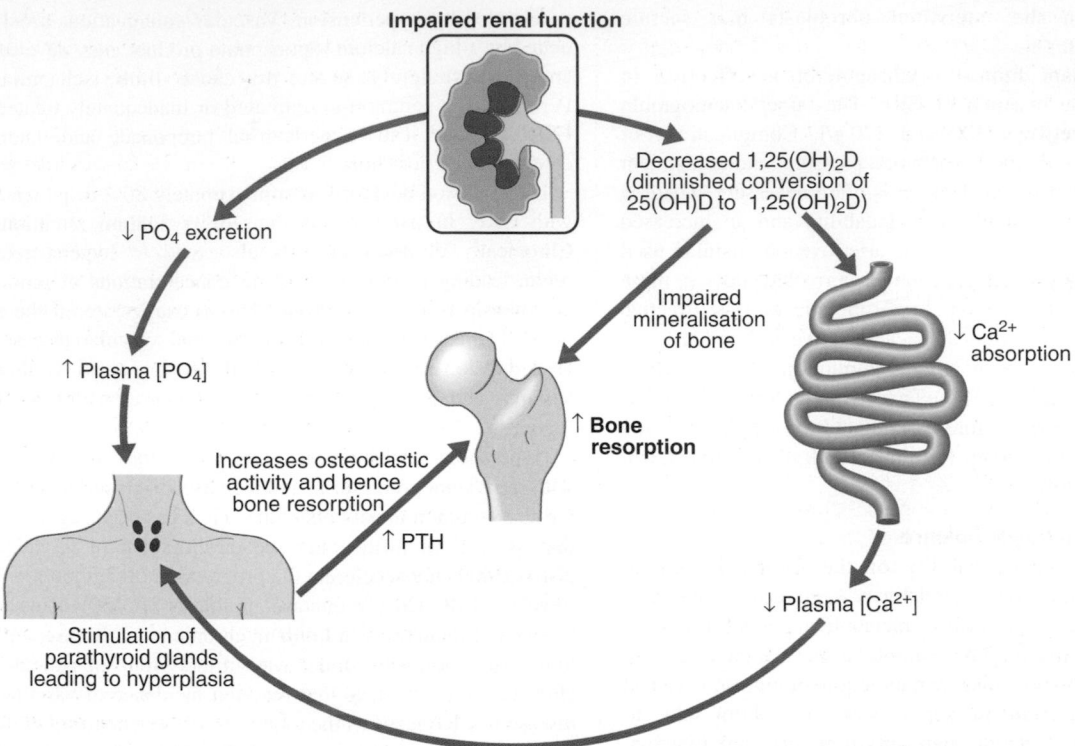

Fig. 17.22 Pathogenesis of renal osteodystrophy. The net result of decreased 1,25(OH)$_2$ cholecalciferol levels and increased parathyroid hormone (PTH) levels in the presence of high [PO$_4$] is bone which exhibits increased osteoclastic activity and increased osteoid as a consequence of decreased mineralisation.

To minimise the effects of CRF on bone, plasma calcium and phosphate should be kept as near to normal as possible. Hypocalcaemia is corrected by giving 1α-hydroxylated synthetic analogues of vitamin D. The dose is adjusted to avoid hypercalcaemia. This will usually prevent or control osteomalacia, although it is sometimes resistant, presumably because of other factors inhibiting bone mineralisation. Calcitriol also binds to a receptor in the parathyroid glands, resulting in decreased PTH gene transcription. New calcimimetic agents also reduce PTH via a direct action on the parathyroid glands.

Hyperphosphataemia is controlled by dietary restriction of foods with high phosphate content (milk, cheese, eggs) and the use of phosphate-binding drugs administered with food. These agents form insoluble complexes with dietary phosphate and prevent its absorption (e.g. calcium carbonate and aluminium hydroxide). Newer polymer-based phosphate binders that are not associated with the problem of unwanted anion (Ca or Al) absorption are becoming available. Secondary hyperparathyroidism is usually prevented or controlled by these measures but, in severe bone disease with autonomous parathyroid function, parathyroidectomy may become necessary.

Myopathy

Generalised myopathy is due to a combination of poor nutrition, hyperparathyroidism, vitamin D deficiency and disorders of electrolyte metabolism. Muscle cramps are common, and quinine sulphate may be helpful. The 'restless leg syndrome', in which the patient's legs are jumpy during the night, may be troublesome and is often improved by clonazepam.

Other adverse effects

Neuropathy results from demyelination of medullated fibres, with the longer fibres being involved at an earlier stage. Sensory neuropathy may cause paraesthesiae. Amitriptyline and gabapentin may provide some symptom relief. Motor neuropathy may present as foot drop. Uraemic autonomic neuropathy may cause delayed gastric emptying, diarrhoea and postural hypotension. Clinical manifestations of neuropathy appear late in the course of CRF but may improve or even resolve once dialysis is established.

In addition to hyperparathyroidism (see above), a number of hormonal abnormalities may be present. In both sexes there is loss of libido and sexual function, related at least in part to hyperprolactinaemia (p. 799). Treatment with dopamine agonists is sometimes useful for amenorrhoea or galactorrhoea in women. The half-life of insulin is prolonged in CRF due to reduced tubular metabolism of insulin; insulin requirements may therefore decline in diabetic patients in end-stage CRF. However, there is also a post-receptor defect in insulin action, leading to relative insulin resistance. This latter abnormality is improved by dialysis treatment.

Gastrointestinal manifestations are common at low GFRs, including anorexia followed by nausea, and vomiting is commonly seen. There is a higher incidence of peptic ulcer disease in uraemic patients and H_2-receptor antagonists or proton pump inhibitors are commonly used.

Depression is common in patients on or approaching renal replacement therapy and support should be provided for both them and their relatives.

RENAL REPLACEMENT THERAPY

The facility to replace some functions of the kidney artificially by dialysis has been available since the 1960s. Such treatment is now routine in patients with acute or chronic renal failure. It does not replace the endocrine and metabolic functions of the kidney, but aims to maintain the plasma biochemistry (uraemic toxins, electrolytes and acid–base status) at acceptable levels. Dialysis can also remove fluid from the circulation (ultrafiltration) to maintain euvolaemia. The major side-effects of dialysis relate to haemodynamic disturbance caused by fluid removal or the extracorporeal circulation of blood, and reactions between blood and components of the dialysis system (bioincompatibility).

The original renal replacement therapy (RRT) was haemodialysis, and this is still the most common form of treatment. A variety of other types have been developed, particularly for unstable patients with ARF (Fig. 17.23).

RENAL REPLACEMENT IN ACUTE RENAL FAILURE

The decision to institute RRT is made on an individual basis, taking account of other aspects of the patient's care. Guideline indications are as follows:

- *Increased plasma urea and creatinine*. Plasma urea > 30 mmol/l (180 mg/dl) and creatinine > 600 μmol/l (6.8 mg/dl) are undesirable. At lower levels, if there is progressive biochemical deterioration and particularly if there is little or no urine output, it may be appropriate to commence dialysis. There is a trend towards earlier institution of dialysis in ARF, although trials of very early dialysis in post-operative or septic patients with oliguria have not shown consistent benefit compared with the more conventional strategy above.
- *Hyperkalaemia*. A plasma potassium > 6 mmol/l is hazardous. Elevated plasma potassium can usually be reduced by medical measures in the short term (Box 16.15, p. 436), but dialysis is often required for definitive control.
- *Metabolic acidosis*. This will often occur together with hyperkalaemia and raise the plasma potassium further.
- *Fluid overload and pulmonary oedema*. In patients with continued urine output, this may be controlled by careful fluid balance and use of diuretics, but in oligo/anuric patients may be an indication for RRT.
- *Uraemic pericarditis/uraemic encephalopathy*. These are features of severe untreated renal failure; they are uncommon in ARF but are strong indications for RRT.

The principal options for RRT in ARF are haemodialysis, high-volume haemofiltration, continuous arteriovenous or venovenous haemofiltration, and peritoneal dialysis.

Intermittent haemodialysis

This modality offers the best rate of small solute clearance. In previously undialysed patients with ARF and elevated plasma urea, haemodialysis should be started gradually because of the risk of confusion and convulsions due to cerebral oedema (dialysis disequilibrium). Typically, 1 hour of treatment should be prescribed. Subsequently, patients with ARF who are haemodynamically stable can be treated by 3–4 hours of haemodialysis on alternate days, or 2–3 hours every day if they are severely catabolic. For patients at risk of bleeding, epoprostenol may be used instead of heparin for anticoagulation but can cause hypotension. For short dialyses or patients with abnormal clotting, it may be possible to avoid anticoagulation.

Haemofiltration

This may be either intermittent, with 15–30 litres of plasma ultrafiltrate exchanged for replacement fluid over 3–5 hours (high-volume haemofiltration), or continuous with 1–2 litres/hour of filtrate replaced (equivalent to a GFR of 15–30 ml/min); higher rates of filtration may be of benefit in patients with sepsis and multi-organ failure. In continuous arteriovenous haemofiltration (CAVH) the extracorporeal blood circuit is driven by the arteriovenous pressure difference. Poor filtration rates and clotting of the filter are common and this treatment has fallen out of favour. Continuous venovenous haemofiltration (CVVH, Fig. 17.24) is pump-driven, providing a reliable extracorporeal circulation. Issues concerning anticoagulation are similar to those for haemodialysis, but may be more problematic since longer or continuous anticoagulation is necessary.

Intermittent haemodiafiltration

This technique combines standard haemodialysis with the good small solute clearance and high ultrafiltration capacity of haemofiltration.

Peritoneal dialysis

In ARF, this technique is rarely used. It is less efficient than haemodialysis, and seldom achieves adequate biochemical control in catabolic patients. It requires an intact peritoneal cavity and is not feasible after recent abdominal surgery.

RENAL REPLACEMENT IN CHRONIC RENAL FAILURE

When patients are known to have progressive CRF (Box 17.29, p. 486) and are under regular clinic review, preparation for RRT should begin at least 12 months before the predicted start date. This involves psychological and social support, assessment of home circumstances and discussion about choice of treatment. The principal decisions required are the choice between haemodialysis and peritoneal dialysis (Box 17.34), and referral for renal transplantation. In view of the historical high incidence of viral transmission in dialysis units, all such patients must be

17

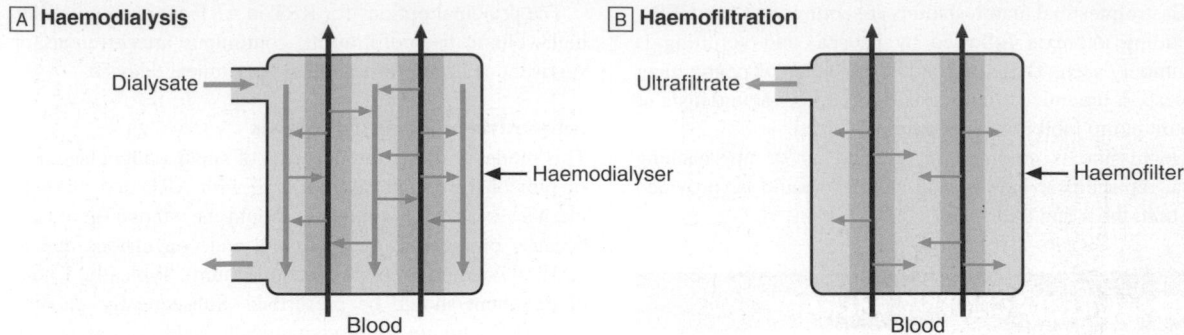

A Haemodialysis

Dialysate →

← Haemodialyser

Blood

- Typical small solute clearance 160 ml/min
- Used in both acute and chronic renal failure

B Haemofiltration

Ultrafiltrate ←

← Haemofilter

Blood

- Typical small solute clearance (2 litres/hr exchanges) 33 ml/min
- ? Less circulatory instability than haemodialysis
- Used mostly in acute renal failure

- **Access to the circulation** for haemodialysis or filtration is required. Arteriovenous fistulae, temporary or semi-permanent tunnelled central venous lines or arterio-venous shunts (e.g. Scribner shunt) may be used. The extracorporeal circuit requires anticoagulation, typically with heparin

C Peritoneal dialysis

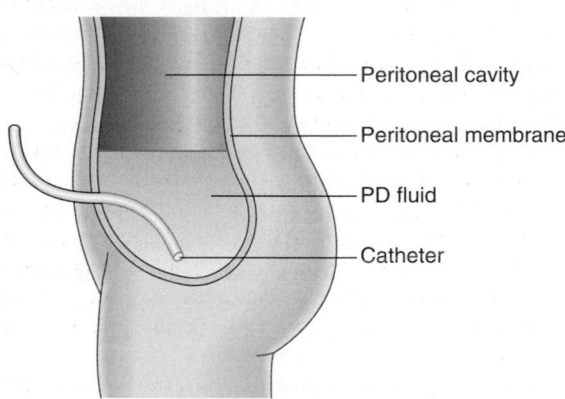

Peritoneal cavity

Peritoneal membrane

PD fluid

Catheter

- **Access to the peritoneal cavity** via 'Tenckhoff' catheter
- **Continuous ambulatory peritoneal dialysis** (CAPD): typically 4 exchanges of 2 litres of fluid a day 4–6 hours apart
- **Automated peritoneal dialysis** (APD): uses a machine to perform exchanges overnight (8–10 hours). Used mostly in chronic renal failure

D Transplantation

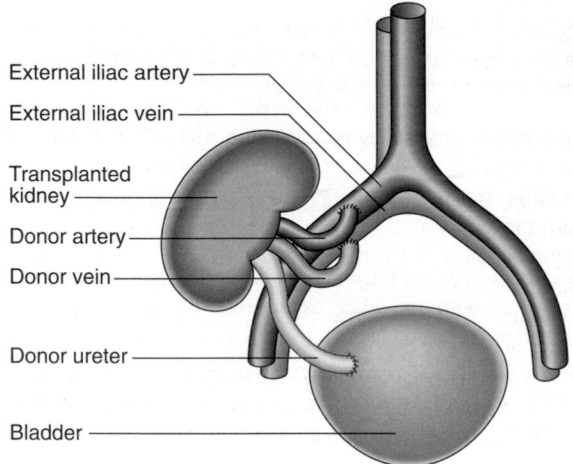

External iliac artery

External iliac vein

Transplanted kidney

Donor artery

Donor vein

Donor ureter

Bladder

- Successful transplantation extends the life expectancy of patients with end-stage CRF
- Requires long-term use of immunosuppressives with attendant risks

E Conservative management

Fig. 17.23 Renal replacement therapy. A In haemodialysis there is diffusion of solutes between plasma and dialysate across a semi-permeable membrane following a concentration gradient. Movement of solutes may be bi-directional and continues as long as the concentration gradient remains. The dialysate composition is chosen to achieve a suitable gradient. Fluid is removed by applying negative pressure to the dialysate side (ultrafiltration). B In haemofiltration there is filtration of water from plasma to ultrafiltrate across a more porous semi-permeable membrane down a pressure gradient with removal of solutes by convection. 'Replacement' fluid of chosen electrolytic composition is added to the circuit after the filter. If fluid removal is required, less is replaced than filtered. C Peritoneal dialysis uses peritoneum as a semi-permeable dialysis membrane. Solutes move down a concentration gradient, and water down an osmotic gradient achieved by using an osmolar compound (typically glucose) in the dialysis fluid. D In transplantation a functioning transplant replaces all of the functions of the failed kidneys. E Some patients may elect not to dialyse and can be actively supported to control the symptoms of ESRF.

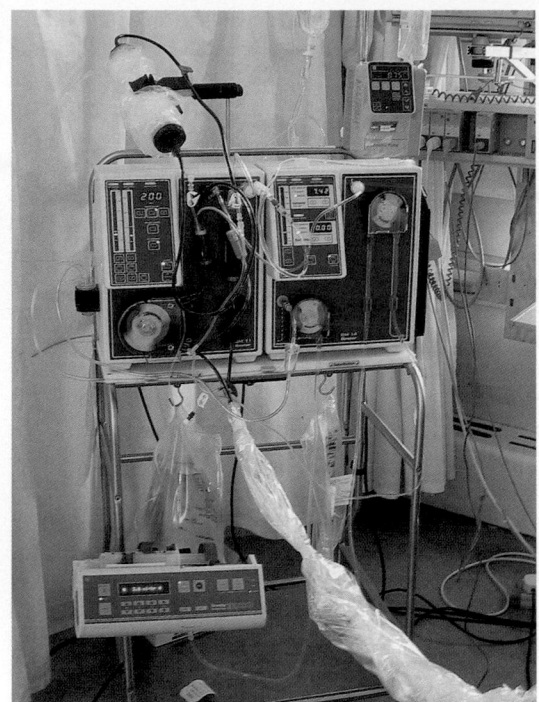

Fig. 17.24 Continuous venovenous haemofiltration (CVVH) on an intensive care unit. In this hypothermic patient the haemofilter and blood lines have been wrapped to reduce heat loss.

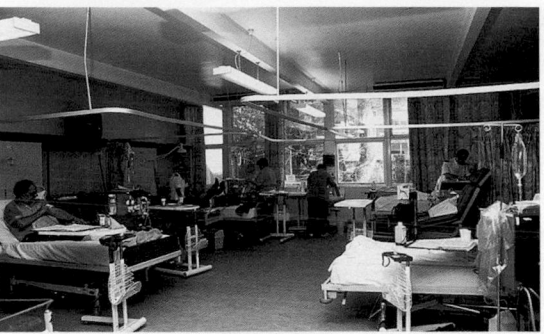

Fig. 17.25 Haemodialysis unit. Six of 19 stations, a mixture of beds and chairs, in an outpatient haemodialysis unit. Each station treats three patients daily and therefore six patients in total (each attending three times weekly).

screened in advance for hepatitis B, hepatitis C and HIV, and have hepatitis B vaccine if they are not immune.

Of patients starting dialysis in the UK, 70% are treated by haemodialysis and 30% by peritoneal dialysis. Mortality figures indicate 78% survival at 1 year (87% counted from day 90 of treatment) and 45% at 5 years. Mortality is strongly influenced by age; patients over 75 have a 15% survival at 5 years, whereas patients aged under 45 have an 83% survival at 5 years. Comorbid conditions such as diabetes mellitus (30% 5-year survival) and generalised vascular disease (34% 5-year survival) also have a strong influence.

Intermittent haemodialysis

This is the standard blood purification therapy in ESRF (Figs 17.25 and 17.26). Haemodialysis is started when the patient has symptomatic advanced renal failure but before the development of serious complications, often with a plasma creatinine of 600–800 µmol/l (6.8–9.0 mg/dl). Vascular access is required; an arteriovenous fistula should be formed, usually in the forearm, when the patient reaches stage 4 kidney disease, so that the fistula has time to develop. After 4–6 weeks, increased pressure in the vein leading from the fistula causes distension and thickening of the vessel wall (arterialisation). Large-bore needles can then be inserted into the vein to provide access for each haemodialysis treatment (Fig. 17.26). Preservation of arm veins is thus very important in patients with progressive renal disease who may require haemodialysis in the future. If this access is not possible, plastic cannulae in central veins can be used for short-term access.

Haemodialysis is usually carried out for 3–5 hours three times weekly. Most patients notice an improvement in symptoms during the first 6 weeks of treatment. Plasma urea

17

17.34 COMPARISON OF HAEMODIALYSIS AND PERITONEAL DIALYSIS	
Haemodialysis	**Peritoneal dialysis**
Efficient 4 hours three times per week usually adequate	Less efficient Four exchanges per day usually required, each taking 30–60 minutes (continuous ambulatory peritoneal dialysis) or 8–10 hours each night (automated peritoneal dialysis)
2–3 days between treatments	A few hours between treatments
Requires visits to hospital (although home treatment possible for some patients)	Performed at home
Requires adequate venous circulation for vascular access	Requires an intact peritoneal cavity without major scarring from previous surgery
Careful compliance with diet and fluid restrictions required between treatments	Diet and fluid less restricted
Fluid removal compressed into treatment periods; may cause symptoms and haemodynamic instability	Slow continuous fluid removal, usually asymptomatic
Infections related to vascular access may occur	Peritonitis and catheter-related infections may occur
Patients are to some extent dependent on others	Patients can take full responsibility for their treatment

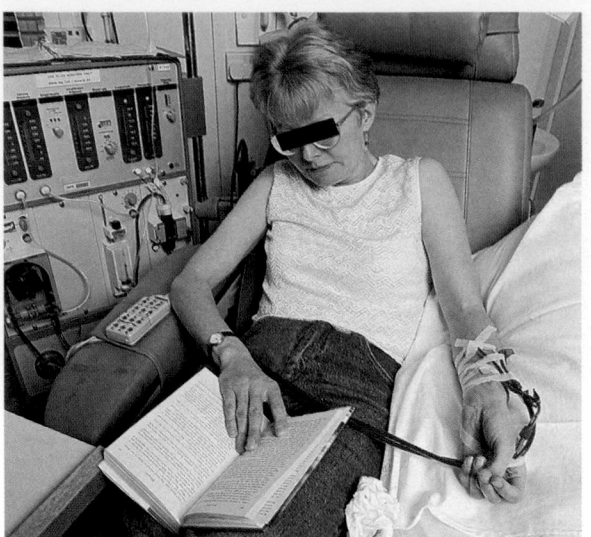

Fig. 17.26 Haemodialysis. A patient receiving haemodialysis through a forearm subcutaneous fistula (a Brescia–Cimino fistula). She subsequently received a live related transplant.

and creatinine are lowered by each treatment but do not return to normal. Some patients are able to carry out their treatment at home. Many patients lead normal and active lives, and patient survival for more than 20 years is commonplace in young patients without extrarenal disease. Box 17.35 summarises some of the problems related to haemodialysis treatment.

Continuous ambulatory peritoneal dialysis (CAPD)

CAPD is a form of long-term dialysis involving insertion of a permanent Silastic catheter into the peritoneal cavity. Two litres of sterile, isotonic dialysis fluid are introduced and left in place for approximately 6 hours. During this time, metabolic waste products diffuse from peritoneal capillaries into the dialysis fluid down a concentration gradient. The

fluid is then drained and fresh dialysis fluid introduced. The inflow fluid is rendered hyperosmolar by the addition of glucose; this results in net removal of fluid from the patient on each cycle (ultrafiltration). This cycle is repeated four times daily, during which time the patient is mobile and able to undertake normal daily activities. CAPD is particularly useful in young children, and in elderly patients with cardiovascular instability. Its long-term use may be limited by episodes of bacterial peritonitis and damage to the peritoneal membrane, but patients have been treated successfully for more than 10 years. Box 17.36 summarises some of the problems related to CAPD treatment.

The use of automated peritoneal dialysis (APD) is now widespread. This system is similar to CAPD but uses a mechanical device to perform the fluid exchanges during the night, leaving the patient free, or with only a single exchange to perform, during the day.

Conservative treatment of stage V chronic kidney disease

Partly as a result of survival data, there is an increasing trend to consider conservative non-dialytic treatment in patients in a high-risk category. Patients are offered full medical, psychological and social support to optimise and sustain their existing renal function for as long as possible, and appropriate palliative care in the terminal phase of their disease. Many of these patients enjoy a good quality of life for several years. It is also appropriate to discontinue dialysis treatment, with the consent of the patient, and to offer conservative therapy and palliative care when quality of life on dialysis is clearly inadequate.

Renal transplantation

Renal transplantation offers the best chance of long-term survival in patients with end-stage renal disease. It can restore normal kidney function and correct all the metabolic abnormalities of CRF. All patients should be considered for transplantation unless there are active contraindications (Box 17.37).

17.35 PROBLEMS WITH HAEMODIALYSIS			
Problem	**Clinical features**	**Cause**	**Treatment**
Hypotension during dialysis	Sudden ↓ BP; often leg cramps; sometimes chest pain	Fluid removal and hypovolaemia	Saline infusion; exclude myocardial infarction; quinine may help cramp
Cardiac arrhythmias	↓ BP; sometimes chest pain	Potassium and acid–base shifts	Check K+ and arterial blood gases; review dialysis prescription; ? stop dialysis
Haemorrhage	Blood loss (overt or occult), ↓ BP	Anticoagulation, vascular access	Stop dialysis; seek source; consider heparin-free treatment
Air embolism	Circulatory collapse, cardiac arrest	Disconnected or faulty lines and equipment malfunction	Stop dialysis
Dialyser hypersensitivity	Acute circulatory collapse	Allergic reaction to dialysis membrane or sterilisant	Stop dialysis; change to different artificial kidney
Emergencies between treatments Pulmonary oedema Systemic sepsis	Breathlessness Rigors, fever, ↓ BP	Fluid overload Usually involves vascular access devices (catheter or fistula)	Ultrafiltration ± dialysis Blood cultures, antibiotics

17.36 PROBLEMS WITH CONTINUOUS AMBULATORY PERITONEAL DIALYSIS (CAPD)

Problem	Clinical features	Cause	Treatment
CAPD peritonitis	Cloudy drainage fluid; abdominal pain and systemic sepsis are variable	Usually entry of skin contaminants via catheter; bowel organisms less common	Culture of peritoneal dialysis fluid Intraperitoneal antibiotics, e.g. tobramycin, vancomycin Catheter removal sometimes required
Catheter exit site infection	Erythema and pus around exit site	Usually skin organisms	Antibiotics; sometimes surgical drainage
Ultrafiltration failure	Fluid overload	Damage to peritoneal membrane, leading to rapid transport of glucose and loss of osmotic gradient	Replace glucose with synthetic poorly absorbed polymers for some exchanges (e.g. icodextrin)
Peritoneal membrane failure	Inadequate clearance of urea etc.	Scarring/damage to peritoneal membrane	Increase exchange volumes; consider automated peritoneal dialysis or switch to haemodialysis

17.37 CONTRAINDICATIONS TO RENAL TRANSPLANTATION

Absolute

- Active malignancy—a period of at least 2 years of complete remission is recommended for most tumours prior to transplantation
- Active vasculitis or anti-GBM disease, with positive serology—at least 1 year of remission is recommended prior to transplantation
- Severe ischaemic heart disease
- Severe occlusive aorto-iliac vascular disease

Relative

- Age—while practice varies, transplants are not routinely offered to very young children (< 1 year) or older people (> 75 years)
- High risk of disease recurrence in the transplant kidney
- Disease of the lower urinary tract—in patients with impaired bladder function, an ileal conduit may be considered
- Significant comorbidity

17.38 RENAL REPLACEMENT THERAPY IN OLD AGE

- **Quality of life:** age itself is not a barrier to good quality of life on RRT.
- **Coexisting cardiovascular disease:** its high prevalence can make dialysis difficult. Older people are more sensitive to fluid balance changes, predisposing to hypotension during dialysis with rebound hypertension between dialyses. The ischaemic heart cannot cope with fluid overload and pulmonary oedema easily develops.
- **Provision of teatment:** only hospital-provided haemodialysis is suitable and older patients require more medical and nursing time.
- **Survival on dialysis:** difficult to predict for an individual patient, but is correlated with age, functional ability and comorbid disease.
- **Withdrawal from dialysis:** a common cause of death in older patients with comorbid disease.
- **Transplantation:** relative risks of surgery and immunosuppression, and limited organ availability exclude most older people from transplantation.
- **Conservative therapy:** i.e. without dialysis but with adequate support, may be a popular option for patients at high risk of complications from dialysis, who have a limited prognosis and little hope of functional recovery.

Kidney grafts may be taken from a cadaver or from a living donor. As described on pages 89–91, matching of a donor to a specific recipient is strongly influenced by immunological factors, since graft rejection is the major cause of failure of the transplant. ABO (blood group) compatibility between donor and recipient is essential, and the degree of matching for major histocompatability (MHC) antigens—particularly HLA–DR—influences the incidence of rejection. T cells are the major cell involved in graft rejection; cytotoxic antibodies against HLA antigens, which may be present pre-transplant (sensitisation), are also important. A cytotoxicity test for these antibodies, and T- and B-cell cross-match tests (donor lymphocytes mixed with patient serum), are performed pre-transplant. Positive tests predict early rejection.

In the transplant operation, the donor vessels are anastomosed to the recipient iliac artery and vein, and the donor ureter to the bladder (Fig. 17.23). Peri-operative problems include:

- *Fluid balance.* Careful matching of input to output is required.
- *Primary graft non-function.* Causes include hypovolaemia, acute tubular necrosis or other pre-existing renal damage, hyperacute rejection, vascular occlusion and urinary tract obstruction.
- *Sepsis* (related to immunosuppression).

Once the graft begins to function, normal or near-normal biochemistry is usually achieved within a few days. All transplant patients require regular life-long clinic follow-up to monitor renal function and immunosuppression.

Management after transplantation

Immunosuppressive therapy is required to prevent rejection. Different therapeutic regimens are used; a commonly used one is triple therapy consisting of prednisolone, plus ciclosporin or tacrolimus and azathioprine. Newer immuno-suppressive drugs such as mycophenolate mofetil and rapamycin are increasing in use. Rejection is treated by short courses of very high-dose corticosteroids in the first instance, although other more potent therapies, such as anti-lymphocyte antibodies or plasma exchange, are used in resistant episodes.

17

Immunosuppression, which must usually be taken throughout the life of the transplant, is associated with an increased incidence of infection, particularly opportunistic infections such as cytomegalovirus and *Pneumocystis carinii* (now *jirovecii*). There is also an increased risk of malignancy, especially of the skin. Approximately 50% of white patients develop skin malignancy by 15 years post-transplant. Lymphomas are rare but may occur early and are often related to infection with herpes viruses, especially Epstein–Barr virus (p. 307).

The prognosis after kidney transplantation has improved significantly. Recent UK statistics for transplants from cadaver donors indicate 96% patient survival and 92% graft survival at 1 year, and 84% patient survival and 76% graft survival at 5 years. Even better figures are obtained with living donor transplantation (92% patient survival and 86% graft survival at 5 years). Living donor operations are becoming more common in the UK and can now be successfully performed with genetically unrelated donors, such as spouses.

Quality of life studies indicate that transplantation offers the best hope of complete rehabilitation and is the most cost-effective treatment for end-stage CRF.

RENAL VASCULAR DISEASES

Diseases which affect renal blood vessels may cause renal ischaemia, leading to acute or chronic renal failure or secondary hypertension. The rising prevalence of atherosclerosis and diabetes mellitus in ageing populations has made renovascular disease an important cause of ESRF.

LARGE-VESSEL DISEASE: RENAL ARTERY STENOSIS

Presentations

Hypertension

Renal artery stenosis classically presents as hypertension if it affects a single kidney or as renal failure if it is bilateral. The hypertension is driven by activation of the renin–angiotensin system in response to renal ischaemia. In atherosclerotic renal artery disease, there is usually evidence of vascular disease elsewhere, particularly in the legs. The selection of hypertensive patients who warrant investigation for secondary hypertension is discussed on page 611. Factors which predict renovascular disease are shown in Box 17.39.

Deterioration of renal function on ACE inhibitors

When renal perfusion pressure drops, the renin–angiotensin–aldosterone system is activated and angiotensin-

mediated glomerular efferent arteriolar vasoconstriction maintains glomerular filtration pressure. ACE inhibitors or angiotensin II receptor antagonists block this physiological response. A drop in GFR (> 20% rise in creatinine) on ACE inhibitors raises the possibility of renal artery stenosis. This is not a sensitive diagnostic test, however.

Flash pulmonary oedema

Repeated episodes of acute pulmonary oedema associated with severe hypertension, occurring without other obvious cause (e.g. myocardial infarction, dysrhythmia, anaemia, thyrotoxicosis) in patients with normal or only mildly impaired renal and cardiac function, can occur in renal artery stenosis. This presentation is characteristic of bilateral renovascular disease because in unilateral disease salt and water retention are partly corrected by increased 'pressure natriuresis' in the normal kidney. Episodes may be precipitated by a sudden increase in blood pressure, e.g. following sympathetic stimulation.

Acute renal infarction

Sudden occlusion of the renal arteries causes acute loin pain, usually with dipstick haematuria. It may be caused by local atherosclerosis (atheroembolic) or by thromboemboli from a distant source, e.g. mural cardiac thrombus. Bilateral occlusion (as in aortic occlusion—look for absent femoral pulses and reduced lower limb perfusion), or acute occlusion of the artery to a single kidney, will cause acute renal failure. Severe hypertension is common but not universal; presumably, some residual renal perfusion is required to generate renin release.

Aetiology

Reduction of renal blood flow is associated with > 70% narrowing of the artery, and commonly with a dilated region more distally (post-stenotic dilatation).

Atherosclerosis is the most common cause, especially in older patients. The characteristic lesion is an ostial stenosis that is associated with atherosclerosis within the aorta and affecting other major branches, particularly the iliac vessels. Renal impairment is not simply related to the degree of stenosis. The picture is often complicated by small-vessel disease in affected kidneys that may be related to subclinical atheroemboli, hypertension or other disease. As the stenosis becomes more severe, global renal ischaemia leads to shrinkage of the affected kidney: ischaemic nephropathy. However, the progression of stenosis is not easily predictable, and in many instances the outcome is determined by coronary, cerebral or other vascular disease. Some patients develop renal failure.

In younger patients (< 50 years), fibromuscular dysplasia is a more likely cause of renal artery stenosis. This is an uncommon congenital disorder of unknown cause affecting the media ('medial fibroplasia'), which narrows the artery but rarely leads to total occlusion. It may be associated with disease in other arteries; for example, those who have carotid artery dissections are more likely to have this appearance in their renal arteries. It most commonly presents with hypertension in patients aged 15–30 years, and in women more frequently than men. Irregular narrowing

17.39 RENAL ARTERY STENOSIS

Renal artery stenosis is more likely if:
- Hypertension is severe, *or* of recent onset, *or* difficult to control
- Kidneys are asymmetrical in size
- Flash pulmonary oedema occurs repeatedly
- There is peripheral vascular disease of lower limbs
- Renal function has deteriorated on ACE inhibitors

17

('beading') affects the distal renal artery, sometimes extending into intrarenal branches.

Rarely, large-vessel vasculitis, particularly Takayasu's arteritis (p. 1140), may involve renal arteries. Medium-sized arteries are more typically affected in polyarteritis nodosa (p. 1140).

Investigations

A number of investigations may be abnormal in patients with renovascular disease, but unfortunately the non-invasive tests described below are insufficiently sensitive to be used for screening in hypertensive patients. Renal function may be impaired and plasma renin activity may be elevated, sometimes with hypokalaemia. Ultrasound may reveal a discrepancy in size between the two kidneys and Doppler ultrasound can identify significant renal artery stenosis. Renal isotope scanning may show delayed uptake of isotope and reduced excretion by an affected kidney, but this is unreliable in the presence of renal impairment. Even if basal perfusion appears normal, administration of a single dose of an ACE inhibitor ('captopril renography') may induce changes in DTPA excretion in a kidney with renal artery stenosis.

The definitive investigation is renal arteriography (Fig. 17.27), but this carries the risk of contrast nephropathy, and significant additional risks in patients with severe atherosclerosis (Box 17.2, p. 462). Non-invasive angiographic techniques such as MR angiography (Fig. 17.27) and spiral CT angiography are being increasingly used. MR angiography is expensive and limited in availability. CT angiography entails large, intravenously administered doses of contrast medium which may be nephrotoxic. Although these techniques can at present give good views of only the main renal arteries, these are the vessels affected in atherosclerosis and are most amenable to intervention. Given the expense and possible risks, angiography should only be undertaken in patients in whom intervention to improve renal perfusion would be contemplated. This is usually limited to young patients and those in whom blood pressure cannot be controlled with antihypertensive agents ('resistant hypertension'), those who have a history of 'flash' pulmonary oedema or accelerated phase ('malignant') hypertension, or those in whom renal function is deteriorating.

Management

Untreated, atheromatous renal artery stenosis will progress to complete arterial occlusion and loss of kidney function in about 15% of cases. This figure is increased with more severe degrees of stenosis. If the progression is gradual, collateral vessels may develop and some function may be preserved, preventing infarction and loss of kidney structure. Conversely, at least 85% of patients with renal artery stenosis will not develop progressive renal impairment, and indeed in many patients the stenosis may be haemodynamically insignificant and not responsible for coexisting essential hypertension. Although investigations such as captopril renography or plasma renin activity have been advocated as predictors of the response to reversal of the stenosis, it remains difficult to predict which patients will respond.

Treatment options are:

- Medical management with blood pressure lowering, low-dose aspirin and lipid-lowering drugs. This will usually have been attempted before angiography is performed.
- Angioplasty, with placement of stents in atherosclerotic disease areas to improve primary patency rates and prevent rapid recurrence.
- Surgical resection of the stenosed segment and re-anastomosis. This is rarely undertaken now for atherosclerotic disease.

Angioplasty is widely used, but there may be substantial risks in patients with atherosclerosis: of contrast nephropathy (Box 17.2, p. 462), of renal artery occlusion and renal infarction, and of atheroemboli (p. 499) from manipulations in a severely diseased aorta. Small-vessel disease distal to the stenosis may preclude substantial functional recovery. The overall effect on blood pressure, on renal function and on patient survival is far from clear, and trials are currently addressing this. Persisting with conservative medical treatment may be appropriate if there is widespread atheromatous disease of the aorta and elsewhere. Surgical mortality is significant in patients with atherosclerosis; when intervention is required, percutaneous procedures are generally preferred.

In non-atheromatous fibromuscular dysplasia, the renal artery stenosis is much more likely to be the cause of the presentation, and angioplasty has a high chance of success in improving blood pressure and protecting renal function.

DISEASES OF SMALL INTRARENAL VESSELS

A number of conditions are associated with acute damage and occlusion of small blood vessels (arterioles and capillaries) in the kidney (Box 17.40). They may be

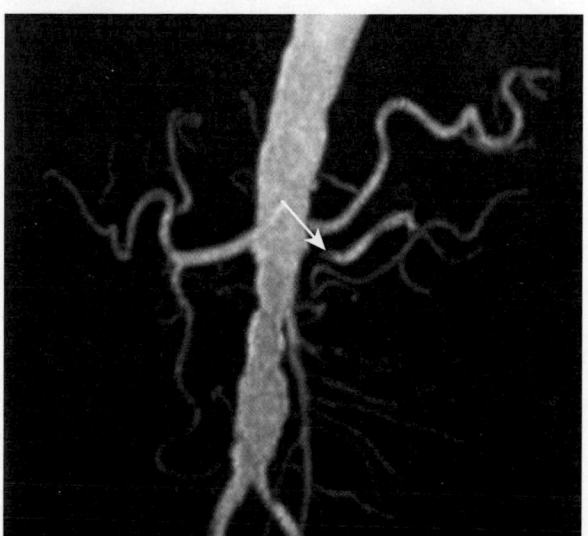

Fig. 17.27   Renal artery stenosis. A magnetic resonance angiogram following injection of contrast. The abdominal aorta is severely irregular and atheromatous. The left renal artery is stenosed (arrow).

17

17.40 MICROVASCULAR DISORDERS ASSOCIATED WITH ACUTE RENAL DAMAGE

- Thrombotic microangiopathy (haemolytic uraemic syndrome and thrombotic thrombocytopenic purpura)
    - Associated with verotoxin-producing *E. coli*
    - Other (familial, drugs, cancer etc.)
- Disseminated intravascular coagulation
- Malignant hypertension
- Small-vessel vasculitis
- Systemic sclerosis (scleroderma)
- Atheroemboli ('cholesterol' emboli)

associated with similar changes elsewhere in the body. A common feature of these syndromes is microangiopathic haemolytic anaemia, in which haemolysis occurs as a consequence of damage incurred to red blood cells during passage through the abnormal vessels; fragmented red cells can be seen on a blood film.

Thrombotic microangiopathy: HUS and TTP

Haemolytic uraemic syndrome (HUS) and thrombotic thrombocytopenic purpura (TTP) are types of thrombotic microangiopathy. Common features include damage to endothelial cells of the microcirculation, which is followed by cell swelling, platelet adherence and thrombosis. A severe microangiopathy causes a marked reduction in the platelet count and anaemia. Other features of intravascular haemolysis (p. 1030)—raised bilirubin and lactate dehydrogenase (LDH), decreased haptoglobins—are also present. A reticulocytosis is often seen. The aetiology of the syndromes may be different, although there is substantial overlap. The kidney microcirculation tends to be most affected in HUS, with involvement of other organs (including the brain) in more severe cases. In TTP the brain is commonly affected and involvement of the kidney may be less severe.

E.coli O157-associated HUS

Thrombotic microangiopathy associated with *E. coli* infection (especially O157 serotypes) is associated with verotoxin-producing organisms (p. 328). Although the bacteria live as commensals in the gut of cattle and other domestic livestock, they can cause haemorrhagic diarrhoea in humans when the infection is contracted from contaminated food products, water or other infected individuals. In a proportion of cases, verotoxin produced by the organisms enters the circulation and binds to specific glycolipid receptors that are expressed on the surface of microvascular endothelial cells. In children, this causes diarrhoea-associated (D+)HUS, although in more severe cases the brain and other organs are also affected. D+HUS is now the most common cause of ARF in children in developed countries. In adults, the disease may more closely resemble TTP. All patients usually recover, often after 5–15 days of dialysis. No specific treatments have been shown to help.

TTP and other HUS

Other causes of thrombotic microangiopathy have a less certain outlook and are more likely to recur (sometimes after renal transplantation). Familial examples may reflect an abnormality of endothelial cell defence against damage or

thrombosis, including deficiency of complement activation inhibitors (associated with familial HUS) or of von Willebrand protease (associated with TTP, p. 1060). The disease may occur post-partum, in response to certain drugs (especially chemotherapy), after bone marrow transplantation, in malignancy and apparently spontaneously. Plasma exchange using fresh frozen plasma is effective in many of these cases, probably by replacing a deficient substance (e.g. the von Willebrand protease).

Disseminated intravascular coagulation

In this condition, consumption of clotting factors and platelets occurs due to uncontrolled thrombosis in the microvasculature, leading to a tendency to haemorrhage from larger vessels (p. 1060). Precipitating conditions include septic shock, in which bacterial endotoxin directly activates the coagulation cascade; obstetric complications; disseminated cancer; massive transfusion; and other causes of coagulation activation or depletion.

Accelerated phase ('malignant') hypertension

Hypertension is described as being in accelerated phase (p. 611) when it causes acute damage to renal and other arterioles. It is often symptomatic, with headache, impaired vision and, finally, manifestations of renal failure (Fig. 17.28). Severe hypertensive retinopathy with papilloedema is almost always present, and it is usually associated with some of the features of microangiopathy described above. In the absence of a previous history, it may be difficult to distinguish these patients from those with HUS and hypertension. Patients usually respond to effective control of blood pressure, although renal function is permanently lost in 20% of cases.

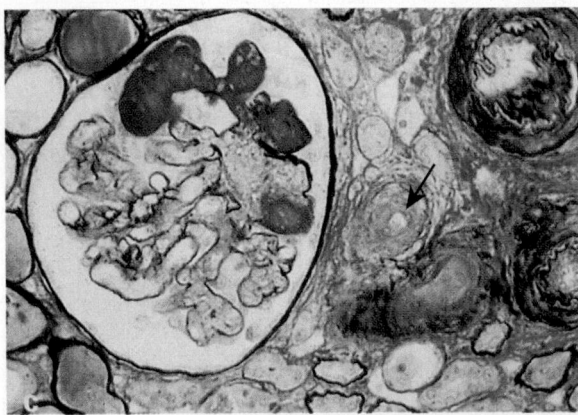

Fig. 17.28 Glomerular capillary thrombosis in malignant hypertension. Similar changes occur in thrombotic microangiopathy. The adjacent arteriole (arrow) shows gross intimal thickening.

Systemic sclerosis (scleroderma)

This connective tissue disease is described on page 1134. Renal involvement is a serious feature, and is characterised by intimal cell proliferation and luminal narrowing of intrarenal arteries and arterioles. Clinically, it usually presents as 'scleroderma renal crisis', with severe hypertension, microangiopathic features and progressive oliguric renal failure. There is intense intrarenal vasospasm, and plasma renin activity is markedly elevated. Use of ACE inhibitors to control the hypertension has improved the 1-year survival from 20% to 75%; however, about 50% of patients continue to require RRT.

Atheroembolic renal disease ('cholesterol' emboli)

This is caused by showers of cholesterol-containing microemboli, arising in atheromatous plaques in major arteries. It occurs in patients with widespread atheromatous disease, usually after interventions such as surgery or arteriography but sometimes after anticoagulation. There is loss of renal function, haematuria and proteinuria, and sometimes eosinophilia and inflammatory features which may mimic a small-vessel vasculitis. Accompanying signs of microvascular occlusion in the lower limbs (e.g. ischaemic toes, livedo reticularis) are common but not invariable (Fig. 17.29). There is no specific treatment.

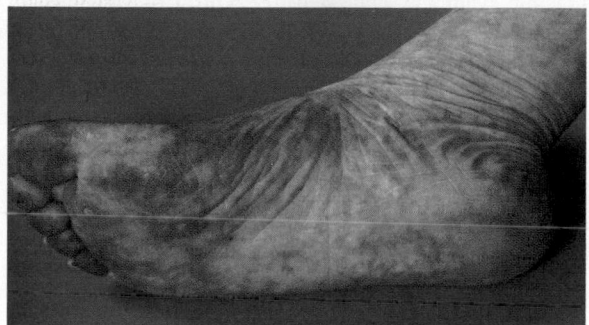

Fig. 17.29   The foot of a patient who suffered extensive atheroembolism following coronary artery stenting.

Small-vessel vasculitis

Renal disease caused by small-vessel vasculitis usually affects the glomeruli, as described in the next section and on page 515.

GLOMERULAR DISEASES

Glomerular diseases account for a significant proportion of acute and chronic renal failure. Glomerular damage may follow a number of insults: immunological injury, inherited abnormality (e.g. Alport's syndrome), metabolic stress (e.g. diabetes mellitus), deposition of extraneous materials (e.g. amyloid), or other direct injury to glomerular cells. The cell types of the glomerulus that may be the target of injury are shown in Figure 17.31 overleaf. The response of the glomerulus to injury varies according to the nature of the insult (Fig. 17.30). At one extreme, specific injury to podocytes, or structural alteration of the glomerulus affecting podocyte function (for example, by scarring or deposition of excess matrix or other material), causes proteinuria and nephrotic syndrome (Box 17.5, p. 467). At the other end of the spectrum, inflammation leads to cell damage and proliferation, breaks form in the GBM and blood leaks into urine. In its extreme form, with acute sodium retention and hypertension, such disease is labelled nephritic syndrome.

GLOMERULONEPHRITIS

Glomerulonephritis literally means 'inflammation of glomeruli' and, although inflammation is not apparent in all varieties ('glomerulopathy' is sometimes used to denote this), the name sticks.

17

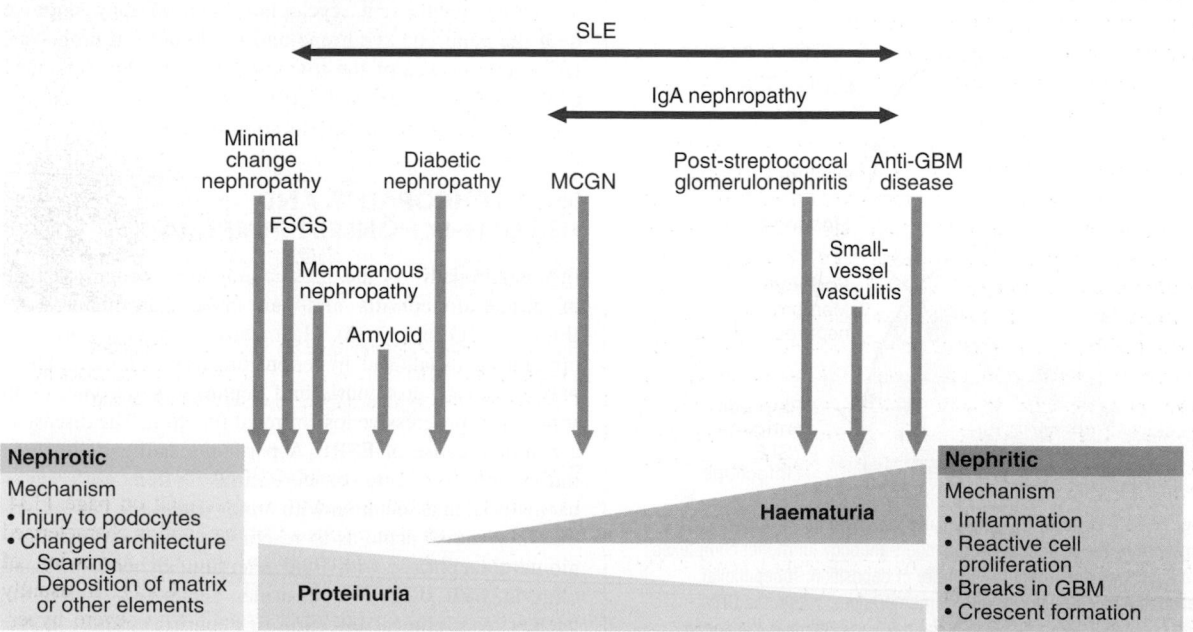

Fig. 17.30   Spectrum of glomerular diseases. (FSGS = focal and segmental glomerulosclerosis; MCGN = mesangiocapillary glomerulonephritis)

Most types of glomerulonephritis seem to be immuno-logically mediated and several respond to immunosuppressive drugs. For some diseases there is direct evidence of this: for example, the anti-GBM antibodies seen in Goodpasture's disease. Deposition of antibody occurs in many types of glomerulonephritis (Box 17.41, overleaf), but frequently the presumed mechanisms involve cellular immunity, which is more difficult to investigate. Although deposition of circulating immune complexes was previously thought to be a common mechanism of glomerulonephritis, it now seems that most granular deposits of immunoglobulin are formed 'in situ' by antibodies which complex about glomerular antigens, or about other antigens ('planted' antigens, e.g. viral or bacterial ones) that have localised in glomeruli (Fig. 17.31).

Classifications of glomerulonephritis are largely histopathological and may appear daunting, but the details are largely a specialist concern. Clinically important types are described in the text. Box 17.41 and Figure 17.32 show additional detail and illustrate the major types.

MINIMAL CHANGE NEPHROPATHY AND PRIMARY FOCAL SEGMENTAL GLOMERULOSCLEROSIS (FSGS)

Patients with minimal change nephropathy and a subgroup of patients with FSGS can be seen as opposite ends of a spectrum of conditions causing idiopathic nephrotic syndrome (Box 17.5, p. 467).

Minimal change disease occurs at all ages but accounts for nephrotic syndrome in most children and about one-quarter of adults. Proteinuria usually remits on high-dose corticosteroid therapy (1 mg/kg prednisolone for

6 weeks), although some patients who respond incompletely or relapse frequently need maintenance corticosteroids, cytotoxic therapy or other agents. Minimal change disease does not progress to CRF; the main problems are those of the nephrotic syndrome and complications of treatment.

FSGS is a histological description (Fig. 17.31) with many causes. The primary FSGS group that present with idiopathic nephrotic syndrome and no other cause of renal disease typically show little response to corticosteroid treatment and often progress to renal failure; the disease frequently recurs after renal transplantation, and sometimes proteinuria recurs almost immediately. However, a proportion of patients with FSGS do respond to corticosteroids (a good prognostic sign). As FSGS is a focal process, abnormal glomeruli may not be seen on renal biopsy if only a few are sampled, leading to an initial diagnosis of minimal change nephropathy. Juxtamedullary glomeruli are more likely to be affected in early disease.

In other patients with the histological appearances of FSGS but lesser proteinuria, focal scarring reflects healing of previous focal glomerular injury, such as haemolytic uraemic syndrome, cholesterol embolism or vasculitis. In others, it seems to represent particular types of nephropathy: for example, those associated with heroin misuse, HIV infection and massive obesity. Associations with numerous other forms of injury and renal disorders are reported. There is no specific treatment for most of these.

MEMBRANOUS NEPHROPATHY

This is the most common cause of nephrotic syndrome in adults. A proportion of cases are associated with known causes (Box 17.41 and Figs 17.32D and F) but most are idiopathic. Of this group, approximately one-third remit spontaneously, one-third remain in a nephrotic state, and one-third show progressive loss of renal function. Short-term treatment with high doses of corticosteroids and alkylating agents (e.g. cyclophosphamide) may improve both the nephrotic syndrome and the long-term prognosis. However, because of the toxicity of these regimens, most nephrologists reserve such treatment for those with severe nephrotic syndrome or deteriorating renal function.

IgA NEPHROPATHY AND HENOCH–SCHÖNLEIN PURPURA

IgA nephropathy is the most commonly recognised type of glomerulonephritis and can present in many ways (Figs 17.32G and 17.33). Haematuria is almost universal, proteinuria usual, and hypertension very common. There may be severe proteinuria and nephrotic syndrome, or in some cases progressive loss of renal function. The disease is a common cause of ESRF. A particular hallmark in some individuals is acute exacerbations, often with gross haematuria, in association with minor respiratory infections. This may be so acute as to resemble acute post-infectious glomerulonephritis, with fluid retention, hypertension and oliguria with dark or red urine. Characteristically, the latency from clinical infection to nephritis is short: a few days or less. These episodes usually subside spontaneously.

17

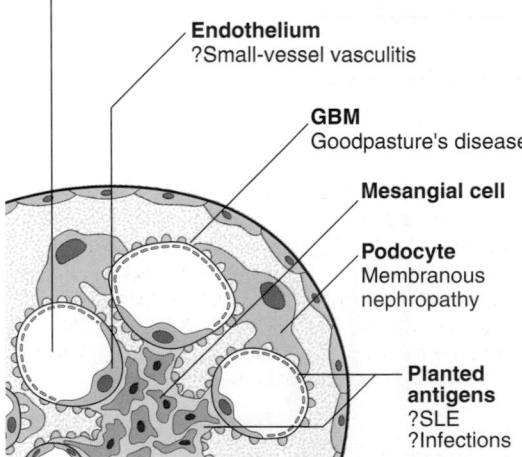

Circulating immune complexes
Cryoglobulinaemia
Serum sickness
?Endocarditis

Endothelium
?Small-vessel vasculitis

GBM
Goodpasture's disease

Mesangial cell

Podocyte
Membranous nephropathy

Planted antigens
?SLE
?Infections

Fig. 17.31 Cells of the glomerulus and targets of immunity and autoimmunity. Antibodies and antigen-antibody (immune) complexes are described according to their site of deposition: subepithelial, between podocyte and GBM; intramembranous, within the GBM; subendothelial, between endothelial cell and GBM; and mesangial, within the mesangial matrix.

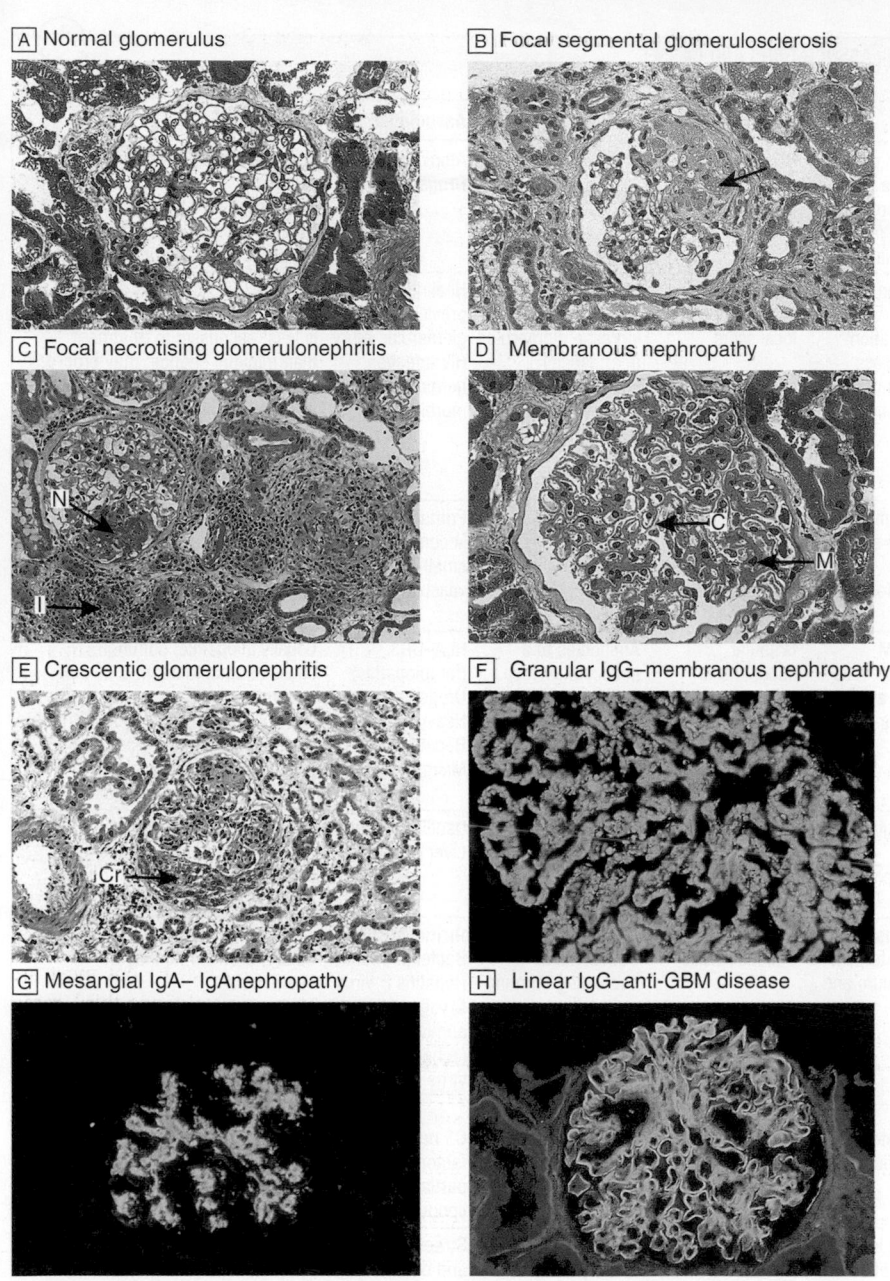

A Normal glomerulus

B Focal segmental glomerulosclerosis

C Focal necrotising glomerulonephritis

D Membranous nephropathy

E Crescentic glomerulonephritis

F Granular IgG–membranous nephropathy

G Mesangial IgA– IgAnephropathy

H Linear IgG–anti-GBM disease

Fig. 17.32   Histopathology of glomerular disease. (A – E light microscopy)
A A normal glomerulus. Note the open capillary loops and thinness of their walls—'should look as if you could cut yourself on them'. B Focal segmental glomerulosclerosis. The portion of the glomerulus arrowed shows loss of capillary loops and cells, which are replaced by matrix. C Focal necrotising glomerulonephritis. A portion of the glomerulus (N = focal necrotising lesion) is replaced by bright pink material with some 'nuclear dust'. Neutrophils may be seen elsewhere in the glomerulus. There is surrounding interstitial inflammation (I). This is most commonly associated with small-vessel vasculitis and may progress to crescentic nephritis (see E). D Membranous nephropathy. The capillary loops (C) are thickened (compare with the normal glomerulus) and there is expansion of the mesangial regions by matrix deposition (M). However, there is no gross cellular proliferation or excess of inflammatory cells. E Crescentic glomerulonephritis. The lower part of Bowman's space is occupied by a semicircular formation ('crescent', Cr) of large pale cells, compressing the glomerular tuft. This is usually seen in aggressive inflammatory types of glomerulonephritis.
Antibody deposition in the glomerulus. (F – H direct immunofluorescence)
F Granular deposits of IgG along the basement membrane in a subepithelial pattern, typical of membranous nephropathy. G IgA deposits in the mesangium, as seen in IgA nephropathy. H Ribbon-like linear deposits of anti-GBM antibodies along the GBM in Goodpasture's disease. Glomerular structure is well preserved in all of these examples.

17

17.41 GLOMERULONEPHRITIS: TYPES, ASSOCIATIONS AND CAUSES

	Histology	Immune deposits	Pathogenesis	Association	Clinical features
Minimal change	Normal, except on electron microscopy, where fusion of podocyte foot processes is seen (occurs in many types of proteinuria)	None	Unknown	Atopy, HLA–DR7 Drugs	Acute and often severe nephrotic syndrome Good response to corticosteroids Dominant cause of idiopathic nephrotic syndrome in childhood
Focal segmental glomerulosclerosis (FSGS)	Segmental scars in some glomeruli No acute inflammation Podocyte foot process fusion seen in primary FSGS with nephrotic syndrome	Non-specific trapping in focal scars	Unknown; in some, circulating factors increase glomerular permeability Injury to podocytes may be a common feature	Healing of previous local glomerular injury HIV infection, heroin misuse, morbid obesity	*Primary FSGS* presents as idiopathic nephrotic syndrome but is less responsive to treatment than minimal change; may progress to renal impairment, can recur after transplantation *Secondary FSGS* presents with variable proteinuria and outcome
Focal segmental (necrotising) glomerulonephritis	Segmental inflammation and/or necrosis in some glomeruli May be crescent formation	Variable according to cause, but typically negative (or 'pauci-immune')	Small-vessel vasculitis	Primary or secondary small-vessel vasculitis	Usually implies presence of systemic disease, and responds to treatment with corticosteroids and cytotoxic agents Check ANCA, ANA
Membranous nephropathy	Thickening of GBM Progressing to increased matrix deposition and glomerulosclerosis	Granular subepithelial IgG	Antibodies to a podocyte surface antigen, with complement-dependent podocyte injury (presumed from animal model)	HLA–DR3 (for idiopathic) Drugs Heavy metals Hepatitis B virus Malignancy	Usually idiopathic; common cause of adult idiopathic nephrotic syndrome One-third progress; may respond to chlorambucil/prednisolone Associated HLA class II allele varies in different populations
IgA nephropathy	Increased mesangial matrix and cells Focal segmental nephritis in acute disease	Mesangial IgA	Unknown	Usually idiopathic Liver disease	Very common disease with range of presentations, but usually including haematuria and hypertension (see text)
Mesangiocapillary glomerulonephritis (MCGN) (= membranoproliferative glomerulonephritis, MPGN)					
Type I	Mesangial cells interpose between endothelium and GBM	Subendothelial	Deposition of circulating immune complexes or 'planted' antigens	Bacterial infection Hepatitis B virus Cryoglobulin-aemia (± hepatitis C virus infection)	Usually proteinuria, may be haematuria Most common pattern found in association with subacute bacterial infection No proven treatments except where cause can be treated
Type II	Mesangial cells interpose between endothelium and GBM	Intramembranous dense deposits	Associated with complement consumption caused by autoantibodies	C3 nephritic factor and partial lipodystrophy	Also known as dense deposit disease
Post-infection	Diffuse (uniformly in all glomeruli) proliferation of endothelial and mesangial cells Infiltration by neutrophils and macrophages May be crescent formation	Subendothelial	Immune response to streptococcal infection Cross-reactive epitopes or other explanation	Streptococcal and other infections	Now rare in developed countries Presents with severe sodium and fluid retention, hypertension, haematuria, oliguria Usually resolves spontaneously
Goodpasture's disease (anti-GBM disease)	Usually crescentic nephritis	Linear IgG along GBM	Autoimmunity to $\alpha 3$ chain of type IV collagen	HLA–DR15 (previously known as DR2)	Associated with lung haemorrhage but either may occur alone Treat with corticosteroids, cyclophosphamide and plasma exchange to remove circulating autoantibodies
Lupus nephritis	Almost any histological type	Always positive and often profuse Pattern varies according to type	Some anti-DNA antibodies also bind to glomerular targets	Complement deficiencies Complement consumption	Very variable presentation, sometimes as renal disease alone without systemic features Responds to cytotoxic therapy in addition to prednisolone

17

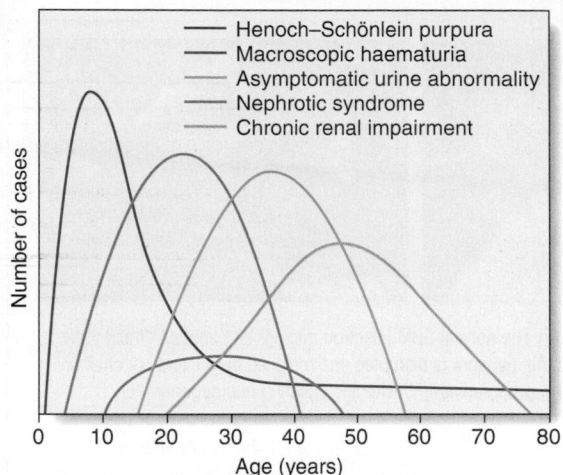

Fig. 17.33 **Clinical presentations of IgA nephropathy in relation to age at diagnosis.** Henoch–Schönlein purpura is most common in childhood but may occur at any age. Macroscopic haematuria is very uncommon over the age of 40 years. The importance of asymptomatic urine abnormality as the presentation of IgA nephropathy will depend on attitudes to routine urine testing and renal biopsy. It is uncertain whether those presenting with chronic renal impairment have a disease distinct from that of those presenting at a younger age with macroscopic haematuria.

In children, and occasionally in adults, a systemic vasculitis occurring in response to similar infections is called Henoch–Schönlein purpura. A characteristic petechial rash (cutaneous vasculitis, typically affecting buttocks and lower legs) and abdominal pain (gastrointestinal vasculitis) usually dominate the clinical picture, with mild glomerulonephritis being indicated by haematuria. When the disease occurs in older children or adults, the glomerulonephritis is usually more prominent. Renal biopsy shows mesangial IgA deposition and appearances indistinguishable from acute IgA nephropathy.

Occasionally, IgA nephropathy progresses rapidly and crescent formation may be seen. The response to immunosuppressive therapy is usually poor. The management of less acute disease is largely directed towards the control of blood pressure in an attempt to prevent or retard progressive renal disease.

GLOMERULONEPHRITIS ASSOCIATED WITH INFECTION

Bacterial infections, usually subacute (typically subacute bacterial endocarditis), may cause a variety of histological patterns of glomerulonephritis, but usually with plentiful immunoglobulin deposition and often with evidence of complement consumption (low serum C3, Box 17.41). In the developed world, hospital-acquired infections are now a common cause of these syndromes. World-wide, glomerulonephritis associated with malaria, hepatitis B, hepatitis C, schistosomiasis, leishmaniasis and other chronic infections is very common. The usual histological patterns are membranous and mesangiocapillary lesions, although many other types may be seen. FSGS associated with HIV

17.42 CAUSES OF GLOMERULONEPHRITIS ASSOCIATED WITH LOW SERUM COMPLEMENT
● Post-infection glomerulonephritis
● Subacute bacterial infection–especially endocarditis
● SLE
● Cryoglobulinaemia
● Mesangiocapillary glomerulonephritis–usually type II

infection is prevalent in black races. Proving a causative relationship between renal disease and infection in individual cases is extremely difficult. Acute and chronic infections may also cause interstitial renal disease (p. 504).

Acute post-infectious glomerulonephritis

This is most common following infection with certain strains of streptococcus and therefore is often called post-streptococcal nephritis, but it can occur following other infections. It is much more common in children than adults but is now rare in the developed world. The latency is usually about 10 days after a throat infection or longer after skin infection, suggesting an immune mechanism rather than direct infection.

An acute nephritis of varying severity occurs. Sodium retention, hypertension and oedema, are particularly pronounced. There is also reduction of GFR, proteinuria, haematuria and reduced urine volume. Characteristically, this gives the urine a red or smoky appearance. There are low serum concentrations of C3 and C4 (Box 17.42) and evidence of streptococcal infection (perform antistreptolysin O (ASO) titre, culture of throat swab, and other swab tests if skin infection is suspected).

Renal function begins to improve spontaneously within 10–14 days, and management by fluid and sodium restriction and use of diuretic and hypotensive agents is usually adequate. Remarkably, the renal lesion in almost all children and most adults seems to resolve completely despite the severity of the glomerular inflammation and proliferation seen histologically.

RAPIDLY PROGRESSIVE GLOMERULONEPHRITIS

This describes an extreme inflammatory nephritis which causes rapid loss of renal function over days to weeks. Renal biopsy shows crescentic lesions often associated with necrotising lesions within the glomerulus (focal segmental (necrotising) glomerulonephritis). It is typically seen in Goodpasture's disease, where there are specific anti-GBM antibodies, and in small-vessel vasculitides (pp. 515 and 1138), but can also be seen in SLE (pp. 515 and 1132) and occasionally IgA and other nephropathies.

INHERITED GLOMERULAR DISEASES

ALPORT'S SYNDROME

A number of uncommon diseases may affect the glomerulus in childhood, but the most important one affecting adults is

17

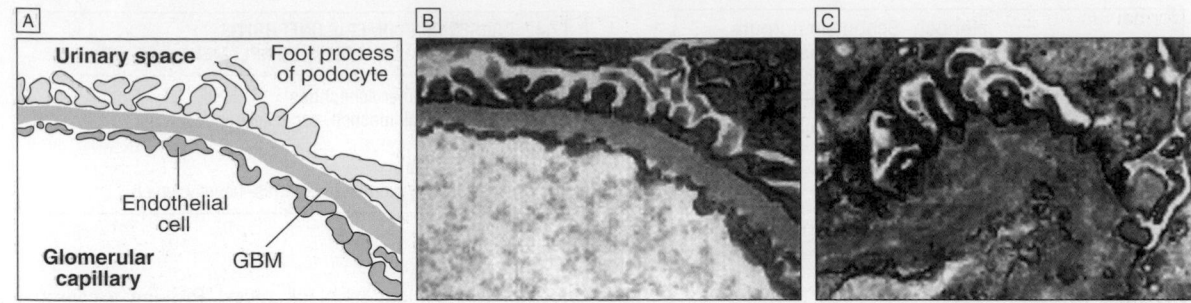

Fig. 17.34 Alport's syndrome. [A] Diagrammatic structure of the normal GBM. [B] The normal GBM (electron micrograph) contains mostly the tissue-specific α3, α4 and α5 chains of type IV collagen. [C] In Alport's syndrome this network is disrupted and replaced by α1 and α2 chains. Although the GBM appears structurally normal in early life, in time thinning appears, progressing to thickening, splitting and degeneration.

Alport's syndrome. Most cases arise from a mutation or deletion of the *COL4A5* gene on the X chromosome which encodes type IV collagen, resulting in inheritance as an X-linked recessive disorder (p. 55). Mutations in *COL4A3* or *COL4A4* genes are less common and cause autosomal recessive disease. The accumulation of abnormal collagen results in a progressive degeneration of the GBM (Fig. 17.34). Affected patients progress from haematuria to ESRF in their late teens or twenties. Female carriers of *COL4A5* mutations usually have haematuria but rarely develop significant renal disease. Some other basement membranes containing the same collagen isoforms are similarly affected, notably in the cochlea, so that Alport's syndrome is associated with sensorineural deafness and ocular abnormalities.

No specific treatment has been devised to slow the progress of this condition, but patients with Alport's syndrome are good candidates for renal replacement therapy as they are young and usually otherwise healthy. Some of these patients develop an immune response to the normal collagen antigens present in the GBM of a transplanted kidney, and in a small minority anti-GBM disease develops and destroys the allograft.

THIN GBM DISEASE

In 'thin GBM' disease there is glomerular bleeding, usually only at the microscopic or stick-test level, without associated hypertension, proteinuria or reduction of GFR. The glomeruli appear normal by light microscopy, but on electron microscopy the GBM is abnormally thin. This autosomal dominant condition accounts for a large proportion of 'benign familial haematuria' and has an excellent prognosis. Some families may be carriers of autosomal recessive Alport's syndrome, but this does not account for all cases.

TUBULO-INTERSTITIAL DISEASES

Acute tubular necrosis is the most common cause of the clinical syndrome of acute renal failure, and is described on page 482. Illustrations of this and other tubulo-interstitial pathologies are shown in Figure 17.35.

INTERSTITIAL NEPHRITIS

A group of inflammatory, inherited and other diseases affect renal tubules and the surrounding interstitium. The clinical presentation is often renal failure, but electrolyte abnormalities are common, especially hyperkalaemia and acidosis. Proteinuria (and albuminuria) is rarely > 1 g/24 hrs but low molecular weight proteinuria (e.g. retinol-binding protein, β_2-microglobulin, lysozyme) with haematuria and pyuria are common.

ACUTE INTERSTITIAL NEPHRITIS (AIN)

Acute inflammation within the tubulo-interstitium is most commonly allergic, particularly to drugs, but other causes include toxins and a variety of systemic diseases and infections (Box 17.43).

Renal biopsies (Fig. 17.35) show intense inflammation, with polymorphonuclear leucocytes and lymphocytes surrounding tubules and blood vessels and invading tubules (tubulitis), and occasional eosinophils (especially in drug-induced disease).

Diagnosis

Only a minority (perhaps 30%) of patients with drug-induced AIN have a generalised drug hypersensitivity

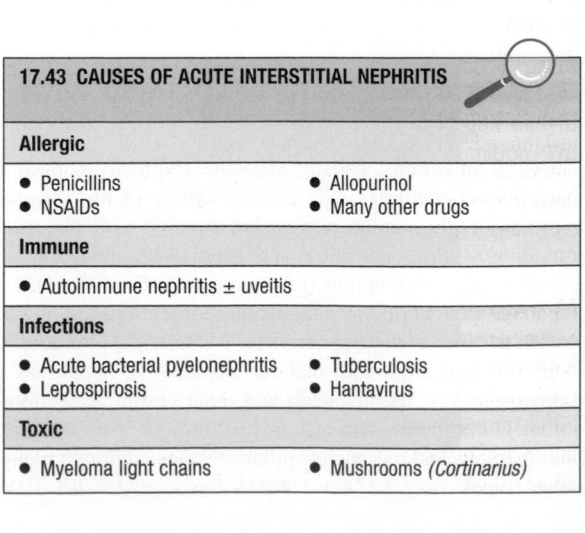

17.43 CAUSES OF ACUTE INTERSTITIAL NEPHRITIS	
Allergic	
• Penicillins	• Allopurinol
• NSAIDs	• Many other drugs
Immune	
• Autoimmune nephritis ± uveitis	
Infections	
• Acute bacterial pyelonephritis	• Tuberculosis
• Leptospirosis	• Hantavirus
Toxic	
• Myeloma light chains	• Mushrooms *(Cortinarius)*

17

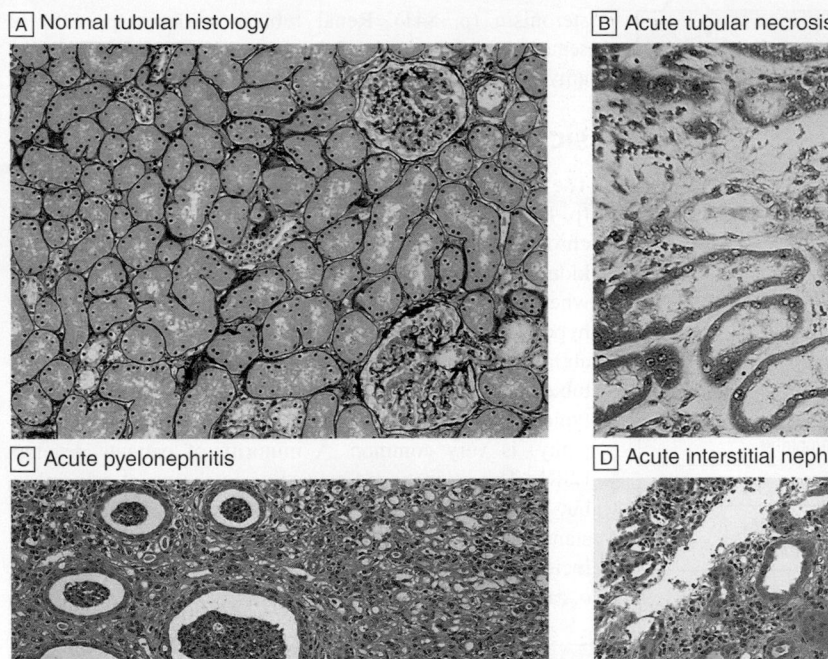

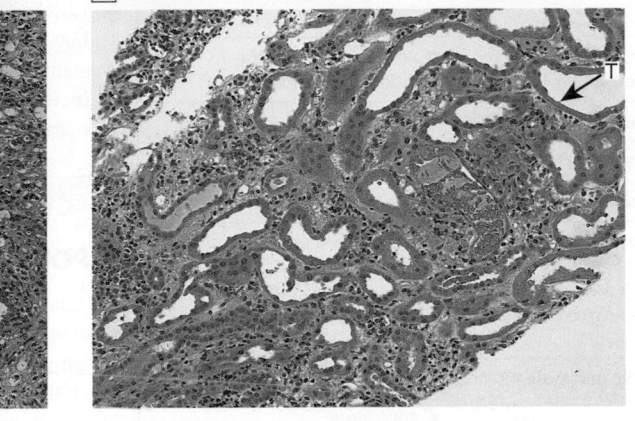

Fig. 17.35 Tubular histopathology. Ⓐ Normal tubular histology. The tubules are back-to-back. Brush borders can be seen on the luminal borders of cells in the proximal tubule. Ⓑ Acute tubular necrosis. There are scattered breaks (B) in tubular basement membranes, swelling and vacuolation of tubular cells, and in places apoptosis and necrosis of tubular cells with shedding of cells into the lumen. During the regenerative phase there is increased tubular mitotic activity. The interstitium (I) is oedematous and infiltrated by inflammatory cells. The glomeruli (not shown) are relatively normal, although there may be endothelial cell swelling and fibrin deposition. Ⓒ Acute bacterial pyelonephritis. A widespread inflammatory infiltrate that includes many neutrophils is seen. Granulocyte casts (G) are forming within some dilated tubules (T). Other tubules are scarcely visible because of the extent of the inflammation and damage. Ⓓ Acute (allergic) interstitial nephritis. In this patient who received an NSAID, an extensive mononuclear cell infiltrate (no neutrophils) involving tubules (T) is seen. This inflammation does not involve the glomeruli (not shown). Sometimes eosinophils are prominent. Transplant rejection looks similar to this.

reaction (e.g. fever, rash, eosinophilia) and dipstick testing of the urine is usually unimpressive. However, leucocyturia is common, and eosinophils are found in the urine in up to 70% of patients. Deterioration of renal function in drug-induced AIN may be dramatic and resemble rapidly progressive glomerulonephritis. Renal biopsy is usually required to confirm the diagnosis. The degree of chronic inflammation in a biopsy is a useful predictor of the eventual outcome for renal function. Many patients are not oliguric despite moderately severe ARF, and AIN should always be considered in patients with non-oliguric ARF.

Management
Some patients with drug-induced AIN recover following withdrawal of the drug alone, but corticosteroids (e.g. prednisolone 1 mg/kg/day) accelerate recovery and may prevent long-term scarring. Dialysis is sometimes necessary, but is usually only short-term. Other specific causes (Box 17.43) should be treated where possible.

CHRONIC INTERSTITIAL NEPHRITIS
Aetiology
Chronic interstitial nephritis (CIN) is caused by a heterogeneous group of diseases, summarised in Box 17.44. However, it is quite common for the condition to be diagnosed late and for no aetiology to be apparent.

Toxic causes of CIN
The combination of interstitial nephritis and tumours of the collecting system is seen in Balkan nephropathy, so called because of where cases are found, and has been controversially attributed to ingestion of fungal toxins, particularly ochratoxin A, present in food made from stored grain. A plant toxin, aristolochic acid, has been blamed for a rapidly progressive syndrome caused by mistaken identity of ingredients in herbal preparations.

Papillary necrosis and analgesic nephropathy
Long-term ingestion (years to decades) of analgesic drugs can cause renal papillary necrosis and CIN. As the papillae

17.44 CAUSES OF CHRONIC INTERSTITIAL NEPHRITIS

Acute interstitial nephritis

- Any of the causes of AIN if persistent

Glomerulonephritis

- Varying degrees of interstitial inflammation occur in association with most types of inflammatory glomerulonephritis

Immune/inflammatory

- Sarcoidosis
- Sjögren's syndrome
- SLE, primary autoimmune
- Chronic transplant rejection

Toxic

- Mushrooms
- Lead
- Chinese herbs
- Balkan nephropathy

Drugs

- All drugs causing AIN
- Lithium toxicity
- Analgesic nephropathy
- Ciclosporin, tacrolimus

Infection

- Consequence of severe pyelonephritis

Congenital/developmental

- Vesico-ureteric reflux—is associated; causation not clear
- Renal dysplasias—often associated with reflux
- Inherited—now well recognised but mechanisms unclear
- Other—Wilson's disease, medullary sponge kidney, sickle-cell nephropathy

Metabolic and systemic diseases

- Hypokalaemia, hyper-calciuria, hyperoxaluria
- Amyloidosis

17

are at the end of the capillary distribution in the kidney, they become ischaemic most easily and may necrose in this condition, in sickle-cell disease and occasionally in diabetes and other conditions. Necrosed papillae may cause ureteric obstruction and renal colic. Papillary necrosis is difficult to identify other than on IVU or retrograde pyelography. In animals, lesions can be induced with almost any NSAID; however, there has been a dramatic fall in the incidence of this disease following withdrawal of phenacetin from compound analgesics. If it is diagnosed, cessation of analgesic intake may arrest progression.

Clinical and biochemical features

Most patients present in adult life with CRF, hypertension and small kidneys. CRF is often moderate (urea < 25 mmol/l or 150 mg/dl) but, because of tubular dysfunction, electrolyte abnormalities are typically more severe (e.g. hyperkalaemia, acidosis). Urinalysis abnormalities are non-specific. A minority of patients present with hypotension, polyuria and features of sodium and water depletion (e.g. low blood pressure and jugular venous pressure)—salt-losing nephropathy. Impairment of urine-concentrating ability and sodium conservation places patients with CIN at risk of superimposed ARF with even moderate salt and water depletion during an acute illness.

Hyperkalaemia may be disproportionate in CIN or in diabetic nephropathy because of hyporeninaemic hypoaldo-

steronism (p. 841). Renal tubular acidosis (p. 438) is seen most often in myeloma, sarcoidosis, cystinosis and amyloidosis.

SICKLE-CELL NEPHROPATHY

The longer survival of patients with sickle-cell disease (p. 1035) means that a larger proportion live to develop chronic complications of microvascular occlusion. In the kidney these changes are most pronounced in the medulla, where the vasa recta are the site of sickling because of hypoxia and hypertonicity. Loss of urinary concentrating ability and polyuria are the earliest changes; distal renal tubular acidosis and impaired potassium excretion are typical. Papillary necrosis (as seen in analgesic nephropathy) is very common. A minority of patients develop ESRF. This is managed according to the usual principles, but response to recombinant erythropoietin is understandably poor. Patients with sickle trait have an increased incidence of unexplained microscopic haematuria, and occasionally overt papillary necrosis.

CYSTIC KIDNEY DISEASES

POLYCYSTIC KIDNEY DISEASE

Adult polycystic kidney disease (PKD) is a common condition (prevalence ~1:1000) that is inherited as an autosomal dominant trait. Small cysts lined by tubular epithelium develop from infancy or childhood and enlarge slowly and irregularly. Surrounding normal kidney tissue is progressively attenuated. Renal failure is associated with grossly enlarged kidneys.

Mutations in PKD1 account for 85% of cases and PKD2 for about 15%. ESRF occurs in ~50% of patients with PKD1 mutations with a mean age of onset of 52 years, but in a minority of patients with PKD2 mutations with a mean age of onset of 69 years. Other genes are responsible rarely.

Clinical features

Common clinical features are shown in Box 17.45. Affected subjects are usually asymptomatic until later life. After the age of 20 there is often insidious onset of hypertension. One or both kidneys may be palpable and the surface may be nodular. There is then a gradual reduction in renal function.

About 30% of patients with PKD have hepatic cysts (Fig. 23.42, p. 988), but disturbance of liver function is rare. Sometimes (almost always in women) this causes massive and symptomatic hepatomegaly, usually concurrent with

17.45 ADULT POLYCYSTIC KIDNEY DISEASE: COMMON CLINICAL FEATURES

- Vague discomfort in loin or abdomen due to increasing mass of renal tissue
- Acute loin pain or renal colic due to haemorrhage into a cyst
- Hypertension
- Haematuria (with little or no proteinuria)
- Urinary tract infection
- Renal failure

renal enlargement, but occasionally with only minor renal involvement.

Berry aneurysms of cerebral vessels are an associated feature, and about 10% of patients have a subarachnoid haemorrhage. This feature appears to be largely restricted to certain families (and presumably specific mutations). Mitral and aortic regurgitation are frequent but rarely severe, and colonic diverticula and abdominal wall hernias may occur.

PKD is not a pre-malignant condition. The rate of renal malignancy is no different from that of other patients with renal failure (but is higher than the general population).

Investigations and screening

The diagnosis is usually based on family history, clinical findings and ultrasound. Ultrasound demonstrates cysts in ~95% of affected patients over the age of 20, but may not detect small developing cysts in younger patients. It is important to identify multiple cysts, not just two or three. Now that the gene defects responsible for PKD have been identified, it is sometimes possible to make a specific genetic diagnosis, but the genes involved are particularly difficult because of their size, the existence of a closely related PKD1 pseudogene, and the wide variety of mutations which affect different families. Occasionally, linkage analysis (p. 51) may be used to exclude the diagnosis in a young adult with normal renal imaging.

Screening for intracranial aneurysms is not generally indicated. Where non-invasive MR angiography is available, some centres screen patients in families with a history of subarachnoid haemorrhage. However, even then, the yield of screening has been low, and the risk–benefit ratio of intervention in asymptomatic aneurysms in this disease is not known.

Management

Nothing has yet been found to alter the rate of progression of renal failure in human PKD, although there are some potentially interesting approaches under investigation. Good control of blood pressure is important because cardio-vascular morbidity and mortality are so common in renal disease, but there is no evidence that control of moderate hypertension retards the development of renal failure in PKD, in contrast to the evidence for glomerular diseases.

Patients with PKD are usually good candidates for dialysis and transplantation. Sometimes kidneys are so large that one or both have to be removed to make space for a renal transplant.

OTHER CYSTIC DISEASES

Medullary cystic diseases

Medullary sponge kidney is characterised by cysts confined to papillary collecting ducts. The disease is not inherited and its cause is unknown. Patients usually present as adults with renal stones. These are often recurrent, and preventive measures (p. 472) need to be implemented if so, but the prognosis is generally good. The diagnosis is made by ultrasound or IVU (Fig. 17.36). Contrast medium is seen to fill dilated or cystic tubules, which are sometimes calcified.

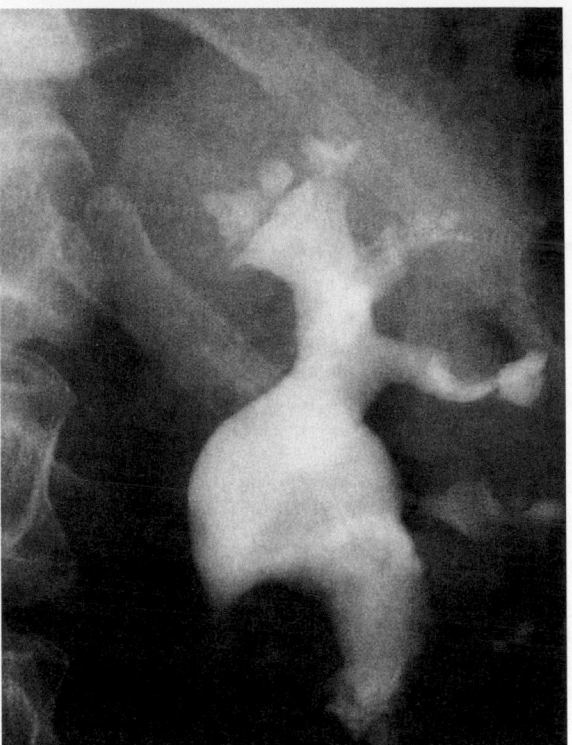

Fig. 17.36 Medullary sponge kidney. Intravenous pyelogram showing contrast medium filling both the collecting system and cavities arising from collecting ducts, especially within papillae of the upper pole. The cavities have been likened to bunches of grapes. A plain abdominal X-ray may show calcification in the same regions.

Medullary cystic kidney diseases are a heterogenous group of inherited disorders, known as nephronophthisis in children. Small cortical cysts are associated with progressive destruction of the nephron. The childhood variants are characterised by thirst and polyuria due to nephrogenic diabetes insipidus, often with a family history of similar disease. Sometimes affected patients are 'salt-losing', which aggravates the degree of renal failure. Even when they are treated appropriately, serious renal failure is usual. The genetic basis of these disorders is emerging; several genes involving multiple mechanisms are involved.

Acquired cystic disease

Patients with a very long history of renal failure (usually on long-term dialysis) often develop multiple renal cysts in their shrunken kidneys: acquired cystic kidney disease. Kidneys are enlarged but not to the size of kidneys in PKD. Acquired cystic disease is associated with increased eryth-ropoietin production, and sometimes with the development of renal cell carcinoma, probably explaining the increased rate of this tumour in dialysis patients.

ISOLATED DEFECTS OF TUBULAR FUNCTION

An increasing number of disorders are now known to be due to specific defects of transporter molecules or other functions in renal tubular cells. Only a few are mentioned here.

Renal glycosuria is a benign autosomal recessive defect of tubular reabsorption of glucose, caused by mutations of the sodium/glucose cotransporter SGLT2. Glucose appears in the urine in the presence of a normal blood glucose concentration.

Cystinuria is a rare condition in which reabsorption of filtered cystine, ornithine, arginine and lysine is defective. It is caused by mutations in the SLC3A1 amino acid transporter gene. The high concentration of cystine in urine leads to cystine stone formation (pp. 471–472).

Other uncommon tubular disorders include vitamin D-resistant rickets (pp. 441 and 1126), in which reabsorption of filtered phosphate is reduced; nephrogenic diabetes insipidus (p. 796), in which the tubules are resistant to the effects of vasopressin; and Bartter's and Gitelman's syndromes, in which there is sodium-wasting and hypokalaemia (p. 434).

The term 'Fanconi syndrome' is used to describe generalised proximal tubular dysfunction. It is not related to Fanconi anaemia. Notable abnormalities include low blood phosphate and uric acid, the finding of glucose and amino acids in urine, and proximal renal tubular acidosis (p. 438). In addition to the causes of interstitial nephritis described above, some congenital metabolic disorders are associated with Fanconi syndrome, notably Wilson's disease, cystinosis and hereditary fructose intolerance.

Renal tubular acidosis describes the common endpoint of a variety of diseases affecting distal (classical or type 1) or proximal (type 2) renal tubular function. These syndromes are described on page 438.

DISEASES OF THE COLLECTING SYSTEM AND URETERS

CONGENITAL ABNORMALITIES

Congenital anomalies of the urinary tract (Fig. 17.37) affect more than 10% of infants and, if not immediately lethal, may lead to complications in later life, including obstructive nephropathy and CRF. About 1 in 500 infants are born with only one kidney. Although usually compatible with normal life, this is often associated with other abnormalities.

A ureterocele (Fig. 17.10, p. 466) occurs behind a pin-hole ureteric orifice when the intramural part of the ureter dilates and bulges into the bladder. It can become very large and cause lower urinary tract obstruction. Incision of the pin-hole opening relieves the obstruction.

Ectopic ureters occur with congenital duplication of one or both kidneys (duplex kidneys). Developmentally, the ureter has two main branches and, if this arrangement persists, the two ureters of the duplex kidneys may drain separately into the bladder. One ureter enters normally on the trigone, while the ectopic ureter (from the upper renal moiety) enters the bladder or, more rarely, the vagina or seminal vesicle.

A ureter that is ectopic and drains into the bladder is liable to have an ineffective valve mechanism so that urine passes

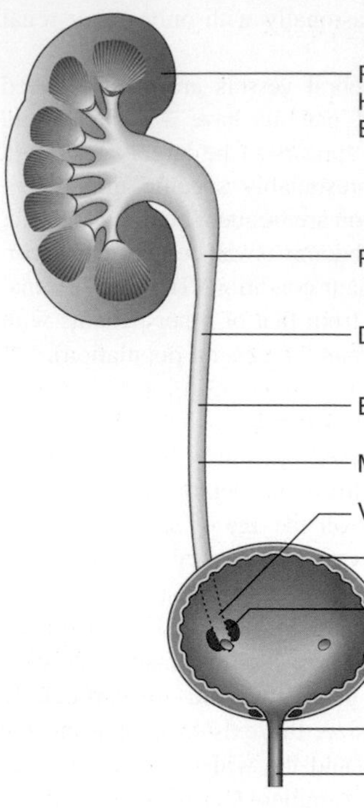
Renal agenesis/dysplasia
Horseshoe kidney
Ectopic kidney
PUJ obstruction
Duplex ureter
Ectopic ureter
Megaureter
Vesico-ureteric reflux
Bladder exstrophy
Ureterocele
Urethral valves
Epispadias, hypospadias

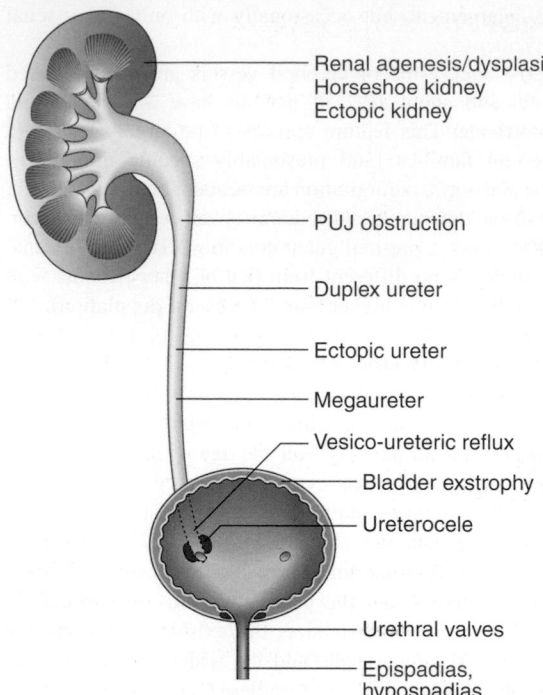

Fig. 17.37 Congenital abnormalities of the urinary tract.

up the ureter on voiding (vesico-ureteric reflux, see below). Reflux can occur in normally sited ureters if the intramural ureter fails to act as a valve. The pressure of refluxing urine behaves as an intermittent obstruction, which in children may lead to serious renal damage. The management of vesico-ureteric reflux and associated reflux nephropathy is outlined below.

In primary obstructive megaureter there is dilatation of the ureter in all but its terminal segment without obvious cause and without vesico-ureteric reflux. Radiographic and pressure/flow studies may be needed to determine whether there is obstruction to urine flow. Narrowing of the ureter and reimplantation may be necessary.

PELVIURETERIC JUNCTION OBSTRUCTION

This causes idiopathic hydronephrosis and results from a functional obstruction at the junction of the ureter and renal pelvis despite normal muscle cells on electron microscopy. The aetiology is obscure. The abnormality is likely to be congenital and is often bilateral. It can be seen in very young children, but gross hydronephrosis may present at any age.

The common presentation is ill-defined renal pain or ache exacerbated by drinking large volumes of liquid. Rarely, it is asymptomatic. Diagnosis is suspected after ultrasound or IVU and confirmed with a diuretic renogram. Treatment is surgical excision of the PUJ and reanastomosis (pyeloplasty). This can now be performed laparoscopically. Less invasive alternatives are also possible, including balloon dilatation and endoscopic pyelotomy, but are less effective.

RETROPERITONEAL FIBROSIS

Fibrosis of the retroperitoneal connective tissues may encircle and compress the ureter(s), causing obstruction. This fibrosis is most commonly idiopathic, but can represent a reaction to infection, radiation or aortic aneurysm, or be caused by cancer or a drug reaction. Patients usually present with ill-defined symptoms of ureteric obstruction. Typically, there is an acute phase response (high CRP and ESR). IVU or CT shows ureteric obstruction with medial deviation of the ureters. Idiopathic retroperitoneal fibrosis responds well to corticosteroids; failure to respond indicates the need for surgery to exclude malignancy and relieve obstruction.

REFLUX NEPHROPATHY (CHRONIC PYELONEPHRITIS)

This is a chronic interstitial nephritis (p. 505) associated with vesico-ureteric reflux (VUR) in early life, and with the appearance of 'scars' in the kidney, as demonstrated by various imaging techniques. The incidence of reflux nephropathy is not known. About 12% of patients in Europe requiring treatment for end-stage renal disease are said to have renal scarring, but diagnostic criteria are imprecise.

Pathogenesis

VUR, in which urine refluxes back from the bladder into the ureter, is closely associated with recurrent UTI in childhood, and until recently it was widely assumed that this relationship was critical to the association of VUR with progressive renal damage. However, antenatal ultrasound has shown that renal scars occur in utero, in the absence of infection. Furthermore, epidemiological surveys and controlled trials have found that efforts to reduce progression to ESRF by surgical or other means have not been effective. Reflux diminishes as the child grows, and usually disappears. It is often not demonstrable in an adult with a scarred kidney.

Susceptibility to VUR has a genetic component, and may be associated with renal dysplasia and other congenital abnormalities of the urinary tract. It can be associated with outflow obstruction, usually caused by urethral valves, but usually occurs in an apparently normal bladder.

Pathology

Abnormalities may be unilateral or bilateral and of any grade of severity. Renal scars are juxtaposed to dilated calyces. Gross scarring of the kidneys, commonly at the poles, is seen, with reduced size and narrowing of the cortex and medulla (Fig. 17.38). In patients who develop heavy proteinuria and hypertension, renal biopsies show glomerulomegaly and focal glomerulosclerosis, probably as a secondary response to reduced nephron number and functional mass.

Clinical features

Usually the renal scarring and dilatation is asymptomatic, and the patient presents at any age with hypertension (sometimes severe), proteinuria or features of CRF. There

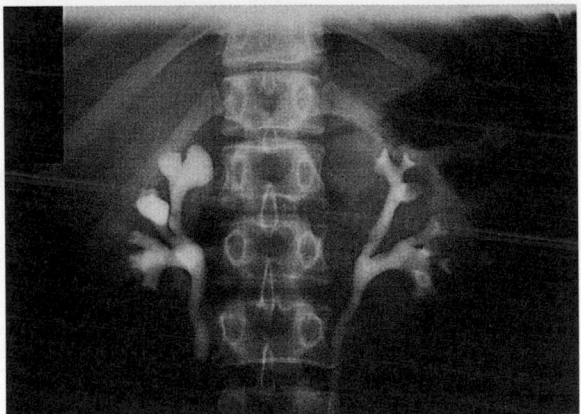

Fig. 17.38 Reflux nephropathy (chronic pyelonephritis). Intravenous urogram revealing clubbing of the calyces which is particularly marked in the upper right pole. The appearances on the left are virtually normal.

may be no history of overt UTI. However, symptoms arising from the urinary tract may be present and include frequency of micturition, dysuria and aching lumbar pain. Urinary white cells and moderate proteinuria (usually < 1 g/24 hrs) are common but not invariable. There is an increased prevalence of renal calculi.

A number of women present with hypertension and/or proteinuria in pregnancy. In some families there is a clear inheritance pattern.

Investigations

Ultrasound is an insensitive technique for identifying focal renal scars, although it will detect major dysplasia and renal dysgenesis, and exclude significant obstruction. Radionuclide DMSA scans are more sensitive (Fig 17.8, p. 464). Longitudinal sectioning by MRI or CT may be useful.

To investigate VUR, radionuclide techniques can also be used as an alternative to micturating cysto-urethrography (MCUG—when the bladder is filled with contrast media through a urinary catheter, and images are taken during and after micturition, Fig. 17.39). However, these techniques are of reduced value, as surgery for VUR is undertaken less often.

Management

Infection, if present, should be treated (Box 17.46); if recurrent, it should be prevented with prophylactic therapy as described for UTI (p. 469). If pyelonephrosis develops or unilateral renal infection or pain persists, nephrectomy or other measures may be indicated. Occasionally, hypertension is cured by the removal of a diseased kidney when the disease is predominantly or entirely unilateral.

As most childhood reflux tends to disappear spontaneously and trials have shown small or no benefits from anti-reflux surgery, such intervention is uncommon, although it may be considered if there is recurrent pyelonephritis or for relief of symptoms. Local treatments (e.g. the subureteric injection of biocompatible material) are also used.

17

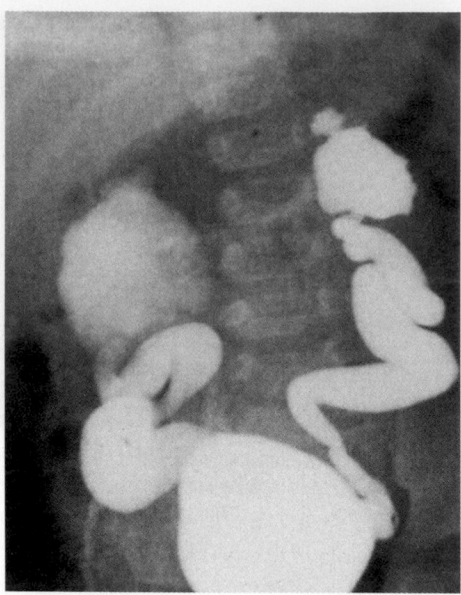

Fig. 17.39 Vesico-ureteric reflux (grade IV) shown by micturating cystogram. The bladder has been filled with contrast medium through a urinary catheter. After micturition there was gross VUR into widely distended ureters and pelvicalyceal systems.

17.46 PROPHYLACTIC ANTIBIOTICS AND VESICO-URETERIC REFLUX | EBM

'Prophylactic antibiotics reduce recurrences of UTI but there is no evidence that they protect against further renal scarring or dysfunction.'

- Smellie JM, et al. Lancet 2001; 357:1329–1333.

For further information: 💻 www.clinicalevidence.org

17

Prognosis

Children and adults with small or unilateral renal scars have a good prognosis, provided renal growth is normal. With significant unilateral scars there is usually compensatory hypertrophy of the contralateral kidney.

In patients with more severe bilateral disease prognosis is predicted by the severity of renal dysfunction, hypertension and proteinuria. If the serum creatinine is normal and hypertension and proteinuria are absent, then the long-term prognosis is usually good.

URINARY TRACT CALCULI AND NEPHROCALCINOSIS

The clinical features vary according to the size, shape and position of the stone, and the nature of any underlying condition. Renal calculi or nephrocalcinosis may be present for years without giving rise to symptoms, and may be discovered during radiological examination for another disorder. More commonly, patients present with pain, recurrent urinary infection or clinical features of urinary tract obstruction. Protein, red cells or leucocytes may appear in the urine.

DISEASES OF THE LOWER GENITOURINARY TRACT

Several pathologies of the lower urinary tract are discussed elsewhere in this chapter, including infection (pp. 467–470), bladder and urethral dysfunction causing incontinence (p. 475), and urinary tract cancer (pp. 511–514). Testicular tumours are discussed on page 771. Chapter 15 also describes diseases affecting the genitalia.

DISEASES OF THE PROSTATE GLAND

BENIGN PROSTATIC HYPERPLASIA

From 40 years of age the prostate increases in volume by 2.4 cm^3 per year on average. The process begins in the periurethral (transitional) zone and involves both glandular and stromal tissue to a variable degree. Associated symptoms are common from 60 years of age, and some 50% of men over 80 years will have lower urinary tract symptoms associated with benign prostatic hyperplasia (BPH).

Clinical features

The primary symptoms of BPH are due to the prostate obstructing the urethra; they consist of hesitancy, poor prolonged flow and a sensation of incomplete emptying. Secondary (irritative) symptoms comprising urinary frequency, urgency of micturition and urge incontinence are not specific to BPH.

Patients may present more dramatically with acute urinary retention when they are suddenly unable to micturate and develop a painful distended bladder. This is often precipitated by excessive alcohol intake, constipation or prostatic infection. It is an emergency and requires the bladder to be drained by a catheter to relieve the retention.

In chronic urinary retention the bladder slowly distends due to inadequate emptying over a long period of time. This condition is characterised by pain-free bladder distension which may result in hydroureter, hydronephrosis and renal failure. Patients with chronic retention can also develop acute retention: so-called acute on chronic retention. They require careful management because of their renal failure.

Investigations

Symptoms are scored on the international prostate symptom score (IPSS, Box 17.47), which serves as a valuable starting point for the assessment of urinary problems. Once a baseline value is established, any improvement/deterioration may be assessed on subsequent visits. Flow rates are accurately measured with a flow meter and prostate volume can be estimated by rectal examination or more accurately by transrectal ultrasound scan (TRUS). Objective assessment of obstruction is only possible by urodynamics (Fig. 17.14, p. 474). Renal function should be assessed and, if appropriate, obstructive nephropathy identified by ultrasound.

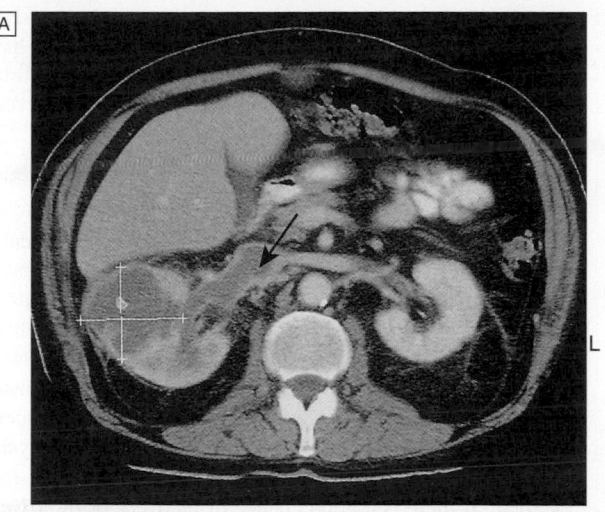
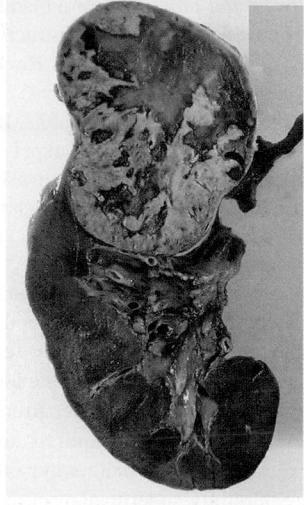

Fig. 17.40 **Renal adenocarcinoma.** A In this CT, the right kidney is expanded by a low-density tumour which fails to take up contrast material. Tumour is shown extending into the renal vein and inferior vena cava (arrow). B Pathology specimen showing typical necrosis.

Investigations

The initial investigation is ultrasound, which allows differentiation between solid tumour and simple renal cysts. Thereafter, a contrast-enhanced CT of the abdomen and chest should be performed for staging (Fig. 17.40A).

Management and prognosis

Radical nephrectomy that includes the perirenal fascial envelope and ipsilateral para-aortic lymph nodes is performed whenever possible. Renal adenocarcinoma is resistant to radiotherapy and chemotherapy but some benefit has been seen with immunotherapy using interferon and interleukin-2. Even when metastases are present, nephrectomy should always be considered; not only may systemic effects disappear, but there may even be regression of any metastases. Solitary metastases tend to remain single for long periods and excision is often worth while.

If the tumour is confined to the kidney, 5-year survival is 75%. This falls to only 5% when there are distant metastases.

TUMOUR SYNDROMES

Some uncommon autosomal dominant inherited conditions are associated with multiple renal tumours in adult life. In tuberous sclerosis (p. 1307), replacement of renal tissue by multiple angiomyolipomas (tubers) may occasionally cause renal failure in adults. Other organs affected include the skin (adenoma sebaceum on the face) and brain (causing seizures and mental retardation). The von Hippel–Lindau syndrome (p. 1238) is associated with multiple renal cysts, renal adenomas and renal adenocarcinoma. Other organs affected include the central nervous system (haemangioblastomas) and the adrenals (phaeochromocytoma).

TUMOURS OF THE RENAL PELVIS, URETERS AND BLADDER

The vast majority of these tumours arise from the urothelium or transitional cell lining. The urothelium is exposed to chemical carcinogens excreted in the urine, such as naphthylamines and benzidine which were extensively used in the chemical and dye industries until their carcinogenic properties were recognised. Almost all tumours are transitional cell carcinomas. Squamous carcinoma may occur in urothelium that has undergone metaplasia, usually following chronic inflammation or irritation due to a stone or schistosomiasis.

The incidence of transitional cell carcinoma in the bladder in the UK is 45 cases per 100 000 population, and is three times more common in men than women. The appearance of a transitional cell tumour ranges from a delicate papillary structure to a solid ulcerating mass (Fig. 17.41). The appearance correlates well with subsequent behaviour, in that papillary tumours are relatively benign cancers while those which ulcerate are much more aggressive.

Clinical features and investigations

More than 80% of patients have haematuria, which is usually visible and painless. It should be assumed that such bleeding is from a tumour until proved otherwise

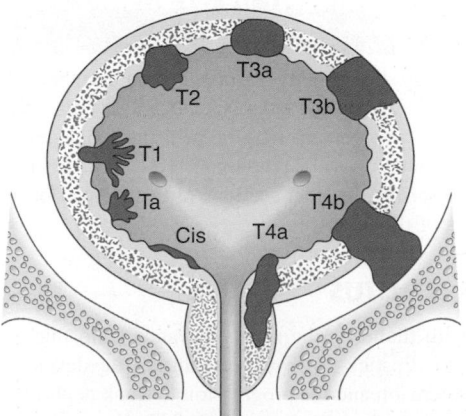

Fig. 17.41 **Transitional cell carcinoma of the bladder.** Stages are shown from carcinoma in situ (Cis) to invasive tumour progressing beyond the bladder and prostate (T4b).

17

(p. 477). A tumour at the lower end of a ureter or a bladder tumour involving the ureteric orifice may cause obstructive symptoms. Examination is usually unhelpful. Rectal examination detects only very advanced tumours.

Investigation of haematuria is described on page 477. If a suspicious defect is seen on IVU in the ureter or renal pelvis, a retrograde ureteropyelogram is required. Solid invasive tumours are staged by CT of the abdomen, pelvis and chest.

Management

Small, large and even multiple superficial bladder tumours can be treated endoscopically by transurethral resection of the tumour(s) (TURT). Intravesical chemotherapy (e.g. epirubicin, mitomycin C) is useful for treating multiple low-grade bladder tumours and for reducing their recurrence rate. Regular 'check' cystoscopies are required and recurrences can usually be controlled by diathermy; only rarely will cystectomy be required for superficial disease.

Untreated patients with carcinoma in situ (Cis) have a high risk of progression to invasive cancer. The tumour responds well to intravesical bacille Calmette–Guérin (BCG) treatment but more aggressive treatment may be needed.

The management of invasive bladder tumours is debated and is largely a matter for specialist urological surgeons, many of whom recommend radical cystectomy with urinary diversion into an incontinent ileal conduit or a continent catheterisable bowel pouch for patients under 70 years of age.

Transitional cell carcinoma of the renal pelvis and ureter is usually treated by nephroureterectomy and regular surveillance of the bladder, but if the tumour is solitary and low-grade it may be treated endoscopically; surveillance remains problematic.

Prognosis

The prognosis of bladder tumours depends on tumour stage and grade. The 5-year survival rate varies from 50–60% in those with superficial tumours to 20–30% for those with deep muscle invasion. Overall, about one-third of patients survive for 5 years.

RENAL INVOLVEMENT IN SYSTEMIC DISORDERS

The kidneys may be directly involved in a number of multisystem diseases or secondarily affected by diseases of other organs. Involvement may be at a pre-renal, renal (glomerular or interstitial) or post-renal level. Many of the diseases are described in other sections of this chapter or in other chapters of the book.

DIABETES MELLITUS

In patients with diabetes, the steady advance from micro-albuminuria to dipstick-positive proteinuria, the development of hypertension and the progression to frank nephrotic syndrome are described on pages 841–843. Few patients require renal biopsy to establish the diagnosis, but atypical features or progression should lead to suspicion that an alternative condition could be present.

Management with ACE inhibitors and other hypotensive agents to slow progression is described on page 842, and has been dramatically effective. In some patients, proteinuria may be eradicated and progression completely halted, even if renal function is abnormal.

HEPATIC–RENAL DISEASE

IgA nephropathy (p. 500) is more common in patients with liver disease. Severe hepatic dysfunction may cause a haemodynamically mediated type of renal failure, hepatorenal syndrome, described on page 949. However, it also predisposes the kidney to develop acute renal failure (acute tubular necrosis) in response to relatively minor insults including bleeding and infection. Patients with such severe hepatic failure are often difficult to treat by dialysis and have a poor prognosis. Where treatment is justified—for example, if there is a good chance of recovery or of a liver transplant—very slow or continuous treatments are less likely to precipitate or exacerbate encephalopathy.

PULMONARY–RENAL DISEASE

The pulmonary–renal syndrome is a dramatic presentation with renal and respiratory failure. Goodpasture's disease and small-vessel vasculitis can cause this presentation (see below).

MALIGNANT DISEASES

Cancer may affect the kidney in many ways (Box 17.51).

17.51 RENAL EFFECTS OF MALIGNANCIES
Direct involvement
• Kidney: hypernephroma (primary adenocarcinoma), lymphoma   • Urinary tract: e.g. urothelial tumours, cervical carcinoma
Immune reaction
• Glomerulonephritis: especially membranous nephropathy   • Systemic vasculitis (rarely): usually ANCA-negative
Metabolic consequences
• Hypercalcaemia (p. 772)   • Uric acid crystal formation in tubules: usually in tumour lysis syndromes
Remote effects of tumour products
• Light chains in myeloma (p. 1052), amyloidosis (p. 79)   • Antibodies in cryoglobulinaemia (p. 1141)

TUBERCULOSIS OF THE KIDNEY AND URINARY TRACT

Tuberculosis of the kidney is secondary to tuberculosis elsewhere (p. 695) and is the result of blood-borne infection. Initially, lesions develop in the renal cortex; these may ulcerate into the renal pelvis and involve the ureters, bladder, epididymis, seminal vesicles and prostate. Calcification in the kidney and stricture formation in the ureter are typical.

17

Clinical features may include symptoms of bladder involvement (frequency, dysuria); haematuria (sometimes macroscopic); malaise, fever, night sweats, lassitude, weight loss; loin pain; associated genital disease; and chronic renal failure as a result of urinary tract obstruction or destruction of kidney tissue.

Neutrophils are present in the urine but routine urine culture may be negative ('sterile pyuria'). Special techniques of microscopy and culture may be required to identify tubercle bacilli and are most usefully performed on early morning urine specimens. Bladder involvement should be assessed by cystoscopy. Radiology of the urinary tract (Box 17.8, p. 468) and a chest X-ray to look for pulmonary tuberculosis are mandatory. Anti-tuberculous chemotherapy follows standard regimes (p. 700). Surgery to relieve urinary tract obstruction or to remove a very severely infected kidney may be required.

SYSTEMIC VASCULITIS

Medium- to large-vessel vasculitis (e.g. classical polyarteritis nodosa, p. 1140) only causes renal disease when arterial involvement leads to hypertension or renal infarction. In contrast, small-vessel vasculitis (p. 1138) commonly affects the kidneys with rapid and profound impairment of glomerular function.

Small-vessel vasculitis

This causes a focal inflammatory glomerulonephritis, usually with focal necrosis (Box 17.41, p. 502 and Fig. 17.32, p. 501), and often causes crescentic changes. It is usually associated with a systemic illness with acute phase response, weight loss and arthralgia, and characteristically in some patients causes pulmonary haemorrhage, which can be life-threatening. However, in other patients it presents as a kidney-limited disorder, with rapidly deteriorating renal function and crescentic nephritis.

The most important causes of this syndrome, microscopic polyangiitis and Wegener's granulomatosis, are usually associated with antibodies to neutrophil granule enzymes (ANCA, p. 1141), but these antibodies are non-specific and cannot be relied upon to make the diagnosis so biopsy of the affected tissue may be required. Henoch–Schönlein purpura (pp. 500 and 1141) is associated with IgA nephropathy and ANCA are usually absent. Vasculitis in other organs may give clues to the underlying systemic disorder and its subtype: for example, ear, nose and throat involvement and lung disease in Wegener's granulomatosis, or rash on the buttocks in Henoch–Schönlein purpura.

Treatment of the primary types of small-vessel vasculitis with cyclophosphamide and corticosteroids is life-saving (p. 1141). Death from extrarenal manifestations of the disease is prevented and renal function can be salvaged in acute disease, even if the glomerulonephritis is so severe as to cause oliguria. In these circumstances, plasma exchange offers additional benefit.

Vasculitis may also be seen in rheumatoid arthritis, SLE and cryoglobulinaemia, although SLE usually involves the kidney in different ways (see below).

SYSTEMIC LUPUS ERYTHEMATOSUS (SLE)

The diverse manifestations of SLE are described on page 1132. Subclinical renal involvement, with low-level haematuria and proteinuria but minimally impaired or normal renal function, is common in SLE. Usually this is due to glomerular disease, although serologically and sometimes clinically overlapping syndromes (e.g. mixed connective tissue disorder, Sjögren's syndrome) may cause interstitial nephritis. As indicated in Box 17.41 (p. 502) and Figure 17.30 (p. 499), SLE can produce almost any histological pattern of glomerular disease and an accordingly wide range of clinical features, ranging from florid rapidly progressive glomerulonephritis to nephrotic syndrome.

Diffuse proliferative lupus nephritis

Typically, patients present with subacute disease and inflammatory features (haematuria, hypertension, variable renal impairment), accompanied by heavy proteinuria that often reaches nephrotic levels. In severely affected patients the most common histological pattern is an inflammatory, diffusely proliferative glomerulonephritis with distinct features to suggest lupus. Controlled trials have shown that the risk of ESRF in this type of disease is significantly reduced by cyclophosphamide treatment, often given as regular intravenous pulses (Box 25.75, p. 1134).

Dialysis and transplantation in SLE

Many patients go into relative remission from SLE once ESRF has developed. This may be because ESRF itself is an immunosuppressed state, as indicated by the higher incidence of bacterial infections in ESRF from all causes. Patients with ESRF caused by SLE are usually good candidates for dialysis and transplantation. Although it may recur in renal allografts, the immunosuppression required to prevent allograft rejection usually controls SLE too.

PREGNANCY

Pregnancy has important physiological effects on the renal system and is associated with a number of distinct disorders. Some conditions are more common in pregnancy, the manifestations of others are modified by the physiological changes of pregnancy, and a few diseases (e.g. pre-eclampsia) are unique to pregnancy.

Physiological adaptations begin in the first few weeks. Peripheral vascular resistance declines, blood volume, cardiac output and GFR increase, and there is usually a reduction in blood pressure and plasma creatinine and urea values in the first trimester. Recordings of baseline blood pressure and urine testing from the first antenatal clinic visit are valuable if problems arise later.

Pregnancy and renal disease

Pyelonephritis is more common during pregnancy, perhaps because of dilatation of the urinary collecting system and ureters, so asymptomatic bacteriuria should be treated (Box 17.52).

Proteinuria caused by glomerular disease is always exacerbated, and nephrotic syndrome may develop without any alteration in the underlying disease in individuals who had only slight proteinuria before pregnancy. This gives a particular risk of venous thromboembolism, which is now the leading cause of maternal deaths in developed countries.

Systemic autoimmune diseases are typically relatively quiescent during pregnancy, but tend to relapse in the first few weeks and months following delivery. Pre-existing renal disease increases the fetal and maternal risk involved in pregnancy, to a degree dependent on the level of renal function, proteinuria and hypertension. Patients with such diseases who may become pregnant should be aware of the extra associated risks. During pregnancy, therapy should not usually be stopped, but blood pressure targets may be modified (after discussion with the patient) and agents altered to those of proven safety.

Pre-eclampsia and related disorders

Pre-eclampsia is a systemic disorder that occurs in or near the third trimester of pregnancy (Box 17.53). Its aetiology is unknown, although a number of risk factors are described (Box 17.54).

Diagnosis

Pre-eclampsia is traditionally defined by the triad of oedema, proteinuria and hypertension. However, oedema is common in late pregnancy, proteinuria is a late sign and, while hypertension is usually present, it may be relative, mild or even absent. Furthermore, all these features occur in

17.53 PRE-ECLAMPSIA AND RELATED DISEASES

Clinical syndromes

- Eclampsia: severe hypertension, encephalopathy and fits
- Disseminated intravascular coagulation
- Thrombotic microangiopathy: may also occur post-partum (post-partum haemolytic uraemic syndrome)
- Acute fatty liver of pregnancy
- 'HELLP' syndrome: haemolysis, elevated liver enzymes, low platelets (thrombotic microangiopathy with abnormal liver function)

Clinical signs

- Hypertension
- Proteinuria
- Oedema
- Other evidence of the clinical syndromes listed above

Investigations

- Uric acid levels increased (before renal impairment apparent)
- Platelets decreased
- Reduced GFR (late)
- Fetus small for dates and growing slowly
- Fetal distress (late)

17.54 RISK FACTORS FOR PRE-ECLAMPSIA

- First pregnancy
- First pregnancy with a new partner or long inter-pregnancy interval
- Pre-eclampsia in previous pregnancies
- Age < 20 years or > 35 years
- Multiple pregnancy (singleton < twin < triplets etc.)
- Pre-existing hypertension
- Pre-existing renal disease

pre-existing renal disease exacerbated by pregnancy. Distinguishing pre-eclampsia from pre-existing renal disease is important. Pre-eclampsia presents progressively, increasing risks to mother and fetus which can be reversed almost immediately by early delivery. In contrast, in pre-existing renal disease, continuing the pregnancy for as long as possible may permit delivery of a healthier, more mature baby. Proteinuria and hypertension in the first trimester of pregnancy suggest pre-existing renal disease.

Management

The only effective management for pre-eclampsia is delivery. The role of antiplatelet therapy (low-dose aspirin) remains controversial. Hypertension is a consequence not the cause of the disorder, and treatment is only justified to lower it from severe and immediately dangerous levels (e.g. higher than 180/110 mmHg). Treating lower levels has been shown to confer no benefit and exposes the fetus to additional drugs. If life-threatening complications are not present and the baby is immature, corticosteroids may be given to induce maturation of fetal lungs, and delivery postponed while mother and baby are closely observed. Magnesium sulphate reduces the incidence of eclamptic convulsions.

Maternal acute renal failure may occur in most of these syndromes, and may result from cortical necrosis (irreversible infarction of the renal cortex).

DRUGS AND THE KIDNEY

PRESCRIBING IN RENAL DISEASE

Many drugs and drug metabolites are excreted by the kidney so the presence of renal impairment alters the required dose and frequency. This is discussed on page 26.

DRUG-INDUCED RENAL DISEASE

The kidney is susceptible to damage by drugs because it is the route of excretion of many water-soluble compounds, including drugs and their metabolites. Some may reach high concentrations in the renal cortex as a result of proximal tubular transport mechanisms. Others are concentrated in the medulla by the operation of the counter-current system. The same applies to certain toxins.

Toxic renal damage may occur by a variety of mechanisms (Box 17.55). Very commonly, drugs contribute

17.55 MECHANISMS AND EXAMPLES OF DRUG- AND TOXIN-INDUCED RENAL DISEASE/DYSFUNCTION

Mechanism	Drug or toxin	Comments
Haemodynamic	NSAIDs	Especially as a co-factor. Via inhibition of prostaglandin synthesis
	ACE inhibitors	Reduce efferent glomerular arteriolar tone. Toxic in the presence of renal artery stenosis and other conditions of renal hypoperfusion
	Radiographic contrast media	Effect mediated via intense vasoconstriction, but this may not be the primary effect of these drugs
Acute tubular necrosis	Aminoglycosides, amphotericin	In most examples there is evidence of direct tubular toxicity, but haemodynamic and other factors probably contribute
	Paracetamol	May occur with or without serious hepatotoxicity
	Others	Drugs often act as one of several co-factors
	Radiographic contrast media	May be secondary to precipitation in tubules
		Furosemide is a co-factor
Loss of tubular/collecting duct function	Lithium	Dose-related, partially reversible loss of concentrating ability
	Cisplatin	
	Aminoglycosides, amphotericin	At lower exposures than cause acute tubular necrosis
Immune (glomerular)	Penicillamine, gold	Membranous nephropathy
	Mercury and heavy metals	Membranous nephropathy
	Penicillamine	Crescentic or focal necrotising glomerulonephritis in association with ANCA and systemic small-vessel vasculitis
	NSAIDs	Minimal change nephropathy
Immune (interstitial)	NSAIDs, penicillins, many others	Acute interstitial nephritis
Chronic interstitial nephritis (alone)	Lithium	As a consequence of acute toxicity. Otherwise controversial
	Ciclosporin, tacrolimus	The major problem with these drugs
	Lead, cadmium	Consequence of chronic toxicity
	Bence Jones protein	Only some light chains are nephrotoxic
	Ochratoxin and other fungal toxins	Produced by *Aspergillus* species. Putative cause of Balkan nephropathy (p. 505)
	Aristolochic acid and other plant toxins	Found in *Aristolochia* clematis. Putative cause of 'Chinese herb' nephropathy
Chronic interstitial nephritis (with papillary necrosis)	Various analgesics (p. 505)	
Obstruction (crystal formation)	Aciclovir	Crystals of the drug form in tubules. Aciclovir is now more common than the original example of sulphonamides
	Chemotherapy	Uric acid crystals forming as a consequence of tumour lysis (typically a first-dose effect in haematological malignancy)
Retroperitoneal fibrosis	Methysergide*, practolol*	Idiopathic is more common (p. 509)

* These drugs are no longer in use in the UK.

as one of multiple insults to the development of acute tubular necrosis. Numerically, reactions to NSAIDs and ACE inhibitors are the most important. Haemodynamic renal impairment, acute tubular necrosis and allergic reactions are usually reversible if recognised early enough. However, other types, especially those associated with extensive fibrosis, are less likely to be reversible.

NSAIDs

As described on page 482, NSAIDs have the predictable effect of impairing renal function in individuals in whom compensatory mechanisms are maintaining renal function (e.g. heart failure, cirrhosis, sepsis and renal impairment of almost any type), and may precipitate acute tubular necrosis in susceptible patients. This is a class effect that is related to alteration of essential prostaglandin-mediated vasodilatation. In addition, idiosyncratic immune reactions may occur: minimal change nephrotic syndrome (p. 500) and acute interstitial nephritis (p. 504), which may occur together. Analgesic nephropathy (p. 505) is an occasional complication of long-term use.

ACE inhibitors

These abolish the compensatory angiotensin II-mediated vasoconstriction of the glomerular efferent arteriole that occurs to maintain glomerular perfusion pressure distal to a renal artery stenosis and in renal hypoperfusion (Fig. 17.1, p. 459). Monitoring of renal function before and after initiation of therapy is essential.

FURTHER INFORMATION

Books and journal articles

Bihl G, Meyers A. Recurrent renal stone disease—advances in pathogenesis and clinical management. Lancet 2001; 358:651–656.

Johnson RJ, Feehally JF, eds. Comprehensive clinical nephrology. 2nd edn. St Louis: Mosby; 2003.

Lameire N, Van Biesen W, Vanholder R. Acute renal failure. Lancet 2005; 365:417–430.

Ronco C, Bellomo R, eds. Critical care nephrology. Dordrecht: Kluwer; 1998.

17

Websites

www.edren.org *Website of the Renal Unit, Royal Infirmary of Edinburgh; information about individual diseases, protocols for immediate in-hospital management and a list of educational resources, including key cases; extensive links to other resources.*

www.ndt-educational.org/guidelines.asp *Website of the European renal association giving agreed European Best Practice Guidelines for the management of anaemia, transplantation and haemodialysis.*

www.nephron.com *The links under 'professional resources' are particularly good and include useful urology links; includes an MDRD (Modification of Diet in Renal Disease study) calculator for estimating GFR from serum creatinine; extensive links to other resources.*

www.renal.org/CKDguide/ckd.html *Website of the UK Renal Association; link to the current guidelines on the detection, referral and management of chronic kidney disease (June 2005).*

17

Cardiovascular disease

CLINICAL EXAMINATION OF THE CARDIOVASCULAR SYSTEM

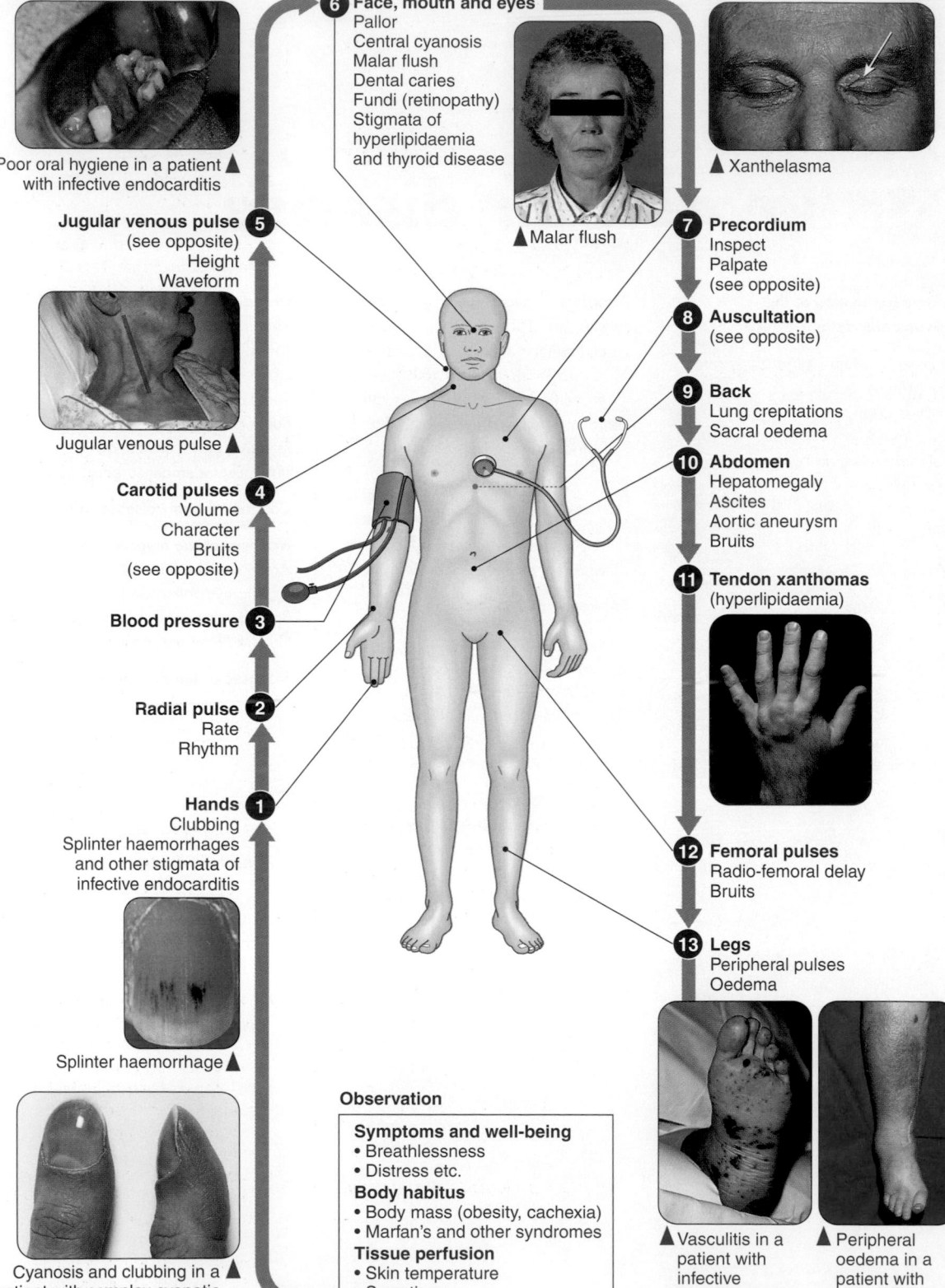

Poor oral hygiene in a patient ▲
with infective endocarditis

6 Face, mouth and eyes
Pallor
Central cyanosis
Malar flush
Dental caries
Fundi (retinopathy)
Stigmata of
hyperlipidaemia
and thyroid disease

▲ Xanthelasma

Jugular venous pulse 5
(see opposite)
Height
Waveform

Jugular venous pulse ▲

▲ Malar flush

7 Precordium
Inspect
Palpate
(see opposite)

8 Auscultation
(see opposite)

9 Back
Lung crepitations
Sacral oedema

Carotid pulses 4
Volume
Character
Bruits
(see opposite)

10 Abdomen
Hepatomegaly
Ascites
Aortic aneurysm
Bruits

11 Tendon xanthomas
(hyperlipidaemia)

Blood pressure 3

Radial pulse 2
Rate
Rhythm

Hands 1
Clubbing
Splinter haemorrhages
and other stigmata of
infective endocarditis

12 Femoral pulses
Radio-femoral delay
Bruits

13 Legs
Peripheral pulses
Oedema

Splinter haemorrhage ▲

Cyanosis and clubbing in a ▲
patient with complex cyanotic
congenital heart disease

Observation

Symptoms and well-being
• Breathlessness
• Distress etc.
Body habitus
• Body mass (obesity, cachexia)
• Marfan's and other syndromes
Tissue perfusion
• Skin temperature
• Sweating
• Urine output

▲ Vasculitis in a
patient with
infective
endocarditis

▲ Peripheral
oedema in a
patient with
congestive
cardiac failure

➍ EXAMINATION OF THE ARTERIAL PULSE

- The character of the pulse is determined by both stroke volume and arterial compliance, and is best assessed by palpating the carotid arteries.
- Aortic regurgitation, anaemia and other causes of a large stroke volume typically produce a bounding pulse with a wide amplitude. (Panel A)
- Aortic stenosis impedes ventricular emptying and may cause a slow rising, weak and delayed pulse. (Panel A)
- Normal sinus rhythm produces a pulse that is regular in time and force. Arrhythmias may cause irregularity. Atrial fibrillation produces a rhythm that is irregular in both time and force. (Panel B)

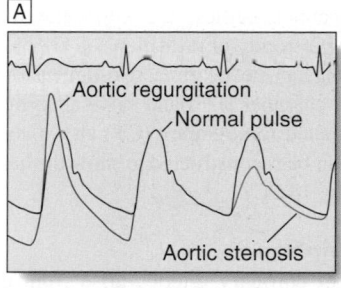

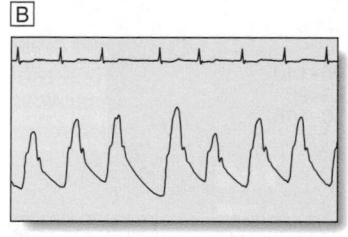

FEATURES THAT DISTINGUISH VENOUS FROM ARTERIAL PULSATION IN THE NECK

- Venous pulse has two peaks in each cardiac cycle (arterial has one).
- Venous pulse varies with respiration (falls on inspiration) and position.
- Abdominal compression causes the venous pulse to rise.
- Venous pulse is not palpable and can be occluded by light pressure.

➎ EXAMINATION OF THE JUGULAR VENOUS PULSE

The internal jugular vein drains directly into the right atrium, and the height of a visible pulsation reflects right atrial pressure. When the patient is placed at 45°, with the head supported and turned a few degrees to the left, the jugular venous pulse (JVP) is visible along the line of the sternocleidomastoid muscle (see opposite).

- The height of the JVP is determined by right atrial pressure and is therefore elevated in right heart failure and reduced in hypovolaemia.
- If the JVP is not easily seen it may be highlighted by gentle pressure on the liver (hepato-jugular reflux).
- In normal sinus rhythm, an a and a v wave approximating to atrial and ventricular systole can be seen.
- The c wave and the x and y descents are subtle and require an experienced observer.
- Tricuspid regurgitation produces giant v waves that coincide with ventricular systole.

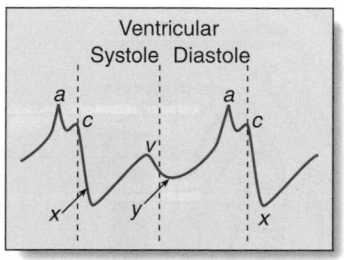

Waveform of the jugular venous pulse.

➐ PALPATION OF THE PRECORDIUM

Technique
- Place heel of hand over left sternal edge and fingertips over apex, then feel the aortic and pulmonary areas by placing fingers in the rib spaces.

Common abnormalities of the apex beat
- Volume overload, e.g. mitral regurgitation: displaced, active, rocking
- Pressure overload, e.g. aortic stenosis: discrete, thrusting
- Dyskinetic, e.g. coronary disease/aneurysm: displaced, incoordinate

Other abnormalities
- Palpable S1 (tapping apex beat—mitral stenosis)
- Palpable P2 (severe pulmonary hypertension)
- Right ventricular hypertrophy (right ventricular heave or lift) felt by heel of hand
- Aortic aneurysm

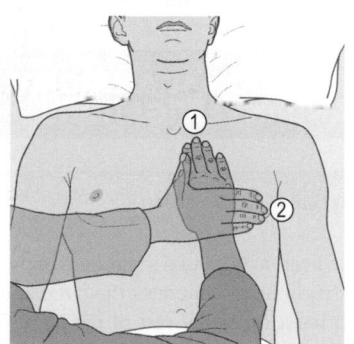

Palpation of the precordium.

➑ AUSCULTATION OF THE HEART

- Use the bell to examine low-pitched noises—first, second, third and fourth heart sounds, mid-diastolic murmurs.
- Use the diaphragm for high-pitched noises—pansystolic murmurs, early diastolic murmurs.
- Time the sounds and murmurs by feeling the carotid pulse; systolic murmurs are synchronous with the pulse.
- Listen to the noises like a piece of music—what tune or cadence can you hear? Analyse each sound separately.

18

The haemodynamic effects of respiration are discussed on page 526.
See pages 557–560 for analysis and interpretation of heart sounds and murmurs.

18

Cardiovascular disease is the most frequent cause of adult death in the Western world; in the UK one-third of men and one-quarter of women will die as a result of ischaemic heart disease. In many developed countries the incidence of ischaemic heart disease has been falling for the last two or three decades, but it is rising in Eastern Europe and on the Indian subcontinent. This has led to predictions that cardiovascular disease will soon become the leading cause of death on all continents. Strategies for the treatment and prevention of heart disease can be highly effective and have been subjected to rigorous evaluation in many randomised controlled trials. The evidence base for the treatment of cardiovascular disease is stronger than for almost any other disease group.

Valvular heart disease is common, but the aetiology varies in different parts of the world. On the Indian subcontinent, it is predominantly due to rheumatic fever, whereas degenerative disease of the aortic valve is the most common problem in developed countries.

Prompt recognition of the development of heart disease is limited by two key factors. Firstly, it is very commonly latent. For example, disease of the coronary arteries can proceed to an advanced stage before the patient notices any symptoms. Secondly, the diversity of symptoms attributable to heart disease is limited and it is common for many different pathologies to present through a common symptomatic pathway.

FUNCTIONAL ANATOMY, PHYSIOLOGY AND INVESTIGATIONS

ANATOMY

The heart acts as two separate pumps operating side by side; the right heart generates the circulation to the lungs and the left heart feeds the rest of the body. The right atrium (RA) drains deoxygenated blood from the superior and inferior venae cavae and discharges blood to the right ventricle (RV), which in turn pumps it into the pulmonary artery. The left atrium (LA) drains oxygenated blood from the lungs through four pulmonary veins and discharges blood into the left ventricle (LV), which in turn pumps it into the aorta (Fig. 18.1). During ventricular contraction (systole), the tricuspid valve in the right heart and the mitral valve in the left heart close, and the pulmonary and aortic valves open. In diastole, the pulmonary and aortic valves close, and the two atrioventricular valves open.

The systolic pressure in the LV is normally at least four times greater than that in the right, and the wall of the LV is usually at least 1 cm thick compared with 2–3 mm for the RV. The atria lie within the mediastinum, anterior to the oesophagus and the descending aorta. The ventricles lie anterior to the atria and taper towards the apex of the heart, which lies to the left of the midline. The RV lies immediately behind the sternum and is not only to the right of but also anterior to the LV.

The normal heart occupies less than 50% of the transthoracic diameter in the frontal plane, as seen on a chest X-ray. On the patient's left, the cardiac silhouette is formed by the aortic arch, the pulmonary trunk, the left atrial appendage and LV. On the right, the RA is joined by superior and inferior venae cavae, and the lower right border is made up by the RV (Fig. 18.2A and B). In disease states or congenital cardiac abnormalities, the silhouette may change as a result of hypertrophy or dilatation.

Echocardiography images the heart in two-dimensional slices so that individual chamber sizes and valve abnormalities can be seen. Computed tomography (CT) also images the heart in slices and can be reconstructed to show the heart in three dimensions (Fig. 18.2C).

The coronary circulation
The left main and right coronary arteries arise from the left and right coronary sinuses, just distal to the aortic

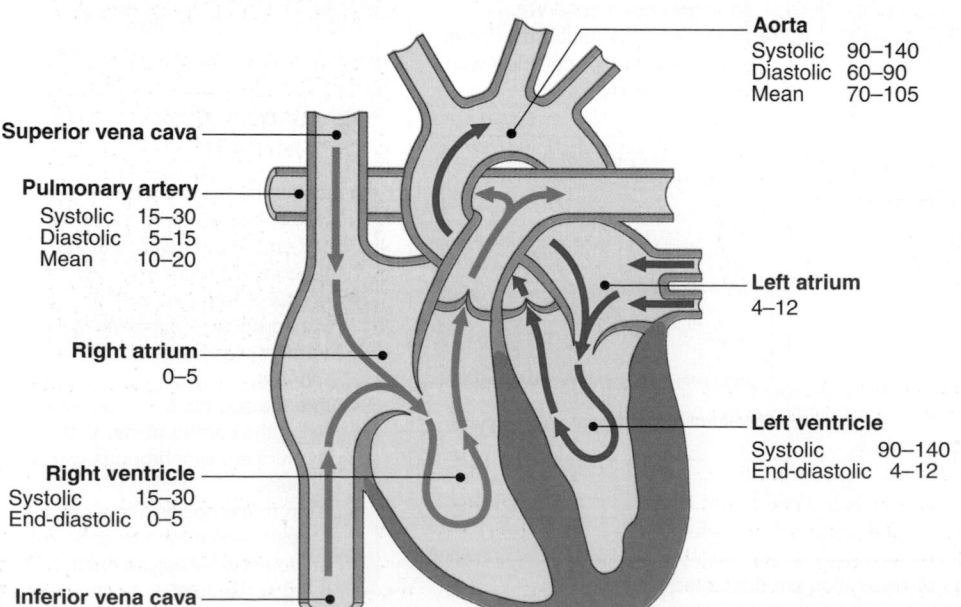

Aorta
Systolic 90–140
Diastolic 60–90
Mean 70–105

Superior vena cava

Pulmonary artery
Systolic 15–30
Diastolic 5–15
Mean 10–20

Left atrium
4–12

Right atrium
0–5

Left ventricle
Systolic 90–140
End-diastolic 4–12

Right ventricle
Systolic 15–30
End-diastolic 0–5

Inferior vena cava

Fig. 18.1 Direction of blood flow through the heart. The blue arrows show unoxygenated blood moving through the right heart to the lungs. The red arrows show oxygenated blood moving from the lungs to the systemic circulation. The normal pressures are shown for each chamber in mmHg.

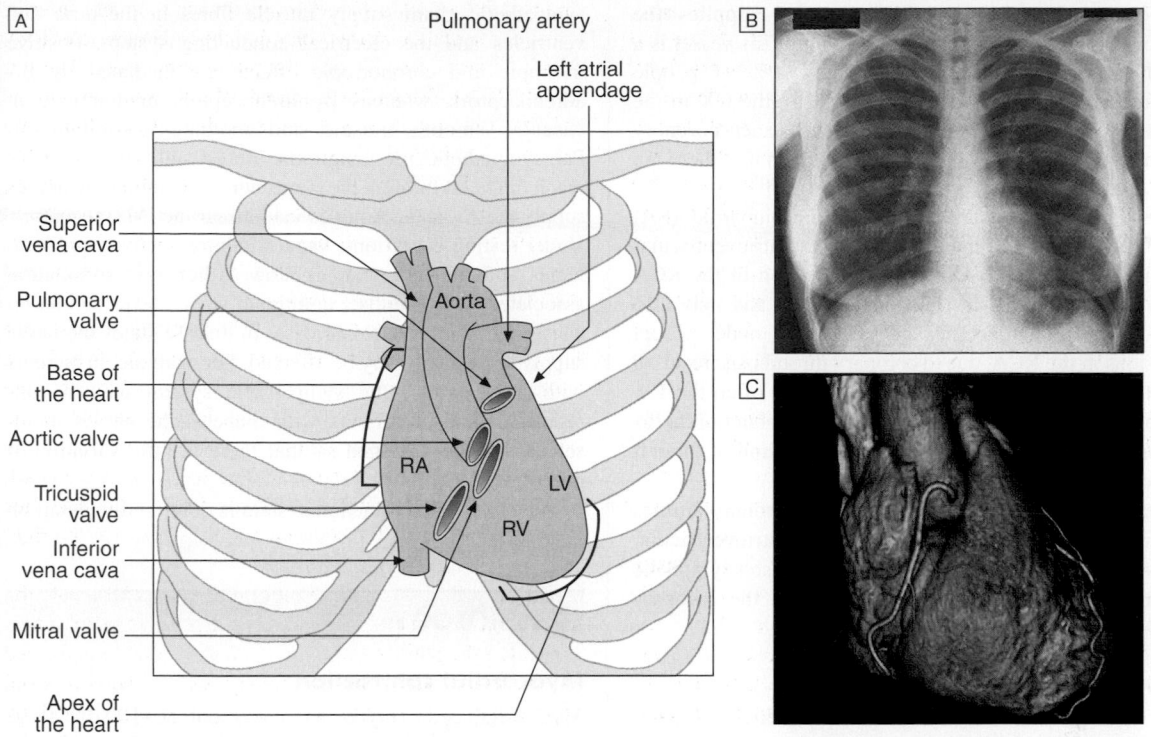

Fig. 18.2   Imaging of the heart. [A] Radiological outline of the heart. The positions of the major cardiac chambers and heart valves are shown. [B] X-ray of the chest showing the silhouette of the heart. [C] Three-dimensional computed tomographic (CT) scan of the heart and great vessels.

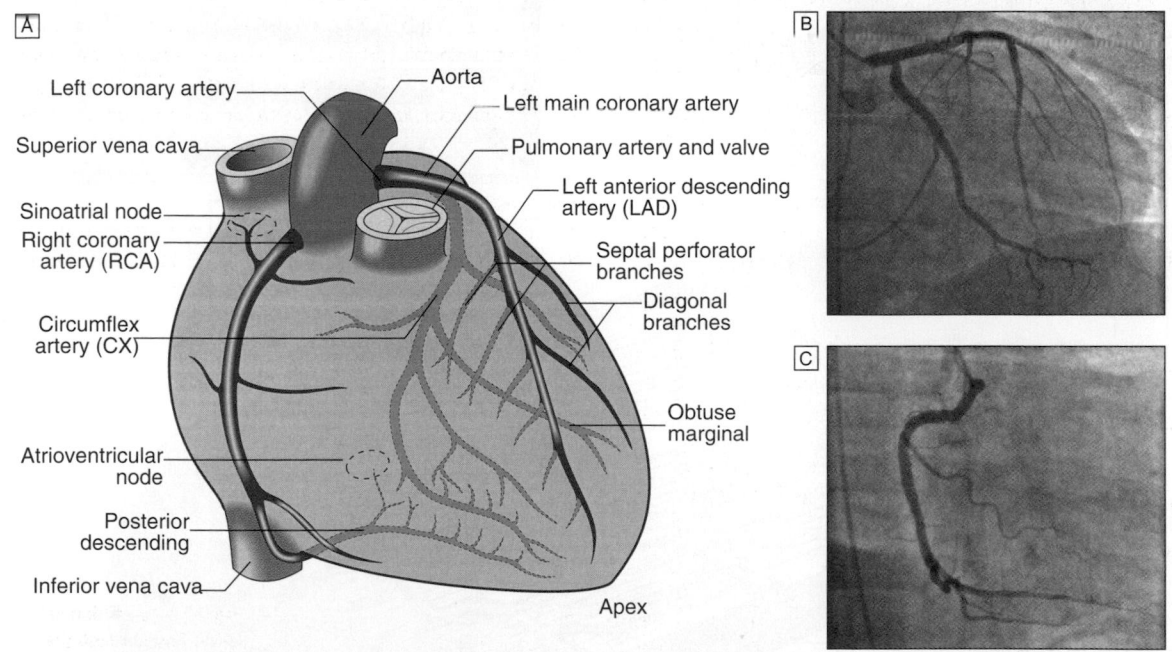

Fig. 18.3   The coronary arteries of the heart. [A] Diagram of the anterior view. [B] Corresponding coronary angiogram of the left coronary artery. [C] Corresponding coronary angiogram of the right coronary artery.

valve (Fig. 18.3). Within 2.5 cm of its origin the left main coronary artery divides into the left anterior descending artery (LAD), which runs in the anterior interventricular groove, and the left circumflex artery (CX), which runs posteriorly in the atrioventricular groove. The LAD gives branches to supply the anterior part of the septum (septal perforators) and the anterior wall and apex of the LV. The CX gives marginal branches that supply the lateral, posterior and inferior segments of the LV. The right coronary artery (RCA) runs in the right atrioventricular groove, giving branches that supply the RA, RV and infero-posterior aspects of the LV. The posterior descending artery runs in the posterior interventricular groove and supplies the inferior part of the interventricular septum. This vessel is a branch of the RCA in approximately 90% of people (dominant right system) and is supplied by the CX in the remainder (dominant left system). The exact coronary anatomy varies greatly from person to person and there are many 'normal variants'.

The right coronary artery supplies the sinoatrial (SA) node in about 60% of individuals, and the atrioventricular (AV) node in about 90%. Proximal occlusion of the RCA therefore often results in sinus bradycardia, and may also cause electrical conduction block of the AV node. Abrupt occlusions in the RCA, due to coronary thrombosis, result in infarction of the inferior part of the LV and often the RV. Abrupt occlusion of the LAD or CX causes infarction in the corresponding territory of the LV, and occlusion of the left main coronary artery is usually fatal.

The venous system mainly follows the coronary arteries but drains to the coronary sinus in the atrioventricular groove, and then to the right atrium. An extensive lymphatic system drains into vessels that travel with the coronary vessels and then into the thoracic duct.

Nerve supply of the heart

The heart is innervated by both sympathetic and parasympathetic fibres. Adrenergic nerves from the cervical sympathetic chain supply muscle fibres in the atria and ventricles and the electrical conducting system. Positive inotropic and chronotropic effects are mediated by β_1-adrenoceptors, whereas β_2-adrenoceptors predominate in vascular smooth muscle and mediate vasodilatation. Parasympathetic pre-ganglionic fibres and sensory fibres reach the heart through the vagus nerves. Cholinergic nerves supply the AV and SA nodes via muscarinic (M2) receptors. Under resting conditions, vagal inhibitory activity predominates and the heart rate is slow. Adrenergic stimulation associated with exercise, emotional stress, fever and so on causes the heart rate to increase. In disease states the nerve supply to the heart may be affected. For example, in patients with heart failure the sympathetic system may be up-regulated, and in patients with diabetes the nerves themselves may be damaged so that there is little variation in heart rate.

The electrical conduction system is described in detail on page 527.

PHYSIOLOGY

Myocardial contraction

Myocardial cells (myocytes) are about 50–100 μm long; each cell branches and interdigitates with adjacent cells. An

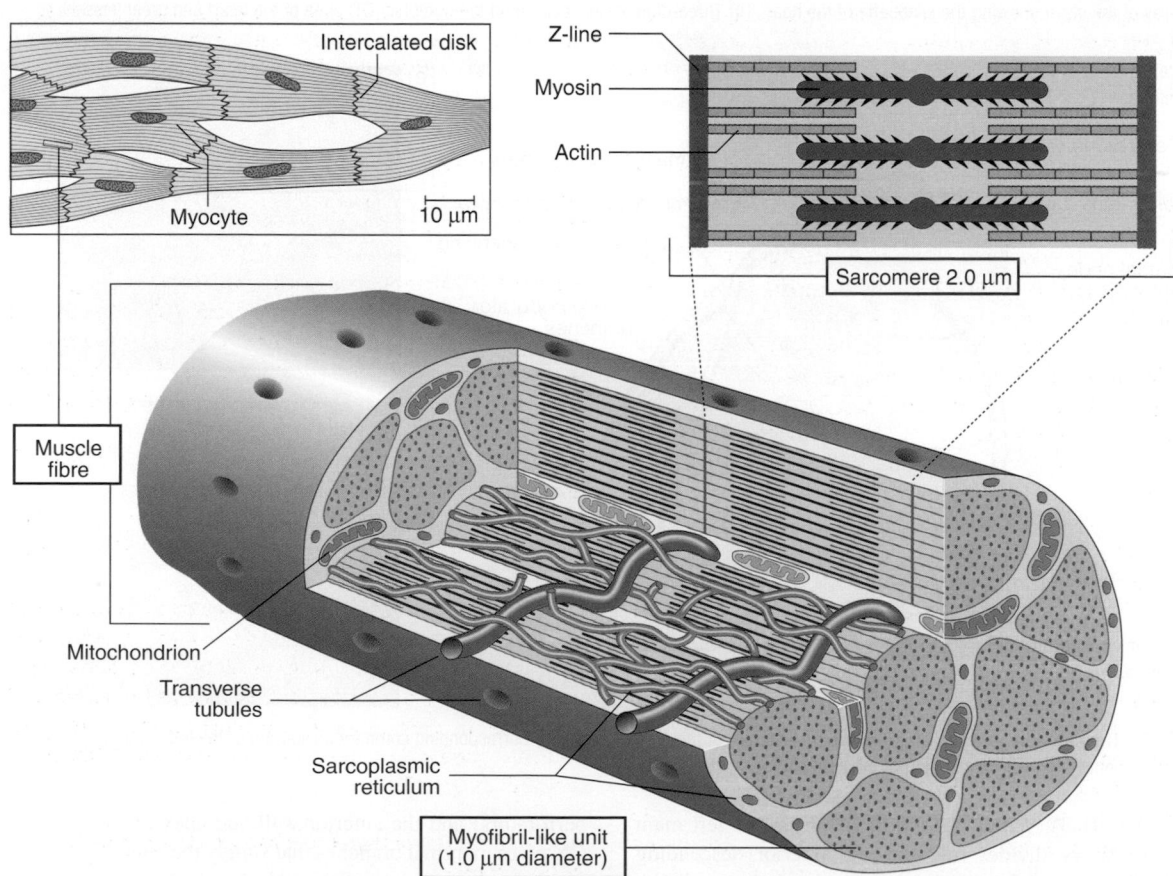

Fig. 18.4 Schematic of myocytes and a muscle fibre. The arrangement of myofibrils, and longitudinal and transverse tubules extending from the sarcoplasmic reticulum are shown. The expanded section shows a schematic of an individual sarcomere with thick filaments composed of myosin and thin filaments composed primarily of actin.

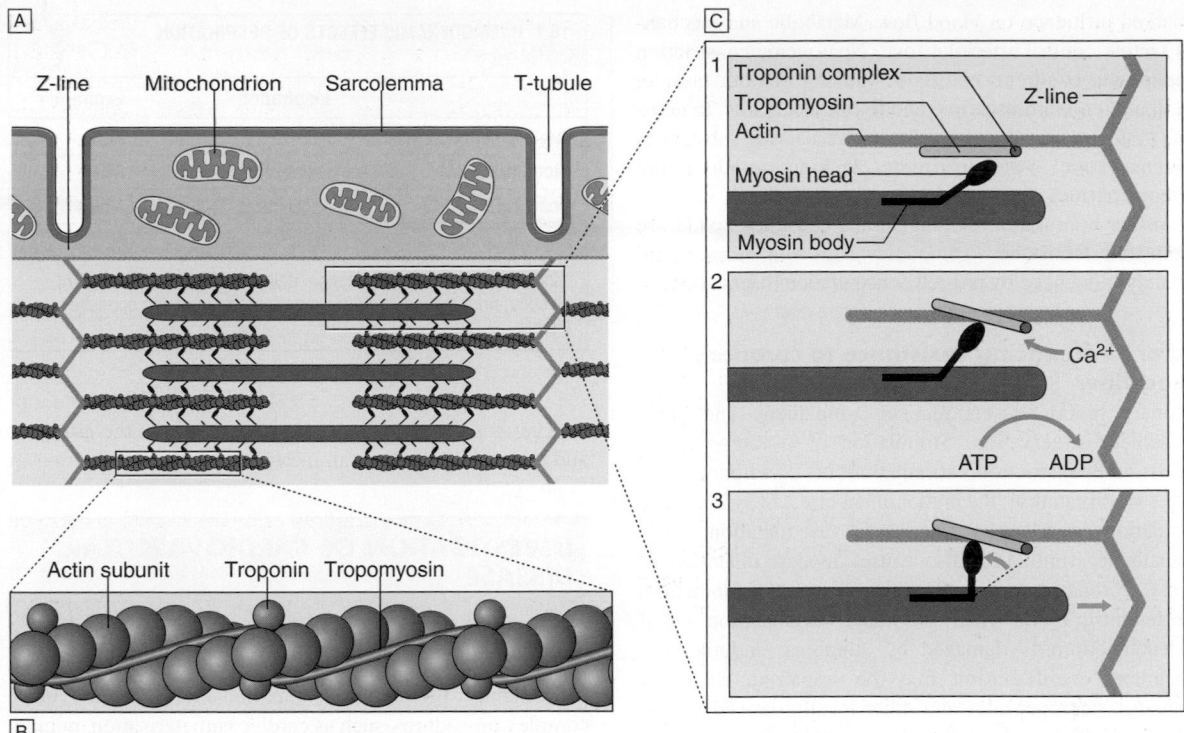

18

Fig. 18.5 **Contraction process within the muscle fibre.** A Schematic of a sarcomere showing the overlapping of actin and myosin filaments. B Enlarged diagram of the structure of an actin filament. C The three stages of contraction resulting in shortening of the sarcomere. (1) The actin binding site is blocked by tropomyosin. (2) ATP-dependent release of calcium ions which bind to troponin, displacing tropomyosin. The binding site is exposed. (ADP = adenosine diphosphate, ATP = adenosine triphosphate) (3) Tilting of the angle of attachment of the myosin head, resulting in fibre shortening.

intercalated disc permits electrical (via gap junctions) and mechanical conduction (via the fascia adherens) to adjacent cells. The basic unit of contraction is the sarcomere (2 µm in length), which is aligned to those of adjacent myofibrils, giving a striated appearance due to the Z-lines (Fig. 18.4). Actin filaments (molecular weight 47 000) are attached at right angles to the Z-lines and interdigitate with thicker parallel myosin filaments (molecular weight 500 000). The cross-links between actin and myosin molecules contain myofibrillar ATPase, which breaks down adenosine triphosphate (ATP) to provide the energy for contraction. Two chains of actin molecules form a helical structure, with a second molecule, tropomyosin, in the grooves of the actin helix, and a further molecule complex, troponin, attached to every seventh actin molecule (Fig. 18.5).

During contraction, shortening of the sarcomere results from the interdigitation of the actin and myosin molecules, without altering the length of either molecule. Contraction is initiated when calcium is made available during the plateau phase of the action potential by calcium ions entering the cell and being mobilised from the sarcoplasmic reticulum. As its concentration rises, calcium binds to troponin, precipitating contraction. The force of cardiac muscle contraction, or inotropic state, is regulated by the influx of calcium ions through 'slow calcium channels'. The extent to which the sarcomere can shorten determines stroke volume of the ventricle. It is maximally shortened in response to powerful inotropic drugs or severe exercise.

However, the enlargement of the heart seen in heart failure is due to slippage of the myofibrils and adjacent cells rather than lengthening of the sarcomere.

Factors influencing cardiac output

Cardiac output is the product of stroke volume and heart rate. Stroke volume is the volume of blood ejected each cardiac cycle, and is dependent upon end-diastolic volume and pressure (preload), myocardial contractility and systolic aortic pressure (afterload).

Stretch of cardiac muscle (arising from an increment in end-diastolic volume) causes an increase in the force of contraction, producing a greater stroke volume. This relationship is known as Starling's Law of the heart (Fig. 18.21, p. 543).

The contractile state of the myocardium is controlled in part by neuro-endocrine factors, such as adrenaline (epinephrine). It is also influenced by various inotropic drugs and their antagonists. The response to a physiological change or to a drug can be predicted on the basis of its combined influence on preload, afterload and contractility (Fig. 18.25, p. 548).

Factors influencing resistance to systemic blood flow

Systemic blood flow is critically dependent upon vascular resistance, which varies with the fourth power of the radius of the resistance vessel. Thus small changes in calibre have

525

a marked influence on blood flow. Metabolic and mechanical factors control arteriolar tone. Neurogenic constriction operates via α-adrenoceptors on vascular smooth muscle, and dilatation via muscarinic and β$_2$-adrenoceptors. In addition, systemic and locally released vasoactive substances influence tone; vasoconstrictors include noradrenaline (norepinephrine), angiotensin II and endothelin-1, whereas adenosine, bradykinin, prostaglandins and nitric oxide are vasodilators. Resistance to blood flow rises with viscosity, and is mainly influenced by red cell concentration (haematocrit).

Factors influencing resistance to coronary blood flow

Coronary blood vessels receive sympathetic and parasympathetic innervation. Stimulation of α-adrenoceptors causes vasoconstriction; stimulation of β$_2$-adrenoceptors causes vasodilatation; the predominant effect of sympathetic stimulation in coronary arteries is vasodilatation. Parasympathetic stimulation also causes modest dilatation of normal coronary arteries. Healthy coronary endothelium releases nitric oxide which promotes vasodilatation, but if the endothelium is damaged by atheroma, endothelium-dependent vasodilatation may be impaired. Systemic hormones, neuropeptides and other locally derived factors such as endothelins also influence arterial tone and coronary flow. A similar balance exists in the systemic circulation where they contribute to the maintenance and regulation of peripheral vascular tone and blood pressure.

As a result of vascular regulation, an atheromatous narrowing (stenosis) in a coronary artery does not limit flow, even during exercise, until the cross-sectional area of the vessel is reduced by at least 70%.

The haemodynamic effects of respiration

There is a fall in intrathoracic pressure during inspiration that tends to promote venous flow into the chest, producing an increase in the flow of blood through the right heart. However, a substantial volume of blood is sequestered in the chest as the lungs expand; the increase in the capacitance of the pulmonary vascular bed usually exceeds any increase in the output of the right heart and there is therefore a reduction in the flow of blood into the left heart during inspiration. In contrast, expiration is accompanied by a fall in venous return to the right heart, a reduction in the output of the right heart, a rise in the venous return to the left heart (as blood is squeezed out of the lungs) and an increase in the output of the left heart.

The net effect of these changes in the normal heart is summarised in Box 18.1.

Pulsus paradoxus

This term is used to describe the dramatic fall in blood pressure during inspiration that is characteristic of tamponade (p. 645) and severe airways obstruction. The phenomenon is an exaggeration of normal. In airways obstruction, it is due to accentuation of the change in intrathoracic pressure with respiration. In cardiac tamponade, however, compression of the right heart prevents the normal increase in flow through the right heart on inspiration, which

18.1 HAEMODYNAMIC EFFECTS OF RESPIRATION		
	Inspiration	Expiration
Jugular venous pressure	Falls	Rises
Blood pressure	Falls (up to 10 mmHg)	Rises
Heart rate	Accelerates	Slows
Second heart sound	Splits*	Fuses*

* Inspiration prolongs RV ejection, delaying P2, and shortens LV ejection, bringing forward A2; expiration produces the opposite effects.

exaggerates the usual drop in venous return to the left heart and produces a marked fall in blood pressure.

INVESTIGATION OF CARDIOVASCULAR DISEASE

Some simple investigations, such as electrocardiography (ECG), chest X-ray and echocardiography, can be conveniently performed at the bedside; however, more complex procedures, such as cardiac catheterisation, nuclear scanning, computed tomography (CT) and magnetic resonance imaging (MRI), require specialist facilities.

ELECTROCARDIOGRAPHY (ECG)

ECG is used to determine the cardiac rhythm and the condition of the conducting tissues. Information is also gained about chamber size and the presence of myocardial ischaemia and infarction, and about the effects of some drugs on the heart.

The fundamental basis for ECG is that the electrical activation of a heart muscle cell causes a depolarisation of its membrane. The depolarisation is propagated along the length of the cell or fibre, and transmitted to adjoining cells. The result is a moving wave front of depolarisation, which passes through the heart and sets up electrical currents; these can be detected by surface electrodes, amplified and displayed as the ECG. From the electrical point of view, the heart acts as if it has only two chambers because the two atria and then the two ventricles contract together. In the electrical conduction system, the sinoatrial (sinus) node is situated at the junction of the superior vena cava and right atrium, and is the origin of the impulses responsible for heart rhythm under normal conditions ('sinus rhythm'). Depolarisation of the sinoatrial node triggers a wave front of depolarisation which travels through the atria. Conduction directly to the ventricles is prevented by the annulus fibrosus, which insulates the atria from the ventricles. The atrioventricular (AV) node, which is normally the only route of conduction from the atria to the ventricles, is situated beneath the right atrial endocardium at the lower end of the interatrial septum; it conducts slowly and regulates the frequency of conduction to the ventricles. The bundle of His passes from the AV node through the annulus fibrosus and divides into right and left bundle branches, which pass down

18

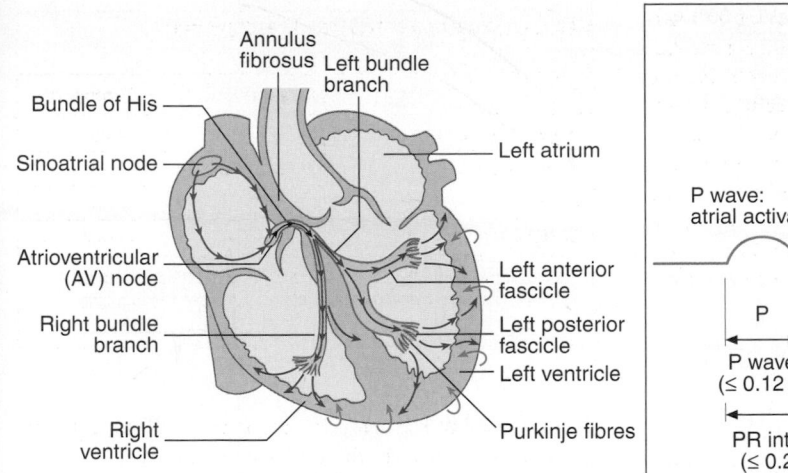

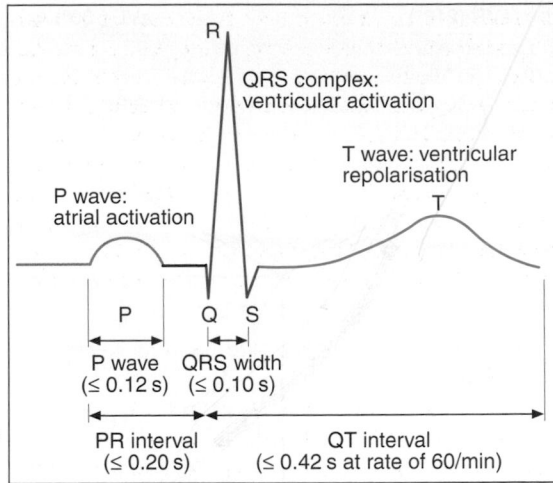

Fig. 18.6   The cardiac conduction system. A Depolarisation starts in the sinoatrial node and spreads through the atria (blue arrows), and then through the AV node (black arrows). Depolarisation then spreads through the bundle of His and the bundle branches to reach the ventricular muscle (red arrows). Repolarisation is in the opposite direction (green arrows). B The components of the ECG correspond to depolarisation and repolarisation as depicted in part A. The upper limit of the normal range for each interval is given in brackets.

the respective sides of the ventricular septum (Fig. 18.6A) and radiate out as the Purkinje network. The left bundle branch is subdivided into anterior and posterior fascicles. Injury to one of the main bundles may manifest on the ECG as right or left bundle branch block, whereas selective injury of one of the left fascicles (hemiblock—p 571) produces deviation of the electrical axis. Abnormalities of cardiac rhythm are discussed on pages 560–578.

The standard 12-lead ECG (Box 18.2)

Normally, cardiac activation starts in the sinoatrial node, but this cannot be detected on the ECG. Depolarisation then spreads through the atria, creating the P wave and triggering atrial contraction. The PR interval represents the delay from the onset of atrial depolarisation to the onset of ventricular depolarisation (Fig. 18.6). Electrical activity then spreads rapidly through the bundle of His and the bundle branches, triggering ventricular contraction and creating the QRS complex. The muscle mass of the ventricles is much larger than that of the atria, and the QRS complex is therefore correspondingly larger than the P wave. Repolarisation is a slower process that occurs from the epicardium to the endocardium, and produces the T wave. The QT interval (Fig. 18.6) represents the total duration of ventricular depolarisation and repolarisation.

The 12-lead ECG is generated from chest and limb electrodes which view the heart from different directions. There are four limb electrodes: one on each wrist and one on each ankle, connected to a central terminal which is electrically neutral. The signal recorded from the electrode on the left arm is augmented relative to the central terminal and is therefore designated lead aVL (Fig. 18.7). Similarly augmented signals are obtained from the right arm (aVR) and left leg (aVF). These leads record the electrical activity of the heart within the frontal plane, with each lead 120° apart. Readings for leads I, II and III (the bipolar

18.2 ECG CONVENTIONS AND INTERVALS
• Depolarisation towards electrode: positive deflection
• Depolarisation away from electrode: negative deflection
• Sensitivity: 10 mm = 1 mV
• Paper speed: 25 mm per second
• Each large (5 mm) square = 0.2 s
• Each small (1 mm) square = 0.04 s
• Heart rate = 1500/R-R interval (mm) (i.e. 300 ÷ number of large squares between beats)

leads) are generated by the difference in potential between two adjacent electrodes. Lead I is the difference between the left arm and the right arm, lead II is the difference between the left leg and the right arm, and lead III is the difference between the left leg and the left arm. By convention lead I is designated as 0° within the frontal plane axis. The other leads are referenced from this point so that aVF becomes +90°, aVL −30° etc.

When depolarisation spreads towards an electrode it produces a positive deflection in that lead; when it moves away a negative deflection is registered. The principal direction of depolarisation in the heart is known as the electrical vector or axis. When the vector is at right angles to a lead, the depolarisation in that lead is equally negative and positive (isoelectric). In the example in Figure 18.7, the QRS complex is isoelectric in aVL, negative in aVR and most strongly positive in lead II; the main vector or axis of depolarisation is therefore 60°. The normal cardiac axis lies between −30° and +90°. Examples of left and right axis deviation are shown in Figures 18.7B and C.

There are six chest leads, V_1–V_6, from electrodes placed on the anterior and lateral side of the chest over the heart. Leads V_1 and V_2 lie approximately over the right ventricle, leads V_3 and V_4 over the interventricular septum, and V_5 and

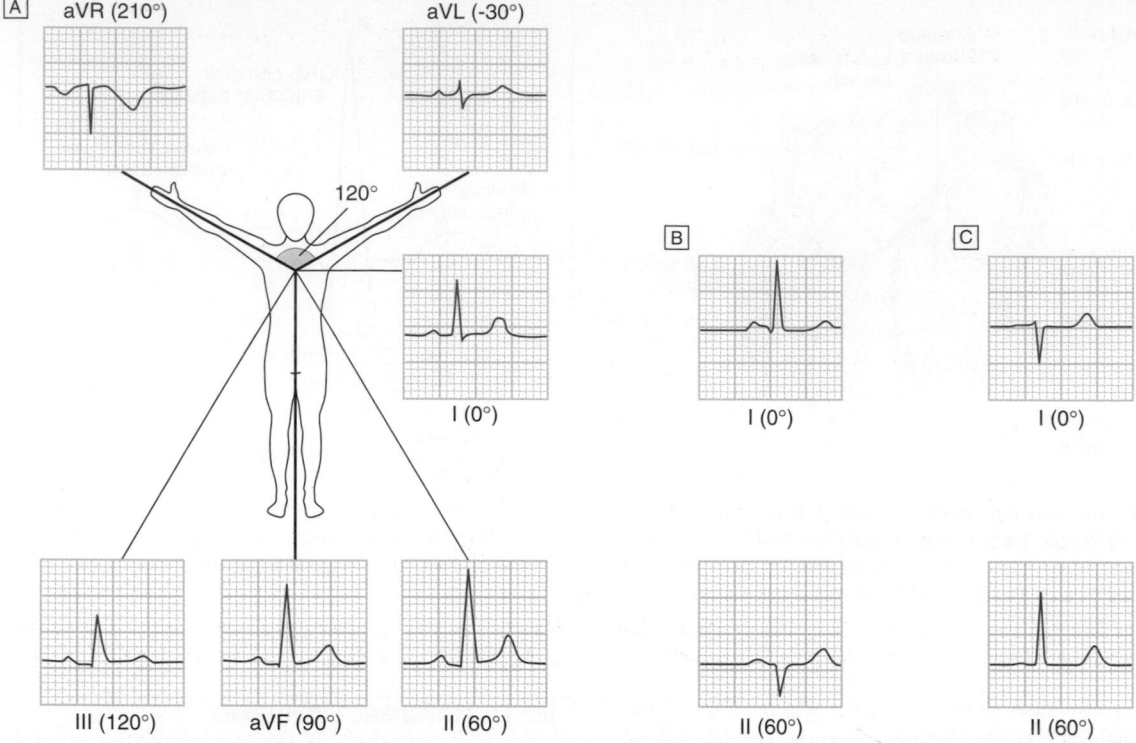

Fig. 18.7   The appearance of the ECG from different leads in the frontal plane. Ⓐ Normal. Ⓑ Left axis deviation, negative deflection in lead II, positive in lead I. Ⓒ Right axis deviation with negative deflection in lead I and positive in lead II.

V_6 over the left ventricle. The left ventricle has the greater muscle mass and contributes the major component of the QRS complex. Depolarisation of the interventricular septum occurs first and moves from left to right; this generates an initial negative deflection in V_6 (Q wave) and an initial positive deflection in V_1 (R wave). The second phase of depolarisation is activation of the body of the left ventricle, which creates a large positive deflection or R wave in V_6 (with reciprocal changes in V_1). The third and final phase of depolarisation involves the right ventricle and produces a small negative deflection or S wave in V_6 (Fig. 18.8).

The ECG in infarction and ischaemia

When an area of the myocardium is ischaemic or undergoing infarction, repolarisation and depolarisation become abnormal relative to the surrounding myocardium. In transmural infarction there is initial ST segment elevation (the current of injury) in the leads facing or overlying the infarct; Q waves (negative deflections) will then appear as the entire thickness of the myocardial wall becomes electrically neutral relative to the adjacent myocardium. The changes occurring in infarction are described in more detail on page 592. Figures 18.73–18.76 (pp. 593–594) are examples of some common patterns of infarction. In myocardial ischaemia the ECG typically shows ST segment depression and/or T wave inversion; it is usually the subendocardium which most readily becomes ischaemic. Other conditions, such as left ventricular hypertrophy and electrolyte disturbances, can cause similar ST and T wave changes.

Exercise (stress) ECG

A 12-lead ECG is recorded during exercise on a treadmill or bicycle ergometer. The limb leads are placed on the shoulders and hips rather than the wrists and ankles. The Bruce Protocol has been well validated and is the most widely used test format for treadmill testing (Box 18.3) Blood pressure is recorded and symptoms assessed regularly throughout the test. Common indications for exercise testing are shown in Box 18.4. A test is 'positive' if anginal pain occurs, blood pressure falls or fails to rise, or there is ST segment shifts of > 1 mm (Fig. 18.61, p. 583). The results of an exercise tolerance test (ETT) are not always conclusive. Some patients with a negative test will have underlying

18.3 THE BRUCE PROTOCOL FOR EXERCISE TOLERANCE TESTING		
	Speed		**Gradient (% incline)**
	(mph)	**(kph)**	
Stage 1	1.7	2.7	10
Stage 2	2.5	4.0	12
Stage 3	3.4	5.4	14
Stage 4	4.2	6.7	16
Stage 5	5.0	8.0	18
Each stage lasts for 3 minutes.			

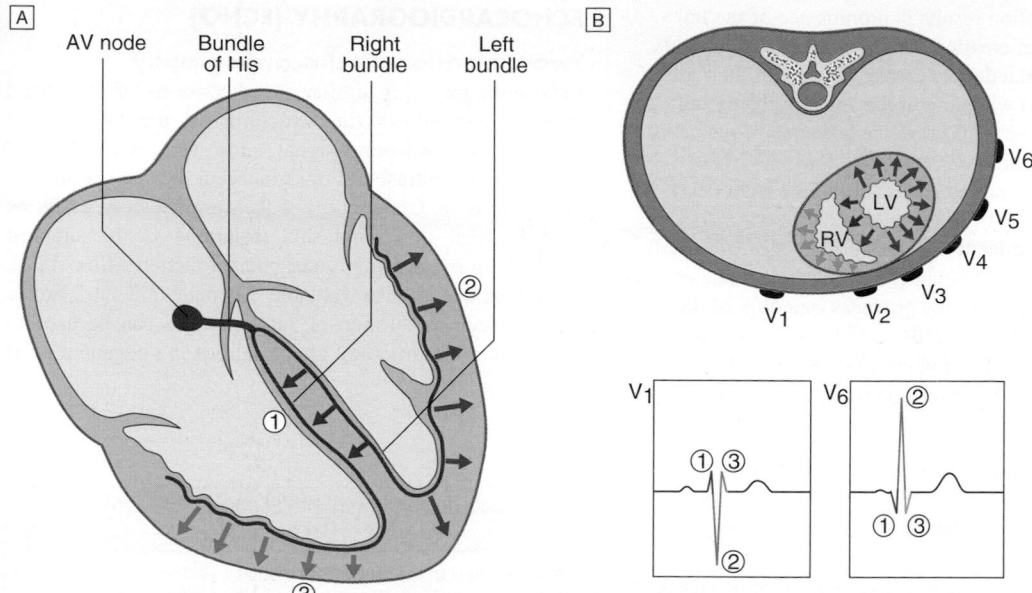

Fig. 18.8 The sequence of activation of the ventricles. [A] Activation of the septum occurs first (red arrows), followed by spreading of the impulse through the left ventricle (blue arrows) and then the right ventricle (green arrows). [B] Normal electrocardiographic complexes from leads V_1 and V_6.

18

18.4 INDICATIONS FOR EXERCISE TESTING

- To confirm the diagnosis of angina
- To evaluate stable angina
- To assess prognosis following myocardial infarction
- To assess outcome after coronary revascularisation, e.g. coronary angioplasty
- To diagnose and evaluate the treatment of exercise-induced arrhythmias

---

18.5 EXERCISE TEST: HIGH-RISK FINDINGS

- Low threshold for ischaemia (i.e. within stage 1 or 2 of the Bruce Protocol)
- Fall in BP on exercise
- Widespread, marked or prolonged ischaemic ECG changes
- Exercise-induced arrhythmia

---

coronary disease (false negative) and, conversely, some with a positive test will not have coronary disease (false positive). Exercise testing is an unreliable population screening tool because in low-risk individuals (e.g. asymptomatic young or middle-aged women) an abnormal response is more likely to represent a false positive than a true positive test. In patients with symptoms suggestive of angina, exercise testing has much better sensitivity and specificity, and is clinically very useful (Box 18.5).

Stress tests are contraindicated in the presence of unstable angina, decompensated heart failure and severe hypertension.

Ambulatory ECG (Holter monitoring)

Continuous recordings of one or more ECG leads may be obtained by attaching them to a small portable solid state or tape recorder for 24 hours or more. This technique is useful for detecting transient episodes of arrhythmia or ischaemia, which seldom occur fortuitously during the short time taken for routine 12-lead ECG recordings (Fig. 18.49, p. 569). A variety of hand-held or implantable patient-activated devices can be used to record the ECG during symptomatic episodes and are particularly suitable for investigating patients with infrequent but potentially serious symptoms. Many of these devices have the facility to transmit ECG recordings to a cardiac centre through the telephone.

RADIOLOGY

A chest X-ray is useful for determining the size and shape of the heart, and the state of the pulmonary blood vessels and lung fields. Most information is given by a posteroanterior (PA) projection taken in full inspiration. Anteroposterior (AP) projections are convenient when the patient is confined to bed (e.g. in intensive care units) but result in magnification of the cardiac shadow because of the divergence of the X-ray beam.

An estimate of overall heart size can be made by comparing the maximum width of the cardiac outline with the maximum internal transverse diameter of the thoracic cavity. This 'cardiothoracic ratio' should be less than 0.5. Enlargement of the cardiac silhouette occurs in pericardial effusion. Apparent or artefactual cardiomegaly may be due to a mediastinal mass or pectus excavatum, and cannot be reliably assessed from an AP film. Cardiomegaly is also not a sensitive marker for detecting left ventricular systolic dysfunction since the cardiothoracic ratio is normal in many affected patients.

Dilatation of individual cardiac chambers can be recognised by the characteristic alterations they cause to the cardiac silhouette:

18

- Left atrial dilatation results in prominence of the left atrial appendage, creating the appearance of a straight left heart border, a double cardiac shadow to the right of the sternum, and widening of the angle of the carina (bifurcation of the trachea) as the left main bronchus is pushed upwards (Fig. 18.9).
- Right atrial enlargement projects from the right heart border towards the right lower lung field.
- Left ventricular dilatation causes prominence of the left lower heart border and enlargement of the cardiac silhouette. LV hypertrophy produces rounding of the left heart border (Fig. 18.10).
- Right ventricular dilatation increases heart size, displaces the apex upwards and straightens the left heart border.

Lateral or oblique projections may be useful in detecting aortic or mitral valve calcification, which may be obscured by the spine on the PA view. However, echocardiography is more sensitive.

The lung fields on the chest X-ray may show congestion and oedema in patients with heart failure (Fig. 18.24, p. 547), and an increase in pulmonary blood flow ('pulmonary plethora') in those with left-to-right shunt. Pleural effusions may also occur in heart failure.

ECHOCARDIOGRAPHY (ECHO)

Two-dimensional echocardiography

Echocardiography is similar to other forms of ultrasound imaging and allows the structures of the heart to be visualised as a two-dimensional 'slice'. Images are obtained by placing the ultrasound transducer on the chest wall, so it is non-invasive. Contraction of the ventricles can easily be seen in 'real time' and this technique is the simplest available for assessing ventricular function (Box 18.6). The technique is also valuable for detecting intracardiac masses, such as thrombi or tumours, and can be used to define complex structural abnormalities in congenital heart disease.

18.6 COMMON INDICATIONS FOR ECHOCARDIOGRAPHY

- Assessment of left ventricular function
- Diagnosis and quantification of severity of valve disease
- Identification of vegetations in endocarditis
- Identification of structural heart disease in atrial fibrillation
- Detection of pericardial effusion
- Identification of structural heart disease in systemic embolism

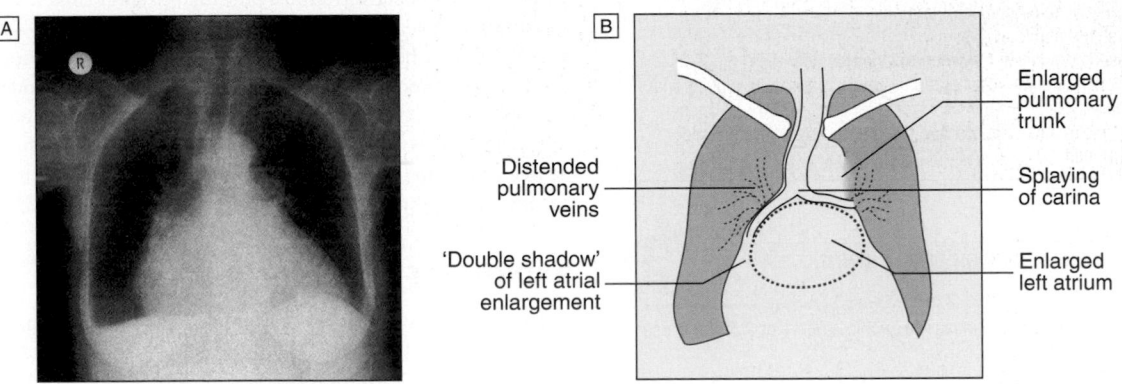

Fig. 18.9   A patient with mitral stenosis and regurgitation indicating enlargement of the left atrium and prominence of the pulmonary artery trunk. [A] Chest X-ray. [B] The major structures.

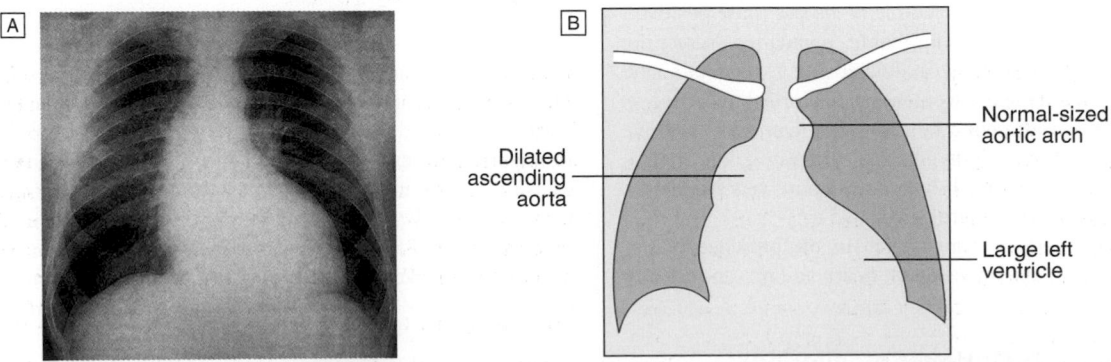

Fig. 18.10   A patient with aortic regurgitation, left ventricular enlargement and dilatation of the ascending aorta. [A] Chest X-ray. [B] The position of major structures.

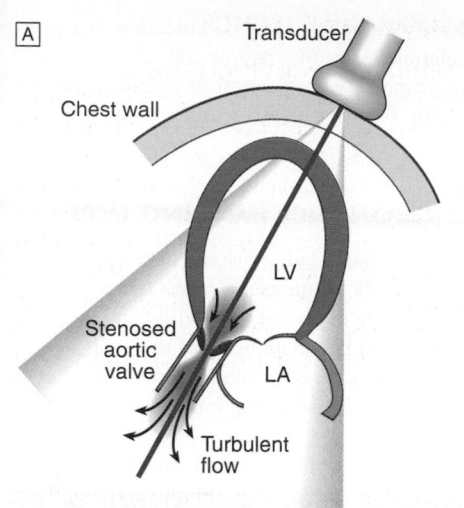

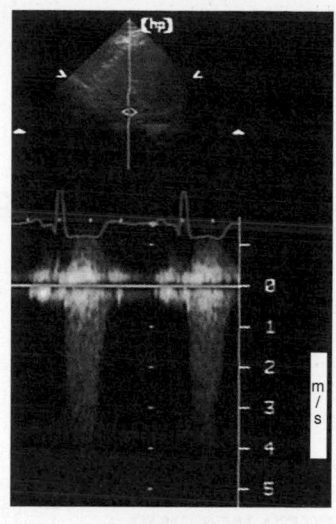

Fig. 18.11 Doppler echocardiography in aortic stenosis. [A] The aortic valve is imaged and a Doppler beam passed directly through the left ventricular outflow tract and the aorta into the turbulent flow beyond the stenosed valve. [B] The velocity of the blood cells is recorded to determine the maximum velocity and hence the pressure gradient across the valve. In this example the peak velocity is approximately 450 cm/sec (4.5 m/sec) indicating severe aortic stenosis (peak gradient of 81 mmHg).

18

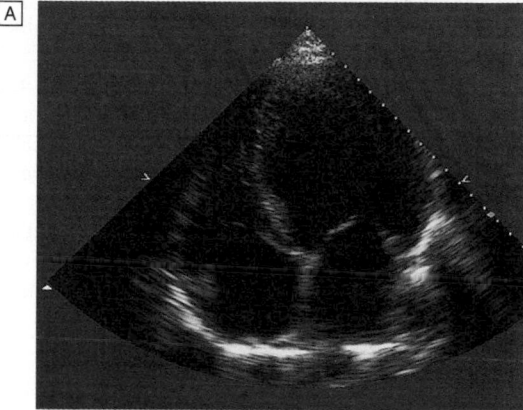

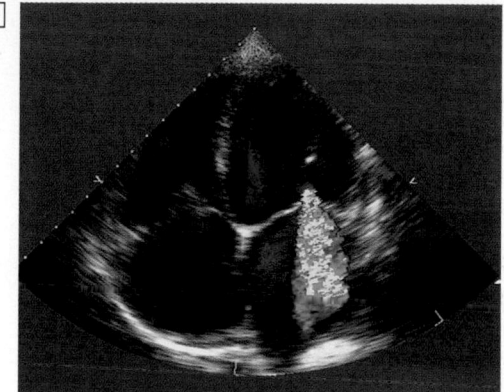

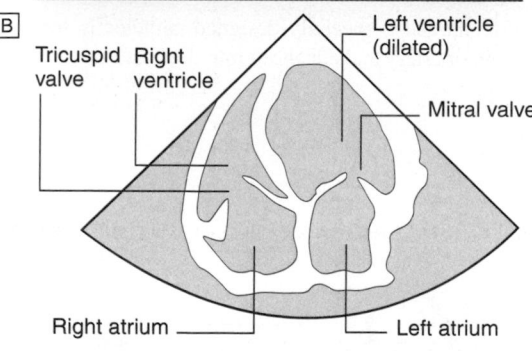

Fig. 18.12 Echocardiographic illustration of the principal cardiac structures in the 'four-chamber' view. [A] Late diastole. [B] The major features. [C] Systole: colour-flow Doppler has been used to demonstrate mitral regurgitation which appears as a flame-shaped (yellow/blue) turbulent jet into the left atrium (p. 621).

Doppler echocardiography

This technique depends on the fundamental principle that sound waves reflected from moving objects, such as intracardiac red blood cells, undergo a frequency shift. The speed and direction of movement of the red cells, and thus of blood, can be detected in the heart chambers and great vessels. The greater the frequency shift, the faster the blood is moving. The derived information can be presented either as a plot of blood velocity against time for a particular point in the heart (Fig. 18.11) or as a colour overlay on a two-dimensional real-time echo picture (colour flow Doppler, Fig. 18.12). Doppler echocardiography is valuable in detecting abnormal directions of blood flow, e.g. aortic or mitral reflux, and in estimating pressure gradients, e.g. the gradient across a stenosed aortic valve (Fig. 18.11). Normal velocities are in the order of 1 m/sec; however, in the presence of a stenosis, flow velocity is increased. For example, in severe aortic stenosis the peak (maximum) aortic velocity may be increased to 5 m/sec. An estimate of the pressure gradient across a valve or lesion is given by the modified Bernoulli equation:

Pressure gradient (mmHg) = 4 × (peak velocity in m/sec)^2

Advanced techniques include three-dimensional echocardiography, intravascular ultrasound (defines vessel wall abnormalities and guides coronary intervention), intra-

18

cardiac ultrasound (provides high-resolution images of cardiac structures) and Doppler tissue imaging (quantifies myocardial contractility and diastolic function).

Transoesophageal echocardiography

In this technique an ultrasound probe in the shape of an endoscope is passed into the oesophagus and positioned immediately behind the left atrium. This produces very clear images; in endocarditis, for example, it is often possible to see vegetations that are too small to be detected by ordinary echocardiography. The high-quality images that can be obtained make the technique particularly valuable for investigating patients with prosthetic (especially mitral) valve dysfunction, congenital abnormalities (e.g. atrial septal defect), aortic dissection, infective endocarditis and systemic embolism.

COMPUTED TOMOGRAPHIC (CT) IMAGING

This is useful for imaging the chambers of the heart, the great vessels, the pericardium and surrounding structures. In practice it is most useful for imaging the aorta in suspected aortic dissection (Fig. 18.84, p. 608). Helical CT has a gantry which is capable of continuous rotation and can acquire images in sub-second scan times. A further development of helical CT has been the introduction of multi-slice technology that is capable of delivering up to 32–64 slices per rotation of the gantry. These images are almost completely devoid of motion artefact.

Non-invasive imaging of the coronary arteries is now a real possibility. The spatial resolution of CT provides images of the proximal coronary arteries that are becoming comparable to conventional coronary arteriography. Coronary artery bypass grafts are also well seen using helical CT (Fig. 18.67, p. 588), and in some centres graft patency is routinely assessed by this technique. It is also possible to identify coronary artery calcification that gives a broad correlation with the degree of atherosclerotic disease. In this respect, quantification of calcified plaques has been used for risk stratification and to guide further investigations.

MAGNETIC RESONANCE IMAGING (MRI)

MRI requires no ionising radiation and can be used to generate multiple 'slices' of the heart. It has many growing applications and is particularly useful for imaging the aorta (Fig. 18.83, p. 608), and the relationship of the great vessels to the cardiac chambers in congenital heart disease. It is also particularly useful in detecting infiltrative conditions affecting the heart.

Physiological data can be obtained from the signal returned from moving blood. Algorithms and software packages are available to help quantify velocities across regurgitant or stenotic valves. It is also possible to perform regional wall-motion analyses. In particular, the right ventricular wall is readily visualised on MRI, unlike echocardiography where it can be difficult to assess.

A significant area of promise for cardiac MRI is in the assessment of myocardial viability. It is possible to demonstrate areas of myocardial hypoperfusion by dynamically scanning patients during injection of an MRI contrast agent, such as gadolinium. This technique can demonstrate areas of ischaemia with significantly better spatial resolution than complementary nuclear medicine techniques, and can be useful in selecting patients for revascularisation procedures.

CARDIAC CATHETERISATION

In this technique a specially designed catheter is inserted into a vein or artery and advanced into the heart under X-ray

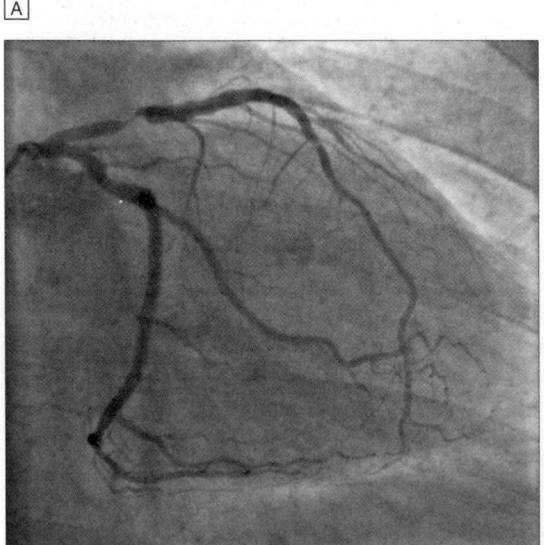

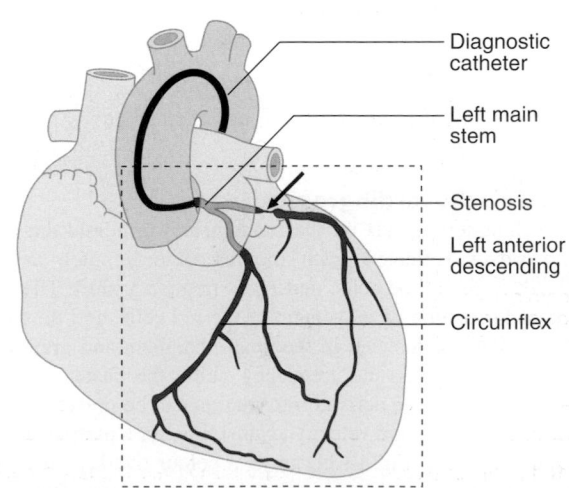

Diagnostic catheter

Left main stem

Stenosis

Left anterior descending

Circumflex

Fig. 18.13 The left anterior descending and circumflex coronary arteries with a stenosis in the left anterior descending vessel. A Coronary artery angiogram. B Schematic of the vessels and branches.

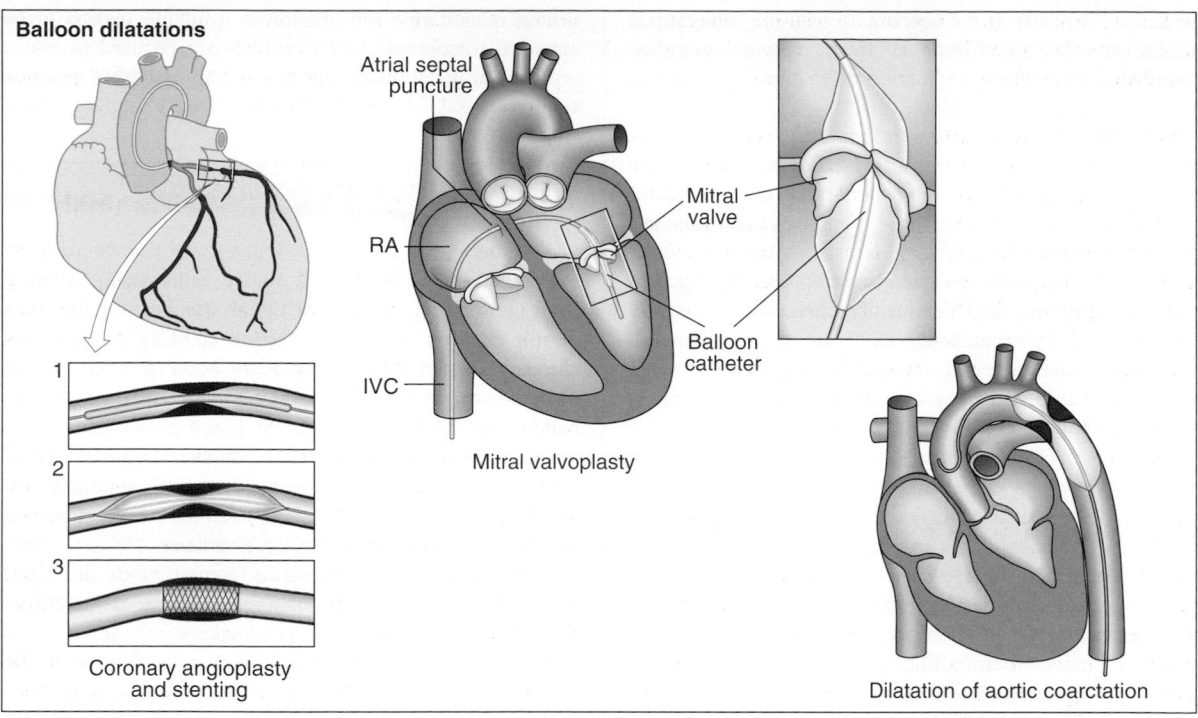

Balloon dilatations

1

2

3

Coronary angioplasty
and stenting

Atrial septal
puncture

RA

IVC

Mitral
valve

Balloon
catheter

Mitral valvoplasty

Dilatation of aortic coarctation

18

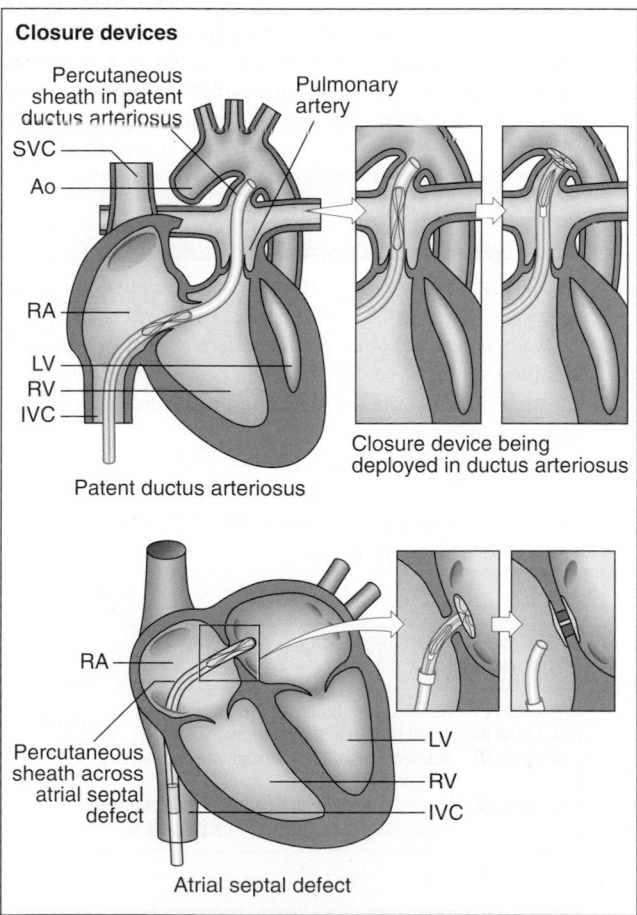

Closure devices

Percutaneous
sheath in patent
ductus arteriosus

Pulmonary
artery

SVC

Ao

RA

LV
RV
IVC

Patent ductus arteriosus

Closure device being
deployed in ductus arteriosus

RA

Percutaneous
sheath across
atrial septal
defect

LV

RV

IVC

Atrial septal defect

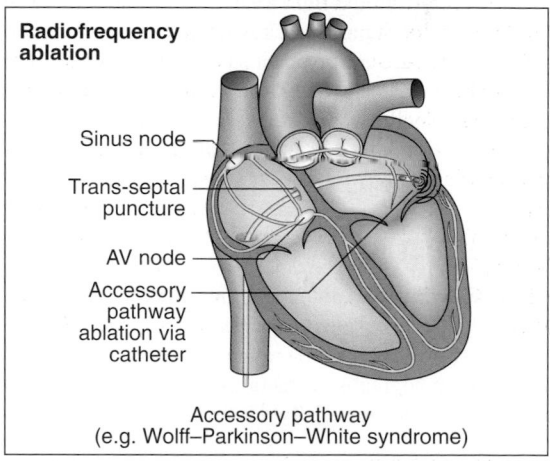

**Radiofrequency
ablation**

Sinus node

Trans-septal
puncture

AV node

Accessory
pathway
ablation via
catheter

Accessory pathway
(e.g. Wolff–Parkinson–White syndrome)

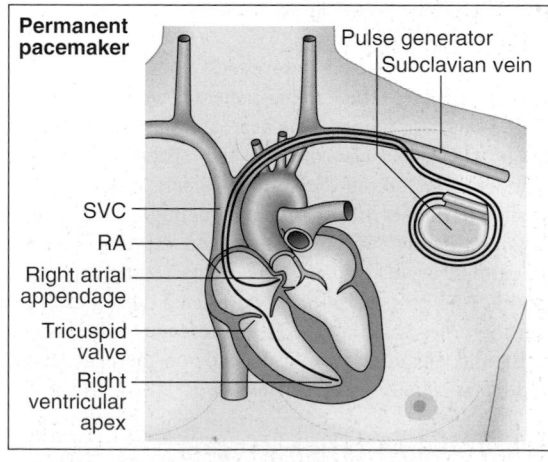

**Permanent
pacemaker**

Pulse generator

Subclavian vein

SVC

RA

Right atrial
appendage

Tricuspid
valve

Right
ventricular
apex

Fig. 18.14   Percutaneous therapeutic procedures in cardiology. (RA = right atrium; RV = right ventricle; LV = left ventricle; Ao = aorta;
SVC = superior vena cava; IVC = inferior vena cava)

18

guidance. This allows the operator to measure intracardiac pressures, take blood samples from individual cardiac chambers and obtain angiograms by injecting contrast media into a chamber or blood vessel.

Left heart catheterisation is mainly used to assess coronary artery disease but is also used to evaluate disease of the mitral valve, aortic valve and aorta. Left ventriculography is used to determine the size and function of the left ventricle; coronary angiography is used to detect stenoses (Fig. 18.13) and guide revascularisation procedures such as balloon angioplasty and stenting. The procedure is usually accomplished by cannulating the heart via the femoral, brachial or radial artery. It can often be completed as a day case, and is safe, with serious complications occurring in fewer than 1 in 1000 cases.

Right heart catheterisation is used to assess pulmonary artery pressure and can also be used to detect intracardiac shunts by measuring oxygen saturation in different chambers. For example, a step up in oxygen saturation from 65% in the right atrium to 80% in the pulmonary artery is indicative of a large left-to-right shunt that might be due to a ventricular septal defect. Cardiac output can also be measured using thermodilution techniques. Left atrial pressure can be measured directly by puncturing the interatrial septum from the right atrium, with a special catheter. However, for most purposes, a satisfactory approximation to left atrial pressure can be obtained by 'wedging' an end-hole or balloon catheter in a branch of the pulmonary artery. Swan–Ganz balloon catheters are often used to monitor pulmonary 'wedge' pressure as a guide to left heart filling pressure in critically ill patients (Fig. 8.2, p. 181).

RADIONUCLIDE IMAGING

The availability of gamma-emitting radionuclides with a short half-life has made it possible to study cardiac function non-invasively. The gamma rays are detected by means of a planar or tomographic camera and permit images of the heart to be reconstructed. Two techniques are available.

Blood pool imaging to assess ventricular function
The isotope is injected intravenously and mixes with the circulating blood. The gamma camera detects the amount of isotope-emitting blood in the heart at different phases of the cardiac cycle, and also the size and 'shape' of the cardiac chambers. By linking the gamma camera to the ECG it is possible to collect information over multiple cardiac cycles, allowing 'gating' of the systolic and diastolic phases of the cardiac cycle; the left (and right) ventricular ejection fraction (the proportion of blood ejected during each beat) can then be calculated. The reference value for left ventricular ejection fraction depends on the exact method used but is usually greater than 60%.

Myocardial perfusion imaging
This technique involves obtaining scintiscans of the myocardium at rest and during stress after the administration of an intravenous radioactive isotope such as [99]technetium tetrofosmin (Fig. 18.62, p. 584). More sophis-

ticated quantitative information is available with positron emission tomography (PET) which can be used to assess myocardial metabolism, but this is only available in a few centres.

THERAPEUTIC PROCEDURES

See Figure 18.14.

Catheters can be passed under radiographic control from the femoral, brachial or radial artery into the heart to permit balloon dilatation and/or stenting of diseased coronary arteries. Coarctation of the aorta (p. 637) can also be treated by dilating the narrowing in the aorta with a large balloon and by stent placement. Stenosed valves (particularly the mitral valve) can sometimes be dilated in a similar way.

Patients with congenital heart defects such as atrial septal defect and patent ductus arteriosus can have these closed by devices delivered to the heart via a catheter.

Pacemakers are implanted to correct bradycardias or atrioventricular block. Implantable cardiac defibrillators have similar capabilities to pacemakers and, in addition, can deliver an internal shock to defibrillate the heart if a catastrophic rhythm such as ventricular fibrillation occurs.

Recurrent arrhythmias can be treated by transcatheter radiofrequency ablation, in which a catheter placed precisely adjacent to an area of abnormal electrical conduction or an excitable focus can deliver an impulse to ablate conduction through that area of the heart.

PRESENTING PROBLEMS IN CARDIOVASCULAR DISEASE

Cardiovascular disease gives rise to a relatively limited range of symptoms. Differential diagnosis therefore often depends on careful analysis of the factors that provoke the symptoms, the subtle differences in how they are described by the patient, the clinical findings and appropriate investigations.

A close relationship between symptoms and exercise is the hallmark of heart disease. The New York Heart Association (NYHA) functional classification is often used to grade disability (Box 18.7).

18.7 NEW YORK HEART ASSOCIATION (NYHA) FUNCTIONAL CLASSIFICATION

- **Class I** No limitation during ordinary activity
- **Class II** Slight limitation during ordinary activity
- **Class III** Marked limitation of normal activities without symptoms at rest
- **Class IV** Unable to undertake physical activity without symptoms; symptoms may be present at rest

CHEST PAIN

Chest pain is a common presentation of cardiac disease, but can also be a manifestation of anxiety or of disease of the lungs, the musculoskeletal system or the gastrointestinal system (Box 18.8, p. 536). Some patients deny 'pain' in favour of 'discomfort' but the significance remains the same.

CHARACTERISTICS OF ISCHAEMIC CARDIAC PAIN

A number of key characteristics help to distinguish cardiac pain from that of other causes (Fig. 18.15). Diagnosis may be difficult and it is often helpful to classify pain as possible, probable or definite ischaemic cardiac pain, based on the balance of evidence (Fig. 18.16).

- *Site of origin of pain*. Cardiac pain is typically located in the centre of the chest because of the derivation of the nerve supply to the heart and mediastinum.
- *Radiation*. Ischaemic cardiac pain, especially when severe, may radiate to the neck, jaw, and upper or even lower arms. Occasionally, cardiac pain may be experienced only at the sites of radiation or in the back. Pain situated over the left anterior chest and radiating laterally may have many causes, including pleural or lung disorders, musculoskeletal problems and anxiety.
- *Character of the pain*. Cardiac pain is typically dull, constricting, choking or 'heavy', and is usually described as squeezing, crushing, burning or aching but not sharp, stabbing, pricking or knife-like. The sensation can be described as breathlessness. Patients often emphasise that it is a discomfort rather than a pain. They typically use characteristic hand gestures (e.g. open hand or clenched fist) when describing ischaemic pain (Fig. 18.15).
- *Provocation*. Anginal pain occurs during (not after) exertion and is promptly relieved (in less than 5 minutes) by resting. The pain may also be brought on or exacerbated by emotion and tends to occur more readily during exertion, after a large meal or in a cold wind. In crescendo or unstable angina, similar pain may be precipitated by minimal exertion and may occur at rest. The increase in venous return or preload induced by lying down may also be sufficient to provoke pain in vulnerable patients (decubitus angina). The pain of myocardial infarction may be preceded by a period of stable or unstable angina but may occur de novo.

  In contrast, pleural or pericardial pain is usually described as a 'sharp' or 'catching' sensation that is exacerbated by breathing, coughing or movement. Pain associated with a specific movement (bending, stretching, turning) is likely to be musculoskeletal in origin.
- *Pattern of onset*. The pain of myocardial infarction typically takes several minutes or even longer to develop; similarly, angina builds up gradually in proportion to the intensity of exertion. Pain that occurs after rather than during exertion is usually musculoskeletal or psychological in origin. The pain of aortic dissection, massive pulmonary embolism or pneumothorax is usually very sudden or instantaneous in onset.
- *Associated features*. The pain of myocardial infarction, massive pulmonary embolism or aortic dissection is

18

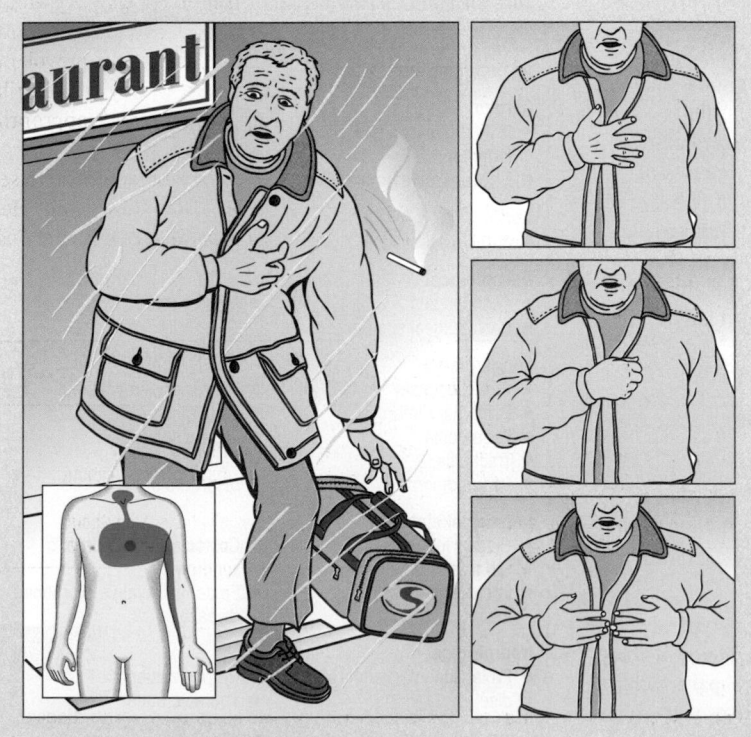

Fig. 18.15 Typical ischaemic cardiac pain. Characteristic hand gestures used to describe cardiac pain. Typical radiation of pain is shown in the schematic.

18

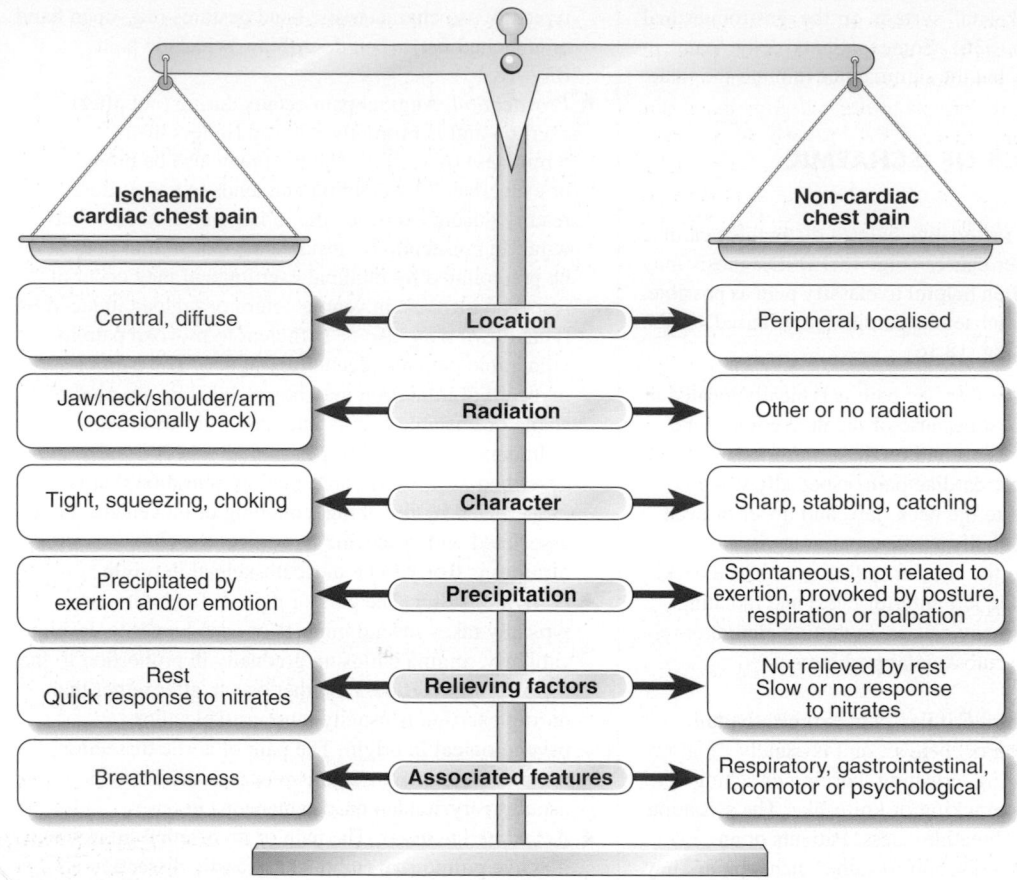

<table>
<tr><td>Ischaemic
cardiac chest pain</td><td></td><td>Non-cardiac
chest pain</td></tr>
<tr><td>Central, diffuse</td><td>Location</td><td>Peripheral, localised</td></tr>
<tr><td>Jaw/neck/shoulder/arm
(occasionally back)</td><td>Radiation</td><td>Other or no radiation</td></tr>
<tr><td>Tight, squeezing, choking</td><td>Character</td><td>Sharp, stabbing, catching</td></tr>
<tr><td>Precipitated by
exertion and/or emotion</td><td>Precipitation</td><td>Spontaneous, not related to
exertion, provoked by posture,
respiration or palpation</td></tr>
<tr><td>Rest
Quick response to nitrates</td><td>Relieving factors</td><td>Not relieved by rest
Slow or no response
to nitrates</td></tr>
<tr><td>Breathlessness</td><td>Associated features</td><td>Respiratory, gastrointestinal,
locomotor or psychological</td></tr>
</table>

Fig. 18.16 Identifying ischaemic cardiac pain: the 'balance' of evidence.

often accompanied by autonomic disturbance including sweating, nausea and vomiting. Breathlessness, due to pulmonary congestion arising from transient ischaemic left ventricular dysfunction, is often a prominent and occasionally the dominant feature of myocardial infarction or angina (angina equivalent). Breathlessness may also accompany any of the respiratory causes of chest pain and may be associated with cough, wheeze or other respiratory symptoms. Classical gastrointestinal symptoms (oesophageal reflux, oesophagitis, peptic ulceration or biliary disease) may provide the clue to the source of non-cardiac chest pain but effort-related 'indigestion' is usually due to heart disease.

THE DIFFERENTIAL DIAGNOSIS OF CHEST PAIN

Conditions that can cause chest pain are shown in Box 18.8. The differential diagnosis of peripheral or pleural chest pain is discussed on page 662.

Psychological aspects of chest pain

Emotional distress is a very common cause of atypical chest pain (p. 249). This diagnosis should be considered if there are features of anxiety or neurosis, and the pain lacks a predictable relationship with exercise. However, it is important to remember that the prospect of heart disease is

---

18.8 COMMON CAUSES OF CHEST PAIN

Anxiety/emotion

Cardiac
- Myocardial ischaemia (angina)
- Myocardial infarction
- Myocarditis
- Pericarditis
- Mitral valve prolapse

Aortic
- Aortic dissection
- Aortic aneurysm

Oesophageal
- Oesophagitis
- Oesophageal spasm
- Mallory–Weiss syndrome

Lungs/pleura
- Bronchospasm
- Pulmonary infarct
- Pneumonia
- Tracheitis
- Pneumothorax
- Pulmonary embolism
- Malignancy
- Tuberculosis
- Connective tissue disorders (rare)

Musculoskeletal
- Osteoarthritis
- Rib fracture/injury
- Intercostal muscle injury
- Costochondritis (Tietze's syndrome)
- Epidemic myalgia (Bornholm disease)

Neurological
- Prolapsed intervertebral disc
- Herpes zoster
- Thoracic outlet syndrome

a frightening experience, particularly when it has been responsible for the death of a close friend or relative; psychological and organic features therefore often coexist. Anxiety may amplify the effects of organic disease and can create a very confusing picture. Patients who believe they are suffering from heart disease are sometimes afraid to take exercise and this may make it difficult to establish their true effort tolerance; assessment may also be complicated by the impact of physical deconditioning.

Myocarditis and pericarditis

These conditions may cause pain that is characteristically felt retrosternally, to the left of the sternum, or in the left or right shoulder, and typically varies in intensity with movement and the phase of respiration. The pain is usually described as 'sharp' and may 'catch' the patient during inspiration or coughing; there is occasionally a history of a prodromal viral illness.

Mitral valve prolapse

Sharp left-sided chest pain that is suggestive of a musculoskeletal problem may be a feature of mitral valve prolapse (p. 621).

Aortic dissection

This pain is severe, sharp and tearing, often felt in or penetrating through to the back, and is typically very abrupt in onset (p. 606).

Oesophageal pain

Oesophageal pain can mimic that of angina very closely, is sometimes precipitated by exercise and may be relieved by nitrates; however, it is usually possible to elicit a history relating chest pain to supine posture or eating, drinking or oesophageal reflux. It often radiates to the back.

Bronchospasm

Patients with reversible airways obstruction, such as asthma, may describe exertional chest tightness that is relieved by rest. This may be difficult to distinguish from ischaemic chest tightness. Bronchospasm may be associated with wheeze, atopy and cough (p. 657).

Musculoskeletal chest pain

This is a common problem that is very variable in site and intensity but does not usually fall into any of the patterns described above. The pain may vary with posture or movement of the upper body and is sometimes accompanied by local tenderness over a rib or costal cartilage. There are numerous causes of chest wall pain, including arthritis, costochondritis, intercostal muscle injury and Coxsackie viral infection (epidemic myalgia or Bornholm disease). Many minor soft tissue injuries are related to everyday activities such as driving, manual work and sport.

INITIAL EVALUATION OF SUSPECTED CARDIAC PAIN

A careful history is crucial to the process of determining whether pain is cardiac or not. Although the physical findings and subsequent investigations may help to confirm the diagnosis, they are of more value in determining the nature and extent of any underlying heart disease, the risk of a serious adverse event and the best course of management.

Stable angina

Effort-related chest pain is the hallmark of stable angina (Fig. 18.17). The reproducibility of the pain and its relationship to physical exertion (and occasionally emotion) are the most important features of the history. The duration of symptoms should be noted because patients with recent-onset angina are at greater risk than those with long-standing and unchanged symptoms.

Physical examination is often normal but may reveal evidence of important risk factors (e.g. xanthoma indicating hyperlipidaemia), left ventricular dysfunction (e.g. dyskinetic apex beat, gallop rhythm), other manifestations of arterial disease (e.g. bruits, signs of peripheral vascular

	Stable angina	Unstable angina
	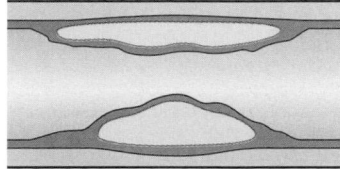	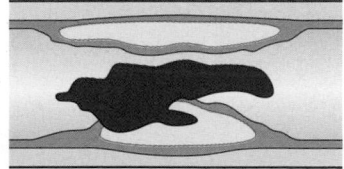
Pathophysiology	• Fixed stenosis	• Dynamic stenosis
Clinical features	• Demand-led ischaemia • Related to effort • Predictable • Symptoms over long term	• Supply-led ischaemia • Symptoms at rest • Unpredictable • Symptoms over short term
Risk assessment	• Symptoms on minimal exertion • Exercise testing Duration of exercise Degree of ECG changes Abnormal BP response	• Frequent or nocturnal symptoms • ECG changes at rest • ECG changes with symptoms • Elevation of troponin

Fig. 18.17 Pathophysiology, clinical features and risk assessment of patients with stable or unstable angina.

18

18

disease) and unrelated conditions that may exacerbate angina (e.g. anaemia, thyroid disease). Stable angina is usually a symptom of coronary artery disease but may be a manifestation of other forms of heart disease, particularly aortic valve disease and hypertrophic cardiomyopathy. In patients with angina in whom a murmur is found, echocardiography can be helpful.

A full blood count, fasting blood glucose, lipids, thyroid function tests and a 12-lead ECG are the most important baseline investigations. Exercise testing may help to confirm the diagnosis and is also used to identify high-risk patients who require further investigation and treatment (p. 528).

Acute coronary syndromes

Prolonged and severe cardiac chest pain may be due to unstable angina (which comprises recent-onset limiting angina, rapidly worsening or crescendo angina, and angina at rest) or acute myocardial infarction; these are known collectively as the acute coronary syndromes. Although there may be a history of antecedent chronic stable angina, an episode of chest pain at rest is often the first presentation of coronary disease. In this situation, the diagnosis depends heavily on an analysis of the character of the pain and its associated features. Physical examination may reveal signs of important comorbidity (e.g. peripheral and/or cerebrovascular disease), autonomic disturbance such as pallor or sweating, and complications such as arrhythmia or heart failure.

Patients presenting with symptoms that are consistent with an acute coronary syndrome require urgent evaluation because these conditions carry a high risk of avoidable complications, such as sudden death and myocardial infarction. Signs of haemodynamic compromise (hypotension, heart failure), ECG changes (ST elevation or depression), and biochemical markers of cardiac damage, such as elevated troponin I and T, are the most powerful indicators of short-term risk. A 12-lead ECG is mandatory and is the most useful method of initial triage (Fig. 18.18). The release

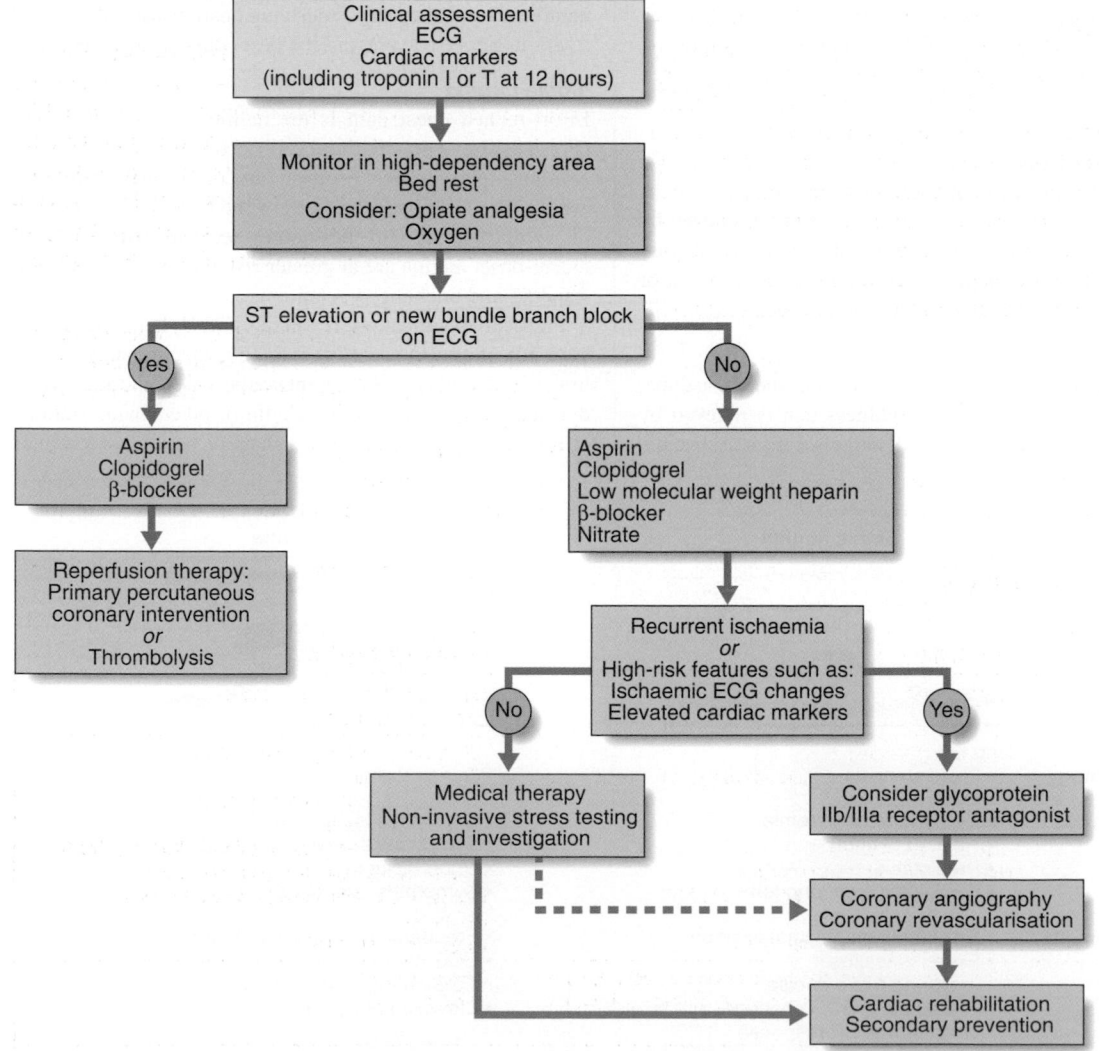

Fig. 18.18 Summary of treatment for unstable angina and non-ST segment elevation myocardial infarction.

of biochemical markers such as creatine kinase, troponin and myoglobin is relatively slow (p. 593) and, although bedside analysis systems are available, these tests are seldom used to guide immediate treatment.

If the diagnosis is unclear, patients with a suspected acute coronary syndrome should be observed in hospital. Repeated ECG recordings are valuable, particularly if a trace can be obtained during an episode of pain. Plasma troponin concentrations should be measured and, if normal, the test should be repeated a minimum of 12 hours after the onset of symptoms. New ECG changes or a positive troponin test confirm the diagnosis of an acute coronary syndrome. The subsequent management of myocardial infarction and unstable angina is described in detail on pages 589–600.

If the pain has not recurred 12 hours after the onset of symptoms, cardiac troponin tests are negative and there are no new ECG changes, the patient may be discharged from hospital. An exercise test helps to confirm or refute a diagnosis of underlying coronary disease at this stage.

BREATHLESSNESS (DYSPNOEA)

Dyspnoea of cardiac origin may vary in severity from an uncomfortable awareness of breathing to a frightening sensation of 'fighting for breath'. The sensation of dyspnoea originates in the cerebral cortex, and although the precise pathways that mediate it remain poorly defined, they include stimuli arising from receptors in the lungs, upper airways and respiratory muscles (Box 18.9 and Ch. 19).

There are several causes of cardiac dyspnoea: acute left heart failure, chronic heart failure, arrhythmia and angina equivalent. The assessment and treatment of heart failure is described on page 542, angina on page 581 and arrhythmias on page 560.

ACUTE LEFT HEART FAILURE

Acute left heart failure may be triggered by a major event such as myocardial infarction in a previously healthy heart, or a relatively minor event such as the onset of atrial fibrillation in a diseased heart. An increase in the left ventricular diastolic pressure causes the pressure in the left atrium, pulmonary veins and pulmonary capillaries to rise. When the hydrostatic pressure of the pulmonary capillaries exceeds the oncotic pressure of plasma (about 25–30 mmHg) fluid moves from the capillaries into alveoli. This stimulates respiration, through a series of autonomic reflexes, producing rapid, shallow respiration. Congestion of the bronchial mucosa may cause wheeze (cardiac asthma).

Acute pulmonary oedema is a terrifying experience and patients will often describe the sensation of 'fighting for breath'. Sitting upright or standing may provide some relief by helping to reduce congestion at the apices of the lungs. The patient may be unable to speak and is typically distressed, agitated, cyanosed, sweaty and pale. Respiration is rapid with recruitment of accessory muscles, coughing and wheezing. Sputum may be profuse, frothy and blood-streaked or pink. Extensive crepitations and rhonchi are usually audible in the chest and there may also be signs of right heart failure.

CHRONIC HEART FAILURE

Chronic heart failure is the most common cardiac cause of chronic dyspnoea. Symptoms may first present on moderately severe exertion, such as walking up a steep hill, and may be described as a difficulty in 'catching my breath'. As heart failure progresses, the dyspnoea is provoked by lesser exertion and ultimately the patient may be breathless walking from room to room, washing, dressing or trying to hold a conversation. Other symptoms of breathlessness may include:

- *Orthopnoea*. Lying down increases the venous return to the heart and may provoke breathlessness in patients with heart failure. The patient may use more pillows to prevent this.
- *Paroxysmal nocturnal dyspnoea*. In patients with severe heart failure, fluid shifts from the interstitial tissues in the peripheries to the circulation within 1–2 hours of

18.9 SOME CAUSES OF DYSPNOEA		
System	Acute dyspnoea at rest	Chronic exertional dyspnoea
Cardiovascular system	*Acute pulmonary oedema	*Chronic congestive cardiac failure Myocardial ischaemia
Respiratory system	*Acute severe asthma *Acute exacerbation of chronic obstructive pulmonary disease *Pneumothorax *Pneumonia *Pulmonary embolus Acute respiratory distress syndrome Inhaled foreign body (especially in the child) Lobar collapse Laryngeal oedema (e.g. anaphylaxis)	*Chronic obstructive pulmonary disease *Chronic asthma Chronic pulmonary thromboembolism Bronchial carcinoma Interstitial lung diseases: sarcoidosis, fibrosing alveolitis, extrinsic allergic alveolitis, pneumoconiosis Lymphatic carcinomatosis (may cause intolerable dyspnoea) Large pleural effusion(s)
Others	Metabolic acidosis (e.g. diabetic ketoacidosis, lactic acidosis, uraemia, overdose of salicylates, ethylene glycol poisoning) Hyperventilation	Severe anaemia Obesity
* Denotes a common cause.		

lying down in bed. Pulmonary oedema may supervene, causing the patient to wake and sit upright, profoundly breathless.

- *Cheyne–Stokes respiration.* This cyclic pattern of respiration is due to impaired responsiveness of the respiratory centre to carbon dioxide and may occur in left ventricular failure. The pattern of slowly diminishing respiration, leading to apnoea, followed by progressively increasing respiration and hyperventilation, may be accompanied by a sensation of breathlessness and panic during the period of hyperventilation. The Cheyne–Stokes cycle length is a function of the circulation time. The condition can also occur in more diffuse cerebral atherosclerosis, stroke or head injury and may be exaggerated by sleep, barbiturates and opiates.

ARRHYTHMIA

Any arrhythmia may cause breathlessness, but usually only does so if the heart is structurally abnormal, such as with the onset of atrial fibrillation in a patient with mitral stenosis.

ANGINA EQUIVALENT

The sensation of breathlessness is a common feature of angina. Patients will sometimes describe chest tightness as 'breathlessness'. However, myocardial ischaemia may also induce true breathlessness by provoking transient left ventricular dysfunction or heart failure. When breathlessness is the dominant or sole feature of myocardial ischaemia it is known as 'angina equivalent'. A history of chest tightness, the close correlation with exercise, and objective evidence of myocardial ischaemia from stress testing may all help to establish the diagnosis.

ACUTE CIRCULATORY FAILURE (CARDIOGENIC SHOCK)

Shock is a loosely defined term used to describe the clinical syndrome that develops when there is critical impairment of tissue perfusion due to some form of acute circulatory failure.

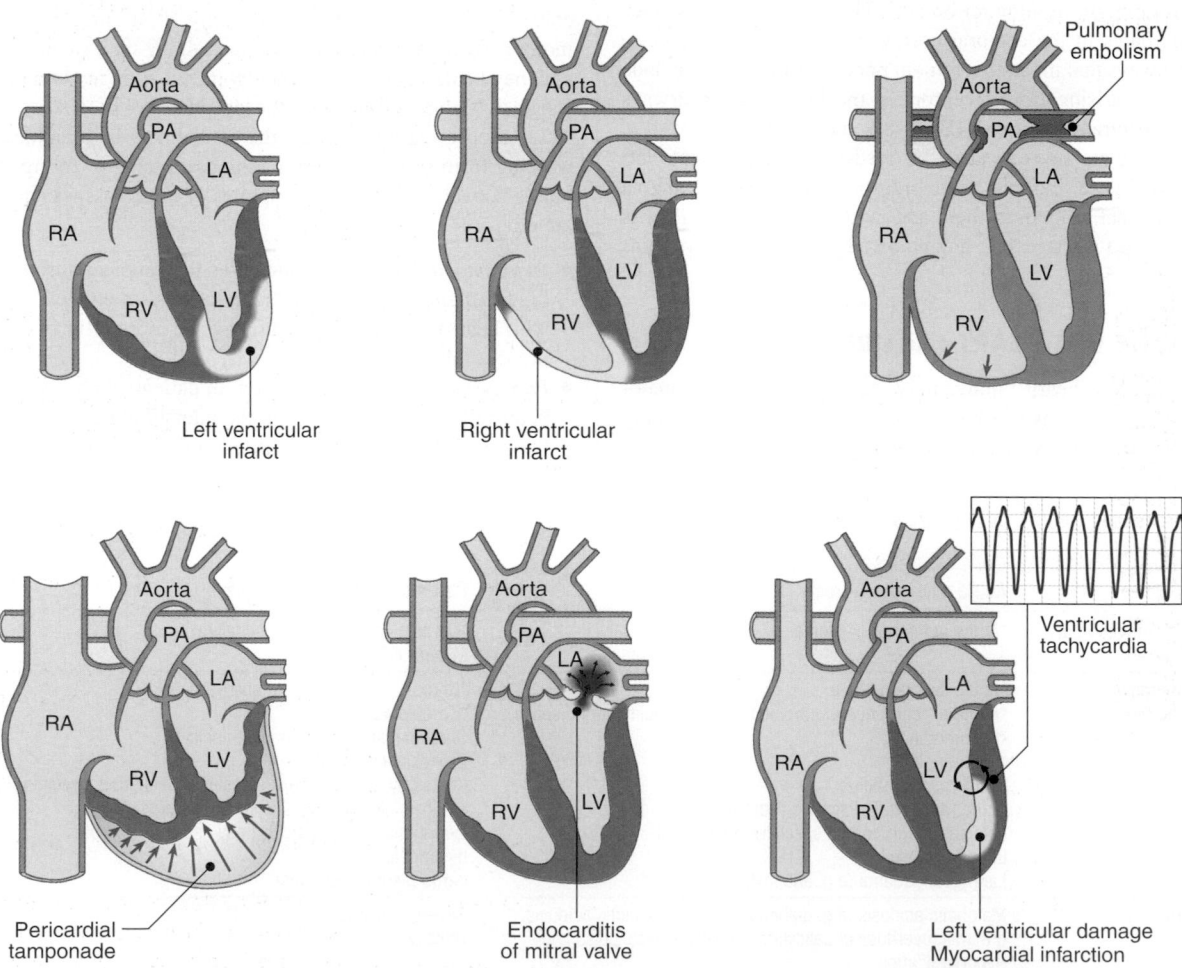

Fig. 18.19   Some examples of the common causes of acute circulatory failure (cardiogenic shock).

There are numerous causes of shock, and the condition is described in detail on page 186. However, the important features of acute heart failure or cardiogenic shock will be described here. Examples of some common causes are illustrated in Figure 18.19. Echocardiography is very helpful when the diagnosis is in doubt.

MYOCARDIAL INFARCTION

Shock in acute myocardial infarction is usually (more than 70% of cases) due to left ventricular dysfunction. However, it may also be due to infarction of the right ventricle and a variety of mechanical complications, including tamponade (due to infarction and rupture of the free wall), an acquired ventricular septal defect (due to infarction and rupture of the septum) and acute mitral regurgitation (due to infarction or rupture of the papillary muscles).

Severe myocardial systolic dysfunction causes a fall in cardiac output, blood pressure and thereby coronary perfusion pressure. Diastolic dysfunction causes a rise in left ventricular end-diastolic pressure, pulmonary congestion and oedema, leading to hypoxia that further worsens myocardial ischaemia. This is further exacerbated by peripheral vasoconstriction. These factors combine to create the 'downward spiral' of cardiogenic shock (Fig. 18.20).

Hypotension, oliguria, confusion and cold, clammy

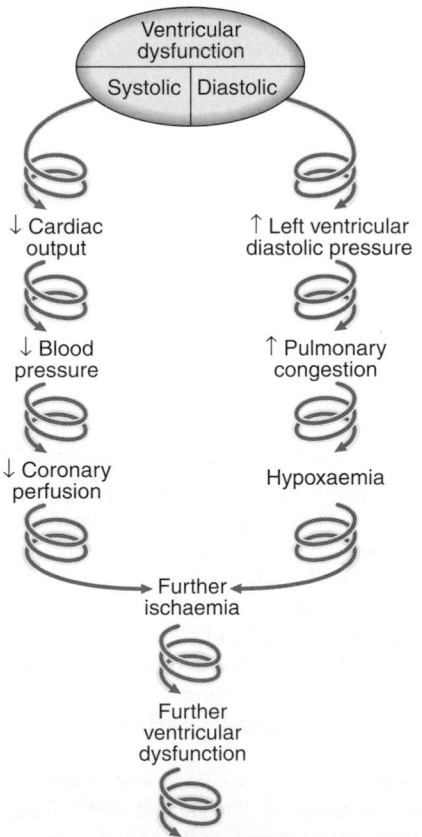

Fig. 18.20 The downward spiral of cardiogenic shock.

peripheries are the manifestations of a low cardiac output, whereas breathlessness, hypoxia, cyanosis and inspiratory crackles at the lung bases are typical features of pulmonary oedema. A chest X-ray (Fig. 18.24, p. 547) may reveal signs of pulmonary congestion when clinical examination is normal. If necessary, a Swan–Ganz catheter can be used to measure the pulmonary artery wedge pressure: an indirect measure of left atrial pressure or preload that guides fluid replacement.

These findings can be used to divide patients with acute myocardial infarction into four haemodynamic subsets (Box 18.10).

18.10 ACUTE MYOCARDIAL INFARCTION: HAEMODYNAMIC SUBSETS
Normal cardiac output. No pulmonary oedema
• The normal state of affairs; carries a good outlook and requires no treatment for heart failure
Normal cardiac output. Pulmonary oedema
• Usually due to moderate left ventricular dysfunction; should be treated with diuretics and vasodilators
Low cardiac output. No pulmonary oedema
• Often caused by a combination of right ventricular infarction and hypovolaemia due to a reduced oral intake of fluids, vomiting and inappropriate diuretic therapy. Such patients are easier to manage if a Swan–Ganz catheter is inserted and i.v. fluids given to raise the left atrial pressure to between 14 and 16 mmHg
Low cardiac output. Pulmonary oedema
• Usually due to extensive left ventricular damage and carries a very poor prognosis. The patient may benefit from treatment with diuretics, vasodilators and inotropes

The viable myocardium surrounding a fresh infarct may contract poorly for a few days and then recover. This phenomenon is known as myocardial stunning and means that it is often worth treating acute heart failure energetically in this setting in the hope that overall cardiac function will improve.

ACUTE MASSIVE PULMONARY EMBOLISM

This may complicate leg or pelvic vein thrombosis and usually presents with sudden collapse. The clinical features are discussed on page 726.

Bedside echocardiography may be very helpful and usually demonstrates a small underfilled vigorous left ventricle with a dilated right ventricle; it is sometimes possible to see thrombus in the right ventricular outflow tract or main pulmonary artery. Spiral CT of the chest with contrast will usually provide a definitive diagnosis and is preferable to invasive pulmonary angiography, which may be hazardous.

Treatment (p. 727) is with high-flow oxygen and anti-coagulation with low molecular weight heparin. Thrombo-lytic therapy is valuable in selected cases with severe haemodynamic compromise, and surgical embolectomy may be needed on rare occasions.

PERICARDIAL TAMPONADE

This is due to a collection of fluid or blood in the pericardial sac, compressing the heart; the effusion may be small and is sometimes less than 100 ml. Sudden deterioration may be due to bleeding into the pericardial space.

Tamponade may complicate any form of pericarditis and is often due to malignant disease (p. 261). Other causes include trauma and rupture of the free wall of the myocardium following myocardial infarction.

The important clinical features are listed in Box 18.11.

18.11 CLINICAL FEATURES OF PERICARDIAL TAMPONADE
• Dyspnoea • Collapse • Tachycardia • Hypotension • Gross elevation of the jugular venous pressure • Soft heart sounds with an early third heart sound • Pulsus paradoxus (a large fall in blood pressure during inspiration when the pulse may be impalpable) • Kussmaul's sign (a paradoxical rise in the jugular venous pressure during inspiration)

An ECG may show features of the underlying disease, such as pericarditis or acute myocardial infarction. When there is a large pericardial effusion, the ECG complexes are small and there may be electrical alternans (a changing axis with alternate beats caused by the heart swinging from side to side in the pericardial fluid). A chest X-ray may show an enlarged globular heart but can look normal. Echocardiography, which may be done at the bedside, is the best way of confirming the diagnosis, and helps to identify the optimum site for aspiration of the fluid.

Prompt recognition of tamponade is important because the patient usually responds dramatically to percutaneous pericardiocentesis (p. 645) or surgical drainage.

VALVULAR HEART DISEASE

Acute left ventricular failure may be due to the sudden onset of aortic regurgitation, mitral regurgitation or prosthetic valve dysfunction. Some of the common causes of these are listed in Box 18.12.

18.12 CAUSES OF ACUTE VALVE FAILURE
Aortic regurgitation
• Aortic dissection • Infective endocarditis
Mitral regurgitation
• Papillary muscle rupture due to acute myocardial infarction • Infective endocarditis • Rupture of chordae due to myxomatous degeneration
Prosthetic valve failure
• Mechanical valves: fracture, jamming, thrombosis, dehiscence • Biological valves: degeneration with cusp tear

The clinical diagnosis of acute valvular dysfunction is sometimes difficult. Murmurs are often unimpressive because there is usually a tachycardia and a low cardiac output. Transthoracic echocardiography will establish the diagnosis in most cases; however, transoesophageal echocardiography is sometimes required, especially in patients with prosthetic mitral valves.

Patients with acute valve failure usually require cardiac surgery and should be referred for urgent assessment in a cardiac centre.

Aortic dissection may cause shock by causing aortic regurgitation, coronary dissection, tamponade or blood loss (p. 606).

MANAGEMENT OF SHOCK

The management of shock is discussed in detail in Chapter 8 (p. 186).

HEART FAILURE

Heart failure is an imprecise term used to describe the state that develops when the heart cannot maintain an adequate cardiac output or can do so only at the expense of an elevated filling pressure. In the mildest forms of heart failure, cardiac output is adequate at rest and becomes inadequate only when the metabolic demand increases during exercise or some other form of stress.

In practice, heart failure may be diagnosed whenever a patient with significant heart disease develops the signs or symptoms of a low cardiac output, pulmonary congestion or systemic venous congestion.

Almost all forms of heart disease can lead to heart failure and it is important to appreciate that, like anaemia, the term refers to a clinical syndrome rather than a specific diagnosis. Good management depends on an accurate aetiological diagnosis, because in some situations a specific remedy may be available, but mainly because the nature of the pathophysiology guides logical drug therapy. The possible mechanisms and some causes of heart failure are shown in Box 18.13.

Heart failure is frequently due to coronary artery disease, tends to affect elderly people and often leads to prolonged disability. The prevalence of heart failure rises from around 1% in the age group 50–59 years to between 5 and 10% of those aged 80–89 years. In the United Kingdom, most patients admitted to hospital with heart failure are more than 65 years old and remain inpatients for a week or more.

Although the outlook depends to some extent on the underlying cause of the problem, heart failure carries a very poor prognosis; approximately 50% of patients with severe heart failure due to left ventricular dysfunction will die within 2 years. Many patients die suddenly from malignant ventricular arrhythmias or myocardial infarction.

Pathophysiology

Cardiac output is a function of the preload (the volume and pressure of blood in the ventricle at the end of diastole), the afterload (the volume and pressure of blood in the

18.13 MECHANISMS OF HEART FAILURE

Cause	Examples	Features
Reduced ventricular contractility	Myocardial infarction (segmental dysfunction)	In coronary artery disease, 'akinetic' or 'dyskinetic' segments contract poorly and may impede the function of the normal segments by distorting their contraction and relaxation patterns
	Myocarditis/cardiomyopathy (global dysfunction)	Progressive ventricular dilatation
Ventricular outflow obstruction (pressure overload)	Hypertension, aortic stenosis (left heart failure) Pulmonary hypertension, pulmonary valve stenosis (right heart failure)	Initially concentric ventricular hypertrophy allows the ventricle to maintain a normal output by generating a high systolic pressure. However, secondary changes in the myocardium and increasing obstruction eventually lead to failure with ventricular dilatation and rapid clinical deterioration
Ventricular inflow obstruction	Mitral stenosis, tricuspid stenosis	Small vigorous ventricle, dilated hypertrophied atrium. Atrial fibrillation is common and often causes marked deterioration because ventricular filling depends heavily on atrial contraction
Ventricular volume overload	LV volume overload (e.g. mitral or aortic regurgitation, arteriovenous fistulae) Ventricular septal defect RV volume overload (e.g. atrial septal defect) Increased metabolic demand (high output)	Dilatation and hypertrophy allow the ventricle to generate a high stroke volume and help to maintain a normal cardiac output. However, secondary changes in the myocardium eventually lead to impaired contractility and worsening heart failure
Arrhythmia	Atrial fibrillation	Tachycardia does not allow for adequate filling of the heart, resulting in reduced cardiac output and back pressure
	Tachycardia cardiomyopathy	Incessant tachycardia causes myocardial fatigue
	Complete heart block	Bradycardia limits cardiac output even if stroke volume is normal
Diastolic dysfunction	Constrictive pericarditis	Marked fluid retention and peripheral oedema, ascites, pleural effusions and elevated jugular veins
	Restrictive cardiomyopathy	Bi-atrial enlargement (restrictive filling pattern and high atrial pressures). Atrial fibrillation may cause deterioration
	Left ventricular hypertrophy and fibrosis	Good systolic function but poor diastolic filling
	Cardiac tamponade	Hypotension, elevated jugular veins, pulsus paradoxus, poor urine output

ventricle during systole) and myocardial contractility. The interaction of these variables is shown in Figure 18.21, which is based on Starling's Law of the heart.

In patients without valvular disease, the primary abnormality in heart failure is impairment of ventricular function leading to a fall in cardiac output. This activates counter-regulatory neurohormonal mechanisms that in normal physiological circumstances would support cardiac function, but in the setting of impaired ventricular function can lead to a deleterious increase in both afterload and preload (Fig. 18.22). A vicious circle may be established because any additional fall in cardiac output will cause further neurohormonal activation and increasing peripheral vascular resistance.

Stimulation of the renin–angiotensin–aldosterone system leads to vasoconstriction, salt and water retention, and sympathetic activation mediated by angiotensin II, which is a potent constrictor of arterioles both in the kidney and systemic circulation (Fig. 18.22). Activation of the sympathetic nervous system may initially maintain cardiac output through an increase in myocardial contractility, heart

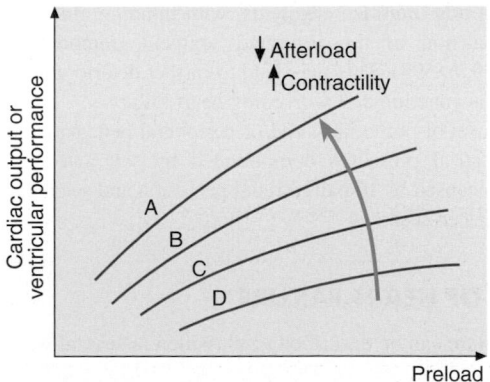

Fig. 18.21 Starling's Law. Normal (A), mild (B), moderate (C) and severe (D) heart failure. Ventricular performance is related to the degree of myocardial stretching. An increase in preload (end-diastolic volume, end-diastolic pressure, filling pressure or atrial pressure) will therefore enhance function; however, overstretching causes marked deterioration. In heart failure the curve moves to the right and becomes flatter. An increase in myocardial contractility or a reduction in afterload will shift the curve upwards and to the left.

18

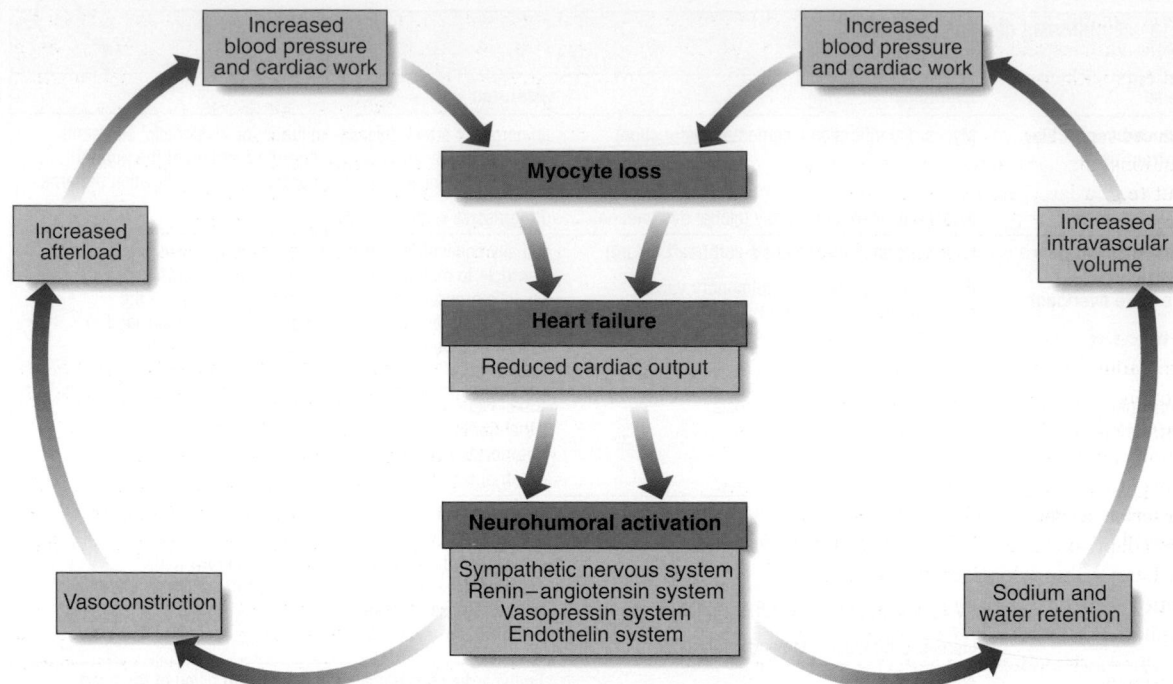

Fig. 18.22   Neurohormonal activation and compensatory mechanisms in heart failure. There is a vicious circle in progressive heart failure.

rate and peripheral vasoconstriction. However, prolonged sympathetic stimulation leads to cardiac myocyte apoptosis, hypertrophy and focal myocardial necrosis. Salt and water retention is promoted by the release of aldosterone, endothelin (a potent vasoconstrictor peptide with marked effects on the renal vasculature) and, in severe heart failure, antidiuretic hormone (ADH). Natriuretic peptides are released from the atria in response to atrial stretch, and act as physiological antagonists to the fluid-conserving effect of aldosterone.

After myocardial infarction, cardiac contractility is impaired and neurohormonal activation may lead to hypertrophy of non-infarcted segments, with thinning, dilatation and expansion of the infarcted segment (remodelling, Fig. 18.79, p. 598). This may lead to further deterioration in ventricular function and worsening heart failure.

The onset of pulmonary and/or peripheral oedema is due to high atrial pressures compounded by salt and water retention caused by impaired renal perfusion and secondary hyperaldosteronism.

TYPES OF HEART FAILURE

Heart failure can be described or classified in several ways.

Left, right and biventricular heart failure
The left side of the heart is a term for the functional unit of the left atrium and left ventricle, together with the mitral and aortic valves; the right heart comprises the right atrium, right ventricle, tricuspid and pulmonary valves.

- *Left-sided heart failure.* There is a reduction in the left ventricular output and/or an increase in the left atrial or

pulmonary venous pressure. An acute increase in left atrial pressure may cause pulmonary congestion or pulmonary oedema; a more gradual increase in left atrial pressure, as occurs with mitral stenosis, may lead to reflex pulmonary vasoconstriction, which protects the patient from pulmonary oedema at the cost of increasing pulmonary hypertension.
- *Right-sided heart failure.* There is a reduction in right ventricular output for any given right atrial pressure. Causes of isolated right heart failure include chronic lung disease (cor pulmonale), multiple pulmonary emboli and pulmonary valvular stenosis.
- *Biventricular heart failure.* Failure of the left and right heart may develop because the disease process (e.g. dilated cardiomyopathy or ischaemic heart disease) affects both ventricles, or because disease of the left heart leads to chronic elevation of the left atrial pressure, pulmonary hypertension and right heart failure.

Forward and backward heart failure
In some patients with heart failure the predominant problem is an inadequate cardiac output (forward failure), whilst other patients may have a normal or near-normal cardiac output with marked salt and water retention causing pulmonary and systemic venous congestion (backward failure).

Diastolic and systolic dysfunction
Heart failure may develop as a result of impaired myocardial contraction (systolic dysfunction) but can also be due to poor ventricular filling and high filling pressures caused by abnormal ventricular relaxation (diastolic dysfunction). The latter is commonly found in patients with left ventricular hypertrophy and occurs in many forms of heart

disease, notably hypertension and ischaemic heart disease. Systolic and diastolic dysfunction often coexist, particularly in patients with coronary artery disease.

High-output failure

Conditions that are associated with a very high cardiac output (e.g. a large arteriovenous shunt, beri-beri (p. 123), severe anaemia or thyrotoxicosis) can occasionally cause heart failure. In such cases, additional causes of heart failure are often present.

Acute and chronic heart failure

Heart failure may develop suddenly, as in myocardial infarction, or gradually, as in progressive valvular heart disease. When there is gradual impairment of cardiac function, a variety of compensatory changes may take place.

The phrase 'compensated heart failure' is sometimes used to describe a patient with impaired cardiac function in whom adaptive changes have prevented the development of overt heart failure. A minor event, such as an intercurrent infection or development of atrial fibrillation, may precipitate overt or acute heart failure in this type of patient (Box 18.14). Acute left heart failure occurs either de novo or as an acute decompensated episode on a background of chronic heart failure, i.e. acute-on-chronic heart failure.

CLINICAL ASSESSMENT

Acute left heart failure

Acute de novo left ventricular failure usually presents with a sudden onset of dyspnoea at rest that rapidly progresses to acute respiratory distress, orthopnoea and prostration. The precipitant, such as acute myocardial infarction, is often apparent from the patient's history.

The patient appears agitated, pale and clammy. The peripheries are cool to the touch and the pulse is rapid. Inappropriate bradycardia or excessive tachycardia should be identified promptly as this may be the precipitant for the acute episode of heart failure. The blood pressure is usually high because of sympathetic nervous system activation, but may be normal or low if the patient is in cardiogenic shock.

The jugular venous pressure is usually elevated, particularly with associated fluid overload or right heart failure. In acute de novo heart failure, there has been no time for ventricular dilatation and the apex is not displaced. Auscultation occasionally identifies the murmur of a catastrophic valvular or septal rupture, or reveals a triple 'gallop' rhythm. Crepitations are heard at the lung bases, consistent with pulmonary oedema.

Acute-on-chronic heart failure will have additional features of long-standing heart failure (see below). Potential precipitants, such as an upper respiratory tract infection or inappropriate cessation of diuretic medication, should be identified.

Chronic heart failure

Patients with chronic heart failure commonly experience a relapsing and remitting course, with periods of stability and episodes of decompensation leading to worsening symptoms that may necessitate hospitalisation.

The clinical picture depends on the nature of the underlying heart disease, the type of heart failure that it has evoked, and the neural and endocrine changes that have developed (Box 18.13, p. 543, and Fig. 18.23).

A low cardiac output causes fatigue, listlessness and a poor effort tolerance; the peripheries are cold and the blood pressure is low. To maintain perfusion of vital organs, blood flow may be diverted away from skeletal muscle and this may contribute to fatigue and weakness. Poor renal perfusion may lead to oliguria and uraemia.

Pulmonary oedema due to left heart failure may present with breathlessness, orthopnoea, paroxysmal nocturnal dyspnoea and inspiratory crepitations over the lung bases.

In contrast, right heart failure produces a high jugular venous pressure, with hepatic congestion and dependent peripheral oedema. In ambulant patients the oedema affects the ankles, whereas in bed-bound patients it collects around the thighs and sacrum. Ascites or pleural effusion can occur in some cases (Fig. 18.23). Heart failure is not the only cause of oedema (Box 18.15).

Chronic heart failure is sometimes associated with marked weight loss (cardiac cachexia) caused by a combination of anorexia and impaired absorption due to gastro-intestinal congestion; poor tissue perfusion due to a low cardiac output; and skeletal muscle atrophy due to immobility. Increased plasma concentrations of tumour necrosis factor-alpha have been found in patients with cardiac cachexia.

18.14 FACTORS THAT MAY PRECIPITATE OR AGGRAVATE HEART FAILURE IN PATIENTS WITH PRE-EXISTING HEART DISEASE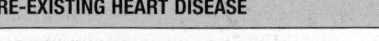

- Myocardial ischaemia or infarction
- Intercurrent illness, e.g. infection
- Arrhythmia, e.g. atrial fibrillation
- Inappropriate reduction of therapy
- Administration of a drug with negative inotropic properties (e.g. β-blocker) or fluid-retaining properties (e.g. non-steroidal anti-inflammatory drugs, corticosteroids)
- Pulmonary embolism
- Conditions associated with increased metabolic demand, e.g. pregnancy, thyrotoxicosis, anaemia
- Intravenous fluid overload, e.g. post-operative i.v. infusion

---

18.15 DIFFERENTIAL DIAGNOSIS OF PERIPHERAL OEDEMA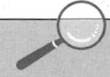

- **Cardiac failure:** right or combined left and right heart failure, pericardial constriction, cardiomyopathy
- **Chronic venous insufficiency:** varicose veins
- **Hypoalbuminaemia:** nephrotic syndrome, liver disease, protein-losing enteropathy; often widespread, can affect arms and face
- **Drugs**
  Sodium retention: fludrocortisone, non-steroidal anti-inflammatory agents
  Increasing capillary permeability: nifedipine, amlodipine
- **Idiopathic:** women > men
- **Chronic lymphatic obstruction**

18

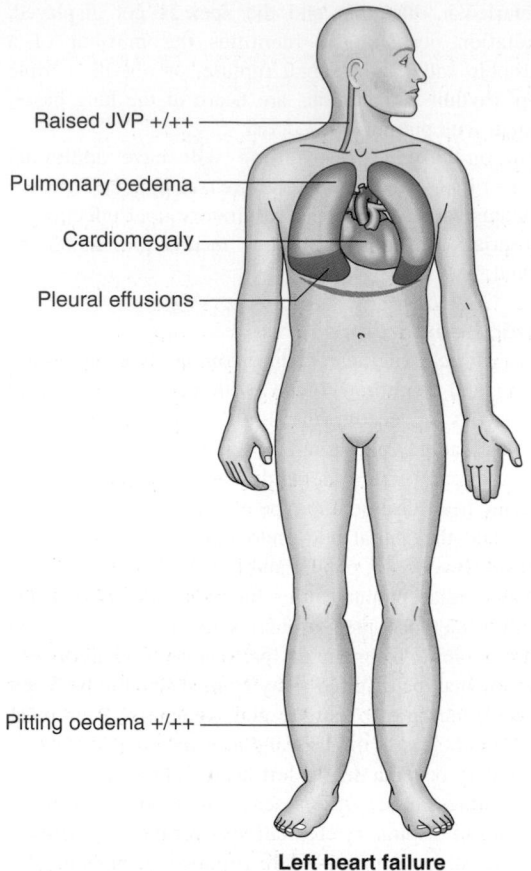

Raised JVP +/++
Pulmonary oedema
Cardiomegaly
Pleural effusions

Pitting oedema +/++

Left heart failure

Raised JVP +++

Hepatomegaly

Ascites

Peripheral pitting
oedema +++

Right heart failure

Fig. 18.23   Left and right heart failure.

COMPLICATIONS

In advanced heart failure a number of non-specific complications may occur:

- *Renal failure* is caused by poor renal perfusion due to a low cardiac output and may be exacerbated by diuretic therapy, ACE inhibitors and angiotensin receptor blockers.
- *Hypokalaemia* may be the result of treatment with potassium-losing diuretics or hyperaldosteronism caused by activation of the renin–angiotensin system and impaired aldosterone metabolism due to hepatic congestion. Most of the body's potassium is intracellular and there may be substantial depletion of potassium stores, even when the plasma potassium concentration is in the normal range.
- *Hyperkalaemia* may be due to the effects of drug treatment, particularly the combination of angiotensin-converting enzyme (ACE) inhibitors and spironolactone (which both promote potassium retention), and renal dysfunction.
- *Hyponatraemia* is a feature of severe heart failure and may be caused by diuretic therapy, inappropriate water retention due to high ADH secretion, or failure of the cell membrane ion pump. It is a poor prognostic sign,
- *Impaired liver function* is caused by hepatic venous congestion and poor arterial perfusion, which frequently

cause mild jaundice and abnormal liver function tests; reduced synthesis of clotting factors may make anticoagulant control difficult.
- *Thromboembolism.* Deep vein thrombosis and pulmonary embolism may occur due to the effects of a low cardiac output and enforced immobility, whereas systemic emboli may be related to arrhythmias, atrial flutter or fibrillation, or intracardiac thrombus complicating conditions such as mitral stenosis or LV aneurysm.
- *Atrial and ventricular arrhythmias* are very common and may be related to electrolyte changes (e.g. hypokalaemia, hypomagnesaemia), the underlying structural heart disease, and the pro-arrhythmic effects of increased circulating catecholamines and some drugs (e.g. digoxin). Sudden death occurs in up to 50% of patients with heart failure and is often due to a ventricular arrhythmia. Frequent ventricular ectopic beats and runs of non-sustained ventricular tachycardia are common findings in patients with heart failure and are associated with an adverse prognosis.

INVESTIGATIONS

Simple tests (e.g. urea, electrolytes, haemoglobin, thyroid function, ECG, chest X-ray) may help to establish the nature and severity of the underlying heart disease and detect any complications. Brain natriuretic peptide (BNP) is elevated in heart failure and can be used as a screening test in breathless patients and those with oedema.

Echocardiography is a very useful investigation and should be considered in all patients with significant heart failure in order to:

- determine the aetiology
- detect hitherto unsuspected valvular heart disease (e.g. occult mitral stenosis) and other conditions that may be amenable to specific remedies
- identify patients who will benefit from long-term therapy with drugs such as ACE inhibitors (see below).

The chest X-ray in left heart failure

A rise in pulmonary venous pressure from left-sided cardiac failure first shows on the chest X-ray (Fig. 18.24) as an abnormal distension of the upper lobe pulmonary veins (with the patient in the erect position). The vascularity of the lung fields becomes more prominent, and the right and left pulmonary arteries dilate. Subsequently, interstitial oedema causes thickened interlobular septa and dilated lymphatics. These are evident as horizontal lines in the costophrenic angles (septal or 'Kerley B' lines). More advanced changes due to alveolar oedema cause a hazy opacification spreading from the hilar regions, and pleural effusions.

MANAGEMENT OF HEART FAILURE

Management of acute pulmonary oedema

This needs urgent treatment:

- Sit the patient up in order to reduce pulmonary congestion.
- Give oxygen (high flow, high concentration). Non-invasive positive pressure ventilation (continuous positive airways pressure, CPAP, of 5–10 mmHg) by a tight-fitting face mask results in a more rapid improvement in the patient's clinical state.
- Administer nitrates (e.g. i.v. glyceryl trinitrate 10–200 µg/min or buccal glyceryl trinitrate 2–5 mg) titrated upwards every 10 minutes, until clinical improvement occurs or systolic blood pressure falls to < 110 mmHg.
- Administer a loop diuretic such as furosemide 50–100 mg i.v.

The patient should initially be kept on strict bed rest with continuous monitioring, including cardiac rhythm, blood pressure and pulse oximetry.

Intravenous opiates may be cautiously used when patients are in extremis. They reduce sympathetically mediated peripheral vasoconstriction but run the risk of respiratory depression and exacerbation of hypoxia and hypercapnia.

18

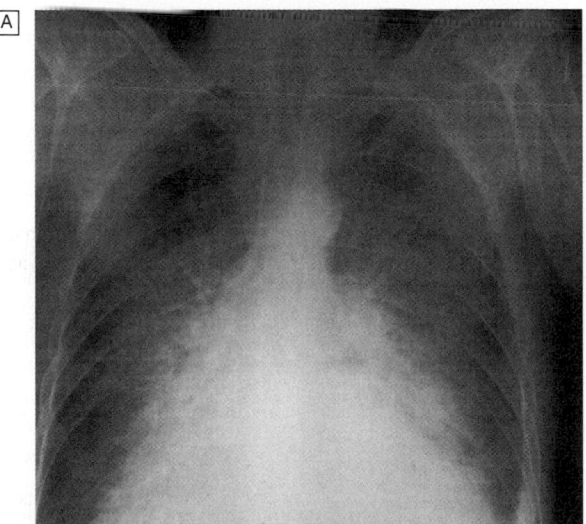

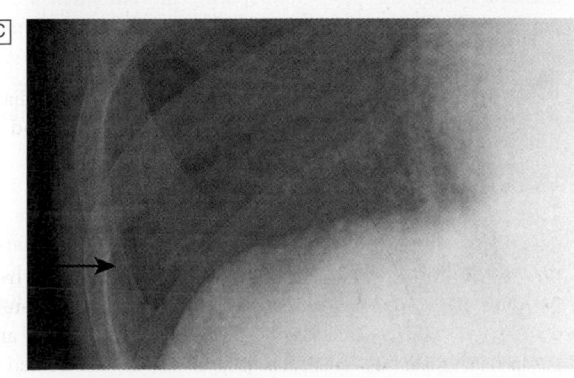

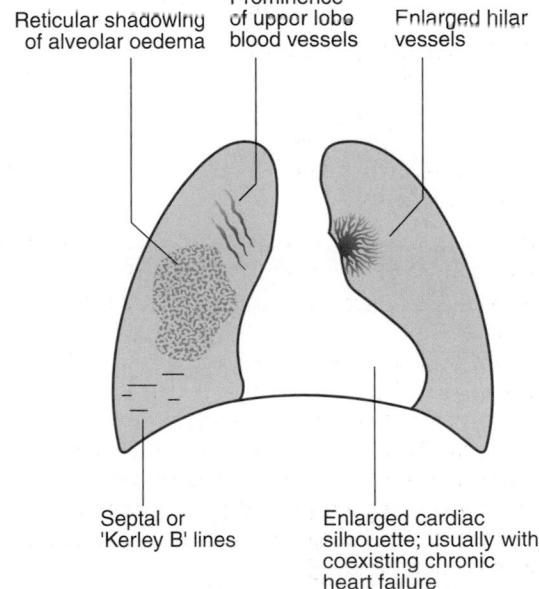

Fig. 18.24   Radiological features of heart failure. [A] Chest X-ray of a patient with pulmonary oedema. [B] Schematic highlighting the radiological features of heart failure. [C] Enlargement of lung base showing septal or 'Kerley B' lines (arrow).

18

If these measures prove ineffective, inotropic agents may be required to augment cardiac output, particularly in hypotensive patients. Insertion of an intra-aortic balloon pump can be very beneficial in patients with acute cardiogenic pulmonary oedema, especially when secondary to myocardial ischaemia.

MANAGEMENT OF CHRONIC HEART FAILURE

General measures

Effective education of patients and their relatives about the causes and treatment of heart failure can help adherence to a management plan (Box 18.16). Some patients may need to weigh themselves daily, and adjust their diuretic therapy accordingly.

In patients with coronary heart disease, secondary preventative measures such as low-dose aspirin and lipid-lowering therapy are required (p. 580).

Drug therapy

Cardiac function can be improved by increasing contractility, optimising preload or decreasing afterload. The effects of these measures are illustrated in Figure 18.22. Drugs that reduce preload are most appropriate in patients with high end-diastolic filling pressures and evidence of pulmonary or systemic venous congestion (backward failure); drugs that reduce afterload or increase myocardial contractility are more useful in patients with signs and symptoms of a low cardiac output (forward failure).

Diuretics

These are usually the first-line treatment. The main types, mode of action and side-effects of these drugs are described

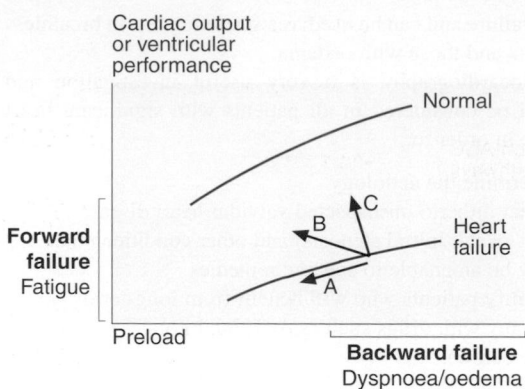

Fig. 18.25 The effect of treatment on ventricular performance curves in heart failure. Diuretics and venodilators (A), angiotensin-converting enzyme (ACE) inhibitors and mixed vasodilators (B), and positive inotropic agents (C).

on page 427. In heart failure, diuretics produce an increase in urinary sodium excretion, leading to a reduction in blood and plasma volume, and may also cause a small but significant degree of arterial and venous dilatation. Diuretic therapy will therefore reduce preload and improve pulmonary and systemic venous congestion; it may also cause a small reduction in afterload and ventricular volume, leading to a fall in wall tension and increased cardiac efficiency.

Although a fall in preload (ventricular filling pressure) tends to reduce cardiac output, the 'Starling curve' in heart failure is flat so there may be a substantial and beneficial fall in filling pressure with little change in cardiac output (Fig. 18.21, p. 543, and Fig. 18.25). Nevertheless, excessive diuretic therapy may cause an undesirable fall in cardiac output, with a rising blood urea, hypotension and increasing lethargy, especially in patients with a marked diastolic component to their heart failure.

In some patients with severe chronic heart failure, particularly in the presence of chronic renal impairment, oedema may persist despite oral loop diuretics. In such patients an intravenous infusion of furosemide 10 mg/hr for example, can initiate a diuresis. Also combining a loop diuretic with a thiazide (e.g. bendroflumethiazide 5 mg daily) or a thiazide-like diuretic (e.g. metolazone 5 mg daily) may prove effective; however, such combinations can produce an excessive diuresis.

Aldosterone receptor antagonists such as spironolactone and eplerenone are potassium-sparing diuretics that are of particular benefit in patients with heart failure. They may cause hyperkalaemia, particularly when used with an ACE inhibitor. They improve long-term clinical outcome in patients with severe heart failure and those with heart failure following acute myocardial infarction.

Vasodilators

The use of vasodilators in acute circulatory failure is described on page 186. These drugs are also valuable in chronic heart failure; venodilators (e.g. nitrates) reduce preload, and arterial dilators (e.g. hydralazine) reduce afterload (Fig. 18.25). However, their use is limited by pharmacological tolerance and hypotension.

18.16 GENERAL MEASURES FOR THE MANAGEMENT OF HEART FAILURE
Education
• Explanation of nature of disease, treatment and self-help strategies
Diet
• Good general nutrition and weight reduction for the obese • Avoidance of high-salt foods and added salt, especially for patients with severe congestive heart failure
Alcohol
• Moderate or eliminate alcohol consumption. Alcohol-induced cardiomyopathy requires abstinence
Smoking
• Stopping
Exercise
• Regular moderate aerobic exercise within limits of symptoms
Vaccination
• Influenza and pneumococcal vaccination should be considered

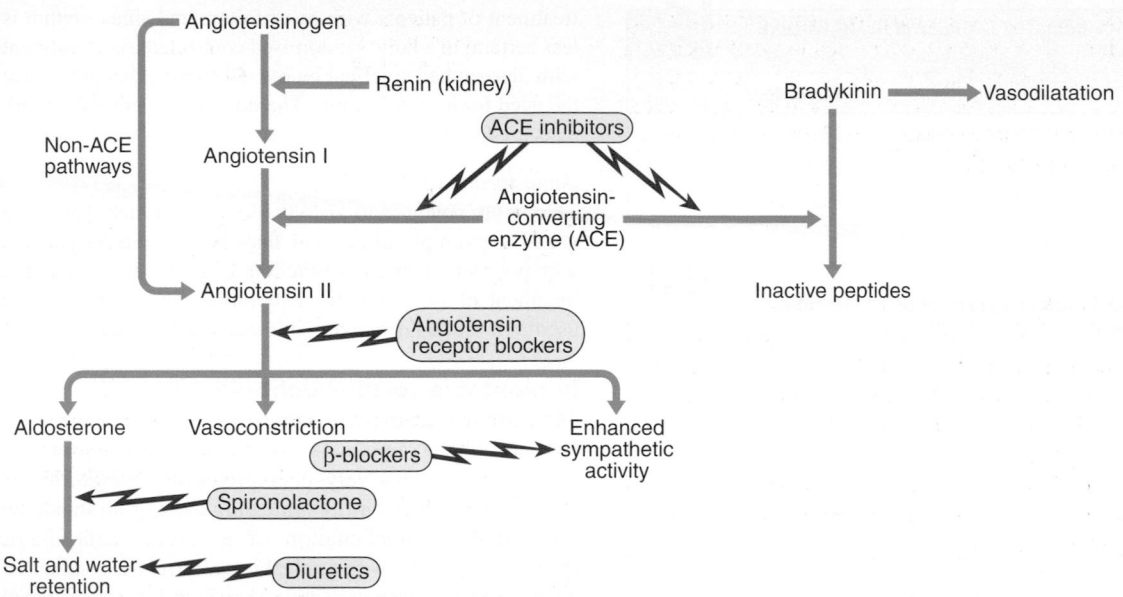

Fig. 18.26 Neurohormonal activation and sites of action of drugs used in the treatment of heart failure.

18

Angiotensin-converting enzyme (ACE) inhibitors

The development of these drugs has been a major advance in the treatment of heart failure. They interrupt the vicious circle of neurohormonal activation that is characteristic of moderate and severe heart failure by preventing the conversion of angiotensin I to angiotensin II, thereby preventing salt and water retention, peripheral arterial and venous vasoconstriction, and activation of the sympathetic nervous system (Fig. 18.26). They also prevent the undesirable activation of the renin–angiotensin system caused by diuretic therapy.

The major benefit of ACE inhibitor therapy in heart failure is a reduction in afterload; however, there may also be an advantageous reduction in preload and a modest increase in the plasma potassium concentration. Treating heart failure, with a combination of a loop diuretic and an ACE inhibitor therefore has many potential advantages.

Clinical trials have shown that in moderate and severe heart failure, ACE inhibitors can produce a substantial improvement in effort tolerance and in mortality. ACE inhibitors can also improve outcome and prevent the onset of overt heart failure in patients with poor residual left ventricular function following myocardial infarction (Boxes 18.17 and 18.18).

Unfortunately, these drugs can cause profound hypotension with postural symptoms and a deterioration in renal function (especially in patients with bilateral renal artery stenosis or pre-existing renal disease). Moreover, there may be a potentially catastrophic fall in blood pressure following the first dose of an ACE inhibitor, particularly if the drug is started in the presence of hypotension, hypovolaemia or hyponatraemia due to prior diuretic therapy, especially in the elderly. In stable patients without hypotension (systolic BP > 100 mmHg), ACE inhibitors can usually be started in the community without problems. However, in other patients it is usually advisable to withhold diuretics for 24

hours before starting treatment with a low dose, while the patient is supine and under observation. If hypotension occurs, this can be counteracted by elevating the foot of the bed and administering intravenous saline. Renal function must be monitored and should be checked 1–2 weeks after starting therapy. Typical starting doses and target doses for commonly used ACE inhibitors are shown in Box 18.19.

Angiotensin receptor blockers

Examples include losartan 50–100 mg once daily, candesartan 4–16 mg daily or valsartan 40–160 mg daily. These drugs act by blocking the action of angiotensin II on

18

18.19 ACE INHIBITOR DOSAGES IN HEART FAILURE

	Starting dose	Target dose
Enalapril	2.5 mg 12-hourly	10 mg 12-hourly
Lisinopril	5 mg daily	20 mg daily
Ramipril	1.25 mg 12-hourly	5 mg 12-hourly

EBM

18.20 ANGIOTENSIN RECEPTOR BLOCKERS (ARBs) AND CHRONIC HEART FAILURE

'Compared with ACE inhibitors, ARBs are better tolerated and have similar efficacy in reducing cardiovascular events. ARBs reduce cardiovascular morbidity and mortality in patients with symptomatic heart failure who are intolerant of ACE inhibitors. NNT_B for 5 years to prevent one death or hospitalisation for heart failure = 8. The addition of an ARB to an ACE inhibitor produces further additional benefit. NNT_B for 5 years to prevent one death or hospitalisation for heart failure = 16.'

- Granger CB, et al. Lancet 2003; 362:772–776.
- McMurray JJV, et al. Lancet 2003; 362:767–771.

the heart, peripheral vasculature and kidney; in heart failure, they produce beneficial haemodynamic changes that are similar to the effects of ACE inhibitors (Fig. 18.26). They have comparable effects on mortality and are a useful alternative for patients who cannot tolerate ACE inhibitors (Box 18.20). Unfortunately, they share all the more serious adverse effects of ACE inhibitors including renal dysfunction.

Beta-adrenoceptor antagonists (β-blockers)

These drugs may help to counteract the deleterious effects of enhanced sympathetic stimulation and reduce the risk of arrhythmias and sudden death. When initiated in standard doses they may precipitate acute-on-chronic heart failure, but when given in small incremental doses (e.g. bisoprolol started at a dose of 1.25 mg daily, and increased gradually over a 12-week period to a target maintenance dose of 10 mg daily) under carefully monitored conditions, they can increase ejection fraction, improve symptoms, reduce the frequency of hospitalisation and reduce mortality in patients with chronic heart failure (Box 18.21).

EBM

18.21 β-BLOCKERS AND TREATMENT OF CHRONIC HEART FAILURE

'Adding oral β-blockers gradually in small incremental doses to standard therapy including ACE inhibitors in people with heart failure reduces the rate of death or hospital admission. NNT_B for 1 year to prevent one death = 21.'

- Lechat P, et al. Circulation 1998; 98:1184–1191.
- McMurray JJV. Heart 1999; 82:14–22.
- Shibola MC, et al. Br J Heart Fail 2002; 4:11 720.

For further information: 💻 www.escardio.org

Digoxin

This should be used as first-line therapy in patients with heart failure and atrial fibrillation, when it usually provides adequate control of the ventricular rate together with a small positive inotropic effect. The role of digoxin in the treatment of patients with heart failure and sinus rhythm is less certain; in a large randomised controlled trial, treatment with digoxin had no effect on overall survival but did reduce the need for hospitalisation. The dosage and side-effects are discussed on page 575.

Amiodarone (p. 573)

This is a potent anti-arrhythmic drug which has little negative inotropic effect and may be valuable in patients with poor left ventricular function. It is only effective in the treatment of symptomatic arrhythmias, and should not be used as a preventative agent in the asymptomatic.

Implantable cardiac defibrillators and resynchronisation therapy

Patients with symptomatic ventricular arrhythmias and heart failure have a very poor prognosis. Irrespective of their response to anti-arrhythmic drug therapy, all should be considered for implantation of a cardiac defibrillator (p. 576). In patients with marked intraventricular conduction delay, prolonged depolarisation may lead to uncoordinated left ventricular contraction. When this is associated with severe symptomatic heart failure, cardiac resynchronisation therapy may be considered. Here, both the left and right ventricles are paced simultaneously in an attempt to generate a more coordinated left ventricular contraction and improve cardiac output.

Revascularisation

Coronary artery bypass surgery or percutaneous coronary intervention may improve function in areas of the myocardium that are 'hibernating' because of inadequate blood supply, and can be used to treat carefully selected patients with heart failure and coronary artery disease. If necessary, 'hibernating' myocardium can be identified by stress echocardiography and specialised nuclear techniques.

Heart transplantation

Cardiac transplantation is an established and very successful form of treatment for patients with intractable heart failure. Coronary artery disease and dilated cardiomyopathy are the most common indications. The introduction of ciclosporin for immunosuppression has improved survival, which now exceeds 90% at 1 year. The use of transplantation is limited by the availability of donor hearts so it is generally reserved for young patients with severe symptoms.

Conventional heart transplantation is contraindicated in patients with pulmonary vascular disease due to long-standing left heart failure, complex congenital heart disease (e.g. Eisenmenger's syndrome) or primary pulmonary hypertension, because the right ventricle of the donor heart may fail in the face of increased pulmonary vascular resistance. However, heart–lung transplantation can be successful for patients with Eisenmenger's syndrome. Lung transplantation has been used for primary pulmonary hypertension.

Although cardiac transplantation usually produces a dramatic improvement in the recipient's quality of life, serious complications may occur:

18.22 CONGESTIVE CARDIAC FAILURE IN OLD AGE

- **Incidence:** rises with age and affects 5–10% of people in their 80s.
- **Common causes:** coronary artery disease, hypertension and calcific degenerative valvular disease.
- **Diastolic dysfunction:** often prominent, particularly in those with a history of hypertension.
- **ACE inhibitors:** improve symptoms and mortality but more frequently associated with postural hypotension and renal impairment than in younger patients.
- **Loop diuretics:** usually required but may be poorly tolerated in those with urinary incontinence and men with prostate enlargement.

- *Rejection.* In spite of routine therapy with ciclosporin A, azathioprine and corticosteroids, episodes of rejection are common and may present with heart failure, arrhythmias or subtle ECG changes; cardiac biopsy is often used to confirm the diagnosis before starting treatment with high-dose corticosteroids.
- *Accelerated atherosclerosis.* Recurrent heart failure is often due to progressive atherosclerosis in the coronary arteries of the donor heart. This is not confined to patients who were transplanted for coronary artery disease and is probably a manifestation of chronic rejection. Angina is rare because the heart has been denervated.
- *Infection.* Opportunistic infection with organisms such as cytomegalovirus or *Aspergillus* remains a major cause of death in transplant recipients.

Ventricular assist devices

Because of the limited supply of donor organs, ventricular assist devices (VADs) have been employed as a bridge to cardiac transplantation, or more recently as potential long-term or 'destination' therapy. They assist cardiac output by using a roller, centrifugal or pulsatile pump that, in some cases, is implantable and portable. These devices withdraw blood through cannulae inserted in the atria or ventricular apex and pump it into the pulmonary artery or aorta. VADs are designed not only to unload the ventricles but also to provide support to the pulmonary and systemic circulations. Their more widespread application is limited by high complication rates (haemorrhage, systemic embolism, infection, neurological and renal sequelae), although some improvements in survival and quality of life have been demonstrated in patients with severe heart failure.

HYPERTENSION

High blood pressure is a trait as opposed to a specific disease and represents a quantitative rather than a qualitative deviation from the norm. Any definition of hypertension is therefore arbitrary.

Systemic blood pressure rises with age, and the incidence of cardiovascular disease (particularly stroke and coronary artery disease) is closely related to average blood pressure at all ages, even when blood pressure readings are within the so-called 'normal range'. Moreover, a series of randomised

controlled trials have demonstrated that antihypertensive therapy can reduce the incidence of stroke and, to a lesser extent, coronary artery disease (Box 18.99, p. 613).

The cardiovascular risks associated with a given blood pressure are dependent upon the combination of risk factors in the specific individual. These include age, gender, weight, physical inactivity, smoking, family history, serum cholesterol, diabetes mellitus and pre-existing vascular disease. Effective management of hypertension therefore requires a holistic approach that is based on the identification of those at highest cardiovascular risk and the adoption of multifactorial interventions, targeting not only blood pressure but all modifiable cardiovascular risk factors.

In light of these observations a practical definition of hypertension is 'the level of blood pressure at which the benefits of treatment outweigh the costs and hazards'. The British Hypertension Society classification of hypertension is provided in Figure 18.86 (p. 612) and is consistent with those defined by the European Society of Hypertension and the World Health Organization—International Society of Hypertension.

APPROACH TO NEWLY DIAGNOSED HYPERTENSION

Hypertension occasionally causes headache but most patients remain asymptomatic. Accordingly, the diagnosis is usually made at routine examination or when a complication arises. A blood pressure check is advisable every 5 years in adults.

The objectives of the initial evaluation of a patient with high blood pressure readings are:

- to obtain accurate and representative measurements of blood pressure
- to identify contributory factors and any underlying cause (secondary hypertension)
- to assess other risk factors and quantify cardiovascular risk
- to detect any complications (target organ damage) that are already present
- to identify comorbidity that may influence the choice of antihypertensive therapy.

These goals can usually be attained by a careful history, clinical examination and some simple investigations. Details of these, along with pathophysiology and management, are discussed on page 608.

SYNCOPE AND PRESYNCOPE

A wide variety of cardiovascular disorders can cause an abrupt fall in cerebral perfusion that may manifest as recurrent or isolated episodes of syncope (sudden loss of consciousness) and presyncope (lightheadedness and near-collapse).

Differential diagnosis

The common causes of blackouts and funny turns are listed in Figure 18.27. Diagnosis may be difficult but

18

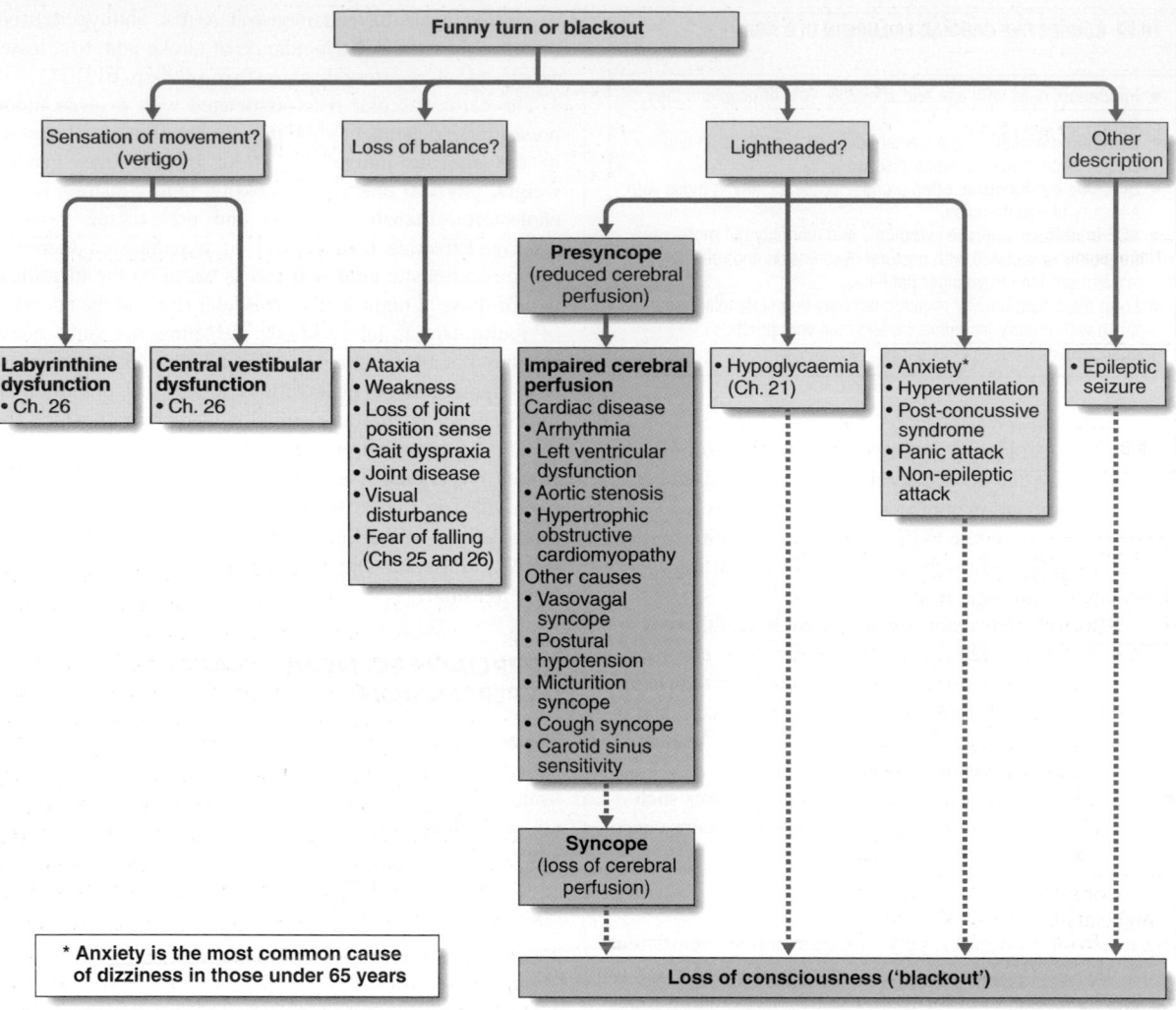

Fig. 18.27 The differential diagnosis of syncope and presyncope.

the probable mechanism of the patient's symptoms can usually be determined by careful analysis of the history. For example, a history of vertigo is suggestive of a labyrinthine or central vestibular disorder (p. 1164).

Whenever possible, an accurate description of the attack should be obtained from the patient and a witness. Particular attention should be paid to possible precipitants or triggers such as medication, exercise and alcohol, the duration of the unconscious period and the recovery phase. Some useful discriminants which can help to identify the likely mechanism of a blackout are listed in Box 18.23. In cardiac syncope, defined as due to arrhythmia or structural heart disease, onset is usually sudden and recovery is usually rapid. In contrast, patients with vasovagal syncope often feel nauseated and unwell for several minutes before and after the episode. Patients with seizures do not exhibit pallor, may have abnormal movements and usually take more than 5 minutes to recover and are often confused on recovery.

A careful history, clinical examination and simple tests will often reveal the cause of recurrent syncope. The pattern and description of the patient's symptoms should indicate the probable mechanism and will therefore determine subsequent investigations (Fig. 18.28).

Arrhythmia

Lightheadedness may occur in association with a wide variety of arrhythmias, but blackouts (Stokes–Adams attacks, p. 571) are usually due to profound bradycardia or malignant ventricular tachyarrhythmias. Ambulatory ECG recordings may help to establish the diagnosis but are of limited value unless the patient experiences typical symptoms while the recorder is in place. Since minor rhythm disturbances are quite common in the healthy population, a close temporal relationship must be demonstrated between the patient's symptoms and a recorded arrhythmia before arriving at a diagnosis. Patient-activated ECG recorders are useful diagnostic aids for patients with recurrent dizziness but are clearly of no value in assessing sudden episodes of collapse. In patients with presyncope or syncope in whom these investigations fail to establish a cause, an implantable 'loop recorder' can be placed beneath the skin of the upper chest under local anaesthetia. This device

18.23 TYPICAL FEATURES OF CARDIAC SYNCOPE, VASOVAGAL SYNCOPE AND SEIZURES

	Cardiac syncope	Vasovagal syncope	Seizures
Premonitory symptoms	Often none Lightheadedness Palpitation Chest pain Breathlessness	Nausea Lightheadedness Sweating	Confusion Hyperexcitability Olfactory hallucinations 'Aura'
Unconscious period	Extreme 'death-like' pallor	Pallor	Prolonged (> 1 min) unconsciousness Motor seizure activity* Tongue-biting Urinary incontinence
Recovery	Rapid recovery (< 1 min) Flushing	Slow Nausea Lightheadedness	Prolonged confusion (> 5 mins) Headache Focal neurological signs

* **N.B.** Cardiac syncope can also cause convulsions by inducing cerebral anoxia.

18

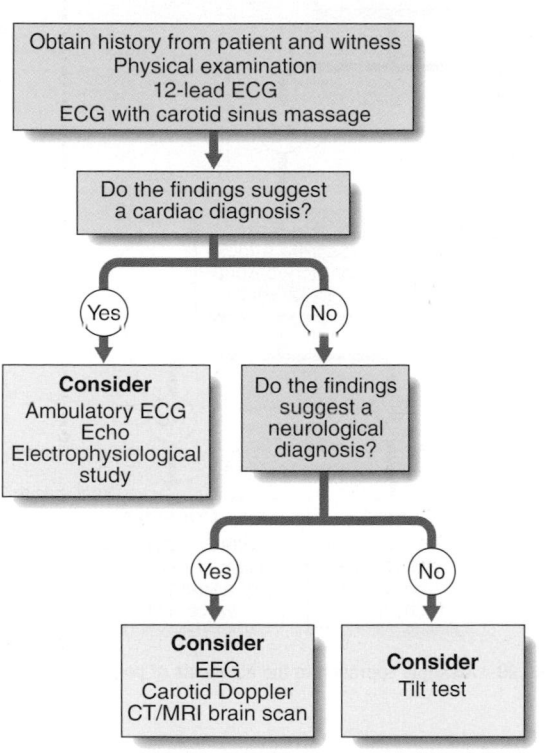

Fig. 18.28 A simple guide to the investigation and diagnosis of recurrent presyncope and syncope.

continuously records an ECG and will store arrhythmic events in its digital memory, which can be later accessed using a telemetry device.

Structural heart disease

Severe aortic stenosis, hypertrophic obstructive cardiomyopathy and severe coronary artery disease can cause lightheadedness or syncope on exertion. This is usually mediated by profound hypotension due to the combination of a reduction in cardiac output and a drop in peripheral vascular resistance, but may also be the consequence of an arrhythmia.

Carotid sinus syndrome

Hypersensitivity of the carotid baroreceptors can cause recurrent episodes of altered consciousness by promoting inappropriate bradycardia and vasodilatation. The diagnosis can be established by monitoring the ECG and blood pressure during carotid sinus massage; however, this should not be attempted in patients with suspected or proven carotid vascular disease as it may cause TIA. A positive cardio-inhibitory response is defined as a sinus pause of 3 seconds or more; a positive vasodepressor response is defined as a fall in systolic blood pressure of more than 50 mmHg. Carotid sinus massage will produce positive findings in about 10% of elderly subjects but fewer than 25% of these individuals will report spontaneous syncope. Symptoms should not therefore be attributed to the hypersensitive carotid sinus syndrome unless they are reproduced by carotid sinus massage. Dual-chamber pacing may relieve symptoms that are due to bradycardia.

Vasovagal syncope

This is usually triggered by a reduction in venous return due to prolonged standing, excessive heat or a large meal. It is mediated by the Bezold–Jarisch reflex, which is characterised by initial sympathetic activation that then leads to vigorous contraction of the relatively underfilled ventricles. This stimulates ventricular mechanoreceptors and in turn produces parasympathetic (vagal) activation and sympathetic withdrawal causing bradycardia, vasodilatation or both. Head-up tilt testing, which involves lying the patient on a table that is then tilted to an angle of 70° for up to 45 minutes while the ECG and blood pressure are monitored, can be used to confirm the diagnosis. A positive test is characterised by profound bradycardia (cardio-inhibitory response) and/or hypotension (vasodepressor response) that is associated with typical symptoms. Treatment is often unnecessary but in severe cases β-blockers (which inhibit the initial sympathetic activation) or disopyramide (a vagolytic agent) may be helpful. A dual-chamber pacemaker can be useful if symptoms are predominantly due to bradycardia. Finally, the subgroup of patients with a urinary sodium excretion of less than 170 mmol/24 hours may respond to salt loading.

Some variants of vasovagal syncope occur in the presence of identifiable triggers (e.g. cough syncope, micturition syncope) and are known collectively as situational syncope.

Postural hypotension

Symptomatic postural hypotension is caused by a failure of the normal compensatory mechanisms. Relative hypovolaemia (often due to excessive diuretic therapy), sympathetic degeneration (diabetes mellitus, Parkinson's disease, ageing) and drug therapy (vasodilators, antidepressants) can all cause or aggravate the problem. Treatment is often ineffective; however, withdrawing unnecessary medication while advising the patient to wear graduated elastic stockings and get up slowly may be helpful. Treatment with fludrocortisone, in an attempt to expand blood volume through sodium and water retention, may also be of value.

PALPITATION

Palpitation is a very common and sometimes frightening symptom. Patients may use the term to describe a wide variety of sensations including an unusually erratic, fast, slow or forceful heart beat and even chest pain or breathlessness. Initial evaluation should concentrate on determining the likely mechanism of the symptom and whether or not there is significant underlying heart disease.

A detailed description of the sensation is essential and patients should be asked to illustrate their experience by tapping out the heart beat on their chest or a table. A provisional diagnosis can usually be made on the basis of a careful and thorough history (Box 18.24 and Fig. 18.29), and investigations are often unnecessary. However, it may be necessary to obtain an ECG recording during an attack of typical palpitation to make a definitive diagnosis.

Recurrent but short-lived bouts of an irregular heart beat are usually due to atrial or ventricular extrasystoles (ectopic beats). Some patients will describe the experience as a 'flip' or a 'jolt' in the chest, while others report dropped or missed beats. Extrasystoles are often more frequent during periods of stress or debility; they may also be triggered by alcohol and some foodstuffs such as strong cheese or chocolate.

Poorly defined attacks of a pounding, forceful and relatively fast (90–120/min) heart beat are a common manifestation of anxiety. This symptom complex may also be a manifestation of other forms of a hyperdynamic circulation, such as anaemia, pregnancy and thyrotoxicosis, and can occur in some forms of valve disease (e.g. aortic regurgitation).

Discrete bouts of a very rapid (> 120/min) heart beat are more likely to be due to a paroxysmal arrhythmia. Atrial, junctional and ventricular tachycardias may all present in this way. In contrast, episodes of atrial fibrillation typically present with a characteristically irregular and chaotic tachycardia.

Palpitation is usually benign and, even if the patient's symptoms are due to an arrhythmia, the outlook is good if there is no underlying structural heart disease. Most cases are due to an awareness of the normal heart beat, a sinus

18.24 THE EVALUATION OF PALPITATION

- Is the palpitation continuous or intermittent?
- Is the heart beat regular or irregular?
- What is the approximate heart rate?
- Do symptoms occur in discrete attacks?
    Is the onset abrupt?
    How do attacks terminate?
- Are there any associated symptoms?
  e.g. Chest pain
       Lightheadedness
       Polyuria (a feature of supraventricular tachycardia, p. 564)
- Are there any precipitating factors, e.g. exercise, alcohol?
- Is there a history of structural heart disease, e.g. coronary artery disease, valvular heart disease?

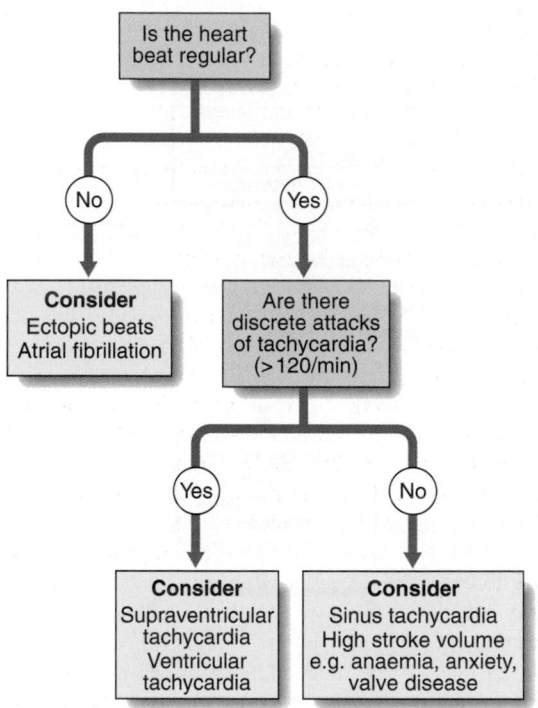

Fig. 18.29 A simple approach to the diagnosis of palpitation.

tachycardia or benign extrasystoles that have been triggered by stress, an intercurrent illness, or the effects of caffeine, alcohol and nicotine, but this may still be unpleasant and frightening. In these situations a careful explanation and reassurance may be all that is required. However, if the patient continues to experience distressing symptoms, a spell of treatment with a low dose of a β-blocker may be helpful.

The diagnosis and management of individual arrhythmias are considered in detail on pages 560–578.

CARDIAC ARREST AND SUDDEN CARDIAC DEATH

Cardiac arrest describes the sudden and complete loss of cardiac output due to asystole, ventricular tachycardia or fibrillation, or loss of mechanical cardiac contraction. The

18.25 COMMON CAUSES OF SUDDEN ARRHYTHMIC DEATH

Coronary artery disease (85%)

- Myocardial ischaemia
- Myocardial infarction (MI)
- Prior MI with myocardial scarring

Structural heart disease (10%)

- Aortic stenosis (p. 623)
- Hypertrophic cardiomyopathy (p. 642)
- Dilated cardiomyopathy (p. 641)
- Arrhythmogenic right ventricular dysplasia (p. 643)
- Congenital heart disease (p. 633)

No structural heart disease (5%)

- Long QT syndrome (p. 568)
- Brugada syndrome (p. 569)
- Wolff–Parkinson–White syndrome (p. 565)
- Adverse drug reactions (torsades de pointes, p. 568)
- Severe electrolyte abnormalities

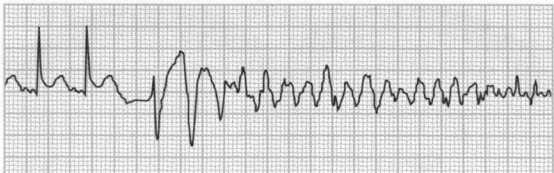

Fig. 18.30 Ventricular fibrillation. A bizarre chaotic rhythm initiated in this case by two ectopic beats in rapid succession.

18

clinical diagnosis is based on the victim being unconscious and pulseless (breathing may take some time to stop completely after cardiac arrest). Death is virtually inevitable unless effective treatment is given promptly.

Sudden cardiac death is usually due to the development of a catastrophic arrhythmia and accounts for 25–30% of deaths from cardiovascular disease, claiming an estimated 70 000 to 90 000 lives each year in the UK. Arrhythmias may complicate many types of heart disease and can sometimes occur in the absence of recognisable structural abnormalities (Box 18.25). Sudden death is also occasionally due to an acute mechanical catastrophe such as cardiac rupture or aortic dissection (p. 606).

Coronary artery disease is the most common condition leading to cardiac arrest. It can cause lethal arrhythmia in several settings. One-third of all people developing myocardial infarction die before reaching hospital, many within an hour of the onset of acute symptoms, and the cardiac rhythm in the majority of these cases is ventricular fibrillation or pulseless ventricular tachycardia. Acute myocardial ischaemia (in the absence of infarction) less often causes these arrhythmias. Patients with a history of previous myocardial infarction are at risk of sudden arrhythmic death due to a combination of scar-related arrhythmia and ischaemia. Patients at greatest risk are those with poor left ventricular function; this risk is reduced by appropriate treatment of heart failure with β-blockers and ACE inhibitors. Some of these patients may be suitable for implantation of a cardiac defibrillator (p. 576).

Aetiology of cardiac arrest

Cardiac arrest may be caused by ventricular fibrillation, pulseless ventricular tachycardia, asystole or pulseless electrical activity.

Ventricular fibrillation and pulseless ventricular tachycardia

These are the most common and most easily treatable cardiac arrest rhythms. Ventricular fibrillation produces rapid, ineffective, uncoordinated movement of the ventricles, which therefore produce no pulse. The ECG (Fig. 18.30) shows chaotic, bizarre, irregular ventricular complexes. Ventricular tachycardia (p. 567) can cause cardiac arrest if the ventricular rate is so rapid that effective mechanical contraction and relaxation cannot occur, or if it occurs in the presence of severe left ventricular impairment. This rhythm may degenerate into ventricular fibrillation. Defibrillation is the only effective treatment for these arrhythmias, and will restore cardiac output in more than 80% of patients if delivered immediately. However, the chances of a successful outcome fall by around 10% with each minute's delay, and by more if basic life support is not given (see below). When cardiac arrest occurs outside hospital, death is inevitable unless a defibrillator can be brought promptly to the patient.

Asystole

This occurs when there is no electrical activity within the ventricles and is usually due to failure of the conducting tissue or massive ventricular damage complicating myocardial infarction. Cardiac massage or a blow to the chest can sometimes restore cardiac activity, although an artificial pacemaker may be needed to prevent further attacks.

Pulseless electrical activity

This occurs when there is no effective cardiac output despite the presence of organised electrical activity. It may be caused by reversible conditions such as hypovolaemia, cardiac tamponade or tension pneumothorax (Fig. 18.33) but is often due to a catastrophic event such as cardiac rupture or massive pulmonary embolism and therefore carries an extremely poor prognosis.

Management of cardiac arrest

The Chain of Survival

This term refers to the sequence of events that are necessary to maximise the chances of a cardiac arrest victim surviving (Fig. 18.31). A victim of cardiac arrest is most likely to survive if all links in the chain are strong, i.e. if the arrest is witnessed, help is called immediately, basic life support is administered by a trained individual, the emergency medical services respond promptly, and defibrillation is achieved within a few minutes. Good training in both basic and advanced life support is essential to the practice of medicine, and should be maintained by regular refresher courses. In recent years, public access defibrillation has been introduced in places of high population density, particularly where traffic congestion may impede the response of emergency services, e.g. railway stations, airports and sports stadia. Designated individuals can respond to a cardiac

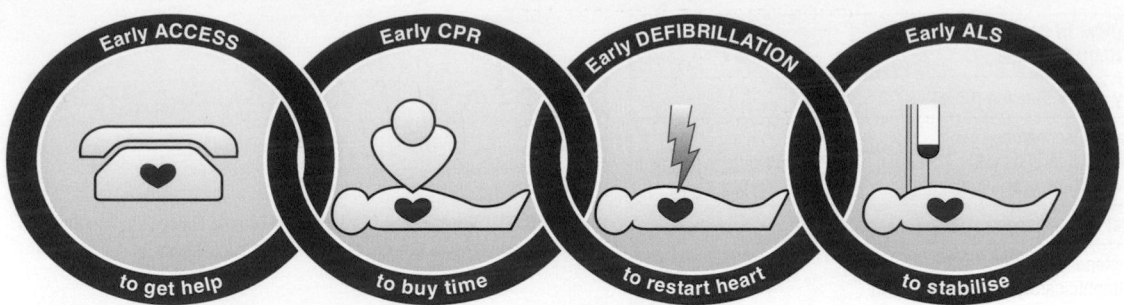

Fig. 18.31   The Chain of Survival in cardiac arrest. (CPR = cardiopulmonary resuscitation; ALS = advanced life support)

arrest using basic life support and an automated external defibrillator.

Basic life support (BLS)

BLS encompasses manoeuvres that attempt to maintain a low level of circulation until more definitive treatment with advanced life support can be given. Management of the collapsed patient requires prompt assessment and restoration of the airway, maintenance of breathing using rescue breathing ('mouth-to-mouth' breathing) and maintenance of the circulation using chest compressions (Fig. 18.32), with the aim of maintaining the circulation until more definitive treatment with advanced life support can be administered.

Advanced life support (ALS)

ALS (Fig. 18.33) aims to restore normal cardiac rhythm by defibrillation when the cause of cardiac arrest is due to a tachyarrhythmia, or to restore cardiac output by correcting other reversible causes of cardiac arrest. ALS can also involve administration of intravenous drugs to support the circulation, and endotracheal intubation to ventilate the lungs. An updated guideline will be released in 2006, and will be placed on the Davidson website (www.studentconsult.com).

If cardiac arrest is witnessed, a precordial thump may sometimes convert ventricular fibrillation or tachycardia to normal rhythm, but this is futile if cardiac arrest has lasted longer than a few seconds.

The priority is to assess the patient's cardiac rhythm by attaching a defibrillator/monitor. Ventricular fibrillation (VF) or pulseless ventricular tachycardia (VT) is treated with immediate defibrillation. In recent years, defibrillators have been developed that produce a biphasic shock, i.e. the polarity of the shock is reversed midway through the delivery. This allows more reliable defibrillation at low shock energies. Thus, defibrillation is firstly with a biphasic shock of 100 joules or 200 joules monophasic. If normal rhythm is not restored, a further shock of 100 joules is given; if unsuccessful, this is followed by a third shock of 150 joules (360 joules if monophasic). If these three shocks are unsuccessful, 1 mg of adrenaline (epinephrine) intravenously and a further 1 minute of cardiopulmonary resuscitation should be given before trying a further sequence of up to three biphasic shocks, each at 150 joules (or 360 joules monophasic).

Ventricular fibrillation of low amplitude, or 'fine VF', may mimic asystole. Therefore, if asystole cannot be confidently diagnosed, the patient should be regarded as having 'fine VF' and defibrillated. If an electrical rhythm is present which would be expected to produce a cardiac output, 'pulseless electrical activity' is present. There are several potentially reversible causes which can be easily remembered as a list of four Hs and four Ts (green box, Fig. 18.33). Pulseless electrical activity is treated by maintaining cardiopulmonary resuscitation (CPR) whilst seeking such causes. Asystole is treated by cardiopulmonary resuscitation, with the additional support of atropine and adrenaline (epinephrine), and sometimes external or transvenous pacing in an attempt to generate an electrical rhythm.

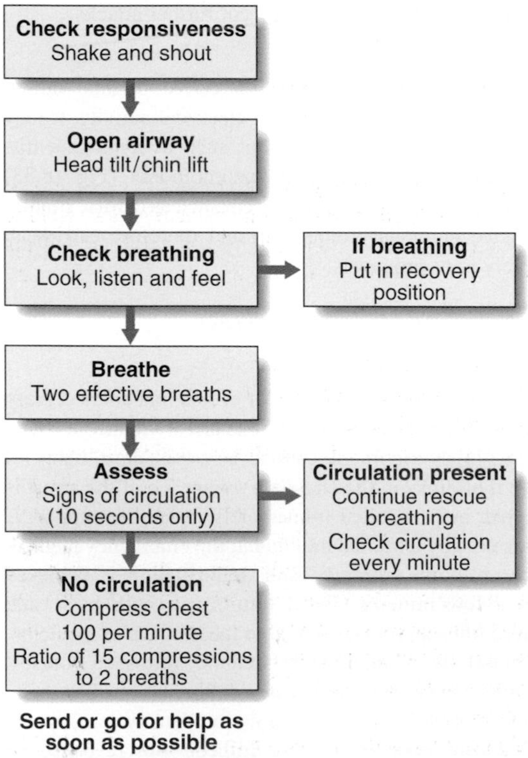

Survivors of cardiac arrest

Patients who survive a cardiac arrest caused by acute myocardial infarction need no specific treatment beyond that given to those recovering from an uncomplicated infarct, since their prognosis is similar (p. 600). Those with reversible causes, such as exercise-induced ischaemia or

Check responsiveness
Shake and shout

↓

Open airway
Head tilt/chin lift

↓

Check breathing
Look, listen and feel → **If breathing**
Put in recovery position

↓

Breathe
Two effective breaths

↓

Assess
Signs of circulation
(10 seconds only) → **Circulation present**
Continue rescue breathing
Check circulation every minute

↓

No circulation
Compress chest
100 per minute
Ratio of 15 compressions to 2 breaths

Send or go for help as soon as possible

Fig. 18.32   Algorithm for adult basic life support. For further information see www.resus.org.uk.

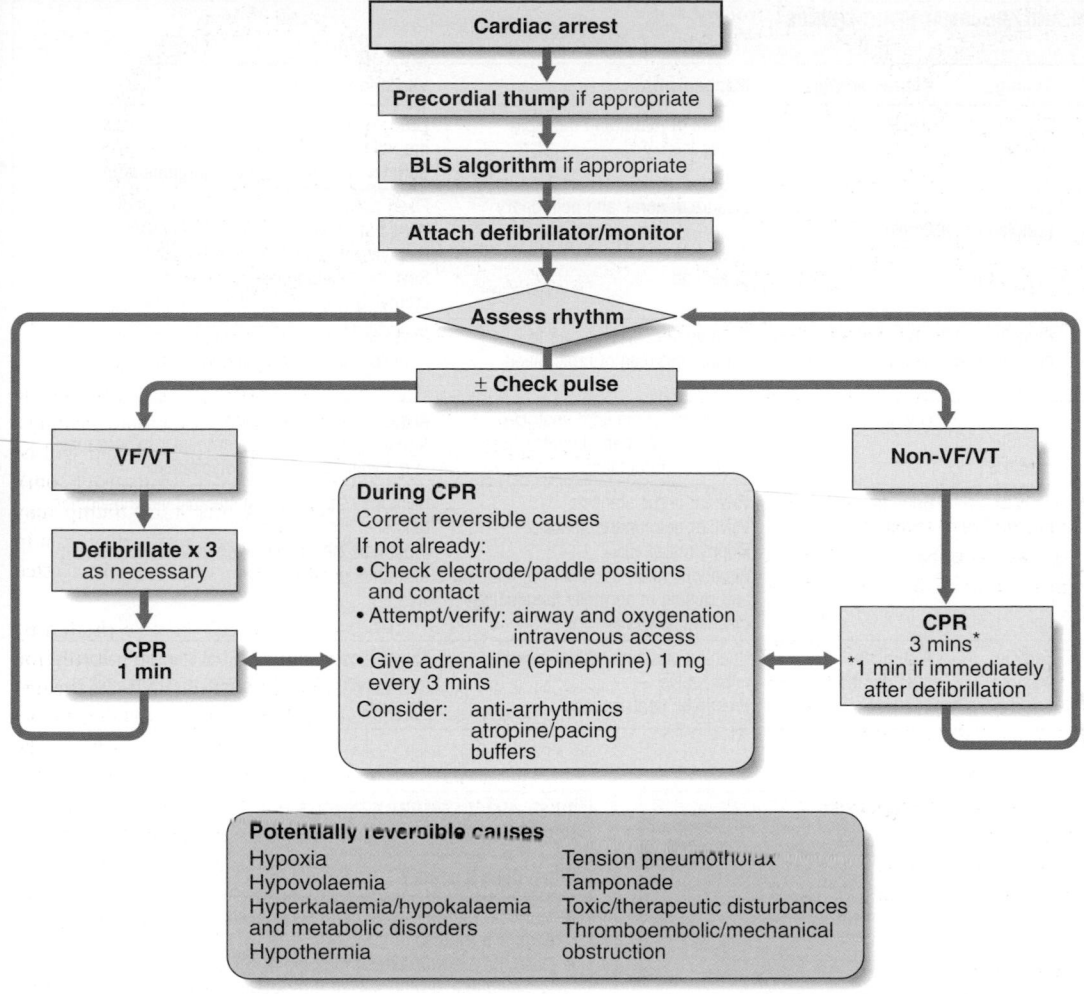

Fig. 18.33 Algorithm for adult advanced life support. For further information see www.resus.org.uk. (BLS = basic life support; VF = ventricular fibrillation; VT = pulseless ventricular tachycardia; CPR = cardiopulmonary resuscitation)

aortic stenosis (p. 623), should have the underlying cause treated if possible. Survivors of VT or VF arrest in whom no reversible cause can be identified may be at risk of another episode and should be considered for anti-arrhythmic therapy or implantation of an implantable cardiac defibrillator (p. 576).

ABNORMAL HEART SOUNDS AND MURMURS

The first clinical manifestation of heart disease may be the discovery of an abnormal sound on auscultation (Box 18.26). Such a finding may be incidental—for example, during a routine childhood examination—or may be prompted by symptoms of heart disease. Clinical evaluation is always helpful but an echocardiogram is often necessary to confirm the nature of an abnormal heart sound or murmur.

Is the sound cardiac?
Additional heart sounds and murmurs demonstrate a consistent relationship to a specific part of the cardiac cycle, but extracardiac sounds (e.g. pleural rub or venous hum) do not. Pericardial friction produces a characteristic scratching or crunching noise, which often has two components corresponding to atrial and ventricular systole and may vary with posture and respiration.

Is the sound pathological?
Pathological sounds and murmurs are the product of turbulent blood flow or rapid ventricular filling due to abnormal loading conditions. Some added sounds are physiological but may also occur in pathological conditions; for example, a third sound is common in young people and in pregnancy but is also a feature of heart failure (Box 18.26). Similarly, a systolic murmur due to turbulence across the right ventricular outflow tract may occur in hyperdynamic states (e.g. anaemia, pregnancy) but may also be due to pulmonary stenosis or an intracardiac shunt leading to volume overload of the right ventricle (e.g. atrial septal defect).

Benign murmurs do not occur in diastole (Box 18.27), and systolic murmurs that radiate or are associated with a thrill are almost always pathological.

18.26 NORMAL AND ABNORMAL HEART SOUNDS

Sound	Timing	Characteristics	Mechanisms	Variable features
First heart sound (S1)	Onset of systole	Usually single or narrowly split	Closure of mitral and tricuspid valves	Loud: hyperdynamic circulation (anaemia, pregnancy, thyrotoxicosis); mitral stenosis Soft: heart failure; mitral regurgitation
Second heart sound (S2)	End of systole	Split on inspiration Single on expiration (p. 526)	Closure of aortic and pulmonary valve A_2 first P_2 second	Fixed wide splitting with atrial septal defect Wide but variable splitting with delayed right heart emptying (e.g. right bundle branch block) Reversed splitting due to delayed left heart emptying (e.g. left bundle branch block)
Third heart sound (S3)	Early in diastole, just after S2	Low pitch, often heard as 'gallop'	From ventricular wall due to abrupt cessation of rapid filling	Physiological: young people, pregnancy Pathological: heart failure, mitral regurgitation
Fourth heart sound (S4)	End of diastole, just before S1	Low pitch	Ventricular origin (stiff ventricle and augmented atrial contraction) related to atrial filling	Absent in atrial fibrillation A feature of severe left ventricular hypertrophy (e.g. hypertrophic cardiomyopathy)
Systolic clicks	Early or mid-systole	Brief, high-intensity sound	Valvular aortic stenosis Valvular pulmonary stenosis Floppy mitral valve Prosthetic heart sounds from opening and closing of normally functioning mechanical valves	Click may be lost when stenotic valve becomes thickened or calcified Prosthetic clicks lost when valve obstructed by thrombus or vegetations
Opening snap (OS)	Early in diastole	High pitch, brief duration	Opening of stenosed leaflets of mitral valve Prosthetic heart sounds	Moves closer to S2 as mitral stenosis becomes more severe. May be absent in calcific mitral stenosis

18.27 FEATURES OF A BENIGN OR INNOCENT HEART MURMUR

- Soft
- Mid-systolic
- Heard at left sternal edge
- No radiation
- No other cardiac abnormalities

Auscultatory evaluation of a heart murmur

Timing, intensity, location, radiation and quality are all useful clues to the origin and nature of a heart murmur (Box 18.28). Radiation of a murmur is determined by the direction of turbulent blood flow and is only detectable when there is a high-velocity jet, e.g. in mitral regurgitation (radiation from apex to axilla) or aortic stenosis (radiation from base to neck). Similarly, the pitch and quality of the sound can help to distinguish the murmur, e.g. the 'blowing' murmur of mitral regurgitation or the 'rasping' murmur of aortic stenosis.

The position of a murmur in relation to the cardiac cycle should be assessed by timing it with the heart sounds, carotid pulse and apex beat; this is a very valuable discriminant (Figs 18.34 and 18.35).

Systolic murmurs associated with ventricular outflow tract obstruction (Box 18.29)

These occur in mid-systole and have a crescendo-decrescendo pattern reflecting the changing velocity of blood flow. Pansystolic murmurs maintain a constant intensity and extend from the first heart sound throughout systole (up to and beyond the second heart sound). They occur when blood leaks from a ventricle into a low-pressure

18.28 AUSCULTATORY FEATURES OF HEART MURMURS
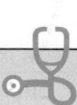

When does it occur?

- Time the murmur using heart sounds, carotid pulse and the apex beat. Is it systolic or diastolic?
- Does the murmur extend throughout systole or diastole or is it confined to a shorter part of the cardiac cycle?

How loud is it? (intensity)

- Grade 1   Very soft (only audible in ideal conditions)
- Grade 2   Soft
- Grade 3   Moderate
- Grade 4   Loud with associated thrill
- Grade 5   Very loud
- Grade 6   Heard without stethoscope

N.B. Diastolic murmurs are sometimes graded 1–4.

Where is it heard best? (location)

- Listen over the apex and base of the heart, including the aortic and pulmonary areas

Where does it radiate?

- Evaluate radiation to the neck, axilla or back

What does it sound like? (pitch and quality)

- Pitch is determined by flow (high pitch indicates high-velocity flow)
- Is the intensity constant or variable?

chamber at an even or constant velocity; mitral regurgitation, tricuspid regurgitation and ventricular septal defect are the only causes of a pansystolic murmur. Late systolic murmurs are unusual but may occur in mitral valve prolapse (if the mitral regurgitation is confined to late

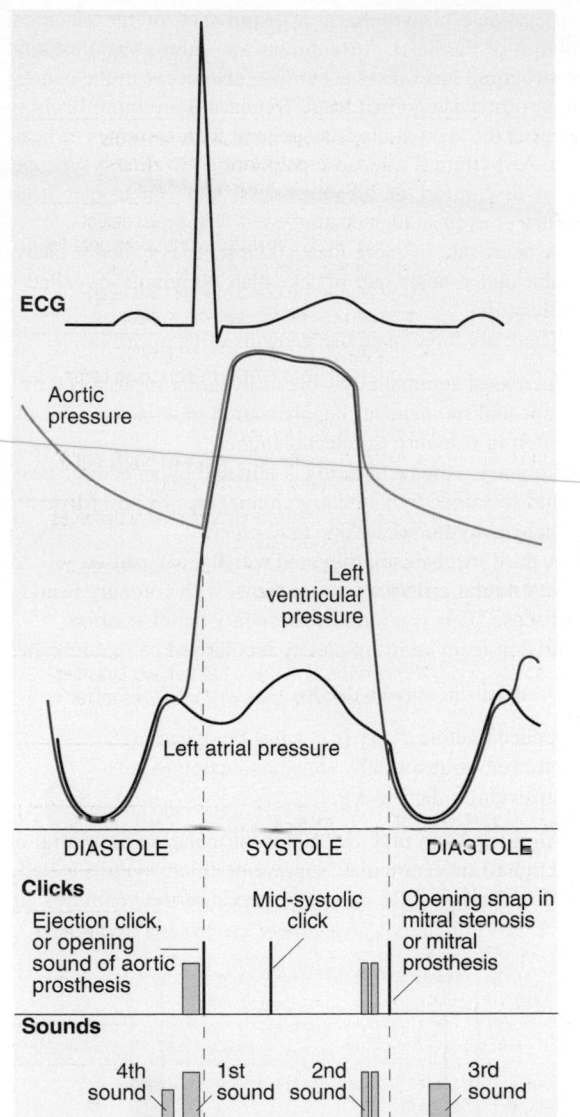

Fig. 18.34 The relationship of the cardiac cycle to the ECG, the left ventricular pressure wave and the position of heart sounds.

systole) and hypertrophic cardiomyopathy (if dynamic obstruction occurs late in systole).

Mid-diastolic murmurs

These are due to accelerated or turbulent flow across the mitral or tricuspid valves. They are low-pitched noises that are often difficult to hear, and should be evaluated with the bell of the stethoscope. A mid-diastolic murmur may be due to mitral stenosis (located at the apex and axilla), tricuspid stenosis (located at the left sternal edge), increased flow across the mitral valve (e.g. the to-and-fro murmur of severe mitral regurgitation) or increased flow across the tricuspid valve (e.g. left-to-right shunt through a large atrial septal defect). Early diastolic murmurs have a soft, blowing quality with a decrescendo pattern and should be evaluated with the diaphragm of the stethoscope; they are due to regurgitation

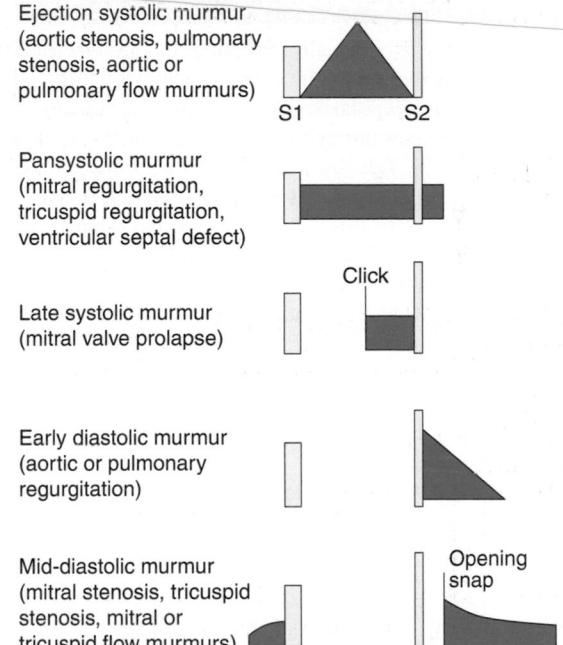

Fig. 18.35 The timing and pattern of cardiac murmurs.

18

18.29 FEATURES OF SOME COMMON SYSTOLIC MURMURS

Condition	Timing and duration	Quality	Location and radiation	Associated features
Aortic stenosis	Mid-systolic	Loud rasping	Base and left sternal edge, radiating to suprasternal notch and carotids	Single second heart sound Ejection click (in young patients) Slow rising pulse Left ventricular hypertrophy (pressure overload)
Mitral regurgitation	Pansystolic	Blowing	Apex, radiating to axilla	Soft first heart sound Third heart sound Left ventricular hypertrophy (volume overload)
Ventricular septal defect (VSD)	Pansystolic	Harsh	Lower left sternal edge, radiating to whole precordium	Thrill Biventricular hypertrophy
Benign	Mid-systolic	Soft	Left sternal edge, no radiation	No other signs of heart disease

18

across the aortic or pulmonary valves and are best heard at the left sternal edge with the patient sitting forwards in held expiration.

Continuous murmurs

These result from a combination of systolic and diastolic flow (e.g. persistent ductus arteriosus) and must be distinguished from extracardiac noises such as bruits from arterial shunts, venous hums (high rates of venous flow in children) and pericardial friction rubs.

The characteristics of specific valve defects and congenital anomalies are described in the relevant sections later in the chapter.

DISORDERS OF HEART RATE, RHYTHM AND CONDUCTION

The heart beat is normally initiated by an electrical discharge from the sinoatrial (sinus) node. The atria and ventricles then depolarise sequentially as electrical depolarisation passes through specialised conducting tissues (Fig. 18.6, p. 527). The sinus node acts as a pacemaker and its intrinsic rate is regulated by the autonomic nervous system; vagal activity slows the heart rate, and sympathetic activity accelerates it via cardiac sympathetic nerves and circulating catecholamines.

If the sinus rate becomes unduly slow, a lower centre may assume the role of pacemaker. This is known as an escape rhythm and may arise in the AV node (nodal rhythm) or the ventricles (idioventricular rhythm).

A cardiac arrhythmia is a disturbance of the electrical rhythm of the heart. Arrhythmias are often a manifestation of structural heart disease but may also occur in the context of an otherwise normal heart. Symptoms are more likely to occur if the arrhythmia is associated with extremes of heart rate. Arrhythmias can cause palpitation, dizziness, syncope, chest discomfort or breathlessness, and can trigger heart failure or even sudden death.

A heart rate of more than 100/minute is called a tachycardia and a heart rate of less than 60/minute is called a bradycardia.

There are three main mechanisms of tachycardia:

- Increased automaticity—the tachycardia is produced by repeated spontaneous depolarisation of an ectopic focus, often in response to catecholamines.
- Re-entry—the tachycardia is initiated by an ectopic beat and sustained by a re-entry circuit (Fig. 18.36). Most tachyarrhythmias are due to re-entry.
- A third mechanism, triggered activity, can cause ventricular arrhythmias in patients with coronary heart disease. This is a form of secondary depolarisation arising from an incompletely repolarised cell membrane.

Bradycardia may be due to:

- reduced automaticity (e.g. sinus bradycardia)
- blocked or abnormally slow conduction (e.g. atrioventricular block).

An arrhythmia may be 'supraventricular' (sinus, atrial or junctional) or ventricular. Supraventricular rhythms usually produce narrow QRS complexes because the ventricles are

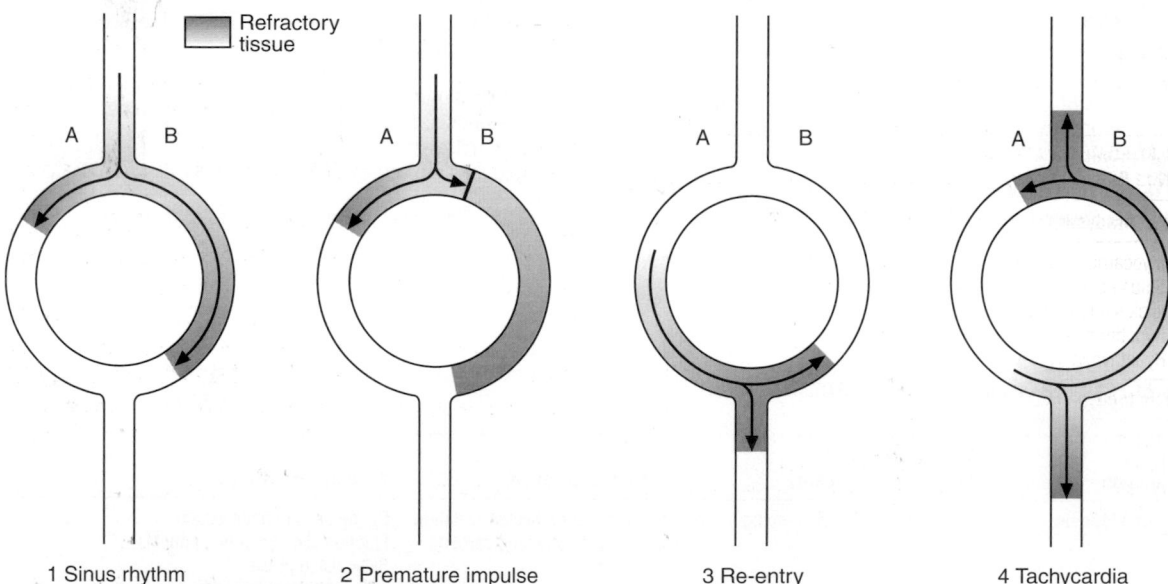

1 Sinus rhythm   2 Premature impulse   3 Re-entry   4 Tachycardia

Fig. 18.36   The mechanism of re-entry. Re-entry can occur when there are two alternative pathways with different conducting properties (e.g. the AV node and an accessory pathway, or an area of normal tissue and an area of ischaemic tissue). In this example, pathway A conducts slowly and recovers quickly while pathway B conducts rapidly and recovers slowly. (1) In sinus rhythm each impulse passes down both pathways before entering a common distal pathway. (2) As the pathways recover at different rates a premature impulse may find pathway A open and B closed. (3) Pathway B may recover while the premature impulse travels selectively down pathway A. The impulse may then travel retrogradely up pathway B, setting up a closed loop or re-entry circuit. (4) This may initiate a tachycardia that will continue until the circuit is interrupted by a change in conduction rates or electrical depolarisation.

depolarised normally through the AV node and bundle of His. In contrast, ventricular rhythms produce broad bizarre QRS complexes because the ventricles are activated in an abnormal sequence. However, occasionally a supraventricular rhythm can produce broad or wide QRS complexes due to coexisting bundle branch block or the presence of accessory conducting tissue (see below).

SINUS RHYTHMS

SINUS ARRHYTHMIA

Phasic alteration of the heart rate during respiration (the sinus rate increases during inspiration and slows during expiration) is a consequence of normal parasympathetic nervous system activity and can be pronounced in children. Absence of this normal variation in heart rate with breathing or with changes in posture may be a feature of autonomic neuropathy (p. 844).

SINUS BRADYCARDIA

A sinus rate of less than 60/min may occur in healthy people at rest and is a common finding in athletes. Some pathological causes are listed in Box 18.30. Asymptomatic sinus bradycardia requires no treatment. Symptomatic sinus bradycardia usually responds to intravenous atropine 0.6–1.2 mg.

SINUS TACHYCARDIA

This is defined as a sinus rate of more than 100/min, and is usually due to an increase in sympathetic activity associated with exercise, emotion, pregnancy or pathology (Box 18.30). Young adults can produce a rapid sinus rate, up to 200/min, during intense exercise.

18.30 SOME PATHOLOGICAL CAUSES OF SINUS BRADYCARDIA AND TACHYCARDIA	
Sinus bradycardia	
• Myocardial infarction	• Cholestatic jaundice
• Sinus node disease (sick sinus syndrome)	• Raised intracranial pressure
• Hypothermia	• Drugs, e.g. β-blocker, digoxin, verapamil
• Hypothyroidism	
Sinus tachycardia	
• Anxiety	• Thyrotoxicosis
• Fever	• Phaeochromocytoma
• Anaemia	• Drugs, e.g. β-adrenoceptor agonists (bronchodilators)
• Heart failure	

ATRIAL TACHYARRHYTHMIAS

ATRIAL ECTOPIC BEATS (EXTRASYSTOLES, PREMATURE BEATS)

These usually cause no symptoms but can give the sensation of a missed beat or an abnormally strong beat. The ECG

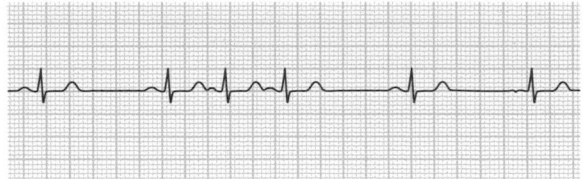

Fig. 18.37 Atrial ectopic beats. The first, second and fifth complexes are normal sinus beats. The third, fourth and sixth complexes are atrial ectopic beats with identical QRS complexes and abnormal (sometimes barely visible) P waves.

(Fig. 18.37) shows a premature but otherwise normal QRS complex; if visible, the preceding P wave has a different morphology because the atria activate from an abnormal site. In most cases these are of no consequence, although very frequent atrial ectopic beats may herald the onset of atrial fibrillation. Treatment is rarely necessary.

ATRIAL TACHYCARDIA

Atrial tachycardia may be a manifestation of increased atrial automaticity, sinoatrial disease or digoxin toxicity. It produces a narrow complex tachycardia with abnormal P-wave morphology, sometimes associated with atrioventricular block if the atrial rate is rapid. It may respond to β-blockers, which reduce automaticity, or class I or III antiarrhythmic drugs (Box 18.42, p. 574). The ventricular response in rapid atrial tachycardias may be controlled by AV node-blocking drugs. Catheter ablation therapy can be offered to patients with recurrent or drug-resistant atrial tachycardia.

ATRIAL FLUTTER

Atrial flutter is characterised by a large (macro) re-entry circuit within the right atrium, usually encircling the tricuspid annulus. The atrial rate is approximately 300/min. It is usually associated with 2:1, 3:1, or 4:1 atrioventricular block (with corresponding heart rates of 150, 100, 75). Rarely, in young patients, every beat is conducted, producing a heart rate of 300/min and haemodynamic collapse. The ECG shows saw-toothed flutter waves (Fig. 18.38). When there is regular 2:1 AV block it may be difficult to identify flutter waves which are buried in the QRS complexes and T-waves. Atrial flutter should always be suspected when there is a narrow complex tachycardia of

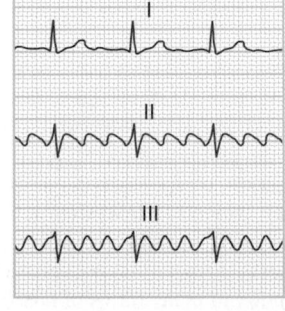

Fig. 18.38 Atrial flutter. Simultaneous recording showing atrial flutter with 3:1 atrioventricular block; flutter waves are only visible in leads II and III.

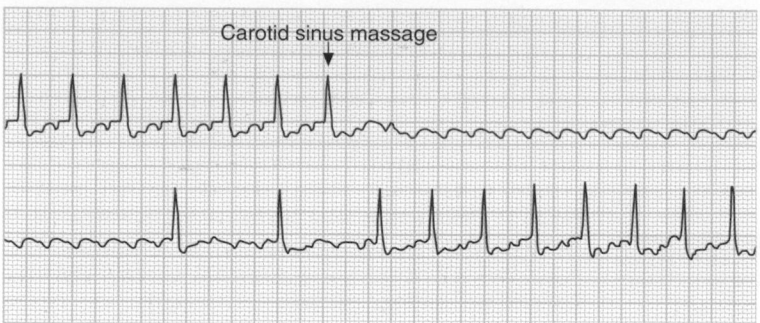

Fig. 18.39 Carotid sinus massage in atrial flutter: continuous trace. In this example, the diagnosis of atrial flutter with 2:1 block was established when carotid sinus massage produced temporary AV block revealing the flutter waves.

150/min. Carotid sinus massage or intravenous adenosine may help to establish the diagnosis by temporarily increasing the degree of AV block and revealing the flutter waves (Fig. 18.39).

Management

Digoxin, β-blockers or verapamil can be used to control the ventricular rate (pp. 572–575). However, in many cases it may be preferable to try and restore sinus rhythm by direct current (DC) cardioversion or drug therapy. Amiodarone, propafenone or flecainide may be effective and can also be used to prevent recurrent episodes of atrial flutter. Flecainide should always be prescribed with an AV node-blocking drug, e.g. a β-blocker. Catheter ablation offers a 90% chance of complete cure and is the treatment of choice for patients with persistent and troublesome symptoms.

ATRIAL FIBRILLATION

Atrial fibrillation (AF) is the most common sustained cardiac arrhythmia, with an overall prevalence of 0.5% in the adult population of the UK. The prevalence rises with age, affecting 2–5% of 70-year-olds and 9% of those aged over 80 years. Atrial fibrillation is characterised by the presence of multiple, interacting re-entry circuits looping around the atria. Episodes are often initiated by salvoes of ectopic beats that can arise from conducting tissue in the pulmonary veins or from diseased atrial tissue. AF is more likely to become sustained in atria that are enlarged, or in which conduction is slow (as is the case in many forms of heart disease). During episodes of AF, the atria beat rapidly, but in an uncoordinated and ineffective manner. The ventricles are activated irregularly at a rate determined by conduction through the AV node. This produces the characteristic 'irregularly irregular' pulse. The ECG (Fig. 18.40) shows normal but irregular QRS complexes; there are no P waves but the baseline may show irregular fibrillation waves.

AF can be classified as paroxysmal (intermittent, self-terminating episodes), persistent (prolonged episodes that can be terminated by electrical or chemical cardioversion) or permanent. In patients seen for the first time with AF it can be difficult to identify which form of the arrhythmia is present. Unfortunately for many patients, paroxysmal AF will become permanent as the underlying disease process that predisposes to AF progresses.

AF may be the first manifestation of many forms of heart

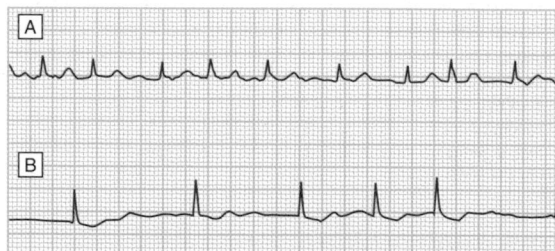

Fig. 18.40 Two examples of atrial fibrillation. The QRS complexes are irregular and there are no P waves. A There is usually a fast ventricular rate, often between 120 and 160/min, at the onset of atrial fibrillation. B In chronic atrial fibrillation the ventricular rate may be much slower due to the effects of medication and AV nodal fatigue.

18.31 COMMON CAUSES OF ATRIAL FIBRILLATION

- Coronary artery disease (including acute myocardial infarction)
- Valvular heart disease, especially rheumatic mitral valve disease
- Hypertension
- Sinoatrial disease
- Hyperthyroidism
- Alcohol
- Cardiomyopathy
- Congenital heart disease
- Chest infection
- Pulmonary embolism
- Pericardial disease
- Idiopathic (lone AF)

disease (Box 18.31), particularly those that are associated with enlargement or dilatation of the atria. Alcohol, hyperthyroidism and chest disease are also common causes of AF, although multiple aetiological factors often coexist such as the combination of alcohol, hypertension and coronary disease. About 50% of all patients with paroxysmal AF and 20% of patients with persistent or permanent AF have otherwise normal hearts: an entity sometimes known as 'lone atrial fibrillation'.

AF can cause palpitation, breathlessness and fatigue. In patients with poor ventricular function or valve disease it may precipitate or aggravate cardiac failure because of loss of atrial function and heart rate control. A fall in blood pressure may cause lightheadedness, and chest pain may occur with underlying coronary disease. However, AF is often completely asymptomatic, in which case it is usually discovered as the result of a routine examination or ECG.

18.32 ATRIAL FIBRILLATION IN OLD AGE

- **Prevalence:** rises with age, reaching more than 10% in those over 80 years of age.
- **Symptoms:** sometimes asymptomatic but often accompanied by diastolic heart failure.
- **Hyperthyroidism:** AF may be the dominant feature of otherwise silent or occult hyperthyroidism.
- **Cardioversion:** followed by high rates (~70% at one year) of recurrent AF.
- **Stroke:** AF is an important cause of cerebral embolism. It is found in 15% of all stroke patients and 2–8% of those with TIAs.
- **Anticoagulation:** although the risk of thromboembolism rises, the hazards of anticoagulation also rise with age because of increased comorbidity, particularly cognitive impairment and falls.
- **Target INR:** if anticoagulation is recommended, in those over 75 years, care should be taken to maintain an INR below 3.0 because of the increased risk of intracranial haemorrhage.
- **Aspirin:** a safer alternative if anticoagulation cannot be recommended, but its benefits in reducing the risk of stroke are less significant and consistent than with warfarin.

AF is associated with a twofold increase in mortality and significant morbidity which are largely attributable to the effects of the underlying heart disease and the risk of cerebral embolism. Careful assessment, risk stratification and therapy can improve the outlook considerably.

Management

Assessment of patients with newly diagnosed AF includes a full history, physical examination, 12-lead ECG, echocardiogram and thyroid function tests. Additional investigations such as exercise testing may be needed to determine the nature and extent of any underlying heart disease. Biochemical evidence of hyperthyroidism is found in a small minority of patients with otherwise unexplained AF.

When AF complicates an acute illness (e.g. chest infection, pulmonary embolism), effective treatment of the primary disorder will usually restore sinus rhythm. Otherwise, the main objectives are to restore sinus rhythm as soon as possible, prevent recurrent episodes of AF, optimise the heart rate during periods of AF, minimise the risk of thromboembolism and treat any underlying disease.

Paroxysmal atrial fibrillation

Occasional attacks that are well tolerated do not necessarily require treatment, but β-blockers are the drug of choice if symptoms are troublesome. Beta-blockers are particularly useful for treating patients with AF associated with ischaemic heart disease, hypertension and cardiac failure. They may prevent AF in those who are prone to episodes during exertion or at times of stress. Class Ic drugs (Box 18.42, p. 574) such as propafenone or flecainide are also effective at preventing episodes but should be avoided in patients with coronary disease or left ventricular dysfunction. Amiodarone is the most effective agent for preventing AF but its side-effects restrict its use to patients in whom other measures fail. Digoxin and verapamil are not effective drugs for preventing paroxysms of AF, although they serve to limit the heart rate when AF occurs by blocking the AV node. Radiofrequency ablation has emerged as a promising treatment for paroxysmal AF in patients who do not have structural heart disease (p. 576). It is usually directed at the ostia of the pulmonary veins from which triggering ectopic beats may emanate. Ablation prevents AF in up to 70% of patients with prior drug-resistant episodes, although anti-arrhythmic drugs often need to be continued afterwards to maintain sinus rhythm. An alternative strategy, suitable for patients with structural heart disease, is 'overdrive' atrial pacing, which helps to maintain sinus rhythm in patients with bradycardia-related AF (which is often a manifestation of sinoatrial disease) and which may suppress the ectopic triggers for AF. This is effective in around 60% of patients treated.

Persistent and permanent atrial fibrillation

There are two options for treating persistent AF:

- attempting to restore and maintain sinus rhythm: rhythm control
- accepting that AF will be permanent and using treatments to control the ventricular rate and to prevent embolic complications: rate control.

Rhythm control. An attempt to restore sinus rhythm is particularly appropriate if the arrhythmia has precipitated troublesome symptoms and there is a modifiable or treatable underlying cause. Electrical cardioversion (p. 575) is initially successful in three-quarters of patients but relapse is frequent (25–50% at 1 month and 70–90% at 1 year). Attempts to restore and maintain sinus rhythm are most successful if AF has been present for < 3 months, the patient is young, and there is no important structural heart disease.

Immediate DC cardioversion, after the administration of intravenous heparin, is appropriate if AF has been present for less than 48 hours. An attempt to restore sinus rhythm by infusing intravenous flecainide (2 mg/kg over 30 minutes, maximum dose 150 mg) is a safe and attractive alternative to electrical cardioversion if there is no underlying structural heart disease. In other situations, DC cardioversion should be deferred until the patient has been established on warfarin, with an international normalised ratio (INR) of between 2.0 and 3.0, for a minimum of 3 weeks, and any underlying problems, such as hyperthyroidism, have been dealt with. Anticoagulation should be maintained for at least 1 month and ideally for 6 months following successful cardioversion; if relapse occurs, a second (or third) cardioversion may be appropriate. Concomitant anti-arrhythmic therapy with drugs such as amiodarone or β-blockers may reduce the risk of recurrence.

Rate control. If sinus rhythm cannot be restored, treatment should be directed towards maintaining an appropriate heart rate. Digoxin, β-blockers or rate-limiting calcium antagonists such as verapamil or diltiazem (pp. 573–575) will reduce the ventricular rate by increasing the degree of AV block. This alone may produce a striking improvement in overall cardiac function, particularly in patients with mitral stenosis. Beta-blockers and rate-limiting calcium antagonists are often more effective than digoxin at controlling the heart rate during exercise and may have additional benefits in patients with hypertension and/or structural heart disease. Combination therapy (e.g. digoxin + atenolol) is often advisable.

18

In exceptional cases, poorly controlled and symptomatic AF can be treated by deliberately inducing complete heart block with transvenous catheter radiofrequency ablation; a permanent pacemaker must be implanted beforehand.

Prevention of thromboembolism

Loss of atrial contraction and left atrial dilatation cause stasis of blood in the left atrium, and may lead to thrombus formation in the left atrial appendage. This predisposes patients to stroke and other forms of systemic embolism. The annual risk of these events in patients with persistent AF is ~5% but it is influenced by many factors (Box 18.33) and may range from less than 1% to 12% (Box 18.34).

Several large randomised trials have shown that treatment with adjusted-dose warfarin (target INR 2.0–3.0) reduces the risk of stroke by about two-thirds, at the cost of an annual risk of bleeding of approximately 1–1.5%, whereas treatment with aspirin reduces the risk of stroke by only one-fifth (Box 18.35). Warfarin is thus indicated for patients with AF who have specific risk factors for stroke. For patients with intermittent AF, the risk of stroke is proportionate to the frequency and duration of AF episodes. Patients with frequent, prolonged (> 24-hour) episodes of AF should be considered for warfarin anticoagulation.

A careful assessment of the risk of embolism will help to define the possible benefits of antithrombotic therapy (Box 18.34), which must be balanced against the potential hazards of treatment. Echocardiography is a valuable aid in risk stratification. Warfarin is indicated in patients at high

---

18.35 ANTICOAGULATION IN ATRIAL FIBRILLATION — EBM

'Anticoagulation with warfarin reduces the risk of ischaemic stroke in non-rheumatic atrial fibrillation by about 62% (absolute risk reduction 2.7% for primary prevention and 8.4% for secondary prevention), while aspirin reduces the risk by only 22% (absolute risk reduction 1.5% for primary prevention and 2.5% for secondary prevention). NNT_B for 1 year (warfarin vs placebo) = 18.'

- Hart RG, et al. Ann Intern Med 1999; 131:492–501.
- Benavente O, et al. Cochrane Library, issue 4, 2000. Oxford: Update Software.

For further information: 🖳 www.sign.ac.uk

---

or very high risk of stroke, unless anticoagulation poses unacceptable risks. Comorbid conditions that may be complicated by bleeding, such as peptic ulcer, uncontrolled hypertension, alcohol misuse, poor drug compliance and potential drug interactions, are all relative contraindications to warfarin. Patients at moderate risk of stroke may be treated with warfarin or aspirin after discussing the balance of risk and benefit with the individual. Young patients (under 65 years) with no evidence of structural heart disease have a very low risk of stroke; they do not require warfarin but may benefit from aspirin treatment.

'SUPRAVENTRICULAR' TACHYCARDIAS

The term 'supraventricular tachycardia' (SVT) is commonly used to describe a range of regular tachycardias that have a similar appearance on an ECG. These tachycardias are usually associated with a narrow QRS complex and are characterised by a re-entry circuit or automatic focus involving the atria. The term SVT is misleading, as in many cases the ventricles also form part of the re-entry circuit, e.g. in patients with atrioventricular re-entrant tachycardia.

AV NODAL RE-ENTRY TACHYCARDIA (AVNRT)

This is due to re-entry in the right atrium and AV node and produces a regular tachycardia with a rate of 140–220/min. It tends to occur in hearts that are otherwise normal, and episodes may last from a few seconds to many hours. The patient is usually aware of a fast heart beat and may feel faint or breathless. Polyuria, mainly due to the release of atrial natriuretic peptide, is sometimes a feature, and cardiac pain or heart failure may occur if there is coexisting structural heart disease. The ECG (Fig. 18.41) usually shows a tachycardia with normal QRS complexes but occasionally there may be rate-dependent bundle branch block.

18.33 RISK FACTORS FOR THROMBOEMBOLISM IN ATRIAL FIBRILLATION

- Previous ischaemic stroke or transient ischaemic attack
- Mitral valve disease
- Age over 65
- Hypertension
- Diabetes mellitus
- Heart failure
- Echocardiographic features of: left ventricular dysfunction, left atrial enlargement or mitral annular calcification

---

18.34 EFFECT OF RISK STATUS AND TREATMENT ON THE ANNUAL RISK OF STROKE IN NON-RHEUMATIC ATRIAL FIBRILLATION

Risk group	Untreated	Aspirin	Warfarin
Very high Previous stroke or transient ischaemic attack	12%	10%	5%
High Age > 65 and one other risk factor (Box 18.33)	6.5%	5%	2.5%
Moderate Age > 65, no other risk factors Age < 65, other risk factors	4%	3%	1.5%
Low Age < 65 and no other risk factors	1.2%	1%	0.5%

N.B. In most studies the annual risk of significant bleeding during warfarin therapy is between 1.0 and 1.5%.

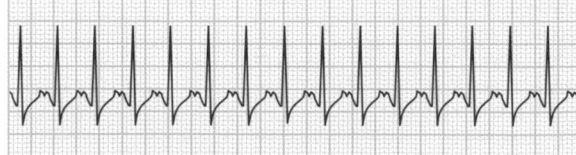

Fig. 18.41 Supraventricular tachycardia. The rate is 180/min and the QRS complexes are normal.

Management

Treatment is not always necessary. However, an attack may be terminated by carotid sinus pressure or other measures that increase vagal tone (e.g. Valsalva manoeuvre). Intravenous adenosine or verapamil will restore sinus rhythm in most cases. Suitable alternative drugs include β-blockers, flecainide and digoxin. In an emergency when there is severe haemodynamic compromise, the tachycardia should be terminated by DC cardioversion (p. 575).

If attacks are frequent or otherwise disabling, prophylactic oral therapy with a β-blocker, verapamil, disopyramide or digoxin may be indicated. Catheter ablation (p. 576) offers a very high chance of complete cure and is usually preferable to long-term drug treatment.

ATRIOVENTRICULAR RE-ENTRANT TACHYCARDIA (AVRT) AND WOLFF–PARKINSON–WHITE SYNDROME

In these conditions there is an abnormal band of conducting tissue which connects the atria and ventricles. It resembles Purkinje tissue in its physiology, in that it conducts very

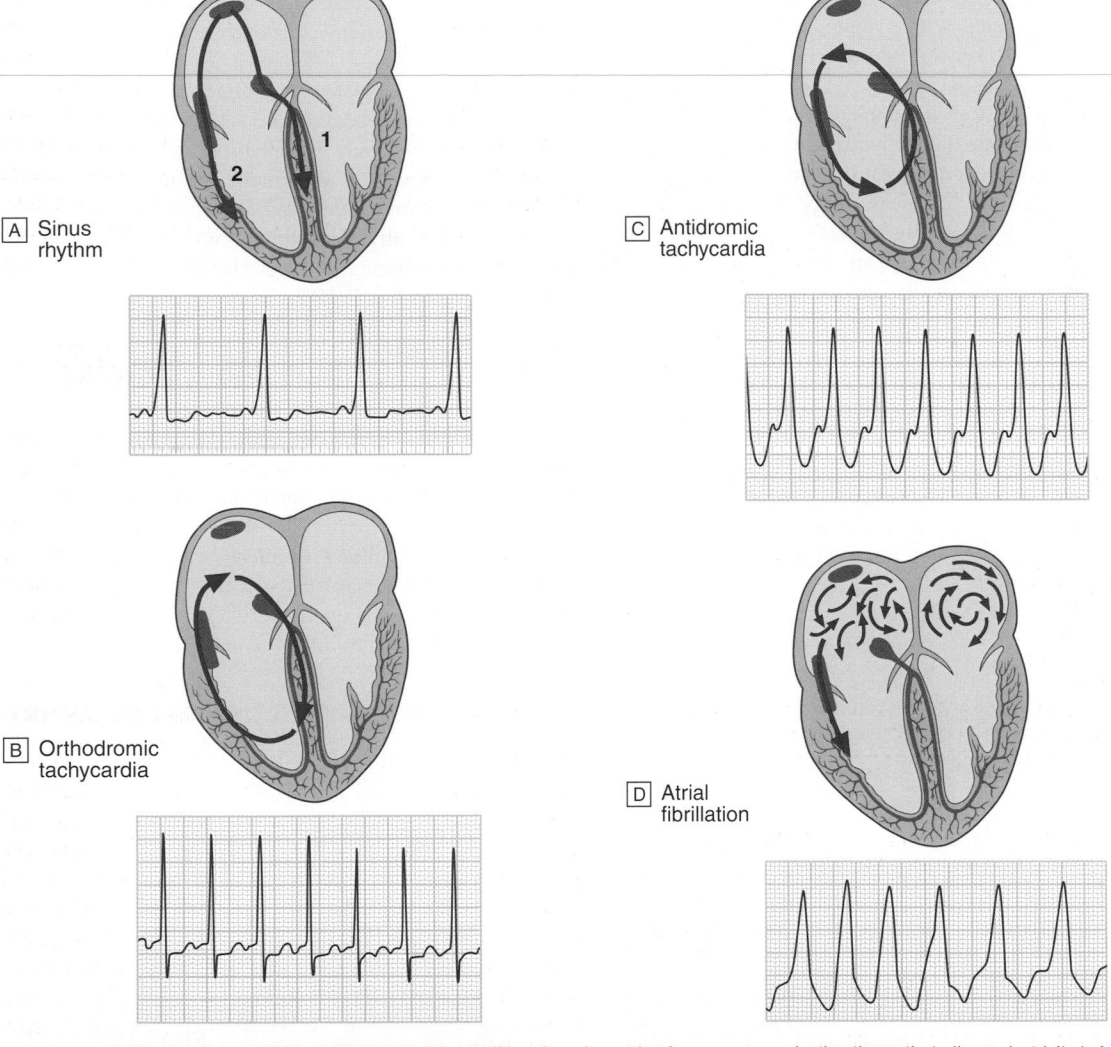

Fig. 18.42 Wolff–Parkinson–White syndrome. In this condition there is a strip of accessory conducting tissue that allows electricity to bypass the AV node and spread from the atria to the ventricles rapidly and without delay. When the ventricles are depolarised through the AV node (1) the ECG is normal, but when the ventricles are depolarised through the accessory conducting tissue (2) the ECG shows a very short PR interval and a broad QRS complex. **A Sinus rhythm.** In sinus rhythm the ventricles are partly depolarised through the AV node, and partly through the accessory pathway, producing an ECG with a short PR interval and broadened QRS complexes; the characteristic slurring of the upstroke of the QRS complex is known as a delta wave. The degree of pre-excitation (the proportion of electricity passing down the accessory pathway) and therefore the ECG appearances may vary a lot, and at times the ECG can look normal. **B Orthodromic tachycardia.** This is the most common form of tachycardia in WPW. The re-entry circuit passes antegradely through the AV node and retrogradely through the accessory pathway, producing a narrow-complex tachycardia that is indistinguishable from other forms of SVT. **C Antidromic tachycardia.** Occasionally, the re-entry circuit passes antegradely through the accessory pathway and retrogradely through the AV node. The ventricles are then depolarised through the accessory pathway, producing a broad-complex tachycardia. **D Atrial fibrillation.** In this rhythm the ventricles are largely depolarised through the accessory pathway, producing an irregular broad-complex tachycardia which is often more rapid than the example shown.

18

rapidly, and is known as an accessory pathway. In around half of cases this pathway only conducts in the retrograde direction (from ventricles to atria) and thus does not alter the appearance of the ECG in sinus rhythm. This is known as a concealed accessory pathway. In the remainder of cases, conduction takes place partly through the AV node and partly through the rapidly conducting accessory pathway during sinus rhythm. Premature activation of ventricular tissue via the pathway produces a short PR interval and a 'slurring' of the QRS complex, called a delta wave (Fig. 18.42A). This is known as a manifest accessory pathway. As the AV node and bypass tract have different conduction speeds and refractory periods, a re-entry circuit can develop, causing tachycardia (Figs 18.42B and 18.42C); when this is associated with symptoms, the condition is known as Wolff–Parkinson–White syndrome. The ECG appearance of this tachycardia may be indistinguishable from that of AVNRT. Carotid sinus pressure or intravenous adenosine can terminate the tachycardia. If atrial fibrillation occurs, it may produce a dangerously rapid ventricular rate because the accessory pathway lacks the rate-limiting properties of the AV node (Fig. 18.42D). This is known as pre-excited atrial fibrillation and may cause collapse, syncope and even death. It should be treated as an emergency, usually with DC cardioversion.

Prophylactic anti-arrhythmic drug therapy is only indicated in symptomatic patients and is aimed at slowing the conduction rate and prolonging the refractory period of the bypass tract, using agents such as flecainide, propafenone or amiodarone (pp. 572–575); digoxin and verapamil shorten the refractory period of the accessory pathway and should be avoided. Catheter ablation (p. 576) of the accessory pathway is the treatment of choice for symptomatic patients.

VENTRICULAR TACHYARRHYTHMIAS

VENTRICULAR ECTOPIC BEATS (EXTRASYSTOLES, PREMATURE BEATS)

The QRS complexes of ventricular ectopic beats are of abnormal morphology because the bundle branches are activated one after the other, rather than simultaneously. The ECG shows premature broad, bizarre QRS complexes which may be unifocal (identical beats arising from a single ectopic focus) or multifocal (varying morphology with multiple foci—Fig. 18.43). 'Couplet' and 'triplet' are terms used to describe two or three successive ectopic beats, whereas a run of alternate sinus and ectopic beats is known as ventricular 'bigeminy'. Ectopic beats produce a low stroke volume because left ventricular contraction occurs before filling is complete. The pulse is therefore irregular, with weak or missed beats (Fig. 18.43). Patients are usually asymptomatic but may complain of an irregular heart beat, missed beats or abnormally strong beats (due to the increased output of the post-ectopic sinus beat). The significance of ventricular ectopic beats (VEBs) depends on the presence or absence of underlying heart disease.

Ventricular ectopic beats in otherwise healthy subjects

VEBs are frequently found in healthy people, and their prevalence increases with age. Ectopic beats in patients with otherwise normal hearts are more prominent at rest, and disappear with exercise. Treatment is not necessary unless the patient is highly symptomatic, in which case β-blockers can be used.

VEBs are sometimes a manifestation of otherwise subclinical heart disease, particularly coronary artery disease.

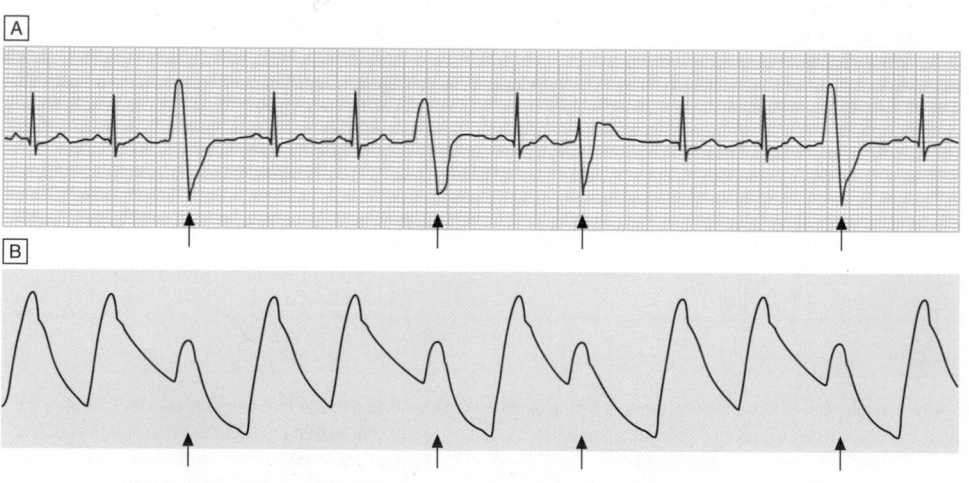

Fig. 18.43 Ventricular ectopic beats. [A] There are broad bizarre QRS complexes (arrows) with no preceding P wave in between normal sinus beats. Their configuration varies, so these are multifocal ectopics. [B] A simultaneous arterial pressure trace is shown. The ectopic beats result in a weaker pulse (arrows), which may be perceived as a 'dropped beat'.

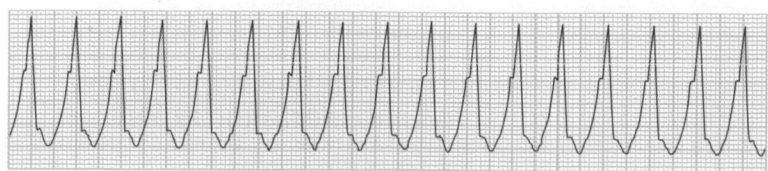

Fig. 18.44 Ventricular tachycardia: rhythm strip. Typical broad bizarre QRS complexes with a rate of 160/min.

There is no evidence that anti-arrhythmic therapy improves prognosis but the discovery of frequent VEBs might reasonably prompt some general cardiac investigations.

Ventricular ectopic beats associated with heart disease

Frequent VEBs often occur during acute myocardial infarction but need no treatment. Persistent frequent (> 10 per hour) ventricular ectopic beats in patients who have survived the acute phase of myocardial infarction indicate a poor long-term outcome. Other than β-blockers, anti-arrhythmic drugs do not improve and may even worsen prognosis.

VEBs are common in patients with heart failure, when they are associated with an adverse prognosis, but again the outlook is no better if they are suppressed with anti-arrhythmic drugs. Effective treatment of the heart failure may suppress the ectopic beats.

VEBs are also a feature of digoxin toxicity, are sometimes found in mitral valve prolapse, and may occur as 'escape beats' in the presence of an underlying bradycardia. Treatment should always be directed at the underlying condition.

VENTRICULAR TACHYCARDIA (VT)

VT most often occurs in patients with coronary heart disease or cardiomyopathies. In these settings it is serious because it may cause haemodynamic compromise or degenerate into ventricular fibrillation (p. 555). It is caused by abnormal automaticity or triggered activity in ischaemic tissue, or by re-entry within diseased ventricular tissue. Patients may complain of palpitation or the symptoms of low cardiac output, such as dizziness, dyspnoea or syncope. The ECG shows tachycardia with broad, abnormal QRS complexes with a rate above 120/min (Fig. 18.44). VT may be difficult to distinguish from supraventricular tachycardia with bundle branch block or pre-excitation (Wolff–Parkinson–White syndrome). Features in favour of a diagnosis of VT are listed in Box 18.36. A 12-lead (Fig. 18.45), intracardiac (Fig. 18.46) or oesophageal ECG may help to establish the

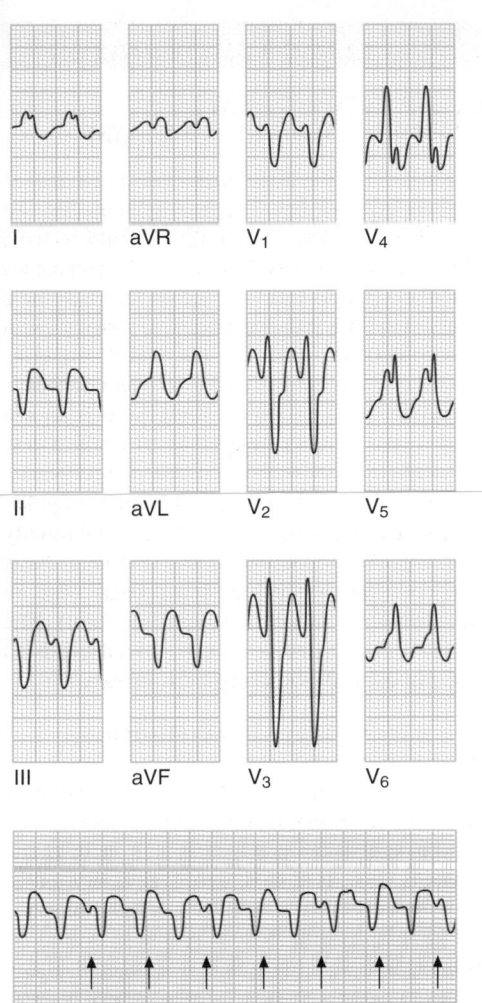

I aVR V₁ V₄

II aVL V₂ V₅

III aVF V₃ V₆

Rhythm strip

Fig. 18.45 Ventricular tachycardia: 12-lead ECG. The morphology of this tachycardia is typical of VT, with very broad QRS complexes and marked left axis deviation. In addition, there is AV dissociation; some P waves are visible and others are buried in the QRS complexes (arrows).

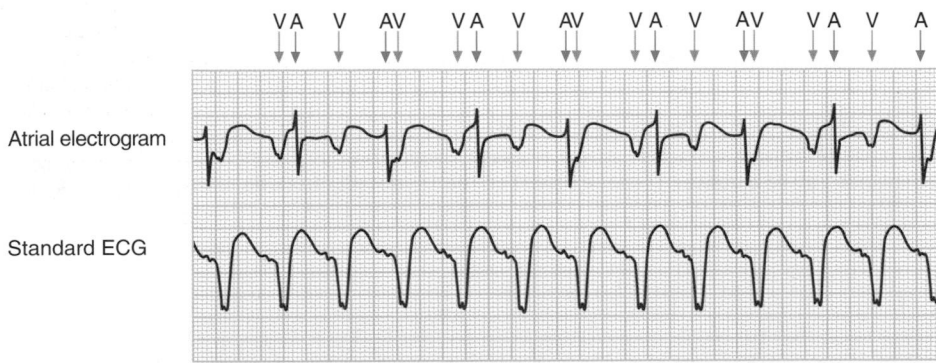

VA V AV VA V AV VA V AV VA V A

Atrial electrogram

Standard ECG

Fig. 18.46 Ventricular tachycardia: intracardiac ECG. A simultaneous recording of an atrial electrogram, obtained by placing a pacing lead in the right atrium, and an ordinary rhythm strip illustrating ventricular tachycardia with AV dissociation. Although the standard ECG shows a broad-complex tachycardia with no visible P waves, dissociated atrial activity is clearly visible in the atrial electrogram. (A = atrial depolarisation; V = ventricular depolarisation)

18

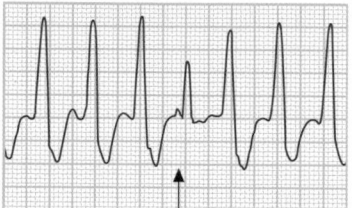

Fig. 18.47   Ventricular tachycardia: fusion beat (arrow). In ventricular tachycardia there is independent atrial and ventricular activity. Occasionally a P wave is conducted to the ventricles through the AV node. This may produce a normal sinus beat in the middle of the tachycardia (a capture beat); however, more commonly the conducted impulse fuses with an impulse from the tachycardia (a fusion beat). This phenomenon can only occur when there is AV dissociation and is therefore diagnostic of ventricular tachycardia.

diagnosis. When there is doubt it is safer to manage the problem as VT, which is by far the most common cause of a broad-complex tachycardia.

The common causes of ventricular tachycardia include acute myocardial infarction, cardiomyopathy and chronic ischaemic heart disease, particularly when it is associated with a ventricular aneurysm or poor left ventricular function.

Patients recovering from myocardial infarction sometimes have periods of idioventricular rhythm ('slow' VT) at a rate only slightly above the preceding sinus rate and less than 120/min. These episodes often reflect reperfusion of the infarct territory and may be a good sign. They are usually self-limiting and asymptomatic, and do not require treatment. Other forms of ventricular tachycardia, if they last for more than a few beats, will require treatment, often as an emergency.

VT occasionally occurs in patients with otherwise healthy hearts ('normal heart VT'), usually because of abnormal automaticity in the right ventricular outflow tract or one of the fascicles of the left bundle branch. In these cases the prognosis is good and catheter ablation can be curative.

Management

Prompt action to restore sinus rhythm is required and in most cases should be followed by prophylactic therapy. DC cardioversion is the treatment of choice if systolic BP is less than 90 mmHg. If the arrhythmia is well tolerated, intravenous amiodarone may be given as a bolus followed by an intravenous infusion (p. 573). Intravenous lidocaine can be used but it can depress left ventricular function, causing hypotension or acute heart failure. Hypokalaemia, hypomagnesaemia, acidosis and hypoxaemia can aggravate the situation and must be corrected.

Beta-blockers may be effective at suppressing VT. Amiodarone can be added if additional control is needed. Class I anti-arrhythmic drugs can be used acutely but are dangerous in the long term in patients with ischaemic heart disease. In patients considered at high risk of arrhythmic death (e.g. those with poor left ventricular function, or in whom VT is associated with haemodynamic compromise), the use of an implantable cardiac defibrillator is recommended. Rarely, surgery or catheter ablation can be used to interrupt the arrhythmia focus or circuit.

TORSADES DE POINTES (TWISTING POINTS)

This form of polymorphic ventricular tachycardia is a complication of prolonged ventricular repolarisation (prolonged QT interval). The ECG shows rapid irregular complexes that oscillate from an upright to an inverted position and seem to twist around the baseline as the mean QRS axis changes (Fig. 18.48). The arrhythmia is usually non-sustained and repetitive but may degenerate into ventricular fibrillation. During periods of sinus rhythm the ECG will usually show a prolonged QT interval.

Some of the common causes are listed in Box 18.37. The arrhythmia is more common in women and is often triggered by a combination of aetiological factors (e.g. multiple medications and hypokalaemia). The congenital long QT syndromes are a family of genetic disorders that are characterised by mutations in genes that code for cardiac sodium or potassium channels.

Treatment should be directed at the underlying cause. Intravenous magnesium (8 mmol over 15 minutes, then 72 mmol over 24 hours) should be given in all cases. Atrial pacing will usually suppress the arrhythmia through rate-dependent shortening of the QT interval. Intravenous isoprenaline is a reasonable alternative to pacing but should be avoided in patients with the congenital long QT syndrome.

Long-term therapy may not be necessary if the underlying cause can be removed. Beta-blockers or left stellate

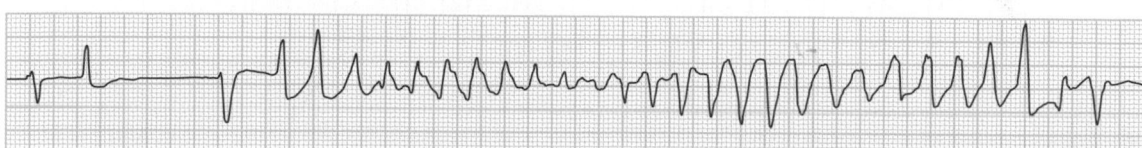

Fig. 18.48   Torsades de pointes. A bradycardia with a long QT interval is followed by polymorphic ventricular tachycardia that is triggered by an R on T ectopic.

18.37 CAUSES OF LONG QT INTERVAL AND TORSADES DE POINTES

Bradycardia

- Bradycardia compounds other factors that cause torsades de pointes

Electrolyte disturbance

- Hypokalaemia
- Hypomagnesaemia
- Hypocalcaemia

Drugs

- Disopyramide (and other class Ia anti-arrhythmic drugs, p. 572)
- Sotalol, amiodarone (and other class III anti-arrhythmic drugs)
- Amitriptyline (and other tricyclic antidepressants)
- Chlorpromazine (and other phenothiazines)
- Erythromycin (and other macrolides)
- … and many more

Congenital syndromes

- Romano–Ward syndrome (autosomal dominant)
- Jervell and Lange–Nielson syndrome (autosomal recessive, associated with congenital deafness)

ganglion block may be of value in patients with a congenital long QT syndrome. An implantable cardiac defibrillator is often advisable.

The Brugada syndrome is a related genetic disorder that may present with polymorphic ventricular tachycardia or sudden death; it is characterised by a defect in sodium channel function, and an abnormal ECG (right bundle branch block and ST elevation in V_1 and V_2, but not usually prolongation of the QT interval).

SINOATRIAL DISEASE (SICK SINUS SYNDROME)

Sinoatrial disease can occur at any age, but is most common in the elderly. The underlying pathology is not understood but may involve fibrosis, degenerative changes and/or ischaemia of the sinoatrial (sinus) node. The condition is characterised by a variety of arrhythmias (Box 18.38) and may present with palpitation, dizzy spells or syncope, due to intermittent tachycardia, bradycardia, or pauses with no atrial or ventricular activity (sinoatrial block or sinus arrest) (Fig. 18.49).

A permanent pacemaker may benefit patients with troublesome symptoms due to spontaneous bradycardias, or those with symptomatic bradycardias induced by drugs required to prevent tachyarrhythmias. Atrial pacing may help to prevent episodes of atrial fibrillation. Permanent pacing does not improve prognosis and is not indicated in patients who are asymptomatic.

18

18.38 COMMON FEATURES OF SINOATRIAL DISEASE

- Sinus bradycardia
- Sinoatrial block (sinus arrest)
- Paroxysmal supraventricular tachycardia
- Paroxysmal atrial fibrillation
- Atrioventricular block

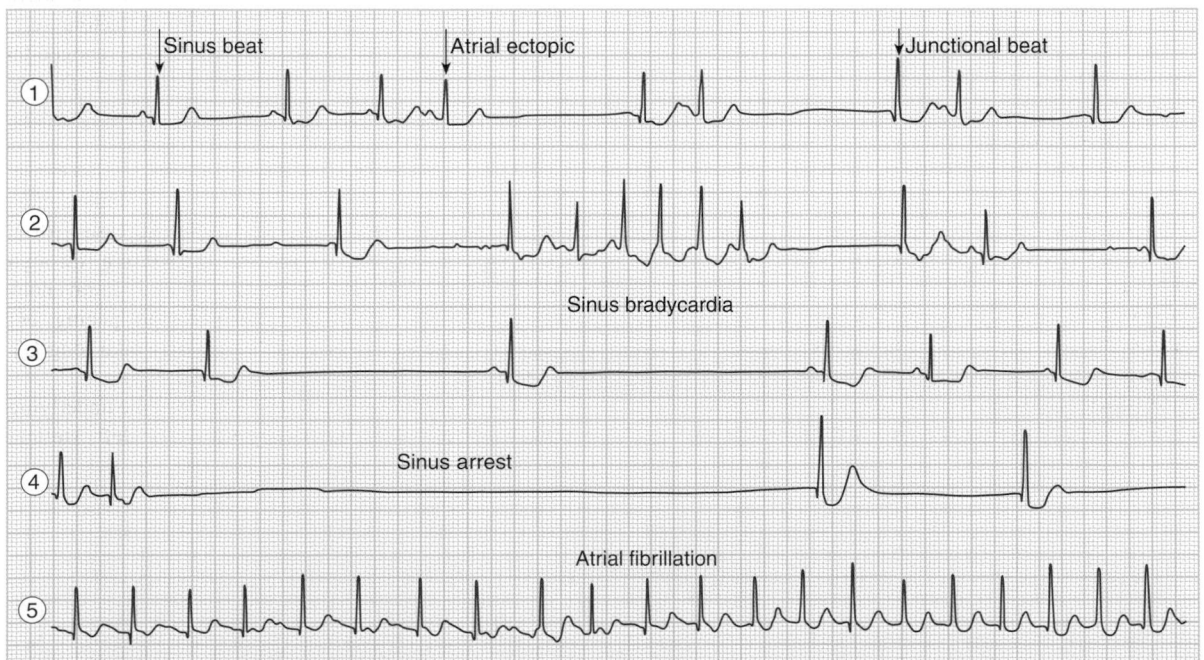

Fig. 18.49 Sinoatrial disease (sick sinus syndrome). A continuous rhythm strip from a 24-hour ECG tape recording illustrating periods of sinus rhythm, atrial ectopics, junctional beats, sinus bradycardia, sinus arrest and paroxysmal atrial fibrillation.

ATRIOVENTRICULAR AND BUNDLE BRANCH BLOCK

ATRIOVENTRICULAR (AV) BLOCK

Atrioventricular conduction is influenced by autonomic activity. AV block can therefore be intermittent and may only be evident when the conducting tissue is stressed by a rapid atrial rate. Accordingly, atrial tachyarrhythmias are often associated with AV block (Fig. 18.39, p. 562).

First-degree AV block
In this condition AV conduction is delayed so the PR interval is prolonged (> 0.20 seconds) (Fig. 18.50). It rarely causes symptoms.

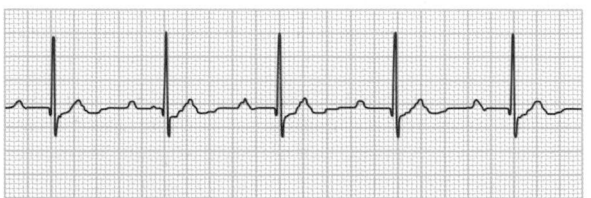

Fig. 18.50 First-degree heart block. The PR interval is prolonged and measures 0.26 seconds.

Second-degree AV block
In this condition dropped beats occur because some impulses from the atria fail to conduct to the ventricles.

In Mobitz type I second-degree AV block (Fig. 18.51) there is progressive lengthening of successive PR intervals culminating in a dropped beat. The cycle then repeats itself. This is known as Wenckebach's phenomenon and is usually due to impaired conduction in the AV node itself. The phenomenon may be physiological and is sometimes observed at rest or during sleep in athletic young adults with high vagal tone.

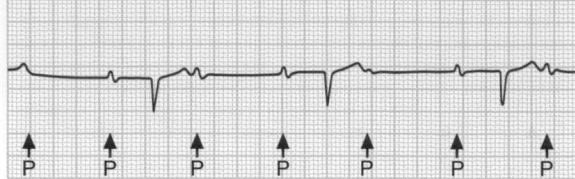

Fig. 18.53 Second-degree atrioventricular block with fixed 2:1 block. Alternate P waves are not conducted. This may be due to Mobitz type I or II block.

In Mobitz type II second-degree AV block (Fig. 18.52) the PR interval of the conducted impulses remains constant but some P waves are not conducted. This is usually caused by disease of the His–Purkinje system and carries a risk of asystole.

In 2:1 AV block (Fig. 18.53) alternate P waves are conducted so it is impossible to distinguish between Mobitz type I and type II block.

Third-degree (complete) AV block
When AV conduction fails completely, the atria and ventricles beat independently (AV dissociation, Fig. 18.54). Ventricular activity is maintained by an escape rhythm arising in the AV node or bundle of His (narrow QRS complexes) or the distal Purkinje tissues (broad QRS complexes). Distal escape rhythms tend to be slower and less reliable.

The aetiology is shown in Box 18.39.

Complete heart block produces a slow (25–50/min), regular pulse that, except in the case of congenital complete heart block, does not vary with exercise. There is usually a compensatory increase in stroke volume with a large volume pulse and systolic flow murmurs. Cannon waves may be visible in the neck and the intensity of the first heart sound varies due to the loss of AV synchrony.

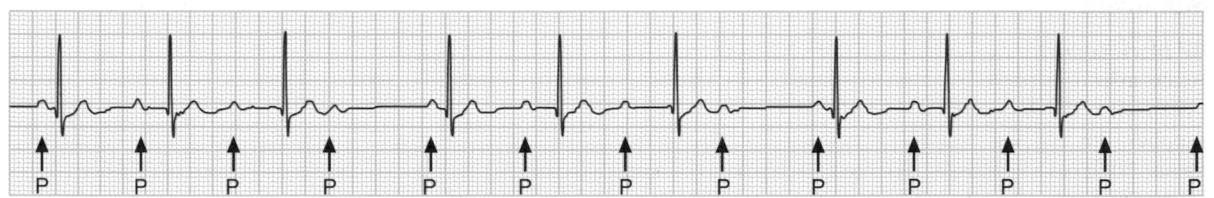

Fig. 18.51 Second-degree atrioventricular block (Mobitz type I—Wenckebach's phenomenon). The PR interval progressively increases until a P wave is not conducted. The cycle then repeats itself. In this example, conduction is at a ratio of 4:3, leading to groupings of three ventricular complexes in a row.

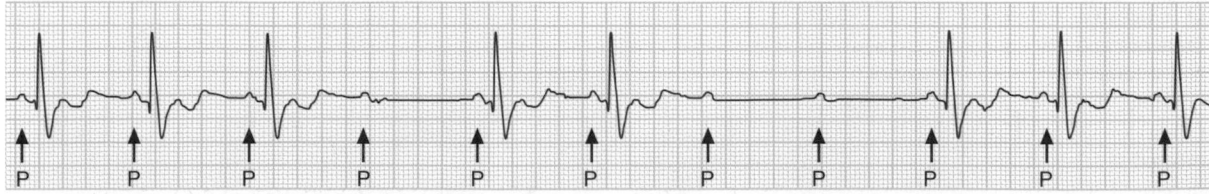

Fig. 18.52 Second-degree atrioventricular block (Mobitz type II). The PR interval of conducted beats is normal but some P waves are not conducted. The constant PR interval distinguishes this from Wenckebach's phenomenon.

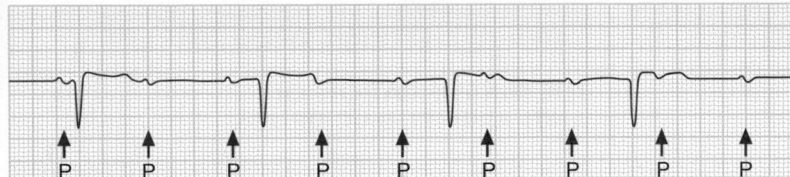

Fig. 18.54 Complete (third-degree) atrioventricular block. There is complete dissociation of atrial and ventricular complexes. The atrial rate is 80/min and the ventricular rate is 38/min.

18

18.39 AETIOLOGY OF COMPLETE HEART BLOCK	
Congenital	
Acquired	

- Idiopathic fibrosis
- Myocardial infarction/ischaemia
- Inflammation
  Acute (e.g. aortic root abscess in infective endocarditis)
  Chronic (e.g. sarcoidosis, p. 715; Chagas disease, p. 355)
- Trauma (e.g. cardiac surgery)
- Drugs (e.g. digoxin, β-blocker)

Stokes–Adams attacks

Episodes of ventricular asystole may complicate complete heart block or Mobitz type II second-degree AV block, and can also occur in patients with sinoatrial disease (Fig. 18.49). This may cause recurrent syncope or 'Stokes–Adams' attacks.

A typical episode is characterised by a sudden loss of consciousness, which frequently occurs without warning and may result in a fall. Convulsions (due to cerebral ischaemia) can occur if there is prolonged asystole. There is pallor and a death-like appearance during the attack, but when the heart starts beating again there is a characteristic flush. In contrast to epilepsy, recovery is rapid.

The carotid sinus syndrome and the vasovagal syndrome (p. 553) may cause similar symptoms.

Management

AV block complicating acute myocardial infarction

Acute inferior myocardial infarction is often complicated by transient AV block because the right coronary artery supplies the AV junction. There is usually a reliable escape rhythm, and if the patient remains well, no treatment is required. Symptomatic second-degree or complete heart block may respond to atropine (0.6 mg i.v., repeated as necessary) or if this fails, a temporary pacemaker. In most cases the AV block will resolve within 7–10 days.

Second-degree or complete heart block complicating acute anterior myocardial infarction is usually a sign of extensive ventricular damage involving both bundle branches and carries a poor prognosis. Asystole may ensue and a temporary pacemaker should be inserted as soon as possible. If the patient presents with asystole, i.v. atropine (3 mg) or i.v. isoprenaline (2 mg in 500 ml 5% dextrose, infused at 10–60 ml/hour) may help to maintain the circulation until a temporary pacing electrode can be inserted. Transcutaneous pacing can provide effective temporary rhythm support.

Chronic AV block

Patients with symptomatic bradyarrhythmias associated with AV block should receive a permanent pacemaker (see below).

Asymptomatic first-degree or Mobitz type I second-degree AV block (Wenckebach's phenomenon) does not require treatment but may be an indication of serious underlying heart disease.

A permanent pacemaker is usually indicated in patients with asymptomatic Mobitz type II second-degree or complete heart block because there is evidence that pacing can improve their prognosis. An exception may be made in young asymptomatic patients with congenital complete heart block who have a mean daytime heart rate of more than 50 per minute.

BUNDLE BRANCH BLOCK AND HEMIBLOCK

Interruption of the right or left branch of the bundle of His delays activation of the appropriate ventricle, broadens the QRS complex (0.12 seconds or more) and produces the characteristic alterations in QRS morphology shown in Figures 18.55 and 18.56.

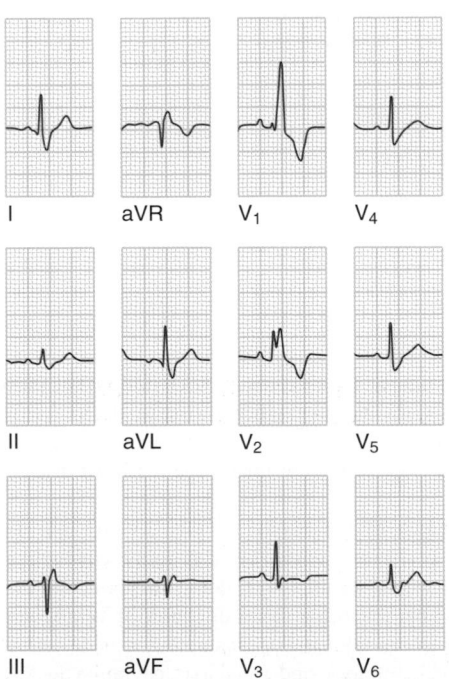

Fig. 18.55 Right bundle branch block. Note the wide QRS complexes with 'M'-shaped configuration in leads V_1 and V_2 and a wide S wave in lead I.

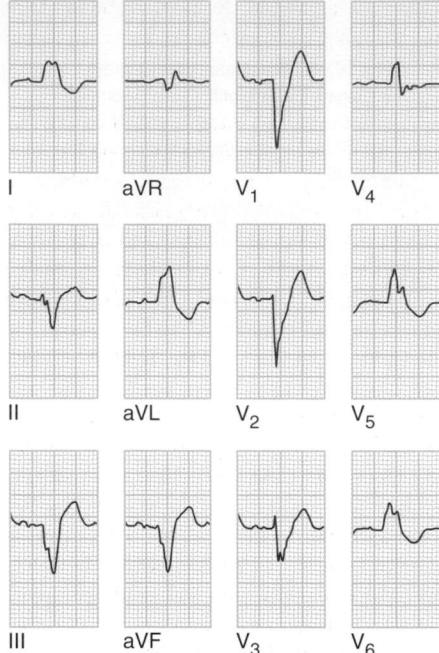

I   aVR V_1 V_4

II   aVL V_2 V_5

III   aVF V_3 V_6

Fig. 18.56 Left bundle branch block. Note the wide QRS complexes with the loss of the Q wave or septal vector in lead I and 'M'-shaped QRS complexes in V_5 and V_6.

18.40 COMMON CAUSES OF BUNDLE BRANCH BLOCK
Right bundle branch block
• Normal variant • Right ventricular hypertrophy or strain, e.g. pulmonary embolism • Congenital heart disease, e.g. atrial septal defect • Coronary artery disease
Left bundle branch block
• Coronary artery disease • Hypertension • Aortic valve disease • Cardiomyopathy

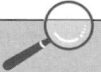

Right bundle branch block (RBBB) can be a common normal variant but left bundle branch block (LBBB) usually signifies important underlying heart disease. Both forms of bundle branch block may be due to conducting tissue disease but are also features of other types of heart disease (Box 18.40).

The left branch of the bundle of His divides into an anterior and a posterior fascicle. Damage to the conducting tissue at this point (hemiblock) does not broaden the QRS complex, but alters the mean direction of ventricular depolarisation (mean QRS axis), causing left axis deviation in left anterior hemiblock and right axis deviation in left posterior hemiblock (Fig. 18.7, p. 528). The combination of right bundle branch and left anterior or posterior hemiblock is known as bifascicular block.

ANTI-ARRHYTHMIC DRUG THERAPY

THE CLASSIFICATION OF ANTI-ARRHYTHMIC DRUGS

Some of the drugs used to treat individual arrhythmias have already been mentioned. These agents may be classified according to their mode or main site of action (Box 18.41 and Fig. 18.57). The main uses, dosages and side-effects of the most widely used drugs are summarised in Box 18.42, and principles of use are outlined in Box 18.43. Identification of ion channel subtypes has led to refinement of drug classifications according to the specific mechanisms targeted.

Class I drugs

Class I drugs act principally by suppressing excitability and slowing conduction in atrial or ventricular muscle.

- *Quinidine* can cause torsades de pointes, hypersensitivity and unpleasant gastrointestinal side-effects; it has been shown to increase mortality in patients with paroxysmal atrial fibrillation and should be avoided.
- *Disopyramide* has weak atropine-like effects and may cause urinary retention or precipitate glaucoma. It has a depressant effect on ventricular function and should be avoided in cardiac failure. If it is used in patients with atrial flutter and AV block, there is a risk of a paradoxical increase in heart rate as the atria slow and 2:1 block changes to 1:1 conduction; this can be prevented by pre-treatment with digoxin.
- *Lidocaine* must be given parenterally and has a very short plasma half-life, so plasma concentration will depend on the rate of infusion. It is mainly used for the urgent treatment or prophylaxis of ventricular tachycardia.

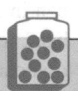

18.41 CLASSIFICATION OF ANTI-ARRHYTHMIC DRUGS ACCORDING TO THEIR EFFECT ON THE INTRACELLULAR ACTION POTENTIAL
Class I—membrane-stabilising agents (sodium channel blockers)

(a) Block Na^+ channel and prolong action potential
   • Quinidine, disopyramide
(b) Block Na^+ channel and shorten action potential
   • Lidocaine, mexiletine
(c) Block Na^+ channel with no effect on action potential
   • Flecanide, propafenone

Class II—β-adrenoceptor antagonists (β-blockers)
• Atenolol, bisoprolol, metoprolol, l-sotalol
Class III—drugs whose main effect is to prolong the action potential
• Amiodarone, d-sotalol
Class IV—slow calcium channel blockers
• Verapamil, diltiazem
N.B. Some drugs (e.g. digoxin and adenosine) have no place in this classification, while others have properties in more than one class, e.g. amiodarone, which has actions in all four classes.

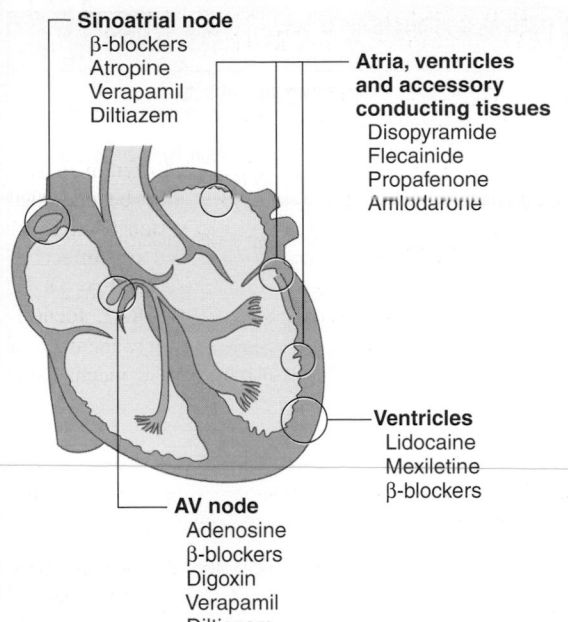

Sinoatrial node
β-blockers
Atropine
Verapamil
Diltiazem

Atria, ventricles and accessory conducting tissues
Disopyramide
Flecainide
Propafenone
Amiodarone

Ventricles
Lidocaine
Mexiletine
β-blockers

AV node
Adenosine
β-blockers
Digoxin
Verapamil
Diltiazem

Fig. 18.57   Classification of anti-arrhythmic drugs by site of action.

- *Mexiletine* can be given intravenously or orally and is used for the treatment or prophylaxis of ventricular arrhythmias. Side-effects include nausea, vomiting, confusion, dizziness, tremor and nystagmus
- *Flecainide* can be given intravenously or orally for the treatment or prophylaxis of supraventricular or ventricular arrhythmias and may be useful in the management of Wolff–Parkinson–White syndrome. Unfortunately, it is a potent myocardial depressant and cannot therefore be used safely in patients with poor left ventricular function. Like all anti-arrhythmic drugs, it can in some circumstances be pro-arrhythmic and has been found to be hazardous in patients with a history of myocardial infarction.
- *Propafenone* is indicated for the treatment or prophylaxis of all tachyarrhythmias and is particularly useful in paroxysmal atrial fibrillation, ventricular tachycardia and the Wolff–Parkinson–White syndrome. Propafenone is a class Ic drug but also has some β-blocker (class II) properties and may precipitate heart failure or heart block in susceptible patients. Important interactions with digoxin, warfarin and cimetidine have been described.

Class II drugs

This group comprises the β-adrenoceptor antagonists (β-blockers). The agents used most commonly are as follows.

- *Atenolol, bisoprolol and metoprolol* are cardioselective β-blockers that are usually well tolerated.
- *Sotalol* is a racemic mixture of two isomers with non-selective β-blocker (mainly l-sotalol) and class III (mainly d-sotalol) activity. It may cause torsades de pointes.
- *Propranolol* is not cardioselective and is subject to extensive first-pass metabolism in the liver. The effective

oral dose is therefore unpredictable and must be titrated after treatment is started with a small dose.

Class III drugs

Class III drugs act by prolonging the plateau phase of the action potential, thus lengthening the refractory period.

Amiodarone is the principal drug in this class, although both disopyramide and sotalol have class III activity. Amiodarone has unusual pharmacokinetics and is effective against a wide variety of atrial and ventricular arrhythmias. It is probably the most effective drug currently available for controlling paroxysmal atrial fibrillation and the arrhythmias associated with the Wolff–Parkinson–White syndrome. Furthermore, it is very useful in preventing episodes of recurrent ventricular tachycardia, particularly in patients with poor left ventricular function. Amiodarone has an extraordinarily long tissue half-life (25–110 days). This means that the onset of action after oral and intravenous therapy is delayed; indeed, it may take several months to reach steady state. For the same reason, the drug's effects may last for weeks or months after treatment has been stopped. Side-effects are frequent (up to one-third of patients), numerous and potentially serious; they include photosensitisation, corneal deposits, gastrointestinal problems, thyroid dysfunction (p. 744), liver disease, pulmonary fibrosis and torsades de pointes. Drug interactions are also common; for example, the effects of digoxin and warfarin are potentiated by amiodarone.

Class IV drugs

These block the 'slow calcium channel' which is particularly important for impulse generation and conduction in atrial and nodal tissue, although it is also present in ventricular muscle.

Verapamil is the most widely used anti-arrhythmic drug in this class; however, diltiazem has similar properties. Intravenous verapamil may cause profound bradycardia and/or hypotension and should not be used in conjunction with oral or intravenous β-blockers.

Other anti-arrhythmic drugs

- *Atropine sulphate* (0.6 mg i.v., repeated if necessary to a maximum of 3 mg) increases the sinus rate and sinoatrial and AV conduction, and is the treatment of choice for severe bradycardia and/or hypotension due to vagal overactivity. It may also be of value in the initial management of symptomatic bradyarrhythmias complicating the early stages of inferior myocardial infarction and cardiac arrest due to asystole. Repeat dosing may be necessary because the drug disappears rapidly from the circulation after parenteral administration. Side-effects include dry mouth, thirst, blurred vision and both atrial and ventricular extrasystoles.
- *Adenosine* must be given intravenously; like carotid sinus massage, it produces transient AV block lasting a few seconds. Accordingly, it may be used to terminate junctional tachycardias when the AV node is part of the re-entry circuit or to help establish the diagnosis in difficult arrhythmias such as atrial flutter with 2:1 AV

18.42 THE MAIN USES, DOSAGES AND SIDE-EFFECTS OF THE MOST WIDELY USED ANTI-ARRHYTHMIC DRUGS

Drug	Main uses	Route	Dose (adult)	Important side-effects
CLASS I				
Disopyramide	Prevention and treatment of atrial and ventricular tachyarrhythmias	I.v. / Oral	2 mg/kg at 30 mg/min then 0.4 mg/kg/hr (max 800 mg/day) / 300–800 mg daily in divided dosage	Myocardial depression, hypotension, dry mouth, urinary retention
Lidocaine	Treatment and short-term prevention of VT and VF	I.v.	Bolus 50–100 mg / 4 mg/min for 30 mins, then 2 mg/min for 2 hrs, then 1 mg/min for 24 hrs	Myocardial depression, confusion, convulsions
Mexiletine	Prevention and treatment of ventricular tachyarrhythmias	I.v. / Oral	Loading dose: 100–250 mg at 25 mg/min then 250 mg in 1 hr then 250 mg in 2 hrs Maintenance therapy: 0.5 mg/min / 200–250 mg 8-hourly	Myocardial depression, GI irritation, confusion, dizziness, tremor, nystagmus, ataxia
Flecainide	Prevention and treatment of atrial and ventricular tachyarrhythmias	I.v. / Oral	2 mg/kg over 10 mins then 1.5 mg/kg/hr for 1 hr then 0.1 mg/kg/hr / 50–100 mg 12-hourly	Myocardial depression, dizziness
Propafenone	Prevention and treatment of atrial and ventricular tachyarrhythmias	Oral	150 mg 8-hourly for 1 week then 300 mg 12-hourly	Myocardial depression, dizziness
CLASS II				
Atenolol	Treatment and prevention of SVT and AF Prevention of VEs and exercise-induced VT	I.v. / Oral	2.5 mg at 1 mg/min repeated at 5 min intervals (max 10 mg) / 25–100 mg daily	Myocardial depression, bradycardia, bronchospasm, fatigue, depression, nightmares, cold peripheries
Bisoprolol		Oral	2.5–10 mg daily	
Metoprolol		I.v. / Oral	5 mg over 2 mins to a maximum of 15 mg / 50–100 mg 8- or 12-hourly	
Sotalol		I.v. / Oral	10–20 mg slowly / 40–160 mg 12-hourly	Sotalol can cause torsades de pointes
CLASS III				
Amiodarone	Serious or resistant atrial and ventricular tachyarrhythmias	I.v. / Oral	5 mg/kg over 20–120 mins then up to 15 mg/kg/24 hrs / Initially 600–1200 mg/day then then 100–400 mg daily	Photosensitivity, skin discoloration, corneal deposits, thyroid dysfunction, alveolitis, nausea and vomiting, hepatotoxicity, peripheral neuropathy, torsades de pointes; potentiates digoxin and warfarin
CLASS IV				
Verapamil	Treatment of SVT, control of AF	I.v. / Oral	5–10 mg over 30 secs / 40–120 mg 8-hourly or 240 mg SR daily	Myocardial depression, hypotension, bradycardia, constipation
OTHER				
Atropine	Treatment of bradycardia and/or hypotension due to vagal overactivity	I.v.	0.6–3 mg	Dry mouth, thirst, blurred vision, atrial and ventricular extrasystoles
Adenosine	Treatment of SVT, aid to diagnosis in unidentified tachycardia	I.v.	3 mg over 2 secs, followed if necessary by 6 mg then 12 mg at intervals of 1–2 mins	Flushing, dyspnoea, chest pain Avoid in asthma
Digoxin	Treatment and prevention of SVT, rate control of AF	I.v. / Oral	Loading dose: 0.5–1 mg (total), 0.5 mg over 30 mins then 0.25–0.5 mg 4- to 8-hourly to maximum total of 1 mg, assessing response before each additional dose / 0.5 mg 6-hourly for 2 doses, then 0.125–0.25 mg daily	GI disturbance, xanthopsia, arrhythmias (Box 18.45)

(VT = ventricular tachycardia; VF = ventricular fibrillation; SVT = supraventricular tachycardia; AF = atrial fibrillation; VE = ventricular ectopic; SR = sustained-release formulation)

18.43 ANTI-ARRHYTHMIC DRUGS: PRINCIPLES OF USE

The drugs used to treat arrhythmias are potentially toxic and should be used carefully according to the following principles:

- Many arrhythmias are benign and do not require specific treatment
- Precipitating or causal factors should be corrected if possible. These may include excess alcohol or caffeine consumption, myocardial ischaemia, hyperthyroidism, acidosis, hypokalaemia and hypomagnesaemia
- If drug therapy is required it is best to use as few drugs as possible
- In difficult cases, programmed electrical stimulation (electrophysiological study) may help to identify the optimum therapy
- When dealing with life-threatening arrhythmias it is essential to ensure that prophylactic treatment is effective. Ambulatory monitoring, exercise testing and programmed electrical stimulation may be of value
- Patients on long-term anti-arrhythmic drugs should be reviewed regularly and attempts made to withdraw therapy if the factors which precipitated the arrhythmias are no longer operative
- For patients with recurrent SVT, radiofrequency ablation is often preferable to long-term drug therapy

18.44 RESPONSE TO INTRAVENOUS ADENOSINE

Arrhythmia	Response
Supraventricular junctional tachycardia	Termination
Atrial fibrillation, atrial flutter	Transient AV block
Ventricular tachycardia	No effect

18.45 DIGOXIN TOXICITY

Extracardiac manifestations

- Anorexia, nausea, vomiting
- Diarrhoea
- Altered colour vision (xanthopsia)

Cardiac manifestations

- Bradycardia
- Multiple ventricular ectopics
- Ventricular bigeminy (alternate ventricular ectopics)
- Atrial tachycardia (with variable block)
- Ventricular tachycardia
- Ventricular fibrillation

block (Fig. 18.38, p. 561) or broad-complex tachycardia (Boxes 18.42 and 18.44).

Adenosine is given as an intravenous bolus according to an ascending dosage schedule. The initial dose is 3 mg given over 2 seconds. If there is no response after 1–2 minutes, 6 mg should be given and if necessary the physician should wait another 1–2 minutes before administering the maximum dose of 12 mg. Patients should be warned that they may experience short-lived and sometimes distressing side-effects of flushing, breathlessness and chest pain. Adenosine can cause bronchospasm and should be avoided in asthmatics; its effects are greatly potentiated by dipyridamole and inhibited by theophylline and other xanthines.

- *Digoxin* is a purified glycoside from the European foxglove, *Digitalis lanata*, which slows conduction and prolongs the refractory period in the AV node. This effect helps to control the ventricular rate in atrial fibrillation and will often interrupt re-entry tachycardias involving the AV node. On the other hand, digoxin tends to shorten refractory periods and enhance excitability and conduction in other parts of the heart (including accessory conduction pathways); it may therefore increase atrial and ventricular ectopic activity and can lead to more complex atrial and ventricular tachyarrhythmias.

Digoxin is largely excreted by the kidneys, and the maintenance dose (Box 18.42) should be reduced in children, the elderly and those with renal impairment. It is widely distributed and has a long tissue half-life (36 hours) so that effects may persist several days after the last dose. Measurements of plasma digoxin concentration are useful in demonstrating that the dose is inadequate and in confirming a clinical impression of toxicity (Box 18.45).

THERAPEUTIC PROCEDURES

EXTERNAL DEFIBRILLATION AND CARDIOVERSION

The heart can be completely depolarised by passing a sufficiently large electrical current through it from an external source. This will interrupt any arrhythmia and produce a brief period of asystole which is usually followed by the resumption of normal sinus rhythm. Defibrillators deliver a direct current (DC), high-energy, short-duration shock via two metal paddles coated with conducting jelly or a gel pad, positioned over the upper right sternal edge and the apex.

Energy applied during a critical period around the peak of the T wave may provoke ventricular fibrillation, so when this technique is used to treat organised rhythms such as atrial fibrillation or ventricular tachycardia, the shock should be synchronised with the ECG and is normally given 0.02 seconds after the peak of the R wave. The precise timing of the discharge is not important in ventricular fibrillation.

In ventricular fibrillation and other emergencies, the energy of the first and second shock should be 100 joules and thereafter 150 joules; there is no need for an anaesthetic if the patient is unconscious. Elective cardioversion requires a general anaesthetic. High-energy shocks may cause chest wall pain post-procedure, so if there is no urgency it is appropriate to begin with a low-amplitude shock (e.g. 25–50 joules), going on to larger shocks if necessary.

Digoxin toxicity increases the risk of untoward arrhythmias after cardioversion so it is conventional practice to withhold the drug for 24 hours before elective cardioversion. Patients with long-standing atrial arrhythmias are at risk of systemic embolism before and after cardioversion, so it is wise to ensure that the patient is adequately anticoagulated for at least 4 weeks either side of the procedure.

IMPLANTABLE CARDIAC DEFIBRILLATORS (ICDs)

These devices resemble a large cardiac pacemaker, and consist of a generator device, and a lead or leads that are implanted into the heart via the subclavian or cephalic vein (Fig. 18.14, p. 533). They can automatically sense and terminate life-threatening ventricular arrhythmias using tiered sequences of treatments. ICDs have all of the functions of a pacemaker (to deal with bradycardias) but in addition can treat ventricular tachyarrhythmias using overdrive pacing, synchronised cardioversion, or defibrillation. ICD implant procedures are subject to similar complications as pacemaker implants (e.g. infection, erosion—see below).

The indications for ICD implantation are expanding as devices become smaller, cheaper and easier to implant, and as trial data establish situations in which this therapy can reduce the risk of sudden arrhythmic death (Box 18.46). These can be divided into 'secondary prevention' indications, for which the ICD is implanted in patients who have already had a potentially life-threatening ventricular arrhythmia, and 'primary prevention' indications, for which the patient is considered to be at significant future risk of arrhythmic death; ICDs may be used prophylactically in selected patients with inherited conditions associated with high risk of sudden cardiac death (e.g. long QT syndrome, hypertrophic cardiomyopathy, arrhythmogenic right ventricular dysplasia, pp. 641–643). Although clinical trials have established benefit in large populations, health-care resource implications may limit widespread implementation.

18.46 KEY INDICATIONS FOR ICD THERAPY
Primary prevention
• After myocardial infarction, if LV ejection fraction < 30%   • Mild to moderate symptomatic heart failure, on optimal drug therapy, with LV ejection fraction < 35%
Secondary prevention
• Survivors of VF or VT cardiac arrest not due to transient or reversible cause   • VT with haemodynamic compromise or significant LV impairment (LV ejection fraction < 35%)

CATHETER ABLATION

Catheter ablation therapy has become the treatment of choice for many patients with recurrent arrhythmias (Fig. 18.14, p. 533). A series of catheter electrodes are inserted into the heart via the venous system, and are used to record the activation sequence of the heart in sinus rhythm, during tachycardia and after pacing manoeuvres. Once the arrhythmia focus or circuit is identified, a steerable catheter is placed into this critical zone (e.g. over an accessory pathway, in Wolff–Parkinson–White syndrome) and the culprit tissue is selectively ablated using heat (via radiofrequency current) or sometimes by freezing (cryoablation). The procedure takes approximately 2 or 3 hours, and does

not require a general anaesthetic. The patient may experience some discomfort during the ablation itself. Serious complications are rare (< 1%) and include inadvertent complete heart block requiring pacemaker implantation, and cardiac tamponade. For many arrhythmias, radiofrequency ablation is a very attractive form of treatment because it offers the prospect of a lifetime cure, thereby eliminating the need for long-term drug therapy.

The technique has revolutionised the management of many arrhythmias and is now the treatment of choice for AV nodal re-entry tachycardia and atrioventricular re-entrant (accessory pathway) tachycardias, where it is curative in more than 90% of cases. Focal atrial tachycardias and atrial flutter can also be eliminated by radiofrequency ablation, although some patients subsequently experience episodes of atrial fibrillation. The applications of the technique are expanding and it can now be used to treat some forms of ventricular tachycardia. Recently, catheter ablation techniques have been developed to prevent atrial fibrillation. This involves ablation at two sites: the ostia of the pulmonary veins, from which ectopic beats may trigger paroxysms of arrhythmia, and in the left atrium itself, where re-entry circuits maintain atrial fibrillation once established. This technique is effective at reducing episodes of atrial fibrillation in around 70–80% of younger patients with structurally normal hearts, and tends to be reserved for patients with drug-resistant atrial fibrillation.

Exceptionally troublesome AF and other refractory atrial tachyarrhythmias can be treated by using radiofrequency ablation to induce complete heart block deliberately; a permanent pacemaker must be implanted as well.

TEMPORARY AND PERMANENT PACEMAKERS

Temporary pacemakers

• *Transcutaneous pacing* is administered by delivering an electrical stimulus that is sufficient to induce cardiac contraction through two large adhesive gel pad electrodes placed over the apex and upper right sternal edge, or over the precordium and back. It is easy and quick to set up, but causes significant discomfort because it induces forceful pectoral and intercostal muscle contraction. Modern external cardiac defibrillators often incorporate a transcutaneous pacing system which can be used as a temporary measure until transvenous pacing is established.

• *Transvenous pacing* is delivered by inserting a bipolar pacing electrode via the internal jugular, subclavian or femoral vein and positioning it at the apex of the right ventricle, using fluoroscopic imaging. The electrode is then connected to an external pulse generator which can be adjusted to alter the energy output or pacing rate. The threshold is the lowest output that will reliably pace the heart and should be less than 1 volt (for pulse width 0.5 milliseconds) at implantation. The generator should be set to deliver an output that is at least twice this figure, and may require daily adjustment because the threshold tends to rise, due to inflammation and oedema around the tip of the electrode.

Temporary pacing may be indicated in the management of transient heart block and other arrhythmias complicating acute myocardial infarction, to maintain an adequate rhythm in other situations of transient or reversible bradycardia (i.e. due to metabolic disturbance or drug overdose), or as a prelude to permanent pacing. Complications include pneumothorax, brachial plexus or subclavian artery injury, local infection or septicaemia (usually *Staphylococcus aureus*), and pericarditis. Failure of the system may be due to lead displacement or a progressive increase in the threshold (exit block). The complication and failure rates increase with time and it is seldom wise to use a temporary pacing system for more than 7 days.

The ECG of right ventricular pacing is characterised by regular broad QRS complexes with a left bundle branch block pattern. Each complex is immediately preceded by a 'pacing spike' (Fig. 18.58). Nearly all pulse generators are used in the 'demand' mode so that a spontaneously occurring QRS complex will inhibit the pacemaker.

Permanent pacemakers

Permanent artificial pacemakers utilise the same principles, but the pulse generator is implanted under the skin. Electrodes can be placed in the right ventricle (usually at the apex), the right atrial appendage or, for atrioventricular sequential (dual chamber) pacing, both (Fig. 18.14, p. 533).

Permanent pacemakers are programmable so the lower rate, output, pacing mode and other parameters can be altered by an external programmer using a telemetry system. This facility allows the cardiologist to prolong the life of the pacemaker by choosing optimum settings and to optimise the pacemaker function to suit an individual patient's needs. For example, programming can be used to increase output in the face of an unexpected increase in threshold, or to increase the lower rate of the pacemaker in a patient with cardiac failure. Pacemakers also store useful diagnostic data, which can be retrieved by telemetry, about the patient's own heart rate trends, and the occurrence of tachyarrhythmias such as ventricular tachycardia.

Atrial pacing may be appropriate for patients with sinoatrial disease without AV block (the pacemaker acts as an external sinus node). Ventricular pacing is the only suitable mode for patients with continuous atrial fibrillation and bradycardia. In dual-chamber pacing the atrial electrode can be used to detect spontaneous atrial activity and trigger ventricular pacing (Fig. 18.58), thereby preserving atrioventricular synchrony and allowing the ventricular rate to increase together with the atrial rate during exercise and other forms of stress. Dual-chamber pacing has many advantages compared with ventricular pacing; these include superior haemodynamics leading to a better effort

18.47 INTERNATIONAL GENERIC PACEMAKER CODE

Chamber paced	Chamber sensed	Response to sensing
0 = none	0 = none	0 = none
A = atrium	A = atrium	T = triggered
V = ventricle	V = ventricle	I = inhibited
D = both	D = both	D = both

tolerance, a lower prevalence of atrial arrhythmias in patients with sinoatrial disease, and avoidance of 'pacemaker syndrome' (a fall in blood pressure and dizziness precipitated by loss of atrioventricular synchrony).

A code is used to signify the pacing mode (Box 18.47). For example, a system that paces the atrium, senses the atrium and is inhibited if it senses spontaneous activity is designated AAI. Most dual-chamber pacemakers are programmed to a mode termed DDD; here, ventricular pacing is triggered by a sensed sinus P-wave, and inhibited by a sensed spontaneous QRS complex. A fourth letter, 'R', is added if the pacemaker has a rate response function (e.g. AAIR = atrial demand pacemaker with rate response function).

Rate-responsive pacemakers are used in patients who are unable to mount an increase in heart rate during exercise. These devices have a sensor (e.g. vibration or respiration) that triggers a rise in heart rate in response to movement or increased respiratory rate. The sensitivity of the sensor is programmable, as is the maximum paced heart rate.

Early complications of permanent pacing include pneumothorax, cardiac tamponade, infection and lead displacement. Late complications include infection (which can usually only be treated satisfactorily by removing the pacing system), erosion of the generator or lead, chronic pain related to the implant site, and lead fracture due to mechanical fatigue.

CARDIAC RESYNCHRONISATION THERAPY (CRT)

This is a new treatment for selected patients with heart failure who are in sinus rhythm and who have left bundle branch block. This conduction defect is associated with an incoordinate left ventricular contraction and can aggravate heart failure in susceptible patients. CRT devices carry an additional lead that is placed via the coronary sinus into one of the veins on the epicardial surface of the left ventricle. Simultaneous septal and left ventricular epicardial pacing resynchronises left ventricular contraction. These devices

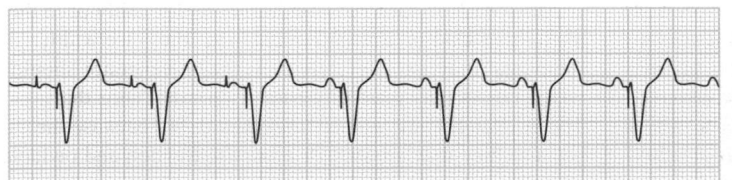

Fig. 18.58 Dual-chamber pacing. The first three beats show atrial and ventricular pacing with narrow pacing spikes in front of each P wave and QRS complex. The last four beats show spontaneous P waves with a different morphology and no pacing spike; the pacemaker senses or tracks these P waves and maintains AV synchrony by pacing the ventricle after an appropriate interval.

18

18

18.48 CARDIAC RESYNCHRONISATION THERAPY (CRT) FOR HEART FAILURE

'CRT improves symptoms and quality of life, and reduces mortality in patients with moderate to severe symptomatic heart failure who are in sinus rhythm, with left bundle branch block and LV ejection fraction ≤ 35%.'

- Cardiac Resynchronisation–Heart Failure (CARE–HF) Study. Cleland J, et al. N Engl J Med 2005; 352:1539–1549.
- COMPANION Study. Bristow MR, et al. N Engl J Med 2004; 350:2140–2150.

improve effort tolerance and reduce the likelihood of hospital admission in properly selected cases (Box 18.48). CRT devices often incorporate a defibrillator function.

ATHEROSCLEROSIS

Atherosclerosis may manifest as coronary heart disease (e.g. angina, myocardial infarction, sudden death), cerebrovascular disease (e.g. stroke and transient ischaemic attack) or peripheral vascular disease (e.g. claudication and critical limb ischaemia). These entities often coexist and the pathogenesis of the disease is similar. Occult coronary artery disease is common in those who present with other forms of atherosclerotic vascular disease, such as intermittent claudication or stroke, and is an important cause of subsequent morbidity and mortality in these patients.

PATHOPHYSIOLOGY

Atherosclerosis is a progressive inflammatory disorder of the arterial wall that is characterised by focal lipid-rich deposits of atheroma that remain clinically silent until they become large enough to impair arterial perfusion or until ulceration or disruption of the lesion results in thrombotic occlusion or embolisation of the affected vessel. These mechanisms are common to the entire vascular tree, and the clinical manifestations of atherosclerosis depend upon the site of the lesion and the vulnerability of the organ supplied.

Atherosclerosis is a disorder that begins early in life; abnormalities of arterial endothelial function have been detected among high-risk children and adolescents (e.g. cigarette smokers and those with familial hyperlipidaemia or hypertension), and early atherosclerotic lesions have been found in the arteries of victims of accidental death in the second and third decades of life. Nevertheless, clinical manifestations often do not appear until the sixth, seventh or eighth decade.

Early atherosclerosis

Fatty streaks tend to occur at sites of altered arterial shear stress, such as bifurcations, and are associated with abnormal endothelial function. They develop when inflammatory cells, predominantly monocytes, bind to receptors expressed by endothelial cells, migrate into the intima, take up oxidised low-density lipoprotein (LDL) from the plasma and become lipid-laden foam cells or macrophages. Extracellular lipid pools appear in the intimal space when these foam cells die and release their contents (Fig. 18.59). In response to cytokines and growth factors produced by the activated macrophages, smooth muscle cells migrate from the media of the arterial wall into the intima, and change from a contractile to a repair phenotype in an attempt to stabilise the atherosclerotic lesion. If they are successful, the lipid core will be covered by smooth muscle cells and matrix, producing a stable atherosclerotic plaque that will remain asymptomatic until it becomes large enough to obstruct arterial flow.

Advanced atherosclerosis

In an established atherosclerotic plaque, macrophages mediate inflammation and smooth muscle cells promote repair; if inflammation predominates, the plaque becomes active or unstable and may be complicated by ulceration and superadded thrombosis. Cytokines such as interleukin-1, tumour necrosis factor-alpha, interferon-gamma, platelet-derived growth factors and matrix metalloproteinases are released by activated macrophages and may cause the intimal smooth muscle cells overlying the plaque to become senescent, resulting in thinning of the protective fibrous cap; they may also digest collagen cross-struts within the plaque. These changes make the lesion vulnerable to the effects of mechanical stress and may lead to erosion, fissuring or rupture of the plaque surface (Fig. 18.59). Any breach in the integrity of the plaque will expose its contents to circulating blood and may trigger platelet aggregation and thrombosis that extends into the atheromatous plaque and the arterial lumen. This type of plaque event may cause partial or complete obstruction at the site of the lesion and/or distal embolisation resulting in infarction or ischaemia of the affected organ. It is the common mechanism that underlies many of the acute manifestations of atherosclerotic vascular disease (e.g. acute lower limb ischaemia, myocardial infarction and stroke).

The number and complexity of arterial plaques increase with age and with systemic risk factors (see below) but the rate of progression of individual plaques is variable. There is a complex and dynamic interaction between mechanical wall stress and atherosclerotic lesions. 'Vulnerable plaques' are characterised by a lipid-rich core, a thin fibrocellular cap, an increase in inflammatory cells, and the release of specific enzymes that degrade matrix proteins. In contrast, stable plaques are typified by a small lipid pool, a thick fibrous cap, calcification and plentiful collagenous cross-struts. Lipid-lowering therapy may help to stabilise vulnerable plaques. Fissuring or rupture tends to occur at sites of maximal mechanical stress, particularly the margins of an eccentric plaque, and may be triggered by a surge in blood pressure (e.g. during exercise or emotional upset). Surprisingly, plaque events are often subclinical and may heal spontaneously; however, this may allow thrombus to be incorporated into the lesion, producing plaque growth and further obstruction to flow in the arterial lumen.

Atherosclerosis may also induce complex changes in the media that lead to arterial remodelling; thus, some arterial segments may slowly constrict (negative remodelling) whilst others may gradually enlarge (positive remodelling). These changes are poorly understood but are important because they may amplify or minimise the degree to which atheroma encroaches into the arterial lumen.

Early atherosclerosis

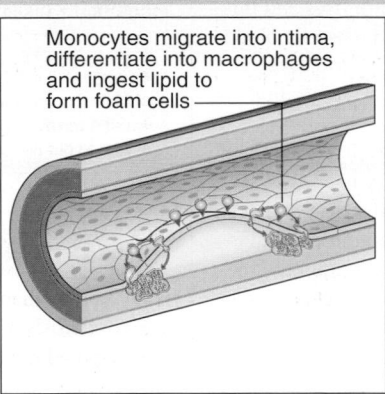

Activated endothelial cells express adhesion molecules and recruit inflammatory cells, predominantly monocytes

Lipid accumulates in intimal space
Abnormal endothelial cell function

Monocytes migrate into intima, differentiate into macrophages and ingest lipid to form foam cells

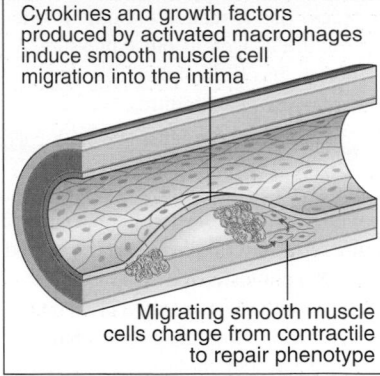

Cytokines and growth factors produced by activated macrophages induce smooth muscle cell migration into the intima

Migrating smooth muscle cells change from contractile to repair phenotype

18

Stable atherosclerotic plaque

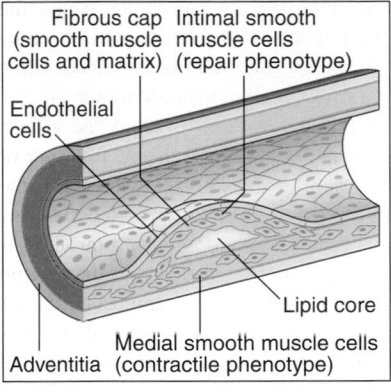

Fibrous cap (smooth muscle cells and matrix)   Intimal smooth muscle cells (repair phenotype)

Endothelial cells

Lipid core

Adventitia   Medial smooth muscle cells (contractile phenotype)

Advanced atherosclerosis

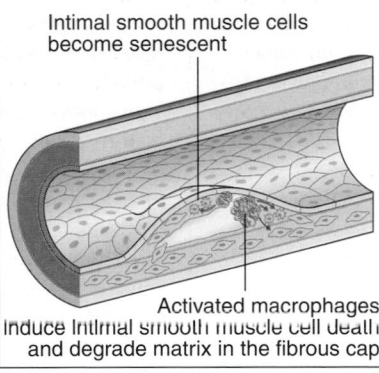

Intimal smooth muscle cells become senescent

Activated macrophages induce intimal smooth muscle cell death and degrade matrix in the fibrous cap

Unstable coronary artery disease

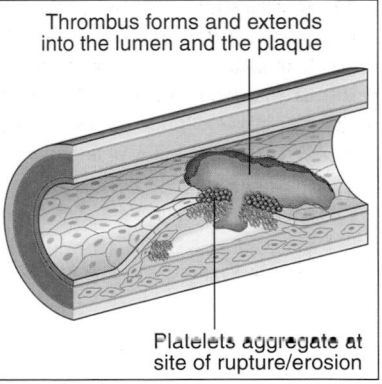

Thrombus forms and extends into the lumen and the plaque

Platelets aggregate at site of rupture/erosion

Fig. 18.59 The pathogenesis of atherosclerosis.

RISK FACTORS

The role and relative importance of many risk factors for the development of coronary, peripheral and cerebrovascular disease have been defined in experimental animal studies, epidemiological studies and clinical interventional trials. Some key factors have emerged but do not explain all the risk; thus, unknown or as yet unconfirmed factors may account for up to 40% of the variation in risk of atheromatous vascular disease from one person to the next.

The impact of genetic risk is illustrated by twin studies; for example, a monozygotic twin of an affected individual has an eightfold increased risk, and a dizygotic twin a fourfold increased risk of dying from coronary heart disease compared to the general population.

The effect of risk factors is multiplicative rather than additive. People with a combination of risk factors (e.g. smoking, hypertension and diabetes) are at greatest risk and assessment should therefore be based on a holistic approach that takes account of all identifiable risk factors. It is also important to distinguish between relative risk (the proportional increase in risk) and absolute risk (the actual chance of an event). Thus, a man of 35 with a plasma cholesterol of 7 mmol/l (~170 mg/dl) who smokes 40 cigarettes a day is relatively much more likely to die from coronary disease within the next decade than a non-smoking woman of the same age with a normal cholesterol, but the absolute likelihood of his dying during this time is still small (high relative risk, low absolute risk).

- *Age and sex.* Age is the most powerful independent risk factor for atherosclerosis. Pre-menopausal women have much lower rates of disease than age- and risk-matched males; however, the gender difference disappears rapidly after the menopause. Randomised controlled trials have demonstrated that hormone replacement therapy has no role in the primary or secondary prevention of coronary heart disease. Indeed, isolated oestrogen therapy appears potentially to cause an increased cardiovascular event rate.
- *Family history.* Atherosclerotic vascular disease often runs in families. This may be due to a combination of shared genetic, environmental and lifestyle (e.g. smoking, exercise and diet) factors. The most common inherited risk characteristics (hypertension, hyperlipidaemia, diabetes) are polygenic. A 'positive' family history is present when clinical problems in first-degree relatives occur at relatively young age, such as < 50 years for men and < 55 years for women.
- *Smoking.* Smoking is probably the most important avoidable cause of atherosclerotic vascular disease; there is a strong, consistent and dose-linked relationship between cigarette smoking and ischaemic heart disease.

18

- *Hypertension* (see below). The incidence of atherosclerosis increases as blood pressure rises and this excess risk is related to both systolic and diastolic blood pressure as well as pulse pressure. Antihypertensive therapy has been shown to reduce coronary mortality, stroke and heart failure.
- *Hypercholesterolaemia* (p. 446). Robust epidemiological data demonstrate that the risk of coronary heart disease and other forms of atherosclerotic vascular disease rises with plasma cholesterol concentration, and in particular the ratio of total cholesterol to high-density lipoprotein (HDL) cholesterol. A much weaker correlation also exists with plasma triglyceride concentration. Extensive large-scale randomised trials have shown that lowering total LDL and cholesterol concentrations reduces the risk of cardiovascular events including death, myocardial infarction and stroke, and also reduces the need for revascularisation.
- *Diabetes mellitus*. This is a potent risk factor for all forms of atherosclerosis and is often associated with diffuse disease that is difficult to treat. Insulin resistance (normal glucose homeostasis with high levels of insulin) is associated with obesity and physical inactivity, and is also a potent risk factor for coronary heart disease (p. 815). Glucose intolerance accounts for a major part of the high incidence of ischaemic heart disease in certain ethnic groups, e.g. South Asians.
- *Haemostatic factors*. Platelet activation and high levels of fibrinogen are associated with an increased risk of coronary thrombosis. Anti-phospholipid antibodies are associated with recurrent arterial thomboses.
- *Physical activity*. Physical inactivity roughly doubles the risk of coronary heart disease and is a major risk factor for stroke. Regular exercise (brisk walking, cycling or swimming for 20 minutes two or three times a week) appears to have a protective effect which may be related to increased HDL cholesterol, lower blood pressure, reduced blood clotting, and collateral vessel development.
- *Obesity* (p. 111). Obesity, particularly if central or truncal, is an independent risk factor, although it is often associated with other adverse factors such as hypertension, diabetes and physical inactivity.
- *Alcohol*. A moderate intake of alcohol (2–4 units a day) appears to offer some protection from coronary disease; however, heavy drinking is associated with hypertension and excess cardiac events.
- *Other dietary factors*. Diets deficient in fresh fruit, vegetables and polyunsaturated fatty acids are associated with an increased risk of vascular disease. Low levels of vitamin C, vitamin E and other antioxidants may enhance the production of oxidised LDL. Hyperhomocysteinaemia is associated with accelerated atherosclerosis including stroke and peripheral vascular disease. Low dietary folate, vitamin B_{12} and vitamin B_6 can elevate homocysteine concentrations.
- *Personality*. Certain personality traits are associated with an increased risk of coronary disease. Nevertheless, there is little or no evidence to support the popular belief that stress is a major cause of coronary artery disease.

18.49 POPULATION ADVICE TO PREVENT CORONARY DISEASE

- Do not smoke
- Take regular exercise (minimum of 20 mins, three times a week)
- Maintain 'ideal' body weight
- Eat a mixed diet rich in fresh fruit and vegetables
- Aim to get no more than 10% of energy intake from saturated fat

PRIMARY PREVENTION

Two complementary strategies can be used to prevent atherosclerosis in apparently healthy but at-risk individuals.

The population strategy aims to modify the risk factors of the whole population through diet and lifestyle advice on the basis that even a small reduction in smoking or average cholesterol, or modification of exercise and diet will produce worthwhile benefits (Box 18.49). Some risk factors for atheroma, such as obesity and smoking, are also associated with a high risk of other diseases and should be actively discouraged through public health measures.

In contrast, the targeted strategy aims to identify and treat high-risk individuals, who usually have a combination of risk factors and can be identified by using composite scoring systems (p. 611 and Appendix). It is important to consider the absolute risk of atheromatous cardiovascular disease that any one individual is facing before contemplating specific antihypertensive or lipid-lowering therapy because this will help to determine whether the possible benefits of intervention are likely to outweigh the expense, inconvenience and possible side-effects of treatment. For example, a 65-year-old man with an average blood pressure of 150/90 mmHg, who smokes and has diabetes, a total:HDL cholesterol of 8 and left ventricular hypertrophy on ECG, will have a 10-year risk of CHD of 68% and a 10-year risk of any cardiovascular event of 90%. Lowering his cholesterol will reduce these risks by 30% and lowering his blood pressure will produce a further 20% reduction; both treatments would obviously be worth while. Conversely, a 55-year-old woman who has an identical blood pressure, is a non-smoker, is not diabetic and has a normal ECG and a total:HDL cholesterol of 6 has a much better outlook, with a predicted CHD risk of 14% and cardiovascular risk of 19% over the next 10 years. Although lowering her cholesterol and blood pressure would also reduce risk by 30% and 20% respectively, the value of both forms of treatment would clearly be questionable.

There is strong observational evidence that moderate to high levels of physical activity reduce the risk of coronary heart disease and stroke (relative risk reduction 30–50%). Observational studies have found that the risk of death and cardiovascular events falls when people stop smoking.

SECONDARY PREVENTION

Patients who already have evidence of atheromatous vascular disease (e.g. peripheral vascular disease or myocardial infarction) are at high risk of another vascular event and can be offered a variety of treatments (Box 18.50) and measures that have been shown to improve their outlook (secondary prevention). The energetic correction of risk factors, particularly smoking, hypertension and hypercholesterolaemia, is particularly important in this patient group because the absolute risk of further vascular events is very high. In the light of recent randomised controlled trials, especially the Heart Protection Study, all patients with coronary heart disease should be given statin therapy irrespective of their serum cholesterol concentration. Blood pressure should be treated to a target of ≤ 130/80 (p. 612). Aspirin and ACE inhibitors are of benefit in all patients with evidence of vascular disease (Boxes 18.51 and 18.52). Beta-blockers will benefit patients with a history of myocardial infarction (see below) or heart failure.

Many clinical events offer an unrivalled opportunity to introduce effective secondary preventive measures. For example, patients who have just survived a myocardial infarction or undergone bypass surgery are usually keen to help themselves and may be particularly receptive to appropriate lifestyle advice, such as weight reduction, stopping smoking etc.

CORONARY HEART DISEASE

Coronary heart disease (CHD) is the most common form of heart disease and the single most important cause of premature death in Europe, the Baltic states, Russia, North and South America, Australia and New Zealand. By 2020 it is estimated that it will be the major cause of death in all regions of the world.

In the UK (population 59 million), 1 in 3 men and 1 in 4 women die from CHD, an estimated 330 000 people have a myocardial infarct each year and approximately 1.3 million people have angina. The death rates from CHD in the UK are amongst the highest in Western Europe (more than 140 000 people) but are falling, particularly in younger age groups; in the last 10 years CHD mortality has fallen by 42% among UK men and women aged 16–64.

Disease of the coronary arteries is almost always due to atheroma and its complications, particularly thrombosis; the common clinical manifestations and pathological correlates of CHD are shown in Box 18.53. Occasionally, the coronary arteries are involved in other disorders such as aortitis, polyarteritis and other connective tissue disorders.

18.53 CORONARY HEART DISEASE: CLINICAL MANIFESTATIONS AND PATHOLOGY

Clinical problem	Pathology
Stable angina	Ischaemia due to fixed atheromatous stenosis of one or more coronary arteries
Unstable angina	Ischaemia caused by dynamic obstruction of a coronary artery due to plaque rupture with superimposed thrombosis and spasm
Myocardial infarction	Myocardial necrosis caused by acute occlusion of a coronary artery due to plaque rupture and thrombosis
Heart failure	Myocardial dysfunction due to infarction or ischaemia
Arrhythmia	Altered conduction due to ischaemia or infarction
Sudden death	Ventricular arrhythmia, asystole or massive myocardial infarction

STABLE ANGINA

Angina pectoris is the symptom complex caused by transient myocardial ischaemia and constitutes a clinical syndrome rather than a disease; it may occur whenever there is an imbalance between myocardial oxygen supply and demand (Box 18.54). Coronary atheroma is by far the most common cause of angina; however, the symptom may also be a manifestation of other forms of heart disease, particularly aortic valve disease and hypertrophic cardiomyopathy.

This section describes the features of 'stable' angina pectoris which occurs when coronary perfusion is impaired by fixed or stable atheroma of the coronary arteries.

18

18

18.54 FACTORS INFLUENCING MYOCARDIAL OXYGEN SUPPLY AND DEMAND

Oxygen demand

Cardiac work
- Heart rate
- Blood pressure
- Myocardial contractility
- Left ventricular hypertrophy
- Valve disease, e.g. aortic stenosis

Oxygen supply

Coronary blood flow
- Duration of diastole
- Coronary perfusion pressure (aortic diastolic minus coronary sinus or right atrial diastolic pressure)
- Coronary vasomotor tone
- Oxygenation
  Haemoglobin
  Oxygen saturation

N.B. Coronary blood flow occurs mainly in diastole.

18.55 ACTIVITIES PRECIPITATING ANGINA

Common
- Physical exertion
- Cold exposure
- Heavy meals
- Intense emotion

Uncommon
- Lying flat (decubitus angina)
- Vivid dreams (nocturnal angina)

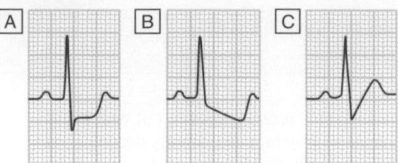

Fig. 18.60 Forms of exercise-induced ST depression. [A] Planar ST depression is usually indicative of myocardial ischaemia. [B] Down-sloping depression also usually indicates myocardial ischaemia. [C] Up-sloping depression, however, may be a normal finding.

18.56 A GUIDE TO RISK STRATIFICATION IN STABLE ANGINA

High risk	Low risk
Post-infarct angina	Predictable exertional angina
Poor effort tolerance	Good effort tolerance
Ischaemia at low workload	Ischaemia only at high workload
Left main or three-vessel disease	Single-vessel or minor two-vessel disease
Poor LV function	Good LV function

N.B. Patients may fall between these categories.

Clinical features

The history is by far the most important factor in making the diagnosis; the features of cardiac pain and the differential diagnosis of chest pain are discussed on pages 534–539.

Stable angina is characterised by central chest pain, discomfort or breathlessness that is precipitated by exertion or other forms of stress (Box 18.55), and is promptly relieved by rest (Figs 18.15 and 18.16, pp. 535–536). Some patients find that the discomfort comes when they start walking, and that later it does not return despite greater effort ('warm-up angina').

Physical examination is frequently negative, but should include a careful search for evidence of valve disease (particularly aortic), important risk factors (e.g. hypertension, diabetes), left ventricular dysfunction (e.g. cardiomegaly, gallop rhythm), other manifestations of arterial disease (e.g. carotid bruits, peripheral vascular disease) and unrelated conditions that may exacerbate angina (e.g. anaemia, thyrotoxicosis).

Investigations

Resting ECG

The ECG may show evidence of previous myocardial infarction but is often normal even in patients with left main or severe three-vessel coronary artery disease. Occasionally, there is T-wave flattening or inversion in some leads, providing non-specific evidence of myocardial ischaemia or damage.

The most convincing ECG evidence of myocardial ischaemia is obtained by demonstrating reversible ST segment depression or elevation, with or without T-wave inversion, at the time the patient is experiencing symptoms (whether spontaneous or induced by exercise testing).

Exercise ECG

An exercise tolerance test (ETT) is usually performed using a standard treadmill or bicycle ergometer protocol (p. 528) while monitoring the patient's ECG, blood pressure and general condition. Planar or down-sloping ST segment depression of 1 mm or more is indicative of ischaemia (Fig. 18.60); up-sloping ST depression is less specific and often occurs in normal individuals.

Exercise testing can be used to confirm or refute a diagnosis of angina and is also a useful means of assessing the severity of coronary disease and identifying high-risk individuals (Box 18.56). For example, the amount of exercise which can be tolerated and the extent and degree of any ST segment change (Fig. 18.61) provide a useful guide to the likely extent of coronary disease.

Exercise testing is not infallible and may produce false positive results in the presence of digoxin therapy, left ventricular hypertrophy, left bundle branch block or Wolff–Parkinson–White syndrome. The predictive accuracy of exercise testing is lower in women than men. The test should be classed as inconclusive (and not negative) if the patient cannot achieve an adequate level of exercise because of locomotor or other non-cardiac problems.

Other forms of stress testing

Myocardial perfusion scanning. This may be helpful in the evaluation of patients with an equivocal or uninterpretable exercise test and those who are unable to exercise; its predictive accuracy is higher than that of the exercise ECG. The technique involves obtaining scintiscans of the myocardium at rest and during stress after the

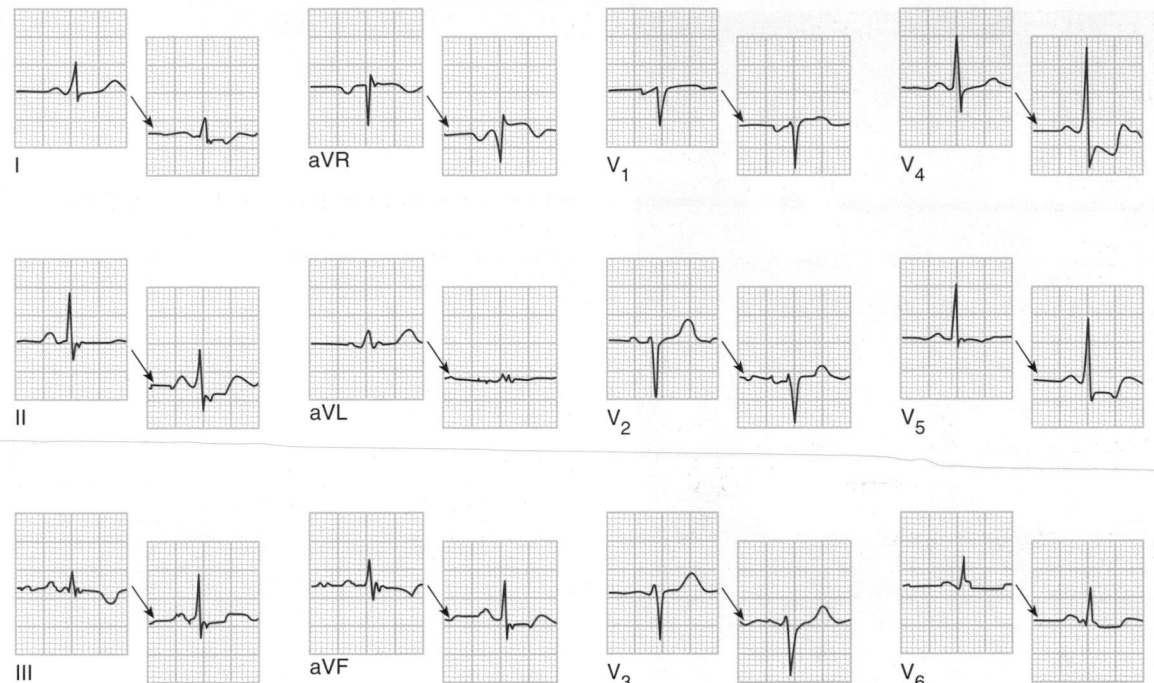

Fig. 18.61 A positive exercise test. The resting 12-lead ECG shows some minor T-wave changes in the inferolateral leads but is otherwise normal. After 3 minutes' exercise on a treadmill there is marked planar ST depression in leads II, V_4 and V_5 (right offset). Subsequent coronary angiography revealed critical three-vessel coronary artery disease.

18

administration of an intravenous radioactive isotope such as [99]technetium tetrofosmin. It may be used in conjunction with conventional exercise testing or some form of pharmacological stress such as a controlled infusion of dobutamine. Thallium and tetrofosmin are taken up by viable perfused myocardium. A perfusion defect present during stress but not rest provides evidence of reversible myocardial ischaemia (Fig. 18.62), whereas a persistent perfusion defect seen during both phases of the study is usually indicative of previous myocardial infarction.

Stress echocardiography. This is an alternative to myocardial perfusion scanning and can achieve similar predictive accuracy (superior to exercise ECG). The technique uses transthoracic echocardiography to identify ischaemic segments of myocardium and areas of infarction. The former characteristically exhibit reversible defects in contractility during exercise or pharmacological stress with a dobutamine infusion; the latter typically do not contract at rest or during stress.

Coronary arteriography

In contrast to the functional information provided by stress testing, coronary arteriography provides detailed anatomical information about the extent and nature of coronary artery disease (Fig. 18.63), and is usually performed with a view to coronary bypass grafting or percutaneous coronary intervention (PCI—p. 586). In some patients, diagnostic coronary angiography may be indicated when non-invasive tests have failed to elucidate the cause of atypical chest pain. The procedure is performed under local anaesthesia and requires specialised radiological equipment, cardiac monitoring and an experienced operating team.

Management

The management of angina pectoris involves:

- a careful assessment of the likely extent and severity of arterial disease
- the identification and control of significant risk factors (e.g. smoking, hypertension, hyperlipidaemia)
- the use of measures to control symptoms
- the identification of high-risk patients and application of treatments to improve life expectancy.

Symptoms alone are a poor guide to the extent of coronary artery disease; exercise or pharmacological stress testing is therefore advisable in all patients who are potential candidates for revascularisation. An algorithm for the investigation and treatment of patients with stable angina is shown in Figure 18.64.

Treatment should start with a careful explanation of the problem and a discussion of the potential lifestyle and medical interventions that may relieve symptoms and improve prognosis (Box 18.57). Anxiety and misconceptions often contribute to disability; for example, some patients avoid all forms of exertion because they believe that each attack of angina is a 'mini heart attack' that results in permanent damage. Effective management of these psychological factors can make a huge difference to the patient's quality of life.

Antiplatelet therapy

Low-dose (75–150 mg) aspirin reduces the risk of adverse events such as myocardial infarction and should be prescribed for all patients with coronary artery disease

583

18

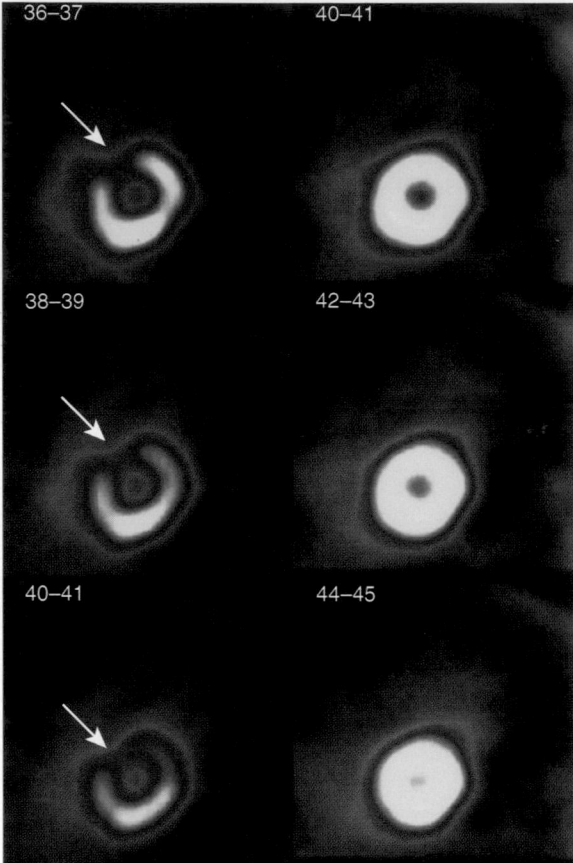

36–37   40–41

38–39   42–43

40–41   44–45

Fig. 18.62   A technetium scan showing reversible anterior myocardial ischaemia. The images are cross-sectional tomograms of the left ventricle. The resting scans (right) show even uptake of technetium and look like doughnuts; during stress (in this case a dobutamine infusion) there is reduced uptake of technetium, particularly along the anterior wall (arrows), and the scans look like crescents (left).

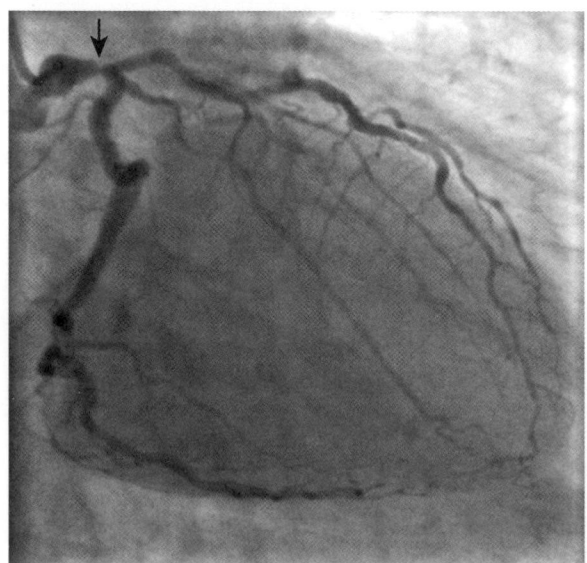

Fig. 18.63   Coronary angiogram from a patient with stable angina. There is severe stenosis of the left main stem (arrow).

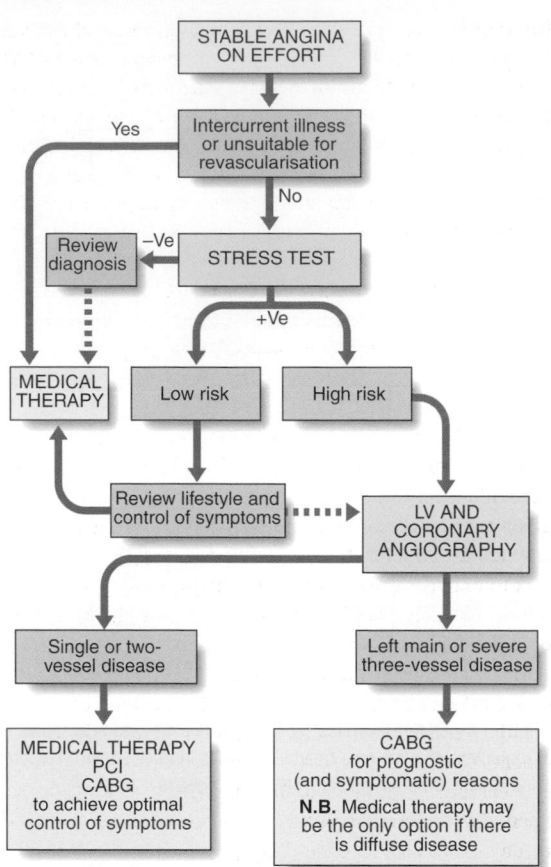

Fig. 18.64   A scheme for the investigation and treatment of stable angina on effort. (PCI = percutaneous coronary intervention; CABG = coronary artery bypass grafting)

18.57 ADVICE TO PATIENTS WITH STABLE ANGINA

- Do not smoke
- Aim at ideal body weight
- Take regular exercise (exercise up to, but not beyond, the point of chest discomfort is beneficial and may promote collateral vessels)
- Avoid severe unaccustomed exertion, and vigorous exercise after a heavy meal or in very cold weather
- Take sublingual nitrate before undertaking exertion that may induce angina

indefinitely (Box 18.52). Clopidogrel (75 mg daily) is an equally effective antiplatelet agent that can be prescribed if aspirin causes troublesome dyspepsia or other side-effects.

Anti-anginal drug treatment

Four groups of drugs are used to help relieve or prevent the symptoms of angina: nitrates, β-blockers, calcium antagonists and potassium channel activators.

Nitrates. These drugs act directly on vascular smooth muscle to produce venous and arteriolar dilatation; their beneficial effects in angina are due to a reduction in myocardial oxygen demand (lower preload and afterload) and an increase in myocardial oxygen supply (coronary vasodilatation).

Sublingual glyceryl trinitrate (GTN) administered from a metered-dose aerosol (400 µg per spray) or as a tablet (300 or 500 µg) allowed to dissolve under the tongue or crunched and retained in the mouth will usually relieve an attack of angina in 2–3 minutes. Unwanted side-effects include headache (which may be more distressing than the angina), symptomatic hypotension and, rarely, syncope. To avoid these symptoms the tablet may be spat out as soon as the angina is relieved.

Patients often need to be reassured that GTN is not habit-forming and will not lose its effect if used repeatedly. They should also be encouraged to use the drug prophylactically before engaging in exercise that is liable to provoke symptoms.

Sublingual GTN has a short duration of action (Box 18.58); however, a variety of alternative nitrate preparations can provide a more prolonged therapeutic effect. GTN can be given transcutaneously as a patch (5–10 mg daily), or as a slow-release buccal tablet (1–5 mg 6-hourly). GTN is subject to extensive first-pass metabolism in the liver and is therefore virtually ineffective when swallowed; however, other nitrates such as isosorbide dinitrate (10–20 mg 8-hourly) and isosorbide mononitrate (20–60 mg once or twice a day) can be given by mouth. Headache is common but tends to diminish if the patient perseveres with the treatment. Continuous nitrate therapy causes pharmacological tolerance and this should be avoided by using a regimen that includes a nitrate-free period of 6–8 hours every day. A variety of once-daily proprietary preparations with a built-in nitrate-free period are available. It is usually advisable to schedule the medication so that drug levels are low during the night when the patient is inactive; however, if nocturnal angina is a prominent symptom, long-acting nitrates can be given at the end of the day instead.

Beta-blockers. These drugs lower myocardial oxygen demand by reducing heart rate, blood pressure and myocardial contractility. Unfortunately, they can exacerbate the symptoms of peripheral vascular disease and may provoke bronchospasm in patients with obstructive airways disease. The properties and side-effects of β-blockers are discussed above (p. 573).

In theory, non-selective β-blockers may aggravate coronary vasospasm by blocking the coronary artery β_2-adrenoceptors and it is usually advisable to use a once-daily cardioselective preparation (e.g. atenolol 50–100 mg daily, slow-release metoprolol 50–200 mg daily, bisoprolol 5–10 mg daily).

A β-blocking drug should not be withdrawn abruptly because this may have a rebound effect and precipitate dangerous arrhythmias, worsening angina or myocardial infarction (the β blocker withdrawal syndrome).

Calcium antagonists. These drugs inhibit the slow inward current caused by the entry of extracellular calcium through the cell membrane of excitable cells, particularly cardiac and arteriolar smooth muscle, and lower myocardial oxygen demand by reducing blood pressure and myocardial contractility.

Dihydropyridine calcium antagonists, such as nifedipine and nicardipine, often cause a reflex tachycardia; this may be counterproductive and it is often best to use these drugs in combination with a β-blocker. In contrast, verapamil and diltiazem are particularly suitable for patients who are not receiving a β-blocker because they inhibit conduction through the AV node and tend to cause a bradycardia or even atrioventricular block in susceptible individuals. The calcium antagonists may reduce myocardial contractility and can aggravate or precipitate heart failure. Other unwanted effects include peripheral oedema, flushing, headache and dizziness.

The dosage and some of the distinguishing features of these drugs are listed in Box 18.59.

Potassium channel activators. This class of drug has arterial and venous dilating properties but does not exhibit the tolerance seen with nitrates. Nicorandil (10–30 mg 12-hourly orally) is the only drug in this class currently available for clinical use.

Although each of these groups of drug has been shown to be superior to placebo in relieving the symptoms of angina, there is little convincing evidence that one group is more

18

18.58 DURATION OF ACTION OF SOME NITRATE PREPARATIONS		
Preparation	Peak action	Duration of action
Sublingual GTN	4–8 mins	10–30 mins
Buccal GTN	4–10 mins	30–300 mins
Transdermal GTN	1–3 hrs	Up to 24 hrs
Oral isosorbide dinitrate	45–120 mins	2–6 hrs
Oral isosorbide mononitrate	45–120 mins	6–10 hrs

18.59 CALCIUM ANTAGONISTS USED FOR THE TREATMENT OF ANGINA		
Drug	Dose	Feature
Nifedipine	5–20 mg 8-hourly*	May cause marked tachycardia
Nicardipine	20–40 mg 8-hourly	May cause less myocardial depression than the other drugs in this group
Amlodipine	2.5–10 mg daily	Ultralong-acting
Verapamil	40–80 mg 8-hourly*	Commonly causes constipation; useful anti-arrhythmic properties (p. 573)
Diltiazem	60–120 mg 8-hourly*	Similar anti-arrhythmic properties to verapamil
* Once- or twice-daily slow-release preparations are available.		

18

effective than another. Moreover, many commonly used combinations of anti-anginal drugs have not been evaluated in well-controlled clinical trials. Nevertheless, it is conventional to start therapy with low-dose aspirin, sublingual GTN and a β-blocker, and then add a calcium channel antagonist or a long-acting nitrate later, if necessary. The goal is the control of angina with minimum side-effects and the simplest possible drug regimen. There is little or no evidence that prescribing multiple anti-anginal drugs is of benefit, and revascularisation should be considered if an appropriate combination of two drugs fails to achieve a symptomatic response.

Invasive treatment

The most widely used invasive options for the treatment of ischaemic heart disease include percutaneous coronary intervention (PCI; including percutaneous transluminal coronary angioplasty, PTCA) and coronary artery bypass graft (CABG) surgery.

Percutaneous coronary intervention (PCI)

This is performed by passing a fine guidewire across a coronary stenosis under radiographic control and using it to position a balloon which is then inflated to dilate the stenosis (Fig. 18.14, p. 533 and Fig. 18.65). A coronary stent is a piece of coated metallic 'scaffolding' that can be deployed on a balloon and used to maximise and maintain dilatation of a stenosed vessel. The routine use of stents in appropriate vessels reduces both acute complications and the incidence of clinically important restenosis (Box 18.60).

PCI provides an effective symptomatic treatment but there is no evidence that it improves survival in patients with chronic stable angina. PCI is mainly used in single or two-vessel disease; stenoses in bypass grafts can be dilated as well as those in the native coronary arteries, and the technique is often used to provide palliative therapy for patients with recurrent angina after CABG. Coronary surgery is usually the preferred option in patients with three-vessel or left main disease, although recent trials have demonstrated that PCI is also feasible in such patients.

The main acute complications of PCI are occlusion of the target vessel or a side branch by thrombus or a loose flap of intima (coronary artery dissection), and consequent myocardial damage. This occurs in about 2–5% of procedures and can often be corrected by deploying a stent; however, emergency CABG is sometimes required. Minor myocardial damage, as indicated by elevation of sensitive intracellular markers (troponins), occurs in up to 10% of

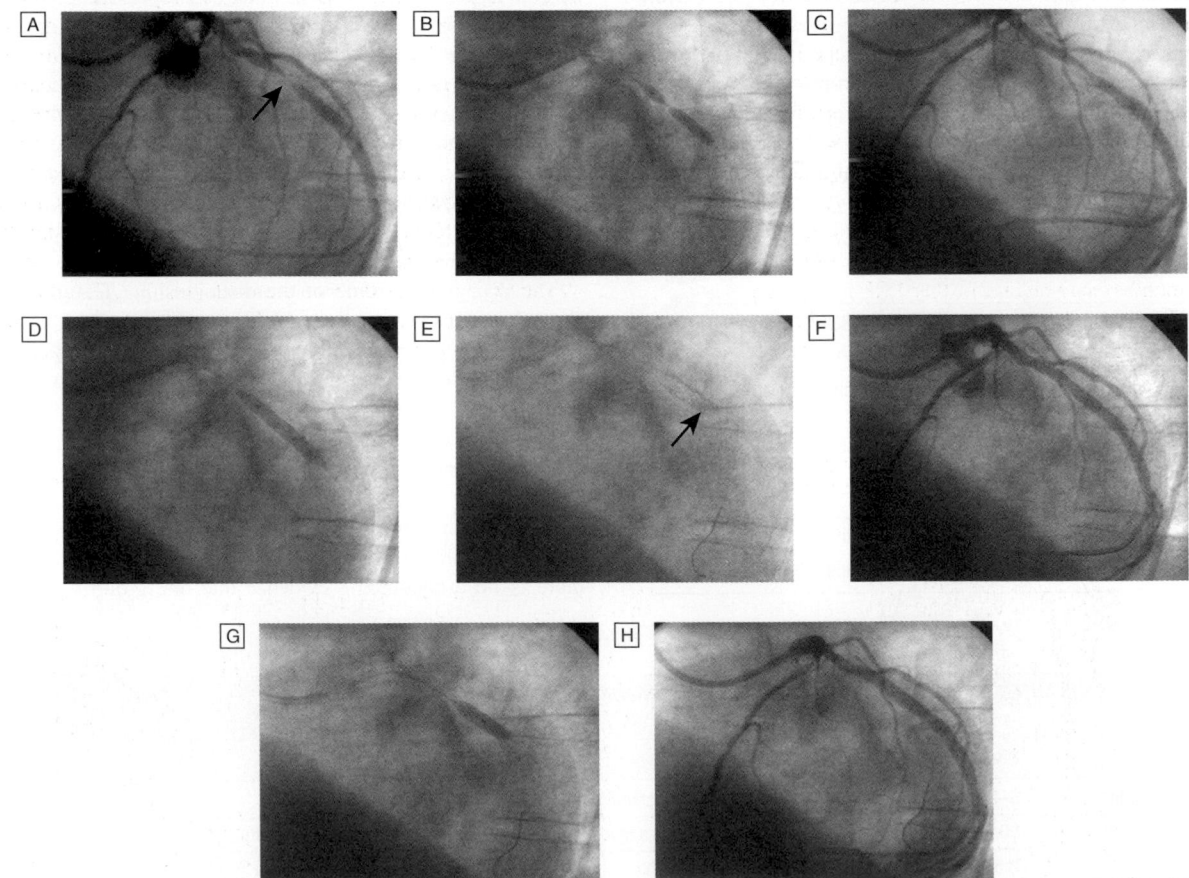

Fig. 18.65 Percutaneous coronary intervention. A sequence of images from a 58-year-old woman with stable angina. **A** Severe stenosis of the circumflex artery (arrow). **B** A balloon has been advanced into the stenosis, over a guidewire, and has been inflated. (Note the waisting caused by the lesion.) **C** Residual stenosis and dissection (tramline shadow—arrow) after balloon dilatation. **D** A stent is deployed on a balloon. **E** The stent is visible on plain fluoroscopy (arrow). **F** Angiogram after stenting. **G** A short balloon is used to dilate the stent at high pressure. **H** Final result.

cases. The main long-term complication of PCI is restenosis (Box 18.61), which occurs in up to one-third of cases; this is due to a combination of elastic recoil and smooth muscle proliferation (neo-intimal hyperplasia) and tends to occur within 3 months. Stenting substantially reduces the risk of restenosis, probably because it allows the operator to achieve more complete dilatation in the first place. Drug-eluting stents can reduce this risk even further by allowing an antiproliferative drug, such as sirolimus or paclitaxel, to elute slowly from the coating and prevent neo-intimal hyperplasia and in-stent restenosis. Recurrent angina (affecting up to 15–20% of patients receiving an intracoronary stent at 6 months) may require further PCI or bypass grafting.

The risk of complications and the likely success of the procedure are closely related to the morphology of the stenoses, the experience of the operator and the presence of important comorbidity (e.g. diabetes, peripheral arterial disease). A good outcome is less likely if the target lesion is complex, long, eccentric or calcified, lies on a bend or within a tortuous vessel, involves a branch or contains acute thrombus.

In combination with aspirin and heparin, adjunctive therapy with potent platelet inhibitors, such as clopidogrel or glycoprotein IIb/IIIa receptor antagonists, has been shown to improve the outcome of PCI, with lower short- and long-term rates of death and myocardial infarction.

Coronary artery bypass grafting (CABG)

The internal mammary arteries, radial arteries or reversed segments of the patient's own saphenous vein can be used to bypass coronary artery stenoses (Figs 18.66 and 18.67). This usually involves major surgery under cardiopulmonary bypass, but in some cases, grafts can be applied to the beating heart: 'off-pump' surgery. The operative mortality is approximately 1.5%, but risks are higher in elderly patients, those with poor left ventricular function and those with significant comorbidity, such as renal failure.

Approximately 90% of patients are free of angina 1 year after surgery, but fewer than 60% of patients are asymptomatic 5 or more years after CABG. Early post-operative angina is usually due to graft failure arising from technical problems during the operation or poor 'run off' due to disease in the distal native coronary vessels. Late recurrence of angina may be due to progressive disease in the native coronary arteries or graft degeneration. Less than 50% of vein grafts are patent 10 years after surgery. However, arterial grafts have a much better long-term patency rate with more than 80% of internal mammary artery grafts patent at 10 years. This has lead many surgeons to consider total arterial revascularisation (TAR) during CABG surgery. Aspirin (75–150 mg daily) and clopidogrel (75 g daily) have both been shown to improve graft patency, and one or other should be prescribed indefinitely if well tolerated. Intensive

18

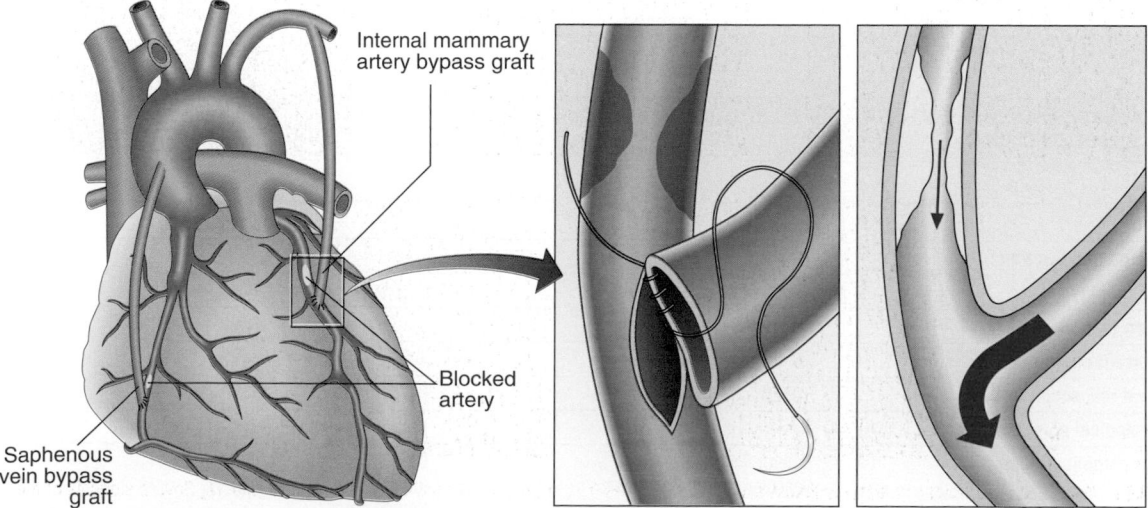

Fig. 18.66 Coronary artery bypass graft surgery. Narrowed or stenosed arteries are bypassed using saphenous vein grafts connected to the aorta, or by utilising the internal mammary artery.

Internal mammary artery bypass graft

Blocked artery

Saphenous vein bypass graft

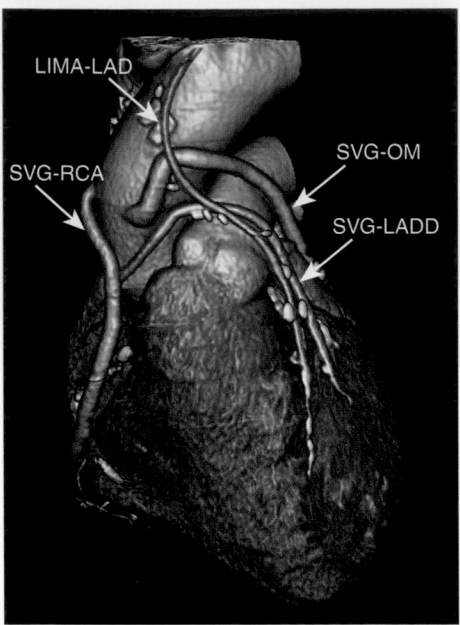

Fig. 18.67 Three-dimensional reconstruction of multislice computed tomography of the heart. The image shows the patent saphenous vein grafts (SVG) to the right coronary artery (RCA), obtuse marginal branch (OM) and diagonal branch (LADD), and left internal mammary artery graft (LIMA) to the left anterior descending (LAD) coronary artery.

18.62 CORONARY ARTERY BYPASS GRAFTING (CABG) FOR STABLE ANGINA `EBM`

'CABG is superior to medical treatment for at least 10 years after surgery in terms of survival. Greatest benefit occurred in those with a significant stenosis in the left main coronary artery or those with three-vessel disease and impaired ventricular function.'

- Yusuf S, et al. Lancet 1994; 344:563–570.
- Davies RF, et al. Circulation 1997; 95:2037–2043.

For further information: 🖥 www.sign.ac.uk

---

lipid-lowering therapy has also been shown to slow the progression of disease in the native coronary arteries and bypass grafts, and to reduce clinical cardiovascular events; serum LDL cholesterol concentrations should therefore be reduced below 3.2 mmol/l (~120 mg/dl). There is substantial excess cardiovascular morbidity and mortality in patients who continue to smoke after bypass grafting. Persistent smokers are twice as likely to die in the 10 years following surgery compared with those who give up at surgery.

CABG has been shown to improve survival in patients with left main coronary stenosis, and symptomatic patients with three-vessel coronary disease (i.e. involving left anterior descending, circumflex and right coronary arteries, Box 18.62) or two-vessel disease involving the proximal left anterior descending coronary artery. Improvement in survival is most marked in those with impaired left ventricular function or positive stress testing prior to surgery and those who have undergone left internal mammary artery grafting.

Neurological complications are common, with a 1–5% risk of perioperative stroke. Between 30% and 80% of patients develop short-term cognitive impairment that is often mild and typically resolves within 6 months. There are also reports of long-term cognitive decline that may be evident in more than 30% of patients at 5 years.

PCI and CABG are compared in Boxes 18.63 and 18.64.

Prognosis

Symptoms are a poor guide to prognosis; nevertheless, the 5-year mortality of patients with severe angina (NYHA class III or IV, p. 534) is nearly double that of patients with mild symptoms. Exercise testing and other forms of stress testing are much more powerful predictors of mortality; for example, in one study, the 4-year mortality of patients with stable angina and a negative exercise test was 1%, compared to more than 20% in those with a strongly positive test.

In general, the prognosis of coronary artery disease is related to the number of diseased vessels (one-, two- or three-vessel coronary artery disease) and the degree of left ventricular dysfunction. A patient with single-vessel disease

---

18.63 COMPARISON OF PERCUTANEOUS CORONARY INTERVENTION (PCI) AND CORONARY ARTERY BYPASS GRAFTING (CABG)

	PCI	CABG
Death	< 0.5%	< 1.5%
Myocardial infarction*	2%	10%
Hospital stay	12–36 hrs	5–8 days
Return to work	2–5 days	6–12 weeks
Recurrent angina	15–20% at 6 months	10% at 1 year
Repeat revascularisation	10–20% at 2 years	2% at 2 years
Neurological complications	Rare	Common (see text)
Other complications	Emergency CABG Vascular damage related to access site	Diffuse myocardial damage Infection (chest, wound) Wound pain

* Defined as CK-MB > 2 × normal, pp. 593–594.

18

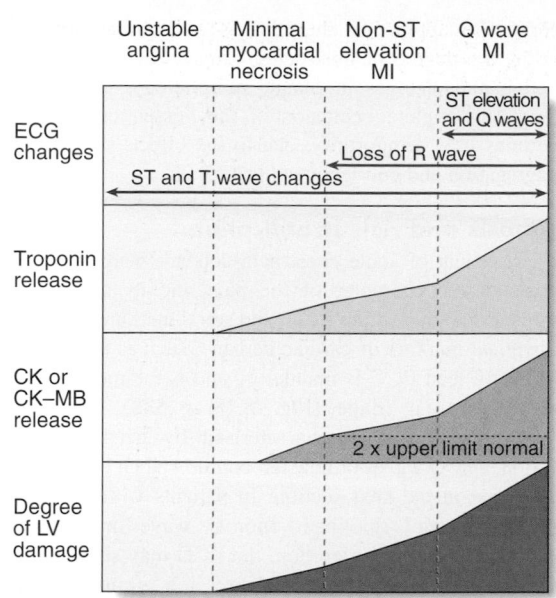

Fig. 18.68 **The spectrum of acute coronary syndromes.** The relation between ECG changes, biochemical markers of damage and the extent of myocardial necrosis. (CK = creatine kinase)

and good LV function has an excellent outlook (5-year survival > 90%), whereas a patient with severe LV dysfunction and extensive three-vessel disease has a poor prognosis (5-year survival < 30%) without revascularisation.

Spontaneous symptomatic improvement due to the development of collateral vessels is common.

ANGINA WITH NORMAL CORONARY ARTERIES

Approximately 10% of patients who report stable angina on effort will be found to have angiographically normal coronary arteries. Many of these patients are women and the mechanism of their symptoms is often difficult to establish. It is important to review the original diagnosis and explore other potential causes.

Coronary artery spasm

Vasospasm in coronary arteries may coexist with atheroma, especially in unstable angina (see below); occasionally (< 1% of all cases of angina), however, vasospasm may occur without angiographically detectable atheroma. This form of angina is sometimes known as variant angina and may be accompanied by spontaneous and transient ST elevation on the ECG (Prinzmetal's angina). Calcium antagonists, nitrates and other coronary vasodilators (e.g. nicorandil) are the most useful therapeutic agents but may be ineffective.

Syndrome X

The constellation of typical angina on effort, objective evidence of myocardial ischaemia on stress testing, and angiographically normal coronary arteries is sometimes known as syndrome X. This disorder is poorly understood but carries a good prognosis and may respond to treatment with anti-anginal therapy.

UNSTABLE ANGINA

Unstable angina is a clinical syndrome that is characterised by new-onset or rapidly worsening angina (crescendo angina), angina on minimal exertion or angina at rest. The condition shares common pathophysiological mechanisms with acute myocardial infarction (Fig. 18.59, p. 579) and the term 'acute coronary syndrome' is used to describe these

disorders collectively. These entities comprise a spectrum of disease that encompasses ischaemia with no myocardial damage, ischaemia with minimal myocardial damage, partial thickness (non-Q wave) myocardial infarction, and full thickness (Q wave) myocardial infarction (Fig. 18.68).

An acute coronary syndrome may present as a new phenomenon or against a background of chronic stable angina. The culprit lesion is usually a complex ulcerated or fissured atheromatous plaque with adherent platelet-rich thrombus and local coronary artery spasm (Fig. 18.69). It is

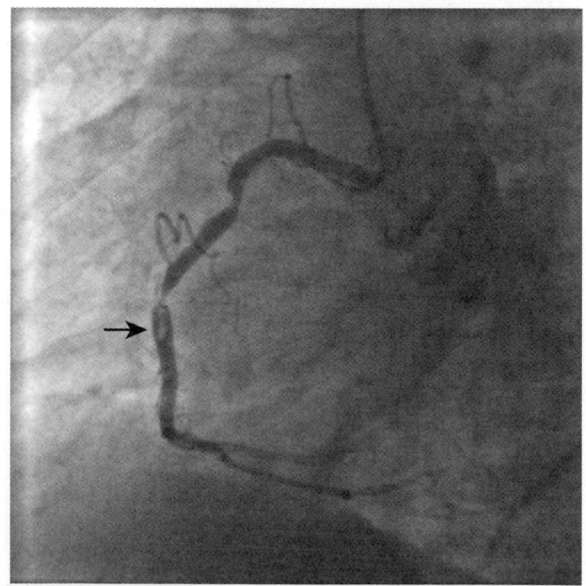

Fig. 18.69 **Right coronary angiogram in a patient with an acute coronary syndrome demonstrating a thrombus filling defect (arrow).**

18

important to appreciate that this is a dynamic process whereby the degree of obstruction may either increase by accretion and changes in plaque morphology, sometimes leading to complete occlusion of the vessel, or regress, sometimes only temporarily, due to the effects of platelet disaggregation and endogenous fibrinolysis.

Diagnosis and risk stratification

The assessment of acute chest pain depends heavily on an analysis of the character of the pain and its associated features, evaluation of the ECG, and serial measurements of biochemical markers of cardiac damage, such as troponin I and T. A 12-lead ECG is mandatory and is the most useful method of initial triage (Fig. 18.18, p. 538). Evolving transmural infarction is characterised by persistent ST elevation, new Q waves or new left bundle branch block, and is discussed in the next section. In patients with unstable angina or partial thickness (non-Q wave or non-ST elevation) myocardial infarction, the ECG may show ST/T wave changes including ST depression, transient ST elevation and T-wave inversion; the T-wave changes are sometimes prolonged.

Approximately 12% of patients with well-characterised unstable angina or non-ST segment elevation myocardial infarction progress to acute infarction or death, and almost one-third will suffer a recurrence of severe ischaemic pain, within 6 months of the index event. The risk markers that are indicative of an adverse prognosis include recurrent ischaemia, extensive ECG changes at rest or during pain, the release of biochemical markers (creatine kinase or troponin, p. 593), arrhythmias and haemodynamic complications (e.g. hypotension, mitral regurgitation) during episodes of ischaemia; those who experience unstable angina following acute myocardial infarction are also at increased risk. Risk stratification is important because it guides the use of more complex pharmacological and interventional treatment (Box 18.65 and Fig. 18.18).

Management

Patients should be admitted urgently to hospital because there is a significant risk of death or acute myocardial infarction during the unstable phase, and appropriate

---

18.66 ORAL ANTIPLATELET AGENTS IN UNSTABLE ANGINA   **EBM**

'Aspirin alone (75–325 mg/day) reduces the risk of death and myocardial infarction in unstable angina ($NNT_B = 20$). The combination of clopidogrel (75 mg daily) and aspirin is superior to aspirin alone (NNT_B for death, MI and stroke = 45).'

- Antithrombotic Trialists Collaboration. BMJ 2002; 324:71–86.
- Clopidogrel in Unstable Angina to prevent Recurrent Events (CURE) trial investigators. N Engl J Med 2001; 345:494–502.

For further information: 💻 www.acc.org

18.67 LOW MOLECULAR WEIGHT HEPARIN IN UNSTABLE ANGINA   **EBM**

'Treating patients with unstable angina with aspirin plus low molecular weight heparin is more effective than aspirin alone in reducing the combined endpoint of death, myocardial infarction, refractory angina and urgent need for revascularisation.'

- Antman EM, et al. for the TIMI IIB (Thrombolysis in Myocardial Infarction) and ESSENCE (Efficacy and Safety of Subcutaneous Enoxaparin in Non-Q-wave Coronary Events) Investigators. TIMI IIB-ESSENCE meta-analysis. Circulation 1999; 100:1602–1608.
- Eikelboom JW, et al. Lancet 2000; 355:1936–1942.

For further information: 💻 www.acc.org

18.68 INTRAVENOUS GLYCOPROTEIN IIb/IIIa INHIBITORS IN ACUTE CORONARY SYNDROMES   **EBM**

'In patients with acute coronary syndromes, antiplatelet treatment with i.v. glycoprotein IIb/IIIa inhibitors reduced the combined endpoint of death or myocardial infarction. Most benefit was seen in the context of percutaneous coronary intervention and there was no convincing evidence of benefit in patients who were treated without revascularisation. (NNT_B (death or MI) = 50; NNT_B (death, MI or revascularisation) = 33).'

- Kong DF, et al. Circulation 1998; 2829–2835.
- Bertrand ME, et al. Eur Heart J 2000; 21:1406–1432.

For further information: 💻 www.nice.org.uk

---

medical therapy can reduce the incidence of adverse events by at least 60%.

The initial treatment should include bed rest, antiplatelet therapy (aspirin 300 mg followed by 75–325 mg daily long-term and clopidogrel 300 mg followed by 75 mg daily for 12 months, Box 18.66), anticoagulant therapy (e.g. unfractionated or fractionated heparin) and a β-blocker (e.g. atenolol 50–100 mg daily or metoprolol 50–100 mg 12-hourly). A dihydropyridine calcium antagonist (e.g. nifedipine or amlodipine) can be added to the β-blocker, but may cause an unwanted tachycardia if used alone; verapamil or diltiazem is therefore the calcium antagonist of choice if a β-blocker is contraindicated. An intravenous infusion of unfractionated heparin (with dose adjusted according to the activated partial thromboplastin time) or weight-adjusted subcutaneous low molecular weight heparin (e.g. enoxaparin 1 mg/kg 12-hourly) should be given (Box 18.67). If pain persists or recurs, infusions of intravenous nitrates (e.g. GTN 0.6–1.2 mg/hr or isosorbide dinitrate 1–2 mg/hr) or buccal nitrates may help, but such patients should also be considered for early revascularisation. Refractory cases or those with haemodynamic compromise should be considered for a glycoprotein IIb/IIIa receptor

---

18.65 UNSTABLE ANGINA: RISK STRATIFICATION ⓘ

	High risk	Low risk
Clinical	Post-infarct angina Recurrent pain at rest Heart failure	No history of MI Rapid resolution of symptoms
ECG	Arrhythmia ST depression Transient ST elevation Persistent deep T-wave inversion	Minor or no ECG changes
Biochemistry	Troponin T > 0.1 µg/l	Troponin T < 0.1 µg/l

N.B. There is a 5- to 10-fold difference in risk between the lowest and highest risk groups.

18

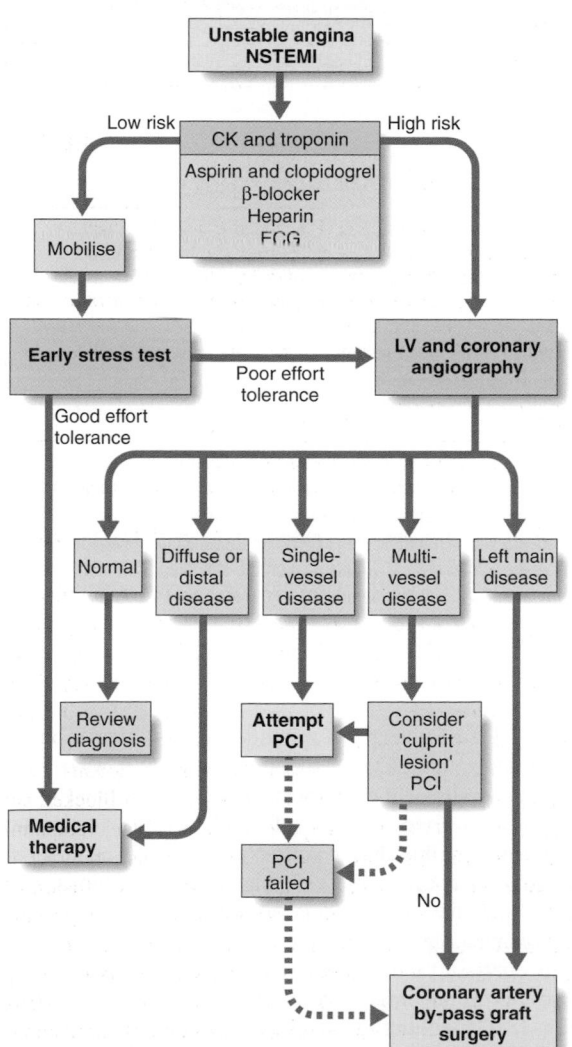

Fig. 18.70   A guide to the investigation and treatment of unstable angina and non-ST segment elevation myocardial infarction (NSTEMI). See Figure 18.18 on page 538, Box 18.65 and text for identification of high- and low-risk patients.

antagonist (e.g. abciximab, tirofiban or eptifibatide), intra-aortic balloon pump or emergency coronary angiography (Box 18.68).

Most low-risk patients stabilise with aspirin, clopidogrel, heparin and anti-anginal therapy, and can be gradually mobilised. If there are no contraindications, exercise testing may be performed prior to or shortly following discharge. Coronary angiography should be considered with a view to revascularisation in all patients at moderate or high risk, including those who fail to settle on medical therapy, those with extensive ECG changes, those with an elevated plasma troponin and those with severe pre-existing stable angina. This often reveals disease that is amenable to PCI (Fig. 18.70); however, if the lesions are not suitable for PCI the patient should be considered for urgent CABG.

MYOCARDIAL INFARCTION

Myocardial infarction (MI) is almost always due to the formation of occlusive thrombus at the site of rupture or erosion of an atheromatous plaque in a coronary artery (Fig. 18.59, p. 579). The thrombus often undergoes spontaneous lysis over the course of the next few days, although by this time irreversible myocardial damage has occurred. Without treatment the infarct-related artery remains permanently occluded in 30% of patients. The process of infarction progresses over several hours and therefore most patients present when it is still possible to salvage myocardium and improve outcome (Fig. 18.71).

CLINICAL FEATURES

Pain is the cardinal symptom of MI, but breathlessness, vomiting, and collapse or syncope are common features (Box 18.70). The pain occurs in the same sites as angina but is usually more severe and lasts longer; it is often described as a tightness, heaviness or constriction in the chest. At its worst, the pain is one of the most severe which can be experienced and the patient's expression and pallor may vividly convey the seriousness of the situation.

Most patients are breathless and in some this is the only symptom. Indeed, some myocardial infarcts pass un-recognised. Painless or 'silent' myocardial infarction is particularly common in older or diabetic patients. If syncope occurs, it is usually due to an arrhythmia or profound hypotension. Vomiting and sinus bradycardia are often due to vagal stimulation and are particularly common in patients with inferior MI. Nausea and vomiting may also be caused or aggravated by opiates given for pain relief. Sometimes infarction occurs in the absence of physical signs.

Sudden death, from ventricular fibrillation or asystole, may occur immediately, and many deaths occur within the first hour. If the patient survives this most critical stage, the liability to dangerous arrhythmias remains, but diminishes as each hour goes by. Thus, it is vital that patients know not to delay calling for help if symptoms occur. The development of cardiac failure reflects the extent of myocardial damage and is the major cause of death in those who survive the first few hours of infarction.

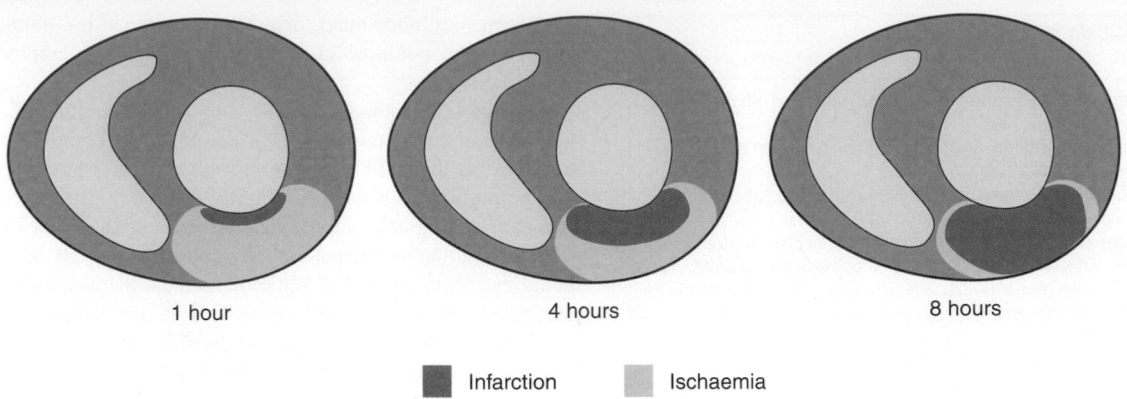

1 hour   **4 hours**   **8 hours**

■ Infarction   ■ Ischaemia

Fig. 18.71 The time course of myocardial infarction. The relative proportion of ischaemic, infarcting and infarcted tissue slowly changes over a period of 12 hours. In the early stages of myocardial infarction a significant proportion of the myocardium in jeopardy is potentially salvageable.

18.70 CLINICAL FEATURES OF MYOCARDIAL INFARCTION

Symptoms

- Prolonged cardiac pain
  Chest, throat, arms, epigastrium or back
- Anxiety and fear of impending death
- Nausea and vomiting
- Breathlessness
- Collapse/syncope

Physical signs

- Signs of sympathetic activation
  Pallor, sweating, tachycardia
- Signs of vagal activation
  Vomiting, bradycardia
- Signs of impaired myocardial function
  Hypotension, oliguria, cold peripheries
  Narrow pulse pressure
  Raised jugular venous pressure
  Third heart sound
  Quiet first heart sound
  Diffuse apical impulse
  Lung crepitations
- Signs of tissue damage
  Fever
- Signs of complications, e.g. mitral regurgitation, pericarditis (see text)

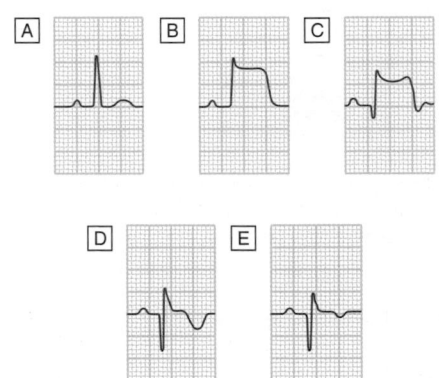

Fig. 18.72 The serial evolution of ECG changes in full thickness myocardial infarction. Ⓐ Normal ECG complex. Ⓑ Acute ST elevation ('the current of injury'). Ⓒ Progressive loss of the R wave, developing Q wave, resolution of the ST elevation and terminal T wave inversion. Ⓓ Deep Q wave and T wave inversion. Ⓔ Old or established infarct pattern; the Q wave tends to persist but the T wave changes become less marked. The rate of evolution is very variable but, in general, stage B appears within minutes, stage C within hours, stage D within days and stage E after several weeks or months. This diagrammatic representation should be compared with the actual ECGs in Figures 18.74, 18.75 and 18.76.

The differential diagnosis is wide and includes most causes of central chest pain or collapse (p. 536).

INVESTIGATIONS

Electrocardiography

The ECG is usually helpful in confirming the diagnosis; however, it may be difficult to interpret if there is bundle branch block or evidence of previous MI. Only rarely is the initial ECG entirely normal, but in up to one-third of cases the initial ECG changes may not be diagnostic.

The earliest ECG change is usually ST elevation; later on there is diminution in the size of the R wave, and in transmural (full thickness) infarction a Q wave begins to develop. One explanation for the Q wave is that the myocardial infarct acts as an 'electrical window', transmitting the changes of potential from within the ventricular cavity and allowing the ECG to 'see' the reciprocal R wave from the other walls of the ventricle. Subsequently, the T wave becomes inverted because of a change in ventricular repolarisation; this change persists after the ST segment has returned to normal. These features are shown in Figure 18.72 and their sequence is sufficiently reliable for the approximate age of the infarct to be deduced.

In contrast to transmural lesions, partial thickness or subendocardial infarction causes ST/T wave changes (Fig. 18.73) without Q waves or prominent ST elevation; this is often accompanied by some loss of the R waves in the leads facing the infarct and is also known as non-Q wave or non-ST elevation myocardial infarction (see above).

The ECG changes are best seen in the leads that 'face' the infarcted area. When there has been anteroseptal infarction,

18

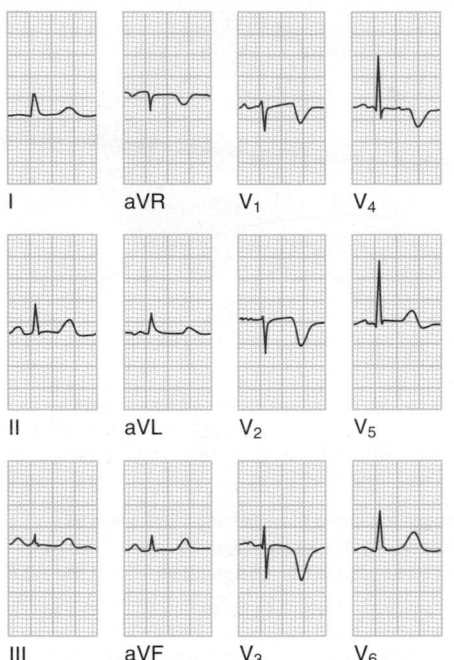

Fig. 18.73 Recent anterior non-ST elevation (partial thickness) infarction. There is deep symmetrical T-wave inversion together with a reduction in the height of the R wave in leads V_1, V_2, V_3 and V_4.

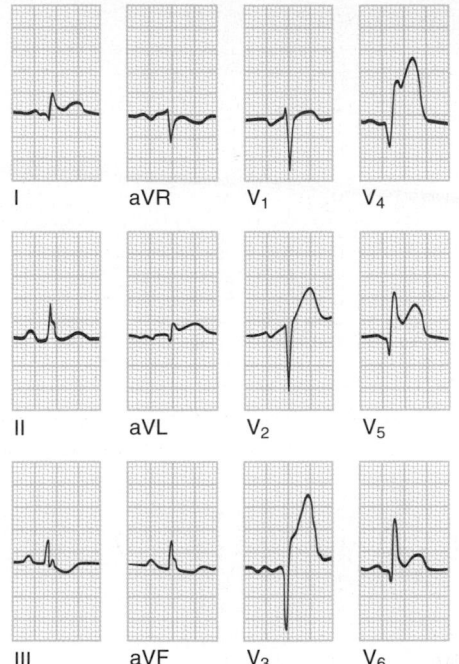

Fig. 18.74 Acute full thickness anterior myocardial infarction. This ECG was recorded from a 48-year-old man who had developed severe chest pain 6 hours earlier. There is ST elevation in leads I, aVL, V_2, V_3, V_4, V_5 and V_6, and there are Q waves in leads V_3, V_4 and V_5. Anterior infarcts with prominent changes in leads V_2, V_3 and V_4 are sometimes called 'anteroseptal' infarcts, as opposed to 'anterolateral' infarcts in which the ECG changes are predominantly found in V_4, V_5 and V_6.

18

abnormalities are found in one or more leads from V_1 to V_4, while anterolateral infarction produces changes from V_4 to V_6, in aVL and in lead I. Inferior infarction is best shown in leads II, III and aVF, while at the same time leads I, aVL and the anterior chest leads may show 'reciprocal' changes of ST depression (Figs 18.74, 18.75 and 18.76). Infarction of the posterior wall of the left ventricle does not cause ST elevation or Q waves in the standard leads, but can be diagnosed by the presence of reciprocal changes (ST depression and a tall R wave in leads V_1–V_4). Some infarctions (especially inferior) also involve the right ventricle; this may be identified by recording from additional leads placed over the right precordium.

Plasma biochemical markers

MI causes a detectable rise in the plasma concentration of enzymes and proteins that are normally concentrated within cardiac cells. The biochemical markers that are most widely used in the detection of MI are creatine kinase (CK), a more sensitive and cardiospecific isoform of this enzyme (CK-MB), and the cardiospecific proteins, troponins T and I. The troponins are also released, to a minor degree, in unstable angina with minimal myocardial damage (Fig. 18.68, p. 589). Serial (usually daily) estimations are particularly helpful because it is the change in plasma concentrations of these markers that is of diagnostic value (Fig. 18.77).

CK starts to rise at 4–6 hours, peaks at about 12 hours and falls to normal within 48–72 hours. CK is also present in skeletal muscle, and a modest rise in CK (but not CK-MB) may sometimes be due to an intramuscular injection, vigorous physical exercise or, in old people particularly, a fall. Defibrillation causes significant release of CK but not

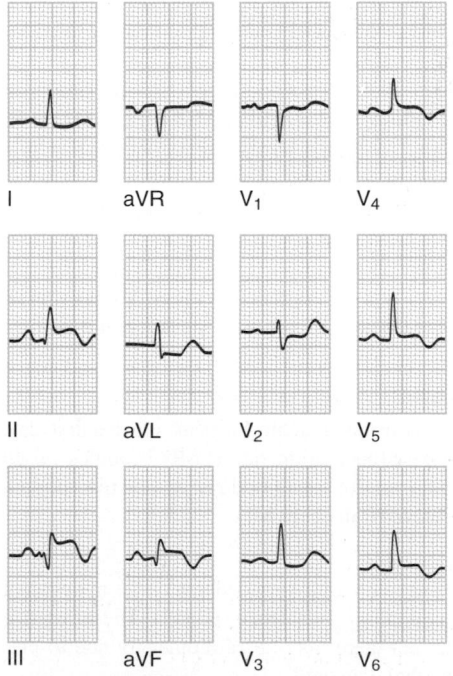

Fig. 18.75 Acute full-thickness inferolateral myocardial infarction. This ECG was recorded from a 55-year-old woman who had developed severe chest pain 4 hours earlier. There is ST elevation in the inferior leads II, III and aVF and the lateral leads V_4, V_5 and V_6. There is also 'reciprocal' ST depression in leads aVL and V_2.

18

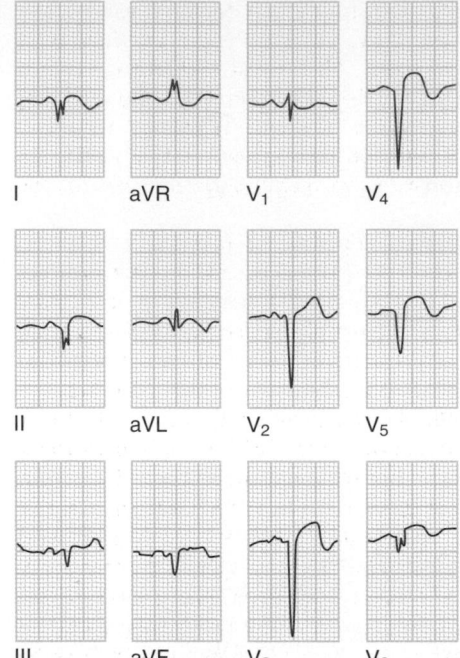

Fig. 18.76 Established anterior and inferior full-thickness infarction. This ECG was recorded from a 70-year-old man who had presented with an acute anterior infarct 2 days earlier and had been treated for an inferior myocardial infarct 11 months before then. There are Q waves in the inferior leads (II, III and aVF) and Q waves with some residual ST elevation in the anterior leads (I and V_2–V_6).

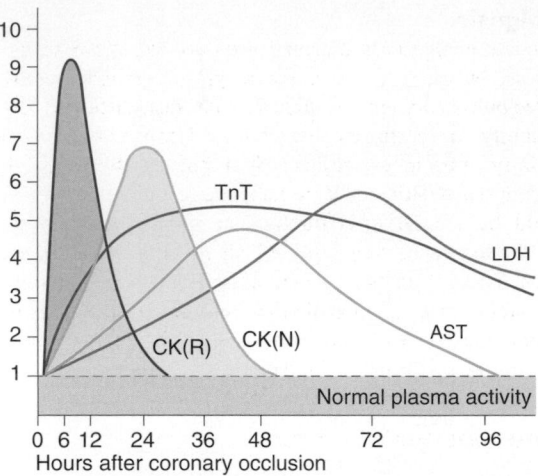

Fig. 18.77 Changes in plasma enzyme concentrations after myocardial infarction. Creatine kinase (CK) and troponin T (TnT) are the first to rise, followed by aspartate aminotransferase (AST) and then lactate (hydroxybutyrate) dehydrogenase (LDH). In patients treated with a thrombolytic agent, reperfusion is usually accompanied by a rapid rise in plasma creatine kinase (curve CK (R)) due to a washout effect; if there is no reperfusion, the rise is less rapid but the area under the curve is often greater (curve CK (N)).

18.71 EARLY MANAGEMENT OF ACUTE MYOCARDIAL INFARCTION

Provide facilities for defibrillation

Immediate measures
- High-flow oxygen
- I.v. access
- ECG monitoring
- 12-lead ECG
- I.v. analgesia (opiates) and antiemetic
- Aspirin 300 mg

Reperfusion
- Primary PCI or thrombolysis

Detect and manage acute complications
- Arrhythmias
- Ischaemia
- Heart failure

CK-MB or troponins. The most sensitive markers of myocardial cell damage are the cardiac troponins T and I, which are released within 4–6 hours and remain elevated for up to 2 weeks.

The American College of Cardiology and the European Society of Cardiology have redefined MI as 'a typical rise in cardiac troponin T or I, or CK-MB, above the 99th centile for normal, with at least one of the following: ischaemic symptoms, development of pathological Q waves on the ECG, ischaemic ECG changes (ST depression or elevation) or coronary artery intervention (e.g. PCI)'. This definition therefore includes non-ST segment elevation MIs as well as those that evolve through ST segment elevation and Q wave development.

Other blood tests
A leucocytosis is usual, reaching a peak on the first day. The erythrocyte sedimentation rate (ESR) becomes raised and may remain so for several days. C-reactive protein (CRP) is also elevated in acute MI.

Chest X-ray
This may demonstrate pulmonary oedema that is not evident on clinical examination (Fig. 18.24, p. 547). The heart size is often normal but there may be cardiomegaly due to pre-existing myocardial damage.

Echocardiography
This can be performed at the bedside and is a very useful technique for assessing left and right ventricular function and for detecting important complications such as mural thrombus, cardiac rupture, ventricular septal defect, mitral regurgitation and pericardial effusion.

EARLY MANAGEMENT

Patients with suspected acute MI require immediate access to medical/paramedical care and defibrillation facilities. In the UK, ambulances are equipped with semi-automatic advisory defibrillators. A patient with severe chest pain also requires urgent medical assessment and analgesia, so it is often appropriate to summon an ambulance and a general practitioner at the same time.

The essentials of the immediate management of acute MI are listed in Box 18.71.

Patients are usually managed in a dedicated cardiac unit because this offers a convenient way of concentrating the necessary expertise, monitoring and resuscitation facilities. If there are no complications, the patient can be mobilised from the second day and discharged from hospital on the fifth or sixth day.

Analgesia

Adequate analgesia is essential not only to relieve severe distress, but also to lower adrenergic drive and thereby reduce pulmonary and systemic vascular resistance and susceptibility to ventricular arrhythmias. Intravenous opiates (initially morphine sulphate 5–10 mg or diamorphine 2.5–5 mg) and antiemetics (initially metoclopramide 10 mg) should be administered through an intravenous cannula and titrated by giving repeated small aliquots until the patient is comfortable. Intramuscular injections should be avoided because the clinical effect may be delayed by poor skeletal muscle perfusion and a painful haematoma may form following thrombolytic therapy.

Acute reperfusion therapy

Thrombolysis

Coronary thrombolysis helps restore coronary patency, preserves left ventricular function and improves survival. Successful thrombolysis leads to reperfusion with relief of pain, resolution of acute ST elevation and sometimes transient arrhythmias (e.g. idioventricular rhythm). The sooner the patient is treated, the better the results will be; any delay will only increase the extent of myocardial damage—'minutes mean muscle'.

Clinical trials have shown that the appropriate use of these drugs can reduce the hospital mortality of myocardial infarction by 25%–50% and follow-up studies have demonstrated that this survival advantage is maintained for at least 10 years. The benefit is greatest in those patients who receive treatment within the first few hours, and choice of agent is less important than speed of treatment. Pre-hospital thrombolysis may be appropriate if transfer times are prolonged (> 30 mins) and the necessary expertise and ECG facilities are available.

Streptokinase, 1.5 million U in 100 ml of saline given as an intravenous infusion over 1 hour, is a widely used regimen. Streptokinase is antigenic and occasionally causes serious allergic manifestations. It may also cause hypotension, which can often be managed by stopping the infusion and restarting at a slower rate. Circulating neutralising antibodies are formed following treatment with streptokinase and may persist for 5 years or more. These antibodies can render subsequent infusions of streptokinase ineffective so it is advisable to use another non-antigenic agent if the patient requires further thrombolysis in the future.

Alteplase (human tissue plasminogen activator or tPA) is a genetically engineered drug that is not antigenic and seldom causes hypotension. The standard regimen is given over 90 minutes (bolus dose of 15 mg, followed by 0.75 mg/kg body weight, but not exceeding 50 mg, over 30 minutes and then 0.5 mg/kg body weight, but not exceeding 35 mg, over 60 minutes). There is evidence that tPA may produce better survival rates than streptokinase, particularly among high-risk patients (e.g. large anterior infarct), but with a slightly higher risk of intracerebral bleeding (10 per 1000 increased survival, but 1 per 1000 more non-fatal stroke).

Newer-generation analogues of tPA have been generated that have a longer plasma half-life and can be given as an intravenous bolus. Large-scale trial data have demonstrated that tenecteplase (TNK) is as effective as alteplase at reducing death and MI whilst conferring similar intracerebral bleeding risks. However, other major bleeding and transfusion risks are lower and the practical advantages of bolus administration may provide opportunities for prompt treatment in the emergency department or in the pre-hospital setting.

Reteplase (rPA) is administered as a double bolus and trial data indicate a similar outcome to that achieved with alteplase, although some of the bleeding risks appear slightly higher. The double bolus administration may provide practical advantages over the infusion of alteplase.

An overview of all the large randomised trials confirms that thrombolytic therapy significantly reduces short-term mortality in patients with suspected MI if it is given within 12 hours of the onset of symptoms and the ECG shows bundle branch block or characteristic ST segment elevation of greater than 1 mm in the limb leads or 2 mm in the chest leads (Box 18.72). Thrombolysis appears to be of little net benefit, and may be harmful in other patient groups, specifically those who present more than 12 hours after the onset of symptoms and those with a normal ECG or ST depression. In patients with ST elevation or bundle branch block, the absolute benefit of thrombolysis plus aspirin is approximately 50 lives saved per 1000 patients treated within 6 hours and 40 lives saved per 1000 patients treated between 7 and 12 hours after the onset of symptoms. The benefit is greatest for patients treated within the first 2 hours. To achieve prompt therapy, patients with suspected myocardial infarction should be assessed as soon as possible. Thrombolytic therapy can be administered before arrival at hospital by paramedical ambulance crews, often supported by telemetry of the ECG to hospital staff.

The major hazard of thrombolytic therapy is bleeding. Cerebral haemorrhage causes 4 extra strokes per 1000 patients treated and the incidence of other major bleeds is between 0.5% and 1%. Accordingly, it may be wise to withhold the treatment if there is a significant risk of serious bleeding. Some potential contraindications to thrombolytic therapy are outlined in Box 18.73.

The potential benefits and risks of thrombolytic therapy must be assessed in every case. For example, it would be reasonable to give thrombolytic therapy to a patient who presents early with evidence of extensive anterior infarction despite a history of active peptic ulceration. On the other hand, the risks of thrombolysis would probably exceed

18

EBM

18.72 THROMBOLYTIC TREATMENT IN ACUTE MYOCARDIAL INFARCTION

'Prompt thrombolytic treatment (within 12 hours, and particularly within 6 hours, of the onset of symptoms) reduces mortality in patients with acute myocardial infarction and ECG changes of ST elevation or new bundle branch block ($NNT_B = 56$). Intracranial haemorrhage is more common in people given thrombolysis with one additional stroke for every 250 people treated.'

- Fibrinolytic Therapy Trialists' (FTT) Collaborative Group. Lancet 1994; 343:311–322.
- Collins R. N Engl J Med 1997; 336:847–860.

For further information: 💻 www.escardio.org

18

18.74 PRIMARY PERCUTANEOUS CORONARY INTERVENTION IN ACUTE MYOCARDIAL INFARCTION

EBM

'Primary PCI is more effective than thrombolysis for the treatment of acute myocardial infarction. Death, non-fatal reinfarction and stroke are reduced from 14% with thrombolytic therapy to 8% with primary PCI.'

- Keeley EC, et al. Lancet 2003; 361:13–20.

For further information: 💻 www.acc.org

the benefits in a patient with a similar history of peptic ulceration who presents late with evidence of limited inferior myocardial infarction.

Primary percutaneous coronary intervention (PCI)

In institutions that are able to offer rapid access (within 3 hours) to a 24-hour catheter laboratory service, percutaneous coronary intervention is the treatment of choice (Fig. 18.78 and Box 18.74). In comparison to thrombolytic therapy, it is associated with a 50% greater reduction in the risk of death, recurrent myocardial infarction or stroke. The widespread use of PCI has been limited by the availability of the resources necessary to achieve this highly specialised emergency service. As a consequence, intravenous thrombolytic therapy remains the first-line reperfusion treatment in many hospitals. For some patients, thrombolytic therapy is contraindicated or fails to achieve coronary arterial reperfusion. Early emergency PCI (within 6 hours of symptom onset) may be considered under such circumstances, particularly where there is evidence of cardiogenic shock.

Maintaining vessel patency

Antiplatelet therapy

Oral administration of 75–300 mg aspirin daily improves survival (30% reduction in mortality) on its own, and complements the effect of thrombolytic therapy (Box 18.75). The first tablet (300 mg) should be given orally within the first 12 hours and the therapy should be continued indefinitely if there are no unwanted effects. In combination with aspirin, the early (within 12 hours) use of clopidogrel 75 mg daily confers a further 10% reduction in mortality with no evidence of increased adverse bleeding events.

Anticoagulants

Subcutaneous heparin (12 500 U twice daily), given in addition to oral aspirin, may prevent reinfarction after successful thrombolysis and reduce the risk of thrombo-

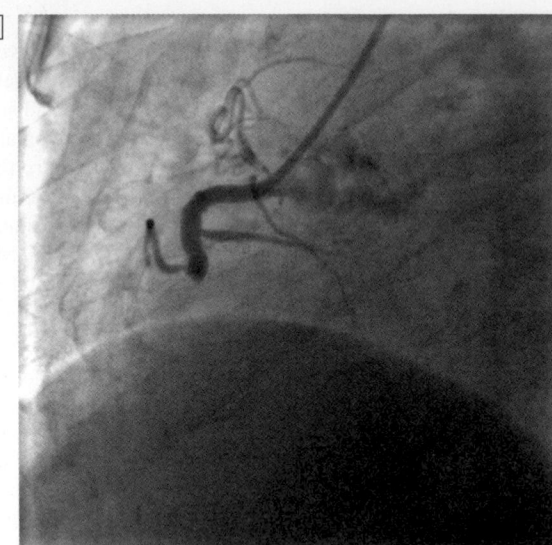

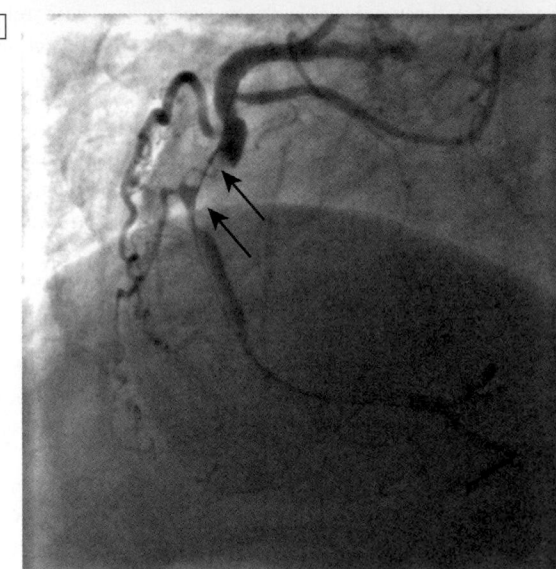

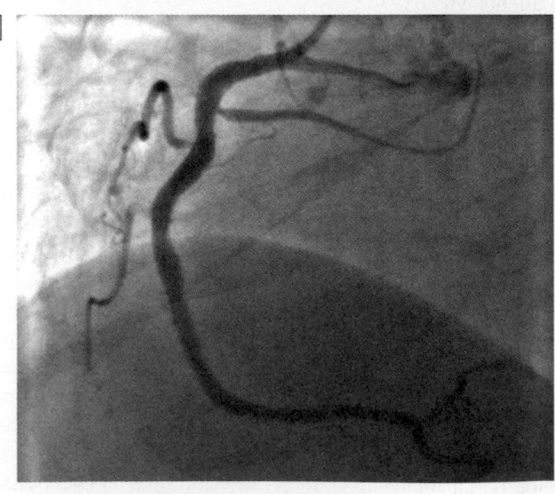

Fig. 18.78 Primary angioplasty. [A] Acute right coronary artery occlusion. [B] Initial angioplasty demonstrates a large thrombus filling defect (arrows). [C] Complete restoration of normal flow following intracoronary stent insertion.

18.75 ASPIRIN IN ACUTE MYOCARDIAL INFARCTION **EBM**

'In acute myocardial infarction, aspirin reduces mortality (NNT_B = 40), reinfarction (NNT_B = 100) and stroke (NNT_B = 300). The optimal dose of aspirin is 160–325 mg acutely, followed by a maintenance dose of 75 mg daily.'

- Second International Study of Infarct Survival (ISIS 2) Collaborative Group. Lancet 1988; ii:349–360.
- Antiplatelet Trialists' Collaboration. BMJ 1994; 308:81–106.

For further information: 🖥 www.escardio.org

18.76 COMMON ARRHYTHMIAS IN ACUTE MYOCARDIAL INFARCTION

- Ventricular fibrillation
- Ventricular tachycardia
- Accelerated idioventricular rhythm
- Ventricular ectopics
- Atrial fibrillation
- Atrial tachycardia
- Sinus bradycardia (particularly after inferior MI)
- Heart block

embolic complications. Clinical trials have shown that this form of therapy, when given for 7 days or until discharge from hospital, produces a small reduction in short-term mortality (approximately 5 lives saved per 1000 patients treated) but also increases the risk of cerebral haemorrhage (0.56% versus 0.4%) and of other bleeding complications (1% versus 0.8%). Intravenous heparin should be given for 48–72 hours following thrombolysis with alteplase, TNK or reteplase. Recent trial data suggest that low molecular weight heparin can be used in place of unfractionated heparin and with similar safety.

A period of treatment with warfarin should be considered if there is persistent atrial fibrillation or evidence of extensive anterior infarction, or if echocardiography shows mobile mural thrombus, because these patients are at increased risk of systemic thromboembolism.

Adjunctive therapy

Beta-blockers

Intravenous β-blockers (e.g. atenolol 5–10 mg or metoprolol 5–15 mg given over 5 minutes) relieve pain, reduce arrhythmias and improve short-term mortality in patients who present within 12 hours of the onset of symptoms, but should be avoided if there is heart failure, atrioventricular block or severe bradycardia. Chronic oral β-blocker therapy improves long-term survival and should be given to all patients who can tolerate it.

Nitrates and other agents

Sublingual glyceryl trinitrate (300–500 μg) is a valuable first-aid measure in threatened infarction, and intravenous nitrates (nitroglycerin 0.6–1.2 mg/hour or isosorbide dinitrate 1–2 mg/hour) are useful for the treatment of left ventricular failure and the relief of recurrent or persistent ischaemic pain.

Large-scale trials have shown that there is no evidence of a survival advantage from the routine use of oral nitrate therapy, oral calcium antagonists or intravenous magnesium in patients with acute MI.

COMPLICATIONS OF INFARCTION

Arrhythmias

Nearly all patients with acute MI have some form of arrhythmia; in many cases this is transient and of no haemodynamic or prognostic significance. Various degrees of atrioventricular block (pp. 570–571) are also common. Some common arrhythmias are listed in Box 18.76;

diagnosis and management are discussed in detail on pages 560–578.

Pain relief, rest and the correction of hypokalaemia can all play a major role in the prevention of arrhythmias.

Ventricular fibrillation

This occurs in about 5–10% of patients who reach hospital, and is thought to be the major cause of death in those who die before receiving medical attention. Prompt defibrillation will usually restore sinus rhythm. Moreover, the prognosis of patients with early ventricular fibrillation (within the first 48 hours) who are successfully and promptly resuscitated in this way is identical to the prognosis of patients with acute MI that is not complicated by ventricular fibrillation. Prompt pre-hospital resuscitation and defibrillation have the potential to save many more lives than thrombolysis.

Atrial fibrillation

This is common, frequently transient and may not require treatment. However, if the arrhythmia causes a rapid ventricular rate with severe hypotension or circulatory collapse, cardioversion by means of an immediate synchronised DC shock should be considered. In other situations, digoxin or β-blockers are usually the treatment of choice. Atrial fibrillation (due to acute atrial stretch) is often a feature of impending or overt left ventricular failure, and therapy may be ineffective if heart failure is not recognised and treated appropriately. Anticoagulation may be required if AF persists.

Sinus bradycardia

This does not usually require treatment, but if there is hypotension or haemodynamic deterioration, atropine (0.6 mg i.v.) may be given.

Atrioventricular block

Atrioventricular block complicating inferior infarction is usually temporary and often resolves following thrombolytic therapy; it may also respond to atropine (0.6 mg i.v. repeated as necessary). However, if there is clinical deterioration due to second-degree or complete atrioventricular block, a temporary pacemaker should be considered. Atrioventricular block complicating anterior infarction is more serious because asystole may suddenly supervene; a prophylactic temporary pacemaker should be inserted (p. 576).

Ischaemia

Post-infarct angina occurs in up to 50% of patients. Most patients have a residual stenosis in the infarct-related vessel despite successful thrombolysis, and this may cause angina if there is still viable myocardium downstream; nevertheless, there is no evidence that routine angioplasty improves

18

outcome after thrombolysis. In some patients, occlusion of a vessel may precipitate angina by disturbing a system of collateral flow that was compensating for disease in another vessel.

Patients who develop angina at rest or on minimal exertion following MI should be managed in the same way as patients with unstable angina who are thought to be at high risk (pp. 590–591). Intravenous nitrates (e.g. nitro-glycerin 0.6–1.2 mg/hour or isosorbide dinitrate 1–2 mg/hour) and either intravenous heparin (1000 U/hour, adjusted according to the thrombin time) or low molecular weight heparin may be helpful, and early coronary angiography with a view to angioplasty of the 'culprit' lesion should be considered. Glycoprotein IIb/IIIa receptor antagonists are of benefit in selected patients, particularly those undergoing PCI.

Acute circulatory failure

Acute circulatory failure usually reflects extensive myo-cardial damage and indicates a bad prognosis. All the other complications of MI are more likely to occur when acute heart failure is present.

The assessment and management of heart failure com-plicating acute MI are discussed in detail on page 548.

Pericarditis

This may occur at any stage of the illness but is particularly common on the second and third days. The patient may recognise that a different pain has developed even though it is at the same site, and that this pain is positional and tends to be worse or is sometimes only present on inspiration. A pericardial rub may be audible. Non-steroidal and steroidal anti-inflammatory drugs should be avoided in the early recovery period as they may increase the risk of aneurysm formation and myocardial rupture. Opiate-based analgesia should be used.

The post-myocardial infarction syndrome (Dressler's syndrome) is characterised by persistent fever, pericarditis and pleurisy, and is probably due to autoimmunity. The symptoms tend to occur a few weeks or even months after the infarct and often subside after a few days; prolonged or severe symptoms may require treatment with high-dose aspirin, an NSAID or even corticosteroids.

Mechanical complications

Part of the necrotic muscle in a fresh infarct may tear or rupture, with devastating consequences:

- Papillary muscle damage may cause acute pulmonary oedema and shock due to the sudden onset of severe mitral regurgitation, which presents with a pansystolic murmur and third heart sound. In the presence of severe valvular regurgitation, the murmur may be quiet or absent. The diagnosis can be confirmed by Doppler echocardiography, and emergency mitral valve replacement may be necessary. Lesser degrees of mitral regurgitation are common and may be transient.
- Rupture of the interventricular septum may cause left-to-right shunting through a ventricular septal defect. This usually presents with sudden haemodynamic

deterioration accompanied by a new loud pansystolic murmur radiating to the right sternal border, but may be difficult to distinguish from acute mitral regurgitation. However, patients with an acquired ventricular septal defect tend to develop right heart failure rather than pulmonary oedema. Doppler echocardiography and right heart catheterisation will confirm the diagnosis. Without prompt surgery, the condition is usually fatal.
- Rupture of the ventricle may lead to cardiac tamponade and is usually fatal (p. 645), although it may rarely be possible to support a patient with an incomplete rupture until emergency surgery is performed.

Embolism

Thrombus often forms on the endocardial surface of freshly infarcted myocardium; this may lead to systemic embolism and occasionally causes a stroke or ischaemic limb.

Venous thrombosis and pulmonary embolism may occur but have become less common with the use of prophylactic anticoagulants and early mobilisation.

Impaired ventricular function, remodelling and ventricular aneurysm

Acute transmural MI is often followed by thinning and stretching of the infarcted segment (infarct expansion); this leads to an increase in wall stress with progressive dilatation and hypertrophy of the remaining ventricle (ventricular remodelling—Fig. 18.79). As the ventricle dilates, it becomes less efficient and heart failure may supervene. Infarct expansion occurs over a few days and weeks but ventricular remodelling may take years; heart failure may therefore develop many years after acute MI. ACE inhibitor therapy reduces late ventricular remodelling and can prevent the onset of heart failure (p. 600 and Box 18.18, p. 549).

A left ventricular aneurysm develops in approximately 10% of patients and is particularly common when there is persistent occlusion of the infarct-related vessel. Heart

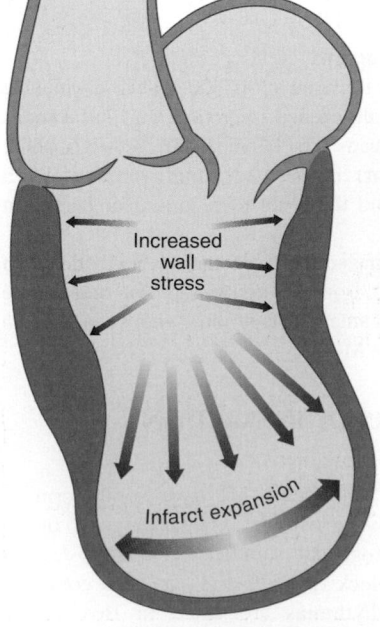

Fig. 18.79 Infarct expansion and ventricular remodelling. Full-thickness myocardial infarction causes thinning and stretching of the infarcted segment (infarct expansion), which leads to increased wall stress with progressive dilatation and hypertrophy of the remaining ventricle (ventricular remodelling).

Increased wall stress

Infarct expansion

failure, ventricular arrhythmias, mural thrombus and systemic embolism are all recognised complications of aneurysm formation. Other clinical features include a paradoxical impulse on the chest wall, persistent ST elevation on the ECG, and sometimes an unusual bulge from the cardiac silhouette on the chest X-ray. Echocardiography is usually diagnostic. Surgical removal of a left ventricular aneurysm carries a high morbidity and mortality but is sometimes necessary.

LATE MANAGEMENT

Patients who have survived an MI are at risk of further ischaemic events; management should therefore aim to identify those at high risk and introduce effective secondary prevention (Box 18.77).

Risk stratification and further investigation

The prognosis of patients who have survived an acute MI is related to the degree of myocardial damage, the extent of any residual myocardial ischaemia and the presence of significant ventricular arrhythmias.

Left ventricular function

The degree of left ventricular dysfunction can be crudely assessed from the physical findings (tachycardia, third heart sound, crackles at the lung bases, elevated venous pressure etc.), the ECG changes and the size of the heart and presence of pulmonary oedema on chest X-ray. However, formal measurements using echocardiography or radionuclide imaging are often valuable.

Ischaemia

Patients with early post-MI ischaemia should be managed in the same way as patients with high-risk unstable angina (pp. 590–591). Patients without spontaneous ischaemia who are suitable candidates for revascularisation should undergo an exercise tolerance test approximately 4 weeks after the infarct; this will help to identify those individuals with significant residual myocardial ischaemia who require further investigation, and may help to boost the confidence of the remainder.

If the exercise test is negative and the patient has a good effort tolerance, the outlook is good, with a 1–4% chance of an adverse event in the next 12 months. In contrast, patients with residual ischaemia in the form of chest pain or ECG changes at low exercise levels are at high risk, with a 15–25% chance of suffering a further ischaemic event in the next 12 months.

Coronary angiography, with a view to angioplasty or bypass grafting, should therefore be considered in any patient with spontaneous ischaemia, significant angina on effort, or a strongly positive exercise tolerance test.

Arrhythmias

The presence of ventricular arrhythmias during the convalescent phase of MI may be a marker of poor ventricular function and may herald sudden death. Although empirical anti-arrhythmic treatment appears to be of no value and even hazardous, selected patients may benefit from sophisticated electrophysiological testing and specific anti-arrhythmic therapy (including implantable cardiac defibrillators, p. 576).

Recurrent ventricular arrhythmias are sometimes manifestations of myocardial ischaemia or impaired LV function and may respond to appropriate treatment directed at the underlying problem.

Secondary prevention

Smoking

The 5-year mortality of patients who continue to smoke cigarettes is double that of those who quit smoking at the time of their infarct. Giving up smoking is the single most effective contribution a patient can make to his or her own future. The success of smoking cessation can be increased by supportive advice and nicotine replacement therapy.

Hyperlipidaemia

Convincing evidence from large-scale randomised clinical trials has demonstrated the importance of lowering serum cholesterol following MI. Lipids should be measured within 24 hours of presentation because there is often a transient fall in blood cholesterol in the 3 months following infarction. Dietary advice should be given but is often ineffective. HMG CoA reductase enzyme inhibitors ('statins') can produce marked reductions in total (and LDL) cholesterol and have been shown to reduce the subsequent risk of death, reinfarction, stroke and the need for revascularisation (Box 18.50, p. 581). Irrespective of serum cholesterol concentrations, all patients should receive statin therapy after MI. Recent evidence suggests that patients with serum LDL cholesterol concentrations greater than 3.2 mmol/l (~120 mg/dl) benefit from more intensive lipid-lowering (e.g. atorvastatin 80 mg daily).

Other risk factors

Maintaining an ideal body weight, taking regular exercise, and achieving good control of hypertension and diabetes may all improve the long-term outlook.

Mobilisation and rehabilitation

There is histological evidence that the necrotic muscle of an acute myocardial infarct takes 4–6 weeks to become replaced with fibrous tissue, and it is conventional to restrict physical activities during this period. When there are no complications, the patient can sit in a chair on the second day, walk to the toilet on the third day, return home in 5 days

---

18.77 LATE MANAGEMENT OF MYOCARDIAL INFARCTION

Risk stratification and further investigation (see text)

Lifestyle modification
- Stop smoking
- Regular exercise
- Diet (weight control, lipid-lowering)

Secondary prevention drug therapy
- Antiplatelet therapy (aspirin and/or clopidogrel)
- β-blocker
- ACE inhibitor
- Statin
- Additional therapy for control of diabetes and hypertension

Rehabilitation

18

and gradually increase activity with the aim of returning to work in 4–6 weeks. The majority of patients may resume driving after 4–6 weeks; however, in most countries, vocational driving licence holders (e.g. heavy goods and public service vehicle) require special assessment.

Emotional problems, such as denial, anxiety and depression, are common, and must be recognised and dealt with accordingly. Many patients are severely and even permanently incapacitated as a result of the psychological rather than the physical effects of MI, and all benefit from thoughtful explanation, counselling and reassurance at every stage of the illness. Many patients mistakenly believe that 'stress' was the cause of their heart attack and may restrict their activity inappropriately. The patient's spouse or partner will also require emotional support, information and counselling.

Formal rehabilitation programmes based on graded exercise protocols with individual and group counselling are often very successful, and in some cases have been shown to improve the long-term outcome.

Drug therapy

Aspirin and clopidogrel

Low-dose aspirin therapy reduces the risk of further infarction and other vascular events by approximately 25% and should be continued indefinitely if there are no unwanted effects. Clopidogrel should be given in combination with aspirin for the first 4 weeks. If patients are intolerant of aspirin, clopidogrel is a suitable alternative.

Beta-blockers

Continuous treatment with an oral β-blocker has been shown to reduce long-term mortality by approximately 25% among the survivors of acute MI (Box 18.78). Unfortunately, a significant minority of patients do not tolerate β-blockers because of bradycardia, atrioventricular block, hypotension or asthma. Patients with heart failure, irreversible chronic obstructive pulmonary disease or peripheral vascular disease derive similar if not greater secondary preventative benefits from β-blocker therapy if they can tolerate it, and should not be denied this treatment.

ACE inhibitors

Several clinical trials have shown that long-term treatment with an ACE inhibitor (e.g. enalapril 10 mg 12-hourly or ramipril 2.5–5 mg 12-hourly) can counteract ventricular remodelling, prevent the onset of heart failure, improve survival and reduce hospitalisation. The benefit of treatment is greatest in those with overt heart failure (clinical or radiological) but extends to patients with asymptomatic LV dysfunction and those with preserved LV function. This form of therapy should therefore be considered in all patients who have sustained a myocardial infarct. Caution must be exercised in hypovolaemic or hypotensive patients because the introduction of an ACE inhibitor may exacerbate hypotension and impair coronary perfusion. In patients intolerant of ACE inhibitor therapy, angiotensin receptor blockers (e.g. valsartan 40–160 mg daily or candesartan 4–16 mg daily) are suitable alternatives and are better tolerated.

Patients with acute MI complicated by heart failure and LV dysfunction appear to benefit from additional aldosterone receptor antagonism (e.g. eplerenone 25–50 mg daily).

Device therapy (p. 576)

Implantable cardiac defibrillators are of benefit in preventing sudden cardiac death in patients who have severe left ventricular impairment (ejection fraction $\leq 30\%$) after MI.

PROGNOSIS

In almost one-quarter of all cases of MI, death occurs within a few minutes without medical care. Half the deaths from MI occur within 24 hours of the onset of symptoms and about 40% of all affected patients die within the first month. The prognosis of those who survive to reach hospital is much better, with a 28-day survival of more than 80%.

Early death is usually due to an arrhythmia but later on the outcome is determined by the extent of myocardial damage. Unfavourable features include poor left ventricular function, atrioventricular block and persistent ventricular arrhythmias. The prognosis is worse for anterior than for inferior infarcts. Bundle branch block and high enzyme levels both indicate extensive myocardial damage. Old age, depression and social isolation are also associated with a higher mortality.

Of those who survive an acute attack, more than 80% live for a further year, about 75% for 5 years, 50% for 10 years and 25% for 20 years.

18.78 β-BLOCKERS IN SECONDARY PREVENTION AFTER MYOCARDIAL INFARCTION `EBM`

'β-blockers reduce the risk of overall mortality ($NNT_B = 48$), sudden death ($NNT_B = 63$) and non-fatal reinfarction ($NNT_B = 56$) in patients after myocardial infarction. The greatest benefit was seen in those at highest risk and about one-quarter of patients suffered adverse events.'

• Yusuf S, et al. Prog Cardiovasc Dis 1985; 27:335–371.
• Beta-blocking Pooling Project research group. Eur Heart J 1988; 9:8–16.

For further information: 💻 www.sign.ac.uk

18.79 MYOCARDIAL INFARCTION IN OLD AGE

• **Atypical presentation:** often with anorexia, fatigue or weakness rather than chest pain.
• **Case fatality:** rises steeply. Hospital mortality exceeds 25% in those over 75 years old, which is five times greater than that seen in those aged less than 55 years.
• **Survival benefit of treatments:** not influenced by age. The absolute benefit of evidence-based treatments may therefore be greatest in older people.
• **Hazards of treatments:** rise with age (e.g. increased risk of intracerebral bleeding after thrombolysis) and is due partly to increased comorbidity.
• **Quality of evidence:** older patients, particularly those with significant comorbidity, were under-represented in many of the RCTs that helped to establish the treatment of myocardial infarction. The balance of risk and benefit for many treatments (e.g. thrombolysis, primary PTCA) in frail older people is therefore uncertain.

CARDIAC RISK OF NON-CARDIAC SURGERY

Non-cardiac surgery, particularly major vascular, abdominal or thoracic surgery, can precipitate serious perioperative cardiac complication such as MI and death in patients with coronary artery and other forms of heart disease. Careful pre-operative cardiac assessment may help to determine the balance of benefit versus risk on an individual patient basis, and identify measures that can be used to minimise the operative risk (Box 18.80).

18.80 MAJOR RISK FACTORS FOR CARDIAC COMPLICATIONS OF NON-CARDIAC SURGERY
• Recent (< 6 months) MI or unstable angina
• Severe stable angina on effort
• Poorly controlled heart failure
• Severe valvular heart disease (especially aortic stenosis)

A hypercoagulable state is part of the normal physiological response to surgery and may promote coronary thrombosis leading to an acute coronary syndrome (unstable angina or MI) in the early post-operative period. Patients with a history of recent PCI, unstable angina or MI are at greatest risk and, whenever possible, elective non-cardiac surgery should be avoided for 3 (and preferably 6) months after such an event. Antiplatelet agents and β-blockers reduce the risk of perioperative MI in patients with coronary artery disease and, where possible, should be prescribed throughout the perioperative period.

Careful attention to fluid balance during and after surgery is particularly important in patients with impaired left ventricular function and valvular heart disease because antidiuretic hormone is released as part of the normal physiological response to surgery, and in these circumstances the over-zealous administration of intravenous fluids can easily precipitate heart failure. Patients with severe valvular heart disease, particularly aortic stenosis and mitral stenosis, are also at increased risk because they may not be able to increase their cardiac output in response to the stress of surgery.

Atrial fibrillation may be triggered by hypoxia, myocardial ischaemia or heart failure (atrial stretch) and is a common post-operative complication in patients with pre-existing heart disease. The arrhythmia usually terminates spontaneously when the precipitating factors have been eliminated but it may be advisable to prescribe digoxin or β-blockers to control the heart rate.

VASCULAR DISEASE

PERIPHERAL ARTERIAL DISEASE

In developed countries, almost all peripheral arterial disease (PAD) is due to atherosclerosis (pp. 578–581). The pathology of PAD is similar to coronary artery disease and the most important risk factors are smoking, diabetes, hyperlipidaemia and hypertension. Plaque rupture is responsible for the most serious manifestations of the disease, and often occurs in a plaque that hitherto has been asymptomatic.

Approximately 20% of middle-aged (55–75 years) people in the UK have PAD but only one-quarter of such individuals will have symptoms. The clinical manifestations depend upon the anatomical site, the presence or absence of a collateral supply, the speed of onset and the mechanism of injury (Box 18.81).

CHRONIC LOWER LIMB ARTERIAL DISEASE

PAD affects the leg eight times more often than the arm. The lower limb arterial tree comprises the aorto-iliac ('inflow'), femoropopliteal and infra-popliteal ('outflow')

18.81 FACTORS INFLUENCING THE CLINICAL MANIFESTATIONS OF PERIPHERAL ARTERIAL DISEASE
Anatomical site
Cerebral circulation   • Transient ischaemic attack (TIA), amaurosis fugax, vertebrobasilar insufficiency
Renal arteries   • Hypertension and renal failure
Mesenteric arteries   • Mesenteric angina, acute intestinal ischaemia
Limbs (legs >> arms)   • Intermittent claudication, critical limb ischaemia, acute limb ischaemia
Collateral supply
• In a patient with a complete circle of Willis, occlusion of one carotid artery may be asymptomatic   • In a patient without cross-circulation, stroke is likely
Speed of onset
• Where PAD develops slowly, a collateral supply will develop   • Sudden occlusion of a previously normal artery is likely to cause severe distal ischaemia
Mechanism of injury
Haemodynamic   • Plaque must reduce arterial diameter by 70% ('critical stenosis') to reduce flow and pressure at rest. On exertion (e.g. walking), a much lesser stenosis may become 'critical'. This mechanism tends to have a relatively benign course due to collateralisation
Thrombotic   • Occlusion of a long-standing critical stenosis may be asymptomatic due to collateralisation. However, acute rupture and thrombosis of a non-haemodynamically significant plaque usually has severe consequences
Atheroembolic   • Symptoms depend upon embolic load and size   • Carotid (TIA, amaurosis fugax or stroke) and peripheral arterial (blue toe/finger syndrome) plaque are common examples
Thromboembolic   • Usually secondary to atrial fibrillation   • The clinical consequences are usually dramatic as the thrombus load is often large and tends to occlude a major, previously healthy, non-collateralised artery suddenly and completely

18

segments. One or more segments may be affected in a variable and asymmetric manner. Lower limb ischaemia presents as two distinct clinical entities: intermittent claudication and critical limb ischaemia. The presence and severity of ischaemia can be determined by clinical examination (Box 18.82) and measurement of the ankle:brachial pressure index (ABPI), the ratio between the (highest systolic) ankle and brachial blood pressures. In health the ABPI is > 1.0, in intermittent claudication typically 0.5–0.9, and in critical limb ischaemia usually < 0.5.

Intermittent claudication

Ischaemic pain of the leg muscles precipitated by walking and relieved by rest is known as intermittent claudication (IC). The pain is usually felt in the calf muscles because the disease tends to affect the superficial femoral artery. However, the pain may be felt in the thigh or buttock if the iliac arteries are involved. Typically, the pain comes on after a reasonably constant 'claudication distance', and rapidly and completely subsides on stopping walking. Resumption of walking leads to a return of the pain. Most patients describe a cyclical pattern of exacerbation and resolution due to the progression of disease and the subsequent development of collaterals.

Approximately 5% of middle-aged men report IC. Provided patients comply with 'best medical therapy' (Box 18.83), only 1–2% per year will deteriorate to a point where amputation and/or revascularisation are required. However, the annual mortality rate exceeds 5%, which is 2–3 times higher than an equivalent non-claudicant population. This excess mortality is due to the fact that IC is nearly always found in association with widespread atherosclerosis.

Indeed, most claudicants succumb to MI or stroke. General measures to reduce cardiovascular mortality, many of which may also improve the functional status of the limb, are central to patient management. Peripheral vasodilators such as cilostazol can improve symptoms in patients with intermittent claudication. Intervention (angioplasty, stenting, endarterectomy or bypass) is usually only considered once best medical therapy has been instituted and given at least 6 months to effect symptomatic improvement, and then only in those patients who are severely disabled or whose livelihood is threatened by their disability.

Critical limb ischaemia

Critical limb ischaemia (CLI) is defined as rest (night) pain, requiring opiate analgesia, and/or tissue loss (ulceration or gangrene), present for more than 2 weeks, in the presence of an ankle blood pressure of less than 50 mmHg (Fig. 18.80). Rest pain and no tissue loss with ankle pressures above 50 mmHg is sometimes known as subcritical limb ischaemia (SCLI). The term severe limb ischaemia (SLI) is often used to describe both entities. Whereas IC is usually due to single-segment plaque, CLI is always due to multi-level disease.

Many patients with CLI have not previously sought medical advice for IC, principally because they often have other comorbidity that prevents them from walking to a point where claudication pain might develop. In contrast

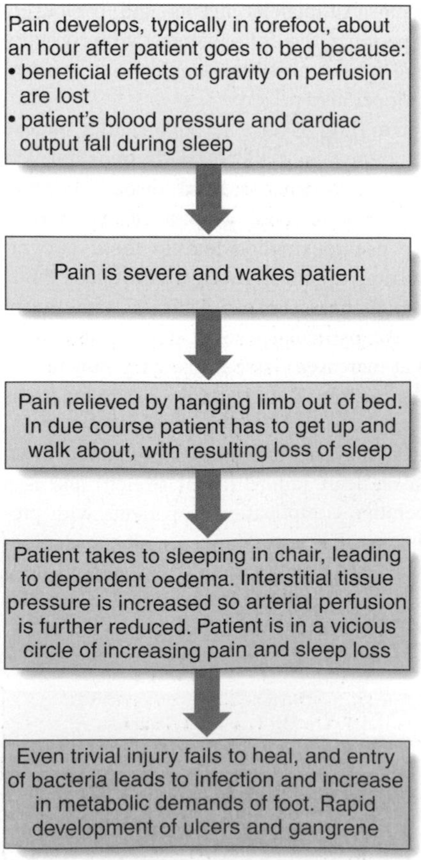

18.82 FEATURES OF CHRONIC LOWER LIMB ISCHAEMIA

- Pulses—diminished or absent
- Bruits—denote turbulent flow but bear no relationship to the severity of the underlying disease
- Reduced skin temperature
- Pallor on elevation and rubor on dependency (Buerger's sign)
- Superficial veins that fill sluggishly and empty ('gutter') upon minimal elevation
- Muscle-wasting
- Skin and nails—dry, thin and brittle
- Loss of hair

18.83 BEST MEDICAL THERAPY FOR PERIPHERAL ARTERIAL DISEASE

- Cessation of smoking
- Regular exercise (in a typical claudicant this would entail 30 minutes of walking three times per week)
- Antiplatelet agent (aspirin 75 mg daily or clopidogrel 75 mg daily)
- Reduction of cholesterol (diet + statin therapy)
- Diagnosis and treatment of diabetes mellitus (all should have fasting glucose measured)
- Diagnosis and treatment of frequently associated conditions (e.g. hypertension, anaemia, heart failure)

All patients with any manifestation of PAD should be considered candidates for best medical therapy.

Pain develops, typically in forefoot, about an hour after patient goes to bed because:
- beneficial effects of gravity on perfusion are lost
- patient's blood pressure and cardiac output fall during sleep

↓

Pain is severe and wakes patient

↓

Pain relieved by hanging limb out of bed. In due course patient has to get up and walk about, with resulting loss of sleep

↓

Patient takes to sleeping in chair, leading to dependent oedema. Interstitial tissue pressure is increased so arterial perfusion is further reduced. Patient is in a vicious circle of increasing pain and sleep loss

↓

Even trivial injury fails to heal, and entry of bacteria leads to infection and increase in metabolic demands of foot. Rapid development of ulcers and gangrene

Fig. 18.80 Progressive night pain and the development of tissue loss.

to IC, patients with CLI are at risk of losing their limb, sometimes their life, in a matter of weeks or months without surgical bypass or endovascular revascularisation. However, treatment is difficult because such patients represent end-stage disease, have severe multi-level disease, are usually elderly and nearly always have significant multi-system comorbidity. Imaging is performed using duplex ultrasonography, and additional more detailed non-invasive imaging can be provided by MRI or CT with intravenous injection of contrast agents. Intra-arterial digital subtraction angiography is mainly used for those patients who are thought suitable for endovascular revascularisation.

Diabetic vascular disease

Approximately 5–10% of patients with PAD have diabetes but this proportion increases to 30–40% in those with CLI. Although critical limb ischaemia was thought to be caused by an obstructive microangiopathy at the capillary level, this is now known to be incorrect, and diabetes is not a contraindication per se to lower limb revascularisation. Nevertheless, the 'diabetic foot' does pose a number of particular problems (Box 18.84 and p. 844). If the blood supply is adequate, then dead tissue can be excised in the expectation that healing will occur, provided infection is controlled and the foot is protected from pressure. However, if ischaemia is also present, the priority is to revascularise the foot, if possible. Sadly, many diabetic patients present late with extensive tissue loss, which accounts for the high amputation rate.

Buerger's disease (thromboangiitis obliterans)

This is an inflammatory obliterative arterial disease that is distinct from atherosclerosis. It is rare in the UK but more common in people from the Mediterranean and North Africa. It is likely that there is a strong genetic element. Buerger's disease usually presents in young (20–30 years) male smokers and characteristically affects the peripheral arteries, giving rise to claudication in the feet or rest pain in the fingers or toes. The condition also affects the veins, and superficial thrombophlebitis is common. Wrist and ankle pulses are usually absent, but brachial and popliteal pulses are characteristically palpable. Arteriography shows narrowing or occlusion of arteries below the knee but relatively healthy vessels above that level.

The condition often remits if the patient stops smoking; sympathectomy and prostaglandin infusions may be helpful. If amputation is required it can often be limited to the digits at first. However, bilateral below-knee amputation is the most frequent outcome if patients continue to smoke.

CHRONIC UPPER LIMB ARTERIAL DISEASE

The subclavian artery is the most common site of disease, which may manifest as:

- *Arm claudication* (rare).
- *Atheroembolism* (blue finger syndrome). Small emboli lodge in digital arteries and may be confused with Raynaud's phenomenon (see below), except that in this case the symptoms are unilateral. Failure to make the diagnosis may eventually lead to amputation.
- *Subclavian steal*. When the arm is used, blood is 'stolen' from the brain via the vertebral artery. This leads to vertebro-basilar ischaemia, which is characterised by dizziness, cortical blindness and/or collapse.

Most subclavian artery disease should be treated by means of angioplasty with or without stenting, as the results are good and surgery (carotid-subclavian bypass) is difficult.

18.84 DIABETIC VASCULAR DISEASE: THE 'DIABETIC FOOT'	
Feature	**Difficulty**
Arterial calcification	Spuriously high ABPI due to incompressible ankle vessels. Inability to clamp arteries for the purposes of bypass surgery. Resistant to angioplasty
Immunocompromise	Prone to rapidly spreading cellulitis, gangrene and osteomyelitis
Multisystem arterial disease	Coronary and cerebral arterial disease increases the risks of intervention
Distal disease	Diabetic vascular disease has a predilection for the calf vessels. Although vessels in the foot are often spared, performing a satisfactory bypass or angioplasty to these small vessels is a technical challenge
Sensory neuropathy	Even severe ischaemia and/or tissue loss may be completely painless. Diabetic patients often present late with extensive destruction of the foot. Loss of proprioception leads to abnormal pressure loads and exacerbates joint destruction (Charcot's joints)
Motor neuropathy	Weakness of the long and short flexors and extensors leads to abnormal foot architecture, abnormal pressure loads, callus formation and ulceration
Autonomic neuropathy	This leads to a dry foot deficient in sweat that normally lubricates the skin and contains antibacterial substances. Scaling and fissuring create a portal of entry for bacteria. Abnormal blood flow in the bones of the ankle and foot may also contribute to osteopenia and bony collapse

18.85 ATHEROSCLEROTIC VASCULAR DISEASE IN OLD AGE

- **Prevalence:** related almost exponentially to age in developed countries, although atherosclerosis is not considered part of the normal ageing process.
- **Statin therapy:** no role in the primary prevention of atherosclerotic disease in those over 75 years, but reduces cardiovascular events in those with established vascular disease, albeit with no reduction in overall mortality.
- **Presentation in the frail:** frequently with advanced multi-system arterial disease, along with a host of other comorbidities.
- **Intervention in the very frail:** in those with extensive disease and limited life expectancy, the risks of surgery may outweigh the benefits, and symptomatic care is all that should be offered.

RAYNAUD'S PHENOMENON AND RAYNAUD'S DISEASE

Raynaud's phenomenon

Cold and sometimes emotional stimuli may trigger vasospasm in the peripheral arteries. Raynaud's phenomenon describes the characteristic sequence of digital pallor due to vasospasm, followed by cyanosis due to the presence of deoxygenated blood, and then rubor due to reactive hyperaemia.

Primary Raynaud's phenomenon

This is also called Raynaud's disease and affects 5–10% of young women in temperate climates. The condition is often familial and usually appears between the ages of 15 and 30 years. It does not progress to ulceration or infarction and significant pain is unusual. No investigation is necessary and the patient should be reassured and advised to avoid exposure to cold, in the first instance. Treatment with a long-acting preparation of nifedipine may also be helpful. The underlying cause is unclear. Sympathectomy is not indicated.

Secondary Raynaud's phenomenon

This is also known as Raynaud's syndrome and tends to occur in older people in association with connective tissue disease (most commonly systemic sclerosis or the CREST syndrome, p. 1134), vibration-induced injury (from the use of power tools) and thoracic outlet obstruction (e.g. cervical rib). In contrast to primary disease the condition is associated with fixed obstruction of the digital arteries; fingertip ulceration and necrosis are often present and pain is usual. The fingers must be protected from cold and trauma, infection requires treatment with antibiotics, and surgery should be avoided if possible. Vasoactive drugs have no clear benefit. Sympathectomy helps for a year or two. Prostacyclin infusions are sometimes beneficial.

ACUTE LIMB ISCHAEMIA

Acute limb ischaemia is most frequently caused by acute thrombotic occlusion of a pre-existing stenotic arterial segment, thromboembolism and trauma, which may be iatrogenic. Apart from paralysis (inability to wiggle toes/fingers) and paraesthesia (loss of light touch over the dorsum of the foot/hand), the so-called 'Ps of acute ischaemia' (Box 18.86) are non-specific for ischaemia and/or inconsistently related to its severity. Pain on squeezing the calf indicates muscle infarction and impending irreversible ischaemia.

All suspected acutely ischaemic limbs must be discussed immediately with a vascular surgeon; a few hours can make the difference between death/amputation and complete recovery of limb function. If there are no contraindications (for example, acute aortic dissection or trauma, particularly head injury), an intravenous bolus of heparin (3000–5000 U) should be administered to limit propagation of thrombus and protect the collateral circulation. Distinguishing thrombosis from embolism is frequently difficult but it is important because treatment and prognosis are different (Box 18.87). Acute limb ischaemia due to thrombosis can usually be

18.86 SYMPTOMS AND SIGNS OF ACUTE LIMB ISCHAEMIA

Symptoms/signs	Comment
Pain Pallor Pulselessness	May be absent in complete acute ischaemia, and can be present in chronic ischaemia
Perishing cold	Unreliable, as the ischaemic limb takes on the ambient temperature
Paraesthesia Paralysis	Important features of impending irreversible ischaemia

18.87 ACUTE LIMB ISCHAEMIA: DISTINGUISHING FEATURES OF EMBOLISM AND THROMBOSIS IN SITU

Clinical features	Embolism	Thrombosis in situ
Severity	Complete (no collaterals)	Incomplete (collaterals)
Onset	Seconds or minutes	Hours or days
Limb	Leg 3:1 arm	Leg 10:1 arm
Multiple sites	Up to 15%	Rare
Embolic source	Present (usually AF)	Absent
Previous claudication	Absent	Present
Palpation of artery	Soft, tender	Hard, calcified
Bruits	Absent	Present
Contralateral leg pulses	Present	Absent
Diagnosis	Clinical	Angiography
Treatment	Embolectomy, warfarin	Medical, bypass, thrombolysis
Prognosis	Loss of life > loss of limb	Loss of limb > loss of life

treated medically in the first instance: intravenous heparin (target APTT 2.0–3.0), antiplatelet agents, high-dose statins, intravenous fluids to avoid dehydration, correction of anaemia, oxygen and sometimes prostaglandins such as iloprost. Careful monitoring is required. Acute limb ischaemia due to embolus will normally result in extensive tissue necrosis within 6 hours unless the limb is revascularised. The indications for thrombolysis remain controversial but, in general, enthusiasm for this treatment is waning. Irreversible ischaemia mandates early amputation or palliative therapy.

CEREBROVASCULAR DISEASE

This is discussed on pages 1200–1212.

RENOVASCULAR DISEASE

This is discussed on pages 496–499.

ISCHAEMIC GUT INJURY

This is discussed on pages 922–923.

DISEASES OF THE AORTA

Three types of condition may affect the aorta: aneurysm, dissection and aortitis (Fig. 18.81).

AORTIC ANEURYSM

An aortic aneurysm is an abnormal dilatation of the aortic wall. Aortic dissection has a different pathology and is considered separately.

Aetiology and types of aneurysm

Non-specific aneurysms

Although there are important clinical and pathological differences between occlusive atheromatous and aneurysmal arterial disease, these conditions share similar risk factors (e.g. smoking and hypertension) and often coexist. Why some patients develop occlusive and others aneurysmal disease remains unclear; however, unlike occlusive disease, what is now termed 'non-specific' aneurysmal disease tends to run in families, and genetic factors are undoubtedly important. The most common site for 'non-specific' aneurysm formation is the infrarenal abdominal aorta. The suprarenal abdominal aorta and a variable length of the descending thoracic aorta may be affected in 10–20% of patients but the ascending aorta is usually spared.

Marfan's syndrome

This connective tissue disorder is inherited as an autosomal dominant trait and is caused by mutations in the fibrillin gene on chromosome 15. There is considerable phenotypic variation but the major features involve the skeleton (arachnodactyly, joint hypermobility, scoliosis, chest deformity and high arched palate), the eyes (dislocation of the lens) and the cardiovascular system (aortic disease and mitral regurgitation). Weakening of the aortic media leads

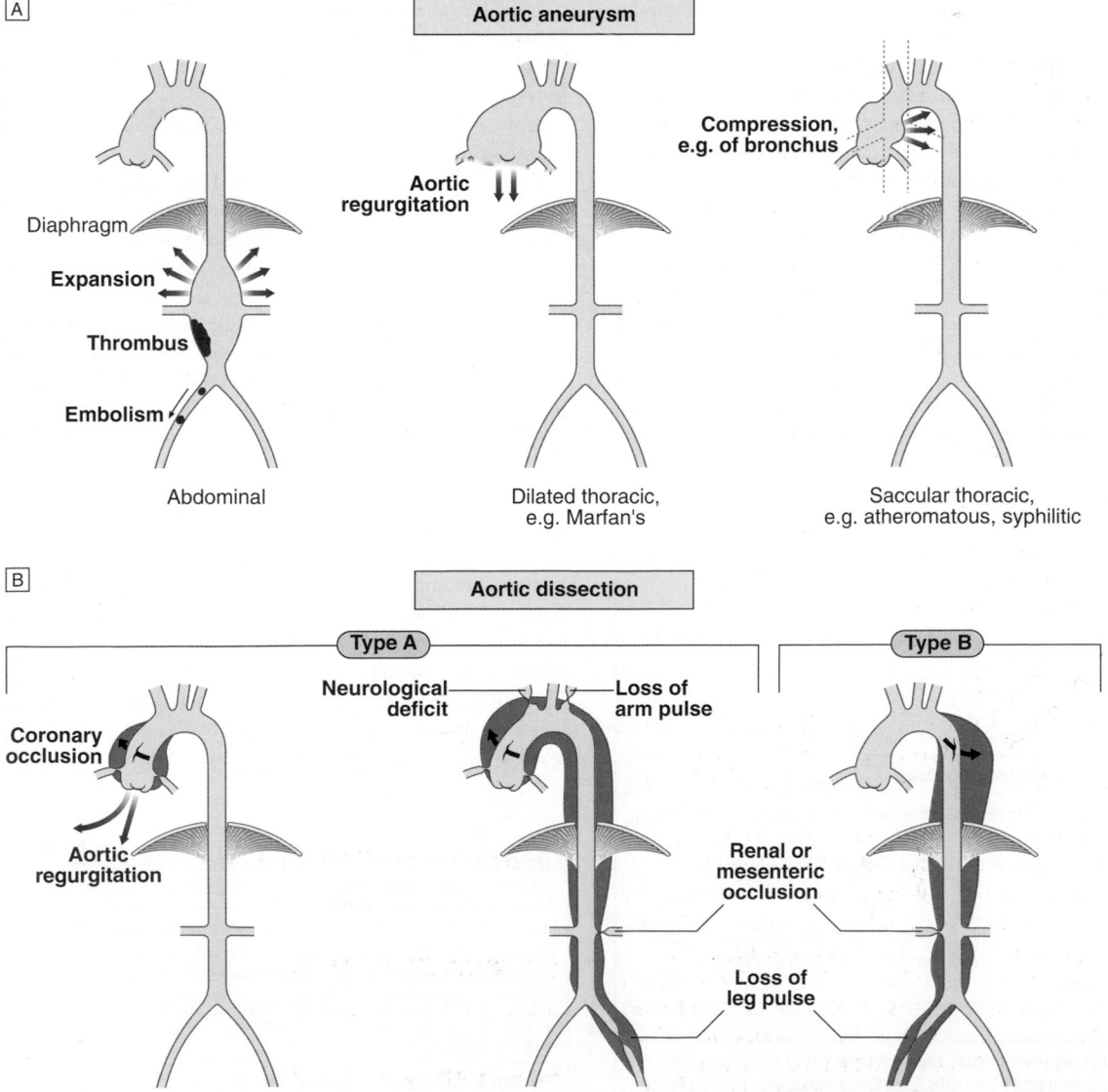

Fig. 18.81 **Types of aortic disease and their complications.** [A] Types of aortic aneurysm. [B] Types of aortic dissection.

18

to progressive dilatation of the ascending aorta that may be complicated by aortic regurgitation and aortic dissection (see below). Pregnancy is particularly hazardous. Chest radiography, echocardiography, MRI or CT may detect aortic dilatation at an early stage and can be used to monitor the disease.

Treatment with β-blockers reduces the rate of aortic dilatation and the risk of rupture. Elective replacement of the ascending aorta may be considered in patients with evidence of progressive aortic dilatation but carries a mortality of 5–10%.

Aortitis

Syphilis is a rare cause of aortitis that characteristically produces saccular aneurysms of the ascending aorta containing calcification. Other conditions that can cause aortitis and aneurysm formation include Takayasu's disease, Reiter's syndrome, giant cell arteritis and ankylosing spondylitis (pp. 1106–1108 and 1139–1140).

Thoracic aneurysms

Thoracic aortic aneurysms may produce chest pain similar to cardiac pain, associated with expansion of the aneurysm. If they extend proximally they may cause aortic valve regurgitation. They can also cause symptoms by compressing the trachea, main bronchus or superior vena cava (Fig. 18.81A). Occasionally, they may erode into the adjacent structures, causing haemorrhage, tamponade and death.

Abdominal aortic aneurysms (AAAs)

AAAs are present in 5% of men aged over 60 years and 80% are confined to the infrarenal segment. Men are affected three times more commonly than women. AAA can present in a number of ways (Box 18.88). The median age at presentation is 65 years for elective and 75 years for emergency cases. About two-thirds of AAAs are sufficiently calcified to show up on a plain abdominal X-ray. Ultrasound is the best way of establishing the diagnosis; an approximate size may be obtained, and the technique can be used to follow up patients with asymptomatic aneurysms that are not yet large enough to warrant surgical repair. CT will provide much more accurate information about the size and extent of the aneurysm, the surrounding structures and whether there is any other intra-abdominal pathology, and is the standard pre-operative investigation; however, it is not suitable for surveillance. Arteriography is usually only indicated if there are concerns about associated lower limb, renal and/or visceral occlusive disease.

Management. Until an asymptomatic AAA has reached a maximum of 5.5 cm in diameter, the risks of surgery generally outweigh the risks of rupture. All symptomatic AAAs should be considered for repair, not only to rid the patient of symptoms but also because pain often predates rupture. Distal embolisation is a strong indication for repair, regardless of size, because otherwise limb loss is common. Most patients with a ruptured AAA do not survive to reach hospital, but if they do and surgery is thought to be appropriate, there must be no delay in getting them to the operating theatre to clamp the aorta.

Open AAA repair is the established treatment of choice in both the elective and the emergency setting, and entails replacing the aneurysmal segment with a prosthetic (usually Dacron) graft. The 30-day mortality for this procedure is approximately 5–8% for elective asymptomatic AAA, 10–20% for emergency symptomatic AAA, and 50% for ruptured AAA. However, patients who survive operation to leave hospital have a long-term survival which approaches that of the normal population. Some AAAs may be treated with a covered stent placed via a femoral arteriotomy under radiological guidance.

AORTIC DISSECTION

In this dramatic condition a breach in the integrity of the aortic wall allows arterial blood to burst into the media of the aorta which is then split into two layers, creating a 'false lumen' alongside the existing or 'true lumen' (Fig. 18.81B). The aortic valve may be damaged and the branches of the aorta may be compromised. Typically, the false lumen eventually re-enters the true lumen, creating a double-

---

18.88 ABDOMINAL AORTIC ANEURYSM: COMMON PRESENTATIONS	

Incidental

- On physical examination, plain X-ray or, most commonly, abdominal ultrasound
- Even large AAAs can be difficult to feel, so many remain undetected until they rupture
- Studies are currently under way to determine whether screening will reduce the number of deaths from rupture (Box 18.89)

Pain

- In the central abdomen, back, loin, iliac fossa or groin

Thromboembolic complications

- Thrombus within the aneurysm sac may be a source of emboli to the lower limbs
- Less commonly, the aorta may undergo thrombotic occlusion

Compression

- Surrounding structures such as the duodenum (obstruction and vomiting) and the inferior vena cava (oedema and deep vein thrombosis)

Rupture

- Into the retroperitoneum, the peritoneal cavity or surrounding structures (most commonly the inferior vena cava, leading to an aortocaval fistula)

EBM

18.89 POPULATION SCREENING AND PREVENTION OF RUPTURED ABDOMINAL AORTIC ANEURYSM

'Ultrasound screening for AAA in men aged 65–75 years, with surgical repair of those AAA that are > 5.5 cm, are rapidly growing or become symptomatic, reduces the community incidence of rupture by approximately 50% and is cost-effective.'

- MASS Study Group. Lancet 2002; 360:1531–1539.
- MASS Study Group. BMJ 2002; 352:1135.

For further information: 💻 www.mrc-bsu.cam.ac.uk/BSUsite/Research/MASS/

barrelled or biluminal aorta, but it may also rupture into the left pleural space or pericardium with fatal consequences.

The primary event is often a spontaneous or iatrogenic tear in the intima of the aorta; multiple tears or entry points are common. On the other hand, many dissections appear to be triggered by a haemorrhage in the media of the aorta which then ruptures through the intima into the true lumen. This form of spontaneous bleeding from the vasa vasorum is sometimes confined to the aortic wall, when it may present as a painful intramural haematoma.

Disease of the aorta and hypertension are the most important aetiological factors but a variety of other conditions may be implicated (Box 18.90). Chronic dissections may lead to aneurysmal dilatation of the aorta, and thoracic aneurysms may be complicated by dissection; it is therefore sometimes difficult to determine which was the primary pathology.

The peak incidence is in the sixth and seventh decades of life but dissection can occur in younger patients, most commonly in association with Marfan's syndrome, pregnancy or trauma; men are twice as frequently affected as women.

Aortic dissection is classified anatomically and for management purposes into type A and type B (Fig. 18.81B), involving or sparing the ascending aorta respectively. Type A dissections account for two-thirds of cases and frequently

also extend into the descending aorta. The pain tends to follow the path of the dissection, migrating from its point of origin and along the dissection tract; involvement of the ascending aorta typically gives rise to anterior chest pain, and the descending aorta intrascapular pain.

Clinical features

The patient usually presents with severe 'tearing' chest pain. The onset of pain is typically very abrupt and collapse is common. If there is aortic regurgitation the aortic valve may need to be repaired or even replaced. Unless there is frank rupture, the patient is invariably hypertensive. There may be asymmetry of the brachial, carotid or femoral pulses, and the signs of aortic reflux may be present in type A dissections. Occlusion of aortic branches may cause a variety of complications including myocardial infarction (coronary), paraplegia (spinal), mesenteric infarction with an acute abdomen (coeliac and superior mesenteric), renal failure (renal) and acute limb (usually leg) ischaemia.

Investigations

The chest X-ray characteristically shows broadening of the upper mediastinum and distortion of the aortic 'knuckle', but these findings are variable and are absent in 10% of cases. A left-sided pleural effusion is common. The ECG may show left ventricular hypertrophy in patients with hypertension, or rarely, changes of acute MI (usually inferior). Doppler echocardiography may show aortic regurgitation, a dilated aortic root and, occasionally, the flap of the dissection. Transoesophageal echocardiography is particularly helpful because transthoracic echocardiography can only image the first 3–4 cm of the ascending aorta (Fig. 18.82). CT and MRI (Figs 18.83 and 18.84) are both highly specific, and angiography of the aortic arch is not usually required unless these techniques are not available.

Management

Assessment and treatment are urgent because the early mortality of acute dissection is approximately 1% per hour. Initial management comprises pain control and anti-hypertensive treatment with labetalol, a combined α- and

18.90 FACTORS THAT MAY PREDISPOSE TO AORTIC DISSECTION

- Hypertension (80% of cases)
- Aortic atherosclerosis
- Non-specific aortic aneurysm
- Aortic coarctation
- Collagen disorders (e.g. Marfan's syndrome, Ehlers–Danlos syndrome)
- Fibromuscular dysplasia
- Previous aortic surgery (e.g. CABG, aortic valve replacement)
- Pregnancy (usually third trimester)
- Trauma
- Iatrogenic (e.g. cardiac catheterisation, intra-aortic balloon pumping)

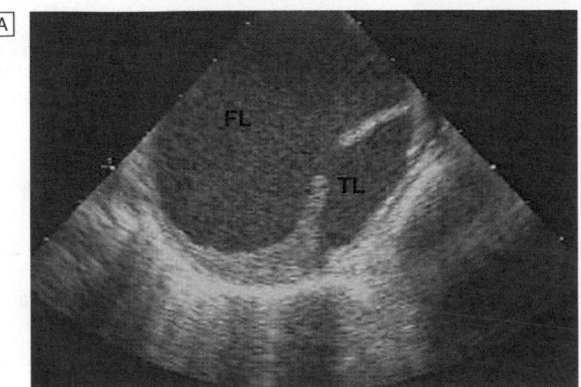

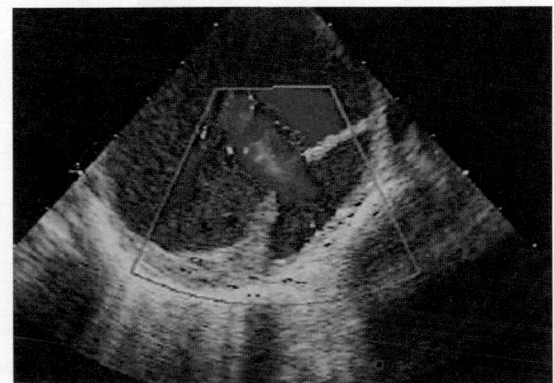

Fig. 18.82 **Echocardiograms from a patient with a chronic aortic dissection demonstrating the communication between the two lumens.** The false lumen (FL) is typically larger than the true lumen (TL) in chronic disease. [A] Transoesophageal echocardiogram. [B] Colour-flow Doppler study.

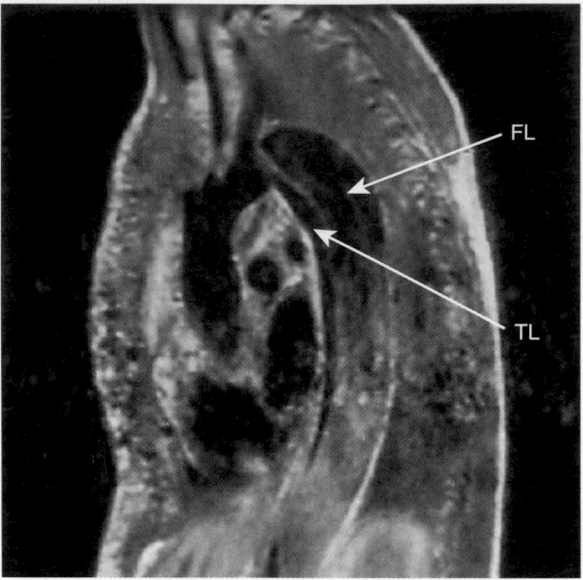

Fig. 18.83 Sagittal view of an MRI scan from a patient with long-standing aortic dissection illustrating a biluminal aorta. There is sluggish flow in the false lumen (FL) which accounts for its grey appearance. (TL = true lumen)

β-blocking drug, to maintain the systolic pressure below 120 mmHg. Type A dissections require emergency surgical repair. Surgery involves replacing the ascending aorta with a Dacron graft. Type B aneurysms can be treated medically unless there is actual or impending external rupture, or vital organ (gut, kidneys) or limb ischaemia.

Percutaneous or minimal access endoluminal repair is possible in some cases and involves either 'fenestrating' (perforating) the intimal flap so that blood can return from the false to the true lumen (so decompressing the former), or implanting a stent graft placed from the femoral artery (Fig. 18.84).

HYPERTENSION

Aetiology
In more than 95% of cases, a specific underlying cause of hypertension cannot be found. Such patients are said to have essential hypertension.

The pathogenesis of essential hypertension is not clearly understood. Different investigators have proposed the kidney, the peripheral resistance vessels and the sympathetic nervous system as the seat of the primary abnormality. In reality the problem is probably multifactorial. Hypertension

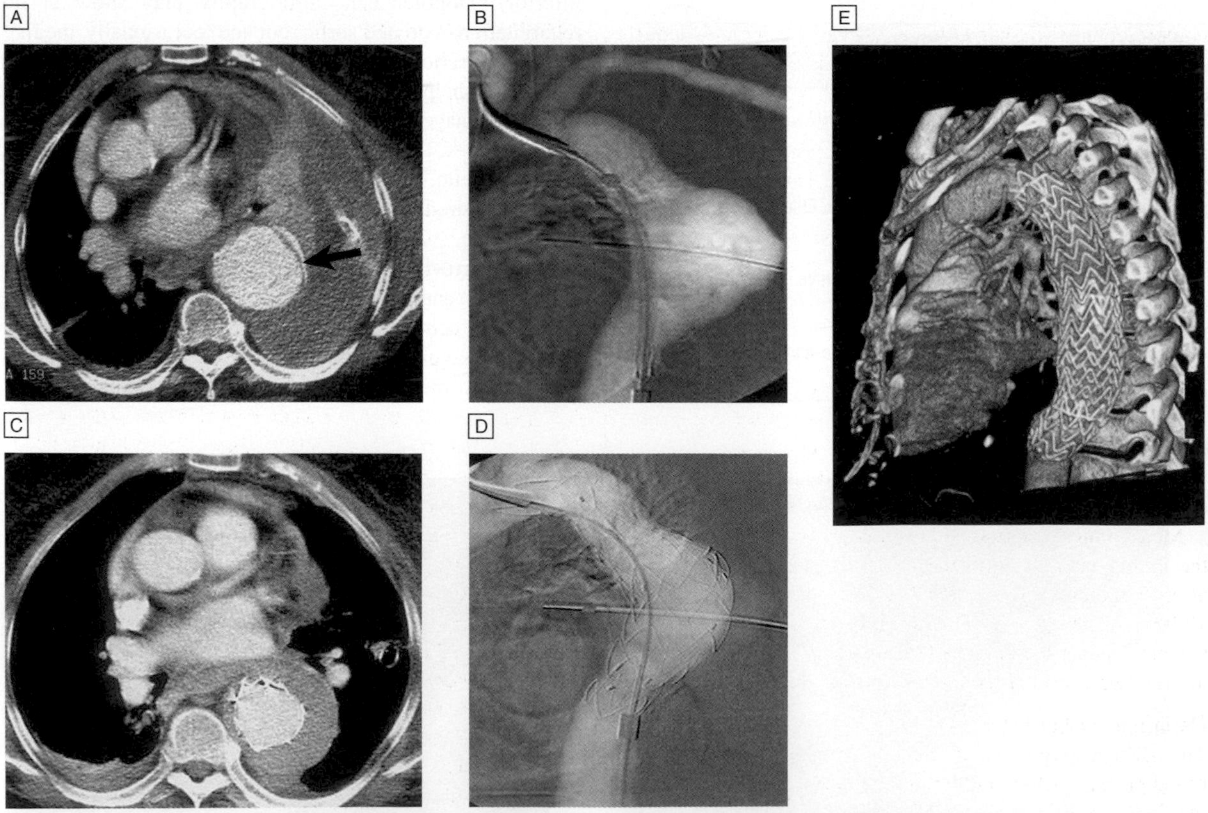

Fig. 18.84 Images from a patient with an acute type B aortic dissection that had ruptured into the left pleural space and was repaired by deploying an endoluminal stent graft. A CT scan illustrating an intimal flap (arrow) in the descending aorta and a large pleural effusion. B Aortogram illustrating aneurysmal dilatation; a stent graft has been introduced from the right femoral artery and is about to be deployed. C CT scan after endoluminal repair. The pleural effusion has been drained but there is a haematoma around the descending aorta. D Aortogram illustrating the stent graft. E Three-dimensional reconstruction of aortic stent graft.

18.91 CAUSES OF SECONDARY HYPERTENSION

Alcohol

Obesity

Pregnancy (pre-eclampsia)

Renal disease (Ch. 17)
- Renal vascular disease
- Parenchymal renal disease, particularly glomerulonephritis
- Polycystic kidney disease

Endocrine disease (Ch. 20)
- Phaeochromocytoma
- Cushing's syndrome
- Primary hyperaldosteronism (Conn's syndrome)
- Hyperparathyroidism
- Acromegaly
- Primary hypothyroidism
- Thyrotoxicosis
- Congenital adrenal hyperplasia due to 11-β-hydroxylase or 17-hydroxylase deficiency
- Liddle's syndrome
- 11-β-hydroxysteroid dehydrogenase deficiency

Drugs
- e.g. Oral contraceptives containing oestrogens, anabolic steroids, corticosteroids, non-steroidal anti-inflammatory drugs, carbenoxolone, sympathomimetic agents

Coarctation of the aorta (p. 637)

18.92 MEASUREMENT OF BLOOD PRESSURE

- Use a machine that has been validated, well maintained and properly calibrated
- Measure sitting BP routinely, with additional standing BP in elderly and diabetic patients and those with possible postural hypotension
- Remove tight clothing from the arm
- Support the arm at the level of the heart
- Use a cuff of appropriate size (the bladder must encompass > two-thirds of the arm)
- Lower the mercury slowly (2 mm per second)
- Read the BP to the nearest 2 mmHg
- Use phase V (disappearance of sounds) to measure diastolic BP
- Take two measurements at each visit

18.93 DEFINITION OF HYPERTENSION

Category	Systolic blood pressure (mmHg)	Diastolic blood pressure (mmHg)
Blood pressure		
Optimal	< 120	< 80
Normal	< 130	< 85
High normal	130–139	85–89
Hypertension		
Grade 1 (mild)	140–159	90–99
Grade 2 (moderate)	160–179	100–109
Grade 3 (severe)	≥ 180	≥ 110
Isolated systolic hypertension		
Grade 1	140–159	< 90
Grade 2	≥ 160	< 90

is more common in some ethnic groups, particularly Black Americans and Japanese, and approximately 40–60% is explained by genetic factors. Important environmental factors include a high salt intake, heavy consumption of alcohol, obesity, lack of exercise and impaired intrauterine growth. There is very little evidence that 'stress' causes hypertension.

In about 5% of unselected cases, hypertension can be shown to be a consequence of a specific disease or abnormality leading to sodium retention and/or peripheral vasoconstriction (secondary hypertension, Box 18.91).

Measurement of blood pressure
A decision to embark upon antihypertensive therapy effectively commits the patient to life-long treatment, so it is vital that the blood pressure (BP) readings on which this decision is based are as accurate as possible.

Measurements should be made to the nearest 2 mmHg, in the sitting position with the arm supported, and repeated after 5 minutes' rest if the first recording is high (Box 18.92). To avoid spuriously high recordings in obese subjects, the cuff should contain a bladder that encompasses at least two-thirds of the circumference of the arm.

Definition of hypertension
The British Hypertension Society has defined ranges of blood pressure which fall within the normal range and those that indicate hypertension (Box 18.93).

Home and ambulatory blood pressure recordings
Exercise, anxiety, discomfort and unfamiliar surroundings can all lead to a transient rise in BP. Sphygmomanometry, particularly when performed by a doctor, can cause an unrepresentative surge in BP which has been termed 'white coat' hypertension, and as many as 20% of patients with apparent hypertension in the clinic may have a 'normal BP' when it is recorded by automated devices used in their own home. The risk of cardiovascular disease in these patients is less than that observed in patients with sustained hypertension but greater than that seen in normotensive subjects.

A series of automated ambulatory BP measurements, obtained over 24 hours or longer, provides a better profile than a limited number of clinic readings. Indeed, ambulatory BP measurements correlate more closely with evidence of target organ damage than casual BP measurements. However, treatment thresholds and targets must be adjusted downwards because ambulatory BP readings are systematically lower (approximately 12/7 mmHg) than clinic measurements (Box 18.98, p. 613); the average ambulatory daytime (not 24-hour or night-time) BP should be used to guide management decisions.

Patients can also measure their own BP at home using a range of variable-quality semi-automatic devices; the real value of such measurements is not well established but similar considerations apply.

Home or ambulatory BP measurements may be particularly helpful in patients with unusually labile blood pressure, those with refractory hypertension, those who may be experiencing symptomatic hypotension, and those in whom white coat hypertension is suspected.

18

History

Family history, lifestyle (exercise, salt intake, smoking habit) and other risk factors should be recorded. A careful history will also identify those patients with drug- or alcohol-induced hypertension and may elicit the symptoms of other causes of secondary hypertension such as phaeochromocytoma (paroxysmal headache, palpitation and sweating) or complications such as coronary artery disease (e.g. angina, breathlessness).

Examination

Radio-femoral delay (coarctation of the aorta, Fig. 18.99, p. 637) enlarged kidneys (polycystic kidney disease), abdominal bruits (renal artery stenosis) and the characteristic facies and habitus of Cushing's syndrome are all examples of physical signs that may help to identify one of the causes of secondary hypertension (Box 18.91). Examination may also reveal features of important risk factors such as central obesity and hyperlipidaemia (tendon xanthomas etc.). Nevertheless, the majority of abnormal signs are due to the complications of hypertension.

Non-specific findings may include left ventricular hypertrophy (apical heave), accentuation of the aortic component of the second heart sound, and a fourth heart sound. The optic fundi are often abnormal (Fig. 18.85) and there may be evidence of generalised atheroma or specific complications such as aortic aneurysm or peripheral vascular disease.

Target organ damage

The adverse effects of hypertension principally involve the blood vessels, central nervous system, retina, heart and kidneys, and can often be detected clinically.

Blood vessels

In larger arteries (over 1 mm in diameter) the internal elastic lamina is thickened, smooth muscle is hypertrophied and fibrous tissue is deposited. The vessels dilate and become tortuous and their walls become less compliant. In smaller arteries (under 1 mm) hyaline arteriosclerosis occurs in the wall, the lumen narrows and aneurysms may develop. Widespread atheroma develops and may lead to coronary and/or cerebrovascular disease, particularly if other risk factors (e.g. smoking, hyperlipidaemia, diabetes) are present.

These structural changes in the vasculature often perpetuate and aggravate hypertension by increasing peripheral vascular resistance and reducing renal function.

Hypertension is also implicated in the pathogenesis of aortic aneurysm and aortic dissection.

Central nervous system

Stroke is a common complication of hypertension and may be due to cerebral haemorrhage or cerebral infarction. Carotid atheroma and transient cerebral ischaemic attacks are more common in hypertensive patients. Subarachnoid haemorrhage is also associated with hypertension.

Hypertensive encephalopathy is a rare condition characterised by high blood pressure and neurological symptoms, including transient disturbances of speech or vision, paraesthesiae, disorientation, fits and loss of consciousness. Papilloedema is common. A CT scan of the brain often shows haemorrhage in and around the basal ganglia; however, the neurological deficit is usually reversible if the hypertension is properly controlled.

Retina

The optic fundi reveal a gradation of changes linked to the severity of hypertension; fundoscopy can, therefore, provide an indication of the arteriolar damage occurring elsewhere (Box 18.94).

18.94 HYPERTENSIVE RETINOPATHY
• **Grade 1** Arteriolar thickening, tortuosity and increased reflectiveness ('silver wiring')
• **Grade 2** Grade 1 plus constriction of veins at arterial crossings ('arteriovenous nipping')
• **Grade 3** Grade 2 plus evidence of retinal ischaemia (flame-shaped or blot haemorrhages and 'cotton wool' exudates)
• **Grade 4** Grade 3 plus papilloedema

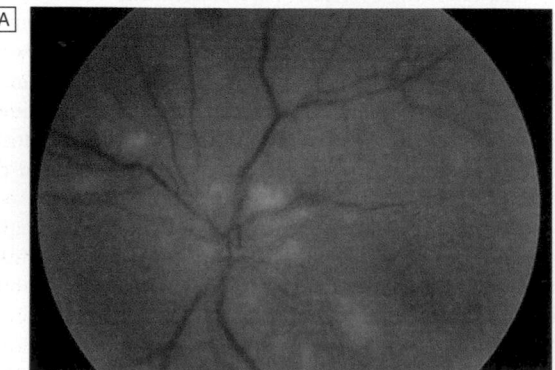
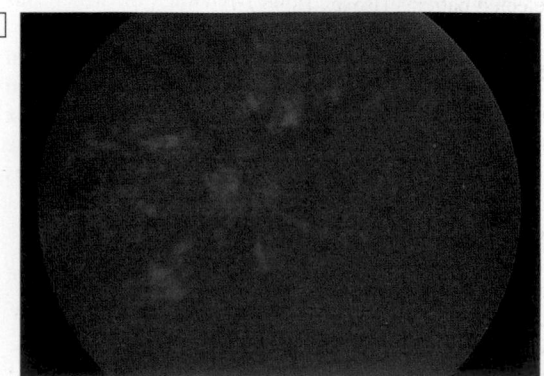

Fig. 18.85 Retinal changes in hypertension. Ⓐ Grade 4 hypertensive retinopathy showing swollen optic disc, retinal haemorrhages and multiple cotton wool spots (infarcts). Ⓑ Central retinal vein thrombosis showing swollen optic disc and widespread fundal haemorrhage, commonly associated with systemic hypertension.

'Cotton wool' exudates are associated with retinal ischaemia or infarction, and fade in a few weeks (Fig. 18.85A). 'Hard' exudates (small, white, dense deposits of lipid) and microaneurysms ('dot' haemorrhages) are more characteristic of diabetic retinopathy (Fig. 21.16, p. 839).

Hypertension is also associated with central retinal vein thrombosis (Fig. 18.85B).

Heart

The excess cardiac mortality and morbidity associated with hypertension are largely due to a higher incidence of coronary artery disease.

High blood pressure places a pressure load on the heart and may lead to left ventricular hypertrophy with a forceful apex beat and fourth heart sound. ECG or echocardiographic evidence of left ventricular hypertrophy is highly predictive of cardiovascular complications and therefore particularly useful in risk assessment.

Atrial fibrillation is common and may be due to diastolic dysfunction caused by left ventricular hypertrophy or the effects of coronary artery disease.

Severe hypertension can cause left ventricular failure in the absence of coronary artery disease, particularly when renal function, and therefore sodium excretion, is impaired.

Kidneys

Long-standing hypertension may cause proteinuria and progressive renal failure (p. 481) by damaging the renal vasculature.

'Malignant' or 'accelerated' phase hypertension

This rare condition may complicate hypertension of any aetiology and is characterised by accelerated microvascular damage with necrosis in the walls of small arteries and arterioles ('fibrinoid necrosis') and by intravascular thrombosis. The diagnosis is based on evidence of high blood pressure and rapidly progressive end organ damage such as retinopathy (grade 3 or 4), renal dysfunction (especially proteinuria) and/or hypertensive encephalopathy (see above). Left ventricular failure may occur and, if this is untreated, death occurs within months.

Investigations

All hypertensive patients should undergo a limited number of investigations. Additional investigations are appropriate in selected patients (Boxes 18.95 and 18.96).

MANAGEMENT

Quantification of cardiovascular risk

The sole objective of antihypertensive therapy is to reduce the incidence of adverse cardiovascular events, particularly coronary heart disease, stroke and heart failure. The relative benefit of antihypertensive therapy (approximately 30% reduction in risk of stroke and 20% reduction in risk of coronary heart disease—Box 18.99) is similar in all patient groups, so the absolute benefit (total number of events prevented) of treatment is greatest in those at highest risk. For example, to extrapolate from the Medical Research Council (MRC) Mild Hypertension Trial (1985), 566 young patients would have to be treated with bendroflumethiazide for 1 year to prevent 1 stroke (the equivalent figure for

18.95 HYPERTENSION: INVESTIGATION OF ALL PATIENTS

• Urinalysis for blood, protein and glucose
• Blood urea, electrolytes and creatinine
    N.B. Hypokalaemic alkalosis may indicate primary
    hyperaldosteronism but is usually due to diuretic therapy
• Blood glucose
• Serum total and high-density lipoprotein (HDL) cholesterol
• 12-lead ECG (left ventricular hypertrophy, coronary artery
  disease)

18.96 HYPERTENSION: INVESTIGATION OF SELECTED PATIENTS

• Chest X-ray: to detect cardiomegaly, heart failure, coarctation of
  the aorta
• Ambulatory BP recording: to assess borderline or 'white coat'
  hypertension
• Echocardiogram: to detect or quantify left ventricular hypertrophy
• Renal ultrasound: to detect possible renal disease
• Renal angiography: to detect or confirm presence of renal artery
  stenosis
• Urinary catecholamines: to detect possible phaeochromocytoma
  (p. 787)
• Urinary cortisol and dexamethasone suppression test: to detect
  possible Cushing's syndrome (p. 779)
• Plasma renin activity and aldosterone: to detect possible primary
  aldosteronism (p. 782)

18

propranolol was 1423 patient years); in the MRC trial of antihypertensive treatment in the elderly (1992), 1 stroke was prevented for every 286 patients treated for 1 year.

A formal estimate of absolute cardiovascular risk may help to determine whether the likely benefits of therapy will outweigh its costs and hazards. This should take account of all the relevant risk factors and not just the blood pressure. A variety of computer programs and risk charts are available for this purpose (a chart issued by the Joint British Societies can be found in the Appendix). Most of the excess morbidity and mortality associated with hypertension is attributable to coronary heart disease and many treatment guidelines are therefore based on estimates of the 10-year coronary heart disease risk. Total cardiovascular risk can be estimated by multiplying coronary heart disease (CHD) risk by 4/3 (i.e. if CHD risk is 30%, cardiovascular risk is 40%).

The value of this approach can be illustrated by comparing two hypothetical cases. A 65-year-old man with an average blood pressure of 150/90 mmHg, who smokes, has diabetes, a total:HDL cholesterol of 8 and ECG changes of left ventricular hypertrophy, will be found to have a 10-year CHD risk of 68% (Joint British Societies risk assessor). Antihypertensive therapy (assuming 20% relative risk reduction) would therefore be expected to prevent 14 coronary events for every 1000 patient years of treatment and would be advisable. In contrast, a 55-year-old woman with exactly the same blood pressure, who does not smoke, is not diabetic, has a total:HDL cholesterol of 6 and a normal ECG, has a predicted 10-year CHD risk of less than 14%; treatment in this case might therefore prevent fewer than 3 events per 1000 patient years of treatment and would be questionable.

Threshold for intervention

Systolic blood pressure and diastolic blood pressure are both powerful predictors of cardiovascular risk. The British Hypertension Society management guidelines therefore utilise both readings, and treatment should be initiated if they exceed the given threshold (Fig. 18.86).

Patients with diabetes or cardiovascular disease are at particularly high risk and the threshold for initiating antihypertensive therapy is therefore lower (≥ 140/90) in these patient groups. The thresholds for treatment in the elderly are the same as for younger patients (Box 18.97).

Treatment targets

In the hypertension optimal treatment (HOT) trial, the optimum blood pressure for reduction of major cardiovascular events was found to be 139/83 mmHg, and even lower in patients with diabetes; moreover, reducing blood pressure below this level caused no harm. Unfortunately, it seems clear that despite best practice, the targets suggested by the British Hypertension Society (Box 18.98) will not be achievable in many patients. In the UK the rule of halves has been observed: only half of all hypertensives are diagnosed,

18.97 HYPERTENSION IN OLD AGE

- **Prevalence:** affects more than half of all people over the age of 60 (including isolated systolic hypertension).
- **Risks:** hypertension is the most important risk factor for MI, heart failure and stroke in older people.
- **Benefit of treatment:** absolute benefit from anti-hypertensives is greatest in older people (at least up to 80 years).
- **Target BP:** similar to that for younger patients.
- **Tolerance of treatment:** antihypertensives are tolerated as well as in younger patients.
- **Drug of choice:** low-dose thiazides, but in the presence of coexistent disease (e.g. gout, diabetes) other agents may be more appropriate.

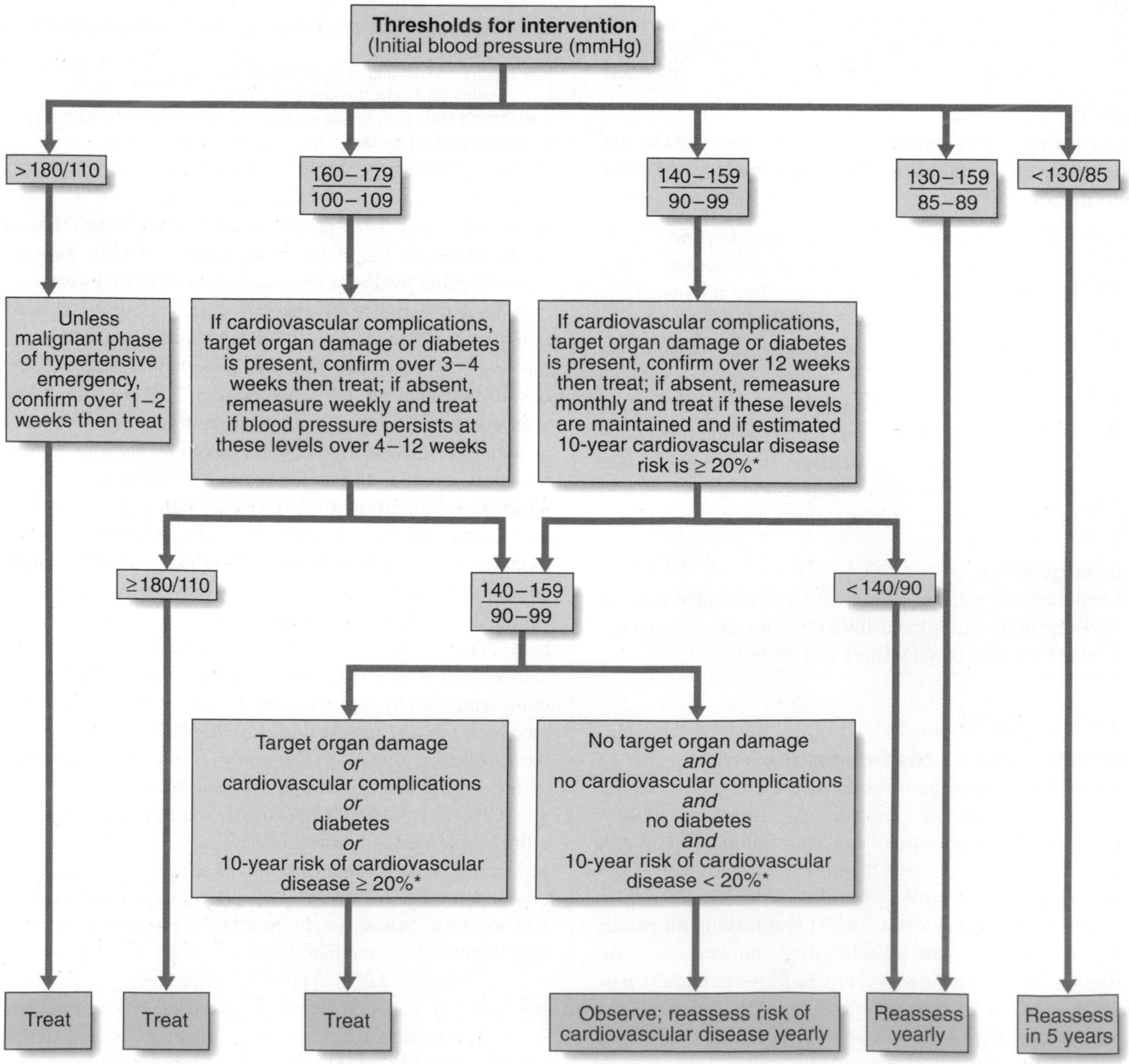

Thresholds for intervention
(Initial blood pressure (mmHg))
>180/110
160–179
100–109
140–159
90–99
130–159
85–89
<130/85
Unless malignant phase of hypertensive emergency, confirm over 1–2 weeks then treat
If cardiovascular complications, target organ damage or diabetes is present, confirm over 3–4 weeks then treat; if absent, remeasure weekly and treat if blood pressure persists at these levels over 4–12 weeks
If cardiovascular complications, target organ damage or diabetes is present, confirm over 12 weeks then treat; if absent, remeasure monthly and treat if these levels are maintained and if estimated 10-year cardiovascular disease risk is ≥ 20%*
≥180/110
140–159
90–99
<140/90
Target organ damage or cardiovascular complications or diabetes or 10-year risk of cardiovascular disease ≥ 20%*
No target organ damage and no cardiovascular complications and no diabetes and 10-year risk of cardiovascular disease < 20%*
Treat
Treat
Treat
Observe; reassess risk of cardiovascular disease yearly
Reassess yearly
Reassess in 5 years

Fig. 18.86 Management of hypertension: British Hypertension Society guidelines. (* Assessed with risk chart for cardiovascular disease.)

18.98 OPTIMAL TARGET BLOOD PRESSURES DURING ANTIHYPERTENSIVE TREATMENT: BRITISH HYPERTENSION SOCIETY GUIDELINES		
	No diabetes	Diabetes
Clinic measurements	< 140/85	< 140/80
Mean day-time ambulatory or home measurement	< 130/80	< 130/75

N.B. Both systolic and diastolic values should be attained.

18

only half of these patients are on treatment, and blood pressure is well controlled in only half of those receiving therapy.

Patients taking antihypertensive therapy require follow-up, typically at 3-month intervals, to monitor blood pressure, minimise side-effects and reinforce lifestyle advice.

Non-drug therapy

Appropriate lifestyle measures may obviate the need for drug therapy in patients with borderline hypertension, reduce the dose and/or the number of drugs required in patients with established hypertension, and directly reduce cardiovascular risk.

Correcting obesity, reducing alcohol intake, restricting salt intake, taking regular physical exercise and increasing consumption of fruit and vegetables can all lower blood pressure. Moreover, quitting smoking, eating oily fish and adopting a diet that is low in saturated fat may produce further reductions in cardiovascular risk.

Antihypertensive drugs

- *Thiazide and other diuretics.* The mechanism of action of these drugs is incompletely understood, and it may take up to a month for the maximum effect to be observed. A daily dose of 2.5 mg bendroflumethiazide or 0.5 mg cyclopenthiazide is appropriate. More potent loop diuretics, such as furosemide 40 mg daily or bumetanide 1 mg daily, have few advantages over thiazides in the treatment of hypertension unless there is substantial renal impairment or they are used in conjunction with an ACE inhibitor.
- *Beta-adrenoceptor antagonists (β-blockers).* Metoprolol (100–200 mg daily), atenolol (50–100 mg daily) and bisoprolol (5–10 mg daily) are cardioselective and therefore preferentially block the cardiac β_1-adrenoceptors, as opposed to the β_2-adrenoceptors that mediate vasodilatation and bronchodilatation.
- *Labetalol and carvedilol.* Labetalol (200 mg–2.4 g daily in divided doses) and carvedilol (6.25–25 mg 12-hourly) are combined β- and α-adrenoceptor antagonists which are sometimes more effective than pure β-blockers. Labetalol can be used as an infusion in malignant phase hypertension.
- *Angiotensin-converting enzyme (ACE) inhibitors.* These drugs (e.g. enalapril 20 mg daily, ramipril 5–10 mg daily or lisinopril 10–40 mg daily) inhibit the conversion of angiotensin I to angiotensin II and are usually well tolerated. They should be used with particular care in

patients with impaired renal function or renal artery stenosis because they can reduce the filtration pressure in the glomeruli and precipitate renal failure. Electrolytes and creatinine should be checked before and 1–2 weeks after commencing therapy. Side-effects include first-dose hypotension, cough, rash, hyperkalaemia and renal dysfunction.

- *Angiotensin receptor blockers.* These drugs (e.g. losartan 50–100 mg daily, valsartan 40–160 mg daily) block the angiotensin II type I receptor and have similar effects to ACE inhibitors but do not cause cough and are better tolerated.
- *Calcium antagonists.* The dihydropyridines (e.g. amlodipine 5–10 mg daily, nifedipine 30–90 mg daily) are effective and usually well-tolerated antihypertensive drugs that are particularly useful in the elderly. Side-effects include flushing, palpitations and fluid retention. The rate-limiting calcium antagonists (e.g. diltiazem 200–300 mg daily, verapamil 240 mg daily) can be useful when hypertension coexists with angina but they may cause bradycardia. The main side-effect of verapamil is constipation.
- *Other drugs.* A variety of vasodilators are used to treat hypertension. These include the α_1-adrenoceptor antagonists (α-blockers), such as prazosin (0.5–20 mg daily in divided doses), indoramin (25–100 mg 12-hourly) and doxazosin (1–16 mg daily), and drugs that act directly on vascular smooth muscle, such as hydralazine (25–100 mg 12-hourly) and minoxidil (10–50 mg daily). Side-effects include first-dose and postural hypotension, headache, tachycardia and fluid retention. Minoxidil also causes increased facial hair and is therefore unsuitable for female patients.

Centrally acting drugs, such as methyldopa (initial dose 250 mg 8-hourly) and clonidine (0.05–0.1 mg 8-hourly), are effective antihypertensive drugs but cause fatigue and are usually poorly tolerated.

Choice of antihypertensive drug

Trials that have compared the major classes of antihypertensive drug (thiazides, β-blockers, calcium antagonists, ACE inhibitors and α-blockers) have shown no consistent or important differences in outcome, efficacy, side-effects or quality of life (Box 18.99). The choice of antihypertensive therapy is therefore usually dictated by cost, convenience, the response to treatment and freedom from side-effects. Nevertheless, comorbid conditions may have an important influence on initial drug selection

EBM

18.99 BENEFIT OF ANTIHYPERTENSIVE DRUG THERAPY

'Diuretics or β-blockers have been shown to reduce the risk of coronary heart disease by 16%, stroke by 38%, cardiovascular death by 21% and all causes of mortality by 13%. The effects of ACE inhibitors and calcium antagonists are similar. NNT_Bs vary greatly according to the absolute baseline risk of cardiovascular disease.'

- Whelton PK, He J. In: Hennekens CH et al. (eds). Clinical Trials in cardiovascular disease: a companion to Brainwald's Heart Disease. Philadelphia: WB Saunders; 1999.
- Blood Pressure Lowering Treatment Trialists' Collaboration. Lancet 2003; 362:1527–1535.

18.100 THE INFLUENCE OF COMORBIDITY ON THE CHOICE OF ANTIHYPERTENSIVE DRUG THERAPY

Class of drug	Compelling indications	Possible indications	Caution	Compelling contraindications
α-blockers	Benign prostatic hypertrophy	–	Postural hypotension, heart failure[1]	Urinary incontinence
Angiotensin-converting enzyme (ACE) inhibitors	Heart failure Left ventricular dysfunction, post-myocardial infarction or established coronary heart disease Type 1 diabetic nephropathy Secondary stroke prevention[4]	Chronic renal disease[2] Type 2 diabetic nephropathy	Renal impairment[2] Peripheral vascular disease[3]	Pregnancy Renovascular disease[2]
Angiotensin II receptor blockers	ACE inhibitor intolerance Type 2 diabetic nephropathy Hypertension with left ventricular hypertrophy Heart failure in ACE-intolerant patients, after myocardial infarction	Left ventricular dysfunction after myocardial infarction Intolerance of other antihypertensive drugs Proteinuric renal disease, chronic renal disease[2] Heart failure	Renal impairment[2] Peripheral vascular disease[3]	Pregnancy
β-blockers	Myocardial infarction, angina Heart failure[5]		Heart failure[5] Peripheral vascular disease Diabetes (except with coronary heart disease)	Asthma or chronic obstructive pulmonary disease Heart block
Calcium channel blockers (dihydropyridine)	Elderly patients, isolated systolic hypertension	Angina	–	–
Calcium channel blockers (rate-limiting)	Angina	Elderly patient	Combination with β-blockade	Heart block, heart failure
Thiazides or thiazide-like diuretics	Elderly patients, isolated systolic hypertension, heart failure, secondary stroke prevention	–	–	Gout[6]

[1] In heart failure when used as monotherapy.
[2] ACE inhibitors or angiotensin II receptor blockers may be beneficial in chronic renal failure and those with renovascular disease but should only be used with caution, close supervision and specialist advice when there is established and significant renal impairment.
[3] Caution with ACE inhibitors and angiotensin II receptor blockers in peripheral vascular disease because of association with renovascular disease.
[4] In combination with a thiazide or thiazide-like diuretic.
[5] Beta-blockers are used increasingly to treat stable heart failure but may worsen acute heart failure.
[6] Thiazides or thiazide-like diuretics may sometimes be necessary to control blood pressure in people with a history of gout, ideally used in combination with allopurinol.

(Box 18.100); for example, a β-blocker might be the most appropriate treatment for a patient with angina unless there is also a history of asthma. Thiazide diuretics and dihydropyridine calcium antagonists are the most suitable drugs for the treatment of high blood pressure in elderly people.

Although some patients can be satisfactorily treated with a single antihypertensive drug, a combination of drugs is often required to achieve optimal blood pressure control. Combination therapy may be desirable for other reasons; for example, low-dose therapy with two or three drugs may produce fewer unwanted effects than treatment with the maximum dose of a single drug. Moreover, some drugs have complementary or synergistic actions (Fig. 18.87); for example, thiazides increase activity of the renin–angiotensin system while ACE inhibitors block it.

The emergency treatment of accelerated phase or malignant hypertension

In accelerated phase hypertension, it is unwise to lower blood pressure too quickly because this may compromise tissue perfusion (due to altered autoregulation) and can cause cerebral damage, including occipital blindness, and precipitate coronary or renal insufficiency. Even in the presence of cardiac failure or hypertensive encephalopathy, a controlled reduction, to a level of about 150/90 mmHg, over a period of 24–48 hours is ideal.

In most patients it is possible to avoid parenteral therapy and bring blood pressure under control with bed rest and oral drug therapy. Intravenous or intramuscular labetalol (2 mg/min to a maximum of 200 mg), intravenous glyceryl trinitrate (0.6–1.2 mg/hour), intramuscular hydralazine (5 or 10 mg aliquots repeated at half-hourly intervals) and intravenous sodium nitroprusside (0.3–1.0 µg/kg body weight per minute) are all effective remedies but require careful supervision, preferably in a high-dependency unit.

Refractory hypertension

The common causes of treatment failure in hypertension are non-adherence with drug therapy, inadequate therapy, and failure to recognise an underlying cause such as renal

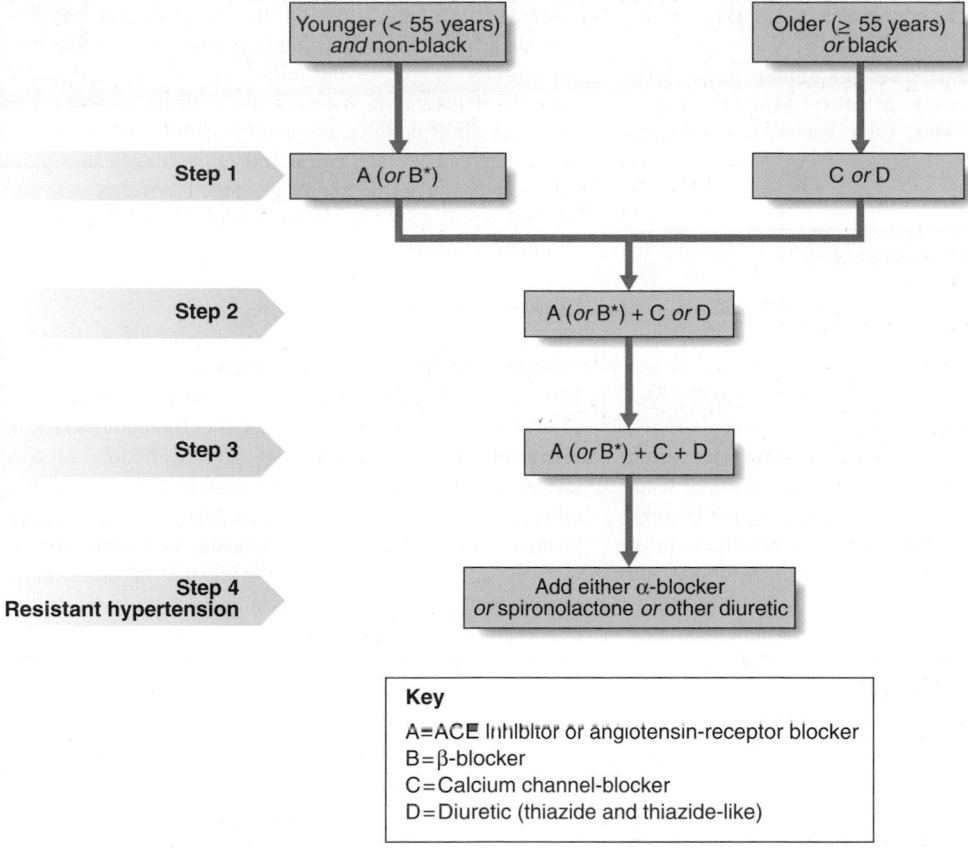

Fig. 18.87 Antihypertensive drug combinations. (* Combination therapy involving B and D may induce more new-onset diabetes compared with other combination therapies.)

artery stenosis or phaeochromocytoma; of these, the first is by far the most prevalent. There is no easy solution to compliance problems, but simple treatment regimens, attempts to improve rapport with the patient and careful supervision may all help.

Adjuvant drug therapy

- *Aspirin.* Antiplatelet therapy is a powerful means of reducing cardiovascular risk but may cause bleeding, particularly intracerebral haemorrhage, in a small number of patients. The benefits of aspirin therapy are thought to outweigh the risks in hypertensive patients aged 50 or over who have well-controlled blood pressure and either target organ damage, diabetes or a 10-year coronary heart disease risk of more than 15%.
- *Statins.* Treating hyperlipidaemia can also produce a substantial reduction in cardiovascular risk. These drugs are strongly indicated in patients who have established vascular disease, or hypertension with a high (> 15% in 10 years) risk of developing coronary heart disease (pp. 449–450).

DISEASES OF THE HEART VALVES

A diseased valve may be narrowed (stenosed) or it may fail to close adequately, and thus permit regurgitation of

---

18.101 PRINCIPAL CAUSES OF VALVE DISEASE

Valve regurgitation

- Congenital
- Acute rheumatic carditis
- Chronic rheumatic carditis
- Infective endocarditis
- Syphilitic aortitis
- Valve ring dilatation (e.g. dilated cardiomyopathy)
- Traumatic valve rupture
- Senile degeneration
- Damage to chordae and papillary muscles (e.g. MI)

Valve stenosis

- Congenital
- Rheumatic carditis
- Senile degeneration

---

blood. The less precise term 'incompetence' may be used synonymously with regurgitation or reflux, but the latter are preferable. The principal causes of valve disease are summarised in Box 18.101.

Doppler echocardiography is the most useful technique for assessing patients with valvular heart disease (p. 531), but it is a very sensitive technique that often detects minor, unimportant and even 'physiological' abnormalities, such as trivial regurgitation of the mitral valve. Disease of the heart valves may progress with time and selected patients require regular review, usually every 1 or 2 years, to ensure that deterioration is detected before complications such as heart

18

failure ensue. Patients with valvular heart disease are susceptible to bacterial endocarditis which can be prevented by good dental hygiene and the use of antibiotic prophylaxis at times of bacteraemia such as dental extraction (p. 633).

The aetiology of individual valve lesions is considered below.

RHEUMATIC HEART DISEASE

ACUTE RHEUMATIC FEVER

Incidence and pathogenesis

Acute rheumatic fever (ARF) usually affects children (most commonly between 5 and 15 years) or young adults, and has become very rare in Western Europe and North America. Nevertheless, it remains endemic in parts of Asia, Africa and South America, with an annual incidence in some countries of more than 100 per 100 000; it is still the most common cause of acquired heart disease in childhood and adolescence.

The condition is triggered by an immune-mediated delayed response to infection with specific strains of group A streptococci that possess antigens which may cross-react with cardiac myosin and sarcolemmal membrane protein.

Antibodies produced against the streptococcal antigens mediate inflammation in the endocardium, myocardium and pericardium as well as the joints and skin. Histologically, fibrinoid degeneration is seen in the collagen of connective tissues. Aschoff nodules are pathognomonic and occur only in the heart. They are composed of multinucleated giant cells surrounded by macrophages and T lymphocytes, and are not seen until the subacute or chronic phases of rheumatic carditis.

Clinical features

ARF is a multisystem disorder that typically follows an episode of streptococcal pharyngitis and usually presents with fever, anorexia, lethargy and joint pains. Symptoms characteristically occur 2–3 weeks after the initial attack of pharyngitis but the patient may give no history of sore throat. Arthritis occurs in approximately 75% of patients; other features include rashes, carditis and neurological changes (Fig. 18.88). The diagnosis, according to the revised Jones criteria, is based upon two or more major manifestations, or one major and two or more minor manifestations; evidence of preceding streptococcal infection is also required (Box 18.102). Only about 25% of patients will have a positive culture for group A streptococcus at the time of diagnosis because there is a

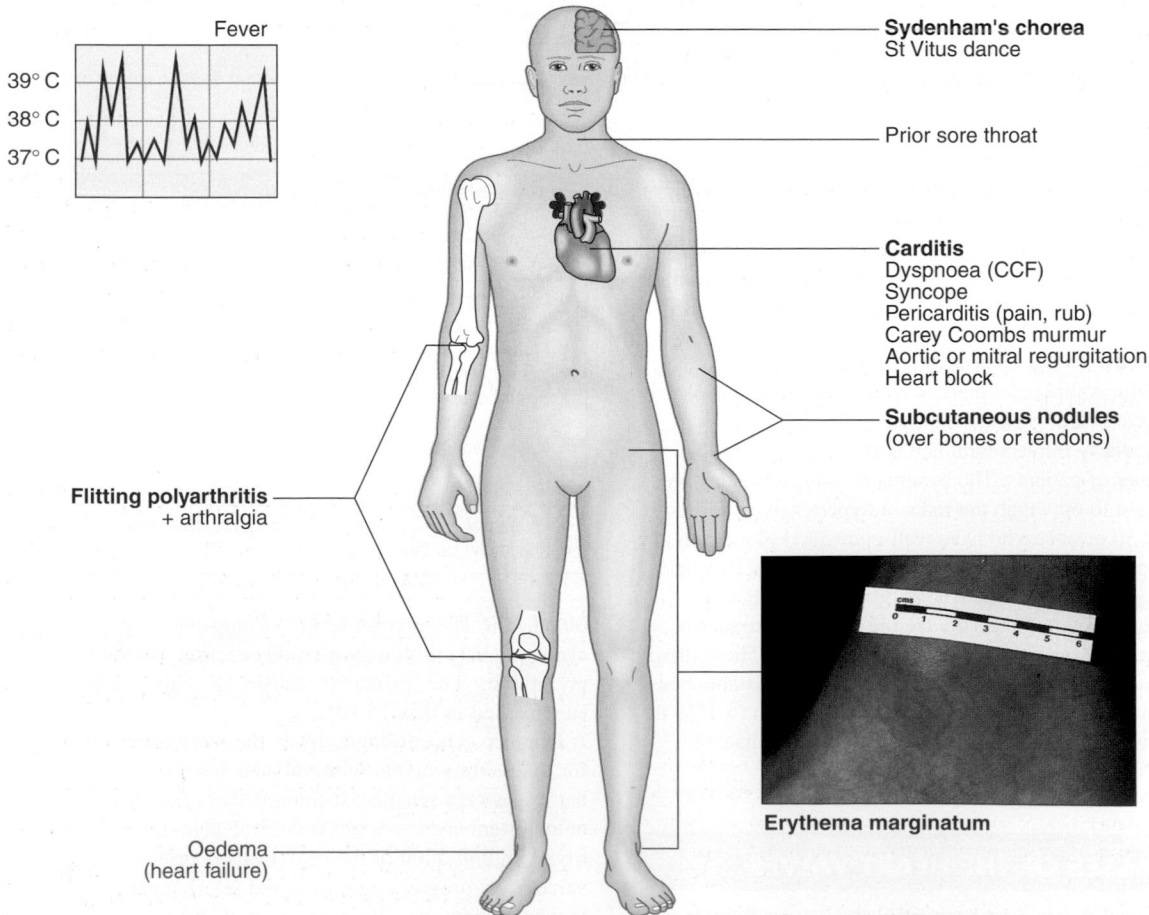

Fever

39° C
38° C
37° C

Sydenham's chorea
St Vitus dance

Prior sore throat

Carditis
Dyspnoea (CCF)
Syncope
Pericarditis (pain, rub)
Carey Coombs murmur
Aortic or mitral regurgitation
Heart block

Subcutaneous nodules
(over bones or tendons)

Flitting polyarthritis
+ arthralgia

Erythema marginatum

Oedema
(heart failure)

Fig. 18.88 **Clinical features of rheumatic fever.** Bold labels indicate Jones major criteria. (CCF = congestive cardiac failure)

18.102 JONES CRITERIA FOR THE DIAGNOSIS OF RHEUMATIC FEVER

Major manifestations

- Carditis
- Polyarthritis
- Chorea
- Erythema marginatum
- Subcutaneous nodules

Minor manifestations

- Fever
- Arthralgia
- Previous rheumatic fever
- Raised ESR or CRP
- Leucocytosis
- First-degree AV block

PLUS

- Supporting evidence of preceding streptococcal infection: recent scarlet fever, raised antistreptolysin 0 or other streptococcal antibody titre, positive throat culture

N.B. Evidence of recent streptococcal infection is particularly important if there is only one major manifestation.

latent period between infection and presentation; serological evidence of recent streptococcal infection with a raised antistreptolysin O (ASO) antibody titre may therefore be helpful. A diagnosis of presumptive ARF can be made without evidence of preceding streptococcal infection in cases of isolated chorea or pancarditis, if other causes for these have been excluded. In cases of established rheumatic heart disease or prior ARF, a diagnosis of ARF can be made based only on the presence of multiple minor criteria and evidence of preceding group A streptococcal pharyngitis.

Carditis

This is a 'pancarditis' that involves the endocardium, myocardium and pericardium to varying degrees; its incidence declines with increasing age, ranging from 90% at 3 years to around 30% in adolescence. Carditis may manifest as breathlessness (due to heart failure or pericardial effusion), palpitations or chest pain (usually due to pericarditis or pancarditis). Other features include tachycardia, cardiac enlargement and new or changed cardiac murmurs. A soft systolic murmur due to mitral regurgitation is very common. A soft mid-diastolic murmur (the Carey Coombs murmur) is typically due to valvulitis, with nodules forming on the mitral valve leaflets. Aortic regurgitation occurs in about 50% of cases but the tricuspid and pulmonary valves are rarely involved in the acute process. Pericarditis may cause chest pain, a pericardial friction rub and precordial tenderness. Cardiac failure may be due to myocardial dysfunction and/or mitral or aortic regurgitation. ECG changes are common and include ST and T wave changes; conduction defects sometimes occur and may cause syncope.

Arthritis

This is usually an early feature that tends to occur when streptococcal antibody titres are high. It is the most common major manifestation and is characterised by acute, painful, asymmetric and migratory inflammation of the large joints (typically the knees, ankles, elbows and wrists). The joints are involved in quick succession and are usually red, swollen and tender for between a day and up to 4 weeks. The

pain characteristically responds to aspirin; if it does not, the diagnosis is in doubt.

Skin lesions

Erythema marginatum occurs in less than 5% of patients. The lesions start as red macules (blotches) which fade in the centre but remain red at the edges and occur mainly on the trunk and proximal extremities but not the face. The resulting red rings or 'margins' may coalesce or overlap (Fig. 18.88).

Subcutaneous nodules occur in 5–7% of patients. They are small (0.5–2.0 cm), firm and painless, and are best felt over extensor surfaces of bone or tendons. Nodules typically appear more than 3 weeks after the onset of other manifestations and are therefore a feature that helps to confirm rather than make the diagnosis.

Other systemic manifestations are rare, but include pleurisy, pleural effusion and pneumonia.

Sydenham's chorea (St Vitus dance)

This is a late neurological manifestation that typically appears at least 3 months after the episode of ARF when all the other signs may have disappeared. It occurs in up to one-third of cases and is more common in females. Emotional lability may be the first feature and is typically followed by purposeless involuntary choreiform movements of the hands, feet or face. Speech may be explosive and halting. Spontaneous recovery usually occurs within a few months. Approximately one-quarter of patients with Sydenham's chorea will go on to develop chronic rheumatic valve disease.

Investigations

These are listed in Box 18.103. The ESR and CRP are non-specific markers of systemic inflammation, and are useful for monitoring progress of the disease. Positive throat swab cultures are obtained in only 10–25% of cases of ARF. ASO titres are normal in about one-fifth of adult cases of rheumatic fever and most cases of chorea. Echocardiography typically shows mitral regurgitation with dilatation of the mitral annulus and prolapse of the anterior mitral leaflet; other common findings are aortic regurgitation and pericardial effusion.

18.103 INVESTIGATIONS IN ACUTE RHEUMATIC FEVER

Evidence of a systemic illness (non-specific)

- Leucocytosis, raised ESR, raised CRP

Evidence of preceding streptococcal infection (specific)

- Throat swab culture: group A β-haemolytic streptococci (also from family members and contacts)
- Antistreptolysin 0 antibodies (ASO titres): rising titres, or levels of > 200 U (adults) or > 300 U (children)

Evidence of carditis

- Chest X-ray: cardiomegaly; pulmonary congestion
- ECG: first- and rarely second-degree heart block; features of pericarditis; T-wave inversion; reduction in QRS voltages
- Echocardiography: cardiac dilatation and valve abnormalities

18

Treatment of the acute attack

A single dose of benzyl penicillin 1.2 million U i.m. or oral phenoxymethylpenicillin 250 mg 6-hourly for 10 days should be given on diagnosis to eliminate any residual streptococcal infection. If the patient is penicillin-allergic, erythromycin or a cephalosporin can be used. Treatment is then directed towards limiting cardiac damage and relieving symptoms.

Bed rest and supportive therapy

Bed rest is important as it lessens joint pain and reduces cardiac workload. The duration of bed rest should be guided by symptoms and markers of inflammation (e.g. temperature, leucocyte count and ESR) and should be continued until these have settled. Patients can then return to normal physical activity, but strenuous exercise should be avoided in those who have had carditis.

Cardiac failure should be treated as necessary. Some patients, particularly those in early adolescence, develop a fulminant form of the disease with severe mitral regurgitation and sometimes concomitant aortic regurgitation. If heart failure does not respond to medical treatment in these cases, valve replacement may be necessary and is often associated with a dramatic decline in rheumatic activity. Atrioventricular block is seldom progressive and pacemaker insertion is rarely needed.

Aspirin

This will usually relieve the symptoms of arthritis rapidly and a prompt response (within 24 hours) helps to confirm the diagnosis. A reasonable starting dose is 60 mg/kg body weight per day, divided into six doses. In adults, 100 mg/kg per day may be needed up to the limits of tolerance or a maximum of 8 g per day. Mild toxic effects include nausea, tinnitus and deafness; more serious ones are vomiting, tachypnoea and acidosis. Aspirin should be continued until the ESR has fallen and then gradually tailed off.

Corticosteroids

These produce more rapid symptomatic relief than aspirin, and are indicated in cases with carditis or severe arthritis. There is no evidence that long-term steroids are beneficial. Prednisolone, 1.0–2.0 mg/kg per day in divided doses, should be continued until the ESR is normal then tailed off.

Secondary prevention

Patients are susceptible to additional attacks of rheumatic fever if further streptococcal infection occurs, and long-term prophylaxis with penicillin should be given as benzyl penicillin 1.2 million U i.m. monthly (if compliance is in doubt) or oral phenoxymethylpenicillin 250 mg 12-hourly. Sulfadiazine or erythromycin may be used if the patient is allergic to penicillin (sulphonamides prevent infection but are not effective in the eradication of group A streptococci). Further attacks of rheumatic fever are unusual after the age of 21, at which age treatment may be stopped. However, treatment should be extended if an attack has occurred in the last 5 years, or the patient lives in an area of high prevalence or has an occupation (e.g. teaching) with high exposure to streptococcal infection. In those with residual heart disease, prophylaxis should continue until 10 years after the last episode or 40 years of age, whichever is longer. Long-term antibiotic prophylaxis prevents another attack of ARF but does not protect against infective endocarditis.

CHRONIC RHEUMATIC HEART DISEASE

Chronic valvular heart disease develops in at least half of those affected by rheumatic fever with carditis. Two-thirds of cases occur in women. Some episodes of rheumatic fever may pass unrecognised and it is only possible to elicit a history of rheumatic fever or chorea in about half of all patients with chronic rheumatic heart disease.

The mitral valve is affected in more than 90% of cases; the aortic valve is the next most frequently affected, followed by the tricuspid and then the pulmonary valve. Isolated mitral stenosis accounts for about 25% of all cases of rheumatic heart disease, and an additional 40% have mixed mitral stenosis and regurgitation.

Valve disease may be symptomatic during fulminant forms of ARF, but may remain asymptomatic for many years.

Pathology

In contrast to the destructive lytic process of ARF, the main pathological process in chronic rheumatic heart disease is progressive fibrosis. The heart valves are predominantly affected but involvement of the pericardium and myocardium may contribute to heart failure and conduction disorders. Fusion of the mitral valve commissures and shortening of the chordae tendineae may lead to mitral stenosis with or without regurgitation. Similar changes in the aortic and tricuspid valves produce distortion and rigidity of the cusps, leading to stenosis and/or regurgitation. Once a valve has been damaged, the altered haemodynamic stresses perpetuate and extend the damage, even in the absence of a continuing rheumatic process.

MITRAL VALVE DISEASE

MITRAL STENOSIS

Aetiology and pathophysiology

Mitral stenosis is almost always rheumatic in origin, although in the elderly it can be caused by heavy calcification of the mitral valve apparatus. There is also a rare form of congenital mitral stenosis.

In rheumatic mitral stenosis, the mitral valve orifice is slowly diminished by progressive fibrosis, calcification of the valve leaflets, and fusion of the cusps and subvalvular apparatus. The flow of blood from left atrium to left ventricle is restricted and left atrial pressure rises, leading to pulmonary venous congestion and breathlessness. There is dilatation and hypertrophy of the left atrium, and left ventricular filling becomes more dependent on left atrial contraction.

Any increase in heart rate shortens diastole when the mitral valve is open, and produces a further rise in left atrial pressure; situations that demand an increase in cardiac output will also increase left atrial pressure. Exercise and pregnancy are therefore poorly tolerated.

The mitral valve orifice is normally about 5 cm² in diastole and may be reduced to 1 cm² or less in severe mitral stenosis. Patients usually remain asymptomatic until the stenosis is approximately 2 cm² or less. At first, symptoms occur only on exercise; however, in severe stenosis, left atrial pressure is permanently elevated and symptoms may occur at rest. Reduced lung compliance, due to chronic pulmonary venous congestion, contributes to breathlessness and a low cardiac output may cause fatigue.

Atrial fibrillation due to progressive dilatation of the left atrium is very common. The onset of atrial fibrillation often precipitates pulmonary oedema because the accompanying tachycardia and loss of atrial contraction frequently lead to marked haemodynamic deterioration with a rapid rise in left atrial pressure. In contrast, a more gradual rise in left atrial pressure tends to cause an increase in pulmonary vascular resistance, which leads to pulmonary artery hypertension that may protect the patient from pulmonary oedema. Pulmonary hypertension may lead to right ventricular hypertrophy and dilatation, tricuspid regurgitation and right heart failure.

Less than 20% of patients remain in sinus rhythm; many of these have a small fibrotic left atrium and severe pulmonary hypertension.

All patients with mitral stenosis, and particularly those with atrial fibrillation, are at risk from left atrial thrombosis and systemic thromboembolism. Prior to the advent of anticoagulant therapy, emboli caused one-quarter of all deaths in this condition.

Clinical features
These are shown in Box 18.104.

Symptoms
Effort-related dyspnoea is usually the dominant symptom. Exercise tolerance typically diminishes very slowly over many years and patients often do not appreciate the extent of their disability. Eventually symptoms occur at rest. Acute pulmonary oedema or pulmonary hypertension can lead to haemoptysis. Systemic embolism may be a presenting feature.

Signs
The forces that open and close the mitral valve increase as left atrial pressure rises. The first heart sound (S1) is therefore often unusually loud and may even be palpable (tapping apex beat). An opening snap may be audible and moves closer to the second sound (S2) as the stenosis becomes more severe and left atrial pressure rises. However, the first heart sound and opening snap may be inaudible if the valve is heavily calcified.

Turbulent flow produces the characteristic low-pitched mid-diastolic murmur and sometimes a thrill (Fig. 18.89). The murmur is accentuated by exercise and during atrial systole (pre-systolic accentuation). Early in the disease, a pre-systolic murmur may be the only auscultatory abnormality, but in patients with symptoms, the murmur usually extends from the opening snap to the first heart sound. Coexisting mitral regurgitation causes a pansystolic murmur which radiates towards the axilla.

If pulmonary hypertension supervenes there may be a right ventricular heave at the left sternal edge (due to right ventricular hypertrophy) and accentuation of the pulmonary component of the second heart sound. Tricuspid regurgitation secondary to right ventricular dilatation causes a systolic murmur and systolic waves in the venous pulse.

The physical signs of mitral stenosis are often found before symptoms develop, and their recognition is of particular importance in pregnancy.

Investigations
The ECG (Box 18.105) may show either the bifid P waves (P mitrale) associated with left atrial hypertrophy, or atrial

18

18.104 CLINICAL FEATURES OF MITRAL STENOSIS

Symptoms

- Breathlessness (pulmonary congestion)
- Fatigue (low cardiac output)
- Oedema, ascites (right heart failure)
- Palpitation (atrial fibrillation)
- Haemoptysis (pulmonary congestion, pulmonary embolism)
- Cough (pulmonary congestion)
- Chest pain (pulmonary hypertension)
- Symptoms of thromboembolic complications (e.g. stroke, ischaemic limb)

Signs

- Atrial fibrillation
- Mitral facies
- Auscultation
  Loud first heart sound, opening snap
  Mid-diastolic murmur
- Signs of raised pulmonary capillary pressure
  Crepitations, pulmonary oedema, effusions
- Signs of pulmonary hypertension
  RV heave, loud P₂

18.105 INVESTIGATIONS IN MITRAL STENOSIS

ECG

- Left atrial hypertrophy (if not in AF)
- Right ventricular hypertrophy

Chest X-ray

- Enlarged left atrium
- Signs of pulmonary venous congestion

Echo

- Thickened immobile cusps
- Reduced valve area
- Reduced rate of diastolic filling of LV

Doppler

- Pressure gradient across mitral valve
- Pulmonary artery pressure
- Left ventricular function

Cardiac catheterisation

- Assessment of coexisting coronary artery disease and mitral regurgitation

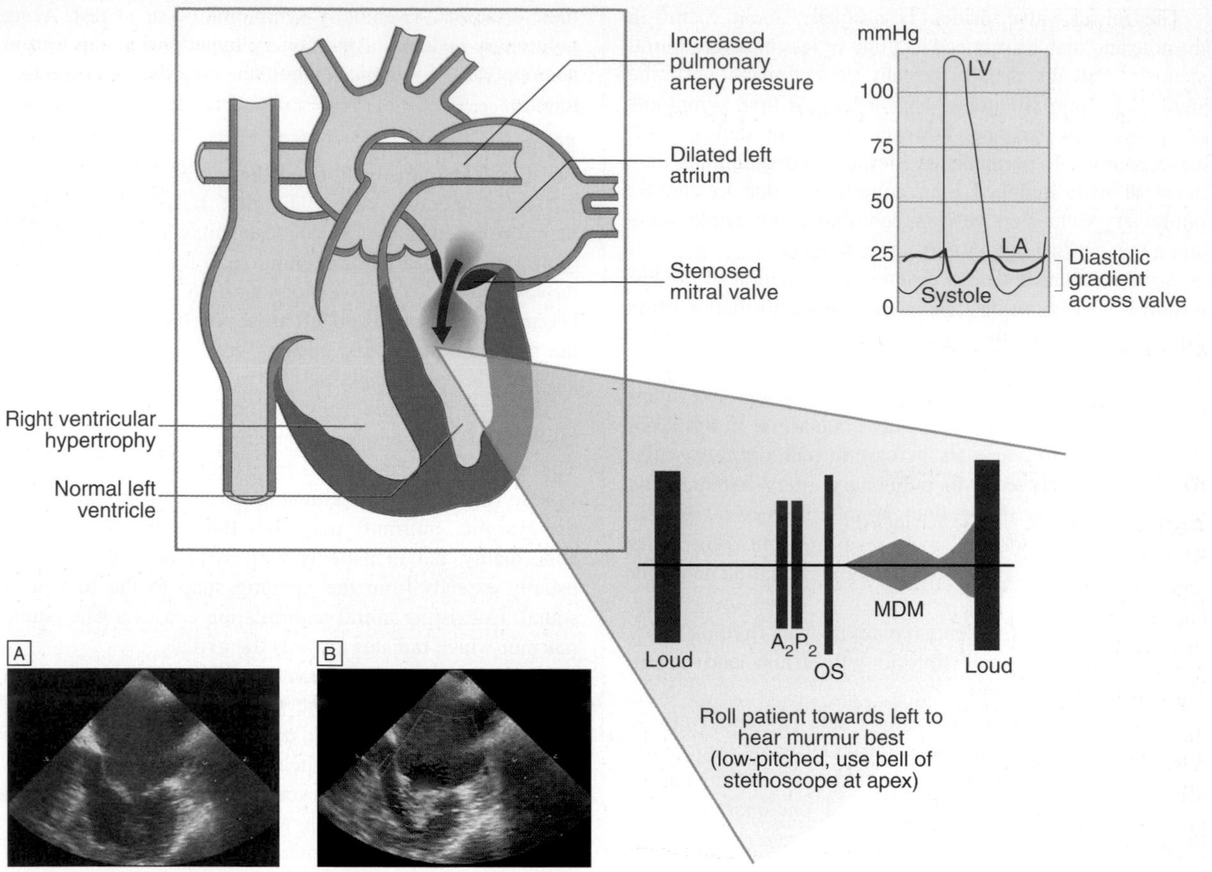

18

Increased
pulmonary
artery pressure

Dilated left
atrium

Stenosed
mitral valve

Right ventricular
hypertrophy

Normal left
ventricle

mmHg

100
LV
75
50
25
LA
Diastolic
gradient
across valve
0
Systole

Loud
A₂P₂
OS
MDM
Loud

Roll patient towards left to
hear murmur best
(low-pitched, use bell of
stethoscope at apex)

A

B

Fig. 18.89 Mitral stenosis: murmur and illustration of the diastolic pressure gradient between left atrium and left ventricle. (Mean gradient is reflected by the area between LA and LV in diastole.) The first heart sound is loud, there is an opening snap (OS) and mid-diastolic murmur (MDM) with pre-systolic accentuation. A Echocardiogram showing reduced opening of the mitral valve in diastole. B Colour Doppler showing turbulent flow.

fibrillation. There may also be evidence of right ventricular hypertrophy (pulmonary hypertension). The chest X-ray (Fig. 18.9, p. 530) may show enlargement of the left atrium and its appendage, enlargement of the main pulmonary artery and enlargement of the upper pulmonary veins and horizontal linear shadows in the costophrenic angles.

Doppler echocardiography provides the definitive evaluation of mitral stenosis (Box 18.105 and Fig. 18.89). Cardiac catheterisation has a role in assessing coexisting mitral regurgitation and coronary artery disease.

Management

Patients with minor symptoms should be treated medically, but the definitive treatment of mitral stenosis is by balloon valvuloplasty, mitral valvotomy or mitral valve replacement. Intervention should be considered if the patient remains symptomatic despite medical treatment or if pulmonary hypertension develops.

Medical management

This consists of anticoagulants to reduce the risk of systemic embolism, a combination of digoxin, β-blockers or rate-limiting calcium antagonists to control the ventricular rate in atrial fibrillation (or to prevent a rapid ventricular rate if atrial fibrillation should develop), diuretics to control

pulmonary congestion, and antibiotic prophylaxis against infective endocarditis (Box 18.125, p. 633).

Mitral balloon valvuloplasty

This is the treatment of choice if the appropriate criteria are fulfilled (Box 18.106 and Fig. 18.14, p. 533). Closed or open mitral valvotomy may be used if the facilities or expertise for valvuloplasty are not available. Patients who have undergone mitral valvuloplasty or valvotomy should receive antibiotic prophylaxis against infective endocarditis and should be followed up at 1–2-yearly intervals because restenosis may occur. Clinical symptoms and signs are a guide to the severity of mitral restenosis, but Doppler echocardiography provides a more accurate assessment.

18.106 CRITERIA FOR MITRAL VALVULOPLASTY

- Significant symptoms
- Isolated mitral stenosis
- No (or trivial) mitral regurgitation
- Mobile, non-calcified valve/subvalve apparatus on echo
- Left atrium free of thrombus

For further information see www.acc.org, which has comprehensive guidelines on valvular heart disease.

18.107 CAUSES OF MITRAL REGURGITATION

- Mitral valve prolapse
- Dilatation of the left ventricle and mitral valve ring (e.g. coronary artery disease, cardiomyopathy)
- Damage to valve cusps and chordae (e.g. rheumatic heart disease, endocarditis)
- Damage to papillary muscle
- Myocardial infarction

Mitral valve replacement

Valve replacement is indicated if there is substantial mitral reflux, or if the valve is rigid and calcified (p. 633).

MITRAL REGURGITATION

Aetiology and pathophysiology

Rheumatic disease is the principal cause of mitral regurgitation in countries where rheumatic fever is common, but elsewhere, including in the UK, other causes are more important (Box 18.107). Mitral regurgitation may also follow mitral valvotomy or valvuloplasty.

Chronic mitral regurgitation causes gradual dilatation of the left atrium with little increase in pressure and therefore relatively few symptoms. Nevertheless, the left ventricle dilates slowly and the left ventricular diastolic and left atrial pressures gradually increase as a result of chronic volume overload of the left ventricle; breathlessness and pulmonary oedema eventually supervene. In contrast, acute mitral regurgitation tends to cause a rapid rise in left atrial pressure (because left atrial compliance is normal) and marked symptomatic deterioration.

Mitral valve prolapse

This is also known as 'floppy' mitral valve and is one of the more common causes of mild mitral regurgitation. It is caused by congenital anomalies or degenerative myxomatous changes and is sometimes a feature of connective tissue disorders such as Marfan's syndrome (p. 605).

In the mildest forms of mitral prolapse, the valve remains competent but bulges back into the atrium during systole, causing a mid-systolic click but no murmur. Occasionally, multiple clicks are audible. In the presence of a regurgitant valve, the click is followed by a late systolic murmur which lengthens as the regurgitation becomes more severe. A click is not always audible and the physical signs may vary with both posture and respiration.

Progressive elongation of the chordae tendineae may lead to increasing mitral regurgitation, and if chordal rupture occurs, regurgitation may suddenly become severe. These complications are rare before the fifth or sixth decade of life.

Haemodynamically significant mitral valve prolapse can predispose to infective endocarditis and requires antibiotic prophylaxis. Mitral valve prolapse is also associated with a variety of typically benign arrhythmias, atypical chest pain and a very small risk of embolic stroke or transient ischaemic attack. Nevertheless, the overall long-term prognosis is good. An echocardiogram of mitral valve prolapse is shown in Figure 18.90.

Other causes of mitral regurgitation

Mitral valve function depends on the chordae tendineae and their papillary muscles; dilatation of the left ventricle distorts the geometry of these and may cause mitral regurgitation. Dilated cardiomyopathy and the impaired ventricular function that results from coronary artery disease are common causes of so-called 'functional' mitral regurgitation. Ischaemia or infarction of the papillary muscles may also cause mitral regurgitation. Endocarditis may lead to distortion or perforation of the valve leaflets and is an important cause of acute mitral regurgitation.

Clinical features

These are summarised in Box 18.108.

The symptoms depend on how suddenly the regurgitation develops. Chronic mitral regurgitation produces a symptom complex that is similar to that of mitral stenosis, but sudden-onset mitral regurgitation usually presents with acute pulmonary oedema.

The regurgitant jet causes an apical systolic murmur (Fig. 18.90) which often radiates into the axilla, and may be accompanied by a thrill. The first heart sound is quiet because valve closure is abnormal. Increased forward flow through the mitral valve may give rise to a loud third heart sound and even a short mid-diastolic murmur. The apex beat feels active and rocking due to left ventricular volume overload and is usually displaced to the left as a result of dilatation of the left ventricle.

18.108 CLINICAL FEATURES OF MITRAL REGURGITATION

Symptoms

- Dyspnoea (pulmonary venous congestion)
- Fatigue (low cardiac output)
- Palpitation (AF, increased stroke volume)
- Oedema, ascites (right heart failure)

Signs

- Atrial fibrillation/flutter
- Cardiomegaly—displaced hyperdynamic apex beat
- Apical pansystolic murmur ± thrill
- Soft S1, apical S3
- Signs of pulmonary venous congestion (crepitations, pulmonary oedema, effusions)
- Signs of pulmonary hypertension and right heart failure

Investigations

These are shown in Box 18.109 and include chest X-ray, ECG and Doppler echocardiography. Atrial fibrillation is common, as a consequence of atrial dilatation. At cardiac catheterisation the severity of mitral regurgitation may be indicated by the size of the v (systolic) waves in the left atrial or PAW pressure trace, or by left ventriculography; however, this is not always reliable, as left atrial compliance may vary. In practice, a common problem lies in deciding on the extent to which cardiac failure is due to mitral regurgitation as opposed to impaired left ventricular function.

18

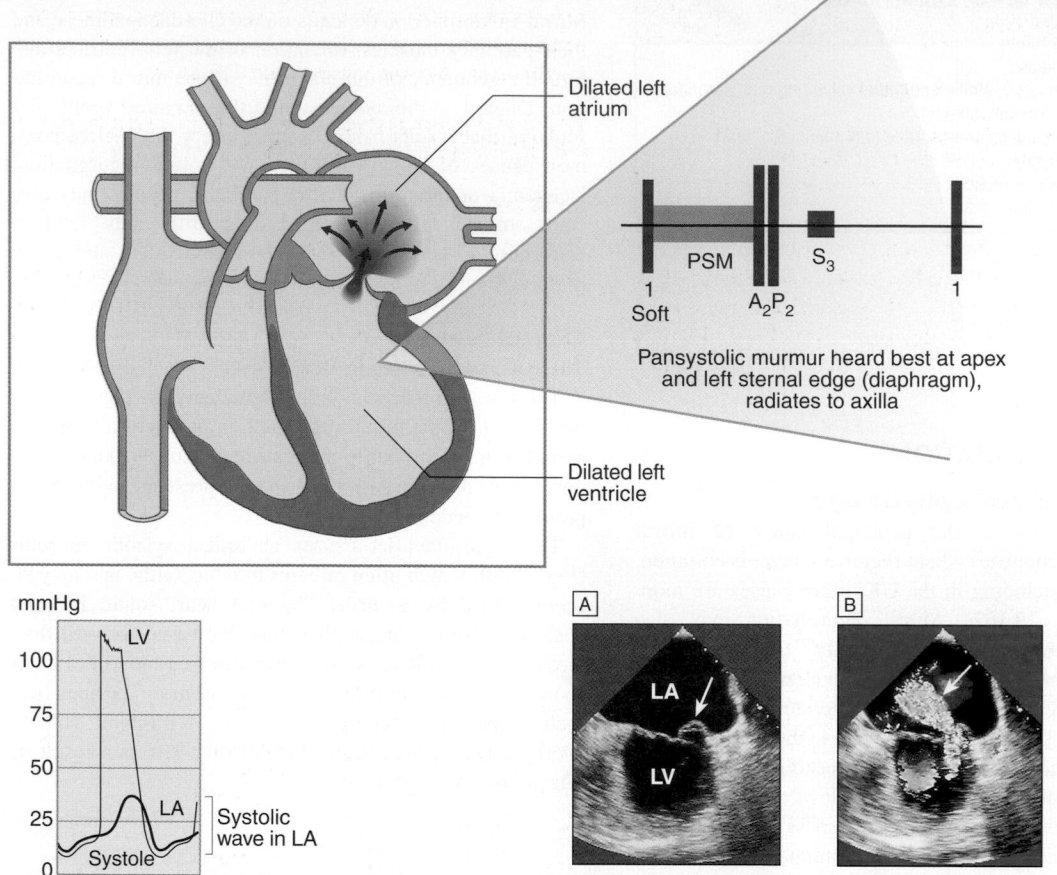

Fig. 18.90 Mitral regurgitation: radiation of the murmur to the axilla and illustration of systolic wave in left atrial pressure. The first sound is normal or soft and merges with a pansystolic murmur (PSM) extending to the second heart sound. A third heart sound occurs with severe regurgitation. The left atrium and ventricle become dilated. **A** A transoesophageal echocardiogram shows an example of mitral valve prolapse, with one leaflet bulging towards the left atrium (LA; arrow). **B** This results in a jet of mitral regurgitation on colour Doppler (arrow).

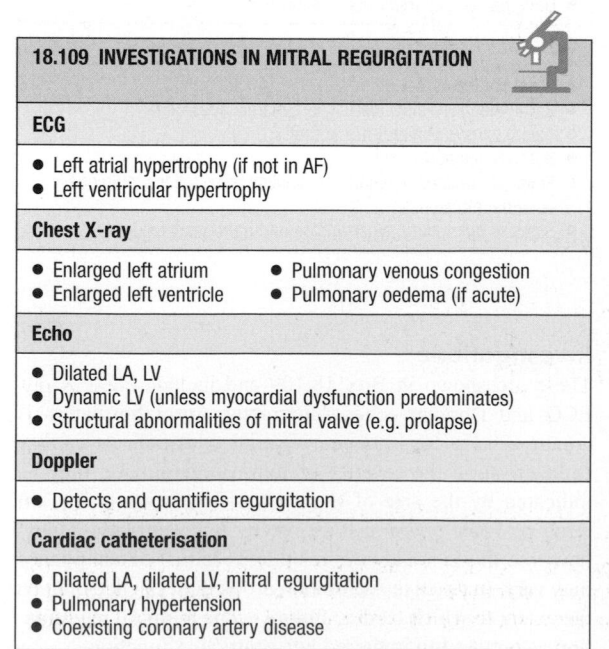

18.109 INVESTIGATIONS IN MITRAL REGURGITATION	
ECG	
● Left atrial hypertrophy (if not in AF) ● Left ventricular hypertrophy	
Chest X-ray	
● Enlarged left atrium ● Enlarged left ventricle	● Pulmonary venous congestion ● Pulmonary oedema (if acute)
Echo	
● Dilated LA, LV ● Dynamic LV (unless myocardial dysfunction predominates) ● Structural abnormalities of mitral valve (e.g. prolapse)	
Doppler	
● Detects and quantifies regurgitation	
Cardiac catheterisation	
● Dilated LA, dilated LV, mitral regurgitation ● Pulmonary hypertension ● Coexisting coronary artery disease	

Management

Mitral regurgitation of moderate severity can be treated medically (Box 18.110). In all patients with mitral regurgitation, high afterload may worsen the degree of regurgitation and hypertension should be treated with vasodilating drugs such as ACE inhibitors. Patients should be reviewed at regular intervals because worsening symptoms, progressive radiological cardiac enlargement or echocardiographic evidence of deteriorating left ventricular function are indications for surgical intervention (mitral valve replacement or repair). Mitral valve repair can be used to treat most forms of mitral valve prolapse and offers many advantages when compared to mitral valve replacement. Indeed, it is now advocated for severe regurgitation even in asymptomatic patients because results are excellent and early repair has been shown to prevent irreversible left ventricular damage. Commonly, mitral regurgitation accompanies the ventricular dilatation and dysfunction that accompany coronary artery disease. If such patients are to undergo coronary bypass graft surgery it is common practice to repair the valve and restore mitral valve function by

18.110 MEDICAL MANAGEMENT OF MITRAL REGURGITATION

- Diuretics
- Vasodilators, e.g. ACE inhibitors (p. 549)
- Digoxin if atrial fibrillation is present
- Anticoagulants if atrial fibrillation is present
- Antibiotic prophylaxis against infective endocarditis

inserting an annuloplasty ring to overcome annular dilatation and to bring the valve leaflets closer together. A common dilemma in patients with ventricular dilatation and mitral regurgitation is to determine which of the two abnormalities is the predominant problem. If, for example,

ventricular dilatation is the underlying cause of mitral regurgitation, then mitral valve repair or replacement may actually worsen ventricular function as the ventricle can no longer empty into the low-pressure left atrium.

AORTIC VALVE DISEASE

AORTIC STENOSIS

Aetiology and pathophysiology

The likely aetiology varies with the age of the patient (Box 18.111). In congenital aortic stenosis, some obstruction may be present from birth or become apparent in infancy. With bicuspid aortic valves, significant obstruction may take

18

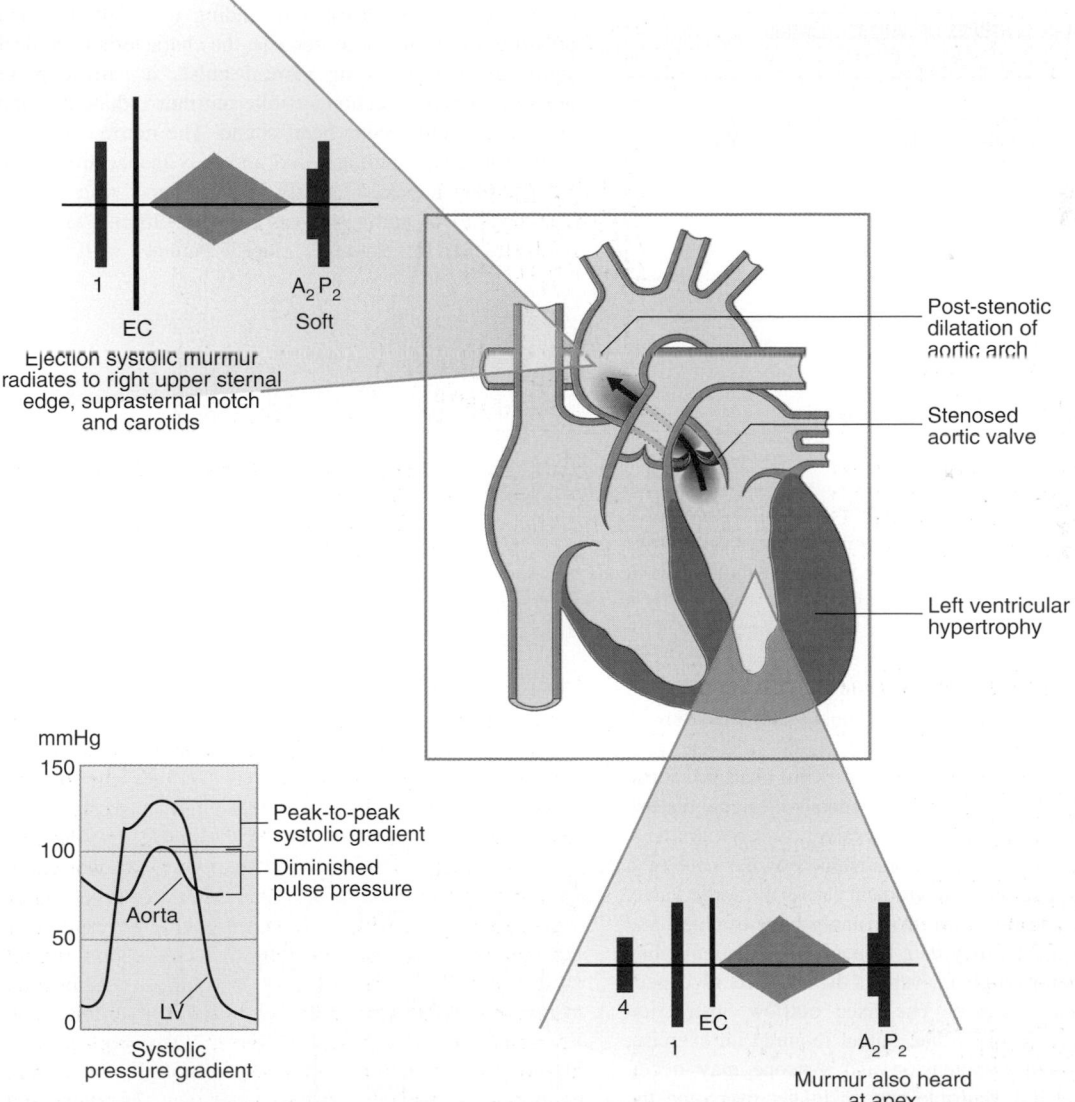

Fig. 18.91 Aortic stenosis. Pressure traces show the systolic gradient between left ventricle and aorta. The carotid pulse is low-volume and slow-rising. The 'diamond shape' murmur may be heard best with the diaphragm in the aortic outflow and also at the apex. The aortic component of the second heart sound (A_2) is quiet or inaudible so that the second sound is single or soft, especially in patients with calcific valves. An ejection click (EC) may be present in young patients with bicuspid aortic valve but not in older patients with calcified valves. Aortic stenosis may lead to left ventricular hypertrophy with a fourth sound at the apex and post-stenotic dilatation of the aortic arch. The typical Doppler signal with aortic stenosis is illustrated in Figure 18.11, page 531.

18

Infants, children, adolescents

- Congenital aortic stenosis
- Congenital subvalvular aortic stenosis
- Congenital supravalvular aortic stenosis

Young adults to middle-aged

- Calcification and fibrosis of congenitally bicuspid aortic valve
- Rheumatic aortic stenosis

Middle-aged to elderly

- Senile degenerative aortic stenosis
- Calcification of bicuspid valve
- Rheumatic aortic stenosis

18.112 CLINICAL FEATURES OF AORTIC STENOSIS

Symptoms

- Mild or moderate aortic stenosis is usually asymptomatic
- Exertional dyspnoea
- Angina
- Exertional syncope
- Sudden death
- Episodes of acute pulmonary oedema

Signs

- Ejection systolic murmur
- Slow-rising carotid pulse
- Narrow pulse pressure
- Thrusting apex beat (LV pressure overload)
- Signs of pulmonary venous congestion (e.g. crepitations)

---

years to develop as the valve becomes fibrotic and calcified as the patient ages. The aortic valve is the second most frequently affected by rheumatic fever, and commonly both the aortic and mitral valves are affected. In the elderly, a structurally normal tricuspid aortic valve may be affected by fibrosis and calcification in a process that histologically is similar to that of atherosclerosis affecting the arterial wall. Haemodynamically significant stenosis develops slowly, typically occurring at the ages of 30–60 in those with rheumatic disease, 50–60 in those with bicuspid aortic valves and 70–90 in those with degenerative calcific disease affecting a normal tricuspid aortic valve.

Cardiac output is initially maintained at the cost of a steadily increasing pressure gradient across the aortic valve. The left ventricle becomes increasingly hypertrophied and coronary blood flow may then be inadequate; patients may therefore develop angina, even in the absence of conco-mitant coronary disease. The fixed outflow obstruction limits the increase in cardiac output required on exercise, and effort-related hypotension and syncope may occur. Eventually the left ventricle can no longer overcome the outflow tract obstruction and pulmonary oedema super-venes. In contrast to mitral stenosis, which tends to progress very slowly, patients with aortic stenosis typically remain asymptomatic for many years but deteriorate rapidly when symptoms develop; thus death usually ensues within 3–5 years of the onset of symptoms.

Clinical features

Symptoms and signs are summarised in Box 18.112 and the characteristic murmur is illustrated in Figure 18.91.

Aortic stenosis is commonly picked up in asymptomatic patients at routine clinical examination, but the three cardinal symptoms are angina, breathlessness and syncope. Angina arises because of the increased demands of the hypertrophied left ventricle working against the high-pressure outflow tract obstruction leading to a mismatch between oxygen demand and supply. Angina may also be due to coexisting coronary artery disease, especially in the elderly where it affects more than 50% of patients. Exertional breathlessness suggests cardiac decompensation as a consequence of the excessive pressure overload placed on the left ventricle. Syncope usually occurs on exertion when cardiac output fails to rise to meet demand because of severe outflow obstruction leading to a fall in blood pressure. In severe aortic stenosis, the characteristic clinical signs are a slow rising carotid pulse, a narrow pulse pressure, a harsh ejection systolic murmur radiating to the neck, and a soft second heart sound. The murmur is often likened to a saw cutting wood and may (especially in the elderly) have a musical quality, like the 'mew' of a seagull. The severity of aortic stenosis may be difficult to gauge clinically as, for example, elderly patients with a non-

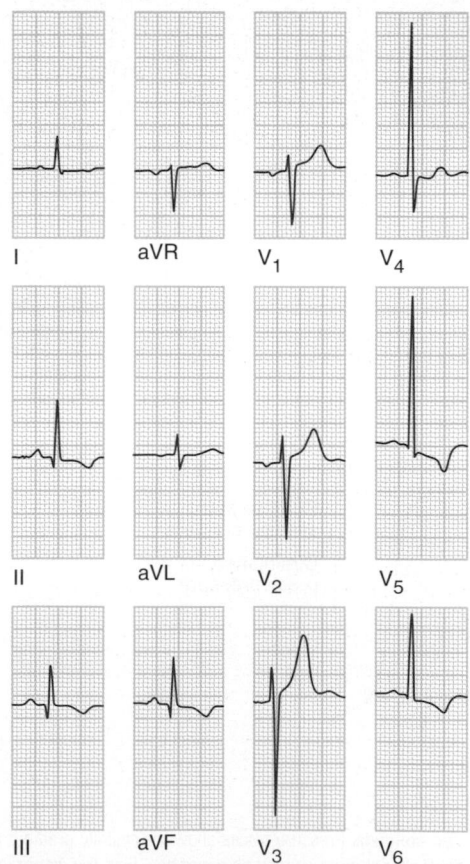

Fig. 18.92 Left ventricular hypertrophy: QRS complexes in limb leads have increased amplitude with a very large R wave in V_5 and S wave in V_2. There is ST depression and T-wave inversion in leads II, III, AVF, V_5 and V_6: a 'left ventricular strain' pattern.

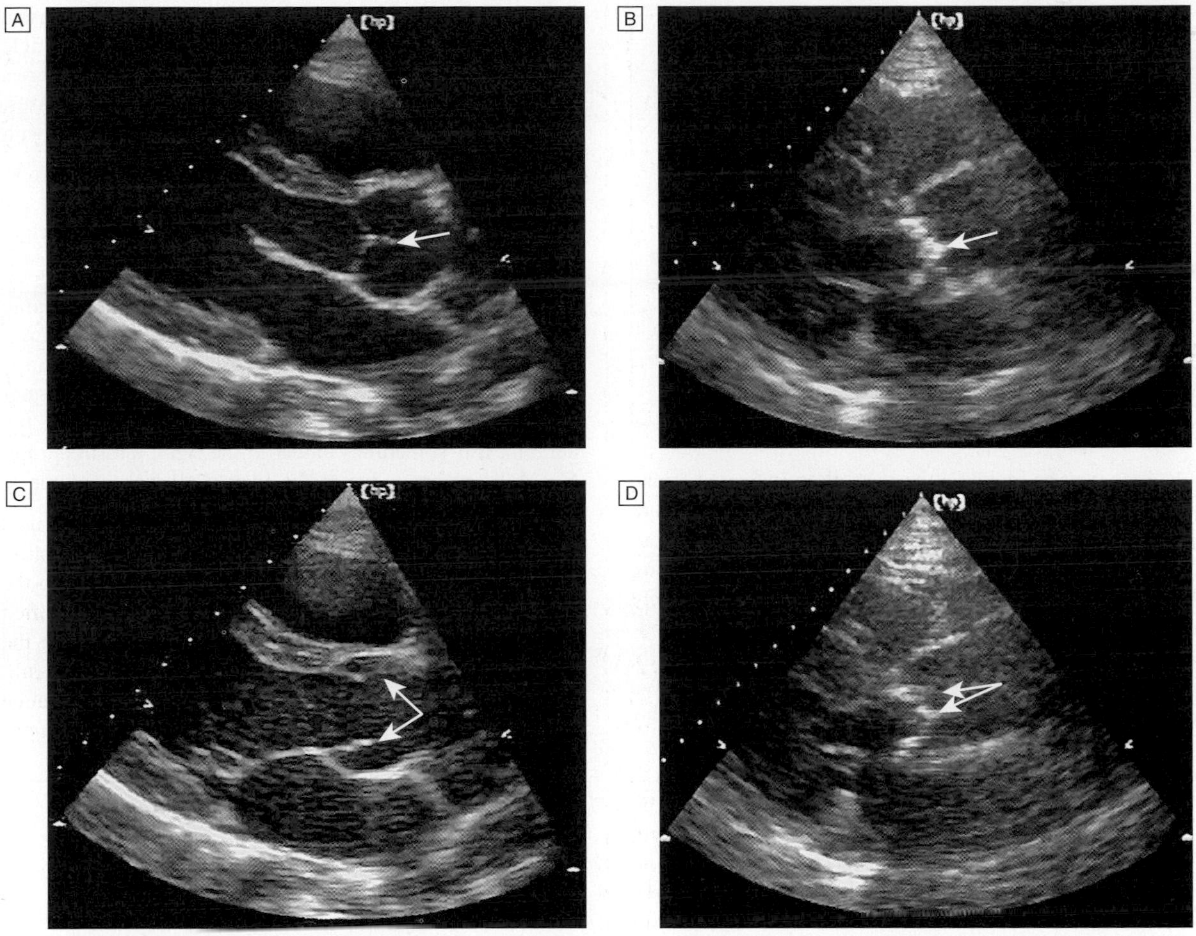

Fig. 18.93 Two-dimensional echocardiogram comparing a normal subject with a patient with calcific aortic stenosis. A Normal subject in diastole; the aortic leaflets are closed and thin, and a point of coaptation is seen (arrow). B Calcific aortic stenosis in diastole; the aortic leaflets are thick and calcified (arrow). C Normal in systole; the aortic leaflets are open (arrows). D Calcific aortic stenosis in systole; the thickened leaflets have barely moved (arrows).

18.113 INVESTIGATIONS IN AORTIC STENOSIS
ECG
• Left ventricular hypertrophy (usually)   • Left bundle branch block
Chest X-ray
• May be normal. Sometimes enlarged left ventricle and dilated ascending aorta on PA view, calcified valve on lateral view
Echo
• Calcified valve with restricted opening, hypertrophied LV (Fig. 18.93)
Doppler
• Measurement of severity of stenosis   • Detection of associated aortic regurgitation
Cardiac catheterisation
• Mainly to identify associated coronary artery disease   • May be used to measure gradient between LV and aorta

compliant 'stiff' arterial system may have an apparently normal carotid upstroke in the presence of severe aortic stenosis. Milder degrees of stenosis may be difficult to distinguish from aortic sclerosis where the valve is thickened or calcified but not obstructed. The patient should be carefully examined for the presence of other valve lesions, particularly in rheumatic valve disease when there is frequently concomitant mitral valve disease.

Investigations

These are shown in Box 18.113. In advanced cases, ECG features of hypertrophy are often gross (Fig. 18.92), and down-sloping ST segments and T inversion ('strain pattern') may be seen in leads reflecting the left ventricle. Nevertheless, especially in the elderly, the ECG can be normal despite severe stenosis. Doppler echocardiography permits calculation of the systolic gradient across the aortic valve, from which the severity of stenosis can be assessed. This may be misleading in patients with an impaired ventricle, as velocities across the aortic valve may be diminished because of a reduced stroke volume. Conversely, in those in whom aortic regurgitation is also present,

18.114 AORTIC STENOSIS IN OLD AGE

- **Incidence:** the most common form of valve disease affecting the very old.
- **Symptoms:** a common cause of syncope, angina and heart failure in the very old.
- **Signs:** because of increasing stiffening in the central arteries, low pulse pressure and a slow rising pulse may not be present.
- **Surgery:** can be successful in those aged 80 or more in the absence of comorbidity, but with a higher operative mortality. The prognosis without surgery is poor once symptoms have developed.
- **Valve replacement type:** a biological valve is often preferable to a mechanical, because this obviates the need for anticoagulation, and the durability of biological valves usually exceeds the patient's anticipated life expectancy.

velocities may be increased because of an increased stroke volume. In these circumstances, aortic valve area is a more accurate assessment of severity and may be calculated from Doppler measurements. CT and MRI are useful in assessing the degree of valve calcification and stenosis, but are only helpful in the minority of patients in whom Doppler echocardiography is difficult. Cardiac catheterisation is usually necessary to assess the coronary arteries before aortic valve replacement.

Management

All patients with asymptomatic aortic stenosis should be kept under review, as the development of angina, syncope, symptoms of low cardiac output or heart failure is an indication for prompt surgery. Those with moderately severe or severe stenosis should be evaluated every 1–2 years with Doppler echocardiography to detect progression in severity; this tends to be more rapid in older patients with heavily calcified valves. Studies of asymptomatic aortic stenosis in older people have revealed a relatively benign prognosis without surgery, and for these patients conservative management is appropriate. Patients with symptomatic severe aortic stenosis should have aortic valve replacement. Old age as such is not a contraindication to valve replacement, and results are very good in experienced centres, even for those in their 80s. To wait too long exposes the patient to the risk of sudden death or irreversible deterioration in ventricular function. Some patients with severe aortic stenosis deny symptoms, and if this could be due to a sedentary lifestyle, a careful exercise test may reveal symptoms on modest exertion. Aortic balloon valvuloplasty is useful in congenital aortic stenosis but is of no long-term value in elderly patients with calcific aortic stenosis.

Anticoagulants are only required in patients who have atrial fibrillation, such as those with coexisting mitral valve disease, or those who have had a valve replacement with a mechanical prosthesis.

AORTIC REGURGITATION

Aetiology and pathophysiology

This condition may be due to disease of the aortic valve cusps or dilatation of the aortic root (Box 18.115).

The left ventricle dilates and hypertrophies to compensate for the regurgitation; the stroke output of the left ventricle may eventually be doubled or trebled and the major arteries are then conspicuously pulsatile. As the disease progresses, left ventricular diastolic pressure rises, at first only with exercise, and breathlessness develops.

Clinical features

Until the onset of breathlessness, the only symptom may be an awareness of the heart beat, particularly when lying on the left side; this results from the increased stroke volume (Box 18.116). Paroxysmal nocturnal dyspnoea is sometimes the first symptom and peripheral oedema, or angina, may occur. The characteristic murmur is illustrated in Figure 18.94. Although it is usually best heard to the left of the sternum, it is sometimes louder to the right; a thrill is rare. A systolic murmur due to the increased stroke volume is

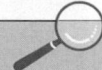

18.115 CAUSES OF AORTIC REGURGITATION

Congenital

- Bicuspid valve or disproportionate cusps

Acquired

- Rheumatic disease
- Infective endocarditis
- Trauma
- Aortic dilatation (Marfan's syndrome, aneurysm, dissection, syphilis, ankylosing spondylitis)

18.116 CLINICAL FEATURES OF AORTIC REGURGITATION (AR)

Symptoms

Mild to moderate AR
- Often asymptomatic
- Awareness of heart beat, 'palpitations'

Severe AR
- Breathlessness
- Angina

Signs

Pulses
- Large-volume or 'collapsing' pulse
- Low diastolic and increased pulse pressure
- Bounding peripheral pulses
- Capillary pulsation in nail beds—Quincke's sign
- Femoral bruit ('pistol shot')—Duroziez's sign
- Head nodding with pulse—de Musset's sign

Murmurs
- Early diastolic murmur
- Systolic murmur (increased stroke volume)
- Austin Flint murmur (soft mid-diastolic)

Other signs
- Displaced, heaving apex beat (volume overload)
- Pre-systolic impulse
- Fourth heart sound
- Pulmonary venous congestion (crepitations)

18

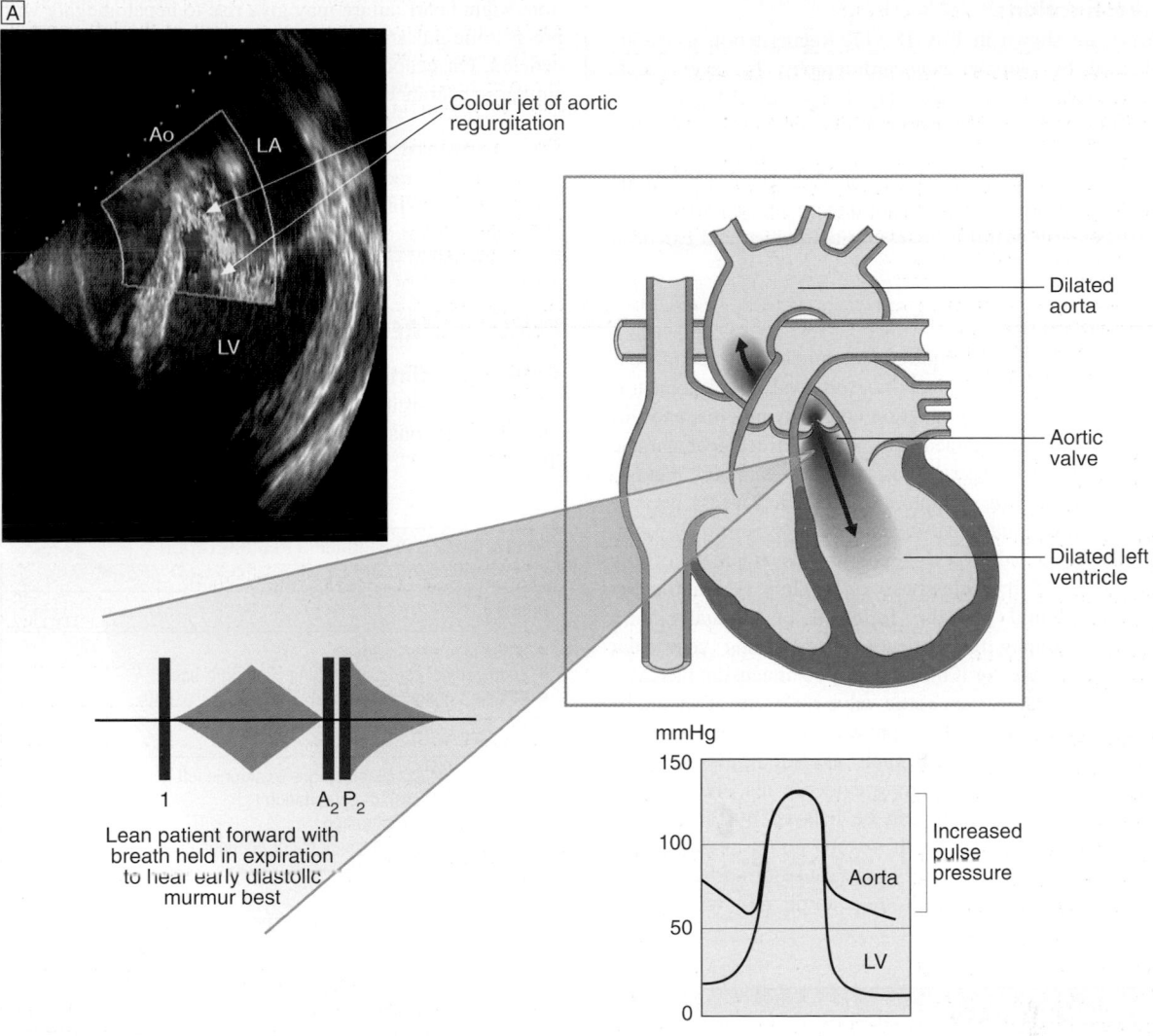

Colour jet of aortic regurgitation

Dilated aorta

Aortic valve

Dilated left ventricle

1   A₂ P₂

Lean patient forward with breath held in expiration to hear early diastolic murmur best

mmHg
150

100

50

0

Aorta

LV

Increased pulse pressure

Fig. 18.94 Aortic regurgitation. The early diastolic murmur is best heard at the left sternal edge and may be accompanied by an ejection systolic murmur due to the enlarged stroke volume ('to and fro' murmur). Aortic regurgitation may lead to dilatation of the aortic arch and left ventricle. [A] An echocardiogram with the regurgitant jet on colour Doppler (arrows). (LV = left ventricle; LA = left atrium; Ao = aorta)

18.117 INVESTIGATIONS IN AORTIC REGURGITATION

ECG

- Initially normal, later LV hypertrophy and T-wave inversion

Chest X-ray

- Cardiac dilatation, maybe aortic dilatation
- Features of left heart failure

Echo

- Dilated left ventricle
- Hyperdynamic left ventricle
- Fluttering anterior mitral leaflet
- Doppler detects reflux

Cardiac catheterisation (may not be required)

- Dilated LV
- Aortic regurgitation
- Dilated aortic root

---

common and does not necessarily indicate stenosis. When the leak is small, the murmur will be heard only if the steps shown in Figure 18.94 are followed; this is of crucial importance in the early detection of infective endocarditis affecting the aortic valve. However, when the leak is large the diagnosis is usually easy. The regurgitant jet causes fluttering and, if severe, partial closure of the anterior mitral leaflet; this may render the mitral valve functionally stenotic leading to a soft mid-diastolic (Austin Flint) murmur.

In acute severe regurgitation (e.g. perforation of aortic cusp in endocarditis) there may be no time for compensatory left ventricular hypertrophy and dilatation to develop and the features of heart failure may predominate. Moreover, in this situation the classical signs of aortic regurgitation may be masked by tachycardia and an abrupt rise in LV end-diastolic pressure; thus, the pulse pressure may be near-normal and the diastolic murmur may be short or even absent.

18

18

Investigations

These are shown in Box 18.117. Regurgitation is readily detected by Doppler echocardiography. In severe acute aortic regurgitation, the rapid rise in LV diastolic pressure may cause premature mitral valve closure. Cardiac catheterisation and aortography can be helpful in assessing the severity of regurgitation, and dilatation of the aorta and the presence of coexisting coronary artery disease. MRI is particularly useful in assessing the degree and extent of aortic dilatation.

Management

Treatment may be required for underlying conditions such as endocarditis or syphilis. Aortic valve replacement is indicated if aortic regurgitation causes symptoms, and this may need to be combined with aortic root replacement and coronary bypass surgery. Those with chronic aortic regurgitation may remain asymptomatic for many years because compensatory ventricular dilatation and hypertrophy occur, but should be advised to report the development of any symptoms of breathlessness or angina. Asymptomatic patients should also be followed up annually with echocardiography for evidence of increasing ventricular size; if this occurs or if the end systolic dimension increases to 55 mm or more, then aortic valve replacement should be undertaken. Systolic blood pressure should be controlled with vasodilating drugs such as nifedipine or ACE inhibitors. There is conflicting evidence that the need for aortic valve replacement can be delayed by their use in asymptomatic patients with severe aortic regurgitation. When aortic root dilatation is the cause of aortic regurgitation (e.g. Marfan's syndrome), aortic root replacement may be necessary.

TRICUSPID VALVE DISEASE

TRICUSPID STENOSIS

Aetiology

Tricuspid stenosis is usually rheumatic in origin, and is therefore seldom seen in developed countries. Clinically evident tricuspid disease occurs in fewer than 5% of patients with rheumatic heart disease and nearly always in association with mitral and aortic valve disease. Isolated rheumatic tricuspid stenosis is very rare. Tricuspid stenosis and regurgitation are also features of the carcinoid syndrome (p. 903).

Clinical features and investigations

Usually the symptoms of the associated mitral and aortic valve disease predominate; however, tricuspid stenosis may cause symptoms of right heart failure including hepatic discomfort and peripheral oedema.

The main clinical feature is a raised jugular venous pressure with a prominent *a* wave, and a slow *y* descent due to the loss of normal rapid RV filling (p. 521). There is also a mid-diastolic murmur usually best heard at the lower left or right sternal edge; this is generally higher-pitched than the murmur of mitral stenosis and is increased by inspira-

tion. Right heart failure may give rise to hepatomegaly with pre-systolic pulsation (large *a* wave), ascites and peripheral oedema. On echocardiography and Doppler, the valve has similar appearances to those of rheumatic mitral stenosis.

Management

In patients who require surgery to other valves, the tricuspid valve is either replaced or valvotomy performed at the time of surgery. Balloon valvuloplasty can be used to treat rare cases of isolated tricuspid stenosis.

TRICUSPID REGURGITATION

Aetiology, clinical features and investigations

Tricuspid regurgitation is common. The most frequent cause is 'functional' as a result of right ventricular dilatation (Box 18.118).

18.118 CAUSES OF TRICUSPID REGURGITATION
Primary
• Rheumatic heart disease • Endocarditis, particularly in injection drug-users • Ebstein's congenital anomaly (Box 18.129, p. 640)
Secondary
• Right ventricular dilatation due to chronic left heart failure ('functional tricuspid regurgitation') • Right ventricular infarction • Pulmonary hypertension (e.g. cor pulmonale)

Symptoms are usually non-specific, and relate to reduced forward flow (tiredness) and venous congestion (oedema, hepatic enlargement). The most prominent sign is a large systolic wave in the jugular venous pulse (a *cv* wave replaces the normal *x* descent). Other features include a pansystolic murmur at the left sternal edge and systolic pulsation of the liver. Echocardiography may reveal dilatation of the right ventricle; if the valve has been affected by rheumatic disease the leaflets will appear thickened, and in endocarditis vegetations may be seen. Ebstein's anomaly (Box 18.129, p. 640) is a congenital abnormality in which the tricuspid valve is displaced towards the right ventricular apex, with consequent enlargement of the right atrium; it is commonly associated with tricuspid regurgitation.

Management

Tricuspid regurgitation due to right ventricular dilatation often improves when the cause of right ventricular overload is corrected, e.g. by diuretic and vasodilator treatment of congestive cardiac failure. Patients with a normal pulmonary artery pressure tolerate isolated tricuspid reflux well, and valves damaged by endocarditis do not always need to be replaced. Patients undergoing mitral valve replacement who have tricuspid regurgitation due to marked dilatation of the tricuspid annulus benefit from repair of the valve with an annuloplasty ring to bring the leaflets closer together. Those with rheumatic damage may require tricuspid valve replacement.

PULMONARY VALVE DISEASE

PULMONARY STENOSIS

Aetiology

This can occur in the carcinoid syndrome but is usually congenital, when it may be isolated or associated with other abnormalities such as Fallot's tetralogy (p. 639).

Clinical features, investigations and management

The principal finding on examination is an ejection systolic murmur, loudest to the left of the upper sternum and radiating towards the left shoulder. There may be a thrill, best felt when the patient leans forward and breathes out. The murmur is often preceded by an ejection sound (click). Delay in right ventricular ejection may cause wide splitting of the second heart sound. Severe pulmonary stenosis is characterised clinically by a loud harsh murmur, an inaudible pulmonary closure sound (P_2), an increased right ventricular heave, prominent *a* waves in the jugular pulse, ECG evidence of right ventricular hypertrophy, and post-stenotic dilatation in the pulmonary artery on the chest X-ray. Doppler echocardiography is the definitive investigation.

Mild to moderate isolated pulmonary stenosis is relatively common, does not usually progress and does not require treatment; it is a low-risk lesion for infective endocarditis.

Severe pulmonary stenosis (resting gradient > 50 mmHg with a normal cardiac output) is treated by percutaneous pulmonary balloon valvuloplasty or, if not available, by surgical valvotomy. Long-term results are very good. Post-operative pulmonary regurgitation is common but benign.

PULMONARY REGURGITATION

Pulmonary regurgitation is rarely an isolated phenomenon and is usually associated with pulmonary artery dilatation due to pulmonary hypertension. It may, for example, complicate mitral stenosis, producing an early diastolic decrescendo murmur at the left sternal edge that is difficult to distinguish from aortic regurgitation (Graham Steell murmur). The pulmonary hypertension may also be secondary to other disease of the left side of the heart, primary pulmonary vascular disease or Eisenmenger's syndrome (p. 635). Trivial pulmonary regurgitation is a frequent Doppler finding in normal individuals that is of no clinical significance.

INFECTIVE ENDOCARDITIS

Infective endocarditis is due to microbial infection of a heart valve (native or prosthetic), the lining of a cardiac chamber or blood vessel, or a congenital anomaly (e.g. septal defect). The causative organism is usually a bacterium, but may be a rickettsia, chlamydia or fungus.

Pathophysiology

Infective endocarditis typically occurs at sites of pre-existing endocardial damage. However, infection with particularly virulent or aggressive organisms (e.g. *Staphylococcus aureus*) can cause endocarditis in a previously normal heart; for example, staphylococcal endocarditis of the tricuspid valve is a common complication of intravenous drug misuse. Many acquired and congenital cardiac lesions are vulnerable to endocarditis, particularly areas of endocardial damage caused by a high-pressure jet of blood, such as ventricular septal defect, mitral regurgitation and aortic regurgitation, many of which are haemodynamically insignificant. In contrast, the risk of endocarditis at the site of many haemodynamically important low-pressure lesions (e.g. a large atrial septal defect) is negligible.

Infection tends to occur at sites of endothelial damage because these areas attract deposits of platelets and fibrin, which are vulnerable to colonisation by blood-borne organisms. The avascular valve tissue and presence of fibrin aggregates help to protect proliferating organisms from host defence mechanisms. When the infection is established, vegetations composed of organisms, fibrin and platelets grow and may become large enough to cause obstruction; they may also break away as emboli. Adjacent tissues are destroyed and abscesses may form; valve regurgitation may develop or increase if the affected valve is damaged by tissue distortion, cusp perforation or disruption of chordae. Extracardiac manifestations such as vasculitis and skin lesions are due to emboli or immune complex deposition. Mycotic aneurysms may develop in arteries at the site of infected emboli. At postmortem it is common to find infarction of the spleen and kidneys, and sometimes an immune glomerulonephritis.

Microbiology

The *viridans* group of streptococci (*Strep. mitis*, *Strep. sanguis*) are commensals in the upper respiratory tract that may enter the blood stream on chewing or teeth-brushing, or at the time of dental treatment, and are common causes of subacute endocarditis (Box 18.119). Other organisms, including *Enterococcus faecalis*, *E. faecium* and *Strep. bovis*, may enter the blood from the bowel or urinary tract. *Strep. milleri* and *Strep. bovis* endocarditis are sometimes associated with large-bowel neoplasms.

Staph. aureus is a common cause of acute endocarditis, originating from skin infections, abscesses or vascular access sites (e.g. intravenous and central lines), or from intravenous drug misuse. It is a highly virulent and invasive organism, usually producing florid vegetations, rapid valve destruction and abscess formation. Other causes of acute endocarditis include *Strep. pneumoniae* and *Strep. pyogenes*.

Post-operative endocarditis after cardiac surgery may affect native or prosthetic heart valves or other prosthetic materials. The most common organism is a coagulase-negative staphylococcus *(Staph. epidermidis)*, which is a normal skin commensal. There is frequently a history of post-operative wound infection with the same organism. *Staph. epidermidis* occasionally causes endocarditis in patients who have not had cardiac surgery and its presence in blood cultures may be erroneously dismissed as contamination. Another coagulase-negative staphylococcus, *Staph. lugdenensis*, has recently been recognised as a cause of rapidly destructive acute endocarditis that is frequently

18

18.119 INFECTIVE ENDOCARDITIS ON NATIVE VALVES: PREVALENCE OF ORGANISMS IN EUROPE AND NORTH AMERICA (% OF CASES)

Bacteria	
• Streptococci	
Viridans group	30–40%
Enterococci	10–15%
Other streptococci	20–25%
• Staphylococci	
Staph. aureus	9–27%
Coagulase-negative	1–3%
• Gram-negative bacilli	
• Haemophilus	Total 3–8%
• Anaerobes	
Other organisms	
• Rickettsiae, fungi	< 2%

associated with multiple emboli and often affects previously normal valves. Unless accurately identified, it may also be overlooked as a contaminant.

In Q fever endocarditis due to *Coxiella burnetii*, the patient often has a history of contact with farm animals. The aortic valve is usually affected and there may be hepatic complications and purpura. Life-long antibiotic therapy may be required.

Gram-negative bacteria of the so-called HACEK group (*Haemophilus* spp; *Actinobacillus actinomycetem–comitans*; *Cardiobacterium hominis*; *Eikenella* spp. and *Kingella kingae*) are slow-growing fastidious organisms that may only be revealed after prolonged culture and may be resistant to penicillin.

Brucella is associated with a history of contact with goats or cattle and often affects the aortic valve.

Yeasts and fungi (*Candida*, *Aspergillus*) may attack previously normal or prosthetic valves, particularly in immuno-compromised patients or those with indwelling intravenous lines. Abscesses and emboli are common, therapy is difficult (surgery is often required) and the mortality is high. Concomitant bacterial infection may be present.

Incidence

The incidence of infective endocarditis in community-based studies ranges from 2–5 cases per 100 000 per annum. In a large British study, the underlying condition was rheumatic heart disease in 24% of patients, congenital heart disease in 19%, and some other cardiac abnormality (e.g. calcified atrial valve, floppy mitral valve) in 25%. The remainder (32%) were not thought to have a pre-existing cardiac abnormality. More than 50% of patients with infective endocarditis are over 60 years of age.

18.120 ENDOCARDITIS IN OLD AGE

- **Symptoms and signs:** may be non-specific, e.g. confusion, weight loss, malaise and weakness, and the diagnosis may not be suspected.
- **Common causative organisms:** often enterococci (from the urinary tract) and *Streptococcus bovis* (from a colonic source).
- **Morbidity and mortality:** much higher.

Clinical features

Possible clinical features and their frequency are shown in Figure 18.95.

The clinical course of endocarditis

Endocarditis occurs as an acute and a more insidious 'subacute' form. However, there is considerable overlap because the clinical pattern is influenced not only by the organism, but also by the site of infection, prior antibiotic therapy and the presence of a valve or shunt prosthesis. Furthermore, the subacute form may abruptly develop acute life-threatening complications such as valve disruption or emboli.

Subacute endocarditis. This should be suspected when a patient known to have congenital or valvular heart disease develops a persistent fever, complains of unusual tiredness, night sweats or weight loss, or develops new signs of valve dysfunction or heart failure. Less often, it presents as an embolic stroke or peripheral arterial embolism. Other features include purpura and petechial haemorrhages in the skin and mucous membranes, and splinter haemorrhages under the fingernails or toe nails. Osler's nodes are painful tender swellings at the fingertips that are probably the product of vasculitis; they are rare. Digital clubbing is a late sign. The spleen is frequently palpable; in *Coxiella* infections the spleen and the liver may be considerably enlarged. Microscopic haematuria is common. The finding of any of these features in a patient with persistent fever or malaise is an indication for re-examination to detect hitherto unrecognised heart disease.

Acute endocarditis. This usually presents as a severe febrile illness with prominent and changing heart murmurs and petechiae. Clinical stigmata of chronic endocarditis are usually absent. Embolic events are common, and cardiac or renal failure may develop rapidly. Abscesses may be detected on echocardiography. Partially treated acute endocarditis behaves like subacute endocarditis.

Post-operative endocarditis. Any unexplained fever in a patient who has had heart valve surgery should be investigated for possible endocarditis. The infection usually affects the valve ring and may resemble subacute or acute endocarditis, depending on the virulence of the organism. Morbidity and mortality are high and redo surgery is often required. The range of organisms is similar to that seen in native valve disease, but when endocarditis occurs during the first few weeks after surgery, it is usually due to infection with a coagulase-negative staphylococcus that was introduced during the perioperative period. A clinical diagnosis of endocarditis can be made on the presence of two major, one major and three minor, or five minor criteria (Box 18.121).

Investigations

Blood culture is the crucial investigation because it may identify the infection and guide antibiotic therapy. Three sets of blood cultures should be taken prior to commencing therapy, and these need not wait for episodes of pyrexia. The first two specimens will detect bacteraemia in 90% of culture-positive cases. Aseptic technique is essential and the risk of contaminants should be minimised by sampling from

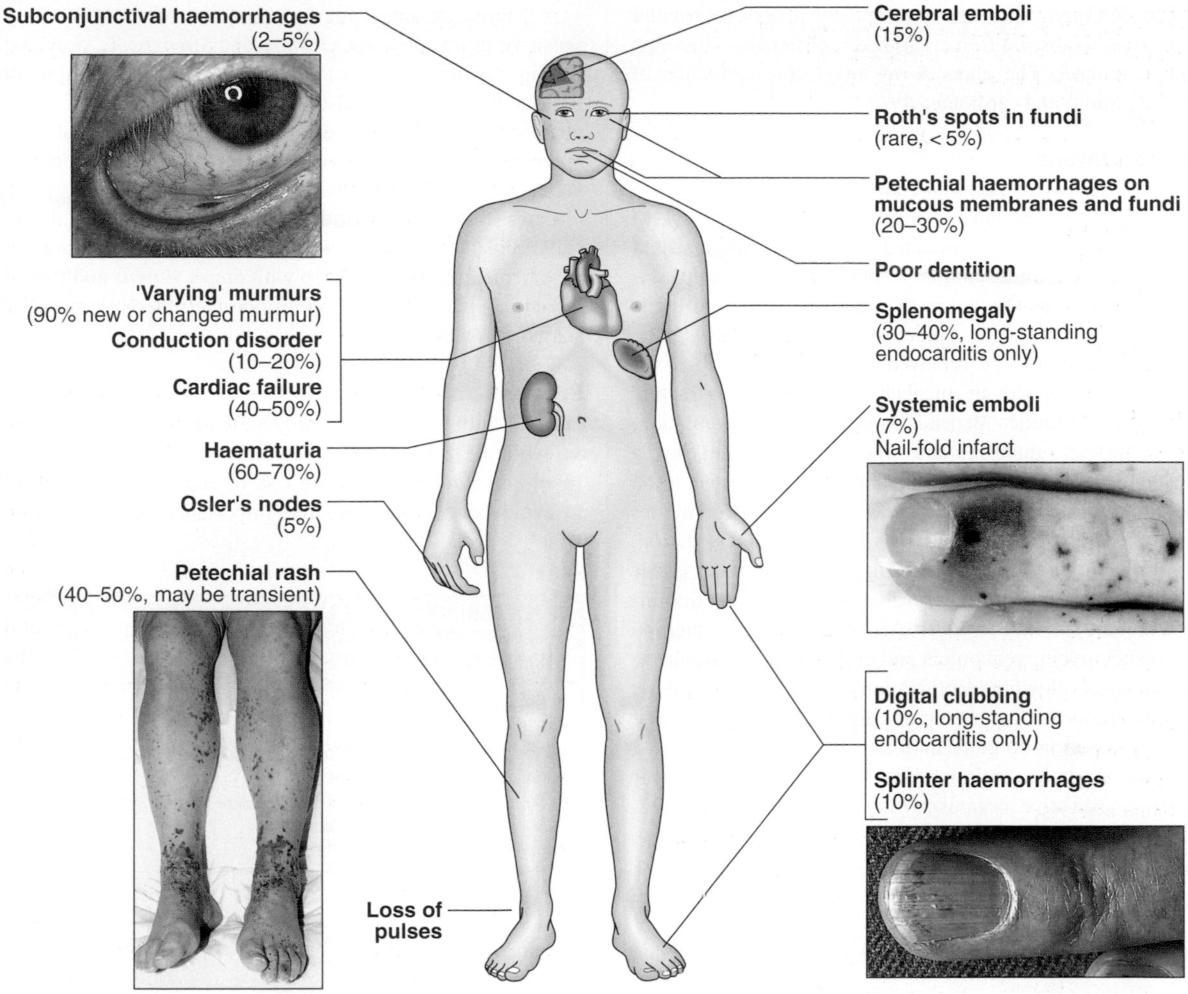

Subconjunctival haemorrhages
(2–5%)

Cerebral emboli
(15%)

Roth's spots in fundi
(rare, < 5%)

Petechial haemorrhages on
mucous membranes and fundi
(20–30%)

Poor dentition

'Varying' murmurs
(90% new or changed murmur)
Conduction disorder
(10–20%)
Cardiac failure
(40–50%)

Splenomegaly
(30–40%, long-standing
endocarditis only)

Haematuria
(60–70%)

Systemic emboli
(7%)
Nail-fold infarct

Osler's nodes
(5%)

Petechial rash
(40–50%, may be transient)

Digital clubbing
(10%, long-standing
endocarditis only)

Splinter haemorrhages
(10%)

Loss of
pulses

Fig. 18.95 **Clinical features which may be present in endocarditis.**

18.121 DIAGNOSIS OF INFECTIVE ENDOCARDITIS (MODIFIED DUKE CRITERIA)

Major criteria

- Positive blood culture
  Typical organism from two cultures
  Persistent positive blood cultures taken > 12 hours apart
  Three or more positive cultures taken over more than 1 hour
- Endocardial involvement
  Positive echocardiographic findings of vegetations
  New valvular regurgitation

Minor criteria

- Predisposing valvular or cardiac abnormality
- Intravenous drug misuse
- Pyrexia ≥ 38°C
- Embolic phenomenon
- Vasculitic phenomenon
- Blood cultures suggestive—organism grown but not achieving major criteria
- Suggestive echocardiographic findings

- **Definite endocarditis:** two major, or one major and three minor, or five minor
- **Possible endocarditis:** one major and one minor, or three minor

---

different venepuncture sites. An in-dwelling line should not be used to take cultures. Aerobic and anaerobic cultures are required.

Echocardiography is the key investigation for detecting and following the progress of vegetations, for assessing valve damage and for detecting abscess formation. Vegetations as small as 2–4 mm can be detected by transthoracic echo, and even smaller ones (1–1.5 mm) can be visualised by transoesophageal echo, which is particularly valuable for identifying abscess formation and investigating patients with prosthetic heart valves. Vegetations may be difficult to distinguish in the presence of an abnormal valve; the sensitivity of transthoracic echo is approximately 65% but that of transoesophageal echo is more than 90%. Failure to detect vegetations does not exclude the diagnosis and should not delay treatment.

Elevation of the ESR, a normocytic, normochromic anaemia and leucocytosis are common but not invariable, and thrombocytopenia may be present. Measurement of serum CRP is more reliable than the ESR in monitoring progress. Proteinuria may occur and microscopic haematuria is usually present.

The ECG may show the development of atrioventricular block (due to abscess formation) and occasionally infarction due to emboli. The chest X-ray may show evidence of cardiac failure and cardiomegaly.

Management

The case fatality of bacterial endocarditis is approximately 20% and even higher in those with prosthetic valve endocarditis and those infected with antibiotic-resistant organisms. A multidisciplinary approach with careful co-operation between the physician, surgeon and bacteriologist increases the chance of a successful outcome. Any source of infection should be removed as soon as possible; for example, a tooth with an apical abscess should be extracted.

Empirical treatment depends on the mode of presentation, the suspected organism, and whether the patient has a prosthetic valve and/or penicillin allergy. For example, if the presentation is acute, flucloxacillin and gentamicin are recommended, and for a subacute or indolent presentation, benzyl penicillin and gentamicin. In those with either penicillin allergy, a prosthetic valve or suspected meticillin-resistant *Staph. aureus* (MRSA) infection, triple therapy with vancomycin, gentamicin and oral rifampicin should be considered. Following identification of the causal organism, determination of the minimum inhibitory concentration (MIC) is essential to guide antibiotic therapy.

Some common antimicrobial treatment regimens for common causative organisms are shown in Box 18.122. For patients allergic to penicillins, a glycopeptide (e.g. vancomycin) may be substituted.

A 2-week treatment regimen may be sufficient for fully sensitive strains of *Strep. viridans* and *Strep. bovis*, provided certain conditions are met (Box 18.123). For the empirical treatment of bacterial endocarditis, penicillin plus gentamicin is the regimen of choice for most patients; however, when staphylococcal infection is suspected, vancomycin plus gentamicin is recommended.

Cardiac surgery (débridement of infected material and valve replacement) is advisable in a substantial proportion of patients, particularly those with *Staph. aureus* and fungal infections (Box 18.124); antimicrobial therapy must be started before surgery.

Prevention

Patients with valvular or congenital heart disease may be susceptible to infective endocarditis. These individuals should be made aware of the risk of endocarditis, the need to avoid bacteraemia and the importance of maintaining

18.123 CONDITIONS TO BE MET FOR THE SHORT-COURSE TREATMENT OF *STREP. VIRIDANS* AND *STREP. BOVIS* ENDOCARDITIS

- Native valve infection
- MIC ≤ 0.1 mg/l
- No adverse prognostic factors (e.g. heart failure, aortic regurgitation, conduction defect)
- No evidence of thromboembolic disease
- No vegetations > 5 mm diameter
- Clinical response within 7 days

18.122 ANTIMICROBIAL TREATMENT OF COMMON CAUSATIVE ORGANISMS IN INFECTIVE ENDOCARDITIS

Organism	Antimicrobial	Dose	Duration Native valve	Duration Prosthetic valve
Viridans streptococci and *Strep. bovis*				
MIC ≤ 0.1 mg/ml	Benzyl penicillin i.v. and gentamicin i.v.	1.2 g 4-hourly 1 mg/kg 8–12-hourly	4 weeks[1] 2 weeks	6 weeks 2 weeks
MIC > 0.1 to < 0.5 mg/ml	Benzyl penicillin i.v. and gentamicin i.v.	1.2 g 4-hourly 1 mg/kg 8–12-hourly	4 weeks 2 weeks	6 weeks 4–6 weeks
MIC ≥ 0.5 mg/ml	Benzyl penicillin i.v. and gentamicin i.v.	1.2 g 4-hourly 1 mg/kg 8–12-hourly	4 weeks 4 weeks	6 weeks 4–6 weeks
Enterococci				
Ampicillin-sensitive	Ampicillin i.v. and gentamicin i.v.[2]	2 g 4-hourly 1 mg/kg 8–12-hourly	4 weeks 4 weeks	6 weeks 6 weeks
Ampicillin-resistant	Vancomycin i.v. and gentamicin i.v.[2]	1 g 12-hourly 1 mg/kg 8–12-hourly	4 week 4 weeks	6 weeks 6 weeks
Staphylococci				
Penicillin-sensitive	Benzyl penicillin i.v.	1.2 g 4-hourly	4 week	6 weeks
Penicillin-resistant Meticillin-sensitive	Flucloxacillin i.v.	2 g 4-hourly (< 85 kg 6-hourly)	4 weeks	6 weeks[3]
Penicillin-resistant Meticillin-resistant	Vancomycin i.v. and gentamicin i.v.	1 g 12-hourly 1 mg/kg 8-hourly	4 weeks 4 weeks	6 weeks[3] 6 weeks[3]

[1] When conditions in Box 18.123 are met, 2 weeks of benzyl penicillin.
[2] In high-level gentamicin resistance, consider streptomycin.
[3] Consider additional rifamipicin 300–600 mg 12-hourly orally for 2 weeks.
(MIC = minimum inhibitory concentration)

18.124 INDICATIONS FOR CARDIAC SURGERY IN INFECTIVE ENDOCARDITIS

- Heart failure due to valve damage
- Failure of antibiotic therapy (persistent or uncontrolled infection)
- Large vegetations on left-sided heart valves with evidence or 'high risk' of systemic emboli
- Abscess formation

N.B. Patients with prosthetic valve endocarditis or fungal endocarditis often require cardiac surgery.

18.125 ANTIBIOTIC PROPHYLAXIS AGAINST ENDOCARDITIS

Procedure	Antibiotic regimen
Dental or upper respiratory tract procedures under local anaesthetic	Amoxicillin 3 g orally 1 hr before
If allergic to or received penicillin in last month	Clindamycin 600 mg orally 1 hr before

N.B. Previous endocarditis: treat as special-risk (see below).

Procedure	Antibiotic regimen
Dental or upper respiratory tract procedures under general anaesthetic	Amoxicillin 1 g i.v. at induction *plus* amoxicillin 0.5 g orally 6 hrs later
If allergic to or received penicillin in last month	Vancomycin 1 g i.v. infusion over at least 100 mins *plus* gentamicin 120 mg i.v. at induction
Special-risk patients, i.e. prosthetic valve or previous endocarditis Genitourinary procedures	Amoxicillin 1 g i.v. *plus* gentamicin 120 mg i.v. at induction *plus* amoxicillin 0.5 g orally 6 hrs later
If allergic to or received penicillin in last month	Vancomycin 1 g i.v. infusion over at least 100 mins *plus* gentamicin 120 mg i.v. at induction

N.B. Obstetric and gynaecological procedures or gastrointestinal surgery/instrumentation—treat only special-risk patients.

18.126 PROSTHETIC HEART VALVES: OPTIMAL ANTICOAGULANT CONTROL

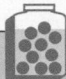

Mechanical valves	Target INR
Ball and cage (e.g. Starr–Edwards) Tilting disc (e.g. Bjork–Shiley)	3.5
Bi-leaflet (e.g. St Jude)	3.0
Biological valves with atrial fibrillation	2.5

All mechanical valves require long-term anticoagulation because they may develop thrombus around the valve, causing obstruction to flow and/or embolism (Box 18.126); the prosthetic clicks may become inaudible if the valve malfunctions. Biological valves have the advantage of not requiring anticoagulants to maintain proper function; however, many patients undergoing valve replacement surgery, especially mitral valve replacement, will have atrial fibrillation that requires anticoagulation anyway. Biological valves are less durable than mechanical valves and may degenerate 7 or more years after implantation, particularly when used in the mitral position. They are more durable in the aortic position and in older patients, and so are particularly appropriate for patients over 65 undergoing aortic valve replacement.

Symptoms or signs of unexplained heart failure in a patient with a prosthetic heart valve may be due to valve dysfunction; biological valve dysfunction is usually associated with the development of a regurgitant murmur. Urgent assessment is required.

CONGENITAL HEART DISEASE

Congenital heart disease usually manifests in childhood but may pass unrecognised and not present until adult life. Defects which are well tolerated, e.g. atrial septal defect, may cause no symptoms until adult life or may be detected incidentally on routine examination or chest X-ray. Congenital defects that were previously fatal in childhood can now be corrected, or at least partially corrected, so that survival to adult life is the norm. Such patients may remain well for many years and subsequently re-present in later life with related problems such as arrhythmia or ventricular dysfunction (Box 18.127).

The fetal circulation

Understanding the fetal circulation helps to understand how some forms of congenital heart disease occur. The fetus has only a small flow of blood through the lungs, as it obviously does not breathe in utero. The fetal circulation therefore allows oxygenated blood from the placenta to pass directly to the left side of the heart through the foramen ovale without having to flow through the lungs (Fig. 18.96).

Congenital defects may arise if the changes from fetal circulation to the extrauterine circulation are not properly completed. Atrial septal defects occur at the site of the foramen ovale. A patent ductus arteriosus may remain if it fails to close after birth. Failure of the aorta to develop at the point of the aortic isthmus and where the ductus

good dental health. Any potential source of infection in susceptible individuals should be treated promptly, and invasive procedures that may cause transient bacteraemia should be accompanied by appropriate antibiotic prophylaxis. The chosen drug regimen should be sufficient to kill the likely organism, and should be given shortly before the anticipated bacteraemia in order to reduce the risk of resistance (Box 18.125).

VALVE REPLACEMENT SURGERY

Diseased heart valves can be replaced with mechanical or biological prostheses. The three most commonly used types of mechanical prosthesis are the ball and cage, tilting single disc and tilting bi-leaflet valves. All generate prosthetic sounds or clicks on auscultation. Pig valves mounted on a supporting stent are the most commonly used biological valves. They generate normal heart sounds. All prosthetic valves used in the aortic position produce a systolic flow murmur.

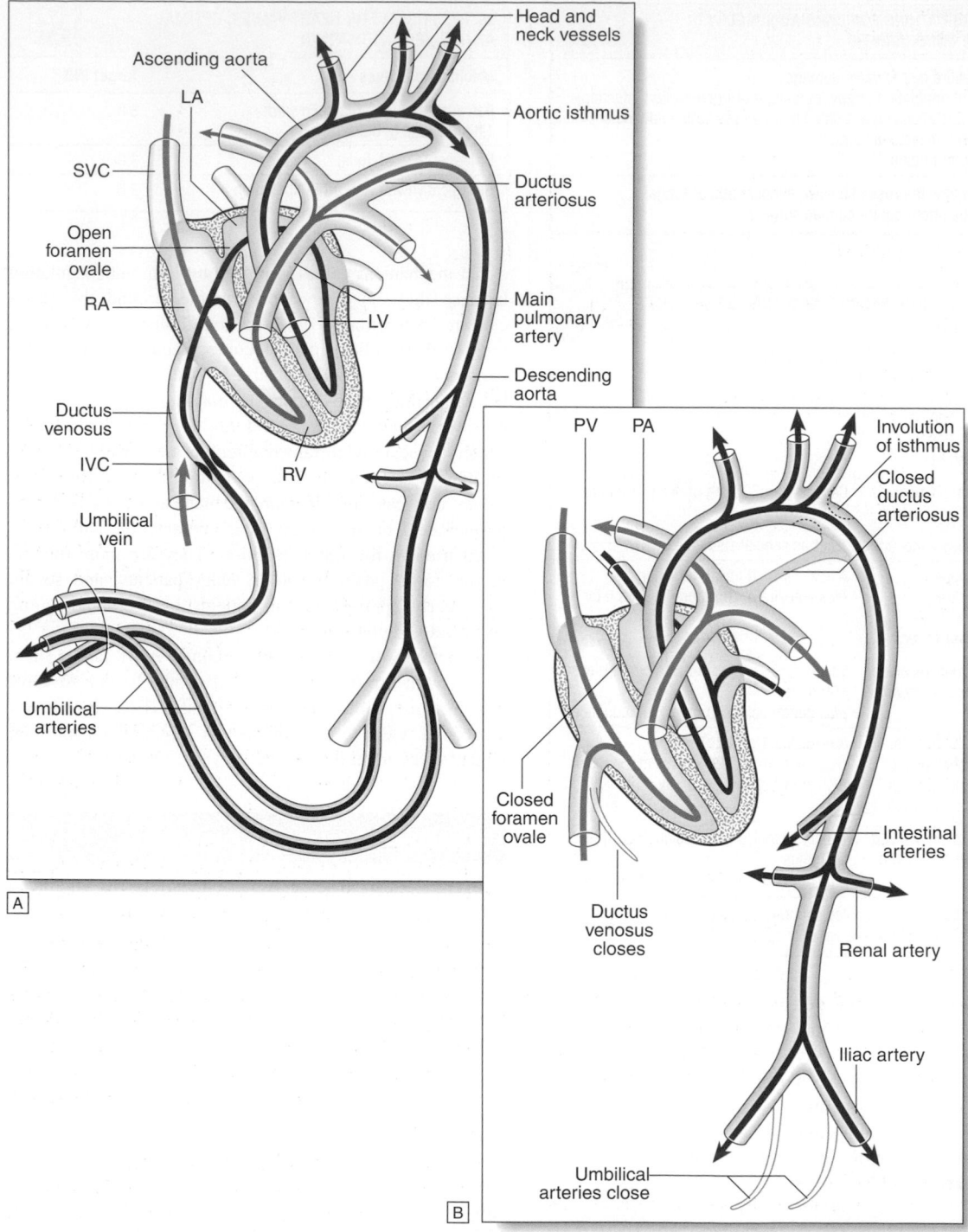

Fig. 18.96   Changes in the circulation at birth. ▲ In the fetus, oxygenated blood comes through the umbilical vein where it enters the inferior vena cava via the ductus venosus (red). The oxygenated blood streams from the right atrium through the open foramen ovale to the left atrium and via the left ventricle into the aorta. Venous blood from the superior vena cava (blue) crosses under the main blood stream into the right atrium and then, partly mixed with oxygenated blood (purple), into the right ventricle and pulmonary artery. The pulmonary vasculature has a high resistance and so little blood passes to the lungs; most blood passes through the ductus arteriosus to the descending aorta. The aortic isthmus is a constriction in the aorta that lies in the aortic arch before the junction with the ductus arteriosus and limits the flow of oxygen-rich blood to the descending aorta. This configuration means that less oxygen-rich blood is supplied to organ systems that take up their function mainly after birth, e.g. the kidneys and intestinal tract. ⓑ At birth, the lungs expand with air and pulmonary vascular resistance falls so that blood now flows to the lungs and back to the left atrium. The left atrial pressure rises above right atrial pressure and the flap valve of the foramen ovale closes. The umbilical arteries and the ductus venosus close. In the next few days, the ductus arteriosus closes under the influence of hormonal changes (particularly prostaglandins) and the aortic isthmus expands.

18.127 PRESENTATION OF CONGENITAL HEART DISEASE THROUGHOUT LIFE

Birth and neonatal period

- Cyanosis
- Heart failure

Infancy and childhood

- Cyanosis
- Heart failure
- Arrhythmia
- Murmur
- Failure to thrive

Adolescence and adulthood

- Heart failure
- Murmur
- Arrhythmia
- Cyanosis due to shunt reversal (Eisenmenger's syndrome)
- Hypertension (coarctation)
- Late consequences of previous cardiac surgery, e.g. arrhythmia, heart failure

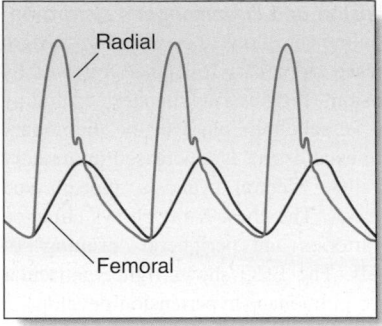

Fig. 18.97 Radio-femoral delay.

18

18.128 INCIDENCE AND RELATIVE FREQUENCY OF CONGENITAL CARDIAC MALFORMATIONS

Lesion	% of all CHD defects
Ventricular septal defect	30
Atrial septal defect	10
Patent ductus arteriosus	10
Pulmonary stenosis	7
Coarctation of aorta	7
Aortic stenosis	6
Tetralogy of Fallot	6
Complete transposition of great arteries	4
Others	20

arteriosus attaches can lead to narrowing or coarctation of the aorta.

In fetal development, the heart develops as a single tube which folds back on itself and then divides into two separate circulations. Failure of septation can lead to some forms of atrial and ventricular septal defect. Failure of alignment of the great vessels with the ventricles contributes to transposition of the great arteries, tetralogy of Fallot and truncus arteriosus.

Aetiology and incidence

The incidence of haemodynamically significant congenital cardiac abnormalities is about 0.8% of live births (Box 18.128). Maternal infection or exposure to drugs or toxins may cause congenital heart disease. Maternal rubella infection is associated with persistent ductus arteriosus, pulmonary valvular and/or artery stenosis, and atrial septal defect. Maternal alcohol misuse is associated with septal defects, and maternal lupus erythematosus with congenital complete heart block. Genetic or chromosomal abnormalities such as Down's syndrome may cause septal defects, and gene defects have also been identified as causing specific abnormalities, e.g. Marfan's (p. 605) and DiGeorge's (deletion in chromosome 22q) syndromes.

Clinical features

Symptoms may be absent, or the child may be breathless or fail to attain normal growth and development. All degrees of severity occur. Some defects are not compatible with extrauterine life, or only for a short time. Clinical signs vary with the anatomical lesion. Murmurs, thrills or signs of cardiomegaly may be present. In coarctation of the aorta, radio-femoral delay may be noted (Fig. 18.97). Tall stature with long limbs and lens dislocation may be obvious in Marfan's syndrome. Features of other congenital conditions such as Down's syndrome, may also be apparent. Cerebrovascular accidents and cerebral abscesses are complications of severe cyanotic congenital disease.

Early diagnosis is important because many types of congenital heart disease are amenable to surgical treatment, but this opportunity may be lost if secondary changes such as pulmonary vascular damage occur.

Central cyanosis and digital clubbing

Central cyanosis of cardiac origin occurs when desaturated blood enters the systemic circulation without passing through the lungs (i.e. a right-to-left shunt). In the neonate, the most common cause is transposition of the great arteries, in which the aorta arises from the right ventricle and the pulmonary artery from the left. In older children, cyanosis is usually the consequence of a ventricular septal defect combined with severe pulmonary stenosis (tetralogy of Fallot) or with pulmonary vascular disease (Eisenmenger's syndrome). Prolonged cyanosis is associated with finger and toe clubbing (p. 520).

Growth retardation and learning difficulties

These may be a feature with large left-to-right shunts at ventricular or great arterial level, but can also occur with other defects, especially if they form part of a genetic syndrome. Major intellectual impairment is uncommon in children with isolated congenital heart disease; however, minor learning difficulties can occur and may also be the consequence of cardiac surgery.

Syncope

In the presence of increased pulmonary vascular resistance or severe left or right ventricular outflow obstruction, exercise may provoke syncope as systemic vascular resistance falls on exercise but pulmonary vascular resistance may rise, worsening right-to-left shunting and cerebral oxygenation.

18

Pulmonary hypertension and Eisenmenger's syndrome

Persistently raised pulmonary flow (e.g. with left-to-right shunt) leads to increased pulmonary resistance followed by pulmonary hypertension. Progressive changes, including obliteration of distal vessels, take place in the pulmonary vasculature and, once established, the increased pulmonary resistance is irreversible. Central cyanosis appears and digital clubbing develops. The chest X-ray shows enlarged central pulmonary arteries and peripheral 'pruning' of the pulmonary vessels. The ECG shows right ventricular hypertrophy. If severe pulmonary hypertension develops, a left-to-right shunt may reverse, resulting in right-to-left shunting and marked cyanosis (Eisenmenger's syndrome). This is more common with large ventricular septal defects or persistent ductus arteriosus than with atrial septal defects. Patients with Eisenmenger's syndrome are at particular risk from abrupt changes in afterload that exacerbate right-to-left shunting, e.g. vasodilatation, anaesthesia, pregnancy.

Pregnancy

During pregnancy, there is a 50% increase in plasma volume, a 40% increase in whole blood volume and a similar increase in cardiac output. Abnormalities causing severe outflow tract obstruction, such as aortic stenosis, are not well tolerated and are associated with significant maternal morbidity and mortality. However, most patients with surgically corrected congenital heart disease, and many with palliated or untreated disease, will tolerate pregnancy well. Pregnancy is particularly hazardous in the presence of conditions associated with cyanosis or severe pulmonary hypertension. For example, maternal mortality in patients with Eisenmenger's syndrome is more than 50% and sterilisation is usually recommended in such patients. There is a 2–5% risk that the offspring of patients with congenital heart disease will be born with cardiac abnormalities; this is greater if the mother rather than the father is affected.

PERSISTENT DUCTUS ARTERIOSUS

Aetiology

During fetal life, before the lungs begin to function, most of the blood from the pulmonary artery passes through the ductus arteriosus into the aorta (Fig. 18.96). Normally the ductus closes soon after birth but sometimes it fails to do so. Persistence of the ductus may be associated with other abnormalities and is more common in females.

Since the pressure in the aorta is higher than that in the pulmonary artery (PA), there will be a continuous arteriovenous shunt, the volume of which depends on the size of the ductus. As much as 50% of the left ventricular output may be recirculated through the lungs, with a consequent increase in the work of the heart (Fig. 18.98).

Clinical features

With small shunts there may be no symptoms for years, but when the ductus is large, growth and development may be retarded. Usually there is no disability in infancy but cardiac failure may eventually ensue, dyspnoea being the first symptom. A continuous 'machinery' murmur is heard with late systolic accentuation, maximal in the second

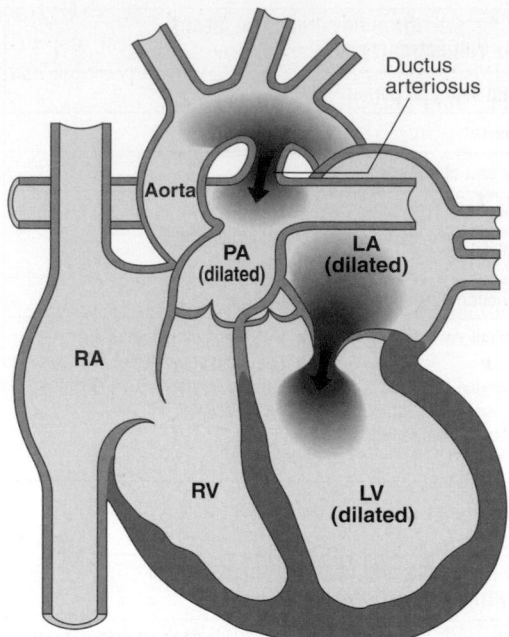

Fig. 18.98 Persistent ductus arteriosus. There is a connection between the aorta and the pulmonary artery with left-to-right shunting and dilatation of the pulmonary artery, left atrium and left ventricle.

left intercostal space below the clavicle (Fig. 18.98). It is frequently accompanied by a thrill. Pulses are increased in volume.

A large left-to-right shunt in infancy may cause a considerable rise in pulmonary artery pressure, and sometimes this leads to progressive pulmonary vascular damage. Enlargement of the pulmonary artery may be detected radiologically. The ECG is usually normal.

Persistent ductus with reversed shunting

If pulmonary vascular resistance increases, pulmonary artery pressure rises and may continue to do so until it equals or exceeds aortic pressure. The shunt through the defect may then reverse, causing central cyanosis (Eisenmenger's syndrome), which may be more apparent in the feet and toes than in the upper part of the body. The murmur becomes quieter, may be confined to systole or may disappear. The ECG shows evidence of right ventricular hypertrophy.

Management

It is now usual practice to close a patent ductus at cardiac catheterisation with an implantable occlusive device (Fig. 18.14, p. 533). Closure should be undertaken in infancy if the shunt is significant and pulmonary resistance not elevated, but this may be delayed until later childhood in those with smaller shunts, for whom closure remains advisable to reduce the risk of endocarditis.

Pharmacological treatment in the neonatal period

When the ductus is structurally intact, a prostaglandin synthetase inhibitor (indometacin or ibuprofen) may be used in the first week of life to induce closure. However, in the presence of a congenital defect with impaired lung perfusion (e.g. severe pulmonary stenosis and left-to-right shunt through the ductus), it may be advisable to improve oxygenation by keeping the ductus open with prostaglandin treatment. Unfortunately, these treatments do not work if the ductus is intrinsically abnormal.

COARCTATION OF THE AORTA

Aetiology
Narrowing of the aorta most commonly occurs in the region where the ductus arteriosus joins the aorta, i.e. at the isthmus just below the origin of the left subclavian artery (Fig. 18.96, p. 634 and Fig. 18.99). The condition is twice as common in males as in females and occurs in 1 in 4000 children. It is associated with other abnormalities, of which the most frequent are bicuspid aortic valve and 'berry' aneurysms of the cerebral circulation (p. 1210). Acquired coarctation of the aorta is rare but may follow trauma or occur as a complication of a progressive arteritis (Takayasu's disease, p. 1140).

Clinical features and investigations
Aortic coarctation is an important cause of cardiac failure in the newborn, but symptoms are often absent when it is detected in older children or adults. Headaches may occur from hypertension proximal to the coarctation, and occasionally weakness or cramps in the legs may result from decreased circulation in the lower part of the body. The blood pressure is raised in the upper body but normal or low in the legs. The femoral pulses are weak, and delayed in comparison with the radial pulse (Fig. 18.97). A systolic murmur is usually heard posteriorly, over the coarctation. There may also be an ejection click and systolic murmur in the aortic area due to a bicuspid aortic valve. As a result of the aortic narrowing, collaterals form, mainly involving the

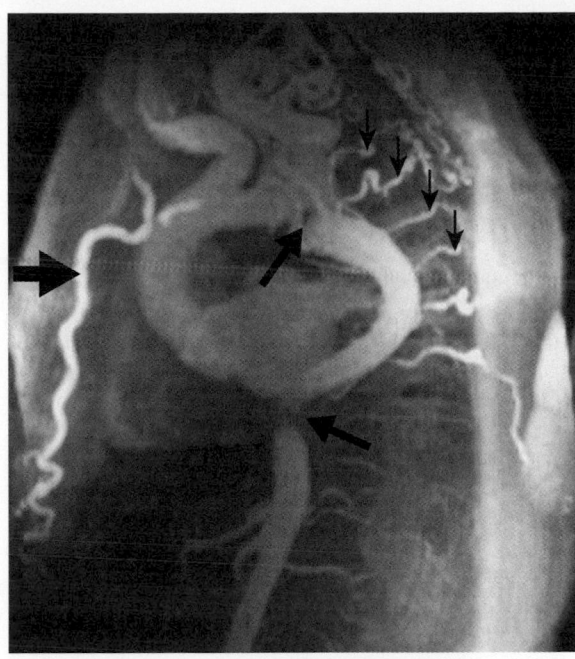

Fig. 18.100 **MRI scan of coarctation of the aorta.** The aorta is severely narrowed just beyond the arch at the start of the descending aorta (upper medium arrow). Extensive collaterals have developed with a large internal mammary artery shown (large arrow), and several intercostal arteries (small arrows). Unusually, in this case there is also a coarctation of the abdominal aorta (lower medium arrow).

periscapular, internal mammary and intercostal arteries. These may result in localised bruits.

Chest X-ray in early childhood is often normal but at a later age may show changes in the contour of the aorta (indentation of the descending aorta, '3 sign') and notching of the under-surfaces of the ribs from collaterals. MRI is ideal for demonstrating the lesion (Fig. 18.100). The ECG may show left ventricular hypertrophy.

Management
In untreated cases, death may occur from left ventricular failure, dissection of the aorta or cerebral haemorrhage. Surgical correction is advisable in all but the mildest cases. If this is done sufficiently early in childhood, persistent hypertension can be avoided. Patients repaired in late childhood or adult life often remain hypertensive or develop recurrent hypertension later in life. Recurrence of stenosis may occur as the child grows, and this may be managed by balloon dilatation, which can also be used as the primary treatment in some cases (Fig. 18.14, p. 533). Coexistent bicuspid aortic valve, which occurs in over 50% of cases, may lead to progressive aortic stenosis or regurgitation and also requires long-term follow-up.

ATRIAL SEPTAL DEFECT

Aetiology
Atrial septal defect is one of the most common congenital heart defects, and occurs twice as frequently in females. Most are 'ostium secundum' defects, involving the fossa

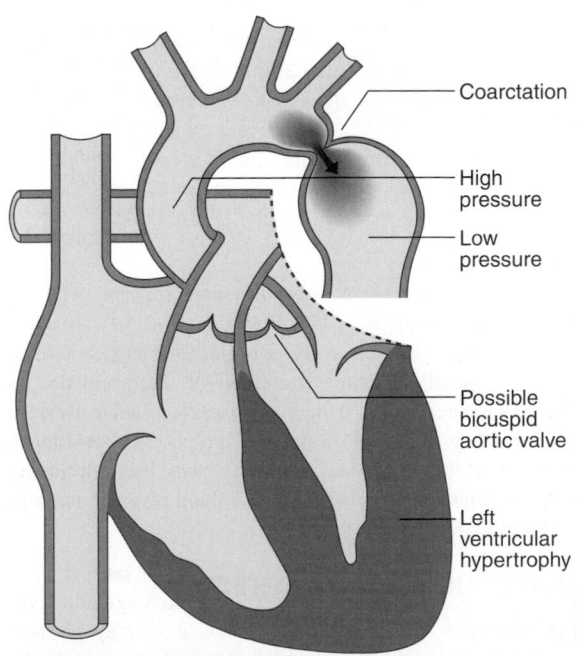

Fig. 18.99 **Coarctation of the aorta.**

- Coarctation
- High pressure
- Low pressure
- Possible bicuspid aortic valve
- Left ventricular hypertrophy

ovalis which in utero was the foramen ovale (Fig. 18.96, p. 634). 'Ostium primum' defects result from a defect in the atrioventricular septum and are associated with a 'cleft mitral valve' (split anterior leaflet).

Since the normal right ventricle is more compliant than the left, a large volume of blood shunts through the defect from the left to the right atrium and then to the right ventricle and pulmonary arteries (Fig. 18.101). As a result there is gradual enlargement of the right side of the heart and of the pulmonary arteries. Pulmonary hypertension and shunt reversal sometimes complicate atrial septal defect, but are less common and tend to occur later in life than with other types of left-to-right shunt.

Clinical features

Most children are free of symptoms for many years and the condition is often detected at routine clinical examination or following a chest X-ray. Dyspnoea, chest infections, cardiac failure and arrhythmias, especially atrial fibrillation, are other possible modes of presentation. The characteristic physical signs are the result of the volume overload of the right ventricle:

- wide fixed splitting of the second heart sound: wide because of delay in right ventricular ejection (increased stroke volume and right bundle branch block) and fixed because the septal defect equalises left and right atrial pressures throughout the respiratory cycle
- a systolic flow murmur over the pulmonary valve.

In children with a large shunt, there may be a diastolic flow murmur over the tricuspid valve. Unlike a mitral flow murmur, this is usually high-pitched.

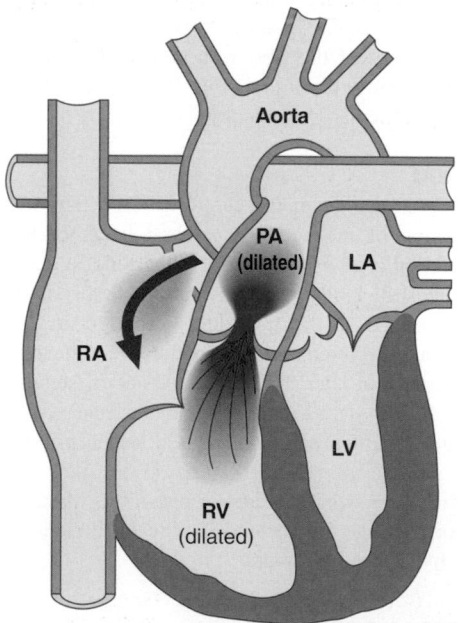

Fig. 18.101 Atrial septal defect. Blood flows across the atrial septum (arrow) from left to right. The murmur is produced by increased flow velocity across the pulmonary valve, as a result of left-to-right shunting and a large stroke volume. The density of shading is proportional to velocity of blood flow.

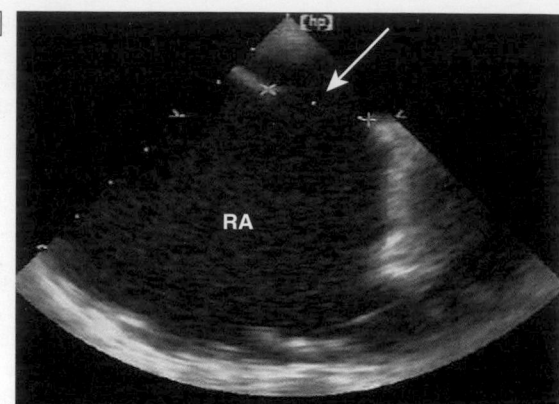

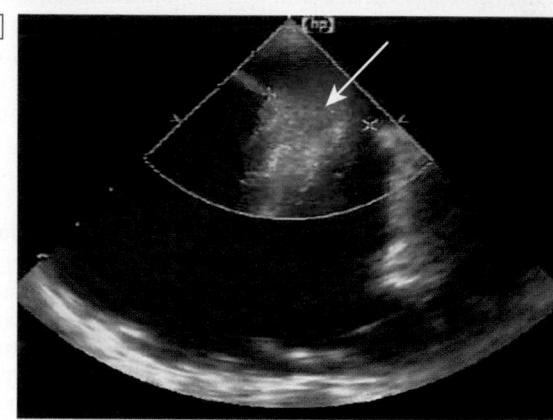

Fig. 18.102 Transoesophageal echocardiogram of an atrial septal defect (ASD). [A] The defect is clearly seen between the left atrium and the right atrium (RA). [B] Doppler colour-flow imaging shows flow across the defect.

The chest X-ray typically shows enlargement of the heart and the pulmonary artery as well as pulmonary plethora. The ECG usually shows incomplete right bundle branch block because right ventricular depolarisation is delayed as a result of ventricular dilatation (with a 'primum' defect there is also left axis deviation). Echocardiography can directly demonstrate the defect and typically shows RV dilatation, RV hypertrophy and pulmonary artery dilatation. The precise size and location of the defect can be shown by transoesophageal echocardiography (Fig. 18.102).

Management

Atrial septal defects in which pulmonary flow is increased 50% above systemic flow (i.e. flow ratio of 1.5:1) are often large enough to be clinically recognisable and should be closed surgically. Closure can also be accomplished at cardiac catheterisation using implantable closure devices (Fig. 18.14, p. 533). The long-term prognosis thereafter is excellent unless pulmonary hypertension has developed. Severe pulmonary hypertension and shunt reversal are both contraindications to surgery.

VENTRICULAR SEPTAL DEFECT

Aetiology

Congenital ventricular septal defect occurs as a result of incomplete septation of the ventricles. Embryologically, the interventricular septum has a membranous and a muscular portion, and the latter is further divided into inflow, trabecular and outflow portions. Most congenital defects are 'perimembranous', i.e. at the junction of the membranous and muscular portions.

Ventricular septal defects are the most common congenital cardiac defect, occurring once in 500 live births. The defect may be isolated or part of complex congenital heart disease. Acquired ventricular septal defect may result from rupture as a complication of acute myocardial infarction, or rarely from trauma.

Clinical features

Flow from the high-pressure left ventricle to the low-pressure right ventricle during systole produces a pansystolic murmur usually heard best at the left sternal edge but radiating all over the precordium (Fig. 18.103). A small defect often produces a loud murmur (maladie de Roger) in the absence of other haemodynamic disturbance. Conversely, a large defect may produce a softer murmur, particularly if pressure in the right ventricle is elevated. This may be found immediately after birth, while pulmonary vascular resistance remains high, or when the shunt is reversed in Eisenmenger's syndrome.

Congenital ventricular septal defect may present as cardiac failure in infants, as a murmur with only minor haemodynamic disturbance in older children or adults, or rarely as Eisenmenger's syndrome. In a proportion of infants, the murmur gets quieter or disappears due to spontaneous closure of the defect.

If cardiac failure complicates a large defect, it is usually absent in the immediate postnatal period and only becomes apparent in the first 4–6 weeks of life. In addition to the murmur, there is prominent parasternal pulsation, tachypnoea and indrawing of the lower ribs on inspiration. The chest X-ray shows pulmonary plethora and the ECG shows bilateral ventricular hypertrophy.

Management

Small ventricular septal defects require no specific treatment apart from endocarditis prophylaxis. Cardiac failure caused by a ventricular septal defect in infancy is initially treated medically with digoxin and diuretics. Persisting failure is an indication for surgical repair of the defect. Percutaneous closure devices are under development.

Doppler echocardiography helps to predict the small septal defects that are likely to close spontaneously. Eisenmenger's syndrome is avoided by monitoring for signs of rising pulmonary resistance (serial ECG and echocardiography) and carrying out surgical repair when appropriate. Surgical closure is contraindicated in fully developed Eisenmenger's syndrome when heart-lung transplantation may be the only effective method of treatment.

Prognosis

Except in the case of Eisenmenger's syndrome, long-term prognosis is very good in congenital ventricular septal defect. Many patients with Eisenmenger's syndrome die in the second or third decade of life, but a few survive to the fifth decade without transplantation.

TETRALOGY OF FALLOT

The four components of the tetralogy are shown in Figure 18.104.

The right ventricle outflow obstruction is most often subvalvular (infundibular), but may be valvular, supravalvular or a combination of these. The ventricular septal defect is usually large and similar in aperture to the aortic

18

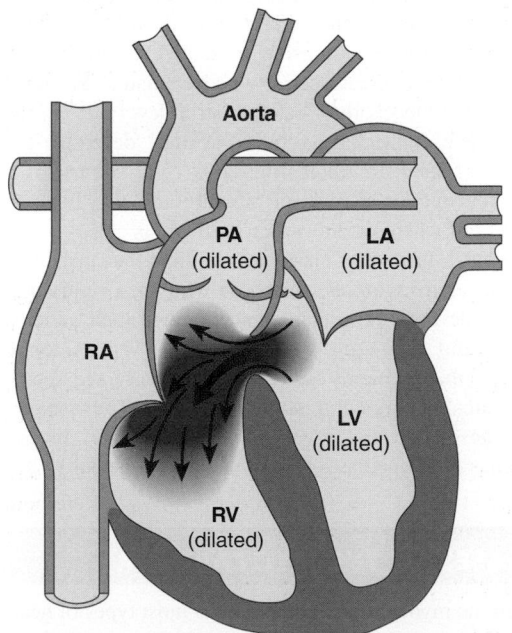

Fig. 18.103 Ventricular septal defect. In this example a large left-to-right shunt (arrows) has resulted in chamber enlargement.

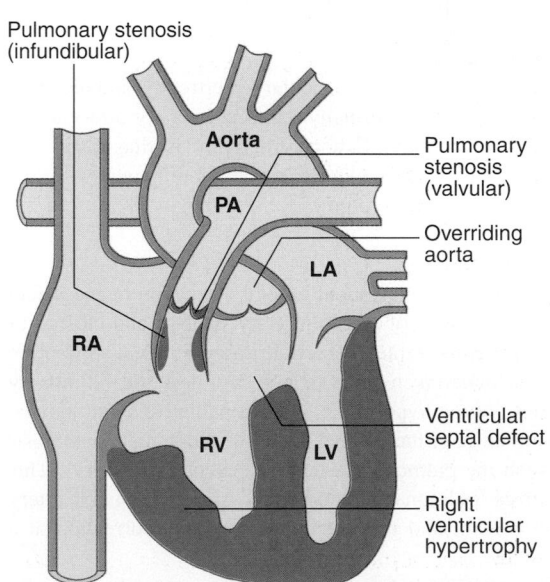

Fig. 18.104 Tetralogy of Fallot. The tetralogy comprises (1) pulmonary stenosis, (2) overriding of the ventricular septal defect by the aorta, (3) a ventricular septal defect and (4) right ventricular hypertrophy.

orifice. The combination results in elevated right ventricular pressure and right-to-left shunting of cyanotic blood across the ventricular septal defect.

Aetiology

The embryological cause is abnormal development of the bulbar septum which separates the ascending aorta from the pulmonary artery, and which normally aligns and fuses with the outflow part of the interventricular septum. The defect occurs in about 1 in 2000 births and is the most common cause of cyanosis in infancy after the first year of life.

Clinical features

Children are usually cyanosed but this may not be present in the neonate because it is only when right ventricular pressure rises to equal or exceed left ventricular pressure that a large right-to-left shunt develops. The subvalvular component of the right ventricle outflow obstruction is dynamic, and may increase suddenly under adrenergic stimulation. The affected child suddenly becomes increasingly cyanosed, often after feeding or a crying attack, and may become apnoeic and unconscious. These attacks are called 'Fallot's spells'. In older children, Fallot's spells are uncommon but cyanosis becomes increasingly apparent, with stunting of growth, digital clubbing and polycythaemia. Some children characteristically obtain relief by squatting after exertion, which increases the afterload of the left heart and reduces the right-to-left shunting. The natural history before the development of surgical correction was variable, but most patients died in infancy or childhood.

On examination the most characteristic feature is the combination of cyanosis with a loud ejection systolic murmur in the pulmonary area (as for pulmonary stenosis). However, cyanosis may be absent in the newborn or in patients with only mild right ventricular outflow obstruction ('acyanotic tetralogy of Fallot').

Investigations

The ECG shows right ventricular hypertrophy, and the chest X-ray shows an abnormally small pulmonary artery and a 'boot-shaped' heart. Echocardiography is diagnostic and demonstrates that the aorta is not continuous with the anterior ventricular septum.

Management

The definitive management is total correction of the defect by surgical relief of the pulmonary stenosis and closure of the ventricular septal defect. Primary surgical correction may be undertaken prior to age 5, unless the pulmonary arteries are too hypoplastic, when a palliative shunt may be performed (e.g. the Blalock–Taussig shunt, an anastomosis between the pulmonary artery and subclavian artery). This improves pulmonary blood flow and pulmonary artery development, and may facilitate definitive correction at a later stage.

The prognosis after total correction is good, especially if the operation is performed in childhood. Follow-up is needed to identify residual shunting, recurrent pulmonary stenosis and rhythm disorders.

18.129 OTHER CAUSES OF CYANOTIC CONGENITAL HEART DISEASE	
Defect	**Features**
Tricuspid atresia	Absent tricuspid orifice, hypoplastic RV, RA to LA shunt, VSD shunt, other anomalies Surgical correction *may* be possible
Transposition of the great vessels	Aorta arises from the morphological RV, pulmonary artery from LV Shunt via atria, ductus and possibly VSD Palliation by balloon atrial septostomy/enlargement Surgical correction possible
Pulmonary atresia	Pulmonary valve atretic and pulmonary artery hypoplastic RA to LA shunt, pulmonary flow via ductus Palliation by balloon atrial septostomy Surgical correction may be possible
Ebstein's anomaly	Tricuspid valve is dysplastic and displaced into RV, right ventricle 'atrialised' Tricuspid regurgitation and RA to LA shunt Wide spectrum of severity Arrhythmias Surgical repair possible, but significant risks

OTHER CAUSES OF CYANOTIC CONGENITAL HEART DISEASE

Other causes of cyanotic congenital heart disease are summarised in Box 18.129. Echocardiography is usually the definitive diagnostic procedure, supplemented if necessary by cardiac catheterisation.

ADULT CONGENITAL HEART DISEASE

There are increasing numbers of children who have had surgical correction of congenital defects and who may have further cardiological problems as adults. For example, those who have undergone correction of coarctation of the aorta may develop hypertension in adult life. Those with transposition of the great arteries who have had a 'Mustard' repair, where blood is re-directed at atrial level leaving the right ventricle connected to the aorta, may develop right ventricular failure in adult life. The right ventricle is unsuited for function at systemic pressures and may begin to dilate and fail when patients are in their 20s or 30s.

Those who have had surgery involving the atria may develop atrial arrhythmias, and those who have ventricular scars may develop ventricular arrhythmias. Such patients require careful follow-up from the teenage years through adult life so that problems can be identified early and appropriate medical or surgical treatment instituted. The management of these adult or 'grown-up' congenital heart disease patients has developed as a cardiological sub-specialty.

DISEASES OF THE MYOCARDIUM

Although the myocardium is involved in most types of heart disease, the terms 'myocarditis' and 'cardiomyopathy' are usually reserved for conditions that primarily affect the heart muscle.

18

ACUTE MYOCARDITIS

This is an acute inflammatory condition that may complicate a wide variety of infections; inflammation may be due to infection of the myocardium or the effects of circulating toxins. Viral infection is the most common cause and the main culprits are the Coxsackie viruses (35 cases per 1000 infections) and influenza viruses A and B (25 cases per 1000 infections). Myocarditis may occur several weeks after the initial viral infection and susceptibility is increased by corticosteroid treatment, immunosuppression, radiation, previous myocardial damage and exercise. Some bacterial and protozoal infections may be complicated by myocarditis; for example, approximately 5% of patients with Lyme disease (*Borrelia burgdorferi*, p. 319) develop myopericarditis, which is often associated with variable degrees of atrioventricular block.

The clinical picture ranges from a symptomless disorder, sometimes recognised by the presence of an inappropriate tachycardia or abnormal ECG, to fulminant heart failure. Myocarditis may be heralded by a 'flu'-like illness. ECG changes are common but non-specific. Biochemical markers of myocardial injury (e.g. troponin I and T, creatine kinase) are elevated in proportion to the extent of damage. Echocardiography may reveal left ventricular dysfunction which is sometimes regional (due to focal myocarditis), and if the diagnosis is uncertain it can be confirmed by endomyocardial biopsy.

In most patients the disease is self-limiting and the immediate prognosis is excellent. However, death may occur, due to a ventricular arrhythmia or rapidly progressive heart failure. Myocarditis has been reported as a cause of sudden and unexpected death in young athletes. There is strong evidence that some forms of myocarditis may lead to chronic low-grade myocarditis or dilated cardiomyopathy (see below); for example, in Chagas disease (p. 355) the patient frequently recovers from the acute infection but goes on to develop a chronic dilated cardiomyopathy 10 or 20 years later.

Specific antimicrobial therapy may be used if a causative organism has been identified; however, this is rare and in most cases only supportive therapy is available. Treatment for cardiac failure or arrhythmias may be required and patients should be advised to avoid intense physical exertion because there is some evidence that this can induce potentially fatal ventricular arrhythmias. Clinical trials have failed to demonstrate any benefit from treatment with corticosteroids and immunosuppressive agents.

CARDIOMYOPATHY

The aetiology of most intrinsic disorders of the myocardium has not been elucidated and a functional classification is therefore the most appropriate means of describing these diseases (Fig. 18.105).

DILATED CARDIOMYOPATHY

This condition is characterised by dilatation and impaired contraction of the left (and sometimes the right) ventricle;

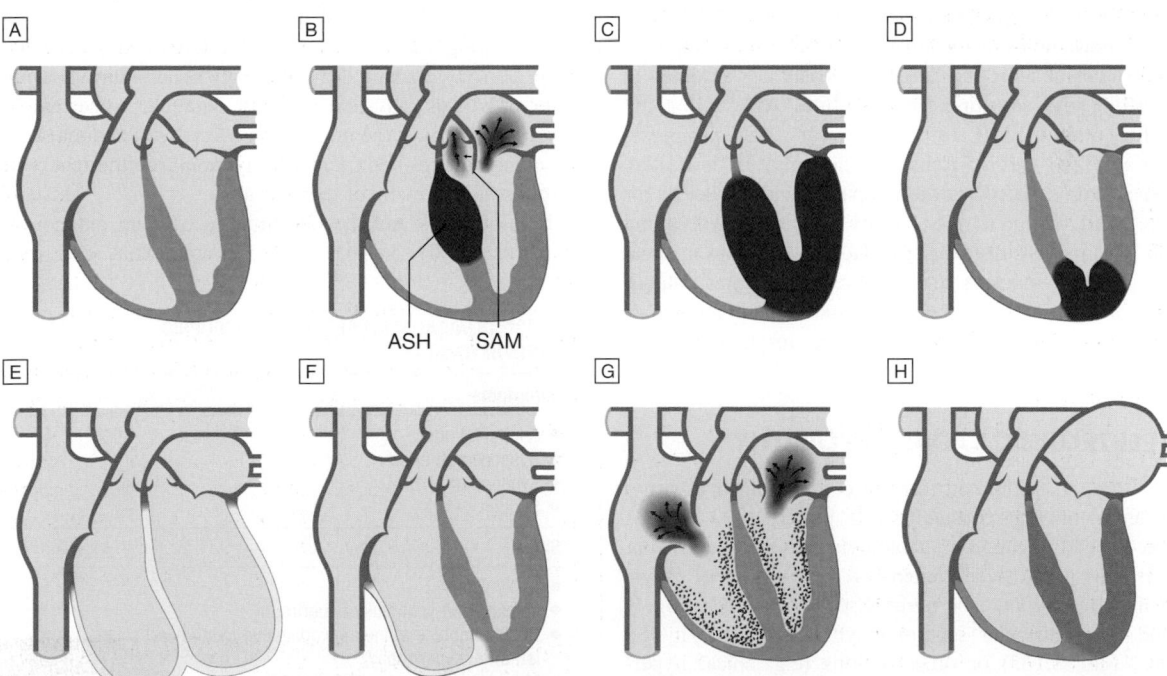

Fig. 18.105   Types of cardiomyopathy. Ⓐ Normal. Ⓑ Hypertrophic cardiomyopathy: asymmetric septal hypertrophy (ASH) with systolic anterior motion of the mitral valve (SAM), causing mitral reflux and dynamic LV outflow tract obstruction. Ⓒ Hypertrophic cardiomyopathy: concentric hypertrophy. Ⓓ Hypertrophic cardiomyopathy: apical hypertrophy. Ⓔ Dilated cardiomyopathy. Ⓕ Arrhythmogenic right ventricular dysplasia. Ⓖ Obliterative cardiomyopathy. Ⓗ Restrictive cardiomyopathy.

left ventricular mass is increased but wall thickness is normal or reduced (Fig. 18.105). The histological changes are variable but include myofibrillary loss, interstitial fibrosis and T-cell infiltrates. The differential diagnosis includes coronary artery disease and some specific disorders of heart muscle (see below), and a diagnosis of dilated cardiomyopathy should only be offered when these conditions have been excluded.

The pathogenesis is not clear but dilated cardiomyopathy probably encompasses a heterogenous group of conditions. Alcohol is an important aetiological factor in a significant proportion of patients. At least 25% of cases are inherited as an autosomal dominant trait and a variety of single gene mutations have been identified. Most of these mutations affect proteins in the cytoskeleton of the myocyte (e.g. dystrophin, lamin A and C, emerin and metavinculin) and many are associated with minor skeletal muscle abnormalities. Most of the X-linked inherited skeletal muscular dystrophies (e.g. Becker and Duchenne, p. 1254) are associated with cardiomyopathy. Finally, a late autoimmune reaction to viral myocarditis is thought to be the main aetiological factor in a substantial subgroup of patients with dilated cardiomyopathy; a similar mechanism is thought to be responsible for the heart muscle disease that occurs in up to 10% of patients with advanced HIV infection.

In North America and Europe, symptomatic dilated cardiomyopathy has an incidence of 20 per 100 000 and a prevalence of 38 per 100 000. Men are affected more than twice as often as women. Most patients present with heart failure or are found to have the condition during routine investigation. Arrhythmia, thromboembolism and sudden death are common and may occur at any stage; sporadic chest pain is a surprisingly frequent symptom. The ECG usually shows non-specific changes but echocardiography is useful in establishing the diagnosis. Treatment is aimed at controlling the resulting heart failure. Although some patients remain well for many years, the prognosis is variable and cardiac transplantation may be indicated. Patients with dilated cardiomyopathy and moderate or severe heart failure may be at risk of sudden arrhythmic death. This risk is substantially reduced by rigorous medical therapy with β-blockers and angiotensin receptor antagonists. Some patients may be considered for implantation of a cardiac defibrillator and/or cardiac resynchronisation therapy.

HYPERTROPHIC CARDIOMYOPATHY

This is the most common form of cardiomyopathy, with a prevalence of approximately 100 per 100 000, and is characterised by inappropriate and elaborate left ventricular hypertrophy with malalignment of the myocardial fibres. The hypertrophy may be generalised or confined largely to the interventricular septum (asymmetric septal hypertrophy, Fig. 18.105) or other regions (e.g. apical hypertrophic cardiomyopathy, a variant which is common in the Far East).

Heart failure may develop because the stiff non-compliant ventricles impede diastolic filling. Septal hypertrophy may also cause dynamic left ventricular outflow tract obstruction (hypertrophic obstructive cardiomyopathy, or HOCM) and mitral regurgitation due to abnormal systolic anterior motion of the anterior mitral valve leaflet. Effort-related symptoms (angina and breathlessness), arrhythmia and sudden death are the dominant clinical problems.

The condition is a genetic disorder with autosomal dominant transmission, a high degree of penetrance and variable expression. In most patients, the disease appears to be due to a single point mutation in one of the genes that encode sarcomeric contractile proteins. There are three common groups of mutation with different phenotypes. Beta-myosin heavy chain mutations are associated with elaborate ventricular hypertrophy. Troponin mutations are associated with little, and sometimes even no hypertrophy but marked myocardial fibre disarray, an abnormal vascular response (e.g. exercise-induced hypotension) and a high risk of sudden death. Myosin-binding protein C mutations tend to present late in life and are often associated with hypertension and arrhythmia.

Symptoms and signs are similar to those of aortic stenosis, except that in hypertrophic cardiomyopathy the character of the arterial pulse is jerky (Box 18.130).

The ECG is usually abnormal and may show the features of left ventricular hypertrophy with a wide variety of often bizarre abnormalities (e.g. pseudo-infarct pattern, deep T-wave inversion). Echocardiography is usually diagnostic; however, diagnosis may be difficult when another cause of left ventricular hypertrophy is present (e.g. physical training—athletes' heart, hypertension) but the degree of hypertrophy is greater than expected. Genetic testing may facilitate diagnosis in the future.

The natural history is variable but clinical deterioration is often slow. The annual mortality from sudden death is 2–3% among adults and 4–6% in children and adolescents (Box 18.131). Sudden death typically occurs during or just after vigorous physical activity; indeed, hypertrophic cardiomyopathy is the most common cause of sudden death in young athletes. Ventricular arrhythmias are thought to be responsible for many of these deaths.

Beta-blockers and the rate-limiting calcium antagonists (e.g. verapamil) can help to relieve angina and sometimes

---

18.130 CLINICAL FEATURES OF HYPERTROPHIC CARDIOMYOPATHY

Symptoms

- Angina on effort
- Dyspnoea on effort
- Syncope on effort
- Sudden death

Signs

- Jerky pulse*
- Palpable left ventricular hypertrophy
- Double impulse at the apex (palpable fourth heart sound due to left atrial hypertrophy)
- Mid-systolic murmur at the base*
- Pansystolic murmur (due to mitral regurgitation) at the apex

* Signs of left ventricular outflow tract obstruction which may be augmented by standing up (reduced venous return), inotropes and vasodilators (e.g. sublingual nitrate).

18.131 RISK FACTORS FOR SUDDEN DEATH IN HYPERTROPHIC CARDIOMYOPATHY

- A history of previous cardiac arrest or sustained ventricular tachycardia
- Recurrent syncope
- An adverse genotype and/or family history
- Exercise-induced hypotension
- Multiple episodes of non-sustained ventricular tachycardia on ambulatory ECG monitoring
- Marked increase in left ventricular wall thickness

prevent syncopal attacks; however, there is no pharmacological treatment that is definitely known to improve prognosis. Arrhythmias are common and often respond to treatment with amiodarone. Outflow tract obstruction can be improved by partial surgical resection (myectomy) or by iatrogenic infarction of the basal septum (septal ablation) using a catheter-delivered alcohol solution. An implantable cardiac defibrillator (ICD) should be considered in patients with clinical risk factors for sudden death (Box 18.131). Digoxin and vasodilators may increase outflow tract obstruction and should be avoided.

ARRHYTHMOGENIC RIGHT VENTRICULAR DYSPLASIA

In this condition, patches of the right ventricular myocardium are replaced with fibrous and fatty tissue (Fig. 18.105). The disease is inherited as an autosomal dominant trait. The prevalence in the UK is thought to be approximately 10 per 100 000. The dominant clinical problems are ventricular arrhythmias, sudden death and right-sided cardiac failure. The ECG typically shows inverted T waves in the right precordial leads. MRI is a useful diagnostic tool and is often used to screen the first-degree relatives of affected individuals. Patients at high risk of sudden death can be offered an ICD.

OBLITERATIVE CARDIOMYOPATHY

This disease involves the endocardium of one or both ventricles and is characterised by thrombosis and elaborate fibrosis with gradual obliteration of the ventricular cavities (e.g. endomyocardial fibroelastosis, Fig. 18.105). The mitral and tricuspid valves may become regurgitant. Heart failure and pulmonary and systemic embolism are prominent features. It can sometimes be associated with eosinophilia (e.g. eosinophilic leukaemia, Churg–Strauss syndrome, p. 1141). In tropical countries, the disease can be responsible for up to 10% of cardiac deaths. Mortality is high (50% at 2 years). Anticoagulation and antiplatelet therapy are usually advisable, and diuretics may help symptoms of heart failure. Surgery (tricuspid and/or mitral valve replacement with decortication of the endocardium) may be helpful in selected cases.

RESTRICTIVE CARDIOMYOPATHY

In this rare condition, ventricular filling is impaired because the ventricles are 'stiff' (Fig. 18.105). This leads to high atrial pressures with atrial hypertrophy, dilatation and later atrial fibrillation. Amyloidosis is the most common cause of restrictive cardiomyopathy in the UK. However, other forms of infiltration (e.g. glycogen storage diseases), idiopathic perimyocyte fibrosis and a familial form of restrictive cardiomyopathy can present with this form of heart disease. Diagnosis can be very difficult and may require complex Doppler echocardiography, CT or MRI, and endomyocardial biopsy. Treatment is symptomatic but the prognosis is usually poor and transplantation may be indicated.

SPECIFIC DISEASES OF HEART MUSCLE

Many forms of specific heart muscle disease produce a clinical picture that is indistinguishable from dilated cardiomyopathy (e.g. connective tissue disorders, sarcoidosis, haemochromatosis, alcoholic heart muscle disease, Box 18.132). In contrast, amyloidosis and eosinophilic heart disease produce symptoms and signs similar to those found in restrictive or obliterative cardiomyopathy, whereas the heart disease associated with Friedreich's ataxia (pp. 1222–1223) can mimic hypertrophic cardiomyopathy.

Treatment and prognosis are determined by the underlying disorder. Abstention from alcohol may lead to a dramatic improvement in patients with alcoholic heart muscle disease.

18.132 SPECIFIC DISEASES OF HEART MUSCLE

Infections

- Viral, e.g. Coxsackie A and B, influenza, HIV
- Bacterial, e.g. diphtheria, *Borrelia burgdorferi*
- Protozoal, e.g. trypanosomiasis

Endocrine and metabolic disorders

- e.g. Diabetes, hypo- and hyperthyroidism, acromegaly, carcinoid syndrome, phaeochromocytoma, inherited storage diseases

Connective tissue diseases

- e.g. Systemic sclerosis, systemic lupus erythematosus (SLE), polyarteritis nodosa

Infiltrative disorders

- e.g. Haemochromatosis, haemosiderosis, sarcoidosis, amyloidosis

Toxin

- e.g. Doxorubicin, alcohol, cocaine, irradiation

Neuromuscular disorders

- e.g. Dystrophia myotonica, Friedreich's ataxia

CARDIAC TUMOURS

Primary cardiac tumours are rare (< 0.2% of autopsies), but the heart and mediastinum may be the site of metastases.

Most primary tumours are benign (75%), and of these the majority are myxomas. The remainder are fibromas, lipomas, fibroelastomas and haemangiomas.

18

ATRIAL MYXOMA

Myxomas most commonly arise in the left atrium as single or multiple polypoid tumours, attached by a pedicle to the interatrial septum. They are usually gelatinous but may be solid and even calcified, with superimposed thrombus.

The tumour may be detected incidentally on echocardiography, or following investigation of pyrexia, syncope, arrhythmias or emboli. Occasionally, the condition presents with malaise and features suggestive of a connective tissue disorder, including a raised ESR.

On examination the first heart sound is usually loud, and there may be a murmur of mitral regurgitation with a variable diastolic sound (tumour 'plop') due to prolapse of the mass through the mitral valve.

The diagnosis is made on echocardiography and treatment is by surgical excision. If the pedicle is removed, fewer than 5% of tumours recur.

DISEASES OF THE PERICARDIUM

The normal pericardial sac contains about 50 ml of fluid, similar to lymph, which lubricates the surface of the heart. The pericardium limits distension of the heart, contributes to the haemodynamic interdependence of the ventricles, and acts as a barrier to infection. Nevertheless, congenital absence of the pericardium does not appear to result in significant clinical or functional limitations.

ACUTE PERICARDITIS

Aetiology

Pericardial inflammation may be due to infection, immunological reaction, trauma or neoplasm (Box 18.133) and sometimes remains unexplained. Pericarditis and myocarditis often coexist, and all forms of pericarditis may produce a pericardial effusion (see below) which, depending on the aetiology, may be fibrinous, serous, haemorrhagic or purulent.

A fibrinous exudate may eventually lead to varying degrees of adhesion formation, whereas serous pericarditis often produces a large effusion of turbid, straw-coloured fluid with a high protein content.

A haemorrhagic effusion is often due to malignant disease, particularly carcinoma of the breast, carcinoma of the bronchus and lymphoma.

18.133 AETIOLOGY OF ACUTE PERICARDITIS	
Common	
• Acute myocardial infarction	• Viral (e.g. Coxsackie B, but often not identified)
Less common	
• Uraemia	• Trauma (e.g. blunt chest injury)
• Malignant disease	• Connective tissue disease (e.g. SLE)
Rare (in UK)	
• Bacterial infection	• Tuberculosis
• Rheumatic fever	

Purulent pericarditis is rare and may occur as a complication of septicaemia, by direct spread from an intrathoracic infection, or from a penetrating injury.

Clinical features

The characteristic pain of pericarditis is retrosternal, radiates to the shoulders and neck and is typically aggravated by deep breathing, movement, a change of position, exercise and swallowing. A low-grade fever is common.

A pericardial friction rub is a high-pitched superficial scratching or crunching noise produced by movement of the inflamed pericardium, and is diagnostic of pericarditis; it is usually heard in systole but may also be audible in diastole and frequently has a 'to-and-fro' quality.

Investigations

The ECG shows ST elevation with upward concavity (Fig. 18.106) over the affected area, which may be widespread. PR interval depression is a very sensitive indicator of acute pericarditis. Later, there may be T-wave inversion, particularly if there is a degree of myocarditis.

Management

The pain is usually relieved by aspirin (600 mg 4-hourly), but a more potent anti-inflammatory agent such as indometacin (25 mg 8-hourly) may be required. Cortico-

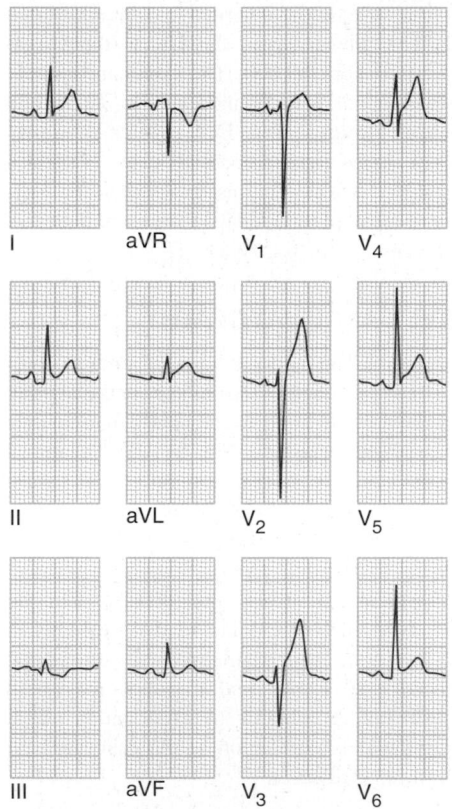

Fig. 18.106 ECG from a young man with viral pericarditis.
Widespread ST elevation (leads I, II, aVL and V_1–V_6) is shown. The upward concave shape of the ST segments (see leads II and V_6) and the unusual distribution of changes (involving anterior and inferior leads) may help to distinguish pericarditis from acute myocardial infarction.

steroids may suppress symptoms but there is no evidence that they accelerate cure.

In viral pericarditis, recovery usually occurs within a few days or weeks, but there may be recurrences (chronic relapsing pericarditis). Purulent pericarditis requires treatment with antimicrobial therapy, paracentesis and, if necessary, surgical drainage.

PERICARDIAL EFFUSION

If a pericardial effusion develops, there is sometimes a sensation of retrosternal oppression. An effusion is difficult to detect clinically; although the heart sounds may become quieter, pericardial friction is not always abolished.

The QRS voltages on the ECG are often reduced in the presence of a large effusion. The QRS complexes may alternate in amplitude due to a to-and-fro motion of the heart within the fluid-filled pericardial sac (electrical alternans). Serial chest X-rays may show a rapid increase in the size of the cardiac shadow over days or even hours, and when there is a large effusion the heart often has a globular or pear-shaped appearance. Echocardiography is the definitive investigation (Fig. 18.107).

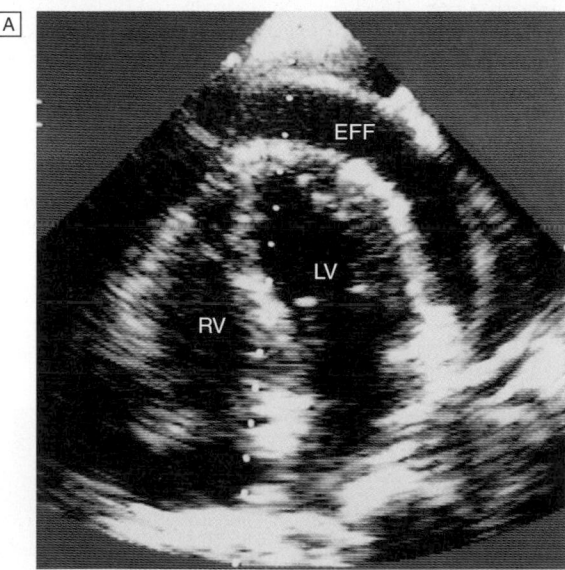

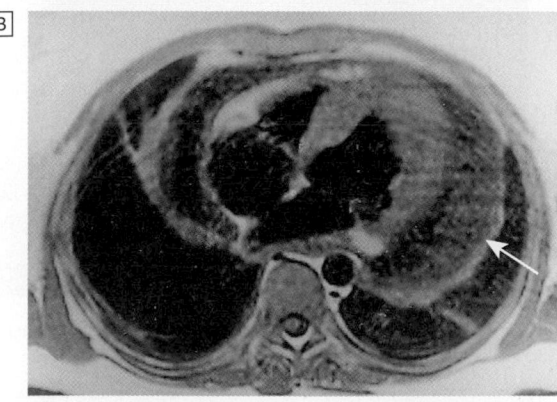

Fig. 18.107 Pericardial effusion. A Echocardiogram (apical view) (effusion is marked EFF). B MRI scan (effusion is marked with an arrow).

Cardiac tamponade

This term is used to describe acute heart failure due to compression of the heart by a large or rapidly developing effusion. Typical physical findings are of a markedly raised jugular venous pulse, hypotension, pulsus paradoxus (p. 526) and oliguria. Atypical presentations may occur when the effusion is loculated as a result of previous pericarditis or cardiac surgery. See also page 542.

Pericardial aspiration

Aspiration of a pericardial effusion may be indicated for diagnostic purposes or for the treatment of cardiac tamponade. It may be accomplished by introducing a needle just medial to the cardiac apex or by inserting a needle below the xiphoid process and directing it towards the left shoulder; the procedure is guided by simultaneous echocardiography. The route of choice will depend on the experience of the operator, the shape of the patient and the position of the effusion. A few millilitres of fluid aspirated through the needle may be sufficient for diagnostic purposes; however, if therapeutic drainage is required, it is safer to use a plastic cannula inserted over a needle or guidewire.

Complications of pericardiocentesis include arrhythmias, damage to a coronary artery, and bleeding with exacerbation of tamponade as a result of injury to the right ventricle. When tamponade is due to cardiac rupture or aortic dissection, pericardial aspiration may precipitate further, potentially fatal bleeding and in these situations emergency surgery is usually the treatment of choice. A viscous, loculated or recurrent effusion may also require formal surgical drainage.

TUBERCULOUS PERICARDITIS

Tuberculous pericarditis may complicate pulmonary tuberculosis but may also be the first manifestation of the infection. In Africa, a tuberculous pericardial effusion is a common feature of AIDS.

The condition typically presents with chronic malaise, weight loss and a low-grade fever. An effusion usually develops and the pericardium may become thick and unyielding, leading to pericardial constriction or tamponade. An associated pleural effusion is often present.

The diagnosis may be confirmed by aspiration of the fluid and direct examination or culture for tubercle bacilli. Treatment requires specific antituberculous chemotherapy (p. 701); in addition, a 3-month course of prednisolone (initial dose 60 mg a day, tapering down rapidly) has been shown to improve outcome.

CHRONIC CONSTRICTIVE PERICARDITIS

Constrictive pericarditis is due to progressive thickening, fibrosis and calcification of the pericardium. In effect, the heart is encased in a solid shell and cannot fill properly; the calcification may extend into the myocardium, so there may also be impaired myocardial contraction.

The condition often follows an attack of tuberculous pericarditis but can also complicate haemopericardium, viral

18.134 CLINICAL FEATURES OF CONSTRICTIVE PERICARDITIS

- Fatigue
- Rapid, low-volume pulse
- Elevated jugular venous pulse (JVP) with a rapid *y* descent
- Kussmaul's sign (a paradoxical rise in the JVP during inspiration)
- Loud early third heart sound or 'pericardial knock'
- Hepatomegaly
- Ascites
- Peripheral oedema
- Pulsus paradoxus (an excessive fall in blood pressure during inspiration), present in some cases

pericarditis, rheumatoid arthritis and purulent pericarditis. It is often impossible to identify the original insult.

Clinical features

The symptoms and signs of systemic venous congestion are the hallmarks of constrictive pericarditis; atrial fibrillation is common and there is often dramatic ascites and hepatomegaly (Box 18.134). Breathlessness is not a prominent symptom because the lungs are seldom congested.

The condition is sometimes overlooked and should be suspected in any patient with unexplained right heart failure and a small heart. A chest X-ray, which may show pericardial calcification (Fig. 18.108), and echocardiography often help to establish the diagnosis. CT and MRI are also useful techniques for imaging the pericardium.

Constrictive pericarditis is often difficult to distinguish from restrictive cardiomyopathy and the final diagnosis may depend on complex echo-Doppler studies and cardiac catheterisation.

Management

Surgical resection of the diseased pericardium can lead to a dramatic improvement but carries a high morbidity and produces disappointing results in up to 50% of patients.

FURTHER INFORMATION

Books and journal articles

Grubb N, Newby D. Churchill's pocketbook of cardiology. 2nd edn. Edinburgh: Churchill Livingstone; 2006.

Newby D, Grubb N. Cardiology: an illustrated colour text. Edinburgh: Churchill Livingstone; 2005.

Sicilian Gambit. The search for novel antiarrhythmic strategies. European Heart Journal 1998; 19(8):1178–96. Review.

Zipes D, Libby P, Bonow R, Braunwald H, eds. Braunwald's heart disease: a textbook of cardiovascular medicine. 7th edn. Philadelphia: WB Saunders; 2005.

Websites

www.acc.org *The website of the American College of Cardiology (ACC) gives free access to guidelines for the evaluation and management of many cardiac conditions.*

www.americanheart.org *The website of the American Heart Association (AHA) gives free access to all the ACC/AHA/ESC guidelines and AHA scientific statements. It is useful for fact sheets for patients about cardiac conditions.*

www.escardio.org *The website of the European College of Cardiology (ESC) provides free access to guidelines for the diagnosis and management of many cardiac conditions. It also provides free access for educational modules for self-directed learning.*

www.nice.org.uk *The evidence-base for cardiology is extensive. The evidence for a number of treatments and procedures in cardiology is reviewed.*

www.sign.ac.uk *Clear and evidence-based guidelines on the management of most common cardiac conditions.*

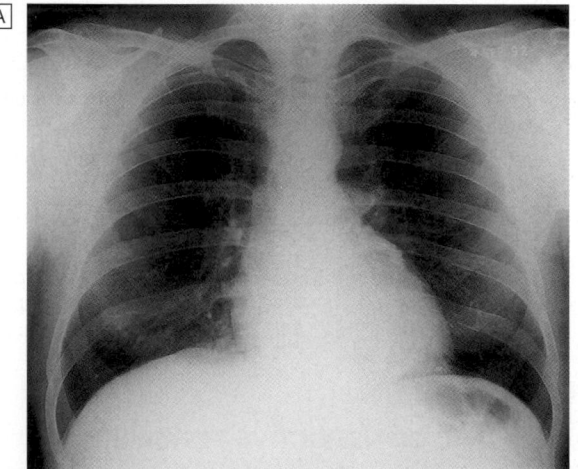
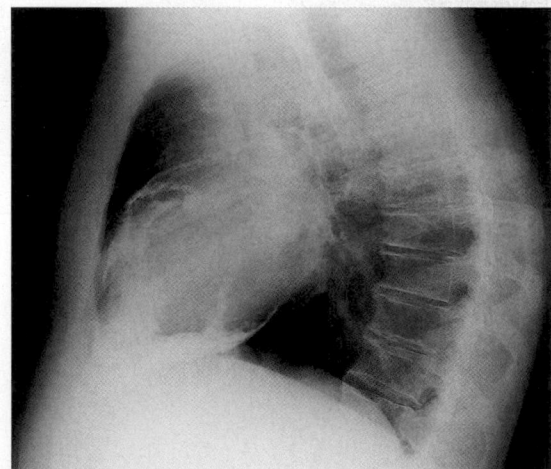

Fig. 18.108   Chest X-rays from a patient with severe heart failure due to chronic constrictive pericarditis. The heart is not enlarged and there is heavy calcification of the pericardium that is most visible on the lateral film. **A** PA X-ray. **B** Lateral X-ray.

J.A. INNES
P.T. REID

Respiratory disease

CLINICAL EXAMINATION OF THE RESPIRATORY SYSTEM

19

Thorax 6 — 10
(see opposite)

Inspection 6
Deformity
(e.g. pectus excavatum)
Scars
Intercostal indrawing
Symmetry of expansion
Hyperinflation
Paradoxical rib movement
(low flat diaphragm)

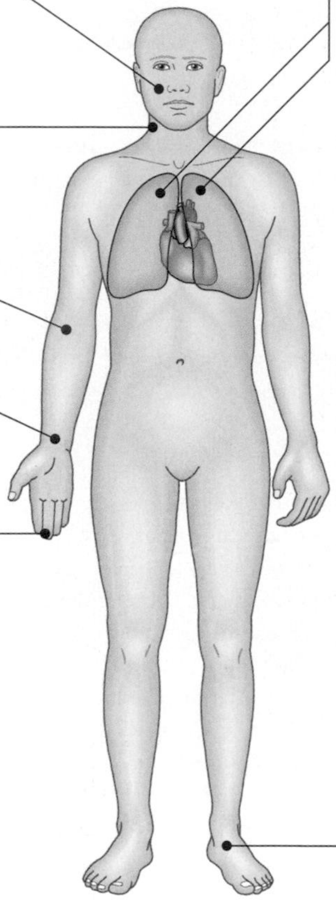

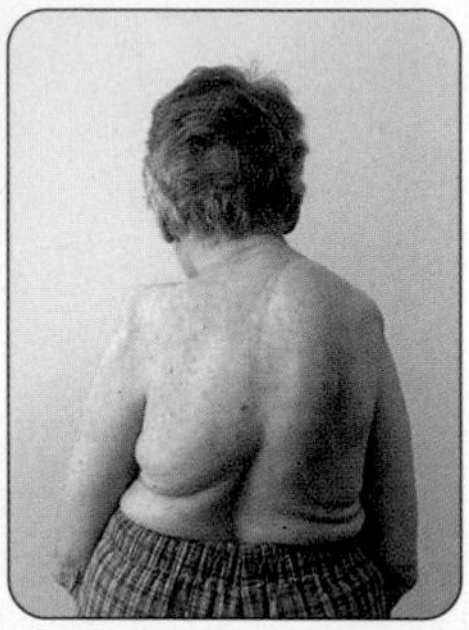

▲ Idiopathic kyphoscoliosis

Face, mouth and eyes 5
Pursed lips?
Central cyanosis?
Anaemia?
Horner's syndrome
(Ch. 26)

Jugular venous pulse 4
Elevated?
Pulsatile?

Blood pressure 3
Arterial paradox?

Radial pulse 2
Rate
Rhythm

Hands 1
Digital clubbing
Tar staining
Peripheral cyanosis
Signs of occupation
CO_2 retention flap

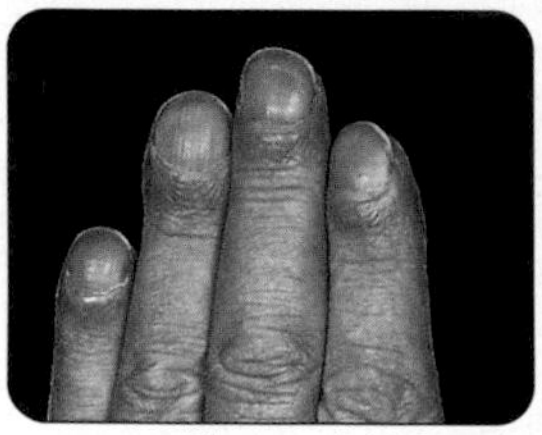

Finger clubbing ▲

7 Palpation
From the front:
Trachea central
Cricosternal distance
Cardiac apex displaced?
Expansion
From behind:
Cervical lymphadenopathy
Expansion

8 Percussion
Resonant? Dull?
'Stony dull' (effusion)

9 Auscultation
Breath sounds:
normal, bronchial, louder or softer?
Added sounds:
wheezes, crackles, rubs
Spoken voice (vocal resonance):
absent (effusion), increased
(consolidation)?
Whispered voice:
whispering pectoriloquy

10 Leg oedema
? Cor pulmonale
? Venous thrombosis

Observation

- Respiratory rate
- Cachexia, fever, rash?
- Sputum (see below)
- Fetor
- Locale
  Oxygen delivery (mask, cannulae)
  Nebulisers
  Inhalers

Sputum

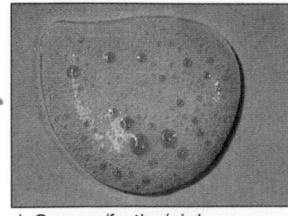
▲ Serous/frothy/pink
Pulmonary oedema

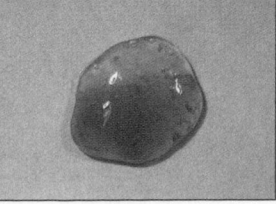
▲ Mucopurulent
Bronchial or pneumonic
infection

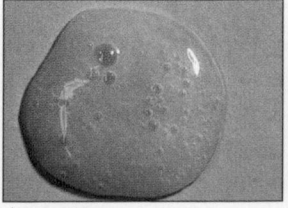
▲ Purulent
Bronchial or pneumonic
infection

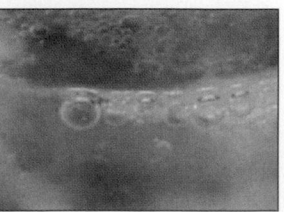
▲ Blood-stained
Cancer, tuberculosis,
bronchiectasis,
pulmonary embolism

6–10 KEY FEATURES ON EXAMINATION OF COMMON RESPIRATORY CONDITIONS

Chronic obstructive pulmonary disease

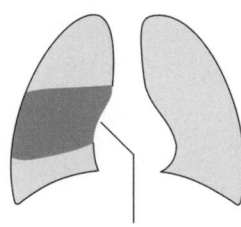

Pursed lip breathing
Central cyanosis
Prolonged expiration

Reduced cricosternal distance

Intercostal indrawing during inspiration

Cardiac apex not palpable
Loss of cardiac dullness on percussion

Use of accessory muscles

Hyperinflated 'barrel' chest

Auscultation
  Reduced breath sounds ± wheeze

Heart sounds loudest in epigastrium

Inward movement of lower ribs on inspiration (low flat diaphragm)

Also: raised JVP, peripheral oedema if cor pulmonale

Pulmonary fibrosis

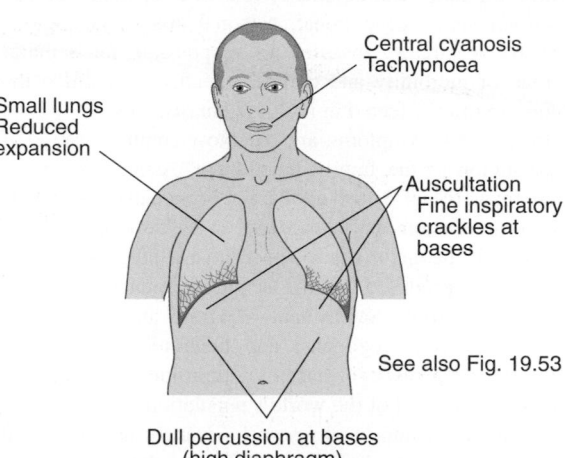

Central cyanosis
Tachypnoea

Small lungs
Reduced expansion

Auscultation
Fine inspiratory crackles at bases

See also Fig. 19.53

Dull percussion at bases
(high diaphragm)

Also: finger clubbing common in idiopathic pulmonary fibrosis; raised JVP and peripheral oedema if cor pulmonale

Right middle lobe pneumonia

Febrile ± rigors
In pain (if pleurisy)
Purulent sputum

Inspection
  Tachypnoea
  Central cyanosis (if severe)
Palpation
  ↓Expansion on R
Percussion
  Dull R midzone and axilla
Auscultation
  Bronchial breath sounds and ↑vocal resonance over consolidation
  Pleural rub if pleurisy

Obscures R heart border on X-ray (Fig. 19.33)

Right upper lobe collapse

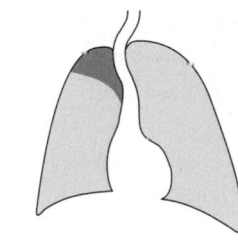

Inspection
  ↓Volume R upper zone
Palpation
  Trachea deviated to R
  ↓Expansion R upper zone
Percussion
  Dull R upper zone
Auscultation
  ↓Breath sounds with central obstruction

X-ray
  Deviated trachea (to R)
  Elevated horizontal fissure
  ↓Volume R hemithorax
  Central (hilar) mass may be seen

Left pneumothorax

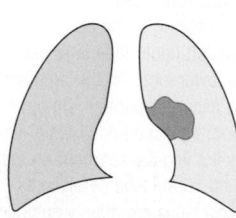

Inspection
  Tachypnoea (pain, deflation reflex)
Palpation
  ↓Expansion L side
Percussion
  Resonant or hyper-resonant on L
Auscultation
  Absent breath sounds on L

'Tension' pneumothorax also causes
  Deviation of trachea to opposite side
  Tachycardia and hypotension

Large right pleural effusion

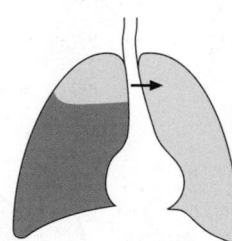

Inspection
  Tachypnoea
Palpation
  ↓Expansion on R
  Trachea and apex may be moved to L
Percussion
  Stony dull
  R mid- and lower zones
Auscultation
  Absent breath sounds and vocal resonance R base
  Crackles above effusion

19

The lungs, with their combined alveolar surface area of around 140 m², are directly open to the external environment. Thus structural, functional or microbiological changes within the lungs can be closely related to epidemiological, environmental, occupational, personal and social factors. Primary respiratory diseases are responsible for a major burden of morbidity and untimely deaths. In addition the lungs are often affected in multisystem diseases.

Respiratory symptoms are the most common cause of presentation to the family practitioner. Asthma occurs in more than 10% of British adults, and bronchial carcinoma is the most common fatal malignancy in the developed world. The lung is the major site of opportunistic infection in those immunocompromised by the acquired immunodeficiency syndrome (AIDS) or by anti-allograft and anti-cancer chemotherapeutic regimens; and tuberculosis (including multiple drug-resistant strains) continues to increase, infecting one-third of the world's population.

A number of important research advances have occurred in recent years. Greater understanding of the genetics and cell biology of the lung has opened the way to novel therapies, including treatments targeting inflammatory mechanisms and the possibility of airway-delivered gene therapy for cystic fibrosis. Finally, recent advances in our understanding of the cellular and molecular mechanisms underlying diseases such as asthma and the acute respiratory distress syndrome (ARDS) are likely to lead to rational, mechanism-based therapy within the foreseeable future.

FUNCTIONAL ANATOMY, PHYSIOLOGY AND INVESTIGATIONS

APPLIED ANATOMY AND PHYSIOLOGY

The conducting airways, from nose to the alveoli, connect the external environment with the extensive, thin and vulnerable alveolar surface. As air is inhaled through the upper airways it is filtered (in the nose), heated to body temperature and fully saturated with water vapour; partial recovery of this heat and moisture occurs on expiration. Total airway cross-section rises steeply from the narrowest point at the glottis to over 300 cm² in the third-generation respiratory bronchioles. As a result, in the trachea and large bronchi airspeed is high and the airway is particularly vulnerable to obstruction by foreign bodies and tumours. Airway patency is maintained by the cough reflex and by reinforcing cartilage rings. Normal breath sounds originate mainly from the rapid turbulent airflow in the larynx and in these central airways.

The multitude of small airways within the lung parenchyma lack structural stiffness and are kept patent in health by radial traction from the network of elastin fibres in surrounding alveolar walls. Airflow is slow and normally silent in these airways, and gas transport occurs largely by diffusion in the final generations. Major bronchial and pulmonary divisions are shown in Figure 19.1. (See also bronchoscopic appearances in Fig. 19.8, p. 655.)

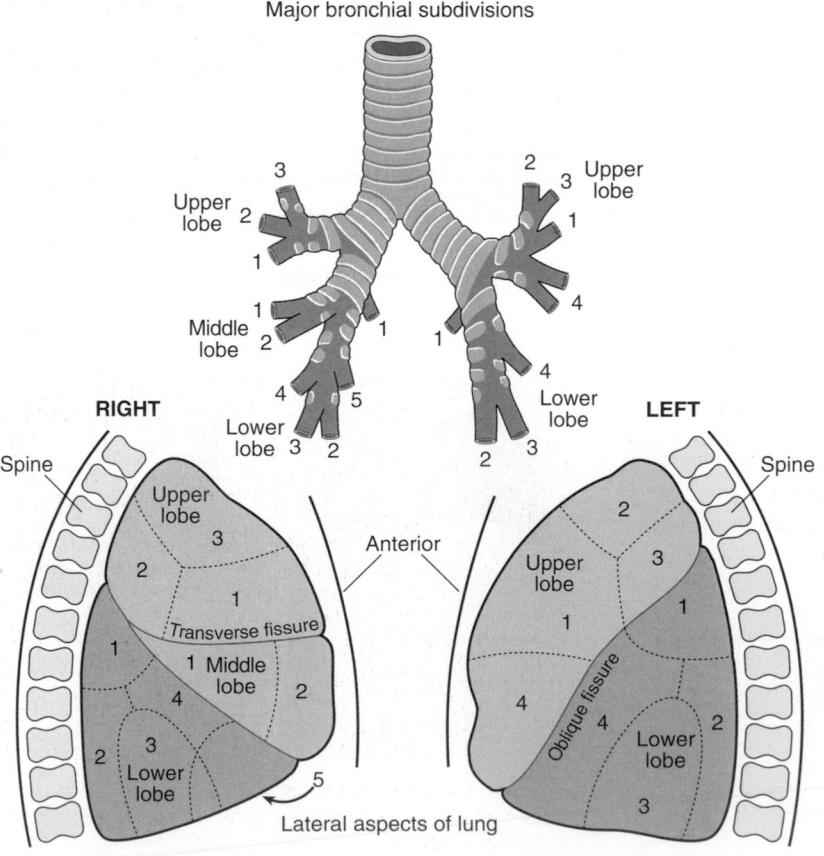

Fig. 19.1 The major bronchial divisions and the fissures, lobes and segments of the lungs. The position of the oblique fissure is such that the left upper lobe is largely anterior to the lower lobe. On the right side the transverse fissure separates the upper from the anteriorly placed middle lobe which is matched by the lingular segment on the left side. The site of the lobe determines whether physical signs are mainly anterior or posterior. Each lobe is composed of two or more bronchopulmonary segments, i.e. the lung tissue supplied by the main branches of each lobar bronchus. BRONCHOPULMONARY SEGMENTS: **Right**—*Upper lobe* (1) Anterior (2) Posterior (3) Apical. *Middle lobe* (1) Lateral (2) Medial. *Lower lobe* (1) Apical (2) Posterior basal (3) Lateral basal (4) Anterior basal (5) Medial basal. **Left**—*Upper lobe* (1) Anterior (2) Apical (3) Posterior (4) Lingular. *Lower lobe* (1) Apical (2) Posterior basal (3) Lateral basal (4) Anterior basal.

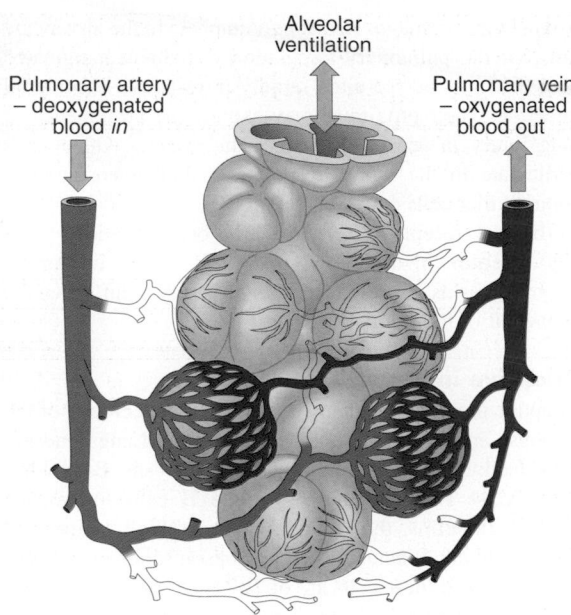

Fig. 19.2 The acinus—the basic gas exchange unit of the lung.

The acinus is the gas exchange unit of the lung (Fig. 19.2) and comprises branching respiratory bronchioles and clusters of alveoli. Here, filtered, moistened and heated air makes close contact with the pulmonary capillaries (gas-to-blood distance < 0.4 μm) and oxygen uptake and CO_2 excretion occurs. The alveoli are lined with flattened epithelial cells (type I pneumocytes), and a few, more cuboidal, type II pneumocytes. The latter produce surfactant, a mixture of phospholipids, which reduces surface tension and counteracts the tendency of alveoli to collapse. Type II pneumocytes can also divide to reconstitute the type I pneumocytes after lung injury.

VENTILATION, PERFUSION, DIFFUSION AND GAS EXCHANGE

Gravity determines the distribution of ventilation and blood flow in the lungs, with most ventilation and perfusion going to dependent zones. Locally, hypoxia constricts pulmonary arterioles and airway CO_2 dilates bronchi, helping to maintain good matching of ventilation and perfusion within pulmonary segments.

Diseases which impair ventilation locally result in some desaturated and CO_2-laden blood entering the pulmonary veins, causing arterial hypoxaemia. Increased ventilation of remaining normal lung units can increase CO_2 excretion, correcting arterial CO_2 to normal, but cannot augment oxygen uptake or correct hypoxaemia, because maximal oxygen uptake in these normal lung units is limited by the capacity of haemoglobin. The resulting pattern of blood gas abnormality is hypoxia with normocapnia, which is sometimes termed 'type I respiratory failure'. Diseases causing this abnormality are listed in Box 19.18 (p. 668) and management of respiratory failure is discussed on page 667.

Hypoxia with hypercapnia (type II respiratory failure) is seen if there is severe generalised ventilation–perfusion mismatch (insufficient normal lung to correct CO_2) or a disease which reduces total ventilation. The latter category includes not just diseases of the lung or chest wall but also diseases affecting any part of the neuromuscular mechanism of ventilation; for example, brain injury, narcotic poisoning, polyneuropathies or myopathies (Box 19.18, p. 668).

In addition to causing ventilation–perfusion mismatch, diseases which destroy or thicken the alveolar capillary membrane (e.g. emphysema or fibrosis) can directly impair gas diffusion.

The pulmonary circulation in health operates at low pressure (approximately 24/9 mmHg), and can accommodate large increases in flow (e.g. during exercise) without much rise in pressure. Pulmonary hypertension may result when pulmonary vessels are destroyed by emphysema, obstructed by thrombus or involved in interstitial inflammation or fibrosis. The right ventricle responds by hypertrophy, with right axis deviation and P pulmonale on the ECG. Pulmonary hypertension with hypoxia and hypercapnia may lead to generalised salt and water retention (cor pulmonale) with elevation of the jugular venous pressure (JVP) and peripheral oedema.

LUNG DEFENCES

UPPER AIRWAY DEFENCES

Most large particles are trapped by nasal hairs, and smaller particles are cleared towards the oropharynx by the columnar ciliated epithelium which covers the turbinates and septum (Fig. 19.3). During cough, expiratory muscle effort against a closed glottis results in high intrathoracic pressure, which is then released explosively. The flexible posterior tracheal wall is pushed inwards by the high pressure, reducing cross-section and maximising the airspeed to achieve effective expectoration. The larynx also acts as a sphincter protecting the airway during swallowing and vomiting.

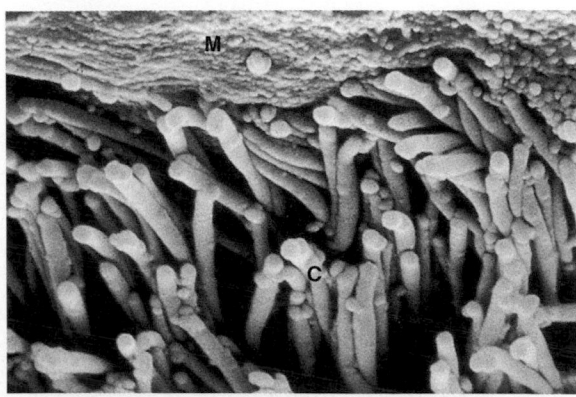

Fig. 19.3 The mucociliary escalator. Scanning electron micrograph of the respiratory epithelium showing large numbers of cilia (C) overlaid by the mucus 'raft' (M).

19

LOWER AIRWAY DEFENCES

The sterility, structure and function of the lower airways are maintained by close cooperation between the innate and adaptive immune responses.

Innate immune defence

The innate response is characterised by a number of non-specific defence mechanisms. Inhaled particulate matter is trapped in airway mucus and cleared by the mucociliary escalator. Cigarette smoke increases mucus secretion but reduces mucociliary clearance and contributes to enhanced propensity for lower respiratory tract infections including pneumonia. Defective mucociliary transport is also a feature of several rare diseases including Kartagener's syndrome, Young's syndrome and ciliary dysmotility syndrome, which are characterised by repeated pulmonary infections and bronchiectasis.

Airway secretions contain an array of antimicrobial peptides, antiproteinases and antioxidants (Box 19.1). Many of these molecules assist with the opsonisation and killing of bacteria and the regulation of the powerful proteolytic enzymes secreted by inflammatory cells. In particular, α_1-antiproteinase (A1Pi) regulates neutrophil elastase and deficiency of A1Pi has been linked to the appearance of premature emphysema.

Professional phagocytes such as macrophages engulf microbes, organic dusts and other particulate matter (Fig. 19.4). Inorganic agents such as asbestos or silica overwhelm the macrophages causing death by necrosis and the release of powerful proteolytic enzymes that cause parenchymal damage. Neutrophil numbers in the airway are low, but the pulmonary circulation contains a marginated pool that may be recruited rapidly in response to bacterial infection. Their proximity may explain the prominence of lung injury in sepsis syndromes and trauma. Other cells participate in the innate response, including eosinophils, natural killer cells and mast cells.

Toll-like receptors have recently been identified as a key receptor involved in mediating innate immunity. Polymorphisms of these receptors are likely to influence the behaviour of the immune response.

Adaptive immune defence

Adaptive immunity is characterised by the specificity of the response and the development of memory. Lung dendritic cells facilitate antigen presentation to T- and B-lymphocytes. CD4 T-helper cells assist the B cells to produce immunoglobulins that neutralise microbial toxins and initiate a highly efficient process of opsonisation and phagocytic killing. If these cells are of Th2 type, they promote the production of IgE and hence predispose to allergy. Other responses lead to the manufacture of IgM, IgG and IgA antibodies.

The innate and adaptive immune responses are co-ordinated by an array of cytokines which are critical in initiating, regulating and terminating the response and in coordinating the repair processes.

INVESTIGATION OF RESPIRATORY DISEASE

A detailed history, thorough examination and basic haematological and biochemical tests usually suggest the

---

19.1 PROTECTIVE AGENTS IN THE EPITHELIAL LUNG FLUID

- Defensins
- Secretory lactoperoxidase A_2
- Lactoperoxidase
- IgA
- Lysozyme
- Lactoferrin
- Surfactant proteins (collectins)
- Antiproteinases: α_1-antiproteinase, secretory leucocyte protease inhibitor (SLPI), elafin
- Antioxidants: glutathione

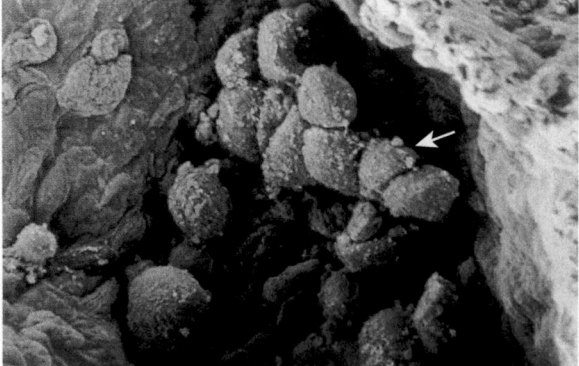

Fig. 19.4 Alveolar macrophages. Scanning electron micrograph showing alveolar macrophages (arrow) patrolling the alveolar spaces of the lung.

19.2 RESPIRATORY FUNCTION IN OLD AGE

- **Reserve capacity**: this is vast so a significant reduction in function can occur with ageing with only minimal effect on normal breathing, although the ability to combat acute intercurrent disease is reduced.
- **Decline in FEV_1**: the FEV_1/FVC ratio falls by around 0.2% per year from 70% at the age of 40–45 years, due to a decline in elastic recoil in the small airways with age. Smoking accelerates this decline threefold on average. Symptoms only occur when FEV_1 drops below 50% of predicted.
- **Increasing ventilation–perfusion mismatch**: the reduction in elastic recoil causes a tendency for the small airways to collapse during expiration, particularly in dependent areas of the lungs, thus reducing ventilation.
- **Reduced ventilatory responses to hypoxia and hypercapnia**: older people may be less tachypnoeic for any given fall in PaO_2 or rise in $PaCO_2$.
- **Impaired defences against infection**: due to reduced numbers of glandular epithelial cells which leads to a reduction in protective mucus.
- **Decline in maximum oxygen uptake**: due to a combination of changes in muscles, and the respiratory and cardiovascular systems. This leads to a reduction in cardiorespiratory reserve and exercise capacity.
- **Loss of chest wall compliance**: due to reduced intervertebral disc spaces and ossification of the costal cartilages; respiratory muscle strength and endurance also decline. These changes only become important in the presence of other respiratory disease.

likely diagnosis and certain key differentials. However, a number of further investigations are usually required to finalise the diagnosis and/or monitor disease activity.

IMAGING

The 'plain' chest X-ray

Chest radiography is performed on the majority of patients suspected of having chest disease. A postero-anterior (PA) film provides information on the lung fields, heart, mediastinum, vascular structures and the thoracic cage. Additional information may be obtained from a lateral film, particularly if pathology is suspected behind the heart shadow or deep in the diaphragmatic sulci. Common abnormalities are summarised in Box 19.3.

Increased shadowing may represent accumulation of fluid, lobar collapse or consolidation. Uncomplicated consolidation should not change the position of the mediastinum and the presence of an air bronchogram provides reassurance that proximal bronchi are patent. Collapse (implying obstruction of the proximal bronchus) is accompanied by loss of volume and displacement of the mediastinum towards the affected side.

The presence of ring shadows (diseased bronchi seen end-on), tramline shadows (diseased bronchi side-on) or tubular shadows (bronchi filled with secretions) suggests bronchiectasis. Nodular, reticular or honeycomb patterns are characteristic of diffuse parenchymal lung diseases. The presence of pleural fluid is suggested by a dense basal shadow which, in the erect patient, ascends towards the axilla. The assessment of a solitary pulmonary nodule is discussed below.

In large pulmonary embolism relative oligaemia may cause a lung field to appear abnormally dark. Increased translucency is seen with emphysematous bullae or a pneumothorax.

Computed tomography (CT)

CT scanning provides detailed images of the pulmonary parenchyma, mediastinum, pleura and bony structures. The contrast can be altered to highlight different structures such as the lung parenchyma, the mediastinal vascular structures or bone. Sophisticated software facilitates 3D reconstruction of the thorax and virtual bronchoscopy.

CT scanning is superior to chest radiography in determining the position and size of a pulmonary lesion and whether calcification or cavitation is present. It is now routinely used in the assessment of patients with suspected lung cancer and facilitates guided percutaneous needle biopsy. Information on tumour stage may be gained by examining the mediastinum, liver and adrenal glands.

High-resolution CT (HRCT) scanning uses thin sections to provide a detailed assessment of the pulmonary parenchyma and is particularly useful in assessing diffuse parenchymal lung disease, identifying bronchiectasis (Fig. 19.5), and assessing the type and extent of emphysema.

CT pulmonary angiography (CTPA) is increasingly used in the diagnosis of pulmonary thromboembolism (Fig. 19.58, p. 727), where it may either confirm the suspected embolism or highlight an alternative diagnosis.

Ultrasound

Ultrasound is sensitive at detecting pleural fluid and may also be used to direct and improve the diagnostic yield from pleural biopsy. Information may also be provided on the anatomy of an empyema cavity and facilitate directed drainage.

19

19.3 COMMON CHEST X-RAY APPEARANCES

Increased lucency

- Consolidation: infection, infarction, inflammation, and rarely bronchoalveolar cell carcinoma
- Lobar collapse: mucus plugging, tumour, compression by lymph nodes
- Solitary nodule: see text
- Multiple nodules: miliary TB, dust inhalation, metastatic malignancy, healed varicella pneumonia, rheumatoid disease
- Ring shadows, tramlines and tubular shadows: bronchiectasis
- Cavitating lesions: tumour, abscess, infarct, pneumonia (*Staphylococcus/Klebsiella*), Wegener's granulomatosis
- Reticular, nodular and reticulonodular shadows: diffuse parenchymal lung disease, infection
- Pleural abnormalities: fluid, plaques, tumour

Increased translucency

- Bullae
- Pneumothorax
- Oligaemia

Hilar abnormalities

- Unilateral hilar enlargement: TB, bronchial carcinoma, lymphoma
- Bilateral hilar enlargement: sarcoid, lymphoma, TB, silicosis

Other abnormalities

- Hiatus hernia
- Surgical emphysema

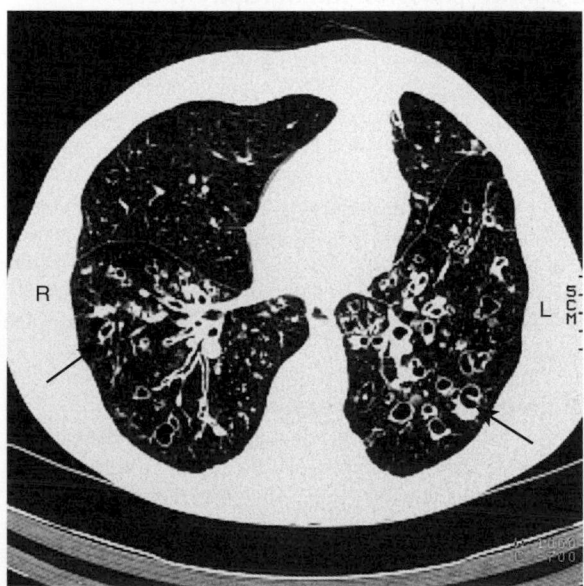

Fig. 19.5 Computed tomography of the thorax. This scan shows extensive dilatation of the bronchi (bronchiectasis) with thickened walls (arrows) in both lower lobes.

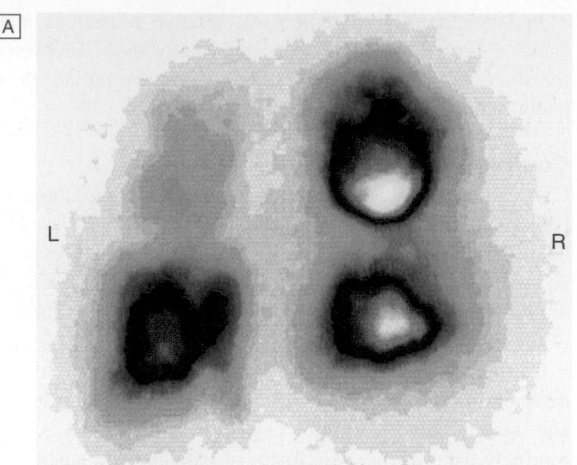
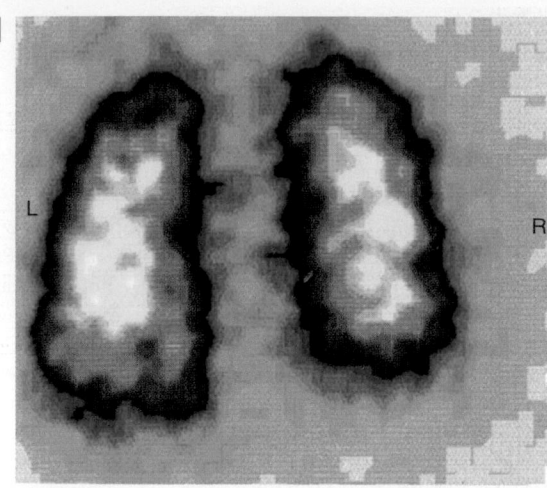

Fig. 19.6 Lung ventilation and perfusion scintigraphy. Ⓐ Multiple perfusion defects present in left upper zone and right midzone of perfusion scan. Ⓑ Normal ventilation scan. The appearances indicate a high probability of recent pulmonary embolism.

Ventilation–perfusion imaging

The main value of this technique is in the detection of pulmonary thromboemboli. Ventilation is assessed by inhalation of ^{133}Xe and perfusion by the injection of macroaggregates of ^{99m}Tc-albumin. A 'filling defect' in the perfusion scan accompanied by preserved ventilation (V̇/Q̇ mismatch) is highly suggestive of a recent pulmonary embolism (Fig. 19.6). However, the applicability of this technique is limited in patients with underlying lung disease in whom as many as 70% of scans may be non-contributory. Ventilation–perfusion scanning is also useful in pre-operative assessment of the functional effects of lung cancer and bullae.

Positron emission tomography (PET)

PET scanners exploit the avid ability of malignant tissue to absorb and metabolise glucose. The radiotracer ^{18}F-fluorodeoxyglucose (FDG) is administered and rapidly taken up by malignant tissue. It is then phosphorylated but cannot be metabolised further, becoming 'trapped' in the cell. PET scanning is useful in the investigation of pulmonary nodules, and in staging mediastinal lymph nodes and distal metastatic disease in patients with lung cancer. The negative predictive value is high; however, the positive predictive value is poor. Co-registration of PET and CT (PET-CT) enhances localisation and characterisation of the metabolic abnormalities.

Pulmonary angiography

Conventional pulmonary angiography is performed by passing contrast medium down a catheter inserted via the femoral vein into the main pulmonary artery (Fig. 19.7). The technique represents the gold standard for the diagnosis of pulmonary embolism but is rarely used, particularly now that CTPA is widely available. It is essential in the investigation of patients with pulmonary hypertension, providing information on pulmonary and right heart pressures.

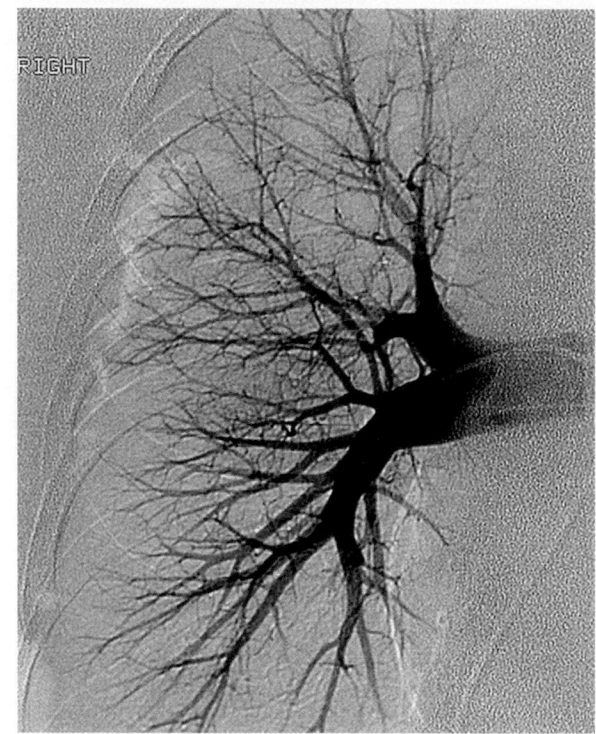

Fig. 19.7 Normal digital subtraction pulmonary angiogram of the right lung.

ENDOSCOPIC EXAMINATION

Laryngoscopy

The larynx may be inspected indirectly with a mirror or directly with a laryngoscope. Fibreoptic instruments allow a magnified view to be obtained.

Bronchoscopy

The trachea (Fig. 19.8) and larger bronchi may be inspected by either a flexible or a rigid bronchoscope. Flexible

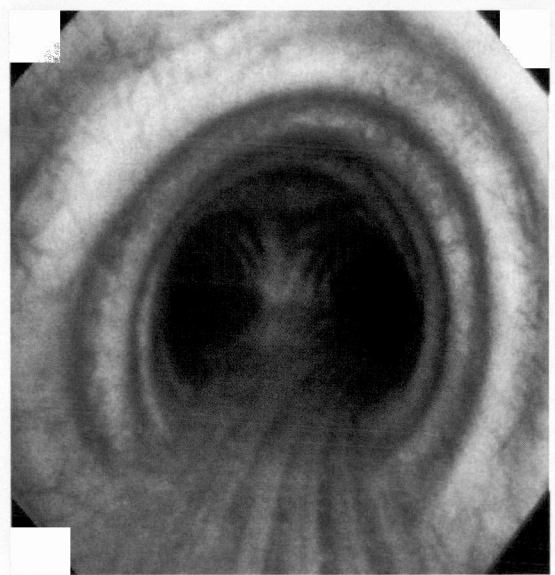

Fig. 19.8 Bronchoscopic appearances of the lower trachea, carina and the right and left main bronchi.

bronchoscopy may be performed under local anaesthesia with sedation as an outpatient. Structural changes, such as distortion or obstruction, can be seen. Abnormal tissue in the bronchial lumen or wall can be biopsied, and bronchial brushings, washings or aspirates can be taken for cytological or bacteriological examination. Small biopsy specimens of lung tissue taken by forceps passed through the bronchial wall (transbronchial biopsies) may reveal sarcoid granulomas or malignant diseases and may be helpful in diagnosing certain bronchocentric disorders (e.g. hypersensitivity pneumonitis, cryptogenic organising pneumonia), but are generally too small to be of diagnostic value in other diffuse parenchymal pulmonary disease (p. 713). Transbronchial needle aspiration (TBNA) may sample mediastinal lymph nodes and assist with staging of lung cancer. Endobronchial ultrasound is currently undergoing assessment as a method of directing and enhancing the diagnostic yield of TBNA.

Rigid bronchoscopy requires general anaesthesia but is more advantageous in certain situations e.g. evaluating massive haemoptysis or removing foreign bodies. In addition, endobronchial laser therapy and endobronchial stenting may be more easily performed with rigid bronchoscopy.

Assessment of the mediastinum

Lymph nodes down to the main carina can be sampled using a mediastinoscope passed through a small incision at the suprasternal notch under general anaesthetic. This procedure is particularly useful in lung cancer as a means of determining whether nodal disease is present. Lymph nodes in the lower mediastinum may be biopsied using an alternative and less invasive method, endoscopic ultrasound (EUS). In this technique an oesophageal endoscope equipped with an ultrasound transducer and biopsy needle is used to aspirate a sample for cytology.

Pleural aspiration and biopsy

Pleural aspiration and biopsy using an Abram's needle is a 'blind' procedure but often provides histological evidence of the cause of a pleural effusion. In difficult cases, video-assisted thoracoscopy may be used to obtain pleural or lung biopsies.

SKIN TESTS

The tuberculin test (p. 700) may be of value in the diagnosis of tuberculosis. Skin hypersensitivity tests are useful in the investigation of allergic diseases.

IMMUNOLOGICAL AND SEROLOGICAL TESTS

The presence of pneumococcal antigen (revealed by counterimmunoelectrophoresis) in sputum, blood or urine may be of diagnostic importance. Exfoliated cells colonised by influenza A virus (p. 688) can be detected by fluorescent antibody techniques. In blood, high or rising antibody titres to specific organisms (such as *Legionella*, *Mycoplasma*, *Chlamydia* or viruses) may eventually clinch a diagnosis suspected on clinical grounds. Precipitating antibodies may be found as a reaction to fungi such as *Aspergillus* (p. 703) or to antigens involved in hypersensitivity pneumonitis (p. 718).

MICROBIOLOGICAL INVESTIGATIONS

Sputum, pleural fluid, throat swabs, blood and bronchial washings and aspirates can be examined for bacteria, fungi and viruses. In some cases, as when *Mycobacterium tuberculosis* is isolated, the information is diagnostically conclusive but in other circumstances the findings must be interpreted in conjunction with the results of clinical and radiological examination.

HISTOPATHOLOGICAL AND CYTOLOGICAL EXAMINATION

Histopathological examination of biopsy material (obtained from pleura, lymph node or lung) often allows a 'tissue diagnosis' to be made. This is of particular importance in suspected malignancy or in elucidating the pathological changes in interstitial lung disease (p. 713). Important causative organisms, such as *M. tuberculosis*, *Pneumocystis carinii* (now *jirovecii*) or fungi, may be identified in bronchial washings, brushings or transbronchial biopsies.

Cytological examination of exfoliated cells in sputum, pleural fluid or bronchial brushings and washings or of fine-needle aspirates from lymph nodes or pulmonary lesions can support a diagnosis of malignancy but if this is indeterminate a tissue biopsy is necessary to confirm the diagnosis. Cellular patterns in bronchial lavage fluid may help to distinguish pulmonary changes due to sarcoidosis (p. 715) from those caused by idiopathic pulmonary fibrosis (p. 714) or hypersensitivity pneumonitis (p. 718).

RESPIRATORY FUNCTION TESTING

Respiratory function tests are used to aid diagnosis, assess functional impairment and monitor treatment or progression

19

19

19.4 ABBREVIATIONS USED IN RESPIRATORY FUNCTION TESTING	
Abbreviation	Stands for
FEV$_1$	Forced expiratory volume in 1 second
FVC	Forced vital capacity
VC	Vital capacity (relaxed)
PEF	Peak (maximum) expiratory flow
TLC	Total lung capacity
FRC	Functional residual capacity
RV	Residual volume
TL$_{CO}$	Gas transfer factor for carbon monoxide
K$_{CO}$	Gas transfer per unit lung volume

of disease. Common abbreviations used in respiratory function testing are shown in Box 19.4.

In diseases characterised by airway narrowing (e.g. asthma, bronchitis and emphysema) maximum expiratory flow is limited by dynamic compression of small intra-thoracic airways, some of which close completely during expiration, limiting the volume which can be expired. Hyperinflation of the chest results, and can become extreme if elastic recoil is also lost due to parenchymal destruction, as in emphysema. In contrast, diseases which cause lung inflammation and/or scarring and fibrosis are characterised by progressive loss of lung volume with normal expiratory flow rates. Gas exchange is impaired by both parenchymal destruction (emphysema) and by interstitial disease, which disrupts the local matching of ventilation and perfusion.

In respiratory function testing, airway narrowing, lung volume and gas exchange capacity are quantified and compared with normal values adjusted for age, gender, height and ethnic origin.

Airway narrowing is assessed by forced expiration into a peak flow meter or a spirometer. Peak flow meters are cheap and convenient for home monitoring (e.g. detection and monitoring of asthma) but values are effort-dependent. The forced expiratory volume in 1 second (FEV$_1$) and vital capacity (VC) are obtained from maximal forced and relaxed expirations into a spirometer. FEV$_1$ is disproportionately reduced in airflow obstruction resulting in FEV$_1$/VC ratios of less than 70%. When airflow obstruction is seen, spirometry should be repeated following inhaled short-acting β$_2$-adrenoceptor agonists (e.g. salbutamol); reversibility to normal is suggestive of asthma (p. 670). To distinguish large airway narrowing (e.g. tracheal stenosis or compression) from small airway narrowing, flow-volume loops are recorded during maximum expiratory and inspiratory efforts (Fig. 19.9).

Lung volume can be measured by dilution of an inhaled inert gas (usually helium) or by determining the pressure/volume relationship of the thorax by body plethysmography. The former method measures the volume of intrathoracic gas which mixes quickly with tidal breaths, while the latter measures total intrathoracic gas volume, including poorly ventilated areas such as bullae.

To measure the capacity of the lungs to exchange gas, patients inhale a test mixture of 0.3% carbon monoxide, which is avidly bound to haemoglobin in pulmonary capillaries. After a short breath-hold, the rate of disappearance of CO into the circulation is calculated from a

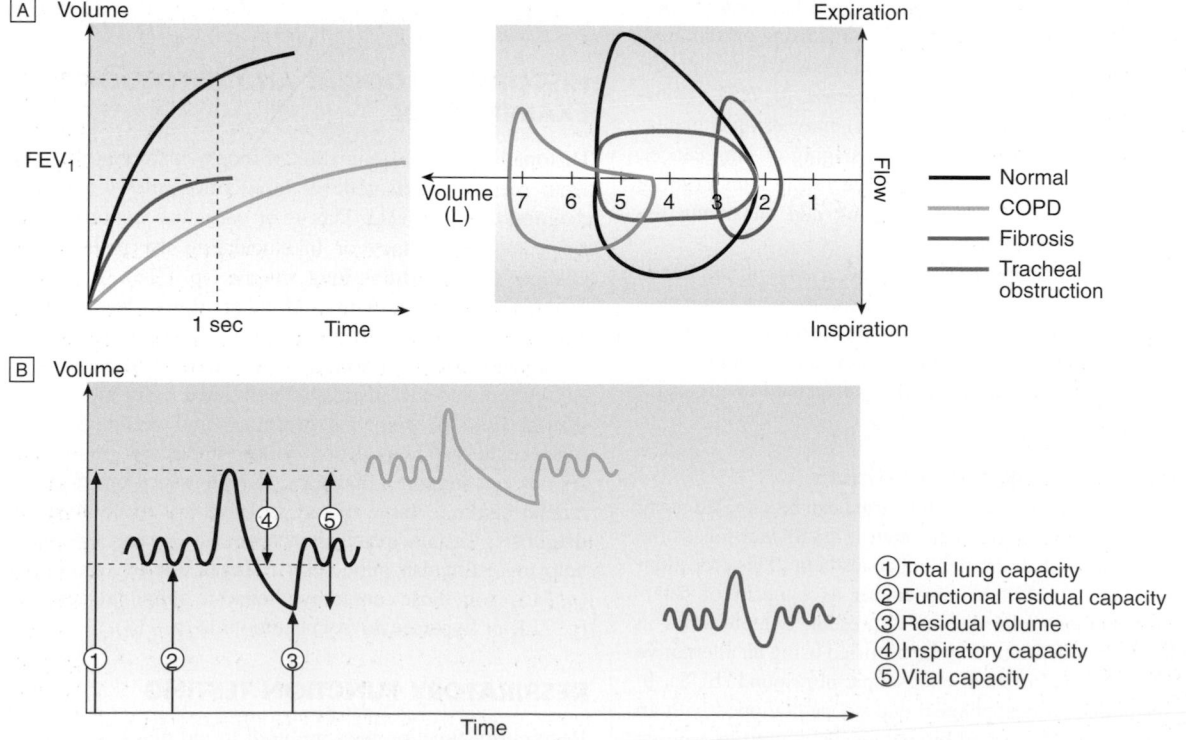

Fig. 19.9 Respiratory function tests in health and disease. A Forced expiration. B Lung volume measurement.

19.5 PATTERNS OF RESPIRATORY FUNCTION ABNORMALITIES IN DISEASE

	Asthma	Chronic bronchitis	Emphysema	Pulmonary fibrosis
FEV_1	↓↓	↓↓	↓↓	↓
VC	↓	↓	↓	↓↓
FEV_1/VC	↓	↓	↓	→/↑
TL_{co}	→	→	↓↓	↓↓
K_{co}	→	→	↓	→/↓
TLC	→/↑	↑	↑↑	↓
RV	→/↑	↑	↑↑	↓

sample of expirate, and expressed as the TL_{co} or carbon monoxide transfer factor. Helium is also included in the test breath to allow calculation of the volume of lung examined by the test breath. Transfer factor expressed per unit lung volume is termed K_{co}. Common respiratory function abnormalities are summarised in Box 19.5.

Arterial blood gases and oximetry

The measurement of hydrogen ion concentration, PaO_2 and $PaCO_2$, and derived bicarbonate concentration of arterial blood is essential in assessing the degree and type of respiratory failure and for measuring acid–base status. Interpretation of results is made easier by blood gas diagrams (e.g. Fig. 19.10), which indicate whether any acidosis or alkalosis is due to acute or chronic respiratory derangements of

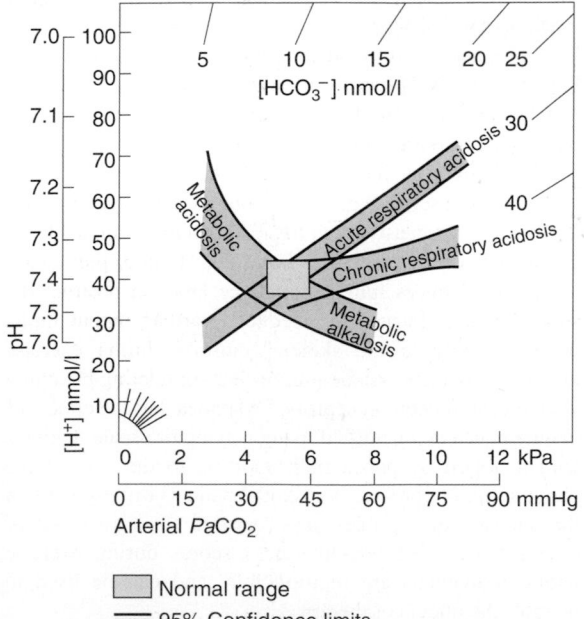

□ Normal range
══ 95% Confidence limits

Fig. 19.10 Changes in blood [H⁺], $PaCO_2$ and plasma [HCO₃⁻] in acid–base disorders. The rectangle indicates limits of normal reference ranges for [H⁺] and $PaCO_2$. The bands represent 95% confidence limits of single disturbances in human blood in vivo. When the point obtained by plotting [H⁺] against $PaCO_2$ does not fall within one of the labelled bands, compensation is incomplete or a mixed disorder is present.

$PaCO_2$, or to metabolic causes. Pulse oximeters allow non-invasive continuous assessment of oxygen saturation in patients who require monitoring in order to assess hypoxaemia and its response to therapy.

Exercise tests

Resting measurements are sometimes unhelpful in early disease or in patients complaining only of exercise-induced symptoms. Exercise testing with spirometry before and after can be helpful in demonstrating exercise-induced asthma. Walk tests include the self-paced 6 minute walk and the externally paced incremental 'shuttle' test. These can provide simple, repeatable assessments of disability and response to treatment. Finally, cardiopulmonary exercise testing using cycle or treadmill exercise with measurement of metabolic gas exchange, ventilation and cardiac responses is useful in distinguishing cardiac limitation from respiratory limitation in the breathless patient.

PRESENTING PROBLEMS IN RESPIRATORY DISEASE

COUGH

Cough is the most frequent symptom of respiratory disease. It is caused by stimulation of sensory nerves in the mucosa of the pharynx, larynx, trachea and bronchi. Acute sensitisation of the normal cough reflex occurs in a number of conditions (see below) and the patient typically reports cough induced by changes in air temperature or exposure to cigarette smoke or perfumes. The characteristics of cough originating at various levels of the respiratory tract are detailed in Box 19.6.

The explosive quality of a normal cough is lost in patients with respiratory muscle paralysis or vocal cord palsy. Paralysis of a single vocal cord gives rise to a prolonged, low-pitched, inefficient 'bovine' cough accompanied by hoarseness. Coexistence of an inspiratory noise (stridor) indicates partial obstruction of a major airway (e.g. laryngeal oedema, tracheal tumour, scarring or compression or an inhaled foreign body) and requires urgent investigation and treatment. Sputum production is common in patients with acute or chronic cough, and its nature and appearance can provide valuable clues as to the aetiology (p. 648).

Causes of cough

Acute or transient cough most commonly relates to viral lower respiratory tract infection, post-nasal drip resulting from rhinitis or sinusitis, aspiration of a foreign body or throat-clearing secondary to laryngitis or pharyngitis. Acute cough occurring in the context of more serious diseases such as pneumonia, aspiration, congestive heart failure or pulmonary embolism is usually easy to diagnose due to the presence of other clinical features. Rarely, cough may also arise following stimulation of the parietal pleura: for example, during the aspiration of a pleural effusion.

Patients with chronic cough present more of a diagnostic challenge, especially those individuals with a normal

19.6 COUGH

Origin	Common causes	Clinical features
Pharynx	Post-nasal drip	History of chronic rhinitis
Larynx	Laryngitis, tumour, Whooping cough, croup	Voice or swallowing altered, harsh or painful cough Paroxysms of cough, often associated with stridor
Trachea	Tracheitis	Raw retrosternal pain with cough
Bronchi	Bronchitis (acute) and COPD Asthma Bronchial carcinoma	Dry or productive, worse in mornings Usually dry, worse at night Persistent (often with haemoptysis)
Lung parenchyma	Tuberculosis Pneumonia Bronchiectasis Pulmonary oedema Interstitial fibrosis	Productive, often with haemoptysis Dry initially, productive later Productive, changes in posture induce sputum production Often at night (may be productive of pink, frothy sputum) Dry, irritant and distressing

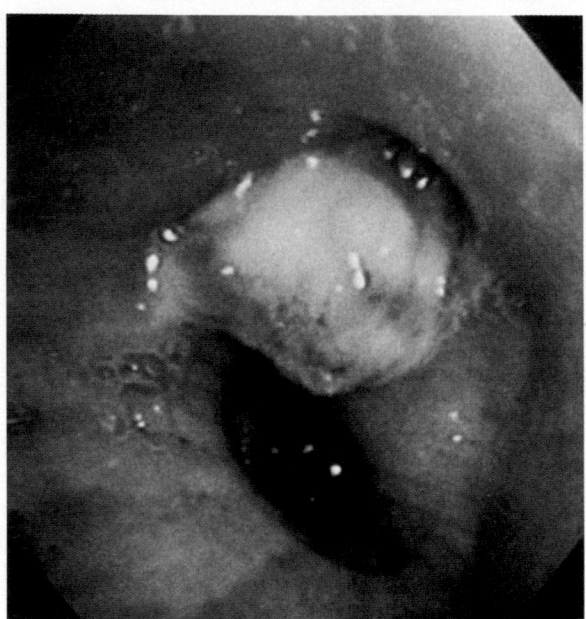

Fig. 19.11 Bronchoscopic appearances of inhaled foreign body (tooth) with a covering mucous film.

examination, chest X-ray and lung function studies. In this context, most cough can be explained by post-nasal drip secondary to nasal or sinus disease; cough-variant asthma (where cough may be the principal or exclusive clinical manifestation) or gastro-oesophageal reflux with aspiration. The latter cause may require ambulatory pH monitoring or a prolonged trial of anti-reflux therapy (p. 880) to diagnose. Ten to fifteen per cent of patients (particularly women) taking angiotensin-converting enzyme (ACE) inhibitors develop drug-induced chronic cough. *Bordetella pertussis* infection in adults can also result in protracted cough and should always be suspected in those in close contact with children. While most patients with a bronchogenic carcinoma have an abnormal chest X-ray on presentation, fibreoptic bronchoscopy or spiral CT of the airways is advisable in most adults with otherwise un-explained cough of recent onset (especially in smokers) as

this may reveal a small endobronchial tumour or unexpected foreign body (Fig. 19.11).

DYSPNOEA

Breathlessness or dyspnoea can be defined as the feeling of an uncomfortable need to breathe. It is unusual among sensations in having no defined receptors, no localised representation in the brain, and multiple causes both in health (e.g. exercise) and in diseases of the lungs, heart or muscles.

Pathophysiology

Physiological stimuli to breathing are summarised in Figure 19.12. Respiratory diseases can stimulate breathing and dyspnoea by stimulating intrapulmonary sensory nerves (e.g. pneumothorax, interstitial inflammation and pulmonary embolus), by increasing the mechanical load on the respiratory muscles (e.g. airflow obstruction or pulmonary fibrosis) or by causing hypoxia, hypercapnia or acidosis, stimulating chemoreceptors. In cardiac failure, pulmonary congestion reduces lung compliance and can obstruct the small airways. In addition, reduced cardiac output limits oxygen supply to the skeletal muscles during exercise causing early lactic acidaemia, further stimulating breathing via the central chemoreceptors. Dyspnoea and the effects of treatment can be quantified using a symptom scale. Patients tend to report dyspnoea in proportion to the sum of the above stimuli to breathe. Individual patients differ greatly in the intensity of breathlessness reported for a given set of circumstances, but breathlessness scores during exercise within individuals are reproducible, and can be used to monitor the effects of therapy.

Differential diagnosis

Patients with dyspnoea present either with chronic dyspnoea on exertion or as an emergency with acute breathlessness (with prominent symptoms even at rest). It is useful therefore to describe the causes of dyspnoea in this fashion (Box 19.7).

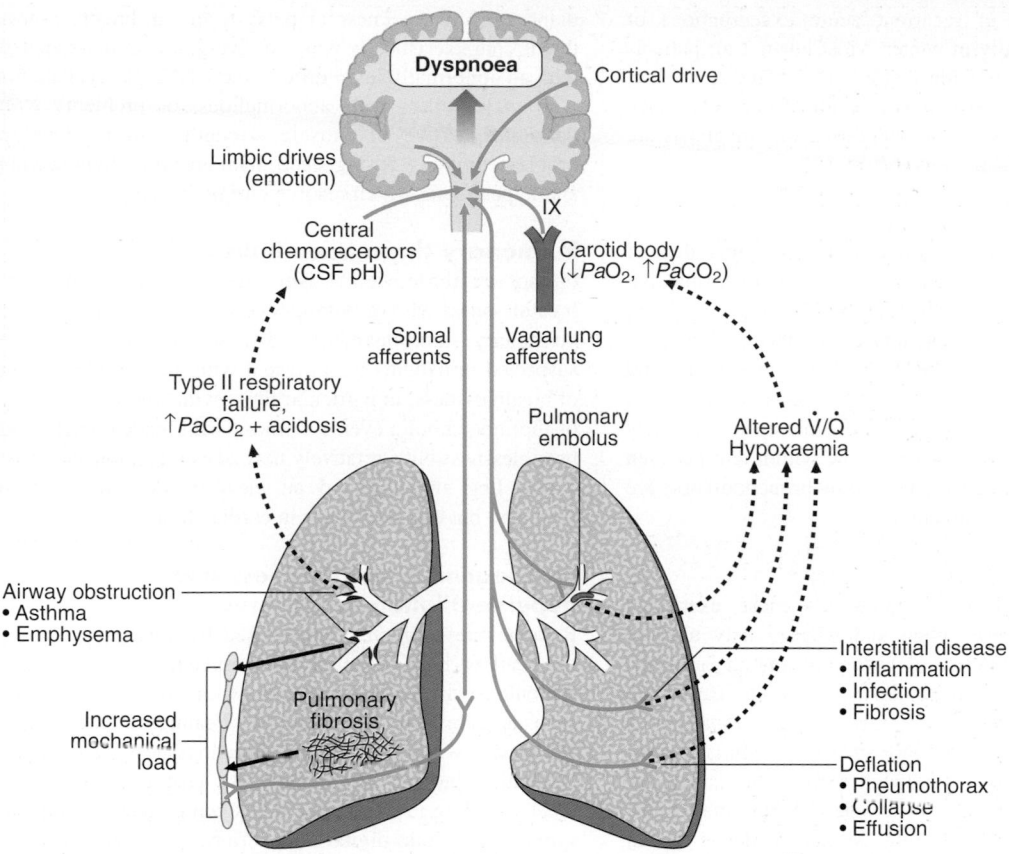

Fig. 19.12   Respiratory stimuli contributing to dyspnoea.

19.7 SOME CAUSES OF DYSPNOEA		
System	**Acute dyspnoea at rest**	**Chronic exertional dyspnoea**
Cardiovascular	*Acute pulmonary oedema (p. 539)	Chronic heart failure (p. 539) Myocardial ischaemia (angina equivalent) (p. 540)
Respiratory	*Acute severe asthma *Acute exacerbation of COPD *Pneumothorax *Pneumonia *Pulmonary embolus Acute respiratory distress syndrome Inhaled foreign body (especially in the child) Lobar collapse Laryngeal oedema (e.g. anaphylaxis)	*COPD *Chronic asthma Bronchial carcinoma Interstitial lung disease (sarcoidosis, fibrosing alveolitis, extrinsic allergic alveolitis, pneumoconiosis) Chronic pulmonary thromboembolism Lymphatic carcinomatosis (may cause intolerable dyspnoea) Large pleural effusion(s)
Others	Metabolic acidosis (e.g. diabetic ketoacidosis, lactic acidosis, uraemia, overdose of salicylates, ethylene glycol poisoning) Psychogenic hyperventilation (anxiety or panic-related)	Severe anaemia Obesity
* Denotes a common cause.		

CHRONIC EXERTIONAL DYSPNOEA

Chronic obstructive pulmonary disease (COPD)

The exertional dyspnoea in COPD typically varies little day to day, but exercise capacity falls steadily over months or years. Patients usually report relief of dyspnoea at rest and overnight, a useful distinction from asthma (see below). On lying flat, however, cranial displacement of the diaphragm by the abdominal contents compromises ventilation resulting in orthopnoea, so many patients choose to sleep propped up. If bronchitis is present, chronic cough and sputum is usual, particularly in the mornings, but sputum may be absent when emphysema predominates. There

19

19

is often a history of recurrent acute exacerbations of breathlessness, usually in winter. Most but not all patients have a significant smoking history. In advanced disease, ankle swelling may develop as a result of cor pulmonale. The features on examination suggesting this diagnosis are illustrated on page 648.

Asthma

Dyspnoea in asthma is associated with episodes of wheeze or chest tightness, varying in severity over time, but usually worse in the morning and often waking the patient overnight. There may be a history of childhood wheeze, or of wheeze or rhinitis provoked by pollens, dusts, household pets or occupational allergens. In exercise-induced asthma, wheeze and chest tightness typically come on immediately after exercise. Variability of peak flow within and between days, and reversal of FEV_1 to normal by bronchodilators are typical findings on investigation.

Heart disease

Impaired left ventricular function can cause exertional dyspnoea. Orthopnoea, cough and wheeze may also be present, as in lung disease. A history of angina or hypertension may be useful in implicating a cardiac cause. On examination, an increase in heart size as judged by a displaced apex beat, a raised JVP and cardiac murmurs may indicate cardiac disease (although these signs can occur in severe cor pulmonale). The chest X-ray may show cardiomegaly and an ECG may provide evidence of left ventricular disease. Arterial blood gases may be of value, since in the absence of an intracardiac shunt or pulmonary oedema the PaO_2 in cardiac disease is usually normal and the $PaCO_2$ is low or normal.

Interstitial or alveolar disease of the lung

A large number of conditions can cause interstitial lung disease (p. 713), which may be difficult to distinguish from infiltrating malignancy and opportunistic lung infection (Box 19.83, p. 713). A detailed history should be obtained, including lifetime occupation and exposure to birds, dusts and other sources of organic agents which may provoke lung disease. Dyspnoea in these conditions is usually relentless and progressive. The chest X-ray nearly always shows interstitial shadowing, but early changes may be very subtle. Pulmonary function tests usually show a restrictive defect (reduced volumes) and reduced gas transfer. Arterial blood gases show hypoxaemia, but the $PaCO_2$ is seldom elevated, even in advanced disease. Desaturation may be detected by oximetry, particularly during exercise testing, which may be valuable in detecting early disease and in monitoring the response to treatment.

Diseases of the chest wall or respiratory muscles

These are usually obvious on history, examination and chest radiography. Other rarer causes of alveolar hypoventilation, e.g. brain-stem defects, primary alveolar hypoventilation and alveolar hypoventilation in gross obesity, may cause disordered breathing and cyanosis, but these conditions are not usually associated with breathlessness. Bilateral diaphragmatic weakness or palsy results in breathlessness that is characteristically worse on lying; it is also associated with an abnormally large drop in the vital capacity. Patients with major chest wall abnormalities, or problems with ventilatory drive or muscle strength tend to develop problems initially during sleep, with nocturnal hypoxaemia and hypercapnia which resolve during the day.

Pulmonary thromboembolism

Pulmonary thromboembolism often presents with acute breathlessness with or without chest pain. However, chronic pulmonary thromboembolic disease (p. 724) should be suspected in patients who present with more gradual onset of breathlessness, in particular those with a previous history of thromboembolic events or those with marked exertional breathlessness but a relatively normal examination and chest X-ray. Leg swelling and an elevated JVP may arouse suspicion but can also occur in cardiac failure.

Psychogenic breathlessness and hyperventilation syndromes

Breathlessness which is not caused by organic disease of the heart or lungs is relatively common. It is particularly difficult to diagnose in patients with coexisting disease, such as asthma or heart disease. Features in the history associated with psychogenic breathlessness and hyperventilation include an 'inability to take a deep enough breath' leading to extra deep sighs being taken. Additional symptoms include digital and perioral paraesthesiae, light headedness, central chest discomfort or even carpopedal spasm due to acute respiratory alkalosis. These additional symptoms may provoke further anxiety and exacerbate hyperventilation. Psychogenic breathlessness rarely disturbs sleep, frequently occurs at rest, may be provoked by stressful situations and may even be relieved by exercise. 'Points' scores such as the Nijmegen questionnaire are used in the assessment of this problem—Box 19.8. Arterial blood gases show normal PO_2, low PCO_2 and alkalosis. This picture is diagnostic and is useful in excluding other lung diseases. Occasionally, formal exercise testing may be required to exclude organic causes with confidence.

Explanation of the cause of the symptoms coupled with reassurance that they do not represent a serious disorder of the heart or lungs often helps patients with hyperventilation. Some patients may benefit from breathing exercises or relaxation therapy.

19.8 SOME FACTORS POINTING TO PSYCHOGENIC HYPERVENTILATION

- 'Inability to take a deep breath'
- Frequent sighing/erratic ventilation at rest
- Short breath-holding time in the absence of severe respiratory disease
- Difficulty in performing/inconsistent spirometry manoeuvres
- High score (over 26) on Nijmegen questionnaire
- Induction of symptoms during submaximal hyperventilation
- Resting end-tidal $CO_2 < 4.5\%$
- Associated digital paraesthesiae

19.9 DIFFERENTIAL DIAGNOSIS OF ACUTE SEVERE DYSPNOEA

Condition	History	Signs	Chest radiography	Arterial blood gases	ECG	Other tests
Pulmonary oedema	Chest pain Orthopnoea Palpitations A previous cardiac history*	Central cyanosis JVP ($\rightarrow$ or $\uparrow$) Sweating* Cool extremities Dullness and crepitations at bases*	Cardiomegaly Upper zone vessel enlargement* Overt oedema/ pleural effusions*	$\downarrow Pa\,O_2$ $\downarrow Pa\,CO_2$	Sinus tachycardia Signs of myocardial infarction/ischaemia* Arrhythmia	Echocardiography* ($\downarrow$ left ventricular function)
Massive pulmonary embolus	Recent surgery or other risk factors Chest pain Previous pleurisy Syncope* Dizziness*	Severe central cyanosis Elevated JVP* Absence of signs in the lung (unless previous pulmonary infarction)* Shock (tachycardia, reduced blood pressure)	May be subtle changes only Prominent hilar vessels Oligaemic lung fields*	$\downarrow\downarrow Pa\,O_2$ $\downarrow Pa\,CO_2$	Sinus tachycardia $S_1Q_3T_3$ pattern $\downarrow T$ (V_1–V_4) Right bundle-branch block	Echocardiography* V/Q scan* CT pulmonary angiography*
Acute severe asthma	History of previous episodes, asthma medications, wheeze*	Tachycardia and pulsus paradoxus Cyanosis (late) JVP $\rightarrow$* $\downarrow\downarrow$ peak flow, rhonchi*	Hyperinflation only (unless complicated by pneumothorax)*	$\downarrow Pa\,O_2$ $\downarrow Pa\,CO_2$ ($Pa\,CO_2$ rises in extremis)	Sinus tachycardia (bradycardia with severe hypoxaemia—late)	
Acute exacerbation of COPD	Previous episodes (admissions)* If in type II respiratory failure may not be distressed	Cyanosis Signs of COPD (p. 649)* Signs of CO_2 retention (warm periphery, flapping tremor, bounding pulses)*	Hyperinflation* Signs of emphysema Signs of events precipitating exacerbation	$\downarrow$ or $\downarrow\downarrow Pa\,O_2$ $Pa\,CO_2 \uparrow$ in type II failure, with $\uparrow$ [H+] and $\uparrow$ bicarbonate	Nil, or signs of right ventricular strain	
Pneumonia	Prodromal illness* Fever* Rigors* Pleurisy*	Fever, confusion Pleural rub* Consolidation* Cyanosis (only if severe)	Pneumonic consolidation*	$\downarrow Pa\,CO_2$ $\downarrow Pa\,O_2$	Tachycardia	$\uparrow$ CRP $\uparrow$ White cell count Sputum and blood culture
Metabolic acidosis	Evidence of diabetes/renal disease* Overdose of aspirin or ethylene glycol*	Fetor (ketones) Hyperventilation without physical signs in heart or lungs* Dehydration* Air hunger (Kussmaul's respiration)	Normal	$Pa\,O_2$ normal* $\downarrow\downarrow Pa\,CO_2$ $\downarrow\downarrow$ pH ($\uparrow$ H+)		
Psychogenic (a diagnosis of exclusion)	Previous episodes	Not cyanosed* No heart signs* No lung signs* Carpopedal spasm	Normal	$Pa\,O_2$ normal* $\downarrow\downarrow Pa\,CO_2$ pH normal or $\uparrow$ (H+ $\downarrow$)*		End-tidal $P\,CO_2$ low at rest and during exercise

* Denotes a valuable discriminatory feature.

ACUTE SEVERE DYSPNOEA

This is one of the most common and dramatic medical emergencies and it is easy for the inexperienced clinician to be disconcerted. Although there are a number of possible causes, attention to the history and a rapid but careful examination will usually suggest a diagnosis which can be confirmed by routine investigations, including chest X-ray, electrocardiogram (ECG) and arterial blood gases. Some specific features that aid in the diagnosis of important causes of acute severe breathlessness are considered in detail in Box 19.9.

History

It is important to ascertain the rate of onset and severity of the breathlessness and whether associated cardiovascular symptoms (chest pain, palpitations, sweating and nausea) or respiratory symptoms (cough, wheeze, haemoptysis, stridor—Fig. 19.13) are present. A previous history of repeated episodes of left ventricular failure, asthma or exacerbations of COPD is valuable. In the severely ill patient it may be necessary to obtain the history from accompanying persons. In children, the possibility of inhalation of a foreign body (Fig. 19.11) or acute epiglottitis should always be considered.

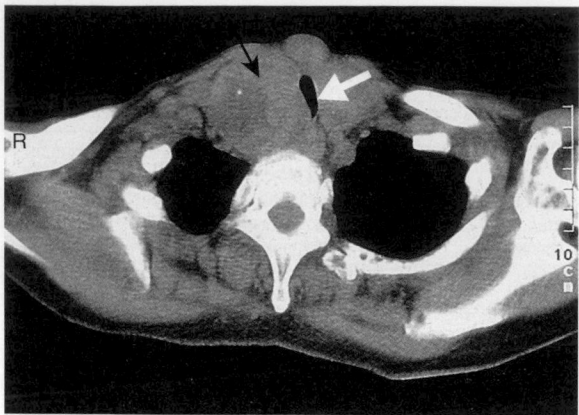

Fig. 19.13 CT showing retrosternal multinodular goitre (small arrow) causing acute severe breathlessness and stridor due to tracheal compression (large arrow).

Clinical assessment of the acutely breathless patient

The following should be assessed and documented immediately: the level of consciousness, degree of central cyanosis, evidence of anaphylaxis (urticaria or angi-oedema), patency of the upper airway, ability to speak (in single words or sentences) and the cardiovascular status (heart rate and rhythm, blood pressure and degree of peripheral perfusion). Pulmonary oedema is suggested by pink frothy sputum and bi-basal crackles, asthma or COPD by wheeze and prolonged expiration, pneumothorax by a silent resonant hemithorax, and pulmonary embolus by severe dyspnoea with normal breath sounds. The peak expiratory flow should be measured whenever possible. Leg swelling may suggest cardiac failure or, if asymmetrical, venous thrombosis. Arterial blood gases, chest X-ray and an ECG should be obtained to confirm the clinical diagnosis, and oxygen given pending results. Urgent endotracheal intubation may become necessary if the conscious level declines or severe respiratory acidosis is present.

CHEST PAIN

Chest pain is a frequent manifestation of both cardiac and respiratory disease and is considered in detail on page 534. Pleural or chest wall involvement by lung disease gives rise to peripheral chest pain which is exacerbated by deep breathing or coughing (Box 19.10). Central chest pain suggests heart disease but occurs with tumours affecting the mediastinum, oesophageal disease (p. 877) or disease of the thoracic aorta (p. 605). Massive pulmonary embolus may cause ischaemic cardiac pain as well as severe breathlessness. Tracheitis produces raw upper retrosternal pain which is worse on coughing. Musculoskeletal chest wall pain is usually exacerbated by movement and associated with local tenderness.

19.10 DIFFERENTIAL DIAGNOSIS OF CHEST PAIN	
Central	
Cardiac	
• Myocardial ischaemia (angina)	• Myocarditis
• Myocardial infarction	• Pericarditis
	• Mitral valve prolapse syndrome
Aortic	
• Aortic dissection	• Aortic aneurysm
Oesophageal	
• Oesophagitis	• Mallory–Weiss syndrome
• Oesophageal spasm	
Massive pulmonary embolus	
Mediastinal	
• Tracheitis	• Malignancy
Anxiety/emotion[1]	
Peripheral	
Lungs/pleura	
• Pulmonary infarct	• Malignancy
• Pneumonia	• Tuberculosis
• Pneumothorax	• Connective tissue disorders
Musculoskeletal[2]	
• Osteoarthritis	• Costochondritis (Tietze's syndrome)
• Rib fracture/injury	
• Intercostal muscle injury	• Epidemic myalgia (Bornholm disease)
Neurological	
• Prolapsed intervertebral disc	• Herpes zoster
	• Thoracic outlet syndrome

[1]May also cause peripheral chest pain.
[2]Can sometimes cause central chest pain.

HAEMOPTYSIS

Coughing up blood, irrespective of the amount, is an alarming symptom and nearly always brings the patient to the doctor. A clear history should be taken to establish that it is true haemoptysis and not haematemesis, gum bleeding or nosebleed. Haemoptysis must always be assumed to have a serious cause until appropriate investigations have excluded these causes (Box 19.11).

Many episodes of haemoptysis are unexplained, even after full investigation, and are likely to be caused by simple bronchial infection. A history of repeated small haemo-ptyses, or blood-streaking of sputum, is highly suggestive of bronchial carcinoma. Fever, night sweats and weight loss suggest tuberculosis. Pneumococcal pneumonia is often the cause of 'rusty'-coloured sputum but can cause frank haemoptysis, as can all the pneumonic infections which lead to suppuration or abscess formation (p. 694). Bronchiectasis (p. 684) and intracavitary mycetoma (p. 704) can cause catastrophic bronchial haemorrhage and in these patients there may be a history of previous tuberculosis or pneumonia in early life. Pulmonary thromboembolism is a common cause of haemoptysis and should always be considered.

Physical examination may reveal additional clues, e.g. finger clubbing in bronchial carcinoma or bronchiectasis; other signs of malignancy such as cachexia, hepatomegaly, lymphadenopathy etc.; fever or signs of consolidation and

19.11 CAUSES OF HAEMOPTYSIS

Bronchial disease

- Carcinoma*
- Bronchiectasis*
- Acute bronchitis*
- Bronchial adenoma
- Foreign body

Parenchymal disease

- Tuberculosis*
- Suppurative pneumonia
- Lung abscess
- Parasites (e.g. hydatid disease, flukes)
- Trauma
- Actinomycosis
- Mycetoma

Lung vascular disease

- Pulmonary infarction*
- Polyarteritis nodosa
- Goodpasture's syndrome (p. 502)
- Idiopathic pulmonary haemosiderosis

Cardiovascular disease

- Acute left ventricular failure*
- Mitral stenosis
- Aortic aneurysm

Blood disorders

- Leukaemia
- Haemophilia
- Anticoagulants

* More common causes.

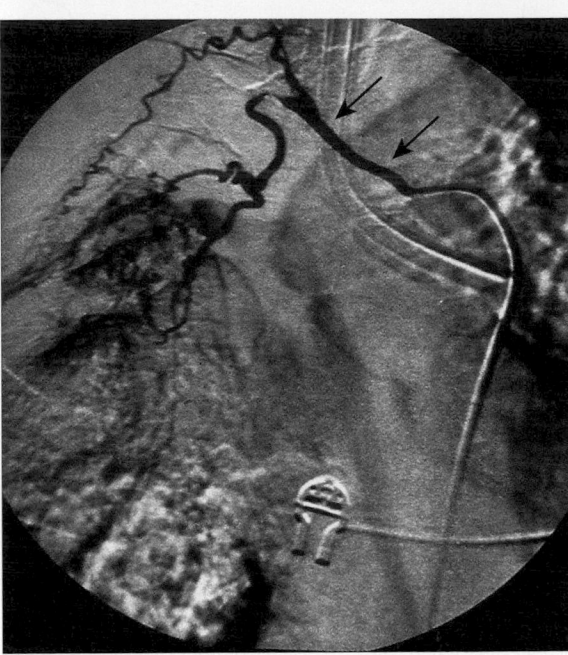

Fig. 19.14 Bronchial artery angiography. An angiography catheter has been passed via the femoral artery and aorta into an abnormally dilated right bronchial artery (arrows). Contrast is seen flowing into the lung. This patient had post-tuberculous bronchiectasis affecting the right upper lobe and presented with massive haemoptysis. Bronchial artery embolisation was successfully carried out.

19

pleurisy in pneumonia or pulmonary infarction; leg signs of deep venous thrombosis in a minority of patients with pulmonary infarction; and signs of systemic diseases including rash, purpura, haematuria, splinter haemorrhages, lymphadenopathy or splenomegaly in the uncommon systemic diseases which may be associated with haemoptysis.

Management

In severe acute haemoptysis, the patient should be nursed upright (or on the side of the bleeding if this is known), given oxygen and haemodynamically resuscitated. Bronchoscopy in the acute phase is difficult and often merely shows blood throughout the bronchial tree. If radiology shows an obvious central cause then rigid bronchoscopy under general anaesthesia may allow intervention to stop bleeding; however the source often cannot be visualised. Intubation with a divided endotracheal tube may allow protected ventilation of the unaffected lung to stabilise the patient. Bronchial arteriography and embolisation (Fig. 19.14), or even emergency pulmonary surgery, can be life-saving in the acute situation.

In the vast majority of cases, however, the haemoptysis itself is not life-threatening and it is possible to follow a logical sequence of investigations which include:

- Chest X-ray, which may give clear evidence of a localised lesion including pulmonary infarction, a tumour (malignant or benign), pneumonia or tuberculosis.
- Full blood count and other haematological tests including clotting screen.

- Bronchoscopy after acute bleeding has settled, which may reveal a central bronchial carcinoma (not visible on the chest X-ray) and permit tissue diagnosis.
- Ventilation–perfusion ($\dot{V}/\dot{Q}$) lung scan, which is helpful in establishing a diagnosis of suspected pulmonary thromboembolic disease. CT pulmonary angiography may be necessary in patients with pre-existing lung disease where interpretation of the $\dot{V}/\dot{Q}$ scan can be difficult.
- CT, which is particularly useful in investigating peripheral lesions seen on the chest X-ray which are not accessible to bronchoscopy and facilitates accurate percutaneous needle biopsy where indicated.

THE SOLITARY RADIOGRAPHIC PULMONARY LESION

The incidental finding of a solitary pulmonary nodule (SPN) on a plain chest X-ray in an adult patient is a common dilemma and the differential diagnosis is broad (Box 19.12). Between 20% and 30% of all cancers present in this way; the incidence increases with age and accounts for over 50% of nodules in patients aged over 50.

Investigations

Radiology

Investigations should commence with a review of previous radiology. A nodule that has been present for more than

19

19.12 THE SOLITARY PULMONARY NODULE

Common causes

- Bronchial carcinoma
- Single metastasis
- Localised pneumonia
- Lung abscess
- Tuberculoma
- Pulmonary infarct

Uncommon causes

- Benign tumours
- Lymphoma
- Arteriovenous malformation
- Hydatid cyst
- Bronchogenic cyst
- Rheumatoid nodule
- Pulmonary sequestration
- Pulmonary haematoma
- Wegener's granuloma
- 'Pseudotumour'—fluid collection in a fissure
- Aspergilloma (usually surrounded by air 'halo')

19.13 CAUSES OF PLEURAL EFFUSION

Common causes

- Pneumonia ('para-pneumonic effusion')
- Tuberculosis
- Pulmonary infarction
- Malignant disease
- Cardiac failure
- Subdiaphragmatic disorders (subphrenic abscess, pancreatitis etc.)

Uncommon causes

- Hypoproteinaemia (nephrotic syndrome, liver failure, malnutrition)
- Connective tissue diseases (particularly systemic lupus erythematosus and rheumatoid arthritis)
- Acute rheumatic fever
- Post-myocardial infarction syndrome
- Meigs' syndrome (ovarian tumour plus pleural effusion)
- Myxoedema
- Uraemia
- Asbestos-related benign pleural effusion

2 years and has not changed can be assumed to be benign. If there are no previous films, or if previous films are normal, a CT scan should be obtained to define the lesion more precisely. Benign disease is favoured by the presence of calcification or fat. A laminated or central deposition of calcification is typical of a granuloma and a 'popcorn' pattern suggestive of a hamartoma. However, CT may detect calcification in some malignant lesions. Features suggestive of malignancy include size > 3 cm or a spiculated appearance, particularly in a smoker. The injection of intravenous contrast medium at the time of the CT provides information regarding the vascularity of the lesion, with malignant tumours tending to show greatest contrast enhancement. CT may also demonstrate hilar and mediastinal lymphadenopathy, important in the staging of a primary bronchial carcinoma. Enhanced imaging techniques that facilitate 3D reconstruction of nodules may allow more accurate topographical assessment but are not widely available. A positive [18]FDG-PET scan (p. 654) is also suggestive of a malignant lesion. False negatives may be seen with carcinoid and bronchiolo-alveolar cell carcinomas.

Invasive procedures

Bronchoscopy is usually unrewarding as the lesion is beyond the vision of the operator. Diagnostic yields from blind washings are typically low and although they may be improved by the use of radiological screening, the technique is cumbersome and time-consuming. Percutaneous needle biopsy under CT guidance has proved to be the most effective procedure for the diagnosis of solitary pulmonary nodules with few complications (pneumothorax and haemorrhage). However, if the lesion has a high probability of malignancy and the patient is fit for surgery, the best option may be to proceed to surgical resection.

Whenever bacterial infection is included in the clinical differential diagnosis, an antibiotic should be given during the period in which the investigations are being performed; the patient should then undergo a repeat X-ray to see whether there has been a reduction in size of the opacity. In elderly patients in whom a primary malignant lesion is suspected, but who are considered unfit for any form of curative treatment, observation by repeat X-ray at intervals of a few weeks may be the most appropriate management decision.

PLEURAL EFFUSION

The accumulation of serous fluid within the pleural space is termed pleural effusion. Accumulations of frank pus (empyema) or blood (haemothorax) represent separate conditions; empyema is considered on page 732. In general, pleural fluid accumulates as a result of either increased hydrostatic pressure or decreased osmotic pressure ('transudative effusion' as seen in cardiac, liver or renal failure), or from increased microvascular pressure due to disease of the pleural surface itself, or injury in the adjacent lung ('exudative effusion'). Some causes of pleural effusion are shown in Boxes 19.13 and 19.14. The cause of the majority of pleural effusions can usually be identified through a thorough history, examination and relevant investigations.

Particular attention should be paid to a recent history of respiratory infection, the presence of heart, liver or renal disease, occupation (e.g. exposure to asbestos), contact with tuberculosis, and risk factors for thromboembolism.

Clinical assessment

Symptoms and signs of pleurisy often precede the development of an effusion, especially in patients with underlying pneumonia, pulmonary infarction or connective tissue disease. However, the onset may be insidious. Breathlessness is the only symptom related to the effusion and its severity depends on the size and rate of accumulation. The physical signs are detailed on page 649.

Investigations

Radiological investigations

The classical appearance of pleural fluid on the erect PA chest film is of a curved shadow at the lung base, blunting the costophrenic angle and ascending towards the axilla. Fluid appears to track up the lateral chest wall. In fact, fluid surrounds the whole lung at this level, but casts a radiological shadow only where the X-ray beam passes tangentially across the fluid against the lateral chest wall.

19.14 PLEURAL EFFUSION: MAIN CAUSES AND FEATURES

Cause	Appearance of fluid	Type of fluid	Predominant cells in fluid	Other diagnostic features
Tuberculosis	Serous, usually amber-coloured	Exudate	Lymphocytes (occasionally polymorphs)	Positive tuberculin test Isolation of *M. tuberculosis* from pleural fluid (20%) Positive pleural biopsy (80%)
Malignant disease	Serous, often blood-stained	Exudate	Serosal cells and lymphocytes Often clumps of malignant cells	Positive pleural biopsy (40%) Evidence of malignant disease elsewhere
Cardiac failure*	Serous, straw-coloured	Transudate	Few serosal cells	Other evidence of left ventricular failure Response to diuretics
Pulmonary infarction*	Serous or blood-stained	Exudate (rarely transudate)	Red blood cells Eosinophils	Evidence of pulmonary infarction Source of embolism Factors predisposing to venous thrombosis
Rheumatoid disease*	Serous Turbid if chronic	Exudate	Lymphocytes (occasionally polymorphs)	Rheumatoid arthritis; rheumatoid factor in serum Cholesterol in chronic effusion; very low glucose in pleural fluid
Systemic lupus erythematosus (SLE)*	Serous	Exudate	Lymphocytes and serosal cells	Other manifestations of SLE Antinuclear factor or anti-DNA in serum
Acute pancreatitis	Serous or blood-stained	Exudate	No cells predominate	High amylase in pleural fluid (greater than in serum)
Obstruction of thoracic duct	Milky	Chyle	None	Chylomicrons

* Effusion often bilateral.

Around 200 ml of fluid is required to be detectable on a PA chest X-ray, but smaller effusions can be identified by ultrasound or CT scanning. Previous scarring or adhesions in the pleural space can cause localised effusions. Pleural fluid localised below the lower lobe ('subpulmonary effusion') simulates an elevated hemidiaphragm. Fluid localised within an oblique fissure may produce a rounded opacity simulating a tumour.

Ultrasonography is more accurate than plain chest radiography at determining the volume of pleural fluid and frequently provides additional helpful information. Visualisation of fluid facilitates safe needle aspiration and guides pleural biopsy increasing the diagnostic yields. The presence of loculation may suggest an evolving empyema or resolving haemothorax. The technique may also distinguish pleural fluid from pleural thickening. CT scanning displays pleural abnormalities more readily than either plain radiography or ultrasound, and may distinguish benign from malignant pleural disease.

Pleural aspiration and biopsy

In some clinical settings (e.g. left ventricular failure) it should not be necessary to sample fluid unless atypical features are present; appropriate treatment should be administered and the effusion re-evaluated. However, in most other circumstances, sampling is necessary to establish a diagnosis. Simple aspiration provides information on the colour and texture of fluid and on appearance alone may immediately suggest an empyema or chylothorax. The presence of blood is consistent with pulmonary infarction or malignancy, but may represent a traumatic tap. Biochemical analysis allows classification into transudate and exudates (Box 19.15) and Gram stain may suggest parapneumonic

19.15 LIGHT'S CRITERIA FOR DISTINGUISHING PLEURAL TRANSUDATE FROM EXUDATE

Pleural fluid is an exudate if one or more of the following criteria are met:
- Pleural fluid protein:serum protein ratio > 0.5
- Pleural fluid LDH: serum LDH ratio > 0.6
- Pleural fluid LDH > two-thirds of the upper limit of normal serum LDH

(LDH = Lactate dehydrogenase)

effusion. The predominant cell type provides useful information and cytological examination is essential. A low pH suggests infection but may also be seen in rheumatoid arthritis, ruptured oesophagus or advanced malignancy.

Combining pleural aspiration with biopsy increases the diagnostic yield. An Abrams needle is most frequently employed. Increased yields are reported when either ultrasound or CT is used to guide the operator. The best results are obtained from video-assisted thoracoscopy, allowing the operator to visualise the pleura and guide the biopsy directly.

Management

Therapeutic aspiration may be required to palliate breathlessness but removing more than 1.5 litres in one episode is inadvisable as there is a small risk of re-expansion pulmonary oedema. An effusion should never be drained to dryness before establishing a diagnosis as further biopsy may be precluded until further fluid accumulates. Treatment of the underlying cause—for example, heart failure, pneumonia, pulmonary embolism or subphrenic abscess—

19

19

will often be followed by resolution of the effusion. The management of pleural effusion in association with pneumonia, tuberculosis and malignancy is dealt with below.

SLEEP-DISORDERED BREATHING

A variety of respiratory disorders manifest themselves during sleep. For example, nocturnal cough and wheeze are characteristic features of asthma, and the hypoventilation that occurs during normal sleep can exacerbate respiratory failure in patients with restrictive lung disease such as kyphoscoliosis, diaphragmatic palsy, muscle weakness (e.g. muscular dystrophy) or intrinsic lung disease (e.g. COPD, pulmonary fibrosis). In contrast, a small but important group of disorders cause problems only during sleep. Patients with such disorders have normal lungs and daytime respiratory function but have either abnormalities of ventilatory drive (central sleep apnoea) or upper airway obstruction (obstructive sleep apnoea) that are manifested during sleep. Of these, the obstructive sleep apnoea/hypopnoea syndrome is by far the most common and important disorder.

THE SLEEP APNOEA/HYPOPNOEA SYNDROME

It is now recognised that 2–4% of the middle-aged population suffer from recurrent upper airway obstruction during sleep. Due to the ensuing sleep fragmentation they experience daytime sleepiness, especially in monotonous situations, and this results in a threefold increased risk of road traffic accidents and a ninefold increased risk of single-vehicle accidents.

Aetiology

The problem results from recurrent occlusion of the pharynx during sleep, usually at the level of the soft palate. On inspiration the pressure in the pharynx is subatmospheric. During wakefulness, upper airway dilating muscles— including palatoglossus and genioglossus—contract actively during each inspiration to preserve airway patency. During sleep, muscle tone declines and the ability of the upper airway dilating muscles to maintain pharyngeal patency falls. In most people sufficient tone persists to result in uncompromised breathing during sleep. In a minority of people, a combination of an anatomically narrow palatopharynx and underactivity of the dilating muscles during sleep results in obstruction of the airway. If the obstruction is incomplete, turbulent flow and vibration occur, resulting in snoring (around 40% of middle-aged men and 20% of middle-aged women snore). If upper airway narrowing progresses to the point of occlusion or near-occlusion, sleeping subjects increase inspiratory effort to try to breathe until the increased effort transiently awakens them, so briefly that they have no recollection, but long enough for the upper airway dilating muscles to open the airway again. Then a series of deep breaths are taken before the subject rapidly returns to sleep, snores and becomes apnoeic once more. This recurrent cycle of apnoea, awakening, apnoea, awakening etc. may repeat itself many hundreds of times

per night and result in severe sleep fragmentation. The awakenings are associated with surges in blood pressure which may increase the risk of sustained hypertension, coronary events and stroke.

Predisposing factors to the sleep apnoea/hypopnoea syndrome include being male, which doubles the risk, probably due to a testosterone effect on the upper airway, and obesity, found in about half the patients, because parapharyngeal fat deposits tend to narrow the throat. Nasal obstruction or a recessed mandible can further exacerbate the problem. Acromegaly and hypothyroidism also predispose individuals to this condition by causing submucosal infiltration and narrowing of the upper airway. The condition is often familial, and in these families the maxilla and mandible are back-set, narrowing the upper airway. Alcohol and sedatives predispose to snoring and apnoeas by relaxing the upper airway dilating muscles.

Clinical assessment

Excessive daytime sleepiness is the principal symptom and snoring is virtually universal. The patient usually feels that he or she has been asleep all night but wakes unrefreshed. Bed partners report loud snoring in all body positions and will often have noticed multiple breathing pauses (apnoeas). Difficulty with concentration, impaired cognitive function and work performance, depression, irritability and nocturia are other features.

Investigations

Provided that the sleepiness does not result from inadequate time in bed or from shift work etc., any person who repeatedly falls asleep during the day when not in bed, who complains that his or her work is impaired by sleepiness, or who is a habitual snorer with multiple witnessed apnoeas should be referred to a sleep or respiratory specialist. A more quantitative assessment of daytime sleepiness can be obtained by questionnaire (Box 19.16).

Overnight studies of breathing, oxygenation and sleep quality are diagnostic (Fig. 19.15) but the level of

---

19.16 EPWORTH SLEEPINESS SCALE

How likely are you to doze off or fall asleep in the situations described below? Use the following scale to choose the most appropriate number for each situation:

0 = would never doze
1 = slight chance of dozing
2 = moderate chance of dozing
3 = high chance of dozing

- Sitting and reading
- Watching TV
- Sitting, inactive in a public place (e.g. a theatre or a meeting)
- As a passenger in a car for an hour without a break
- Lying down to rest in the afternoon when circumstances permit
- Sitting and talking to someone
- Sitting quietly after a lunch without alcohol
- In a car, while stopped for a few minutes in the traffic

Normal subjects average 5.9 (SD 2.2) and patients with severe obstructive sleep apnoea average 16.0 (SD 4.4)

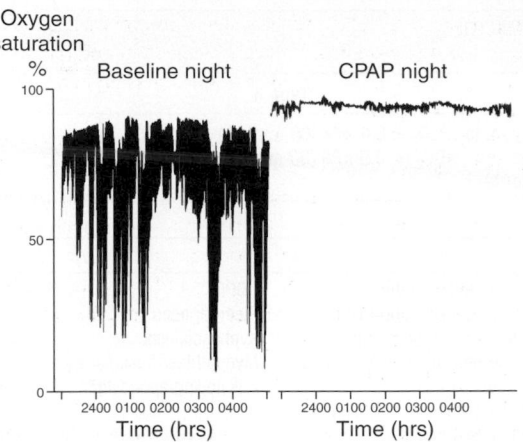

Fig. 19.15 Sleep apnoea/hypopnoea syndrome: overnight oxygen saturation trace. The left-hand panel shows the trace of a 46-year-old patient during a night when he slept without continuous positive airway pressure (CPAP) and had 53 apnoeas plus hypopnoeas/hour, 55 brief awakenings/hour and marked oxygen desaturation. The right-hand panel shows the next night when he slept with a CPAP of 10 cm H_2O delivered through a tight-fitting nasal mask which abolished his breathing irregularity and awakenings and improved his oxygenation.

19.17 DIFFERENTIAL DIAGNOSIS OF PERSISTENT SLEEPINESS
Lack of sleep
<ul><li>Inadequate time in bed</li><li>Extraneous sleep disruption (e.g. babies/children)</li><li>Shift work</li><li>Excessive caffeine intake</li><li>Physical illness (e.g. pain)</li></ul>
Sleep disruption
<ul><li>Sleep apnoea/hypopnoea syndrome</li><li>Periodic limb movement disorder (recurrent limb movements during non-REM sleep, frequent nocturnal awakenings)</li></ul>
Sleepiness with relatively normal sleep
<ul><li>Narcolepsy</li><li>Idiopathic hypersomnolence (rare)</li><li>Neurological lesions (e.g. hypothalamic or upper brain-stem infarcts or tumours)</li><li>Drugs</li></ul>
Psychological/psychiatric
<ul><li>Depression</li></ul>

19

complexity of investigations will vary depending on the probability of diagnosis, differential diagnosis and resources. The current threshold for diagnosing the sleep apnoea/hypopnoea syndrome is 15 apnoeas/hypopnoeas per hour of sleep, where an apnoea is a 10-second or longer breathing pause and a hypopnoea a 10-second or longer 50% reduction in breathing.

Differential diagnosis

A number of other conditions can cause daytime sleepiness but these can usually be excluded by a careful history (Box 19.17). Narcolepsy is a rare cause of sleepiness, occurring in 0.05% of the population (p. 1177), and is associated with cataplexy (when muscle tone is lost in fully conscious people in response to emotional triggers, p. 1177), hypnagogic hallucinations (hallucinations at sleep onset) and sleep paralysis. Idiopathic hypersomnolence occurs in younger individuals and is characterised by long nocturnal sleeps.

Management

In a few patients advice to avoid evening alcohol and lose weight suffices, but most need to use continuous positive airway pressure (CPAP) delivered by a nasal mask every night at home. CPAP keeps the throat open by keeping the upper airway pressure above atmospheric. The pressure for CPAP is set in the laboratory to the lowest that will prevent apnoeas, hypopnoeas and awakenings. The effect is often dramatic (Fig. 19.15) and CPAP results in improvements in symptoms, daytime performance, quality of life and survival. Unfortunately, 30–50% of patients are poorly compliant or do not tolerate such therapy. Mandibular advancement devices worn within the mouth are an alternative approach which is effective in some patients. There is no evidence that palatal surgery has any role in the management of this condition, but surgical treatment of nasal obstruction may be helpful.

RESPIRATORY FAILURE

The term respiratory failure is used when pulmonary gas exchange fails to maintain normal arterial oxygen and carbon dioxide levels. Its classification into type I and type II relates to the absence or presence of hypercapnia (raised $PaCO_2$). The physiological basis of respiratory failure is described on page 651. Some causes of respiratory failure and its characteristic blood gas abnormalities are shown in Box 19.18.

Management

Prompt diagnosis and management of the underlying cause is crucial to the management of patients with respiratory failure. Occasionally, rapid reversal of the precipitating event—e.g. tracheostomy for laryngeal obstruction, fixation of ribs in a flail chest injury, reversal of narcotic poisons, nebulised bronchodilators in acute severe asthma or tube drainage of a tension pneumothorax—will restore good gas exchange. In acute left ventricular failure, in massive pulmonary embolism and when pulmonary infarction or pneumonia is the cause of pleural pain, treatment with opiates is entirely appropriate, but these drugs depress respiratory drive and should never be used in asthma or COPD, except immediately prior to and during assisted mechanical ventilation.

Common to all cases is the need to restore adequate arterial oxygen levels, for which oxygen therapy with or without mechanically assisted ventilation is important. The consequences of untreated severe hypoxaemia include systemic hypotension, pulmonary hypertension,

19.18 RESPIRATORY FAILURE: UNDERLYING CAUSES AND BLOOD GAS ABNORMALITIES

	Type I		Type II	
	Hypoxia (PaO_2 < 8.0 kPa (60 mmHg)) Normal or low $PaCO_2$ (< 6.6 kPa (50 mmHg))		Hypoxia (PaO_2 < 8.0 kPa (60 mmHg)) Raised $PaCO_2$ (> 6.6 kPa (50 mmHg))	
	Acute	Chronic	Acute	Chronic
H^+	→ or ↑	→	↑	→ or ↑
Bicarbonate	→	→	→	↑
Causes	Acute asthma Pulmonary oedema Pneumonia Lobar collapse Pneumothorax Pulmonary embolus ARDS	Emphysema Lung fibrosis Lymphangitis carcinomatosa Right-to-left shunts Brain-stem lesion	Acute severe asthma Acute exacerbation COPD Upper airway obstruction Acute neuropathies/paralysis Narcotic drugs Primary alveolar hypoventilation Flail chest injury	COPD Sleep apnoea Kyphoscoliosis Myopathies/muscular dystrophy Ankylosing spondylitis

polycythaemia, tachycardia, and cerebral dysfunction ranging from confusion to coma.

Oxygen therapy

The delivery of oxygen to tissue mitochondria depends on several factors including: inspired oxygen concentration (FiO_2); alveolar ventilation; ventilation–perfusion distribution within the lung; haemoglobin and concentrations of agents such as carbon monoxide which may bind to haemoglobin; influences on the oxygen–haemoglobin dissociation curve (p. 184); cardiac output; and distribution of capillary blood flow within the tissues.

Oxygen therapy improves hypoxaemia by increasing alveolar PO_2 in poorly ventilated lung units. However, in conditions where desaturated blood is completely bypassing aerated lung (e.g. a right to left cardiac shunt, or a completely consolidated lobe), increasing FiO_2 has little or no effect on arterial PO_2. Indeed, when a shunt is present, careful measurement of arterial PO_2 when breathing 100% oxygen allows calculation of the percentage of the cardiac output flowing through the shunt.

Normally, high-flow oxygen (35–60%) is appropriate treatment in respiratory failure (e.g. severe asthma, pulmonary oedema or pneumonia) because respiratory drive is high. A small percentage of patients with severe chronic COPD and type II respiratory failure develop abnormal tolerance of raised CO_2 and may become dependent on hypoxic drive to breathe. In these patients only, lower concentrations of oxygen (24–28%) may be needed to avoid precipitating worsening respiratory depression (see below).

Toxic effects of oxygen

100% oxygen is both irritant and toxic if inhaled for more than a few hours. Premature infants develop retrolental fibroplasia and blindness if exposed to excessive concentrations. In adults, pulmonary oxygen toxicity (manifested by pulmonary oedema and free radical damage leading ultimately to fibrosis) would not be expected to occur unless the patient had been treated with inappropriately high concentrations of oxygen for more than 24 hours.

Administration of oxygen

Oxygen should always be prescribed in writing with clearly specified flow rates or concentrations.

- *High concentrations*, such as 40–60% oxygen via a high-flow mask, are particularly useful in acute type I respiratory failure such as commonly occurs in pneumonia, asthma or pulmonary oedema. When high-flow masks are used for prolonged periods, the oxygen should be humidified by passing it over warm water.
- *Low concentrations*. Venturi masks (24% or 28%), are the most accurate method of delivering controlled oxygen therapy in type II respiratory failure. However, once patients are stable, if a low concentration of oxygen is required continuously for more than a few hours, 1–2 litres per minute delivered via nasal cannulae allows patients to eat and to undergo physiotherapy etc. while continuing to receive oxygen. It is important to realise that the actual percentage of oxygen received from nasal cannulae will vary widely depending on minute ventilation, nasal blockage and any tendency to mouth-breathe. Humidification is not necessary with low-flow masks or nasal cannulae, as a high proportion of atmospheric air is mixed with oxygen.
- *Chronic oxygen delivery* from cylinders delivered to the home, or more conveniently from an oxygen concentrator, is often given via a low-concentration mask or nasal cannulae (for indications, see Box 19.33, p. 682). Portable oxygen may increase exercise tolerance in some patients with chronic hypoxic lung disease, and lightweight portable cylinders with oxygen-sparing devices may allow previously housebound patients to resume outdoor activities. Exercise testing is helpful in selecting patients who benefit from this treatment.

Monitoring of response to therapy

In patients with acute respiratory failure, close monitoring is essential and arterial blood gases taken on presentation should be repeated within 20 minutes to establish that treatment has achieved acceptable PaO_2 levels. If hypoxia persists despite appropriate oxygen therapy, progressive hypercapnia ($PaCO_2$ > 6.6 kPa (50 mmHg)) with acute respiratory acidosis develops or the patient becomes exhausted, an early decision should be made about whether it is appropriate to support ventilation temporarily by means of non-invasive ventilation or formal intubation and mechanical ventilation (p. 194). Very ill patients may require immediate ventilatory support on presentation.

CHRONIC AND 'ACUTE ON CHRONIC' TYPE II RESPIRATORY FAILURE

The most common cause of chronic type II respiratory failure is COPD. Here CO_2 retention may occur on a chronic basis, the acidaemia being corrected by renal retention of bicarbonate, which results in the plasma pH remaining within the normal range. This 'compensated' pattern, which is also seen in some patients with chronic neuromuscular disease or kyphoscoliosis, is maintained until there is a further pulmonary insult (Box 19.18), such as an exacerbation of COPD which precipitates an episode of 'acute on chronic' respiratory failure.

The further acute increase in $PaCO_2$ results in acidaemia and worsening hypercapnia, and may lead to drowsiness and eventually to coma. The principal aim of treatment in acute on chronic type II respiratory failure is to achieve a safe PaO_2 (> 7.0 kPa (52 mmHg)) without increasing $PaCO_2$ and acidosis, while identifying and treating the precipitating condition (Box 19.19). These patients usually have severe pre-existing lung disease, and only a small insult may be required to tip the balance towards severe respiratory failure. Moreover, in contrast to acute severe asthma, a patient with 'acute on chronic' type II respiratory failure due to COPD

19.19 ASSESSMENT AND MANAGEMENT OF 'ACUTE ON CHRONIC' TYPE II RESPIRATORY FAILURE

Initial assessment

N.B. Patient may not appear distressed despite being critically ill
- Conscious level (response to commands, ability to cough)
- CO_2 retention (warm periphery, bounding pulses, flapping tremor)
- Airways obstruction (wheeze, prolonged expiration, hyperinflation, intercostal indrawing, pursed lips)
- Cor pulmonale (peripheral oedema, raised JVP, hepatomegaly, ascites)
- Background functional status and quality of life
- Signs of precipitating cause (Box 19.18)

Investigations

- Arterial blood gases (severity of hypoxaemia, hypercapnia, acidaemia, bicarbonate)
- Chest X-ray

Management

- Maintenance of airway
- Treatment of specific precipitating cause (Box 19.18)
- Frequent physiotherapy ± pharyngeal suction
- Nebulised bronchodilators
- Controlled oxygen therapy
    Start with 24% controlled-flow mask
    Aim for a PaO_2 > 7 kPa (52 mmHg) (a PaO_2 < 5 (37 mmHg) is dangerous)
- Antibiotics
- Diuretics

Progress

- If $PaCO_2$ continues to rise or patient cannot achieve a safe PaO_2 without severe hypercapnia and acidaemia, respiratory stimulants (e.g. doxapram) or mechanical ventilatory support may be required

may not feel overtly distressed despite being critically ill with severe hypoxaemia, hypercapnia and acidaemia.

Management

In the initial assessment it is important to evaluate the patient's conscious level, the ability to cough effectively and the accompanying respiratory drive. This may give a preliminary indication of whether the patient will be able to tolerate non-invasive ventilation and whether physiotherapy will be helpful to clear retained secretions. Initial treatment includes low-concentration controlled oxygen therapy (24–28% oxygen with careful monitoring of blood gases), physiotherapy, bronchodilators, broad-spectrum antibiotics and diuretics (p. 683). The risks of worsening hypercapnia and coma must be balanced against those of severe hypoxaemia, which include potentially fatal arrhythmias or severe cerebral complications. The aim of oxygen therapy in this patient group is not necessarily to achieve a normal PaO_2; even a small increase will often have a greatly beneficial effect on tissue oxygen delivery since the PaO_2 values of these patients are often on the steep part of the oxygen saturation curve (p. 184). It is important to remember that while physical signs of CO_2 retention (confusion, flapping tremor, bounding pulses etc.) can be helpful if present, they are often unreliable, so there is no substitute for arterial blood gases in the assessment of initial severity and response to treatment. If controlled oxygen treatment causes a further increase in the $PaCO_2$ associated with a reduction in pH, non-invasive or invasive ventilatory support (p. 193) may be required. In this patient group the decision regarding intubation for mechanical ventilation can be particularly complex and difficult. Ideally, an early decision should be made, based mainly on whether there is a potentially remediable precipitating condition and whether the patient is likely to regain an acceptable quality of life.

Doxapram (1.5–4 mg/min) by slow intravenous infusion should only be used as a respiratory stimulant where non-invasive ventilation is not available or is poorly tolerated, or in those with reduced respiratory drive. Even in these circumstances this agent provides only minor and transient improvements in arterial blood gas parameters.

MECHANICALLY ASSISTED VENTILATION

Patients with initially severe respiratory failure (type I or type II) or those who fail to improve despite optimal medical therapy may require mechanical ventilation. The various types of non-invasive (via a face or nasal mask) or invasive (via an endotracheal tube) ventilation are detailed on page 193.

In many patients with respiratory failure, intubation and intermittent positive pressure ventilation (IPPV) with full sedation is appropriate. For specific groups of patients, however, non-invasive ventilation (NIV) has proved to be of great value in the treatment of respiratory failure. NIV is particularly effective as long-term treatment in respiratory failure due to skeletal deformity, neuromuscular disease and central alveolar hypoventilation. It is also effective in 'acute on chronic' type II respiratory failure due to an exacerbation of COPD where it reduces the need for

19

19.20 SOME INDICATIONS FOR LUNG TRANSPLANTATION	
Parenchymatous lung disease	
• Cystic fibrosis • Emphysema • Pulmonary fibrosis	• Langerhans cell histiocytosis • Lymphangioleiomyomatosis • Obliterative bronchiolitis
Pulmonary vascular disease	
• Primary pulmonary hypertension • Thromboembolic pulmonary hypertension	• Veno-occlusive disease • Eisenmenger's syndrome (p. 635)

intubation and shortens hospital stay. It can also be used in weaning such patients from IPPV ventilation.

LUNG TRANSPLANTATION

Lung transplantation is now an established treatment for carefully selected patients with advanced lung disease unresponsive to medical treatment (Box 19.20). Single-lung transplantation may be used for older patients with emphysema and patients with intrapulmonary restrictive disorders such as lung fibrosis. It is contraindicated in patients with chronic bilateral pulmonary infection, such as cystic fibrosis and bronchiectasis, where bilateral lung transplantation is the favoured option. Combined transplantation of the heart and lungs remains necessary for the treatment of patients with advanced congenital heart disease such as Eisenmenger's syndrome and is preferred by some surgeons for the treatment of primary pulmonary hypertension unresponsive to prostanoid therapy. Although prognosis is good with modern immunosuppressive drugs, the availability of lung transplants remains limited due to shortage of donor lungs. More recently, living lobar transplantation has been introduced.

OBSTRUCTIVE PULMONARY DISEASES

ASTHMA

Asthma is characterised by chronic airway inflammation and increased airway hyper-responsiveness leading to symptoms of wheeze, cough, chest tightness and dyspnoea. It is characterised functionally by the presence of airflow obstruction which is variable over short periods of time, or is reversible with treatment.

Epidemiology

The prevalence of asthma increased steadily over the latter part of the last century in countries with a Western lifestyle and is also increasing in developing countries. Current estimates suggest that 300 million people world-wide suffer from asthma and an additional 100 million may be diagnosed with asthma by 2025. In childhood, asthma is more common in boys, but following puberty females are more frequently affected. The socio-economic impact of asthma is enormous, particularly when poor control leads to days lost from school or work, hospital admissions and, for some patients, a premature death.

Aetiology

The aetiology of asthma is complex, and multiple environmental and genetic determinants are implicated (Fig. 19.16).

The hygiene hypothesis proposes that decreased infections in early life bias the immune system towards an allergic phenotype. T lymphocytes may differentiate into two distinct subsets: Th1 and Th2. In infancy, a shift occurs from the in utero Th2 bias towards a Th1 response necessary for fighting viral and bacterial infection. A reduction in childhood infections favours persistence of a Th2 bias (characterised by cytokines such as interleukins 4, 5 and 13), directing the immune system towards an allergic type of response. In support of this hypothesis, day care attendance (which presumably increases exposure to childhood infections) is associated with lower rates of atopy, wheeze and asthma in later childhood. Other infections, however, such as respiratory syncytial virus, appear to increase the risk of developing asthma and the validity of this hypothesis (including the ability to distinguish Th1 and Th2 cells clearly in humans) has been challenged.

The association between atopy—a propensity to produce IgE—and asthma suggests that sensitisation and exposure to allergens is an important risk factor. Warm, humid, centrally heated homes favour multiplication of house dust mites and this may contribute to childhood asthma. Many patients with asthma appear sensitised to pets such as cats and dogs;

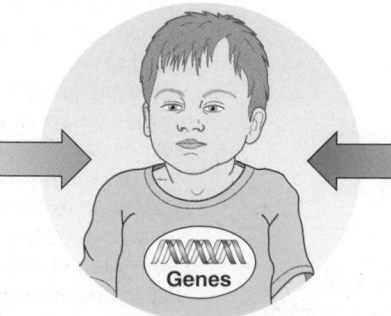

May protect against asthma
Living on farm
Large families
Childhood infections, including parasites
Predominance of lactobacilli in gut flora
Exposure to pets in early life

May predispose to asthma
Childhood infections, e.g. respiratory syncytial virus
Allergen exposure, e.g. house dust mite, household pets
Indoor pollution
Dietary deficiency of antioxidants
Exposure to pets in early life

Genes

Fig. 19.16 Factors implicated in the development of, or protection from, asthma.

however, the relationship between pet exposure and the development of asthma is complex, with some studies suggesting that pet exposure in early life may protect against asthma. Growing up on a farm appears to be protective for atopy and asthma, but the mechanism remains uncertain.

Dietary intake may be important. Milk fat and anti-oxidants such as vitamin E and selenium may protect against the development of asthma in children; however, in other studies early exposure to cows' milk protein has been linked to the development of atopy and asthma. Interest in probiotics as a potential therapy has been fuelled by observations that higher levels of *Lactobacillus* in the gut may protect against the development of atopic disease.

The increase in asthma may also be linked to the rise of obesity in Western society through mechanical mechanisms such as gastro-oesophageal reflux. Shared genetic traits, modification of the immune system by diet, or alteration of airway responsiveness by hormones are, however, alternative explanations.

The rapid rise in asthma is inconsistent with a genetic explanation; however, the development of asthma, the course of the disease and the response to treatment appear to be under genetic as well as environmental control. In common with other complex disease phenotypes, it is unlikely that a single asthma gene will emerge.

Pathophysiology

The inhalation of an allergen in a sensitised atopic asthmatic patient results in a two-phase bronchoconstrictor response (Fig. 19.17). The inhaled allergen rapidly interacts with mucosal mast cells via an IgE-dependent mechanism, resulting in the release of mediators such as histamine and the cysteinyl leukotrienes with resulting broncho-constriction. In persistent asthma a chronic and complex inflammatory response ensues, which is characterised by an influx of numerous inflammatory cells, the transformation and participation of airway structural cells, and the secretion of an array of cytokines, chemokines and growth factors (Fig. 19.18 and Box 19.21).

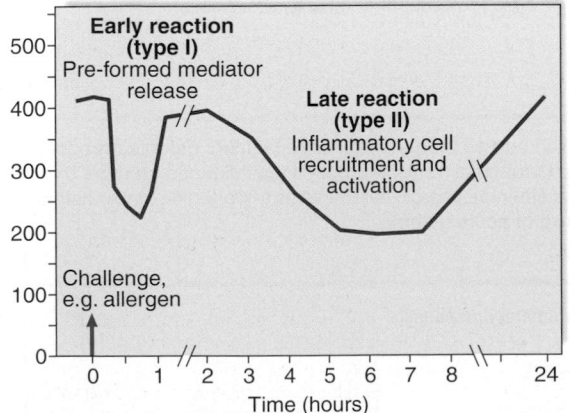

Peak flow (l/min)

Fig. 19.17 Changes in peak flow following allergen challenge. A similar biphasic response is observed following a variety of different challenges. Occasionally an individual will develop an isolated late response with no early reaction.

19.21 CARDINAL PATHOPHYSIOLOGICAL FEATURES OF ASTHMA
Airflow limitation
• Usually reverses spontaneously or with treatment
Airway hyper-reactivity
• Exaggerated bronchoconstriction to a wide range of non-specific stimuli, e.g. exercise, cold air
Airway inflammation
• Eosinophils, lymphocytes, mast cells, neutrophils; associated oedema, smooth muscle hypertrophy and hyperplasia, thickening of basement membrane, mucous plugging and epithelial damage.

Airway hyper-reactivity (AHR) is integral to the diagnosis of asthma and appears to be related, but not exclusively so, to airway inflammation. Other factors are likely to be important including the behaviour of airway smooth muscle, the degree of airway narrowing and the influence of neurogenic mechanisms.

With increasing severity and chronicity of the disease, remodelling of the airway occurs, leading to fibrosis of the airway wall, fixed narrowing of the airway and a reduced response to bronchodilator medication.

Clinical features

Asthma is not a uniform disease but a dynamic clinical syndrome with a variety of features. Typical symptoms include recurrent episodes of wheezing, chest tightness, breathlessness and cough. Common precipitants include exercise, particularly in cold weather, exposure to airborne allergens or pollutants, and viral upper respiratory tract infections (beware the cold that 'goes to the chest' or takes more than 10 days to clear). Patients with mild intermittent asthma are usually asymptomatic between exacerbations which occur during viral respiratory tract infections or after exposure to allergens. In persistent asthma the pattern is one of chronic wheeze and breathlessness.

Asthma characteristically displays a diurnal pattern, with symptoms and PEF being worse in the early morning. Particularly when asthma is poorly controlled, symptoms such as cough and wheeze disturb sleep and have led to the use of the term 'nocturnal asthma'. Cough may be the dominant symptom in some patients and the lack of wheeze or breathlessness may lead to a delay in reaching the diagnosis of so-called 'cough-variant asthma'.

In some circumstances the appearance of asthma relates to the use of medications. Beta-adrenoceptor antagonists (β-blockers—even when administered topically as eye drops) may induce bronchospasm. Aspirin and other non-steroidal anti-inflammatory drugs are associated with asthma in about 10% of patients. This is believed to reflect a shift in the metabolism of arachidonic acid from the cyclo-oxygenase pathway generating prostaglandins, towards the lipo-oxygenase pathway generating cysteinyl leukotrienes. Aspirin-sensitive asthma is often associated with rhino-sinusitis and nasal polyps.

Occupational asthma is now the most common form of occupational respiratory disorder and accounts for around

19

Mast cell

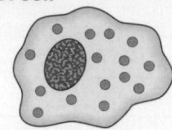

Cross-linking of IgE that binds to high affinity Fcε receptors leads to release of a variety of mediators key to the early-phase response including histamine, mast cell proteases and leukotrienes. Stores and secretes a range of pro-inflammatory cytokines

Eosinophil

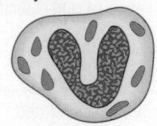

Appearance in sputum predates and predicts asthma exacerbations. Presence in airway suggests corticosteroid responsiveness. Charcot–Leyden crystals found in sputum derived from eosinophil products. Eosinophil granules contain an array of proteases, including major basic protein, with the potential to disrupt airway epithelium

T lymphocyte

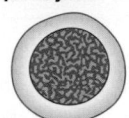

Coordinates the recruitment and behaviour of other inflammatory cells. Th2 cells secrete cytokines that promote the allergic response. Increased numbers of activated T cells present during asthma exacerbations. Patients with corticosteroid-resistant asthma have shown in vitro T-cell corticosteroid resistance

Neutrophil

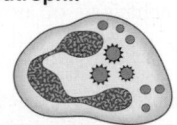

Identified in increased numbers in the airways of patients with severe and near-fatal asthma. Also a feature in some forms of occupational asthma. Predominance in sputum may predict poor response to inhaled corticosteroids

Macrophage

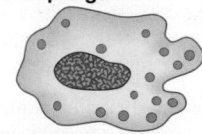

Secretes chemicals likely to be relevant to injury and repair including the secretion of growth factors that may be involved in airway wall remodelling

Epithelium

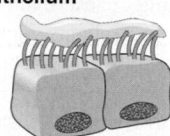

Epithelial integrity disrupted, facilitating increased antigen translocation. Creola bodies (clumps of shed epithelial cells) and Curschmann's spirals (strips of desquamated epithelium) seen in biopsies from asthmatic patients. Participates in inflammatory response by secreting pro-inflammatory cytokines and growth factors. Increased mucus secretion and reduced mucociliary clearance. Subepithelial basement membrane thickened

Airway smooth muscle

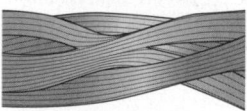

Undergoes hypertrophy and hyperplasia contributing to airway wall remodelling. Altered function contributes to airway hyper-reactivity. Secretes pro-inflammatory cytokines and growth factors

Endothelium

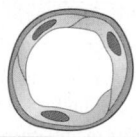

Increased microvascular permeability contributes to increased mucus secretion. Expression of adhesion molecules promotes recruitment of inflammatory cells

Neuronal dysfunction

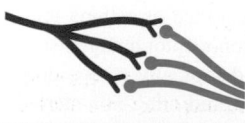

Non-adrenergic non-cholinergic (NANC) nerves promote bronchodilatation; defects proposed as a potential mechanism of increased bronchial tone. Neuropeptides influence function of inflammatory cells. Remains unclear whether cholinergic mechanisms important in stable asthma but increased cholinergic tone a feature of acute asthma

Fig. 19.18   The cellular and structural components to the asthmatic inflammatory response.

5% of all adult-onset asthma. This should be considered in all adult asthmatics of working age, particularly if symptoms improve during time away from work, e.g. weekends or holidays. Atopic individuals and smokers appear to be at increased risk. Early diagnosis and removal from exposure leads to a significantly improved prognosis and may result in cure. The recognition of occupational asthma has important medico-legal implications and should prompt screening of the workplace as other employees may also have developed the disease.

An important minority of patients appear to have a particularly severe form of asthma; this appears to be more common in women. Allergic triggers appear to be less important and airway neutrophilia predominates.

Investigations

The diagnosis of asthma is made on the basis of a compatible clinical history combined with the demonstration of variable airflow obstruction (Box 19.22).

Pulmonary function tests

Peak flow meters are inexpensive and widely available, and provide a simple and straightforward method of confirming the diagnosis. Ideally patients should be instructed to record peak flow readings after rising in the morning and before retiring in the evening. A diurnal variation in PEF (the lowest values typically being recorded in the morning) of more than 20% is considered diagnostic and the magnitude of variability provides some indication of disease severity (Fig. 19.19). A trial of corticosteroids (e.g. 30 mg daily for 2 weeks) may be useful in documenting the improvement in PEF seen in patients with asthma.

The measurement of FEV_1 and VC by spirometry allows the demonstration of airflow obstruction, and following the administration of a bronchodilator, confirms the diagnosis when a 15% (and 200 ml) improvement in FEV_1 is noted (Fig. 19.20). Spirometry is also particularly helpful in monitoring the severity of airflow obstruction in patients with impaired lung function.

Enhanced bronchoconstriction (AHR) to a variety of direct and indirect stimuli including exercise, cold air, dusts, smoke and chemicals such as histamine and methacholine, is an integral part of the definition of asthma, and may be helpful in patients presenting with normal lung function (Fig. 19.21). For patients whose symptoms are prominently related to exercise, an exercise test may be followed by a drop in PEF or FEV_1 (Fig. 19.22). AHR is sensitive but non-specific: it therefore has a high negative predictive value but positive results may be seen in other conditions such as COPD, bronchiectasis and CF. Challenge tests using adenosine are being developed and may prove more specific.

19.22 MAKING A DIAGNOSIS OF ASTHMA

Compatible clinical history *plus either/or*:
- $FEV_1 \geq 15\%$ (and 200 ml) increase following administration of a bronchodilator/trial of corticosteroids
- > 20% diurnal variation on ≥ 3 days in a week for 2 weeks on PEF diary
- $FEV_1 \geq 15\%$ decrease after 6 mins of exercise

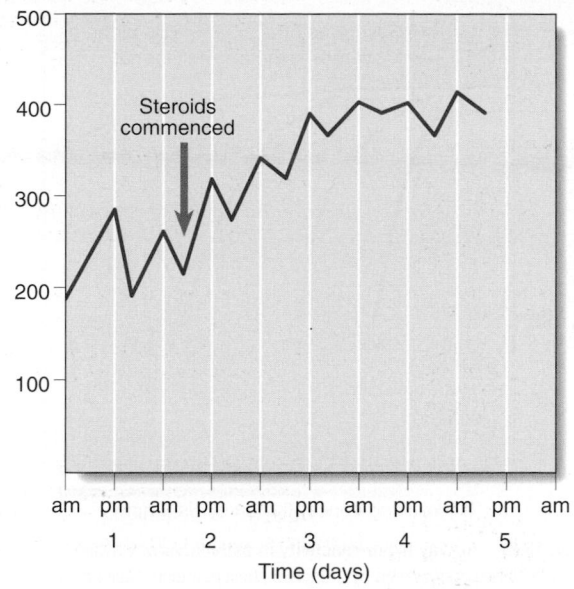

Fig. 19.19 Serial recordings of peak expiratory flow (PEF) in a patient with asthma. Note the sharp overnight fall (morning dip) and subsequent rise during the day. In this example corticosteroids have been commenced, followed by a subsequent improvement in PEF rate and loss of morning dipping.

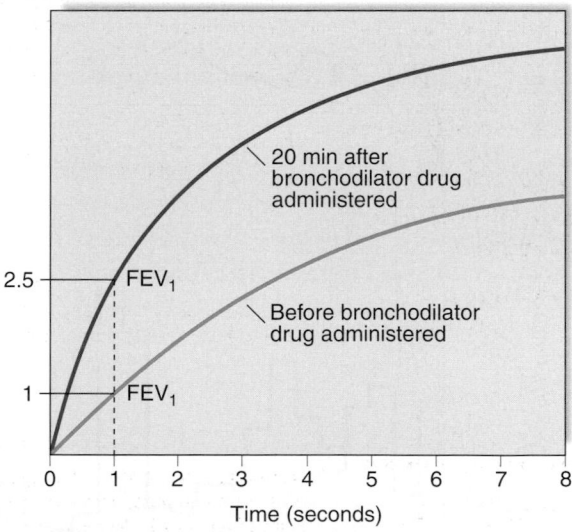

Fig. 19.20 Reversibility test. Forced expiratory manoeuvres before and 20 minutes after inhalation of a β_2-adrenoceptor agonist. Note the increase in FEV_1 from 1.0 to 2.5 litres.

The diagnosis of occupational asthma can be particularly difficult and it is often best to seek specialist assistance. Two-hourly recordings of peak flow, preferably including a period of time away from work, may establish the diagnosis but are often difficult to undertake (Fig. 19.23). Bronchial provocation tests with the suspected agent may be required.

19

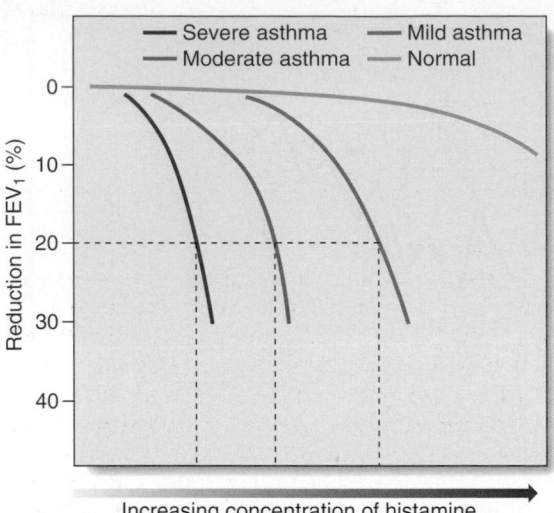

Fig. 19.21 **Airway hyper-reactivity in asthma.** Airway hyper-reactivity is demonstrated by bronchial challenge tests based on the administration of sequentially increasing concentrations of either histamine or methacholine. The reactivity of the airways is expressed as the concentration or dose of either chemical required to produce a certain decrease (usually 20%) in the FEV_1 (PC_{20} or PD_{20} respectively).

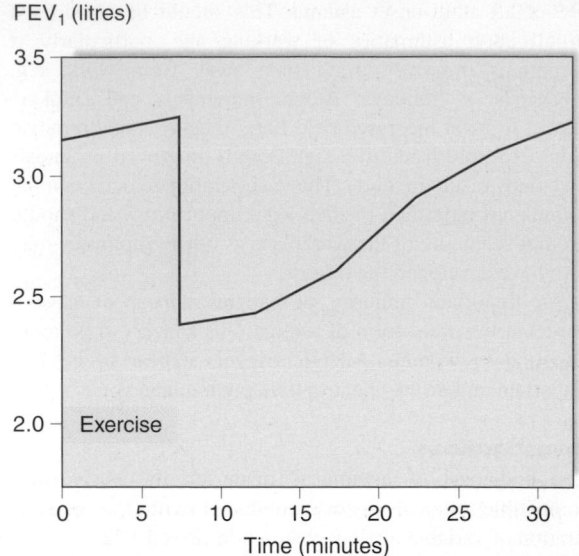

Fig. 19.22 **Exercise-induced asthma.** Serial recordings of forced expiratory volume in 1 second (FEV_1) in a patient with bronchial asthma before and after 6 minutes of strenuous exercise. Note initial slight rise on completion of exercise, followed by sudden fall and gradual recovery. Adequate warm-up exercise or pre-treatment with a β_2-adrenoceptor agonist, nedocromil sodium or a leukotriene antagonist (e.g. montelukast sodium) often protects against exercise-induced symptoms.

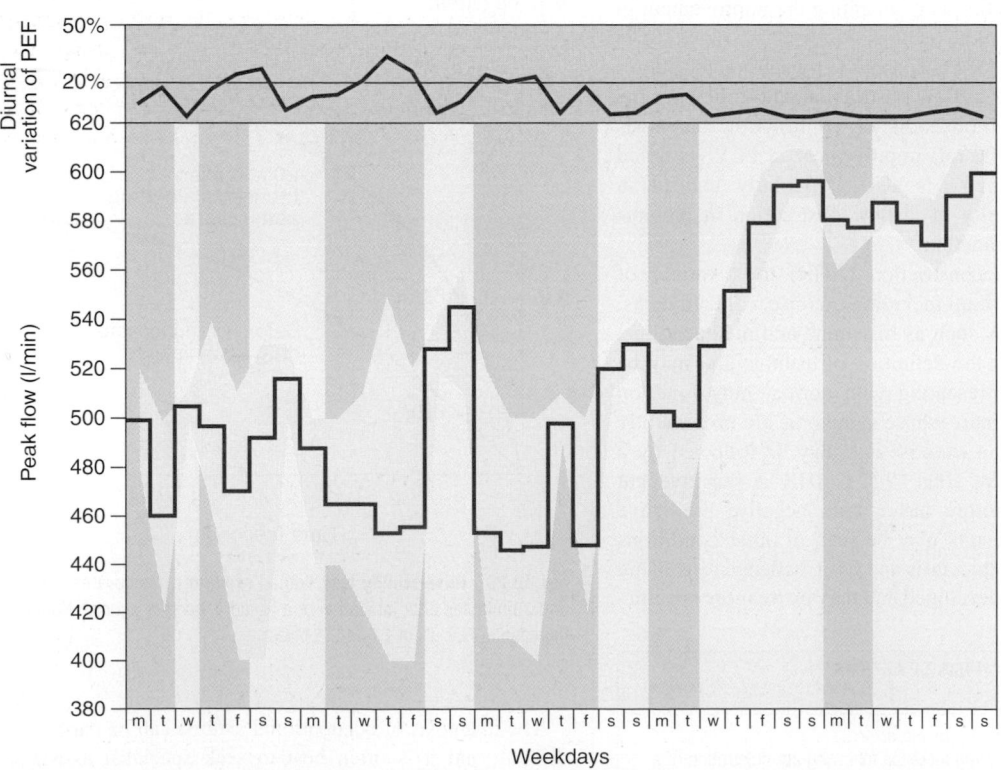

Fig. 19.23 **Peak flow readings in occupational asthma.** Subjects with suspected occupational asthma are asked to perform 2-hourly serial peak flows at and away from work. The maximum, mean and minimum values are plotted for each day. Days at work are displayed in the shaded areas. The diurnal variation is displayed at the top of the figure. In this example, a period away from work is followed by a marked improvement in peak flow readings and a reduction in diurnal variation.

Skin prick tests or the measurement of specific IgE may confirm sensitivity to the suspected agent.

Radiological examination

Radiological examination is generally unhelpful in establishing the diagnosis but may point to alternative diagnoses. Acute asthma is accompanied by hyperinflation, and lobar collapse may be seen if mucus has occluded a large bronchus. Flitting infiltrates, on occasion accompanied by lobar collapse, suggest asthma complicated by allergic bronchopulmonary aspergillosis (ABPA). An HRCT scan may be useful to detect bronchiectasis.

Measurement of allergic status

An elevated sputum or peripheral blood eosinophil count may be observed and the serum total IgE is typically elevated in atopic asthma. Skin prick tests are simple and provide a rapid assessment of atopy. Similar information may be provided by the measurement of allergen-specific IgE.

Assessment of airway inflammation

Induced sputum and exhaled breath allow the non-invasive assessment of airway inflammation and may prove useful in the diagnosis of asthma and assist in the monitoring of disease activity.

Management

Principles of management

In the majority of patients with asthma, the disease can be effectively managed in primary care by partnerships between doctors, nurses and, most importantly, patients themselves. The goals of asthma therapy have been endorsed by several sets of guidelines (Box 19.23). Management may be directed towards achieving these goals by following a stepwise approach (Fig. 19.24).

19.23 THE GOALS OF ASTHMA MANAGEMENT

- Achieve and maintain control of symptoms
- Prevent asthma exacerbations
- Maintain pulmonary function as close to normal as possible
- Avoid adverse effects from asthma medications
- Prevent development of irreversible airflow limitation
- Prevent asthma mortality

Patient education

The variable nature of asthma suggests that encouraging patients to take responsibility for control of their disease should lead to improved clinical outcomes. Patient education should begin at the time of diagnosis and be revisited in subsequent consultations. Patients (or their carers) should be taught about the relationship between symptoms and inflammation, the importance of key symptoms such as nocturnal waking, the different types of medication and the use of PEF to guide management decisions. Written action plans may prove helpful in developing these skills.

Avoidance of aggravating factors

This is particularly important in the management of occupational asthma, when removal from the offending agent is one of the few instances when asthma may be cured or substantially improved. Similarly, the identification of sensitisation to a household pet suggests that asthma control may be improved by removing the animal from the home, although it may take several years before dander levels fall substantially. House dust mite exposure may be minimised by replacing carpets with floorboards and using mite-impermeable bedding. However, to date improvements in asthma control following such measures have been difficult to demonstrate. Many patients are sensitised to several

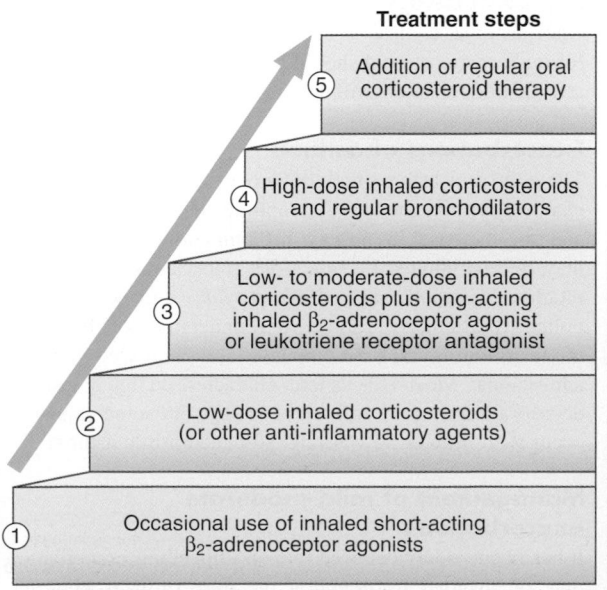

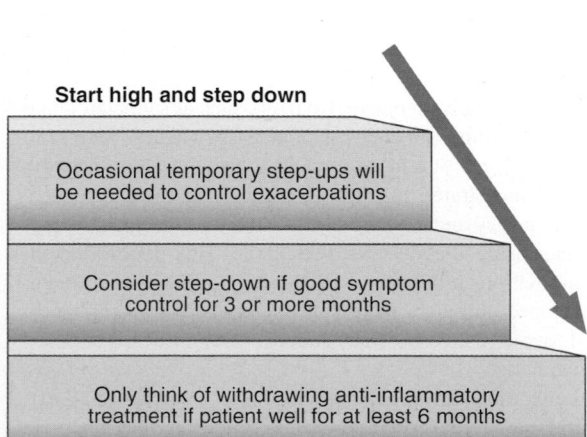

Fig. 19.24   Concept of step-up and step-down drug treatment in asthma.

antigens making avoidance strategies almost impossible. Measures to reduce fungal exposure and eliminate cockroaches may be applicable in specific circumstances and medications known to precipitate or aggravate asthma should be avoided. Patients should be advised not to smoke.

A stepwise approach to the management of asthma

Step 1: Occasional use of inhaled short-acting β_2-adrenoreceptor agonist bronchodilators

For patients with mild intermittent asthma (symptoms less than once a week for 3 months and fewer than two nocturnal episodes/month), it is usually sufficient to prescribe an inhaled short-acting β_2-agonist to be used on an as required basis. However, many patients, and their physicians, underestimate the severity of asthma and these patients should be carefully supervised. A history of a severe exacerbation should lead to a reclassification of the patient's condition as persistent asthma.

Step 2: Introduction of regular preventer therapy

Regular anti-inflammatory therapy (preferably inhaled corticosteroids—ICS) should be started in addition to inhaled β_2-agonists taken on an as required basis in any patient who:

- has experienced an exacerbation of asthma in the last 2 years
- uses inhaled β_2-agonists three times a week or more
- reports symptoms three times a week or more
- is awakened by asthma one night per week.

A reasonable starting dose is 400 µg beclometasone dipropionate (BDP) or equivalent per day in adults. BDP and budesonide (BUD) are approximately equivalent in clinical practice, although there may be variations with different delivery devices. Fluticasone and mometasone provide equal clinical activity to BDP/BUD at half the dosage.

Step 3: Add-on therapy

If the patient remains poorly controlled despite regular use of ICS, a thorough review of the patient should be made with particular regard to adherence and inhaler technique. A further increase in the dose of ICS may benefit some patients but in general, add-on therapy should be considered beyond an ICS dose of 800 µg/day BDP (or equivalent) in adults.

Long-acting β_2-agonists (LABAs), such as salmeterol and formoterol (duration of action of at least 12 hours), represent the first choice of add-on therapy as they have consistently been demonstrated to improve asthma control and reduce the frequency and severity of exacerbations when compared to increasing the dose of ICS alone (Box 19.24). Fixed combination inhalers of ICS and LABAs have been developed; these are more convenient, increase compliance and avoid concerns that patients may use LABAs as monotherapy.

Leukotriene receptor antagonists (e.g. montelukast 10 mg daily) are a relatively new class of agent that may be delivered orally and may reduce exacerbations. Theophyllines may be useful in some patients but their unpredictable

---

19.24 LONG-ACTING β_2-ADRENORECEPTOR AGONISTS IN CHRONIC ASTHMA	EBM

'In patients whose asthma is poorly controlled despite regular inhaled corticosteroids, addition of a long-acting β_2-adrenoreceptor agonist improves symptoms and lung function and prevents exacerbations.'

- Greening AP, et al. Lancet 1994; 334:219–224.
- Pauwels RA, et al. N Engl J Med 1997; 387:1405–1411.

For further information: 🖥 www.brit-thoracic.org.uk

---

metabolism, propensity for drug interactions and prominent side-effect profile have limited their use.

Step 4: Poor control on moderate dose of inhaled steroid and add-on therapy: addition of a fourth drug

In adults the dose of ICS may be increased to 2000 µg BDP/BUD daily. A nasal corticosteroid preparation should be used in patients with prominent upper airway symptoms. Oral therapy with leukotriene receptor antagonists, theophyllines or a slow-release β_2-agonist may be considered. If the trial of add-on therapy is ineffective it should be discontinued. Oral itraconazole should be contemplated in patients with ABPA. New therapies such as monoclonal antibodies directed against IgE may prove helpful and further studies are awaited.

Step 5: Continuous or frequent use of oral steroids

At this stage prednisolone therapy (usually administered as a single daily dose in the morning) should be prescribed in the lowest amount necessary to control symptoms. Patients on long-term corticosteroid tablets (> 3 months) or receiving more than three or four courses per year will be at risk of systemic side-effects. Osteoporosis can be prevented in this group of patients using bisphosphonates. Steroid-sparing therapies such as methotrexate, ciclosporin or oral gold may be considered but should be overseen by a specialist and are accompanied by significant side-effects.

Step-down therapy

Once asthma control is established, the dose of inhaled (or oral) corticosteroid should be titrated to the lowest dose at which effective control of asthma is maintained.

Exacerbations of asthma

The course of asthma may be punctuated by exacerbations characterised by increased symptoms, deterioration in PEF and an increase in airway inflammation. Exacerbations may be precipitated by infections (most commonly viral), moulds (*Alternaria* and *Cladosporium*) and on occasion pollen (particularly following thunderstorms). Increases in air pollution are accompanied by increased hospital admissions. Most attacks are characterised by a gradual deterioration over several hours to days but some appear to occur with little or no warning: so-called brittle asthma.

Management of mild–moderate exacerbations

It has been widely believed that an impending exacerbation may be avoided by doubling the dose of ICS; however, recent studies have failed to confirm this. Short courses of 'rescue' oral corticosteroids (prednisolone 30–60 mg daily) are therefore often required to regain control of symptoms. Tapering of the dose to withdraw treatment is not necessary unless given for more than 3 weeks.

Indications for 'rescue' courses include:

- symptoms and PEF progressively worsening day by day
- fall of PEF below 60% of the patient's personal best recording
- onset or worsening of sleep disturbance by asthma
- persistence of morning symptoms until midday
- progressively diminishing response to an inhaled bronchodilator
- symptoms severe enough to require treatment with nebulised or injected bronchodilators.

Management of acute severe asthma

Initial assessment

The features of acute asthma are listed in Box 19.25. An immediate assessment of patients (Fig. 19.25) should include their ability to speak, pulse rate, respiratory rate, BP and SaO_2. Measurement of PEF is mandatory unless the patient is too ill to cooperate and is most easily interpreted when expressed as a percentage of the predicted normal or of the previous best value obtained on optimal treatment. Arterial blood gas analysis is essential to determine the $PaCO_2$, a normal or elevated level being particularly dangerous. A chest X-ray is not immediately necessary unless pneumothorax is suspected.

19.25 IMMEDIATE ASSESSMENT OF ACUTE SEVERE ASTHMA
Acute severe asthma
- PEF 33–50% predicted (< 200 l/min) - Respiratory rate ≥ 25/min - Heart rate ≥ 110/min - Inability to complete sentences in 1 breath
Life-threatening features
- PEF 33–50% predicted (< 100 l/min) - SpO_2 < 92% or PaO_2 < 8 kPa (60 mmHg) (especially if being treated with oxygen) - Normal $PaCO_2$ - Silent chest - Cyanosis - Feeble respiratory effort - Bradycardia or arrhythmias - Hypotension - Exhaustion - Confusion - Coma
Near-fatal asthma
- Raised $PaCO_2$ and/or requiring mechanical ventilation with raised inflation pressures

Oxygen. High concentrations of oxygen (humidified if possible) should be administered to maintain the oxygen saturation above 92% in adults. The presence of a high $PaCO_2$ should not be taken as an indication to reduce oxygen concentration but is a warning sign of a severe or

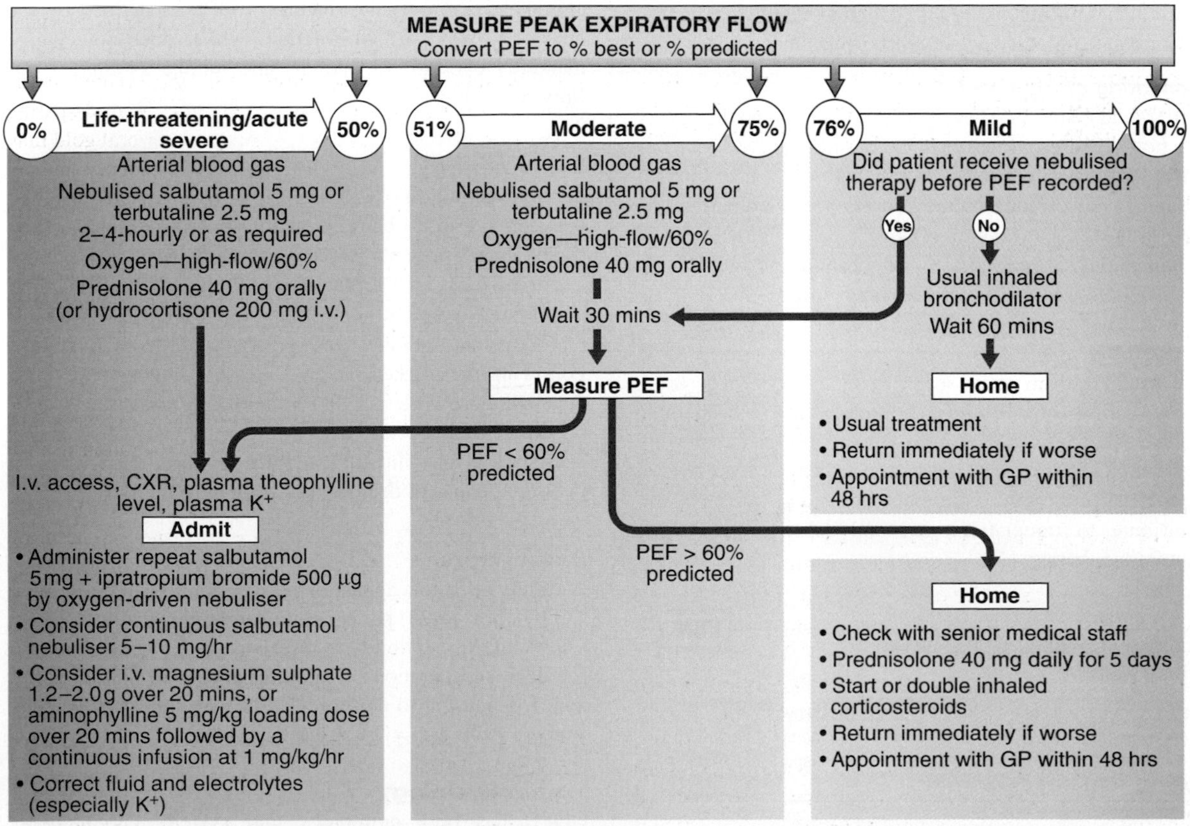

19

MEASURE PEAK EXPIRATORY FLOW
Convert PEF to % best or % predicted

0% — Life-threatening/acute severe — 50%

Arterial blood gas
Nebulised salbutamol 5 mg or terbutaline 2.5 mg
2–4-hourly or as required
Oxygen—high-flow/60%
Prednisolone 40 mg orally
(or hydrocortisone 200 mg i.v.)

I.v. access, CXR, plasma theophylline level, plasma K^+

Admit

- Administer repeat salbutamol 5 mg + ipratropium bromide 500 μg by oxygen-driven nebuliser
- Consider continuous salbutamol nebuliser 5–10 mg/hr
- Consider i.v. magnesium sulphate 1.2–2.0 g over 20 mins, or aminophylline 5 mg/kg loading dose over 20 mins followed by a continuous infusion at 1 mg/kg/hr
- Correct fluid and electrolytes (especially K^+)

51% — Moderate — 75%

Arterial blood gas
Nebulised salbutamol 5 mg or terbutaline 2.5 mg
Oxygen—high-flow/60%
Prednisolone 40 mg orally

Wait 30 mins

Measure PEF

PEF < 60% predicted

PEF > 60% predicted

76% — Mild — 100%

Did patient receive nebulised therapy before PEF recorded?

Yes / No

No → Usual inhaled bronchodilator
Wait 60 mins

Home

- Usual treatment
- Return immediately if worse
- Appointment with GP within 48 hrs

Home

- Check with senior medical staff
- Prednisolone 40 mg daily for 5 days
- Start or double inhaled corticosteroids
- Return immediately if worse
- Appointment with GP within 48 hrs

Fig. 19.25 Immediate treatment of patients with acute severe asthma.

life-threatening attack. Failure to achieve appropriate oxygenation is an indication for assisted ventilation.

High doses of inhaled bronchodilators. Short-acting β_2-agonists represent the agent of first choice. In hospital they are most conveniently administered via a nebuliser driven by oxygen but delivery of multiple doses of salbutamol via a metered dose inhaler through a spacer device provides equivalent bronchodilation and may be considered in primary care. Ipratropium bromide provides additional bronchodilator therapy and should be added to salbutamol in patients with acute severe or life-threatening attacks.

Systemic corticosteroids. Systemic corticosteroids reduce the inflammatory response and hasten the resolution of exacerbations. They should be administered to all patients with an acute severe attack. They can usually be administered orally (prednisolone 30–60 mg), but intravenous hydrocortisone 200 mg may be used in patients who are unable to swallow or vomiting.

Intravenous fluids. There are no controlled trials to support the use of intravenous fluids but many patients are dehydrated due to high insensible water loss and will probably benefit from hydration therapy. Potassium supplements may be necessary because repeated doses of salbutamol can lower serum potassium.

Subsequent management
If patients fail to improve, a number of further options may be considered. Intravenous magnesium may provide additional bronchodilation in patients whose presenting PEF is < 30% predicted (Box 19.26). Some patients appear to benefit from the use of intravenous aminophylline but careful monitoring is required. Intravenous leukotriene receptor antagonists may soon become available.

Monitoring of treatment
PEF should be recorded every 15–30 minutes and then every 4–6 hours. Pulse oximetry should ensure that SaO_2 remains > 92% but repeat arterial blood gases are necessary if the initial $PaCO_2$ measurements were normal or raised, the PaO_2 was < 8 kPa (60 mmHg), or the patient deteriorates.

Indications for endotracheal intubation and intermittent positive pressure ventilation are shown in Box 19.27.

Prognosis
The outcome from acute severe asthma is generally good. Death from asthma is fortunately rare but a considerable number of deaths occur in young people and many are preventable. Failure to recognise the severity of an attack, on the part of either the assessing physician or the patient, contribute to under-treatment and delay in delivering appropriate therapy.

19.26 INTRAVENOUS MAGNESIUM IN ACUTE ASTHMA   **EBM**

'Intravenous magnesium added to standard therapy in the management of acute asthma is of insufficient benefit to justify its routine use, although it reduced admission to hospital in a subset of patients with severe exacerbations.'

- Rowe BH, et al. (Cochrane Review). Cochrane Library, issue 2, 2001. Oxford: Update Software.

19.27 INDICATIONS FOR ASSISTED VENTILATION IN ACUTE SEVERE ASTHMA

- Coma
- Respiratory arrest
- Deterioration of arterial blood gas tensions despite optimal therapy
  PaO_2 < 8 kPa (60 mmHg) and falling
  $PaCO_2$ > 6 kPa (45 mmHg) and rising
  pH low and falling (H^+ high and rising)
- Exhaustion, confusion, drowsiness

Prior to discharge patients should be stable on discharge medication (nebulised therapy should have been discontinued for at least 24 hours) and the PEF should have reached 75% of predicted or personal best. The acute attack provides an opportunity to look for and address any trigger factors, for the delivery of asthma education and the provision of a written self-management plan. The patient should be offered an appointment with a GP or asthma nurse within 2 working days of discharge and follow-up at a specialist hospital clinic within a month.

CHRONIC OBSTRUCTIVE PULMONARY DISEASE (COPD)

COPD is a heterogeneous condition embracing several overlapping pathological processes including chronic bronchitis, chronic bronchiolitis (small airway disease) and emphysema. Many patients also exhibit a systemic component characterised by impaired nutrition, weight loss and skeletal muscle dysfunction. COPD is defined by the presence of airways obstruction, which does not change markedly over several months and, unlike asthma, is not fully reversible.

Epidemiology
The prevalence of COPD in the UK is estimated to be between 1 and 2% but is probably greater because airflow limitation is present in 10% of the general population. Exacerbations of COPD account for 10% of hospital admissions in the UK and with around 30 000 deaths/year it represents the sixth most common cause of death in the UK. Following the marked increase in tobacco consumption in developing countries COPD is gaining global importance; if current trends continue, it will become the fifth leading cause of lost disability-adjusted life years and the third most important cause of death world-wide by 2020.

Risk factors
A variety of factors appear to increase the risk of developing COPD (Box 19.28) but cigarette smoking remains the most important. Susceptibility to cigarette smoke varies but both the dose and duration of smoking appear to be important, and it is unusual to develop COPD with less than 10 pack years (1 pack year = 20 cigarettes/day/year).

Pathophysiology
COPD has both pulmonary and systemic components (Fig. 19.26). An enlargement of mucus-secreting glands and

19.28 RISK FACTORS FOR DEVELOPMENT OF COPD

Exposures

- Tobacco smoke—accounts for 95% of cases in UK
- Biomass solid fuel fires
- Occupation—coal miners and those who work with cadmium
- Outdoor and indoor air pollution
- Low socioeconomic status
- Low birth weight—may reduce maximally attained lung function in young adult life
- Lung growth—insults including childhood infections or maternal smoking may affect growth of lung during childhood, resulting in a lower maximally attained lung function in adult life
- Infections—recurrent infection may accelerate decline in FEV_1. Persistence of adenovirus in lung tissue may alter local inflammatory response predisposing to lung damage. HIV infection associated with emphysema
- Cannabis smoking (controversial)

Host factors

- Genetic factors—α_1-antiproteinase deficiency
- Airway hyper-reactivity

an increased number of goblet cells in the larger airways contribute to enhanced secretion of airway mucus that manifests as chronic bronchitis. Loss of elastic tissue surrounding the smaller airways, accompanied by inflammation and fibrosis in the airway wall and mucus accumulation within the airway lumen, results in airflow limitation, further increased by enhanced cholinergic tone.

Premature airway closure leads to gas trapping and hyperinflation, which in turn decrease pulmonary and chest

wall compliance. During exercise, the time available for expiration shortens, resulting in progressive hyperinflation. Increased $\dot{V}/\dot{Q}$ mismatch increases the dead space volume and limits maximal sustainable ventilation. Flattening of the diaphragmatic muscles and an increasingly horizontal alignment of the intercostal muscles place the respiratory muscles at a mechanical disadvantage. The work of breathing is therefore markedly increased, first on exercise but then, as the disease advances, at rest.

In the alveolar capillary units the unopposed action of proteases and oxidants results in destruction of the alveoli and the appearance of emphysema (Fig. 19.27). Emphysema may be classified by the pattern of the enlarged airspaces: centriacinar, panacinar and periacinar. Bullae form in some individuals. This results in impaired gas exchange and respiratory failure.

Clinical features

COPD should be suspected in any patient over the age of 40 years who presents with symptoms of persistent cough and sputum production and/or breathlessness. Depending on the presentation important differential diagnoses include asthma, tuberculosis, bronchiectasis and congestive cardiac failure. Chronic severe asthma may be difficult to distinguish from COPD.

Cough is usually the first symptom but seldom prompts the patient to consult a doctor. It is characteristically accompanied by small amounts of mucoid sputum. Chronic bronchitis is formally defined when a cough and sputum occur on most days for at least 3 consecutive months for at least 2 successive years. Haemoptysis may complicate

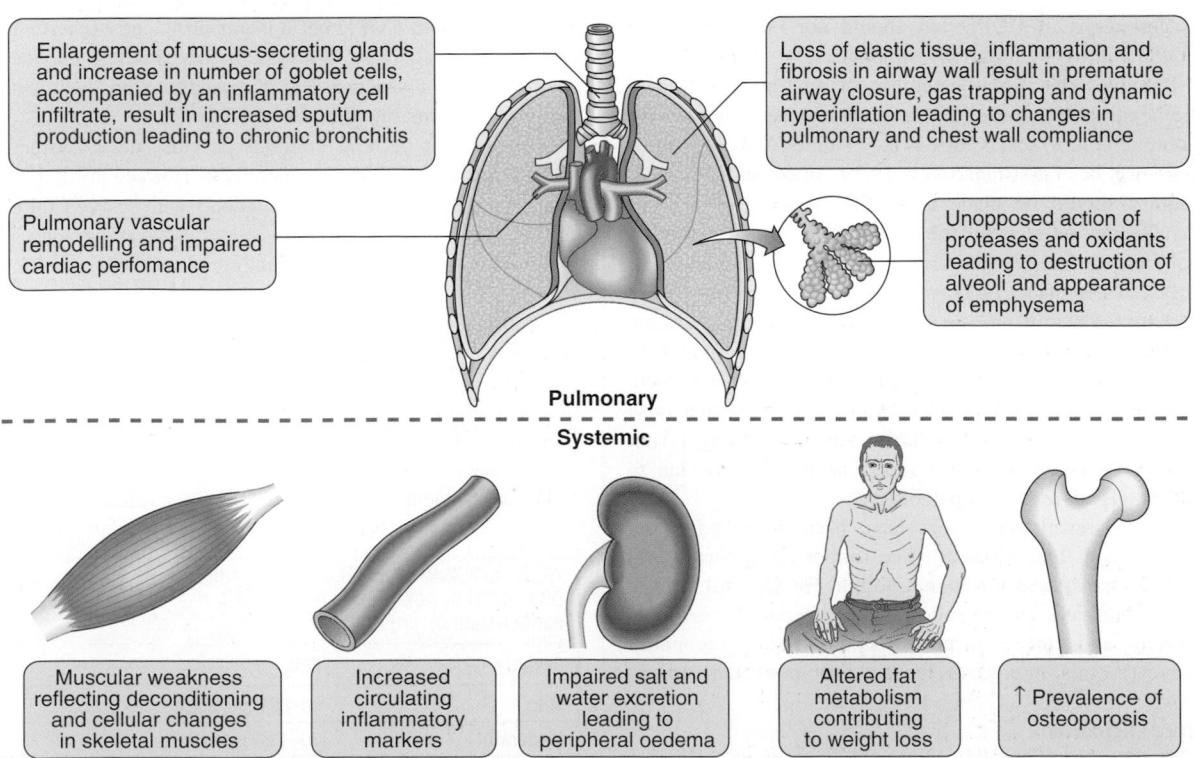

Fig. 19.26 **The pulmonary and systemic features of COPD.**

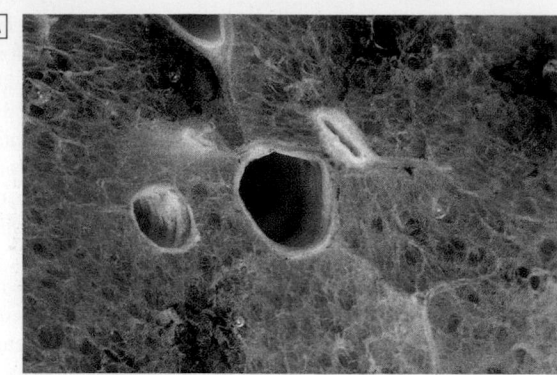
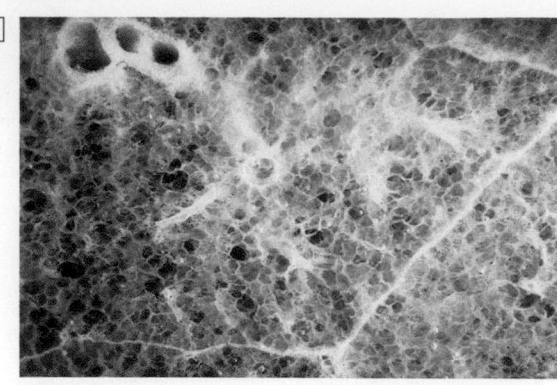

Fig. 19.27 The pathology of emphysema. [A] Normal lung. [B] Emphysematous lung showing gross loss of the normal surface area available for gas exchange.

19

19.29 MODIFIED MRC DYSPNOEA SCALE	
Grade	**Degree of breathlessness related to activities**
0	No breathlessness except with strenuous exercise
1	Breathlessness when hurrying on the level or walking up a slight hill
2	Walks slower than contemporaries on level ground because of breathlessness or has to stop for breath when walking at own pace
3	Stops for breath after walking about 100 m or after a few minutes on level ground
4	Too breathless to leave the house, or breathless when dressing or undressing

exacerbations of COPD but should not be attributed to COPD without thorough investigation.

Breathlessness usually heralds the first presentation to the health professional. The level should be quantified for future reference; scales such as the modified MRC dyspnoea scale may be of assistance (Box 19.29). In advanced disease, enquiry should be made as to the presence of oedema (which may be seen for the first time during an exacerbation) and morning headaches indicative of hypercapnia.

Physical signs (p. 649) are non-specific, correlate poorly with lung function, and are seldom obvious until the disease is advanced. The presence of pitting oedema should be documented and the body mass index (BMI) recorded. Crackles may accompany infection but if persistent raise the possibility of bronchiectasis. Finger clubbing is not consistent with COPD and should alert the physician to potentially more serious pathology.

Two classical phenotypes have been described: 'pink puffers' and 'blue bloaters'. The former are typically thin and breathless, and maintain a normal $PaCO_2$ until the late stage of disease. The latter develop (or tolerate) hypercapnia earlier and may develop oedema and secondary polycythaemia. In practice, these phenotypes often overlap.

Investigations

Although there are no reliable radiographic signs that correlate with the severity of airflow limitation, a chest X-ray is essential to identify alternative diagnoses such as cardiac failure, other complications of smoking such as lung cancer, and the presence of large bullae. A blood count is useful to exclude anaemia or document polycythaemia, and in younger patients with predominantly basal emphysema, α_1-antiproteinase should be assayed.

The diagnosis of COPD requires objective demonstration of airflow obstruction by spirometry and is established when the post-bronchodilator FEV_1 is less than 80% of the predicted value and accompanied by $FEV_1/FVC < 70\%$. The presence of an $FEV_1/FVC < 70\%$ in the presence of an FEV_1 of 80% or more suggests the presence of mild disease. Particular attention should be paid to vital capacity, as this is dependent on the technique and effort employed by the patient. The severity of COPD may be defined in relation to the post-bronchodilator FEV_1 (Box 19.30). A low peak flow is consistent with COPD but it is not sufficiently specific to confirm the diagnosis, is unable to discriminate between obstructive and restrictive disorders, and may underestimate the severity of airflow limitation in COPD.

Measurement of lung volumes provides an assessment of hyperinflation. This is generally performed by helium dilution technique; however, in patients with severe COPD, and in particular large bullae, body plethysmography is preferred because the use of helium may underestimate lung volumes. The presence of emphysema is suggested by a low gas transfer. Exercise tests provide an objective assessment of exercise tolerance and provide a baseline on which to judge the response to bronchodilator therapy or rehabilitation programmes; they may also be valuable when assessing prognosis. Pulse oximetry may prompt referral for a domiciliary oxygen assessment if less than 93%.

The assessment of health status provides valuable clinical

19.30 ASSESSMENT OF SEVERITY OF AIRFLOW OBSTRUCTION ACCORDING TO FEV₁ AS A PERCENTAGE OF PREDICTED VALUE	
Severity	**FEV₁**
Mild	50–80% predicted
Moderate	30–49% predicted
Severe	< 30% predicted

information but currently available questionnaires are too cumbersome for day-to-day practice.

CT is likely to play an increasing role in the assessment of COPD as it allows the detection, characterisation and quantification of emphysema (Fig. 19.28) and is more sensitive than the chest X-ray at detecting bullae.

Management

The management of COPD (Fig. 19.29) has been the subject of unjustified pessimism. It is usually possible to improve breathlessness, reduce the frequency and severity of exacerbations, and improve health status and prognosis.

Smoking cessation

Every attempt should be made to highlight the role of smoking in the development and progress of the disease and encourage, advise and assist the patient toward smoking cessation. On cessation (p. 98), patients should be warned to expect an apparent worsening of chest symptoms and reassured that this is temporary. Cessation is difficult but highly rewarding and remains the only intervention proven to decelerate the decline in FEV_1 (Fig. 19.30 and Box 19.31).

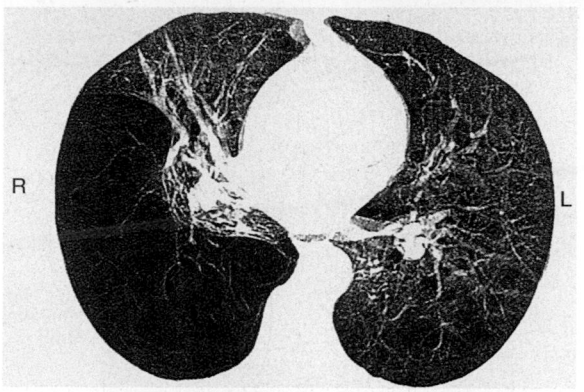

Fig. 19.28 Gross emphysema. High-resolution CT showing emphysema most evident in the right lower lobe.

19

Bronchodilators

Bronchodilator therapy is central to the management of breathlessness in patients with COPD. The inhaled route is preferred and a number of different agents delivered by a variety of devices are available. Choice should be informed

Smoking	• Offer help to stop smoking at every opportunity • Combine pharmacotherapy with appropriate support as part of a programme
Breathlessness and exercise limitation	• Use short-acting bronchodilator p.r.n. (β_2-agonist or anticholinergic) • If still symptomatic, try combined therapy with a short-acting β_2-agonist and a short-acting anticholinergic • If still symptomatic, use a long-acting bronchodilator (β_2-agonist or anticholinergic) • In moderate or severe COPD: If still symptomatic, consider a trial of a combination of a long-acting β_2-agonist and inhaled corticosteroid. **Discontinue if no benefit after 4 weeks** • If still symptomatic, consider adding theophylline • Offer pulmonary rehabilitation to all patients who consider themselves functionally disabled (usually MRC grade 3 and above) • Consider referral for surgery: bullectomy, LVRS, transplantation
Frequent exacerbations	• Offer pneumococcal and annual influenza vaccination • Give self-management advice • Optimise bronchodilator therapy with one or more long-acting bronchodilator (β_2-agonist or anticholinergic) • Add inhaled corticosteroids if FEV_1 50% and two or more exacerbations in a 12-month period (N.B. These will usually be used with long-acting bronchodilators)
Respiratory failure	• Assess for appropriate oxygen: LTOT, ambulatory, short burst • Consider referral for assessment for long-term domiciliary NIV
Cor pulmonale	• Need for oxygen • Use diuretics
Abnormal BMI	• Refer for dietetic advice • Give nutritional supplements if BMI is low
Chronic productive cough	• Consider trial of mucolytic therapy • Continue if symptomatic improvement
Anxiety and depression	• Be aware of these and screen most physically disabled patients • Treat with conventional pharmacotherapy

Stop therapy if ineffective (applies to Breathlessness and exercise limitation section)

Fig. 19.29 Summary of management of COPD.

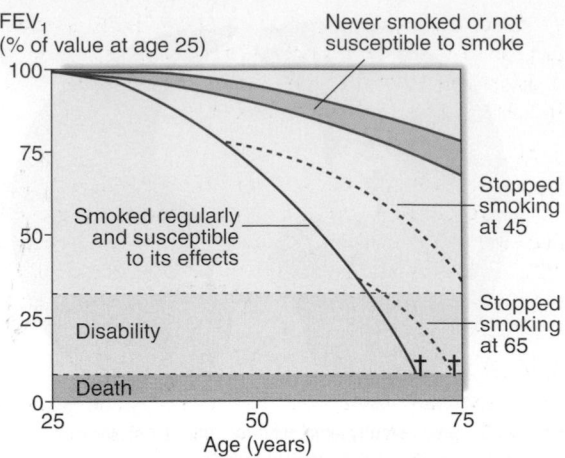

Fig. 19.30 Model of annual decline in FEV₁ with accelerated decline in susceptible smokers. When smoking is stopped, subsequent loss is similar to that in healthy non-smokers.

19.31 BENEFITS OF SMOKING CESSATION IN COPD | EBM

'The Lung Health Study showed that smoking cessation was associated with improvements in lung function and a reduction in respiratory symptoms in patients with mild-to-moderate COPD.'

- Scanlon PD, et al. Am J Respir Crit Care Med 2000; 161:381–390.
- Kanner RE, et al. Am J Med 1999; 106:410–416.

---

by patient preference and inhaler assessment. Short-acting bronchodilators may be used for patients with mild disease but longer-acting bronchodilators are more appropriate for patients with moderate to severe disease. It is important to realise that significant improvements in breathlessness may be reported despite minimal changes in FEV₁, probably reflecting improvements in lung emptying that reduce dynamic hyperinflation and ease the work of breathing.

Oral bronchodilator therapy may be contemplated in patients who cannot use inhaled devices efficiently. Theophylline preparations improve breathlessness and quality of life, but their use has been limited by side-effects, unpredictable metabolism and drug interactions. Bambuterol—a pro-drug of terbutaline—is used on occasion. Orally active highly selective phosphodiesterase inhibitors are currently being developed.

Corticosteroids

Inhaled corticosteroids (ICS) reduce the frequency and severity of exacerbations; they are currently recommended in patients with severe disease (FEV₁ < 50%) who report two or more exacerbations requiring antibiotics or oral steroids per year. Regular use is associated with a small improvement in FEV₁, but there is no impact on the accelerated decline in lung function. The combination of ICS with long-acting β₂-agonists produces further improvement in breathlessness and reduces the frequency and severity of exacerbations.

Oral corticosteroids are useful during exacerbations but maintenance therapy contributes to osteoporosis and impaired skeletal muscle function and should be avoided. Oral

corticosteroid trials may assist in the diagnosis of asthma but do not predict response to inhaled steroids in COPD.

Pulmonary rehabilitation

Exercise should be encouraged at all stages and patients reassured that breathlessness, whilst distressing, is not dangerous. Multidisciplinary programmes that incorporate physical training, disease education and nutritional counselling reduce symptoms, improve health status and enhance confidence. Most programmes include two to three sessions per week, last between 6 and 12 weeks, and are accompanied by demonstrable and sustained improvements.

Oxygen therapy

Long-term domiciliary oxygen therapy (LTOT) has been shown to improve survival, prevent progression of pulmonary hypertension, decrease the incidence of secondary polycythaemia, and improve neuropsychological health (Box 19.32). It is most conveniently provided by an oxygen concentrator via nasal prongs and patients should be instructed to use oxygen for a minimum of 15 hours/day; greater benefits are seen in patients who receive > 20 hours/day. The aim of therapy is to increase the PaO_2 to at least 8 kPa (60 mmHg) or SaO_2 at least 90% (Box 19.33). Ambulatory oxygen therapy should be considered in patients who desaturate on exercise and show objective improvement in exercise capacity and/or dyspnoea with oxygen. Oxygen flow rates should be adjusted to maintain SaO_2 above 90%. Short-burst oxygen therapy is widely prescribed but is expensive and of unproven benefit.

19.32 LONG-TERM DOMICILIARY OXYGEN THERAPY (LTOT) | EBM

'LTOT (used for ≥ 15 hrs/day) in patients with COPD and chronic severe hypoxaemia improves survival, reduces secondary polycythaemia and prevents progression of primary pulmonary hypertension.'

- Crokett AJ, et al. (Cochrane Review). Cochrane Library, issue 4, 2000. Oxford: Update Software

For further information: 💻 www.brit-thoracic.org.uk

19.33 PRESCRIPTION OF LONG-TERM OXYGEN THERAPY (LTOT) IN COPD

Arterial blood gases measured in clinically stable patients on optimal medical therapy on at least two occasions 3 weeks apart
- PaO_2 < 7.3 kPa (55 mmHg) irrespective of $PaCO_2$ and FEV₁ < 1.5 litres
- PaO_2 7.3–8 kPa (55–60 mmHg) plus pulmonary hypertension, peripheral oedema or nocturnal hypoxaemia
- Patient stopped smoking

Use at least 15 hours/day at 2–4 litres/min to achieve a PaO_2 > 8 kPa (60 mmHg) without unacceptable rise in $PaCO_2$

Surgical intervention

Selected patients with COPD may benefit from surgical intervention. Young patients with minimal airflow limitation and a lack of generalised emphysema, but in whom large bullae compress surrounding normal lung tissue, may be considered for bullectomy. Lung volume reduction surgery

19

(LVRS) removes peripheral emphysematous lung tissue reducing hyperinflation and decreasing the work of breathing. In carefully selected patients LVRS results in improvements in FEV_1, lung volumes, exercise tolerance and quality of life. Effects last for at least 2 years but long-term outcomes are unknown. Both bullectomy and LVRS can be performed thorascopically, minimising morbidity. Lung transplantation may benefit highly selected patients with advanced disease but is limited by shortages in donor organs.

Other measures

Patients with COPD should be offered an annual influenza vaccination and, as appropriate, pneumococcal vaccination. Obesity, poor nutrition, depression and social isolation should be identified and, if possible, improved. Mucolytic therapy (e.g. acetylcysteine 200 mg orally 8-hourly for 8 weeks in the first instance) may be recommended in patients with chronic cough and sputum production and should be continued if symptomatic benefit is reported.

Prognosis

COPD has a variable natural history. The prognosis is inversely related to age and directly related to the post-bronchodilator FEV_1. Additional poor prognostic indicators include weight loss (survival is negatively correlated with BMI) and pulmonary hypertension. A recent study has suggested that a composite score comprising the body mass index (B), the degree of airflow obstruction (O), a measurement of dyspnoea (D) and exercise capacity (E) may assist in predicting death from respiratory and other causes (Box 19.34).

Acute exacerbations of COPD

Acute exacerbations of COPD are characterised by an increase in symptoms and deterioration in lung function and health status. They become more common as the disease progresses and may be caused by bacteria, viruses or a change in air quality. They may be accompanied by the development of respiratory failure and/or fluid retention and represent an important cause of death.

Many patients can be managed at home with the use of increased bronchodilator therapy, a short course of oral corticosteroids, and if appropriate, antibiotics. The presence of cyanosis, peripheral oedema or an alteration in consciousness should prompt referral to hospital. In other patients consideration of comorbidity and social circumstances may influence decisions regarding placement.

Oxygen therapy

In patients with an exacerbation of severe COPD, high concentrations of oxygen may cause respiratory depression and worsening acidosis (p. 668). Controlled oxygen at 24% or 28% should be used with the aim of maintaining a $PaO_2 > 8$ kPa (60 mmHg) (or an $SaO_2 > 90\%$) without worsening acidosis.

Bronchodilators

Nebulised short-acting β_2-agonists combined with an anticholinergic agent should be administered. Provided patients are properly supervised it is usually safe to drive nebulisers with oxygen, but if concern exists regarding oxygen sensitivity nebulisers may be driven by compressed air and supplemental oxygen delivered by nasal cannula.

Corticosteroids

Oral prednisolone reduces symptoms and improves lung function. Currently doses of 30 mg for 10 days are recommended but shorter courses may be acceptable. Prophylaxis against osteoporosis should be considered in patients who receive repeated courses of steroids.

Antibiotic therapy

The role of bacteria in exacerbations remains controversial and there is little evidence for the routine administration of antibiotics. They are currently recommended for patients reporting an increase in sputum purulence, sputum volume or breathlessness. In most cases simple regimens are advised such as an aminopenicillin or a macrolide. Co-amoxiclav is only required in regions where β-lactamase-producing organisms are known to be common.

Non-invasive ventilation

If, despite the above measures, the patient remains tachypnoeic and acidotic ($H^+ \geq 45$, pH < 7.35), then NIV should be commenced (p. 669). Several studies have shown that its use is associated with reduced requirements for mechanical ventilation and reductions in mortality (Box 19.35). It is not useful in patients who cannot protect their airway. Mechanical ventilation may be contemplated in those with a reversible cause for deterioration (e.g. pneumonia), or when no prior history of respiratory failure has been noted.

Additional therapy

There has been a vogue for using an infusion of intravenous aminophylline but evidence for benefit is limited and

---

19.34 COMPONENTS USED TO COMPUTE BMI, DEGREE OF AIRFLOW OBSTRUCTION AND DYSPNOEA, AND EXERCISE CAPACITY (BODE) INDEX

Variable	Points on BODE index			
	0	1	2	3
FEV_1	≥ 65	50–64	36–49	≤ 35
Distance walked in 6 min (m)	≥ 350	250–349	150–249	≤ 149
MMRC dyspnoea scale	0–1	2	3	4
Body mass index	> 21	≤ 21		

A patient with a BODE score of 0–2 has a mortality rate of around 10% at 52 months whereas a patient with a BODE score of 7–10 has a mortality rate of around 80% at 52 months

---

19.35 NON-INVASIVE VENTILATION IN COPD EXACERBATIONS   **EBM**

'Early non-invasive ventilation of patients with mild to moderate respiratory acidosis during an acute exacerbation of COPD reduces the need for endotracheal intubation, the length of hospital stay and the in-hospital mortality.'

- Brochard L, et al. N Engl J Med 1995; 333:817–822.
- Plant PK, et al. Lancet 1999; 355:1931–1935.

19.36 OBSTRUCTIVE PULMONARY DISEASE IN OLD AGE

- **Asthma**: may appear de novo in old age and airflow obstruction should not always be assumed to be due to COPD.
- **PEF recordings**: older people with poor vision have difficulty reading PEF meters.
- **Perception of bronchoconstriction**: less than in younger patients, so an older patient's description of symptoms is not a reliable indicator of severity.
- **Stopping smoking**: the benefits on the rate of loss of lung function decline with age but remain valuable up to the age of 80.
- **Metered dose inhalers**: most older people cannot use these because of difficulty coordinating and triggering the device. Even mild cognitive impairment virtually precludes their use. Frequent demonstration and reinstruction in the use of all devices are required.
- **Mortality rates for acute asthma**: higher in old age, partly because patients underestimate the severity of bronchoconstriction and also develop a lower degree tachycardia and pulsus paradoxus for the same degree of bronchoconstriction.
- **Treatment decisions**: advanced age in itself is not a barrier to intensive care or mechanical ventilation in an acute episode of asthma or COPD, but this decision can be difficult and should be shared with the patient (if possible), the relatives and the GP.

19.37 CAUSES OF BRONCHIECTASIS

Congenital

- Cystic fibrosis
- Ciliary dysfunction syndromes
  Primary ciliary dyskinesia (immotile cilia syndrome)
  Kartagener's syndrome (sinusitis and transposition of the viscera)
- Primary hypogammaglobulinaemia (p. 897)

Acquired—children

- Pneumonia (complicating whooping cough or measles)
- Primary TB
- Inhaled foreign body

Acquired—adults

- Suppurative pneumonia
- Pulmonary TB
- Allergic bronchopulmonary aspergillosis complicating asthma (p. 703)
- Bronchial tumours

attention must be paid to the risk of inducing arrhythmias and drug interactions. The use of the respiratory stimulant doxapram has been largely superseded by the development of NIV, but it may be useful for a limited period in selected patients with a low respiratory rate. Diuretics should be administered if peripheral oedema has developed.

Discharge

Discharge from hospital may be contemplated once the patient is clinically stable on his or her usual maintenance medication. The provision of a nurse-led 'hospital at home' team providing short-term nebuliser loan improves discharge rates and provides additional support for the patient.

BRONCHIECTASIS

Bronchiectasis is the term used to describe abnormal dilatation of the bronchi. It is usually acquired but may result from an underlying genetic or congenital defect of airway defences.

Aetiology and pathogenesis

Bronchiectasis is usually caused by chronic inflammation and infection in airways. Box 19.37 shows the common causes, of which TB is the most common world-wide.

Localised bronchiectasis may be due to bronchial distension resulting from the accumulation of pus beyond an obstructing bronchial lesion, such as enlarged tuberculous hilar lymph nodes, a bronchial tumour or an inhaled foreign body (e.g. an aspirated peanut).

Pathology

The bronchiectatic cavities may be lined by granulation tissue, squamous epithelium or normal ciliated epithelium.

There may also be inflammatory changes in the deeper layers of the bronchial wall and hypertrophy of the bronchial arteries. Chronic inflammatory and fibrotic changes are usually found in the surrounding lung tissue.

Clinical features

The symptoms of bronchiectasis are summarised in Box 19.38.

Physical signs in the chest may be unilateral or bilateral. If the bronchiectatic airways do not contain secretions and there is no associated lobar collapse, there are no abnormal physical signs. When there are large amounts of sputum in the bronchiectatic spaces numerous coarse crackles may be heard over the affected areas. When collapse is present the

19.38 SYMPTOMS OF BRONCHIECTASIS

Due to accumulation of pus in dilated bronchi

- Chronic productive cough usually worse in mornings and often brought on by changes of posture. Sputum often copious and persistently purulent in advanced disease. Halitosis is a common accompanying feature

Due to inflammatory changes in lung and pleura surrounding dilated bronchi

- Fever, malaise and increased cough and sputum volume when spread of infection causes pneumonia, which may be associated with pleurisy. Recurrent pleurisy in the same site often occurs in bronchiectasis

Haemoptysis

- Can be slight or massive and is often recurrent. Usually associated with purulent sputum or an increase in sputum purulence. Can, however, be the only symptom in so-called 'dry bronchiectasis'

General health

- When disease is extensive and sputum persistently purulent a decline in general health occurs with weight loss, anorexia, lassitude, low-grade fever, and failure to thrive in children. In these patients digital clubbing is common

character of the physical signs depends on whether or not the proximal bronchus supplying the collapsed lobe is patent (breath sounds are diminished if the airway is obstructed). Advanced disease may lead to scarring with associated overlying bronchial breathing.

Investigations

Bacteriological and mycological examination of sputum

In addition to common respiratory pathogens, sputum culture may reveal *Pseudomonas aeruginosa*, fungi such as *Aspergillus* and various *Mycobacteria*. Frequent cultures are necessary to ensure appropriate treatment of resistant organisms.

Radiological examination

Bronchiectasis, unless very gross, is not usually apparent on a chest X-ray. In advanced disease, thickened airway walls, cystic bronchiectatic spaces, and associated areas of pneumonic consolidation or collapse may be visible. CT is much more sensitive, and shows thickened dilated airways (Fig. 19.5, p. 653).

Assessment of ciliary function

A screening test can be performed in patients suspected of having a ciliary dysfunction syndrome by assessing the time taken for a small pellet of saccharin placed in the anterior chamber of the nose to reach the pharynx, when the patient can taste it. This time should not exceed 20 minutes and is greatly prolonged in patients with ciliary dysfunction. Ciliary beat frequency may also be assessed using biopsies taken from the nose. Structural abnormalities of cilia can be detected by electron microscopy.

Management

In patients with airflow obstruction, inhaled bronchodilators and corticosteroids should be used to enhance airway patency.

Physiotherapy

Patients should be instructed how to perform regular daily physiotherapy to keep the dilated bronchi empty of secretions. Efficiently performed, this is of great value both in reducing the amount of cough and sputum and in preventing recurrent episodes of bronchopulmonary infection. Patients should adopt a position in which the lobe to be drained is uppermost. Deep breathing followed by forced expiratory manoeuvres (the 'active cycle of breathing' technique) is of help in allowing secretions in the dilated bronchi to gravitate towards the trachea, from which they can be cleared by vigorous coughing. 'Percussion' of the chest wall with cupped hands may help to dislodge sputum, and a number of mechanical devices are available which cause the chest wall to oscillate, thus achieving the same effect. The optimum duration and frequency of physiotherapy depends on the amount of sputum but 5–10 minutes once or twice daily is a minimum for most patients.

Antibiotic therapy

The policy governing the use of antibiotics in most patients with bronchiectasis is the same as that in COPD (p. 683). Some present difficult therapeutic problems because of secondary infection with bacteria such as staphylococci and Gram-negative bacilli, in particular *Pseudomonas* species. In these circumstances antibiotic therapy should be guided by the microbiological results but frequently requires the use of oral ciprofloxacin (250–750 mg 12-hourly) or ceftazidime by intravenous injection or infusion (1–2 g 8-hourly).

Surgical treatment

Surgery is only indicated in a small proportion of cases. These are usually young patients in whom the bronchiectasis is unilateral and confined to a single lobe or segment as demonstrated by CT. Unfortunately, many of the patients in whom medical treatment proves unsuccessful are also unsuitable for pulmonary resection because of either extensive bronchiectasis or coexisting chronic lung disease. In progressive forms of bronchiectasis resection of destroyed areas of lung which are acting as a reservoir of infection should only be considered as a last resort.

Prognosis

The disease is progressive when associated with ciliary dysfunction and cystic fibrosis, and eventually causes respiratory failure. In other patients the prognosis can be relatively good if postural drainage is performed regularly and antibiotics are used judiciously.

Prevention

As bronchiectasis commonly starts in childhood following measles, whooping cough or a primary tuberculous infection, it is essential that these conditions receive adequate prophylaxis and treatment. The early recognition and treatment of bronchial obstruction are also particularly important.

CYSTIC FIBROSIS

Genetics, pathogenesis and epidemiology

Cystic fibrosis (CF) is the most common fatal autosomal recessive disease in Caucasians, with a carrier rate of 1 in 25 and an incidence of about 1 in 2500 live births (pp. 45–46). CF is the result of mutations affecting a gene (on the long arm of chromosome 7) coding for a chloride channel known as cystic fibrosis transmembrane conductance regulator (*CFTR*), which controls salt and water movement across epithelial cell membranes. The most common *CFTR* mutation in northern European and American populations is ΔF508, but over 800 mutations of this gene have now been identified. The genetic defect causes increased sodium chloride content in sweat and increased resorption of sodium and water from respiratory epithelium (Fig. 19.31). Relative dehydration of the airway epithelium is thought to predispose to chronic bacterial infection and ciliary dysfunction. The gene defect also causes disorders in the gut epithelium, pancreas, liver and reproductive tract (see below).

Neonatal screening for CF is now routine in the UK, and should prevent delayed diagnosis and improve outcomes. Prenatal screening by amniocentesis may be offered to those known to be at high risk.

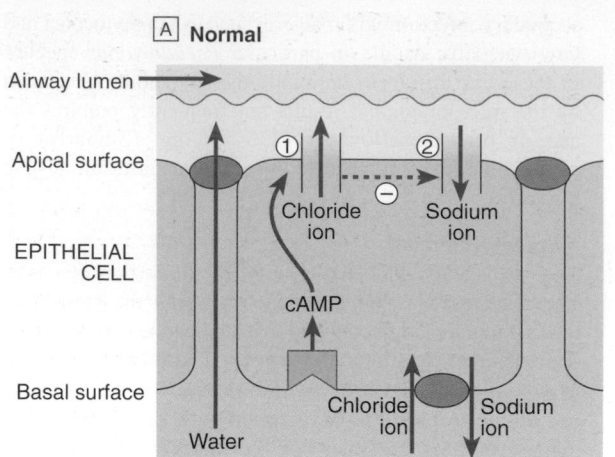
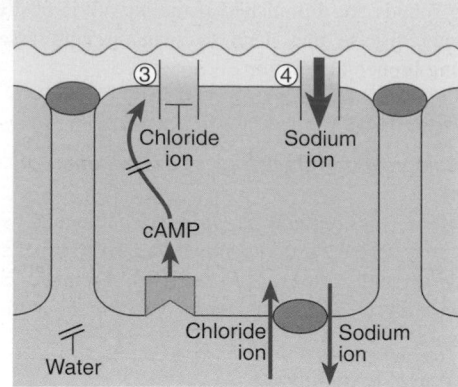

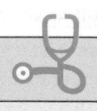 β₂-adrenoceptor

Fig. 19.31 Cystic fibrosis: basic defect in the pulmonary epithelium. A The CF gene codes for a chloride channel (1) in the apical (luminal) membrane of epithelial cells in the conducting airways. This channel is normally controlled by cyclic adenosine monophosphate (cAMP) and indirectly by β-adrenoceptor stimulation. It is one of several apical ion channels which together control the quantity and solute content of airway-lining fluid. Normal channels appear to inhibit the adjacent epithelial sodium channels (2). B In CF, one of many CF gene defects causes absence or defective function of this chloride channel (3). This leads to reduced chloride secretion and loss of inhibition of sodium channels with excessive sodium resorption (4) and dehydration of the airway lining. The resulting abnormal airway-lining fluid is believed to predispose to infection by mechanisms which are not fully understood.

Clinical features

The lungs are macroscopically normal at birth, however bronchiolar inflammation and infections usually lead to bronchiectasis in childhood. At this stage, the lungs are most commonly infected with *Staphylococcus aureus*; however, the majority of patients have *Pseudomonas aeruginosa* infection by the time they reach adolescence. Recurrent exacerbations of bronchiectasis, initially in the upper lobes but subsequently throughout both lungs, cause progressive lung damage resulting ultimately in death from respiratory failure. Other clinical manifestations of the gene defect include intestinal obstruction, exocrine pancreatic failure with malabsorption, diabetes and hepatic cirrhosis. Most men with CF are infertile due to failure of development of the vas deferens, but microsurgical sperm aspiration and in vitro fertilisation are now possible. Other clinical manifestations of CF are summarised in Box 19.39. Interestingly, genotype is a poor predictor of severity of disease in most individuals; even siblings with matching genotypes may have quite different phenotypes. This suggests that other 'modifier genes' (as yet unidentified) influence clinical outcome.

Management

Treatment of CF lung disease

The management of CF lung disease is that of severe bronchiectasis (see above). All patients with CF who produce sputum should have regular chest physiotherapy, which should be performed more frequently during exacerbations. While infections with *Staph. aureus* can often be managed with oral antibiotics, intravenous treatment (often self-administered at home through a sub-

19.39 COMPLICATIONS OF CYSTIC FIBROSIS	
Respiratory	
• Infective exacerbations of bronchiectasis • Spontaneous pneumothorax • Haemoptysis • Nasal polyps	• Respiratory failure • Cor pulmonale • Lobar collapse due to secretions
Gastrointestinal	
• Malabsorption and steatorrhoea • Distal intestinal obstruction syndrome	• Biliary cirrhosis and portal hypertension • Gallstones
Others	
• Diabetes (25% of adults) • Delayed puberty • Male infertility • Stress incontinence	• Psychosocial problems • Osteoporosis • Arthropathy

cutaneous vascular port) is usually needed for *Pseudomonas* species. Nebulised antibiotic therapy, mainly with colomycin or tobramycin is used between exacerbations in an attempt to suppress chronic *Pseudomonas* infection (Box 19.40). Unfortunately, the bronchi of many CF patients eventually become colonised with pathogens which are resistant to most antibiotics. Resistant strains of *P. aeruginosa*, *Stenotrophomonas maltophilia* and *Burkholderia cepacia* are the main culprits, and may require prolonged treatment with unusual combinations of antibiotics. *Aspergillus* and 'atypical mycobacteria' are also frequently found in the sputum of CF patients, but in most cases these behave as

19

19.40 NEBULISED ANTIPSEUDOMONAL ANTIBIOTICS IN CYSTIC FIBROSIS

'Nebulised antipseudomonal antibiotics improve lung function and prevent both infective exacerbation and hospitalisation in cystic fibrosis patients with *Pseudomonas aeruginosa*.'

- Ramsey BW, et al. N Engl J Med 1999; 340:23–30.
- Ryan G, et al. (Cochrane Review). Cochrane Library, issue 4, 2000. Oxford: Update Software.

benign 'colonisers' of the bronchiectatic airways and do not require specific therapy. Some patients have coexistent asthma, which is treated with inhaled bronchodilators and corticosteroids; allergic bronchopulmonary aspergillosis (p. 703) also occasionally occurs in CF.

Treatment with nebulised recombinant human deoxyribonuclease (DNase) has been available since 1994. The aim of this therapy is to liquify the CF sputum by breaking up the excess of viscous DNA derived from disintegrated inflammatory cells. Trials have shown a significant improvement in pulmonary function and a reduction in the number of infective exacerbations in a subgroup of patients. Careful monitoring of response to treatment is appropriate as this treatment is very expensive. Recently it has been shown that oral macrolides such as azithromycin also reduce exacerbations and improve lung function in patients with *Pseudomonas* colonisation.

For advanced CF lung disease, home oxygen and non-invasive ventilation may be necessary to treat respiratory failure. Ultimately, lung transplantation can produce dramatic improvements but is limited by donor organ availability.

Treatment of non-respiratory manifestations of CF

There is a clear link between good nutrition and prognosis in CF. Malabsorption is treated with oral vitamins and pancreatic enzyme supplements and the increased calorie requirements of CF patients are met by supplemental feeding including nasogastric or gastrostomy tube feeding if required. Diabetes eventually appears in about 25% of patients and often requires insulin therapy. Osteoporosis secondary to malabsorption and chronic ill health should be sought and treated.

The prognosis of CF has greatly improved in the last decade, mainly because of better control of bronchial sepsis and nutritional support. The median survival of patients with CF born in the 1990s is now predicted to be at least 40 years.

The potential for somatic gene therapy

The discovery of the CF gene and the fact that the lethal defect is located in the respiratory epithelium (which is accessible by inhaled therapy) presents an exciting opportunity for gene therapy. Manufactured normal CF gene can be 'packaged' within a viral or liposome vector and delivered to the respiratory epithelium to correct the genetic defect. Initial trials in the nasal and bronchial epithelium have shown some effect, and further trials of nebulised bronchial delivery are planned. Improved gene transfer efficiency is needed before this will become a practical clinical treatment.

INFECTIONS OF THE RESPIRATORY SYSTEM

Infections of the upper and lower respiratory tract continue to be a major cause of morbidity and mortality throughout the world, with patients at the extremes of age or with pre-existing lung disease or immune suppression being at particular risk. Viruses are the most frequent cause of upper respiratory illnesses, with bacteria being responsible for the majority of community- and hospital-acquired pneumonia in adults. Organisms such as *Mycoplasma*, *Coxiella* and *Chlamydia* are less common causes of severe pneumonia. Pulmonary infection by *Mycobacterium tuberculosis*, atypical mycobacteria and fungi results in diseases of a more chronic type. These are described separately.

UPPER RESPIRATORY TRACT INFECTIONS

The clinical features, complications and management of the common and most important upper respiratory tract infections are summarised in Box 19.41. The vast majority of these illnesses, of which acute coryza (common cold) is by far the most common, are caused by viruses (Box 19.42). Immunity is short-lived and virus-specific. Other viral infections include acute laryngitis and acute laryngo-tracheobronchitis. Bacterial infection is the usual cause of acute tonsillitis, otitis media and epiglottitis.

Most patients with upper respiratory tract infections recover rapidly and specific investigation is indicated only in more severe illness. The possibility of acute epiglottitis, which represents a medical emergency, must be considered at all times (Box 19.41). Viruses can be isolated from exfoliated cells collected on throat swabs, and may be identified retrospectively by serological tests. Certain viruses can be identified in exfoliated cells by the fluorescent antibody technique, allowing the pathogen to be identified more rapidly. Throat swabs may also be helpful if streptococcal pharyngitis is suspected, and examination of the blood will identify infectious mononucleosis (p. 307). Radiographic examination may be required if an underlying chronic infection involving the sinuses is suspected.

PNEUMONIA

Pneumonia is defined as an acute respiratory illness associated with recently developed radiological pulmonary shadowing which may be segmental, lobar or multilobar. The clinical context in which a pneumonia develops is highly suggestive of the likely organism(s) involved and hence the immediate choice of antibiotics; pneumonias are therefore usually classified as community-acquired, hospital-acquired (nosocomial), or those occurring in immunocompromised hosts or patients with underlying damaged lung (including suppurative and aspirational pneumonias). 'Lobar pneumonia' is a radiological and pathological term referring to homogeneous consolidation of one or more lung lobes, often with associated pleural

19

19.41 THE COMMON AND MOST IMPORTANT UPPER RESPIRATORY TRACT INFECTIONS: CLINICAL FEATURES, COMPLICATIONS AND MANAGEMENT

Infection	Clinical features	Complications	Management
Acute coryza (common cold)	Rapid onset. Burning and tickling sensation in nose. Sneezing. Sore throat. Blocked nose with watery discharge. Discharge usually green/yellow after 24–48 hrs. Nasal allergy can give rise to similar clinical features	Sinusitis. Lower respiratory tract infection (bronchitis/pneumonia). Hearing impairment, otitis media (due to blockage of eustachian tubes)	Most do not require treatment. Paracetamol 0.5–1 g 4–6-hourly for relief of systemic symptoms. Nasal decongestant in some cases. Antibiotics not necessary in uncomplicated coryza
Acute laryngitis	Often a complication of acute coryza. Dry sore throat. Hoarse voice or loss of voice. Attempts to speak cause pain. Initially, painful and unproductive cough. Stridor in children (croup) because of inflammatory oedema leading to partial obstruction of a small larynx	Complications rare. Chronic laryngitis. Downward spread of infection may cause tracheitis, bronchitis or pneumonia	Rest voice. Paracetamol 0.5–1 g 4–6-hourly for relief of discomfort and pyrexia. Steam inhalations may be of value. Antibiotics not necessary in simple acute laryngitis
Acute laryngo-tracheobronchitis (croup)*	Initial symptoms like common cold. Sudden paroxysms of cough accompanied by stridor and breathlessness. Contraction of accessory muscles and indrawing of intercostal spaces. Cyanosis and asphyxia in small children, if appropriate treatment not given	Asphyxia. Death. Superinfection with bacteria, especially *Streptococcus pneumoniae* and *Staphylococcus aureus*. Viscid secretions may occlude bronchi	Inhalations of steam and humidified air/high concentrations of oxygen. Endotracheal intubation or tracheostomy to relieve laryngeal obstruction and allow clearing of bronchial secretions. Intravenous antibiotic therapy for seriously ill (co-amoxiclav or erythromycin). Maintain adequate hydration
Acute epiglottitis	Fever and sore throat, rapidly leading to stridor because of swelling of epiglottis and surrounding structures (usually infection with *Haemophilus influenzae*). Stridor and cough in absence of much hoarseness may distinguish acute epiglottitis from other causes of stridor	Death from asphyxia which may be precipitated by attempts to examine the throat—*avoid using a tongue depressor or any instrument* unless facilities for endotracheal intubation or tracheostomy are immediately available	Intravenous antibiotic therapy essential. Co-amoxiclav or chloramphenicol. Other measures as for acute laryngotracheobronchitis
Acute bronchitis and tracheitis	Often follows acute coryza. Initially irritating unproductive cough accompanied by retrosternal discomfort of tracheitis. Chest tightness, wheeze and breathlessness when bronchi become involved. Tracheitis causes pain on coughing. Sputum is initially scanty or mucoid. After a day or so sputum becomes mucopurulent, more copious and, in tracheitis, often blood-stained. Acute bronchial infection may be associated with a pyrexia of 38–39°C and a neutrophil leucocytosis. Spontaneous recovery occurs over a few days	Bronchopneumonia. Exacerbation of chronic bronchitis which often results in type II respiratory failure in patients with severe COPD. Acute exacerbation of bronchial asthma	Specific treatment rarely necessary in previously healthy individuals. Cough may be eased by pholcodine 5–10 mg 6–8-hourly. In patients with COPD (p. 678) and asthma (p. 670) aggressive treatment of exacerbations may be required. Amoxicillin 250 mg 8-hourly should be given to previously healthy patients who are thought to be developing bronchopneumonia (see also p. 687)
Influenza (a specific acute illness caused by a group of myxoviruses—two common types, A and B)	Sudden onset of pyrexia associated with generalised aches and pains, anorexia, nausea and vomiting. Degree of ill health ranges from mild to rapidly fatal. Usually harsh unproductive cough. Most patients do not develop complications and acute symptoms subside within 3–5 days, but may be followed by 'post-influenzal asthenia' which can persist for several weeks. During epidemics the diagnosis is usually easy. Sporadic cases may have to be diagnosed by virus isolation, fluorescent antibody techniques or serological tests for specific antibodies	Tracheitis, bronchitis, bronchiolitis and bronchopneumonia. Secondary bacterial invasion by *Strep. pneumoniae*, *H. influenzae* and *Staph. aureus* may occur. Toxic cardiomyopathy may cause sudden death (rare). Encephalitis, demyelinating encephalopathy and peripheral neuropathy are also rare complications	Bed rest is advisable until fever has subsided. Paracetamol 0.5–1 g 4–6-hourly can be used to relieve headache and generalised pains. Pholcodine 5–10 mg 6–8-hourly may be given to suppress cough. Specific treatment for pneumonia (p. 691) may be necessary

* Whooping cough (caused by *Bordetella pertussis*) is often considered a disease of non-immunised children but it also occurs in sporadic 'epidemics' in middle life when immunisation effectiveness has waned. After a short, febrile tracheobronchitis (which itself is responsive to antibiotics), severe episodic paroxysmal coughing bouts, associated with laryngospasm and often leading to intercostal muscle tears or fractured ribs, may persist for many weeks

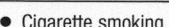

19.42 RESPIRATORY INFECTIONS CAUSED BY VIRUSES	
Clinical syndrome	**Usual cause (other causes in parentheses)**
Epidemic influenza	Influenza A and B
'Influenza-like' illness	Adenoviruses, rhinoviruses (enteroviruses)
Sore throat	Adenoviruses (enteroviruses, parainfluenza viruses, influenza A and B in partially immune)
Common cold (coryza)	Rhinoviruses (coronaviruses, enteroviruses, adenoviruses, respiratory syncytial virus)
'Feverish' cold	Rhinoviruses, enteroviruses (influenza A and B, parainfluenza viruses, respiratory syncytial virus)
Croup	Parainfluenza 1, 2, 3 (rhinoviruses, enteroviruses)
Bronchitis	Rhinoviruses, adenoviruses (influenza A and B)
Bronchiolitis	Respiratory syncytial virus (parainfluenza 3)
Pneumonia	Influenza A and B, chickenpox (respiratory syncytial virus, parainfluenza, measles and adenoviruses)

19.43 FACTORS THAT PREDISPOSE TO PNEUMONIA	
• Cigarette smoking	• Old age
• Upper respiratory tract infections	• Recent influenza infection
• Alcohol	• Pre-existing lung disease
• Corticosteroid therapy	

19

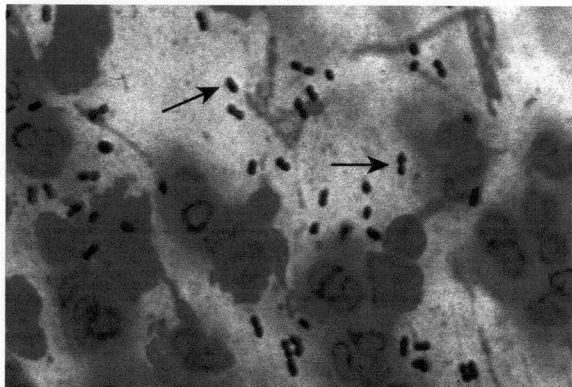

Fig. 19.32 Gram stain of sputum showing Gram-positive diplococci characteristic of *Strep. pneumoniae* (arrows).

inflammation; bronchopneumonia refers to more patchy alveolar consolidation associated with bronchial and bronchiolar inflammation often affecting both lower lobes.

COMMUNITY-ACQUIRED PNEUMONIA (CAP)

UK figures suggest that an estimated 5–11/1000 adults suffer from CAP each year, accounting for around 5–12% of all lower respiratory tract infections. The incidence varies with age, being much higher in the very young and the elderly. Pneumonia accounts for almost one-fifth of childhood deaths world-wide, with approximately 2 million children under 5 dying each year. Most patients may be safely managed at home, but hospital admission is necessary in 20–40% of patients (5–10% of whom require intensive care). The mortality rate of adults managed at home is very low (< 1%); hospital death rates are typically between 5 and 10% and may be as high as 50% in severe illness.

CAP is usually spread by droplet infection and most cases occur in previously healthy individuals. Several factors can impair the effectiveness of local defences and predispose to CAP (Box 19.43). Once the organism settles in the alveoli, an inflammatory response ensues. The classical pathological response evolves through the phases of congestion, red and then grey hepatisation, and finally resolution with little or no scarring.

Clinical features

Pneumonia typically presents as an acute illness in which systemic features such as fever, rigors, shivering and vomiting often predominate. The appetite is usually lost and headache frequently reported. Pulmonary symptoms include cough, which at first is characteristically short, painful and dry, but later accompanied by the expectoration of mucopurulent sputum. Rust-coloured sputum may be seen in patients with *Streptococcus pneumoniae*, and the occasional patient may report haemoptysis. Pleuritic chest pain may be a presenting feature and on occasion may be referred to the shoulder or anterior abdominal wall. Upper abdominal tenderness is sometimes apparent in patients with lower lobe pneumonia or if there is associated hepatitis. Less typical presentations may be seen in the very young and the elderly.

The majority of cases of CAP are due to infection with *Strep. pneumoniae* (Fig. 19.32). Thereafter the most likely alternatives depend on the age of the patient and the clinical circumstances. For example, *Mycoplasma pneumoniae* and *Chlamydia pneumoniae* are common in young adults but seldom reported in the elderly, whereas *Haemophilus influenzae* should be considered in elderly patients but is rarely reported in young adults. In younger children, viral infections predominate. A history of foreign travel may suggest *Legionella* infection and recent influenza may predispose to *Staph. aureus* (although most cases of post-influenza pneumonia are caused by *Strep. pneumoniae*). Other clinical features may provide clues to the likely infecting organism(s). However, in day-to-day practice these have limited predictive value (Box 19.44). The term 'atypical pneumonia' has recently been abandoned.

Investigations

The main objectives of investigating patients with a clinically based diagnosis of pneumonia are:

- to obtain radiological confirmation of the diagnosis
- to exclude other conditions that may mimic pneumonia (Box 19.45)
- to obtain a microbiological diagnosis
- to assess the severity of pneumonia
- to identify the development of complications.

19

19.44 COMMON CLINICAL FEATURES OF COMMUNITY-ACQUIRED PNEUMONIA

Organism	Clinical features
Common organisms	
Streptococcus pneumoniae	Most common in winter. All age groups but particularly young to middle-aged. Rapid onset, high fever, pleuritic chest pain, herpes labialis, 'rusty' sputum. Bacteraemia is more common in women and patients with diabetes and COPD
Chlamydia pneumoniae	Young to middle-aged, large-scale epidemics, or sporadic, often mild, self-limiting disease. Headaches and a longer duration of symptoms before hospital admission. Usually diagnosed on serology
Mycoplasma pneumoniae	Children and young adults. Common in autumn. Epidemics occur every 3–4 years. Rare complications include haemolytic anaemia, Stevens–Johnson syndrome, erythema nodosum, myocarditis, pericarditis, meningoencephalitis, Guillain–Barré syndrome
Legionella pneumophila	Middle to old age, recent foreign travel, local epidemics around point source, e.g. cooling tower. A variety of features are said to be more common such as headache, confusion, malaise, myalgia, high fever and diarrhoea. Laboratory results include hyponatraemia, elevated liver enzymes, hypoalbuminaemia and elevated creatine kinase. Chest X-ray appearances may be slow to resolve
Uncommon organisms	
Haemophilus influenzae	Often underlying lung disease (COPD, bronchiectasis)
Staphylococcus aureus	Coexistent debilitating illness and often preceded by influenza. Radiographic features include multilobar shadowing, cavitation, pneumatoceles and abscesses. Dissemination to other organs may cause osteomyelitis, endocarditis or brain abscesses. Mortality up to 30%
Chlamydia psittaci	Contact with birds, especially recently imported exotic birds: parrots, domestic ducks and turkeys. Malaise, low-grade fever, protracted illness, hepatosplenomegaly
Coxiella burnetii (Q fever)	Male sex, farm or abattoir contact. Chronic course, influenza-like illness, dry cough, high fever, conjunctivitis, hepatomegaly, endocarditis
Klebsiella	More common in men and alcoholics. Upper lobe involvement typical. Low platelet count and leucopenia
Actinomyces israelii	Mouth commensal. Cervicofacial, abdominal or pulmonary infection, empyema, chest wall sinuses, pus with sulphur granules
Primary viral pneumonias	Influenza, parainfluenza and measles can cause pneumonia commonly complicated by bacterial infection. Respiratory syncytial virus seen mainly in infancy. Varicella can cause severe pneumonia healing with multiple nodular shadows that may calcify

19.45 DIFFERENTIAL DIAGNOSIS OF PNEUMONIA

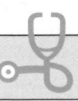

- Pulmonary infarction
- Pulmonary/pleural TB
- Pulmonary oedema (can be unilateral)
- Pulmonary eosinophilia (p. 723)
- Malignancy: bronchoalveolar cell carcinoma (p. 711)
- Rare disorders: cryptogenic organising pneumonia/bronchiolitis obliterans organising pneumonia (COP/BOOP)

Radiological examination

A chest X-ray is not essential but a confident diagnosis necessitates chest radiography. In lobar pneumonia, a homogeneous opacity localised to the affected lobe or segment usually appears within 12–18 hours from the onset of the illness (Fig. 19.33). Radiological examination is also helpful if a complication such as parapneumonic effusion, intrapulmonary abscess formation, or empyema is suspected.

Microbiological investigations

Many cases of CAP can be managed successfully without identification of the organism, particularly if there are no features that indicate severe disease. Thus, the extent of microbiological investigations should be guided by the clinical circumstances. A full range of microbiological tests should be performed on patients with severe CAP (Box 19.46). The identification of *Legionella pneumophila* has important public health implications and requires notification. In patients who do not respond to initial therapy, microbiological investigations may lead to the appropriate modification of therapy. Microbiology also provides useful epidemiological information.

Assessment of gas exchange

Pulse oximetry provides a simple non-invasive method of measuring arterial oxygen saturation (SaO_2), and assists in monitoring response to oxygen therapy. An arterial blood gas should be sampled in those with $SaO_2 < 92\%$ or with features of severe pneumonia to assess whether the patient has evidence of ventilatory failure or acidosis.

General blood tests

The white cell count is often only marginally raised or may even be normal in patients with pneumonia caused by atypical organisms, whereas a neutrophil leucocytosis of more than $15 \times 10^9/l$ favours a bacterial aetiology. A very high ($> 20 \times 10^9/l$) or low ($< 4 \times 10^9/l$) white cell count may be seen in severe pneumonia. The urea and electrolytes and liver function tests should also be checked. The C-reactive protein (CRP) is typically elevated.

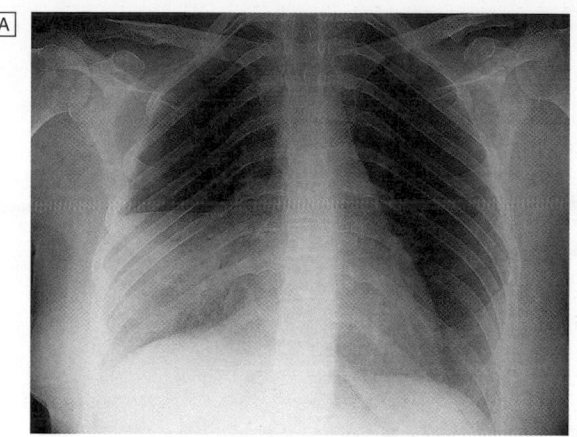
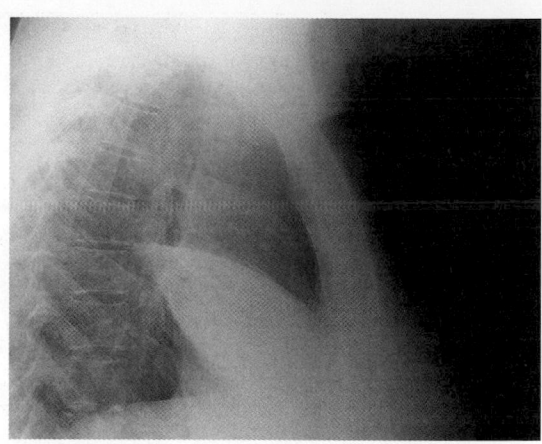

Fig. 19.33 Pneumonia of the right middle lobe. [A] Postero-anterior (PA) view: consolidation in right middle lobe with characteristic opacification beneath the horizontal fissure and loss of normal contrast between the right heart border and lung. [B] Lateral view: consolidation confined to the anteriorly situated middle lobe.

19

19.46 MICROBIOLOGICAL INVESTIGATIONS IN PATIENTS WITH COMMUNITY-ACQUIRED PNEUMONIA

All patients

- Sputum—direct smear by Gram (Fig. 19.32) and Ziehl–Neelsen stains. Culture and antimicrobial sensitivity testing
- Blood culture—frequently positive in pneumococcal pneumonia
- Serology—acute and convalescent titres to diagnose *Mycoplasma*, *Chlamydia*, *Legionella* and viral infections. Pneumococcal antigen detection in serum

Severe community-acquired pneumonia

The above tests *plus* consider:
- Tracheal aspirate, induced sputum, bronchoalveolar lavage, protected brush specimen or percutaneous needle aspiration. Direct fluorescent antibody stain for *Legionella* and viruses
- Serology—*Legionella* antigen in urine. Pneumococcal antigen in sputum and blood. Immediate IgM for *Mycoplasma*
- Cold agglutinins—positive in 50% of patients with *Mycoplasma*

Selected patients

- Throat/nasopharyngeal swabs—helpful in children or during influenza epidemic
- Pleural fluid—should always be sampled when present in more than trivial amounts, preferably with ultrasound guidance

---

Assessment of disease severity

A relatively straightforward scoring system has been proposed that guides antibiotic and admission policies and gives useful prognostic information (Fig. 19.34).

Management

Patients with CAP should be advised to rest, and if appropriate, avoid smoking. The severity of the illness should be defined and regularly re-evaluated by nursing observation. Attention is then paid to oxygenation, fluid balance and antibiotic therapy. In certain circumstances, such as prolonged illness, nutritional support may be required.

Oxygen

Oxygen should be administered to all patients with tachypnoea, hypoxaemia, hypotension or acidosis with the aim of maintaining the $PaO_2 \geq 8$ kPa (60 mmHg) or $SaO_2 \geq 92\%$. High concentrations (> 35%), preferably humidified, should be used in all patients who do not have hypercapnia associated with COPD. Assisted ventilation should be considered at an early stage in those who remain hypoxaemic despite adequate oxygen therapy. NIV may have a limited role but should only be used under close supervision as many patients continue to deteriorate. Indications for ITU referral are summarised in Box 19.47.

Fluid balance

An adequate oral intake of fluid should be encouraged but intravenous fluids should be considered in those with severe illness, elderly patients and those whose systemic features include vomiting. Inotropic support may be required in patients with shock (p. 193).

Antibiotic treatment

If possible, culture specimens should be sent prior to starting antibiotics but treatment should not be unduly delayed and in patients with severe illness should be commenced as soon as the clinical diagnosis is made. The choice of antibiotic is guided by clinical context, severity assessment, local knowledge of antibiotic resistance patterns, and at times epidemiological information. Current regimens are detailed

---

19.47 INDICATIONS FOR REFERRAL TO ITU

- CURB score 4–5 failing to respond rapidly to initial management
- Persisting hypoxia ($PaO_2 < 8$ kPa (60 mmHg)) despite high concentrations of oxygen
- Progressive hypercapnia
- Severe acidosis
- Shock
- Depressed consciousness

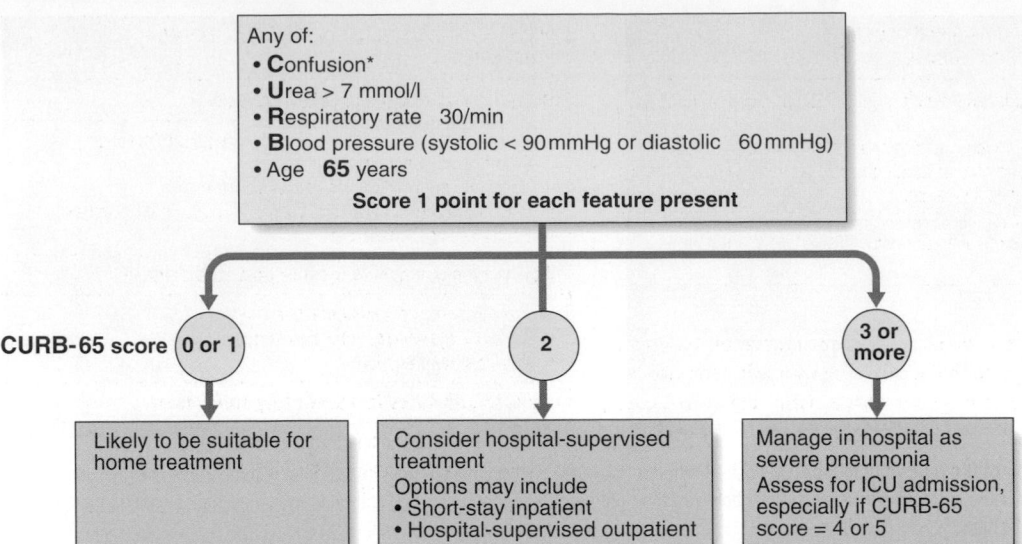

Any of:
• **C**onfusion*
• **U**rea > 7 mmol/l
• **R**espiratory rate   30/min
• **B**lood pressure (systolic < 90 mmHg or diastolic   60 mmHg)
• Age   **65** years
Score 1 point for each feature present

CURB-65 score (0 or 1)   (2)   (3 or more)

Likely to be suitable for home treatment

Consider hospital-supervised treatment
Options may include
• Short-stay inpatient
• Hospital-supervised outpatient

Manage in hospital as severe pneumonia
Assess for ICU admission, especially if CURB-65 score = 4 or 5

Fig. 19.34 Hospital CURB-65. * Defined as a Mental Test Score of 8 or less, or new disorientation in person, place or time. (A urea of 7 mmol/l ≅ 20 mg/dl.)

19.48 ANTIBIOTIC TREATMENT FOR COMMUNITY-ACQUIRED PNEUMONIA (CAP)

Uncomplicated CAP

• Amoxicillin 500 mg 8-hourly orally
• *If patient is allergic to penicillin*
  Clarithromycin 500 mg 12-hourly orally *or*
  Erythromycin 500 mg 6-hourly orally
• *If Staphylococcus is cultured or suspected*
  Flucloxacillin 1–2 g 6-hourly i.v. *plus*
  Clarithromycin 500 mg 12-hourly i.v.
• *If Mycoplasma or Legionella is suspected*
  Clarithromycin 500 mg 12-hourly orally or i.v. *or*
  Erythromycin 500 mg 6-hourly orally or i.v. *plus*
  Rifampicin 600 mg 12-hourly i.v. in severe cases

Severe CAP

• Clarithromycin 500 mg 12-hourly i.v. *or*
  Erythromycin 500 mg 6-hourly i.v. *plus*
• Co-amoxiclav 1.2 g 8-hourly i.v. *or*
  Ceftriaxone 1–2 g daily i.v. *or*
  Cefuroxime 1.5 g 8-hourly i.v. *or*
  Amoxicillin 1 g 6-hourly i.v. *plus* flucloxacillin 2 g 6-hourly i.v.

19.49 COMPLICATIONS OF PNEUMONIA

• Para-pneumonic effusion—common
• Empyema—page 732
• Retention of sputum causing lobar collapse
• Development of thromboembolic disease
• Pneumothorax—particularly with *Staph. aureus*
• Suppurative pneumonia/lung abscess—see below
• ARDS, renal failure, multi-organ failure
• Ectopic abscess formation (*Staph. aureus*)
• Hepatitis, pericarditis, myocarditis, meningoencephalitis
• Pyrexia due to drug hypersensitivity

Physiotherapy

Formal physiotherapy is not indicated in patients with CAP but assisted coughing is important in patients who suppress cough because of pleural pain. The administration of analgesic drugs should be coordinated with this form of physiotherapy to optimise patient cooperation.

Complications

Most patients respond promptly to antibiotic therapy. However, fever may persist for several days and the chest X-ray often takes several weeks or even months to resolve, especially in the elderly. Delayed recovery suggests either that a complication has occurred (such as an empyema, Box 19.49) or that the diagnosis is incorrect (Box 19.45). Alternatively, the pneumonia may be secondary to a proximal bronchial obstruction or recurrent aspiration.

Discharge and follow-up

Discharge from hospital should only be contemplated when patients are clinically stable with no more than one of the following clinical signs: temperature > 37.8°C, heart rate > 100/min, respiratory rate > 24/min, systolic BP < 90 mmHg, SaO_2 < 90%, inability to maintain oral intake

---

in Box 19.48. In most patients with uncomplicated pneumonia a 7–10-day course is adequate, although treatment is usually required for longer in patients with *Legionella*, staphylococcal or *Klebsiella* pneumonia. Oral antibiotics are usually adequate unless the patient has a severe illness, impaired consciousness, loss of swallowing reflex or functional or anatomical reasons for malabsorption.

Treatment of pleural pain

It is important to relieve pleural pain in order to allow the patient to breathe normally and cough efficiently. Mild analgesics such as paracetamol are rarely adequate; however, opiates must be used with extreme caution in patients with poor respiratory function.

19

and abnormal mental status. As the appearance of the chest X-ray typically lags behind clinical recovery, it need not be repeated before discharge in those who have made a satisfactory clinical recovery. Clinical review by GP or hospital should be arranged at around 6 weeks and a chest X-ray obtained if there are persistent symptoms, physical signs or reasons to suspect underlying malignancy.

Prevention

Influenza vaccination is recommended to those at high risk of mortality from influenza or pneumonia. Pneumococcal vaccination is followed by a good antibody response but the efficacy in preventing pneumonia in high-risk groups remains uncertain (Box 19.50).

HOSPITAL-ACQUIRED PNEUMONIA

Hospital-acquired or nosocomial pneumonia refers to a new episode of pneumonia occurring at least 2 days after admission to hospital. The term includes post-operative and certain forms of aspiration pneumonia, and pneumonia or bronchopneumonia developing in patients with chronic lung disease, general debility or those receiving assisted ventilation.

Aetiology

The factors predisposing to the development of pneumonia in a hospitalised patient are listed in Box 19.51. The elderly are particularly at risk and this condition now occurs in 2–5% of all hospital admissions.

The most important distinction between hospital- and community-acquired pneumonia is the difference in the spectrum of pathogenic organisms, with the majority of hospital-acquired infections caused by Gram-negative bacteria. These include *Escherichia*, *Pseudomonas* and *Klebsiella* species. Infections caused by *Staph. aureus* (including multidrug-resistant—MRSA—forms) are also common in hospital, and anaerobic organisms are much more likely than in pneumonia acquired in the community. This profile of organisms in part reflects the high rate of colonisation of the nasopharynx of hospital patients with Gram-negative bacteria, together with poor host defences and general inability of the severely ill or semiconscious patient to clear upper airway and respiratory tract secretions.

Clinical features

The clinical features and investigation of patients with hospital-acquired pneumonia are very similar to CAP (pp. 689–690). In the elderly or debilitated patient who

19.51 FACTORS PREDISPOSING TO NOSOCOMIAL PNEUMONIA

Reduced host defences against bacteria

- Reduced immune defences (e.g. corticosteroid treatment, diabetes, malignancy)
- Reduced cough reflex (e.g. post-operative)
- Disordered mucociliary clearance (e.g. anaesthetic agents)
- Bulbar or vocal cord palsy

Aspiration of nasopharyngeal or gastric secretions

- Immobility or reduced conscious level
- Vomiting, dysphagia, achalasia or severe reflux
- Nasogastric intubation

Bacteria introduced into lower respiratory tract

- Endotracheal intubation/tracheostomy
- Infected ventilators/nebulisers/bronchoscopes
- Dental or sinus infection

Bacteraemia

- Abdominal sepsis
- Intravenous cannula infection
- Infected emboli

19.52 RESPIRATORY INFECTION IN OLD AGE

- **Increased risk of and from respiratory infection**: because of reduced immune responses, increased closing volumes, reduced respiratory muscle strength and endurance, altered mucus layer, poor nutritional status and the increased prevalence of chronic lung disease.
- **Predisposing factors**: other medical conditions may predispose to infection, e.g. swallowing difficulties due to stroke increase the risk of aspiration pneumonia.
- **Atypical presentation**: classical symtoms and signs are less likely, and older patients often present with atypical symptoms, especially confusion.
- **Mortality**: the vast majority of deaths from pneumonia in developed countries occur in older people.
- **Influenza**: has a much higher complication rate, morbidity and mortality. Vaccination significantly reduces morbidity and mortality in old age but uptake is poor.
- **Tuberculosis**: most cases in old age represent reactivation of previous, often unrecognised disease and may be precipitated by steroid therapy, diabetes mellitus and the factors above. Cryptic miliary TB is an occasional alternative presentation. Older people more commonly suffer adverse effects from antituberculous chemotherapy and require close monitoring.

develops acute bronchopneumonia (or 'hypostatic pneumonia') symptoms of acute bronchitis are followed after 2 or 3 days by increased cough and sputum purulence associated with a rise in temperature. Breathlessness and central cyanosis may then appear, but pleural pain is uncommon. In the early stages the physical signs are those of acute bronchitis followed by the development of crackles. There is a neutrophil leucocytosis and the chest X-ray shows mottled opacities in both lung fields, chiefly in the lower zones.

Management

Adequate Gram-negative coverage is usually obtained with:

- a third-generation cephalosporin (e.g. cefotaxime) plus an aminoglycoside (e.g. gentamicin) or

19

- meropenem or
- a monocyclic β-lactam (e.g. aztreonam) plus flucloxacillin.

Aspiration pneumonia can be treated with co-amoxiclav 1.2 g 8-hourly plus metronidazole 500 mg 8-hourly. The nature and severity of most hospital-acquired pneumonias dictate that these antibiotics are all given intravenously, at least initially.

Physiotherapy is of particular importance in the immobile and elderly, and adequate oxygen therapy, fluid support and monitoring are essential. The mortality from hospital-acquired pneumonia is high (approximately 30%).

SUPPURATIVE AND ASPIRATIONAL PNEUMONIA (INCLUDING PULMONARY ABSCESS)

Suppurative pneumonia is the term used to describe a form of pneumonic consolidation in which there is destruction of the lung parenchyma by the inflammatory process. Although microabscess formation is a characteristic histological feature of suppurative pneumonia, it is usual to restrict the term 'pulmonary abscess' to lesions in which there is a large localised collection of pus, or a cavity lined by chronic inflammatory tissue, from which pus has escaped by rupture into a bronchus.

Suppurative pneumonia and pulmonary abscess may be produced by infection of previously healthy lung tissue with *Staph. aureus* or *Klebsiella pneumoniae*. These are, in effect, primary bacterial pneumonias associated with pulmonary suppuration. More frequently, suppurative pneumonia and pulmonary abscess develop after the inhalation of septic material during operations on the nose, mouth or throat under general anaesthesia, or of vomitus during anaesthesia or coma. In such circumstances gross oral sepsis may be a predisposing factor. Additional risk factors for aspiration pneumonia include bulbar or vocal cord palsy, achalasia or oesophageal reflux and alcoholism. Aspiration into the lungs of acid gastric contents can give rise to a severe haemorrhagic pneumonia often complicated by the acute respiratory distress syndrome (ARDS, p. 187). Injection drug-users are at particular risk of developing haematogenous lung abscess, often in association with endocarditis affecting the pulmonary and tricuspid valves.

Bacterial infection of a pulmonary infarct or of a collapsed lobe may also produce a suppurative pneumonia or a lung abscess. The organism(s) isolated from the sputum include *Strep. pneumoniae*, *Staph. aureus*, *Strep. pyogenes*, *H. influenzae* and, in some cases, anaerobic bacteria. In many cases, however, no pathogen can be isolated, particularly when antibiotics have been given.

The clinical features of a suppurative pneumonia are summarised in Box 19.53.

Chest X-ray features

There is a homogeneous lobar or segmental opacity consistent with consolidation or collapse. A large, dense opacity, which may later cavitate and show a fluid level, is the characteristic finding when a frank lung abscess is present. Occasionally, a pre-existing emphysematous bulla

19.53 CLINICAL FEATURES OF SUPPURATIVE PNEUMONIA
Symptoms
• Cough productive of large amounts of sputum which is sometimes fetid and blood-stained
• Pleural pain common
• Sudden expectoration of copious amounts of foul sputum occurs if abscess ruptures into a bronchus
Clinical signs
• High remittent pyrexia
• Profound systemic upset
• Digital clubbing may develop quickly (10–14 days)
• Chest examination usually reveals signs of consolidation; signs of cavitation rarely found
• Pleural rub common
• Rapid deterioration in general health with marked weight loss can occur if disease not adequately treated

becomes infected and appears as a cavity containing an air-fluid level.

Management

In many patients oral treatment with amoxicillin 500 mg 6-hourly is effective. If an anaerobic bacterial infection is suspected (e.g. from fetor of the sputum), oral metronidazole 400 mg 8-hourly should be added. Antibacterial therapy should be modified according to the results of microbiological examination of the sputum. Prolonged treatment for 4–6 weeks may be required in some patients with lung abscess. Removal or treatment of any obstructing endobronchial lesion is essential.

In contrast to uncomplicated CAP, physiotherapy is of great value, especially when large abscess cavities have formed. It may not be possible to drain lower lobe cavities without postural coughing.

In most patients there is a good response to treatment and although residual fibrosis and bronchiectasis are common sequelae, these seldom give rise to serious morbidity. Abscesses that fail to resolve despite optimal medical therapy require surgical intervention.

PNEUMONIA IN THE IMMUNOCOMPROMISED PATIENT

Pulmonary infection is common in patients receiving immunosuppressive drugs and in those with diseases causing defects of cellular or humoral immune mechanisms. However, it is important to appreciate that the majority of infections are caused by the same common pathogens that cause pneumonia in non-immunocompromised individuals (Box 19.54). That said, Gram-negative bacteria, especially *Pseudomonas aeruginosa*, are more of a problem than Gram-positive organisms, and unusual organisms or those normally considered to be of low virulence or non-pathogenic may become 'opportunistic' pathogens. Importantly infection is often due to more than one organism.

Clinical features

The patient usually presents with fever, cough, breathlessness and infiltrates on the chest X-ray. Patients may

19.54 COMMON CAUSES OF IMMUNE SUPPRESSION-ASSOCIATED LUNG INFECTION

	Causes	Infecting organisms
Defective phagocytic function	Acute leukaemia Cytotoxic drugs Agranulocytosis	Gram-positive bacteria including *Staph. aureus* Gram-negative bacteria Fungi, e.g. *Candida albicans* and *Aspergillus fumigatus*

Defects in cell-mediated immunity	Immunosuppressive drugs
	Cytotoxic chemotherapy
	Lymphoma
	Thymic aplasia
		Viruses
		   Cytomegalovirus
		   Herpesvirus
		   Adenovirus
		   Influenza
		Fungi
		   Pneumocystis carinii (now *jirovecii*)
		   C. albicans
		   A. fumigatus

Defects in antibody production	Multiple myeloma Chronic lymphocytic leukaemia	*Haemophilus influenzae* *Mycoplasma pneumoniae*

develop non-specific symptoms, and a high index of suspicion is required to determine the site and nature of the infection. In general, the onset of symptoms tends to be less rapid in patients with opportunistic organisms such as *Pneumocystis carinii* (now *jirovecii*) and mycobacterial infections (p. 389). In *P. jirovecii* pneumonia symptoms of cough and breathlessness can be present several days or weeks before the onset of systemic symptoms or the appearance of radiographic abnormality.

Diagnosis

The initial diagnostic approach should be similar to that for other pneumonias. Some patients who cannot produce sputum can be induced to do so by the inhalation of nebulised hypertonic saline. If the patient is fit for bronchoscopy, the use of bronchoalveolar lavage, bronchial brushings or transbronchial biopsies may help in establishing the diagnosis. Lung biopsy offers the greatest chance of establishing a diagnosis if examination of sputum or bronchoalveolar lavage fluid has not revealed a pathogen. This, however, is a relatively high-risk and invasive procedure and should be reserved for patients in whom less invasive procedures fail to establish a diagnosis and in whom there has been no response to broad-spectrum antibiotic treatment.

Management

Whenever possible, treatment should be based on an established aetiological diagnosis. In practice, however, the cause of the pneumonia is frequently not known when treatment has to be started. Hence, broad-spectrum antibiotic therapy is required (e.g. a third-generation cephalosporin, or a quinolone, plus an antistaphylococcal antibiotic, or an antipseudomonal penicillin plus an aminoglycoside); treatment is thereafter tailored according to the results of investigations and the clinical response. The management of *P. jirovecii* infection is detailed on page 390.

SEVERE ACUTE RESPIRATORY DISTRESS SYNDROME (SARS)

SARS rose to prominence in late 2002 when a series of cases in the Guangdong Province, China, was followed by an international outbreak. The illness is characterised by the presence of a high fever (> 38°C), malaise and muscle aches and later a dry cough with shortness of breath or difficulty in breathing. A history of travel within 10 days of onset of symptoms to an area with documented or suspected community transmission of SARS or close contact within 10 days of onset of symptoms with a person known to be a suspect SARS case is typical. The chest X-ray is usually indicative of pneumonia. SARS has recently been attributed to the Corona virus (Urbani SARS-associated coronavirus); however, additional viruses, or other factors may be involved. The optimum method of treating SARS remains uncertain and is largely supportive, including mechanical ventilation. The role of antibacterial, antiviral and immunomodulatory therapy is still under research.

TUBERCULOSIS

Epidemiology

Tuberculosis (TB) is caused by infection with *Mycobacterium tuberculosis* (MTB), which is part of a complex of organisms including *M. bovis* (reservoir cattle) and *M. africanum* (reservoir human).

The introduction of social and environmental measures and highly effective chemotherapy led to optimism that TB could be eradicated. However, in the latter part of the last century a number of factors converged contributing to the re-emergence of TB as a major threat to world health (Box 19.55). Current estimates suggest that around one-third of the world's population has latent tuberculosis and that between 2002 and 2020 an estimated 1000 million people will become newly infected, 150 million will contract disease, and 36 million will die. Unfortunately the majority of these cases are likely to occur in the world's poorest nations, who struggle to cover the costs associated with management and control programmes.

19.55 REASONS FOR THE INCREASING INCIDENCE OF TB

Developed countries

- Immigration from high-prevalence areas
- Human immunodeficiency virus (HIV)
- Social deprivation (homelessness, poverty)
- Increasing proportion of elderly
- Drug resistance

Developing countries

- Ineffective control programmes
- Lack of access to health care
- Poverty, civil unrest
- HIV
- Population increase
- Drug resistance

Pathology and pathogenesis

M. bovis infection arises from drinking non-sterilised milk from infected cows; otherwise, *M. tuberculosis* is spread by the inhalation of aerosolised droplet nuclei from other infected patients. The smallest particles (1–5 μm) enter the periphery of the lung and are engulfed by macrophages. In response to antigen presentation, CD4+ T lymphocytes produce an array of cytokines, including interferon-gamma (IFN-γ), that drive the recruitment of monocytes and direct the formation of granulomas limiting the replication and spread of the organism. Classical tuberculous granulomas display central caseous necrosis.

The formation of a mass of granulomas surrounding an area of caseation leads to the appearance of the primary lesion in the lung, referred to as the 'Ghon focus'. The combination of a primary lesion and regional lymph node involvement is termed the 'Ghon complex'. If the bacilli spread (either by lymph or blood) before immunity is established, secondary foci may be established in other organs including lymph nodes, serous membranes, meninges, bones, liver, kidneys and lungs. These foci resolve once an immune response is mounted and the organisms gradually lose viability. However, 'latent bacilli' may persist for many years.

In most cases, infection of a healthy individual is subclinical and indicated only by the appearance of a cell-mediated, delayed-type hypersensitivity reaction to tuberculin (demonstrated by tuberculin skin testing). However, if the organism cannot be contained, primary progressive disease ensues (Fig. 19.35). The estimated lifetime risk of developing disease after primary infection is 10%, with roughly half of this risk occurring in the first 2 years after infection. Factors predisposing to TB are summarised in Box 19.56.

The timetable of tuberculosis is shown in Box 19.57.

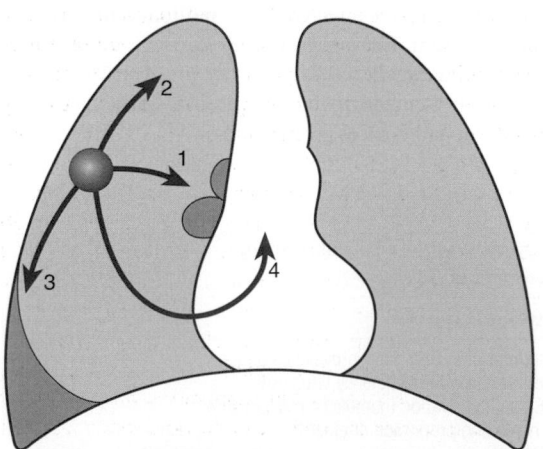

Fig. 19.35   Primary pulmonary TB. (1) Spread from the primary focus to hilar and mediastinal lymph glands to form the 'primary complex', which in most cases heals spontaneously. (2) Direct extension of the primary focus—'progressive pulmonary tuberculosis'. (3) Spread to the pleura—tuberculous pleurisy and pleural effusion. (4) Blood-borne spread: *few bacilli*—pulmonary, skeletal, renal, genitourinary infection often months or years later; *massive spread*—miliary tuberculosis and meningitis.

19.56 FACTORS INCREASING THE RISK OF TB

Patient-related

- Age (children > young adults < elderly)
- First-generation immigrants from high-prevalence countries
- Close contacts of patients with smear-positive pulmonary tuberculosis
- Overcrowding: prisons, collective dormitories
- Chest radiographic evidence of self-healed tuberculosis
- Primary infection < 1 year previously

Associated diseases

- Immunosuppression—HIV, infliximab, high-dose corticosteroids, cytotoxic agents
- Malignancy (especially lymphoma and leukaemia)
- Type 1 diabetes mellitus
- Chronic renal failure
- Silicosis
- Gastrointestinal disease associated with malnutrition (gastrectomy, jejuno-ileal bypass, cancer of the pancreas, malabsorption)
- Deficiency of vitamin D or A

19.57 TIMETABLE OF TB

Time from infection	Manifestations
3–8 weeks	Primary complex, positive tuberculin skin test
3–6 months	Meningeal, miliary and pleural disease
Up to 3 years	Gastrointestinal, bone and joint, and lymph node disease
Around 8 years	Renal tract disease
From 3 years onwards	Post-primary disease due to reactivation or reinfection

Clinical features: pulmonary disease

Primary pulmonary TB

Primary TB refers to the infection of a previously uninfected (tuberculin-negative) individual. A few patients develop a self-limiting febrile illness but clinical disease only occurs if there is a hypersensitivity reaction or progressive infection (Box 19.58). Progressive primary disease may appear during the course of the initial illness or after a latent period of weeks or months.

Miliary TB

Blood-borne dissemination gives rise to miliary TB which may present acutely but more frequently is characterised by 2–3 weeks of fever, night sweats, anorexia, weight loss and a dry cough. Hepatosplenomegaly may be present and the presence of a headache may indicate co-existent tuberculous meningitis. Auscultation of the chest is frequently normal, although with more advanced disease widespread crackles are evident. Fundoscopy may show choroidal tubercles. The classical appearances on chest X-ray are those of fine 1–2 mm lesions ('millet seed') distributed throughout the lung fields, although occasionally the appearances are

19.58 FEATURES OF PRIMARY TUBERCULOSIS

Infection (4–8 weeks)

- Influenza-like illness
- Skin test conversion
- Primary complex

Disease

- Lymphadenopathy (hilar—often unilateral, paratracheal or mediastinal)
    Collapse (especially right middle lobe)
    Consolidation (especially right middle lobe)
    Obstructive emphysema
    Cavitation (rare)
- Pleural effusion
- Endobronchial
- Miliary
- Meningitis
- Pericarditis

Hypersensitivity

- Erythema nodosum
- Phlyctenular conjunctivitis
- Dactylitis

19.59 CRYPTIC TB

- Age over 60 years
- Intermittent low-grade pyrexia of unknown origin
- Unexplained weight loss, general debility (hepatosplenomegaly in 25–50%)
- Normal chest X-ray
- Blood dyscrasias; leukaemoid reaction, pancytopenia
- Negative tuberculin skin test
- Confirmation by biopsy (granulomas and/or acid-fast bacilli demonstrated) of liver or bone marrow

19.60 CLINICAL PRESENTATIONS OF PULMONARY TB

- Chronic cough, often with haemoptysis
- Pyrexia of unknown origin
- Unresolved pneumonia
- Exudative pleural effusion
- Asymptomatic (diagnosis on chest X-ray)
- Weight loss, general debility
- Spontaneous pneumothorax

19.61 CHRONIC COMPLICATIONS OF PULMONARY TB

Pulmonary

- Massive haemoptysis
- Cor pulmonale
- Fibrosis/emphysema
- Atypical mycobacterial infection
- Aspergilloma
- Lung/pleural calcification
- Obstructive airways disease
- Bronchiectasis
- Bronchopleural fistula

Non-pulmonary

- Empyema necessitans
- Laryngitis
- Enteritis*
- Anorectal disease*
- Amyloidosis
- Poncet's polyarthritis

* From swallowed sputum.

19

coarser. Anaemia and leucopenia may be present. An unusual presentation seen in the elderly is 'cryptic' miliary TB (Box 19.59).

Post-primary pulmonary TB

Pulmonary TB is the most frequent form of post-primary disease. The onset is typically insidious and develops slowly over several weeks. Systemic symptoms include fever, night sweats, malaise, loss of appetite and weight, and are accompanied by progressive pulmonary symptoms (Box 19.60). Very occasionally this form of TB may present with one of the complications listed in Box 19.61. The earliest radiographical change is typically an ill-defined opacity situated in one of the upper lobes. Disease often involves two or more areas of lung and may be bilateral. As disease progresses, consolidation, collapse and cavitation develop to varying degrees (Fig. 19.36). The presence of a miliary pattern or cavitation indicates active disease although there is a wide differential. In extensive disease, collapse may be marked and result in significant displacement of the trachea and mediastinum. Occasionally, a caseous lymph node may drain into an adjoining bronchus, resulting in tuberculous pneumonia.

Clinical features: extrapulmonary disease

Extrapulmonary tuberculosis accounts for about 20% of cases in HIV-negative individuals and is more common in HIV-positive individuals. The most common sites affected are lymph nodes, bones and serous membranes but the most serious forms of spread are disseminated TB and tuberculous meningitis.

Lymphadenitis

Lymph nodes are the most common extrapulmonary site of disease. Cervical and mediastinal glands are affected most frequently, followed by axillary and inguinal; in 5% of patients more than one region is involved. Disease may represent primary infection, spread from contiguous sites or reactivation. Supraclavicular lymphadenopathy is usually the result of spread from mediastinal disease. The nodes are usually painless and initially mobile but become matted together with time. When caseation and liquefaction occur, the swelling becomes fluctuant and may discharge through the skin with the formation of a 'collar-stud' abscess and sinus formation. Approximately half of patients fail to show any constitutional features such as fevers or night sweats. The tuberculin test (p. 700) is usually strongly positive. During or after treatment, paradoxical enlargement, development of new nodes and suppuration may all occur but without evidence of continued infection; rarely surgical excision is necessary. In non-immigrant children in the UK, most mycobacterial lymphadenitis is caused by opportunistic mycobacteria, especially of the M. avium complex.

Gastrointestinal tuberculosis

TB can affect any part of the bowel and patients may present with a wide range of symptoms and signs (Fig. 19.37). Upper gastrointestinal tract involvement is rare and is usually an unexpected histological finding in an endoscopic

19

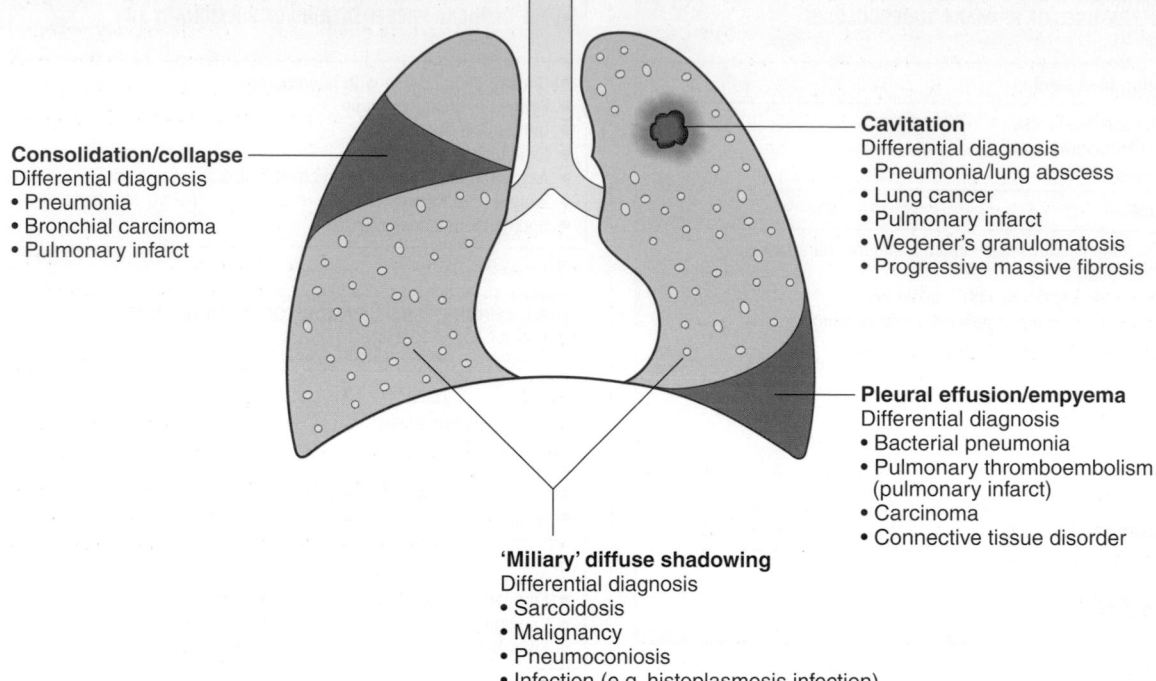

Consolidation/collapse
Differential diagnosis
• Pneumonia
• Bronchial carcinoma
• Pulmonary infarct

Cavitation
Differential diagnosis
• Pneumonia/lung abscess
• Lung cancer
• Pulmonary infarct
• Wegener's granulomatosis
• Progressive massive fibrosis

Pleural effusion/empyema
Differential diagnosis
• Bacterial pneumonia
• Pulmonary thromboembolism
  (pulmonary infarct)
• Carcinoma
• Connective tissue disorder

'Miliary' diffuse shadowing
Differential diagnosis
• Sarcoidosis
• Malignancy
• Pneumoconiosis
• Infection (e.g. histoplasmosis infection)

Fig. 19.36   Chest X-ray: major manifestations and differential diagnosis of pulmonary TB. Less common manifestations include pneumothorax, ARDS (p. 187), cor pulmonale and localised emphysema.

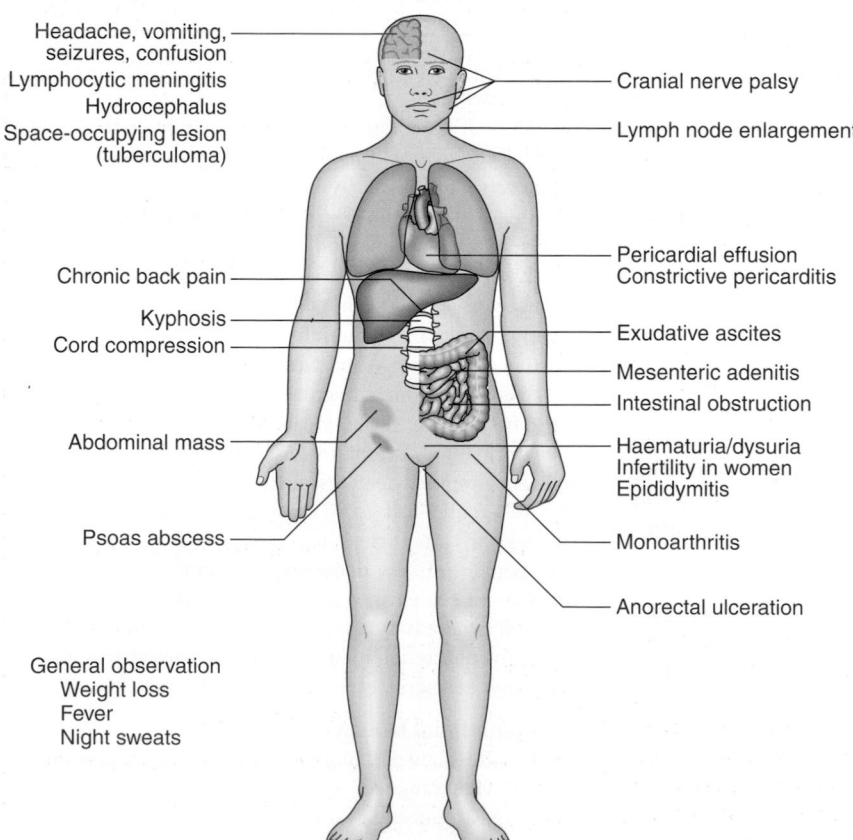

Headache, vomiting, seizures, confusion
Lymphocytic meningitis
Hydrocephalus
Space-occupying lesion (tuberculoma)

Cranial nerve palsy

Lymph node enlargement

Pericardial effusion
Constrictive pericarditis

Chronic back pain

Kyphosis
Cord compression

Exudative ascites

Mesenteric adenitis
Intestinal obstruction

Haematuria/dysuria
Infertility in women
Epididymitis

Abdominal mass

Psoas abscess

Monoarthritis

Anorectal ulceration

General observation
  Weight loss
  Fever
  Night sweats

Fig. 19.37   Systemic presentations of extrapulmonary tuberculosis.

or laparotomy specimen. Ileocaecal disease accounts for approximately half of abdominal TB cases. Fever, night sweats, anorexia and weight loss are usually prominent and a right iliac fossa mass may be palpable. Up to 30% of cases present with an acute abdomen. Ultrasound or CT may reveal thickened bowel wall, abdominal lymphadenopathy, mesenteric thickening or ascites. Barium enema and small bowel enema reveal narrowing, shortening and distortion of the bowel with caecal involvement predominating. Diagnosis rests on obtaining histology by either colonoscopy or mini-laparotomy. The main differential diagnosis is Crohn's disease (p. 910). Tuberculous peritonitis is characterised by abdominal distension, pain and constitutional symptoms. The ascitic fluid is exudative and cellular with a predominance of lymphocytes. Laparoscopy reveals multiple white 'tubercles' over the peritoneal and omental surfaces. Low-grade hepatic dysfunction is common in miliary disease when biopsy reveals granulomas. Occasionally, patients may be frankly icteric with a mixed hepatic/cholestatic picture.

Pericardial disease

Disease occurs in two main forms (Fig. 19.37 and p. 644): pericardial effusion and constrictive pericarditis. Fever and night sweats are rarely prominent and the presentation is usually insidious with breathlessness and abdominal swelling. Pulsus paradoxus, a raised JVP, hepatomegaly, prominent ascites and the absence of peripheral oedema are common to both types of disease. Pericardial effusion is associated with increased pericardial dullness and a globular enlarged heart on chest X-ray. Constriction is associated with atrial fibrillation (< 20%), elevation of the JVP, an early third heart sound and pericardial calcification in 25%. Diagnosis is on clinical, radiological and echocardiographic grounds. The pericardial effusion is blood-stained in 85% of cases. Coexistent pulmonary disease is very rare, with the exception of pleural effusion. Open pericardial biopsy can be performed in patients with effusion where there is doubt about the diagnosis. The addition of corticosteroids has been shown to be beneficial when added to antituberculosis treatment (see below) for both forms of pericardial disease.

Central nervous system disease

Meningeal disease represents the most important form of central nervous system TB. Unrecognised and untreated, it is rapidly fatal. Even when appropriate treatment is prescribed, mortality rates of 30% have been reported whilst survivors may be left with neurological sequelae. Clinical features, investigations and management are dealt with on page 1228.

Bone and joint disease

The spine is the most common site for bony TB (Pott's disease), which usually presents with chronic back pain and typically involves the lower thoracic and lumbar spine (Fig. 19.37). The infection starts as a discitis and then spreads along the spinal ligaments to involve the adjacent anterior vertebral bodies, causing angulation of the vertebrae with subsequent kyphosis. Paravertebral and psoas abscess formation is common and the disease may present with a large (cold) abscess in the inguinal region. CT is

valuable in gauging the extent of disease, the amount of cord compression, and the site for needle biopsy or open exploration if required. The major differential diagnosis is malignancy, which tends to affect the vertebral body and leave the disc intact. Important complications include spinal instability or cord compression.

TB can affect any joint, but most frequently involves the hip or knee. Presentation is usually insidious with pain and swelling; fever and night sweats are uncommon. Radiological changes are often non-specific but, as disease progresses, reduction in joint space and erosions appear.

Genitourinary disease

Fever and night sweats are rare with renal tract TB and patients are often only mildly symptomatic for many years. Haematuria, frequency and dysuria are often present, with sterile pyuria found on urine microscopy and culture. In women, infertility from endometritis, or pelvic pain and swelling from salpingitis or a tubo-ovarian abscess occur occasionally. In men, genitourinary TB may present as epididymitis or prostatitis.

Diagnosis

See Box 19.62.

Mycobacterial infection is usually confirmed by direct microscopy (Ziehl–Neelsen or auramine staining) and culture of samples. It has been estimated that 5000–10 000 acid-fast bacilli must be present in sputum for a patient to be smear-positive, whereas only 10–100 viable organisms are required for sputum to be culture-positive. A stain-positive sputum sample requires confirmation by use of standard culture methods (growth characteristics, pigment production

---

19.62 DIAGNOSIS OF TB

Specimen

Respiratory
- Sputum* (induced with nebulised hypertonic saline if not expectorating)
- Gastric washing* (mainly used for children)
- Bronchoalveolar lavage
- Transbronchial biopsy

Non-respiratory
- Fluid examination (cerebrospinal, ascitic, pleural, pericardial, joint)
- Tissue biopsy (from affected site; also bone marrow/liver may be diagnostic in patients with disseminated disease)

Diagnostic test

- Circumstantial (ESR, CRP, anaemia etc.)
- Tuberculin skin test (low sensitivity/specificity; useful only in primary or deep-seated infection)
- Stain
  - Ziehl–Neelsen
  - Auramine fluorescence
- Nucleic acid amplification
- Culture
  - Solid (Löwenstein–Jensen, Middlebrook)
  - Liquid (e.g. BACTEC)
- Response to empirical antituberculous drugs (usually seen after 5–10 days)

* 3 × early morning samples.

19

and biochemical tests) or molecular DNA technology (hybridisation probes, polymerase chain reaction). Following decontamination, samples should be cultured on a solid medium (Löwenstein–Jensen or Middlebrook). However, as the organism grows slowly, simultaneous culture in liquid culture media (BACTEC or MGIT) should be performed to expedite the testing of drug sensitivities (typically within 7–21 days). Where multiple drug-resistant TB (MDRTB) is suspected, molecular tools may be employed to test for the presence of the rpo gene, currently associated with around 95% of rifampicin-resistant cases. Rapid tests for other forms of drug resistance are under development. If a cluster of cases suggests a common source, fingerprinting of isolates with restriction-fragment length polymorphism (RFLP) or DNA amplification can help confirm this.

Control and prevention

BCG (the Calmette–Guérin bacillus) is a live attenuated vaccine derived from *M. bovis* (pp. 138–139), used to stimulate protective immunity and prevent the dissemination of MTB in an infected host. Reports on the efficacy of BCG are variable (20–60%) but it appears to be most effective in preventing disseminated disease, including tuberculous meningitis, in children. Vaccination policies vary worldwide according to incidence and health-care resources. In the UK vaccination is recommended for the following tuberculin skin test-negative groups:

- contacts < 2 years old
- immigrants from countries where TB is endemic
- infants in high-prevalence ethnic groups
- health-care workers at high risk.

Only those who do not respond to an initial tuberculin skin test are vaccinated. Grade 3–4 tuberculin skin test responders should be referred for clinical and radiological examination. Tuberculin skin testing is usually performed using the Heaf or Mantoux technique (Box 19.63 and Fig. 19.38). Some countries do not use BCG because they value the diagnostic sensitivity of the tuberculin skin test as a measure of recent primary infection. Occasional complications include a local BCG abscess and disseminated infection in immunocompromised persons. BCG should not be administered to HIV-positive individuals.

The identification of latent TB is an integral component of control and cases are commonly identified using the tuberculin skin test. An otherwise asymptomatic contact with a positive tuberculin skin test but a normal chest X-ray may be treated with chemoprophylaxis to prevent infection progressing to clinical disease. Chemoprophylaxis is also recommended for children aged less than 16 years identified during contact tracing to have a strongly positive tuberculin test, children aged less than 2 years in close contact with smear-positive pulmonary disease, those in whom recent tuberculin conversion has been confirmed, and babies of mothers with pulmonary TB. It should also be considered for HIV-infected close contacts of a patient with smear-positive disease. Rifampicin and isoniazid for 3 months, or isoniazid for 6 months are all effective.

Tuberculin skin testing may be associated with false-

19.63 SKIN TESTING IN TUBERCULOSIS: TESTS USING PURIFIED PROTEIN DERIVATIVE (PPD)
Heaf test

• Read at 3–7 days
• Multipuncture method
    Grade 1: 4–6 papules
    Grade 2: Confluent papules forming ring
    Grade 3: Central induration
    Grade 4: >10 mm induration

Mantoux test
• Read at 2–4 days • Using 10 tuberculin units   Positive when induration 5–14 mm (equivalent to Heaf grade 2) and > 15 mm (Heaf grade 3–4)
False negatives
• Severe TB (25% of cases negative) • Newborn and elderly • HIV (if CD4 count < 200 cells/ml) • Recent infection (e.g. measles) or immunisation • Malnutrition • Immunosuppressive drugs • Malignancy • Sarcoidosis

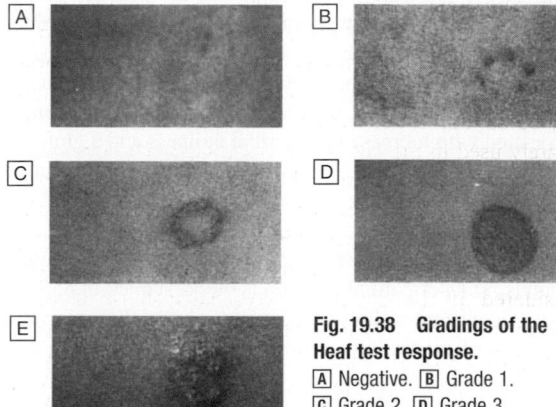

Fig. 19.38 Gradings of the Heaf test response.
A Negative. B Grade 1.
C Grade 2. D Grade 3.
E Grade 4.

positive reactions in those who have had a BCG and in areas where non-tuberculous mycobacteria exposure is high. These limitations may be overcome by the development of whole blood IFN-γ assays against specific mycobacterial antigens such as early secretory antigenic target (ESAT-6).

Contact screening is a legal requirement in many countries. These programmes are vital to TB control and provide valuable epidemiological information. The aim of contact tracing is to identify the probable index case, other cases infected by the same index patient (with or without evidence of disease), and close contacts who should receive BCG vaccination or chemotherapy. Approximately 10–20% of close contacts of patients with smear-positive pulmonary TB and 2–5% of those with smear-negative, culture-positive disease have evidence of tuberculosis infection.

Chemotherapy

A variety of highly effective short-course regimens are available; choice depends on local health resources and

19.64 TREATMENT OF TUBERCULOSIS AS RECOMMENDED BY THE WORLD HEALTH ORGANIZATION

Category of tuberculosis		Initial phase*	Continuation phase
1	New cases of smear-positive pulmonary TB Severe extrapulmonary TB Severe smear-negative pulmonary TB Severe concomitant HIV disease	2 months $H_3R_3Z_3E_3$ *or* 2 months $H_3R_3Z_3S_3$ 2 months HRZE *or* 2 months HRZS	4 months H_3R_3 4 months HR 6 months HE[†]
2[§]	Previously treated smear-positive pulmonary TB Relapse Treatment failure Treatment after default	2 months $H_3R_3Z_3E_3S_3$/1 month $H_3R_3Z_3E$ 2 months HRZES/1 month HRZE	5 months $H_3R_3E_3$ 5 months HRE
3[‡]	New cases of smear-negative pulmonary TB Less severe extrapulmonary TB	2 months $H_3R_3Z_3E_3$ 2 months HRZE	4 months H_3R_3 4 months HR 6 months HE[†]

*The subscript after the letter refers to the number of doses per week; daily has no subscript. H = isoniazid; R = rifampicin; Z = pyrazinamide; E = ethambutol; S = streptomycin.

[†]A continuation phase of 6 months HE has a higher failure and relapse rate than a continuation phase of 4 months of HR but can be used for mobile patients and those with a limited access to health services; the HE regimen can also be used concomitantly with antiretroviral treatment of HIV-infected patients.

[§]Treatment should be guided by sensitivity testing.

[‡]Ethambutol may be omitted in the initial phase of category 3 patients if disease is non-cavitary, smear-negative pulmonary TB, or if patients are known to have a drug-susceptible organism, or for young children with primary TB.

19

infrastructure (Box 19.64). They are based on the principle of an initial intensive phase (which rapidly reduces the bacterial population), followed by a continuation phase to destroy any remaining bacteria. Initial therapy with four drugs has become standard in the UK, although ethambutol may be omitted under certain circumstances. Streptomycin is rarely used in the UK, but it is an important component of short-course treatment regimens in developing nations. Six months of therapy is appropriate for all patients with new-onset, uncomplicated pulmonary or extrapulmonary disease. However, 9–12 months of therapy should be considered if the patient is HIV-positive, or if drug intolerance occurs and a second-line agent is substituted. Meningitis should be treated for a minimum of 12 months. Pyridoxine should be prescribed in pregnant women and malnourished patients.

Most patients can be treated at home. Admission to hospital should be considered where there is uncertainty about the diagnosis, intolerance of medication, questionable compliance, a background of adverse social conditions or a significant risk of MDRTB (culture-positive after 2 months on treatment, contact with known MDRTB). Such patients should be treated in appropriate isolation facilities. Where drug resistance is not expected patients can be assumed to be non-infectious after 2 weeks of appropriate therapy.

In choosing a suitable drug regimen, it is important to bear in mind underlying comorbidity (renal and hepatic dysfunction, eye disease, peripheral neuropathy and HIV status), as well as the potential for drug interactions. Baseline liver function and regular monitoring are important for patients treated with standard therapy including rifampicin, isoniazid and pyrazinamide, as all of these agents are potentially hepatotoxic. Mild asymptomatic increases in transaminases are seen in around 20% of patients but serious liver damage is rare. Patients treated with rifampicin should be advised that their urine, tears and

other secretions will develop a bright orange/red coloration, and women on the oral contraceptive pill must be warned that its efficacy will be reduced and alternative contraception may be necessary. Ethambutol should be used with caution in patients with renal failure, with appropriate dose reduction and monitoring of drug levels. Adverse drug reactions occur in about 10% of patients, but are significantly more common where there is HIV co-infection (Box 19.65).

Corticosteroids reduce inflammation and limit tissue damage and are currently recommended when treating pericardial or meningeal disease, and in children with endobronchial disease. They may also confer benefit in TB of the ureter, pleural effusions and extensive pulmonary disease, and can suppress hypersensitivity drug reactions. Surgery is still occasionally required (e.g. for massive haemoptysis, loculated empyema, constrictive pericarditis, lymph node suppuration, spinal disease with cord compression), but usually only after a full course of antituberculosis treatment.

Directly observed therapy (DOT)

Poor adherence to therapy is a major factor in prolonged infectious illness, risk of relapse, and the emergence of resistance. Directly observed therapy, in which supervised therapy is administered two or three times each week, has been advocated as a method of improving adherence and has become particularly important as a means of improving the control of TB in resource-poor nations. In the UK, it is currently only recommended for patients thought unlikely to be adherent to therapy: homeless, alcohol or drug users, drifters, seriously mentally ill patients and those with a history of non-compliance (Box 19.66).

TB and HIV/AIDS

Globally, approximately 9% of all new TB cases in adults are attributable to HIV infection. The proportion is much

19.65 MAIN ADVERSE REACTIONS OF FIRST-LINE ANTITUBERCULOUS DRUGS

	Isoniazid	Rifampicin	Pyrazinamide	Streptomycin	Ethambutol
Mode of action	Cell wall synthesis	DNA transcription	Unknown	Protein synthesis	Cell wall synthesis
Major adverse reactions	Peripheral neuropathy[1] Hepatitis[2] Rash	Febrile reactions Hepatitis Rash Gastrointestinal disturbance	Hepatitis Gastrointestinal disturbance Hyperuricaemia	8th nerve damage Rash	Retrobulbar neuritis[3] Arthralgia
Less common adverse reactions	Lupoid reactions Seizures Psychoses	Interstitial nephritis Thrombocytopenia Haemolytic anaemia	Rash Photosensitisation Gout	Nephrotoxicity Agranulocytosis	Peripheral neuropathy Rash

[1] The risk of peripheral neuropathy may be reduced by prescribing pyridoxine.
[2] Hepatitis is more common in patients with a slow acetylator status and in alcoholics.
[3] Reduced visual acuity and colour vision may be reported with higher doses and are usually reversible.

19

19.66 DIRECTLY OBSERVED THERAPY IN THE TREATMENT OF TB

EBM

'Systematic review does not show that DOTS is more efficacious than self-administered treatment.'

- Volmik J, et al. (Cochrane Review). Cochrane Library, issue 1, 2005. Oxford: Update Software.

19.67 PREDNISOLONE FOR HIV-POSITIVE PATIENTS WITH TUBERCULOUS PERICARDITIS

EBM

'Addition of prednisolone to standard antituberculous chemotherapy reduced mortality, and led to a faster resolution of physical signs and greater improvement in physical activity.'

- Hakim JG, et al. Heart 2000; 84:183–199.

---

greater in sub-Saharan Africa, but is about 4% in the UK. The close links between HIV and TB, and the potential for both diseases to overwhelm health-care funding in resource-poor nations have been recognised with the promotion of programmes that link detection and treatment of TB with detection and treatment of HIV.

The clinical features vary according to the CD4 count, with low counts favouring atypical presentations; for example, tuberculous pericardial effusion is a common manifestation of HIV in Africa. Extrapulmonary disease appears to be more common (Box 19.67). The appearance of the chest X-ray may be highly variable with greater incidence of lymphadenopathy, pleural effusion, paren-chymal changes, consolidation and miliary disease but significantly less cavitation and atelectasis.

Chemotherapy regimens may be complicated by an increased potential for drug interactions between anti-tuberculous agents and antiretroviral therapy, and an increased incidence of drug-related adverse events—in particular, the use of thioacetazone should be avoided as it is associated with an increased risk of severe, and in some cases fatal, skin reaction. Apparent temporary exacerbations (worsening of symptoms or chest X-ray shortly after starting therapy), sometimes seen in HIV-negative patients, are more common.

Multidrug-resistant TB

The re-emergence of TB has been accompanied by a marked increase in drug-resistant strains, particularly in the poorest countries, and is closely linked to inadequate treatment. Cure is possible but prolonged treatment with less effective, more toxic and more expensive therapies is often necessary. Infection with MDRTB substantially increases the risk of treatment failure, further acquired resistance and death. Molecular probes for rifampicin resistance may be helpful.

Prognosis

Following successful completion of chemotherapy, cure should be anticipated in the majority of patients. There is a small (< 5%) and unavoidable risk of relapse. Most recurrences occur within 5 months and usually have the same drug susceptibility. In the absence of treatment a patient with smear-positive TB will remain infectious for an average of 2 years; in 1 year, 25% of untreated cases will die. A few patients die unexpectedly soon after commencing therapy and it is possible that some of these individuals have subclinical hypoadrenalism that is unmasked by a rifampicin-induced increase in steroid metabolism. HIV-positive patients have higher mortality rates and a modestly increased risk of relapse.

Opportunistic mycobacterial infection

Other species of environmental mycobacteria (often termed 'atypical') may cause human disease (Box 19.68). The sites commonly involved are the lungs, lymph nodes, skin and soft tissues. These mycobacteria are low-grade pathogens (with the exception of *M. malmoense* and *M. ulcerans*), tending to cause disease in the setting of immunocom-promise or scarred lungs. *M. kansasii*, *M. avium* complex (MAC), *M. malmoense* and *M. xenopi* are the species that most often cause lung disease. Most patients are middle-aged to elderly men, over half of whom have COPD, old TB, or both. With the advent of HIV, disseminated infection with MAC has become common when severe immunodeficiency exists (CD4 count < 50 cells/ml—p. 390).

The organisms appear as acid-fast bacilli in the sputum and chest X-ray appearances are similar to classical pulmonary TB; hence clinical uncertainty may exist until cultures become available. Disease is diagnosed when cultures from ≥ 2 specimens, taken more than 7 days apart, are present in a patient with chest radiography typical of

19.68 SITE-SPECIFIC OPPORTUNISTIC MYCOBACTERIAL DISEASE

Pulmonary

- *M. xenopi*
- *M. kansasii*
- *M. malmoense*
- MAC

Lymph node

- MAC
- *M. malmoense*
- *M. fortuitum*
- *M. chelonei*

Soft tissue/skin

- *M. leprae*
- *M. ulcerans* (prevalent in Africa, northern Australia and South-east Asia)
- *M. marinum*
- *M. fortuitum*
- *M. chelonei*

Disseminated

- MAC (HIV-associated)
- *M. haemophilum*
- *M. genavense*
- *M. fortuitum*
- *M. chelonei*
- BCG

(MAC = *Mycobacterium avium* complex—*M. scrofulaceum*, *M. intracellulare* and *M. avium*)

19.69 FACTORS THAT PREDISPOSE TO FUNGAL DISEASE

Systemic factors

- Metabolic disorders—diabetes mellitus
- Chronic alcoholism
- HIV and AIDS
- Corticosteroids and other immunosuppressant medication
- Radiotherapy

Local factors

- Tissue damage by suppuration or necrosis
- Alteration of normal bacterial flora by antibiotic therapy

19.70 CLASSIFICATION OF BRONCHOPULMONARY ASPERGILLOSIS

- Atopic (allergic) asthma (p. 670)
- Allergic bronchopulmonary aspergillosis (asthmatic pulmonary eosinophilia)
- Extrinsic allergic alveolitis (*Aspergillus clavatus*)
- Intracavitary aspergilloma
- Invasive pulmonary aspergillosis

mycobacterial infection. More rapid discriminating systems are under development including DNA probes, high-performance liquid chromatography (HPLC), PCR restriction enzyme analysis (PRA) and 16S rRNA gene sequence analysis. In vitro tests (with the exception of *M. kansasii*) are usually unhelpful in predicting treatment response. Nine months' treatment with rifampicin and ethambutol is usually adequate for *M. kansasii*, but 2 years is recommended for MAC, *M. malmoense* and *M. xenopi*. There is no requirement for notification in the UK as the diseases are not normally communicable.

RESPIRATORY DISEASES CAUSED BY FUNGI

The majority of fungi encountered by humans are harmless saprophytes but in certain circumstances some species may cause disease by infecting human tissue, promoting damaging allergic reactions or producing toxins (Box 19.69). 'Mycosis' is the term applied to disease caused by fungal infection.

ASPERGILLOSIS

Most cases of bronchopulmonary aspergillosis are caused by *Aspergillus fumigatus*, but other members of the genus (*A. clavatus*, *A. flavus*, *A. niger* and *A. terreus*) occasionally cause disease. The conditions associated with *Aspergillus* species are listed in Box 19.70.

ALLERGIC BRONCHOPULMONARY ASPERGILLOSIS (ABPA)

ABPA is caused by a hypersensitivity reaction to *A. fumigatus* involving the bronchial wall and peripheral parts of the lung. It is more common in the autumn and winter and is usually associated with asthma. ABPA can occur in non-asthmatic patients and is a recognised complication of cystic fibrosis. It is one of the causes of pulmonary eosinophilia (p. 723).

Clinical features

Common manifestations include fever, breathlessness, cough productive of bronchial casts and worsening of asthmatic symptoms, but the diagnosis may also be suggested by abnormalities on routine chest X-rays of patients whose asthmatic symptoms are no worse than usual. ABPA may be associated with a persistent vigorous inflammatory response leading to bronchiectasis (characteristically proximal) and, when present, the symptoms and complications of that disease often overshadow those of asthma.

Investigations

Radiographic features include transient diffuse pulmonary infiltrates and lobar or segmental pulmonary collapse. Permanent radiographic changes of bronchiectasis ('tramline', ring and 'gloved-finger' shadows) are seen predominantly in the upper lobes in patients with advanced disease.

The classical features are shown in Box 19.71. Not all are required to make a confident diagnosis.

19.71 FEATURES OF ALLERGIC BRONCHOPULMONARY ASPERGILLOSIS

- Asthma (in the majority of cases)
- Proximal bronchiectasis (inner two-thirds of chest CT field)
- Positive skin test to an extract of *A. fumigatus*
- Elevated total serum IgE > 417 KU/l or 1000 ng/ml
- Elevated serum IgE-*A. fumigatus* or IgG-*A. fumigatus*
- Peripheral blood eosinophilia > 0.5×10^9/litre
- Presence or history of chest X-ray abnormalities
- Fungal hyphae of *A. fumigatus* on microscopic examination of sputum

19

Management

Exacerbations, particularly when associated with new chest X-ray changes, should be treated promptly with prednisolone 40–60 mg daily and physiotherapy. If persistent lobar collapse is a feature, bronchoscopy should be performed to remove impacted mucus and ensure prompt reinflation.

The optimum maintenance therapy for ABPA is uncertain. Regular therapy with low-dose oral corticosteroid therapy (prednisolone 7.5–10 mg daily) is prescribed to suppress the immunopathological responses and prevent progression to tissue damage; some advocate high-dose inhaled corticosteroids. Therapy with itraconazole may be beneficial in some patients.

INTRACAVITARY MYCETOMA

Inhaled air-borne spores of fungi may lodge and germinate in areas of damaged lung tissue forming a fungal ball (mycetoma). These may form in any area of damaged lung but the upper lobes are most frequently involved, reflecting the fact that mycetomas readily form in tuberculous cavities (Fig. 19.39). Less common causes include damage from a lung abscess cavity, a bronchiectatic space, pulmonary infarct, sarcoid, ankylosing spondylitis or even a cavitated tumour. As *A. fumigatus* is the most common organism identified, the term 'aspergilloma' is often used, but other fungi may be implicated.

Clinical features

The range of presentation is varied. Mycetomas are often asymptomatic, being identified on chest X-ray as a dense

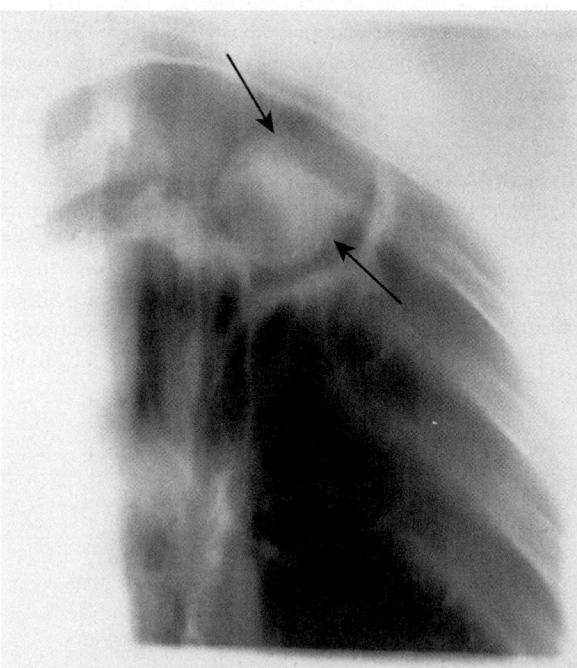

Fig. 19.39 Mycetoma in left upper lobe cavity. Mycetoma demonstrated using conventional tomography. Rounded fungal ball (arrows) separated from the wall of the cavity by a 'halo' of air.

rounded shadow in the upper lobe. However, in some patients they may be responsible for recurrent haemoptysis, which may be severe and life-threatening. Non-specific systemic features such as lethargy and weight loss may also be reported.

Diagnosis

The development of a mycetoma produces a tumour-like opacity on X-ray, but can usually be distinguished from a peripheral bronchial carcinoma by the presence of a crescent of air between the fungal ball and the upper wall of the cavity (Fig. 19.39). HRCT provides greater clarity and often demonstrates the presence of multiple mycetomas. Serum precipitins to *A. fumigatus* can be demonstrated in virtually all patients. Sputum microscopy typically demonstrates scanty hyphal fragments, and is usually positive on culture. Less than 50% of patients exhibit skin hypersensitivity to extracts of *A. fumigatus*.

Management

Treatment is often disappointing. Selected patients with good respiratory reserve may benefit from surgery, particularly those who experience massive haemoptysis. However, surgical resection may be accompanied by significant morbidity and mortality. Bronchial artery embolisation provides a palliative approach to haemoptysis. Specific antifungal therapy is of no value.

INVASIVE PULMONARY ASPERGILLOSIS

Invasion of previously healthy lung tissue by *A. fumigatus* is uncommon but can produce a serious and often fatal condition, which usually occurs in patients who are immunocompromised by either drugs or disease.

Clinical features

Spread of the disease to the lungs is usually rapid, with the production of consolidation, necrosis and cavitation. There is grave systemic disturbance. The formation of multiple abscesses is associated with the production of copious amounts of purulent sputum which is often blood-stained.

A much more indolent form of invasive pulmonary aspergillosis is now recognised.

Diagnosis

Invasive pulmonary aspergillosis should be suspected in any patient thought to have severe suppurative pneumonia (p. 694) that has not responded to antibiotic therapy. The diagnosis can be established by the demonstration of abundant fungal elements in stained smears of sputum. Serum precipitins can be demonstrated in some, but not all, patients.

Management

Invasive aspergillosis carries a high mortality rate but if the diagnosis is established at an early stage, antifungal therapy can be successful. Amphotericin 0.25–1 mg/kg daily by slow intravenous infusion over 6 hours should be given in combination with flucytosine 150–200 mg/kg daily by mouth or by intravenous infusion, in four divided doses. The combination of flucytosine and amphotericin prevents resistance to flucytosine developing and allows a smaller daily dose of amphotericin to be used. Liposomal amphotericin is recommended when toxicity precludes the use of conventional amphotericin. Itraconazole has also been used successfully in the treatment of invasive aspergillosis.

Histoplasmosis, coccidioidomycosis, blastomycosis and cryptococcosis
See pages 374–375.

TUMOURS OF THE BRONCHUS AND LUNG

Lung cancer is the most common cancer world-wide, accounting for 1.2 million new cases annually in 2000, and causing 18% of all cancer deaths. Tobacco use is the major preventable cause; however, just as tobacco use and cancer rates are beginning to fall in some developed countries, both smoking and lung cancer are rising in Eastern Europe and in many developing countries (Box 19.72). The great majority of tumours in the lung are primary bronchial carcinomas. In contrast to many other tumours, the prognosis of primary

19.72 THE BURDEN OF LUNG CANCER
• Strikes 900 000 men and 330 000 women each year
• 18% of all cancer deaths
• More than threefold increase in deaths since 1950
• Rising rates in women: female lung cancer deaths outnumber male in some Nordic countries
• Has overtaken breast cancer in several countries, making it the most common cause of cancer death in men and women
• An estimated 100 million people died in the 20th century from tobacco-associated diseases

lung carcinoma remains poor, with an average of 20% surviving at 1 year and 5% at 5 years. Carcinomas of other organs, in particular the breast, kidney, uterus, ovary, testes and thyroid, may give rise to metastatic pulmonary deposits, as may an osteogenic or other sarcoma.

PRIMARY TUMOURS OF THE LUNG

Aetiology
Cigarette smoking is by far the most important single factor in the causation of lung cancer. It is thought to be directly responsible for at least 90% of lung carcinomas, the risk being directly proportional to the amount smoked and to the tar content of cigarettes. For example, the death rate from the disease in heavy smokers is 40 times that in non-smokers. Risk falls slowly after smoking cessation, but remains above the risk in non-smokers for many years. The effect of 'passive' smoking is more difficult to quantify but is currently believed to be a factor in 5% of all lung cancer deaths. Exposure to naturally occurring radon is another known risk. The incidence of lung cancer is also slightly higher in urban than in rural dwellers; this may reflect differences in atmospheric pollution (including tobacco smoke) or occupation since a number of industrial products (e.g. asbestos, beryllium, cadmium and chromium) are associated with lung cancer.

BRONCHIAL CARCINOMA

The incidence of bronchial carcinoma increased dramatically during the 20th century (Fig. 19.40). In women, smoking prevalence and deaths from lung cancer continue to increase, and more women now die of lung cancer than breast cancer in the USA and the UK.

19

Males

Rate per 100 000

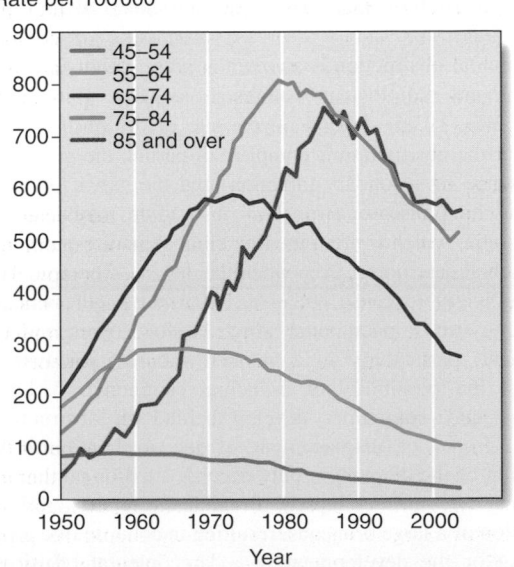

Females

Rate per 100 000

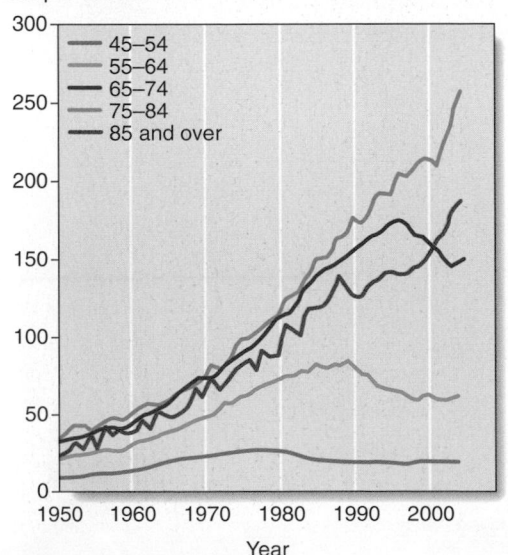

Fig. 19.40 Mortality trends from lung cancer in England and Wales, 1950–2004 by age and year of death. A Males. B Females. Note the decline in mortality from lung cancer in men towards the end of this period, reflecting a change in smoking habit.

Pathology

Bronchial carcinomas arise from the bronchial epithelium or mucous glands. The common cell types are listed in Box 19.73.

When the tumour arises in a large bronchus, symptoms arise early, but tumours originating in a peripheral bronchus can attain a very large size without producing symptoms. Peripheral squamous tumours may undergo central necrosis and cavitation, and may have similar radiographic features to a lung abscess (Fig. 19.41). Bronchial carcinoma may involve the pleura either directly or by lymphatic spread and may extend into the chest wall, invading the intercostal nerves or the brachial plexus and causing severe pain. The primary tumour, or tumour within lymph node metastases, may spread into the mediastinum and invade or compress the pericardium, oesophagus, superior vena cava, trachea, phrenic or left recurrent laryngeal nerves. Lymphatic spread to supraclavicular and mediastinal lymph nodes is also frequently observed. Blood-borne metastases occur most commonly in liver, bone, brain, adrenals and skin. Even a small primary tumour may cause widespread metastatic deposits and this is a particular characteristic of small-cell-type lung cancers.

19.73 COMMON CELL TYPES OF BRONCHIAL CARCINOMA	
Cell type	%
Squamous	35
Adenocarcinoma	30
Small-cell	20
Large-cell	15

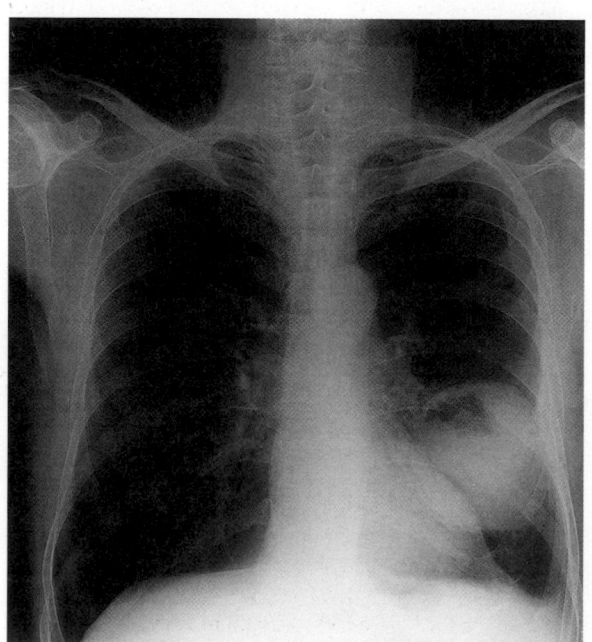

Fig. 19.41 Large cavitated bronchial carcinoma in left lower lobe.

19.74 NON-METASTATIC EXTRAPULMONARY MANIFESTATIONS OF BRONCHIAL CARCINOMA	
Endocrine (Ch. 20)	
• Inappropriate antidiuretic hormone (ADH) secretion causing hyponatraemia • Ectopic adrenocorticotrophic hormone (ACTH) secretion	• Hypercalcaemia due to secretion of parathyroid hormone (PTH)-related peptides • Carcinoid syndrome (p. 903) • Gynaecomastia
Neurological (Ch. 26)	
• Polyneuropathy • Myelopathy • Cerebellar degeneration	• Myasthenia (Lambert–Eaton syndrome, p. 1252)
Other	
• Digital clubbing • Hypertrophic pulmonary osteoarthropathy • Nephrotic syndrome	• Polymyositis and dermatomyositis • Eosinophilia

Clinical features

Lung cancer presents in many different ways. Most commonly, symptoms reflect local involvement of the bronchus, but may also arise from spread to the chest wall or mediastinum, from distant blood-borne spread or, less commonly, as a result of a variety of non-metastatic paraneoplastic syndromes (Box 19.74).

Cough is the most common early symptom; it is often dry but sputum may be purulent if there is secondary infection. A change in the character of the 'regular' cough of a smoker, particularly if it is associated with other new respiratory symptoms, should always alert the clinician to the possibility of bronchial carcinoma.

Haemoptysis is a common symptom, especially in tumours arising in central bronchi. Occasionally, central tumours invade large vessels, causing massive haemoptysis which may be fatal. Repeated episodes of scanty haemoptysis or blood-streaking of sputum in a smoker are highly suggestive of bronchial carcinoma and should always be investigated.

Bronchial obstruction is a common presentation, and the clinical and radiological manifestations (Figs 19.42 and 19.43, Box 19.75) depend on the site of the obstruction, whether the obstruction is complete or partial, the presence or absence of secondary infection, and the extent of pre-existing lung disease. Bronchial obstruction may lead to pneumonia, which is often the first clinical manifestation of a bronchial carcinoma, even when the degree of obstruction is insufficient to cause collapse. Recurrent pneumonia at the same site or pneumonia which is slow to respond to treatment, particularly in a smoker, should immediately suggest the possibility of bronchial carcinoma. A lung abscess may sometimes develop behind an obstructive lesion. Signs of displacement of the mediastinum or elevation of the diaphragm only occur if a major portion of the lung becomes collapsed. Breathlessness may reflect occlusion of a large bronchus, resulting in collapse of a lobe or lung or the development of a large pleural effusion. Stridor (a harsh inspiratory noise) occurs when the lower trachea, carina or main bronchi are narrowed by the primary

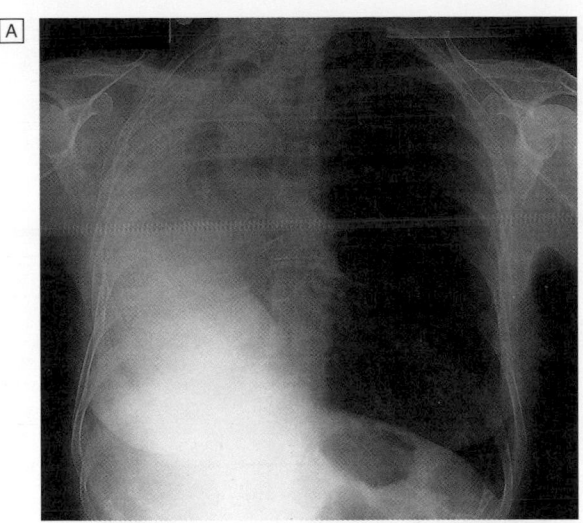

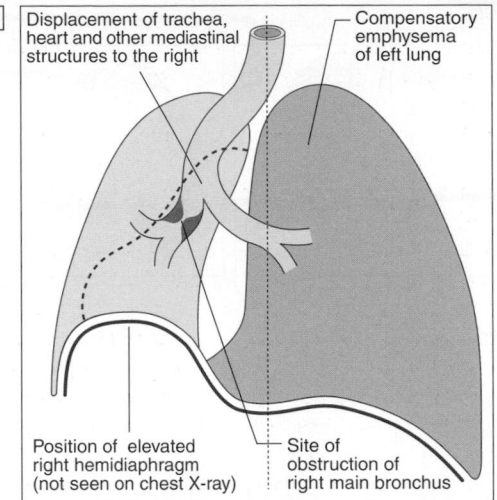

Displacement of trachea, heart and other mediastinal structures to the right

Compensatory emphysema of left lung

Position of elevated right hemidiaphragm (not seen on chest X-ray)

Site of obstruction of right main bronchus

Fig. 19.42 Collapse of the right lung: effects on neighbouring structures. A Chest X-ray. B Artist's impression.

19

19.75 CAUSES OF LARGE BRONCHUS OBSTRUCTION

Common

- Bronchial carcinoma or adenoma (Box 19.79, p. 711)
- Enlarged tracheobronchial lymph nodes (malignant or tuberculous)
- Inhaled foreign bodies (especially right lung and in children)
- Bronchial casts or plugs consisting of inspissated mucus or blood clot (especially asthma, cystic fibrosis, haemoptysis, debility)
- Collections of mucus or mucopus retained in the bronchi as a result of ineffective expectoration (especially post-operative following abdominal surgery)

Rare

- Aortic aneurysm
- Giant left atrium
- Pericardial effusion
- Congenital bronchial atresia
- Fibrous bronchial stricture (e.g. following TB or bronchial surgery/lung transplant)

tumour or by compression from malignant enlargement of the subcarinal and paratracheal lymph nodes.

Pleural pain usually indicates malignant invasion of the pleura, although it can occur with distal infection. Involvement of the intercostal nerves may cause pain in the chest along the appropriate nerve root distribution. Bronchial carcinoma in the apex of the lung ('superior sulcus tumour') may cause Horner's syndrome (ipsilateral partial ptosis, enophthalmos, a small pupil and hypohidrosis of the face) due to involvement of the sympathetic chain at or above the stellate ganglion, and/or Pancoast's syndrome (pain in the shoulder and inner aspect of the arm) caused by involvement of the lower part of the brachial plexus. Mediastinal spread may result in dysphagia.

The patient may also present with symptoms due to blood-borne metastases, such as focal neurological defects, epileptic seizures, personality change, jaundice, bone pain or skin nodules. Lassitude, anorexia and weight loss usually indicate the presence of metastatic spread. Finally, the patient may present with symptoms referable to the presence of a number of non-metastatic extrapulmonary manifestations (Box 19.74). The most frequently encountered endocrine syndromes (inappropriate antidiuretic hormone (ADH) secretion and ectopic adrenocorticotrophic hormone (ACTH) secretion) are usually associated with small-cell lung cancer. Hypercalcaemia due to secretion of parathyroid hormone (PTH)-like peptides is usually caused by squamous cell carcinoma. Associated neurological syndromes may occur with any type of bronchial carcinoma.

Physical signs

Examination is usually normal unless there is significant bronchial obstruction, or the tumour has spread to the pleura, mediastinum or supraclavicular nodes. A tumour obstructing a large bronchus produces the physical signs of collapse (or occasionally obstructive emphysema) and may give rise to pneumonia that is characterised by a relative absence of physical signs and a slow response to treatment. A monophonic or unilateral wheeze which fails to clear with coughing suggests the presence of a fixed bronchial obstruction, and the presence of stridor indicates obstruction at or above the main carina. A hoarse voice associated with an ineffectual or 'bovine' cough usually indicates left recurrent laryngeal nerve palsy. Phrenic nerve paralysis causes unilateral diaphragmatic palsy and hence dullness to percussion and absent breath sounds at a lung base. Involvement of the pleura may produce a pleural rub or signs of pleural effusion (p. 649). Bronchial carcinoma is also the most common cause of the superior vena cava syndrome, which presents initially as bilateral engorgement of the jugular veins and later as oedema affecting the face, neck, arms and conjunctivae. Digital clubbing is often seen and may be associated with a syndrome called hypertrophic pulmonary osteoarthropathy (HPOA), characterised by periostitis of the long bones, most commonly the distal tibia, fibula, radius and ulna. This gives rise to pain and tenderness over the affected bones and often pitting oedema over the

19

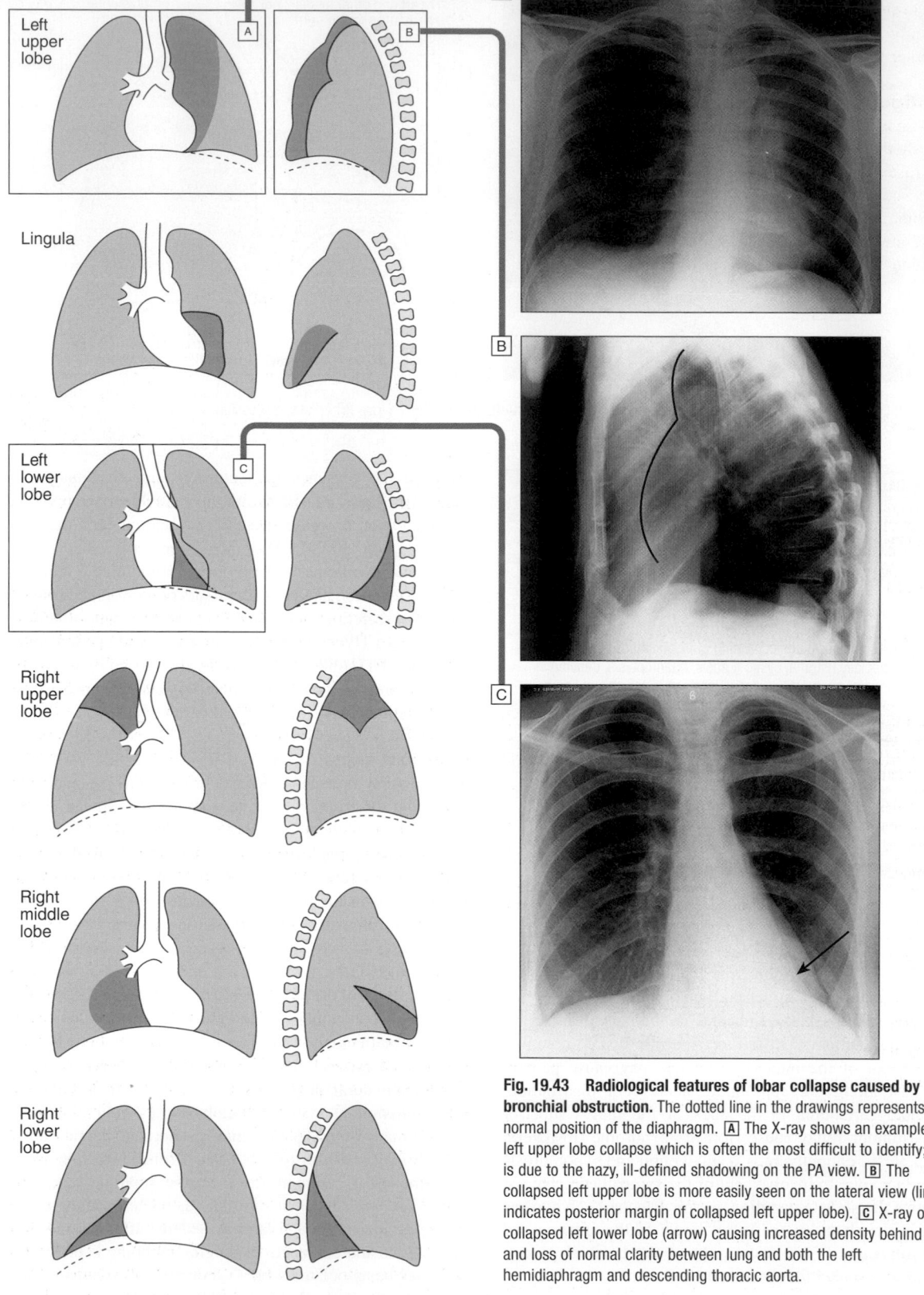

Left
upper
lobe

Lingula

Left
lower
lobe

Right
upper
lobe

Right
middle
lobe

Right
lower
lobe

Fig. 19.43 Radiological features of lobar collapse caused by bronchial obstruction. The dotted line in the drawings represents the normal position of the diaphragm. [A] The X-ray shows an example of left upper lobe collapse which is often the most difficult to identify; this is due to the hazy, ill-defined shadowing on the PA view. [B] The collapsed left upper lobe is more easily seen on the lateral view (line indicates posterior margin of collapsed left upper lobe). [C] X-ray of collapsed left lower lobe (arrow) causing increased density behind heart and loss of normal clarity between lung and both the left hemidiaphragm and descending thoracic aorta.

anterior aspect of the shin. X-rays of the painful bones show subperiosteal new bone formation. HPOA, while most frequently associated with bronchial carcinoma, can occur with other tumours.

Investigations

The main aims of investigation are to confirm the diagnosis, establish the histological cell type and define the extent of the disease.

The common radiological features of bronchial carcinoma are illustrated in Figure 19.44 and Box 19.76. Further investigation to obtain a histological diagnosis and determine operability is nearly always indicated.

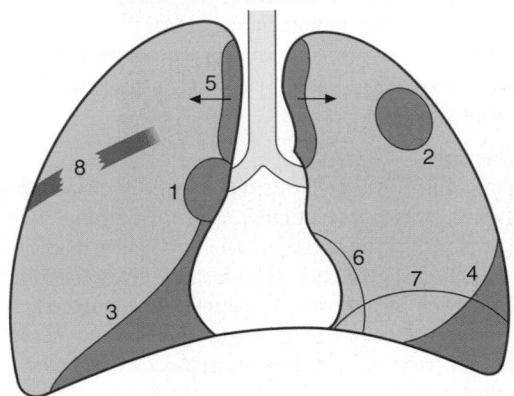

Fig. 19.44 Common radiological presentations of bronchial carcinoma.

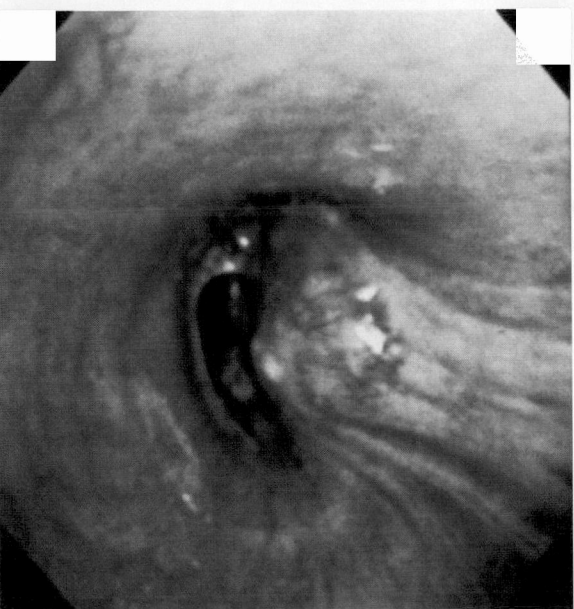

Fig. 19.45 Bronchoscopic view of a bronchogenic carcinoma. There is distortion of mucosal folds, partial occlusion of the airway lumen and abnormal tumour tissue.

19.76 COMMON RADIOLOGICAL PRESENTATIONS OF BRONCHIAL CARCINOMA
❶ **Unilateral hilar enlargement**
• Central tumour. Hilar glandular involvement. Beware—peripheral tumour in apical segment of a lower lobe can look like an enlarged hilar shadow on the PA X-ray
❷ **Peripheral pulmonary opacity** (p. 663)
• Usually irregular but well circumscribed. May have irregular cavitation within it. Can be very large
❸ **Lung, lobe or segmental collapse**
• Usually caused by tumour within the bronchus causing occlusion. Lung collapse can be produced by compression of the main bronchus by enlarged lymph glands
❹ **Pleural effusion**
• Usually indicates tumour invasion of pleural space; very rarely a manifestation of infection in collapsed lung tissue distal to a bronchial carcinoma
❺–❼ **Broadening of mediastinum, enlarged cardiac shadow, elevation of a hemidiaphragm**
• Paratracheal lymphadenopathy may cause widening of the upper mediastinum. A malignant pericardial effusion will cause enlargement of the cardiac shadow. If a raised hemidiaphragm is caused by phrenic nerve palsy, screening will show it to move paradoxically upwards when patient sniffs
❽ **Rib destruction**
• Direct invasion of the chest wall or blood-borne metastatic spread can cause osteolytic lesions of the ribs

Around three-quarters of primary lung tumours can be visualised directly using a flexible bronchoscope. Bronchial biopsies and brush samples can be taken for pathological examination and a direct assessment can be made of operability as judged by the proximity of central tumours to the main carina (Fig. 19.45). If tumour is not visible at bronchoscopy, bronchial washings and brushings can be taken from the radiologically affected lung segment, but the diagnostic yield is much lower. For peripheral lesions not accessible to the bronchoscope, percutaneous needle biopsy under CT or ultrasound guidance is a more reliable way to obtain a histological diagnosis but carries a small risk of iatrogenic pneumothorax. In patients who are not fit enough for bronchoscopy, sputum cytology can be a valuable diagnostic aid (Fig. 19.46). Pleural biopsy is indicated in all patients with pleural effusions. When plain films or CT suggest mediastinal involvement by tumour, tissue samples can be obtained by needle aspiration through the bronchial wall at bronchoscopy, through the oesophagus using endoscopic ultrasound guidance, or by mediastinoscopy under general anaesthetic. Not infrequently, thoracoscopy or thoracotomy is required to obtain a definitive histological diagnosis. In patients with metastatic disease the diagnosis can often be confirmed by needle aspiration or biopsy of affected lymph nodes, skin lesions, liver or bone marrow.

After establishing a histological diagnosis, investigations should focus on determining whether the tumour is operable. This requires excluding involvement of central mediastinal structures or spread of tumour to distant sites and ensuring that the patient's respiratory and cardiac function is sufficient to allow surgical treatment (Box 19.77). The propensity of small-cell lung cancer to metastasise early dictates that patients with this tumour type are usually not suitable for surgical intervention. Head CT, radionuclide

19

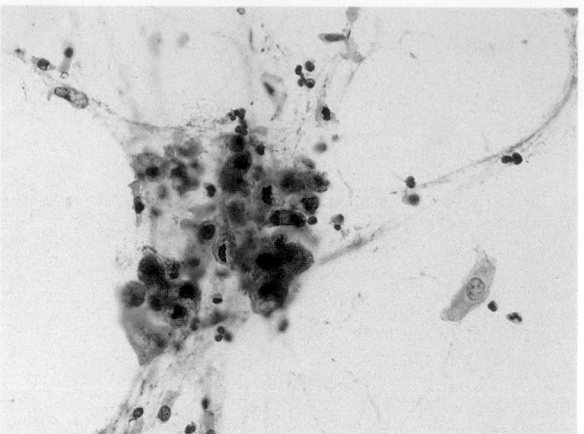

Fig. 19.46 Sputum sample showing a cluster of carcinoma cells.
There is keratinisation, showing orangeophilia of the cytoplasm, and
non-keratinised forms are also seen. The nuclei are large and
'coal-black' in density. These are the features of squamous cell
bronchogenic carcinoma.

**19.77 CONTRAINDICATIONS TO SURGICAL
RESECTION IN BRONCHIAL CARCINOMA**

- Distant metastasis (M1)
- Invasion of central mediastinal structures including heart, great
  vessels, trachea and oesophagus (T4)
- Malignant pleural effusion (T4)
- Contralateral mediastinal nodes (N3)
- $FEV_1 < 0.8$ litres
- Severe or unstable cardiac or other medical condition

N.B. In otherwise fit individuals, direct extension of tumour into the
chest wall, diaphragm, mediastinal pleura or pericardium or to
within 2 cm of the main carina does not exclude surgery. Though
surgically resectable, patients with N2 (ipsilateral mediastinal) nodes
may require neoadjuvant or adjuvant therapy (see text).

---

bone scanning, liver ultrasound and bone marrow biopsy can
be reserved for patients with clinical, haematological or
biochemical evidence of tumour spread to such sites.

Management

Surgical resection carries the best hope of long-term
survival; however, some patients treated with radical
radiotherapy also achieve prolonged remission or cure.
Unfortunately, in the majority of cases (over 85%) surgery is
not possible or is inappropriate due to extensive spread
or co-morbidity, and such patients can only be offered
palliative therapy. Radiotherapy, and in some cases
chemotherapy, can relieve distressing symptoms.

Surgical treatment

Careful staging and assessment of the patient's respiratory
reserve and cardiac status are essential prerequisites to
surgery. This, coupled with improvements in surgical and
post-operative care, now offers 5-year survival rates of over
75% in stage I disease (N0, tumour confined within visceral
pleura) and 55% in stage II disease, which includes
resection in patients with ipsilateral peribronchial or hilar
node involvement.

Radiotherapy

While much less effective than surgery, radical radiotherapy
can offer long-term survival in selected patients with
localised disease in whom comorbidity precludes surgery.
The greatest value of radiotherapy, however, is in the
palliation of distressing complications such as superior vena
caval obstruction, recurrent haemoptysis, and pain caused
by chest wall invasion or by skeletal metastatic deposits.
Obstruction of the trachea and main bronchi can also be
relieved temporarily. Radiotherapy can be used in conjunction with chemotherapy in the treatment of small-cell
carcinoma and is particularly efficient at preventing the
development of brain metastases in patients who have had
a complete response to chemotherapy. Continuous hyper-
fractionated accelerated radiotherapy (CHART), in which a
similar total dose is given in smaller but more frequent
fractions, may offer better survival prospects than
conventional schedules.

Chemotherapy

The treatment of small-cell carcinoma with combinations
of cytotoxic drugs, sometimes in combination with
radiotherapy, can increase the median survival of patients
with this highly malignant type of bronchial carcinoma from
3 months to well over a year. Combination chemotherapy
leads to better outcomes than single-agent treatment. In
particular, oral etoposide leads to more toxicity and worse
survival than standard combination chemotherapy. Regular
cycles of therapy, including combinations of i.v. cyclophosphamide, doxorubicin and vincristine or i.v. cisplatin and
etoposide, are commonly used. Nausea and vomiting are
common side-effects and are best treated with $5\text{-}HT_3$
receptor antagonists (p. 266).

The use of combinations of chemotherapeutic drugs
requires considerable medical skill and expertise and it is
recommended that such treatment should only be given
by teams of expert clinicians and nurses. In general,
chemotherapy is less effective in non-small-cell bronchial
cancers. However, recent studies in such patients using
platinum-based chemotherapy regimens have shown a 30%
response rate associated with a small increase in survival
(Box 19.78).

Neoadjuvant and adjuvant chemotherapy

In non-small-cell carcinoma, there is early evidence that
chemotherapy given before surgery may increase survival
and can effectively 'down-stage' disease with limited nodal
spread. Post-operative chemotherapy is also useful when
operative samples show nodal involvement by tumour.

Laser therapy and stenting

Laser treatment via a fibreoptic bronchoscope is essentially
palliative, the aim being to clear tumour tissue occluding

EBM

**19.78 PALLIATIVE CHEMOTHERAPY IN
STAGE IV NON-SMALL CELL LUNG CANCER**

'Adding chemotherapy containing cisplatin improves survival
compared to either radical radiotherapy or supportive care alone.'

For further information: 🖥 www.cochrane.org

19.79 RARER TYPES OF LUNG TUMOUR				
Tumour	**Status**	**Histology**	**Typical presentation**	**Prognosis**
Adenosquamous carcinoma	Malignant	Tumours with areas of unequivocal squamous and adeno-differentiation	Peripheral or central lung mass	Stage-dependent
Carcinoid tumour (p. 903)	Low-grade malignant	Neuroendocrine differentiation	Bronchial obstruction, cough	95% 5-year survival with resection
Bronchial gland adenoma	Benign	Salivary gland differentiation	Tracheobronchial irritation/obstruction	Local resection curative
Bronchial gland carcinoma	Low-grade malignant	Salivary gland differentiation	Tracheobronchial irritation/obstruction	Local recurrence occurs
Hamartoma	Benign	Mesenchymal cells, cartilage	Peripheral lung nodule	Local resection curative
Bronchoalveolar carcinoma	Malignant	Tumour cells line alveolar spaces	Alveolar shadowing, productive cough	Variable, worse if multifocal

19

major airways and allow re-aeration of collapsed lung. The best results are achieved in tumours of the main bronchi. Endobronchial stents can be used to maintain airway patency in the face of extrinsic compression by malignant nodes.

General aspects of management

The best outcomes are obtained when lung cancer is managed in specialist centres by multidisciplinary teams including oncologists, thoracic surgeons, respiratory physicians and specialist nurses. As in other forms of carcinoma, effective communication, pain relief and attention to diet are important (Ch. 11). Lung tumours can cause clinically significant depression and anxiety, and these may need specific therapy. The management of non-metastatic endocrine manifestations is described in Chapter 20. The management of malignant pleural effusions is outlined on page 665.

Prognosis

The overall prognosis in bronchial carcinoma is very poor, with around 80% of patients dying within a year of diagnosis and less than 6% of patients surviving 5 years after diagnosis. The best prognosis is with well-differentiated squamous cell tumours which have not metastasised and are amenable to surgical treatment.

The clinical features and prognosis of other less common benign and malignant tumours of the lung are given in Box 19.79.

SECONDARY TUMOURS OF THE LUNG

Blood-borne metastatic deposits in the lungs may be derived from many primary tumours (p. 705). The secondary deposits are usually multiple and bilateral. Often there are no respiratory symptoms and the diagnosis is made by radiological examination. Breathlessness may occur if a considerable amount of lung tissue has been replaced by metastatic tumour. Endobronchial deposits are uncommon but can cause haemoptysis and lobar collapse.

19.80 LUNG CANCER IN OLD AGE

- **Incidence**: ageing is a major risk factor for the development of lung cancer.
- **Late presentation**: older patients tend to present with more advanced disease.
- **Investigation**: older patients are less likely to be referred for bronchoscopy than younger patients, although it is well tolerated and safe even in the very old. The only older patients who should not be referred are those with other significant pathology who are not fit for intensive investigation and intervention.
- **Outcomes**: 5-year survival rates for older patients who undergo surgery for squamous cell carcinoma are little different to those for younger patients. High-intensity chemotherapy regimens for small-cell carcinoma have high levels of toxicity in old age without significant survival benefits.

LYMPHANGITIC SPREAD OF CARCINOMA IN THE LUNG

Lymphatic infiltration may develop in patients with carcinoma of the breast, stomach, bowel, pancreas or bronchus. This grave condition causes severe and rapidly progressive breathlessness associated with marked hypoxaemia. The chest X-ray shows diffuse pulmonary shadowing radiating from the hilar regions, often associated with septal lines, and CT scans show characteristic polygonal thickened interlobular septa.

TUMOURS OF THE MEDIASTINUM

The mediastinum can be divided into four major compartments with reference to the lateral chest X-ray (Fig. 19.47):

- superior mediastinum—above a line drawn between the lower border of the 4th thoracic vertebra and the upper end of the body of the sternum
- anterior mediastinum—in front of the heart
- middle mediastinum—between the anterior and posterior compartments
- posterior mediastinum—behind the heart.

A variety of conditions can present radiologically as a mediastinal mass (Box 19.81).

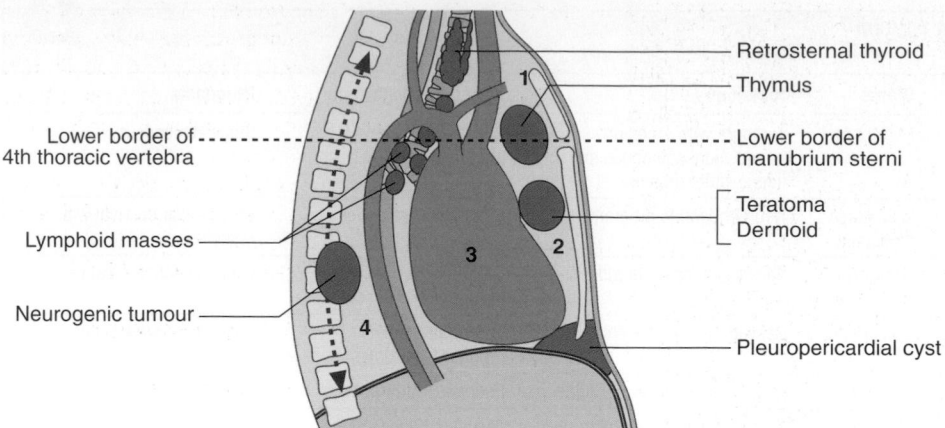

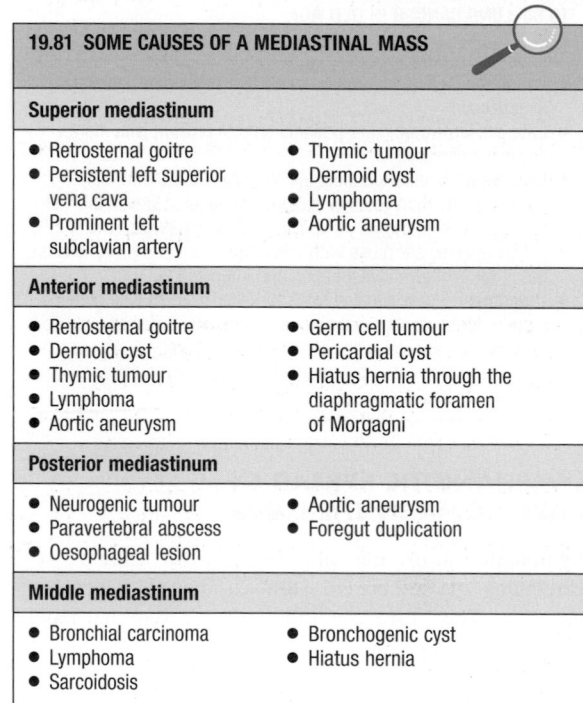

Fig. 19.47 The divisions of the mediastinum described in the diagnosis of mediastinal masses. (1) Superior mediastinum. (2) Anterior mediastinum. (3) Middle mediastinum. (4) Posterior mediastinum. Sites of the more common mediastinal tumours are also illustrated.

19.81 SOME CAUSES OF A MEDIASTINAL MASS

Superior mediastinum

- Retrosternal goitre
- Persistent left superior vena cava
- Prominent left subclavian artery
- Thymic tumour
- Dermoid cyst
- Lymphoma
- Aortic aneurysm

Anterior mediastinum

- Retrosternal goitre
- Dermoid cyst
- Thymic tumour
- Lymphoma
- Aortic aneurysm
- Germ cell tumour
- Pericardial cyst
- Hiatus hernia through the diaphragmatic foramen of Morgagni

Posterior mediastinum

- Neurogenic tumour
- Paravertebral abscess
- Oesophageal lesion
- Aortic aneurysm
- Foregut duplication

Middle mediastinum

- Bronchial carcinoma
- Lymphoma
- Sarcoidosis
- Bronchogenic cyst
- Hiatus hernia

19.82 SYMPTOMS AND SIGNS PRODUCED BY MALIGNANT INVASION OF THE STRUCTURES OF THE MEDIASTINUM

Trachea and main bronchi

- Stridor, breathlessness, cough, pulmonary collapse

Oesophagus

- Dysphagia, oesophageal displacement or obstruction on barium swallow examination

Phrenic nerve

- Diaphragmatic paralysis

Left recurrent laryngeal nerve

- Paralysis of left vocal cord giving rise to hoarseness and 'bovine' cough

Sympathetic trunk

- Horner's syndrome

Superior vena cava

- SVC obstruction results in non-pulsatile distension of neck veins, subconjunctival oedema, and oedema and cyanosis of head, neck, hands and arms. Dilated anastomotic veins on chest wall

Pericardium

- Pericarditis and/or pericardial effusion

Benign tumours and cysts arising within the mediastinum are frequently diagnosed when radiological examination of the chest is undertaken for some other reason. In general, they do not invade vital structures but may cause symptoms by compressing the trachea or occasionally the superior vena cava. A dermoid cyst may very occasionally rupture into a bronchus.

Malignant mediastinal tumours are distinguished by their power to invade as well as compress structures such as bronchi and lungs (Box 19.82). As a result, even a small malignant tumour can produce symptoms, although more commonly the tumour has attained a considerable size before this happens. Included in this category are mediastinal lymph node metastases, lymphomas, leukaemia, malignant thymic tumours and germ-cell tumours. Aortic and innominate aneurysms have destructive features resembling those of malignant mediastinal tumours.

Investigations

Radiological examination

A benign mediastinal tumour generally appears as a sharply circumscribed opacity situated mainly in the mediastinum but often encroaching on one or both lung fields (Fig. 19.48). A malignant mediastinal tumour seldom has a clearly defined margin and often presents as a general broadening of the mediastinal shadow. CT (or MRI) is the investigation of choice for mediastinal tumours.

Endoscopic investigation

Bronchoscopy may reveal a primary bronchial carcinoma causing mediastinal tumour by secondary lymphatic spread. The posterior mediastinum can be imaged by transoesophageal ultrasound, and needle biopsies of lymph node masses

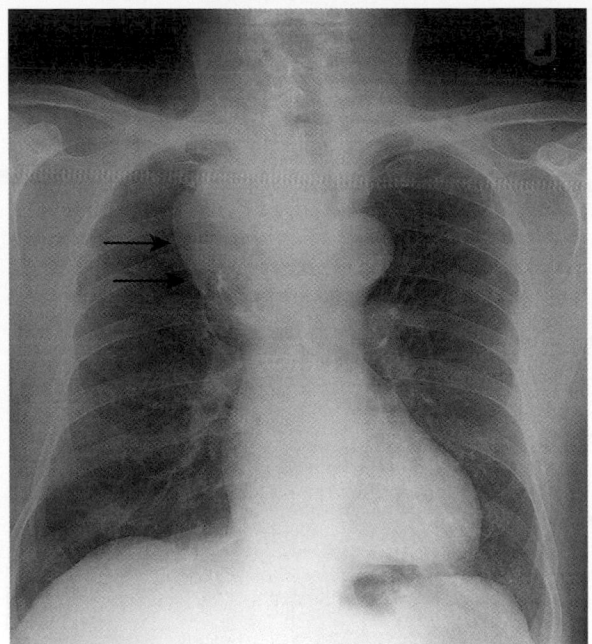

Fig. 19.48 Large mass (intrathoracic goitre—arrows) extending from right upper mediastinum.

may be obtained under ultrasound guidance through the endoscope.

Surgical exploration

If enlarged lymph nodes are suspected in the anterior mediastinum, tissue from these nodes can be removed for histological examination by mediastinoscopy. However, surgical exploration of the chest with removal of part or all of the tumour is often required to obtain a histological diagnosis.

Management

Benign mediastinal tumours should be removed surgically because most produce symptoms sooner or later. Some of them, particularly cysts, may become infected, while others, especially neural tumours, have the potential to undergo malignant transformation. The operative mortality is low provided there is not a relative contraindication to surgical treatment, such as coexisting cardiovascular disease, COPD or extreme age.

INTERSTITIAL AND INFILTRATIVE PULMONARY DISEASES

DIFFUSE PARENCHYMAL LUNG DISEASE

Overview

The diffuse parenchymal lung diseases (DPLDs) are a heterogeneous group of conditions associated with diffuse thickening of the alveolar walls with inflammatory cells and exudates (e.g. the acute respiratory distress syndrome—ARDS), granulomas (e.g. sarcoidosis), alveolar haemor-

rhage (e.g. Goodpasture's syndrome, p. 503), and/or fibrosis (e.g. fibrosing alveolitis). Lung disease may occur in isolation, or as part of a systemic connective tissue disorder — for example, in rheumatoid arthritis and systemic lupus erythematosus. The DPLDs are rare and poorly understood. However, although the presentation and natural history differ, they are frequently considered collectively as they share similar symptoms, physical signs, radiological changes and disturbances of pulmonary function. The classification of DPLD is shown in Figure 19.49.

Diagnosis of interstitial lung disease: a general approach

Establishing a diagnosis is important because:

- Firstly, there are prognostic implications; for example, sarcoidosis is frequently self-limiting, whereas idiopathic pulmonary fibrosis (IPF) is most often fatal.
- Secondly, establishing a specific diagnosis will avoid inappropriate treatment; for example, the powerful immunosuppressive regimens used for some cases of IPF would be undesirable if the underlying condition was asbestosis or hypersensitivity pneumonitis.
- Thirdly, some DPLDs can be expected to respond better than others to treatment, e.g. a good symptomatic response to corticosteroids could be predicted in sarcoidosis, whereas the prognosis would need to be more guarded in IPF.
- Finally, a lung biopsy taken when the patient is already established on empirical immunosuppressive therapy is not only associated with a higher morbidity and mortality, but the interpretation of the tissue obtained is more difficult. It is desirable, therefore, to be confident about the diagnosis before starting any therapy.

Diagnosis often presents a considerable clinical challenge (Box 19.83), necessitating meticulous attention to the history and physical signs and a cooperative approach from teams of clinicians, radiologists and pathologists.

History

The duration of disease may sometimes be difficult to ascertain. Gradually progressive shortness of breath on exertion may be the only symptom, and hence the patient may not present clinically until there is extensive lung pathology. History-taking should include a thorough and

19.83 CONDITIONS WHICH MIMIC INTERSTITIAL LUNG DISEASES	
Infection	
• Viral pneumonia	• TB
• *Pneumocystis jirovecii*	• Parasites, e.g. filariasis
• *Mycoplasma pneumoniae*	• Fungal infection
Malignancy	
• Leukaemia and lymphoma	• Multiple metastases
• Lymphatic carcinomatosis	• Bronchoalveolar carcinoma
Pulmonary oedema	
Aspiration pneumonitis	

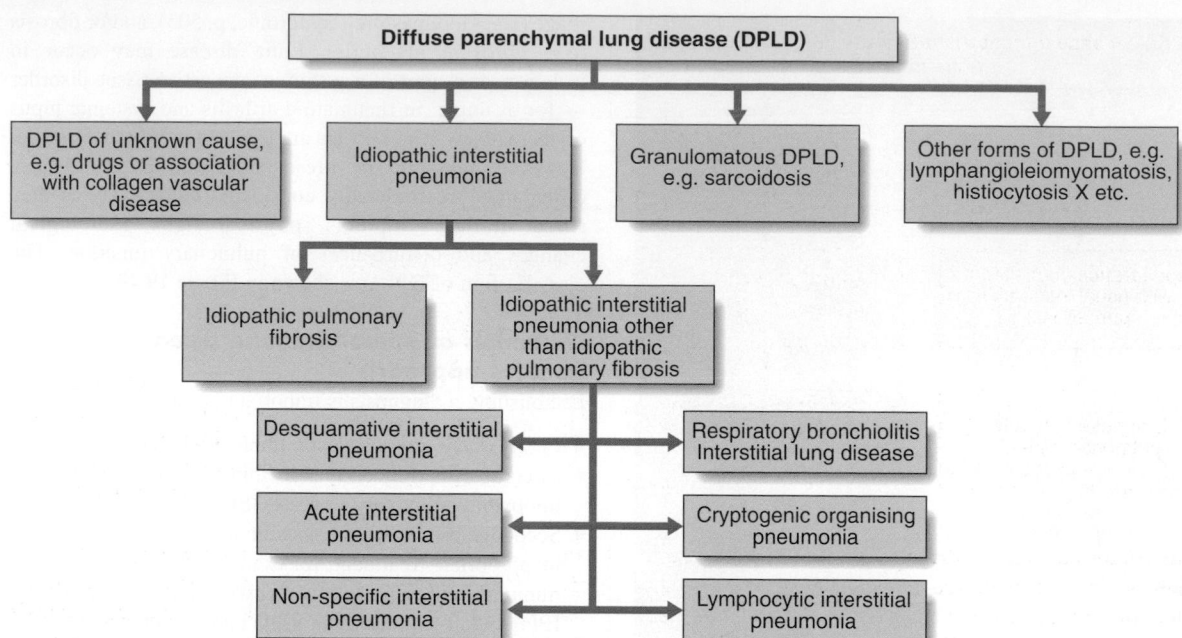

Fig. 19.49 **Classification of diffuse parenchymal lung disease.**

comprehensive search for exposure to organic and inorganic dusts. A 'lifetime' occupational history is essential and should include hobbies that may involve similar exposures. Contact with birds at home or in the working environment is the cause of the most common form of hypersensitivity pneumonitis (HP). The smoking status should be recorded and a drug history that includes over-the-counter prescriptions should be obtained. A history of rashes, joint pains or renal disease may suggest an underlying connective tissue disorder or vasculitis (Ch. 25). The presence of any comorbid disease should be ascertained such as collagen vascular disease, immunodeficiency, HIV or malignancy. In exceptional cases there is a family history of DPLD.

Physical signs

In many cases, especially in early disease, there are few, if any, physical signs. In advanced disease, tachypnoea and cyanosis may be evident at rest and there may be signs of pulmonary hypertension and right heart failure (p. 542). Finger clubbing may be prominent, particularly in IPF or asbestosis. There may be restriction of lung expansion and showers of end-inspiratory crackles posteriorly and laterally. Extrapulmonary signs, including lymphadenopathy or uveitis, may be present in sarcoidosis (Box 19.85) and arthropathies or rashes may occur when a DPLD is a manifestation of a connective tissue disorder (p. 722).

Investigations

Some blood tests may be useful in indicating systemic disease or providing crude indices of disease activity (Box 19.84). Pulmonary function tests typically show a restrictive pattern with diminished lung volumes and a reduced gas transfer, although an elevated gas transfer may be seen in

19.84 INVESTIGATIONS IN DPLD

Laboratory investigations

- Full blood count—lymphopenia in sarcoid; eosinophilia in pulmonary eosinophilias and drug reactions; neutrophilia in hypersensitivity pneumonitis
- Ca^{2+}—may be elevated in sarcoid
- Lactate dehydrogenase (LDH)—may provide non-specific indicator of disease activity in DPLD
- Serum ACE—non-specific indicator of disease activity in sarcoid
- ESR and CRP may be non-specifically raised
- Autoimmune screen and rheumatoid factor may suggest collagen vascular disease

Radiology

- Chest X-ray
- High-resolution CT scan
- Gallium scanning

Pulmonary function

- Spirometry, lung volumes, gas transfer, exercise tests

Bronchoscopy

- Bronchoalveolar lavage—infection, differential cell counts
- Bronchial biopsy may be useful in sarcoid

Lung biopsy (in selected cases)

- Transbronchial biopsy useful in sarcoid and differential of malignancy or infection
- Video-assisted thoracoscopy (VATS)

Others

- Liver biopsy
- Urinary calcium excretion may be useful in sarcoid

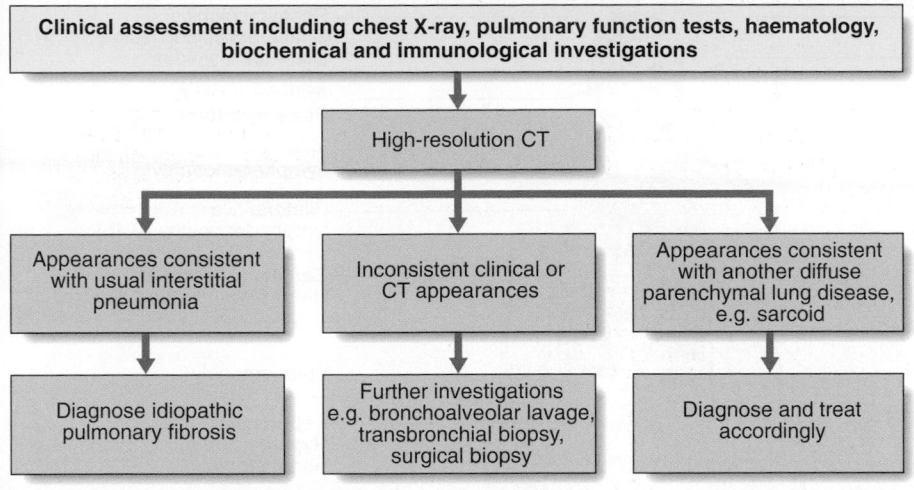

Fig. 19.50 Algorithm for the investigation of patients with interstitial lung disease following initial clinical and chest X-ray examination.

cases of alveolar haemorrhage. The chest X-ray typically shows a fine reticular, reticulonodular or even nodular pattern of infiltration at the bases and periphery with cystic areas and honeycombing in advanced disease. However, plain radiography is insensitive and may not appear abnormal until disease is advanced. HRCT is more sensitive and specific and has become extremely valuable in detecting early interstitial lung disease, assessing the extent and type of involvement and guiding further investigations and management (Fig. 19.50).

Bronchoscopy is useful in certain circumstances. Increased numbers of lymphocytes in the bronchoalveolar lavage (BAL) may suggest either sarcoid or hypersensitivity pneumonitis, whereas a neutrophilia is more suggestive of IPF. Analysis of BAL may suggest important differential diagnoses such as infection or malignancy, and in rare instances may be diagnostic when iron-laden macrophages are seen in pulmonary haemosiderosis or copious lipo-proteinaceous material is retrieved in pulmonary alveolar proteinosis (Box 19.97, p. 725). Transbronchial biopsies may establish the diagnosis in sarcoidosis and in some conditions which mimic ILDs, such as lymphatic carcinomatosis and certain infections. However, it is less specific in heterogeneous disorders such as IPF where video-assisted thoracoscopy (VATS), or a limited thoracotomy, may be required to obtain a more representative sample.

SARCOIDOSIS

Sarcoidosis is a multisystem granulomatous disorder. The condition is more commonly seen in colder parts of Northern Europe where the incidence is approximately 40/10 000. In North America it tends to be more common, and more aggressive, in Afro-Caribbean populations. The aetiology remains uncertain. Links with atypical mycobacteria and viruses remain speculative; there is some evidence of familial clustering and genetic factors are undoubtedly important. Sarcoidosis appears less commonly in smokers.

Pathology
The mediastinal and superficial lymph glands, lungs, liver, spleen, skin, eyes, parotid glands and phalangeal bones

are most frequently affected, but all tissues may be involved (Figs 19.51 and 19.52). The characteristic histological feature is a non-caseating epithelioid granuloma; fibrosis is seen in up to 20% of cases of pulmonary sarcoidosis. Disturbances in calcium metabolism reflect increased formation of calcitrol (1,25-dihydroxyvitamin D_3) by alveolar macrophages and may lead to hypercalciuria, hypercalcaemia and, rarely, nephrocalcinosis.

Clinical features
Sarcoidosis is considered under the diagnostic term of DPLD as over 90% of cases affect the lungs, but the presentation can be quite variable (Box 19.85). Löfgren's syndrome—an acute illness characterised by erythema nodosum, peripheral arthropathy, uveitis, bilateral hilar lymphadenopathy (BHL), lethargy and occasionally fever— is often seen in young women. Alternatively, BHL may be detected in an otherwise asymptomatic individual undergoing a chest X-ray for other purposes. Pulmonary disease may also present in a more insidious manner with cough, exertional breathlessness and radiographic infiltrates; chest auscultation is often surprisingly unremarkable. Fibrosis occurs in some patients and may cause a silent loss of lung function (Box 19.86). Pleural disease is uncommon and finger clubbing is not a feature. Complications such as bronchiectasis, aspergilloma, pneumothorax, pulmonary hypertension and cor pulmonale have been reported but are fortunately rare. The overall mortality is low (1–5%).

19.85 PRESENTATION OF SARCOIDOSIS

- Asymptomatic—abnormal routine chest X-ray (c. 30%) or abnormal liver function tests
- Respiratory and constitutional symptoms (20–30%)
- Erythema nodosum and arthralgia (20–30%)
- Ocular symptoms (5–10%)
- Skin sarcoid (including lupus pernio) (5%)
- Superficial lymphadenopathy (5%)
- Other (1%), e.g. hypercalcaemia, diabetes insipidus, cranial nerve palsies, cardiac arrhythmias, nephrocalcinosis

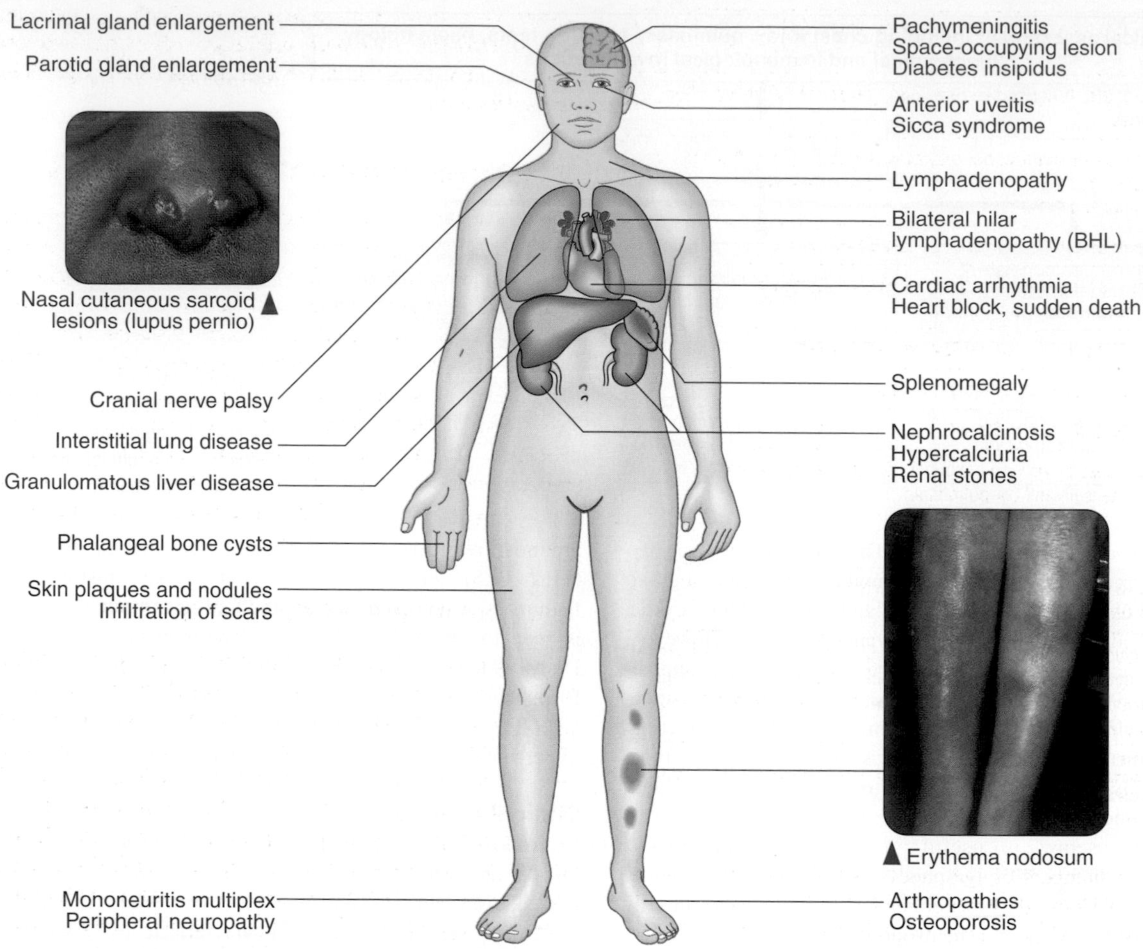

Lacrimal gland enlargement

Parotid gland enlargement

Nasal cutaneous sarcoid ▲
lesions (lupus pernio)

Cranial nerve palsy

Interstitial lung disease

Granulomatous liver disease

Phalangeal bone cysts

Skin plaques and nodules
Infiltration of scars

Mononeuritis multiplex
Peripheral neuropathy

Pachymeningitis
Space-occupying lesion
Diabetes insipidus

Anterior uveitis
Sicca syndrome

Lymphadenopathy

Bilateral hilar
lymphadenopathy (BHL)

Cardiac arrhythmia
Heart block, sudden death

Splenomegaly

Nephrocalcinosis
Hypercalciuria
Renal stones

▲ Erythema nodosum

Arthropathies
Osteoporosis

Fig. 19.51 **The range of possible systemic involvement in sarcoidosis.**

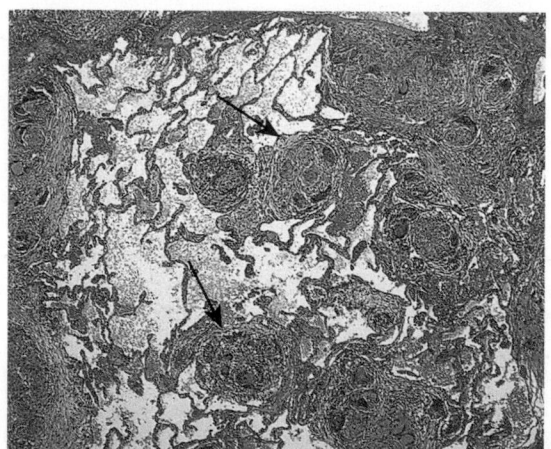

Fig. 19.52 **Histology of sarcoidosis in the lung, showing non-caseating granulomas (arrows).**

Investigations

Lymphopenia is characteristic and liver function tests may be mildly deranged. The serum calcium may be elevated and must be checked. Serum angiotensin-converting enzyme (ACE) may provide a non-specific marker of disease activity and can assist in monitoring the clinical course. Chest radiography has been used to stage sarcoid (Box 19.86). In patients with pulmonary infiltrates pulmonary function may show a restrictive defect accompanied by impaired gas exchange. Exercise tests may reveal oxygen desaturation. Bronchoscopy may demonstrate a 'cobblestone' appearance of the mucosa, and bronchial and transbronchial biopsy usually show non-caseating granulomas. The broncho-alveolar lavage fluid typically contains an increased CD4:CD8 T-cell ratio. Characteristic HRCT appearances include reticulonodular opacities that follow a perilymphatic distribution centred on bronchovascular bundles and the subpleural areas.

The occurrence of erythema nodosum in women in the 2nd–3rd decade with BHL on chest X-ray is often sufficient for a confident diagnosis without recourse to a tissue biopsy. However, when there is real doubt, the diagnosis should be confirmed by histological examination of the involved organ.

Management

The majority of patients enjoy spontaneous remission and, if there is no evidence of organ damage, it is appropriate to withhold therapy for 4–6 months. Patients who present with acute illness and erythema nodosum should receive NSAIDs and on occasion a short course of corticosteroids. Systemic

19.86 CHEST X-RAY CHANGES IN SARCOIDOSIS

Stage I: BHL (usually symmetrical); paratracheal nodes often enlarged

- Often asymptomatic, but may be associated with erythema nodosum and arthralgia. The majority of cases resolve spontaneously within 1 year

Stage II: BHL and parenchymal infiltrates

- Patients may present with breathlessness or cough. The majority of cases resolve spontaneously

Stage III: parenchymal infiltrates without BHL

- Disease less likely to resolve spontaneously

Stage IV: pulmonary fibrosis

- Can cause progression to ventilatory failure, pulmonary hypertension and cor pulmonale

---

19.87 SYSTEMIC CORTICOSTEROIDS IN PULMONARY SARCOIDOSIS

EBM

'Oral glucocorticoids administered for 6–24 months improve chest X-ray appearances and symptoms but there is little evidence of an improvement in lung function and there are no data from follow-up beyond 2 years.'

- Gibson GJ, et al. Thorax 1996; 51:238–247.
- Paramathayan NS, et al. (Cochrane Review). Cochrane Library, issue 2, 2005. Oxford: Update Software.

---

corticosteroids are also indicated in the presence of hypercalcaemia, pulmonary impairment, and renal impairment (Box 19.87). Topical steroids may be useful in uveitis but inhaled corticosteroids have no proven benefit in lung disease. Features suggesting a less favourable outlook include: age > 40, Afro-Caribbean ethnic origin, persistent symptoms for more than 6 months, the involvement of more than three organs, lupus pernio and a stage III/IV chest X-ray. In patients with severe disease both methotrexate and azathioprine have been used successfully and selected patients may be referred for consideration of single lung transplantation.

IDIOPATHIC INTERSTITIAL PNEUMONIAS

The idiopathic interstitial pneumonias (IIPs) are characterised by varying patterns of inflammation and fibrosis in the lung parenchyma, and comprise a number of clinico-pathological entities that are sufficiently different from one another to be considered as separate diseases. The most important of these is idiopathic pulmonary fibrosis (IPF). The other diseases include desquamative interstitial pneumonia (DIP), acute interstitial pneumonia (AIP), non-specific interstitial pneumonia (NSIP), respiratory bronchiolitis–interstitial lung disease (RB-ILD), cryptogenic organising pneumonia (COP) and lymphocytic interstitial pneumonia (LIP) (Box 19.88).

IDIOPATHIC PULMONARY FIBROSIS

This term has replaced cryptogenic fibrosing alveolitis and refers to a specific form of DPLD characterised by pathological (or radiological) evidence of usual interstitial pneumonia (UIP). The aetiology remains unknown: speculation has included exposure to infectious agents such as Epstein–Barr virus, occupational dusts such as metal or wood dusts, prior use of antidepressants, and a possible role for chronic gastro-oesophageal reflux. Familial cases are rare but genetic factors that control the inflammatory and fibrotic response are likely to be important. The disease displays a strong association with cigarette smoking.

Clinical features

IPF is generally a disease of the elderly, being uncommon before the age of 50 years. It usually presents with

---

19.88 DIFFERENTIAL DIAGNOSES OF THE INTERSTITIAL PNEUMONIAS

Clinical diagnosis	Notes
Usual interstitial pneumonia	See text
Non-specific interstitial pneumonia (NSIP)	Median age 40–50 years. No association with smoking. Prognosis variable. Hunt for collagen vascular disease, hypersensitivity pneumonitis, drug-induced pneumonitis, infection or HIV
Respiratory bronchiolitis–interstitial lung disease	More common in men and smokers. Usually presents in the forties or fifties. Smoking cessation may lead to improvement. Natural history remains unclear
Acute interstitial pneumonia	Often preceded by viral URTI. Severe exertional dyspnoea, widespread pneumonic consolidation and diffuse alveolar damage (DAD) on biopsy. Prognosis is often poor
Desquamative interstitial pneumonia (DIP)	More common in men and smokers. Presents in forties or fifties. Insidious onset of dyspnoea. Clubbing in 50%. Biopsy shows increased macrophages in the alveolar space, septal thickening and type II pneumocyte hyperplasia. Prognosis is generally good
Cryptogenic organising pneumonia (may be referred to bronchiolitis obliterans organising pneumonia—BOOP)	Presents as clinical and radiological pneumonia. Systemic features and markedly raised ESR common. Finger clubbing is characteristically absent. Biopsy shows a florid proliferation of immature collagen (Masson bodies) and fibrous tissue. Response to corticosteroids is classically dramatic
Lymphocytic interstitial pneumonia (LIP)	More common in women, slow onset over years. Investigate for associations of collagen vascular disease or HIV. Unclear whether corticosteroids helpful or not

insidiously progressive disabling breathlessness and a non-productive cough. Constitutional symptoms are unusual but arthralgia may be reported. Finger clubbing may be observed in 25–50% of cases and late inspiratory crackles likened to the unzipping of Velcro are classically heard at the lung bases. In advanced cases central cyanosis is detectable and patients may develop features of right heart failure.

Investigations

Blood tests are of little value. Rheumatoid factor and antinuclear factor can be detected in 30–50% of patients. The erythrocyte sedimentation rate (ESR) and lactate dehydrogenase (LDH) are elevated in most cases. Pulmonary function tests show a restrictive defect with reduced lung volumes and gas transfer. However, lung volumes may be preserved in patients with concomitant emphysema. Dynamic tests are useful to demonstrate arterial hypoxaemia on exercise in patients with early disease, but as IPF advances, arterial hypoxaemia and hypocapnia are present at rest. Virtually all patients have an abnormal chest X-ray at presentation with lower zone bi-basal reticular and reticulonodular opacities. A 'honeycomb' appearance may be seen in advanced disease but is non-specific (Box 19.97, p. 725). HRCT may be diagnostic, demonstrating a patchy, predominantly peripheral, subpleural and basal reticular pattern with subpleural cysts (honeycombing) and/or traction bronchiectasis (Fig. 19.53), and is particularly useful in early disease when chest X-ray changes may be indistinct. Patients with typical clinical features and HRCT appearances consistent with UIP do not require lung biopsy, particularly if other known causes of interstitial lung disease have been excluded. However, BAL and transbronchial biopsy may be used to exclude alternative diagnoses.

Management

A median survival of 3 years is typical and survival beyond 5 years unusual. However, the rate of disease progression varies considerably from death within a few months to survival with minimal symptoms for many years. The pattern of serial lung function may be helpful in predicting survival; relative preservation of lung function is a predictor of longer survival and desaturation on exercise heralds a poor prognosis. High numbers of fibroblastic foci on biopsy have been associated with a poor outcome.

Treatment options remain limited. Prednisolone therapy (0.5 mg/kg) combined with azathioprine (2–3 mg/kg) is currently recommended to patients who are highly symptomatic or have rapidly progressive disease, have a predominantly 'ground-glass' appearance on CT or have a sustained fall of > 15% in their FVC or gas transfer over a 3–6-month period. However, response rates are notoriously poor and side-effects guaranteed. Should objective evidence of improvement be demonstrated, the prednisolone dose may be gradually reduced to a maintenance dose of 10–12.5 mg daily. New therapies are urgently required and the potential of novel therapies such as IFN-γ or acetylcysteine is being explored. Lung transplantation (p. 670) should be considered in young patients with advanced disease. Oxygen may be provided for palliation of breathlessness but opiates may be required for relief of severe dyspnoea.

LUNG DISEASES DUE TO ORGANIC DUSTS

A wide range of organic agents may cause respiratory disorders (Box 19.89). Disease results from a local immune response to animal proteins (e.g. bird fancier's lung) or fungal antigens in mouldy vegetable matter. The most common presentation has been termed hypersensitivity pneumonitis.

HYPERSENSITIVITY PNEUMONITIS (HP)

Hypersensitivity pneumonitis (also called extrinsic allergic alveolitis) results from the inhalation of certain types of organic dust which give rise to a diffuse immune complex

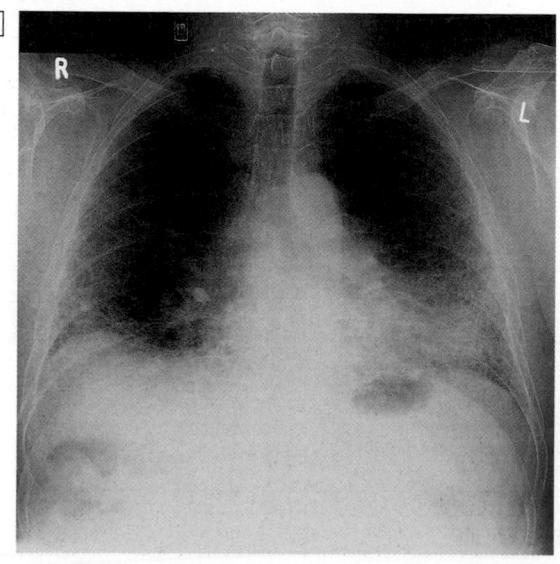

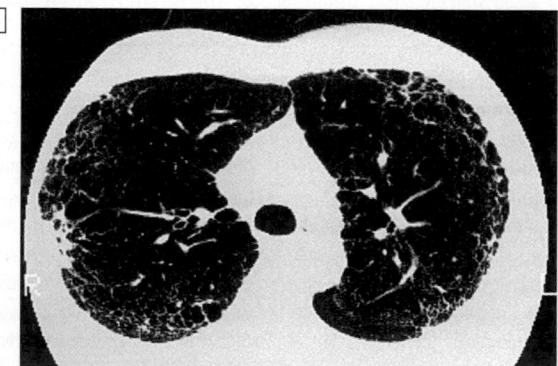

Fig. 19.53 Idiopathic pulmonary fibrosis. [A] Chest X-ray showing bilateral, predominantly lower zone and peripheral coarse reticulonodular shadowing and small lungs. [B] The CT scan shows honeycombing and scarring which is most marked peripherally.

19.89 SOME EXAMPLES OF LUNG DISEASES CAUSED BY ORGANIC DUSTS

Disorder	Source	Antigen/agent
Farmer's lung*	Mouldy hay, straw, grain	*Micropolyspora faeni* *Aspergillus fumigatus*
Bird fancier's lung*	Avian excreta, proteins and feathers	Avian serum proteins
Malt worker's lung*	Mouldy maltings	*Aspergillus clavatus*
Byssinosis	Textile industries	Cotton, flax, hemp dust
Inhalation ('humidifier') fever	Contamination of air conditioning	Thermophilic actinomycetes
Cheese worker's lung*	Mouldy cheese	*Aspergillus clavatus* *Penicillium casei*
Maple bark stripper's lung*	Bark from stored maple	*Cryptostroma corticale*

* Denotes lung disease presenting as hypersensitivity pneumonitis.

19

reaction in the walls of the alveoli and bronchioles. Some examples are provided in Box 19.89. In the UK, 50% of reported cases of HP occur in farm workers; bird fanciers represent another important group.

Pathogenesis and pathology

The pathology of hypersensitivity pneumonitis suggests that both type III and type IV immunological mechanisms may be involved (p. 80). Precipitating IgG antibodies may be detected in the serum and a type III Arthus reaction is believed to occur in the lung where the precipitation of immune complexes results in activation of complement and an inflammatory response in the alveolar walls characterised by the influx of mononuclear cells and foamy histiocytes. The presence of poorly formed non-caseating granulomas in the alveolar walls provides some evidence that type IV responses are also important. Chronic forms of the disease may be accompanied by a fibrotic response in the lung. For reasons that remain uncertain, there is a lower incidence of hypersensitivity pneumonitis in smokers compared to non-smokers.

Clinical features

The acute form of the disease should be suspected when anyone who is regularly or intermittently exposed to organic dust complains, within a few hours of re-exposure to the same dust, of influenza-like symptoms. These include headache, myalgia, malaise, pyrexia, dry cough and breathlessness. Chest auscultation reveals widespread end-inspiratory crackles and squeaks. In cases attributable to chronic low-level exposure (as may be the case with an indoor pet bird) the onset is often more insidious with progressive breathlessness, and established fibrosis may be present by the time the disease is recognised. If unchecked, the disease may progress to cause severe respiratory disability, hypoxaemia, pulmonary hypertension, cor pulmonale and eventually death.

Investigations

The chest X-ray shows diffuse micronodular shadowing that is classically more pronounced in the upper zones. HRCT in patients with acute disease shows bilateral areas of consolidation superimposed on small centrilobar nodular opacities and air-trapping on expiration. In more chronic disease, features of fibrosis with linear opacities and architectural distortion predominate. Pulmonary function tests show a restrictive ventilatory defect with reduced lung volumes and impaired gas transfer. The PaO_2 is reduced and in the presence of over-ventilation the $PaCO_2$ is often below normal.

The diagnosis of HP is usually based on the characteristic clinical and radiological features, together with the identification of a potential source of antigen at the patient's home or place of work (Box 19.90). Reduction in the carbon monoxide transfer factor is the most sensitive functional abnormality. The diagnosis may be supported by a positive precipitin test or by more sensitive serological tests based on the enzyme-linked immunosorbent assay (ELISA) technique. However, it is also important to recognise that the great majority of farmers with positive precipitins do not have farmer's lung, and up to 15% of pigeon breeders may have positive serum precipitins yet remain healthy. Where the diagnosis is suspected but the cause is not readily apparent, it may be helpful to visit the patient's home or workplace. Occasionally, such as when a new agent is suspected, it may be necessary to prove the diagnosis by a provocation test; if positive, inhalation of the relevant antigen is followed after 3–6 hours by pyrexia and a reduction in VC and gas transfer factor. Bronchoalveolar lavage fluid usually shows an increase in the number of CD8+ T lymphocytes. Open lung biopsy may be necessary to establish a diagnosis.

19.90 PREDICTIVE FACTORS IN THE IDENTIFICATION OF HYPERSENSITIVITY PNEUMONITIS

- Exposure to a known offending antigen
- Positive precipitating antibodies to offending antigen
- Recurrent episodes of symptoms
- Inspiratory crackles on examination
- Symptoms occurring 4–8 hours after exposure
- Weight loss

19

Management

Whenever possible, the patient should cease exposure to the inciting agent. However, in some cases this may be difficult to achieve, either because of implications for livelihood (e.g. farmers) or addiction to hobbies (e.g. pigeon breeders). Dust masks with appropriate filters may minimise exposure and may be combined with methods of reducing levels of antigen (e.g. drying hay before storage). In acute cases prednisolone should be given for 3–4 weeks, starting with an oral dose of 40 mg per day. Severely hypoxaemic patients may require high-concentration oxygen therapy initially. Most patients recover completely, but the development of interstitial fibrosis causes permanent disability when there has been prolonged exposure to antigen.

BYSSINOSIS

Not all inhaled organic dusts cause interstitial infiltration. In byssinosis the initial lesion caused by cotton dust inhalation is acute bronchiolitis associated with symptoms and signs of generalised airflow obstruction, more in keeping with asthma. Initially, symptoms tend to recur after the weekend break ('Monday fever') but eventually become continuous. There is usually no radiological abnormality. Recovery usually follows removal from the dust hazard. Smokers have a greater incidence of byssinosis than non-smokers.

INHALATION ('HUMIDIFIER') FEVER

Inhalation fever is characterised by self-limiting fever and breathlessness following exposure to organism-contaminated water from humidifiers or air-conditioning systems. An identical syndrome can also develop after disturbing an accumulation of mouldy hay, compost or mulch.

LUNG DISEASES DUE TO INORGANIC DUSTS

In certain occupations, the inhalation of inorganic dusts, fumes or other noxious substances may give rise to specific

---

19.91 INTERSTITIAL LUNG DISEASE IN OLD AGE

- **Idiopathic pulmonary fibrosis**: the most common interstitial lung disease, with a worse prognosis.
- **Chronic aspiration pneumonitis**: must always be considered in elderly patients presenting with bilateral basal shadowing on a chest X-ray.
- **Wegener's granulomatosis**: a rare condition but more common in old age. Renal involvement is more common at presentation and upper respiratory problems are fewer.
- **Asbestosis**: symptoms may only appear in old age because of the prolonged latent period between exposure and disease.
- **Drug-induced interstitial lung disease**: more common, presumably because of the increased chance of exposure to multiple drugs.
- **Rarer interstitial disease**: sarcoidosis, idiopathic pulmonary haemosiderosis, alveolar proteinosis and eosinophilic pneumonia rarely present.
- **Increased dyspnoea**: coexistent muscle weakness, chest wall deformity (e.g. thoracic kyphosis) and deconditioning may all exacerbate dyspnoea associated with interstitial lung disease.
- **Open lung biopsy**: often inappropriate in the very frail. A diagnosis therefore frequently depends on clinical and HRCT findings alone.

19.92 SOME LUNG DISEASES CAUSED BY INORGANIC GASES AND FUMES

Cause	Occupation	Disease
Irritant gases (chlorine, ammonia, phosgene, nitrogen dioxide)	Various (industrial accidents)	Acute lung injury ARDS
Cadmium	Welding and electroplating	COPD
Isocyanates (e.g. epoxy resins, paints)	Plastic, paints; manufacture of epoxy resins and adhesives	Bronchial asthma Eosinophilic pneumonia

---

19.93 SOME LUNG DISEASES CAUSED BY EXPOSURE TO INORGANIC DUSTS

Cause	Occupation	Description	Characteristic pathological features
Coal dust **Silica**	Coal mining Mining, quarrying, stone dressing, metal grinding, pottery, boiler scaling	Coal worker's pneumoconiosis Silicosis	Focal and interstitial fibrosis, centrilobular emphysema, progressive massive fibrosis
Asbestos	Demolition, ship breaking, manufacture of fireproof insulating materials and brake-pads, pipe and boiler lagging	Asbestos-related disease	Interstitial fibrosis, pleural disease, carcinoma of larynx and bronchus
Iron oxide	Arc welding	Siderosis	Mineral deposition only
Tin oxide	Tin mining	Stannosis	Tin-laden macrophages
Beryllium	Aircraft, atomic energy and electronics industries	Berylliosis	Granulomas, interstitial fibrosis

pathological changes in the lungs. Industrial inorganic gases and fumes can cause acute respiratory diseases including pulmonary oedema and asthma (Box 19.92). Generally, prolonged exposure to inorganic dusts (Box 19.93) leads to diffuse pulmonary fibrosis (the pneumoconioses), although berylliosis causes an interstitial granulomatous disease similar to sarcoidosis. The dusts themselves cause little direct damage to the lung parenchyma and the pathological result depends largely on the inflammatory and fibrotic responses to the particular dust. The fibrogenic properties of mineral dusts vary, silica being markedly fibrogenic whereas iron and tin are almost inert. The most important types of pneumoconiosis are coal worker's pneumoconiosis, silicosis and asbestosis. It must also be emphasised that in many types of pneumoconiosis a long period of dust exposure is required before radiological changes appear, and these may precede clinical symptoms. A detailed occupational history is essential not only to avoid missing a case of occupational lung disease but also to allow appropriate advice to be given to the patient, and if relevant, the employer and legal advisors. Many countries encourage the registration of cases of occupational lung disease.

COAL WORKER'S PNEUMOCONIOSIS

Prolonged inhalation of coal dust overwhelms the alveolar macrophages, which aggregate to form macules in or near the centre of the secondary pulmonary lobule. A fibrotic reaction ensues, resulting in the appearance of scattered discrete fibrotic lesions that constitute simple coal worker's pneumoconiosis (SCWP). This can be divided into three categories on the basis of the size and extent of nodularity on the chest X-ray. However, it does not cause pulmonary function abnormalities nor does it give rise to symptoms or progress following cessation of exposure.

Complicated pneumoconiosis invariably develops against a background of simple pneumoconiosis. In this form of the disease, large dense masses appear mainly in the upper lobes (also known as progressive massive fibrosis, PMF). Cavitation may occur, raising important differential diagnoses such as lung cancer, TB and Wegener's granuloma-

tosis (p. 1141). In contrast to SCWP, PMF is usually associated with cough, production of sputum, that may be black (melanoptysis) and breathlessness. It may progress to respiratory failure after cessation of exposure and right ventricular failure has been described.

Caplan's syndrome describes the coexistence of rheumatoid arthritis and rounded fibrotic nodules 0.5–5 cm in diameter. These are mainly in the periphery of the lung fields and show pathological features similar to a rheumatoid nodule including central necrosis, palisading histiocytes, and a peripheral rim of lymphocytes and plasma cells. This syndrome may also occur in other types of pneumoconiosis.

SILICOSIS

Silicosis results from the inhalation of crystalline or free silica, usually in the form of quartz. The clinical and radiological features are similar to those of coal worker's pneumoconiosis with multiple well-circumscribed 3–5 mm nodular opacities predominantly in the mid- and upper zones. As the disease progresses some of these may coalesce, particularly in the upper lobes. Enlargement of the hilar glands with an 'egg-shell' pattern of calcification is said to be characteristic but is uncommon and non-specific. Patients may be at increased risk of TB—silicotuberculosis.

Silica is highly fibrogenic and the disease is usually progressive (even when exposure ceases). The patient should, therefore, be removed from the offending environment as soon as possible.

Intense exposure to very fine crystalline silica dust can cause a more acute disease similar to alveolar proteinosis (Box 19.97, p. 725) with over-production of surfactant by type II alveolar pneumocytes.

ASBESTOSIS

The main types of the fibrous mineral asbestos are chrysotile (white asbestos), which accounts for 90% of the world's production, crocidolite (blue asbestos) and amosite

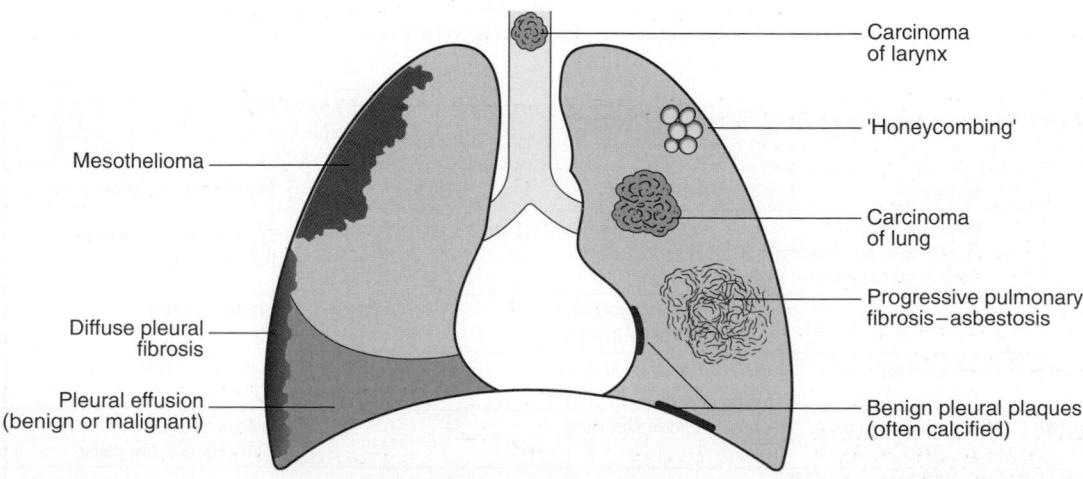

Fig. 19.54 Asbestosis: the range of possible effects on the respiratory tract.

(brown asbestos). Exposure occurs in a variety of occupations (Box 19.93) and is a recognised risk factor for several respiratory diseases (Fig. 19.54), including carcinoma of the lung and larynx. Asbestos-related pleural disease is described on page 735. The law in many countries now enforces improvements in standards of industrial hygiene and provides compensation for asbestos-related disease.

Asbestosis is a diffuse interstitial fibrosis of the lungs that may or may not be associated with fibrosis of the parietal or visceral layer of the pleura. The condition seldom develops less than 20 years after the start of exposure and usually follows substantial and prolonged asbestos exposure over many years. The risk increases with the amount inhaled.

Asbestos fibres are cleared by mucociliary clearance, by pulmonary macrophages and by dissolution. Incomplete phagocytosis of fibres by macrophages triggers a fibrotic process that is typically most marked in the lower lobes. Patients usually present with exertional breathlessness and fine, late inspiratory crackles over the lower zones. Digital clubbing (reported in 40% of patients) is an adverse prognostic feature. The chest X-ray shows bi-basal reticular nodular shadowing and asbestos-related pleural disease is usually present. HRCT scanning is more sensitive than plain radiography and typically shows basal, subpleural, curvilinear opacities, band-like opacities and occasionally 'honeycombing'. Pulmonary function tests typically show a restrictive defect with decreased lung volumes and reduced gas transfer factor.

The diagnosis is usually established by a history of substantial asbestos exposure with the clinical, radiological and pulmonary function abnormalities described above. Asbestos bodies may be identified in sputum or BAL and confirm asbestos exposure. Lung biopsy is rarely necessary but may be required to exclude other causes of interstitial lung disease. If a history of exposure is uncertain, asbestos fibre counts may be performed on lung biopsy material.

Management

No specific treatment is available. Asbestosis usually progresses very slowly. In advanced cases respiratory failure and cor pulmonale may develop and should be treated appropriately. About 40% of patients (who usually smoke) develop carcinoma of the lung and 10% may develop mesothelioma. Patients should be provided with appropriate legal advice if asbestos exposure occurred as a result of negligent exposure. Asbestos-related deaths in the UK should be reported to the Procurator Fiscal or Coroner.

LUNG DISEASES DUE TO SYSTEMIC INFLAMMATORY DISEASE

THE ACUTE RESPIRATORY DISTRESS SYNDROME

See page 187.

RESPIRATORY INVOLVEMENT IN CONNECTIVE TISSUE DISORDERS

Fibrosing alveolitis is a recognised complication of most connective tissue diseases. The clinical features are usually indistinguishable from IPF (p. 717) and the response to immunosuppressive drugs is similarly unpredictable. Connective tissue disorders may also cause disease of the pleura, diaphragm and chest wall muscles (Box 19.94 and Ch. 25). Pulmonary hypertension and cor pulmonale may result from advanced pulmonary fibrosis associated with connective tissue disorders and is particularly common in patients with systemic sclerosis.

Indirect associations between connective tissue disorders and respiratory complications include those due to disease in other organs, e.g. thrombocytopenia causing haemoptysis; pulmonary toxic effects of drugs used to treat the connective tissue disorder (e.g. gold and methotrexate); and secondary infection due to the disease itself, neutropenia or immunosuppressive drug regimens.

Rheumatoid disease

Pulmonary fibrosis is the most common pulmonary manifestation (rheumatoid lung). The clinical features, investigations, treatment and prognosis are similar to those of IPF, although a rare variant of localised upper lobe fibrosis and cavitation has been described.

Pleural effusion is common, especially in men with seropositive disease. Effusions are usually small and unilateral but can be large and bilateral. Most resolve spontaneously. Biochemical testing shows an exudative effusion (Box 19.14, p. 665) with markedly reduced glucose

19.94 RESPIRATORY COMPLICATIONS OF CONNECTIVE TISSUE DISORDERS				
Disorder	**Airways**	**Parenchyma**	**Pleura**	**Diaphragm and chest wall**
Rheumatoid arthritis	Bronchitis, obliterative bronchiolitis, bronchiectasis, crico-arytenoid arthritis, stridor	Fibrosing alveolitis, nodules, upper lobe fibrosis, infections	Pleurisy, effusion, pneumothorax	Poor healing of intercostal drain sites
Systemic lupus erythematosus	–	Fibrosing alveolitis, 'vasculitic' infarcts	Pleurisy, effusion	'Shrinking lungs'
Systemic sclerosis	Bronchiectasis	Pulmonary fibrosis, aspiration pneumonia	–	'Hidebound chest'
Dermatomyositis/ polymyositis	Bronchial carcinoma	Fibrosing alveolitis	–	Intercostal and diaphragmatic myopathy
Rheumatic fever	–	Pneumonia	Pleurisy, effusion	–

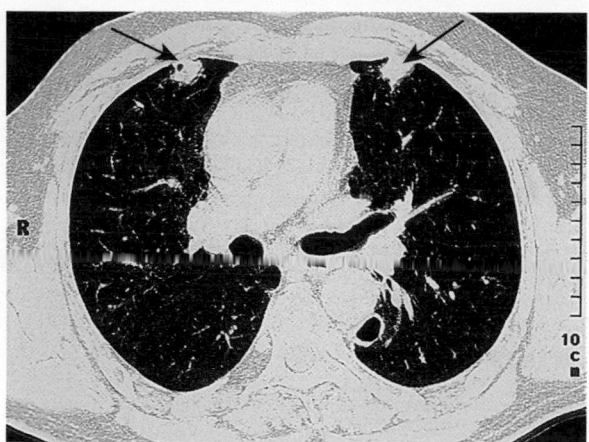

Fig. 19.55 Rheumatoid (necrobiotic) nodules. Thoracic CT just below the level of the main carina showing the typical appearance of peripheral, pleural-based nodules. The nodule in the left lower lobe shows characteristic cavitation.

19.95 PULMONARY EOSINOPHILIA

Extrinsic (cause known)

- Helminths
  e.g. *Ascaris, Toxocara, Filaria*
- Drugs
  Nitrofurantoin, para-aminosalicylic acid (PAS), sulfasalazine, imipramine, chlorpropamide, phenylbutazone
- Fungi
  e.g. *Aspergillus fumigatus* causing allergic bronchopulmonary aspergillosis (p. 703)

Intrinsic (cause unknown)

- Cryptogenic eosinophilic pneumonia
- Churg–Strauss syndrome (diagnosed on the basis of four or more of the following features: asthma, peripheral blood eosinophilia $>1.5 \times 10^9/l$ (or > 10% of a total white cell count), mononeuropathy or polyneuropathy, pulmonary infiltrates, paranasal sinus disease or eosinophilic vasculitis on biopsy of an affected site)
- Hypereosinophilic syndrome
- Polyarteritis nodosa (p. 1140; rare)

19

levels and raised LDH. Effusions that fail to resolve spontaneously may respond to a short course of oral prednisolone (30–40 mg daily) but some become chronic.

Rheumatoid pulmonary nodules are usually asymptomatic and detected incidentally on chest X-rays. They are usually multiple and subpleural in site (Fig. 19.55). Solitary nodules can mimic primary bronchial carcinoma and when multiple the differential diagnoses include pulmonary metastatic disease. Cavitation raises the possibility of TB and predisposes to pneumothorax. The combination of rheumatoid nodules and pneumoconiosis is known as Caplan's syndrome (p. 721).

Bronchitis and bronchiectasis are both more common in rheumatoid patients. Rarely, the potentially fatal condition called obliterative bronchiolitis may develop. Bacterial lower respiratory tract infection is common. Treatments given for rheumatoid arthritis may also be relevant: corticosteroid therapy predisposes to infections, methotrexate may cause pulmonary fibrosis, and anti-TNF therapy has been associated with the reactivation of TB.

Systemic lupus erythematosus

Pulmonary fibrosis is a relatively uncommon manifestation of systemic lupus erythematosus (SLE). An acute alveolitis may rarely be associated with diffuse alveolar haemorrhage. This condition is life-threatening and requires immunosuppression. Pleuropulmonary involvement is more common in lupus than in any other connective tissue disorder and may be a presenting problem, when it is sometimes attributed incorrectly to infection or pulmonary embolism. Up to two-thirds of patients have repeated episodes of pleurisy, with or without effusions. Effusions may be bilateral and may also involve the pericardium.

Some patients with SLE present with exertional dyspnoea and orthopnoea but without overt signs of pulmonary fibrosis. The chest X-ray reveals elevated diaphragms, and pulmonary function testing shows reduced lung volumes. This condition has been described as 'shrinking lungs' and has been attributed to diaphragmatic myopathy.

Antiphospholipid syndrome is associated with an increased risk of venous and pulmonary thromboembolism and these patients require life-long anticoagulation.

Systemic sclerosis

Most patients with systemic sclerosis eventually develop diffuse pulmonary fibrosis; at necropsy more than 90% have evidence of lung fibrosis. In some patients it is indolent, but when progressive, as in IPF, the median survival time is around 4 years. Pulmonary fibrosis is rare in the CREST variant of progressive systemic sclerosis but isolated pulmonary hypertension may develop.

Other pulmonary complications include recurrent aspiration pneumonias secondary to oesophageal disease. Rarely, sclerosis of the skin of the chest wall may be so extensive and cicatrising as to restrict chest wall movement—the so-called 'hidebound chest'.

PULMONARY EOSINOPHILIA AND VASCULITIDES

This term is applied to a group of disorders of different aetiology in which lesions in the lungs produce a chest X-ray abnormality associated with pulmonary eosinophilia, with or without a peripheral blood eosinophilia. There is no satisfactory classification of this disparate group, but they can be divided into two main categories (Box 19.95).

Some causes of extrinsic pulmonary eosinophilia are also given in Box 19.95. The most common disorder of this type in developed countries is allergic bronchopulmonary aspergillosis (p. 703); in tropical countries the presence of microfilariae in the pulmonary capillaries (p. 363) has to be considered.

ACUTE EOSINOPHILIC PNEUMONIA

Acute eosinophilic pneumonia is a rare febrile illness of less than 5 days' duration characterised by infiltrates on the chest

19

X-ray and hypoxic respiratory failure. Bronchoalveolar lavage demonstrates > 25% eosinophils. The condition responds to corticosteroids.

CRYPTOGENIC EOSINOPHILIC PNEUMONIA

Cryptogenic eosinophilic pneumonia usually presents with malaise, fever, breathlessness and unproductive cough. It is more common in middle-aged females. The classical chest X-ray appearance has been likened to the photographic negative of pulmonary oedema with bilateral, peripheral and predominantly upper lobe parenchymal shadowing. Unless corticosteroids have been given, the peripheral blood eosinophil count is almost always very high, and the ESR and total serum IgE are elevated. BAL reveals a high proportion of eosinophils in the lavage fluid. Response to prednisolone (20–40 mg daily) is usually dramatic. Prednisolone treatment can usually be withdrawn after a few weeks without relapse, but long-term low-dose therapy is occasionally necessary to control the disease.

LUNG DISEASES DUE TO IRRADIATION AND DRUGS

RADIOTHERAPY

When radiotherapy is administered to patients with cancer of the lung, breast, spine and oesophagus, normal lung tissue may be included in the radiotherapy field. Acute radiation pneumonitis is typically seen within 6–12 weeks and causes cough and dyspnoea. This may resolve spontaneously but responds to corticosteroid treatment. Chronic interstitial fibrosis may present several months later with symptoms of exertional dyspnoea and cough. Established post-irradiation fibrosis does not usually respond to corticosteroid treatment. The pulmonary effects of radiation (p. 264) are exacerbated by treatment with cytotoxic drugs, oxygen delivery and previous radiotherapy.

DRUGS

Drugs may cause a number of parenchymal reactions, including ARDS (Box 19.96), eosinophilic reactions and diffuse interstitial inflammation/scarring. Drugs can also cause other lung disorders including asthma, haemorrhage (e.g. anticoagulants, penicillamine) and occasionally pleural effusions and pleural thickening (e.g. hydralazine, isoniazid, methysergide). An ARDS-like syndrome of acute non-cardiogenic pulmonary oedema may present with dramatic onset of breathlessness, severe hypoxaemia and signs of alveolar oedema on the chest X-ray. This syndrome has been reported most frequently in cases of opiate overdose in drug addicts (p. 214) but also after salicylate overdose, and there are occasional reports of its occurrence after therapeutic doses of drugs including hydrochlorothiazides and some cytotoxic drugs.

Pulmonary fibrosis may occur in response to a variety of drugs, but is seen most frequently with bleomycin, methotrexate, amiodarone and nitrofurantoin. Eosinophilic pulmonary reactions can also be caused by drugs. The pathogenesis may be an immune reaction similar to that in hypersensitivity pneumonitis, which specifically attracts large numbers of eosinophils into the lungs. This type of reaction is well described as a rare reaction to a variety of antineoplastic agents (e.g. bleomycin), antibiotics (e.g. sulphonamides), sulfasalazine and the anticonvulsants phenytoin and carbamazepine. Patients usually present with breathlessness, cough and fever. The chest X-ray characteristically shows patchy shadowing. Most cases resolve completely on withdrawal of the drug, but if the reaction is severe, rapid resolution can be obtained with corticosteroids.

RARE INTERSTITIAL LUNG DISEASES

See Box 19.97.

PULMONARY VASCULAR DISEASE

VENOUS THROMBOEMBOLISM

Deep venous thrombosis (DVT, p. 1061) and pulmonary embolism (PE) can be considered under the heading of venous thromboembolism (VTE). The majority (75%) of pulmonary emboli arise from the propagation of lower limb

---

19.96 DRUG-INDUCED RESPIRATORY DISEASE

Non-cardiogenic pulmonary oedema (ARDS)

- Hydrochlorothiazide
- Thrombolytics (streptokinase)
- I.v. β-adrenoceptor agonists (e.g. treatment of premature labour)
- Aspirin and opiates (in overdose)

Non-eosinophilic alveolitis

- Amiodarone, flecainide, gold, nitrofurantoin, cytotoxic agents—especially bleomycin, busulfan, mitomycin C, methotrexate

Pulmonary eosinophilia

- Antimicrobials (nitrofurantoin, penicillin, tetracyclines, sulphonamides, nalidixic acid)
- Antirheumatic agents (gold, aspirin, penicillamine, naproxen)
- Cytotoxic drugs (bleomycin, methotrexate, procarbazine)
- Psychiatric drugs (chlorpromazine, dosulepin, imipramine)
- Anticonvulsants (carbamazepine, phenytoin)
- Others (sulfasalazine, nadolol)

Pleural disease

- Bromocriptine, amiodarone, methotrexate, methysergide
- Via induction of SLE—phenytoin, hydralazine, isoniazid

Asthma

- Via pharmacological mechanism (β-blockers, cholinergic agonists, aspirin and NSAIDs)
- Idiosyncratic reaction (tamoxifen, dipyridamole)

19.97 RARE INTERSTITIAL LUNG DISEASES

Disease	Presentation	Chest X-ray	Course
Idiopathic pulmonary haemosiderosis	Haemoptysis, breathlessness, anaemia	Bilateral infiltrates often perihilar Diffuse pulmonary fibrosis	Rapidly progressive in children Slow progression or remission in adults Death from massive pulmonary haemorrhage or cor pulmonale and respiratory failure
Alveolar proteinosis	Breathlessness and cough Occasionally fever, chest pain and haemoptysis	Diffuse bilateral shadowing, often more pronounced in the hilar regions Air bronchogram	Spontaneous remission in one-third Whole lung lavage or granulocyte macrophage-colony stimulating factor (GM-CSF) therapy may be effective
Langerhans cell histiocytosis (histiocytosis X)	Breathlessness, cough, pneumothorax	Diffuse interstitial shadowing progressing to honeycombing	Progressive leading to respiratory failure Poor response to immunosuppressive therapy Smoking cessation is important and may result in significant improvement
Neurofibromatosis	Breathlessness and cough in a patient with multiple organ involvement with neurofibromas including skin	Bilateral reticular nodular shadowing of diffuse interstitial fibrosis	Slow progression to death from respiratory failure Poor response to corticosteroid therapy
Alveolar microlithiasis	May be asymptomatic Breathlessness and cough	Diffuse calcified micronodular shadowing more pronounced in the lower zones	Slowly progressive to cor pulmonale and respiratory failure May stabilise in some
Lymphangio-leiomyomatosis	Haemoptysis, breathlessness, pneumothorax and chylous effusion in females	Diffuse bilateral shadowing CT shows characteristic thin-walled cysts with well-defined walls throughout both lungs	Progressive to death within 10 years Oestrogen ablation and progesterone therapy of doubtful value Lung transplantation
Pulmonary tuberous sclerosis	Very similar to lymphangioleiomyomatosis except occasionally occurs in men		

19.98 CATEGORISATION OF PULMONARY THROMBOEMBOLI

	Acute massive PE	Acute small/medium PE	Chronic PE
Pathophysiology	Major haemodynamic effects: $\downarrow$ cardiac output; acute right heart failure	Occlusion of segmental pulmonary artery $\rightarrow$ infarction $\pm$ effusion	Chronic occlusion of pulmonary microvasculature, right heart failure
Symptoms	Faintness or collapse, central chest pain, apprehension, severe dyspnoea	Pleuritic chest pain, restricted breathing, haemoptysis	Exertional dyspnoea. Late symptoms of pulmonary hypertension or right heart failure
Signs	Major circulatory collapse: tachycardia, hypotension, $\uparrow$ JVP, right ventricular gallop rhythm, split P_2 Severe cyanosis $\downarrow$ Urinary output	Tachycardia Pleural rub, raised hemidiaphragm, crackles, effusion (often blood-stained) Low-grade fever	May be minimal early in disease Later—RV heave, loud, split P_2 Terminal—right heart failure
Chest X-ray	Usually normal. May be subtle oligaemia	Pleuropulmonary opacities, pleural effusion, linear shadows, raised hemidiaphragm	Enlarged pulmonary artery trunk, enlarged heart, prominent RV
ECG	$S_1Q_3T_3$ anterior T-wave inversion Right bundle branch block (RBBB)	Sinus tachycardia	RV hypertrophy and strain
Arterial blood gases	Markedly abnormal with $\downarrow$ PaO_2 and $\downarrow$ $PaCO_2$. Metabolic acidosis	May be normal or $\downarrow$ $PaCO_2$	Exertional $\downarrow$ PaO_2 or desaturation on formal exercise testing
Alternative diagnoses	Myocardial infarction; pericardial tamponade; aortic dissection	Pneumonia, pneumothorax, musculoskeletal chest pain	Other causes of pulmonary hypertension

DVT. Amniotic fluid, placenta, air, fat, tumour (especially choriocarcinoma), and septic emboli (from endocarditis affecting the tricuspid or pulmonary valves) are rare.

VTE is common; PE occurs in around 1% of all patients admitted to hospital and accounts for around 5% of in-hospital deaths. It is a common mode of death in patients with cancer and stroke and remains the most common cause of death in pregnancy.

19

19.99 RISK FACTORS FOR VENOUS THROMBOEMBOLISM

Surgery

- Major abdominal/pelvic surgery
- Hip/knee surgery
- Post-operative intensive care

Obstetrics

- Pregnancy/puerperium

Cardiorespiratory disease

- COPD
- Congestive cardiac failure
- Other disabling disease

Lower limb problems

- Fracture
- Varicose veins
- Stroke/spinal cord injury

Malignant disease

- Abdominal pelvic
- Advanced/metastatic
- Concurrent chemotherapy

Miscellaneous

- Increasing age
- Previous proven VTE
- Immobility
- Thrombotic disorders (Ch. 24)
- Trauma

Clinical features

The varied clinical presentation, non-specific nature of the physical signs and the lack of sensitive and specific diagnostic tests can make the diagnosis of PE difficult (Box 19.98). It is often helpful to consider three questions:

- Is the clinical presentation consistent with PE?
- Does the patient have risk factors for PE?
- Is there any alternative diagnosis that can explain the patient's presentation?

The clinical features of PE depend largely upon the size of embolism and co-morbidity. They encompass a spectrum from cardiovascular collapse to small emboli with few or no haemodynamic consequences. A recognised risk factor is present in between 80% and 90% of patients (Box 19.99).

Investigations

All patients with suspected PE should have a chest X-ray, ECG and arterial blood gas analysis. These tests may also help to exclude important differential diagnoses.

Chest radiography

Pulmonary embolism may give rise to a variety of radiographic appearances (Fig. 19.56) but these are usually non-specific. Normal radiographic appearances in an acutely breathless and hypoxaemic patient should raise the suspicion of PE as should bilateral changes in a patient presenting with unilateral pleuritic chest pain. However, the most important role of the chest X-ray is to exclude key differential diagnoses such as heart failure, pneumonia, pneumothorax or tumour.

Electrocardiography

ECG changes in PE are common but are usually non-specific. The most common findings are a sinus tachycardia and anterior T-wave inversion; larger emboli may cause right heart strain revealed by an $S_1Q_3T_3$ pattern, ST-segment and T-wave changes, or the appearance of right bundle branch block. The ECG is also useful in excluding other important differential diagnoses such as acute myocardial infarction and pericarditis.

Arterial blood gases

Pulmonary embolism is characterised by ventilation–perfusion mismatch and reduced cardiac output with a low mixed venous oxygen saturation and hyperventilation. Arterial blood gases typically show a reduced PaO_2 and a normal or low $PaCO_2$, but are normal in a significant minority. A metabolic acidosis may be seen in acute massive PE with cardiovascular collapse.

D-dimer and other circulating markers

D-dimer is a specific degradation product released into the circulation when cross-linked fibrin undergoes endogenous fibrinolysis (p. 1009). The presence of a low D-dimer (< 500 ng/ml measured by ELISA) has a high negative predictive value and provides a useful screening

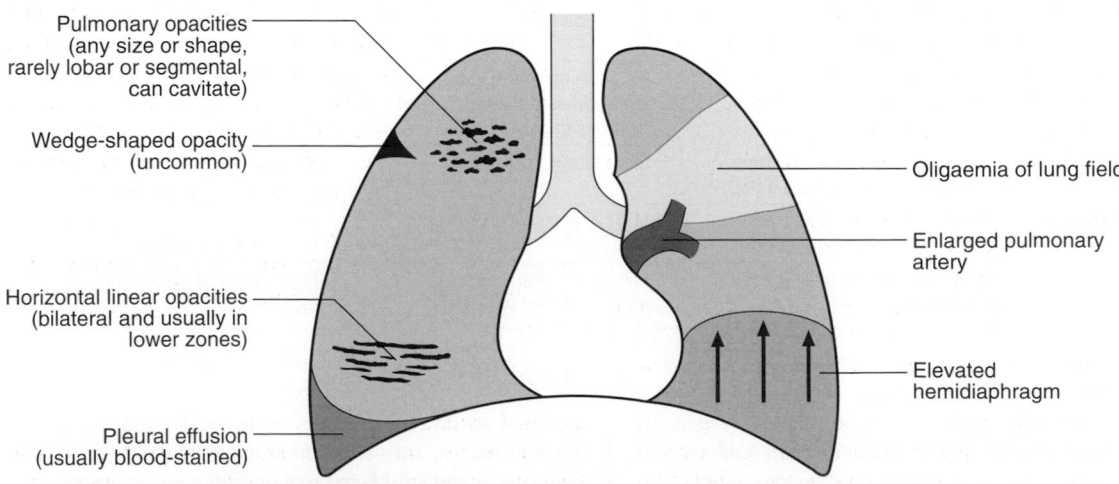

Pulmonary opacities
(any size or shape,
rarely lobar or segmental,
can cavitate)

Wedge-shaped opacity
(uncommon)

Horizontal linear opacities
(bilateral and usually in
lower zones)

Pleural effusion
(usually blood-stained)

Oligaemia of lung field

Enlarged pulmonary
artery

Elevated
hemidiaphragm

Fig. 19.56   Features of pulmonary thromboembolism/infarction on chest X-ray.

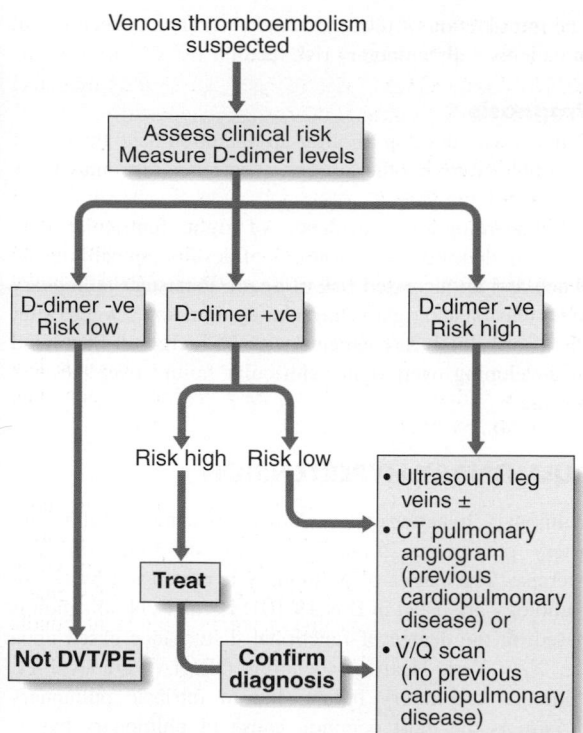

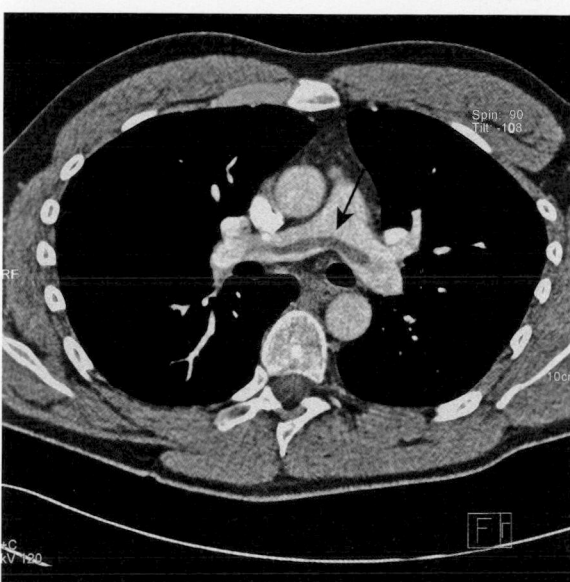

Fig. 19.58 CT pulmonary angiogram. The arrow points to a saddle embolism in the bifurcation of the pulmonary artery.

Fig. 19.57 Algorithm for the investigation of patients with suspected pulmonary thromboembolism. Clinical risk is based on the presence of risk factors for VTE and the probability of another diagnosis.

test (Fig. 19.57). However, a suggestive clinical picture in a high-risk patient must be investigated further even when the D dimer level is normal. Non-specific elevation of the D-dimer is observed in a number of conditions other than PE including myocardial infarction, pneumonia and sepsis. Elevated levels are therefore of limited value. Other circulating markers that reflect right ventricular micro-infarction such as troponin I or pro-brain natriuretic peptide, may prove useful.

Imaging

Ventilation–perfusion scanning has been the most popular method of attempting to confirm the presence of PE (p. 651). The sensitivity and specificity of $\dot{V}/\dot{Q}$ scanning is greatly increased when interpretation is informed by clinical probability. A normal $\dot{V}/\dot{Q}$ scan virtually excludes PE and a low probability scan in the presence of a low clinical probability makes PE unlikely. Similarly, the presence of a high probability scan in a patient with a high clinical probability almost certainly establishes the diagnosis of PE. $\dot{V}/\dot{Q}$ scans are most useful in patients with normal pulmonary architecture. However, PE often presents as an important differential in patients with pre-existing chronic cardiopulmonary pathology (such as COPD or congestive cardiac failure) and in these cases the majority of scans (70%) are indeterminate.

The development of rapid acquisition helical CT scanners has popularised the use of CT pulmonary angiography (CTPA, Fig. 19.58) and has largely replaced conventional

pulmonary angiography. CTPA may not only exclude PE but highlight an alternative diagnosis. Limited resolution may hinder the detection of small peripheral emboli but further advances in CT scanning are likely to improve this. The utility of contrast-enhanced magnetic resonance scanning is also being explored. Both CT and MRI may allow simultaneous visualisation of the pelvic and leg veins.

Colour Doppler ultrasound of the leg veins remains the investigation of choice in patients with clinical DVT, but may also be applied to patients suspected of PE, particularly if there are clinical signs in a limb, as many will have identifiable proximal thrombus in the leg veins.

Echocardiography

Bedside echocardiography is extremely helpful in the differential diagnosis and assessment of acute circulatory collapse (p. 540). Acute dilatation of the right heart is usually present in massive PE, and thrombus (embolism in transit) may be visible. Alternative diagnoses including left ventricular failure, aortic dissection and pericardial tamponade can usually be established with confidence.

Echocardiography is also useful for patients who present with unexplained pulmonary hypertension, providing a simple means of determining pulmonary artery pressure and excluding treatable conditions such as mitral stenosis.

Pulmonary angiography

Pulmonary angiography represents the 'gold standard' for the diagnosis of PE, but has been largely superseded by CTPA.

Management

General measures

Prompt recognition and treatment is potentially life-saving. Oxygen should be given to all hypoxaemic patients in a concentration necessary to restore arterial oxygen saturation

19

to over 90%. Opiates may be necessary to relieve pain and distress but should be used with great caution in the hypotensive patient. Diuretics and vasodilators should also be avoided; indeed, hypotension should be treated by giving intravenous fluid or plasma expander. Inotropic agents are of limited value since in massive PE the hypoxic dilated right ventricle is near maximally stimulated by endogenous catecholamines. Resuscitation by external cardiac massage may be successful in the moribund patient by dislodging and breaking up a large central embolus.

Anticoagulation

Anticoagulation should be commenced immediately in patients with a high or intermediate probability of PE but can usually be safely withheld from patients with a low clinical probability pending further investigation. Low molecular weight heparin administered subcutaneously is as effective as intravenous unfractionated heparin and it is easier to administer (Box 19.100). The dose is standardised for the weight of the patient and does not require monitoring by tests of coagulation. Heparin is effective in reducing mortality in PE by reducing the propagation of clot and the risk of further emboli. It should be administered for at least 5 days and anticoagulation continued using oral warfarin. Heparin should not be discontinued until the international normalised ratio (INR) is greater than 2.

The optimum duration of warfarin therapy is not clear. Current guidelines suggest that patients with an underlying prothrombotic risk or a history of previous emboli should be anticoagulated for life. Those with an identifiable and reversible risk factor require 3 months of therapy, although 6 weeks may be sufficient for some. Six months of therapy is currently recommended for idiopathic VTE. However, long-term, low-intensity warfarin therapy (target INR 1.5–2.0) appears to be associated with reduced risk of bleeding and may prevent recurrent thromboembolism (p. 1061).

Thrombolytic therapy

Thrombolysis appears to improve outcome when acute massive PE is accompanied by shock but it is not clear whether there is any advantage of thrombolysis over heparin in patients with a normal blood pressure. Patients with PE appear to have a high risk of intracranial haemorrhage and must be screened carefully for haemorrhagic risk.

Caval filters

Patients who experience recurrent PE despite adequate anticoagulation, or those patients in whom anticoagulation is contraindicated, may benefit from insertion of a filter in the inferior vena cava below the origin of the renal vessels.

The introduction of retrievable caval filters has been useful in patients with temporary risk factors.

Prognosis

Patients who develop PE after an operation have the lowest recurrence rate; in other groups, recurrence rates may be as high as 9% per year.

Echocardiographic evidence of right ventricular dysfunction identifies patients at risk of developing cardiogenic shock and an increased risk of death. Persistent pulmonary hypertension and right ventricular dysfunction 6 weeks after PE identify high-risk patients with an increased likelihood of developing overt right ventricular failure over the next 5 years.

PULMONARY HYPERTENSION

Pulmonary hypertension is defined as a mean pulmonary artery pressure > 25 mmHg at rest or 30 mmHg with exercise. The causes of pulmonary hypertension by site of pathology are listed in Box 19.101. Further classification is based on the degree of functional disturbance based upon the New York Heart Association (NYHA) grades I–IV. Although respiratory failure due to intrinsic pulmonary disease is the most common cause of pulmonary hypertension, severe pulmonary hypertension may occur as a

---

19.101 CLASSIFICATION OF PULMONARY HYPERTENSION

Pulmonary arterial hypertension

- Primary pulmonary hypertension: sporadic and familial
- Related to: collagen vascular disease (limited cutaneous systemic sclerosis), congenital systemic to pulmonary shunts, portal hypertension, HIV infection, exposure to various drugs or toxins, and persistent pulmonary hypertension of the newborn

Pulmonary venous hypertension

- Left-sided atrial or ventricular heart disease
- Left-sided valvular heart disease
- Pulmonary veno-occlusive disease
- Pulmonary capillary haemangiomatosis

Pulmonary hypertension associated with disorders of the respiratory system and/or hypoxaemia

- COPD
- DPLD
- Sleep-disordered breathing
- Alveolar hypoventilation disorders
- Chronic exposure to high altitude
- Neonatal lung disease
- Alveolar capillary dysplasia

Pulmonary hypertension caused by chronic thromboembolic disease

- Thromboembolic obstruction of the proximal pulmonary arteries
- In situ thrombosis
- Sickle cell disease

Miscellaneous

- Inflammatory conditions
- Extrinsic compression of central pulmonary veins

EBM

19.100 SUBCUTANEOUS LOW MOLECULAR WEIGHT HEPARINS IN ACUTE VENOUS THROMBOEMBOLISM (VTE)

'Low molecular weight heparins administered subcutaneously in a weight-adjusted dosage are the treatment of choice for acute VTE.'

- Columbus investigators. N Engl J Med 1997; 337:657–662.
- Simonneau G, et al. N Engl J Med 1997; 337:663–669.

primary disorder or as a result of chronic repeated thromboembolic events.

Primary pulmonary hypertension (PPH) is a rare but important disease that affects young people, predominantly women, aged between 20 and 30 years. PPH is usually sporadic or associated with an underlying cause. Familial disease is rare but the gene responsible has recently been identified as a member of the TGF-β superfamily, BMPR2, which encodes the type II bone morphogenetic protein receptor. Up to 30% of patients with sporadic pulmonary hypertension have also been found to have mutations in this gene. Pathological features include hypertrophy of both the media and intima of the vessel wall, and a clonal expansion of endothelial cells which take the appearance of plexiform lesions. There is marked narrowing of the vessel lumen and this, together with the frequently observed in situ thrombosis, leads to an increase in pulmonary vascular resistance and pulmonary hypertension.

Clinical features

The diagnosis of pulmonary hypertension is often made late due to the non-specific nature of the presenting symptoms which include breathlessness, chest pain and syncope. Important signs include elevation of the JVP (with a prominent 'a' wave if in sinus rhythm), a parasternal heave (RV hypertrophy), accentuation of the pulmonary component of the second heart sound and an early diastolic murmur due to pulmonary regurgitation.

Investigations

The assessment of patients with pulmonary hypertension should be undertaken in centres with specialist expertise. Transthoracic echocardiography provides a non-invasive assessment of pulmonary artery pressure and a useful means of monitoring the condition. Right heart catheterisation is required to determine whether vasodilatation can reduce pulmonary artery pressure and may therefore be of therapeutic value.

Management

Treatment options for PPH have been limited and the prognosis remains poor. The median survival from time of diagnosis (without heart–lung transplantation) is 2–3 years. All patients should be anticoagulated with warfarin as this has been demonstrated to improve prognosis in severe pulmonary hypertension. Oxygen, diuretics and digoxin should be prescribed as appropriate. Selected patients with pulmonary arterial hypertension who respond to an acute vasodilator test may benefit from therapy with high-dose calcium channel blockers. The use of prostaglandins such as epoprostenol (prostacyclin) as endogenous vasodilators or iloprost therapy, has dramatically improved exercise performance, symptoms and prognosis. Therapy can be administered as a continuous intravenous infusion through a central venous catheter or via a nebuliser. The use of the PDE5 inhibitor, sildenafil, and the oral endothelin antagonist, bosentan, is currently being investigated. Pulmonary thromboendarterectomy should be contemplated in patients with chronic proximal pulmonary thromboembolic disease and heart–lung transplantation considered in selected patients.

DISEASES OF THE NASOPHARYNX, LARYNX AND TRACHEA

DISEASES OF THE NASOPHARYNX

ALLERGIC RHINITIS

This is a disorder in which there are episodes of nasal congestion, watery nasal discharge and sneezing. It may be seasonal or perennial.

Aetiology

Allergic rhinitis is due to an immediate hypersensitivity reaction in the nasal mucosa. Seasonal antigens include pollens from grasses, flowers, weeds or trees. Grass pollen is responsible for hay fever, the most common type of seasonal allergic rhinitis in northern Europe, which is at its peak between May and July. Allergic rhinitis due to pollens is, however, a world-wide problem which may be aggravated during harvest seasons.

Perennial allergic rhinitis may be a specific reaction to antigens derived from house dust, fungal spores or animal dander but similar symptoms can be caused by physical or chemical irritants—for example, pungent odours or fumes, including strong perfumes, cold air and dry atmospheres. The term 'vasomotor rhinitis' is often used because in this context the term 'allergic' is a misnomer.

Clinical features

In the seasonal type there are frequent sudden attacks of sneezing, with profuse watery nasal discharge and nasal obstruction. These attacks last for a few hours and are often accompanied by smarting and watering of the eyes and conjunctival infection. In the perennial variety the symptoms are similar but more continuous and generally less severe. Skin hypersensitivity tests with the relevant antigen

---

19.102 THROMBOEMBOLIC DISEASE IN OLD AGE

- **Risk**: rises by a factor of 2.5 over the age of 60 years.
- **HRT**: in women aged over 60 years, hormone replacement therapy increases the risk of thromboembolism by a factor of 2–4.
- **Prophylaxis for venous thromboembolism**: should be considered in all older patients who are immobile as a result of acute illness, except when this is due to acute stroke.
- **Association with cancer**: the prevalence of cancer among those with DVT increases with age, but the relative risk of malignancy with DVT falls; therefore intensive investigation is not justified if initial assessment reveals no evidence of an underlying neoplasm.
- **Warfarin**: older patients are more sensitive to the anticoagulant effects of warfarin, partly due to the concurrent use of other drugs and the presence of other pathology. Life-threatening or fatal bleeds on warfarin are significantly more common in those aged over 80 years.
- **Chronic immobilty**: long-term anticoagulant therapy is not required as there is no associated increase in thromboembolism.

are usually positive in seasonal allergic rhinitis and are thus of diagnostic value, but they are less useful in perennial rhinitis.

Management

The following symptomatic measures, singly or in combination, are usually effective in both seasonal and perennial allergic rhinitis:

- an antihistamine drug such as loratadine 10 mg daily by mouth
- sodium cromoglicate nasal spray, one metered dose of a 2% solution into each nostril 4–6-hourly
- beclometasone dipropionate or budesonide aqueous nasal spray, one or two doses of 50 µg into each nostril 12-hourly.

In patients whose symptoms are very severe and seriously interfere with school, business or social activities, systemic corticosteroids are occasionally indicated, but side-effects limit their usefulness. Vasomotor rhinitis is often difficult to treat, but may respond to ipratropium bromide, administered into each nostril 6–8-hourly.

Prevention

In the seasonal type an attempt should be made to reduce exposure to pollen—for example, by avoiding country districts and staying indoors with windows closed when pollen counts are reported to be high. The prevention of perennial rhinitis consists of avoiding, as far as possible, exposure to any identifiable aetiological factor but this is often difficult.

LARYNGEAL DISORDERS

Acute infections have already been described (Box 19.41, p. 688). Other disorders of the larynx include chronic laryngitis, laryngeal tuberculosis, laryngeal paralysis and laryngeal obstruction. Tumours of the larynx are relatively common. For detailed information on these conditions, the reader should refer to a textbook of diseases of the ear, nose and throat.

CHRONIC LARYNGITIS

The common causes of this condition are listed in Box 19.103.

Clinical features

The chief symptoms are hoarseness or loss of voice (aphonia). There is irritation of the throat and a spasmodic cough. The disease pursues a chronic course frequently uninfluenced by treatment, and the voice may become permanently impaired.

Differential diagnosis

The causes of chronic hoarseness are listed in Box 19.104.

In some patients a chest X-ray may bring to light an unsuspected bronchial carcinoma or pulmonary TB. If no such abnormality is found, laryngoscopy should be performed, usually by a specialist in otolaryngology.

19.103 SOME CAUSES OF CHRONIC LARYNGITIS
• Repeated attacks of acute laryngitis
• Excessive use of the voice, especially in dusty atmospheres
• Heavy tobacco smoking
• Mouth-breathing from nasal obstruction
• Chronic infection of nasal sinuses

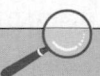

19.104 CAUSES OF CHRONIC HOARSENESS
If hoarseness persists for more than a few days, consider:
• Tumour of the larynx
• TB
• Laryngeal paralysis
• Inhaled corticosteroid treatment

Management

The voice must be rested completely. This is particularly important in public speakers. Smoking should be prohibited. Some benefit may be obtained from frequent inhalations of medicated steam.

LARYNGEAL PARALYSIS

Aetiology

Paralysis is due to interference with the motor nerve supply of the larynx. It is nearly always unilateral and, because of the intrathoracic course of the left recurrent laryngeal nerve, usually left-sided. One or both recurrent laryngeal nerves may be damaged at thyroidectomy or by carcinoma of the thyroid. Rarely, the vagal trunk itself is involved by tumour, aneurysm or trauma.

Clinical features

Hoarseness

This always accompanies laryngeal paralysis, whatever its cause. Paralysis of organic origin is seldom reversible but when only one vocal cord is affected hoarseness may improve or even disappear after a few weeks, as the unparalysed cord compensates by crossing the midline to approximate with the paralysed cord on phonation.

'Bovine cough'

A characteristic feature of organic laryngeal paralysis is a cow-like cough, which lacks the explosive quality of normal coughing because of the failure of the cords to close the glottis. Sputum clearance may also be impaired. A normal cough in patients with partial loss of voice or aphonia virtually excludes laryngeal paralysis.

Stridor

Stridor is occasionally present but is seldom severe, except when laryngeal paralysis is bilateral.

Diagnosis

Laryngoscopy is necessary to establish the diagnosis of laryngeal paralysis with certainty. The paralysed cord lies in the so-called 'cadaveric' position, midway between abduction and adduction.

Management

The cause of laryngeal paralysis should be treated if that is possible. In unilateral paralysis the voice may be improved by the injection of Teflon into the affected vocal cord. In bilateral organic paralysis, tracheal intubation, tracheostomy or a plastic operation on the larynx may be necessary.

PSYCHOGENIC HOARSENESS AND APHONIA

Psychogenic causes of hoarseness or complete loss of voice may be suggested by associated symptoms in the history (p. 236). However, laryngoscopy may be necessary to exclude a physical cause of the abnormality. In psychogenic aphonia only the voluntary movement of adduction of the vocal cords is seen to be impaired.

LARYNGEAL OBSTRUCTION

Laryngeal obstruction is more liable to occur in children than in adults because of the smaller size of the glottis. Some important causes are given in Box 19.105.

Clinical features

Sudden complete laryngeal obstruction by a foreign body produces the clinical picture of acute asphyxia—violent but ineffective inspiratory efforts with indrawing of the intercostal spaces and the unsupported lower ribs, accompanied by cyanosis. Unrelieved, the condition progresses rapidly to coma and death within a few minutes. When, as in most cases, the obstruction is incomplete at first, the main clinical features are progressive breathlessness accompanied by stridor and cyanosis. Urgent treatment to prevent complete obstruction is needed.

Management

Transient laryngeal obstruction due to exudate and spasm, which may occur with acute laryngitis in children (p. 688) and with whooping cough, is potentially dangerous but can usually be relieved by steam inhalation. Laryngeal obstruction from all other causes carries a high mortality and demands prompt treatment.

Relief of obstruction by mechanical measures

When a foreign body causes laryngeal obstruction in children it can often be dislodged by turning the patient head downwards and squeezing the chest vigorously. In adults this is often impossible, but a sudden forceful compression of the upper abdomen (Heimlich manoeuvre) may be effective. In other circumstances the cause of the obstruction should be investigated by direct laryngoscopy, which may also permit the removal of an unsuspected foreign body or the insertion of a tube past the obstruction into the trachea. Tracheostomy must be performed without delay if these procedures fail to relieve obstruction, but except in dire emergencies this operation should be performed in an operating theatre by a surgeon.

Treatment of the cause

In cases of diphtheria, antitoxin should be administered, and for other infections the appropriate antibiotic should be given. In angioedema complete laryngeal occlusion can usually be prevented by treatment with adrenaline (epinephrine) 0.5–1 mg (0.5–1 ml of 1:1000) intramuscularly, chlorphenamine maleate 10–20 mg by slow intravenous injection and intravenous hydrocortisone sodium succinate 200 mg.

TRACHEAL DISORDERS

ACUTE TRACHEITIS

See Box 19.41, page 688.

TRACHEAL OBSTRUCTION

External compression by enlarged mediastinal lymph nodes containing metastatic deposits, usually from a bronchial carcinoma, is a more frequent cause of tracheal obstruction than the uncommon primary benign or malignant tumours. Rarely, the trachea may be compressed by an aneurysm of the aortic arch, a retrosternal goitre (Fig. 19.13, p. 662) or in children by tuberculous mediastinal lymph nodes. Tracheal stenosis is an occasional complication of tracheostomy, prolonged intubation, Wegener's granulomatosis or trauma.

Clinical features

Stridor can be detected in every patient with severe tracheal narrowing. Endoscopic examination of the trachea should be undertaken without delay to determine the site, degree and nature of the obstruction.

Management

Localised tumours of the trachea can be resected, but reconstruction after resection may be technically difficult. Endobronchial laser therapy, bronchoscopically placed tracheal stents, chemotherapy and radiotherapy are alternatives to surgery. The choice of treatment depends upon the nature of the tumour and the general health of the patient. Benign tracheal strictures can sometimes be dilated but may have to be resected.

TRACHEO-OESOPHAGEAL FISTULA

This may be present in newborn infants as a congenital abnormality. In adults it is usually due to malignant lesions in the mediastinum, such as carcinoma or lymphoma, eroding both the trachea and oesophagus to produce a communication between them. Swallowed liquids enter

---

19.105 CAUSES OF LARYNGEAL OBSTRUCTION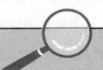

- Inflammatory or allergic oedema, or exudate
- Spasm of laryngeal muscles
- Inhaled foreign body
- Inhaled blood clot or vomitus in an unconscious patient
- Tumours of the larynx
- Bilateral vocal cord paralysis
- Fixation of both cords in rheumatoid disease

19

the trachea and bronchi through the fistula and provoke coughing.

Management

Surgical closure of a congenital fistula, if undertaken promptly, is usually successful. There is usually no curative treatment for malignant fistulae, and death from overwhelming pulmonary infection rapidly supervenes.

DISEASES OF THE PLEURA, DIAPHRAGM AND CHEST WALL

DISEASES OF THE PLEURA

PLEURISY

Pleurisy is not a diagnosis but simply a term used to describe the result of any disease process involving the pleura and giving rise to pleuritic pain or evidence of pleural friction. Pleurisy is a common feature of pulmonary infection and infarction; it may also occur in malignancy.

Clinical features

Pleural pain is the characteristic symptom. On examination rib movement is restricted and a pleural rub may be present. This may only be heard in deep inspiration or near the pericardium (pleuro-pericardial rub). The other clinical features depend upon the nature of the disease causing the pleurisy. Loss of the pleural rub and diminution in the chest pain may indicate recovery or herald the development of a pleural effusion.

Every patient should have a chest X-ray but a normal X-ray does not exclude a pulmonary cause for the pleurisy. A preceding history of cough, purulent sputum and pyrexia is presumptive evidence of a pulmonary infection which may not have been severe enough to produce a radiographic abnormality or which may have resolved before the chest X-ray was taken.

Management

The primary cause of pleurisy must be treated. The symptomatic treatment of pleural pain is described on page 692.

PLEURAL EFFUSION

See page 664.

EMPYEMA

This term describes the presence of pus in the pleural space. The pus may be as thin as serous fluid or so thick that it is impossible to aspirate even through a wide-bore needle. Microscopically, neutrophil leucocytes are present in large numbers. The causative organism may or may not be isolated from the pus. An empyema may involve the whole pleural space or only part of it ('loculated' or 'encysted' empyema) and is almost invariably unilateral.

Aetiology

Empyema is always secondary to infection in a neighbouring structure, usually the lung. The principal infections liable to produce empyema are the bacterial pneumonias and TB. Over 40% of patients with community-acquired pneumonia develop an associated pleural effusion ('para-pneumonic' effusion) and about 15% of these become secondarily infected. Other causes are infection of a haemothorax and rupture of a subphrenic abscess through the diaphragm. Despite the widespread availability of effective antibacterial therapy for patients with pneumonia, empyema continues to be a significant cause of morbidity and mortality even in developed countries. All too often, this reflects a delay in the diagnosis or instigation of appropriate therapy.

Pathology

Both layers of pleura are covered with a thick, shaggy inflammatory exudate. The pus in the pleural space is often under considerable pressure and if the condition is not adequately treated pus may rupture into a bronchus causing a bronchopleural fistula and pyopneumothorax, or track through the chest wall with the formation of a subcutaneous abscess or sinus.

The only way in which an empyema can heal is by eradication of the infection, obliteration of the empyema space and apposition of the visceral and parietal pleural layers. This cannot occur unless re-expansion of the compressed lung is secured at an early stage by removal of all the pus from the pleural space. This cannot take place if:

- the visceral pleura becomes grossly thickened and rigid due to delayed treatment or inadequate drainage of the infected pleural fluid
- the pleural layers are kept apart by air entering the pleura through a bronchopleural fistula
- there is underlying disease in the lung, such as bronchiectasis, bronchial carcinoma or pulmonary TB preventing re-expansion.

In all these circumstances an empyema tends to become chronic, and healing is unlikely without surgical intervention.

Clinical features

An empyema should be suspected in patients with pulmonary infection if there is persistence or recurrence of pyrexia despite the administration of a suitable antibiotic. In other cases the illness produced by the primary infective lesion may be so slight that it passes unrecognised and the first definite clinical features are due to the empyema itself.

Once an empyema has developed, two separate groups of clinical features are found. These are shown in Box 19.106.

Investigations

Radiological examination

The appearances are often indistinguishable from those of pleural effusion. When air is present in addition to pus (pyopneumothorax), a horizontal 'fluid level' marks the interface between the liquid and air. Ultrasound shows the

19

19.106 CLINICAL FEATURES OF EMPYEMA

Systemic features

- Pyrexia, usually high and remittent
- Rigors, sweating, malaise and weight loss
- Polymorphonuclear leucocytosis, high CRP

Local features

- Pleural pain; breathlessness; cough and sputum usually because of underlying lung disease; copious purulent sputum if empyema ruptures into a bronchus (bronchopleural fistula)
- Clinical signs of fluid in the pleural space

19.107 CLASSIFICATION OF PNEUMOTHORAX

Spontaneous

Primary
- Without evidence of overt lung disease. Air escapes from the lung into the pleural space through rupture of a small subpleural emphysematous bulla or pleural bleb, or the pulmonary end of a pleural adhesion

Secondary
- Underlying lung disease, most commonly COPD and TB; also seen in asthma, lung abscess, pulmonary infarcts, bronchogenic carcinoma, all forms of fibrotic and cystic lung disease

Traumatic
- Iatrogenic (e.g. following thoracic surgery or biopsy) or non-iatrogenic

19

position of the fluid, the extent of pleural thickening and whether fluid is in a single collection or multiloculated by fibrin and debris. In addition to showing the pleura, CT can be useful in assessing the underlying lung parenchyma and patency of the major bronchi.

Aspiration of pus

This confirms the presence of an empyema. Ultrasound or CT is recommended to identify the optimal place to undertake aspiration, which is best performed using a wide-bore needle. The pus is frequently sterile when antibiotics have already been given; the distinction between tuberculous and non-tuberculous disease can be difficult and often requires pleural histology and culture.

Management

Treatment of non-tuberculous empyema

When the patient is acutely ill and the pus is thin an intercostal tube should be inserted under ultrasound or CT guidance into the most dependent part of the empyema space and connected to a water-seal drain system. If the initial aspirate reveals turbid fluid or frank pus, or if loculations are seen on ultrasound, the tube should be put on suction (5–10 cm H_2O) and flushed regularly with 20 ml normal saline. Although intrapleural fibrinolytic therapy is widely used in such situations, trial evidence of its benefit is conflicting. Finally, an antibiotic directed against the organism causing the empyema should be given for 2–4 weeks.

An empyema can often be aborted if these measures are started early. If, however, the intercostal tube is not providing adequate drainage, which can happen when the pus is thick or loculated, surgical intervention is required. The empyema cavity is cleared of pus and adhesions, and a wide-bore tube inserted to allow optimal drainage. Surgical 'decortication' of the lung may also be required if gross thickening of the visceral pleura has developed and is preventing re-expansion of the lung.

Treatment of tuberculous empyema

Antituberculosis chemotherapy must be started immediately (p. 701) and the pus in the pleural space aspirated through a wide-bore needle until it ceases to reaccumulate. Intercostal tube drainage is often required. In many patients no other treatment is necessary but surgery is occasionally required to ablate a residual empyema space.

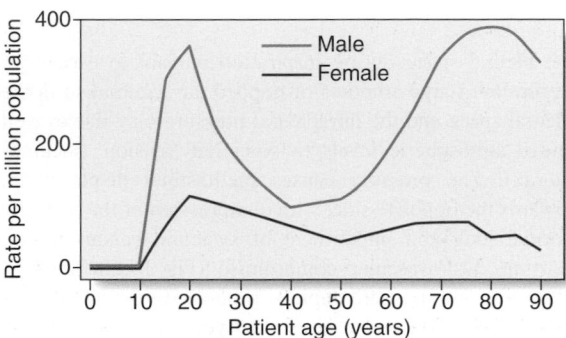

Fig. 19.59 Bimodal age distribution for hospital admissions for pneumothorax in England. The incidence of primary spontaneous pneumothorax peaks in males aged 15–30. Secondary spontaneous pneumothorax occurs mainly in males > 55 years.

SPONTANEOUS PNEUMOTHORAX

Pneumothorax is the presence of air in the pleural space, which can either occur spontaneously, or result from iatrogenic injury or trauma to the lung or chest wall (Box 19.107). Primary spontaneous pneumothorax occurs in patients with no history of lung disease. It principally affects males aged 15–30 (Fig. 19.59) in whom smoking, tall stature and the presence of apical subpleural blebs are additional risk factors. Secondary pneumothorax affects patients with pre-existing lung disease, is most common in older patients, and is associated with the highest mortality rates.

Clinical features

The commonest symptoms are sudden-onset unilateral pleuritic chest pain or breathlessness. In those with underlying chest disease, breathlessness can be severe and may not resolve spontaneously. In patients with a small pneumothorax the physical examination may be normal. A larger pneumothorax (> 15% of the hemithorax) results in decreased or absent breath sounds (p. 649). The combination of absent breath sounds and resonant percussion note is diagnostic of pneumothorax.

If the communication between the airway and the pleura is small, it can act as a one-way valve allowing air to enter

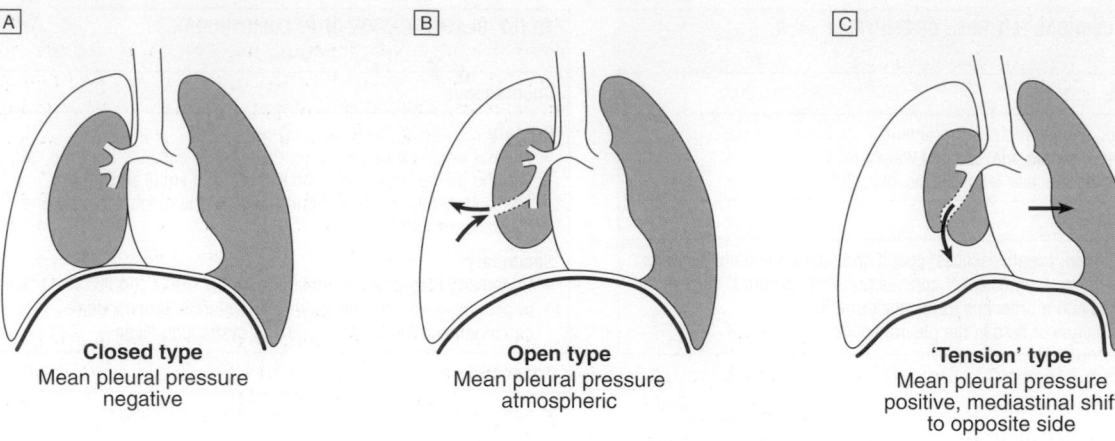

Fig. 19.60   Types of spontaneous pneumothorax. A Closed type. B Open type. C 'Tension' (valvular) type.

the pleural space during inspiration but not to escape on expiration. Large amounts of trapped air accumulate in the pleural space and the intrapleural pressure may rise to well above atmospheric levels (a so-called 'tension' pneumothorax). The pressure causes mediastinal displacement towards the opposite side, with compression of the opposite normal lung and impairment of systemic venous return, causing cardiovascular compromise (Fig. 19.60C). Clinically, the findings are rapidly progressive breathlessness associated with a marked tachycardia, hypotension, cyanosis and tracheal displacement away from the side of the silent hemithorax. Occasionally, 'tension' pneumothorax may occur without mediastinal shift if malignant disease or scarring has splinted the mediastinum.

Where the communication between the lung and pleural space seals off as the lung deflates and does not reopen, the pneumothorax is referred to as 'closed' (Fig. 19.60A). In such circumstances the mean pleural pressure remains negative, spontaneous reabsorption of air and re-expansion of the lung occur over a few days or weeks, and infection is uncommon. This contrasts with an 'open' pneumothorax, where the communication fails to seal and air continues to transfer freely between the lung and pleural space (Fig. 19.60B). An example of the latter is a bronchopleural fistula which, if large, can also facilitate the transmission of infection from the air passages into the pleural space, leading to empyema. An open pneumothorax is commonly seen following rupture of an emphysematous bulla, tuberculous cavity or lung abscess into the pleural space.

Investigations

The chest X-ray shows the sharply defined edge of the deflated lung with complete translucency (no lung markings) between this and the chest wall (Fig. 19.61). Care must be taken to differentiate between a large pre-existing emphysematous bulla and a pneumothorax to avoid misdirected attempts at aspiration. Where doubt exists, CT is useful in distinguishing bullae from pleural air. X-rays also show the extent of any mediastinal displacement and give information regarding the presence or absence of pleural fluid and underlying pulmonary disease.

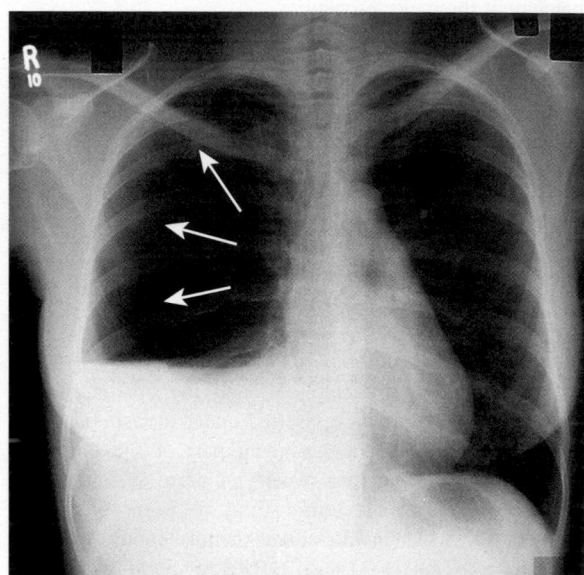

Fig. 19.61   Haemopneumothorax. Chest X-ray of a patient with a right traumatic haemopneumothorax showing the characteristic visceral pleural line displaced from the chest wall (arrows), together with free fluid within the pleural cavity (not seen in patients with uncomplicated spontaneous pneumothorax).

Management

Primary pneumothorax where the lung edge is less than 2 cm from the chest wall and the patient is not breathless normally resolves without intervention. In young patients presenting with a moderate or large spontaneous primary pneumothorax, percutaneous needle aspiration of air is a simple and well-tolerated alternative to intercostal tube drainage, with a 60–80% chance of avoiding the need for a chest drain (Fig. 19.62). In patients with underlying chronic lung disease, however, even a small secondary pneumothorax may cause respiratory failure; hence all such patients require intercostal tube drainage and inpatient observation. When needed, intercostal drains should be inserted in the 4th, 5th or 6th intercostal space in the mid-axillary line following blunt dissection through to the parietal pleura.

19

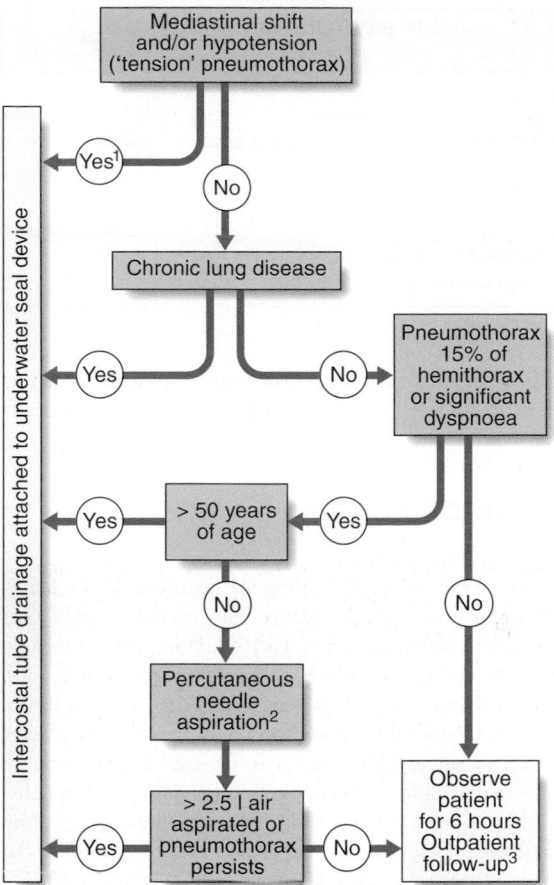

Fig. 19.62   Management of spontaneous pneumothorax.
(1) Immediate decompression is required prior to insertion of intercostal drain. (2) Aspirate in the 2nd intercostal space anteriorly in the mid-clavicular line using a 16 F cannula; discontinue if resistance is felt, the patient coughs excessively, or > 2.5 litres of air are removed. (3) Beware: the post-aspiration chest X-ray is not a reliable indicator of whether a pleural leak remains and hence all patients should be told to attend again immediately in the event of noticeable deterioration.

The tube should be advanced in an apical direction, connected to an underwater seal or one-way Heimlich valve, and secured firmly to the chest wall. Clamping of the drain is potentially dangerous and never indicated. The drain should be removed 24 hours after the lung has fully reinflated and bubbling stopped. Continued bubbling after 5–7 days is an indication for surgery. If bubbling in the underwater bottle stops prior to full reinflation, the tube is either blocked, kinked or displaced. All patients should receive supplemental oxygen as this accelerates the rate at which air is reabsorbed by the pleura.

Patients with a closed pneumothorax should not fly as the trapped gas expands at altitude. After complete resolution, there is no clear evidence on how long patients should avoid flying, although guidelines suggest that a wait of 1–2 weeks, with confirmation of full inflation prior to flight, is prudent. Patients should also be advised to stop smoking and be informed about the risks of a recurrent pneumothorax.

Recurrent spontaneous pneumothorax

After primary spontaneous pneumothorax, recurrence occurs within a year of either aspiration or tube drainage in approximately 25% of patients, and should prompt definitive treatment. Surgical pleurodesis is recommended in all patients following a second pneumothorax (even if ipsilateral) and should be considered following the first episode of secondary pneumothorax if low respiratory reserve makes recurrence hazardous. Pleurodesis can be achieved by pleural abrasion or parietal pleurectomy at thoracotomy or thoracoscopy. Patients who plan to continue activities where pneumothorax would be particularly dangerous (e.g. flying or diving) should also undergo definitive treatment after the first episode of a primary spontaneous pneumothorax.

ASBESTOS-RELATED PLEURAL DISEASE

Benign pleural plaques

These areas of pleural thickening do not produce clinical symptoms and are usually identified on routine chest X-ray. They are often calcified and in the early stage are best seen on oblique films. They are most commonly observed on the diaphragm and anterolateral pleural surfaces (Fig. 19.63).

Benign pleural effusion

This is considered to be a specific asbestos-related entity and may be associated with pleural pain, fever and leucocytosis. The pleural liquid may be blood-stained, and differentiation of this benign condition from a malignant effusion caused by mesothelioma can be difficult. The disease is self-limiting but may cause diffuse pleural fibrosis, which sometimes leads to breathlessness.

Diffuse pleural fibrosis

Diffuse pleural fibrosis is an important pleural manifestation of asbestos fibre inhalation and can restrict chest expansion

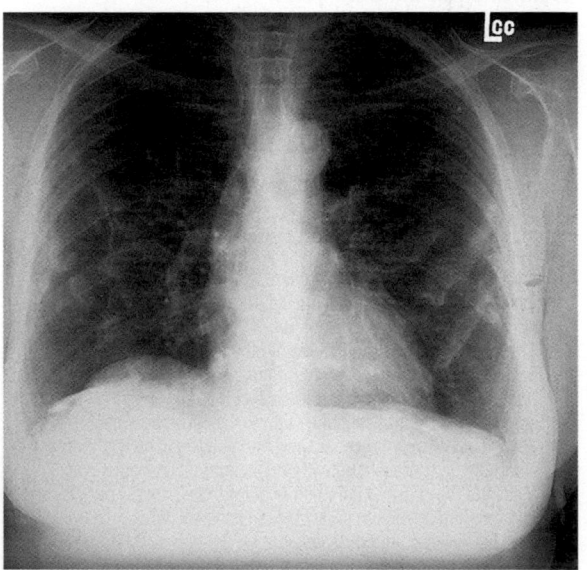

Fig. 19.63   Asbestos-related benign pleural plaques. Chest X-ray showing extensive calcified pleural plaques ('candle wax' appearance), particularly marked on the diaphragm and lateral pleural surfaces.

and cause breathlessness. The restrictive defect caused by diffuse pleural fibrosis tends to progress and, like asbestosis and mesothelioma, qualifies a patient for industrial injury benefit in many countries.

Mesothelioma

Mesothelioma is a malignant tumour affecting the pleura (pleural mesothelioma) or, less commonly, the peritoneum (peritoneal mesothelioma). Although all fibre types are implicated, crocidolite appears to be the most potent cause of mesothelioma. A time lag of 20 years or more between asbestos exposure and the development of mesothelioma is typical. The incidence of this tumour has increased markedly over the past 20 years and this trend is predicted to continue until 2010. Asbestos exposure is also a recognised risk factor for the development of bronchogenic carcinoma.

Clinical presentation is frequently with chest pain. A pleural effusion, often blood-stained, may develop and cause breathlessness. Histological diagnosis is difficult and generous (often surgical) pleural biopsies are needed. Surgical resection is rarely successful and most tumours are resistant to chemotherapy. Radiotherapy is, however, effective in preventing tumour growth through previous chest drain or biopsy sites. There is no curative treatment and chest wall pain is often difficult to control.

DISEASES OF THE DIAPHRAGM

CONGENITAL DISORDERS

Diaphragmatic hernias

Congenital defects of the diaphragm can allow herniation of abdominal viscera. Posteriorly situated hernias through the foramen of Bochdalek are more common than anterior hernias through the foramen of Morgagni.

Eventration of the diaphragm

Abnormal elevation or bulging of one hemidiaphragm, more often the left, results from total or partial absence of muscular development of the septum transversum. Most eventrations are asymptomatic and are detected by chance

---

19.108 PLEURAL DISEASE IN OLD AGE

- **Spontaneous pneumothorax**: invariably associated with underlying lung disease in old age, and has a significant mortality. Surgical or chemical pleurodesis is advised in all such patients.
- **Rib fracture**: a common cause of pleural-type pain. It may be spontaneous (due to coughing), traumatic or pathological. Underlying osteomalacia may contribute to poor healing, especially in the housebound with no exposure to sunlight.
- **TB**: should always be considered and actively excluded in any elderly patient presenting with a unilateral pleural effusion.
- **Mesothelioma**: more common in older than younger people due to a long latency between asbestos exposure (often > 20 years) and the development of disease.
- **Analgesia:** frail older people are particularly sensitive to the respiratory depressant effects of opiate-based analgesia and careful monitoring is required when using these agents for pleural pain.

19.109 CAUSES OF ELEVATION OF A HEMIDIAPHRAGM

- Phrenic nerve paralysis
- Eventration of the diaphragm
- Decrease in volume of one lung (e.g. lobectomy, unilateral pulmonary fibrosis)
- Severe pleuritic pain
- Pulmonary infarction
- Subphrenic abscess
- Large volume of gas in the stomach or colon
- Large tumours or cysts of the liver

---

on X-ray in adult life, but severe respiratory distress can be caused in infancy if the diaphragmatic muscular defect is extensive.

ACQUIRED DISORDERS

Diaphragmatic paralysis

Phrenic nerve damage leading to paralysis of a hemi-diaphragm may be idiopathic but is most often due to bronchial carcinoma (Box 19.109). Other causes include disease of cervical vertebrae, tumours of the cervical cord, shingles, trauma including road traffic and birth injuries, surgery and stretching of the nerve by mediastinal masses and aortic aneurysms. Paralysis of one hemidiaphragm results in loss of approximately 20% of ventilatory capacity, but this is not usually noticed by otherwise healthy individuals. Diagnosis is suggested by elevation of the hemidiaphragm on chest X-ray and is confirmed by using screening ultrasound to demonstrate paradoxical upward movement of the paralysed hemidiaphragm on sniffing.

Bilateral diaphragmatic weakness occurs in peripheral neuropathies of any type including Guillain–Barré syndrome, in disorders affecting the anterior horn cells, e.g. poliomyelitis (pp. 1249 and 1230), in muscular dystrophies and in connective tissue disorders such as SLE and polymyositis (pp. 1132 and 1136).

Other acquired diaphragmatic disorders

Hiatus hernia is common (p. 878). Diaphragmatic rupture is usually caused by a crush injury and may not be detected until years later. Respiratory disorders which cause pulmonary hyperinflation, e.g. emphysema, and those which result in small stiff lungs, e.g. diffuse pulmonary fibrosis, decrease diaphragmatic efficiency and predispose to fatigue. Severe skeletal deformity, such as kyphosis, causes gross distortion of diaphragmatic muscle configuration and gross mechanical disadvantage.

DEFORMITIES OF THE CHEST WALL

THORACIC KYPHOSCOLIOSIS

Abnormalities of alignment of the dorsal spine and their consequent effects on thoracic shape may be caused by:

- congenital abnormality
- vertebral disease, including TB, osteoporosis and ankylosing spondylitis

- trauma
- neuromuscular disease such as poliomyelitis.

Simple kyphosis causes less pulmonary embarrassment than kyphoscoliosis.

Kyphoscoliosis, if severe, restricts and distorts expansion of the chest wall, causing maldistribution of ventilation and blood flow in the lungs and impaired diaphragmatic function. Patients with severe deformity may develop type II respiratory failure (initially manifest during sleep), pulmonary hypertension and right ventricular failure; such patients can often be successfully treated with nocturnal and, if necessary, daytime non-invasive ventilatory support (p. 669).

PECTUS EXCAVATUM

In pectus excavatum (funnel chest) the body of the sternum, usually only the lower end, is curved backwards. The heart is displaced to the left and may be compressed between the sternum and the vertebral column; only rarely is there associated disturbance of cardiac function. The deformity may restrict chest expansion and reduce vital capacity. Operative correction is usually only indicated for cosmetic reasons.

PECTUS CARINATUM

Pectus carinatum (pigeon chest) is frequently caused by severe asthma during childhood. Very occasionally, this deformity can be produced by rickets or be idiopathic.

FURTHER INFORMATION

Books and journal articles
American Thoracic Society and European Respiratory Society. Multidisciplinary consensus classification of the idiopathic interstitial pneumonias. American Journal of Respiratory and Critical Care Medicine 2002; 165:277–304.

Fergusson R, Hill A, MacKay T, et al., eds. The year in respiratory medicine. Oxford: Clinical. *A series of books published yearly summarising many of the most important publications in respiratory medicine for that year.*

Gibson GJ, Geddes DM, Costabel U, et al. Respiratory medicine. 3rd edn. London: WB Saunders; 2003.

Goldhaber SZ. Pulmonary embolism. Lancet 2004; 9417:1295–1305. *An up-to-date review of the literature on pulmonary embolism.*

National Collaborating Centre for Chronic Conditions. Chronic obstructive pulmonary disease. National clinical guideline on management of chronic obstructive pulmonary disease in adults in primary and secondary care. Thorax 2004; 59:suppt 1.

Nunn A, ed. Nunn's applied respiratory physiology. 6th edn. Oxford: Butterworth–Heinemann, 2005. *A comprehensive, clinically orientated textbook of respiratory physiology.*

Workshop report. Global strategy for asthma management and prevention. Updated October 2004. *Evidence-based guidelines for asthma management and prevention, with citations from the scientific literature.*

World Health Organization. Tuberculosis: a manual for medical students. WHO/CDS/TB/99.272. *A comprehensive overview of tuberculosis and its management. This document can be accessed through the WHO tuberculosis website.*

Websites
www.agius.com *A useful website compiled by Professor Agius to gain more information on health, work and the environment.*
www.asthma.org.uk *National Asthma Campaign.*
www.brit-thoracic.org.uk *Website of the British Thoracic Society providing access to guidelines on a wide range of respiratory conditions.*
www.bsaci.org *British Society for Allergy and Clinical Immunology.*
www.ersnet.org *European Respiratory Society.*
www.ginasthma.com *Global Initiative for Asthma website providing a comprehensive overview of asthma.*
www.goldcopd.com *Global Initiative for Chronic Obstructive Lung Disease website containing a comprehensive overview of COPD.*
www.lunguk.org *British Lung Foundation.*
www.sign.ac.uk *Royal College website containing guidelines on many respiratory diseases including asthma, sleep apnoea and lung cancer.*
www.thoracic.org *American Thoracic Society.*
www.who.int *World Health Organization.*

19

M.W.J. STRACHAN

B.R. WALKER

Endocrine disease

CLINICAL EXAMINATION IN ENDOCRINE DISEASE

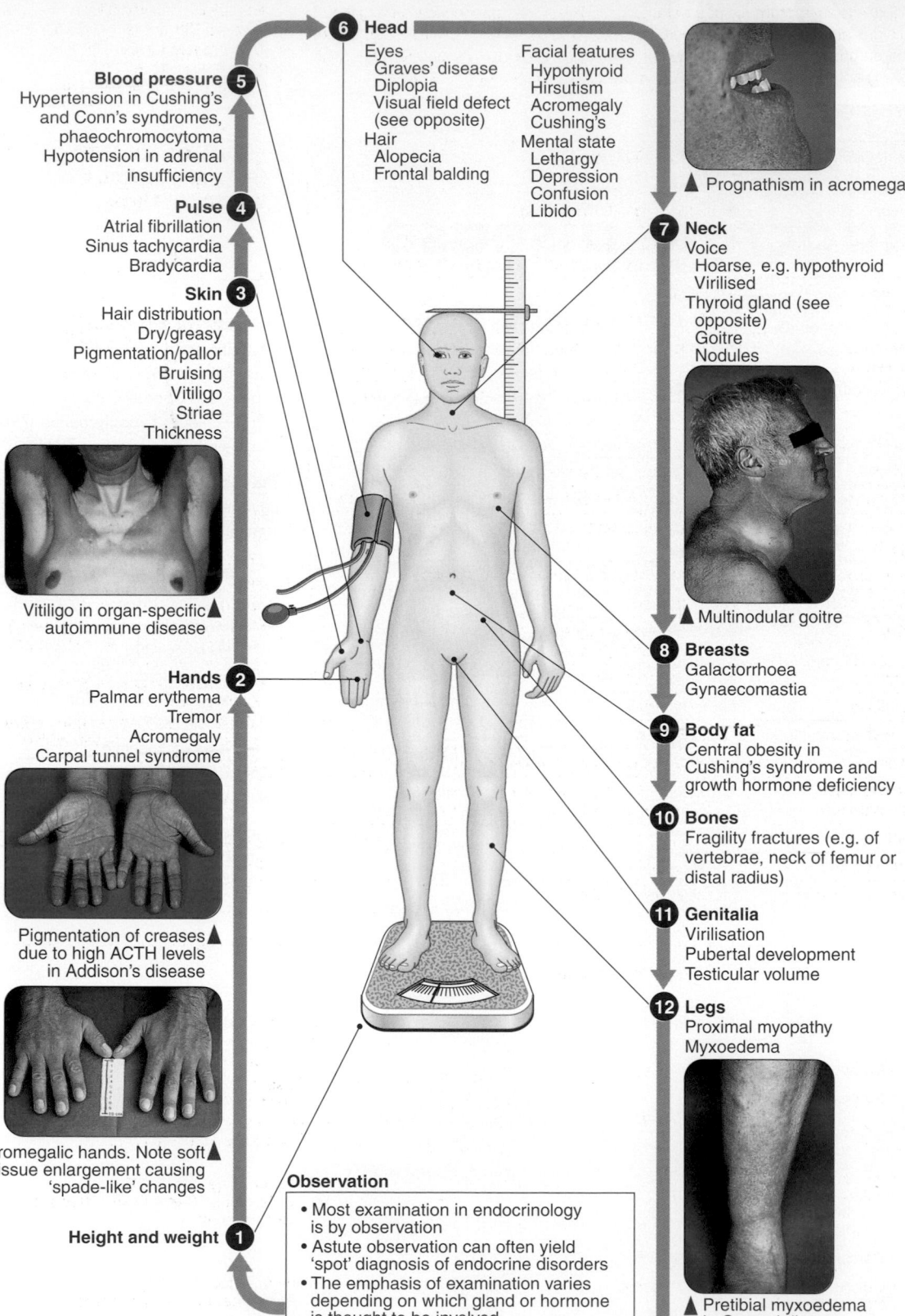

6 Head

Eyes
  Graves' disease
  Diplopia
  Visual field defect
  (see opposite)
Hair
  Alopecia
  Frontal balding

Facial features
  Hypothyroid
  Hirsutism
  Acromegaly
  Cushing's
Mental state
  Lethargy
  Depression
  Confusion
  Libido

▲ Prognathism in acromegaly

5 Blood pressure
Hypertension in Cushing's
and Conn's syndromes,
phaeochromocytoma
Hypotension in adrenal
insufficiency

4 Pulse
Atrial fibrillation
Sinus tachycardia
Bradycardia

7 Neck
Voice
  Hoarse, e.g. hypothyroid
  Virilised
Thyroid gland (see
  opposite)
  Goitre
  Nodules

3 Skin
Hair distribution
Dry/greasy
Pigmentation/pallor
Bruising
Vitiligo
Striae
Thickness

Vitiligo in organ-specific ▲
autoimmune disease

▲ Multinodular goitre

8 Breasts
Galactorrhoea
Gynaecomastia

2 Hands
Palmar erythema
Tremor
Acromegaly
Carpal tunnel syndrome

9 Body fat
Central obesity in
Cushing's syndrome and
growth hormone deficiency

10 Bones
Fragility fractures (e.g. of
vertebrae, neck of femur or
distal radius)

Pigmentation of creases ▲
due to high ACTH levels
in Addison's disease

11 Genitalia
Virilisation
Pubertal development
Testicular volume

12 Legs
Proximal myopathy
Myxoedema

Acromegalic hands. Note soft ▲
tissue enlargement causing
'spade-like' changes

1 Height and weight

Observation

• Most examination in endocrinology
  is by observation
• Astute observation can often yield
  'spot' diagnosis of endocrine disorders
• The emphasis of examination varies
  depending on which gland or hormone
  is thought to be involved

▲ Pretibial myxoedema
in Graves' disease

Patients with endocrine disease present in many ways, and to many different specialists, reflecting the diverse effects of hormone deficiency and excess. Presenting symptoms are often non-specific (below) and long-standing. In many patients, endocrine disease is asymptomatic and detected only by routine biochemical testing (right). Clinical signs are also diverse (opposite) and the emphasis of the clinical examination depends on the gland or hormone which is thought to be abnormal. Diabetes mellitus (Ch. 21) and thyroid disease are the most common endocrine diseases.

COMMON ASYMPTOMATIC BIOCHEMICAL ABNORMALITIES

- Subclinical hypothyroidism (raised TSH, normal T_4—p. 752)
- Hyperglycaemia (Ch. 21)
- Hypercalcaemia (p. 772)
- Hyperprolactinaemia (p. 799)

COMMON PRESENTING SYMPTOMS OF ENDOCRINE DISEASE

Symptom	Most likely endocrine disorder(s)
Lethargy and depression	Hypothyroidism, diabetes mellitus, hyperparathyroidism, hypogonadism, adrenal insufficiency, Cushing's syndrome
Weight gain	Hypothyroidism, Cushing's syndrome
Weight loss	Thyrotoxicosis, adrenal insufficiency, diabetes mellitus
Amenorrhoea/ oligomenorrhoea	Menopause, polycystic ovarian syndrome, hyperprolactinaemia, thyrotoxicosis, premature ovarian failure, Cushing's syndrome
Polyuria and polydipsia	Diabetes mellitus, diabetes insipidus, hyperparathyroidism, Conn's syndrome
Heat intolerance	Thyrotoxicosis, menopause
Palpitations	Thyrotoxicosis, phaeochromocytoma
Thyroid nodule	Solitary thyroid nodule, dominant nodule in multinodular goitre
Generalised thyroid enlargement	Simple goitre (nodular or diffuse), Graves' disease, Hashimoto's thyroiditis
Pain over thyroid	Haemorrhage into nodule, de Quervain's thyroiditis
Prominence of eyes	Graves' disease
Hirsutism	Idiopathic, polycystic ovarian syndrome, congenital adrenal hyperplasia, Cushing's syndrome
Galactorrhoea	Hyperprolactinaemia
Loss of libido	Male hypogonadism
Visual dysfunction	Pituitary tumour
Headache	Acromegaly, pituitary tumour, phaeochromocytoma
Muscle weakness (usually proximal)	Thyrotoxicosis, Cushing's syndrome, hypokalaemia (e.g. Conn's syndrome), hyperparathyroidism, hypogonadism
Paraesthesiae and tetany	Hypoparathyroidism
Recurrent ureteric colic	Hyperparathyroidism
Coarsening of features	Acromegaly, hypothyroidism

❻ EXAMINATION OF THE VISUAL FIELDS BY CONFRONTATION

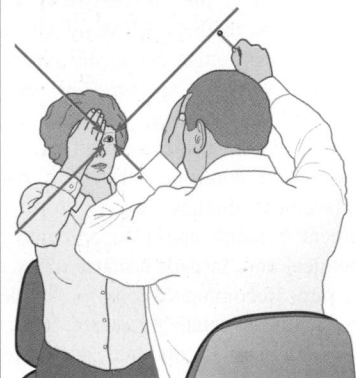

- Sit opposite patient
- You and patient cover opposite eyes
- Bring red pin (or wiggling finger) slowly into view from extreme of your vision, as shown
- Ask patient to say 'now' when it comes into view
- Continue to move pin into centre of vision and ask patient to tell you if it disappears
- Repeat in each of four quadrants
- Repeat in other eye

A bitemporal hemianopia is the classical finding in pituitary macroadenomas (p. 797)

20

❼ EXAMINATION OF THE THYROID GLAND

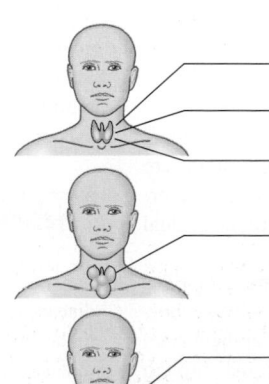

- **Inspect** from front to side

- **Palpate** from behind
  Thyroid moves on swallowing
  Cervical lymph nodes
  Tracheal deviation

- **Auscultate** for bruit
  Ask patient to hold breath
  If present, check for radiating murmur

- **Percuss** for retrosternal thyroid

- Consider systemic signs of thyroid dysfunction (Box 20.6)

Abnormal findings

Diffuse soft goitre with bruit
Graves' disease (p. 754)

Diffuse firm goitre
Hashimoto's thyroiditis (p. 757)

Diffuse tender goitre
Subacute thyroiditis (p. 757)

Multinodular goitre (p.759)
± Retrosternal extension, tracheal compression

Solitary nodule (p. 753)
Adenoma, cyst or carcinoma

Cervical lymphadenopathy
Suggests carcinoma

Endocrinology concerns the synthesis, secretion and action of hormones. These are chemical messengers which have diverse molecular structures, are released from endocrine glands and coordinate the activities of many different cells. Endocrine disease, therefore, has a wide range of manifestations affecting many other major organs. This chapter describes the principles of endocrinology before dealing with diseases of each gland in turn.

Some endocrine diseases are common, particularly those of the thyroid gland, reproductive system and β cells of the pancreas (Ch. 21). For example, thyroid dysfunction occurs in more than 10% of the population in areas with iodine deficiency, e.g. the Himalayas, and 4% of women aged 20–50 years in the UK. Many rare endocrine syndromes present a particular diagnostic challenge to primary care clinicians who may see very few such patients during their working lives. These are described later in the chapter.

Few endocrine therapies have been evaluated by randomised controlled trials, in part because hormone replacement therapy (e.g. with thyroxine) has obvious clinical benefits and placebo-controlled trials would be unethical and, in part, because many endocrine syndromes are rare. Recommendations for 'evidence-based medicine' are, therefore, relatively scarce. They relate mainly to use of therapy that is 'optional' and/or recently available, e.g. oestrogen replacement in post-menopausal women and growth hormone replacement.

FUNCTIONAL ANATOMY, PHYSIOLOGY AND INVESTIGATIONS

MAJOR ENDOCRINE FUNCTIONS AND ANATOMY

Although some endocrine glands (e.g. parathyroid glands and pancreas) respond directly to metabolic signals, most are controlled by hormones released from the pituitary gland. Anterior pituitary hormone secretion is controlled in turn by substances produced in the hypothalamus and released into portal blood which drains directly down the pituitary stalk (Fig. 20.1). Posterior pituitary hormones are synthesised in the hypothalamus and transported down nerve axons to be released from the posterior pituitary. Hormone release in the hypothalamus and pituitary is regulated by numerous stimuli of nervous, metabolic, physical or hormonal origin, in particular feedback control by hormones produced by the target glands (thyroid, adrenal cortex and gonads). These integrated endocrine systems are called 'axes', and are listed in Figure 20.2. The characteristics of each axis are described in relation to individual glands later in this chapter.

A wide variety of molecules act as hormones. Peptides (e.g. insulin), glycoproteins (e.g. thyroid-stimulating hormone, TSH) and amines (e.g. noradrenaline/norepinephrine) act on specific cell surface receptors which signal through G-proteins and/or enzymes on the cytosolic side of the plasma membrane. Other hormones (e.g. steroids, triiodothyronine and vitamin D) bind to specific intracellular

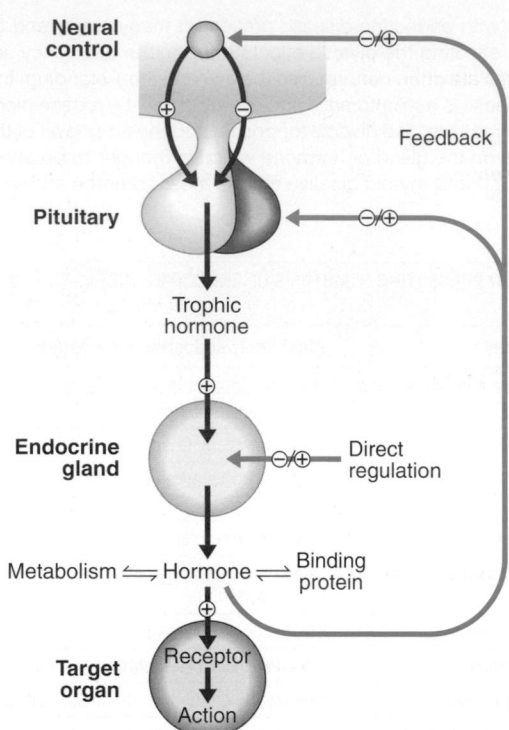

Fig. 20.1 An archetypal endocrine axis. Regulation by negative feedback and direct control is shown along with the equilibrium between active circulating free hormone and bound or metabolised hormone.

receptors which in turn bind to response elements on DNA to regulate gene transcription (p. 39).

The classical model of endocrine function involves hormones which are synthesised in endocrine glands, are released into the circulation, and act at sites distant from those of secretion (as in Fig. 20.1). However, additional levels of complex regulation have now been recognised. Thus, most major organs also secrete hormones or contribute to the peripheral metabolism and activation of prohormones; many hormones act on adjacent cells (paracrine system, e.g. neurotransmitters), or even back on the cell of origin (autocrine system); and the sensitivity of target tissues is regulated in a tissue-specific fashion. The clinical implications of this complexity of hormone action are only now being appreciated, and have led to the development of new therapies (e.g. 5α-reductase inhibitors which prevent activation of androgens within prostate; and aromatase inhibitors which prevent oestrogen generation in breast cancer).

ENDOCRINE PATHOLOGY

For each endocrine axis or major gland in this chapter, diseases can be classified as shown in Box 20.1. Note that pathology arising within the gland is often called 'primary' disease (e.g. primary hypothyroidism in Hashimoto's thyroiditis) while abnormal stimulation of the gland is often called 'secondary' disease (e.g. secondary hypothyroidism in patients with pituitary tumour and TSH deficiency). In

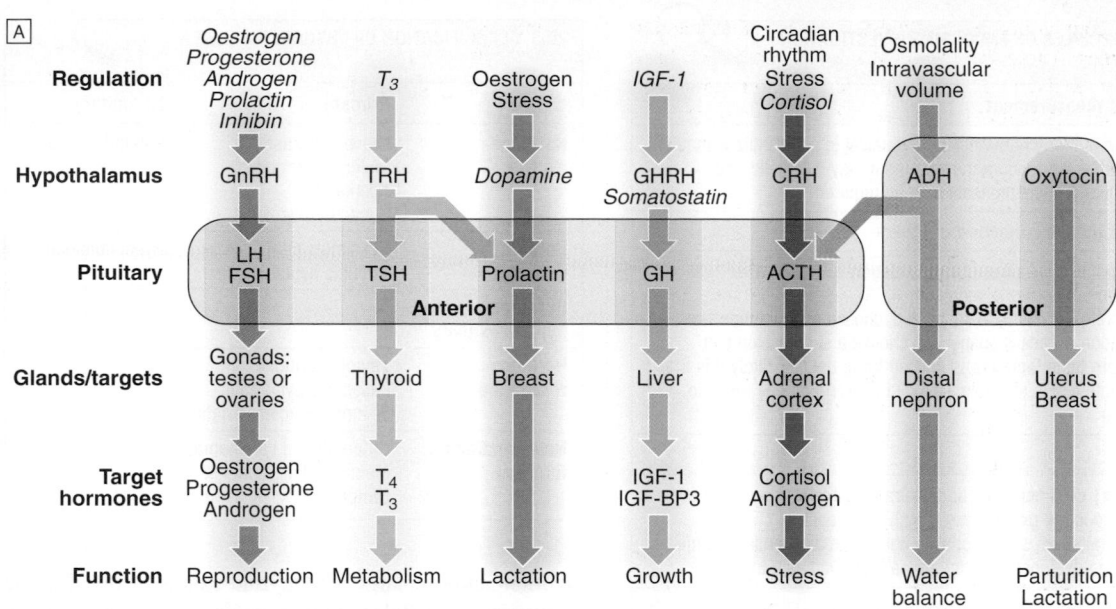

A

Regulation	Oestrogen Progesterone Androgen Prolactin Inhibin	T_3	Oestrogen Stress	IGF-1	Circadian rhythm Stress Cortisol	Osmolality Intravascular volume	
Hypothalamus	GnRH	TRH	Dopamine	GHRH Somatostatin	CRH	ADH	Oxytocin
Pituitary	LH FSH	TSH	Prolactin	GH	ACTH		
	Anterior					Posterior	
Glands/targets	Gonads: testes or ovaries	Thyroid	Breast	Liver	Adrenal cortex	Distal nephron	Uterus Breast
Target hormones	Oestrogen Progesterone Androgen	T_4 T_3		IGF-1 IGF-BP3	Cortisol Androgen		
Function	Reproduction	Metabolism	Lactation	Growth	Stress	Water balance	Parturition Lactation

20

B

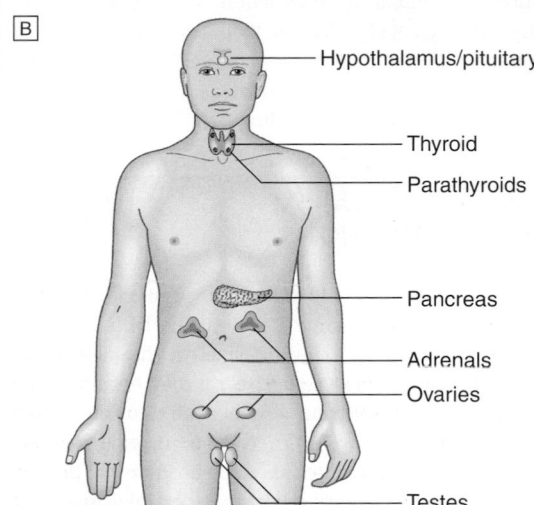

- Hypothalamus/pituitary
- Thyroid
- Parathyroids
- Pancreas
- Adrenals
- Ovaries
- Testes

Fig. 20.2 The principal endocrine 'axes' and glands. A Endocrine axes. Some major endocrine glands are not controlled by the pituitary. These include the parathyroid glands (regulated by calcium concentrations, p. 771), the adrenal zona glomerulosa (regulated by the renin–angiotensin system, p. 777) and the endocrine pancreas (Ch. 21 and p. 789). Italics show negative regulation. (ACTH = adrenocorticotrophic hormone; ADH = antidiuretic hormone, arginine vasopressin; CRH = corticotrophin-releasing hormone; FSH = follicle-stimulating hormone; GH = growth hormone; GHRH = growth hormone-releasing hormone; GnRH = gonadotrophin-releasing hormone; IGF-1 = insulin-like growth factor-1; IGF-BP3 = IGF-binding protein-3; LH = luteinising hormone; T_3 = triiodothyronine; T_4 = thyroxine; TRH = thyrotrophin-releasing hormone; TSH = thyroid-stimulating hormone) **B** Endocrine glands.

20.1 CLASSIFICATION OF ENDOCRINE DISEASE

Hormone excess

- Primary gland over-production
- Secondary to excess trophic substance

Hormone deficiency

- Primary gland failure
- Secondary to deficient trophic hormone

Hormone hypersensitivity

- Failure of inactivation of hormone
- Target organ over-activity/hypersensitivity

Hormone resistance

- Failure of activation of hormone
- Target organ resistance

Non-functioning tumours

addition to these gland-specific disorders, there are two pathologies which affect multiple glands (p. 802): organ-specific autoimmune diseases (which are common) and multiple endocrine neoplasia syndromes (which are rare).

INVESTIGATION OF ENDOCRINE DISEASE

An understanding of biochemical investigations is important in endocrinology. Most hormones can be measured in blood, but the circumstances in which the sample is taken are often crucial, especially for hormones with pulsatile secretion (e.g. growth hormone) or marked physiological variation (e.g. diurnal variation of cortisol, or monthly variation of sex steroids in pre-menopausal women). Other investigations (e.g. imaging and biopsy) are usually reserved for patients who present with a tumour (e.g. in thyroid or pituitary) or in whom the biochemical diagnosis has already been made.

20.2 PRINCIPLES OF ENDOCRINE INVESTIGATION

Timing of measurement

- Release of many hormones is rhythmical (e.g. pulsatile, circadian or monthly), so random measurement may be invalid and sequential or dynamic tests may be required

Choice of dynamic biochemical tests

- Abnormalities are often characterised by loss of normal regulation of hormone secretion
- If hormone deficiency is suspected, choose a stimulation test
- If hormone excess is suspected, choose a suppression test
- The more tests there are to choose from, the less likely it is that any single test is infallible, so avoid interpreting one result in isolation

Imaging

- Secretory cells also take up substrates, which can be labelled
- Most endocrine glands have a high prevalence of 'incidentalomas', so do not scan unless the biochemistry confirms endocrine dysfunction or the primary problem is a tumour

Biopsy

- Many endocrine tumours are difficult to classify histologically (e.g. adrenal carcinoma and adenoma)

The principles of investigation are shown in Box 20.2. The choice of test is often pragmatic; some tests are intellectually attractive, but clinical studies have shown them to have poor predictive value (e.g. the metyrapone test in Cushing's syndrome); local access to reliable sampling facilities and laboratory measurements is an important consideration. Specific tests are described in relation to individual glands in the following sections. Approximate adult reference values for hormone concentrations are given in the Appendix.

PRESENTING PROBLEMS IN ENDOCRINE DISEASE

As illustrated above (p. 741), endocrine diseases present in many different ways. Classical syndromes are described in relation to individual glands in the following sections. The most common classical presentations are of thyroid disease, reproductive disorders and hypercalcaemia. In addition, endocrine diseases are often part of the differential diagnosis of common complaints discussed in other chapters of this book, including electrolyte abnormalities (Ch. 16), hypertension (Ch. 18), obesity (Ch. 5) and osteoporosis (Ch. 25). Although diseases of the adrenal glands, hypothalamus and pituitary are relatively rare, their diagnosis often relies on astute clinical observation in a patient with non-specific complaints, so it is important that clinicians are familiar with their key features.

THE THYROID GLAND

Diseases of the thyroid are classified in Box 20.3. These are common, affecting some 5% of the population,

20.3 CLASSIFICATION OF THYROID DISEASE

	Primary	Secondary
Hormone excess	Graves' disease Multinodular goitre Adenoma Subacute thyroiditis	Pituitary TSHoma
Hormone deficiency	Hashimoto's thyroiditis Atrophic hypothyroidism	Hypopituitarism
Hormone hypersensitivity	–	
Hormone resistance	Thyroid hormone resistance syndrome 5'-monodeiodinase deficiency	
Non-functioning tumours	Differentiated carcinoma Medullary carcinoma Lymphoma	

predominantly females. The thyroid axis is involved in the regulation of cellular differentiation and metabolism in virtually all nucleated cells, so that disorders of thyroid function have diverse manifestations. In addition, structural diseases in the thyroid gland, such as goitre, commonly occur without abnormal thyroid function.

FUNCTIONAL ANATOMY, PHYSIOLOGY AND INVESTIGATIONS

Thyroid physiology is illustrated in Figure 20.3. The parafollicular C cells secrete calcitonin, which is of no apparent physiological significance in humans. The follicular epithelial cells synthesise thyroid hormones by incorporating iodine into the amino acid tyrosine on the surface of thyroglobulin (Tg), a protein secreted into the colloid of the follicle. Iodide is a key substrate for thyroid hormone synthesis; a dietary intake in excess of 100 µg/day is required to maintain thyroid function in adults. The thyroid secretes predominantly thyroxine (T_4), and only a small amount of triiodothyronine (T_3); approximately 85% of T_3 in blood is produced from T_4 by a family of monodeiodinase enzymes which are active in many tissues including liver, muscle, heart and kidney. T_4 can be regarded as a pro-hormone, since it has a longer half-life in blood than T_3 (~1 week compared with ~18 hours) and binds and activates thyroid hormone receptors less effectively than T_3. T_4 can also be converted to the inactive metabolite, reverse T_3.

T_3 and T_4 circulate in plasma almost entirely (> 99%) bound to transport proteins, mainly thyroxine-binding globulin (TBG). It is the unbound or free hormones which diffuse into tissues and exert diverse metabolic actions. While it is possible to measure the concentration of total or free T_3 and T_4 in plasma, the advantage of the free hormone measurements is that they are not influenced by changes in the concentration of binding proteins; in pregnancy, for example, TBG levels are increased and total T_3 and T_4 may be raised, but free thyroid hormone levels are normal.

Production of T_3 and T_4 in the thyroid is stimulated by thyrotrophin (thyroid-stimulating hormone, TSH), a

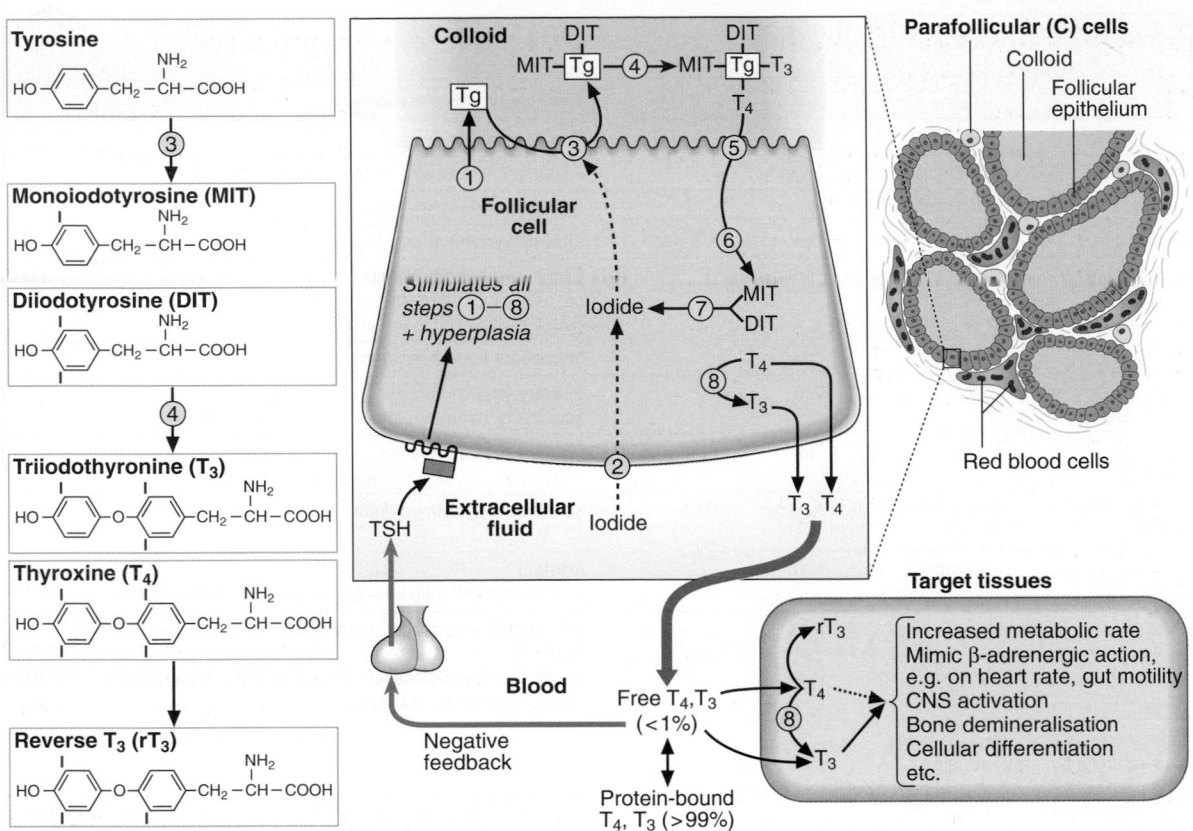

Fig. 20.3 Structure and function of the thyroid gland. (1) Thyroglobulin (Tg) is synthesised and secreted into the colloid of the follicle. (2) Inorganic iodide (I⁻) is actively transported into the follicular cell ('trapping'). (3) Iodide is transported on to the colloidal surface by a transporter (pendrin, defective in Pendred's syndrome) and 'organified' by the thyroid peroxidase enzyme, which incorporates it into the amino acid tyrosine on the surface of Tg to form monoiodotyrosine (MIT) and diiodotyrosine (DIT). (4) Iodinated tyrosines couple to form T_3 and T_4. (5) Tg is endocytosed. (6) Tg is cleaved by proteolysis to free the iodinated tyrosine and thyroid hormones. (7) Iodinated tyrosine is dehalogenated to recycle the iodide. (8) T_4 is converted to T_3 by 5′-monodeiodinase.

glycoprotein released from the thyrotroph cells of the anterior pituitary in response to the hypothalamic tripeptide, thyrotrophin-releasing hormone (TRH, p. 743). A circadian rhythm of TSH secretion can be demonstrated with a peak at 0100 hrs and trough at 1100 hrs, but the variation is small so that thyroid function can be assessed reliably from a single blood sample taken at any time of day and does not usually require any dynamic stimulation or suppression tests. There is a negative feedback of thyroid hormones on the hypothalamus and pituitary such that in thyrotoxicosis, when plasma concentrations of T_3 and T_4 are raised, TSH secretion is suppressed. Conversely, in hypothyroidism due to disease of the thyroid gland, low T_3 and T_4 are associated with high circulating TSH levels. The anterior pituitary is very sensitive to minor changes in thyroid hormone levels within the normal range. Although the reference range for free T_4 is 10–27 pmol/l (0.7–2.10 ng/dl), a rise or fall of 5 pmol/l in an individual in whom the level is usually 20 pmol/l would be associated on the one hand with undetectable TSH, and on the other hand with a raised TSH. For this reason, TSH is usually regarded as the most useful investigation of thyroid function. However, interpretation of TSH values without considering thyroid hormone levels may be misleading in patients with pituitary disease.

Moreover, TSH may take several weeks to 'catch up' with T_4 and T_3 levels, e.g. after prolonged suppression of TSH in thyrotoxicosis is relieved by antithyroid therapy. Common patterns of abnormal thyroid function test results and their interpretation are shown in Box 20.4.

Other modalities commonly employed in the investigation of thyroid disease include measurement of antibodies against the TSH receptor or other thyroid antigens (Box 20.7, p. 749), radioisotope imaging, fine needle aspiration biopsy and ultrasound. Their use is described below.

PRESENTING PROBLEMS IN THYROID DISEASE

The most common presentations of thyroid disease are thyrotoxicosis (i.e. hyperthyroidism), hypothyroidism and goitre (i.e. enlargement of the thyroid). In addition, ready access to accurate tests of thyroid function and an increasing tendency to screen certain populations (e.g. elderly, hospitalised) have led to the identification of patients with abnormal results who are either asymptomatic or have non-specific complaints such as tiredness and weight gain.

20.4 PATTERNS OF THYROID FUNCTION TEST RESULTS

TSH	T_4	T_3	Most likely interpretation(s)
Undetectable	Raised	Raised	**Primary thyrotoxicosis**
Undetectable	Normal[1]	Raised	**Primary T_3-toxicosis**
Undetectable	Normal[1]	Normal[1]	**Subclinical thyrotoxicosis**
Undetectable	Raised	Low, normal or raised[2]	**Sick euthyroidism/non-thyroidal illness**
Undetectable	Low	Low	**Secondary hypothyroidism** i.e. pituitary or hypothalamic disease **Transient thyroiditis in evolution**
Normal	Low	Low[3]	**Secondary hypothyroidism**
Mildly elevated 5–20 mU/l	Low	Low[3]	**Primary hypothyroidism** **Secondary hypothyroidism**
Elevated > 20 mU/l	Low	Low[3]	**Primary hypothyroidism**
Mildly elevated 5–20 mU/l	Normal[4]	Normal[3]	**Subclinical hypothyroidism**
Elevated 20–500 mU/l	Normal	Normal	**Artefact** Endogenous IgG antibodies which interfere with TSH assay
Elevated	High	High	**Non-compliance with T_4 replacement**—recent 'loading' dose **Secondary thyrotoxicosis**—TSH-secreting pituitary tumour **Thyroid hormone resistance**

[1]Usually upper part of reference range.
[2]Depending on the assay system.
[3]T_3 is not a sensitive indicator of hypothyroidism and should not be requested.
[4]Usually lower part of normal range.

THYROTOXICOSIS

Aetiology

Causes of thyrotoxicosis are outlined in Box 20.5. In order to prescribe appropriate treatment it is clearly important to establish the aetiology and one approach is shown in Figure 20.4. In most patients, the thyrotoxicosis is due to Graves' disease, multinodular goitre or autonomously functioning thyroid nodule (toxic adenoma). The prevalence of thyroid-itis varies around the world according to likelihood of viral infections and therapy with amiodarone or iodine.

Clinical assessment

Manifestations of thyrotoxicosis are shown in Box 20.6 and key discriminatory features are highlighted in Figure 20.4. The most common symptoms are weight loss with a normal or increased appetite, heat intolerance, palpitations, tremor and irritability. Tachycardia, palmar erythema and lid lag are common signs. Not all patients have a palpable goitre, but experienced clinicians can discriminate the diffuse soft goitre of Graves' disease from the irregular enlargement of a multinodular goitre. All causes of thyrotoxicosis can cause lid retraction and lid lag due to potentiation of sympathetic innervation of the levator palpebrae muscles, but only Graves' disease causes other features of ophthalmopathy, including periorbital oedema, conjunctival irritation, exophthalmos and diplopia. Pretibial myxoedema (p. 740) and the rare thyroid acropachy (a periosteal hypertrophy

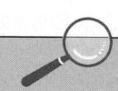

20.5 CAUSES OF THYROTOXICOSIS AND THEIR RELATIVE FREQUENCIES

Cause	Frequency[1] (%)
Graves' disease	76
Multinodular goitre	14
Autonomously functioning solitary thyroid nodule	5
Thyroiditis Subacute (de Quervain's)[2] Post-partum[2]	3 0.5
Iodide-induced Drugs (e.g. amiodarone)[2] Radiographic contrast media[2] Iodine prophylaxis programme[2]	1 – –
Extrathyroidal source of thyroid hormone Factitious hyperthyroidism[2] Struma ovarii[2,3]	0.2 –
TSH-induced TSH-secreting pituitary adenoma Choriocarcinoma and hydatidiform mole[4]	0.2 –
Follicular carcinoma ± metastases	0.1

[1]In a series of 2087 patients presenting to the Royal Infirmary, Edinburgh, over a 10-year period.
[2]Characterised by a negligible radio-iodine uptake test result.
[3]i.e. Ovarian teratoma containing thyroid tissue.
[4]Human chorionic gonadotrophin has thyroid-stimulating activity.

20

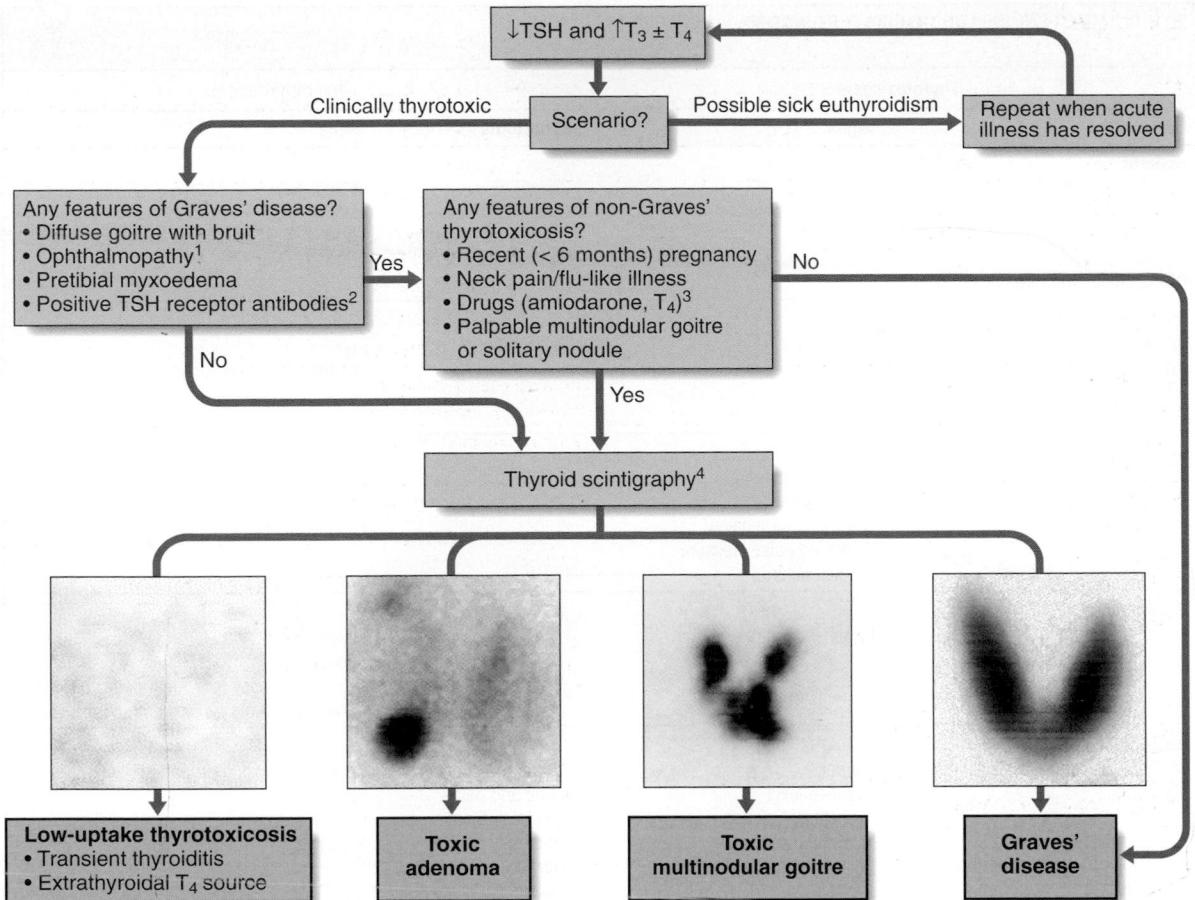

Fig. 20.4 Establishing the differential diagnosis in thyrotoxicosis. (1) Graves' ophthalmopathy refers to clinical features of exophthalmos, and periorbital and conjunctival oedema, not simply the lid lag and lid retraction which can occur in all forms of thyrotoxicosis. (2) TSH receptor antibodies are very rare in patients without autoimmune thyroid disease, but only occur in 80–95% of patients with Graves' disease; a positive test is therefore confirmatory, but a negative test does not exclude Graves' disease. Other thyroid antibodies (e.g. anti-peroxidase and anti-thyroglobulin antibodies) are unhelpful in the differential diagnosis since they occur frequently in the population and are found with several of the disorders which cause thyrotoxicosis. (3) Scintigraphy is not necessary in most cases of drug-induced thyrotoxicosis. (4) [99m]Technetium pertechnetate scans of patients with thyrotoxicosis. In Graves' disease there is diffuse uptake of isotope. In multinodular goitre there is relatively low, patchy uptake within the nodules; such an appearance is not always associated with a palpable thyroid. In a toxic adenoma there is lack of uptake of isotope by normal dormant gland due to suppression of serum TSH. In low-uptake thyrotoxicosis, most commonly due to a viral, post-partum or iodine-induced thyroiditis, there is negligible isotope detected in the region of the thyroid, although uptake is apparent in nearby salivary glands (not shown here).

indistinguishable from finger clubbing, p. 648) are also specific to Graves' disease.

Investigations

It is important to confirm the presence of thyrotoxicosis biochemically by more than one test of thyroid function in view of the likely need for prolonged medical treatment or destructive therapy. Serum T_3 and T_4 are elevated in the majority, but T_4 is in the upper part of the normal range and T_3 raised (T_3 toxicosis) in 5% of patients. In primary thyrotoxicosis, serum TSH is undetectable at less than 0.05 mU/l. Further tests, which may be required to establish the aetiology of thyrotoxicosis, include measurement of TSH receptor antibodies (TRAb, elevated in Graves' disease, Box 20.7) and isotope scanning (Fig. 20.4).

Other non-specific abnormalities are common (Box 20.8). An ECG may demonstrate atrial fibrillation (p. 562).

Radio-iodine uptake tests measure the proportion of isotope which is trapped in the whole gland, but have been largely superseded by [99m]technetium scintigraphy scans which also measure trapping, are quicker to perform with a lower dose of radioactivity, and provide a higher resolution image.

In low-uptake thyrotoxicosis, the cause is usually a transient thyroiditis (p. 757). Occasionally, patients induce 'factitious thyrotoxicosis' by consuming excessive amounts of a thyroid hormone preparation, most often thyroxine. The exogenous thyroxine suppresses pituitary TSH secretion and hence iodine uptake, serum thyroglobulin and release of endogenous thyroid hormones. The T_4:T_3 ratio (typically 30:1 in conventional thyrotoxicosis) is increased to above 70:1 because circulating T_3 in factitious thyrotoxicosis is derived exclusively from the peripheral monodeiodination of T_4 and not from thyroid secretion. The combination of

20

20

20.6 CLINICAL FEATURES OF THYROID DYSFUNCTION

Thyrotoxicosis		Hypothyroidism	
Symptoms	Signs	Symptoms	Signs
General			
Weight loss despite normal or *increased appetite*	*Weight loss*	*Weight gain*	*Weight gain*
Heat intolerance	Goitre with bruit[1]	*Cold intolerance*	Hoarse voice
Fatigue, apathy[2]		*Fatigue, somnolence*	Goitre
Osteoporosis (fracture, loss of height)		Hoarseness	
Gastrointestinal			
Diarrhoea, steatorrhoea, *hyperdefecation*		Constipation	Ileus[3]
Anorexia[2]			Ascites[3]
Vomiting[3]			
Cardiorespiratory			
Palpitations	*Sinus tachycardia*		Bradycardia
Dyspnoea on exertion	Atrial fibrillation		Hypertension
Angina	Systolic hypertension/ increased pulse pressure		Pericardial and pleural effusions[3]
Ankle swelling			
Exacerbation of asthma[3]	Cardiac failure		
Haematological			
	Lymphadenopathy[3]		Macrocytosis
			Anaemia
			Iron deficiency (pre-menopausal women)
			Normochromic
Neuromuscular			
Anxiety, *irritability, emotional lability,* psychosis	Tremor	*Carpal tunnel syndrome*	Delayed relaxation of tendon reflexes
Tremor	Hyper-reflexia	Aches and pains	Cerebellar ataxia[3]
Muscle weakness	Ill-sustained clonus	Muscle stiffness	Myotonia[3]
Periodic paralysis (predominantly in Chinese)	Proximal myopathy	Deafness	
	Bulbar myopathy[2]	Depression	
		Psychosis (myxoedema madness)[3]	
Dermatological			
Sweating	*Palmar erythema*	*Dry skin*	Myxoedema
Pruritis	Pretibial myxoedema[1]	*Dry hair*	Purplish lips
Alopecia	Finger clubbing (thyroid acropachy)[1]	Alopecia	Malar flush
	Spider naevi[3]		Carotenaemia
	Onycholysis[3]		Vitiligo
	Pigmentation[3]		Erythema ab igne (Granny's tartan)
	Vitiligo[1]		
Reproductive			
Amenorrhoea/oligomenorrhoea	Gynaecomastia	*Menorrhagia*	
Infertility, spontaneous abortion		Infertility	
Loss of libido, impotence		Galactorrhoea[3]	
		Impotence[3]	
Ocular			
Grittiness, red eyes	*Lid retraction, lid lag*		Periorbital oedema/myxoedema
Excessive lacrimation	Chemosis[1]		Loss of lateral eyebrows
Diplopia[1]	Exophthalmos[1]		
Loss of acuity[1]	Periorbital oedema[1]		
	Corneal ulceration[1]		
	Ophthalmoplegia[1]		
	Papilloedema[1]		

Italics indicate the most common features, irrespective of the cause.
[1]Features of Graves' disease only.
[2]Features found particularly in elderly patients.
[3]Rare features.

20.7 PREVALENCE OF THYROID AUTOANTIBODIES (%)

	Antibodies to:		
	Thyroid peroxidase[1]	Thyroglobulin	TSH receptor[2]
Normal population	8–27	5–20	0
Graves' disease	50–80	50–70	80–95
Autoimmune hypothyroidism	90–100	80–90	10–20
Multinodular goitre	~30–40	~30–40	0
Transient thyroiditis	~30–40	~30–40	0

[1] Thyroid peroxidase antibodies are the principal component of what was previously measured as thyroid 'microsomal' antibodies.
[2] TSH receptor antibodies (TRAb) can be agonists (stimulatory, causing Graves' thyrotoxicosis) or antagonists ('blocking', causing hypothyroidism).

20.8 NON-SPECIFIC LABORATORY ABNORMALITIES IN THYROID DYSFUNCTION*

Thyrotoxicosis

- Serum enzymes
  Raised alanine aminotransferase, γ-glutamyl transferase, and alkaline phosphatase from liver and bone
- Raised bilirubin
- Mild hypercalcaemia
- Glycosuria
  Associated diabetes mellitus
  'Lag storage' glycosuria (p. 815)

Hypothyroidism

- Serum enzymes
  Raised creatine kinase, aspartate aminotransferase, lactate dehydrogenase
- Hypercholesterolaemia
- Anaemia
  Normochromic normocytic or macrocytic
- Hyponatraemia

*These abnormalities are not useful in differential diagnosis so the tests should be avoided and any further investigation undertaken only if abnormalities persist when the patient is euthyroid.

negligible iodine uptake, high T_4:T_3 ratio and a low or undetectable thyroglobulin is diagnostic and has made what was often a difficult diagnosis much simpler.

Management

Definitive treatment of thyrotoxicosis depends on the underlying cause, as described on pages 754–756, and may include antithyroid drugs, radioactive iodine or surgery. In all patients with thyrotoxicosis a non-selective β-adrenoceptor antagonist (β-blocker), such as propranolol (160 mg daily) or nadolol (40–80 mg daily), will alleviate but not abolish symptoms within 24–48 hours. Beta-blockers cannot be recommended for long-term treatment, but they are extremely useful in the short term, e.g. for patients awaiting hospital consultation or following ^{131}I therapy.

Atrial fibrillation in thyrotoxicosis

Thyrotoxicosis is an important cause of atrial fibrillation; in one series of patients presenting with atrial fibrillation

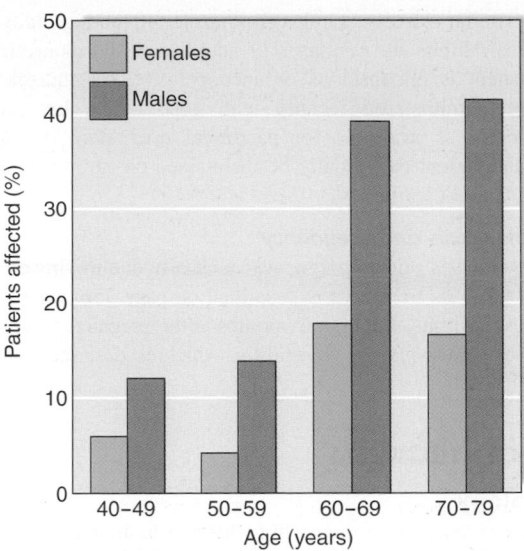

Fig. 20.5 Age-related incidence of atrial fibrillation in patients with thyrotoxicosis.

the prevalence of thyrotoxicosis was 26%, while atrial fibrillation is present in about 10% of all patients with thyrotoxicosis. The incidence increases with age so that almost half of all males with thyrotoxicosis over the age of 60 are affected (Fig. 20.5). Moreover, subclinical thyrotoxicosis (p. 752) is a risk factor for atrial fibrillation. Characteristically, the ventricular rate is little influenced by digoxin, but responds to the addition of a β-blocker. Thrombo-embolic vascular complications are particularly common in thyrotoxic atrial fibrillation so that anticoagulation with warfarin is required, unless contraindicated. Once thyroid hormone and TSH concentrations have been returned to normal, atrial fibrillation will spontaneously revert to sinus rhythm in ~50% of patients. In the remainder, cardioversion will restore sinus rhythm in up to 50%.

Thyrotoxic crisis ('thyroid storm')

This is a rare and life-threatening increase in the severity of the clinical features of thyrotoxicosis. The most prominent signs are fever, agitation, confusion, tachycardia or atrial fibrillation and, in the older patient, cardiac failure. It is a medical emergency and, despite early recognition and treatment, the mortality rate is 10%. Thyrotoxic crisis is most commonly precipitated by infection in a patient with previously unrecognised or inadequately treated thyrotoxicosis. It may also develop shortly after subtotal thyroidectomy in an ill-prepared patient or within a few days of ^{131}I therapy when acute irradiation damage may lead to a transient rise in serum thyroid hormone levels.

Patients should be rehydrated and given a broad-spectrum antibiotic. Propranolol is rapidly effective orally (80 mg 6-hourly) or intravenously (1–5 mg 6-hourly). Sodium ipodate (500 mg per day orally) will restore serum T_3 levels to normal in 48–72 hours. This is a radiographic contrast medium which not only inhibits the release of thyroid hormones, but also reduces the conversion of T_4 to T_3 and is, therefore, more effective than potassium iodide or Lugol's solution. Dexamethasone (2 mg 6-hourly) and amiodarone

749

have similar effects. Oral carbimazole 40–60 mg daily (p. 755) inhibits the synthesis of new thyroid hormone. If the patient is unconscious or uncooperative, carbimazole can be administered rectally with good effect, but no preparation is available for parenteral use. After 10–14 days the patient can usually be maintained on carbimazole alone.

Thyrotoxicosis and pregnancy

Thyrotoxicosis during pregnancy is usually due to Graves' disease and its treatment is described on page 756. Thyrotoxicosis within the first 6 months after pregnancy may be due to post-partum thyroiditis, which is described on page 758.

HYPOTHYROIDISM

Aetiology

The prevalence of primary hypothyroidism is 1:100, but increases to 5:100 if patients with subclinical hypothyroidism (normal T_4, raised TSH) are included. The female:male ratio is approximately 6:1. There are various causes of primary hypothyroidism (Box 20.9), but autoimmune disease (Hashimoto's thyroiditis) and thyroid failure following ^{131}I or surgical treatment of thyrotoxicosis account for

over 90% of cases in those parts of the world which are not significantly iodine-deficient.

Clinical assessment

Clinical features depend on the duration and severity of the hypothyroidism. In the patient in whom complete thyroid failure has developed insidiously over months or years many of the clinical features listed in Box 20.6 are likely to be present. A consequence of prolonged hypothyroidism is the infiltration of many body tissues by the mucopoly-saccharides, hyaluronic acid and chondroitin sulphate, resulting in a low-pitched voice, poor hearing, slurred speech due to a large tongue, and compression of the median nerve at the wrist (carpal tunnel syndrome). Infiltration of the dermis gives rise to non-pitting oedema (i.e. myxoedema) which is most marked in the skin of the hands, feet and eyelids. The resultant periorbital puffiness is often striking and, when combined with facial pallor due to vasoconstriction and anaemia, or a lemon-yellow tint to the skin due to carotenaemia, purplish lips and malar flush, the clinical diagnosis is simple. Most cases of hypothyroidism are not so obvious, however, and unless the diagnosis is positively entertained in the middle-aged woman complaining of tiredness, weight gain, depression or carpal tunnel syndrome, an opportunity for early treatment will be missed.

In establishing the underlying aetiology and appropriate therapy, the key discriminatory features in the history and examination are highlighted in Figure 20.6. Care must be taken to identify patients with transient hypothyroidism, in whom life-long thyroxine therapy is inappropriate. This is often observed during the first 6 months after subtotal thyroidectomy or ^{131}I treatment of Graves' disease, in the post-thyrotoxic phase of subacute thyroiditis and in post-partum thyroiditis. In these conditions thyroxine treatment is not always necessary as the patient is usually asymptomatic during the short period of thyroid failure.

Investigations

In the most common form of hypothyroidism, namely primary hypothyroidism resulting from an intrinsic disorder of the thyroid gland, serum T_4 is low and TSH elevated, usually in excess of 20 mU/l. Serum T_3 concentrations do not discriminate reliably between euthyroid and hypothyroid patients and should not be measured. In the rare secondary hypothyroidism there is atrophy of an inherently normal thyroid gland caused by failure of TSH secretion in a patient with hypothalamic or anterior pituitary disease, e.g. pituitary macroadenoma. Serum T_4 is low but TSH may be low, normal or even slightly elevated (p. 746). Other non-specific abnormalities are shown in Box 20.8. In severe prolonged hypothyroidism the electrocardiogram classically demonstrates sinus bradycardia with low voltage complexes and ST segment and T wave abnormalities. Measurement of thyroid peroxidase antibodies is helpful, but further investigations are rarely required (Fig. 20.6).

Management

As illustrated in Figure 20.6, most patients do not require specialist review and will require life-long thyroxine therapy. It is customary to start slowly and a dose of 50 μg

20.9 CAUSES OF HYPOTHYROIDISM		
Causes	Anti-TPO anti-bodies[1]	Goitre[2]
Autoimmune		
Hashimoto's thyroiditis	++	±
Spontaneous atrophic hypothyroidism	–	–
Graves' disease with TSH receptor-blocking antibodies	+	±
Iatrogenic		
Radioactive iodine ablation	+	±
Thyroidectomy	+	–
Drugs		
Carbimazole, methimazole, propylthiouracil	+	±
Amiodarone	+	±
Lithium	–	±
Transient thyroiditis		
Subacute (de Quervain's) thyroiditis	+	±
Post-partum thyroiditis	+	±
Iodine deficiency		
e.g. In mountainous regions	–	++
Congenital		
Dyshormonogenesis	–	++
Thyroid aplasia	–	–
Infiltrative		
Amyloidosis, Riedel's thyroiditis, sarcoidosis etc.	+	++
Secondary hypothyroidism		
TSH deficiency	–	–

[1] As shown in Box 20.7, thyroid autoantibodies are common in the healthy population, so might be present in anyone. ++ high titre; + more likely to be detected than in the healthy population; – not especially likely.
[2] Goitre: – absent; ± may be present; ++ characteristic.

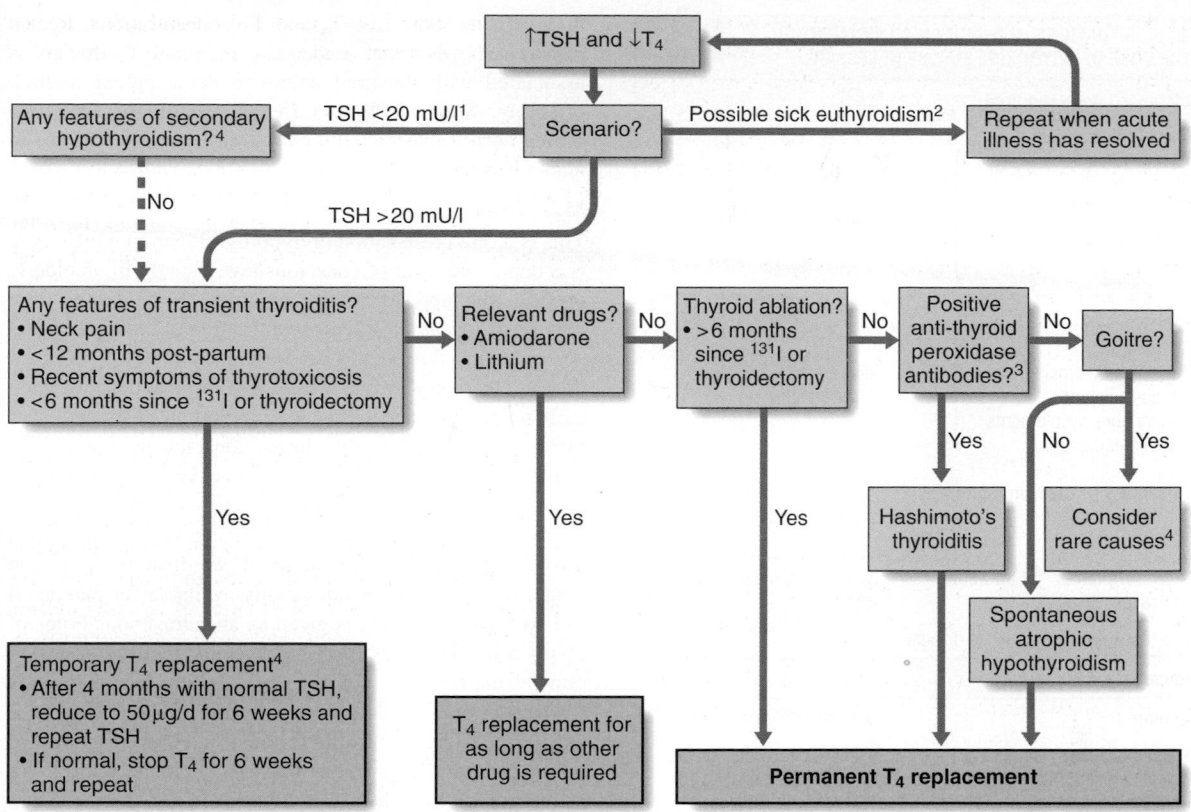

Fig. 20.6 **An approach to adults with suspected primary hypothyroidism.** This scheme ignores congenital causes of hypothyroidism (Box 20.9) such as thyroid aplasia and dyshormonogenesis (associated with nerve deafness in Pendred's syndrome), which are usually diagnosed in childhood. (1) Immunoreactive TSH may be detected at normal or even modestly elevated levels in patients with pituitary failure; unless T_4 is only marginally low then TSH should be > 20 mU/l to confirm the diagnosis of primary hypothyroidism (p. 757). (2) The usual abnormality in sick euthyroidism is a low TSH, but any pattern can occur. (3) Thyroid peroxidase antibodies are highly sensitive, but not very specific for autoimmune thyroid disease (Boxes 20.7 and 20.9). (4) Specialist advice is most appropriate where indicated. Secondary hypothyroidism is rare, but is suggested by deficiency of pituitary hormones or by clinical features of pituitary tumour such as headache or visual field defect (p. 797). Rare causes of hypothyroidism with goitre include infiltration of the thyroid (Box 20.9).

20

per day should be given for 3 weeks, increasing thereafter to 100 µg per day for a further 3 weeks and finally to a maintenance dose, usually 100–150 µg per day. Thyroxine has a half-life of 7 days so it should always be taken as a single daily dose and at least 6 weeks should pass before repeating thyroid function tests and adjusting the dose, usually in increments of 25 µg per day. Patients feel better within 2–3 weeks. Reduction in weight and periorbital puffiness occurs quickly, but the restoration of skin and hair texture and resolution of any effusions may take 3–6 months.

The correct dose of thyroxine in the long term is that which restores serum TSH to within the reference range. To achieve this, serum T_4 will usually be in the upper part of the normal range or even slightly raised, because the T_3 required for receptor activation is derived exclusively from conversion of T_4 within the target tissues without the usual contribution from thyroid secretion. Some physicians advocate combined replacement with T_4 and T_3 but this approach remains controversial and no ideal preparation exists (Box 20.10). Some patients remain symptomatic despite normalisation of TSH and may wish to take extra thyroxine which suppresses TSH values. However, there is

---

EBM

20.10 THERAPY WITH T_3 IN ADDITION TO T_4 IN HYPOTHYROIDISM

'One RCT showed that combined $T_3 + T_4$ has beneficial effects on neuropsychological tests compared with T_4 alone. However, these findings were not replicated in more recent RCTs, no satisfactory combined synthetic preparation is available and the potency of animal thyroid extract is too variable.'

- Bunevicius R, et al. N Engl J Med 1999; 340:420–429.
- Clyde PW, et al. JAMA 2003; 290:2952–2958.
- Sawha AM, et al. J Clin Endocrine Metab 2004; 88:4551–4555.

For further information: 💻 www.thyroid.org (the American Thyroid Association)

---

evidence that suppressed TSH is a risk factor for osteoporosis and atrial fibrillation (p. 752; subclinical thyrotoxicosis) so this approach cannot be recommended.

It is important to measure thyroid function every 1–2 years once the dose of thyroxine is stabilised. This encourages patient compliance with therapy and allows adjustment for variable underlying thyroid activity and other changes in thyroxine requirements (Box 20.11). In some poorly compliant patients, thyroxine is taken diligently or even in excess for a few days prior to a clinic visit, resulting

20.11 SITUATIONS IN WHICH AN ADJUSTMENT OF THE DOSE OF THYROXINE MAY BE NECESSARY

Increased dose required	
Use of other medication Phenobarbital Phenytoin Carbamazepine Rifampicin Sertraline* Chloroquine*	Increase T_4 clearance
Colestyramine Sucralfate Aluminium hydroxide Ferrous sulphate Dietary fibre supplements Calcium carbonate	Interfere with intestinal T_4 absorption
Pregnancy or oestrogen therapy	Increases concentration of serum thyroxine-binding globulin
After surgical or ^{131}I ablation of Graves' disease	Reduces thyroidal secretion with time
Malabsorption, e.g. coeliac disease	
Decreased dose required	
Ageing	Decreases T_4 clearance
Graves' disease developing in patient with long-standing primary hypothyroidism	Switch from production of blocking to stimulating TSH receptor antibodies
*Mechanism not fully established.	

in the seemingly anomalous combination of a high serum T_4 and high TSH (Box 20.4, p. 746).

Thyroxine replacement in ischaemic heart disease

Hypothyroidism and ischaemic heart disease are both common, so inevitably they will sometimes occur together. Although angina may remain unchanged in severity or paradoxically disappear with restoration of metabolic rate, exacerbation of myocardial ischaemia, infarction and sudden death are well-recognised complications of thyroxine replacement, even using doses as low as 25 µg per day. In patients with known ischaemic heart disease, thyroxine should be introduced at low dose and increased very slowly under specialist supervision. It has been suggested that T_3 has an advantage over T_4, since T_3 has a shorter half-life and any adverse effect will reverse more quickly, but the more distinct peak in hormone levels after each dose of T_3 is a disadvantage. Approximately 40% of patients with angina cannot tolerate full replacement therapy despite the use of β-blockers and vasodilators; coronary artery surgery or balloon angioplasty can be performed safely in such patients and, if successful, allow full replacement dosage of thyroxine in the majority.

Hypothyroidism in pregnancy

Most pregnant women with primary hypothyroidism require an increase in the dose of thyroxine of ~50 µg daily to maintain normal TSH levels. This may reflect increased metabolism of thyroxine by the placenta and increased serum thyroxine-binding globulin during pregnancy, resulting in an increase in the total thyroid hormone pool to maintain the same free T_4 and T_3 concentrations. Recent research suggests that inadequate maternal T_4 therapy is associated with impaired cognitive development in their offspring. Serum TSH and free T_4 should be measured during each trimester and the dose of thyroxine adjusted to maintain a normal TSH.

Myxoedema coma

This is a rare presentation of hypothyroidism in which there is a depressed level of consciousness, usually in an elderly patient who appears myxoedematous. Body temperature may be as low as 25°C, convulsions are not uncommon and cerebrospinal fluid (CSF) pressure and protein content are raised. The mortality rate is 50% and survival depends upon early recognition and treatment of hypothyroidism and other factors contributing to the altered consciousness level, e.g. drugs such as phenothiazines, cardiac failure, pneumonia, dilutional hyponatraemia and respiratory failure.

Myxoedema coma is a medical emergency and treatment must begin before biochemical confirmation of the diagnosis. Thyroxine is not usually available for parenteral use so triiodothyronine is given as an intravenous bolus of 20 µg followed by 20 µg 8-hourly until there is sustained clinical improvement. In survivors there is a rise in body temperature within 24 hours and, after 48–72 hours, it is usually possible to substitute oral thyroxine in a dose of 50 µg per day. Unless it is apparent that the patient has primary hypothyroidism, e.g. thyroidectomy scar or goitre, the thyroid failure should be assumed to be secondary to hypothalamic or pituitary disease and treatment given with hydrocortisone 100 mg i.m. 8-hourly, pending the results of T_4, TSH and cortisol concentrations (p. 793). Other measures include slow rewarming (p. 101), cautious use of intravenous fluids, broad-spectrum antibiotics and high-flow oxygen. Occasionally, assisted ventilation may be necessary.

ASYMPTOMATIC ABNORMAL THYROID FUNCTION TEST RESULTS

One of the most common problems in medical practice is how to manage patients with abnormal thyroid function test results who have no obvious signs or symptoms of thyroid disease. For practical purposes these can be divided into three categories.

Subclinical thyrotoxicosis

The serum TSH is undetectable and the serum T_3 and T_4 lie in the upper parts of their respective reference ranges. This combination is most often found in older patients with multinodular goitre. These patients are at increased risk of atrial fibrillation and osteoporosis and hence the consensus view is that such patients have mild thyrotoxicosis and require therapy, usually with ^{131}I (p. 756). Otherwise, annual review is essential as the conversion rate to overt thyrotoxicosis with elevated T_4 and/or T_3 concentrations is 5% each year.

Subclinical hypothyroidism

The serum TSH is raised and the serum T_3 and T_4 concentrations are usually in the lower part of their respective reference ranges. It may persist for many years, although there is a risk of progression to overt thyroid failure, particularly if antibodies to thyroid peroxidase are present in the serum (Box 20.7, p. 749) or if the TSH rises above 10 mU/l. In patients with non-specific symptoms a trial of thyroxine therapy may be appropriate. In those with positive autoantibodies or TSH > 10 mU/l it is better to treat the thyroid failure early rather than risk loss to follow-up and subsequent presentation with profound hypothyroidism. Thyroxine should be given in a dose sufficient to restore the serum TSH concentration to normal (p. 750).

Non-thyroidal illness ('sick euthyroidism')

In patients with systemic illness (e.g. myocardial infarction, pneumonia) there is decreased peripheral conversion of T_4 to T_3 and alterations of binding proteins and their affinity for thyroid hormones. In addition, serum TSH concentrations may be subnormal as a result of the illness itself or the use of drugs such as dopamine or corticosteroids. The most common combination is a low serum TSH, raised T_4 and normal or low T_3, but many patterns of thyroid function tests can be seen, dependent upon the type of assay used. During convalescence, serum TSH concentrations may increase to levels found in primary hypothyroidism. It follows that biochemical assessment of thyroid function should not be undertaken in patients with non-thyroidal illness, unless there is good evidence of concomitant thyroid disease, e.g. goitre, exophthalmos. If an abnormal result is found, treatment should only be given with specialist advice and the tests should be repeated after recovery.

THYROID ENLARGEMENT

Palpable thyroid enlargement is common, affecting about 5% of the population, although it is the minority who seek medical attention, often because a friend or relative has noticed a lump in the neck. Multinodular goitres and solitary nodules sometimes present with acute painful enlargement due to haemorrhage into a nodule. There are several causes of thyroid enlargement (Box 20.12), ranging from the soft diffuse goitre of puberty and youth to the multinodular

goitre of middle age and beyond (p. 759), and the solitary nodule which can present at any age. Whereas diffuse and multinodular goitre are almost invariably benign, there is a 1:20 chance of malignancy in the truly solitary lesion.

Palpation of the neck (including the thyroid gland and any lymph nodes) will allow discrimination of the following distinct groups of patients. Thyroid function tests should always be performed.

Diffuse goitre

In the absence of thyrotoxicosis (p. 746) or hypothyroidism (p. 750) a diffuse goitre rarely needs further investigation or treatment unless it is very large and causing cosmetic symptoms or compression of other local structures (resulting in stridor or dysphagia). The presence of autoantibodies may support the diagnosis of Graves' disease (p. 754) or Hashimoto's thyroiditis (p. 757), while their absence in a younger patient suggests a simple goitre (p. 759). Thyroxine therapy is sometimes justified in an attempt to shrink the goitre (Box 20.12).

Multinodular goitre

This condition is described on page 759. It is usually necessary to confirm the clinical diagnosis using ^{99m}Tc scintigraphy (Fig. 20.4, p. 747) or ultrasonography. Sometimes one of the nodules is much larger than any other (a 'dominant' nodule); if such a nodule is 'cold' on isotope scanning it may be investigated in the same way as a truly solitary nodule since the risk of malignancy is not negligible in such lesions.

Solitary thyroid nodule

It is important to determine whether the nodule is benign, e.g. cyst or colloid nodule, or malignant. It is rarely possible to make this distinction on clinical grounds alone, although the presence of cervical lymphadenopathy increases the likelihood of malignancy. However, a solitary nodule presenting in childhood or adolescence, particularly if there is a past history of head and neck irradiation, or presenting in the elderly should raise the suspicion of a primary thyroid malignancy (pp. 760–761). Very occasionally, a secondary deposit from a renal, breast or lung carcinoma presents as a painful, rapidly growing solitary thyroid nodule.

Investigations

Serum T_3, T_4 and TSH should be measured in all patients with a solitary thyroid nodule. The finding of undetectable TSH is very suggestive of an autonomously functioning thyroid follicular adenoma, which can only be confirmed by thyroid isotope scanning (Fig. 20.4, p. 747), and is for practical purposes always benign.

For euthyroid patients, the most useful investigation is fine needle aspiration of the nodule. This is performed in the outpatient clinic using a standard 21-gauge venepuncture needle and a 20 ml syringe, usually making several passes through different parts of the lesion. Aspiration may be therapeutic in the small proportion of patients in whom the swelling is a pure cyst, although recurrence on more than one occasion is an indication for surgery. Cytological examination will differentiate benign (80%) from suspicious

---

20.12 CAUSES OF THYROID ENLARGEMENT

Diffuse goitre
- Simple goitre[1] (p. 759)
- Hashimoto's thyroiditis[1] (p. 757)
- Graves' disease (p. 754)
- Drugs
  Iodine, amiodarone (p. 758), lithium
- Iodine deficiency (endemic goitre)[1] (p. 758)
- Transient thyroiditis[2] (p. 757)
- Suppurative thyroiditis[2]
- Dyshormonogenesis[1] (p. 762)
- Infiltrative
  Amyloidosis, sarcoidosis etc
- Riedel's thyroiditis[2] (p. 761)

Multinodular goitre (p. 759)

Solitary nodule
- Simple cyst
- Colloid nodule
- Follicular adenoma (p. 760)
- Papillary carcinoma (p. 760)
- Follicular carcinoma (p. 760)
- Medullary cell carcinoma (p. 761)
- Anaplastic carcinoma
- Lymphoma
- Metastasis

[1] Goitre likely to shrink with thyroxine therapy.
[2] Usually tender.

---

or definitely malignant nodules (20%), of which 25–50% are confirmed as cancer at surgery. The advantage of fine needle aspiration over isotope scanning is that a much higher proportion of patients avoid surgery; isotope scanning identifies suspicious 'cold nodules', but most of these are benign. The limitations of fine needle aspiration are that it cannot differentiate between follicular adenoma and carcinoma and that in 10–20% of cases an inadequate specimen is obtained. Ultrasound-guided needle aspiration can be helpful in increasing the quality of specimens.

Management

Solitary nodules with a solid component in which cytology either is inconclusive or shows malignant cells are treated by surgical excision. Those in which malignancy is confirmed by formal histology are then treated as described on page 761. Benign lesions are sometimes excised, e.g. if they are growing, but the majority of patients can be reassured.

AUTOIMMUNE THYROID DISEASE

Thyroid diseases are amongst the most prevalent antibody-mediated autoimmune diseases and are associated with other organ-specific autoimmunity (Ch. 4 and p. 803). Autoantibodies may produce inflammation and destruction of thyroid tissue resulting in hypothyroidism, goitre (in Hashimoto's thyroiditis) or sometimes even transient thyrotoxicosis ('Hashitoxicosis'), or they may stimulate the TSH receptor to cause thyrotoxicosis (in Graves' disease). There is overlap between these conditions, since some patients have multiple autoantibodies.

GRAVES' DISEASE

The most common manifestation is thyrotoxicosis with or without a diffuse goitre. The clinical features and differential diagnosis are described on pages 746–748. Graves' disease also causes ophthalmopathy and rarely pretibial myxoedema (p. 740). These features usually occur in thyrotoxic patients, but can occur in the absence of thyroid dysfunction. Graves' disease can occur at any age but is unusual before puberty and most commonly affects women aged 30–50 years.

Graves' thyrotoxicosis

Pathophysiology

The thyrotoxicosis results from the production of IgG antibodies directed against the TSH receptor on the thyroid follicular cell, which stimulate thyroid hormone production and, in the majority, goitre formation. These antibodies are termed thyroid-stimulating immunoglobulins or TSH receptor antibodies (TRAb) and can be detected in the serum of 80–95% of patients with Graves' disease. The concentration of TRAb in the serum is presumed to fluctuate to account for the natural history of Graves' thyrotoxicosis (Fig. 20.7). The ultimate thyroid failure seen in some patients is thought to result from the presence of blocking antibodies against the TSH receptor, and from tissue destruction by cytotoxic antibodies and cell-mediated immunity.

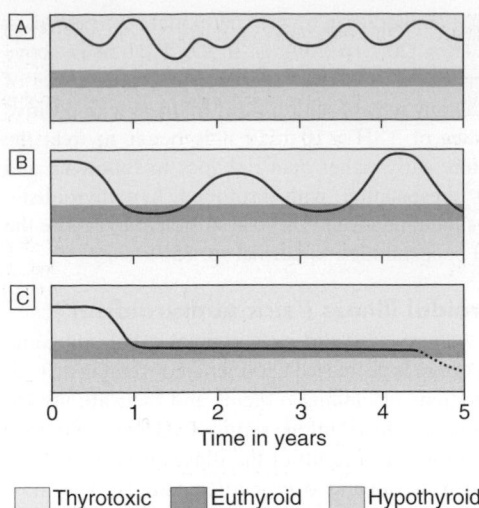

Fig. 20.7 **Natural history of the thyrotoxicosis of Graves' disease.** Ⓐ and Ⓑ The majority (60%) of patients have either prolonged periods of hyperthyroidism of fluctuating severity, or periods of alternating relapse and remission. Ⓒ It is the minority who experience a single short-lived episode followed by prolonged remission and, in some cases, by the eventual onset of hypothyroidism.

In Caucasians there is an association of Graves' disease with HLA-B8, DR3 and DR2, and with inability to secrete the water-soluble glycoprotein form of the ABO blood group antigens. Family studies show that 50% of monozygotic twins are concordant for thyrotoxicosis, as opposed to 5% of dizygotic twins.

The trigger for the development of thyrotoxicosis in genetically susceptible individuals may be infection with viruses or bacteria, although there is no proof. Certain strains of the gut organisms *Escherichia coli* and *Yersinia enterocolitica* possess cell membrane TSH receptors; antibodies to these microbial antigens may cross-react with the TSH receptors on the host thyroid follicular cell. In regions of iodine deficiency (p. 758), iodine supplementation may result in the development of thyrotoxicosis, but only in those with pre-existing subclinical Graves' disease. Smoking is weakly associated with Graves' thyrotoxicosis, but strongly linked with the development of ophthalmopathy.

Management

Symptoms of thyrotoxicosis respond to β-blockade (p. 749) but definitive treatment requires control of thyroid hormone secretion. The different options are compared in Box 20.13. If it were possible to predict with confidence the natural history of the thyrotoxicosis in an individual patient at presentation, it would be appropriate to give an antithyroid drug for 12–18 months to those in whom a single episode was anticipated, and to advise destructive therapy with ^{131}I or surgery for those likely to experience recurrent disease. Unfortunately, such a prediction is not possible, although persistent thyrotoxicosis is more likely in patients who are male, have large goitres, severe thyrotoxicosis and persistently high TRAb titres. For patients under 40 years of age many centres adopt the empirical approach of

20.13 COMPARISON OF TREATMENTS FOR THE THYROTOXICOSIS OF GRAVES' DISEASE

Management	Common indications	Contraindications	Disadvantages/complications
Antithyroid drugs e.g. carbimazole, propylthiouracil	First episode in patients < 40 yrs	Breastfeeding (propylthiouracil suitable)	Hypersensitivity rash 2% Agranulocytosis 0.2% > 50% relapse rate usually within 2 years of stopping drug
Subtotal thyroidectomy	Large goitre Poor drug compliance, especially in young patients Recurrent thyrotoxicosis after course of antithyroid drugs in young patients	Previous thyroid surgery Dependence upon voice, e.g. opera singer, lecturer[1]	Hypothyroidism (~25%) Transient hypocalcaemia (10%) Permanent hypoparathyroidism (1%) Recurrent laryngeal nerve palsy[1] (1%)
Radio-iodine	Patients > 40 yrs[2] Recurrence following surgery irrespective of age Other serious comorbidity	Pregnancy or planned pregnancy within 6 months of treatment Active Graves' ophthalmopathy[3]	Hypothyroidism, approx. 40% in first year, 80% after 15 years Most likely treatment to result in exacerbation of ophthalmopathy[3]

[1]It is not only vocal cord palsy due to recurrent laryngeal nerve damage which alters the voice following thyroid surgery; the superior laryngeal nerves are frequently transected and result in minor changes in voice quality.
[2]In certain parts of the world, ^{131}I is used more liberally and prescribed for young women in the 20–40 age group.
[3]The extent to which radio-iodine exacerbates ophthalmopathy is controversial and practice varies; some use prednisolone for 4 months to reduce this risk (Box 20.15).

20

prescribing a course of carbimazole and recommending surgery if relapse occurs, while ^{131}I is employed as first or second-line treatment in those aged over 40. A number of observational studies have linked therapeutic ^{131}I with increased incidence of some malignancies, particularly of the thyroid and gastrointestinal tract, but the results have been inconsistent; the association may be with Graves' disease rather than its therapy, and the magnitude of the effect, if any, is small. Experience from the Chernobyl disaster suggests that younger people are more sensitive to radiation-induced thyroid cancer. In many centres, however, ^{131}I is used more extensively, even in young patients.

Antithyroid drugs. The most commonly used are carbimazole and its active metabolite, methimazole (not available in the UK). Propylthiouracil is equally effective. These drugs reduce the synthesis of new thyroid hormones by inhibiting the iodination of tyrosine (Fig. 20.3, p. 745). Carbimazole also has an immunosuppressive action, leading to a reduction in serum TRAb concentrations, but this is not enough to influence the natural history of the thyrotoxicosis significantly (Box 20.14).

Antithyroid drugs are introduced at high doses, e.g. carbimazole 40–60 mg daily or prophylthiouracil 400–600 mg daily. There is subjective improvement within 10–14 days and the patient is usually clinically and biochemically euthyroid at 3–4 weeks, when the dose can be reduced. The maintenance dose is determined by measurement of T_4 and TSH, attempting to keep both hormones

within their respective reference ranges. In most patients carbimazole can be taken as a single daily dose and is continued for 12–18 months in the hope that during this period permanent remission will occur. Unfortunately, thyrotoxicosis recurs in at least 50%, usually within 2 years of stopping treatment. Rarely, despite good drug compliance, T_4 and TSH levels fluctuate between those of thyrotoxicosis and hypothyroidism at successive review appointments, presumably due to rapidly changing concentrations of TRAb. In such patients satisfactory control can be achieved by blocking thyroid hormone synthesis with carbimazole 30–40 mg daily and adding T_4 100–150 μg daily as replacement therapy when the patient is euthyroid.

The adverse effects of antithyroid drugs develop within 7–28 days of starting treatment. Rash is common. Agranulocytosis is rare and cannot be predicted by routine measurement of white blood cell count, but fortunately is reversible. Patients should be warned to stop the drug and contact their medical attendant (for a full blood count) immediately should a severe sore throat or fever develop. Cross-sensitivity between the antithyroid drugs is unusual and another member of the group can be substituted with good effect.

Subtotal thyroidectomy. Patients must be rendered euthyroid with antithyroid drugs before operation. Potassium iodide, 60 mg 8-hourly orally, is often added for 2 weeks before surgery to inhibit thyroid hormone release and reduce the size and vascularity of the gland, making surgery technically easier. Complications of surgery are rare (Box 20.13). One year after surgery, 80% of patients are euthyroid, 15% are permanently hypothyroid and 5% remain thyrotoxic. Thyroid failure within 6 months of operation may be temporary. Long-term follow-up of patients treated surgically is necessary, as the late development of hypothyroidism and recurrence of thyrotoxicosis are well recognised.

20.14 ANTITHYROID DRUG THERAPY IN GRAVES' DISEASE **EBM**

'Remission rates in patients with Graves' disease are not improved by combining thyroxine with antithyroid drugs (block and replace therapy).'

● McIver B, et al. N Engl J Med 1996; 334:220–224.

20

Radioactive iodine. [131]I is administered orally as a single dose and is trapped and organified in the thyroid (Fig. 20.3, p. 745). Although it will decay within the thyroid in a few weeks, the effects of its radiation are long-lasting, with cumulative effects on follicular cell survival and replication. The variable radio-iodine uptake and radiosensitivity of the gland means that the choice of dose is empirical; in most centres 185–370 MBq (5–10 mCi) is given orally. This regimen is effective in 75% of patients within 4–12 weeks. During the lag period, symptoms can be controlled by a β-blocker or, in more severe cases, by carbimazole. However, carbimazole reduces the efficacy of ^{131}I therapy because it prevents organification of ^{131}I in the gland, and so should be avoided until 48 hours after radio-iodine administration. If thyrotoxicosis persists after 12–24 weeks, a further dose of ^{131}I should be employed. The disadvantage of ^{131}I treatment is that the majority of patients eventually develop hypothyroidism and long-term follow-up is, therefore, necessary.

Thyrotoxicosis in pregnancy

The coexistence of pregnancy and thyrotoxicosis is unusual as anovulatory cycles are common in thyrotoxic patients and autoimmune disease tends to remit during pregnancy, when the maternal immune response is suppressed. Thyroid function tests must be interpreted in the knowledge that thyroid-binding globulin, and hence total T_4 and T_3 levels, are increased in pregnancy and that TSH normal ranges may be lower; a fully suppressed TSH with elevated free thyroid hormone levels indicates thyrotoxicosis. The thyrotoxicosis is almost always caused by Graves' disease. Both mother and fetus must be considered, since maternal thyroid hormones, TRAb and antithyroid drugs can all cross the placenta to some degree, exposing the fetus to risks of thyrotoxicosis, iatrogenic hypothyroidism and goitre.

Thyrotoxicosis is treated with antithyroid drugs which cross the placenta and also treat the fetus, whose thyroid gland is exposed to the action of maternal TRAb. Propylthiouracil may be preferable to carbimazole since the latter has been associated with a skin defect in the child known as aplasia cutis. In order to avoid fetal hypothyroidism and goitre, it is important to use the smallest dose of antithyroid drug (optimally less than 150 mg propylthiouracil per day) which will maintain maternal (and presumably fetal) free hormones and TSH within their respective normal ranges. Frequent review of mother and fetus (using ultrasonography and heart rate monitoring) is important. TRAb levels can be measured in the third trimester to predict the likelihood of neonatal thyrotoxicosis. When TRAb levels are not elevated, the antithyroid drug can be discontinued 4 weeks before the expected date of delivery to avoid any possibility of fetal hypothyroidism at the time of maximum brain development. After delivery, if antithyroid drug is required and the patient wishes to breastfeed, then propylthiouracil (p. 755) is the drug of choice as it is excreted in the milk to a much lesser extent than carbimazole.

If subtotal thyroidectomy is necessary because of poor drug compliance or drug hypersensitivity, it is most safely performed in the second trimester. Radioactive iodine is absolutely contraindicated as it invariably induces fetal hypothyroidism.

Graves' ophthalmopathy

This condition is immunologically mediated, but the auto-antigen that causes the local accumulation of lymphocytes has not been identified. Within the orbit (and the dermis) there is cytokine-mediated proliferation of fibroblasts which secrete hydrophilic glycosaminoglycans. The resulting increased interstitial fluid content, combined with a chronic inflammatory cell infiltrate, causes marked swelling and ultimately fibrosis of the extraocular muscles (Fig. 20.8) and a rise in retrobulbar pressure. The eye is displaced forwards (proptosis, exophthalmos) and in more severe cases there is optic nerve compression.

Ophthalmopathy, like thyrotoxicosis (Fig. 20.7), typically follows an episodic course and it is helpful to distinguish patients with active inflammation (periorbital oedema and conjunctival inflammation with changing orbital signs) from those in whom the inflammation has 'burnt out' leaving stable orbital dysfunction. Eye disease is detectable in ~50% of patients when first seen with thyrotoxicosis, but active inflammatory episodes may occur long before or long after thyrotoxic episodes (exophthalmic Graves' disease). It is more common in cigarette smokers and is exacerbated by

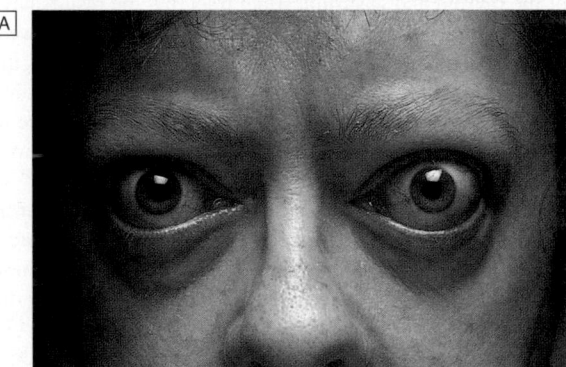

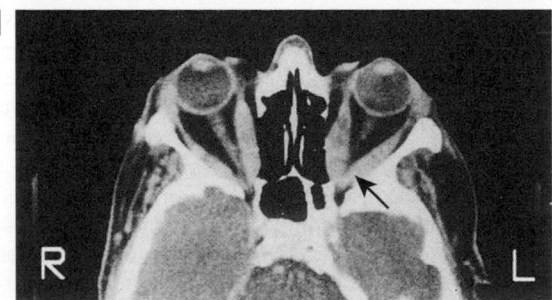

Fig. 20.8 Graves' disease. Ⓐ Bilateral ophthalmopathy in a 42-year-old man. The main symptoms were diplopia in all directions of gaze and reduced visual acuity in the left eye. The periorbital swelling is due to retrobulbar fat prolapsing into the eyelids, and increased interstitial fluid as a result of raised intraorbital pressure.
Ⓑ Transverse CT of the orbits, showing the enlarged extraocular muscles. This is most obvious at the apex of the left orbit (arrow), where compression of the optic nerve caused reduced visual acuity.

poor control of thyroid function, especially hypothyroidism. The most frequent presenting symptoms are related to increased exposure of the cornea, resulting from proptosis and lid retraction. There may be excessive lacrimation made worse by wind and bright light, a 'gritty' sensation in the eye, and pain due to conjunctivitis or corneal ulceration. In addition, there may be reduction of visual acuity and/or visual fields as a consequence of corneal oedema or optic nerve compression. Other signs of optic nerve compression include reduced colour vision and a relative afferent pupillary defect (p. 1193). If the extraocular muscles are involved and do not act in concert, diplopia results.

The majority of patients require no treatment other than reassurance. Methylcellulose eye drops and gel counter the gritty discomfort of dry eyes, and tinted glasses or side shields attached to spectacle frames reduce the excessive lacrimation triggered by sun or wind. Severe inflammatory episodes are treated with oral glucocorticoids (e.g. prednisolone 60 mg daily) and sometimes orbital irradiation (Box 20.15). Loss of visual acuity is an indication for urgent surgical decompression of the orbit. In 'burnt out' disease, surgery to the eyelids and/or ocular muscles may improve conjunctival exposure, cosmetic appearance and diplopia.

20.15 EFFECTS OF ^{131}I AND PREDNISOLONE IN GRAVES' OPHTHALMOPATHY **EBM**

'The deterioration of ophthalmopathy, which occurs in some patients following ^{131}I therapy, can be prevented by prednisolone therapy.'

- Bartalena L, et al. N Engl J Med 1989; 321:1349–1352.

Pretibial myxoedema

This infiltrative dermopathy occurs in fewer than 10% of patients with Graves' disease and has similar pathological features as occur in the orbit. It takes the form of raised pink-coloured or purplish plaques on the anterior aspect of the leg, extending on to the dorsum of the foot (p. 740). The lesions may be itchy and the skin may have a 'peau d'orange' appearance with growth of coarse hair; less commonly, the face and arms may be affected. Treatment is rarely required, but in severe cases topical glucocorticoids may be helpful.

HASHIMOTO'S THYROIDITIS

The nomenclature of autoimmune hypothyroidism can be confusing. Some authorities reserve the term 'Hashimoto's thyroiditis' for patients with positive thyroid peroxidase autoantibodies and a firm goitre who may or may not be hypothyroid, and use the term 'spontaneous atrophic hypothyroidism' for hypothyroid patients without a goitre in whom TSH receptor-blocking antibodies may be more important than antiperoxidase antibodies. However, these syndromes can both be considered as variants of Hashimoto's thyroiditis since both are characterised by destructive lymphoid infiltration of the thyroid, ultimately leading to a varying degree of fibrosis which accounts for the varying degree of thyroid enlargement. In association with the lymphoid thyroid infiltration there is an increased risk of thyroid lymphoma (p. 761), although this is an exceedingly rare complication.

Hashimoto's thyroiditis increases in incidence with age and affects ~3.5 per 1000 women and 0.8 per 1000 men each year. Many present with a small or moderately sized diffuse goitre, which is characteristically firm or rubbery in consistency. The goitre may be soft, however, and impossible to differentiate from simple goitre (p. 759) by palpation alone. Around 25% of patients are hypothyroid at presentation. In the remainder, serum T_4 is normal and TSH normal or raised, but these patients are at risk of developing overt hypothyroidism in future years. Thyroid peroxidase antibodies are present in the serum in > 90% of patients with Hashimoto's thyroiditis. In those under the age of 20 years, antinuclear factor (ANF) may also be positive.

Thyroxine therapy is indicated not only for hypothyroidism (p. 750), but also sometimes for goitre shrinkage. In this context, the dose of thyroxine should be sufficient to suppress serum TSH to low but detectable levels.

TRANSIENT THYROIDITIS

SUBACUTE (DE QUERVAIN'S) THYROIDITIS

In its classical painful form, subacute thyroiditis is a virus-induced (e.g. Coxsackie, mumps or adenovirus) transient inflammation of the thyroid gland. There is pain in the region of the thyroid that may radiate to the angle of the jaw and the ears, and is made worse by swallowing, coughing and movement of the neck. The thyroid is usually palpably enlarged and tender. Systemic upset is common. Affected patients are usually females aged 20–40 years.

Painless transient thyroiditis also occurs, sometimes after viral infection and sometimes in patients with underlying autoimmune disease.

In both painless and painful varieties, inflammation in the thyroid gland is associated with release of colloid and stored thyroid hormones, but also with damage to follicular cells and impaired synthesis of new thyroid hormones. As a result, T_4 and T_3 levels are raised for 4–6 weeks until the pre-formed colloid is depleted. Thereafter, there is usually a period of hypothyroidism of variable severity before the follicular cells recover and normal thyroid function is restored within 4–6 months (Fig. 20.9). In the thyrotoxic phase, the iodine uptake is low because the damaged follicular cells are unable to trap iodine and because endogenous TSH secretion is suppressed. Low-titre thyroid autoantibodies appear transiently in the serum, and the erythrocyte sedimentation rate (ESR) is usually raised. High titre autoantibodies suggest an underlying autoimmune pathology and risk of recurrence and ultimate progression to hypothyroidism.

The pain and systemic upset usually respond to simple measures such as non-steroidal anti-inflammatory drugs (NSAIDs). Occasionally, however, it may be necessary to prescribe prednisolone 40 mg daily for 3–4 weeks. The thyrotoxicosis is mild and treatment with propranolol or nadolol is usually adequate. Antithyroid drugs are of

20

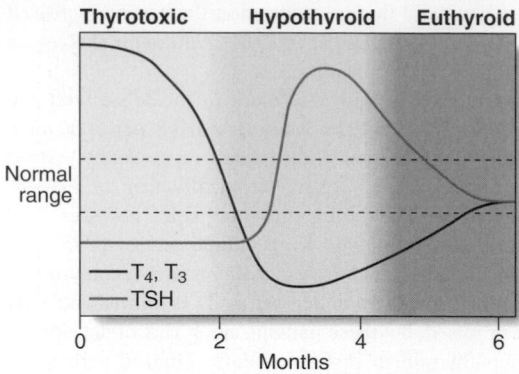

Fig. 20.9 Thyroid function tests in an episode of transient thyroiditis. This pattern might be observed in classical subacute (de Quervain's) thyroiditis, painless thyroiditis or post-partum thyroiditis. The duration of each phase varies between patients. Note that the lower limit of detection of TSH is close to the lower limit of the normal range.

no benefit because thyroid hormone synthesis is impaired rather than enhanced. Careful monitoring of thyroid function and symptoms is required so that thyroxine can be prescribed temporarily in the hypothyroid phase. Care must be taken to identify patients presenting with hypothyroidism who are in the later stages of a transient thyroiditis, since they are unlikely to require life-long thyroxine therapy (p. 750).

POST-PARTUM THYROIDITIS

The maternal immune response, which is modified during pregnancy to allow survival of the fetus, is enhanced after delivery and may unmask previously unrecognised subclinical autoimmune thyroid disease. Surveys have shown that transient biochemical disturbances of thyroid function, i.e. thyrotoxicosis, hypothyroidism and thyrotoxicosis followed by hypothyroidism (Fig. 20.9), occur in 5–10% of women within 6 months of delivery. Those affected are likely to have antithyroid peroxidase antibodies in the serum in early pregnancy. Symptoms of thyroid dysfunction are rare and there is no association between postnatal depression and abnormal thyroid function tests. However, symptomatic thyrotoxicosis presenting for the first time within 6 months of childbirth is likely to be due to post-partum thyroiditis and the diagnosis is confirmed by a negligible radio-isotope uptake. The clinical course and treatment are similar to painless subacute thyroiditis (see above). Post-partum thyroiditis tends to recur after subsequent pregnancies and eventually patients progress over a period of years to permanent hypothyroidism.

IODINE-ASSOCIATED THYROID DISEASE

IODINE DEFICIENCY

In certain mountainous parts of the world, such as the Andes, the Himalayas and central Africa, where there is dietary iodine deficiency, thyroid enlargement is common (more than 10% of the population) and is known as endemic

goitre. Most patients are euthyroid and have normal or raised TSH levels. In general, the more severe the iodine deficiency, the greater the incidence of hypothyroidism. Iodine supplementation programmes have abolished this condition in most developed regions.

IODINE-INDUCED THYROID DYSFUNCTION

The administration of iodine has complex effects on thyroid function. Pharmacological excess of iodine inhibits thyroid hormone release; this is the basis for its utility in the acute treatment of thyroid storm (p. 749) and prior to sub-total thyroidectomy (p. 755). In addition, iodine administration can initially enhance, and subsequently inhibit, iodination of tyrosine and hence thyroid hormone synthesis (Fig. 20.3, p. 745). The resulting effect of iodine on thyroid function varies according to whether the patient has an iodine-deficient diet or underlying thyroid disease. In iodine-deficient parts of the world, transient thyrotoxicosis may be precipitated by prophylactic iodinisation programmes. In iodine-sufficient areas, thyrotoxicosis can be precipitated by radiographic contrast medium or expectorants in individuals who have underlying thyroid disease predisposing to thyrotoxicosis, such as multinodular goitre or Graves' disease in remission. Induction of thyrotoxicosis by iodine is called the Jod–Basedow effect. Chronic excess iodine administration can, however, result in hypothyroidism. Increased iodine within the thyroid gland down-regulates iodine trapping so that uptake is low in all circumstances.

AMIODARONE

The anti-arrhythmic agent amiodarone has a structure that is analogous to thyroxine (Fig. 20.10) and contains huge amounts of iodine; a 200 mg dose contains 75 mg iodine, compared with a daily dietary requirement of just 125 µg. In addition to the effects of the iodine, amiodarone has a cytotoxic effect on thyroid follicular cells and inhibits conversion of T_4 to T_3. Most patients receiving amiodarone have normal thyroid function, but up to 20% develop hypothyroidism or thyrotoxicosis. The ratio of T_4:T_3 is elevated and TSH provides the best indicator of thyroid function.

The thyrotoxicosis has been classified as either:

- type I—a Jod–Basedow effect in patients with underlying thyroid disease, or
- type II—thyroiditis due to cytotoxicity, resulting in a transient thyrotoxicosis.

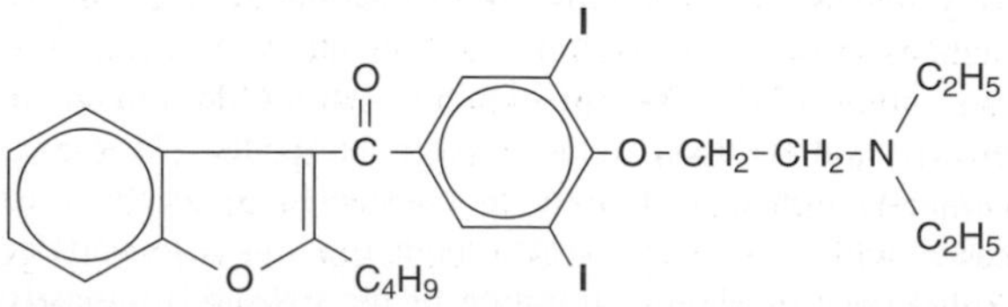

Fig. 20.10 The structure of amiodarone. Note the similarities with thyroxine (Fig. 20.3).

These patterns can overlap and be difficult to distinguish clinically, as iodine uptake is low in both. Measurement of interleukin-6 may help, as concentrations are usually much greater in type II hyperthyroidism.

In hypothyroid patients, thyroxine can be given while amiodarone is continued. Treatment of thyrotoxicosis is more difficult. Excess iodine renders the gland completely resistant to radio-iodine. Antithyroid drugs may be effective in high doses in patients with the type I form, but are ineffective in type II thyrotoxicosis. Potassium perchlorate can be used to displace iodide from the gland and prednisolone has also been advocated. If the cardiac state allows, amiodarone should be discontinued, but it has a long half-life (50–60 days) so its effects are long-lasting.

To minimise the risk of type I hyperthyroidism, thyroid function should be measured in all patients prior to commencement of amiodarone therapy. Amiodarone should be avoided if TSH is suppressed. Thyroid function should be monitored regularly in all patients taking amiodarone.

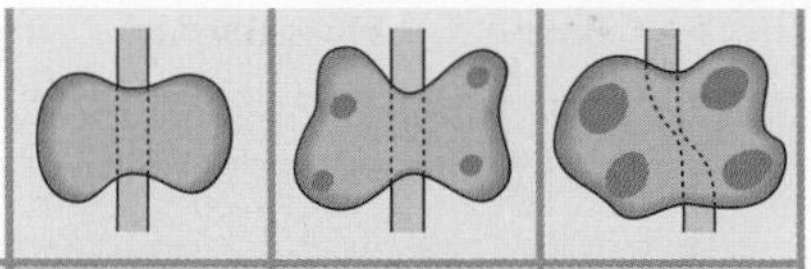

SIMPLE AND MULTINODULAR GOITRE

These terms describe diffuse or multinodular enlargement of the thyroid, which occurs sporadically and is of unknown aetiology.

SIMPLE DIFFUSE GOITRE

This form of goitre usually presents between the ages of 15 and 25 years, often during pregnancy, and tends to be noticed, not by the patient, but by friends and relatives. Occasionally, there is a tight sensation in the neck, particularly when swallowing. The goitre is soft and symmetrical and the thyroid is enlarged to two or three times its normal size. There is no tenderness, lymphadenopathy or overlying bruit. Concentrations of T_3, T_4 and TSH are normal and no thyroid autoantibodies are detected in the serum. No treatment is necessary and in most cases the goitre regresses. In some, however, the unknown stimulus to thyroid enlargement persists and, as a result of recurrent episodes of hyperplasia and involution during the following 10–20 years, the gland becomes multinodular with areas of autonomous function.

MULTINODULAR GOITRE

The natural history is shown in Figure 20.11. Patients with thyroid enlargement in the absence of thyroid dysfunction or positive autoantibodies (i.e. with 'simple goitre', see above) as young adults may progress to develop nodules. These nodules grow at varying rates and secrete thyroid hormone 'autonomously', thereby suppressing TSH-dependent growth and function in the rest of the gland. Ultimately, complete suppression of TSH occurs in about 25% of cases, with T_4 and T_3 levels often within the normal range (subclinical thyrotoxicosis, p. 752) but sometimes elevated (toxic multinodular goitre, Fig. 20.4, p. 747). Opinions differ as to whether the nodules represent multiple adenomas or

Age (in years)	15–25	35–55	> 55
Goitre	Diffuse	Nodular	Nodular
Tracheal compression/ deviation	No	Minimal	Yes
T_3, T_4	Normal	Normal	Raised
TSH	Normal	Normal or undetectable	Undetectable

Fig. 20.11 Natural history of simple goitre.

focal hyperplasia. There are reports that the prevalence of foci of thyroid cancer is increased in multinodular goitres, but for practical purposes patients can be reassured that it is a benign condition and malignancy need only be considered in patients with a large 'dominant' nodule that is 'cold' (i.e. does not take up radioisotope).

Clinical features and investigations

Multinodular goitre is usually diagnosed in patients presenting with thyrotoxicosis, a large goitre with or without tracheal compression, or sudden painful swelling caused by haemorrhage into a nodule or cyst. The goitre is nodular or lobulated on palpation and may extend retrosternally; however, not all mutinodular goitres causing thyrotoxicosis are easily palpable. Very large goitres may cause mediastinal compression with stridor (Fig. 20.12), dysphagia and obstruction of the superior vena cava. Hoarseness due to recurrent laryngeal nerve palsy can occur, but is far more suggestive of thyroid carcinoma.

The diagnosis is confirmed by a radioisotope thyroid scan (Fig. 20.4, p. 747) and/or ultrasonography. In patients with large goitres a flow-volume loop is a good screening test for significant tracheal compression (Fig. 20.12). If intervention is contemplated, a chest X-ray may be helpful, but CT or MRI of the thoracic inlet is optimal to quantify the degree of tracheal displacement or compression and the extent of retrosternal extension. In those with a 'dominant', 'cold' nodule, fine needle aspiration is indicated to exclude thyroid cancer.

Management

If the goitre is small, no treatment is necessary but annual review should be arranged as the natural history is progression to a toxic multinodular goitre. Partial thyroidectomy is indicated for large goitres which cause mediastinal compression or which are cosmetically unattractive. [131]I can result in a significant reduction in thyroid size and may be of value in elderly patients (Box 20.16). Unfortunately, recurrence 10–20 years later is not uncommon. Thyroxine is

20

759

20

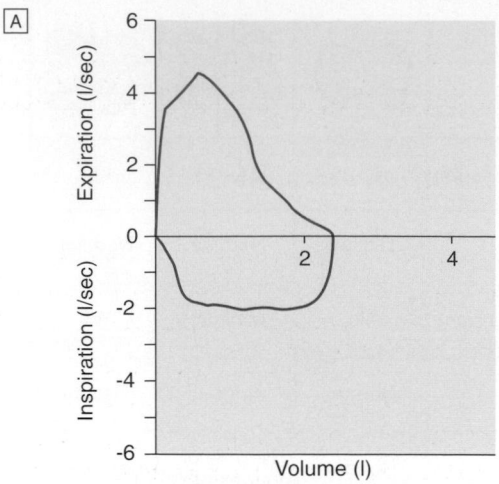

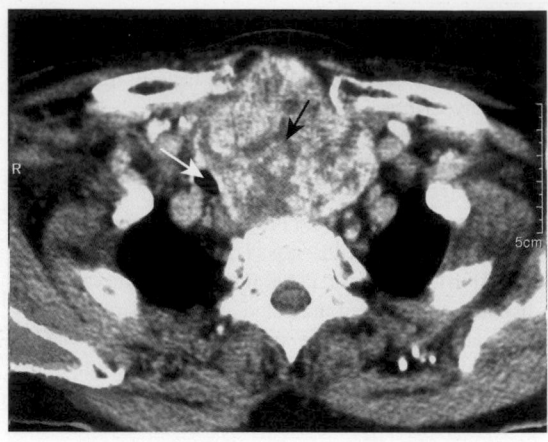

Fig. 20.12 Multinodular goitre with retrosternal extension and tracheal compression. [A] A flow-volume loop (p. 656) showing a square-shaped inspiratory curve indicating extrathoracic airflow obstruction. [B] A CT scan of the upper mediastinum showing a large retrosternal goitre (black arrow) with deviation and compression of the trachea (white arrow).

20.16 MEDICAL THERAPY TO SHRINK NON-TOXIC MULTINODULAR GOITRE   **EBM**

'One RCT showed that ^{131}I, but not thyroxine therapy, reduced thyroid volume in patients with large multinodular goitres and normal thyroid function.'

● Wesche MFT, et al. J Clin Endocrinol Metab 2001; 86:998–1005.

---

of no benefit in shrinking multinodular goitres and may serve only to aggravate any associated thyrotoxicosis.

In toxic multinodular goitre treatment is usually with ^{131}I. The iodine uptake is lower than in Graves' disease so a higher dose is employed (555–1850 MBq, 15–50 mCi) and hypothyroidism is less common. In thyrotoxic patients with a large goitre, partial thyroidectomy may be indicated. Long-term treatment with antithyroid drugs is not usually appropriate as relapse is invariable after drug withdrawal.

Asymptomatic patients with subclinical thyrotoxicosis (p. 752) are increasingly being treated with ^{131}I on the grounds that a suppressed TSH is a risk factor for atrial fibrillation and, particularly in post-menopausal women, osteoporosis.

THYROID NEOPLASIA

Patients with thyroid tumours usually present with a solitary nodule (p. 753). Most are benign and a few of these, called 'toxic adenomas', secrete excess thyroid hormones. Primary thyroid malignancy is rare, accounting for less than 1% of all carcinomas, and has an incidence of 25 per million per annum. As shown in Box 20.17, it can be classified according to the cell type of origin. With the exception of medullary carcinoma, thyroid cancer is more common in females.

TOXIC ADENOMA

The presence of a toxic solitary nodule is the cause of less than 5% of all cases of thyrotoxicosis. The nodule is a follicular adenoma, which autonomously secretes excess thyroid hormones and inhibits endogenous TSH secretion with subsequent atrophy of the rest of the thyroid gland. The adenoma is usually greater than 3 cm in diameter.

Most patients are female and over 40 years of age. Although many nodules are palpable, the diagnosis can be made with certainty only by isotope scanning (Fig. 20.4, p. 747). The thyrotoxicosis is usually mild and in almost 50% of patients the plasma T_3 alone is elevated (T_3 thyrotoxicosis). ^{131}I (555–1110 MBq, 15–30 mCi) is highly effective and is an ideal treatment since the atrophic cells surrounding the nodule do not take up iodine and so receive little or no radiation. For this reason, permanent hypothyroidism is unusual. A surgical hemithyroidectomy is an alternative.

DIFFERENTIATED CARCINOMA

Papillary carcinoma

This is the most common of the malignant thyroid tumours and accounts for 90% of irradiation-induced thyroid cancer. It may be multifocal and spread is to regional lymph nodes. Some patients present with cervical lymphadenopathy and no apparent thyroid enlargement; in such instances, the primary lesion may be less than 10 mm in diameter.

Follicular carcinoma

This is always a single encapsulated lesion. Spread to cervical lymph nodes is rare. Metastases are blood-borne and are most often found in bone, lungs and brain.

Management

This is usually by total thyroidectomy followed by a large dose of ^{131}I (3000 MBq, ~80 mCi) in order to ablate any remaining thyroid tissue, normal or malignant. Thereafter, long-term treatment with thyroxine in a dose sufficient to suppress TSH (usually 150–200 µg daily) is important, as there is evidence that growth of differentiated thyroid

20.17 MALIGNANT THYROID TUMOURS

Origin of tumour	Type of tumour	Frequency (%)	Usual age of presentation (years)	Approximate 20-year survival (%)
Follicular cells	Differentiated carcinoma			
	Papillary	70	20–40	95
	Follicular	10	40–60	60
	Undifferentiated carcinoma			
	Anaplastic	5	> 60	< 1
Parafollicular C cells	Medullary carcinoma	5–10	> 40*	50
Lymphocytes	Lymphoma	5–10	> 60	10

* Patients with medullary carcinoma as part of multiple endocrine neoplasia type 2 (p. 802) may present in childhood.

carcinomas is TSH-dependent. Follow-up is by measurement of serum thyroglobulin, which should be undetectable in patients whose normal thyroid has been ablated and who are taking a suppressive dose of thyroxine. Detectable thyroglobulin is suggestive of tumour recurrence or metastases, which may be detected by whole-body scanning with ^{131}I and may respond to further radio-iodine therapy. For meaningful results, isotope scanning requires serum TSH concentrations to be elevated (> 20 mU/l). In the past this was achieved by stopping thyroxine for 4–6 weeks, inducing symptomatic hypothyroidism. The availability of recombinant human TSH now allows measurement of stimulated thyroglobulin and radio-iodine uptake without the need to stop thyroxine therapy.

Prognosis

Most patients have an excellent prognosis when treated appropriately. Those under 50 years of age with papillary carcinoma can anticipate a near-normal life expectancy if the tumour is less than 2 cm in diameter, confined to the thyroid and cervical nodes, and of low-grade malignancy histologically. Even for patients with distant metastases at presentation, the 10-year survival is approximately 40%.

ANAPLASTIC CARCINOMA AND LYMPHOMA

These two conditions are difficult to distinguish clinically but are distinct cytologically and histologically. Patients are usually elderly women in whom there is rapid thyroid enlargement over 2–3 months. The goitre is hard and symmetrical. There is usually stridor due to tracheal compression and hoarseness due to recurrent laryngeal nerve palsy. There is no effective treatment of anaplastic carcinoma, although radiotherapy may afford temporary relief of mediastinal compression. The prognosis for lymphoma, which may arise from pre-existing Hashimoto's thyroiditis, is better. External irradiation often produces dramatic goitre shrinkage and, when combined with chemotherapy, may result in survival for 5 years or more.

MEDULLARY CARCINOMA

This tumour arises from the parafollicular C cells of the thyroid. In addition to calcitonin, the tumour may secrete

5-hydroxytryptamine (5-HT, serotonin), various peptides of the tachykinin family, ACTH and prostaglandins. As a consequence carcinoid syndrome (p. 791) and Cushing's syndrome (p. 779) may occur.

Patients usually present in middle age with a firm thyroid mass. Cervical lymphadenopathy is common, but distant metastases are rare initially. Serum calcitonin levels are raised and are useful in monitoring response to treatment. Despite the very high levels of calcitonin found in some patients, hypocalcaemia is extremely rare.

Treatment is by total thyroidectomy with removal of affected cervical nodes. Since the C cells do not concentrate iodine, there is no role for ^{131}I therapy. Prognosis is very variable, some patients surviving 20 years or more and others less than 1 year.

Medullary carcinoma of the thyroid may occur sporadically, or in families as part of the multiple endocrine neoplasia (MEN) type 2 syndrome (p. 802).

RIEDEL'S THYROIDITIS

This is not a form of thyroid cancer, but the presentation is similar and the differentiation can usually only be made by thyroid biopsy. It is an exceptionally rare condition of unknown aetiology in which there is extensive infiltration of the thyroid and surrounding structures with fibrous tissue. There may be associated mediastinal and retroperitoneal fibrosis. Presentation is with a slow-growing goitre which is irregular and stony-hard. There is usually tracheal and oesophageal compression necessitating partial thyroidectomy. Other recognised complications include recurrent laryngeal nerve palsy, hypoparathyroidism and eventually hypothyroidism.

CONGENITAL THYROID DISEASE

Early treatment with thyroxine is essential to prevent irreversible brain damage in children with congenital hypothyroidism. Routine screening of TSH levels in blood spot samples obtained 5–7 days after birth (as part of the Guthrie test) has revealed an incidence of approximately 1 in 3000, resulting from thyroid agenesis, ectopic or hypoplastic glands, or dyshormonogenesis. Congenital hypothyroidism is thus six times more common than phenylketonuria. It is now possible to start thyroid replacement therapy within 2 weeks of birth. Developmental assessment of infants treated at this early stage has revealed no differences between cases and controls in most children.

Dyshormonogenesis

Several autosomal recessive defects in thyroid hormone synthesis have been described; the most common results from deficiency of the intrathyroidal peroxidase enzyme. Homozygous individuals present with congenital hypothyroidism; heterozygotes present in the first two decades of life with goitre, normal thyroid hormone levels and a raised TSH. The combination of dyshormonogenetic goitre and nerve deafness is known as Pendred's syndrome and is due to mutations in pendrin, the protein which transports iodide to the luminal surface of the follicular cell (Fig. 20.3, p. 745).

Thyroid hormone resistance

This is a rare disorder in which the pituitary and hypothalamus are resistant to feedback suppression of TSH by T_3, sometimes due to mutations in the thyroid hormone receptor β or due to defects in monodeiodinase activity. The result is high levels of TSH, T_4 and T_3, often with a moderate goitre which may not be noted until adulthood. Thyroid hormone signalling is highly complex and involves different isozymes of both monodeiodinases and thyroid hormone receptors in different tissues. For that reason, other tissues may or may not share the resistance to thyroid hormone and there may be features of thyrotoxicosis (e.g. tachycardia). This condition can be difficult to distinguish from an equally rare TSH-producing pituitary tumour (Box 20.4, p. 746); administration of TRH results in elevation of TSH in thyroid hormone resistance and not in TSHoma, but an MRI scan of the pituitary may be necessary to exclude a macroadenoma (p. 797).

20.18 THE THYROID GLAND IN OLD AGE

Thyrotoxicosis
- **Causes**: commonly due to multinodular goitre.
- **Symptoms**: apathy, anorexia, proximal myopathy, atrial fibrillation and cardiac failure predominate.
- **Non-thyroidal illness**: thyroid function tests are performed more frequently in the elderly but interpretation may be altered by intercurrent illness.

Hypothyroidism
- **Symptoms**: non-specific features such as physical and mental slowing are often attributed to increasing age and the diagnosis is delayed.
- **Thyroxine dose**: to avoid exacerbating latent or established heart disease, the starting dose should be 25 μg daily. Thyroxine requirements fall with increasing age and few patients need > 100 μg daily.
- **Other medication** (Box 20.11, p. 752): this may interfere with absorption or metabolism of thyroxine, necessitating an increase in dose.

THE REPRODUCTIVE SYSTEM

Clinical practice in reproductive medicine is shared between several specialties, including gynaecology, urology, paediatrics, psychiatry and endocrinology. The following section focuses on aspects that are commonly managed by endocrinologists.

FUNCTIONAL ANATOMY, PHYSIOLOGY AND INVESTIGATIONS

The physiology of male and female reproductive function is illustrated in Figures 20.13 and 20.14. Pathways of synthesis of sex steroids are shown in Figure 20.19 (p. 778).

The male

In the male, the testis subserves two principal functions: synthesis of testosterone by the interstitial Leydig cells under the control of luteinising hormone (LH), and spermatogenesis by Sertoli cells under the control of follicle-stimulating hormone (FSH) (but also requiring adequate testosterone). Negative feedback suppression of LH is mediated principally by testosterone, while secretion of

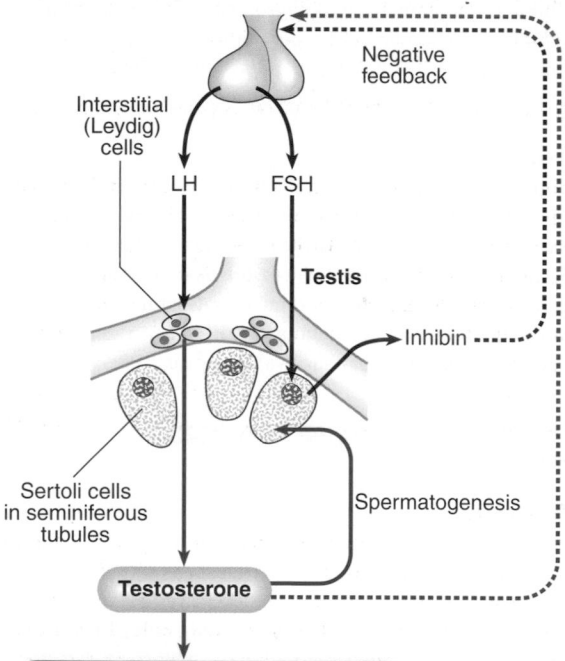

Fig. 20.13 Male reproductive physiology.

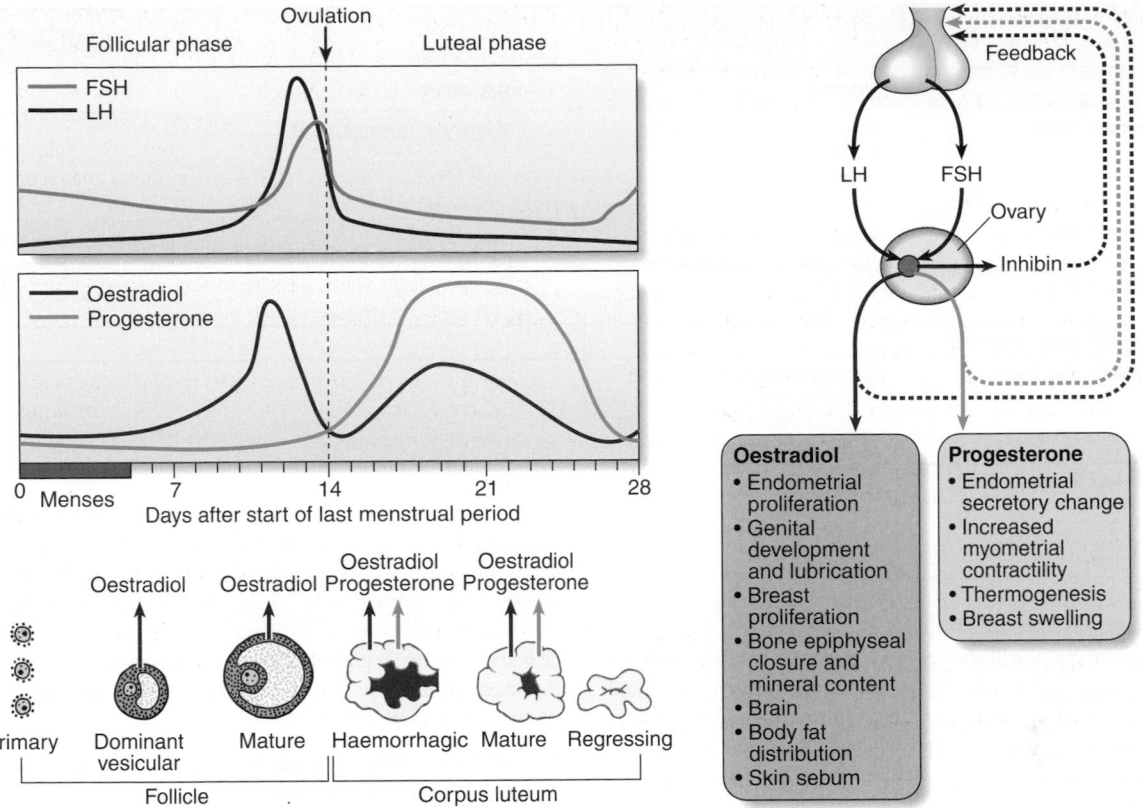

Fig. 20.14 Female reproductive physiology and the normal menstrual cycle.

another hormone by the testis, inhibin, suppresses FSH. The axis can be assessed easily by a random blood sample for testosterone, LH and FSH. Testosterone is largely bound in plasma to sex hormone-binding globulin, and this can also be measured to calculate the 'free androgen index' or the 'bioavailable' testosterone. Testicular function can also be tested by semen analysis.

There is no equivalent of the menopause in men, although testosterone concentrations decline slowly from the fourth decade onwards.

The female

In the female, physiology is complicated by variations in function during the normal menstrual cycle. FSH produces growth and development of ovarian follicles during the first 14 days after the menses. This leads to a gradual increase in oestradiol production from granulosa cells, which initially suppresses FSH secretion (negative feedback) but then, above a certain level, stimulates an increase in both the frequency and amplitude of gonadotrophin-releasing hormone (GnRH) pulses, resulting in a marked increase in LH secretion (positive feedback). The mid-cycle 'surge' of LH induces ovulation. After release of the ovum the follicle differentiates into a corpus luteum which secretes progesterone. Withdrawal of progesterone results in menstrual bleeding. Circulating levels of oestrogen and progesterone in pre-menopausal women are, therefore, critically dependent on the time of the cycle. The most useful 'test' of ovarian function is a careful menstrual

history. In addition, ovulation can be confirmed by measuring plasma progesterone levels during the luteal phase ('Day 21 progesterone') or by tracking changes in oestrogen and progesterone metabolites in urine specimens collected at weekly intervals.

The cessation of menstruation (the menopause) occurs, in most developed countries, at a median age of 50.8 years. In the 5 years before there is a gradual increase in the number of anovulatory cycles; this is referred to as the climacteric. Oestrogen and inhibin secretion falls and negative feedback results in increased pituitary secretion of LH and FSH (typically to levels > 30 U/l).

The pathophysiology of male and female reproductive dysfunction is summarised in Box 20.19.

PRESENTING PROBLEMS IN REPRODUCTIVE DISEASE

DELAYED PUBERTY

Genetic factors have a major influence in determining the timing of the onset of puberty, e.g. the age of menarche (the onset of menstruation) is often comparable within sibling and mother–daughter pairs and within ethnic groups. However, because there is also a threshold for body weight that acts as a trigger for normal puberty, the onset of puberty can be moderated by other factors including nutritional

20.19 CLASSIFICATION OF DISEASES OF THE REPRODUCTIVE SYSTEM

	Primary	Secondary
Hormone excess	Polycystic ovarian syndrome Granulosa cell tumour Leydig cell tumour Teratoma	Pituitary gonadotrophinoma
Hormone deficiency	Menopause Hypogonadism (Box 20.20) Turner's syndrome Klinefelter's syndrome	Hypopituitarism Kallmann's syndrome (isolated GnRH deficiency) Severe systemic illness, including anorexia nervosa
Hormone hypersensitivity	–	

Hormone resistance	Androgen resistance syndromes
	   Complete ('testicular feminisation')
	   Partial (Reifenstein's syndrome)
	5α-reductase type 2 deficiency	

Non-functioning tumours	Ovarian cysts Carcinoma Teratoma Seminona	

20

status and chronic illness (p. 108). Puberty may be considered delayed if the onset of the physical features of sexual maturation has not occurred by a chronological age that is 2.5 standard deviations above the national average, i.e. in the UK by the age of 14 years in boys and in girls by the age of 13 years.

Aetiology

The differential diagnosis is considered in Box 20.20. The key issue in the assessment of an affected child is to determine whether the delay in puberty is simply because the 'clock is running slow' (constitutional delay of puberty)

20.20 CAUSES OF DELAYED PUBERTY AND HYPOGONADISM

Constitutional delay

Hypogonadotrophic hypogonadism
- Structural hypothalamic/pituitary disease—Box 20.54
- Functional gonadotrophin deficiency
  Chronic systemic illness (e.g. asthma, malabsorption, coeliac disease, cystic fibrosis, renal failure)
  Psychological stress
  Anorexia nervosa
  Excessive physical exercise
  Hyperprolactinaemia
  Other endocrine disease (e.g. Cushing's syndrome, primary hypothyroidism)
- Isolated gonadotrophin deficiency
  Kallmann's syndrome

Hypergonadotrophic hypogonadism
- Chemotherapy/radiotherapy to gonads
- Trauma/surgery to gonads
- Autoimmune gonadal failure
- Mumps
- Tuberculosis
- Haemochromatosis
- Steroid biosynthetic defects
- Anorchidism/cryptorchidism in males
- Klinefelter's syndrome (47XXY, male phenotype)
- Turner's syndrome (45XO, female phenotype)

or because there is pathology in the hypothalamus/pituitary (hypogonadotrophic hypogonadism) or the gonads (hypergonadotrophic hypogonadism).

Constitutional delay of puberty

This is the most common cause of delayed puberty. Affected children are healthy and have usually been more than 2 standard deviations below the mean height for their age throughout childhood. There is often a history of delayed puberty in siblings or parents. 'Bone age' can be estimated by X-rays of epiphyses, usually in the wrist and hand; in constitutional delay, bone age is lower than chronological age and can be extrapolated to predict when a child is likely to enter puberty. Constitutional delay of puberty should be considered as a normal variant as puberty will commence spontaneously. However, affected children can experience significant psychological distress because of their lack of physical development, particularly when compared with their peers.

Hypogonadotrophic hypogonadism

This may be due to structural, inflammatory or infiltrative disorders of the pituitary and/or hypothalamus which are discussed on page 794 and in Box 20.54 (p. 795). In such circumstances, other pituitary hormones, such as growth hormone, are also likely to be deficient.

'Functional' gonadotrophin deficiency is caused by a variety of factors including low body weight, chronic systemic illness (as a consequence of the disease itself or secondary malnutrition), endocrine disorders, and profound psychosocial stress.

Isolated gonadotrophin deficiency is usually due to a genetic abnormality that affects the synthesis of either GnRH or gonadotrophins. The most common form is Kallmann's syndrome, which has been linked with a variety of genetic abnormalities with different modes of inheritance. All forms are associated with GnRH deficiency and a high proportion of affected individuals have agenesis or hypoplasia of the olfactory bulbs, resulting in anosmia or hyposmia. If isolated gonadotrophin deficiency is left untreated, the epiphyses fail to fuse, resulting in tall stature with disproportionately long arms and legs relative to trunk height (eunuchoid habitus).

Cryptorchidism (undescended testes) and gynaecomastia are commonly observed in all forms of hypogonadotrophic hypogonadism.

Hypergonadotrophic hypogonadism

Hypergonadotrophic hypogonadism associated with delayed puberty is usually due to sex chromosome abnormalities, i.e. Klinefelter's syndrome in boys and Turner's syndrome in girls. These disorders are discussed on pages 770–771. Other causes of primary gonadal failure are shown in Box 20.20.

Clinical assessment

A general history and physical examination is required, with particular reference to previous or current medical disorders, social circumstances and family history. Body proportions, sense of smell and pubertal stage should be carefully documented and, in boys, the presence or absence of testes in the scrotum noted. Current weight and height may be plotted on centile charts along with parental heights. Previous growth measurements in childhood, which can usually be obtained from the school health records, are extremely useful. Children with constitutional delay have usually always been small, but have maintained a normal growth velocity that is appropriate for bone age. Poor linear growth, i.e. 'crossing of the centiles', is more likely to be associated with acquired pathology.

Investigations

Key measurements are LH and FSH, testosterone (in boys), oestradiol (in girls), full blood count, renal function, liver function, thyroid function and coeliac disease autoantibodies (p. 894). Chromosome analysis is performed if gonadotrophin concentrations are elevated. If gonadotrophin concentrations are low, then the differential diagnosis lies between constitutional delay and hypogonadotrophic hypogonadism. A plain X-ray of the wrist may be compared with a set of standard films to obtain a bone age. Further tests may be unnecessary if the blood tests are normal and the child has all the clinical features of constitutional delay. If hypogonadotrophic hypogonadism is suspected, neuro-imaging and further investigations will be required as described on page 793.

Management

Puberty can be induced using low doses of oral oestrogen in girls (e.g. ethinylestradiol 2 µg daily) or testosterone in boys (e.g. depot testosterone ester injections 50 mg i.m. each month). Higher doses carry a risk of early fusion of epiphyses. This therapy should be given in a specialist clinic where the progress of puberty and growth can be carefully monitored. In children with constitutional delay, this 'priming' therapy can be discontinued when endogenous puberty is established, usually in less than a year. In children with hypogonadism, the underlying cause should be treated and reversed if possible. If hypogonadism is permanent,

then sex hormone doses are gradually increased during puberty and full adult replacement doses given when development is complete.

SECONDARY AMENORRHOEA

Primary amenorrhoea describes a patient who has never menstruated; this usually occurs as a manifestation of delayed puberty, but may also be a consequence of anatomical defects of the female reproductive system, e.g. endometrial hypoplasia or vaginal agenesis. Secondary amenorrhoea describes the cessation of menstruation. The causes of this common presentation are shown in Box 20.21. In non-pregnant women, secondary amenorrhoea is almost invariably a consequence of either ovarian or hypothalamic/pituitary dysfunction. Premature ovarian failure (premature menopause) is defined, arbitrarily, as occurring before 40 years of age. Rarely, endometrial adhesions (Asherman's syndrome) can form after uterine curettage, surgery or infection, e.g. tuberculosis or schistosomiasis.

20.21 CAUSES OF SECONDARY AMENORRHOEA
Physiological   • Pregnancy   • Menopause
Hypogonadotrophic hypogonadism—Box 20.20
Ovarian dysfunction   • Hypergonadotrophic hypogonadism—Box 20.20   • Polycystic ovarian syndrome   • Androgen-secreting tumours
Uterine dysfunction   • Asherman's syndrome

Clinical assessment

Associated clinical features depend on the age of the patient and are a guide to the underlying cause. Hypothalamic/pituitary disease and premature ovarian failure result in oestrogen deficiency, which causes a variety of symptoms usually associated with the menopause (Box 20.22). If there is weight loss, then this may be primary as in anorexia nervosa (p. 248), or secondary to underlying disease such as tuberculosis or malabsorption. Weight gain may suggest

20.22 SYMPTOMS OF OESTROGEN DEFICIENCY	
Vasomotor effects	
• Hot flushes	• Sweating
Psychological	
• Anxiety • Irritability	• Emotional lability
Genitourinary	
• Dyspareunia • Urgency of micturition	• Vaginal infections

20

hypothyroidism, Cushing's syndrome or, very rarely, a hypothalamic lesion. Hirsutism, obesity and long-standing irregular periods suggest the polycystic ovarian syndrome (PCOS, p. 769). The presence of other autoimmune disease raises the possibility of autoimmune premature ovarian failure. The breasts should be examined for galactorrhoea and a vaginal examination performed, particularly if disease of the uterus is suspected.

Investigations

Pregnancy should be excluded in women of reproductive age by measuring human chorionic gonadotrophin (hCG) in a sample of urine. LH, FSH, oestradiol, prolactin, testosterone, T_4 and TSH should be measured in blood which, in the absence of a menstrual cycle, can be taken at any time. Investigation of hyperprolactinaemia is described on page 800. High levels of LH and FSH with low or low normal oestradiol suggest primary ovarian failure. Ovarian autoantibodies may be positive when there is an underlying autoimmune aetiology, and a karyotype should be performed in younger women to exclude mosaic Turner's syndrome. Elevated LH, prolactin and testosterone with normal oestradiol is common in PCOS. Low levels of LH, FSH and oestradiol suggest hypothalamic or pituitary disease.

There is some overlap in gonadotrophin and oestrogen concentrations between women with hypogonadotrophic hypogonadism and PCOS. If there is doubt as to the underlying cause of secondary amenorrhoea, then the response to 5 days of treatment with an oral progestogen (e.g. medroxyprogesterone acetate 10 mg 12-hourly) can be assessed. In women with PCOS, the progestogen will cause maturation of the endometrium and menstruation will occur a few days after the progestogen is stopped. In women with hypogonadotrophic hypogonadism, menstruation does not occur following progestogen withdrawal because the endometrium is atrophic as a result of oestrogen deficiency. If doubt persists in distinguishing oestrogen deficiency from a uterine abnormality, the capacity for menstruation can be tested with 1 month of treatment with cyclical oestrogen and progestogen (usually administered as the combined oral contraceptive pill).

Assessment of bone mineral density, e.g. by dual energy X-ray absorptiometry (DEXA) scan (pp. 1122–1124), is appropriate in patients with low androgen and oestrogen levels.

Management

Where possible, the underlying cause should be treated. For example, women with functional amenorrhoea due to excessive exercise and low weight should be encouraged to reduce their exercise and regain some weight. The management of structural pituitary and hypothalamic disease is described on page 798 and PCOS on page 769.

In oestrogen-deficient women, oestrogen replacement therapy is necessary to treat symptoms and/or to prevent osteoporosis. Oestrogen should not be given 'unopposed' (i.e. without progesterone) to a woman with a uterus as there is then a risk of endometrial cancer. In pre-menopausal females, the treatment is cyclical oestrogen therapy on days

---

20.23 HORMONE REPLACEMENT THERAPY (HRT) IN POST-MENOPAUSAL WOMEN	EBM

'Administering HRT for 5 years to 10 000 women aged 50–79 years prevents 5 hip fractures and 6 cases of colorectal cancer, while inducing 8 extra cases of breast cancer, 8 of pulmonary embolism, 7 of coronary heart disease and 8 of stroke. The risks increase with age.'

- Writing Group for the Women's Health Initiative Investigators. JAMA 2002; 288:321–333.

1–21 and progestogen on days 14–21. This is administered most conveniently as an oral contraceptive pill. If oestrogenic side-effects (fluid retention, weight gain, hypertension and thrombosis) are a concern, then lower-dose oral or transdermal oestrogen hormone replacement therapy (HRT) may be more appropriate.

The timing of the discontinuation of oestrogen replacement therapy is still a matter of debate. In post-menopausal females, HRT relieves menopausal symptoms and prevents osteoporotic fractures, but is associated with adverse effects (Box 20.23). Many authorities now recommend that women with oestrogen deficiency should take replacement therapy until the age of 50 years and only continue it beyond this age if there are unacceptable symptoms of oestrogen deficiency on discontinuation.

Oestrogen replacement therapy does not stimulate ovulation. Women with hypogonadotrophic hypogonadism who wish fertility are usually given injections of gonadotrophins (daily recombinant FSH until there is adequate follicular development, followed by an injection of hCG to induce follicular rupture). If there is a hypothalamic cause for the hypogonadism, then pulsatile GnRH therapy with a portable infusion pump is an alternative. (The pituitary GnRH receptors respond to pulsatile stimulation; continuous administration of GnRH or its analogues will suppress rather than stimulate LH and FSH secretion.) Monitoring of follicular growth by transvaginal ultrasonography and blood oestradiol levels is mandatory because of the risk of multiple ovulation and the hyperstimulation syndrome, characterised by capillary leak with circulatory shock, pleural effusions and ascites.

MALE HYPOGONADISM

The clinical features of both hypo- and hypergonadotrophic hypogonadism include loss of libido, lethargy with muscle weakness, and decreased frequency of shaving. Patients may also present with gynaecomastia, infertility, delayed puberty and/or anaemia of chronic disease. The causes of hypogonadism are listed in Box 20.20.

Investigations

Male hypogonadism is confirmed by demonstrating a low serum testosterone level. The distinction between hypo- and hypergonadotrophic hypogonadism is by measurement of random LH and FSH. Patients with hypogonadotrophic hypogonadism should be investigated as described for pituitary disease on pages 792–794. Patients with hypergonadotrophic hypogonadism should have the testes examined for

20.24 OPTIONS FOR ANDROGEN REPLACEMENT THERAPY

Route of administration	Preparation	Dose	Frequency	Comments
Intramuscular	Testosterone enantate	50–250 mg	Every 3–4 weeks	Produces peaks and troughs of testosterone levels which are outside the physiological range and may be symptomatic
Intramuscular	Testosterone undecanoate	1000 mg	Every 3 months	Smoother profile than testosterone enantate, less frequent injections
Subcutaneous	Testosterone pellets	600–800 mg	Every 4–6 months	Smoother profile than testosterone enantate, but implantation causes scarring and infection
Transdermal	Testosterone patch	5–10 mg	Daily	Very stable testosterone levels, but high incidence of skin hypersensitivity
Transdermal	Testosterone gel	50–100 mg	Daily	Very stable testosterone levels; transfer of gel can occur following skin-to-skin contact with another person
Oral	Testosterone undecanoate	40–120 mg	12-hourly	Very variable testosterone levels and risk of hepatotoxicity
Oral	Buccal testosterone	30 mg	12-hourly	Stable testosterone levels, may cause gum irritation

20

cryptorchidism or atrophy and a karyotype performed (to identify Klinefelter's syndrome).

Management

Testosterone replacement is indicated in hypogonadal men to prevent osteoporosis, and restore muscle power and libido. Routes of testosterone administration are shown in Box 20.24. First-pass hepatic metabolism of testosterone is highly efficient so bioavailability of ingested preparations is poor. Doses of systemic testosterone can be titrated against symptoms; circulating testosterone levels may provide only a rough guide to dosage because they may be highly variable (Box 20.24). It is prudent to avoid testosterone administration in men with androgen-dependent prostatic carcinoma; prostate-specific antigen (PSA) should be measured before commencing testosterone therapy in men older than 50 years and monitored periodically thereafter.

Testosterone replacement inhibits spermatogenesis. Men with hypogonadotrophic hypogonadism who wish fertility are usually given injections of hCG several times a week (recombinant FSH may also be required in men with hypogonadism of pre-pubertal origin). The duration of gonadotrophin therapy depends on the duration and cause of hypogonadism. If there is a hypothalamic cause, then pulsatile GnRH therapy is an alternative. Extraction of sperm from the epididymis, in vitro fertilisation and intracytoplasmic sperm injection (ICSI) are being used increasingly to try to achieve fertility in men with primary testicular disease.

GYNAECOMASTIA

Gynaecomastia is the presence of glandular breast tissue in males. Normal breast development in women is oestrogen-dependent, while androgens oppose this effect. Gynaecomastia results from an imbalance between androgen and oestrogen activity, which may reflect androgen deficiency or oestrogen excess. Causes are listed in Box 20.25. The most common are physiological, i.e. in the newborn baby (due to maternal and placental oestrogens), in pubertal boys (in whom oestradiol concentrations reach adult levels

20.25 CAUSES OF GYNAECOMASTIA

Idiopathic

Physiological

Drug-induced
- Cimetidine
- Digoxin
- Anti-androgens, e.g. cyproterone acetate, spironolactone
- Some exogenous anabolic steroids, e.g. diethylstilbestrol

Hypogonadism (Box 20.20)

Androgen resistance syndromes

Oestrogen excess
- Liver failure (impaired steroid metabolism)
- Oestrogen-secreting tumour, e.g. of testis
- hCG-secreting tumour, e.g. of testis or lung

before testosterone) and in elderly men (due to decreasing testosterone concentrations). Prolactin excess does not directly cause gynaecomastia (p. 799).

Clinical assessment

A drug history is important. Gynaecomastia is often asymmetrical and palpation may allow breast tissue to be distinguished from the prominent adipose tissue around the nipple that is often observed in obesity. Features of hypogonadism should be sought (see above) and the testes examined for evidence of cryptorchidism, atrophy or a tumour.

Investigations

If a clinical distinction between gynaecomastia and adipose tissue cannot be made, then ultrasonography or mammography is required. A random blood sample should be taken for testosterone, LH, FSH, oestradiol, prolactin and hCG. Elevated oestrogen concentrations are found in testicular tumours and hCG-producing neoplasms.

Management

An adolescent with gynaecomastia who is progressing normally through puberty may be reassured that the gynaecomastia will usually resolve once development is complete. If puberty does not proceed in a harmonious manner, then there may be an underlying abnormality that requires investigation (p. 763). Gynaecomastia may cause significant psychological distress, especially in adolescent boys, and surgical excision may be justified for cosmetic reasons. There are various surgical approaches which include liposuction and open excision via a small incision around the nipple. Androgen replacement will usually improve gynaecomastia in hypogonadal males and any other identifiable underlying cause should be addressed if possible.

HIRSUTISM

Hirsutism refers to the excessive growth of thick terminal hair in an androgen-dependent distribution in women (upper lip, chin, chest, back, lower abdomen, thigh, forearm) and is one of the most common presentations of endocrine disease. It should be distinguished from hypertrichosis, which is generalised excessive growth of vellus hair. The aetiology of androgen excess is shown in Box 20.26.

Clinical assessment

The severity of hirsutism is subjective. Some women suffer profound embarrassment from a degree of hair growth which others would not consider remarkable. Important observations are a drug and menstrual history, calculation of body mass index, measurement of blood pressure, examination for virilisation (clitoromegaly, deep voice,

male-pattern balding, breast atrophy), and associated features including acne vulgaris or Cushing's syndrome (p. 781). Hirsutism of recent onset associated with virilisation is suggestive of an androgen-secreting tumour, but this is rare.

Investigations

A random blood sample should be taken for testosterone, prolactin, LH and FSH. If there are clinical features of Cushing's syndrome, an overnight 1 mg dexamethasone suppression test should be performed (p. 782).

If testosterone levels are elevated above twice the upper limit of the normal female range, especially if this is associated with low LH and FSH, then causes other than idiopathic hirsutism and PCOS are more likely, and the source of the androgen excess should be established. Congenital adrenal hyperplasia due to 21-hydroxylase deficiency is diagnosed by a short ACTH stimulation test with measurement of 17OH-progesterone (p. 51). In patients with androgen-secreting tumours, serum testosterone does not suppress following dexamethasone (either as an overnight or a 48-hour low-dose suppression test) or oestrogen (30 µg daily for 7 days). The tumour should then be sought by CT or MRI of the adrenals and ovaries.

Management

This depends on the cause (Box 20.26). Similar options are available for the treatment of PCOS and idiopathic hirsutism. These are described below.

20.26 CAUSES OF HIRSUTISM			
Cause	Clinical features	Investigation findings	Treatment
Idiopathic	Often familial Mediterranean or Asian background	Normal	Cosmetic measures Anti-androgens
Polycystic ovarian syndrome (Box 20.28)	Obesity Oligomenorrhoea or secondary amenorrhoea Infertility	LH:FSH ratio > 2.5:1 Minor elevation of androgens* Mild hyperprolactinaemia	Weight loss Cosmetic measures Anti-androgens (Insulin-sensitising drugs may be useful)
Congenital adrenal hyperplasia (95% 21-hydroxylase deficiency)	Pigmented History of salt-wasting in childhood, ambiguous genitalia, or adrenal crisis when stressed Jewish background	Elevated androgens* which suppress with dexamethasone Abnormal rise in 17OH-progesterone with ACTH	Glucocorticoid replacement administered in reverse rhythm to suppress early morning ACTH
Exogenous androgen administration	Athletes Virilised	Low LH and FSH Analysis of urinary androgens may detect drug of misuse	Stop steroid misuse
Androgen-secreting tumour of ovary or adrenal cortex	Rapid onset Virilisation: clitoromegaly, deep voice, balding, breast atrophy	High androgens* which do not suppress with dexamethasone or oestrogen Low LH and FSH CT or MRI usually demonstrates a tumour	Surgical excision
Cushing's syndrome	Clinical features of Cushing's syndrome (p. 779)	Normal or mild elevation of adrenal androgens* See investigations, page 781	Treat the cause (p. 782)

*e.g. Serum testosterone levels in women: < 2 nmol/l (< 58 ng/dl) is normal; 2–5 nmol/l (58–144 ng/dl) is minor elevation; > 5 nmol/l (> 144 ng/dl) is high and requires further investigation.

20.27 REPRODUCTIVE MEDICINE IN OLD AGE

- **Post-menopausal osteoporosis:** a major public health issue due to the high incidence of associated fragility fractures, especially of hip.
- **Hormone replacement therapy:** should only be prescribed above the age of 50 for the short-term relief of symptoms of oestrogen deficiency.
- **Sexual activity:** many older people remain sexually active.
- **'Male menopause':** does not occur, although testosterone concentrations do fall with age. Testosterone therapy in mildly hypogonadal men may be of benefit for body composition, muscle and bone. Large randomised trials are required to determine whether benefits outweigh potentially harmful effects on the prostate and the cardiovascular system.
- **Androgens in older women:** hirsutism and balding occur. In the rare patients in whom androgen levels are elevated this may be pathological, e.g. from an ovarian tumour.

20.28 FEATURES OF POLYCYSTIC OVARIAN SYNDROME

Mechanisms*	Manifestations
Pituitary dysfunction	High serum LH High serum prolactin
Anovulatory menstrual cycles	Oligomenorrhoea Secondary amenorrhoea Cystic ovaries Infertility
Androgen excess	Hirsutism Acne
Obesity	Hyperglycaemia Elevated oestrogens
Insulin resistance	Dyslipidaemia Hypertension

*These mechanisms are interrelated—it is not known which, if any, is primary. PCOS probably represents the common endpoint of several different pathologies.

POLYCYSTIC OVARIAN SYNDROME (PCOS)

PCOS describes a constellation of clinical and biochemical features, for which the aetiology remains poorly understood. It is probably the common endpoint of a heterogeneous group of pathologies, characterised by loss of coordinate control of the menstrual cycle. PCOS often affects several family members and is aggravated by obesity. Clinical and biochemical features are shown in Box 20.28, although patients vary in the severity of each feature. Some definitions of PCOS require the demonstration of multiple cysts in the ovaries, which are most readily detected by transvaginal ultrasound. However, the presence of ovarian cysts does not usually alter management, and does not always predict other features of PCOS, so ultrasound examination is arguably not a cost-effective test in this setting.

Management
This depends on the clinical problem.

Infertility
This may be treated under specialist supervision with clomifene or exogenous gonadotrophins. Although patients with PCOS may have amenorrhoea, HRT is not required to prevent osteoporosis as circulating levels of oestrogens and androgens are elevated rather than low. The high oestrogen concentrations can cause endometrial hyperplasia and so it is usual to administer progestogens on a cyclical basis to induce a regular withdrawal bleed and thereby reduce the risk of endometrial neoplasia.

Hirsutism
For hirsutism, most patients will have used cosmetic measures such as shaving, bleaching and waxing before consulting a doctor. Electrolysis and laser treatment are

20.29 ANTI-ANDROGEN THERAPY

Mechanism of action	Drug	Dose	Hazards
Androgen receptor antagonists	Cyproterone acetate	2, 50 or 100 mg on days 1–11 of 28-day cycle with ethinylestradiol 30 µg on days 1–21	Hepatic dysfunction Feminisation of male fetus Progesterone receptor agonist Dysfunctional uterine bleeding
	Spironolactone	100–200 mg daily	Electrolyte disturbance Carcinogenic in rats
	Flutamide	Not recommended	Hepatic dysfunction
5α-reductase inhibitors (prevent conversion of testosterone to active dihydrotestosterone)	Finasteride	5 mg daily	Limited clinical experience; possibly less efficacious than other treatments
Suppress ovarian steroid production and elevate sex hormone-binding globulin	Oestrogen	See combination with cyproterone acetate above or Conventional oestrogen-containing contraceptive	Venous thromboembolism Hypertension Weight gain Dyslipidaemia Increased breast and endometrial carcinoma
Suppress adrenal androgen production	Exogenous glucocorticoid to suppress ACTH	e.g. Hydrocortisone 5 mg at 0900 hrs and dexamethasone 0.5 mg at 2200 hrs	Cushing's syndrome

effective for small areas, e.g. upper lip and chest hair, but are expensive. Eflornithine cream inhibits ornithine decarboxylase in hair follicles and may reduce hair growth when applied on a daily basis to affected areas of the face. Weight loss is a vital step in obese patients with PCOS; this enhances insulin sensitivity, reduces the peripheral conversion of androgens to oestrogens by the aromatase enzyme in adipose tissue, and reduces metabolic clearance of cortisol, thereby reducing ACTH-dependent adrenal androgen secretion.

If these conservative measures have been tried and have failed, then anti-androgen therapy may be employed, as shown in Box 20.29. The life cycle of each hair follicle is at least 3 months and so no improvement is likely to be noticed before this time, when previous follicles have all shed their hair and replacement hair growth has been suppressed. In addition, insulin-sensitising drugs such as the thiazolidinediones and biguanides (Ch. 21) may have a role but require specialist supervision. Unless the patient has lost weight, the hirsutism will return if therapy is discontinued. The patient should be aware that prolonged exposure to some of these agents may not be desirable, that they should be discontinued in advance of pregnancy, and that the prescription should be reviewed at least every 6 months.

TURNER'S SYNDROME

Turner's syndrome affects approximately 1 in 2500 females. The syndrome is classically associated with a 45XO karyotype, but other cytogenetic abnormalities may be responsible, including mosaic forms (e.g. 45XO/46XX or 45XO/46XY) and partial deletions of an X chromosome.

Clinical features
These are shown in Figure 20.15.

Individuals with Turner's syndrome invariably have short stature from an early age and this is often the initial presenting symptom. It is probably due to the absence of one copy of a *SHOX* gene, located on chromosome X and Y, which codes a protein that is predominantly found in bone fibroblasts.

The genital tract and external genitalia in Turner's syndrome are female in character, since this is the default developmental outcome in the absence of testes. Ovarian tissue develops normally until the third month of gestation, but thereafter there is gonadal dysgenesis with accelerated degeneration of oocytes and increased ovarian stromal fibrosis, resulting in 'streak ovaries'. The inability of the ovarian tissue to produce oestrogen results in loss of negative feedback and elevation of FSH and LH concentrations.

There is a wide variation in the spectrum of associated somatic abnormalities. The severity of the phenotype is, in part, related to the underlying cytogenetic abnormality. Mosaic individuals may have only mild short stature and may enter puberty spontaneously before developing gonadal failure.

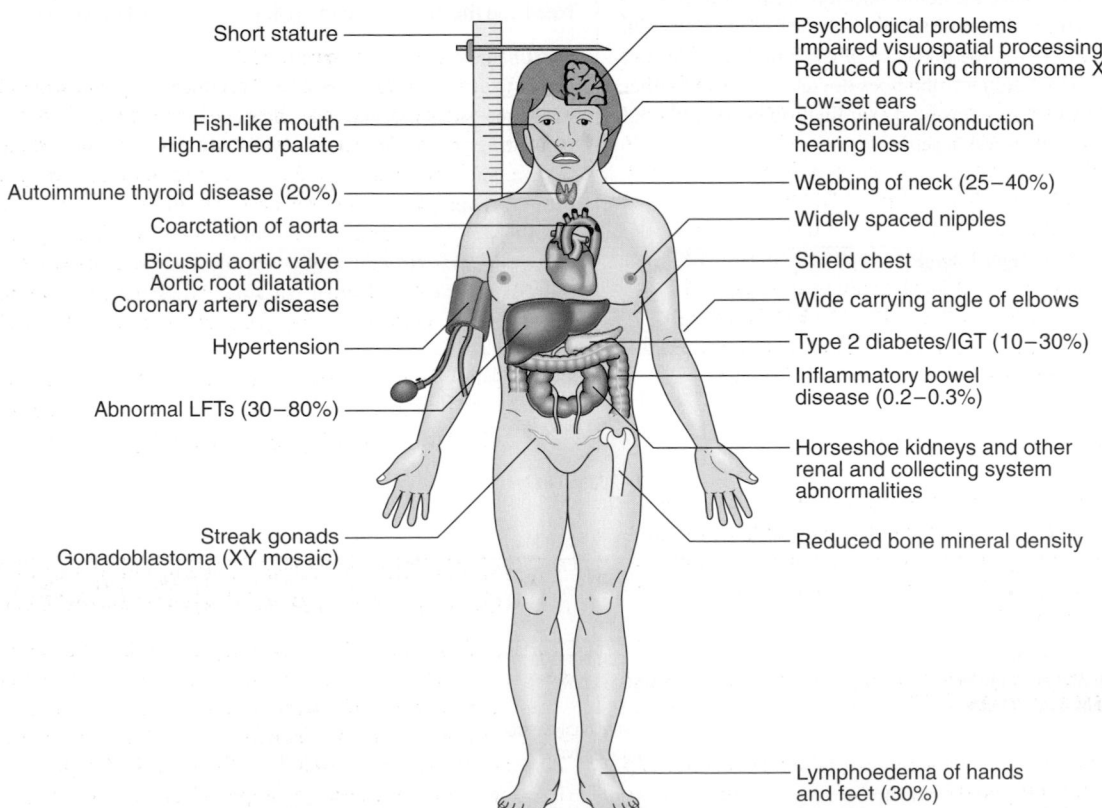

Fig. 20.15 Clinical features of Turner's syndrome (45XO). (IGT = impaired glucose tolerance)

Diagnosis and management

The diagnosis of Turner's syndrome is confirmed by karyotype analysis. Short stature, although not directly due to growth hormone deficiency, responds to high doses of growth hormone. Prophylactic gonadectomy is recommended for individuals with 45XO/45XY mosaicism because there is an increased risk of gonadoblastoma. Pubertal development is induced with oestrogen therapy, but will result in fusion of the epiphyses and cessation of growth. Therefore, the timing of pubertal induction needs to be carefully planned. Adults with Turner's syndrome require long-term oestrogen replacement therapy and should be monitored periodically for the development of aortic root dilatation and other somatic complications.

KLINEFELTER'S SYNDROME

Klinefelter's syndrome affects approximately 1 in 1000 males and is usually associated with a 47XXY karyotype. However, other cytogenetic variants may be responsible, especially 46XY/47XXY mosaicism. The principal pathological abnormality is dysgenesis of the seminiferous tubules. This is evident from infancy (and possibly even in utero) and progresses with age. By adolescence, hyalinisation and fibrosis are present within the seminiferous tubules and Leydig cell function is impaired, resulting in hypogonadism.

Clinical features

The diagnosis of Klinefelter's syndrome is typically made in adolescents who have presented with gynaecomastia and failure to progress normally through puberty. Affected individuals usually have small, firm testes. Tall stature is apparent from early childhood, reflecting characteristically long leg length associated with 47XXY, and may be exacerbated by androgen deficiency with lack of epiphyseal closure in puberty. Other clinical features may include learning difficulties and behavioural disorders, as well as an increased risk of breast cancer and type 2 diabetes in later life. The spectrum of clinical features is wide and some individuals, especially those with 46XY/47XXY mosaicism, may pass through puberty normally and be identified only when undergoing investigation for infertility.

Diagnosis and management

Klinefelter's syndrome is suggested by the typical phenotype in a patient with hypergonadotrophic hypogonadism and is confirmed by karyotype analysis. Individuals with clinical and biochemical evidence of androgen deficiency require androgen replacement as described on page 767.

TESTICULAR TUMOURS

Tumours of the testes are uncommon, with a prevalence of 5 cases per 100 000 population, and occur mainly in young men between the age of 20 and 40 years. They often secrete tumour markers which provide good indices for both diagnosis and prognosis. Seminoma and teratoma account for 85% of all tumours of the testis. Leydig cell tumours are less common.

Seminomas arise from seminiferous tubules and represent a relatively low-grade malignancy. Metastases occur mainly via the lymphatics and may involve the lungs.

Teratomas arise from primitive germinal cells. They may contain cartilage, bone, muscle, fat and a variety of other tissues, and are classified according to the degree of differentiation. Well-differentiated tumours are the least aggressive; at the other extreme, trophoblastic teratoma is highly malignant. Occasionally, teratoma and seminoma occur together.

Leydig cell tumours are usually small and benign, but secrete oestrogens leading to presentation with gynaecomastia (p. 767).

Clinical features and investigations

The common presentation is incidental discovery of a painless testicular lump although some patients complain of a testicular ache. Teratomas tend to occur in a younger age group than seminomas.

All suspicious scrotal lumps should be imaged by ultrasound which provides a high degree of accuracy. Serum levels of the 'tumour markers' α-fetoprotein (AFP) and β-human chorionic gonadotrophin (β-hCG) are increased in extensive disease. Oestradiol may be elevated, suppressing the levels of LH, FSH and testosterone. Accurate staging is based on CT of the lungs, liver and retroperitoneal area.

Management and prognosis

The primary treatment is surgical orchidectomy. Subsequent treatment depends on the histological type and stage. Radiotherapy is the treatment of choice for early-stage seminoma. Teratoma confined to the testes may be managed conservatively, but more advanced cancers are treated with chemotherapy, usually the combination of bleomycin, etoposide and cisplatin. Follow-up is by CT and assessment of AFP and β-hCG. Retroperitoneal lymph node dissection is now only performed for residual or recurrent nodal masses.

The 5-year survival rate for patients with seminoma is 90–95%. For teratomas the 5-year survival varies between 60% and 95%, depending on tumour type, stage and volume.

THE PARATHYROID GLANDS

Parathyroid hormone (PTH) is a key controller of calcium metabolism, which interacts with vitamin D in kidney and bone. Consequences of altered vitamin D in gut and renal disease are discussed in Chapters 22 and 17, respectively. Other metabolic bone disease is discussed in Chapter 25. Here, the investigation of hypercalcaemia and hypocalcaemia and disorders of the parathyroid glands are discussed.

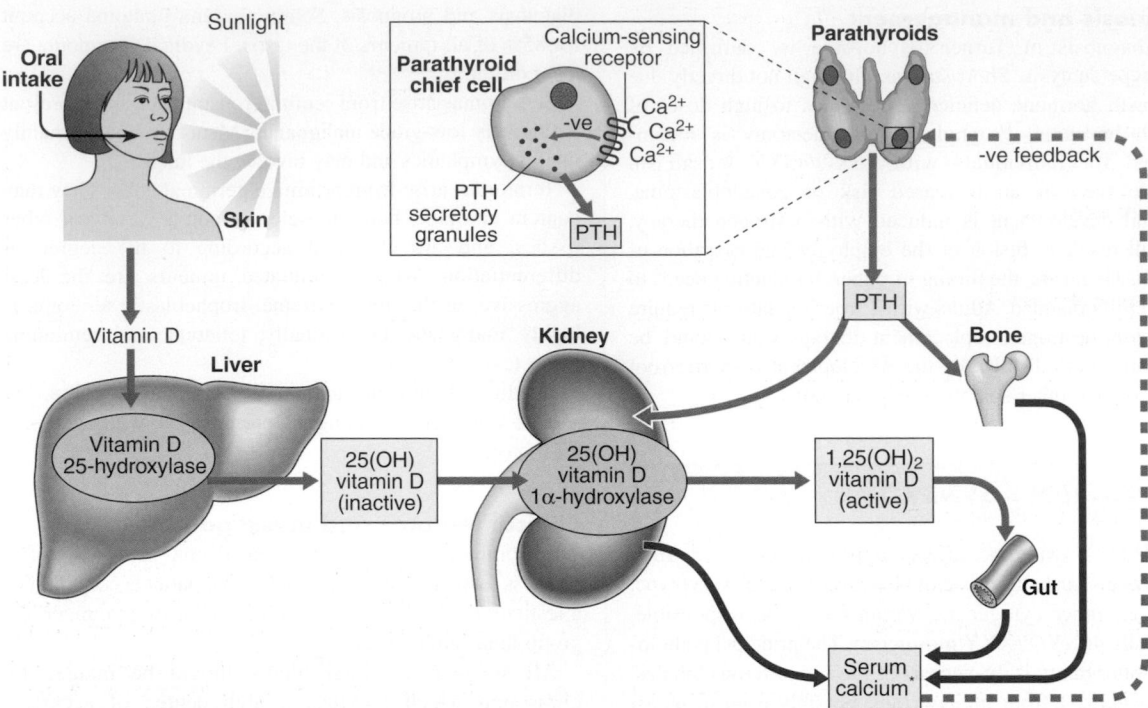

Fig. 20.16 Outline of calcium homeostasis showing interactions between parathyroid hormone (PTH), vitamin D and calcium. *Calcium in serum exists as 50% ionised (Ca^{2+}), 10% non-ionised or complexed with organic ions such as citrate and phosphate, and 40% protein-bound, mainly to albumin. It is the ionised calcium concentration which regulates PTH production.

FUNCTIONAL ANATOMY, PHYSIOLOGY AND INVESTIGATIONS

The four parathyroid glands lie behind the lobes of the thyroid. The parathyroid chief cells respond directly to changes in calcium concentrations via a G-protein-coupled cell surface receptor (the calcium-sensing receptor) located on the surface of parathyroid chief cells (Fig. 20.16). PTH is a single-chain polypeptide of 84 amino acids that is secreted in response to a fall in plasma ionised calcium concentration. PTH interacts with vitamin D and its metabolites in regulating calcium absorption and excretion, as shown in Figure 20.16.

PTH has direct effects that promote reabsorption of calcium from renal tubules and bone. PTH also has indirect effects, mediated by increasing renal conversion of 25-hydroxycholecalciferol (i.e. 25-hydroxy-vitamin D) to the more potent hormone 1,25-dihydroxycholecalciferol, which results in increased calcium absorption from food. PTH plays a central role in regulating calcium homeostasis because vitamin D and dietary calcium are rarely deficient. Moreover, 99% of total body calcium is in bone, but this pool is in dynamic equilibrium with the extracellular fluid by processes of bone resorption and deposition. The initial effect of PTH on bone is to stimulate osteolysis, returning calcium from bone to the extracellular fluid. Prolonged exposure of bone to PTH is associated with increased osteoclastic activity, extensive bone remodelling and osteoblastic repair.

Investigation of calcium metabolism is usually straightforward. Most laboratories measure total calcium in serum. About 50% of circulating calcium is bound to organic ions such as citrate or phosphate and to proteins. Total calcium measurements need to be corrected if the serum albumin is low, by adjusting the value for calcium upwards by 0.1 mmol/l (0.4 mg/dl) for each 5 g/l reduction in albumin below 40 g/l. The differential diagnosis of disorders of calcium metabolism requires measurement of phosphate, alkaline phosphatase and sometimes PTH (for which the blood sample has to be processed rapidly).

Calcitonin is secreted from the parafollicular C cells of the thyroid gland. Although calcitonin is a useful tumour marker in medullary carcinoma of thyroid (p. 761) and can be administered therapeutically in Paget's disease of bone (p. 1129), its release from the parathyroid is of no clinical relevance to calcium homeostasis in humans.

Disorders of the parathyroid glands are summarised in Box 20.30.

PRESENTING PROBLEMS IN PARATHYROID DISEASE

HYPERCALCAEMIA

Hypercalcaemia is one of the most common biochemical abnormalities and is often detected during routine biochemical analysis in asymptomatic patients. However, it can present with chronic symptoms as described below, and

20.30 CLASSIFICATION OF DISEASES OF THE PARATHYROID GLANDS

	Primary	Secondary
Hormone excess	Primary hyperparathyroidism (adenoma, hyperplasia, occasionally carcinoma) Tertiary hyperparathyroidism	Secondary hyperparathyroidism
Hormone deficiency	Post-surgical Autoimmune Autosomal dominant hypoparathyroidism	
Hormone hypersensitivity	–	
Hormone resistance	Pseudohypoparathyroidism Familial hypocalciuric hypercalcaemia	
Non-functioning tumours	Parathyroid carcinoma	

20.31 CAUSES OF HYPERCALCAEMIA

With normal or elevated (i.e. inappropriate) PTH levels

- Primary or tertiary hyperparathyroidism
- Lithium-induced hyperparathyroidism
- Familial hypocalciuric hypercalcaemia

With low (i.e. suppressed) PTH levels

- Malignancy (e.g. lung, breast, renal, ovarian, colonic and thyroid carcinoma, lymphoma, multiple myeloma)
- Elevated 1,25(OH)$_2$ vitamin D (e.g. vitamin D intoxication, sarcoidosis, HIV)
- Thyrotoxicosis
- Paget's disease with immobilisation
- Milk-alkali syndrome
- Thiazide diuretics
- Glucocorticoid deficiency

Clinical assessment

Symptoms and signs of hypercalcaemia include polyuria and polydipsia, renal colic, lethargy, anorexia, nausea, dyspepsia and peptic ulceration, constipation, depression, drowsiness and impaired cognition. Patients with malignant hypercalcaemia can have a rapid onset of symptoms and may have clinical features that help to localise the tumour.

Patients with primary hyperparathyroidism may have a chronic, non-specific history. Their symptoms are described by the adage 'bones, stones and abdominal groans'. However, about 50% of patients with primary hyperparathyroidism are asymptomatic. In others, symptoms may go unrecognised until patients present with renal calculi (5% of first stone formers and 15% of recurrent stone formers have primary hyperparathyroidism). Hypertension is common in hyperparathyroidism. Parathyroid tumours are almost never palpable. A family history of hypercalcaemia raises the possibility of FHH or MEN (p. 802).

Investigations

Low plasma phosphate and elevated alkaline phosphatase support a diagnosis of primary hyperparathyroidism or malignancy. High plasma phosphate and alkaline phosphatase accompanied by renal impairment suggest tertiary hyperparathyroidism (p. 490). Hypercalcaemia may cause nephrocalcinosis and renal tubular impairment resulting in hyperuricaemia and hyperchloraemia.

The most discriminant investigation is the measurement of PTH using a specific immunoradiometric assay. If PTH is normal or elevated and urinary calcium is elevated, then hyperparathyroidism is confirmed. Low urine calcium excretion indicates likely FHH and this can often be confirmed by screening family members for hypercalcaemia. Genetic analysis of the calcium-sensing receptor is also possible.

If PTH is low and no other cause is apparent, then malignancy with or without bony metastases is likely. PTH-related peptide, which is often responsible for the hypercalcaemia associated with malignancy, is not detected by modern PTH assays, but can be measured by a specific assay (although this is not usually necessary). Unless the source is obvious, the patient should be screened for malignancy with a chest X-ray, isotope bone scan, myeloma

occasionally patients present as an acute emergency with severe hypercalcaemia and dehydration.

Causes of hypercalcaemia are listed in Box 20.31. Of these, primary hyperparathyroidism and malignant hypercalcaemia are by far the most common. Familial hypocalciuric hypercalcaemia (FHH) is a rare but important catch for the unwary. This autosomal dominant disorder is caused by an inactivating mutation in one of the alleles of the calcium-sensing receptor, which reduces the ability of the parathyroid gland to 'sense' ionised calcium concentrations. As a result, higher than normal calcium levels are required to suppress PTH secretion. Marginal elevations in serum calcium levels are typically observed in affected individuals, with PTH concentrations that are 'inappropriately' at the upper end of the normal range, or even slightly elevated. In addition, a reduced sensitivity of calcium-sensing receptors in the kidney tubules leads to increased calcium reabsorption and hypocalciuria. An individual with FHH is almost always asymptomatic and without complications, but may end up having an unnecessary (and ineffective) parathyroidectomy if misdiagnosed as having primary hyperparathyroidism. Lithium may also cause hyperparathyroidism by reducing the sensitivity of the calcium-sensing receptor.

20.32 TREATMENT OF SEVERE HYPERCALCAEMIA OF MALIGNANCY

Rehydration with normal saline

- To replace as much as a 4–6 l deficit
- May need monitoring with central venous pressure in old age or renal impairment

Bisphosphonates, e.g. disodium pamidronate 90 mg i.v. over 4 hours

- Causes a fall in calcium which is maximal at 2–3 days and lasts a few weeks
- Unless the cause is removed, follow up with an oral bisphosphonate

Additional rapid therapy may be required in very ill patients

- Forced diuresis with saline and furosemide
- Glucocorticoids, e.g. prednisolone 40 mg daily
- Calcitonin
- Haemodialysis

Treat the cause

---

screen (Ch. 24), serum angiotensin-converting enzyme (elevated in sarcoidosis), and further imaging as appropriate.

Management

Treatment of severe hypercalcaemia and primary hyperparathyroidism is described in Box 20.32 and on page 776, respectively. FHH does not require any specific intervention.

HYPOCALCAEMIA

Aetiology

Hypocalcaemia is much less common than hypercalcaemia. Its differential diagnosis is shown in Box 20.33. Although almost all laboratories routinely report total serum calcium concentrations, it is the ionised concentration which is biologically important. The most common cause of hypocalcaemia is a low serum albumin with normal ionised calcium concentration. Correction of total serum calcium concentration for serum albumin is described in Box 20.33. Conversely, ionised calcium may be low in the face of normal total serum calcium if the serum is alkalotic—for example, as a result of hyperventilation. Magnesium depletion should also be considered as a possible contributing factor, particularly in patients with malabsorption, on diuretic therapy or with a history of alcohol excess.

The most common cause of hypoparathyroidism is damage to the parathyroid glands (or their blood supply) during thyroid surgery, although this complication is only permanent in 1% of thyroidectomies. Transient hypocalcaemia develops in 10% of patients 12–36 hours following subtotal thyroidectomy for Graves' disease. Rarely, hypoparathyroidism can occur as a result of infiltration of the glands, e.g. in haemochromatosis (p. 974) and Wilson's disease (p. 975).

There are a number of rare congenital or inherited forms of hypoparathyroidism. One form is associated with autoimmune polyendocrine syndrome type 1 (p. 803) and another with DiGeorge syndrome (p. 47). Autosomal dominant hypoparathyroidism is the mirror image of familial hypocalciuric hypercalcaemia (FHH, p. 773); an activating mutation in the calcium-sensing receptor results in hypocalcaemia, PTH concentrations that are 'inappropriately' low and hypercalciuria.

In pseudohypoparathyroidism there is tissue resistance to the effects of PTH, such that PTH concentrations are markedly elevated. The PTH receptor is normal but there are defective post-receptor mechanisms. There are several different subtypes, but in the most common form (type 1a)

20.33 DIFFERENTIAL DIAGNOSIS OF HYPOCALCAEMIA

	Total serum calcium concentration	Ionised serum calcium concentration	Serum phosphate concentration	Serum PTH concentration	Comments
Hypoalbuminaemia	↓	→	→	→	Adjust calcium upwards by 0.1 mmol/l (0.4 mg/dl) for every 5 g/l reduction in albumin below 40 g/l
Alkalosis Respiratory, e.g. hyperventilation Metabolic, e.g. Conn's syndrome	→	↓	→	→ or ↑	Chapter 16
Vitamin D deficiency	↓	↓	↓	↑	Chapter 25
Chronic renal failure	↓	↓	↑	↑	Due to impaired vitamin D hydroxylation Serum creatinine ↑
Hypoparathyroidism	↓	↓	↑	↓	See text
Pseudohypoparathyroidism	↓	↓	↑	↑	Characteristic phenotype
Acute pancreatitis	↓	↓	→ or ↓	↑	Usually clinically obvious Serum amylase ↑
Hypomagnesaemia	↓	↓	Variable	↓ or →	Treatment of hypomagnesaemia may correct hypocalcaemia

features include short stature, short 4th metacarpals and metatarsals, rounded face, obesity and subcutaneous calcification. The term 'pseudo-pseudohypoparathyroidism' is used to describe patients with these clinical features in whom serum calcium and PTH concentrations are normal. The inheritance of these disorders is an example of genetic imprinting (p. 54): inheritance of the gene defect from a mother with pseudohypoparathyroidism results in pseudo-hypoparathyroidism in the offspring, but inheritance from the father results in pseudo-pseudohypoparathyroidism.

Clinical assessment
Tetany occurs in all syndromes in which ionised calcium concentrations are low. Additional features are specific to different aetiologies.

Tetany
Low ionised calcium concentrations cause increased excitability of peripheral nerves. In the absence of alkalosis, tetany usually occurs in adults only if total serum calcium is < 2.0 mmol/l (8 mg/dl). Children are more sensitive than adults.

In children, a characteristic triad of carpopedal spasm, stridor and convulsions occurs, although one or more of these may be found independently of the others. The hands in carpal spasm adopt a characteristic position. The meta-carpophalangeal joints are flexed, the interphalangeal joints of the fingers and thumb are extended, and there is opposition of the thumb ('main d'accoucheur'). Pedal spasm is much less frequent. Stridor is caused by spasm of the glottis. Adults complain of tingling in the hands and feet and around the mouth. Less often there is painful carpopedal spasm, while stridor and fits are rare.

Latent tetany may be present when signs of overt tetany are lacking. It is best recognised by eliciting Trousseau's sign; inflation of a sphygmomanometer cuff on the upper arm to more than the systolic blood pressure is followed by carpal spasm within 3 minutes. A less specific sign of hypo-calcaemia is that described by Chvostek, in which tapping over the branches of the facial nerve as they emerge from the parotid gland produces twitching of the facial muscles.

Other features
Hypocalcaemia causes papilloedema and prolongation of the ECG QT interval, which may predispose to ventri-cular arrhythmias. Prolonged hypocalcaemia and hyper-phosphataemia (as in hypoparathyroidism) may cause calcification of the basal ganglia, grand mal epilepsy, psychosis and cataracts. Hypocalcaemia associated with hypophosphataemia, as in vitamin D deficiency, causes rickets in children and osteomalacia in adults (p. 1126).

Management
To control tetany, alkalosis can be reversed acutely if arterial PCO_2 is increased by rebreathing expired air in a paper bag or administering 5% CO_2 in oxygen. Injection of 20 ml of a 10% solution of calcium gluconate slowly into a vein will raise the serum calcium concentration immediately. An intramuscular injection of 10 ml may also be given to obtain a more prolonged effect. In severe cases of alkalotic tetany, intravenous calcium gluconate often relieves the spasm,

while specific treatment of the alkalosis, which will vary with the cause, is being applied (p. 440). Intravenous magnesium is required to correct the hypocalcaemia associated with hypomagnesaemia.

Persistent hypoparathyroidism and pseudohypo-parathyroidism are treated with oral calcium salts and vitamin D analogues, either 1α-hydroxycholecalciferol (alfacalcidol) or 1,25-dihydroxycholecalciferol (calcitriol). This therapy needs careful monitoring because of the risks of iatrogenic hypercalcaemia, hypercalciuria and nephrocalcinosis.

PRIMARY HYPERPARATHYROIDISM

It is customary to distinguish three categories of hyper-parathyroidism, as shown in Box 20.34. In primary hyperparathyroidism there is autonomous secretion of PTH, usually by a single parathyroid adenoma varying in size from a few millimetres to several centimetres in diameter. Secondary hyperparathyroidism is present when there is increased PTH secretion to compensate for prolonged hypocalcaemia and is associated with hyperplasia of all parathyroid tissue. Its effect is to restore serum calcium levels at the expense of the stores of calcium in bone. In a very small proportion of cases of secondary hyperpara-thyroidism, continuous stimulation of the parathyroids results in adenoma formation and autonomous PTH secretion. This is known as tertiary hyperparathyroidism.

Primary hyperparathyroidism is the most common of the parathyroid disorders with a prevalence of about 1 in 800. It is two to three times more common in women than men and 90% of patients are over 50 years of age. It also occurs in all of the familial MEN syndromes, as described on page 802, when hyperplasia or multiple adenomas of all four parathyroid glands rather than a solitary adenoma are more likely. Its clinical presentation is described under hypercalcaemia on page 773.

Skeletal and radiological changes
Classical hyperparathyroid bone disease is now rare due to earlier diagnosis and treatment. Osteitis fibrosa results from increased bone resorption by osteoclasts with fibrous

20.34 HYPERPARATHYROIDISM		
Type	Serum calcium	PTH
Primary Single adenoma (90%) Multiple adenomas (4%) Nodular hyperplasia (5%) Carcinoma (1%)	Raised	Not suppressed
Secondary Chronic renal failure Malabsorption Osteomalacia and rickets	Low	Raised
Tertiary	Raised	Not suppressed

replacement in the lacunae. This may present as bone pain and tenderness, fracture and deformity. Chondrocalcinosis is due to deposition of calcium pyrophosphate crystals within articular cartilage. It typically affects the menisci at the knees and can result in secondary degenerative arthritis or predispose to attacks of acute pseudogout (p. 1115).

There are characteristic changes on plain X-rays. In the early stages there is demineralisation, with subperiosteal erosions and terminal resorption in the phalanges. A 'pepper-pot' appearance may be seen on lateral X-rays of the skull. In nephrocalcinosis, scattered opacities may be visible within the renal outline. There may be soft tissue calcification in arterial walls, soft tissues of the hands and the cornea.

Reduced bone mineral density is now the most common skeletal manifestation of hyperparathyroidism. This is usually not evident radiographically and requires assessment by DEXA scanning.

Localisation of parathyroid tumours

If primary hyperparathyroidism is confirmed biochemically, imaging to locate the adenoma or differentiate adenomas from hyperplasia has traditionally not been necessary. In over 90% of patients an experienced surgeon will locate the adenoma without difficulty. If surgical exploration has been unsuccessful, ^{99m}Tc-sestamibi scanning (Fig. 20.17), ultrasonography, CT and selective neck vein catheterisation with PTH measurements have proved useful in localising the adenoma. There is now an increasing trend to perform ^{99m}Tc-sestamibi scanning prior to initial surgery to allow a more targeted resection through a small incision.

Management

Treatment of severe hypercalcaemia in hyperparathyroidism is shown in Box 20.32. Hypercalcaemia in patients with primary hyperparathyroidism responds less well to glucocorticoids and bisphosphonates than in those with malignancy. Urgent neck surgery is occasionally required, but strenuous attempts should be made to replace fluid deficits and lower the serum calcium concentration before administering an anaesthetic.

Most patients do not require urgent treatment. Currently, the only long-term therapy is surgery, with excision of a solitary parathyroid adenoma or debulking of hyperplastic glands. Some surgeons transplant part of a hyperplastic gland to the forearm where it can be accessed for further debulking at a later date. Post-operative hypocalcaemia is not uncommon during the first 2 weeks while residual suppressed parathyroid tissue recovers.

The selection of patients with primary hyperparathyroidism who require surgery is not always straightforward. Surgery is indicated for young patients (< 50 years) and those with clear-cut symptoms or documented complications such as peptic ulceration, renal stones, renal impairment or osteopenia. However, a large number of patients have only vague symptoms or are asymptomatic. They can be reviewed every 6–12 months, with assessment of symptoms, renal function, serum calcium and bone mineral density. They should be encouraged to maintain a high oral fluid intake to avoid renal stones.

Drugs that enhance the sensitivity of the calcium-sensing receptor (calcimimetics) are being developed and, in the future, may offer an alternative to surgery in hyperparathyroidism.

20.35 THE PARATHYROID GLANDS IN OLD AGE
• **Osteoporosis:** always exclude osteomalacia and hyperparathyroidism by checking vitamin D and calcium concentrations.
• **Primary hyperparathyroidism:** more common with age. Older people can often be observed without surgical intervention.
• **Hypercalcaemia:** may cause confusion.
• **Vitamin D deficiency:** common because of poor diet and limited exposure to the sun.

THE ADRENAL GLANDS

The adrenals function as several separate endocrine glands within one anatomical structure. The adrenal medulla is an extension of the sympathetic nervous system which secretes catecholamines. Most of the adrenal cortex is made up of cells which secrete cortisol and adrenal androgens, and form part of the hypothalamic–pituitary–adrenal axis. The small outer glomerulosa of the cortex secretes aldosterone under the control of the renin–angiotensin system. These functions

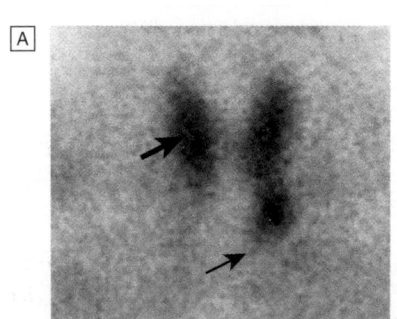

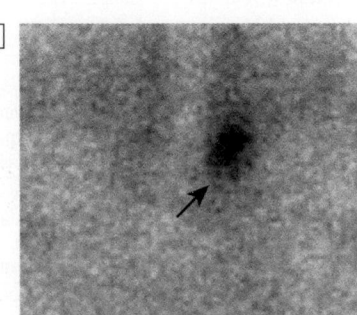

Fig. 20.17 ^{99m}Tc-sestamibi scan of a patient with primary hyperparathyroidism secondary to a parathyroid adenoma. A After 1 hour, there is uptake in the thyroid gland (thick arrow) and the enlarged left inferior parathyroid gland (thin arrow). B After 3 hours, uptake is evident only in the parathyroid.

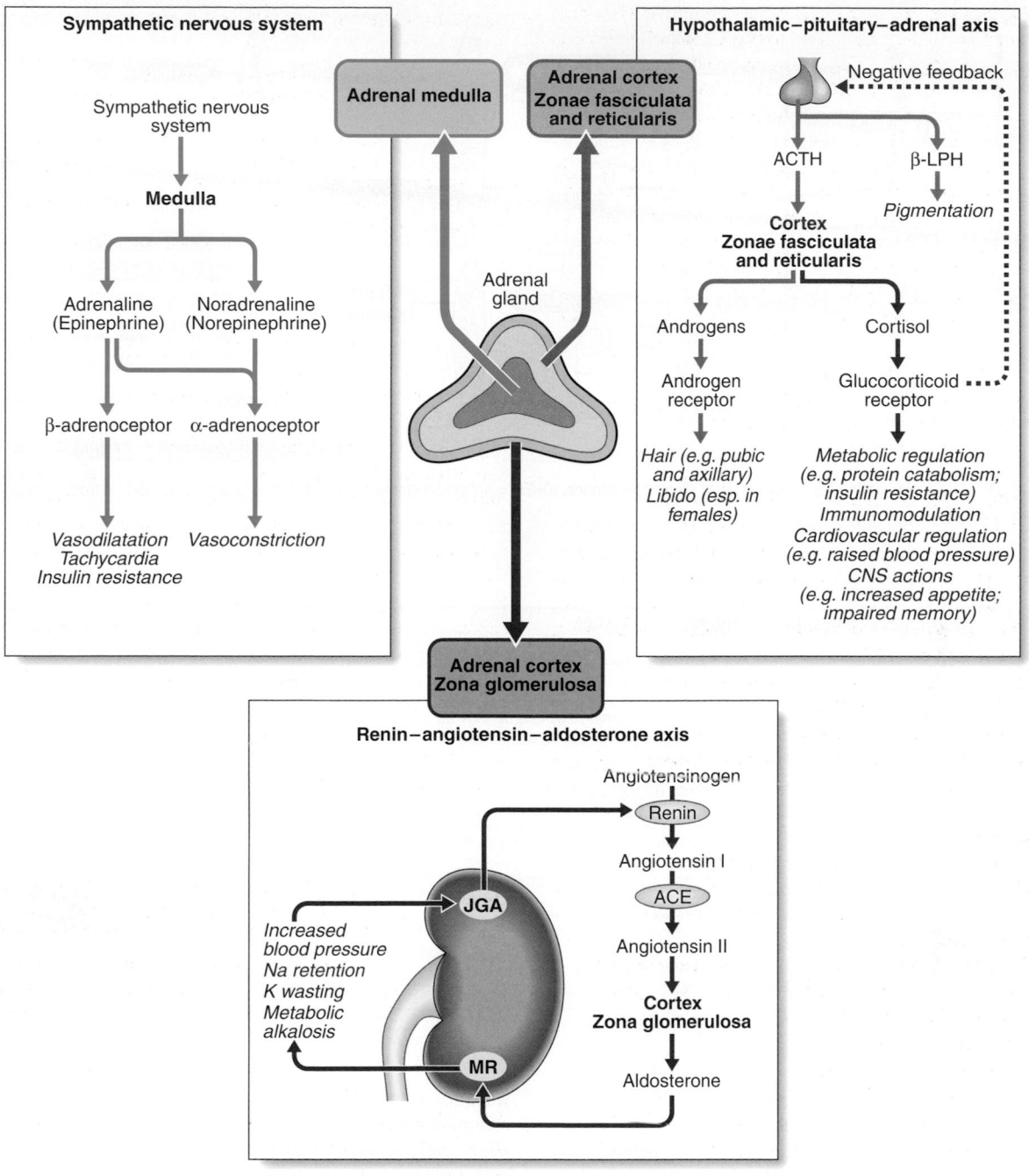

Fig. 20.18 Structure and function of the adrenal glands. (ACE = angiotensin-converting enzyme; JGA = juxtaglomerular apparatus; MR = mineralocorticoid receptor; β-LPH = β-lipotrophic hormone, a fragment of the ACTH precursor peptide pro-opiomelanocortin which contains melanocyte-stimulating hormone activity)

20

are important in the integrated control of cardiovascular, metabolic and immune responses to stress.

Subtle alterations in adrenal function may be important in common diseases, including hypertension, obesity and type 2 diabetes mellitus. However, classical syndromes of adrenal hormone deficiency and excess are relatively rare.

FUNCTIONAL ANATOMY, PHYSIOLOGY AND INVESTIGATIONS

Adrenal anatomy and function are shown in Figure 20.18. Histologically, the cortex is divided into three zones, but these function as two units (zona glomerulosa and zonae

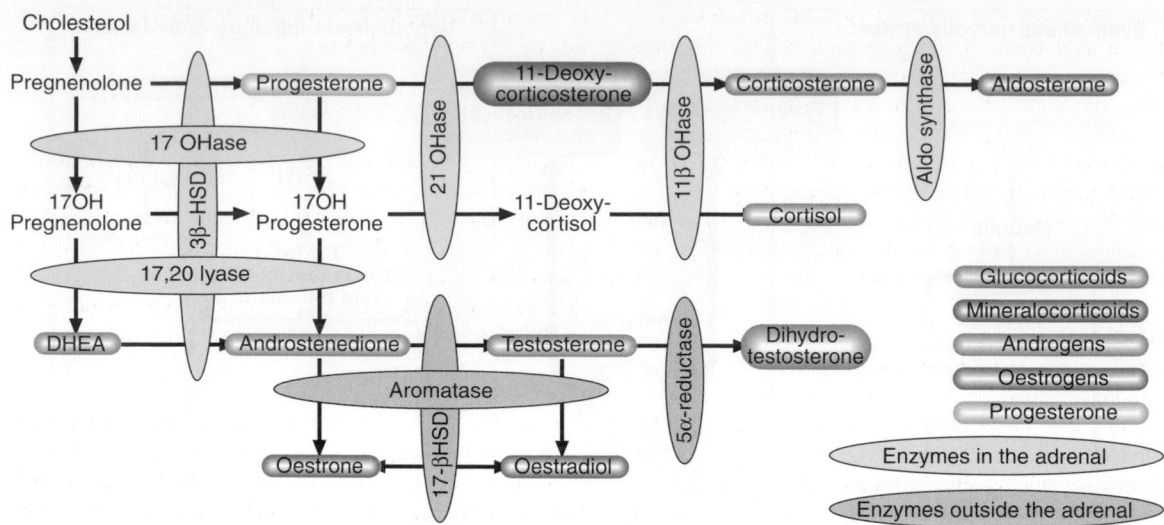

Fig. 20.19   The major pathways of synthesis of steroid hormones. (DHEA = dehydroepiandrosterone; OHase = hydroxylase; HSD = hydroxysteroid dehydrogenase)

20.36 CLASSIFICATION OF DISEASES OF THE ADRENAL GLANDS		
	Primary	**Secondary**
Hormone excess	Non-ACTH-dependent Cushing's syndrome (Box 20.37) Primary hyperaldosteronism (Box 20.46, p. 786) Phaeochromocytoma	ACTH-dependent Cushing's syndrome Secondary hyperaldosteronism
Hormone deficiency	Addison's disease (Box 20.39, p. 782) Congenital adrenal hyperplasia	Hypopituitarism
Hormone hypersensitivity	11β-hydroxysteroid dehydrogenase type 2 deficiency Liddle's syndrome	
Hormone resistance	Pseudohypoaldosteronism Glucocorticoid resistance syndrome	
Non-functioning tumours	Adenoma Carcinoma (usually functioning) Metastatic tumours	

fasciculata/reticularis) which produce corticosteroids in response to humoral stimuli. Pathways for the biosynthesis of corticosteroids are shown in Figure 20.19. Investigation of adrenal function is described under specific diseases below. Pathologies are classified in Box 20.36.

Glucocorticoids

Cortisol is the major glucocorticoid in humans. Levels are highest in the morning on waking and lowest in the middle of the night. Cortisol rises dramatically during stress, including any illness. This elevation protects key metabolic functions (e.g. maintaining cerebral glucose supply during starvation) and puts an important 'brake' on potentially damaging inflammatory responses to infection and injury. The clinical importance of cortisol deficiency is, therefore, most obvious at times of stress.

In the circulation, more than 95% of cortisol is bound to protein, principally cortisol-binding globulin. It is the free fraction which is biologically active via glucocorticoid receptors which regulate the transcription of many genes in many cells. Cortisol can also activate mineralocorticoid receptors, but it does not normally do so because most cells containing mineralocorticoid receptors also express an enzyme, 11β-hydroxysteroid dehydrogenase type 2 (11β-HSD2), which converts cortisol to its inactive metabolite, cortisone. Loss of this protection of mineralocorticoid receptors by inhibition of 11β-HSD2 (e.g. by liquorice) results in cortisol acting like aldosterone as a potent sodium-retaining steroid.

Mineralocorticoids

Aldosterone is the body's most important sodium-retaining hormone, acting via mineralocorticoid receptors. Sodium is retained at the expense of increased excretion of potassium. Increased potassium in the lumen of the distal nephron also results in increased exchange with protons and metabolic alkalosis. The principal stimulus to aldosterone secretion is angiotensin II, a peptide produced by activation of the renin–angiotensin system (Fig. 20.18). Renin secretion from the juxtaglomerular apparatus in the kidney is stimulated by low perfusion pressure in the afferent arteriole, low sodium filtration leading to low sodium concentrations at the macula densa, or increased sympathetic nerve activity. As a result, renin is increased in hypovolaemia and renal artery stenosis, and renin concentrations when standing are about double those when lying down.

Catecholamines

In humans, only a small proportion of circulating noradrenaline (norepinephrine) is derived from the adrenal medulla; much more is released from other nerve endings. The methyltransferase enzyme responsible for the conversion of noradrenaline to adrenaline (epinephrine) is induced by glucocorticoids. Blood flow in the adrenal is centripetal so that the medulla is bathed in high concentrations of cortisol and is the major source of circulating adrenaline. However, in the absence of functioning adrenal medullae, e.g. after bilateral adrenalectomy, there appear to be no clinical consequences attributable to deficiency of circulating catecholamines.

Adrenal androgens

Adrenal androgens are secreted in response to ACTH and are the most abundant steroids in the blood stream. They are probably important in the initiation of puberty (the adrenarche). The adrenals are also the major source of androgens in adult females and may be important in female libido.

PRESENTING PROBLEMS IN ADRENAL DISEASE

Adrenal diseases are rare, but they often need to be considered because they are encountered in the context of common complaints. Classical syndromes of adrenal disease are described below.

CUSHING'S SYNDROME

Cushing's syndrome is caused by excessive activation of glucocorticoid receptors. By far the most common cause is iatrogenic, due to prolonged administration of synthetic glucocorticoids such as prednisolone. Non-iatrogenic Cushing's syndrome is rare, although it presents by many diverse routes and is often a 'spot diagnosis' made by an astute clinician.

Aetiology

Causes are shown in Box 20.37. Amongst endogenous causes, pituitary-dependent cortisol excess (by convention, called Cushing's disease) accounts for ~80% of cases. Both Cushing's disease and adrenal tumour are four times more common in women than men. In contrast, ectopic ACTH syndrome (often due to a small-cell carcinoma of the bronchus) is more common in men.

Clinical assessment

The diverse manifestations of glucocorticoid excess are indicated in Figure 20.20. Many of these are not specific to Cushing's syndrome and, because spontaneous Cushing's syndrome is rare, the positive predictive value of any one feature alone is low. Moreover, some common disorders can be confused with Cushing's syndrome because they are associated with alterations in cortisol secretion: for example, obesity and depression (Box 20.37). Features which have the best predictive value in favour of Cushing's syndrome in an obese patient are bruising, myopathy and hypertension. Any clinical suspicion of cortisol excess is best resolved by further investigation.

In all patients with features of Cushing's syndrome it is vital to exclude iatrogenic causes. Even inhaled or topical glucocorticoid administration can induce Cushing's syndrome in susceptible individuals. A careful drug history must be taken before embarking on complex investigations.

Some clinical features are more common in ectopic ACTH syndrome. Unlike pituitary tumours secreting ACTH, ectopic tumours have no residual negative feedback sensitivity to cortisol, and both ACTH and cortisol levels are usually higher than with other causes. Very high ACTH levels are associated with marked pigmentation. Very high cortisol levels overcome the barrier of 11β-HSD2 in the kidney and cause hypokalaemic alkalosis. Hypokalaemia aggravates both myopathy and hyperglycaemia (by inhibiting insulin secretion). When the tumour secreting ACTH is malignant (e.g. small-cell lung carcinoma), then the onset is usually rapid and may be associated with cachexia. For these reasons, the classical features of Cushing's syndrome are less common in ectopic ACTH syndrome, and if present suggest that a less aggressive tumour (e.g. bronchial carcinoid) is responsible.

In Cushing's disease, the pituitary tumour is usually a microadenoma (< 10 mm in diameter); hence other features of a pituitary macroadenoma (hypopituitarism, visual failure or disconnection hyperprolactinaemia, p. 797) are rare.

20.37 CLASSIFICATION OF CUSHING'S SYNDROME

ACTH-dependent

- Pituitary adenoma secreting ACTH (i.e. Cushing's disease)
- Ectopic ACTH syndrome (e.g. bronchial carcinoid, small-cell lung carcinoma, pancreatic neuro-endocrine tumour)
- Iatrogenic (ACTH therapy)

Non-ACTH-dependent

- Iatrogenic (chronic glucocorticoid therapy, e.g. for asthma)
- Adrenal adenoma
- Adrenal carcinoma

Pseudo-Cushing's syndrome, i.e. cortisol excess as part of another illness

- Alcohol excess (biochemical and clinical features)
- Major depressive illness (biochemical features only, some clinical overlap, p. 240)
- Primary obesity (mild biochemical features, some clinical overlap)

20

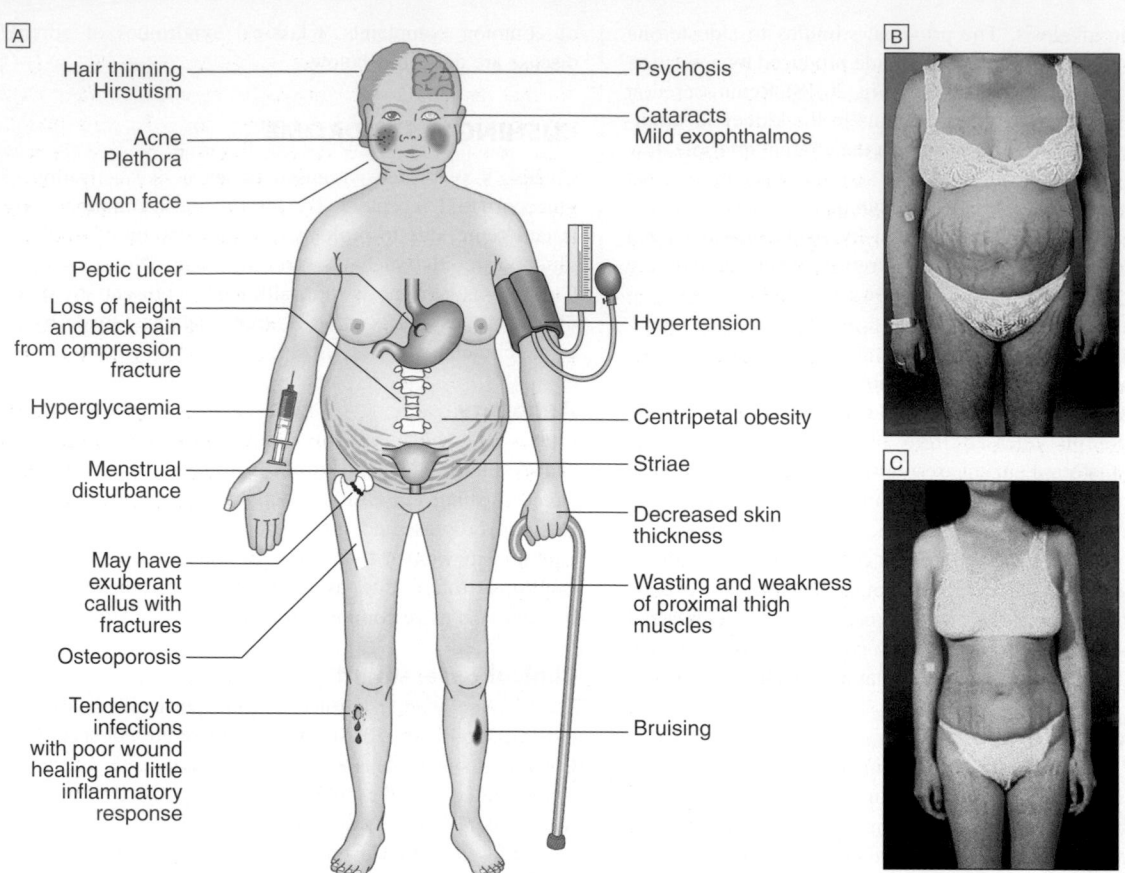

Fig. 20.20 **Cushing's syndrome.** A Clinical features common to all causes. B A patient with Cushing's disease before treatment. C The same patient 1 year after the successful removal of an ACTH-secreting pituitary microadenoma by trans-sphenoidal surgery.

20.38 TESTS FOR CUSHING'S SYNDROME		
Test	**Protocol**	**Interpretation**
Urine free cortisol	24-hr timed collection (some centres use overnight collections corrected for creatinine)	Normal range depends on assay
Overnight dexamethasone suppression test	1 mg orally at midnight; measure plasma cortisol at 0800–0900 hrs	Plasma cortisol < 60 nmol/l (< 2.2 µg/dl) excludes Cushing's
Diurnal rhythm of plasma cortisol	Sample for cortisol at 0900 hrs and at 2300 hrs (requires acclimatisation to ward for at least 48 hrs)	Evening level > 75% of morning level in Cushing's
Low-dose dexamethasone suppression test	0.5 mg 6-hourly for 48 hrs; sample 24-hr urine cortisol during second day and 0900-hr plasma cortisol after 48 hrs	Urine cortisol < 100 nmol/day (36 µg/day) or plasma cortisol < 60 nmol/l (< 2.2 µg/dl) excludes Cushing's
Insulin tolerance test	Box 20.56, page 796	Peak plasma cortisol > 120% of baseline excludes Cushing's
High-dose dexamethasone suppression test	2 mg 6-hourly for 48 hrs; sample 24-hr urine cortisol at baseline and during second day	Urine cortisol < 50% of basal suggests pituitary-dependent disease; > 50% of basal suggests ectopic ACTH syndrome
Corticotrophin-releasing hormone test	100 µg ovine CRH i.v. and monitor plasma ACTH and cortisol for 2 hrs	Peak plasma cortisol > 120% and/or ACTH > 150% of basal values suggests pituitary-dependent disease; lesser responses suggest ectopic ACTH syndrome
Inferior petrosal sinus sampling	Catheters placed in both inferior petrosal sinuses and simultaneous sampling from these and peripheral blood for ACTH; may be repeated 10 minutes after peripheral CRH injection	ACTH concentration in either petrosal sinus > 200% peripheral ACTH suggests pituitary-dependent disease; < 150% suggests ectopic ACTH syndrome

Investigations

The large number of tests available for Cushing's syndrome reflects the fact that no single test is infallible and several are needed to establish the diagnosis. It is useful to divide investigations into those which establish whether the patient has Cushing's syndrome, and those which are used subsequently to elucidate the aetiology.

A recommended sequence of investigations is shown in Figure 20.21 and the interpretation of these tests is shown in Box 20.38. Some additional tests are useful in all cases of Cushing's syndrome, including plasma electrolytes, glucose, glycosylated haemoglobin and bone mineral density measurement.

In iatrogenic Cushing's syndrome, cortisol levels are low unless the patient is taking a corticosteroid (such as prednisolone) which cross-reacts in immunoassays with cortisol.

Does the patient have Cushing's syndrome?

Plasma cortisol levels are highly variable in healthy subjects so that patients with Cushing's syndrome often have daytime values within the normal range. For this reason, there is no place for a random measurement of daytime plasma cortisol in the clinic in either supporting or refuting the diagnosis. Cushing's syndrome is confirmed by the demonstration of increased secretion of cortisol (measured in urine) that fails to suppress with relatively low doses of dexamethasone (measured in plasma or urine) (Box 20.38). Loss of diurnal variation, with elevated evening plasma cortisol, is also characteristic of Cushing's syndrome, but samples are awkward to obtain.

Dexamethasone is used for suppression testing because, unlike prednisolone, it does not cross-react in radioimmunoassays for cortisol. However, metabolism of dexamethasone may be altered by drugs, e.g. enzyme inducers such as

20

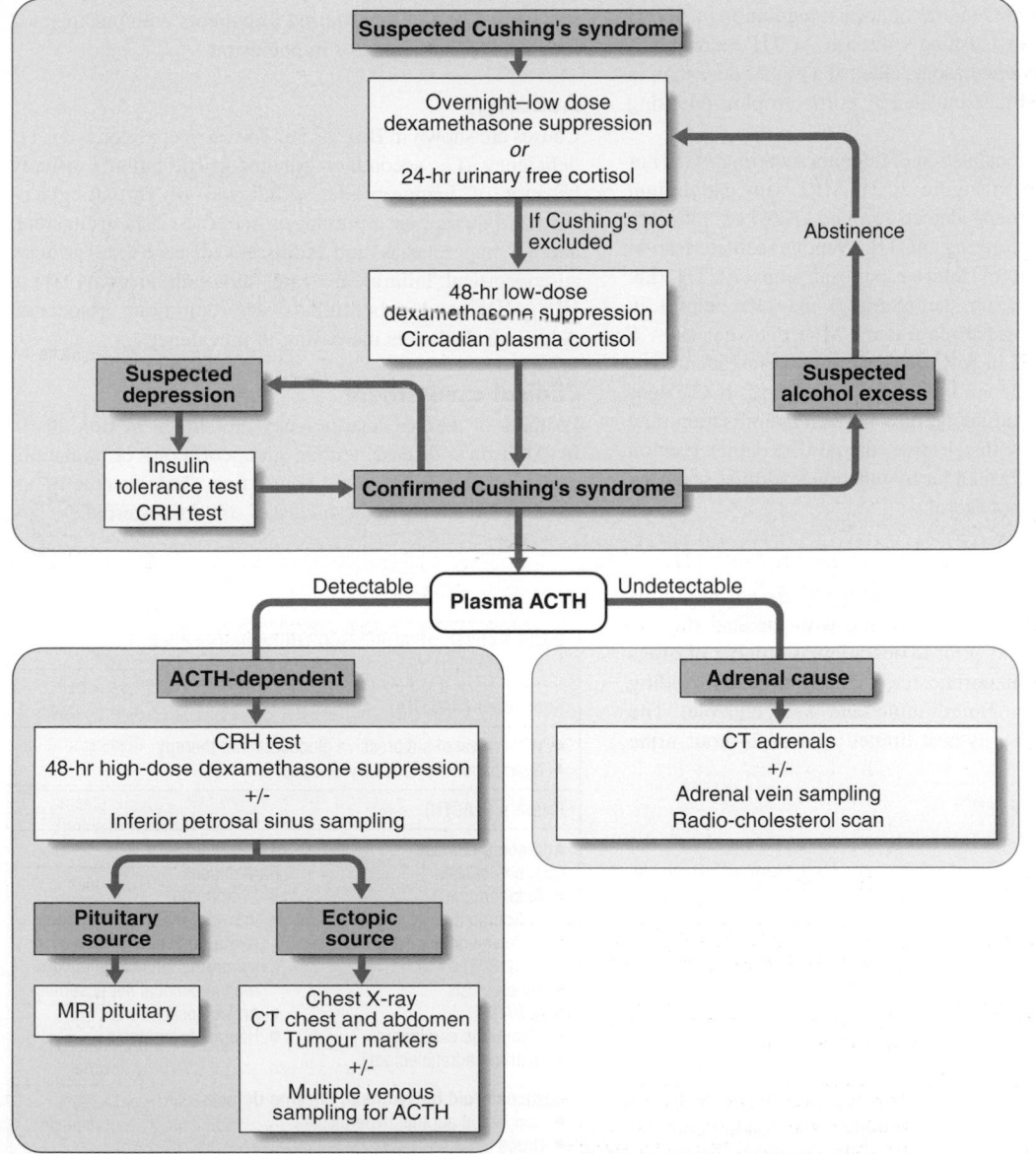

Fig. 20.21 **Sequence of investigations in suspected spontaneous Cushing's syndrome.** (CRH = corticotrophin-releasing hormone)

oestrogen or phenytoin. Also, the hypothalamic–pituitary–adrenal axis may 'escape' from suppression by dexamethasone if a more potent influence such as psychological stress supervenes.

There is a rare syndrome of cyclical Cushing's syndrome in which the excessive secretion of cortisol is episodic. If there is a strong clinical suspicion of Cushing's syndrome but initial screening tests are normal, then weekly 24-hour urine cortisol measurements for up to 3 months are sometimes justified.

What is the cause of the Cushing's syndrome?

Once the presence of Cushing's syndrome is confirmed, measurement of plasma ACTH is the key to establishing the differential diagnosis. In the presence of excess cortisol secretion, an undetectable ACTH indicates an adrenal tumour, while any detectable ACTH is pathological. Tests to discriminate pituitary from ectopic sources of ACTH rely on the fact that pituitary tumours, but not ectopic tumours, retain some features of normal regulation of ACTH secretion. Thus, in Cushing's disease ACTH secretion is suppressed by dexamethasone, albeit at a higher dose than in health, and ACTH is stimulated by corticotrophin-releasing hormone (CRH).

Techniques for localisation of tumours secreting ACTH or cortisol are listed in Figure 20.21. MRI with gadolinium contrast enhancement detects around 70% of pituitary microadenomas secreting ACTH. Venous catheterisation with measurement of inferior petrosal sinus ACTH (i.e. draining directly from the pituitary) may be helpful in confirming Cushing's disease if the MRI does not show a microadenoma. CT or MRI detects most adrenal adenomas. Adrenal carcinomas are usually large (> 5 cm). If CT does not demonstrate a unilateral tumour, then lateralisation may be possible either with selective adrenal vein catheterisation and sampling for cortisol, or by functional adrenal scanning using ^{131}iodo-norcholesterol.

Management

Untreated Cushing's syndrome has a 50% 5-year mortality. Most patients are treated surgically with medical therapy given for a few weeks prior to operation. A number of drugs are used to inhibit corticosteroid biosynthesis, including metyrapone, aminoglutethimide and ketoconazole. The dose of these agents is best titrated against 24-hour urine free cortisol.

Cushing's disease

Trans-sphenoidal surgery with selective removal of the adenoma is the treatment of choice. Experienced surgeons can identify microadenomas which were not detected by MRI and cure about 80% of patients. If the operation is unsuccessful then bilateral adrenalectomy is an alternative.

If bilateral adrenalectomy is used in patients with pituitary-dependent Cushing's syndrome, then there is a risk that the pituitary tumour will grow in the absence of the negative feedback suppression previously provided by elevated cortisol levels. This can result in Nelson's syndrome, with an aggressive pituitary macroadenoma and very high ACTH levels causing pigmentation. Nelson's syndrome can be prevented by pituitary irradiation.

Adrenal tumours

Adrenal adenomas are removed via laparoscopy or a loin incision. Adrenal carcinomas are resected if possible, the tumour bed irradiated and the patient given the adrenolytic drug mitotane. Cytotoxic chemotherapy may retard disease progression in patients with metastases.

Ectopic ACTH syndrome

Localised tumours causing this syndrome (e.g. bronchial carcinoid) should be removed. During treatment or palliation of non-resectable malignancies, it is important to reduce the severity of the Cushing's syndrome using medical therapy (see above).

ADRENAL INSUFFICIENCY

Adrenal insufficiency results from inadequate secretion of cortisol and/or aldosterone. It is potentially fatal and notoriously variable in its presentation. A high index of suspicion is therefore required in patients with unexplained fatigue, hyponatraemia or hypotension.

Aetiology

Causes are shown in Box 20.39. The most common is ACTH deficiency (i.e. secondary adrenocortical failure), usually because of inappropriate withdrawal of chronic glucocorticoid therapy or a pituitary tumour (p. 797). Congenital adrenal hyperplasias and Addison's disease (i.e. primary adrenocortical failure) are rare, although in areas where HIV/AIDS and tuberculosis are common, associated Addison's disease is increasing in prevalence.

Clinical assessment

Features of adrenal insufficiency are shown in Box 20.40. In Addison's disease, either glucocorticoid or mineralocorticoid deficiency may come first, but eventually all patients fail to secrete both classes of corticosteroid.

20.39 CAUSES OF ADRENOCORTICAL INSUFFICIENCY

Secondary (↓ACTH)

- Withdrawal of suppressive glucocorticoid therapy
- Hypothalamic or pituitary disease

Primary (↑ACTH)

Addison's disease

Common causes	Rare causes

• Autoimmune
   Sporadic
   Polyglandular syndromes
   (p. 803)
	• Lymphoma
	• Intra-adrenal haemorrhage
	   (Waterhouse–Friedrichsen
	   syndrome following
	   meningococcal septicaemia)

• Tuberculosis	• Amyloidosis
• HIV/AIDS	• Haemochromatosis
• Metastatic carcinoma	
• Bilateral adrenalectomy	

Corticosteroid biosynthetic enzyme defects
- Congenital adrenal hyperplasias
- Drugs
   Aminoglutethimide, metyrapone, ketoconazole, etomidate etc.

20.40 CLINICAL AND BIOCHEMICAL FEATURES OF ADRENAL INSUFFICIENCY

	Glucocorticoid insufficiency	Mineralocorticoid insufficiency	ACTH excess	Adrenal androgen insufficiency
Withdrawal of exogenous glucocorticoid	+	−	−	+
Hypopituitarism	+	−	−	+
Addison's disease	+	+	+	+
Congenital adrenal hyperplasia (21 OHase deficiency)	+	+	+	−

Clinical features	Weight loss
	Malaise
	Weakness
	Anorexia
	Nausea
	Vomiting
	Gastrointestinal—diarrhoea or constipation
	Postural hypotension
	Shock
	Hypoglycaemia
	Hyponatraemia (dilutional)
	Hypercalcaemia
		Hypotension
		Shock
		Hyponatraemia (depletional)
		Hyperkalaemia
			Pigmentation
			  Sun-exposed areas
			  Pressure areas, e.g. elbows, knees
			  Palmar creases, knuckles
			  Mucous membranes
			  Conjunctivae
			  Recent scars
				Decreased body hair and loss of libido, especially in female

20

Patients may present with chronic features and/or in acute circulatory shock. With a chronic presentation, initial symptoms are often misdiagnosed (e.g. as chronic fatigue syndrome or depression). Adrenocortical insufficiency should also be considered in patients with hyponatraemia, even in the absence of symptoms (p. 429).

Features of an acute adrenal crisis include circulatory shock with severe hypotension, hyponatraemia, hyperkalaemia and, in some instances, hypoglycaemia and hypercalcaemia. Muscle cramps, nausea, vomiting, diarrhoea and unexplained fever may be present. The crisis is often precipitated by intercurrent disease, surgery or infection.

Vitiligo occurs in 10–20% of patients with autoimmune Addison's disease (p. 1280).

Investigations

In patients presenting with chronic illness, the investigations below should be performed before any treatment. In patients with suspected acute adrenal crisis treatment should not be delayed pending results. A random blood sample should be stored for measurement of cortisol. It may be appropriate to spend 30 minutes performing a short ACTH stimulation test (Box 20.41) before administering hydrocortisone, but investigations may need to be delayed until after recovery.

Assessment of glucocorticoids

Random plasma cortisol is usually low in patients with adrenal insufficiency, but it may be within the normal range yet inappropriately low for a seriously ill patient. Random measurement of plasma cortisol cannot therefore be used to confirm or refute the diagnosis, unless the value is high, i.e. > 460 nmol/l (> ~170 µg/dl).

More useful is the short ACTH stimulation test (also called the tetracosactide or short Synacthen test) described in Box 20.41. Cortisol levels fail to increase in response to exogenous ACTH in patients with primary or secondary

20.41 ACTH STIMULATION TEST

Use

- Diagnosis of primary or secondary adrenal insufficiency
- Assessment of hypothalamic–pituitary–adrenal axis in patients taking suppressive glucocorticoid therapy
- Relies on ACTH-dependent adrenal atrophy in secondary adrenal insufficiency, so may not detect acute ACTH deficiency (e.g. in pituitary apoplexy, p. 798)

Dose

- 250 µg $ACTH_{1-24}$ (Synacthen) by i.m. injection at any time of day

Blood samples

- 0 and 30 minutes for plasma cortisol
- 0 minutes also for ACTH (on ice) if Addison's disease is being considered (i.e. patient not known to have pituitary disease or to be taking exogenous glucocorticoids)

Results

- Normal subjects plasma cortisol > 460 nmol/l (~170 µg/dl)* either at baseline or at 30 minutes
- Incremental change in cortisol is not a criterion

* The exact cortisol concentration depends on the cortisol assay being used.

adrenal insufficiency. These can be distinguished by measurement of ACTH (which is low in ACTH deficiency and high in Addison's disease). If an ACTH assay is unavailable, then a long ACTH stimulation test can be used (1 mg depot ACTH i.m. daily for 3 days); in secondary adrenal insufficiency there is a progressive increase in plasma cortisol with repeated ACTH administration, whereas in Addison's disease cortisol remains less than 700 nmol/l (25.4 µg/dl) at 8 hours after the last injection.

In a patient who is already receiving glucocorticoids, the short ACTH stimulation test can be performed first thing in the morning, > 12 hours after the last dose of glucocorticoid, or the treatment can be changed to a synthetic steroid such as dexamethasone (0.75 mg daily), which does not cross-react in the plasma cortisol immunoassay.

Assessment of mineralocorticoids

Plasma electrolyte measurements are insufficient to assess mineralocorticoid secretion in patients with suspected Addison's disease. Hyponatraemia occurs in both aldosterone and cortisol deficiency (Box 20.40 and p. 429). Hyperkalaemia is common, but not universal, in aldosterone deficiency. Plasma renin activity and aldosterone should be measured in the supine position. In mineralocorticoid deficiency, plasma renin activity is high, with plasma aldosterone being either low or in the lower part of the normal range.

Other tests to establish the cause

Patients with unexplained secondary adrenocortical insufficiency should be investigated as described in the section on pituitary disease on page 794. In patients with elevated ACTH, further tests are required to establish the cause of Addison's disease. In those who have autoimmune adrenal failure, antibodies can often be measured against steroid-secreting cells (adrenal and gonad), thyroid antigens, pancreatic β cells and parietal cells. Thyroid function tests, full blood count (to screen for pernicious anaemia), plasma calcium, glucose and tests of gonadal function (p. 762) should be performed. Other causes of adrenocortical disease are usually obvious clinically, particularly if health is not fully restored by corticosteroid replacement therapy. Tuberculosis causes adrenal calcification, visible on plain X-ray or ultrasound scan. A chest X-ray and early morning urine for culture should also be taken. An HIV test may be appropriate if risk factors for infection are present (p. 379). Imaging of the adrenals by CT or MRI to identify metastatic malignancy may also be appropriate.

Management

Patients with adrenocortical insufficiency always need glucocorticoid replacement therapy and usually, but not always, mineralocorticoid. Adrenal androgen replacement for women is not usually employed. Other treatments depend on the underlying cause.

Glucocorticoid replacement

Cortisol (hydrocortisone) is the drug of choice. In the past, cortisone acetate was given, but this has to be converted to cortisol in the liver and in some patients this process may be impaired. In someone who is not critically ill, cortisol should be given by mouth, 15 mg on waking and 5 mg at ~1800 hrs. The dose may need to be adjusted for the individual patient, but this is subjective. Excess weight gain usually indicates over-replacement, whilst persistent lethargy or hyperpigmentation may be due to an inadequate dose. Measurement of plasma cortisol levels is unhelpful, because the dynamic interaction between cortisol and glucocorticoid receptors is not predicted by measurements such as the maximum or minimum plasma cortisol level after each dose. Advice to patients dependent on glucocorticoid replacement is given in

20.42 ADVICE TO PATIENTS ON GLUCOCORTICOID REPLACEMENT
Intercurrent stress
● e.g. Febrile illness—double dose of hydrocortisone
Surgery
● Minor operation—hydrocortisone 100 mg i.m. with pre-medication ● Major operation—hydrocortisone 100 mg 6-hourly for 24 hours, then 50 mg i.m. 6-hourly until ready to take tablets
Vomiting
● Must have parenteral hydrocortisone if unable to take by mouth
Steroid card
● Patient should carry this at all times. Should give information regarding diagnosis, steroid, dose and doctor
Bracelet
● Patients should be encouraged to buy one of these and have it engraved with the diagnosis and a reference number for a central database

Box 20.42. These are physiological replacement doses which should not cause Cushingoid side-effects.

An adrenal crisis is a medical emergency and requires intravenous hydrocortisone succinate 100 mg and intravenous fluid (normal saline and 10% dextrose for hypoglycaemia). Parenteral hydrocortisone should be continued (100 mg i.m. 6-hourly) until gastrointestinal symptoms abate before starting oral therapy. The precipitating cause should be sought and, if possible, treated.

Mineralocorticoid replacement

Aldosterone is not readily available and fludrocortisone (i.e. 9α-fluoro-hydrocortisone) is the mineralocorticoid used. The halogen group prevents fludrocortisone from being metabolised by 11β-HSD2 and thereby confers a longer half-life and access to mineralocorticoid receptors. The usual dose is 0.05–0.1 mg daily. Adequacy of replacement can be assessed objectively by measurement of blood pressure, plasma electrolytes and plasma renin activity.

In adrenal crisis, however, rapid replacement of sodium deficiency is more important than administration of fludrocortisone. Intravenous saline should be infused as required to normalise haemodynamic indices. In severe hyponatraemia (< 125 mmol/l) caution should be exercised to avoid too rapid normalisation, which risks pontine demyelination (p. 429).

PROBLEMS WITH GLUCOCORTICOID THERAPY

The remarkable anti-inflammatory properties of glucocorticoids have led to their use in a wide variety of clinical conditions described elsewhere in this book, but the hazards are significant. Equivalent doses of commonly used glucocorticoids are listed in Box 20.43. Topical preparations (dermal, rectal and inhaled) can also be absorbed into the systemic circulation. Although this rarely occurs to a sufficient degree to produce clinical features of Cushing's syndrome, it can result in significant suppression of endogenous ACTH and cortisol secretion (p. 779).

20.43 EQUIVALENT DOSES OF GLUCOCORTICOIDS

- Hydrocortisone: 20 mg
- Cortisone acetate: 25 mg
- Prednisolone: 5 mg
- Dexamethasone: 0.5 mg

Side-effects of glucocorticoid therapy

The side-effects of glucocorticoid therapy are illustrated in Figure 20.20 (p. 780). These effects are related to dose, which should, therefore, be kept to a minimum. Some patients will have pre-existing disease that is exacerbated by glucocorticoid therapy; particular care is required in patients with diabetes mellitus or glucose intolerance to avoid symptomatic hyperglycaemia. Rapid changes in cortisol levels can also lead to marked mood disturbance, either depression or mania (p. 240), and insomnia.

Even though the drug is being used for its anti-inflammatory effect, this may produce problems. Thus, signs of perforation of a viscus may be masked and the patient may show no febrile response to an infection. Gastric erosions are more common, probably because of impaired prostaglandin synthesis. Hence, the combination of corticosteroid with analgesic drugs such as aspirin may lead to haemorrhage from the stomach or duodenum. Latent tuberculosis may be reactivated and patients on corticosteroids should be advised to avoid contact with varicella zoster if they are not immune.

Osteoporosis is a particularly important problem because, for a given bone mineral density, the fracture risk appears to be greater in glucocorticoid-induced osteoporosis than in post-menopausal osteoporosis. Therefore, people aged over 65 or with a previous osteoporotic fracture or known to have low bone mineral density should commence bone-protective therapy when systemic glucocorticoids are prescribed (if the intended duration of steroid therapy is > 3 months) (Box 20.44).

20.44 PROLONGED GLUCOCORTICOID THERAPY IN THE PREVENTION OF OSTEOPOROSIS — EBM

'Bisphosphonates, calcium + vitamin D, and calcitonin increase bone mineral density in patients with glucocorticoid-induced osteoporosis.'

- Bone and Tooth Society, National Osteoporosis Society, Royal College of Physicians. Glucocorticoid-induced osteoporosis: guidelines for prevention and treatment. London: RCP 2002.

Withdrawal of glucocorticoid therapy

All glucocorticoid therapy, even if inhaled or applied topically, can suppress the hypothalamic–pituitary–adrenal axis (HPA). In practice, this is only likely to result in a crisis due to adrenal insufficiency on withdrawal of treatment if glucocorticoids have been administered orally or systemically for longer than 3 weeks, if repeated courses have been prescribed within the previous year, or if the dose is higher than the equivalent of 40 mg prednisolone per day. In these circumstances, the drug, when it is no longer required for the underlying condition, must be withdrawn slowly at a rate

20.45 THE ADRENAL GLANDS IN OLD AGE

- **Presentation:** adrenocortical insufficiency is often insidious and difficult to spot.
- **Anti-inflammatory glucocorticoid therapy:** especially hazardous in older people, who are already relatively immunocompromised and susceptible to osteoporosis, hyperglycaemia etc.
- **'Physiological' glucocorticoid replacement therapy:** increased risk of adrenal crisis, because compliance may not be so good and there is a greater incidence of intercurrent illness. Patient education with regular reinforcement of principles described in Box 20.42 is crucial.

dictated by the duration of treatment. If glucocorticoid therapy has been prolonged, then it may take many months for the HPA to recover. All patients must be advised to avoid sudden drug withdrawal. They should be issued with a steroid card and/or wear an engraved bracelet (Box 20.42).

Recovery of the HPA is aided if there is no exogenous glucocorticoid present during the nocturnal surge in ACTH secretion, i.e. if the glucocorticoid is given in the morning. Giving ACTH to stimulate adrenal recovery is of no value as the pituitary remains suppressed.

In patients who have received glucocorticoids for longer than a few weeks, it is often valuable to confirm that the HPA is recovering during glucocorticoid withdrawal. Once the dose of glucocorticoid is reduced to a minimum (e.g. 4 mg prednisolone or 0.5 mg dexamethasone per day), then measure plasma cortisol at 0900 hrs before the next dose. If this is detectable, then perform an ACTH stimulation test (p. 783) to confirm that glucocorticoids can be withdrawn completely.

ENDOCRINE HYPERTENSION

The general principles of the investigation and management of hypertension are discussed in Chapter 18. While the majority of patients with hypertension have either no discernible cause (essential hypertension) or underlying renal parenchymal or reno-vascular disease (p. 496), a small percentage have an underlying endocrine disorder. The precise proportion is variable depending upon the diagnostic criteria applied (see below). Most cases of endocrine hypertension are related to mineralocorticoid excess; catecholamine excess (phaeochromocytoma) is much rarer and is considered on page 787. Cushing's syndrome (p. 779), hyperparathyroidism (p. 775), acromegaly (p. 801) and thyroid dysfunction (p. 748) also raise blood pressure.

Mineralocorticoid excess

Indications to test for mineralocorticoid excess in hypertensive patients include hypokalaemia (including hypokalaemia induced by thiazide diuretics), poor control of blood pressure with conventional therapy, or presentation at a young age.

Aetiology

Causes of excessive activation of mineralocorticoid receptors are shown in Box 20.46. Most often this results

20

20.46 CAUSES OF MINERALOCORTICOID EXCESS

With renin high and aldosterone high (secondary hyperaldosteronism)

- Inadequate renal perfusion, e.g. diuretic therapy, cardiac failure, liver failure, nephrotic syndrome, renal artery stenosis
- Renin-secreting renal tumour (very rare)

With renin low and aldosterone high (primary hyperaldosteronism)

- Adrenal adenoma secreting aldosterone (Conn's syndrome)
- Idiopathic bilateral adrenal hyperplasia
- Glucocorticoid-suppressible hyperaldosteronism (rare)

With renin low and aldosterone low (non-aldosterone-dependent activation of mineralocorticoid pathway)

- Ectopic ACTH syndrome
- Liquorice misuse (inhibition of 11β-HSD2)
- Liddle's syndrome
- 11-deoxycorticosterone-secreting adrenal tumour
- Rare forms of congenital adrenal hyperplasia and 11β-HSD2 deficiency

from enhanced secretion of renin (secondary hyperaldosteronism) in response to inadequate renal perfusion and hypotension. Secondary hyperaldosteronism may be associated with hypertension in renovascular disease and in very rare renin-secreting renal tumours. Less commonly, mineralocorticoid excess and hypertension occur in the face of suppressed renin secretion (primary hyperaldosteronism and rare disorders of mineralocorticoid action).

The prevalence of primary hyperaldosteronism is controversial. If only hypertensive patients with hypokalaemia are investigated, then fewer than 1% of patients with hypertension will be found to have primary hyperaldosteronism. Around half of these have an adrenal adenoma secreting aldosterone (Conn's syndrome). However, recent studies in which hypertensive patients have been screened using aldosterone/renin ratios (see below) suggest that the prevalence may be as high as 5%. Most of these 'extra' patients have bilateral adrenal hyperplasia rather than Conn's syndrome and many have normal plasma potassium. Although mineralocorticoid receptor antagonists might be the antihypertensive agent of choice in such patients, it remains to be determined whether investigation of all hypertensive patients for bilateral adrenal hyperplasia is worthwhile.

Glucocorticoid-suppressible hyperaldosteronism is a rare autosomal dominant disorder caused by translocation of two homologous genes, such that the ACTH-regulated promoter of one gene (11β-hydroxylase) is linked with the coding exons of another (aldosterone synthase, Fig. 20.19, p. 778). The result is inappropriate secretion of aldosterone from the adrenal in response to normal levels of ACTH, despite suppression of renin and angiotensin II levels.

In a few conditions, the mineralocorticoid receptor pathway in the distal nephron is activated even though aldosterone levels are low. Either the receptors are activated by cortisol (ectopic ACTH syndrome or 11β-HSD2 deficiency) or 11-deoxycorticosterone (rare congenital adrenal hyperplasias or tumours), or post-receptor mechanisms are inappropriately activated (e.g. the epithelial sodium channel in Liddle's syndrome).

Clinical assessment

Many patients are asymptomatic, but they may have features of sodium retention or potassium loss. Sodium retention may cause oedema, while hypokalaemia causes muscle weakness (or even paralysis, especially in Chinese), polyuria (secondary to renal tubular damage which produces nephrogenic diabetes insipidus) and occasionally tetany (because of associated metabolic alkalosis and low ionised calcium).

Investigations

Biochemical. Plasma electrolytes may show hypokalaemia and elevated bicarbonate. Plasma sodium is usually towards the upper end of the normal range in primary mineralocorticoid excess, but is characteristically low in secondary hyperaldosteronism (because low plasma volume stimulates ADH release and high angiotensin II levels stimulate thirst).

The key measurements are plasma renin activity and aldosterone (Box 20.46). Almost all antihypertensive drugs interfere with these hormones (e.g. β-blockers inhibit, whilst thiazide diuretics stimulate renin secretion), so these should be stopped for at least 6 weeks beforehand. If this is not possible, then antihypertensives which have minimal effects on the renin–angiotensin system, such as calcium antagonists and α-blockers, should be employed.

If renin is low and aldosterone levels are high, then Conn's adenoma can be differentiated from bilateral adrenal hyperplasia by tests of aldosterone response to angiotensin II; in Conn's adenoma aldosterone does not rise on standing or with furosemide administration. In the rare circumstance when renin and aldosterone are both low, further tests include measurement of urinary cortisol and its metabolites, and 11-deoxycorticosterone.

Localisation. The only cause of primary hyperaldosteronism which is usually treated by surgery is Conn's adenoma. Abdominal CT is often the only test required to localise the tumour (Fig. 20.22), but it is important to recognise that non-functioning adrenal adenomas are present in about 20% of patients with essential hypertension, and adrenal CT should only be performed when the biochemistry supports the diagnosis of adrenal tumour. If the scan is inconclusive, then adrenal vein catheterisation with measurement of aldosterone (and cortisol to confirm positioning of the catheters) or ^{131}iodo-norcholesterol scanning may be helpful.

Management

Mineralocorticoid receptor antagonists (spironolactone or eplerenone) are valuable in treating both hypokalaemia and hypertension in all forms of mineralocorticoid excess. High doses of spironolactone (up to 400 mg/day) may be required. Up to 20% of males develop gynaecomastia on spironolactone. Amiloride (10–40 mg/day), which blocks the epithelial sodium channel regulated by aldosterone, or eplerenone can be used when such problems arise. Glucocorticoid-suppressible hyperaldosteronism is treated by suppression of ACTH, e.g. with dexamethasone.

20

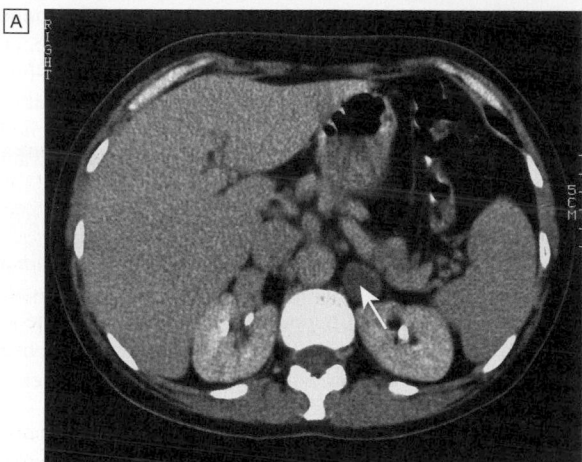

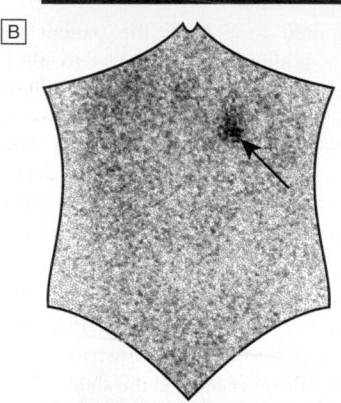

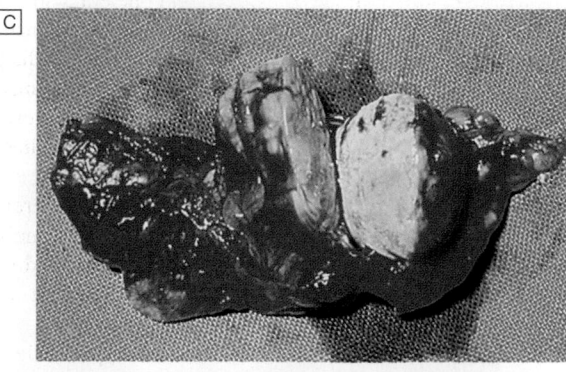

Fig. 20.22 Conn's adenoma. [A] CT scan of left adrenal adenoma (arrow). [B] ^{131}Iodo-norcholesterol scan showing uptake in left adrenal adenoma (arrow). [C] The tumour is 'canary yellow' because of intracellular lipid accumulation.

In patients with Conn's adenoma, medical therapy is usually given for a few weeks to normalise whole-body electrolyte balance before unilateral adrenalectomy. Laparoscopic surgery cures the biochemical abnormality but hypertension remains in as many as 70% of cases, probably because of irreversible damage to the systemic microcirculation.

INCIDENTAL ADRENAL MASS

It is not uncommon for a mass in the adrenal gland to be identified on a CT or MRI scan of the abdomen that has been performed for another indication. Such lesions are known as adrenal 'incidentalomas'. They are present in up to 10% of adults and the prevalence increases with age.

Aetiology

Eighty-five per cent of adrenal incidentalomas are non-functioning adrenal adenomas. The remainder are functional tumours of the adrenal cortex (secreting cortisol, aldosterone or androgens), phaeochromocytomas, primary and secondary carcinomas, hamartomas and other rare disorders including granulomatous infiltrations.

Clinical assessment and investigations

Patients with an adrenal incidentaloma are usually asymptomatic. However, clinical signs and symptoms of excess glucocorticoids (p. 781), mineralocorticoids (p. 786), catecholamines (see below) and, in women, androgens (p. 779) should be sought. Investigations should include a 24-hour urine collection for catecholamines and urine free cortisol and, in women, measurement of serum testosterone, dehydroepiandrosterone and androstenedione concentrations. Patients with hypertension should be investigated for mineralocorticoid excess as described above. CT-guided biopsy may be performed when an unusual diagnosis is suspected (either by clinical findings or on CT appearances) and in patients with known extra-adrenal malignancy, in whom it may sometimes be important to determine whether an adrenal mass is a metastatic lesion or not. Adrenal biopsy is not useful in distinguishing an adrenal adenoma from an adrenal carcinoma.

Management

Functional lesions and tumours > 5 cm in diameter are usually removed by laparoscopic adrenalectomy. In patients with non-functioning lesions < 5 cm in diameter the risk of malignancy is low and excision is only required if serial imaging suggests tumour growth.

PHAEOCHROMOCYTOMA

This is a rare tumour of chromaffin tissue that secretes catecholamines and is responsible for less than 0.1% of cases of hypertension. There is a useful 'rule of tens' in this condition: ~10% are malignant, ~10% are extra-adrenal (i.e. elsewhere in the sympathetic chain) and ~10% are familial.

Clinical features

These depend on the pattern of catecholamine secretion and are listed in Box 20.47.

Some patients present with a complication of hypertension, e.g. stroke, myocardial infarction, left ventricular failure, hypertensive retinopathy or accelerated-phase hypertension. The apparent paradox of postural hypotension between episodes is explained by 'pressure natriuresis' during hypertensive episodes so that intravascular volume is reduced. There may be features of the familial syndromes associated with phaeochromocytoma including neurofibromatosis (p. 1237), von Hippel–Lindau syndrome (p. 1238) and MEN type 2 (p. 802).

20.47 CLINICAL FEATURES OF PHAEOCHROMOCYTOMA

- Hypertension (usually paroxysmal; often postural drop of blood pressure)
- Paroxysms of:
  Pallor (occasionally flushing)
  Palpitations
  Sweating
  Headache
  Anxiety (fear of death—angor animi)
- Abdominal pain, vomiting
- Constipation
- Weight loss
- Glucose intolerance

Investigations

Excessive secretion of catecholamines can be confirmed by measuring the hormones (adrenaline/epinephrine, noradrenaline/norepinephrine and dopamine) in plasma or their metabolites (e.g. vanillyl-mandelic acid, VMA; conjugated metanephrine and normetanephrine) in urine. However, catecholamine secretion is usually paroxysmal and sometimes the paroxysms are infrequent. Therefore, false-negative results may be obtained if samples are collected during a period when symptoms or hypertension are absent.

Increased urinary catecholamine excretion occurs in stressed patients (e.g. after myocardial infarction or major surgery) and is induced by some drugs (notably β-blockers and antidepressants). For this reason, a suppression test may be valuable. Normal adrenomedullary secretion is suppressed by administration of drugs which interfere with sympathetic outflow, such as clonidine or pentolonium tartrate. In phaeochromocytoma these drugs do not suppress plasma catecholamines. Provocative tests of catecholamine release should not be used.

Recent studies suggest that the prevalence of germ-line mutations in patients with phaeochromocytoma justifies genetic screening (of RET, NF-1, VHL, PGL and succinyl dehydrogenase genes), even in patients with no relevant family history or features of a familial syndrome.

Localisation

Phaeochromocytomas are usually identified by abdominal CT or MRI (Fig. 20.23). Difficulty can arise with the localisation of extra-adrenal tumours. Scintigraphy using meta-iodobenzyl guanidine (MIBG) can be useful. Selective venous sampling with measurement of plasma noradrenaline (norepinephrine) may be required.

Management

Medical therapy is required to prepare the patient for surgery, preferably for a minimum of 6 weeks to allow restoration of normal plasma volume. The most useful drug in the face of very high circulating catecholamines is the α-blocker phenoxybenzamine (10–20 mg orally 6–8-hourly) because it is a non-competitive antagonist, unlike prazosin or doxazosin. If α-blockade produces a marked tachycardia, then a β-blocker (e.g. propranolol) or combined α- and β-antagonist (e.g. labetalol) can be added. On no account should the β-antagonist be given before the α-antagonist, as it may cause a paradoxical rise in blood pressure due to unopposed α-mediated vasoconstriction.

During surgery sodium nitroprusside and the short-acting α-antagonist phentolamine are useful in controlling hypertensive episodes which may result from anaesthetic induction or tumour mobilisation. Post-operative hypotension may occur and require volume expansion and, very

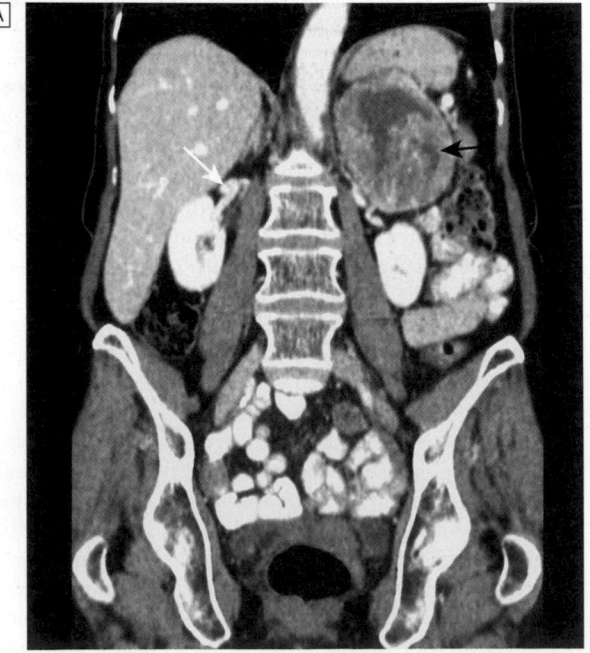
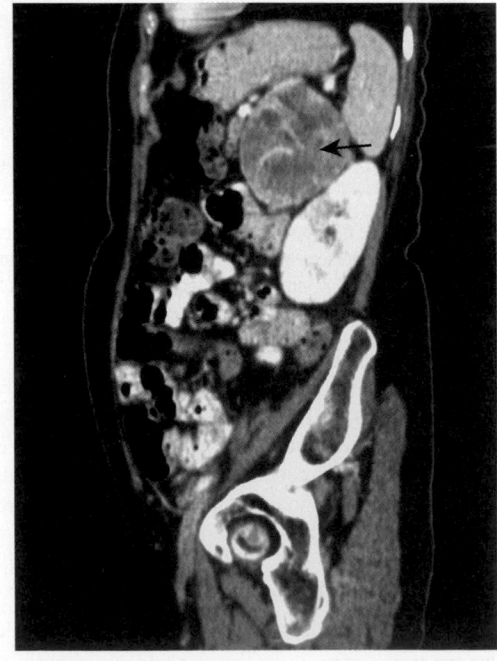

Fig. 20.23 CT scan of abdomen showing large left adrenal phaeochromocytoma. A Coronal view. B Sagittal view. The normal right adrenal (white arrow) contrasts with the large heterogeneous phaeochromocytoma arising from the left adrenal gland (black arrows).

occasionally, noradrenaline (norepinephrine) infusion. This is uncommon if the patient has been prepared adequately with phenoxybenzamine.

CONGENITAL ADRENAL HYPERPLASIA

Aetiology and clinical features

Defects in the cortisol biosynthetic pathway result in insufficiency of hormones 'distal' to the block, with impaired negative feedback and increased ACTH secretion. ACTH then stimulates the production of steroids 'proximal' to the enzyme block. This produces adrenal hyperplasia and a combination of clinical features that depend on the severity and site of the defect in biosynthesis. All of these enzyme abnormalities are inherited as autosomal recessive traits.

The most common enzyme defect is 21-hydroxylase deficiency. This results in impaired synthesis of cortisol and aldosterone and accumulation of 17OH-progesterone, which is then diverted to form adrenal androgens (Fig. 20.19, p. 778). In about one-third of cases this defect is severe and presents in infancy with features of glucocorticoid and mineralocorticoid deficiency (Box 20.40, p. 783) and androgen excess (i.e. ambiguous genitalia in girls). In the other two-thirds, mineralocorticoid secretion is adequate, but there may be features of cortisol insufficiency and/or ACTH and androgen excess (including precocious pseudo-puberty; Box 20.26, p. 768). Sometimes the mildest enzyme defects are not apparent until adult life, when females may present with amenorrhoea and/or hirsutism (p. 768). This is called 'non-classical' or 'late-onset' congenital adrenal hyperplasia.

Defects of all the other enzymes in Figure 20.19 (p. 778) have been described, but are much rarer. Both 17-hydroxylase and 11β-hydroxylase deficiency may produce hypertension due to excess production of 11-deoxycortico-sterone, a mineralocorticoid.

Investigations

High levels of plasma 17OH-progesterone are found in 21-hydroxylase deficiency. In late-onset cases this may only be demonstrated after ACTH administration. To avoid salt-wasting crises in infancy, 17OH-progesterone can be routinely measured in heel prick blood spot samples taken from all infants in the first week of life. Assessment is otherwise as described for adrenal insufficiency on page 782.

In siblings of affected children, antenatal genetic diagnosis can be made by amniocentesis or chorionic villus sampling. This allows prevention of virilisation of affected female fetuses by administration of dexamethasone to the mother.

Management

The aim is to replace deficient corticosteroids, and also suppress ACTH and hence adrenal androgen production. In contrast with glucocorticoid replacement therapy in other forms of cortisol deficiency (p. 779), it is usual to give 'reverse' treatment, i.e. a larger dose of a long-acting synthetic glucocorticoid just before going to bed to suppress the early morning ACTH peak, and a smaller dose in the morning. A careful balance is required between adequate suppression of adrenal androgen excess and excessive glucocorticoid replacement resulting in features of Cushing's syndrome. In children, growth velocity is the most useful measurement since either under- or over-replacement with glucocorticoids suppresses growth. In adults, clinical features (menstrual cycle, hirsutism, weight gain, blood pressure) and biochemical profiles (plasma renin activity and 17OH-progesterone levels) provide a guide.

Patients with late-onset 21-hydroxylase deficiency may not require corticosteroid replacement. If hirsutism is the main problem, anti-androgen therapy may be just as effective (p. 768).

THE ENDOCRINE PANCREAS AND GASTROINTESTINAL TRACT

A series of hormones are secreted from cells distributed throughout the gastrointestinal tract and pancreas. Functional anatomy and physiology are described in Chapters 21 and 22. Pathology of these hormones is listed in Box 20.48. They account for one extremely common condition, diabetes mellitus (Ch. 21), and a handful of rare conditions.

20

20.48 CLASSIFICATION OF ENDOCRINE DISEASES OF THE PANCREAS AND GASTROINTESTINAL TRACT		
	Primary	**Secondary**
Hormone excess	Insulinoma Gastrinoma (Zollinger–Ellison syndrome) Carcinoid syndrome (secretion of 5-HT, etc.) Glucagonoma VIPoma Somatostatinoma	Hypergastrinaemia of achlorhydria
Hormone deficiency	Diabetes mellitus	
Hormone hypersensitivity	Rare, e.g. pseudoacromegaly	
Hormone resistance	Insulin resistance syndromes (e.g. type 2 diabetes mellitus, lipodystrophy, leprechaunism)	
Non-functioning tumours	Pancreatic carcinoma Pancreatic neuro-endocrine tumour	

PRESENTING PROBLEMS IN ENDOCRINE PANCREATIC DISEASE

SPONTANEOUS HYPOGLYCAEMIA

Hypoglycaemia most commonly occurs as a side-effect of treatment with insulin or sulphonylurea drugs in people with diabetes mellitus. In non-diabetic individuals, symptomatic hypoglycaemia is rare, but it is not uncommon to detect venous blood glucose concentrations below 3.0 mmol/l (54 mg/dl) in asymptomatic individuals. For this reason, and because the symptoms of hypoglycaemia are non-specific, a hypoglycaemic disorder should only be diagnosed if all three conditions of Whipple's triad are met (Fig. 20.24). There is, therefore, no specific blood glucose concentration at which spontaneous hypoglycaemia can be said to occur, although the lower the blood glucose concentration is below 3.0 mmol/l, the more likely it is to have pathological significance.

Some causes of spontaneous hypoglycaemia are shown in Figure 20.24, but the list of potential causes is long. Traditionally, hypoglycaemic disorders were classified as being either 'fasting' or 'post-prandial' ('reactive'), depending on whether low blood glucose concentrations occurred in the absence of food or following a meal. However, there is little evidence to support the existence of 'reactive hypoglycaemia' as the cause of symptoms (including in the 'late dumping syndrome' in post-gastrectomy patients, p. 888). For practical purposes, spontaneous hypoglycaemia need only be investigated if it occurs on fasting.

Clinical assessment

Clinical features of hypoglycaemia are described in the section on insulin-induced hypoglycaemia on page 823. Like insulin-treated diabetic patients with recurrent hypoglycaemia, patients with chronic spontaneous hypoglycaemia often have attenuated autonomic responses, and may present with a wide variety of features of neuroglycopenia, including odd behaviour and convulsions. Symptoms are almost always episodic, and key questions include whether they are more frequent on fasting or exercise, and whether they are relieved by consumption of refined carbohydrate. Hypoglycaemia should be considered in all comatose patients, even if there is an apparently obvious cause, such as hemiplegic stroke or alcohol intoxication.

Investigations

Does the patient have a hypoglycaemic disorder?

In an acute presentation (confusion, coma, convulsions), suspected hypoglycaemia is usually tested first of all with capillary blood glucose strips and automated meters. However, while these are sufficient to exclude hypoglycaemia, they are relatively inaccurate in the hypoglycaemic range. Hypoglycaemia should, therefore, always be confirmed by formal laboratory blood glucose measurement. At the same time, a blood sample should be immediately chilled on ice and centrifuged for later measurement of alcohol, insulin, C-peptide and, if appropriate, sulphonylurea levels. Taking these samples during an acute presentation prevents subsequent unnecessary dynamic tests and is of medico-legal importance in cases where poisoning is suspected.

In patients attending an outpatient clinic with episodic symptoms suggestive of hypoglycaemia, establishing the existence of a hypoglycaemic disorder is more challenging. The main diagnostic test is the prolonged (72-hour) fast. If symptoms of hypoglycaemia develop during the fast, then blood samples should be taken to confirm hypoglycaemia and for later measurement of insulin and C-peptide. Hypoglycaemia is then corrected with oral or intravenous glucose and Whipple's triad completed by confirmation of the resolution of symptoms. The absence of clinical and biochemical evidence of hypoglycaemia during a prolonged fast excludes the diagnosis of a hypoglycaemic disorder.

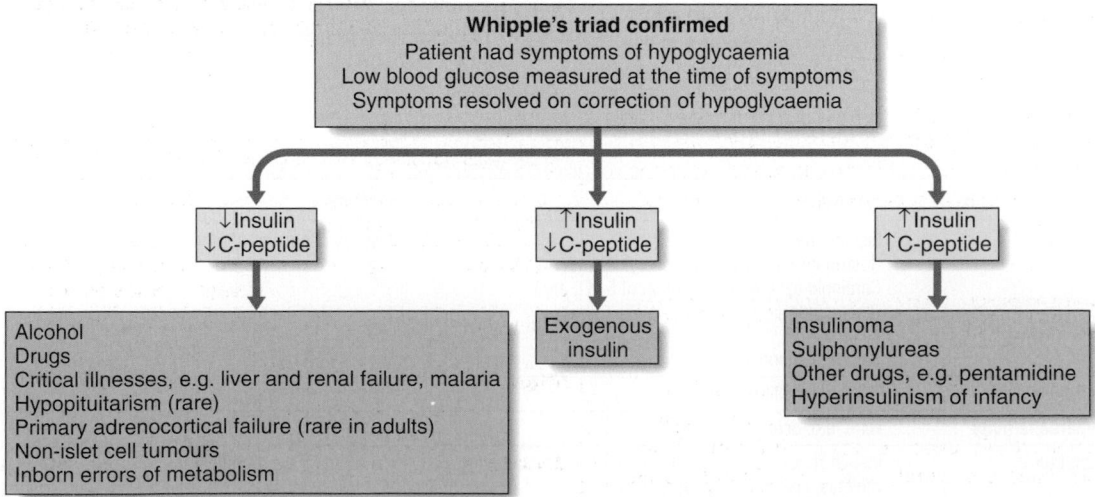

Fig. 20.24 Differential diagnosis of spontaneous hypoglycaemia. Measurement of insulin and C-peptide concentrations during an episode is helpful in determining the underlying cause.

The diagnosis of 'reactive hypoglycaemia' was classically established by a prolonged glucose tolerance test, but this test is now discredited because of its high false-positive rate.

What is the cause of the hypoglycaemia?

In the acute setting, the underlying diagnosis is often obvious. Alcohol excess is the most common cause of spontaneous hypoglycaemia in the UK, but other drugs, for example salicylates, quinine and pentamidine, may also be implicated. Hypoglycaemia is one of many metabolic derangements which occur in patients with hepatic failure, renal failure, sepsis or malaria.

Hypoglycaemia in the absence of insulin, or any insulin-like factor, in the blood indicates impaired gluconeogenesis and/or availability of glucose from glycogen in the liver. Hypoglycaemia associated with high insulin and low C-peptide concentrations is indicative of administration of exogenous insulin, either factitiously or feloniously; the low C-peptide indicates that pancreatic secretion of pro-insulin is suppressed. Adults with high insulin and C-peptide concentrations during an episode of hypoglycaemia are most likely to have an insulinoma, but sulphonylurea ingestion should also be considered (particularly in health-care professionals). Insulinomas in the pancreas are usually small (< 5 mm diameter), but can often be identified by CT, MRI, or endoscopic or laparoscopic ultrasound. Scanning should include the liver since around 10% of insulinomas are malignant. Rarely, large non-pancreatic tumours, such as sarcomas, may cause recurrent hypoglycaemia because of their ability to produce excess insulin-like growth factor-2.

Management

Treatment of acute hypoglycaemia should be initiated as soon as laboratory blood samples have been taken, but should not be deferred until the formal laboratory confirmation is obtained. Intravenous dextrose (10% or 50%) is effective in the short term, and should be followed on recovery with oral carbohydrate. Continuous dextrose infusion may be necessary, especially in sulphonylurea poisoning. Intramuscular glucagon (1 mg) stimulates hepatic glucose release, but is ineffective in patients with depleted glycogen reserves (e.g alcohol excess, liver disease) and may paradoxically exacerbate sulphonylurea-induced hypoglycaemia.

Chronic recurrent hypoglycaemia in insulin-secreting tumours can be treated by diet (regular oral carbohydrate consumption) combined with inhibitors of insulin secretion (diazoxide, thiazide diuretics or somatostatin analogues). Insulinomas are usually resected.

NEURO-ENDOCRINE TUMOURS

Neuro-endocrine tumours (NETs) constitute a heterogeneous group of neoplasms that originate from neuro-endocrine cells. NETs arise in many different organs including the pancreas, small and large bowel, lung, adrenals (phaeochromocytoma, p. 787) and thyroid (medullary carcinoma, p. 761). Although there is a wide spectrum of malignant potential, NETs generally grow slowly and metastasise late in their clinical course. Most NETs occur sporadically, but a proportion are associated with genetic cancer syndromes such as MEN 1, MEN 2 and neurofibromatosis type 1 (pp. 802 and 1237). NETs commonly secrete a variety of hormones ectopically into the circulation.

Carcinoid tumours

These may arise in the thymus, bronchi and throughout the gastrointestinal tract, but are most commonly observed in the small bowel. They present due to local mass effects, e.g. small bowel obstruction, appendicitis, pain from hepatic metastases, or because of symptoms related to hormone excess. This includes ectopic secretion of ACTH, causing Cushing's syndrome (p. 779), or 5-HT, causing 'carcinoid syndrome'. Carcinoid syndrome (Box 20.49) only occurs when the vasoactive hormones reach the systemic circulation. In the case of gastrointestinal carcinoids, this invariably means that the tumour has metastasised to the liver, as hormones secreted by the primary tumour into the portal vein are metabolised by the liver.

Pancreatic neuro-endocrine tumours

The majority of pancreatic NETs are non-secretory, but when hormones are produced symptoms may ensue (Box 20.50). The tumours may be single or multifocal (the latter typically occurring in the context of MEN 1).

Investigations

The investigation of suspected Cushing's syndrome (p. 779) and insulinoma are described above. Chromogranin A is produced by most NETs and may be measured in a fasting blood sample along with the other hormones listed

20.49 CLINICAL FEATURES OF THE CARCINOID SYNDROME
• Flushing
• Wheezing
• Diarrhoea
• Facial telangiectasia
• Cardiac involvement (tricuspid regurgitation, pulmonary stenosis, right ventricular endocardial plaques) leading to heart failure

20.50 PANCREATIC NEURO-ENDOCRINE TUMOURS		
Tumour	**Hormone**	**Effects**
Gastrinoma	Gastrin	Peptic ulcer and steatorrhoea (Zollinger–Ellison syndrome)
Insulinoma	Insulin	Recurrent hypoglycaemia (see above)
VIPoma	Vasoactive intestinal peptide (VIP)	Watery diarrhoea and hypokalaemia
Glucagonoma	Glucagon	Diabetes mellitus, necrolytic migratory erythema
Somatostatinoma	Somatostatin	Diabetes mellitus and steatorrhoea

in Box 20.50. 5-HT excess is diagnosed by measuring concentrations of its metabolite, 5-hydroxyindoleacetic acid (5-HIAA), in a 24-hour urine collection. NETs may be localised by ultrasound, CT, MRI and, in the case of pancreatic tumours, endoscopic ultrasound. Scintigraphy with a radiolabelled somatostatin analogue may help in localisation, particularly of carcinoids and gastrinomas.

Management

Treatment of solitary tumours is by surgical resection. If metastatic or multifocal primary disease is present, then surgery is usually not indicated, unless there is, for example, gastrointestinal obstruction. Diazoxide may reduce insulin secretion in insulinomas (see above) and high doses of proton pump inhibitors suppress acid production in gastrinomas. Somatostatin analogues reduce the symptoms associated with 5-HT, glucagon and vasoactive intestinal peptide (VIP) excess. Other treatment modalities, such as cytotoxic chemotherapy, targeted radionucleide therapy with ^{131}I-MIBG (which may be taken up by NET metastases) and resection/embolisation of hepatic metastases, have a more limited role.

20.51 DISORDERS OF THE ENDOCRINE PANCREAS IN OLD AGE

- **Spontaneous hypoglycaemia**: may present with focal neurological abnormality. Blood glucose should be checked in all patients with acute neurological symptoms and signs, especially stroke, as these will reverse with early treatment of hypoglycaemia.

THE HYPOTHALAMUS AND THE PITUITARY GLAND

Diseases of the hypothalamus and pituitary are rare, with an annual incidence of ~1:50000. The pituitary plays a central role in several major endocrine axes, so that investigation and treatment invariably involves several other glands.

FUNCTIONAL ANATOMY, PHYSIOLOGY AND INVESTIGATIONS

The anatomy of the pituitary is shown in Figure 20.25 and its numerous functions are shown in Figure 20.2 (p. 743). The pituitary gland is enclosed in the sella turcica and bridged over by a fold of dura mater called the diaphragma sellae, with the sphenoidal air sinuses below and the optic chiasm above. The cavernous sinuses are lateral to the pituitary fossa and contain the 3rd, 4th and 6th cranial nerves and the internal carotid arteries. The gland is composed of two lobes, anterior and posterior, and is connected to the hypothalamus by the infundibular stalk, which has portal vessels carrying blood from the median eminence of the hypothalamus to the anterior lobe and nerve fibres to the posterior lobe.

Diseases of the hypothalamus and pituitary are classified in Box 20.52. By far the most common disorder is an adenoma of the anterior pituitary gland.

Investigations

Although pituitary disease presents with diverse manifestations (see below), the approach to the patient is similar in

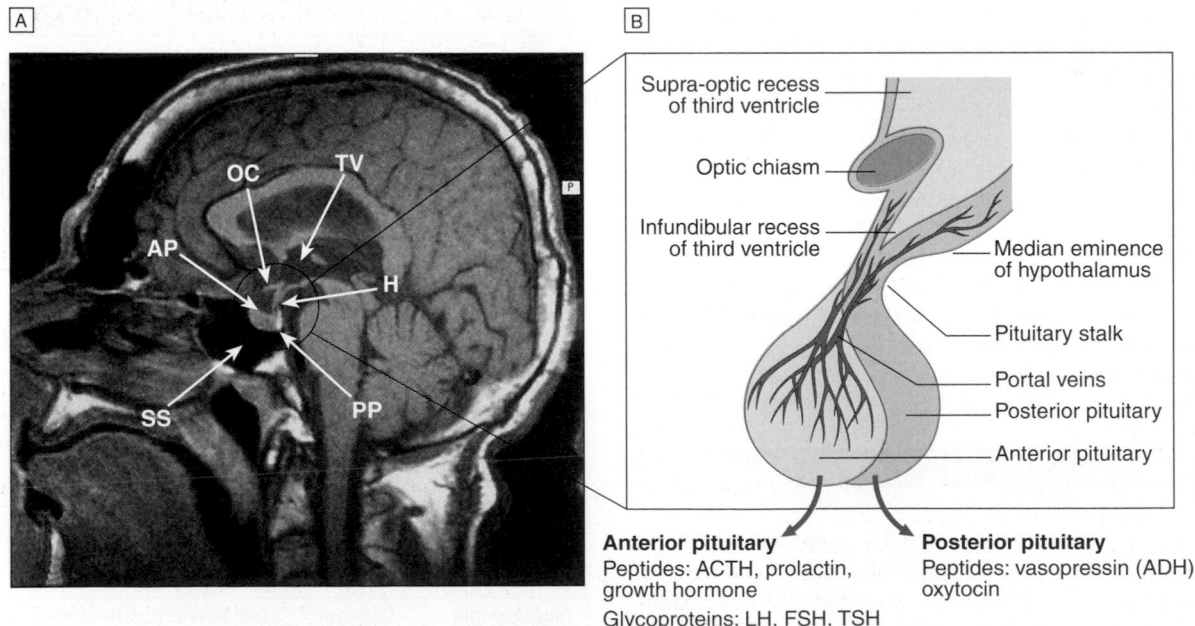

Fig. 20.25 **Anatomical relationships and function of the pituitary and hypothalamus.** See also Figure 20.2 (p. 743). **A** MRI. (SS = sphenoid sinus; AP = anterior pituitary; OC = optic chiasm; TV = third ventricle; H = hypothalamus; PP = posterior pituitary) **B** Close-up of the central area of the MRI.

Anterior pituitary
Peptides: ACTH, prolactin, growth hormone
Glycoproteins: LH, FSH, TSH

Posterior pituitary
Peptides: vasopressin (ADH), oxytocin

20.52 CLASSIFICATION OF DISEASES OF THE PITUITARY AND HYPOTHALAMUS

	Primary	Secondary
Hormone excess		
Anterior pituitary	Prolactinoma Acromegaly Cushing's disease Rare TSH-, LH- and FSHomas	Disconnection hyperprolactinaemia
Hypothalamus and posterior pituitary	Syndrome of inappropriate antidiuretic hormone (SIADH; p. 430)	
Hormone deficiency		
Anterior pituitary	Hypopituitarism	e.g. GnRH deficiency (Kallmann's syndrome)
Hypothalamus and posterior pituitary	Cranial diabetes insipidus	
Hormone hypersensitivity	–	–
Hormone resistance	Growth hormone resistance (Laron dwarfism) Nephrogenic diabetes insipidus	
Non-functioning tumours	Pituitary adenoma Craniopharyngioma Metastatic tumours	

all cases. Clinical assessment is described below. Investigations follow the outline in Box 20.53.

Anterior pituitary gland

Tests for hormone excess vary according to the hormone in question. For example, prolactin is not secreted in pulsatile fashion, although it rises with significant psychological stress. Assuming that the patient was not distressed by venepuncture, a random measurement of serum prolactin is sufficient to diagnose hyperprolactinaemia. In contrast, growth hormone is secreted in a pulsatile fashion. A high random level does not confirm acromegaly; the diagnosis is only confirmed by failure of growth hormone to be suppressed (by the insulin-induced rise in insulin-like growth factor-1) during an oral glucose tolerance test. Similarly, in suspected ACTH-dependent Cushing's disease (p. 779), random measurement of plasma cortisol is unreliable and the diagnosis is usually made by a dexamethasone suppression test.

The means of testing for hypopituitarism also differs between hormones. A common test, which is still employed in some centres, involves the simultaneous administration of thyrotrophin-releasing hormone (TRH), gonadotrophin-releasing hormone (GnRH) and insulin (to induce hypoglycaemic stress and stimulate ACTH and growth hormone). However, this is a potentially hazardous procedure and there is evidence that assessment of the target glands for most of these hormones provides equally reliable results. Details of each test are given in the sections on individual glands elsewhere in this chapter and in Box 20.53.

Local complications of a large pituitary tumour most commonly reflect compression of the optic pathway. The resulting visual field defect can be documented by formal charting (e.g. a Goldman's perimetry chart, p. 798). Viewing the pituitary gland by MRI reveals 'abnormalities' of the pituitary fossa in as many as 10% of 'healthy' middle-aged people. It should therefore be performed only if there is a

20.53 INVESTIGATION OF PATIENTS WITH PITUITARY AND HYPOTHALAMIC DISEASE

Identify pituitary hormone deficiency

ACTH deficiency
- Short ACTH stimulation test (Box 20.41, p. 783)
- Insulin tolerance test (Box 20.56, p. 796)—only if uncertainty in interpretation of short ACTH stimulation test (e.g. acute presentation)

LH/FSH deficiency
- In the male, measure random serum testosterone, LH and FSH
- In the pre-menopausal female, ask if menses are regular
- In the post-menopausal female, measure random serum LH and FSH (which would normally be > 30 mU/l)

TSH deficiency
- Measure random serum thyroxine
- Note that TSH is often detectable in secondary hypothyroidism, due to inactive TSH isoforms in the blood

Growth hormone deficiency
(Only investigate if growth hormone replacement therapy is being contemplated; p. 796)
- Measure immediately after exercise
- Consider other stimulatory tests (Box 20.55, p. 795)

Cranial diabetes insipidus
(Only investigate if patient complains of polyuria/polydipsia, which may be masked by ACTH or TSH deficiency)
- Exclude other causes of polyuria with blood glucose, potassium and calcium measurements
- Water deprivation test (Box 20.59, p. 797) or 5% saline infusion test

Identify hormone excess

- Measure random serum prolactin
- Investigate for acromegaly (glucose tolerance test) or Cushing's syndrome (p. 779) if there are clinical features

Establish the anatomy and diagnosis

- Consider visual field testing
- Image the pituitary and hypothalamus by MRI or CT

clear biochemical abnormality or in a patient who presents with clinical features of pituitary tumour (see below). A pituitary tumour may be classified as either a macro-adenoma (> 10 mm diameter) or a microadenoma (< 10 mm diameter). Microadenomas are not associated with hypopituitarism or compression of local structures and are only treated if they are secreting excess hormones. Functional imaging (e.g. with a radio-labelled somatostatin analogue) is rarely used.

Surgical biopsy is usually only performed as part of a therapeutic operation. Conventional staining identifies pituitary tumours as either chromophobe, acidophil or basophil. Classically, acidophil tumours are associated with growth hormone or prolactin excess, basophil tumours are associated with ACTH hypersecretion, and chromophobe tumours are non-functioning. However, many chromophobe tumours are associated with hormonal excess. Immuno-histochemistry using antisera against the pituitary hormones is more valuable in identifying the hormone(s) secreted by specific pituitary cells. It is not possible for histology to identify the rare pituitary tumours that regrow rapidly and invade local structures.

Posterior pituitary and hypothalamus

Patients with hypothalamic disease are at risk of anterior pituitary dysfunction and require assessment as above. In addition, these patients may have posterior pituitary dysfunction. Note that the posterior pituitary is rarely affected by pituitary tumours, and dysfunction most commonly occurs following pituitary surgery. In practice, the only posterior

pituitary function requiring investigation is deficiency of vasopressin resulting in diabetes insipidus (p. 796).

PRESENTING PROBLEMS IN HYPOTHALAMIC AND PITUITARY DISEASE

Clinical features of pituitary disease are shown in Figure 20.26. Younger women with pituitary disease most commonly present with secondary amenorrhoea (p. 765) or galactorrhoea (in hyperprolactinaemia). Post-menopausal women and men of any age are less likely to report symptoms of hypogonadism and so are more likely to present late with larger tumours causing visual field defects. Pituitary tumours may be discovered as an incidental finding on a CT or MRI scan; the increasing use of neuroimaging has made this a more common route of presentation.

ANTERIOR PITUITARY HORMONE DEFICIENCY

The term 'hypopituitarism' means the combined deficiency of any of the anterior pituitary hormones. This most commonly results from the destructive effects of a pituitary macroadenoma, but other causes are shown in Box 20.54.

Clinical assessment

The presentation is highly variable and depends on the underlying lesion and the pattern of resulting hormone

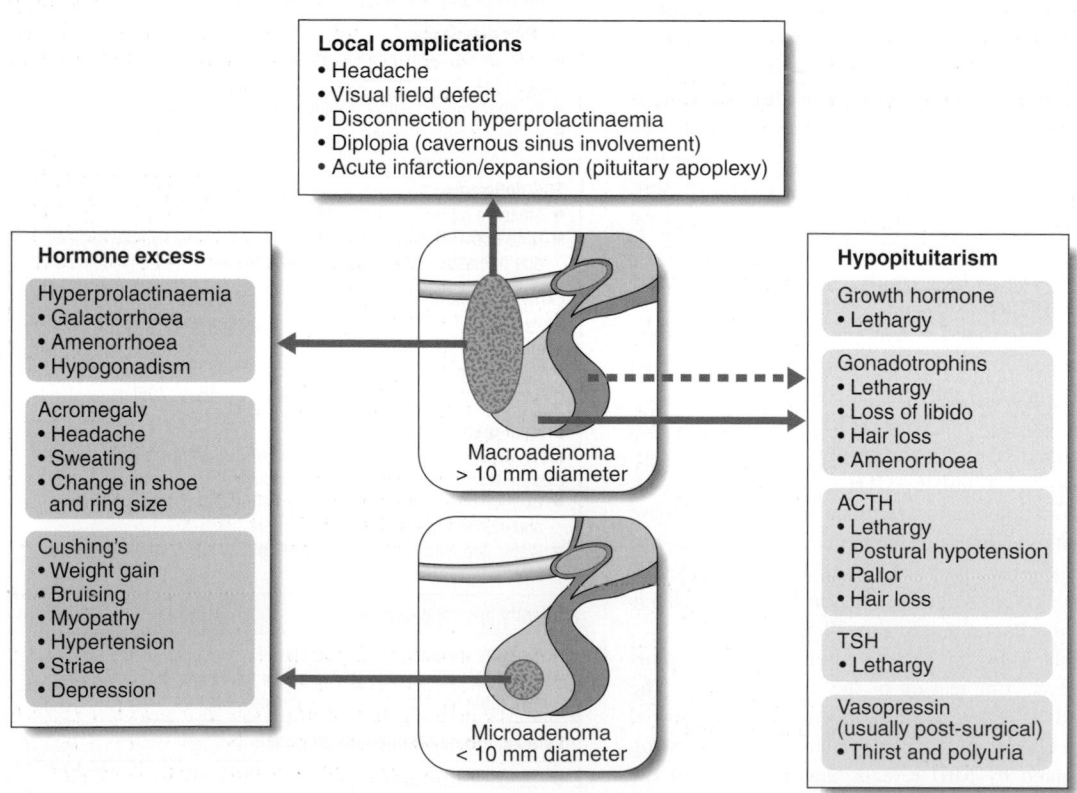

Fig. 20.26   Common symptoms and signs to consider in a patient with suspected pituitary disease.

20.54 CAUSES OF ANTERIOR PITUITARY HORMONE DEFICIENCY
Structural
• Primary pituitary tumour 　Adenoma* 　Carcinoma (exceptionally rare) • Secondary tumour (including leukaemia and lymphoma) • Craniopharyngioma* • Meningioma* • Chordoma • Germinoma (pinealoma) • Arachnoid cyst • Rathke's cleft cyst • Langerhans cell histiocytosis • Haemorrhage (apoplexy)
Inflammatory/infiltrative
• Sarcoidosis • Lymphocytic hypophysitis • Infections, e.g. pituitary abscess, TB, syphilis, encephalitis • Haemochromatosis
Congenital deficiencies
• GnRH (Kallmann's syndrome)*—gonadotrophin-releasing hormone • GHRH*—growth hormone-releasing hormone • TRH—thyrotrophin-releasing hormone • CRH—corticotrophin-releasing hormone
Functional*
• Chronic systemic illness • Anorexia nervosa • Excessive exercise
Other
• Head injury* • (Para-)sellar surgery* • (Para-)sellar radiotherapy* • Post-partum necrosis (Sheehan's syndrome)
* Denotes the most common causes of pituitary hormone deficiency.

deficiency. With progressive lesions of the pituitary there is a characteristic sequence of loss of pituitary hormone secretion. Growth hormone secretion is often the earliest to be lost. In adults, this produces lethargy, muscle weakness and increased fat mass, but these features are not obvious in isolation. Next, gonadotrophin (LH and FSH) secretion becomes impaired with, in the male, loss of libido and, in the female, oligomenorrhoea or amenorrhoea. Later, in the male there may be gynaecomastia and decreased frequency of shaving. In both sexes axillary and pubic hair eventually become sparse or even absent and the skin becomes characteristically finer and wrinkled. Chronic anaemia may also occur.

The next hormone to be lost is usually ACTH, resulting in symptoms of cortisol insufficiency. In contrast to primary adrenal insufficiency (p. 782), angiotensin II-dependent zona glomerulosa function is not lost and hence aldosterone secretion maintains normal plasma potassium. However, there may be postural hypotension and a dilutional hyponatraemia for three reasons:

• Failure of vasoconstriction in the absence of cortisol results in pooling of blood in the legs on standing.

• Antidiuretic hormone (ADH) release is enhanced by hypotension and cortisol deficiency.
• Cortisol is required for normal water excretion by the kidney.

In contrast to the pigmentation of Addison's disease, a striking degree of pallor is usually present, principally because of lack of stimulation of melanocytes by β-lipotrophic hormone (β-LPH, a fragment of the ACTH precursor peptide) in the skin.

Finally, TSH secretion is lost with consequent secondary hypothyroidism. This contributes further to apathy and cold intolerance. In contrast to primary hypothyroidism, frank myxoedema is rare, presumably because the thyroid retains some autonomous function.

The onset of all of the above symptoms is notoriously insidious. However, patients sometimes present acutely unwell with adrenocortical insufficiency. This may be precipitated by a mild infection or injury, or may occur secondary to pituitary apoplexy (p. 798).

Investigations
The strategy of investigation of pituitary disease is described in Box 20.53. In acutely unwell patients, the priority is to diagnose and treat cortisol deficiency (p. 782). Other tests can be undertaken later. Specific dynamic tests for diagnosing hormone deficiency are described in Boxes 20.41 (ACTH, p. 783) and 20.55 (growth hormone). More specialised biochemical tests, such as insulin tolerance tests (Box 20.56), GnRH and TRH tests, are rarely required. All patients with biochemical evidence of pituitary hormone deficiency should have an MRI or CT scan to identify pituitary or hypothalamic tumours. If a tumour is not identified, then further investigations are indicated to exclude infectious or infiltrative causes.

20.55 TESTS OF GROWTH HORMONE SECRETION
GH levels are commonly undetectable, so a choice from the range of 'stimulation' tests is required: • 1 hour after going to sleep • Frequent sampling during sleep • Post-exercise • Insulin-induced hypoglycaemia • Arginine (may be combined with GHRH) • Glucagon • Clonidine
Note that in pre-pubertal patients, priming with sex steroid is required before 'stimulation' tests are performed.

Management
Treatment of acutely ill patients is similar to that described for adrenocortical insufficiency on page 779, except that sodium depletion is not an important component to correct. Chronic hormone replacement therapies are described below. Once the cause of hypopituitarism is established, specific treatment—of a pituitary macroadenoma, for example (p. 797)—may be required.

20

20.56 INSULIN TOLERANCE TEST

Use

- Assessment of the hypothalamic–pituitary–adrenal axis
- Assessment of growth hormone deficiency
- Indicated when there is doubt from other tests in Box 20.53
- Usually performed in specialist centres, especially in children
- Intravenous glucose and hydrocortisone must be available for resuscitation

Contraindications

- Ischaemic heart disease
- Epilepsy
- Severe hypopituitarism (0800 hrs plasma cortisol < 180 nmol/l or 6.6 μg/dl)

Dose

- 0.15 U/kg body weight soluble insulin i.v.

Aim

- To produce adequate hypoglycaemia (tachycardia and sweating—with blood glucose < 2.2 mmol/l (40 mg/dl))

Blood samples

- 0, 30, 45, 60, 90, 120 minutes for blood glucose, plasma cortisol and growth hormone

Results

- Normal subjects GH > 20 mU/l (6.7 ng/ml)*
- Normal subjects cortisol > 550 nmol/l (~20.2 μg/dl)*

* The precise cut-off figure for a satisfactory cortisol and GH response depends on the assay used and so varies between centres.

Cortisol replacement

Hydrocortisone (another name for cortisol) should be given if there is ACTH deficiency. Suitable doses are described in the section on adrenal disease (p. 784). Mineralocorticoid replacement is not required.

Thyroid hormone replacement

Thyroxine 100–150 μg once daily should be given as described on page 750. Unlike in primary hypothyroidism, measuring TSH is not helpful in adjusting the replacement dose, because patients with hypopituitarism often secrete glycoproteins which are measured in the TSH assays, but are not bioactive. The aim is to maintain serum T_4 in the upper part of the reference range. It is dangerous to give thyroid replacement to patients with adrenal insufficiency without first giving glucocorticoid therapy, since this may precipitate adrenal crisis.

Sex hormone replacement

This is indicated if there is gonadotrophin deficiency in men of any age and in women under the age of 50 to restore normal sexual function and to prevent osteoporosis (pp. 766–767).

Growth hormone replacement

Growth hormone (GH) is administered, by daily subcutaneous self-injection, to young patients with GH deficiency, renal failure or Turner's syndrome to assist them in attaining their growth potential. Until recently, GH was discontinued

EBM

20.57 GROWTH HORMONE REPLACEMENT IN ADULT HYPOPITUITARISM

'GH improves quality of life, exercise capacity, lipid profile and body fat distribution, although results are inconsistent between trials and between patients.'

- Carroll PV, et al. J Clin Endocrinol Metab 1998; 83:382–395.

For further information: 💻 www.nice.org.uk

once the epiphyses had fused, and was not given to adults. However, although hypopituitary adults receiving 'full' replacement with hydrocortisone, thyroxine and sex steroids are usually much improved by these therapies, they often remain lethargic and unwell compared with a healthy population. Some studies suggest that some of these patients feel better, and have objective improvements in their fat/muscle mass ratios and other metabolic parameters, if they are also given GH replacement (Box 20.57). Growth hormone therapy may also help young adults to achieve a higher peak bone mineral density. The principal side-effect is sodium retention, manifest as peripheral oedema or carpal tunnel syndrome. For this reason, GH replacement is started at a low dose, with monitoring of the response by measurement of serum insulin-like growth factor-1 (IGF-1) levels.

DIABETES INSIPIDUS

This uncommon disorder is characterised by the persistent excretion of excessive quantities of dilute urine, and by thirst. It can be classified as cranial diabetes insipidus, in which there is deficient production of ADH by the

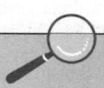

20.58 CAUSES OF DIABETES INSIPIDUS

Cranial

Structural hypothalamic or high stalk lesion
- Box 20.54

Idiopathic

Genetic defect
• Dominant	• Recessive (DIDMOAD syndrome—association of diabetes insipidus with diabetes mellitus, optic atrophy, deafness)

Nephrogenic

Genetic defect
• V2 receptor mutation	• Cystinosis
• Aquaporin-2 mutation	

Metabolic abnormality
• Hypokalaemia	• Hypercalcaemia

Drug therapy
• Lithium	• Demeclocycline

Poisoning
- Heavy metals

Chronic kidney disease
• Polycystic kidney disease	• Infiltrative disease
• Sickle-cell anaemia	

hypothalamus, and nephrogenic diabetes insipidus, in which the renal tubules are unresponsive to ADH.

Aetiology

Causes of diabetes insipidus are listed in Box 20.58.

Clinical assessment

The most marked symptoms are polyuria and polydipsia. The patient may pass 5–20 litres or more of urine in 24 hours. This is of low specific gravity and osmolality. If the patient has an intact thirst mechanism, is conscious and has access to oral fluids, then he or she can maintain adequate fluid intake. However, in an unconscious patient or a patient with damage to the hypothalamic thirst centre, diabetes insipidus is potentially lethal. If there is associated cortisol deficiency, then diabetes insipidus may not be manifest until glucocorticoid replacement therapy is given. The differential diagnosis of diabetes insipidus includes diabetes mellitus and primary polydipsia, a condition that is seen most often in patients with established psychiatric disease.

Investigations

Diabetes insipidus is confirmed if, in the face of elevated plasma osmolality (i.e. > 300 mOsm/kg), either ADH is not measurable in serum or the urine is not maximally concentrated (i.e. is < 600 mOsm/kg). Sometimes, random simultaneous samples of blood and urine will confirm the diagnosis, or refute the diagnosis by demonstrating a urine osmolality > 600 mOsm/kg. More often, a dynamic test is required. Most centres use a water deprivation test, described in Box 20.59. An alternative is to infuse hypertonic saline (5%

saline) and measure ADH secretion in response to increasing plasma osmolality. Thirst can also be assessed during these tests on a visual analogue scale. Anterior pituitary function and suprasellar anatomy should be assessed in patients with cranial diabetes insipidus as indicated in Box 20.53.

In primary polydipsia the urine may be excessively dilute because of chronic diuresis which 'washes out' the solute gradient across the loop of Henle, but plasma osmolality is low rather than high. DDAVP (see below) should not be administered to patients with primary polydipsia, since it will prevent excretion of water and risks severe water intoxication if the patient continues to drink fluid to excess.

In nephrogenic diabetes insipidus appropriate further tests include plasma electrolytes, calcium and investigation of the renal tract (Chs 16 and 17).

Management

Treatment of cranial diabetes insipidus is with des-amino-des-aspartate-arginine vasopressin (desmopressin, DDAVP), an analogue of ADH with a longer half-life. DDAVP is usually administered via the mucous membrane of the nose, either as a metered dose spray or using a manual aerosol device. It is also available as tablets, although bioavailability of peptides after oral administration is very low and rather unpredictable. In sick patients, DDAVP is given by intramuscular injection. The dose of DDAVP required to keep the patient in water balance must be determined by measuring plasma sodium concentrations and/or osmolality. The principal hazard is excessive treatment resulting in water intoxication and hyponatraemia. Inadequate treatment results in thirst and a compensatory increase in fluid intake in the conscious patient. The ideal dose prevents nocturia, but allows a degree of polyuria from time to time before the next dose (e.g. DDAVP nasal dose 5 µg in the morning and 10 µg at night).

Polyuria in nephrogenic diabetes insipidus is improved by thiazide diuretics (e.g. bendroflumethiazide 2.5–5 mg/day), amiloride (5–10 mg/day) and NSAIDs (e.g. indometacin 15 mg 8-hourly), although the last of these carries a risk of reducing glomerular filtration rate.

PITUITARY AND (PARA-)SELLAR TUMOURS

Pituitary and hypothalamic disease may present as a space-occupying lesion that has been identified within the pituitary fossa or the suprasellar space by CT or MRI. Such a lesion may simply be an incidental discovery during neuroimaging for another indication (e.g. the investigation of cerebrovascular disease) or may come to attention during the investigation of one or more mass effects it has caused.

Sellar and para-sellar tumours produce a variety of mass effects, depending on their size and location. The most common, but least specific, is headache, which may be the consequence of stretching of the diaphragma sellae. Compression of the neural connections between the retina and occipital cortex may lead to a visual field defect. Although the classical abnormalities associated with compression of the optic chiasm are bitemporal hemianopia (Fig. 20.27) or upper quadrantanopia, any type of visual

---

20

20.59 WATER DEPRIVATION TEST

Use

- To establish a diagnosis of diabetes insipidus, and differentiate cranial from nephrogenic causes

Protocol

- No coffee, tea or smoking on the test day
- Free fluids until 0730 hrs on the morning of the test, but discourage patients from 'stocking up' with extra fluid in anticipation of fluid deprivation
- No fluids from 0730 hrs
- Attend at 0830 hrs for body weight, plasma and urine osmolality
- Record body weight, urine volume, urine and plasma osmolality and thirst score on a visual analogue scale every 2 hours for up to 8 hours
- Stop the test if the patient loses 3% of body weight
- If plasma osmolality reaches > 300 mOsm/kg and urine osmolality < 600 mOsm/kg, then administer DDAVP (see text) 2 µg i.m.

Interpretation

- Diabetes insipidus is confirmed by a plasma osmolality > 300 mOsm/kg with a urine osmolality < 600 mOsm/kg
- Cranial diabetes insipidus is confirmed if urine osmolality rises by at least 50% after DDAVP
- Nephrogenic diabetes insipidus is confirmed if DDAVP does not concentrate the urine
- Primary polydipsia is suggested by low plasma osmolality at the start of the test

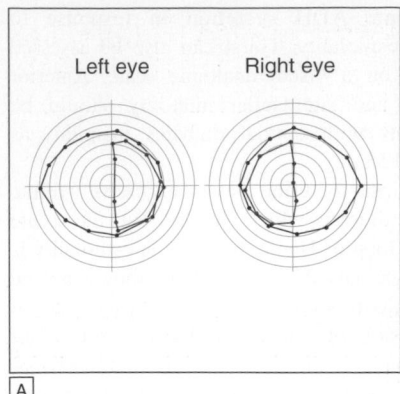

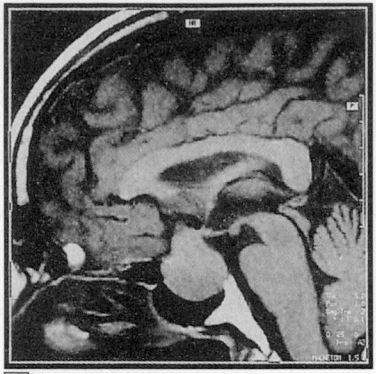

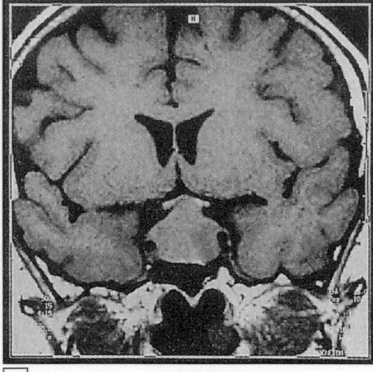

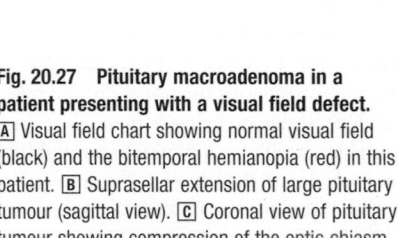

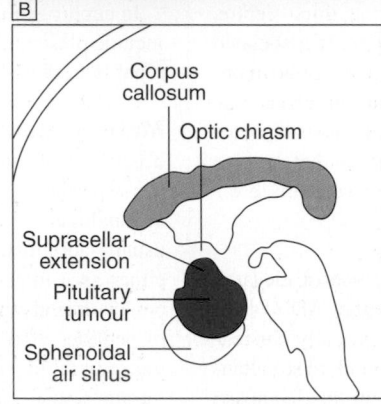

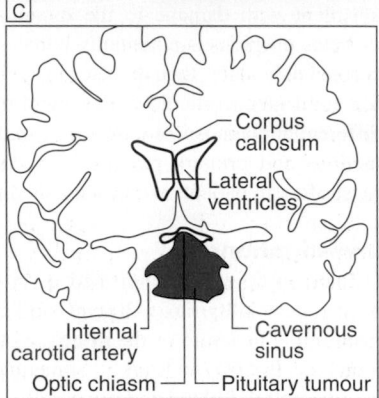

Fig. 20.27 Pituitary macroadenoma in a patient presenting with a visual field defect. A Visual field chart showing normal visual field (black) and the bitemporal hemianopia (red) in this patient. B Suprasellar extension of large pituitary tumour (sagittal view). C Coronal view of pituitary tumour showing compression of the optic chiasm.

field defect can result from suprasellar extension of a tumour because it may compress the optic nerve (unilateral loss of acuity or scotoma) or the optic tract (homonymous hemianopia). Optic atrophy may be apparent on ophthalmoscopy. Lateral extension of a sellar mass into the cavernous sinus with subsequent compression of the 3rd, 4th or 6th cranial nerves may cause diplopia and strabismus.

Occasionally pituitary tumours infarct or there is bleeding into cystic lesions. This is termed 'pituitary apoplexy' and may result in sudden expansion with local compression symptoms and acute-onset hypopituitarism. Non-haemorrhagic infarction can also occur in a normal pituitary gland; predisposing factors include obstetric haemorrhage (Sheehan's syndrome), diabetes mellitus and raised intracranial pressure.

Aetiology and investigations

A wide variety of disorders can present as a mass in the region of the pituitary and hypothalamus (Box 20.54, p. 795), but the majority of intrasellar tumours are pituitary macroadenomas (most commonly non-functioning adenomas, Fig. 20.27), most suprasellar masses are craniopharyngiomas (Fig. 20.30, p. 803), and para-sellar masses are most commonly meningiomas. Some lesions have distinctive neuroradiological features, but often a precise diagnosis requires surgical biopsy. This is usually only performed as part of a therapeutic procedure, e.g. to resect or debulk a tumour that is compressing or threatening the optic chiasm. All patients with (para-)sellar space-occupying lesions should have pituitary function assessed as described in Box 20.53 (p. 793).

20.60 THERAPEUTIC MODALITIES FOR HYPOTHALAMIC AND PITUITARY TUMOURS				
	Surgery	**Radiotherapy**	**Medical**	**Comment**
Non-functioning pituitary macroadenoma	1st line	2nd line	–	
Prolactinoma	2nd line	2nd line	1st line Dopamine agonists	Dopamine agonists usually cause macroadenomas to shrink
Acromegaly	1st line	2nd line	2nd line Somatostatin analogues Dopamine agonists GH receptor antagonists	Medical therapy does not reliably cause macroadenomas to shrink
Cushing's disease	1st line	2nd line	–	Radiotherapy is used in children and to prevent Nelson's syndrome
Craniopharyngioma	1st line	2nd line	–	

Management

Modalities of treatment of common pituitary and hypothalamic tumours are shown in Box 20.60. Associated hypopituitarism should be treated as described on pages 795–796.

If there is evidence of pressure on visual pathways, then urgent treatment is required. The chances of recovery of a visual field defect are proportional to the duration of symptoms; full recovery is unlikely if the defect has been present for longer than 4 months. It is crucial that serum prolactin is measured before emergency surgery is performed. If the prolactin is > 5000 mU/l, then the lesion may be a macroprolactinoma and a therapeutic trial of a dopamine agonist for just a few days may successfully shrink the lesion and make surgery unnecessary (p. 800).

Most operations on the pituitary are performed by the trans-sphenoidal approach. The pituitary fossa is approached via the sphenoid sinus from an incision under the upper lip or through the nose. Transfrontal surgery via a craniotomy is reserved for suprasellar tumours. It is uncommon to be able to resect large lesions completely. All operations on the pituitary carry a risk of damaging normal endocrine function; this risk increases with the size of the primary lesion.

Pituitary function (Box 20.53, p. 793) should be retested 4–6 weeks following surgery. The purpose of this is primarily to detect the development of any new hormone deficits following surgery; rarely, the surgical treatment of a sellar lesion can result in recovery of hormone secretion that was deficient pre-operatively.

Following surgery, imaging is repeated usually after a few months and, if there is any residual mass and the histology confirms a radiosensitive tumour, external radiotherapy may be given to reduce the risk of recurrence. Radiotherapy is not useful in patients requiring urgent therapy because it takes many months or years to be effective and there is a risk of acute swelling of the mass. Radiotherapy carries a lifelong risk of hypopituitarism (50–70% in the first 10 years) and annual pituitary function tests are obligatory. There is also concern that radiotherapy, which is delivered through the temporal lobes, might impair cognitive function and even induce primary brain tumours, but these side-effects have not been quantified reliably and are likely to be rare.

Non-functioning tumours are followed up by repeated imaging at intervals that depend on the size of the lesion and on whether or not radiotherapy has been administered. For smaller lesions that are not causing mass effects therapeutic surgery may not be indicated and the lesion may simply be monitored by serial neuroimaging without a clearcut diagnosis having been established.

HYPERPROLACTINAEMIA

Hyperprolactinaemia is a common biochemical abnormality. The cardinal features are galactorrhoea and hypogonadism. Galactorrhoea describes lactation without breastfeeding. The quantity of milk produced is variable, and it may be observed only by manual expression. Prolactin stimulates milk secretion but not breast development, so that galactorrhoea almost never occurs in men, and is only possible in those in whom gynaecomastia is induced by hypogonadism (p. 766).

20.61 CAUSES OF HYPERPROLACTINAEMIA
Physiological
• Stress (e.g. post-seizure)
• Pregnancy
• Lactation
• Nipple stimulation
• Sleep
• Coitus
• Exercise
• Baby crying
Drugs
Dopamine antagonists
• Antipsychotics (phenothiazines and butyrophenones)
• Antidepressants
• Antiemetics (e.g. metoclopramide, domperidone)
Dopamine-depleting drugs
• Reserpine
• Methyldopa
Oestrogens
• Oral contraceptive pill
Pathological
Common
• Disconnection hyperprolactinaemia (e.g. non-functioning pituitary macroadenoma)
• Prolactinoma (usually microadenoma)
• Primary hypothyroidism
• Polycystic ovarian syndrome
• Macroprolactinaemia
Uncommon
• Hypothalamic disease
• Pituitary tumour secreting prolactin and growth hormone
• Renal failure
Rare
• Chest wall reflex (e.g. post-herpes zoster)
• Ectopic source

Aetiology

The differential diagnosis of hyperprolactinaemia is shown in Box 20.61. Many drugs, especially dopamine antagonists, will elevate prolactin concentrations. Pituitary tumours can cause hyperprolactinaemia not only by their ability to secrete prolactin (prolactinomas), but also if they are large enough to compress the infundibular stalk and thus interrupt the tonic inhibitory effect of hypothalamic dopamine on prolactin secretion ('disconnection' hyperprolactinaemia).

Prolactinoma. Most prolactinomas in pre-menopausal women are microadenomas, because the symptoms of prolactin excess usually result in early presentation. In men and post-menopausal women, however, the presentation is often much more insidious and the tumours are almost invariably macroadenomas at the time of diagnosis.

Macroprolactinaemia. This is a recently recognised cause of hyperprolactinaemia. Macroprolactin (or 'big, big prolactin') is prolactin bound to an IgG antibody. Many prolactin assays do not distinguish macroprolactin from monomeric (i.e. unbound) prolactin. Identification requires gel filtration chromatography or polyethylene glycol precipitation techniques. Macroprolactin cannot cross blood vessel walls to reach prolactin receptors in target tissues

20

and so is less likely to cause the classical symptoms of hyperprolactinaemia.

Clinical assessment

In women, in addition to galactorrhoea, the hypogonadism associated with hyperprolactinaemia causes secondary amenorrhoea and anovulation with infertility (p. 765). In men there is decreased libido, reduced shaving frequency and lethargy (p. 766). Important points in the history include drug use, recent pregnancy and menstrual history. Unilateral galactorrhoea may be confused with nipple discharge, and careful breast examination to exclude malignancy or fibrocystic disease is important. Further assessment should address the features in Figure 20.26 (p. 794).

Investigations

The presence of macroprolactin should be sought in all patients with hyperprolactinaemia. If macroprolactin is identified and monomeric prolactin concentrations are not elevated, then further investigation is not necessary if the patient has no signs or symptoms of pituitary disease. Pregnancy should be excluded in all women of child-bearing potential.

The upper limit of normal for many assays of serum prolactin is ~500 mU/l (~14 ng/ml). In non-pregnant and non-lactating patients, monomeric prolactin concentrations of 500–1000 mU/l are likely to be induced by stress or drugs, and a repeat measurement is indicated. Levels between 1000 and 5000 mU/l are likely to be due to either drugs, a microprolactinoma or 'disconnection' hyperprolactinaemia. Levels above 5000 mU/l are highly suggestive of a macroprolactinoma, and the higher the level, the bigger the tumour. Some macroprolactinomas cause levels over 100 000 mU/l.

Patients with prolactin excess should have tests of gonadal function (p. 762), and T_4 and TSH measured to exclude primary hypothyroidism causing TRH-induced prolactin excess. Unless the prolactin falls after withdrawal of relevant drug therapy, a serum prolactin of > 1000 mU/l is an indication for MRI or CT scan of the hypothalamus and pituitary. Patients with a macroadenoma also need tests for hypopituitarism (Box 20.53).

Management

If possible, the underlying cause should be corrected (e.g. cessation of offending drugs, levothyroxine replacement in primary hypothyroidism). If this is not possible, then in almost all cases of hyperprolactinaemia, dopamine agonist therapy (Box 20.62) will normalise prolactin levels with return of gonadal function. If gonadal function does not return despite effective lowering of prolactin, then there may be associated gonadotrophin deficiency or, in the female, the onset of the menopause. Troublesome physiological galactorrhoea can also be treated with dopamine agonists.

Prolactinomas

As shown in Box 20.60, several therapeutic modalities can be employed in the management of prolactinomas.

Medical. Dopamine agonist drugs are first-line therapy for the majority of patients and likely to be prescribed long-term (Box 20.62). However, it is possible to withdraw dopamine agonist therapy without recurrence of hyperprolactinaemia after 5–10 years of treatment in some patients with a microadenoma. Also, after the menopause, suppression of prolactin is only required in microadenomas if galactorrhoea is troublesome, since hypogonadism is then physiological and tumour growth unlikely. In patients with macroadenomas, drugs can only be withdrawn after curative surgery or radiotherapy and under close supervision.

In general, patients with a macroadenoma should avoid drugs that stimulate prolactin, including oestrogens (Box 20.61).

Surgical. Dopamine agonists not only lower prolactin levels, but shrink the majority of prolactin-secreting macroadenomas. Thus, surgical decompression is not usually necessary unless the macroadenoma is cystic. However, in patients who are intolerant of dopamine agonists, microadenomas can be removed selectively by trans-sphenoidal surgery with a cure rate of about 80%. The cure rate for surgery in macroadenomas is substantially lower.

Radiotherapy. External irradiation may be required for some macroadenomas to prevent regrowth if dopamine agonists are stopped.

Pregnancy. Hyperprolactinaemia often presents with infertility, so dopamine agonist therapy is often followed by

20.62 DOPAMINE AGONIST THERAPY: DRUGS USED TO TREAT PROLACTINOMAS			
	Oral dose*	Advantages	Disadvantages
Bromocriptine	2.5–15 mg/day 8–12-hourly	Available for parenteral use Short half-life; useful in treating infertility Proven long-term efficacy	Ergotamine-like side-effects (nausea, headache, postural hypotension, constipation) Frequent dosing so poor compliance
Cabergoline	250–1000 µg/week 2 doses/week	Long-acting, so missed doses less important Reported to have fewer ergotamine-like side-effects	Limited data on safety in pregnancy
Quinagolide	50–150 µg/day Once daily	A non-ergot with few side-effects in patients intolerant of the above	Untested in pregnancy
Pergolide			An older drug with bromocriptine-like side-effects; no longer used
* Tolerance develops for the side-effects. All of these agents, especially bromocriptine, must be introduced at low dose and increased slowly. If several doses of bromocriptine are missed, the process must start again.			

pregnancy. Patients with microadenomas are advised to withdraw dopamine agonist therapy as soon as pregnancy is confirmed. In contrast, macroprolactinomas may enlarge rapidly under oestrogen stimulation and these patients should continue dopamine agonist therapy and need measurement of prolactin levels and visual fields during pregnancy. All patients should be advised to report headache or visual disturbance promptly. Bromocriptine is the dopamine agonist that is most commonly used in pregnancy as there are long-term data about its safety.

ACROMEGALY

Acromegaly is caused by growth hormone (GH) secretion from a pituitary tumour, usually a macroadenoma.

Clinical features
If GH hypersecretion occurs before epiphyses have fused, then gigantism will result. More commonly, GH excess occurs in adult life, after epiphyseal closure, and acromegaly ensues. If hypersecretion starts in adolescence and persists into adult life, then the two conditions may be combined. The clinical features are shown in Figure 20.28. The most common complaints are headache and sweating. Additional

features include those of any pituitary tumour (Fig. 20.26, p. 794).

Investigations
The clinical diagnosis must be confirmed by measuring GH levels during an oral glucose tolerance test (Fig. 20.29). In normal subjects, plasma GH suppresses to below 2 mU/l. In acromegaly, it does not suppress and in about 50% of patients there is a paradoxical rise. The rest of pituitary function should be investigated as described in Box 20.53 (p. 793). Prolactin concentrations are elevated in about 30% of patients due to co-secretion of prolactin from the tumour.

The diagnosis of acromegaly is more difficult in patients with insulin deficiency, either type 1 or long-standing type 2 diabetes mellitus. GH may fail to suppress following a glucose load in these patients because inadequate insulin secretion results in failure of glucose to stimulate IGF-1 from the liver. It is IGF-1 that, in turn, suppresses GH secretion. This is important, because acromegaly can cause diabetes mellitus by exacerbating insulin resistance. However, in diabetic patients without acromegaly, IGF-1 concentrations are low, while in acromegalic patients they are high.

Additional tests in acromegaly may include screening for colonic neoplasms with colonoscopy.

20

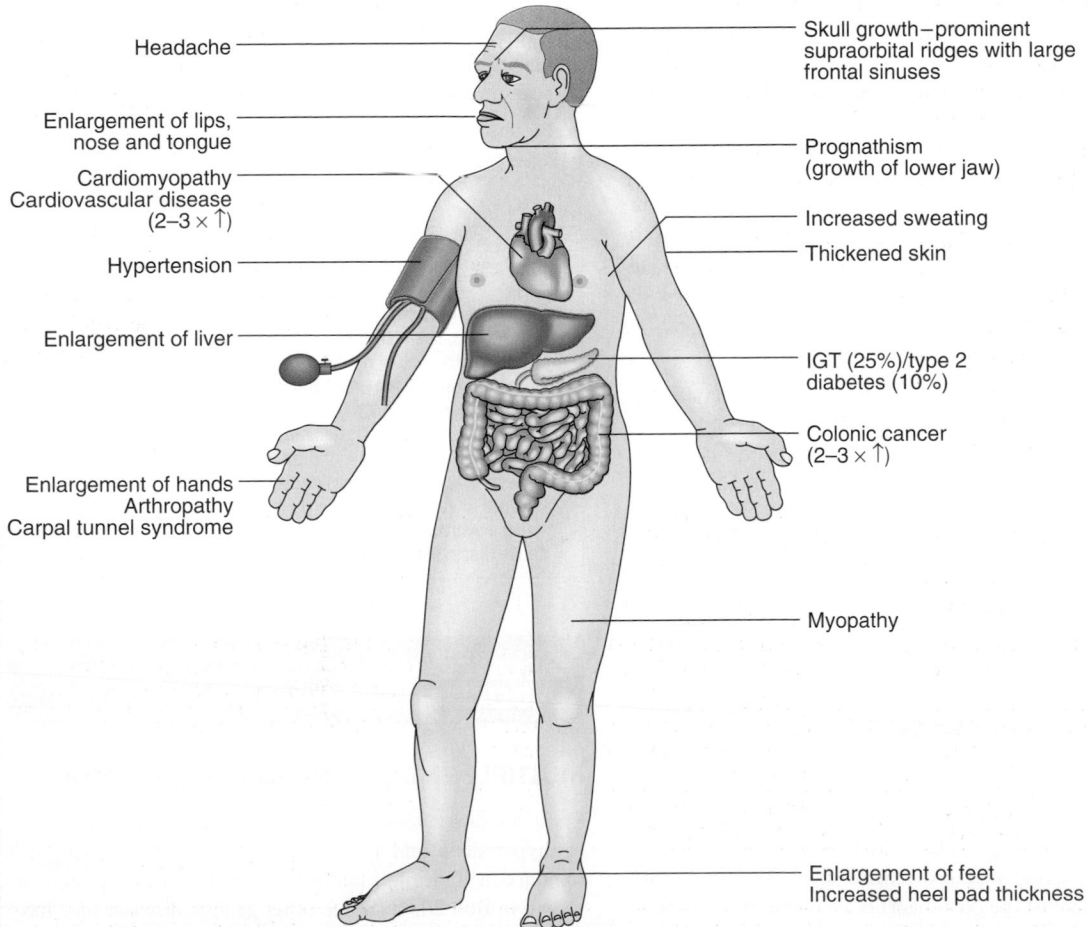

Headache

Enlargement of lips, nose and tongue

Cardiomyopathy Cardiovascular disease (2–3 × ↑)

Hypertension

Enlargement of liver

Enlargement of hands Arthropathy Carpal tunnel syndrome

Skull growth–prominent supraorbital ridges with large frontal sinuses

Prognathism (growth of lower jaw)

Increased sweating

Thickened skin

IGT (25%)/type 2 diabetes (10%)

Colonic cancer (2–3 × ↑)

Myopathy

Enlargement of feet Increased heel pad thickness

Fig. 20.28 Clinical features of acromegaly. (IGT = impaired glucose tolerance)

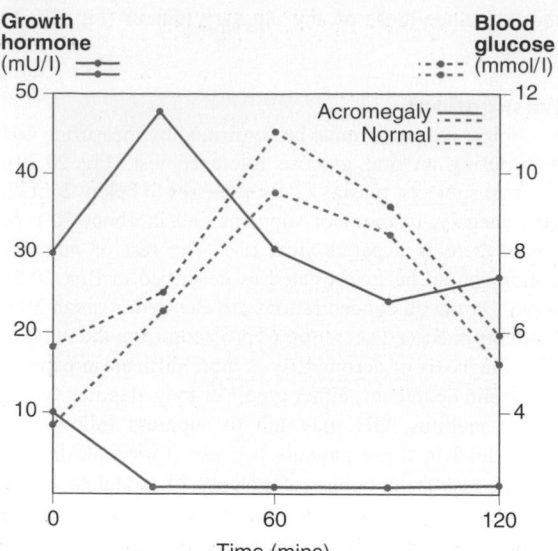

Fig. 20.29 Oral glucose tolerance tests in a normal subject and a patient with acromegaly with measurement of blood glucose and plasma growth hormone. Note the suppression of growth hormone secretion of < 2 mU/l in the normal subject, and failure to suppress (sometimes accompanied by paradoxical elevation) in acromegaly. Glucose tolerance may also be impaired in acromegaly. (Conversion of GH in mU/l to ng/ml depends on the assay used. To convert glucose in mmol/to mg/dl multiply by 18.)

Management

Therapeutic modalities are described in Box 20.60 (p. 798).

Surgical

Trans-sphenoidal surgery is usually the first line of treatment and may result in cure of GH excess, especially in patients with microadenomas. More often, surgery serves to debulk the tumour and further second-line therapy is required, according to post-operative imaging and glucose tolerance test results.

Radiotherapy

External radiotherapy is usually employed as second-line treatment if acromegaly persists after surgery, to stop tumour growth and lower GH levels. However, GH levels fall slowly (over many years) and there is a risk of hypopituitarism.

Medical

In patients with persisting acromegaly after surgery, most centres employ medical therapy to lower GH levels to < 5 mU/l. Medical therapy may be discontinued after several years in patients who have received radiotherapy. Somatostatin analogues (e.g. octreotide or lanreotide) can be administered as slow-release injections every few weeks. In some centres, somatostatin analogues are used as primary therapy for acromegaly, as they can cause modest tumour shrinkage in a proportion of patients. Dopamine agonists are less potent in lowering GH but may be helpful, especially in patients with associated prolactin excess. A peptide GH receptor antagonist (pegvisomant) is available for daily self-injection in patients whose GH concentrations fail to suppress following somatostatin analogue therapy (Box 20.63).

CRANIOPHARYNGIOMA

Craniopharyngiomas are benign tumours that develop in cell rests of Rathke's pouch, and may be located within the sella turcica, or commonly in the suprasellar space. They are often cystic and/or calcified (Fig. 20.30). In young people, they are diagnosed more commonly than pituitary adenomas. They may present with pressure effects on adjacent structures, hypopituitarism and/or cranial diabetes insipidus. In addition, other clinical features that are directly related to hypothalamic damage may also occur. These include hyperphagia and obesity (Fig. 20.30), loss of the sensation of thirst and disturbance of temperature regulation.

Craniopharyngiomas can rarely be reached by the trans-sphenoidal route and so surgery may involve a craniotomy, with a relatively high risk of hypothalamic damage and other complications. Surgery is unlikely to be curative, and radiotherapy is usually given, although there is uncertainty about its efficacy. Unfortunately, craniopharyngiomas often recur, requiring repeated surgery. They often cause considerable morbidity, usually from hypothalamic obesity, water balance problems and/or visual failure.

20.64 THE PITUITARY AND HYPOTHALAMUS IN OLD AGE

• **Late presentation:** often with large tumours causing visual disturbance, because early symptoms are not recognised (e.g. amenorrhoea, sexual dysfunction).
• **Coincidentally discovered pituitary tumours:** may not require surgical intervention if the visual apparatus is not involved, because of slow growth. Radiotherapy alone is sometimes employed simply to prevent further growth.
• **Hyperprolactinaemia:** less impact in post-menopausal women who are already 'physiologically' hypogonadal. Macroprolactinomas, however, require treatment because of their potential to cause mass effects.

DISEASES AFFECTING MULTIPLE ENDOCRINE GLANDS

MULTIPLE ENDOCRINE NEOPLASIA (MEN)

These are rare autosomal dominant syndromes characterised by hyperplasia and formation of adenomas or malignant tumours in multiple glands. They fall into two groups, as shown in Box 20.65. Some other genetic diseases also have an increased risk of endocrine tumours; for example, phaeochromocytoma is associated with von Hippel–Lindau

20

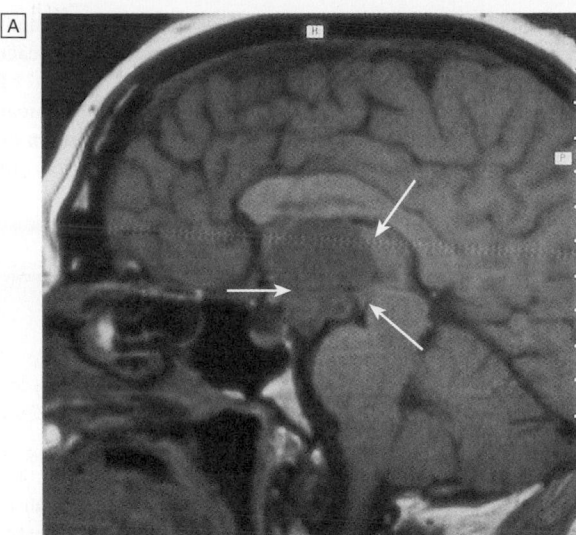

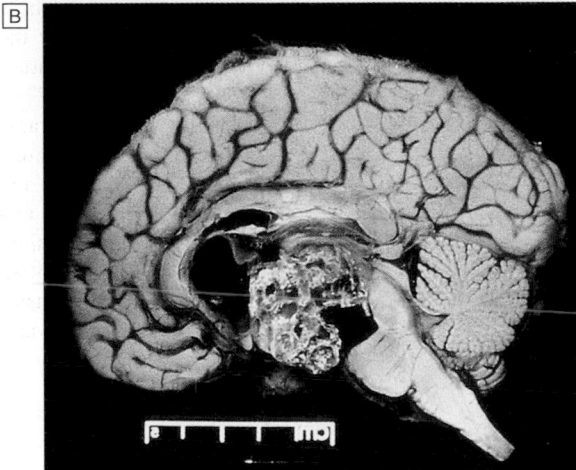

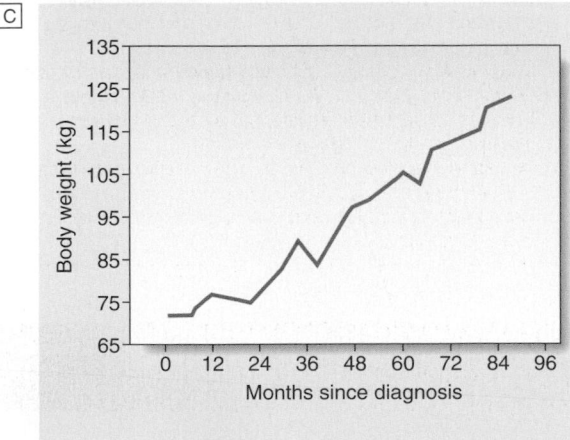

Fig. 20.30 Craniopharyngioma. A This developmental tumour characteristically presents in younger patients and is often cystic and calcified, as shown in this MRI (arrows). B Pathology specimen. C Hypothalamic damage is manifest as diabetes insipidus and loss of satiety, leading to relentless weight gain, as in this young woman following successful surgical resection and irradiation of her craniopharyngioma.

20.65 MULTIPLE ENDOCRINE NEOPLASIA (MEN) SYNDROMES

MEN 1 (Werner's syndrome)

- Primary hyperparathyroidism
- Pituitary tumours
- Pancreatic neuro-endocrine tumours (e.g. insulinoma, gastrinoma)

MEN 2 (Sipple's syndrome)

- Primary hyperparathyroidism
- Medullary carcinoma of thyroid
- Phaeochromocytoma

In addition, in MEN 2b syndrome there are phenotypic changes (including marfanoid habitus, skeletal abnormalities, abnormal dental enamel, multiple mucosal neuromas)

20

syndrome (p. 1238) and neurofibromatosis type 1 (p. 1237).

MEN syndromes should be considered in all patients with two or more of the relevant disorders (e.g. hypercalcaemia and pituitary tumour) and in patients with solitary tumours who report other endocrine tumours in their family.

Important advances have been made in recent years to establish the genetic causes of these syndromes. MEN 1 results from inactivating mutations in 'menin', a tumour suppressor gene on chromosome 11. In MEN 2, mutations in the RET proto-oncogene on chromosome 10 cause constitutive activation of a membrane-associated tyrosine kinase. RET controls the development of cells which migrate from the neural crest, and different mutations causing loss of function of the RET kinase are associated with Hirschsprung's disease (p. 931). Genetic testing can be performed on relatives of affected individuals, after appropriate counselling (p. 50).

Individuals who carry mutations associated with MEN should be entered into a surveillance programme. In MEN 1, this typically involves annual history, examination and measurements of serum calcium, gastrointestinal hormones and prolactin; MRI of the pituitary is performed at less frequent intervals. In individuals with MEN 2, annual history, examination and measurement of serum calcium and urinary catecholamine metabolites is performed. In addition, because the penetrance of medullary carcinoma of the thyroid is 100% in individuals with a RET mutation, prophylactic thyroidectomy is performed in early childhood.

AUTOIMMUNE POLYENDOCRINE SYNDROMES (APS)

Two distinct autoimmune polyendocrine syndromes are known: APS types 1 and 2 (Box 20.66).

APS type 2 (Schmidt's syndrome) is by far the more common and is typically observed in women between the ages of 20 and 60. It is usually defined as the occurrence in the same individual of two or more autoimmune endocrine disorders, some of which are listed in Box 20.66. The mode of inheritance is autosomal dominant with incomplete penetrance and there is a strong association with HLA-DR3 and CTLA-4. APS type 2 may be further subdivided depending on the precise combination of endocrine disorders observed but this is of limited value.

20.66 AUTOIMMUNE POLYENDOCRINE SYNDROMES (APS)*	
Type 1 (APECED)	
• Addison's disease	• Chronic mucocutaneous
• Hypoparathyroidism	candidiasis
• Type 1 diabetes	• Nail dystrophy
• Primary hypothyroidism	• Dental enamel hypoplasia
Type 2 (Schmidt's syndrome)	
• Addison's disease	• Type 1 diabetes
• Primary hypothyroidism	• Vitiligo
• Graves' disease	• Coeliac disease
• Pernicious anaemia	• Myasthenia gravis
• Primary hypogonadism	

* In both types of APS, the precise pattern of disease varies between affected individuals.

presentation of self-antigens to thymocytes in utero, which is essential for the deletion of thymocyte clones that react against self-antigens and hence for the development of immune tolerance (Ch. 4). The most common clinical features are described in Box 20.66, although the pattern of presentation is variable and other autoimmune disorders are observed.

APS type 1, which is also termed autoimmune polyendo-crinopathy–candidiasis–ectodermal dystrophy (APECED), is much rarer and is inherited in an autosomal recessive fashion. It is caused by mutations in the autoimmune regulator gene (AIRE). AIRE is responsible for the

FURTHER INFORMATION

Books and journal articles

deGroot L, Jameson JL. Endocrinology. 4th edn. London: WB Saunders; 2000.

Larson PR, Kronenberg HM, Melmed S, Polonsky KS. Williams Textbook of endocrinology. 10th edn. Philadelphia: WB Saunders; 2003.

Trainer PJ, Besser GM. The Bart's endocrine protocols. Edinburgh: Churchill Livingstone; 1995. *Detailed protocols for dynamic endocrine tests.*

Websites

www.endocrinology.org *Website of the British Society for Endocrinology; useful links to other resources.*

www.endo-society.org *Website of the American Endocrine Society; useful links to other resources.*

21

B.M. FRIER
M. FISHER

Diabetes mellitus

CLINICAL EXAMINATION OF THE PATIENT WITH DIABETES

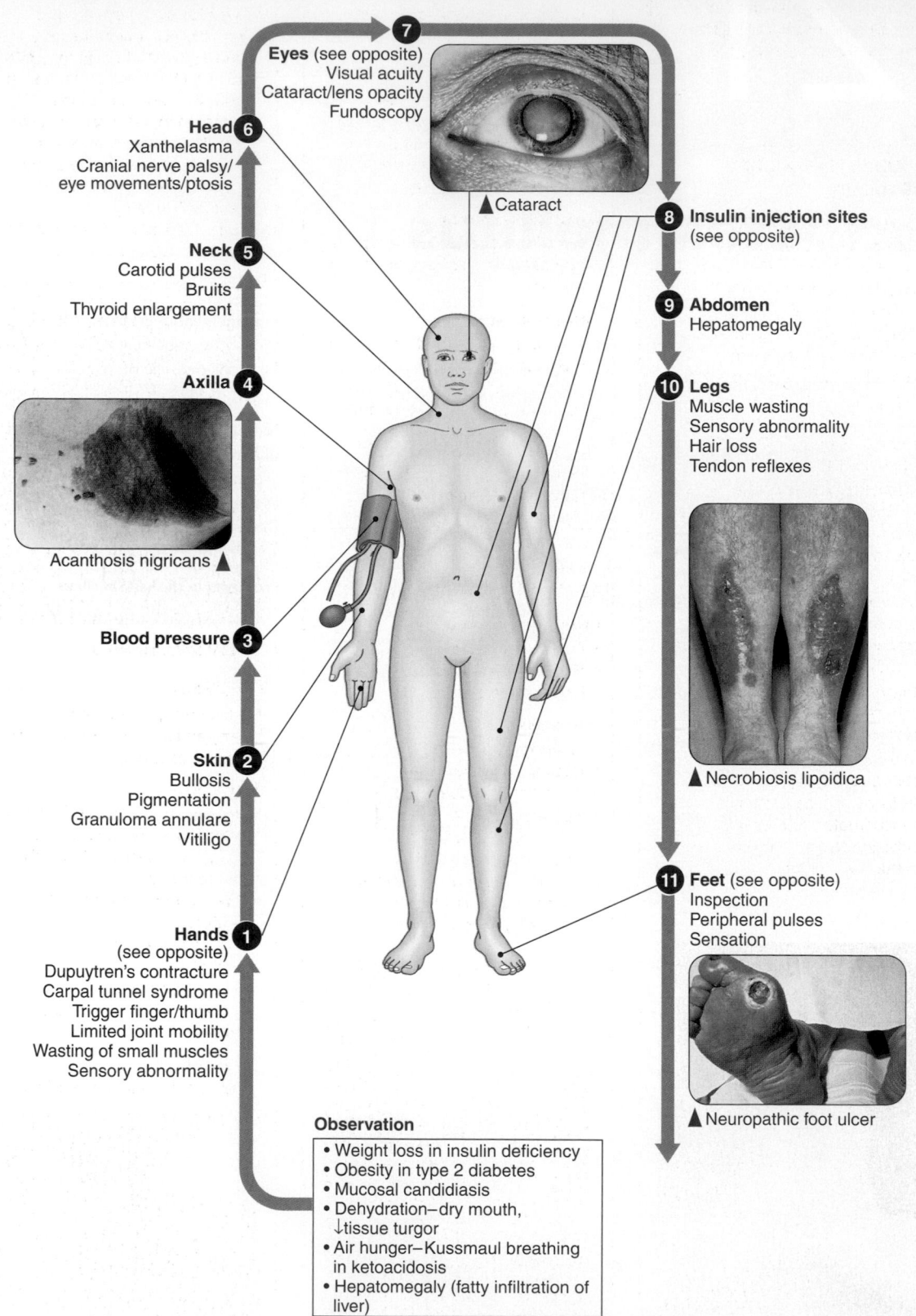

7 Eyes (see opposite)
Visual acuity
Cataract/lens opacity
Fundoscopy

▲ Cataract

6 Head
Xanthelasma
Cranial nerve palsy/
eye movements/ptosis

5 Neck
Carotid pulses
Bruits
Thyroid enlargement

4 Axilla

Acanthosis nigricans ▲

3 Blood pressure

2 Skin
Bullosis
Pigmentation
Granuloma annulare
Vitiligo

1 Hands
(see opposite)
Dupuytren's contracture
Carpal tunnel syndrome
Trigger finger/thumb
Limited joint mobility
Wasting of small muscles
Sensory abnormality

8 Insulin injection sites
(see opposite)

9 Abdomen
Hepatomegaly

10 Legs
Muscle wasting
Sensory abnormality
Hair loss
Tendon reflexes

▲ Necrobiosis lipoidica

11 Feet (see opposite)
Inspection
Peripheral pulses
Sensation

▲ Neuropathic foot ulcer

Observation
- Weight loss in insulin deficiency
- Obesity in type 2 diabetes
- Mucosal candidiasis
- Dehydration—dry mouth,
  ↓tissue turgor
- Air hunger—Kussmaul breathing
  in ketoacidosis
- Hepatomegaly (fatty infiltration of
  liver)

21

Diabetes can affect almost every system in the body. In routine clinical practice, examination of the patient with diabetes is focused on examination of the ❶ hands, ❸ blood pressure, ❼ eyes, ❽ insulin injection sites and ⑪ feet.

❶ EXAMINATION OF THE HANDS

- Limited joint mobility (sometimes called 'cheiroarthropathy') may be present; this is the inability to extend (to 180°) the metacarpophalangeal or interphalangeal joints of at least one finger bilaterally. The effect can be demonstrated in the 'prayer sign'. It causes painless stiffness in the hands, and occasionally affects the wrists and shoulders.
- Dupuytren's contracture (p. 1080) is common in diabetes and may include nodules or thickening of the skin and knuckle pads.
- Carpal tunnel syndrome (p. 1248) is common in diabetes and presents with wrist pain radiating into the hand.
- Trigger finger (flexor tenosynovitis) may be present in people with diabetes.
- Muscle-wasting/sensory changes may be present as features of a peripheral sensorimotor neuropathy, although this is more common in the lower limbs.

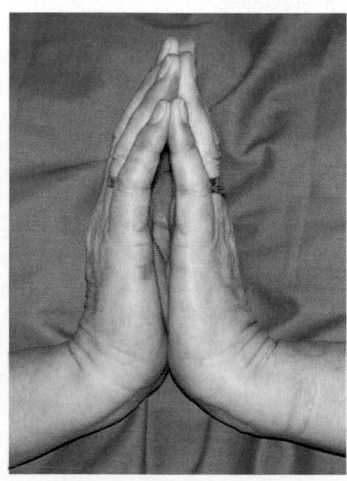

'Prayer sign'.

❼ EXAMINATION OF THE EYES

Visual acuity

- Distance vision using Snellen chart at 6 metres.
- Near vision using standard reading chart.
- Impaired visual acuity may indicate the presence of diabetic eye disease, and serial decline may suggest development or progression in severity.

Lens opacification

- Look for the red reflex using the ophthalmoscope held 30 cm from the eye.

Fundal examination

- The pupils must be dilated with a mydriatic (e.g. tropicamide) and examined in a darkened room.
- Features of diabetic retinopathy (p. 838) should be noted, including evidence of previous laser treatment which leaves photocoagulation scars.

❽ INSULIN INJECTION SITES

Main areas used

- Anterior abdominal wall
- Upper thighs/buttocks
- Upper outer arms

Inspection

- Bruising
- Lumps (lipodystrophy)
- Subcutaneous fat deposition (lipohypertrophy)
- Subcutaneous fat loss (lipoatrophy; associated with injection of unpurified animal insulins—now rare)
- Erythema, infection (rare)

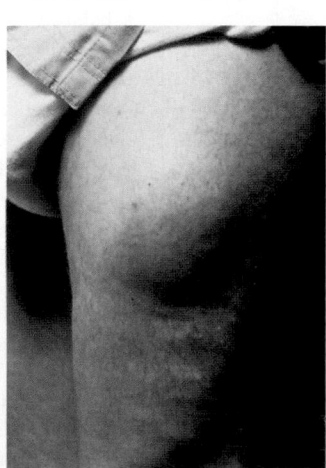

Lipohypertrophy.

⑪ EXAMINATION OF THE FEET

Inspection

- Look for evidence of callus formation on weight-bearing areas, clawing of the toes (a feature of neuropathy), loss of the plantar arch, discoloration of the skin (ischaemia), localised infection and the presence of ulcers.
- Deformity of the feet may be present, especially in Charcot neuroarthropathy.
- Fungal infection may affect skin between toes, and nails.

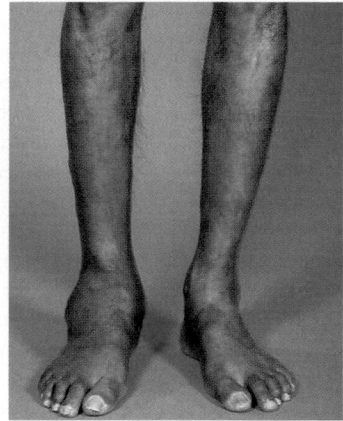

Charcot neuroarthropathy.

Circulation

- Peripheral pulses, skin temperature and capillary refill should be tested.

Sensation

- Light touch: use monofilaments.
- Vibration sense: use 128 Hz tuning fork over big toe/malleoli.
- Pin-prick: use pin.
- Pain: pressure over Achilles tendon.
- Proprioception: test position of big toe.
- Test for distal anaesthesia/ hyperaesthesia in stocking distribution.

Reflexes

- Test plantar and ankle reflexes.

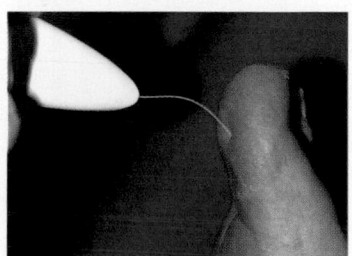

Monofilaments.

21

Diabetes mellitus is a clinical syndrome characterised by hyperglycaemia due to absolute or relative deficiency of insulin. This can arise in many different ways (Box 21.3, p. 810) but is most commonly due to autoimmune type 1 diabetes or to adult-onset type 2 diabetes. Lack of insulin affects the metabolism of carbohydrate, protein and fat, and can cause a significant disturbance of water and electrolyte homeostasis. Death may result from acute metabolic decompensation, while long-standing metabolic derangement is frequently associated with functional and structural changes in the cells of the body, with those of the vascular system being particularly susceptible. These changes lead to the development of clinical 'complications' of diabetes which characteristically affect the eye, the kidney and the nervous system.

The distribution of blood glucose concentration in populations is unimodal, with no clear division between normal and abnormal values. Hyperglycaemia represents an independent risk factor for the development of disease of both small and large blood vessels. Diagnostic criteria for diabetes (p. 817) have been selected to identify those who have a degree of hyperglycaemia which, if untreated, is associated with a significant risk of microvascular disease, and in particular diabetic retinopathy. Less severe hyperglycaemia is called 'impaired glucose tolerance'. This is not associated with substantial risk of microvascular disease, but is associated with increased risk of large vessel disease (e.g. atheroma leading to myocardial infarction) and with a greater risk of developing diabetes in future. The implication of these criteria is that there is no such thing as 'mild' diabetes not requiring effective treatment.

Diabetes occurs world-wide and the incidences of both type 1 and type 2 diabetes are rising; it is estimated that, in the year 2000, 171 million people had diabetes, and this is expected to double by 2030 (Fig. 21.1). This global pandemic principally involves type 2 diabetes, to which several factors contribute, including greater longevity,

21.1 THE CURRENT COST OF DIABETES IN THE UK

- 10–30% reduction in life expectancy
- Most common cause of blindness in age group 20–65 years
- 1000 patients per annum reach end-stage renal failure
- Lower limb amputation rate increased 25-fold
- Use of hospital beds increased sixfold
- 5–7% of total National Health Service budget

obesity, unsatisfactory diet, sedentary lifestyle and increasing urbanisation. Many cases of type 2 diabetes remain undetected. However, the prevalence of both types of diabetes varies considerably around the world, and is related to differences in genetic and environmental factors. The prevalence of known diabetes in Britain is around 2–3%, but is higher in the Middle and Far East (e.g. 12% in the Indian subcontinent). A pronounced rise in the prevalence of type 2 diabetes occurs in migrant populations to industrialised countries, as in Asian and Afro-Caribbean immigrants to the UK. Type 2 diabetes is now being observed in children and adolescents, particularly in some ethnic groups, such as Hispanic and Afro-Americans.

Type 1 diabetes is more common in Caucasian populations, and in northern Europe its prevalence in children has doubled in the last 20 years, with a particular increase in children under 5 years of age. In Europe and North America the ratio of type 2 to type 1 is approximately 7:3.

Diabetes is a major burden upon health-care facilities in all countries. Estimated costs in the UK are shown in Box 21.1.

FUNCTIONAL ANATOMY, PHYSIOLOGY AND INVESTIGATIONS

NORMAL GLUCOSE AND FAT METABOLISM

In humans, blood glucose is tightly regulated by homeostatic mechanisms and maintained within a narrow range. A balance is preserved between the entry of glucose into the circulation from the liver, supplemented by intestinal absorption after meals, and glucose uptake by peripheral tissues, particularly skeletal muscle. A continuous supply of glucose is essential for the brain, which cannot oxidise free fatty acids and relies upon glucose as its principal metabolic fuel.

When intestinal glucose absorption declines between meals, hepatic glucose output is increased in response to low insulin levels and increased levels of the counter-regulatory hormones, glucagon and adrenaline (epinephrine). The liver produces glucose by gluconeogenesis and glycogen breakdown. The main substrates for gluconeogenesis are glycerol and amino acids, as shown in Figure 21.2.

After meals, blood insulin levels rise. Insulin is an anabolic hormone with profound effects on the metabolism of carbohydrate, fat and protein (Box 21.2). Insulin is secreted from pancreatic β cells (Fig. 21.3) into the

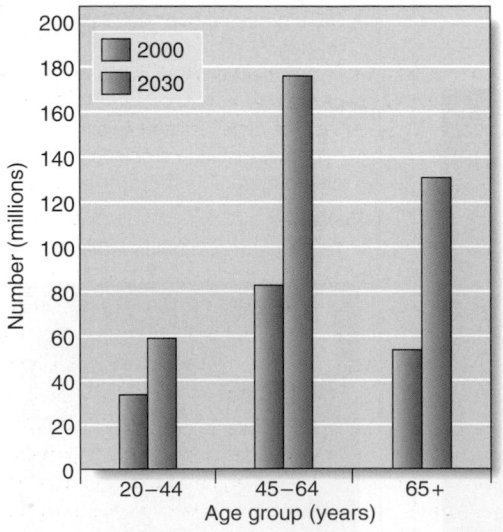

Fig. 21.1 World-wide estimated number of adults with diabetes by age group and year.

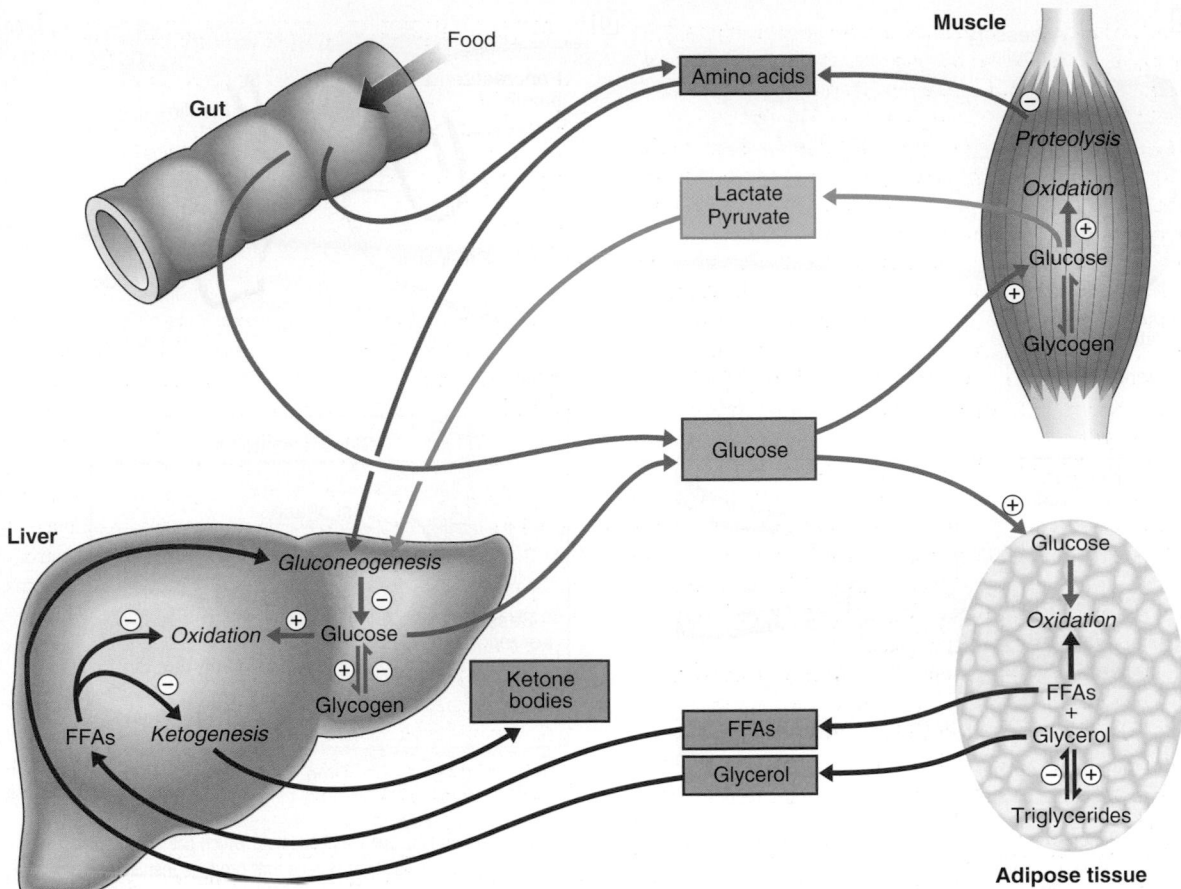

Fig. 21.2   Major metabolic pathways of fuel metabolism and the actions of insulin. $\oplus$ indicates stimulation and $\ominus$ indicates suppression by insulin. In response to a rise in blood glucose, e.g. after a meal, insulin is released, suppressing gluconeogenesis and promoting glycogen synthesis and storage. It promotes the peripheral uptake of glucose, particularly in skeletal muscle, and encourages storage (as muscle glycogen) and protein synthesis. It also promotes lipogenesis and suppresses lipolysis. The release of intermediate metabolites including amino acids (glutamine, alanine), 3-carbon intermediates in oxidation (lactate, pyruvate) and free fatty acids (FFAs) is controlled by insulin. In the absence of insulin, e.g. during fasting, these processes are reversed and favour gluconeogenesis in liver from glycogen, glycerol, amino acids and other 3-carbon precursors.

21.2 METABOLIC ACTIONS OF INSULIN

Increase (anabolic effects)	Decrease (anticatabolic effects)
Carbohydrate metabolism	
Glucose transport (muscle, adipose tissue)	Gluconeogenesis
Glucose phosphorylation	Glycogenolysis
Glycogenesis	
Glycolysis	
Pyruvate dehydrogenase activity	
Pentose phosphate shunt	
Lipid metabolism	
Triglyceride synthesis	Lipolysis
Fatty acid synthesis (liver)	Lipoprotein lipase (muscle)
Lipoprotein lipase activity (adipose tissue)	Ketogenesis
	Fatty acid oxidation (liver)
Protein metabolism	
Amino acid transport	Protein degradation
Protein synthesis	

portal circulation, with a brisk increase in response to a rise in blood glucose. Some characteristics of normal insulin secretion are shown in Figure 21.3. Insulin lowers blood glucose by suppressing hepatic glucose production and stimulating glucose uptake in skeletal muscle and fat, mediated by the glucose transporter, GLUT 4.

Adipocytes (and the liver) synthesise triglyceride from non-esterified ('free') fatty acids (FFAs) and glycerol. Insulin stimulates lipogenesis and inhibits lipolysis, so preventing fat catabolism. Lipolysis, mediated by triglyceride lipase, is stimulated by catecholamines and liberates FFAs which can be oxidised by many tissues. Their partial oxidation in the liver provides energy to drive gluconeogenesis and also produces ketone bodies (acetoacetate, which can be reduced to 3-hydroxybutyrate or decarboxylated to acetone) which are generated in hepatocyte mitochondria. Ketone bodies are organic acids which, when formed in small amounts, are oxidised and utilised as metabolic fuel. However, the rate of utilisation of ketone bodies by peripheral tissues is limited, and when the rate of

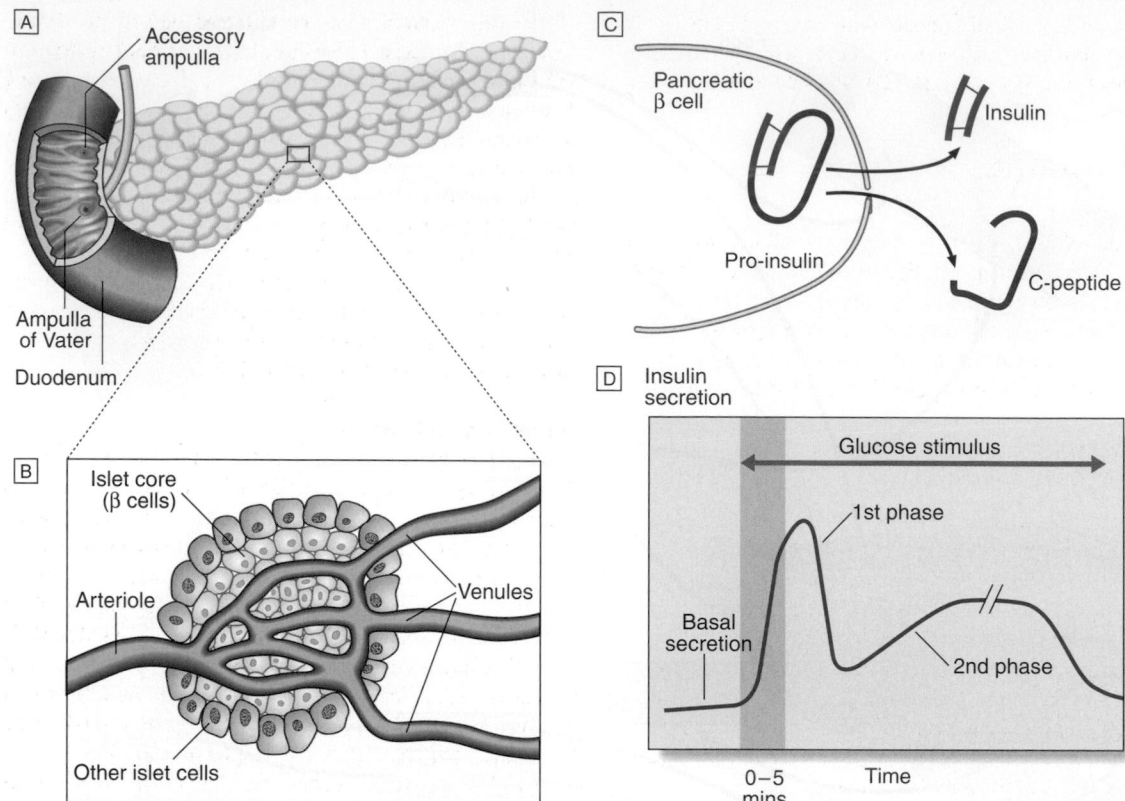

Fig. 21.3 Pancreatic structure and endocrine function. [A] The normal adult pancreas contains about 1 million islets which are scattered throughout the exocrine parenchyma. Histology is shown in Figure 21.4. [B] The core of each islet consists of β cells that produce insulin, and is surrounded by a cortex of endocrine cells that produce other hormones including glucagon (α cells), somatostatin (δ cells) and pancreatic polypeptide (PP cells). [C] Pro-insulin in the pancreatic β cell is cleaved to release insulin and equimolar amounts of inert C-peptide (connecting peptide). Measurement of C-peptide can be used to assess endogenous insulin secretory capacity. [D] An acute first phase of insulin secretion occurs in response to an elevated blood glucose, followed by a sustained second phase.

production by the liver exceeds their removal, hyper-ketonaemia results. Ketogenesis is regulated by the supply of FFAs reaching the liver and is therefore enhanced by insulin deficiency and release of the counter-regulatory hormones that stimulate lipolysis.

AETIOLOGY AND PATHOGENESIS OF DIABETES

In both of the common types of diabetes, environmental factors interact with genetic susceptibility to determine which people develop the clinical syndrome, and the timing of its onset. However, the underlying genes, precipitating environmental factors and pathophysiology differ substantially between type 1 and type 2 diabetes (Box 21.3). Type 1 diabetes was previously termed 'insulin-dependent diabetes mellitus' (IDDM) and is invariably associated with profound insulin deficiency requiring replacement therapy. Type 2 diabetes was previously termed 'non-insulin-dependent diabetes mellitus' (NIDDM) because patients retain the capacity to secrete some insulin but exhibit impaired sensitivity to insulin (insulin resistance) and can usually be treated without insulin replacement therapy.

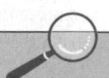

21.3 AETIOLOGICAL CLASSIFICATION OF DIABETES MELLITUS

Type 1 diabetes
- Immune-mediated
- Idiopathic

Type 2 diabetes

Other specific types
- Genetic defects of β-cell function (Box 21.8, p. 815)
- Genetic defects of insulin action
- Pancreatic disease (e.g. pancreatitis, pancreatectomy, neoplastic disease, cystic fibrosis, haemochromatosis, fibrocalculous pancreatopathy)
- Excess endogenous production of hormonal antagonists to insulin (e.g. growth hormone—acromegaly; glucocorticoids—Cushing's syndrome; glucagon—glucagonoma; catecholamines—phaeochromocytoma; thyroid hormones—thyrotoxicosis)
- Drug-induced (e.g. corticosteroids, thiazide diuretics, phenytoin)
- Viral infections (e.g. congenital rubella, mumps, Coxsackie virus B)
- Uncommon forms of immune-mediated diabetes
- Associated with genetic syndromes (e.g. Down's syndrome; Klinefelter's syndrome; Turner's syndrome; DIDMOAD (Wolfram's syndrome)—diabetes insipidus, diabetes mellitus, optic atrophy, nerve deafness; Friedreich's ataxia; myotonic dystrophy)

Gestational diabetes

However, up to 20% of patients with type 2 diabetes will ultimately develop profound insulin deficiency requiring replacement therapy so that IDDM and NIDDM were misnomers.

TYPE 1 DIABETES

Pathology

Type 1 diabetes is a slowly progressive T cell-mediated autoimmune disease (p. 80). Family studies have produced evidence that destruction of the insulin-secreting cells in the pancreatic islets takes place over many years. Hyperglycaemia accompanied by the classical symptoms of diabetes occurs only when 70–90% of β cells have been destroyed.

The pathological picture in the pre-diabetic pancreas in type 1 diabetes is characterised by:

- 'insulitis' (Fig. 21.4)—that is, infiltration of the islets with mononuclear cells containing activated macrophages, helper cytotoxic and suppressor T lymphocytes, natural killer cells and B lymphocytes
- the initial patchiness of this lesion with, until a very late stage, lobules containing heavily infiltrated islets seen adjacent to unaffected lobules
- the striking β-cell specificity of the destructive process, with the glucagon and other hormone-secreting cells in the islet invariably remaining intact.

Islet cell antibodies can be detected before the clinical development of type 1 diabetes, have a variable predictive value as a marker of disease, and disappear with increasing duration of diabetes (Fig. 21.4). At present these antibodies are not suitable for screening or diagnostic purposes, but glutamic acid decarboxylase (GAD) antibodies may have a role in identifying late-onset type 1 diabetes in middle-aged people (latent autoimmune diabetes in adults—LADA) in whom type 2 diabetes might otherwise be suspected.

Type 1 diabetes is associated with other autoimmune disorders (Ch. 4), including thyroid disease (p. 744), coeliac disease (p. 894), Addison's disease (p. 782), pernicious anaemia (p. 1028) and vitiligo (p. 1280).

Genetic predisposition

Genetic factors account for about one-third of the susceptibility to type 1 diabetes, the inheritance of which is polygenic. Over 20 different regions of the human genome show some linkage with type 1 diabetes but most interest has focused on the human leucocyte antigen (HLA) region within the major histocompatibility complex on the short arm of chromosome 6; this locus is designated IDDM 1. The HLA haplotypes *DR3* and/or *DR4* are associated with increased susceptibility to type 1 diabetes in Caucasians and are in 'linkage disequilibrium', i.e. they tend to be transmitted together, with the neighbouring alleles of the *HLA-DQA1* and *DQB1* genes. The latter may be the main

21

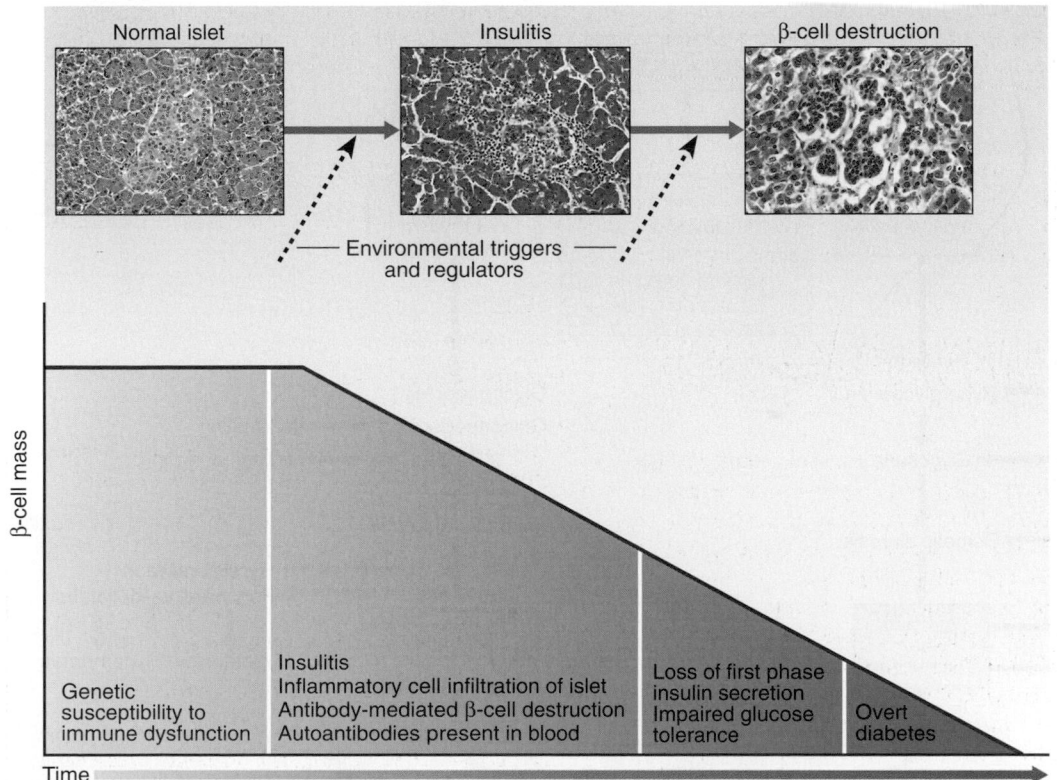

Fig. 21.4 Pathogenesis of type 1 diabetes. Proposed sequence of events in the development of type 1 diabetes. Environmental triggers are described in the text.

determinants of the genetic susceptibility, since these HLA class II genes code for proteins on the surface of cells which present foreign and self-antigens to T lymphocytes. Defective presentation of autoantigens derived from pancreatic islet β cells probably underlies the development of autoimmunity (p. 80).

Environmental factors

Although genetic susceptibility appears to be a prerequisite for the development of type 1 diabetes, the concordance rate between monozygotic twins is less than 40% (Box 21.4), and environmental factors have an important role in promoting clinical expression of the disease. It has been proposed that reduced exposure to microorganisms in early childhood limits maturation of the immune system and increases susceptibility to autoimmune disease (the 'hygiene hypothesis').

The evidence that viral infection might cause some forms of type 1 diabetes is derived from studies where virus particles known to cause cytopathic or autoimmune damage to β cells have been isolated from the pancreas. Several viruses have been implicated, including mumps, Coxsackie B4, retroviruses, rubella (in utero), cytomegalovirus and Epstein–Barr virus.

Circumstantial evidence supports the proposition that dietary factors may influence the development of type 1 diabetes. Bovine serum albumin (BSA), a major constituent of cow's milk, has been implicated in triggering type 1 diabetes, since children who are given cow's milk early in infancy are more likely to develop type 1 diabetes than those who are breastfed. BSA may cross the neonatal gut and raise antibodies which, because of the close homology between BSA and a heat-shock protein expressed by β cells, could cross-react with and cause damage to β-cell components.

Various nitrosamines (found in smoked and cured meats) and coffee have been proposed as potentially diabetogenic toxins.

Stress may precipitate type 1 diabetes by stimulating the secretion of counter-regulatory hormones and possibly by modulating immune activity.

Metabolic disturbances in type 1 diabetes

Patients with type 1 diabetes present when progressive β-cell destruction has crossed a threshold at which adequate insulin secretion and normal blood glucose levels can no longer be sustained. Above a certain level, high glucose levels may be toxic to the remaining β cells so that profound insulin deficiency rapidly ensues. Profound insulin deficiency is associated with the metabolic sequelae shown in Figure 21.5. Hyperglycaemia leads to glycosuria and

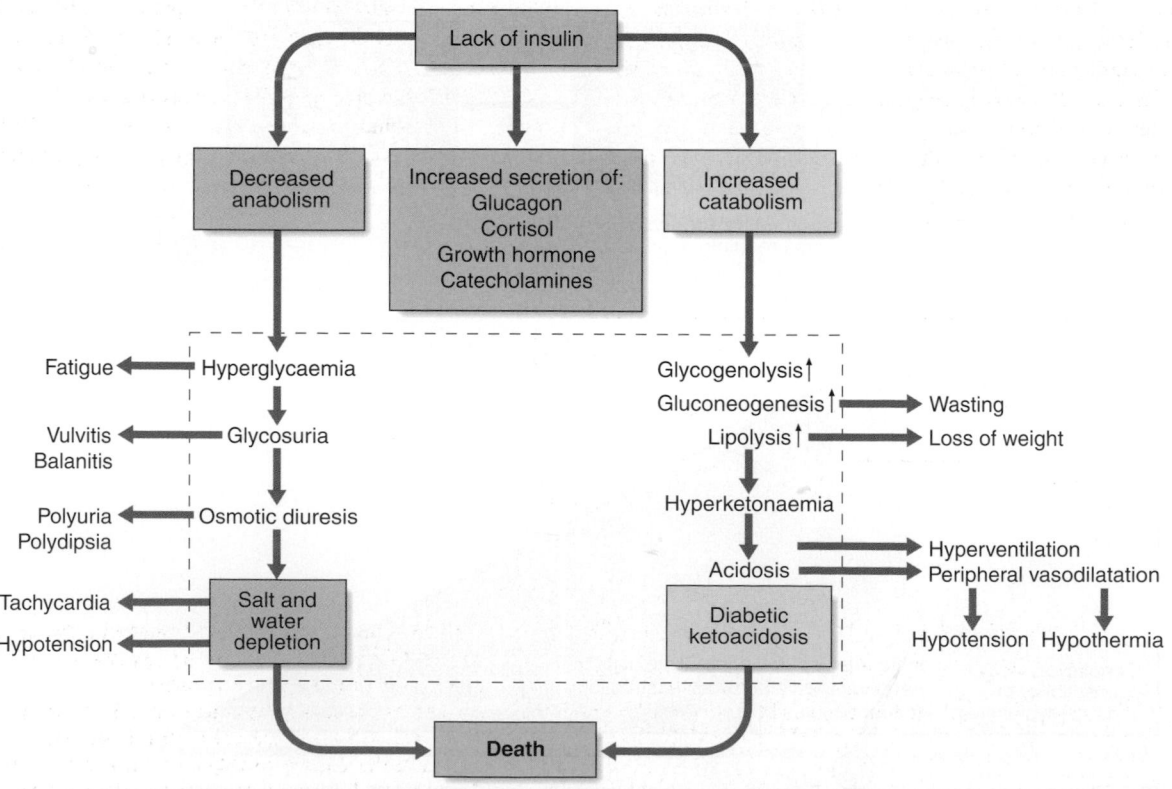

Fig. 21.5 **Pathophysiological basis of the symptoms and signs of uncontrolled diabetes mellitus.**

dehydration, which in turn induces secondary hyperaldosteronism (p. 786). Unrestrained lipolysis and proteolysis result in weight loss, increased gluconeogenesis and ketogenesis. When generation of ketone bodies exceeds the capacity for their metabolism, ketoacidosis results. Elevated blood H^+ ions drive K^+ out of the intracellular compartment, while secondary hyperaldosteronism encourages urinary loss of K^+. Thus patients usually present with quite short histories (typically a few weeks) of hyperglycaemic symptoms (thirst, polyuria, fatigue and infections) and weight loss, and may have developed ketoacidosis (p. 820).

TYPE 2 DIABETES

Pathology

Type 2 diabetes is a more complex condition than type 1 diabetes because there is a combination of resistance to the actions of insulin in liver and muscle together with impaired pancreatic β-cell function leading to 'relative' insulin deficiency. The natural history is shown in Figure 21.6. Insulin resistance appears to come first, and leads to elevated insulin secretion in order to maintain normal blood glucose levels. However, in susceptible individuals the pancreatic β cells are unable to sustain the increased demand for insulin and a slowly progressive insulin deficiency develops.

Insulin resistance

In patients with type 2 diabetes excessive production of glucose in the liver and under-utilisation of glucose in skeletal muscle result from resistance to the action of insulin. A characteristic feature of type 2 diabetes is that it is often associated with other medical disorders, particularly central (visceral) obesity, hypertension and dyslipidaemia (characterised by elevated levels of small dense LDL cholesterol and triglycerides, and a low level of HDL cholesterol). It has been suggested that coexistence of this cluster of conditions, all of which predispose to cardiovascular disease, is a specific entity (the 'insulin resistance syndrome' or 'metabolic syndrome'), with a predisposition to insulin resistance being the primary defect and the

presence of obesity being a powerful amplifier of the insulin resistance. The primary cause of insulin resistance remains unclear but this is a major focus of current research.

Intra-abdominal 'central' adipose tissue is metabolically active, and releases large quantities of FFAs which may induce insulin resistance because they compete with glucose as a fuel supply for oxidation in peripheral tissues such as muscle. In addition, adipose tissue releases a number of hormones (e.g. steroids such as cortisol and a variety of peptides, called 'adipokines' because they are structurally similar to immunological 'cytokines') which act on specific receptors to influence sensitivity to insulin in other tissues. Because visceral adipose tissue drains into the portal vein, central obesity may have a particularly potent influence on insulin sensitivity in the liver, and thereby adversely affect gluconeogenesis and hepatic lipid metabolism.

Exercise is another important determinant of insulin sensitivity. Inactivity is associated with down-regulation of insulin-sensitive kinases and may also increase the accumulation of FFAs within skeletal muscle. Sedentary people are therefore more insulin-resistant than active people with the same degree of obesity. Moreover, exercise allows non-insulin-dependent glucose uptake into muscle, reducing the 'demand' on the pancreatic β cells to produce insulin.

Pancreatic β-cell failure

In the early stages of type 2 diabetes there is only moderate reduction in the total mass of pancreatic islet tissue. Some pathological changes are typical of type 2 diabetes, the most consistent of which is deposition of amyloid. An attractive, but as yet unproven, hypothesis to explain β-cell destruction in type 2 diabetes is that the polypeptide amylin is secreted together with insulin, so that in the presence of insulin resistance the excessive demand for insulin secretion also results in the formation of excess amylin which forms insoluble fibrils of amyloid and ultimately destroys β cells.

While β-cell numbers are typically reduced by 20–30% in type 2 diabetes, α-cell mass is unchanged and glucagon secretion is increased, which may contribute to the hyperglycaemia.

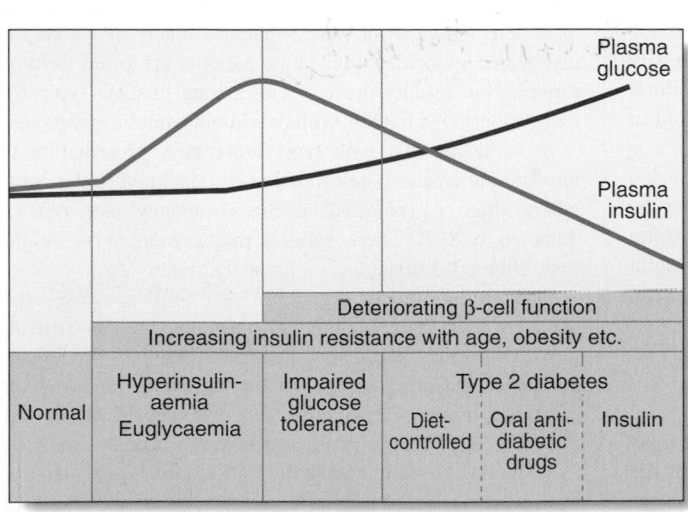

Fig. 21.6 Natural history of type 2 diabetes. In the early stage of the disorder the response to progressive insulin resistance is an increase in insulin secretion by the pancreatic cells, causing hyperinsulinaemia. Eventually the β cells are unable to compensate adequately and blood glucose rises, producing hyperglycaemia. With further β-cell failure (type 2 diabetes) glycaemic control deteriorates and treatment requirements escalate.

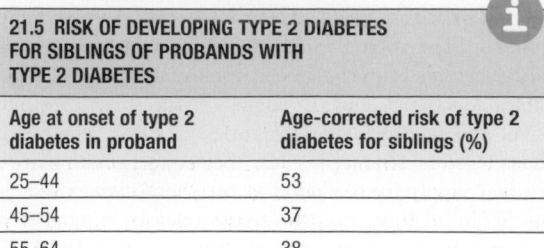

21.5 RISK OF DEVELOPING TYPE 2 DIABETES FOR SIBLINGS OF PROBANDS WITH TYPE 2 DIABETES

Age at onset of type 2 diabetes in proband	Age-corrected risk of type 2 diabetes for siblings (%)
25–44	53
45–54	37
55–64	38
65–80	31

21.6 DIAGNOSIS OF DIABETES MELLITUS IN OLD AGE

- **Prevalence**: increases with age, affecting approximately 10% of people over 65 years. Half of these people are unaware that they have the disorder. Impaired glucose-induced insulin secretion and resistance to insulin-mediated glucose disposal contribute to this high prevalence.
- **Glycosuria**: the renal threshold for glucose rises with age, so glycosuria may not develop until the blood glucose concentration is markedly raised.
- **Pancreatic carcinoma**: may present in old age with the development of diabetes, in association with weight loss and diminished appetite.

Genetic predisposition

Genetic factors are important in the aetiology of type 2 diabetes, as shown by marked differences in susceptibility in different ethnic groups and by studies in monozygotic twins where concordance rates for type 2 diabetes approach 100%. However, many genes are involved and the chance of developing diabetes is also influenced very powerfully by environmental factors (Box 21.5). Over 200 candidate susceptibility genes have been investigated, but at the time of writing consistent association of variants in candidate genes with type 2 diabetes has been found with only three gene polymorphisms. These polymorphisms each increase susceptibility by around 20% and are contained in the genes for PPARγ, the Kir6.2 subunit of the β-cell K_{ATP} channel, and the protease, calpain 10. Genome-wide searches have identified additional regions that contain susceptibility loci on chromosome 1q, 12q and 20q but the underlying genes have not been identified.

Environmental factors

Epidemiological studies provide evidence that type 2 diabetes is associated with overeating, especially when combined with obesity and underactivity. Other more direct studies have shown that middle-aged people with diabetes eat significantly more and are fatter and less active than their non-diabetic siblings. However, although the majority of middle-aged diabetic people are obese, only a minority of obese people develop diabetes. Obesity probably acts as a diabetogenic factor (through increasing resistance to the action of insulin, p. 809) only in those who are genetically predisposed both to insulin resistance and to β-cell failure. The risk of developing type 2 diabetes increases tenfold in people with a body mass index > 30 kg/m² (p. 111).

In addition to the effect of total calorie content on obesity, the constituents of the diet and the style of eating may be important. Sweet foods rich in refined carbohydrate consumed frequently may increase the demand for insulin secretion, while high-fat foods may increase FFAs and exacerbate insulin resistance.

Other risk factors

Age

Type 2 diabetes is principally a disease of the middle-aged and elderly (Box 21.6). In the UK, it affects 10% of the population over 65, and over 70% of all cases of diabetes occur after the age of 50 years.

Pregnancy

During normal pregnancy, insulin sensitivity is reduced through the action of placental hormones and this affects glucose tolerance. The insulin-secreting cells of the pancreatic islets may be unable to meet this increased demand in women genetically predisposed to develop diabetes. The term 'gestational diabetes' refers to hyperglycaemia occurring for the first time during pregnancy (p. 826). Repeated pregnancy may increase the likelihood of developing irreversible diabetes, particularly in obese women; 80% of women with gestational diabetes ultimately develop permanent diabetes.

Metabolic disturbances in type 2 diabetes

Patients with type 2 diabetes have a slow onset of 'relative' insulin deficiency. Relatively small amounts of insulin are required to suppress lipolysis, and some glucose uptake is maintained in muscle, so that unrestrained lipolysis and proteolysis do not occur and weight loss and ketoacidosis are rare. Glycosuria occurs when the blood glucose concentration exceeds the renal threshold (the capacity of renal tubules to reabsorb glucose from the glomerular filtrate) at approximately 10 mmol/l (180 mg/dl). The severity of the classical 'osmotic' symptoms of polyuria and polydipsia is related to the degree of glycosuria. In type 2 diabetes, hyperglycaemia develops slowly over months or years and the renal threshold for glucose rises, so that osmotic symptoms are usually mild. This is one reason for the large number of undetected cases of type 2 diabetes, many of which are discovered coincidentally. Thus, patients are often asymptomatic, but usually present with a long history (typically many months) of fatigue, with or without osmotic symptoms.

In some patients with type 2 diabetes, presentation is late and pancreatic β-cell function has declined to the point where there is profound insulin deficiency (see type 1 diabetes, p. 812). These patients may present with weight loss, although ketoacidosis remains extremely rare.

Intercurrent illness, e.g. with infections, increases the production of counter-regulatory hormones such as cortisol, growth hormone and catecholamines. This can precipitate an acute exacerbation of insulin resistance and insulin deficiency and result in more severe hyperglycaemia and dehydration (see hyperosmolar non-ketotic coma, p. 823).

A number of other metabolic abnormalities, particularly dyslipidaemia, are common in patients with type 2 diabetes (see above and Box 21.7).

21.7 FEATURES OF THE INSULIN RESISTANCE (METABOLIC) SYNDROME*

- Hyperinsulinaemia
- Type 2 diabetes or impaired glucose tolerance
- Hypertension
- Low HDL cholesterol; elevated triglycerides
- Central (visceral) obesity
- Microalbuminuria
- Increased fibrinogen
- Increased plasminogen activator inhibitor-1
- Elevated plasma uric acid
- Increased sympathetic neural activity

*This constellation of features has also been called Reaven's syndrome and syndrome X, and is strongly associated with atherosclerosis. This is manifested by macrovascular disease (coronary, cerebral, peripheral) and an excess mortality.

OTHER FORMS OF DIABETES

Other causes of diabetes are shown in Box 21.3 (p. 810). In most cases there is an obvious cause of destruction of pancreatic β cells. Some acquired disorders, notably other endocrine diseases such as acromegaly (p. 801) or Cushing's syndrome (p. 779), can precipitate type 2 diabetes in susceptible individuals.

A number of unusual genetic diseases are associated with diabetes. In rare families, diabetes is caused by single gene defects with autosomal dominant inheritance (Boxes 21.3 and 21.8). These uncommon subtypes typically present as 'maturity-onset diabetes of the young' (MODY) and constitute less than 5% of all cases of diabetes. Determining the molecular genetic aetiology can help to define the prognosis, optimal treatment, and risk of diabetes in relatives. Patients with mutations in *HNF1-α*, the most common cause of MODY, have a greater hypoglycaemic response to sulphonylureas than patients with type 2 diabetes.

INVESTIGATIONS

URINE TESTING

Glucose

Testing the urine for glucose is a common procedure for detecting diabetes, using sensitive glucose-specific dipsticks. If possible, testing should be performed on urine passed 1–2 hours after a meal since this will detect more cases of diabetes than a fasting specimen. Glycosuria always warrants further assessment by blood testing (see below).

The greatest disadvantage of using urinary glucose as a diagnostic or screening procedure is the individual variation in renal threshold for glucose (Fig. 21.7). The most common cause of glycosuria is a low renal threshold, which is common during pregnancy and in young people. Renal glycosuria is a benign condition unrelated to diabetes. Some drugs may interfere with urine glucose tests. Estimation of the blood glucose concentration, using an accurate laboratory method rather than a side-room technique, is therefore essential in making the diagnosis (Box 21.9).

In some individuals a rapid but transitory rise of blood glucose follows a meal and the concentration exceeds the normal renal threshold; during this time glucose will be present in the urine. This response to an oral glucose load is benign and is described as a 'lag storage' blood glucose curve, although alimentary glycosuria is a better term (Fig. 21.7). It may occur in normal people or after gastric surgery, when it is caused by rapid gastric emptying and more rapid absorption of glucose into the circulation, and is sometimes observed in patients with hyperthyroidism, peptic ulceration or hepatic disease.

Glycosuria is common in normal pregnancy (because the renal threshold for glucose falls secondary to an increase in the glomerular filtration rate), and in late pregnancy lactose appears in the urine. However, the finding of any sugars in the urine of a pregnant woman should never be ignored and in all cases blood glucose should be measured to identify gestational diabetes. Since even minimal hyperglycaemia in pregnancy is associated with increased perinatal mortality and morbidity, it is important to detect and treat these cases effectively (p. 826).

Ketones

Ketone bodies can be identified by the nitroprusside reaction, which is primarily specific for acetoacetate. The test is conveniently carried out using tablets or dipsticks for ketones. Ketonuria may be found in normal people who

21.8 SINGLE GENE DEFECTS OF PANCREATIC β-CELL FUNCTION CAUSING MATURITY-ONSET DIABETES OF THE YOUNG (MODY)*

	Gene	Distribution	Clinical features	Complications
MODY 1	Hepatic nuclear factor 4 alpha (HNF4-α)	Rare	Similar to HNF1-α but age at diagnosis may be later	Frequent
MODY 2	Glucokinase (GCK)	10–65%	Mild hyperglycaemia from birth, stable and managed by diet alone	Rare
MODY 3	Hepatic nuclear factor 1 alpha (HNF1-α) Transcription factor-1 (TCF-1)	20–75%	Diabetes presents during adolescence	Frequent
MODY 4	Insulin promoter factor 1 (IPF1)	Rare	Presentation before 25 years is unusual	Unknown
MODY 5	Hepatic nuclear factor 1 beta (HNF1-β) Transcription factor-2 (TCF-2)	Rare	Early-onset diabetes	Kidney disease, renal cysts, proteinuria, renal failure
MODY 6	NEUROD1/β2	Rare	Little known	Unknown

*Further information: www.ex.ac.uk/diabetesgenes/mody/

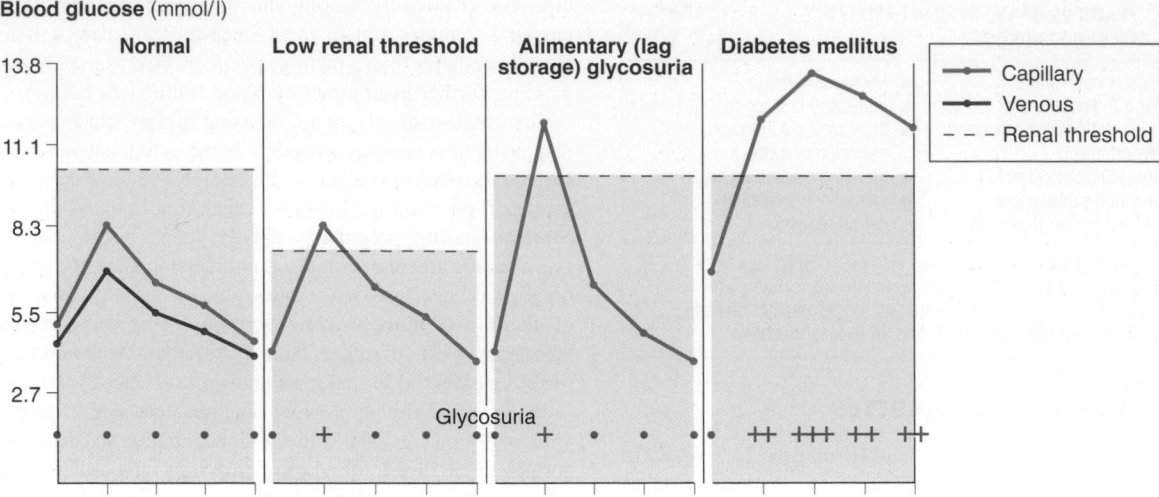

Fig. 21.7   The glucose tolerance test: blood glucose curves after 75 g glucose by mouth. (To convert glucose in mmol/l to mg/dl, multiply by 18.)

have been fasting or exercising strenuously for long periods, who have been vomiting repeatedly, or who have been eating a diet high in fat and low in carbohydrate. Ketonuria is therefore not pathognomonic of diabetes but, if associated with glycosuria, the diagnosis of diabetes is highly likely. In diabetic ketoacidosis (p. 820), ketones can be detected in plasma using dipsticks.

Protein

Dipstick testing for albumin is a standard procedure to identify the presence of renal disease (or urinary infection) in people with diabetes. This will detect urinary albumin greater than 300 mg/l. Smaller amounts of urinary albumin (microalbuminuria) can be measured and these provide indicators of the risk of developing diabetic nephropathy and/or macrovascular disease (Box 21.51, p. 842).

BLOOD TESTING

Glucose

Laboratory glucose testing in blood relies upon enzymatic reaction (glucose oxidase) and is cheap, usually automated and highly reliable. However, variation in blood glucose depends on whether the patient has eaten recently, so it is important to consider the circumstances in which the blood sample was taken. The criteria for the diagnosis of diabetes are considered below.

Blood glucose can also be measured with colorimetric or other testing sticks, which are often read with a portable electronic meter. These are used for capillary (fingerprick) testing to monitor diabetes treatment (p. 807).

Glucose concentrations are lower in venous than in arterial or capillary (fingerprick) blood. Whole blood glucose concentrations are lower than plasma concentrations because red blood cells contain relatively little glucose. In general, venous plasma values are the most reliable for diagnostic purposes.

Glycated haemoglobin

Glycated haemoglobin provides an accurate and objective measure of glycaemic control over a period of weeks to months. This can be utilised as an assessment of glycaemic control in a patient with known diabetes, but is not sufficiently sensitive to make a diagnosis of diabetes and is usually within the normal range in patients with impaired glucose tolerance.

In diabetes, the slow non-enzymatic covalent attachment of glucose to haemoglobin (glycation) increases the amount in the HbA_1 (HbA_{1c}) fraction relative to non-glycated adult haemoglobin (HbA_0). These fractions can be separated by chromatography; laboratories may report glycated haemo-globin as total glycated haemoglobin (GHb), HbA_1 or HbA_{1c}. In many countries HbA_{1c} is now the preferred measurement. The rate of formation of HbA_{1c} is directly proportional to the ambient blood glucose concentration; a rise of 1% in HbA_{1c} corresponds to an approximate average increase of 2 mmol/l in blood glucose. Although HbA_{1c} concentration reflects the integrated blood glucose control over the life-span of the erythrocyte (120 days), half of the erythrocytes are replaced in 60 days and HbA_{1c} is weighted by changes in glycaemic control occurring in the month before measurement (representing 50% of the HbA_{1c} concentra-tion). As HbA_{1c} is affected more by recent than by earlier events, a large shift in blood glucose control is rapidly accompanied by a change in HbA_{1c}, detectable within 2–3 weeks.

Various assay methods can be used to measure HbA_{1c}, precluding direct comparison of HbA_{1c} values between laboratories. While international consensus on a suitable reference method and standardisation of methodology is awaited, a local non-diabetic reference range must be ascer-tained; results can be aligned with the reference range used in the Diabetes Control and Complications Trial (DCCT).

HbA_{1c} estimates may be erroneously diminished in anaemia or during pregnancy, and may be difficult to

21

interpret with some assay methods in patients who have uraemia or a haemoglobinopathy. In clinical practice, HbA$_{1c}$ is usually measured once or twice yearly to assess glycaemic control, permitting appropriate changes in treatment and identifying inconsistency with the patient's record of home blood glucose monitoring. HbA$_{1c}$ also provides an index of risk for developing diabetic complications.

Glycated serum proteins ('fructosamine') can be measured and, because of their shorter half-life, give an indication of glycaemic control over the preceding 2 weeks. Other than in diabetic pregnancy, this is generally too short a period to make clinical decisions on therapeutic management.

Blood lipids

The concentration of serum lipids—total cholesterol, low-density and high-density lipoprotein (LDL and HDL) cholesterol and triglyceride—is another important index of overall metabolic control in diabetic patients and should be measured at diagnosis and regularly thereafter. Ideally, the triglyceride concentration should be measured in the fasting state (p. 446).

PRESENTING PROBLEMS IN DIABETES MELLITUS

NEWLY DISCOVERED HYPERGLYCAEMIA

Hyperglycaemia is a very common biochemical abnormality. It is frequently detected on routine biochemical analysis of asymptomatic patients, following routine dipstick testing of urine showing glycosuria, or during severe illness ('stress hyperglycaemia'). Alternatively, hyperglycaemia may present with the chronic symptoms described in Box 21.12 on next page. Occasionally, patients present as an emergency with acute metabolic decompensation (see below). The key goals are to establish whether the patient has diabetes, what type of diabetes it is and how it should be treated.

Establishing the diagnosis of diabetes

When diabetes is suspected, the diagnosis may be confirmed by a random blood glucose concentration greater than 11.0 mmol/l (199 mg/dl) (Box 21.9). When random blood glucose values are elevated but are not diagnostic of diabetes, glucose tolerance is usually assessed either by a fasting blood glucose estimation or by the oral glucose tolerance test (OGTT) (Box 21.10).

The diagnostic criteria for diabetes mellitus (and normality) recommended by the World Health Organization (WHO) in 2000 are shown in Boxes 21.9 and 21.11. The values are based on the threshold for risk of developing microvascular disease. Patients who do not meet the criteria for diabetes may have 'impaired glucose tolerance' (IGT, Box 21.11) or 'fasting hyperglycaemia' (sometimes called 'impaired fasting glucose', when the fasting glucose is between 6.1 and 6.9 mmol/l (110–125 mg/dl)). These patients have increased risks of progression to frank diabetes with time and of macrovascular atheromatous disease. Lowering the definition of impaired fasting glucose to 5.6 mmol/l has been proposed; this would triple the prevalence of this condition.

21.9 DIAGNOSIS OF DIABETES

Patient complains of symptoms suggesting diabetes

- Test urine for glucose and ketones
- Measure random or fasting blood glucose. Diagnosis confirmed by*:
  Fasting plasma glucose ≥ 7.0 mmol/l (126 mg/dl)
  Random plasma glucose ≥ 11.1 mmol/l (200 mg/dl)

Indications for oral glucose tolerance test (Box 21.11)

- Fasting plasma glucose 6.1–7.0 mmol/l (110–126 mg/dl)
- Random plasma glucose 7.8–11.0 mmol/l (140–199 mg/dl)

N.B. HbA$_{1c}$ (see above) is not used for diagnosis.
* In asymptomatic patients two samples are required to confirm diabetes.

21.10 ORAL GLUCOSE TOLERANCE TEST (OGTT)

- Unrestricted carbohydrate diet for 3 days before test
- Fasted overnight (for at least 8 hrs)
- Rest before test (30 mins); no smoking; seated for duration of test
- Plasma glucose measured before, and 2 hrs after, 75 g glucose load

21.11 ORAL GLUCOSE TOLERANCE TEST: WHO DIAGNOSTIC CRITERIA				
	Glucose concentrations			
	Venous plasma mmol/l (mg/dl)	Venous whole blood mmol/l (mg/dl)	Capillary plasma mmol/l (mg/dl)	Capillary whole blood mmol/l (mg/dl)
Diabetes				
Fasting	≥ 7.0 (≥ 126)	≥ 6.1 (≥ 110)	≥ 7.0 (≥ 126)	≥ 6.1 (≥ 110)
2 hrs after glucose load	≥ 11.1 (≥ 200)	≥ 10.0 (≥ 180)	≥ 12.2 (≥ 220)	≥ 11.1 (≥ 200)
Impaired glucose tolerance				
Fasting	< 7.0 (< 126)	< 6.1 (< 110)	< 7.0 (< 126)	< 6.1 (< 110)
2 hrs after glucose load	7.8–11.0 (140–199)	6.7–9.9 (120–179)	8.9–12.1 (160–219)	7.8–11.0 (140–199)

21

In some people, an abnormal result is observed under conditions which impose a burden on the pancreatic β cells, e.g. during pregnancy, infection, myocardial infarction or other severe stress, or during treatment with diabetogenic drugs such as corticosteroids. This 'stress hyperglycaemia' usually disappears after the acute illness has resolved, but blood glucose should be remeasured.

The diagnostic criteria for diabetes in pregnancy are more stringent than those recommended for non-pregnant subjects. Pregnant women with abnormal glucose tolerance should be referred urgently to a specialist unit for full evaluation.

When a diagnosis of diabetes is confirmed, other investigations should include urea, creatinine, electrolytes, liver and thyroid function tests, lipids, and urine testing for protein or microalbuminuria.

Clinical assessment

Hyperglycaemia causes a wide variety of symptoms (Box 21.12). The clinical features of the two main types of diabetes are compared in Box 21.13. The classical symptoms of thirst, polyuria, nocturia and rapid weight loss are prominent in type 1 diabetes, but are often absent in patients with type 2 diabetes, many of whom are asymptomatic or have non-specific complaints such as chronic fatigue and malaise. Uncontrolled diabetes is associated with an increased susceptibility to infection and patients may present with skin sepsis (boils) and genital candidiasis, and complain of pruritus vulvae or balanitis. A history of pancreatic disease (Box 21.3, p. 810), particularly in patients with a history of alcohol excess, makes insulin deficiency more likely although such patients may develop incidental classical type 2 diabetes.

While the distinction between type 1 and type 2 diabetes is usually obvious, overlap occurs particularly in age at onset, duration of symptoms and family history. A few young people have a form of diabetes designated 'maturity-onset diabetes of the young' (MODY; Box 21.8, p. 815); there is usually a remarkably strong family history of early-onset diabetes. Classical type 2 diabetes is increasingly recognised in obese sedentary young people, including children. Some middle-aged and elderly people present with typical autoimmune type 1 diabetes. Others with apparent type 2 diabetes have evidence of autoimmune activity against pancreatic β cells, and may have a slowly evolving variant of type 1 diabetes (latent autoimmune diabetes in adults—LADA). Some patients with type 2 diabetes have advanced pancreatic β-cell failure at the time of presentation, and rapidly require treatment with insulin. For these reasons, the final diagnosis of the type of diabetes may sometimes be delayed until the natural history or responsiveness to different therapies becomes apparent with time.

The physical signs in patients with type 2 diabetes at diagnosis depend on the mode of presentation. More than 70% are overweight, and obesity may be central (truncal or abdominal). Hypertension is present in at least 50% of patients with type 2 diabetes. Although hyperlipidaemia is also common, skin lesions such as xanthelasma and eruptive xanthomas are rare.

Management

The methods of treatment of diabetes are: dietary/lifestyle modification, oral anti-diabetic agents and insulin by injection. These are described in detail on pages 829–835. In patients with suspected type 1 diabetes, urgent therapy with insulin is required and prompt referral to a specialist is usually required. In patients with suspected type 2 diabetes, the first line of therapy involves advice about dietary and lifestyle modification. Oral anti-diabetic drugs are added only in those who do not achieve good glycaemic control with dietary modification alone, or who have more severe symptomatic hyperglycaemia at diagnosis (e.g. $HbA_{1c} > 10\%$).

In parallel with treatment of hyperglycaemia, other risk factors for complications of diabetes need to be addressed, including treatment of hypertension (p. 608) and dyslipidaemia (p. 443) and advice on smoking cessation (p. 97).

Educating patients

It is essential that people with diabetes understand their condition and learn to handle all aspects of their management as comprehensively and quickly as possible. Ideally this can be achieved by a multidisciplinary team (doctor, dietitian, specialist nurse and podiatrist) in the outpatient setting. However, patients requiring insulin need daily

21.12 SYMPTOMS OF HYPERGLYCAEMIA	

- Thirst, dry mouth
- Polyuria
- Nocturia
- Tiredness, fatigue
- Recent change in weight
- Blurring of vision
- Pruritus vulvae, balanitis (genital candidiasis)
- Nausea; headache
- Hyperphagia; predilection for sweet foods
- Mood change, irritability, difficulty in concentrating, apathy

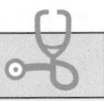

21.13 COMPARATIVE CLINICAL FEATURES OF TYPE 1 AND TYPE 2 DIABETES

	Type 1	Type 2
Typical age at onset	< 40 years	> 50 years
Duration of symptoms	Weeks	Months to years
Body weight	Normal or low	Obese
Ketonuria	Yes	No
Rapid death without treatment with insulin	Yes	No
Autoantibodies	Yes	No
Diabetic complications at diagnosis	No	25%
Family history of diabetes	Uncommon	Common
Other autoimmune disease	Common	Uncommon

advice at first and, if this is not practicable, admission to hospital may be necessary.

Those requiring insulin need to learn how to measure their dose of insulin accurately with an insulin syringe or pen device, to give their own injections and to adjust the dose themselves on the basis of blood glucose values and other factors such as exercise, illness and episodic hypoglycaemia. They must therefore have a working knowledge of diabetes, be familiar with the symptoms of hypoglycaemia (Box 21.23, p. 823), and have ready access to medical advice when the need arises. Information should be provided about driving (statutory regulations and practical advice, Box 21.14). Provision of such education is time-consuming but only in this way can patients safely undertake normal activities while maintaining good control.

It is a sensible precaution for diabetic patients who are taking insulin or an oral anti-diabetic drug to carry a card stating their name and address, the fact that they have diabetes, the nature and dose of any insulin or other drugs they may be taking, and the name, address and telephone number of their family doctor and any specialist diabetes clinic they attend.

Self-assessment of glycaemic control

Semi-quantitative pre-prandial urine testing to assess blood glucose control has major limitations, particularly in people with type 1 diabetes, but also in those with type 2 diabetes where a raised renal threshold for glucose may mask persistent hyperglycaemia. Negative urine tests fail to distinguish between normal and low blood glucose levels, which is a serious disadvantage since the aim of treatment is a normal blood glucose level while avoiding hypo-glycaemia. However, urine glucose testing with visually read strips is inexpensive and may suffice for many people with type 2 diabetes treated with diet alone or in those taking oral therapy who have stable glycaemic control.

Many patients (particularly those treated with insulin) should be taught to perform capillary blood glucose

---

21.15 BLOOD GLUCOSE (BG) TESTING AND DIABETES

Treatment with insulin

- Regular BG monitoring should be performed by all people treated with insulin to adjust the insulin dose and detect hypoglycaemia
- Daily pre-prandial and bedtime measurements are usually recommended
- Target BG levels are typically 5–8 mmol/l (~90–145 mg/dl), although these may be lower (e.g. in gestational diabetes) or higher (e.g. in impaired awareness of hypoglycaemia)

Treatment with antidiabetic drugs

- BG monitoring is optional in many patients with stable type 2 diabetes; patient preference usually decides
- BG monitoring is most useful in patients taking sulphonylureas (risk of hypoglycaemia), during intercurrent illness and prescription of corticosteroids, and during changes in therapy
- BG is usually measured before breakfast (typical target 4–7 mmol/l (~72–126 mg/dl) and 2 hours after food (typical target 4–10 mmol/l (~72–180 mg/dl))

21

---

measurements using blood glucose test strips, read either visually or with a glucose meter (Box 21.15). The principal advantage of home self-monitoring of blood glucose is that information is available immediately and permits the well-informed and motivated patient to make appropriate adjustments in treatment (particularly in insulin dose) on a day-to-day basis. Thus changes in routine can be accommodated, ketoacidosis avoided, compliance with diet encouraged and near-normal metabolism achieved while avoiding frequent and disabling hypoglycaemia. Blood glucose monitoring has a significant cost and may not be justified in many patients with type 2 diabetes. Single random blood glucose estimations obtained at routine clinic visits are of limited value and profiles measured in hospital may be unrepresentative of normal circumstances. Continuous blood glucose monitoring methodology is available but not yet applicable to routine monitoring.

Advice to patients with IGT

These patients have an increased risk of progression to type 2 diabetes (Fig. 21.6, p. 813) and increased risk of macrovascular disease. There is evidence that the lifestyle advice recommended for patients with type 2 diabetes will reduce the risk of progression in IGT. Patients with IGT should be monitored, e.g. with annual fasting blood glucose. Other cardiovascular risk factors should be treated aggressively.

LONG-TERM SUPERVISION OF DIABETES

Diabetes is a complex disorder which progresses in severity with time, so people with diabetes should be seen at regular intervals for the remainder of their lives, either at a specialist diabetic clinic or in primary care where facilities are available and staff are trained in diabetes care. A checklist

---

21.14 DIABETES AND DRIVING

- In the UK, diabetes requiring tablet or insulin therapy has to be declared to the Driver and Vehicle Licensing Agency. In many countries ordinary driving licences are 'period-restricted' for insulin-treated drivers, with vocational licences (large goods vehicles and public service vehicles) being refused. Licensing regulations vary between countries
- The main risk to driving performance is hypoglycaemia. Visual impairment and other complications may occasionally cause problems
- Insulin-treated diabetic drivers should be advised to:
    - Check blood glucose before driving and 2-hourly during long journeys
    - Keep an accessible supply of fast-acting carbohydrate in the vehicle
    - Take regular snacks or meals during long journeys
    - Stop driving if hypoglycaemia develops
    - Refrain from driving until 45–60 minutes after treatment of hypoglycaemia (delayed recovery of cognitive function)
    - Carry identification in case of injury

21.16 CHECKLIST FOR FOLLOW-UP OF PATIENTS WITH DIABETES MELLITUS

Body weight (body mass index)

Urinalysis
- Analyse fasting specimen for glucose, ketones, albumin (both macro- and microalbuminuria)

Glycaemic control
- Glycated haemoglobin (HbA$_{1c}$)
- Inspection of home blood glucose monitoring record

Hypoglycaemic episodes
- Number of severe (requiring assistance for treatment) and frequency of mild (self-treated) episodes
- Time of day when 'hypos' experienced
- Nature and intensity of symptoms
- Ability to identify onset (awareness)

Blood pressure

Eye examination
- Visual acuities (near and distance)
- Ophthalmoscopy (with pupils dilated)
- Digital photography

Lower limbs
- Peripheral pulses
- Tendon reflexes
- Perception of vibration sensation, light touch and proprioception

Feet
- Callus skin indicating pressure areas
- Nails
- Need for podiatry
- Ulceration
- Deformity

---

for follow-up visits is given in Box 21.16. The frequency of visits is very variable, ranging from weekly during pregnancy to annually in the case of patients with well-controlled type 2 diabetes.

Therapeutic goals

The aim of treatment is to relieve the symptoms of hyperglycaemia and to achieve as near normal metabolism as is practicable. The nearer the body weight approaches the ideal level and the closer the blood glucose is kept to normal, the more the total metabolic profile is improved and the lower the incidence of vascular disease and specific diabetic complications. Excellent glycaemic control may also retard the progression of pancreatic β-cell failure (Fig. 21.6, p. 813).

The recommended target HbA$_{1c}$ is 7% or less, to minimise the risk of vascular complications. However, this may be difficult to achieve and to maintain, particularly with increasing duration of diabetes. Type 2 diabetes progresses in severity with time, with evidence of a gradual rise in HbA$_{1c}$ despite escalation in treatment. Strict glycaemic control in type 1 diabetes increases the risk of hypoglycaemia. Glycaemic targets should therefore be appropriate to the age and physical condition of the patient—strict control may be inappropriate in the very young, the elderly, people with several comorbidities or cancer, and those with advanced diabetic complications. Blood glucose targets depend similarly on individual requirements, but fasting

blood glucose values below 6 mmol/l (108 mg/dl) are desirable in type 2 diabetes. Pre-prandial values between 5 and 8 mmol/l would be ideal in patients with type 1 diabetes, in whom values below 4 mmol/l should be avoided. The importance of measuring post-prandial glucose is debatable, and multiple times of testing (> 4/day) are seldom practical.

In people with type 2 diabetes, treatment of hypertension and dyslipidaemia is often required. Treatment can be determined by assessment of cardiovascular risk and targets are adjusted to individual circumstances. The target for blood pressure is usually < 140/80 mmHg. The target levels for lipids are usually a total cholesterol < 5.0 mmol/l (~ 190 mg/dl) and LDL cholesterol < 3.0 mmol/l (~ 115 mg/dl). Similar targets would be appropriate in type 1 diabetes, with modification depending on age and the presence of microalbuminuria.

DIABETIC KETOACIDOSIS

Ketoacidosis is a major medical emergency and remains a serious cause of morbidity, principally in people with type 1 diabetes. A significant number of newly diagnosed diabetic patients present in ketoacidosis. In established diabetes a common course of events is that patients develop an intercurrent infection, lose their appetite, and either stop or drastically reduce their dose of insulin in the mistaken belief that under these circumstances less insulin is required. Any form of stress, particularly that produced by infection, may precipitate severe ketoacidosis, even in patients with type 2 diabetes. No obvious precipitating cause can be found in many cases.

The average mortality in developed countries is 5–10% and is higher in the elderly. Although some deaths from ketoacidosis are associated with severe medical conditions such as acute myocardial infarction or septicaemia, others are the consequence of delays in diagnosis and management errors.

Pathogenesis

A clear understanding of the biochemical basis and pathophysiology of this problem is essential for its efficient treatment.

The cardinal biochemical features of diabetic keto-acidosis are:

- hyperglycaemia
- hyperketonaemia
- metabolic acidosis.

The hyperglycaemia causes a profound osmotic diuresis leading to dehydration and electrolyte loss, particularly of sodium and potassium. Ketosis results from insulin deficiency, exacerbated by elevated catecholamines and other stress hormones, resulting in unrestrained lipolysis and supply of free fatty acids for hepatic ketogenesis (Fig. 21.5). When this exceeds the capacity to metabolise acidic ketones, these accumulate in blood. The resulting metabolic acidosis forces hydrogen ions into cells, displacing potassium ions, which may be lost in urine or through vomiting.

21.17 AVERAGE LOSS OF FLUID AND ELECTROLYTES IN ADULT DIABETIC KETOACIDOSIS OF MODERATE SEVERITY

- Water: 6 litres
- Sodium: 500 mmol
- Chloride: 400 mmol
- Potassium: 350 mmol

}
- 3 litres extracellular —replace with saline
- 3 litres intracellular —replace with dextrose

21.18 CLINICAL FEATURES OF DIABETIC KETOACIDOSIS

Symptoms

- Polyuria, thirst
- Weight loss
- Weakness
- Nausea, vomiting
- Leg cramps
- Blurred vision
- Abdominal pain

Signs

- Dehydration
- Hypotension (postural or supine)
- Cold extremities/peripheral cyanosis
- Tachycardia
- Air hunger (Kussmaul breathing)
- Smell of acetone
- Hypothermia
- Confusion, drowsiness, coma (10%)

The average loss of fluid and electrolytes in moderately severe diabetic ketoacidosis in an adult is shown in Box 21.17. About half the deficit of total body water is derived from the intracellular compartment and occurs comparatively early in the development of acidosis with relatively few clinical features; the remainder represents loss of extracellular fluid sustained largely in the later stages. It is at this time that marked contraction of the size of the extracellular space occurs, with haemoconcentration, a decreased blood volume, and finally a fall in blood pressure with associated renal ischaemia and oliguria.

Every patient in diabetic ketoacidosis is potassium-depleted, but the plasma concentration of potassium gives very little indication of the total body deficit. Plasma potassium may even be raised initially due to disproportionate loss of water and catabolism of protein and glycogen. However, soon after insulin treatment is started there is likely to be a precipitous fall in the plasma potassium due to dilution of extracellular potassium by administration of intravenous fluids, the movement of potassium into cells as a result of treatment with insulin, and the continuing renal loss of potassium.

The magnitude of the hyperglycaemia does not correlate with the severity of the metabolic acidosis; moderate elevation of blood glucose may be associated with life-threatening ketoacidosis. In some cases, hyperglycaemia predominates and acidosis is minimal, with patients presenting in a hyperosmolar state (p. 823).

Clinical assessment

The clinical features of ketoacidosis are listed in Box 21.18. In the fulminating case the striking features are those of salt and water depletion, with loss of skin turgor, furred tongue and cracked lips, tachycardia, hypotension and reduced intra-ocular pressure. Breathing may be deep and sighing, the breath is usually fetid, and the sickly-sweet smell of acetone may be apparent. Mental apathy, confusion or a reduced conscious level may be present. The state of consciousness is very variable in patients with diabetic ketoacidosis; coma is uncommon. A patient with dangerous ketoacidosis requiring urgent treatment may walk into the consulting room. For this reason the term 'diabetic ketoacidosis' is to be preferred to 'diabetic coma', which implies that there is no urgency until unconsciousness supervenes. In fact, it is imperative that energetic treatment is started at the earliest possible stage.

Abdominal pain is sometimes a feature of diabetic ketoacidosis, particularly in children. Serum amylase may be elevated but rarely indicates coexisting pancreatitis. Although leucocytosis invariably occurs, this represents a stress response and does not necessarily indicate infection;

pyrexia may not be present initially because of vasodilatation secondary to acidosis.

Investigations (Box 21.19)

The following are important but should not delay the institution of intravenous fluid and insulin replacement:

- urea and electrolytes, blood glucose, plasma bicarbonate
- arterial blood gases to assess the severity of acidosis (the severity of ketoacidosis can be assessed rapidly by measuring the plasma bicarbonate—less than 12 mmol/l indicates severe acidosis; the hydrogen ion concentration gives a more precise measure but requires arterial blood)
- urinalysis for ketones (a meter is available to quantify ketones in plasma, and a test strip can be used as a semi-quantitative guide to the plasma concentration of acetoacetate and acetone)
- ECG
- infection screen: full blood count, blood and urine culture, C-reactive protein, chest X-ray.

Management

Diabetic ketoacidosis is a medical emergency which should be treated in hospital, preferably in a high-dependency area. Regular clinical and biochemical review is essential,

21.19 MONITORING IN DIABETIC KETOACIDOSIS[1]

Laboratory	Baseline	1 hr	2 hr	3 hr	6 hr	12 hr	24 hr
Glucose[2]	✓		✓	✓	✓	✓	✓
Urea, electrolytes	✓		✓	✓	✓	✓	✓
Creatinine	✓				✓	✓	✓
Bicarbonate	✓		✓	✓	✓	✓	✓
Blood gases	(✓)			✓[3]		✓[3]	

[1]The following should be monitored hourly: pulse, blood pressure, respiratory rate, urine output, capillary blood glucose.
[2]A capillary blood glucose measurement of > 17 mmol/l (~300 mg/dl) using a meter or visually read glucose strips can be very misleading since the actual blood glucose concentration is often considerably higher when measured precisely in the laboratory; therefore an accurate measurement should be made at an early stage.
[3]If no clinical improvement. Blood gases at baseline not necessary if plasma bicarbonate is > 15 mmol/l.

particularly during the first 24 hours of treatment. Treatment must be monitored closely (Box 21.19). Guidelines for the management of ketoacidosis are shown in Boxes 21.20 and 21.21.

The principal components of treatment are:

- the administration of short-acting (soluble) insulin
- fluid replacement
- potassium replacement
- the administration of antibiotics if infection is present.

21.20 MANAGEMENT OF DIABETIC KETOACIDOSIS

Fluid replacement

- 0.9% saline (NaCl) i.v.
    1 litre over 30 minutes
    1 litre over 1 hr
    1 litre over 2 hrs
    1 litre over next 2–4 hrs
- When blood glucose < 15 mmol/l (270 mg/dl)
    Switch to 5% dextrose, 1 litre 8-hourly
    If still dehydrated, continue 0.9% saline and add 5% dextrose
    1 litre per 12 hrs
- Typical requirement is 6 litres in first 24 hrs but avoid fluid overload in elderly patients
- Subsequent fluid requirement should be based on clinical response including urine output

Insulin

- 50 units soluble insulin in 50 ml 0.9% saline i.v. via infusion pump
    6 units/hr initially
    3 units/hr when blood glucose < 15 mmol/l (270 mg/dl)
    2 units/hr if blood glucose declines < 10 mmol/l (180 mg/dl)
- Check blood glucose hourly initially—if no reduction in first hour, rate of insulin infusion should be increased
- Aim for fall in blood glucose of 3–6 mmol/l (~55–110 mg/dl) per hour

Potassium

- None in first litre of i.v fluid unless < 3.0 mmol/l
- If plasma potassium < 3.5 mmol/l, give 40 mmol added potassium
    Give in 1 litre of fluid
    Avoid infusion rate of > 20 mmol/hr
- If plasma potassium is 3.5–5.0 mmol/l, give 20 mmol added potassium
- If plasma potassium is > 5.0 mmol/l, or patient is anuric, give no added potassium

---

21.21 ADDITIONAL PROCEDURES IN THE MANAGEMENT OF DIABETIC KETOACIDOSIS

- Catheterisation if no urine passed after 3 hrs
- Nasogastric tube to keep stomach empty in unconscious or semiconscious patients, or if vomiting is protracted
- Central venous line if cardiovascular system compromised, to allow fluid replacement to be adjusted accurately
- Plasma expander if systolic BP is < 90 mmHg or does not rise with i.v. saline
- Antibiotic if infection demonstrated or suspected
- ECG monitoring in severe cases

Insulin

If an intravenous infusion of insulin (Box 21.20) is not possible, a loading dose of 10–20 units of soluble insulin can be given by intramuscular injection, immediately followed by 5 units hourly thereafter or, alternatively, a fast-acting insulin analogue can be given hourly by subcutaneous injection (initially 0.3 units/kg body weight, then 0.1 units/kg hourly). The blood glucose concentration should fall by 3–6 mmol/l (55–110 mg/dl) per hour. A more rapid fall in blood glucose should be avoided, as hypoglycaemia can be precipitated and the serious complication of cerebral oedema may develop, particularly in children. If blood glucose does not fall within 2 hours of commencing treatment, the dose of insulin should be doubled until a satisfactory response is obtained. Ketosis, dehydration, acidaemia, infection and stress combine to produce severe insulin resistance in some cases but most will respond to a low-dose insulin regimen. When the blood glucose concentration has fallen to 10–15 mmol/l (180–270 mg/dl) the dose of insulin should be reduced to 1–4 units hourly. The half-life of intravenous insulin is short (2.5 minutes) so the insulin infusion should not be interrupted. Restoration of the usual insulin regimen, by subcutaneous injection, should not be instituted until the patient is able to eat and drink normally. 'Sliding scales' of insulin administration (in which insulin is prescribed according to blood glucose levels immediately before injection) should not be used.

Fluid replacement

Intravenous fluid replacement is required since, even when the patient is able to swallow, fluids given by mouth may be poorly absorbed. The extracellular fluid deficit should be replenished by infusing isotonic saline (0.9% NaCl). Early and rapid rehydration is essential, otherwise the administered insulin will not reach the poorly perfused tissues. If the plasma sodium is greater than 155 mmol/l, 0.45% saline may be given initially instead of 0.9%.

The intracellular water deficit must be replaced by using 5% or 10% dextrose and not by more saline. It is best given when the blood glucose concentration approaches normal. An accurate record of fluid balance must be maintained.

Potassium

As the plasma potassium is often high at presentation, treatment with intravenous potassium chloride should be started cautiously (Box 21.20) and carefully monitored. Sufficient should be given to maintain a normal plasma concentration and large amounts may be required (100–300 mmol in the first 24 hours). Cardiac rhythm should be monitored in severe cases because of the risk of electrolyte-induced cardiac arrhythmia.

Bicarbonate

In patients who are severely acidotic ($[H^+] > 100$ nmol/l, pH < 7.0) the infusion of sodium bicarbonate (300 ml 1.26% over 30 minutes into a large vein) should be considered, with the simultaneous administration of potassium. Its use is controversial, however, and should only be considered in exceptional circumstances. Complete correction of the acidosis should not be attempted.

Antibiotics

Infections must be carefully sought and vigorously treated since it may not be possible to abolish ketosis until they are controlled. The management of diabetic ketoacidosis may be complicated by the development of other conditions (Box 21.22) which require active therapy.

NON-KETOTIC HYPEROSMOLAR DIABETIC COMA

This condition is characterised by severe hyperglycaemia (> 50 mmol/l (900 mg/dl)) without significant hyperketonaemia or acidosis. Severe dehydration and pre-renal uraemia are common. It usually affects elderly patients, many with previously undiagnosed diabetes. Mortality is high (40%). Treatment differs from ketoacidosis in two main respects. Firstly, these patients are usually relatively sensitive to insulin and approximately half the dose of insulin recommended for the treatment of ketoacidosis should usually be employed (3 units/hr). Secondly, the plasma osmolality should be measured or, less accurately, calculated using the following formula based on plasma values in mmol/l:

$$\text{Plasma osmolality} = 2[Na^+] + 2[K^+] + [\text{glucose}] + [\text{urea}] \text{ (all mmol/l)}$$

The normal value is 280–300 mmol/kg and the conscious level is depressed when it is high (> 340 mmol/kg). The patient should be given 0.45% saline until the osmolality approaches normal, when isotonic (0.9%) saline should be substituted. The rate of fluid replacement should be regulated on the basis of the central venous pressure, and plasma sodium concentration checked frequently. Thromboembolic complications are common, and prophylactic subcutaneous low molecular weight heparin is recommended.

LACTIC ACIDOSIS

In coma due to lactic acidosis the patient is likely to be taking metformin for type 2 diabetes and is very ill and overbreathing but not as profoundly dehydrated as is usual in coma due to ketoacidosis. The patient's breath does not smell of acetone, and ketonuria is mild or even absent, yet the plasma bicarbonate and pH are markedly reduced ($H^+ > 63$ mmol/l, pH < 7.2) and the anion gap is increased (p. 437). The diagnosis is confirmed by a high (usually > 5.0 mmol/l) concentration of lactic acid in the blood.

Treatment is with intravenous sodium bicarbonate sufficient to raise the arterial pH to above 7.2, along with insulin and glucose. Despite energetic treatment, the mortality in this condition is > 50%. Sodium dichloroacetate may be given to lower blood lactate.

HYPOGLYCAEMIA

When hypoglycaemia (blood glucose < 3.5 mmol/l (63 mg/dl)) occurs in a person with diabetes it is a result of treatment and not a manifestation of the disease itself. It occurs often in those treated with insulin, occasionally in those taking a sulphonylurea drug, and rarely with metformin. When hypoglycaemia develops in non-diabetic people, it is called 'spontaneous' hypoglycaemia, the causes and investigation of which are described on page 790. The risk of hypoglycaemia is the most important single factor limiting the attainment of near-normal glycaemia; fear of hypoglycaemia is common among patients and their relatives.

Clinical assessment

Common symptoms of hypoglycaemia are listed in Box 21.23. They comprise two main groups: those related to acute activation of the autonomic nervous system and those secondary to glucose deprivation of the brain (neuroglycopenia). Symptoms of hypoglycaemia are idiosyncratic and differ with age. The ability to recognise their onset is an important aspect of the initial education of diabetic patients treated with insulin. Mood changes such as tense tiredness, irritability and anger also occur, and behavioural changes are common in children.

Impaired awareness of symptoms

In most instances the patient has no difficulty in recognising the symptoms of hypoglycaemia and can take appropriate remedial action. In certain circumstances (e.g. during sleep, lying supine or when distracted by other activities) warning symptoms are not always perceived by the patient, so that appropriate action is not taken and neuroglycopenia with reduced consciousness ensues. If short-acting insulin is administered to a non-diabetic person, symptoms of hypoglycaemia are usually experienced when the venous or capillary blood glucose falls to 2.5–3.0 mmol/l (45–54 mg/dl). In diabetic patients who are chronically hyperglycaemic the same symptoms may develop at a higher blood glucose level; conversely, patients who have strict glycaemic control (HbA$_{1c}$ within the non-diabetic range) or who are exposed to frequent hypoglycaemia may not experience any symptoms even when the blood glucose is well below 2.5 mmol/l. The glycaemic thresholds for the onset of symptoms and counter-regulatory hormonal secretion are altered in patients with impaired awareness of hypoglycaemia, in that blood glucose has to fall to a much lower level to trigger these responses. This results from cerebral adaptation to recurrent exposure to hypoglycaemia.

The prevalence of impaired perception of the onset of symptoms of hypoglycaemia and modification of the symptom profile increases with the duration of insulin treatment, and almost 50% of patients with type 1 diabetes are affected after 20 years of diabetes. This chronic form of impaired hypoglycaemia awareness may not be reversible; frequency of severe hypoglycaemia is increased sixfold, and intensive insulin therapy should be avoided. In affected patients the usual therapeutic goals need to be modified and frequent self-monitoring of blood glucose is mandatory. Therapy-induced impaired awareness of hypoglycaemia is usually reversible if glycaemic control is relaxed and hypoglycaemia avoided.

Deficient counter-regulatory hormonal responses

In response to a falling blood glucose, there is normally suppression of endogenous insulin secretion (absent in type 1 diabetes) and a brisk secretion of counter-regulatory hormones which antagonise the blood glucose-lowering effect of insulin. Glucagon and adrenaline (epinephrine) are the most potent of these. Hypoglycaemia-induced secretion of glucagon becomes impaired in most people within 5 years of developing type 1 diabetes. After several years many also develop a defective adrenaline response to hypoglycaemia so that if hypoglycaemia develops, glucose recovery may be seriously compromised. Autonomic neuropathy may contribute to the deficient adrenaline response, but those who develop deficient counter-regulatory responses may also have impaired central activation of neuro-endocrine secretion. Counter-regulatory deficiency is closely associated with impaired awareness of hypoglycaemia, suggesting a common pathogenetic mechanism within the brain.

Causes, morbidity and prevention

Risk factors and causes of hypoglycaemia in patients taking insulin or a sulphonylurea drug are listed in Box 21.24. Severe hypoglycaemia, defined as any episode requiring the assistance of another person for recovery, can result in serious morbidity (Box 21.25) and has a recognised mortality of 2–4% in insulin-treated patients. The unrecognised mortality may be higher. Occasionally, sudden death occurs during sleep in otherwise healthy young patients with

21.24 HYPOGLYCAEMIA: COMMON CAUSES AND RISK FACTORS

Causes of hypoglycaemia

- Missed, delayed or inadequate meal
- Unexpected or unusual exercise
- Alcohol
- Errors in oral hypoglycaemic agent or insulin dose/schedule/ administration
- Poorly designed insulin regimen, particularly if predisposing to nocturnal hyperinsulinaemia
- Lipohypertrophy at injection sites causing variable insulin absorption
- Gastroparesis due to autonomic neuropathy
- Malabsorption, e.g. coeliac disease
- Unrecognised other endocrine disorder, e.g. Addison's disease
- Factitious (deliberately induced)
- Breastfeeding by diabetic mother

Risk factors for severe hypoglycaemia

- Strict glycaemic control
- Impaired awareness of hypoglycaemia
- Age (very young and elderly)
- Increasing duration of diabetes
- Sleep
- C-peptide negativity
- History of previous hypoglycaemia
- Renal impairment
- Angiotensin-converting enzyme (ACE) genotype

21.25 MORBIDITY OF SEVERE HYPOGLYCAEMIA IN DIABETIC PATIENTS

CNS

- Impaired cognitive function
- Coma
- Convulsions
- Transient ischaemic attack, stroke
- Intellectual decline
- Brain damage (rare)
- Focal neurological lesions (rare)

Heart

- Cardiac arrhythmias
- Myocardial ischaemia

Eye

- Vitreous haemorrhage
- ? Worsening of retinopathy

Other

- Hypothermia
- Accidents (including road traffic accidents) with injury

type 1 diabetes ('dead-in-bed syndrome'); hypoglycaemia-induced cardiac arrhythmia or acute respiratory arrest with impaired baroreflex sensitivity has been implicated.

Severe hypoglycaemia is very disruptive and impinges on many aspects of the patient's life, including employment, driving (Box 21.14, p. 819), travel (Box 21.26), sport and personal relationships. The incidences of most common causes of hypoglycaemia can all be reduced by adequate patient education. Exercise-induced hypoglycaemia (Fig. 21.8) occurs in people with well-controlled, insulin-treated diabetes because of hyperinsulinaemia and the absence of the capacity to decrease secretion of endogenous insulin, a key factor in the normal adaptation to exercise. If strenuous or protracted exercise is anticipated, the preceding

21

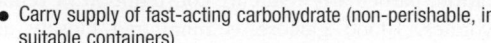

21.26 MEASURES FOR AVOIDANCE AND TREATMENT OF HYPOGLYCAEMIA DURING TRAVEL

- Carry supply of fast-acting carbohydrate (non-perishable, in suitable containers)
    - Screwtop plastic bottles for glucose drinks
    - Packets of powdered glucose (for use in hot, humid climates)
    - Confectionery (foil wrapping in hot climates)
- Companions should carry additional oral carbohydrate, and glucagon
- Frequent blood glucose testing (carry spare meter; visually read strips)
- Use fast-acting insulin analogues for long-distance air travel

dose of insulin should be reduced (the degree of reduction varying widely in individuals but often being substantial) and extra carbohydrate ingested. People treated with insulin should carry some form of fast-acting glucose (glucose drink, tablets or confectionery) at all times.

The incidence of nocturnal hypoglycaemia in patients with type 1 diabetes is difficult to establish but is certainly high. As nocturnal hypoglycaemia does not usually waken the sleeping patient, and the usual warning symptoms are not perceived, it is often undetected. However, on direct questioning, patients may admit to poor quality of sleep, morning headaches, 'hangover', chronic fatigue and vivid dreams or nightmares. Sometimes a partner may observe sweating (which may be profuse), restlessness, twitching or even convulsions. The only reliable way to identify this problem is to measure the blood glucose during the night. Unfortunately, many insulin regimens in current use produce inappropriate nocturnal hyperinsulinaemia. When an intermediate-acting depot insulin such as isophane (p. 834) is taken before the main evening meal between 1700 and 1900 hrs, its peak action will coincide with the period of maximum sensitivity to insulin, namely 2300–0200 hrs. Short-acting insulin administered before a late evening meal (after 2000 hrs) can cause hypoglycaemia after retiring to bed. With a basal-bolus regimen (p. 835) the times of maximum risk of biochemical hypoglycaemia are between 2300 and 0200 hrs and between 0500 and 0700 hrs. To reduce the risk of nocturnal hypoglycaemia, administration of the evening dose of depot intermediate-acting insulin should be deferred until bedtime (after 2300 hrs) or a fast-acting insulin analogue used for the evening meal. It is a sensible precaution for patients to measure the blood glucose before they go to bed and to eat a carbohydrate snack if the reading is less than 6.0 mmol/l (~110 mg/dl).

Management

Treatment of acute hypoglycaemia depends on the severity of the hypoglycaemia and whether the patient is conscious and able to swallow. Treatment may simply require oral carbohydrate if hypoglycaemia is recognised early. If the adult patient is unable to swallow, intravenous glucose (30–50 ml of 20–50% dextrose) or glucagon (1 mg by intramuscular injection) should be administered. The recommended dose of intravenous dextrose in children is 0.2 g/kg. A commercial viscous glucose gel solution can be applied into the buccal cavity; jam or honey may be just as effective but should not be used if the person is unconscious.

As soon as the patient is able to swallow, glucose should be given orally. Full recovery may not occur immediately and reversal of cognitive impairment may not be complete until 60 minutes after normoglycaemia is restored. Further, when hypoglycaemia has occurred in a patient using a long- or intermediate-acting insulin or a long-acting sulphonylurea, such as glibenclamide, the possibility of recurrence should be anticipated and to prevent this a 10% dextrose infusion, titrated to the patient's blood glucose, may be necessary.

The development of cerebral oedema should be considered in patients who fail to regain consciousness after blood glucose is restored to normal. Other causes of impaired consciousness, such as alcohol intoxication, a post-ictal state or cerebral haemorrhage, should be excluded. Cerebral oedema has a high mortality and morbidity, and requires urgent treatment with mannitol and high-dose oxygen.

Following recovery, it is important to try to identify a cause and make appropriate adjustments to the patient's therapy. Unless the reason for a hypoglycaemic episode is clear, the patient should reduce the next dose of insulin by 10–20% and seek medical advice about further adjustments in dose. Patient education on the potential causes and risks

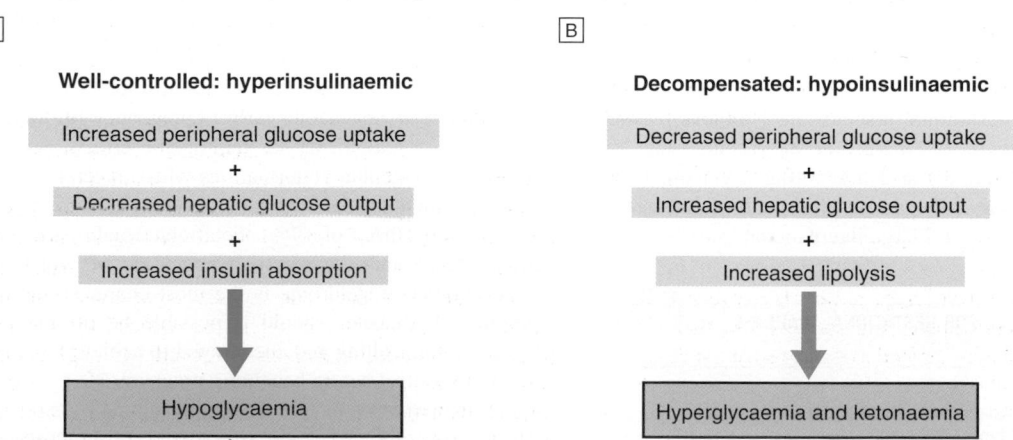

Fig. 21.8 The effect of exercise in diabetic patients being treated with insulin. A Well-controlled hyperinsulinaemic patients. B Decompensated hypoinsulinaemic patients.

of inducing hypoglycaemia and on its treatment, including the need to have an accessible supply of glucose (and glucagon) and to perform regular blood glucose monitoring, are fundamental to the prevention of this potentially dangerous side-effect of treatment. Relatives and friends also need to be familiar with the symptoms and signs of hypoglycaemia and should be instructed as to how this should be managed (including how to give an intramuscular injection of glucagon).

The management of self-poisoning with oral anti-diabetic agents is given on page 211.

DIABETES IN PREGNANCY

GESTATIONAL DIABETES

Glucose metabolism changes during normal pregnancy, reflecting altered glucose handling by the mother and nutritional demands of the developing fetus. In normal women marked insulin resistance develops, particularly by the second half of pregnancy. Fasting glucose decreases slightly, while blood glucose may be increased post-prandially.

Gestational diabetes is defined as diabetes with first onset or recognition during pregnancy. While this includes women with pre-existing (or clinically undetected) type 1 or type 2 diabetes, the majority can expect to be restored to normal glucose tolerance immediately after pregnancy. Risk factors for gestational diabetes are shown in Box 21.27. The presence of hyperglycaemia has a number of important implications for mother and child.

Definition

Controversy surrounds the definition of gestational diabetes and the most appropriate screening method for its detection. There is a continuous relationship between maternal blood glucose and risk of adverse perinatal outcomes so there is no threshold that clearly defines risk. A further concern is that the diagnosis of gestational diabetes per se increases the likelihood of undesirable outcomes, such as caesarean section. In addition, there is some evidence from women with pre-existing diabetes that over-intensive management may cause a detrimental limitation of fetal growth. The WHO suggests that all women meeting criteria for impaired glucose tolerance or diabetes after a 75 g OGTT should be classified as having gestational diabetes. European criteria for diagnosis of gestational diabetes are a venous plasma glucose > 5.5 mmol/l (99 mg/dl) in the fasting state or > 9.0 mmol/l (162 mg/dl) at 2 hours after a glucose load. The role of intensive management of gestational diabetes is being examined in several large international trials.

21.27 RISK FACTORS FOR GESTATIONAL DIABETES

- Obesity
- Ethnicity (South Asian, black, Hispanic, Native American)
- Family history of type 2 diabetes
- Previous glucose abnormalities in pregnancy
- Previous macrosomia

Implications for the mother

Gestational diabetes is managed where possible by dietary modification, particularly reducing consumption of refined carbohydrates. Blood glucose is monitored closely and insulin is introduced if glycaemic control is unsatisfactory.

Gestational diabetes is associated with an increased risk of later development of type 2 diabetes. The risk is as high as 50% at 5 years in certain ethnic groups such as Hispanic women in the USA but is lower in Caucasian populations. Women with gestational diabetes should have glucose tolerance re-assessed after pregnancy (generally at 6 weeks post-partum). If post-partum glucose tolerance has returned to normal (fasting glucose < 6.1 mmol/l (110 mg/dl) and 2 hour glucose < 7.8 mmol/l (140 mg/dl)) advice on lifestyle changes should be given to minimise the long term risk of developing type 2 diabetes. Where glucose intolerance persists after pregnancy in a patient with a strong family history of diabetes, the presence of one of the rare autosomal dominant forms of diabetes (MODY, p. 815) should be considered.

Implications for the fetus

A clear relationship exists between maternal blood glucose and perinatal morbidity for the baby. Maternal glucose crosses the placenta and is an important fuel for the developing fetus. An elevated maternal blood glucose promotes fetal insulin production which stimulates growth. Maternal hyperglycaemia is therefore associated with increased fetal size (fetal macrosomia), which may complicate labour and delivery, resulting in a higher caesarean section rate. Reduction of maternal blood glucose by insulin therapy can reduce fetal growth.

PREGNANCY IN WOMEN WITH ESTABLISHED TYPE 1 DIABETES

Historically, pregnancy in patients with diabetes was associated with a very high incidence of morbidity for mother and child. In the 1940s and 1950s perinatal mortality rates were of the order of 40–50% and maternal mortality could be as high as 5%. Dramatic improvements in these outcomes for mother and child have been driven by the introduction of home monitoring of blood glucose, dietetic advice, modern intensive regimens for insulin delivery using either multiple injections or infusion pumps, improved obstetrical management and the support of a multidisciplinary team.

Maternal hyperglycaemia early in pregnancy (in the first 6 weeks of development) has teratogenic effects, with an increase in congenital abnormalities when maternal HbA$_{1c}$ is greater than 4 standard deviations above the normal mean (generally an HbA$_{1c}$ of ~7%). Fetal abnormalities include cardiac, renal and skeletal malformations, of which the caudal regression syndrome is the most characteristic. All women with diabetes should if possible be offered pre-pregnancy counselling and encouraged to achieve excellent glycaemic control before becoming pregnant.

Later in pregnancy maternal hyperglycaemia is associated with macrosomia, reflecting oversupply of glucose and other fuels to the developing fetus and secondary increases in fetal insulin production. Fetal macrosomia increases

21

21.28 MANAGEMENT OF PREGNANCY IN WOMEN WITH ESTABLISHED DIABETES

- Pregnancy should be planned
- Folic acid supplementation begins before conception
- Maintain strict glycaemic control, i.e. HbA$_{1c}$ close to the non-diabetic range by use of 3–4 injections of insulin daily
- Do not strive for normoglycaemia at the expense of hypoglycaemia. Check blood glucose during the night periodically
- Check overnight sample of urine for ketones regularly; increase intake of carbohydrate and dose of insulin to abolish ketonuria

the risk of birth injury during delivery, and of subsequent neonatal hypoglycaemia. Offspring of mothers with diabetes are also at increased risk of polycythaemia, hyperbilirubinaemia and hypocalcaemia.

Ideally mothers should attempt to maintain near-normal glycaemia through all of pregnancy (Box 21.28), but this is often difficult to achieve. Insulin requirements of women with type 1 diabetes rise considerably. As in all patients with diabetes treated with insulin, strict glycaemic control increases the risk of hypoglycaemia and careful glucose monitoring is esssential. Pregnancy is also associated with an increased potential for ketosis. Ketoacidosis during pregnancy is dangerous for the mother and is associated with a high rate (10–35%) of fetal mortality. Finally, because pregnancy is associated with a worsening of diabetic complications, most notably retinopathy, careful eye screening is required throughout pregnancy.

While the outlook for mother and child has been vastly improved, pregnancy outcomes are still not equivalent to those of non-diabetic mothers. Perinatal mortality rates remain 3–4 times those of the non-diabetic population (at around 30–40 per 1000 pregnancies) and the rate of congenital malformation is increased 5–6-fold.

HYPERGLYCAEMIA IN ACUTE MYOCARDIAL INFARCTION

Hyperglycaemia is often found in patients who have sustained an acute myocardial infarction. In some, this represents stress hyperglycaemia, some have previously undiagnosed diabetes, and many have established diabetes. Many patients with stress hyperglycaemia will have impaired glucose tolerance on a subsequent OGTT. There is much that can be done to reduce mortality from myocardial infarction in those with diabetes (Box 21.29). Hyperglycaemia should be treated with insulin and, in patients with type 2 diabetes, oral anti-diabetic agents should be stopped in the peri-infarct period. A study from Sweden suggested that conversion to insulin therapy in type 2 patients with acute myocardial infarction might reduce the long-term mortality from coronary heart disease, but this has not been confirmed in a recent larger study.

SURGERY AND DIABETES

Surgery, whether performed electively or in an emergency, causes catabolic stress and secretion of counter-regulatory

21.29 TREATMENTS TO REDUCE MORTALITY FROM MYOCARDIAL INFARCTION IN PEOPLE WITH DIABETES

Primary prevention of myocardial infarction
- Strict glycaemic control
- Aggressive control of hypertension
- Cholesterol reduction with a statin

Immediate measures in acute myocardial infarction
- Thrombolysis/fibrinolysis
- Aspirin
- ACE inhibitor
- β-blocker
- ? Intravenous insulin

Secondary prevention of myocardial infarction
- Aspirin
- β-blocker
- ACE inhibitor
- Cholesterol reduction with a statin
- Intensive subcutaneous insulin or anti-diabetic medication

21

hormones both in normal and in diabetic subjects. This results in increased glycogenolysis, gluconeogenesis, lipolysis, proteolysis and insulin resistance. In the non-diabetic person these metabolic effects lead to a secondary increase in the secretion of insulin, which exerts a restraining and controlling influence. In diabetic patients there is either absolute deficiency of insulin (type 1 diabetes) or insulin secretion is delayed and impaired (type 2 diabetes), so that in untreated or poorly controlled diabetes the uptake of metabolic substrate is significantly reduced, catabolism is increased and ultimately metabolic decompensation in the form of diabetic ketoacidosis may develop in both types of diabetes. Starvation will exacerbate this process by increasing lipolysis. In addition, hyperglycaemia impairs phagocytic function (leading to reduced resistance to infection) and wound healing. Thus surgery must be carefully planned and managed in the diabetic patient, with particular emphasis on good metabolic control and avoidance of hypoglycaemia, which is particularly dangerous in the unconscious or semiconscious patient.

Pre-operative assessment
Careful pre-operative assessment is mandatory and is summarised in Box 21.30. Much of this can be done as an outpatient but, if cardiovascular or renal function is

21.30 PRE-OPERATIVE ASSESSMENT IN DIABETIC PATIENTS

- Assess cardiovascular and renal function
- Check for features of neuropathy, particularly autonomic
- Assess glycaemic control
  Measure HbA$_{1c}$
  Monitor pre-prandial and bedtime blood glucose
- Review treatment of diabetes
  Modify insulin regimen if necessary: use intermediate and short-acting insulins
  Stop metformin and long-acting sulphonylureas; replace with insulin if necessary

impaired, there are signs of neuropathy (particularly autonomic), diabetic control is poor or alterations need to be made to the patient's usual treatment, then admission to hospital some days before operation will be required.

Perioperative management

The management of diabetic patients undergoing surgery requiring general anaesthesia is summarised in Figure 21.9. Post-operatively, a glucose/insulin/potassium infusion should be continued until the patient's intake of food is adequate, when the normal insulin or tablet regimen can be resumed. If the intravenous infusion has to be continued for more than 24 hours, plasma electrolytes and urea should be measured and urinary ketones checked daily. If the infusion is prolonged, the concentration of potassium may require adjustment, and if dilutional hyponatraemia occurs, a parallel saline infusion may be necessary. If fluids need to be restricted, e.g. in patients with cardiovascular or renal disease, the rate of infusion can be halved by using a 20% dextrose solution and doubling the concentration of insulin and potassium. The insulin requirement is likely to be higher than that indicated in Figure 21.9 in patients with hepatic disease, obesity or sepsis and in those being treated with corticosteroids or undergoing cardiopulmonary bypass surgery.

Surgical emergencies

If the patient is significantly hyperglycaemic and/or ketoacidotic, this should be corrected first with an intra-venous infusion of saline and/or dextrose plus insulin, 6 units per hour, and potassium as required. Subsequently, treatment is as described in Figure 21.9.

Emergency surgery in a patient with well-controlled insulin-treated diabetes depends on when the last sub-cutaneous injection of insulin was given. If this was recent, an infusion of dextrose alone may be sufficient, but frequent monitoring is essential.

CHILDREN, ADOLESCENTS AND YOUNG ADULTS

Diabetes in children or teenagers is generally ketosis-prone, insulin-deficient type 1 diabetes, but cases of type 2 diabetes in obese children are now occurring, and the possibility of a diagnosis of MODY (p. 815) should be considered, especially when there is a strong family history of diabetes. The management of diabetes in children and adolescents presents particular challenges which should be addressed in specialised clinics. Insulin therapy and diet require appropriate modification to accommodate the normal physiological changes associated with growth and puberty and the physical and emotional problems associated with adolescence. Adherence to prescribed treatment may be erratic, and a deterioration in glycaemic control is common during adolescence.

Wide fluctuations in blood glucose and frequent metabolic emergencies are sometimes observed in a few

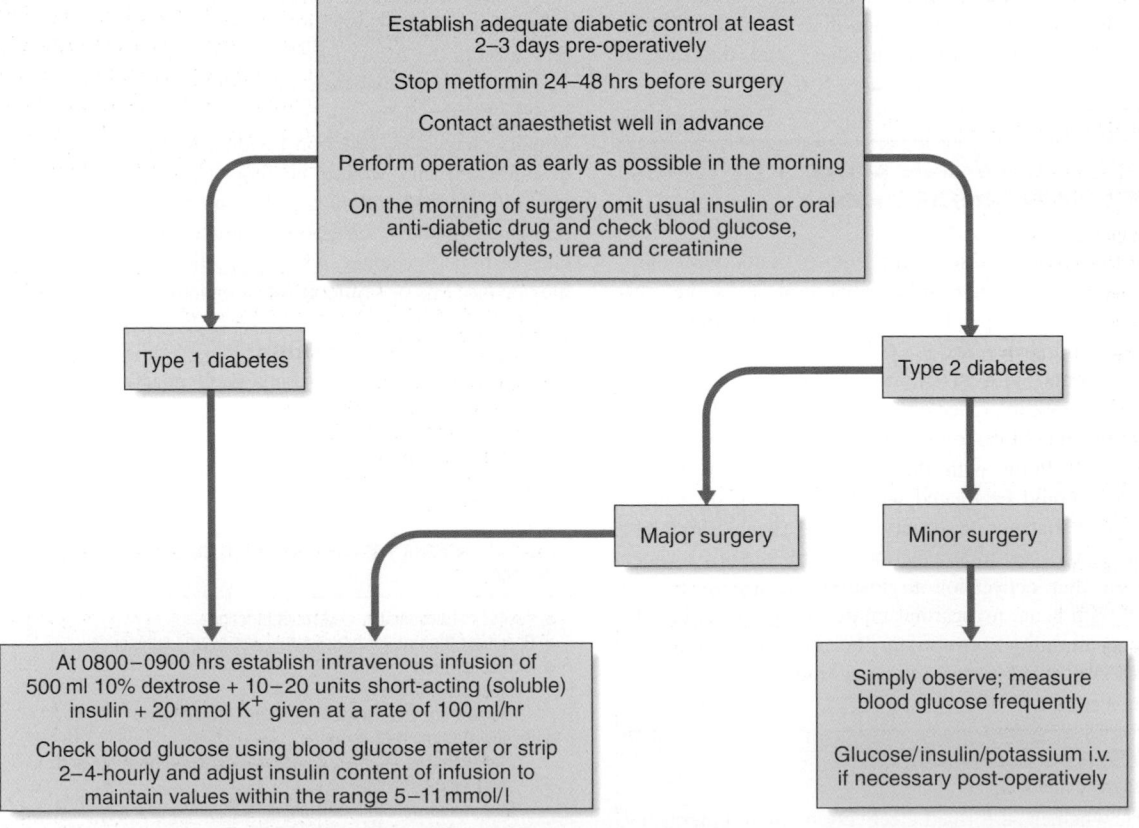

Fig. 21.9 Management of diabetic patients undergoing surgery and general anaesthesia. (Glucose of 5–11 mmol/l ≡ 90–199 mg/dl.)

adolescents and young adults, but use of the term 'brittle diabetes' should be discouraged, as this is not considered to be a pathological entity. Studies have shown that this problem (mostly affecting young women) is associated with persistent manipulation of therapy (stopping insulin or taking excessive doses) to induce recurrent diabetic ketoacidosis or severe hypoglycaemia requiring hospital admission. This attention-seeking behaviour may be a manifestation of psychological disturbance, is factitious (p. 251), and is not a specific phenomenon peculiar to some aspect of diabetes or its management in susceptible individuals.

COMPLICATIONS OF DIABETES

The development of a foot ulcer, renal impairment, sensory loss or retinopathy in a patient with long-standing diabetes would be recognised as a long-term complication of the disorder, but manifestations of a diabetic complication may be the presenting finding in a patient who is not known to have diabetes (Box 21.31). Thus, diabetes may be first suspected when a patient visits an optometrist or podiatrist. Between 20% and 25% of patients with type 2 diabetes have evidence of established diabetic complications at the time of initial diagnosis. Diabetes may be detected for the first time when a patient presents with hypertension or a vascular event such as an acute myocardial infarction or stroke. Blood glucose should therefore be checked in all patients presenting with such pathology. The detailed investigation and management of diabetic complications are described on pages 836–846.

21.31 COMPLICATIONS OF DIABETES
Microvascular/neuropathic
Retinopathy, cataract
• Impaired vision
Nephropathy
• Renal failure
Peripheral neuropathy
• Sensory loss
• Motor weakness
Autonomic neuropathy
• Postural hypotension
• Gastrointestinal problems (gastroparesis; altered bowel habit)
Foot disease
• Ulceration
• Arthropathy
Macrovascular
Coronary circulation
• Myocardial ischaemia/infarction
Cerebral circulation
• Transient ischaemic attack
• Stroke
Peripheral circulation
• Claudication
• Ischaemia

MANAGEMENT OF DIABETES

Three methods of treatment are available for diabetic patients: diet and lifestyle advice alone, oral anti-diabetic drugs, and insulin. Approximately 50% of new cases of diabetes can be controlled adequately by diet alone, 20–30% will need an oral anti-diabetic medication, and 20–30% will require insulin. Regardless of aetiology, the type of treatment is determined by the adequacy of residual β-cell function. However, this cannot be determined easily by measurement of circulating plasma insulin concentration because a level which is adequate in one patient may be inadequate in another, depending upon insulin sensitivity. In clinical practice the age and weight of the patient at diagnosis are closely related to the adequacy of insulin secretion and usually indicate the type of treatment required (Fig. 21.10). However, in each individual the regimen adopted is effectively chosen by therapeutic trial and should be reviewed regularly.

The importance of lifestyle changes such as taking regular exercise, observing a healthy diet and reducing alcohol consumption should not be under-estimated in improving glycaemic control, but many people, particularly the middle-aged and elderly, find them difficult to sustain. Patients should also be encouraged to stop smoking.

The ideal management for diabetes would allow the patient to lead a completely normal life, to remain not only symptom-free but in good health, to achieve a normal metabolic state and to escape the long-term complications of diabetes. This is achievable to a variable degree. Setting individual goals for each patient is discussed on page 820. Although a few diabetic patients die from acute metabolic complications (ketoacidosis and hypoglycaemia), the major problem is the excess mortality and serious morbidity suffered as a result of the long-term complications of diabetes (pp. 836–846); the factors associated with these are listed in Box 21.32.

21.32 FACTORS ASSOCIATED WITH INCREASED MORTALITY AND MORBIDITY IN PEOPLE WITH DIABETES
• Duration of diabetes
• Early age at onset of disease
• High glycated haemoglobin (HbA_{1c})
• Raised blood pressure
• Proteinuria; microalbuminuria
• Dyslipidaemia
• Obesity

DIETARY MANAGEMENT

Dietary measures are required in the treatment of all people with diabetes. The aims are shown in Box 21.33. People with diabetes should have access to dietitians at diagnosis, review and at times of treatment change. Nutritional advice should be tailored to individuals and take account of their age and lifestyle.

21

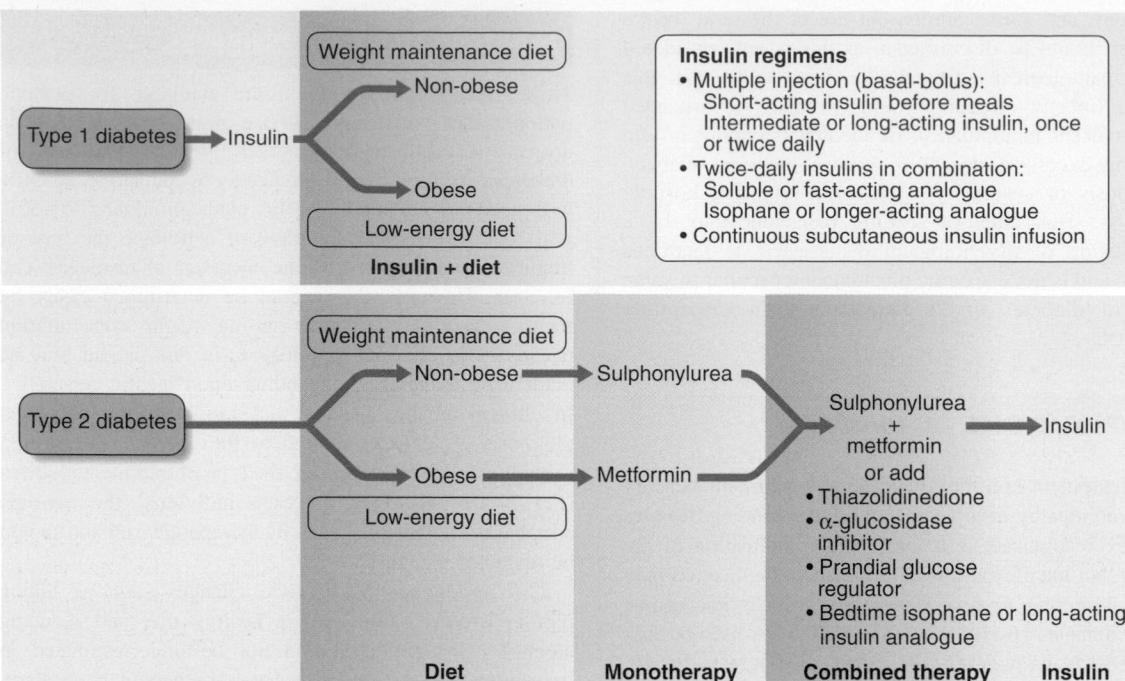

Fig. 21.10 Long-term treatment of diabetes. The treatment required by any individual can usually be determined by considering age and weight at diagnosis, and other features of types 1 and 2 diabetes described on pages 811–814.

21.33 AIMS OF DIETARY MANAGEMENT

- Achieve good glycaemic control
- Reduce hyperglycaemia and avoid hypoglycaemia
- Assist with weight management
- Reduce the risk of micro- and macrovascular complications
- Ensure adequate nutritional intake
- Avoid 'atherogenic' diets or those that aggravate complications, e.g. high protein intake in nephropathy

---

21.34 RECOMMENDED COMPOSITION OF DIET FOR PEOPLE WITH DIABETES

	Percentage of energy intake
Carbohydrate	45–60%
Sucrose	Up to 10%
Fat (total)	< 35%
n-6 Polyunsaturated	< 10%
n-3 Polyunsaturated	Eat oily fish once or twice weekly
Monounsaturated	10–20%
Saturated	< 10%
Protein	10–15% (do not exceed 1 g/kg body weight)

COMPOSITION OF THE DIET

Recommendations for the dietary management of diabetes are summarised in Box 21.34, and emphasise the proportion of energy to be derived from carbohydrate and monounsaturated fat.

Carbohydrate

Traditionally, people with diabetes, especially type 1 diabetes, have been advised to maintain a regular intake of carbohydrate in meals throughout the day. 'Exchanges' (10 g portions) or 'lines' were used previously to enable patients to calculate their carbohydrate intake, but fell into disuse. However, a knowledge of the carbohydrate content of meals remains fundamental to self-management of insulin-treated diabetes. The development of modern insulin regimens, particularly using insulin analogues or continuous subcutaneous insulin infusion (CSII), has allowed greater flexibility in the timing and carbohydrate content of meals. It is now possible to match the amount of carbohydrate in a meal with a dose of short-acting insulin using methods such as DAFNE (Dose Adjustment For Normal Eating), although

this form of intensive dietary management is demanding and requires adequate resources for patient education. Application of similar dietary principles enables motivated individuals with type 1 diabetes to achieve and maintain good glycaemic control, while avoiding post-prandial hyper- and hypoglycaemia.

For people with type 2 diabetes, avoidance of refined carbohydrate and restriction of total intake is important, and the 'plate model' (Fig. 21.11) may provide a simple visual aid to show the proportions of carbohydrate and other food groups for selection at mealtimes. It is adaptable, and can be used as a teaching tool to promote healthy eating.

Glycaemic index

Both the amount and source of carbohydrate determine post-prandial glucose (p. 109). The glycaemic index (GI) of a carbohydrate-containing food is a measure of the change in blood glucose following its ingestion. The increase in blood glucose (from the fasting level) in the 2 hours after

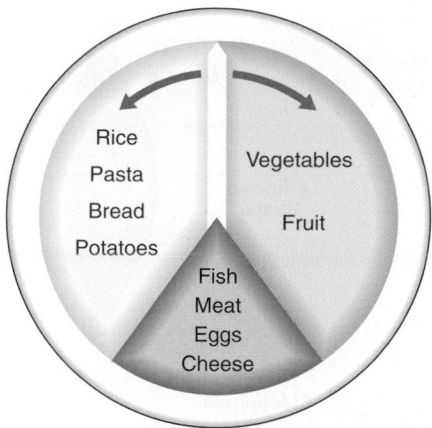

Fig. 21.11 A 'plate model' for meal planning. The plate is divided into three sections. The smallest section (one-fifth of total area) is for the meat, fish, eggs or cheese, and the remainder divided in roughly equal proportions between the staple food (rice, pasta, potatoes, bread etc.) and vegetables or fruit.

ingestion of a particular food is compared with the response to a reference food (glucose or white bread) containing an equivalent amount of carbohydrate. Different foods can be ranked by their effect on post-prandial glycaemia. GI should not be confused with 'glycaemic load' which is the product of the glycaemic index of the food and the amount of carbohydrate in a serving. Consumption of foods with a low GI is encouraged because they produce a slow, gradual rise in blood glucose. Examples include starchy foods such as basmati rice, spaghetti, noodles, granary bread, and beans and lentils. However, different methods of food processing and preparation can influence the GI of foods, as can the ripeness of some foods and differences in strains of rice. In addition, GI is limited to assessing the effect of consuming types of carbohydrate, and does not address the total amount consumed.

Fat

The intake of total fat should be restricted to less than 35% of energy intake, with less than 10% as saturated fat, and 10–20% from monounsaturated fat through consumption of oils and spreads made from olive, rapeseed or groundnut oils (Box 21.34). Monounsaturated fats are promoted as the main source of dietary fat as this will benefit the plasma lipid profile (reduction in total and LDL cholesterol, without lowering HDL cholesterol). Polyunsaturated fats should provide no more than 10% of total fat intake. This type of fat tends to reduce total and LDL cholesterol, but also lowers HDL cholesterol. The ω-3 fatty acids, which are found predominantly in oily fish such as salmon, mackerel, sardines and herring, have been shown to assist with secondary prevention of cardiovascular disease.

WEIGHT MANAGEMENT

Therapy for obesity is described on pages 113–117. In patients with diabetes, weight management is a key factor, as a high percentage of people with type 2 diabetes are overweight or obese, and many anti-diabetic medications

and insulin encourage weight gain. Obesity, particularly abdominal obesity with increased waist circumference, also predicts insulin resistance and cardiovascular risk.

Weight loss can be achieved through a reduction in energy intake and an increase in energy expenditure through physical activity. Very low calorie diets (VLCDs) of < 800 kcals/day can produce rapid initial results, but such energy deficit diets are difficult to sustain, do not promote good food choices or the behavioural changes that are required for long-term weight maintenance, and may cause nutritional deficiencies. Some people find group motivation in a slimming club to be helpful when attempting to lose weight, although care must be taken to ensure that the advice provided at the group sessions is appropriate for diabetes management. Patients on oral anti-diabetic agents, and especially those on insulin, may need to adjust their therapy when changing their diet.

In addition to reducing calorie intake, overweight patients should be strongly encouraged to take regular exercise, in the form of walking, swimming or cycling, for approximately 30 minutes daily, as this improves insulin sensitivity and the lipid profile and lowers blood pressure.

ALCOHOL

Alcohol can be consumed in moderation unless there is a coexisting medical problem that requires abstinence. As alcohol suppresses gluconeogenesis, it can precipitate or protract hypoglycaemia, particularly in patients taking insulin or sulphonylureas. In the UK the weekly recommended limits are a maximum of 14 units for women and 21 units for men, a unit being defined as half pint of beer/lager, a measure of spirits or a small glass of wine. Drinks containing alcohol can be a substantial (and often overlooked) source of calories and total intake may have to be reduced to assist weight reduction.

SALT

People with diabetes should follow the advice given to the general population: namely, to reduce sodium intake to no more than 6 g daily. Further restriction of sodium intake (to less than 3 g daily) is important in treating hypertensive diabetic patients.

DIABETIC FOODS AND SWEETENERS

Low-calorie and sugar-free drinks are useful for patients with diabetes. These drinks usually contain non-nutritive sweeteners. Many 'diabetic foods' contain sorbitol and are usually expensive, high in calories, and may cause gastrointestinal side-effects. As a result, these foods are not recommended as part of the diabetic diet.

ORAL ANTI-DIABETIC DRUGS

Various drugs are effective in reducing hyperglycaemia in patients with type 2 diabetes (Fig. 21.12). Although their mechanisms of action are different, most depend upon a supply of endogenous insulin and they therefore have no

21

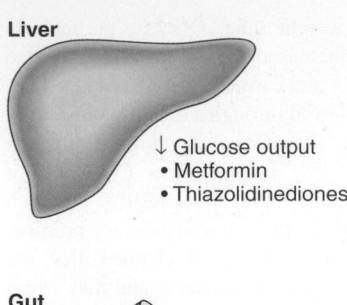
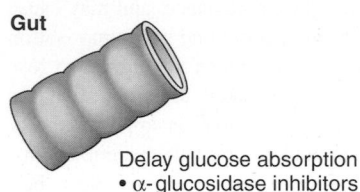
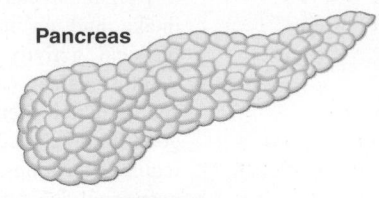
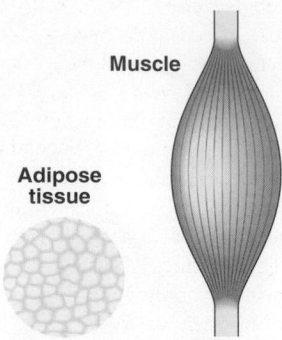

Liver

↓ Glucose output
• Metformin
• Thiazolidinediones

Gut

Delay glucose absorption
• α-glucosidase inhibitors

Pancreas

Insulin replacement
• Insulin

↑ Insulin secretion
• Sulphonylureas
• Meglitinides
• Amino acid derivatives

Muscle

Adipose tissue

↑ Peripheral glucose uptake
• Metformin
↑ Insulin sensitivity
• Thiazolidinediones

Fig. 21.12   Principal modes and sites of action of pharmacological treatments for type 2 diabetes.

21.35 EFFECTS OF HYPOGLYCAEMIC DRUGS USED IN THE TREATMENT OF TYPE 2 DIABETES

	Insulin	Sulphonyl-ureas	Metformin	Acarbose	Thiazolidine-diones	Meglitinides and amino acid derivatives
Reduce basal glycaemia	Yes	Yes	Yes	Slight	Yes	?
Reduce post-prandial glycaemia	Yes	Yes	Yes	Yes	Yes	Yes
Raise plasma insulin	Yes	Yes	No	No	No	Yes
Increase body weight	Yes	Yes	No	No	Yes	Yes
Improve lipid profile	Yes	No	Slight	Slight	Variable	No
Risk of hypoglycaemia	Yes	Yes	No	No	No	Yes
Tolerability	Good	Good	Moderate	Moderate	Good	Good

hypoglycaemic effect in patients with type 1 diabetes. The sulphonylureas and the biguanides have been the mainstay of treatment for many years and have the strongest evidence of preventing complications of diabetes. However, newer agents include the insulin-enhancing agents, the thiazolidinediones, the α-glucosidase inhibitors, which delay carbohydrate digestion and absorption of glucose, and the prandial glucose regulators which stimulate endogenous insulin secretion. Adherence to prescribed medication is best when few drugs are used, preferably with once-daily administration. The effects of these drugs are compared in Box 21.35.

SULPHONYLUREAS

Mechanism of action

The principal effect of sulphonylureas is to stimulate the release of insulin from the pancreatic β cell (insulin secretagogue). They act through a sulphonylurea receptor which is linked to a K⁺ channel on the β-cell surface. K⁺ transport triggers insulin secretion.

Indications for use

Sulphonylureas are valuable in the treatment of non-obese patients with type 2 diabetes who fail to respond to dietary measures alone. Although sulphonylureas will lower the blood glucose concentration of obese patients with type 2 diabetes, such patients should be treated energetically in the first instance by dietary measures with or without metformin, since treatment with sulphonylureas is often associated with an increase in weight which will increase insulin resistance and eventually aggravate the total disability. This leads to secondary failure to respond to the drugs, and progression to treatment with insulin.

The main differences between the individual compounds lie in their potency, duration of action and cost. Tolbutamide, the mildest of the first-generation sulphonylureas, is very well tolerated. Its duration of action is relatively short, it is usually administered 8- or 12-hourly, and is a useful drug in the elderly in whom the risk and the consequences of inducing hypoglycaemia are greater. Chlorpropamide has a biological half-life of about 36 hours and is taken once daily, but may cause severe and prolonged hypoglycaemia. It is now rarely used.

Of the second-generation sulphonylureas, gliclazide and glipizide cause few side-effects, but glibenclamide is prone to induce severe hypoglycaemia and should be avoided in the elderly. Newer long-acting preparations such as glimepiride and a modified-release form of gliclazide can be administered once daily with no apparent increased risk of hypoglycaemia. The dose-response of all sulphonylureas is most effective at low dosage; little additional hypoglycaemic benefit is obtained when the dose is increased to maximal levels. Several drugs can potentiate the hypoglycaemic effect of sulphonylureas by displacing them from their plasma protein-binding sites, e.g. salicylates, phenylbutazone and antifungal agents.

People with type 2 diabetes who fail to respond to initial treatment with sulphonylureas are considered 'primary treatment failures'. The incidence of primary treatment failure depends mainly on the criteria for initial selection and compliance with diet. Patients with 'secondary failure' (i.e. after a period of satisfactory glycaemic control) are not a homogeneous group; they include some with late-onset type 1 diabetes who develop an absolute deficiency of insulin, some with type 2 diabetes whose β-cell failure is advanced, and others who are not adhering to the recommended diet. The most common precipitant of secondary treatment failure is decreasing care with diet, and is usually associated with weight gain. Weight loss suggests worsening β-cell function. With continuing follow-up, 'secondary failure' affects 3–10% of patients each year.

BIGUANIDES

Metformin is the only biguanide available. The long-term benefit of metformin was shown in the United Kingdom Prospective Diabetes Study (UKPDS, p. 838), but it is still less widely used than the sulphonylureas because of a higher incidence of side-effects, particularly gastrointestinal symptoms.

Mechanism of action

The mechanism of action of metformin has not been precisely defined. It has no hypoglycaemic effect in non-diabetic individuals, but in diabetes, insulin sensitivity and peripheral glucose uptake are increased, perhaps through activation of a cAMP-regulated kinase in muscle. There is some evidence that it also impairs glucose absorption by the gut and inhibits hepatic gluconeogenesis. Although secretion of some endogenous insulin is mandatory for its glucose-lowering action, it does not increase insulin secretion and seldom causes hypoglycaemia.

Indications for use

Administration of metformin is not associated with a rise in body weight and it is therefore preferred for the obese patient. In addition, as the glucose-lowering effect of metformin is synergistic with that of the sulphonylurea drugs, the two can be combined when either alone has proved inadequate. Metformin is given with food, 8- or 12-hourly. The usual starting dose is 500 mg 12-hourly, with a gradual increase as required to a maximum of 1 g 8-hourly. Its use is contraindicated in patients with impaired renal or hepatic function and in those who take alcohol in excess in whom the risk of lactic acidosis is significantly increased. It should be discontinued, at least temporarily, if any other serious medical condition develops, especially one causing severe shock or hypoxaemia. In such circumstances, treatment with insulin should be substituted.

ALPHA-GLUCOSIDASE INHIBITORS

The α-glucosidase inhibitors delay carbohydrate absorption in the gut by selectively inhibiting disaccharidases. Acarbose or miglitol is available and is taken with each meal. Both lower post-prandial blood glucose and modestly improve overall glycaemic control. They can be combined with a sulphonylurea. The main side-effects are flatulence, abdominal bloating and diarrhoea.

THIAZOLIDINEDIONES

Mechanism of action

These drugs (also called TZD drugs, 'glitazones' or PPARγ agonists) bind and activate peroxisome proliferator-activated receptor-γ, a nuclear receptor present mainly in adipose tissue that regulates the expression of several genes involved in metabolism, and work by enhancing the actions of endogenous insulin. Their effects are partly direct (in the adipose cells) and partly indirect (by altering release of 'adipokines' such as adiponectin and resistin which alter insulin sensitivity in the liver). Plasma insulin concentrations are not increased and hypoglycaemia is not a problem.

Indications for use

Rosiglitazone or pioglitazone are usually prescribed as second-line therapy with sulphonylureas in patients intolerant of metformin, or as third-line therapy in combination with sulphonylurea and metformin. However, their use as monotherapy and in combination with insulin is likely to increase.

They are most likely to be effective in patients with the most severe insulin resistance (e.g. in abdominal obesity) and there is evidence that they redistribute fat away from the abdomen and towards subcutaneous depots. However, body weight and total body fat are increased by thiazolidinediones.

Thiazolidinediones have few side-effects. The first drug of this class, troglitazone, had to be withdrawn because of hepatotoxicity and newer thiazolidinediones should be avoided in patients with liver dysfunction, but it appears that this effect was specific to troglitazone. An important side-effect of all thiazolidinediones is sodium and fluid retention, which is most likely if they are combined with insulin. Thiazolidinediones must be avoided in patients with cardiac failure.

MEGLITINIDES AND AMINO ACID DERIVATIVES

These drugs are called prandial glucose regulators. Repaglinide directly stimulates endogenous insulin secretion and is taken immediately before food. It is less likely to cause hypoglycaemia than sulphonylureas. Nateglinide has a similar mode of action, restores first-phase insulin secretion, and is prescribed with metformin.

COMBINED ORAL ANTI-DIABETIC THERAPY AND INSULIN

In diabetic patients who are requiring increasing doses of a sulphonylurea or biguanide, either alone or in combination

21

with each other or with a thiazolidinedione, the introduction of a single dose of an intermediate- or long-acting insulin (usually isophane), administered at bedtime, may improve glycaemic control and delay the development of overt pancreatic β-cell failure. The exogenous insulin suppresses hepatic glucose output during the night and lowers fasting blood glucose. This treatment is ineffective in diabetic patients who have no residual endogenous insulin secretion. The combination of bedtime isophane insulin with metformin has been shown to be the regimen least likely to promote weight gain. For patients who are approaching secondary failure to oral medication, this provides a simple and effective introduction to self-treatment with insulin with little risk of hypoglycaemia.

INCRETIN MIMETICS

A new class of therapeutic agents is being developed for treatment of type 2 diabetes. The secretion of insulin in response to a rise in blood glucose is greater when glucose is given by mouth, rather than by intravenous infusion. In part this is caused by secretion of gut hormones, or incretins, which potentiate glucose-induced insulin secretion. Glucagon-like peptide (GLP-1) is an incretin hormone which stimulates insulin secretion in a glucose-dependent manner, thus hypoglycaemia is unlikely. In addition, GLP-1 suppresses glucagon secretion, delays gastric emptying, reduces appetite and encourages weight loss. It has to be given by injection. As GLP-1 is rapidly degraded by the enzyme, dipeptidyl peptidase IV, inhibitors of this enzyme will have to be given to prolong its biological effect. Alternatively, long-acting GLP-1 analogues are being developed. These include liraglutide and exenatide (synthetic exendin-4). These preparations will probably be used in combination with other anti-diabetic medication, have to be given by subcutaneous injection and may cause nausea.

INSULIN

Manufacture and formulation

Insulin was discovered in 1921 and transformed the management of type 1 diabetes, until then a fatal disorder. Until the 1980s insulin was obtained by extraction and purification from pancreata of cows and pigs (bovine and porcine insulins) and some people continue to use animal insulins. The use of recombinant DNA technology has enabled large-scale production of human insulin. Recently, rDNA and protein engineering techniques that alter the amino acid sequence of insulin have been used to produce 'monomeric' analogues of insulin, which are more rapidly absorbed from the site of injection (e.g. insulin lispro or aspart).

The duration of action of short-acting, unmodified insulin ('soluble' or 'regular' insulin), which is a clear solution, can be extended by the addition of protamine and zinc at neutral pH (isophane or NPH insulin) or excess zinc ions (lente insulins). These modified 'depot' insulins are cloudy preparations. Pre-mixed formulations containing short-

21.36 DURATION OF ACTION (IN HOURS) OF INSULIN PREPARATIONS			
Insulin	Onset	Peak	Duration
Rapid-acting (insulin analogues— lispro, aspart, glulisine)	< 0.5	0.5–2.5	3–4.5
Short-acting (soluble (regular))	0.5–1	1–4	4–8
Intermediate-acting (isophane (NPH), lente)	1–3	3–8	7–14
Long-acting (bovine ultralente)	2–4	6–12	12–30
Long-acting (insulin analogues— glargine, detemir)	1–2	None	18–24

acting and isophane insulins in various proportions are available. The time characteristics of insulins are shown in Box 21.36.

In many countries, the insulin concentration in available formulations has been standardised at 100 units/ml.

Insulin delivery

Insulin is injected subcutaneously into the anterior abdominal wall, upper arms, outer thighs and buttocks (Box 21.37). Accidental intramuscular injection often occurs in children and thin adults. The rate of absorption of insulin may be influenced by many factors other than the insulin formulation, including the site, depth and volume of injection, skin temperature (warming), local massage and exercise. Absorption is delayed from areas of lipohypertrophy at injection sites (p. 807), which results from the local trophic action of insulin, so repeated injection at the same site should be avoided. Other routes of administration (intravenous and intraperitoneal) are reserved for specific circumstances.

Insulin is administered using a disposable plastic syringe with a fine needle (which can be reused several times) in preference to the traditional glass syringe and metal needle which require repeated sterilisation. Pen injectors with insulin in cartridge form are popular and convenient and are also available as pre-loaded disposable pens. They do not necessarily improve glycaemic control but may increase compliance.

'Open-loop' systems are battery-powered portable pumps providing continuous subcutaneous or intravenous infusion of insulin, delivered at variable rates without reference to the blood glucose concentration. In practice, the 'loop' is closed by the patient performing blood glucose estimations, and the use of these devices requires a high degree of patient

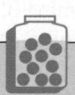

21.37 TECHNIQUE OF INSULIN INJECTION

- Needle sited at right angle to the skin
- Subcutaneous (not intramuscular) injection (depth of injection, needle size)
- Delivery devices—glass syringe (requires resterilisation), plastic syringe (disposable), pen device, infusion pump

motivation. These increasingly sophisticated systems can achieve excellent glycaemic control but will not be adopted for widespread therapeutic use until they are less expensive and incorporate a miniaturised glucose sensor.

Short-acting insulin has to be injected at least 30 minutes before a meal to allow adequate time for absorption. Many patients find this inconvenient and ignore this requirement. However, the rapidly absorbed fast-acting insulin analogues can be administered immediately before food, or even after meals, and their peak action coincides more closely with the post-prandial rise in blood glucose (Box 21.36).

Once absorbed into the blood stream, insulin has a half-life of a few minutes. It is removed mainly by the liver and also the kidneys; plasma insulin concentrations are elevated in patients with liver disease or renal failure. The rate of clearance is also affected by binding to insulin antibodies (associated with the use of animal insulins).

Alternative routes of insulin delivery have been investigated, and intra-pulmonary insulin by inhalation will soon be available, principally for treatment of type 2 diabetes.

Insulin regimens

Various insulin regimens are used in the treatment of diabetes. The choice of regimen depends on the desired degree of glycaemic control, the patient's lifestyle and his or her ability to adjust the insulin dose. Most people require two or more injections of insulin daily. Once-daily injections rarely achieve satisfactory glycaemic control and are reserved either for some elderly patients or for those who retain substantial endogenous insulin secretion and have a low insulin requirement.

Twice-daily administration of a short-acting and intermediate-acting insulin (usually soluble and isophane insulins), given in combination before breakfast and the evening meal, is the simplest regimen and is still commonly used. Individual requirements vary considerably but usually two-thirds of the total daily requirement of insulin is given in the morning in a ratio of 1:2, short:intermediate-acting insulins. The remaining third is given in the evening, and doses are adjusted according to blood glucose monitoring.

Several pre-mixed formulations are available containing different proportions of soluble and isophane insulins (e.g. 30:70 and 50:50). These are of value in patients who have difficulty mixing insulins, but are inflexible as the individual components cannot be adjusted independently.

Multiple injection regimens are popular, with short-acting insulin being taken before each meal, and intermediate-acting insulin being injected at bedtime (basal-bolus regimen). This type of regimen allows greater freedom of timing of meals and is of value to individuals with variable day-to-day activities, but snacks may have to be taken between meals to prevent hypoglycaemia. The use of pen injectors has improved the acceptability of multiple injection regimens. The time-action profile of different insulin regimens, compared to the secretory pattern of insulin in the non-diabetic state, is shown in Figure 21.13. Fast-acting insulin analogues may be used before meals, and are particularly useful if the evening meal is late, as they do

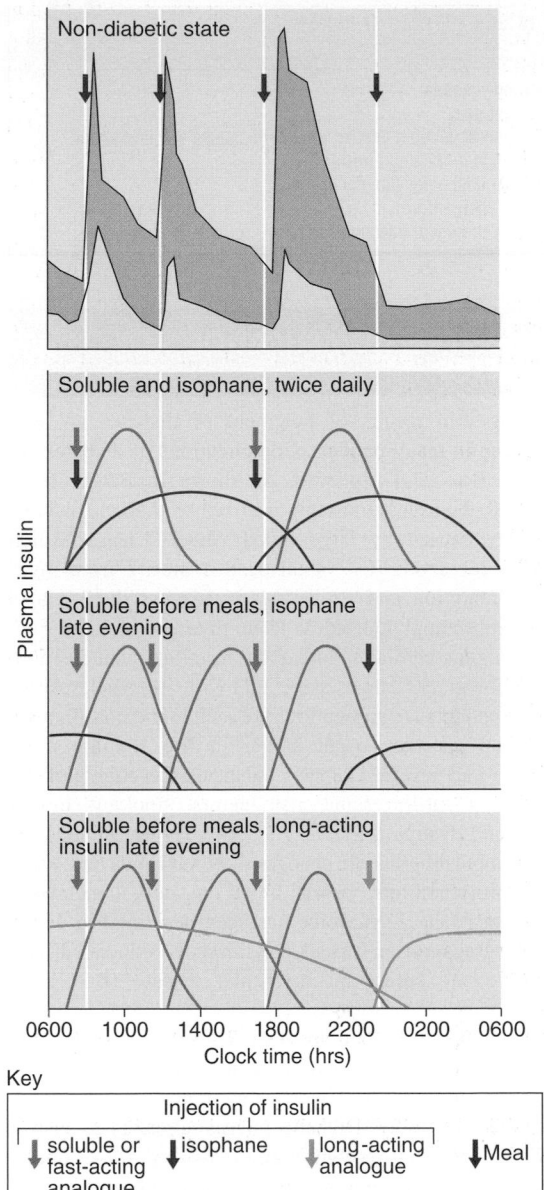

Fig. 21.13 Profiles of plasma insulin associated with different insulin regimens. The schematic profiles are compared with the insulin responses (mean ± standard deviation) observed in non-diabetic adults, shown in the top panel (shaded area). These are theoretical patterns of plasma insulin and may differ considerably in magnitude and duration of action between individuals.

not induce nocturnal hyperinsulinaemia. However, a long interval between meals allows the blood glucose to rise, and may require injection of additional isophane insulin before breakfast. A common problem is fasting hyperglycaemia ('the dawn phenomenon') caused by the release of counter-regulatory hormones during the night as part of the normal circadian rhythm, which increases insulin requirement before wakening.

The complications of insulin therapy are listed in Box 21.38; the most important of these is hypoglycaemia (p. 823).

835

21.38 SIDE-EFFECTS OF INSULIN THERAPY

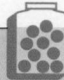

- Hypoglycaemia
- Weight gain
- Peripheral oedema (insulin treatment causes salt and water retention in the short term)
- Insulin antibodies (animal insulins)
- Local allergy (rare)
- Lipodystrophy at injection sites

21.39 MORTALITY IN DIABETES

	Mortality ratio (diabetics vs matched non-diabetic controls)
Overall	2.6
Coronary heart disease Cerebrovascular disease Peripheral vascular disease	2.8
All other causes, including renal failure	2.7

LONG-TERM COMPLICATIONS OF DIABETES

The long-term results of treatment of diabetes are disappointing in many patients. Complications of diabetes are listed in Box 21.31 (p. 829). As shown in Boxes 21.39 and 21.40, the excess mortality incurred by diabetic patients is mainly caused by large blood vessel disease, which accounts for about 70% of all deaths, mostly from myocardial infarction and stroke. Macrovascular disease also causes substantial morbidity from myocardial infarction, stroke, angina, cardiac failure and intermittent claudication. The pathological changes associated with atherosclerosis in diabetic patients are similar to those seen in the non-diabetic population but they occur earlier in life and are more extensive and severe. Diabetes enhances the effects of the other major cardiovascular risk factors: smoking, hypertension and dyslipidaemia (Fig. 21.14). Hyperinsulinaemia may promote atherogenic changes in blood lipids and blood coagulability and raise arterial blood pressure. A metabolic (insulin resistance) syndrome has been described in which the co-segregation of various conditions is associated with premature and severe macrovascular disease (Box 21.7, p. 815).

Disease of small blood vessels is a specific complication of diabetes and is termed diabetic microangiopathy. It contributes to mortality by causing renal failure due to diabetic nephropathy. Diabetic microangiopathy is also a cause of substantial morbidity and disability: for example, blindness due to diabetic retinopathy, difficulty in walking, chronic ulceration of the feet, and bowel and bladder dysfunction due to autonomic neuropathy. A graded relationship has been demonstrated between the duration and degree of sustained hyperglycaemia, however caused and at whatever age it develops, and the risk of microvascular disease.

Pathophysiology

Some of the numerous biochemical and functional abnormalities found in long-standing, poorly controlled diabetes are listed in Box 21.41 and Figure 21.15.

The histopathological hallmark of diabetic microangiopathy is thickening of the capillary basement membrane, with associated increased vascular permeability throughout the body. The development of the characteristic clinical syndromes of diabetic retinopathy, nephropathy, neuropathy and atherosclerosis is thought to result from the local response to the generalised vascular injury. For example, in the wall of large vessels, increased permeability of

21.40 CAUSES OF DEATH IN PEOPLE WITH DIABETES*

- Cardiovascular disease — 70%
- Renal failure — 10%
- Cancer — 10%
- Infections — 6%
- Diabetic ketoacidosis — 1%
- Other — 3%

* These figures are approximate.

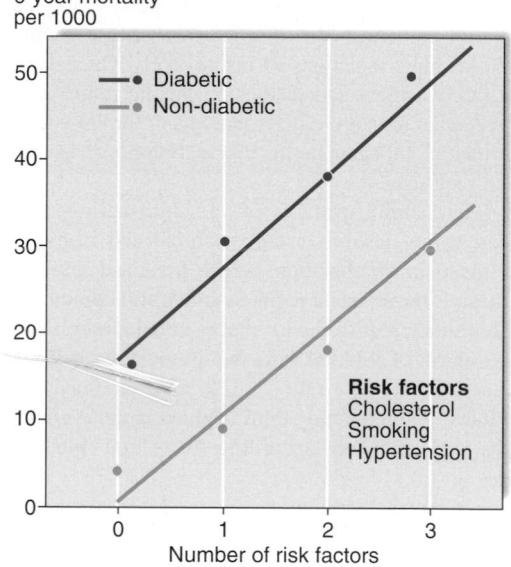

Fig. 21.14 Diabetes mellitus as a risk factor for coronary heart disease (CHD). Three major factors—smoking, hypertension and raised cholesterol—are associated with risk of CHD in the general population. The presence of diabetes mellitus produces an increment in risk in addition to these conventional factors.

arterial endothelium, particularly when combined with hyperinsulinaemia and hypertension, will increase the deposition of atherogenic lipoproteins.

The precise mechanisms linking hyperglycaemia to the pathological changes underlying the clinical syndromes are not yet fully defined. However, it is thought that increased metabolism of glucose to sorbitol via the polyol pathway is of central importance in pathogenesis, since haemodynamic, vascular permeability and structural changes in capillaries

21.41 PATHOGENESIS OF DIABETIC VASCULAR AND NEUROPATHIC COMPLICATIONS: POSSIBLE MECHANISMS

Biochemical consequences of hyperglycaemia

- Non-enzymatic glycation
- Oxidative-reductive stress
- Increased polyol pathway activity
- Intracellular *myo*-inositol depletion
- Increased diacylglycerol synthesis
- Increased protein kinase C activity

Functional abnormalities

- Haemodynamic disturbances
- Haemorrheological and coagulation abnormalities
- Microvascular hypertension
- Endothelial dysfunction
- Increased capillary permeability

are prevented in diabetic animals by treatment with a variety of structurally different aldose-reductase inhibitors which inhibit this process. Other putatively important mechanisms are listed in Box 21.41.

Preventing diabetes complications

Glycaemic control

The possibility of reversing early microvascular disease by improving metabolic control has been examined in several prospective randomised controlled clinical trials involving patients with early background retinopathy and minimal proteinuria. None of these studies produced any evidence of reversal of either retinopathy or nephropathy, and in some cases retinopathy worsened abruptly soon after control was improved. Despite this, in the long term the rate of progression of both retinopathy and nephropathy was

reduced by continuing better control. These studies stimulated a search for markers of early reversible retinal, renal and neural dysfunction, and shifted the emphasis in the management of diabetes to primary prevention of complications.

The Diabetes Control and Complications Trial (DCCT) was a large study that lasted 9 years in type 1 diabetic patients to answer the question: are diabetic complications preventable? The trial demonstrated a 60% overall reduction in the risk of developing diabetic complications in those on intensive therapy with strict glycaemic control (mean HbA_{1c} around 7%), compared with those on conventional therapy (mean HbA_{1c} around 9%—Box 21.42). No single factor other than glycaemic control had a significant effect on outcome.

The conclusions which can be drawn are:

- Diabetic complications are preventable.
- The aim of treatment should be 'near-normal' glycaemia.

In the patients with strict glycaemic control in the DCCT, weight gain was common and severe hypoglycaemic episodes occurred three times more often. Although there

21.42 GLYCAEMIC CONTROL IN TYPE 1 DIABETES **EBM**

'In patients with type 1 diabetes, strict glycaemic control (mean HbA_{1c} 7%) reduced the development of retinopathy and other microvascular complications by 76% compared with conventional therapy (mean HbA_{1c} 9%).'

- Diabetes Control and Complications Trial Research Group. N Engl J Med 1993; 329:977–986.

For further information: 🖥 www.diabetes.niddk.nih.gov/dm/pubs/control/

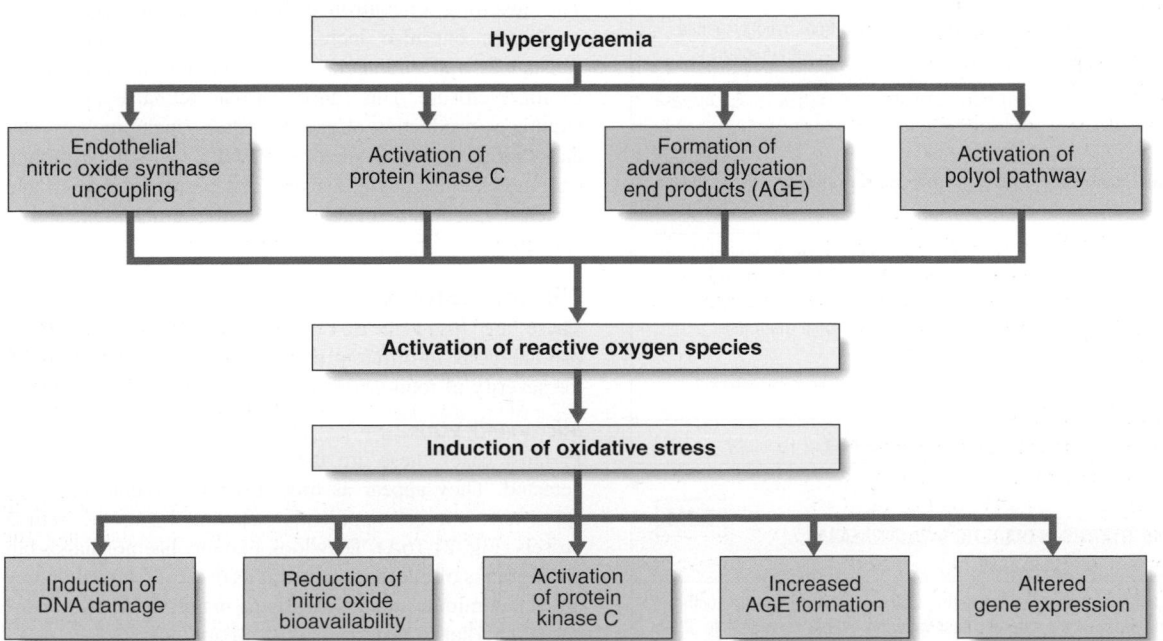

Fig. 21.15 The roles of hyperglycaemia-induced accumulation of reactive oxygen species and oxidative stress in causation of diabetic vascular complications. The induction of oxidative stress causes haemodynamic changes and endothelial and vascular dysfunction, leading to vascular damage.

was no detectable increase in deaths, major macrovascular events or neurological/cognitive defects, this increased risk of hypoglycaemia may alter the risk:benefit ratio of good control in certain patients. Thus less intensive treatment may be indicated in:

- those with impaired awareness of hypoglycaemia
- those with severe macrovascular disease (particularly if they have a past history of myocardial infarction or cerebrovascular accident)
- those at the extremes of life (very young children and the frail elderly, Box 21.43).

A large study of patients with type 2 diabetes, the UKPDS, has shown that the frequency of diabetic complications is lower and progression is slower with good glycaemic control and effective treatment of hypertension, irrespective of the type of therapy used (Box 21.44).

Control of other risk factors

Randomised controlled trials have shown that aggressive management of lipids (Box 21.45) and blood pressure (Box 21.46) limits the complications of diabetes. ACE inhibitors are valuable in improving outcome in heart disease (Box 21.47) and in preventing diabetic nephropathy (p. 841). This often results in the use of multiple medications, with the potential problem of patients' adherence to therapy.

21.43 DIABETES MANAGEMENT IN OLDER PEOPLE

- **Glycaemic control**: the optimal degree of glycaemic control in older people has yet to be determined. Strict glycaemic control should be avoided in the very frail patient.
- **Cognitive and affective function**: may benefit from improving glycaemic control.
- **Hypoglycaemia**: older people have reduced symptomatic awareness of hypoglycaemia and limited knowledge of symptoms, and are at greater risk of and from hypoglycaemia.
- **Mortality**: the mortality rate of older people with diabetes is more than double that of age-matched non-diabetic people, largely because of increased deaths from cardiovascular disease.

21.44 GLYCAEMIC CONTROL IN TYPE 2 DIABETES **EBM**

'In patients with type 2 diabetes, intensive glycaemic control (mean HbA$_{1c}$ 7%) with oral anti-diabetic agents or insulin reduced the development of microvascular complications, particularly retinopathy, by 25% compared with conventional treatment (mean HbA$_{1c}$ 8%).'

- UK Prospective Diabetes Study (UKPDS) Group. Lancet 1998; 352:837–853 and 854–865.

For further information: 🖳 www.dtu.ox.ac.uk

21.45 STATINS IN DIABETIC DYSLIPIDAEMIA **EBM**

'In diabetic patients with existing vascular disease, therapy with a statin reduced the rate of major vascular events from 38% to 33%, and in patients with no cardiovascular disease from 14% to 9%.'

- Collins R, et al. Lancet 2003; 361:2005–2016.

For further information: 🖳 www.ctsu.ox.ac.uk

21.46 CONTROL OF BLOOD PRESSURE IN TYPE 2 DIABETES **EBM**

'Tight blood pressure control (< 140/80 mmHg) reduced the development of microvascular and macrovascular complications by 24% compared with less tight blood pressure control.'

- UK Prospective Diabetes Study (UKPDS) Group. BMJ 1998; 317:703–713.

For further information: 🖳 www.dtu.ox.ac.uk

21.47 ANGIOTENSIN-CONVERTING ENZYME INHIBITORS IN DIABETIC CARDIOVASCULAR DISEASE **EBM**

'In diabetic patients with existing cardiovascular disease or high cardiovascular risk, ACE inhibitors reduced subsequent cardiovascular events from 20% to 15%.'

- Heart Outcomes Prevention Evaluation (HOPE) Study Investigators. Lancet 2000; 355:253–259.

For further information: 🖳 www.diabetes-mellitus.org

DIABETIC RETINOPATHY

Diabetic retinopathy is one of the most common causes of blindness in adults between 30 and 65 years of age in developed countries. Retinal photocoagulation is an effective treatment, particularly if it is given at a relatively early stage when the patient is usually symptomless. This means that regular examination of the fundi, with the pupils fully dilated, is mandatory in all diabetic patients.

Pathogenesis

Hyperglycaemia increases retinal blood flow and metabolism and has direct effects on retinal endothelial cells and pericyte loss, which impairs vascular autoregulation. The resulting uncontrolled blood flow initially dilates capillaries but also increases production of vasoactive substances and endothelial cell proliferation, resulting in capillary closure. This causes chronic retinal hypoxia and stimulates production of growth factors, including vascular endothelial growth factor (VEGF), which stimulate endothelial cell growth (causing new vessel formation) and increase vascular permeability (causing retinal leakage and exudation).

Clinical features

These are listed in Box 21.48. They occur in varying combinations in different patients and are used to classify the severity of retinopathy as shown in Box 21.49.

Microaneurysms

In most cases these are the earliest clinical abnormality detected. They appear as tiny, discrete, circular, dark red spots near to, but apparently separate from, the retinal vessels (Fig. 21.16A). They look like tiny haemorrhages but photographs of injected preparations of retina show that they are in fact minute aneurysms arising mainly from the venous end of capillaries near areas of capillary closure.

Haemorrhages

These most characteristically occur in the deeper layers of the retina and hence are round and regular in shape and

21.48 CLINICAL FEATURES OF DIABETIC RETINOPATHY

- Microaneurysms
- Retinal haemorrhages
- Exudates
- Cotton wool spots
- Venous changes
- Neovascularisation
- Pre-retinal haemorrhage
- Vitreous haemorrhage
- Fibrosis

described as 'blot' haemorrhages (Fig. 21.16A). The smaller ones may be difficult to differentiate from microaneurysms and the two are often grouped together as 'dots and blots'. Superficial flame-shaped haemorrhages in the nerve fibre layer may also occur, particularly if the patient is hypertensive.

Exudates

These are characteristic of diabetic retinopathy. They vary in size from tiny specks to large confluent patches and tend to occur particularly in the perimacular area (Fig. 21.16B). They result from leakage of plasma from abnormal retinal capillaries and overlie areas of neuronal degeneration. The terms 'hard' exudates and 'soft' exudates (i.e. cotton wool spots) are no longer recommended.

Cotton wool spots

These are similar to those seen in hypertension, and also occur particularly within five disc diameters of the optic disc (Fig. 21.16E). They represent arteriolar occlusions causing retinal ischaemia and hence are a feature of pre-proliferative diabetic retinopathy; they are most often seen in rapidly

advancing retinopathy or in association with uncontrolled hypertension.

Intraretinal microvascular abnormalities

Intraretinal microvascular abnormalities (IRMA) are dilated, tortuous capillaries which represent the remaining patent capillaries in an area where most have been occluded and are a feature of severe pre-proliferative retinopathy.

Neovascularisation

This may arise from the venous circulation either on the optic disc or in the retina in response to an ischaemic retina. The earliest appearance is that of fine tufts of delicate vessels forming arcades on the surface of the retina (Fig. 21.16F). As they grow, they may extend forwards onto the posterior surface of the vitreous. They are fragile and leaky and are liable to rupture, causing haemorrhage which may be pre-retinal ('sub-hyaloid') or into the vitreous. Serous products leaking from these new vessel systems stimulate a connective tissue reaction, called gliosis. This first appears as a white, cloudy haze among the network of new vessels. As it extends, the new vessels may be obliterated and the surrounding retina covered by a dense white sheet. At this stage, bleeding is less common but retinal detachment can occur due to contraction of adhesions between the vitreous and the retina.

Venous changes

These include venous dilatation (an early feature probably representing increased blood flow), 'beading' (sausage-like changes in calibre) and increased tortuosity including

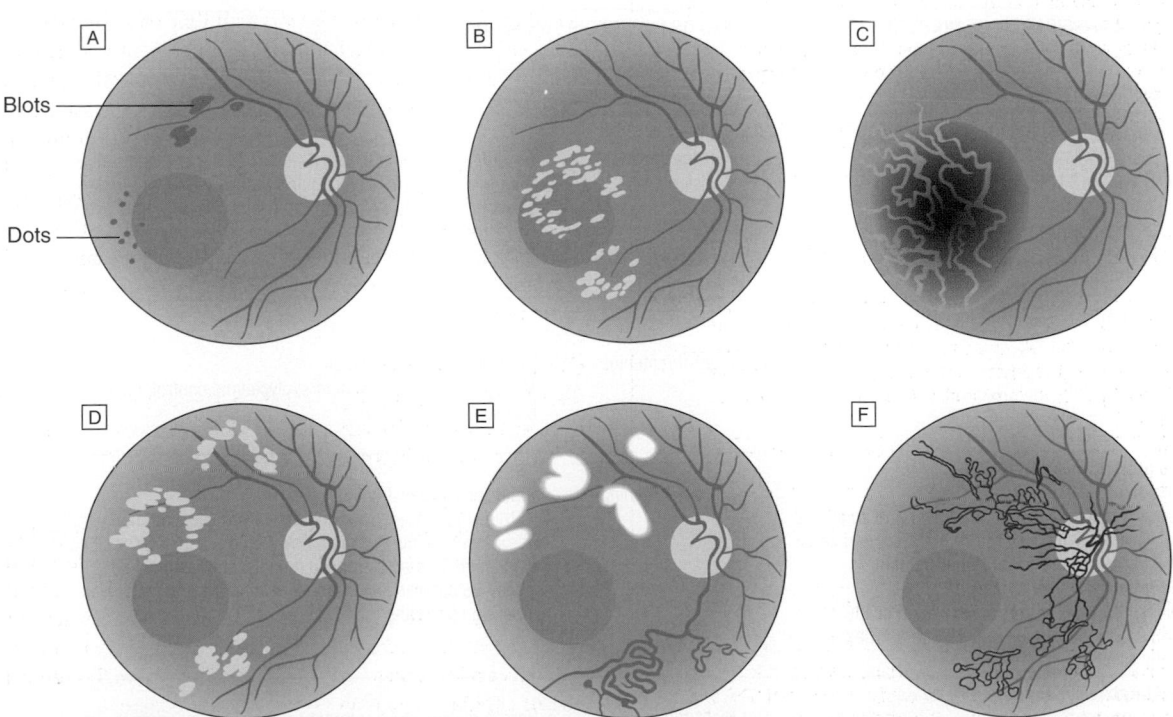

Fig. 21.16 Diagrammatic representation of diabetic eye disease. A Background diabetic retinopathy showing microaneurysms and blot haemorrhages. B Background retinopathy showing exudates. C Maculopathy showing oedema. D Maculopathy with exudates. E Pre-proliferative retinopathy showing venous changes and cotton wool spots. F Proliferative retinopathy showing neovascularisation.

'oxbow lakes' or loops. These latter changes indicate widespread capillary non-perfusion and are a feature of advanced pre-proliferative retinopathy.

Rubeosis iridis

The more severe types of retinopathy may be accompanied by the development of new vessels on the anterior surface of the iris: 'rubeosis iridis'. These vessels may obstruct the drainage angle of the eye and the outflow of aqueous fluid, causing secondary glaucoma.

Classification

A classification of diabetic retinopathy, based on prognosis for vision and indications for specialist referral, is shown in Box 21.49.

Microaneurysms, abnormalities of the veins, and small blot haemorrhages and exudates situated in the periphery will not interfere with vision unless they are associated with oedema and thickening in the macular area. Macular oedema cannot be detected by direct ophthalmoscopy but should be suspected if there is impairment of visual acuity in association with mild peripheral non-proliferative retinopathy and no other obvious pathology.

New vessels may be symptomless until sudden visual loss occurs from a pre-retinal or vitreous haemorrhage. Although these frequently resolve, the risk of recurrence is high, and the more frequent the haemorrhage, the slower and less complete the recovery. Fibrous tissue may seriously interfere with vision by obscuring the retina and/or causing further retinal haemorrhage or detachment.

Prevention

Glycaemic and blood pressure control

Good glycaemic control, particularly in the early years following the development of diabetes, reduces the risk of developing retinopathy. Early diagnosis followed by effective treatment is particularly important for those with type 2 diabetes, 25% of whom present with established retinopathy. In others, retinopathy is diagnosed only when the patient is referred for a specialist opinion after years of ineffective treatment of type 2 diabetes.

Hyperglycaemia promotes retinal hyperperfusion, so a rapid reduction in blood glucose may cause an initial deterioration of retinopathy by causing relative ischaemia. Improvement in glycaemic control should therefore be effected gradually. The rate of progression of retinopathy is still significantly slower in intensively treated patients than in matched control subjects over an 18-month period.

Blood pressure lowering is of proven benefit in hypertensive patients. Elevated plasma cholesterol is a risk factor for diabetic retinopathy, but evidence for the beneficial use of a statin is awaited.

Screening

Regular screening for retinopathy is essential in all diabetic patients but is particularly important in those with risk factors. These include early onset, long duration of diabetes, hypertension, poor glycaemic control, pregnancy, use of the oral contraceptive pill, smoking, excessive alcohol consumption and evidence of microangiopathy elsewhere,

21.49 CLASSIFICATION OF DIABETIC RETINOPATHY BASED ON PROGNOSIS FOR VISION		
Type of retinopathy	Prognosis	Action required

Non-proliferative 'background' retinopathy without maculopathy
Venous dilatation
Peripheral
  Microaneurysms
  Blot haemorrhages
  Exudates
	No immediate threat to vision	Maximise control of blood glucose, lipids and blood pressure
		Give advice to stop smoking and reduce intake of alcohol
		Observe carefully, i.e. fundoscopy with dilated pupils every 6–12 months
		Refer for specialist opinion if rate of progression increases significantly

Maculopathy
Macula
  Exudation
  Haemorrhage
  Ischaemia
Macular oedema
	Sight-threatening	Refer for specialist opinion
		Medical review of risk factors, glycaemic control, blood pressure and lipid levels

Pre-proliferative retinopathy Venous loops and beading Clusters/sheets of microaneurysms and small blot haemorrhages and/or large retinal haemorrhages Intraretinal microvascular abnormalities Multiple cotton wool spots Macular oedema with reduced visual acuity Perimacular exudates ± retinal haemorrhages of any size	Sight-threatening	Refer for specialist opinion At this stage rapid lowering of the blood glucose may result in abrupt worsening of retinopathy with the appearance of cotton wool spots and an increased number of haemorrhages; it may be safer to lower the blood glucose gradually over a period of months
Proliferative retinopathy Pre-retinal haemorrhage Neovascularisation Fibrosis Exudative maculopathy	Sight-threatening	Urgent review and treatment by specialist mandatory

particularly neuropathy and proteinuria. Screening should be undertaken by trained personnel in an organised and audited programme. The preferred screening option is a digital imaging photographic system, with reference if necessary to an ophthalmologist examination by slit lamp biomicroscopy. The problem remains that many people with diabetes do not attend for screening and receive no regular supervision.

Management

Severe non-proliferative and proliferative retinopathy is treated with retinal photocoagulation, which has been shown to reduce severe visual loss by 85% (50% in patients with maculopathy). Photocoagulation is used:

- to destroy areas of retinal ischaemia (since it is thought that this plays a major role in the development of neovascularisation)
- to seal leaking microaneurysms and reduce macular oedema
- to gliose new vessels directly on the retinal surface (but not on the optic disc).

Argon laser photocoagulation is the usual form of laser used for pan-retinal photocoagulation and for treatment of macular oedema. This simple procedure can be carried out with topical anaesthesia and in skilled hands carries little risk; it can be very effective. Pan-retinal photocoagulation results in new vessel elimination, with vision being maintained in up to 90% of patients who have new vessels on the retina and/or disc; macular oedema (Fig. 21.16C) is also successfully treated in many patients with focal laser therapy. Patients must be reviewed regularly to check for further development of new vessels and/or maculopathy. Extensive bilateral photocoagulation can cause significant visual field loss, which may interfere with driving ability and reduce night vision.

Vitrectomy may be used in selected cases with advanced diabetic eye disease where visual loss is due to recurrent vitreous haemorrhage which has failed to clear, or retinal detachment resulting from retinitis proliferans.

Rubeosis iridis is managed by early pan-retinal photocoagulation.

OTHER CAUSES OF VISUAL LOSS IN PEOPLE WITH DIABETES

Around 50% of visual loss in people with type 2 diabetes is due to causes other than diabetic retinopathy. These include cataract, age-related macular degeneration, retinal vein occlusion, retinal arterial occlusion, non-arteritic ischaemic optic neuropathy and glaucoma. Some of these conditions are to be expected in this group as they relate to cardiovascular risk factors (e.g. hypertension, hyperlipidaemia, smoking) which are prevalent in people with type 2 diabetes.

Cataract

Cataract is a permanent lens opacity and is the most common cause of visual deterioration in the elderly population. The lens thickens and opacifies with age, and the increased metabolic insult to the lens in people with diabetes causes these changes to accelerate and occur prematurely.

Very rarely, a type of cataract specific to diabetes, called a 'snow-flake' cataract, occurs in young patients with poorly controlled diabetes. This does not usually affect vision but tends to make fundal examination difficult.

The indications for cataract extraction are similar to those for the non-diabetic population and depend on the degree of visual impairment. An additional indication in diabetes is when adequate assessment of the fundus, or laser treatment to the retina, is prevented. The usual method of extraction is by phakoemulsification, with implantation of an intra-ocular lens.

DIABETIC NEPHROPATHY

Diabetic nephropathy is an important cause of morbidity and mortality, and is now among the most common causes of end-stage renal failure (ESRF) in developed countries. As it is found with other microvascular and macrovascular complications, management is frequently difficult and the benefits of prevention are substantial.

About 30% of patients with type 1 diabetes have developed diabetic nephropathy after 20 years, but the risk after this time falls to less than 1% per year, and from the outset the risk is not equal in all patients (Box 21.50). Epidemiological data have suggested that the overall incidence is declining as standards of glycaemic and blood pressure control have improved.

The pattern of progression of renal abnormalities in diabetes is shown schematically in Figure 21.17. Pathologically, the first changes (seen at the time of microalbuminuria) are thickening of the glomerular basement membrane and accumulation of matrix material in the mesangium. Subsequently, nodular deposits (Fig. 21.18) are characteristic, and glomerulosclerosis worsens (heavy proteinuria develops) until glomeruli are progressively lost and renal function deteriorates.

Diagnosis and screening

Microalbuminuria (Box 21.51) is an important indicator of risk of developing overt diabetic nephropathy, although it is also found in other conditions. It is therefore most reliable as an indicator of diabetic nephropathy within the first 10 years of type 1 diabetes (the majority will progress to overt nephropathy within a further 10 years), and less reliable in older patients with type 2 diabetes, in whom it may be accounted for by other diseases. In particular, the presence of microalbuminuria in patients with type 2 diabetes is associated with an increased risk of macrovascular

21.50 RISK FACTORS FOR DEVELOPING DIABETIC NEPHROPATHY
- Poor control of blood glucose
- Long duration of diabetes
- Presence of other microvascular complications
- Ethnicity (e.g. Asian races, Pima Indians)
- Pre-existing hypertension
- Family history of diabetic nephropathy
- Family history of hypertension

21

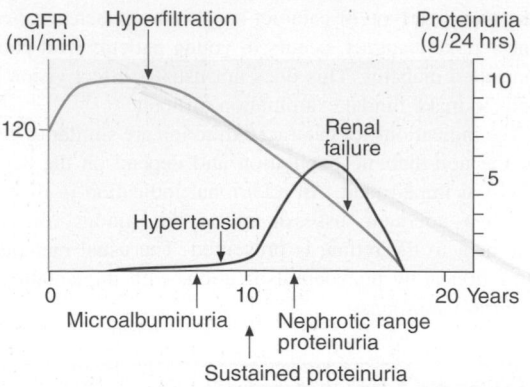

Fig. 21.17 Natural history of diabetic nephropathy. In the first few years of type 1 diabetes mellitus there is hyperfiltration which declines fairly steadily to return to a normal value at approximately 10 years (blue line). After about 10 years there is sustained proteinuria and by approximately 14 years it has reached the nephrotic range (red line). Renal function continues to decline, with the end stage being reached at approximately 16 years.

21

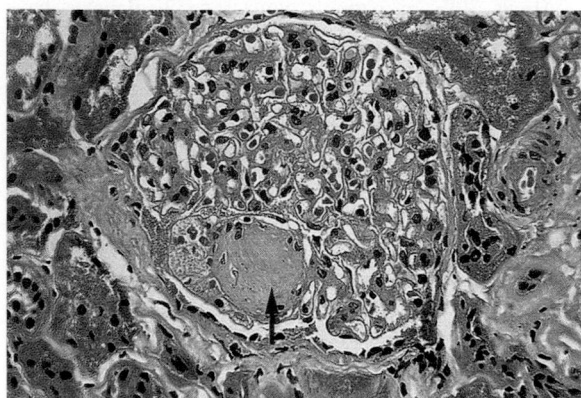

Fig. 21.18 Nodular diabetic glomerulosclerosis. There is thickening of basement membranes and mesangial expansion, and a Kimmelstiel–Wilson nodule (arrow).

21.51 SCREENING FOR MICROALBUMINURIA

- Identifies nephropathy in type 1 and type 2 diabetes; independent predictor of macrovascular disease in type 2 diabetes
- Risk factors include increased blood pressure, poor glycaemic control, smoking
- Random urine sample can estimate urinary albumin:creatinine ratio (3–30 mg/mmol (27–270 µg/mg)) (abnormal values: male > 2.5, female > 3.5)
- If possible confirm with an albumin excretion rate (AER) of 20–200 µg/min (30–300 mg/24 hrs); requires timed collection of urine (overnight or 24 hrs)

Who to screen

- Patients with type 1 diabetes annually from 5 years after diagnosis
- Patients with type 2 diabetes annually from time of diagnosis

Abnormal tests

- Exclude recent (24 hrs) vigorous exercise, fever, heart failure, urine infection, prostatitis, menstruation
- Confirm observation twice within 3–6 months
- Look for blood pressure above target levels

---

disease. Progressively increasing albuminuria, or albuminuria accompanied by hypertension, is much more likely to be due to early diabetic nephropathy.

Management

If there is evidence of incipient nephropathy, vigorous efforts should be made to reduce the risk of progression by:

- improved control of blood glucose
- aggressive reduction of blood pressure
  —institution of angiotensin-converting enzyme inhibitor (ACE-I) therapy (Box 21.52)
  —aggressive cardiovascular risk factor reduction (Box 21.53).

ACE inhibitors have been shown to provide greater benefit than equal blood pressure reduction achieved with other drugs (p. 613). Recent studies have shown similar benefits from angiotensin II receptor antagonists in patients with type 2 diabetes (Box 21.54). There may be particular problems with the use of either in diabetic nephropathy because of hyperkalaemia (p. 434) and renal artery stenosis (p. 496). Non-dihydropyridine calcium antagonists (diltiazem, verapamil) may be suitable alternatives in these circumstances.

Diabetic control becomes difficult as renal impairment progresses. Treatment with metformin should be abandoned when creatinine is higher than 150 µmol/l (1.7 mg/dl) as the risk of lactic acidosis is increased. Long-acting sulphonylureas should be replaced by short-acting agents that are metabolised rather than excreted.

Renal replacement therapy (p. 491) may benefit diabetic patients at an earlier stage than other patients with ESRF, although it may carry additional difficulties. Renal

---

EBM

21.52 ANGIOTENSIN-CONVERTING ENZYME INHIBITORS IN MICROALBUMINURIA

'In patients with type 1 diabetes and microalbuminuria, ACE inhibitor treatment reduced the progression to established proteinuria by 69%, regardless of whether blood pressure was elevated or not.'

- Microalbuminuria Captopril Study Group. Diabetologia 1996; 39:587–593.

EBM

21.53 MULTI-RISK FACTOR INTERVENTION IN TYPE 2 DIABETES

'In type 2 patients with microalbuminuria, intensive treatment (including control of glycaemia and hypertension, with use of ACE inhibitors, statins and aspirin) reduced the risk of cardiovascular disease by 53%, of nephropathy by 61%, and of retinopathy by 58% compared with conventional treatment.'

- Gaede P, et al. N Engl J Med 2003; 348:383–393.

EBM

21.54 ANGIOTENSIN RECEPTOR BLOCKERS IN MICROALBUMINURIA

'In type 2 patients with microalbuminuria, angiotensin receptor blockers reduced the development of persistent proteinuria from 15% to 5%. ACE inhibitors have similar benefits.'

- Parving HH, et al. N Engl J Med 2001; 345:870–878.

transplantation can dramatically improve the life of many, although macrovascular disease causing cardiac failure and peripheral vascular disease, and microvascular disease causing neuropathy and retinopathy show continued progression. The progression of recurrent diabetic nephropathy in the allograft is usually too slow to be a serious problem. Coronary heart disease is the major cause of death. Pancreatic transplantation (generally carried out at the same time as renal transplantation) can produce insulin independence and can slow or reverse microvascular disease, but the supply of organs is very limited and this is available to few. For further information on management, see Chapter 17.

DIABETIC NEUROPATHY

This is a relatively early and common complication affecting approximately 30% of diabetic patients. Although in a few patients it can cause severe disability, it is symptomless in the majority. Like retinopathy, it occurs secondary to metabolic disturbance, and prevalence is related to the duration of diabetes and the degree of metabolic control. Although there is evidence that the central nervous system is affected in long-term diabetes, the clinical impact of diabetes is mainly manifest in the peripheral nervous system.

The main pathological features are listed in Box 21.55. They can occur in motor, sensory and autonomic nerves.

Classification

Various classifications of diabetic neuropathy have been proposed. One is shown in Box 21.56 but motor, sensory and autonomic nerves may be involved in varying combinations so that clinically mixed syndromes usually occur.

21.55 DIABETIC NEUROPATHY: HISTOPATHOLOGY

- Axonal degeneration of both myelinated and unmyelinated fibres
   Early: axon shrinkage
   Later: axonal fragmentation; regeneration
- Thickening of Schwann cell basal lamina
- Patchy, segmental demyelination
- Thickening of basement membrane and microthrombi in intraneural capillaries

21.56 CLASSIFICATION OF DIABETIC NEUROPATHY

Somatic

- Polyneuropathy
   Symmetrical, mainly sensory and distal
   Asymmetrical, mainly motor and proximal (including amyotrophy)
- Mononeuropathy (including mononeuritis multiplex)

Visceral (autonomic)

- Cardiovascular
- Gastrointestinal
- Genitourinary
- Sudomotor
- Vasomotor
- Pupillary

Clinical features

Symmetrical sensory polyneuropathy

This is frequently asymptomatic. The most common signs found on physical examination are diminished perception of vibration sensation distally, 'glove-and-stocking' impairment of all other modalities of sensation, and loss of tendon reflexes in the lower limbs. Sensory abnormalities dominate the clinical presentation. Symptoms include paraesthesiae in the feet and, rarely, in the hands, pain in the lower limbs (dull, aching and/or lancinating, worse at night, and mainly felt on the anterior aspect of the legs), burning sensations in the soles of the feet, cutaneous hyperaesthesia and an abnormal gait (commonly wide-based), often associated with a sense of numbness in the feet. Muscle weakness and wasting develop only in advanced cases, but subclinical motor nerve dysfunction is common. The toes may be clawed with wasting of the interosseous muscles, which results in increased pressure on the plantar aspects of the metatarsal heads with the development of callus skin at these and other pressure points. Electrophysiological tests (p. 1153) demonstrate slowing of both motor and sensory conduction, and tests of vibration sensitivity and thermal thresholds are abnormal.

A diffuse small-fibre neuropathy causes altered perception of pain and temperature and is associated with symptomatic autonomic neuropathy; characteristic features include foot ulcers and Charcot neuroarthropathy.

Asymmetrical motor diabetic neuropathy

Sometimes called diabetic amyotrophy, this presents as severe and progressive weakness and wasting of the proximal muscles of the lower (and occasionally the upper) limbs. It is commonly accompanied by severe pain, mainly felt on the anterior aspect of the leg, and hyperaesthesia and paraesthesiae. Sometimes there may also be marked loss of weight ('neuropathic cachexia'). The patient may look extremely ill and be unable to get out of bed. Tendon reflexes may be absent on the affected side(s). Sometimes there are extensor plantar responses and the cerebrospinal fluid protein is often raised. This condition is thought to involve acute infarction of the lower motor neurons of the lumbosacral plexus. Other lesions involving this plexus, such as neoplasms and lumbar disc disease, must be excluded. Although recovery usually occurs within 12 months, some deficits become permanent. Management is mainly supportive.

Mononeuropathy

Either motor or sensory function can be affected within a single peripheral or cranial nerve. Unlike the gradual progression of distal symmetrical and autonomic neuropathies, mononeuropathies are severe and of rapid onset; they eventually recover. The nerves most commonly affected are the 3rd and 6th cranial nerves, resulting in diplopia, and the femoral and sciatic nerves. Rarely, involvement of other single nerves results in paresis and paraesthesiae in the thorax and trunk (truncal radiculo-pathies).

Nerve compression palsies commonly affect the median nerve, giving the clinical picture of carpal tunnel syndrome, and less commonly the ulnar nerve. Lateral popliteal nerve compression occasionally causes foot drop.

Autonomic neuropathy

This is not necessarily associated with peripheral somatic neuropathy. Either parasympathetic or sympathetic nerves may be predominantly affected in one or more visceral system (Box 21.56). The symptoms and signs arising from autonomic neuropathy are listed in Box 21.57. Tests of autonomic function are listed in Box 21.58. The development of autonomic neuropathy is less clearly related to poor metabolic control than somatic neuropathy, and improved control rarely results in amelioration of symptoms. Within 10 years of developing overt symptoms of autonomic neuro-

pathy, 30–50% of patients are dead—many from sudden cardiorespiratory arrest, the cause of which is unknown. Patients with postural hypotension (a drop in systolic pressure of ≥ 20 mmHg on standing from the supine position) have the highest subsequent mortality.

Erectile dysfunction

Erectile failure (impotence) affects 30% of diabetic males and is often multifactorial. Although neuropathy and vascular causes are common, psychological factors, including depression, anxiety and reduced libido, may be partly responsible. Alcohol and antihypertensive drugs such as thiazide diuretics and β-adrenoceptor antagonists (β-blockers) may cause sexual dysfunction and, rarely, patients may have an endocrine cause such as testosterone deficiency or hyperprolactinaemia. For further information, see page 1200.

Management

Management of peripheral sensorimotor and autonomic neuropathies is outlined in Box 21.59.

THE DIABETIC FOOT

The foot is a frequent site for complications in patients with diabetes and for this reason foot care is particularly important.

Tissue necrosis in the feet is a common reason for hospital admission in diabetic patients. Such admissions tend to be prolonged and may end with amputation.

Aetiology

Foot ulceration occurs as a result of trauma (often trivial) in the presence of neuropathy and/or peripheral vascular disease (p. 601), with infection occurring as a secondary phenomenon following disruption of the protective epidermis. In most cases all three components are involved but sometimes neuropathy or ischaemia may predominate. The clinical features of these two types of foot are compared in Box 21.60. Ischaemia alone accounts for a minority of foot ulcers in diabetic patients, with most being either neuropathic or neuro-ischaemic in type.

The main factors involved in the development of foot ulceration are shown in Figure 21.19. The most common cause of ulceration is a plaque of callus skin beneath which tissue necrosis occurs. This eventually breaks through to the surface.

Management

The main components of medical management are listed in Box 21.61. Removal of callus skin with a scalpel is usually best done by a podiatrist who has specialist training and experience in diabetic foot problems. Effective treatment of local infection with appropriate antibiotics is essential, and may have to be continued for protracted periods; osteomyelitis may be extremely difficult to eradicate. Charcot neuroarthropathy with disorganisation of joints may cause serious deformity. Angiography may be necessary if the foot is ischaemic or ulcers are very slow to heal. Measures to improve glycaemic control may also promote healing.

21.57 CLINICAL FEATURES OF AUTONOMIC NEUROPATHY

Cardiovascular

- Postural hypotension
- Resting tachycardia
- Fixed heart rate

Gastrointestinal

- Dysphagia, due to oesophageal atony
- Abdominal fullness, nausea and vomiting, unstable glycaemia, due to delayed gastric emptying ('gastroparesis')
- Nocturnal diarrhoea ± faecal incontinence (p. 932)
- Constipation, due to colonic atony

Genitourinary

- Difficulty in micturition, urinary incontinence, recurrent infection, due to atonic bladder
- Erectile dysfunction and retrograde ejaculation

Sudomotor

- Gustatory sweating
- Nocturnal sweats without hypoglycaemia
- Anhidrosis; fissures in the feet

Vasomotor

- Feet feel cold, due to loss of skin vasomotor responses
- Dependent oedema, due to loss of vasomotor tone and increased vascular permeability
- Bullous formation

Pupillary

- Decreased pupil size
- Resistance to mydriatics
- Delayed or absent reflexes to light

21.58 TESTS OF CARDIOVASCULAR AUTONOMIC FUNCTION

Simple cardiovascular reflex tests

- Heart rate variation during deep breathing
- Heart rate response to standing
- Heart rate changes during the Valsalva manoeuvre
- Blood pressure response to standing
- Blood pressure response to sustained hand grip

Other tests

- Baroreflex sensitivity using power spectral analysis of heart rate
- Time-domain analysis of heart rate and blood pressure variations
- MIBG (meta-iodobenzylguanidine) scan of the heart

21

21.59 MANAGEMENT OPTIONS FOR PERIPHERAL SENSORIMOTOR AND AUTONOMIC NEUROPATHIES

Condition	Management
Pain and paraesthesiae from peripheral somatic neuropathies	Intensive insulin therapy (strict glycaemic control) Tricyclic antidepressants (amitriptyline, imipramine) Anticonvulsants (gabapentin, carbamazepine, phenytoin, pregabalin) Substance P depleter capsaicin—topical Opiates (tramadol, oxycodone) Membrane stabilisers (mexiletine, intravenous lidocaine) Antioxidant (α-lipoic acid)
Postural hypotension	Support stockings Fludrocortisone α-adrenoceptor agonist (midodrine) Non-steroidal anti-inflammatory drugs (NSAIDs)
Gastroparesis	Dopamine antagonists (metoclopramide, domperidone) Erythromycin
Diarrhoea (p. 869)	Loperamide Broad-spectrum antibiotics Clonidine Octreotide
Constipation	Stimulant laxatives (senna)
Atonic bladder	Intermittent self-catheterisation (p. 1199)
Excessive sweating	Anticholinergic drugs (propantheline, poldine) Clonidine Topical antimuscarinic agent (glycopyrrolate cream)
Erectile dysfunction (impotence)	Phosphodiesterase type 5 inhibitors (sildenafil, vardenafil, tadalafil)—oral Dopamine agonist (apomorphine)—sublingual Prostaglandin E1 (alprostadil)—injected into corpus cavernosum, or intra-urethral administration of pellets (MUSE) Vacuum tumescence devices Implanted penile prosthesis Psychological counselling; psychosexual therapy

21

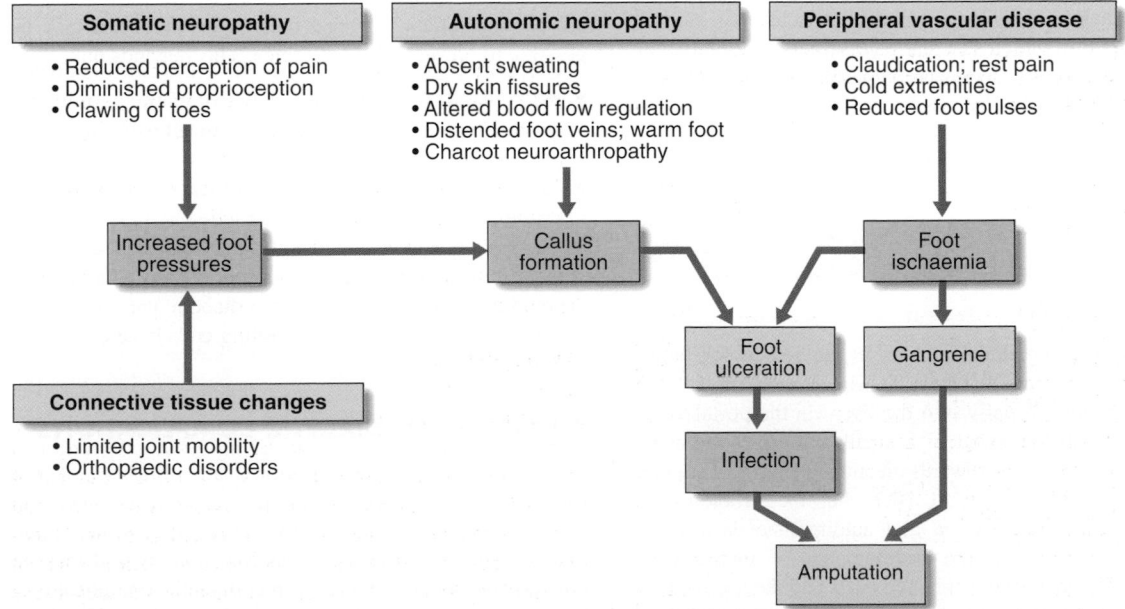

Fig. 21.19 Pathways leading to foot ulceration and amputation in diabetic foot disease. Inter-relationships of aetiological factors and principal clinical features are shown.

21.60 CLINICAL FEATURES OF THE DIABETIC FOOT

	Neuropathy	Ischaemia
Symptoms	None Paraesthesiae Pain Numbness	None Claudication Rest pain
Structural damage	Ulcer Sepsis Abscess Osteomyelitis Digital gangrene Charcot joint	Ulcer Sepsis Gangrene

21.61 MANAGEMENT OF DIABETIC FOOT ULCERS

- Remove callus skin
- Treat infection
- Avoid weight-bearing
- Ensure good glycaemic control
- Control oedema
- Undertake angiogram to assess feasibility of vascular reconstruction where indicated

21.62 DIABETIC FOOT: PRACTICE POINTS

- Prevention is the most effective way of dealing with the problem of tissue necrosis in the diabetic foot
- A podiatrist is an integral part of the diabetes team to ensure regular and effective podiatry and to educate patients in care of the feet
- Specially manufactured and fitted orthotic footware is required to prevent recurrence of ulceration and protect the feet of patients with Charcot neuroarthropathy

Amputation may be unavoidable if there is extensive tissue and/or bony destruction or intractable ischaemic pain at rest in a limb in which vascular reconstruction has failed or is impossible due to extensive large blood vessel disease. Further information is given on the management of peripheral arterial disease on page 603. Preventative measures are shown in Box 21.62.

PROSPECTS IN DIABETES MELLITUS

MANAGEMENT

There are exciting developments in the search for better methods of treating diabetes. Transplantation of isolated pancreatic islets (usually into the liver via the portal vein) has been safely achieved in a small number of humans. Progress is being made towards meeting the needs of supply, purification and storage of islets but the problems of bioincompatibility, rejection and autoimmune destruction remain. Nevertheless, the development of methods of inducing tolerance to transplanted islets and the use of stem cells or transformation of hepatocytes to make insulin by genetic engineering mean that this may still prove the most promising approach in the long term.

Whole pancreas transplantation presents particular problems relating to the exocrine pancreatic secretions, and long-term immunosuppression is necessary. While results are steadily improving, they remain less favourable than for renal transplantation. Xenotransplantation with a porcine pancreas may be an alternative approach. However, it is questionable whether it will ever be considered justifiable to perform transplantation in young diabetic patients before vascular disease is clinically apparent.

Alternative methods and routes of insulin delivery are being sought other than subcutaneous injection which has the disadvantage of delivering insulin into the systemic and not the portal circulation. A wider range of insulin analogues is being developed, inhaled insulin will soon be available commercially and other routes of delivery including oral and transcutaneous (utilising patch technology) are being explored. Several novel oral drugs are being evaluated, including dual PPAR $-\alpha/\gamma$ agonists that act like a thiazolidinedione and fibrate combined, a cannabinoid-receptor-1 inhibitor (rimonabant) and a soluble analogue of amylin, both of which combat obesity and diabetes.

PRIMARY PREVENTION OF DIABETES

From a public health standpoint the only cost-effective way of dealing with diabetes is to prevent it.

Type 2 diabetes is associated with an affluent lifestyle and is likely to arise in genetically predisposed individuals who eat too much and exercise too little. Effective health education has shown promising results in the primary prevention of type 2 diabetes, while screening for diabetes (particularly in high-risk groups such as the first-degree relatives of known cases) and more vigorous and early treatment of impaired glucose tolerance could reduce the incidence of serious vascular disease in these patients.

In type 1 diabetes, the fact that the islet insulin-secreting cells are destroyed slowly over several years before clinical presentation offers the hope that, in the future, it may be possible to prevent type 1 diabetes. This depends on:

- the availability of accurate, predictive markers for the development of clinical diabetes in genetically predisposed individuals
- an understanding of the precise sequence of events leading to pancreatic β-cell destruction
- the development of methods of intervention based on specifically targeted immunomodulation which could be applied early in the pre-diabetic period before most of the insulin-secreting cells have been destroyed.

TREATMENT OF DIABETIC COMPLICATIONS

Treatment with aminoguanidine, an inhibitor of the formation of advanced glycation end-products, has been shown to prevent damage to the retina, kidney, nerve and artery in diabetic animals. It has low toxicity and may be utilised for humans with chronic diabetic complications. Protein kinase C inhibitors have been shown to limit diabetic retinopathy and nephropathy in humans and are undergoing clinical trial.

FURTHER INFORMATION

Books and journal articles

De Fronzo R, Ferrannini E, Keen H, eds. International textbook of diabetes. 3rd edn. Chichester: John Wiley; 2004.

Fisher M, ed. Heart disease and diabetes. London: Martin Dunitz; 2003.

Frier BM, Fisher BM, eds. Hypoglycaemia in clinical diabetes. Chichester: John Wiley; 1999.

Pickup J, Williams G, eds. Textbook of diabetes. 3rd edn. Oxford: Blackwell Scientific; 2002.

Websites

www.cdc.gov/diabetes *Diabetes Public Health Resource*.

www.diabetes.org *American Diabetes Association*.

www.diabetes.org.uk *Diabetes UK*.

www.diabetologists-abcd.org.uk *Association of British Clinical Diabetologists*.

www.idf.org *International Diabetes Federation*.

www.jdrf.org *Juvenile Diabetes Research Foundation*.

www.joslin.org *Joslin Diabetes Center*.

www.mendosa.com/faq.htm *Online Diabetes Resources*.

www.ndei.org *National Diabetes Education Initiative*.

www.sign.ac.uk *Scottish Intercollegiate Guidelines Network*.

21

K.R. PALMER
I.D. PENMAN
S. PATERSON-BROWN

Alimentary tract and pancreatic disease

CLINICAL EXAMINATION OF THE GASTROINTESTINAL TRACT

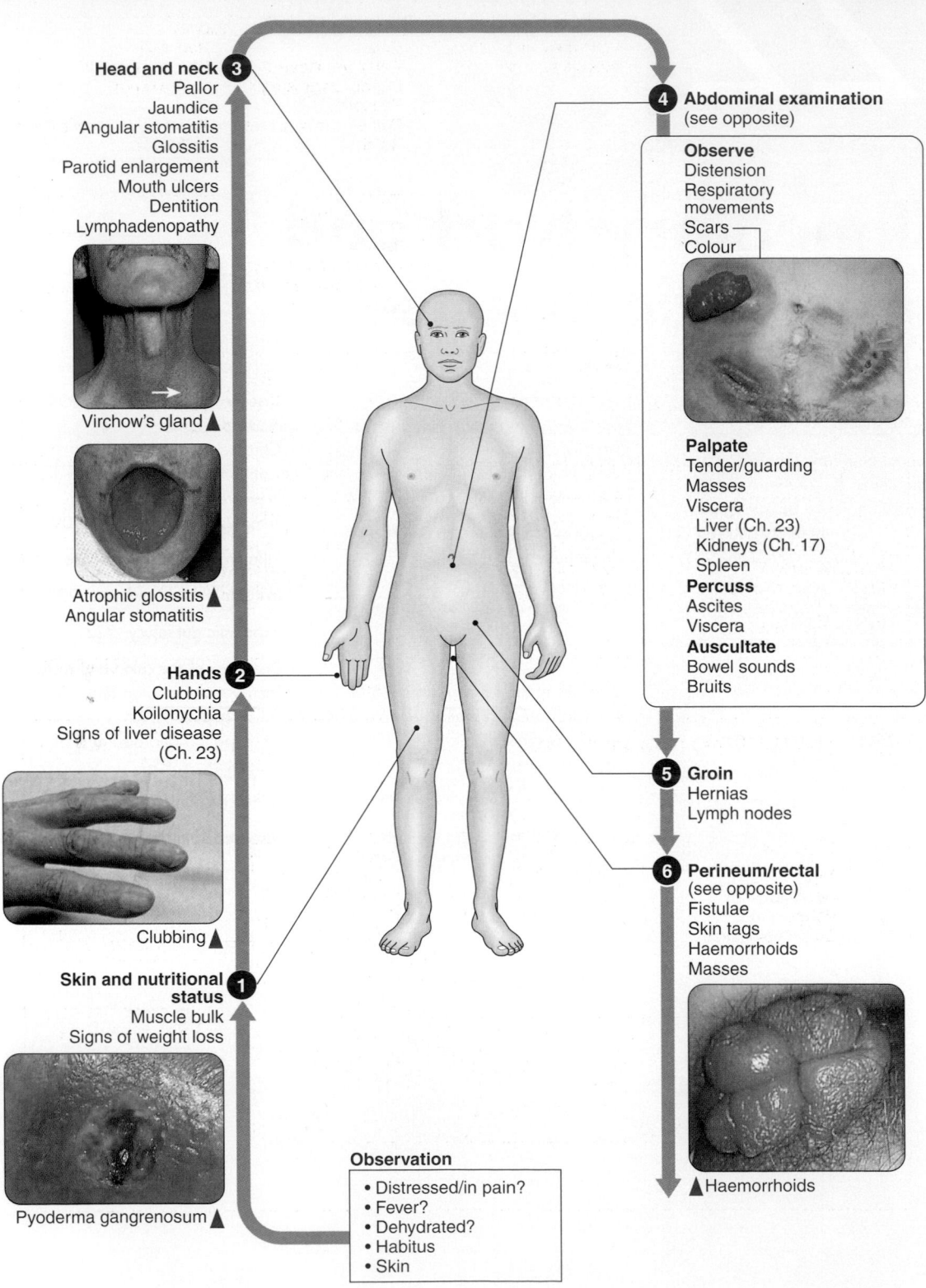

Head and neck 3
Pallor
Jaundice
Angular stomatitis
Glossitis
Parotid enlargement
Mouth ulcers
Dentition
Lymphadenopathy

Virchow's gland ▲

Atrophic glossitis ▲
Angular stomatitis

Hands 2
Clubbing
Koilonychia
Signs of liver disease
(Ch. 23)

Clubbing ▲

**Skin and nutritional
status 1**
Muscle bulk
Signs of weight loss

Pyoderma gangrenosum ▲

Observation
• Distressed/in pain?
• Fever?
• Dehydrated?
• Habitus
• Skin

4 Abdominal examination
(see opposite)

Observe
Distension
Respiratory
movements
Scars
Colour

Palpate
Tender/guarding
Masses
Viscera
  Liver (Ch. 23)
  Kidneys (Ch. 17)
  Spleen
Percuss
Ascites
Viscera
Auscultate
Bowel sounds
Bruits

5 Groin
Hernias
Lymph nodes

6 Perineum/rectal
(see opposite)
Fistulae
Skin tags
Haemorrhoids
Masses

▲ Haemorrhoids

4 ABDOMINAL EXAMINATION: POSSIBLE FINDINGS

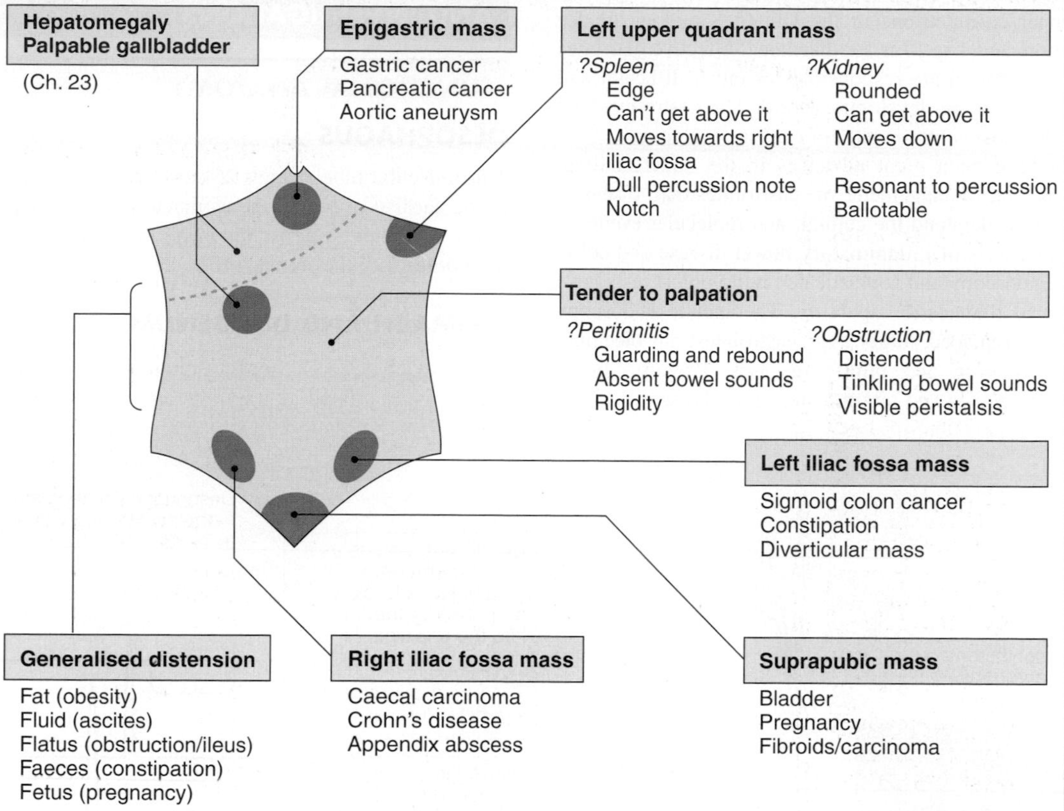

Hepatomegaly
Palpable gallbladder

(Ch. 23)

Epigastric mass

Gastric cancer
Pancreatic cancer
Aortic aneurysm

Left upper quadrant mass

?Spleen
   Edge
   Can't get above it
   Moves towards right
   iliac fossa
   Dull percussion note
   Notch

?Kidney
   Rounded
   Can get above it
   Moves down

   Resonant to percussion
   Ballotable

Tender to palpation

?Peritonitis
   Guarding and rebound
   Absent bowel sounds
   Rigidity

?Obstruction
   Distended
   Tinkling bowel sounds
   Visible peristalsis

Left iliac fossa mass

Sigmoid colon cancer
Constipation
Diverticular mass

Generalised distension

Fat (obesity)
Fluid (ascites)
Flatus (obstruction/ileus)
Faeces (constipation)
Fetus (pregnancy)

Right iliac fossa mass

Caecal carcinoma
Crohn's disease
Appendix abscess

Suprapubic mass

Bladder
Pregnancy
Fibroids/carcinoma

22

6 RECTAL EXAMINATION: COMMON FINDINGS

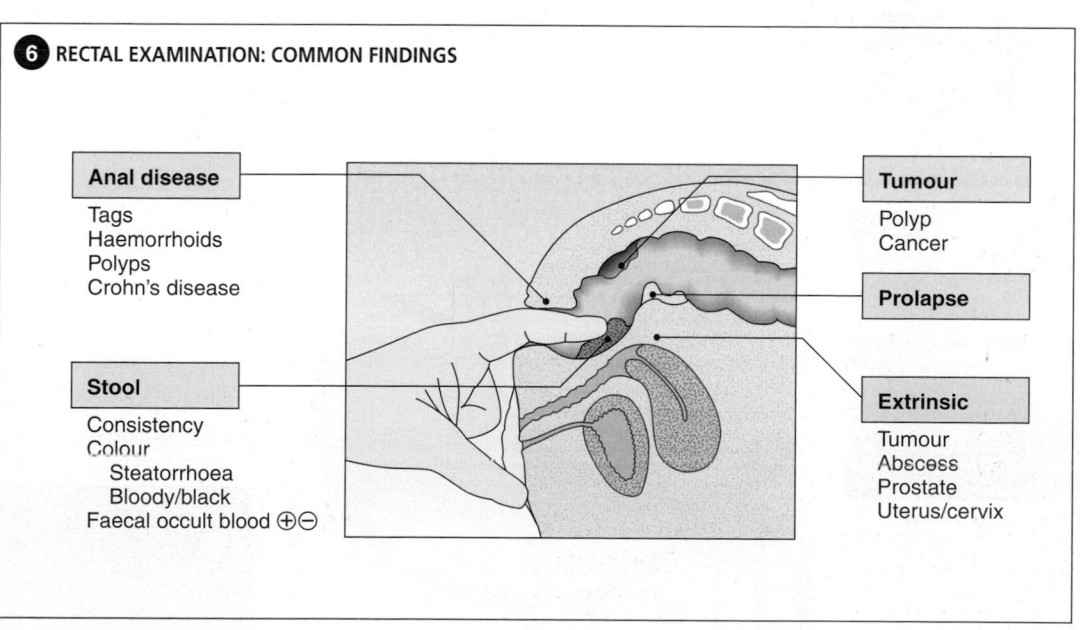

Anal disease

Tags
Haemorrhoids
Polyps
Crohn's disease

Stool

Consistency
Colour
   Steatorrhoea
   Bloody/black
Faecal occult blood ⊕⊖

Tumour

Polyp
Cancer

Prolapse

Extrinsic

Tumour
Abscess
Prostate
Uterus/cervix

Diseases of the gastrointestinal tract are a major cause of morbidity and mortality. Approximately 10% of all general practitioner consultations in the United Kingdom are for indigestion, and 1 in 14 is for diarrhoea. Infective diarrhoea and malabsorption are responsible for much ill health and many deaths in the developing world. The gastrointestinal tract is the most common site for cancer development.

There have been great advances in the understanding, diagnosis and management of gastrointestinal diseases. We largely understand the cellular and molecular events in the pathogenesis of inflammatory bowel disease and colon cancer. Endoscopy and sophisticated radiological tests have transformed diagnostic capability. Therapeutic endoscopy has largely replaced surgery for gastrointestinal bleeding, tumour palliation and biliary diseases. Powerful drugs alleviate dyspepsia and inflammatory bowel disease.

FUNCTIONAL ANATOMY, PHYSIOLOGY AND INVESTIGATIONS

FUNCTIONAL ANATOMY

OESOPHAGUS

This muscular tube extends 25 cm from the cricoid cartilage to the cardiac orifice of the stomach. It has an upper and a lower sphincter. A peristaltic swallowing wave propels the food bolus into the stomach (Fig. 22.1).

STOMACH AND DUODENUM (Fig. 22.2)

The stomach acts as a 'hopper', retaining and grinding food, then actively propelling it into the upper small bowel.

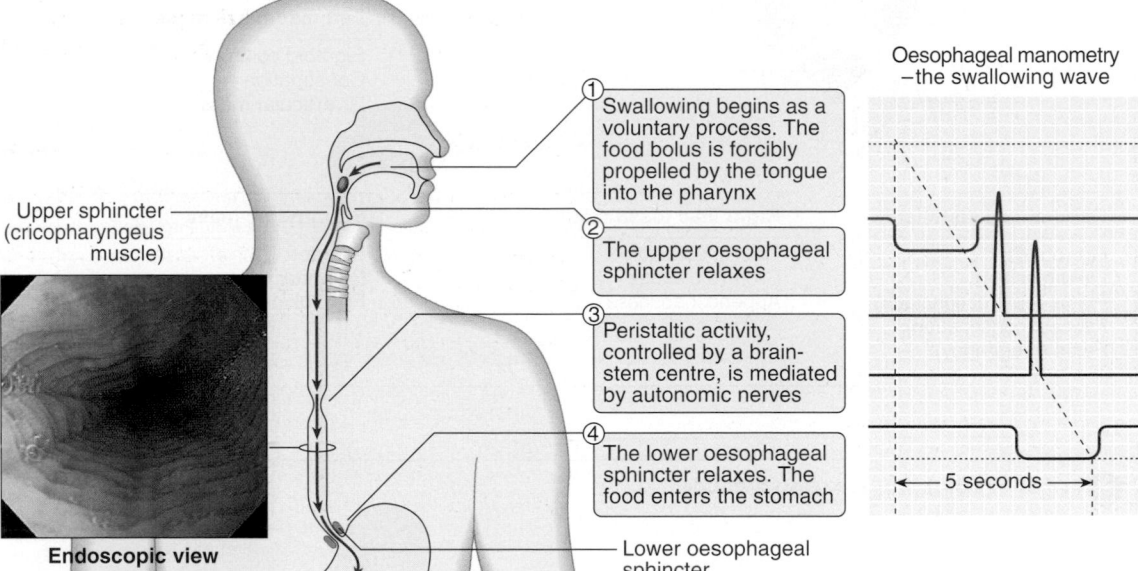

Fig. 22.1 **The oesophagus: anatomy and function.** The swallowing wave.

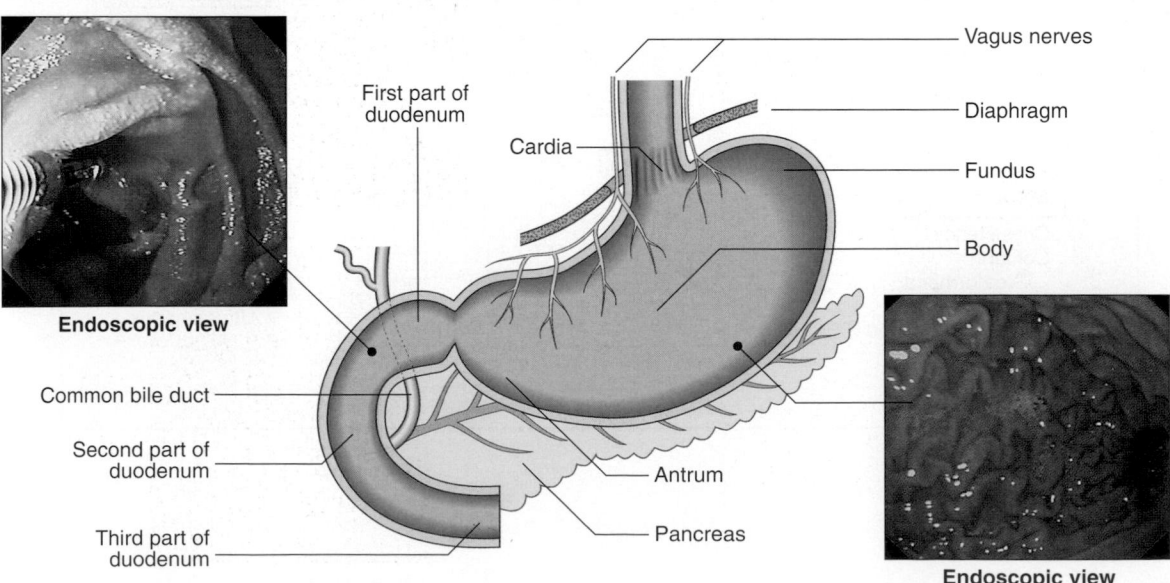

Fig. 22.2 Normal gastric and duodenal anatomy.

Enterochromaffin-like (ECL) cell

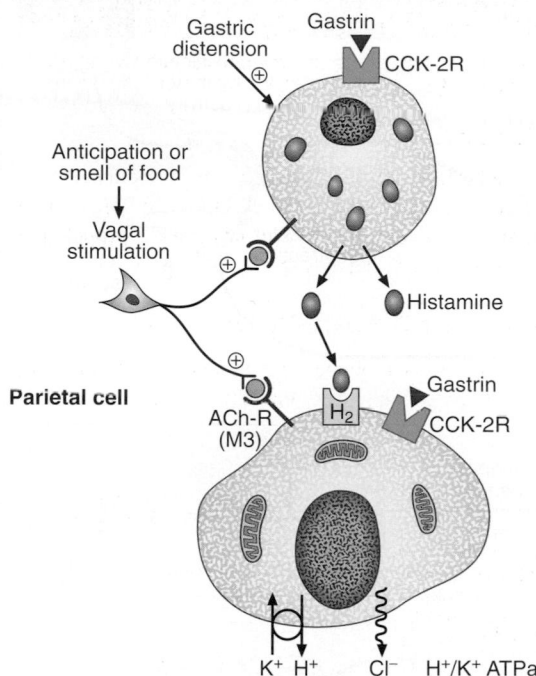

Fig. 22.3   Control of acid secretion. Gastrin released from antral G cells in response to food stimulates histamine release from ECL cells by binding to cholecystokinin (CCK-2) receptors. These are also present on parietal cells. Histamine binds to H_2 receptors on parietal cells and, ultimately, hydrogen ions are secreted in exchange for potassium ions from the apical membrane. Chloride ions passively diffuse to maintain electroneutrality. Cholinergic (vagal) activity and gastric distension also stimulate acid secretion; somatostatin, vasoactive intestinal polypeptide (VIP) and gastric inhibitory polypeptide (GIP) inhibit it.

Gastric secretion

Hydrogen ions, accompanied by chloride ions, are secreted in response to the activity of the hydrogen-potassium ATPase ('proton pump') from the apical membrane of the parietal cells (Fig. 22.3). Acid sterilises the upper gastrointestinal tract and converts pepsinogen to pepsin. Pepsinogen is secreted by chief cells. The glycoprotein intrinsic factor, secreted in parallel with acid, is necessary for vitamin B_{12} absorption.

Gastrin and somatostatin

The hormone gastrin is produced by G cells in the antrum. Somatostatin is secreted from D cells throughout the stomach. Gastrin stimulates whilst somatostatin suppresses acid secretion.

Protective factors

Bicarbonate ions and mucus together protect the gastro-duodenal mucosa from the ulcerative properties of acid and pepsin.

SMALL INTESTINE

The small bowel extends from the ligament of Treitz to the ileocaecal valve (Fig. 22.4). In the fasted state, muscular activity is absent for at least 80% of the time. Every 1–2 hours a wave of peristaltic activity, called the migrating motor complex, passes down the small bowel. Entry of food into the gastrointestinal tract stimulates small bowel peristaltic activity.

Functions of the small intestine are:

- digestion
- absorption—the products of digestion, water, electrolytes and vitamins

22

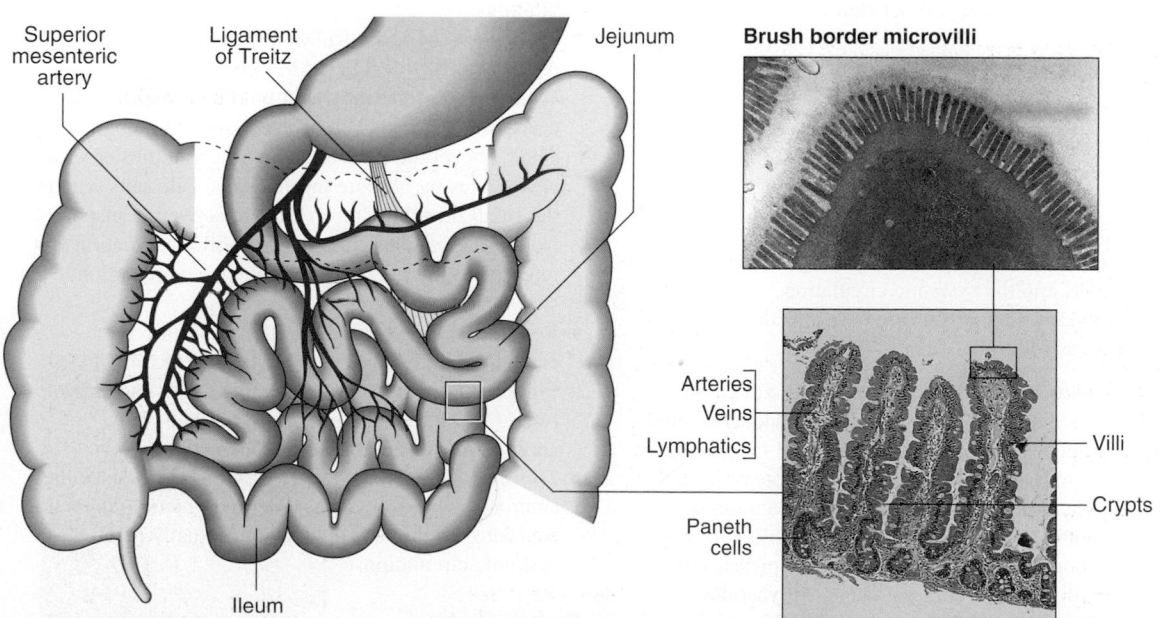

Fig. 22.4   Small intestine: anatomy. Epithelial cells are formed in crypts and differentiate as they migrate to the tip of the villi to form enterocytes (absorptive cells) and goblet cells.

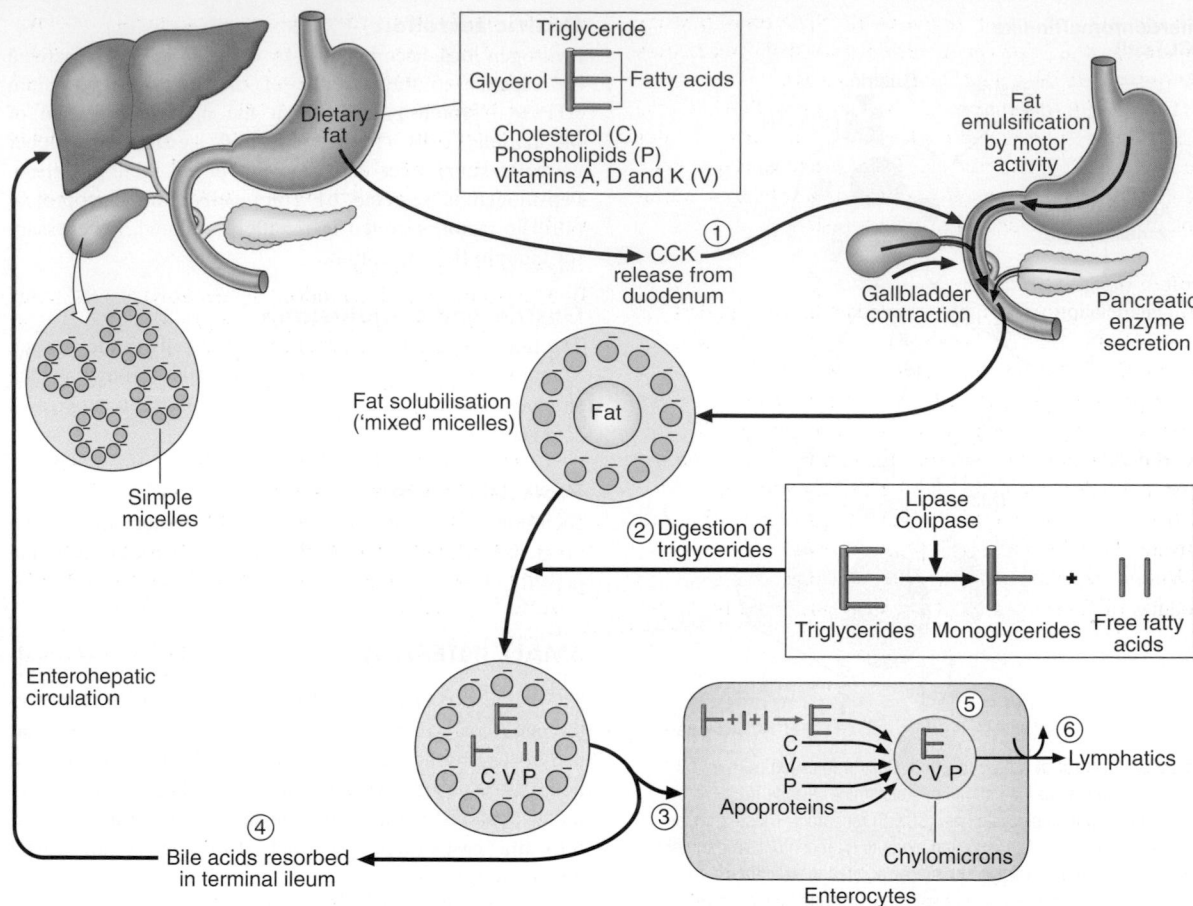

Fig. 22.5 Fat digestion.

- protection against ingested toxins—immunological, mechanical, enzymatic and peristaltic.

Digestion and absorption

Fat (Fig. 22.5)

Dietary lipids comprise long chain triglycerides, cholesterol esters, lecithin and the fat-soluble vitamins A, D, K and E. Lipids are insoluble in water and undergo lipolysis and incorporation into mixed micelles before they can be absorbed into enterocytes where they are processed and pass via lymphatics into the systemic circulation.

Fat absorption and digestion are best considered as a step-wise process as follows:

- *Luminal phase* (Fig. 22.5, step 1). Fatty acids cause cholecystokinin (CCK) release from the duodenum and upper jejunum. CCK stimulates release of the pancreatic enzymes amylase, lipase, colipase and proteases. CCK also stimulates gallbladder contraction and promotes sphincter of Oddi relaxation, resulting in bile inflow to the small bowel. Pancreatic lipase, in the presence of its cofactor colipase, cleaves long chain triglycerides, yielding fatty acids and monoglycerides (Fig. 22.5, step 2). These are solubilised by interacting with bile salts and phospholipids to form mixed micelles. Mixed

micelles also contain cholesterol and fat-soluble vitamins.
- *Absorption*. Mixed micelles diffuse to the brush border of the enterocytes (Fig. 22.5, step 3). Long chain fatty acids there bind to fatty acid-binding proteins and are transported into the cell. Cholesterol, short chain fatty acids, phospholipids and fat-soluble vitamins enter the enterocytes by obscure mechanisms. Bile salts remain in the small intestinal lumen and are actively transported from the terminal ileum into the portal circulation and returned to the liver (the enterohepatic circulation, step 4).
- *Re-esterification* (Fig. 22.5, step 5). Within the enterocyte, fatty acids are re-esterified to form triglycerides. Triglycerides combine with cholesterol ester, fat-soluble vitamins, phospholipids and apoproteins to form chylomicrons.
- *Transport* (Fig. 22.5, step 6). Chylomicrons leave the enterocytes by exocytosis, enter mesenteric lymphatics, pass into the thoracic duct, and eventually reach the systemic circulation.

Carbohydrates

Dietary carbohydrate largely comprises the polysaccharide starch, some sucrose and lactose. Starch is hydrolysed by salivary and pancreatic amylases to alpha-limit dextrins containing 4–8 glucose molecules; to the disaccharide maltose; and to the trisaccharide maltotriose.

Disaccharides are digested by enzymes fixed to the microvillous membrane to form the monosaccharides glucose, galactose and fructose. Glucose and galactose enter the cell by an energy-requiring process involving a carrier protein. Fructose enters by simple diffusion.

Protein (Fig. 22.6)

Intragastric digestion by pepsin is quantitatively modest but nevertheless important because the resulting polypeptides and amino acids stimulate CCK release from the mucosa of the proximal jejunum. CCK stimulates secretion of the proenzymes trypsinogen, chymotrypsinogen, proelastases and procarboxypeptidases from the pancreas. On exposure to brush border enterokinase, inert trypsinogen is converted to the active proteolytic enzyme trypsin. Trypsin then activates the other pancreatic proenzymes.

Within the intestinal lumen, trypsin digests proteins to produce oligopeptides, peptides and amino acids. Oligo-peptides are further hydrolysed by brush border enzymes to yield dipeptides, tripeptides and amino acids. These small peptides and the amino acids are actively transported into the enterocytes where intracellular peptidases further digest peptides to amino acids. Intracellular amino acids are actively transported across the basal cell membrane of the enterocyte into the portal circulation and thence to the liver.

Water and electrolytes

Both absorption and secretion of electrolytes and water occur throughout the intestine. Net transport is the difference between absorption and secretion; in health, absorption predominates. Electrolytes and water are transported by two pathways:

- *the paracellular route*, in which passive flow through tight junctions between cells is a consequence of osmotic, electrical or hydrostatic gradients
- *the transcellular route* across apical and basolateral membranes by energy-requiring specific active transport carriers (pumps).

22

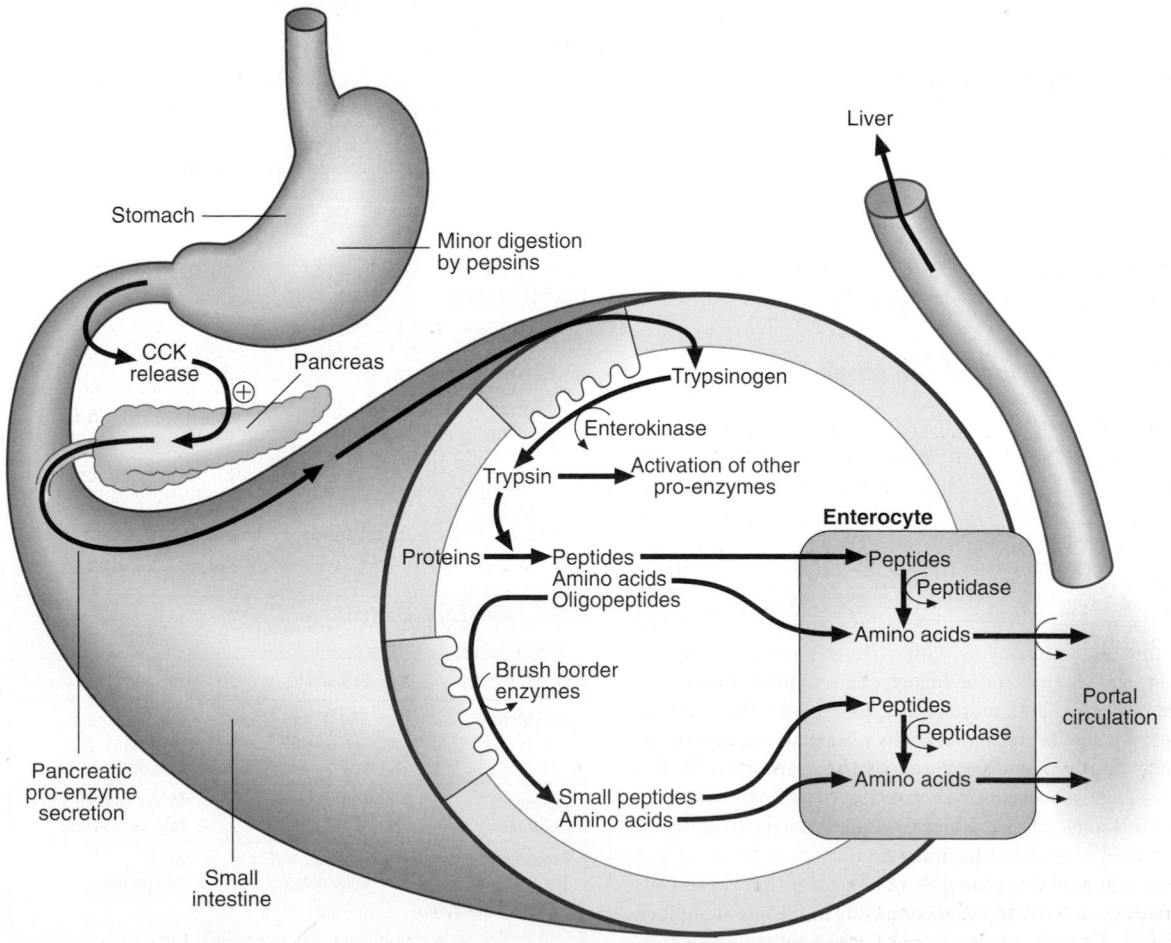

Fig. 22.6 Protein digestion.

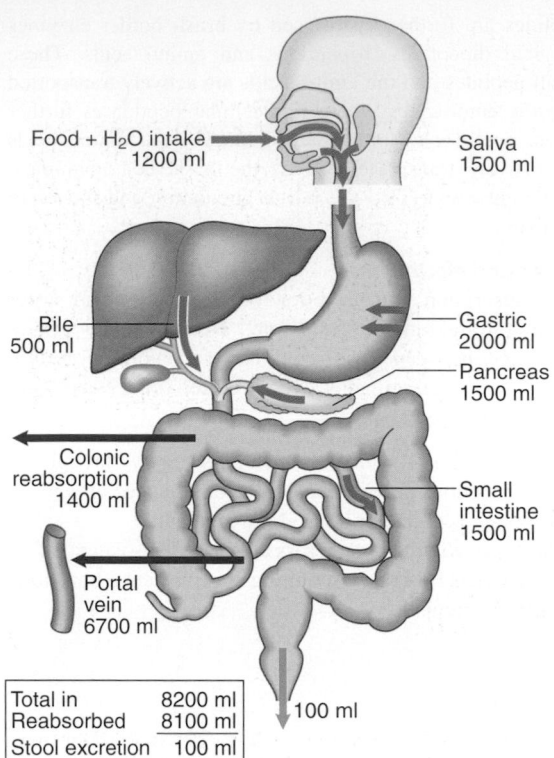

Food + H₂O intake 1200 ml
Saliva 1500 ml
Bile 500 ml
Gastric 2000 ml
Pancreas 1500 ml
Colonic reabsorption 1400 ml
Small intestine 1500 ml
Portal vein 6700 ml
100 ml

Total in	8200 ml
Reabsorbed	8100 ml
Stool excretion	100 ml

Fig. 22.7   Fluid homeostasis in the gastrointestinal tract.

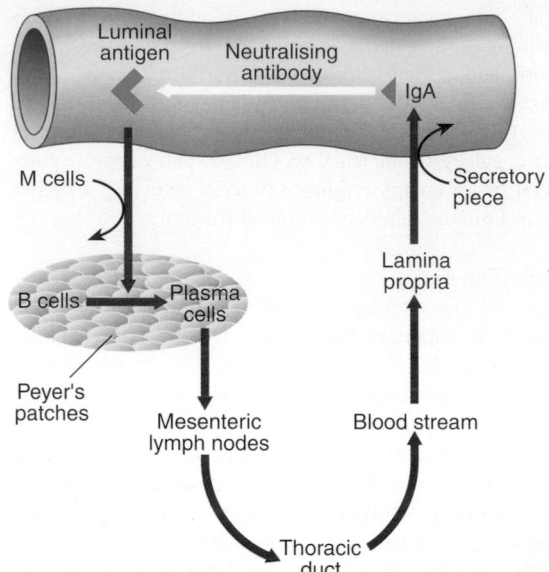

Fig. 22.8   Migration of gut lymphoid tissue in response to antigen exposure.

Fluid balance is carefully maintained and, of the 8 litres of fluid entering the gastrointestinal tract daily, only 100 ml is normally excreted in stools (Fig. 22.7).

Vitamins and trace elements
Water-soluble vitamins are absorbed throughout the intestine. The absorption of folic acid, vitamin B_{12}, calcium and iron is described on pages 1027–1029.

Protective function of the small intestine

Immunology
B and T lymphocytes, macrophages and mast cells are found throughout the gastrointestinal mucosa. Mucosa-associated lymphoid tissue (MALT) constitutes 25% of the total lymphatic tissue of the body.

Luminal macromolecules and viral particles are transported by specialised (M) cells to Peyer's patches (Fig. 22.8). These comprise lymphoid follicles with a well-defined structure. B lymphocytes within Peyer's patches differentiate to plasma cells following exposure to the antigens, and these cells migrate to mesenteric lymph nodes, thence to the blood stream via the thoracic duct and then return to the lamina propria of the gut, bronchial tree and other lymph nodes. They subsequently release IgA which is transported into the lumen of the intestine after linkage to secretory piece. This neutralises the antigen.

The role of T lymphocytes is less clear, but these cells probably help localise the plasma cells to the site of antigen exposure as well as producing inflammatory mediators. Macrophages phagocytose foreign materials and secrete a

range of cytokines which mediate inflammation. Activation of mast cell surface IgE receptors leads to degranulation and release of other molecules involved in inflammation.

Mucosal barrier
The epithelium of the gastrointestinal tract constitutes a barrier to luminal contents. This barrier comprises mucus, secreted by goblet cells, the membranes of the enterocytes and the tight junctions between them. These cells are constantly renewed, those of the small intestine every 48 hours.

PANCREAS

The exocrine pancreas (Box 22.1) is necessary for the digestion of fat, protein and carbohydrate. Inactive pro-enzymes are secreted from acinar cells in response to circulating gastrointestinal hormones (Fig. 22.9) and are then activated by trypsin. Bicarbonate-rich fluid is secreted from ductular cells to produce an optimum alkaline pH for enzyme activity.

22.1 PANCREATIC ENZYMES		
Enzyme	**Substrate**	**Product**
Amylase	Starch and glycogen	Limit dextrans Maltose Maltriose
Lipase Colipase	Triglycerides	Monoglycerides and free fatty acids
Proteolytic enzymes Trypsinogen Chymotrypsinogen Proelastase Procarboxypeptidases	Proteins and polypeptides	Short polypeptides

22

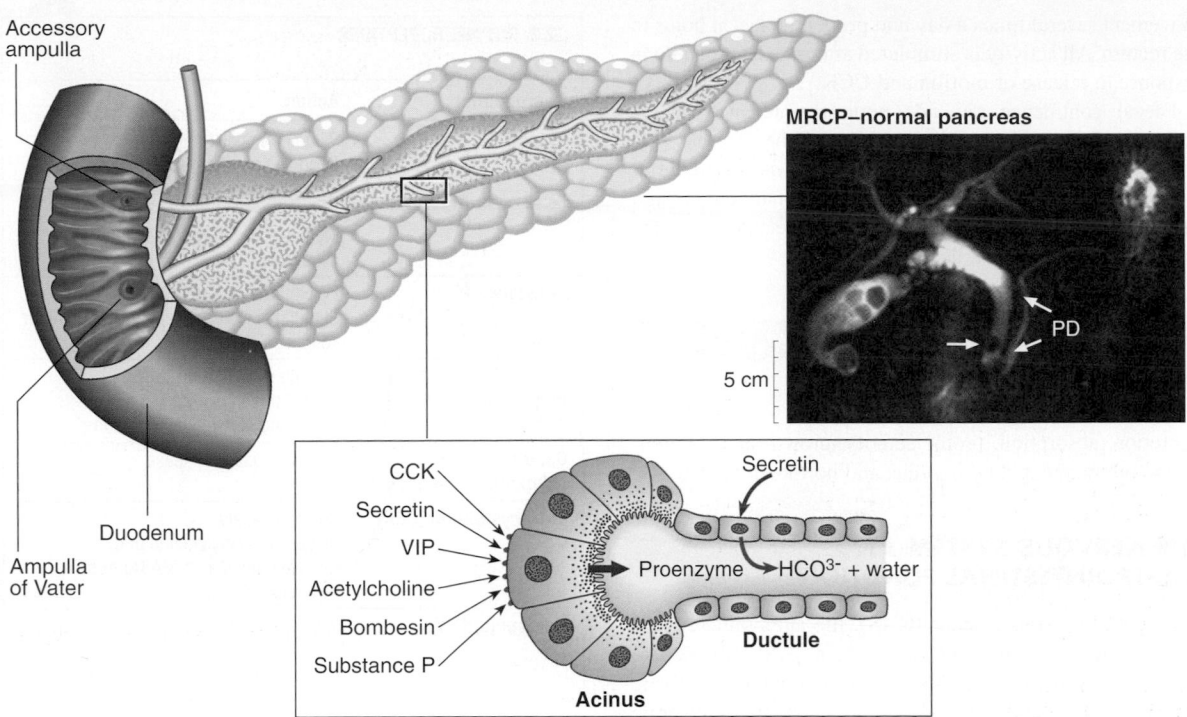

Fig. 22.9 Pancreatic structure and function. Ductular cells secrete alkaline fluid in response to secretin. Acinar cells secrete digestive enzymes from zymogen granules in response to a range of secretagogues. The photograph shows a normal pancreatic duct (PD) and side branches as defined at magnetic resonance cholangiopancreatography (MRCP). Note the incidental calculi in the gallbladder and common bile duct (arrow).

22

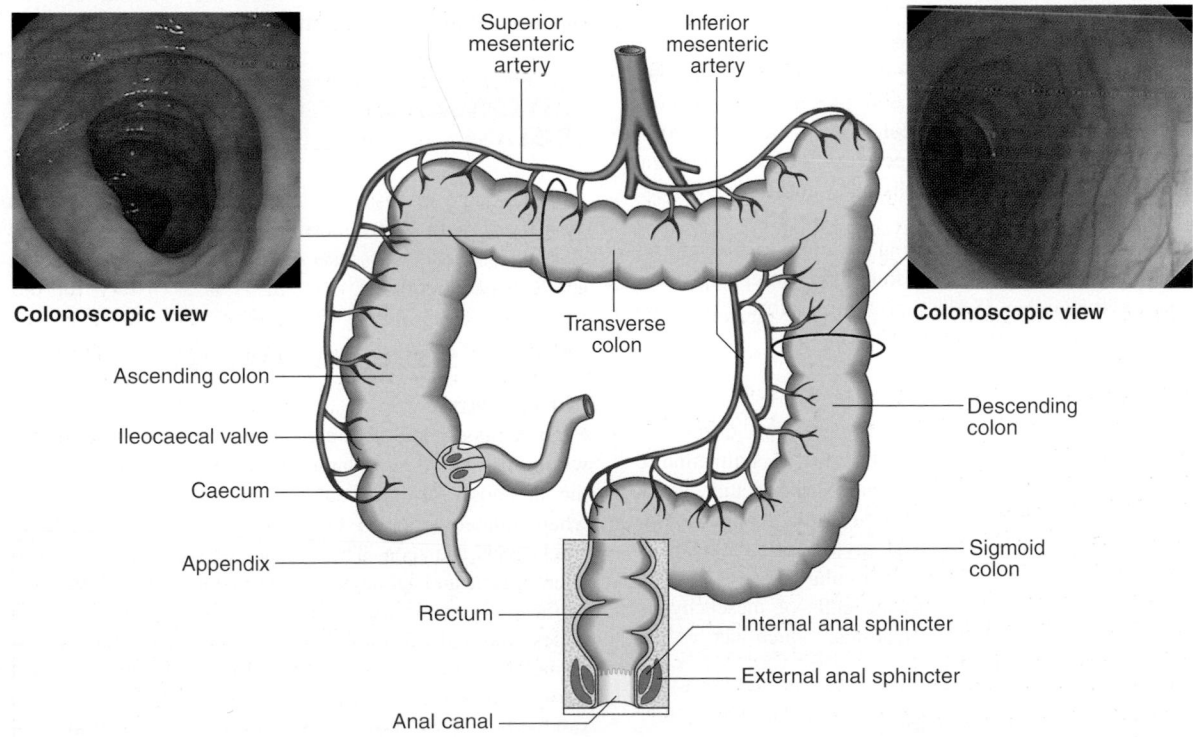

Fig. 22.10 The normal colon, rectum and anal canal.

COLON

The colon (Fig. 22.10) absorbs water and electrolytes. It also acts as a storage organ and has contractile activity. Two types of contraction occur. The first of these is segmentation (ring contraction), which leads to mixing but not propulsion; this facilitates absorption of water and electrolytes. Propulsive (peristaltic contraction) waves cause mass movement several times a day and propel the faecal bolus to the rectum. All activity is stimulated after meals, probably in response to release of motilin and CCK.

Faecal continence depends upon maintenance of the anorectal angle and tonic contraction of the external anal sphincters. Relaxation of these muscles, increased intra-abdominal pressure from a Valsalva manoeuvre and contraction of abdominal muscles, with relaxation of the anal sphincters, result in defecation.

CONTROL OF GASTROINTESTINAL FUNCTION

Secretion, absorption, motor activity, growth and differentiation are modulated by nervous and hormonal factors.

THE NERVOUS SYSTEM AND GASTROINTESTINAL FUNCTION

The central nervous system (CNS), the autonomic system (ANS) and the enteric nervous system (ENS) interact to regulate gut function. The ANS comprises: parasympathetic pathways (vagal and sacral efferent), which are cholinergic and generally increase smooth muscle tone and promote sphincter relaxation; and sympathetic pathways, which release noradrenaline (norepinephrine), reduce smooth muscle tone and stimulate sphincter contraction.

The enteric nervous system

This comprises two major networks intrinsic to the gut wall. The myenteric (Auerbach's) plexus in the smooth muscle layer regulates motor control; and the submucosal (Meissner's) plexus exerts secretory control over the epithelium, enteroendocrine cells and submucosal vessels. Although connected centrally via the ANS, the ENS can function autonomously, using a variety of transmitters including acetylcholine, noradrenaline (norepinephrine), 5-hydroxytryptamine (5-HT, serotonin), nitric oxide and calcitonin gene-related peptide (CGRP).

Peristalsis

Peristalsis is a reflex triggered by gut wall distension, which consists of a wave of circular muscle contraction to propel contents from the oesophagus to the rectum. It can be influenced by innervation but functions independently. It results from a basic electrical rhythm originating from the interstitial cells of Cajal in the circular layer of intestinal smooth muscle. These are stellate cells of mesenchymal origin with smooth muscle features, which act as the 'pacemaker' of the gut.

Migrating motor complexes

Migrating motor complexes (MMC) are powerful waves of contraction spreading from the stomach to the ileum and occurring at a frequency of about 5 per minute every 90 minutes or so, between meals and during fasting. They may serve to sweep intestinal contents distally in preparation for the next meal and are inhibited by eating.

22.2 GUT NEUROPEPTIDES	
Neuropeptide	**Action**
Opioids	Pain perception Decrease motility, regulate sphincter activity Increase acid secretion Modulate electrolyte and water absorption
Substance P	Propagates peristaltic activity Stimulates lower oesophageal sphincter Pain modulation
Vasoactive intestinal polypeptide (VIP)	Smooth muscle relaxation Vasodilatation Water and electrolyte secretion
Gastrin-releasing polypeptide (bombesin)	Mediates gastrin release
Cholecystokinin (CCK)	Controls satiety Release of acetylcholine and γ-aminobutyric acid (GABA) from myenteric plexus
Neuropeptide Y	Vasocontraction of splanchnic circulation Reduces small bowel secretions

GUT HORMONES

The origin, action and control of the major gut hormones, peptides and non-peptide signalling transmitters are summarised in Boxes 22.2 and 22.3.

INVESTIGATION OF GASTROINTESTINAL DISEASE

A wide range of tests are available for the investigation of patients with gastrointestinal symptoms. These can be classified broadly into tests of structure, tests of infection and tests of function.

TESTS OF STRUCTURE: IMAGING

Plain X-rays

Plain X-rays of the abdomen show the distribution of gas within the small and large intestines and are useful in the diagnosis of intestinal obstruction or paralytic ileus where dilated loops of bowel and (in the erect position) fluid levels are seen. The outlines of soft tissues such as liver, spleen and kidneys may be visible, and calcification of these organs as well as pancreas, blood vessels, lymph nodes and calculi may be detected. Abdominal X-rays do not help in cases of gastrointestinal bleeding. A chest X-ray shows the diaphragm, and erect films may detect subdiaphragmatic free air in cases of perforation. Unexpected pulmonary problems such as pleural effusions will also be revealed.

Contrast studies

Barium sulphate is inert and provides good mucosal coating and excellent opacification. It can, however, solidify and

22

22.3 GUT HORMONES

Hormone	Origin	Stimulus	Action
Gastrin	Stomach (G cell)	Products of protein digestion Suppressed by acid and somatostatin	Stimulates gastric acid secretion Stimulates growth of gastrointestinal mucosa
Somatostatin	Throughout GI tract (D cell)	Fat ingestion	Inhibits gastrin and insulin secretion Decreases acid secretion Decreases absorption Inhibits pancreatic secretion
CCK	Duodenum and jejunum (I cells); also ileal and colonic nerve endings	Products of protein digestion Fat and fatty acids Suppressed by trypsin	Stimulates pancreatic enzyme secretion Gallbladder contraction Sphincter of Oddi relaxation Satiety Decreases gastric acid secretion Reduces gastric emptying Regulates pancreatic growth
Secretin	Duodenum and jejunum (S cells)	Duodenal acid Fatty acids	Stimulates pancreatic fluid and bicarbonate secretion Decreases acid secretion Reduces gastric emptying
Motilin	Duodenum, small intestine and colon (Mo cells)	Fasting Dietary fat	Regulates peristaltic activity including migrating motor complexes (MMC)
Gastric inhibitory polypeptide (GIP)	Duodenum (K cells) and jejunum	Glucose and fat	Stimulates insulin release (also known as glucose-dependent insulinotrophic polypeptide) Inhibits acid secretion
Pancreatic polypeptide	Duodenum and jejunum	Protein digestive products Gastric distension	Inhibits pancreatic secretions
Enteroglucagon	Ileum and colon	Unknown	Modulates insulin release Trophic effect
Neurotensin	Ileum and colon	Fatty acids	May inhibit ileal motility in response to fat
Peptide YY	Ileum and colon	Intestinal fat	Decreases pancreatic and gastric secretion
VIP	Nerve fibres throughout GI tract	Unknown	Vasodilator Smooth muscle relaxation Water and electrolyte secretion
Ghrelin	Stomach	Fasting; eating inhibits	May regulate food intake
Guanylin	Small intestine	Unknown	Chloride secretion

22

impact proximal to an obstructive lesion. Water-soluble contrast is used to opacify bowel prior to abdominal computed tomography and in cases of suspected perforation but is less radio-opaque and is also irritant if aspirated into the lungs. Contrast studies are carried out under fluoroscopic control, which allows assessment of motility and correct patient positioning. The double contrast technique improves mucosal visualisation by using gas to distend the barium-coated intestinal surface.

Barium studies are useful for detecting filling defects, which may be intraluminal (e.g. food or faeces), intramural (e.g. carcinoma) or extramural (e.g. lymph nodes). Strictures, erosions, ulcers and motility disorders can all be detected.

The major uses and limitations of various contrast studies are shown in Box 22.4 and Figure 22.11.

Ultrasound, computed tomography (CT) and magnetic resonance imaging (MRI)

These are increasingly used in the evaluation of intra-abdominal disease. They are non-invasive and offer detailed images of the abdominal contents. Their main applications are summarised in Box 22.5 and Figure 22.12.

Endoscopy

Video endoscopy has replaced fibreoptic endoscopes. Images are displayed on a colour monitor. Endoscopes have controls to allow steering of the tip and also possess channels for suction and insufflation of air and water. Accessories can be passed down the endoscope to allow both diagnostic and therapeutic procedures, some of which are illustrated in Figure 22.13.

Upper gastrointestinal endoscopy

This is performed under light intravenous benzodiazepine sedation, or using only local anaesthetic throat spray after the patient has fasted for at least 4 hours. With the patient in the left lateral position the entire oesophagus (excluding pharynx), stomach and first two parts of duodenum can be seen. Indications, contraindications and complications are given in Box 22.6.

22

22.4 CONTRAST RADIOLOGY IN THE INVESTIGATION OF GASTROINTESTINAL DISEASE

	Barium swallow	Barium meal	Barium follow-through	Barium enema
Indications	Dysphagia Heartburn Chest pain Possible motility disorder	Dyspepsia Epigastric pain Anaemia Vomiting Possible perforation (non-ionic contrast)	Diarrhoea and abdominal pain of small bowel origin Possible obstruction by strictures etc.	Altered bowel habit Rectal bleeding Anaemia
Major uses	Strictures Hiatus hernia Gastro-oesophageal reflux and motility disorders, e.g. achalasia	Gastric or duodenal ulcers Gastric cancer Outlet obstruction Gastric emptying disorders	Malabsorption Crohn's disease	Neoplasia Diverticulosis Strictures, e.g. ischaemic Megacolon
Limitations	Risk of aspiration Poor mucosal detail Unable to biopsy	Low sensitivity for early cancer Unable to biopsy or assess *Helicobacter pylori*	Time-consuming Radiation exposure	Difficult in frail elderly or incontinent patients Uncomfortable Sigmoidoscopy also necessary to evaluate rectum Possibly misses polyps < 1 cm Less useful in inflammatory bowel disease

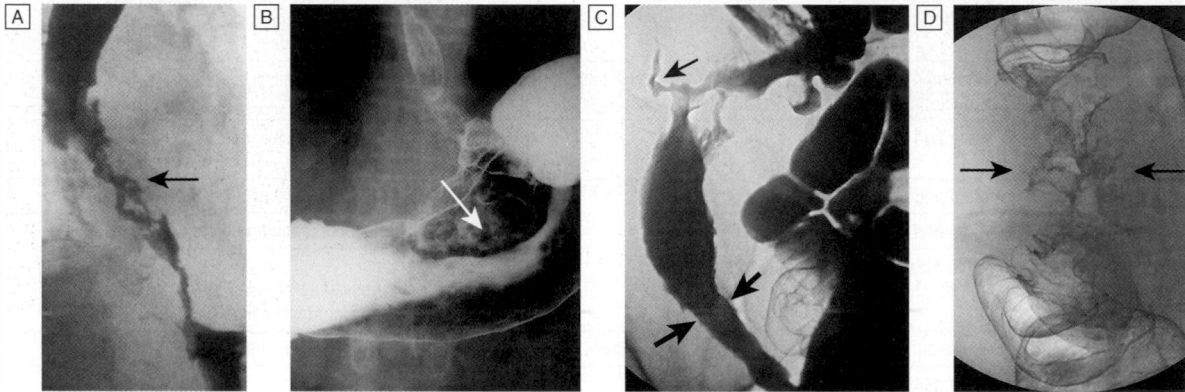

Fig. 22.11   Examples of contrast radiology. ⒜ A long irregular stricture (arrow) caused by oesophageal cancer. ⒝ A polypoid carcinoma demonstrated as a filling defect arising from the gastric body (arrow). ⒞ A long Crohn's stricture in the terminal ileum (large arrows) and also an adjacent fistulous tract (small arrow). ⒟ Colon cancer demonstrated as an 'apple core' stricture in the ascending colon (arrows).

Enteroscopy and capsule endoscopy

Using a longer endoscope (enteroscope) it is possible to visualise a large portion of the small intestine. Enteroscopy is of special value in the assessment of obscure, recurrent gastrointestinal bleeding. Capsule endoscopes contain a light source and lens which, after being swallowed, transmit images from the entire small intestine to a data recorder. Images are then processed by computer software to localise the site of any detected abnormalities. Capsule endoscopy is principally used in the investigation of suspected small bowel bleeding, tumours or ulceration.

Sigmoidoscopy and colonoscopy

Sigmoidoscopy can be carried out either in the outpatient clinic using a 20 cm rigid plastic sigmoidoscope or in the

endoscopy suite using a 60 cm flexible instrument following bowel preparation. When sigmoidoscopy is combined with proctoscopy, accurate detection of haemorrhoids, ulcerative colitis and distal colorectal neoplasia is possible. After full bowel cleansing it is possible to examine the entire colon and often the terminal ileum using a longer colonoscope. Indications, contraindications and complications of colonoscopy are listed in Box 22.7.

Endoscopic retrograde cholangiopancreatography (ERCP)

Using a side-viewing duodenoscope, it is possible to cannulate the main pancreatic duct and common bile duct. ERCP visualises the ampulla of Vater and produces radiological images of the biliary tree and pancreas. Diagnostic ERCP has largely been replaced by magnetic

22.5 ULTRASOUND SCANNING, CT AND MRI IN GASTROENTEROLOGY

Investigation	Ultrasound	CT	MRI
Major uses	Abdominal masses, e.g. cysts, tumours, abscesses Organomegaly Ascites Biliary tract dilatation Gallstones Guided needle aspiration and biopsy of lesions	Assessment of pancreatic disease Hepatic tumour deposits Tumour staging Assessment of vascularity of lesions	Hepatic tumour staging Magnetic resonance cholangiopancreatography (MRCP) Pelvic/perianal disease Crohn's fistulae
Limitations	Low sensitivity for small lesions Little functional information Operator-dependent Gas and obesity may obscure view	Expensive High radiation dose May understage some tumours, e.g. oesophago-gastric	Role in gastrointestinal disease not fully established Limited availability Time-consuming 'Claustrophobic' for some Contraindicated in presence of metallic prosthesis, cardiac pacemaker

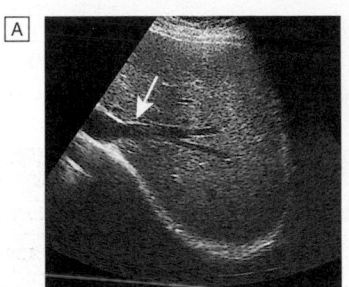
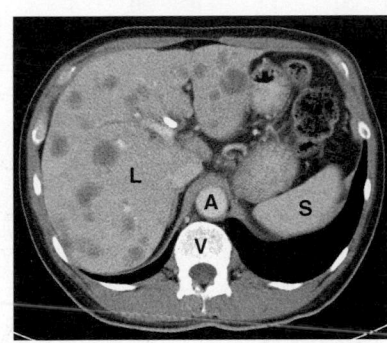
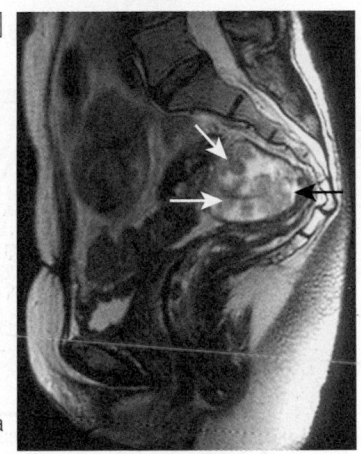

Fig. 22.12   Examples of ultrasound, CT and MRI. [A] Ultrasound of normal liver with hepatic veins entering the inferior vena cava (arrow). [B] CT showing multiple low-density metastatic tumour deposits in the liver. (L = liver; V = vertebra; A = aorta; S = spleen) [C] MRI (sagittal image) showing a large villous adenoma at the rectosigmoid junction (arrows).

22

22.6 UPPER GASTROINTESTINAL ENDOSCOPY

Indications

- Dyspepsia over 55 years of age or with alarm symptoms
- Atypical chest pain
- Dysphagia
- Vomiting
- Weight loss
- Acute or chronic gastrointestinal bleeding
- Suspicious barium meal
- Duodenal biopsies in the investigation of malabsorption

Contraindications

- Severe shock
- Recent myocardial infarction, unstable angina, cardiac arrhythmia*
- Severe respiratory disease*
- Atlantoaxial subluxation*
- Possible visceral perforation

* These are 'relative' contraindications; in experienced hands, endoscopy can be safely performed.

Complications

- Cardiorespiratory depression due to sedation
- Aspiration pneumonia
- Perforation
- Bleeding
- Infective endocarditis (use antibiotic prophylaxis in those with previous endocarditis or a prosthetic heart valve)

22.7 COLONOSCOPY

Indications*

- Suspected inflammatory bowel disease
- Chronic diarrhoea
- Altered bowel habit
- Rectal bleeding or anaemia
- Assessment of abnormal barium enema
- Colorectal cancer screening
- Colorectal adenoma follow-up
- Therapeutic procedures

* Colonoscopy is not useful in the investigation of constipation.

Contraindications

- Severe, active ulcerative colitis
- As for upper gastrointestinal endoscopy

Complications

- Cardiorespiratory depression due to sedation
- Perforation
- Bleeding
- Infective endocarditis (use antibiotic prophylaxis in those with previous endocarditis or a prosthetic heart valve)

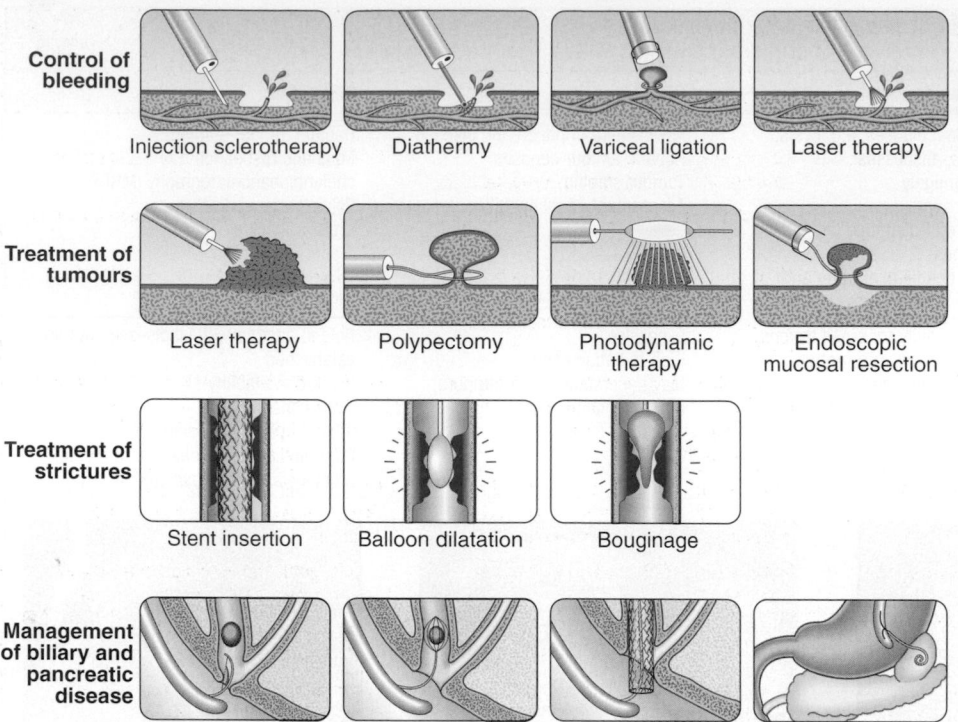

Fig. 22.13 Examples of therapeutic techniques in endoscopy.

Control of bleeding: Injection sclerotherapy · Diathermy · Variceal ligation · Laser therapy · Endoscopic clipping

Treatment of tumours: Laser therapy · Polypectomy · Photodynamic therapy · Endoscopic mucosal resection

Treatment of strictures: Stent insertion · Balloon dilatation · Bouginage

Management of biliary and pancreatic disease: Sphincterotomy · Basket retrieval · Stent insertion · Pseudocyst drainage

22

22.8 ENDOSCOPY IN OLD AGE

- **Tolerance**: endoscopic procedures are generally well tolerated even in very old people.
- **Side-effects from sedation**: older people are more sensitive, and respiratory depression, hypotension and prolonged recovery times are more common.
- **Bowel preparation for colonoscopy**: can be difficult in frail, immobile people. Sodium phosphate-based preparations can cause dehydration or hypotension and should be avoided in those with underlying cardiac or renal failure.
- **Antiperistaltic agents**: hyoscine should be avoided in those with glaucoma and can also cause tachyarrhythmias. Glucagon is preferred if an antiperistaltic agent is needed.

22.9 REASONS FOR BIOPSY OR CYTOLOGICAL EXAMINATION

- Suspected malignant lesions
- Assessment of mucosal abnormalities
- Diagnosis of infection (e.g. *Candida*, *H. pylori*, *Giardia lamblia*)
- Measurement of enzyme contents (e.g. disaccharidases)
- Analysis of genetic mutations (e.g. oncogenes, tumour suppressor genes)

resonance cholangiopancreatography (MRCP), which provides comparable images of the biliary tree and pancreas. MRCP complements CT and endoscopic ultrasound (EUS) in the evaluation of obstructive jaundice, biliary pain and suspected pancreatic disease, and therapeutic ERCP is then used to treat a range of biliary and pancreatic diseases, identified by these non-invasive imaging techniques. These include removal of common bile duct stones, stenting of biliary strictures and resolution of pancreatic duct disruption. Therapeutic ERCP is technically demanding and carries a significant risk of pancreatitis (3–5%), haemorrhage (4% after sphincterotomy) and perforation (1%).

Histology

Biopsy material obtained during endoscopy or percutaneously can provide useful information (Box 22.9).

TESTS OF INFECTION

Bacterial cultures

Stool cultures are essential in the investigation of diarrhoea, especially when it is acute or bloody, to identify pathogenic organisms (Ch. 13).

Serology

Detection of antibodies plays a limited role in the diagnosis of gastrointestinal infection caused by organisms such as *H. pylori*, *Salmonella* species and *Entamoeba histolytica*.

Breath tests

Non-invasive breath tests for *H. pylori* infection are discussed on page 864. Breath tests for suspected small intestinal bacterial overgrowth are discussed on page 897.

TESTS OF FUNCTION

A number of dynamic tests can be used to investigate aspects of gut function, including digestion, absorption, inflammation and epithelial permeability. Some of the more

22.10 DYNAMIC TESTS OF GASTROINTESTINAL FUNCTION

Process	Test	Principle	Comments
Absorption Fat	^{14}C-triolein breath test	Measurement of $^{14}CO_2$ in breath after oral ingestion of radio-labelled fat	Fast and non-invasive but not quantitative
	3-day faecal fat	Quantification of stool fat while patient ingests 100 g/day fat. Normally < 20 mmol/day	Non-invasive but slow and unpleasant for all
Lactose	Lactose H_2 breath test	Measurement of breath H_2 content after 50 g oral lactose. Undigested sugar is metabolised by colonic bacteria in hypolactasia, and expired hydrogen is measured	Non-invasive and accurate. May provoke pain and diarrhoea in sufferers
Bile acids	^{75}SeHCAT test	Isotopic quantification of 7-day whole-body retention of oral dose ^{75}Se-labelled homocholyltaurine (> 15% = normal, < 5% = abnormal)	Accurate and specific but requires two visits and involves radiation. Can be equivocal. Serum 7α-hydroxycholestenone is as sensitive and specific
Pancreatic exocrine function	Pancreolauryl test	Pancreatic esterases cleave fluoroscein dilaurate after oral ingestion. Fluoroscein is absorbed and quantified in urine	Accurate and avoids duodenal intubation. Takes 2 days. Accurate urine collection essential
	Faecal chymotrypsin or elastase	Immunoassay of pancreatic enzymes on stool sample	Simple, quick and avoids urine collection. Does not detect mild disease
Mucosal inflammation/ permeability	^{51}Cr-EDTA	Urinary quantification of label after oral dose. More is absorbed through 'leaky' mucosa	Relatively non-invasive and accurate but involves radioactivity. Limited availability
	Sugar tests (lactulose: rhamnose)	Small intestine absorbs mono- but not disaccharides unless inflamed. Urinary excretion of oral dose of two sugars expressed as ratio (normal < 0.04)	Non-invasive test of small bowel mucosal integrity (e.g. coeliac, Crohn's). Accurate urine collection essential
	Calprotectin	A protein secreted non-specifically by neutrophils into the colon in response to inflammation or neoplasia	Useful screening test for colonic disease

22

commonly used ones are listed in Box 22.10. In the assessment of suspected malabsorption, blood tests (full blood count, erythrocyte sedimentation rate (ESR), folate, B_{12}, iron status, albumin, calcium and phosphate) are essential, and endoscopy is undertaken to obtain mucosal biopsies.

Gastrointestinal motility

A range of diverse radiological, manometric and radio-isotopic tests exist for investigation of gut motility but many are research tests of limited value in daily clinical practice.

Oesophageal motility

A careful barium swallow can give useful information about oesophageal motility. Videofluoroscopy, with joint assessment by a speech and language therapist and a radiologist, may be necessary in difficult cases. Oesophageal manometry (Fig. 22.1, p. 852), often in conjunction with 24-hour pH measurements, is of value in diagnosing cases of refractory gastro-oesophageal reflux, achalasia and noncardiac chest pain.

Gastric emptying

Delayed gastric emptying (gastroparesis) causes persistent nausea, vomiting, bloating or early satiety. Endoscopy and barium studies are often normal. Normal gastric emptying rates for solids are highly variable but approximately 50% leaves the stomach by 90 minutes ($t^1/_2$). Calculating the amount of radioisotope retained in the stomach after a test meal containing solids and liquids labelled with different isotopes (Box 22.11) may reveal the diagnosis.

Small intestinal transit

This is much more difficult to quantify and is seldom necessary in clinical practice. Barium follow-through examination can give a rough estimate by noting the time taken for contrast to reach the terminal ileum (normally 90 minutes or less). Orocaecal transit can be assessed by the lactulose-hydrogen breath test. Lactulose is a disaccharide which normally reaches the colon intact; here, breakdown by colonic bacteria results in hydrogen production. The time at which this occurs, as measured in expired air, is a measure of orocaecal transit.

Colonic and anorectal motility

A plain abdominal X-ray taken on day 5 after ingestion of different-shaped inert plastic pellets on days 1–3 gives an estimate of whole gut transit time. The test is useful in the evaluation of chronic constipation when the position of any retained pellets can be observed, and helps to differentiate cases of slow transit from those due to obstructed defecation. The mechanism of defecation and anorectal function can be assessed by anorectal manometry, electrophysiological tests and defecating proctography.

RADIOISOTOPE TESTS

Many different radioisotope tests are used (Box 22.11). In some, structural information is obtained, e.g. localisation of a Meckel's diverticulum or distribution of activity in inflammatory bowel disease. Others use radioisotopes for

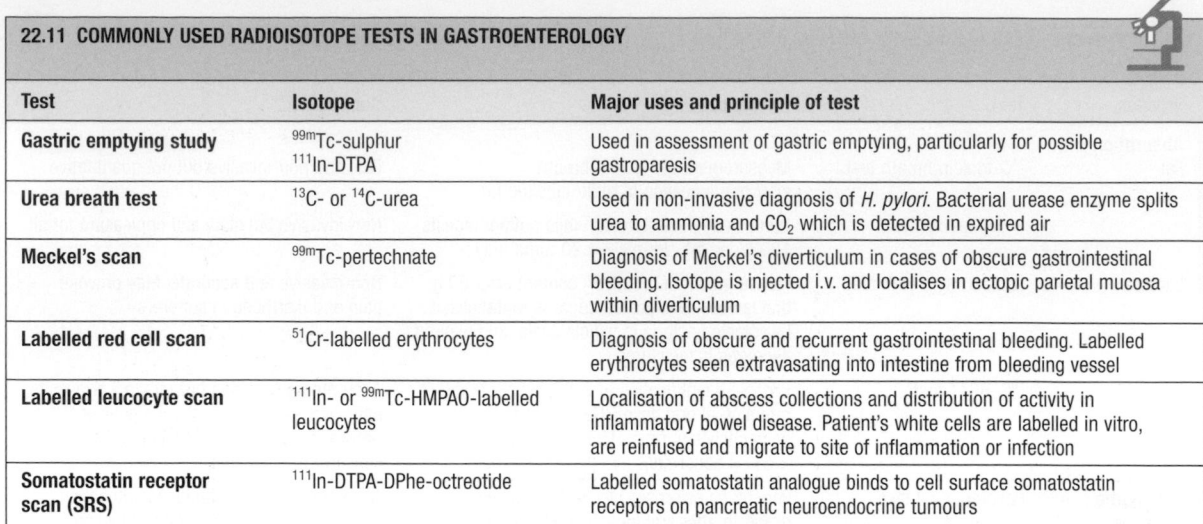

22.11 COMMONLY USED RADIOISOTOPE TESTS IN GASTROENTEROLOGY

Test	Isotope	Major uses and principle of test
Gastric emptying study	99mTc-sulphur 111In-DTPA	Used in assessment of gastric emptying, particularly for possible gastroparesis
Urea breath test	13C- or 14C-urea	Used in non-invasive diagnosis of *H. pylori*. Bacterial urease enzyme splits urea to ammonia and CO_2 which is detected in expired air
Meckel's scan	99mTc-pertechnate	Diagnosis of Meckel's diverticulum in cases of obscure gastrointestinal bleeding. Isotope is injected i.v. and localises in ectopic parietal mucosa within diverticulum
Labelled red cell scan	51Cr-labelled erythrocytes	Diagnosis of obscure and recurrent gastrointestinal bleeding. Labelled erythrocytes seen extravasating into intestine from bleeding vessel
Labelled leucocyte scan	111In- or 99mTc-HMPAO-labelled leucocytes	Localisation of abscess collections and distribution of activity in inflammatory bowel disease. Patient's white cells are labelled in vitro, are reinfused and migrate to site of inflammation or infection
Somatostatin receptor scan (SRS)	111In-DTPA-DPhe-octreotide	Labelled somatostatin analogue binds to cell surface somatostatin receptors on pancreatic neuroendocrine tumours

22

functional information, e.g. rates of gastric emptying or ability to reabsorb bile acids. Yet others are tests of infection and rely on the presence of bacteria to hydrolyse a radio-labelled test substance followed by detection of the radio-isotope in expired air (e.g. urea breath test for *H. pylori*).

PRESENTING PROBLEMS IN GASTROINTESTINAL DISEASE

DYSPHAGIA

Dysphagia is defined as difficulty in swallowing. It may coexist with heartburn or vomiting but should be distinguished from both globus sensation (in which anxious people feel a lump in the throat without organic cause) and odynophagia (pain during swallowing, usually from gastro-oesophageal reflux or candidiasis).

Dysphagia has oropharyngeal and oesophageal causes (Fig. 22.14). Oropharyngeal disorders result from neuro-muscular dysfunction affecting the initiation of swallowing by the pharynx and upper oesophageal sphincter (e.g. bulbar or pseudobulbar palsy and myasthenia gravis). Patients with oropharyngeal dysphagia have difficulty initiating swallowing and develop choking, nasal regurgitation or tracheal aspiration. Drooling, dysarthria, hoarseness and cranial nerve or other neurological signs may be present. Oesoph-ageal causes include structural disease (benign or malignant strictures) and dysmotility of the oesophagus. Patients with oesophageal disease complain of food 'sticking' after swallowing, although the level at which this is felt correlates poorly with the true site of obstruction. Swallowing of liquids is normal until strictures become extreme.

Investigations
Dysphagia implies significant disease and should always be promptly investigated. Endoscopy is the investigation of choice because it facilitates biopsy and dilatation of suspicious strictures. If no abnormality is found, then barium swallow, with videofluoroscopic swallowing assessment, will detect most motility disorders. In a few cases oesophageal manometry is required. The algorithm (Fig. 22.14) summarises a diagnostic approach to dysphagia and lists the major causes.

DYSPEPSIA

Dyspepsia ('indigestion') is a collective term for any symptoms thought to originate from the upper gastro-intestinal tract. It encompasses many different symptoms and disorders (Box 22.12), including some arising outside

22.12 CAUSES OF DYSPEPSIA

Upper gastrointestinal disorders

- Peptic ulcer disease
- Acute gastritis
- Gallstones
- Motility disorders, e.g. oesophageal spasm
- 'Functional' (non-ulcer dyspepsia and irritable bowel syndrome)

Other gastrointestinal disorders

- Pancreatic disease (cancer, chronic pancreatitis)
- Hepatic disease (hepatitis, metastases)
- Colonic carcinoma

Systemic disease

- Renal failure
- Hypercalcaemia

Drugs

- Non-steroidal anti-inflammatory drugs (NSAIDs)
- Iron and potassium supplements
- Corticosteroids
- Digoxin

Others

- Alcohol
- Psychological, e.g. anxiety, depression

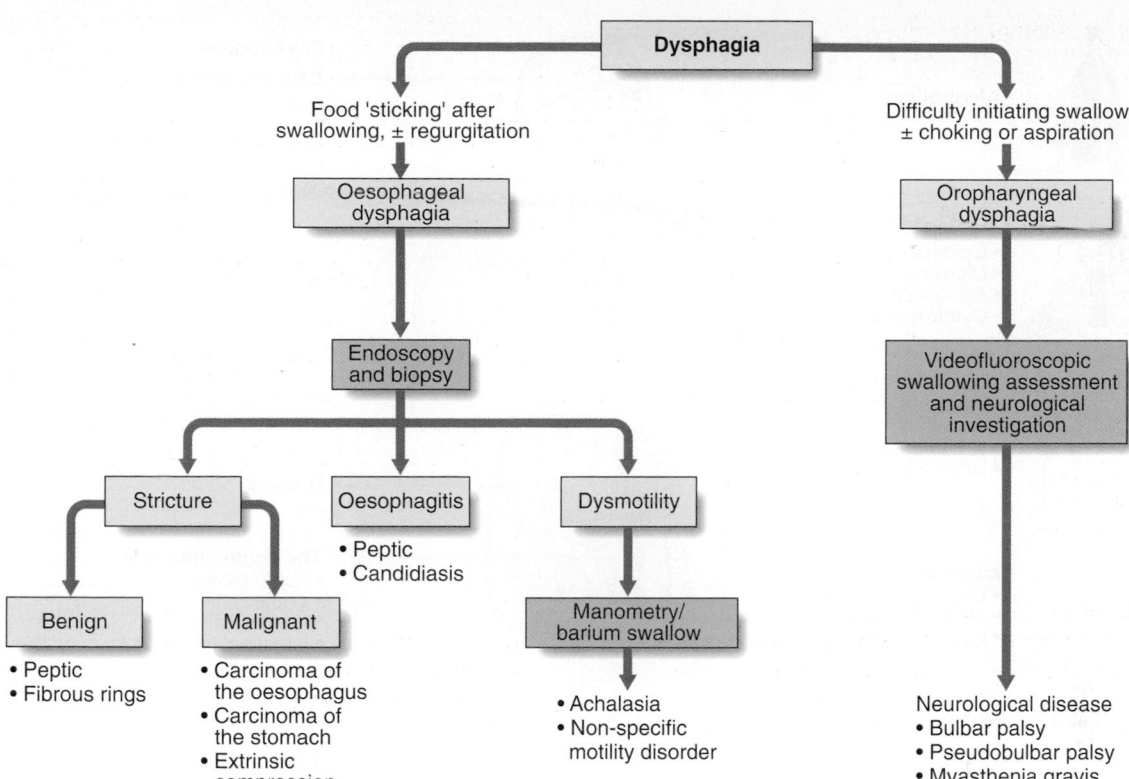

Fig. 22.14 Investigation of dysphagia.

22

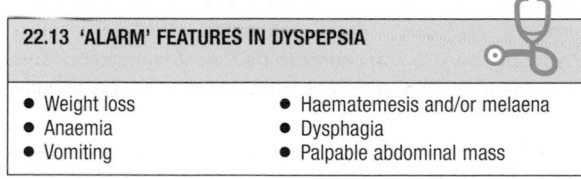

22.13 'ALARM' FEATURES IN DYSPEPSIA
• Weight loss   • Haematemesis and/or melaena
• Anaemia   • Dysphagia
• Vomiting   • Palpable abdominal mass

the digestive system. Heartburn and other 'reflux' symptoms are separate entities and are considered elsewhere.

Although symptoms often correlate poorly with the underlying diagnosis, a careful history is important to:

- elicit symptoms classical of specific disorders, e.g. peptic ulcer
- detect 'alarm' features requiring urgent investigation (Box 22.13)
- detect atypical symptoms more suggestive of other disorders, e.g. myocardial ischaemia.

Dyspepsia is extremely prevalent, affecting up to 80% of the population at some time, and very often no abnormality is discovered during investigation, especially in younger patients. Patients with 'alarm' symptoms, those over 55 years old with new dyspepsia, and younger patients unresponsive to empirical treatment require prompt investigation to exclude serious gastrointestinal disease.

Examination may reveal important findings such as evidence of anaemia, weight loss, lymphadenopathy, abdominal masses or signs of liver disease. An algorithm for the investigation of dyspepsia is outlined in Figure 22.15.

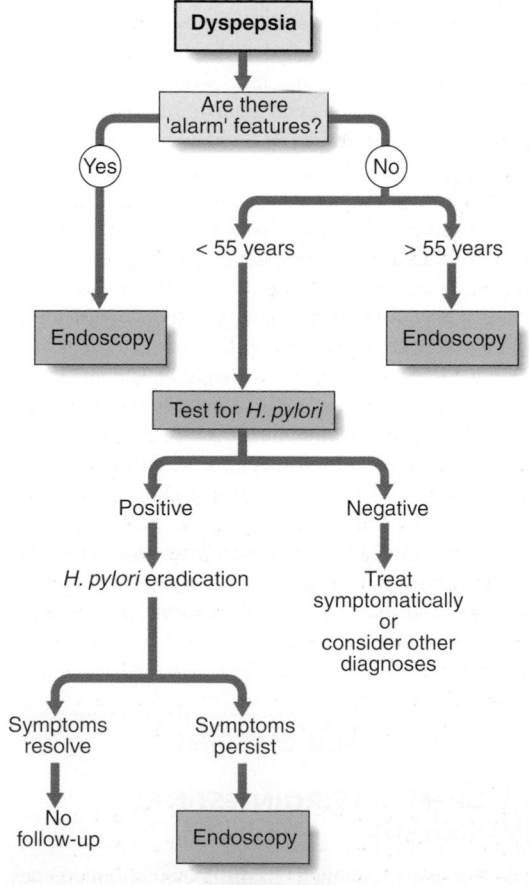

Fig. 22.15 Investigation of dyspepsia.

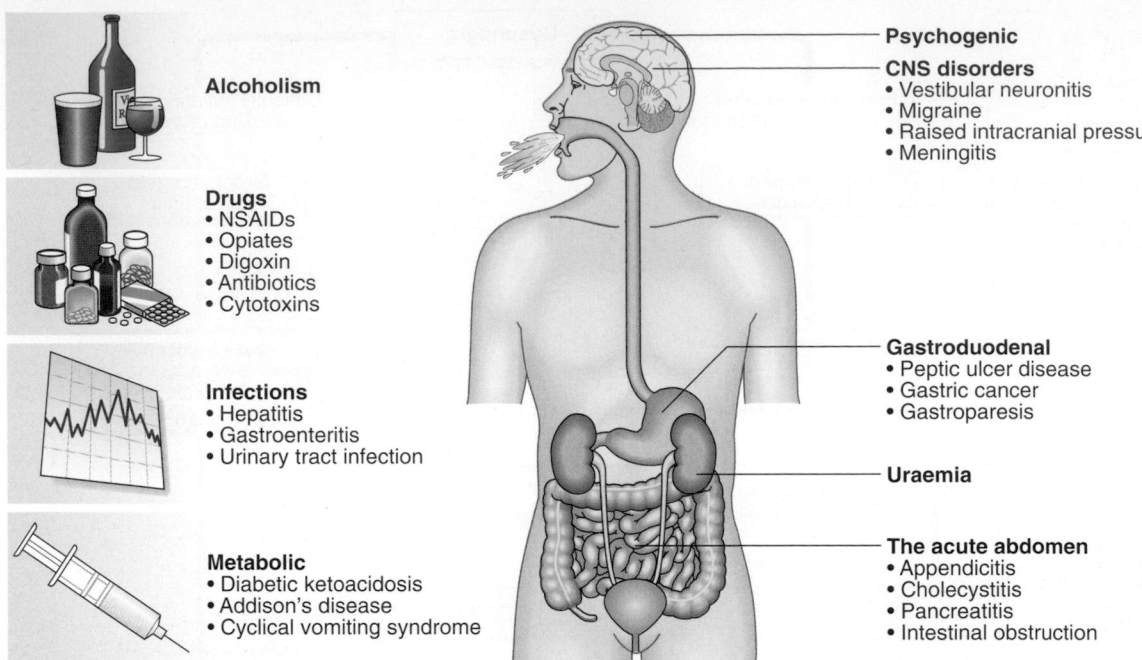

Fig. 22.16 Causes of vomiting.

VOMITING

Vomiting is a highly integrated and complex reflex involving both autonomic and somatic neural pathways. Synchronous contraction of the diaphragm, intercostal muscles and abdominal muscles raises intra-abdominal pressure and, combined with relaxation of the lower oesophageal sphincter, results in forcible ejection of gastric contents.

Vomiting is usually associated with nausea, retching, salivation, anorexia or dyspepsia. It is important to distinguish true vomiting from regurgitation and to elicit whether the vomiting is acute or chronic (recurrent), as the underlying causes may differ. Associated symptoms of abdominal pain, fever, diarrhoea, relationship to food, drug ingestion, headache, vertigo and weight loss should be sought.

Examination may reveal signs of dehydration, fever and infection. Evidence of abdominal masses, peritonitis or intestinal obstruction must be sought, as should neurological signs including papilloedema, nystagmus, photophobia and neck stiffness. Other findings may suggest alcoholism, pregnancy or bulimia as the underlying diagnosis. The diagnostic approach will be dictated by the history and examination. The major causes of vomiting are shown in Figure 22.16.

GASTROINTESTINAL BLEEDING

ACUTE UPPER GASTROINTESTINAL HAEMORRHAGE

This is the most common gastrointestinal emergency, accounting for 50–120 admissions to hospital per 100 000 of the population each year in the United Kingdom. Common causes are shown in Figure 22.17.

Clinical assessment

Haematemesis may be red with clots when bleeding is profuse, or black ('coffee grounds') when less severe. Syncope may occur and is due to hypotension from intravascular volume depletion. Symptoms of anaemia suggest chronic bleeding.

Melaena is the term used to describe the passage of black, tarry stools containing altered blood; this is usually due to bleeding from the upper gastrointestinal tract, although haemorrhage from the right side of the colon is occasionally responsible. The characteristic appearance is the result of the action of digestive enzymes and of bacteria upon haemoglobin. Severe acute upper gastrointestinal bleeding can sometimes cause maroon or bright red stool.

Management

1. Intravenous access
The first step is to gain intravenous access using at least one large-bore cannula.

2. Initial clinical assessment
- *Define circulatory status.* Severe bleeding causes tachycardia with hypotension and oliguria. The patient is cold and sweating, and may be agitated.
- *Seek evidence of liver disease.* Jaundice, cutaneous stigmata, hepatosplenomegaly and ascites may be present in decompensated cirrhosis.
- *Define comorbidity.* The presence of cardiorespiratory, cerebrovascular or renal disease is important, both because these may be worsened by acute bleeding and because these diseases increase the hazards of endoscopy and surgical operations.

22

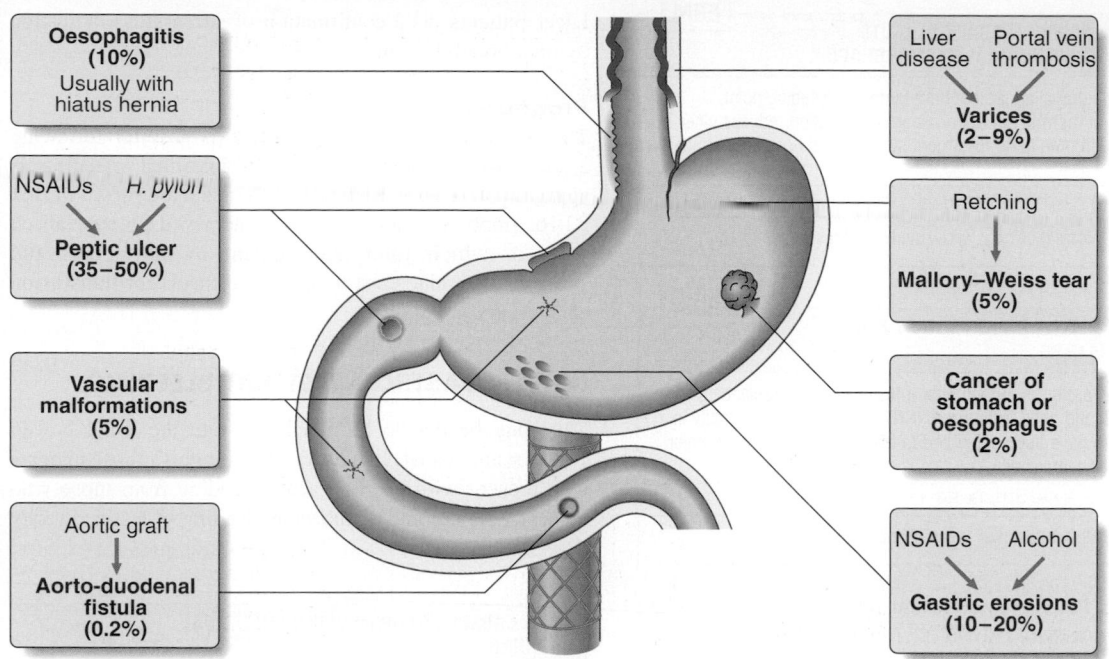

Fig. 22.17 Causes of acute upper gastrointestinal haemorrhage. (Frequency in parentheses.)

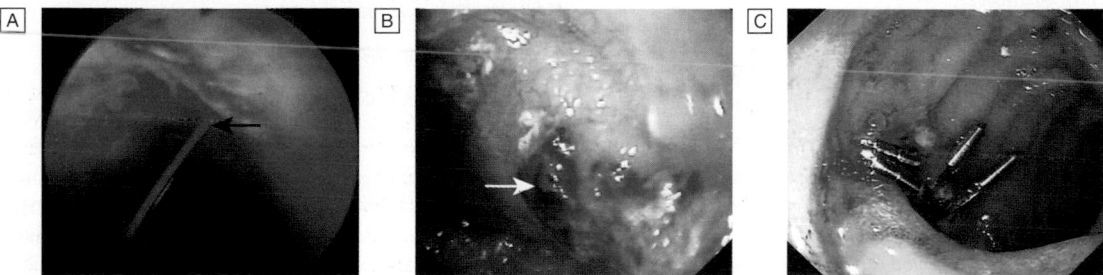

Fig. 22.18 Major stigmata of recent haemorrhage and endoscopic treatment **A** Active spurting haemorrhage (arrow) from a duodenal ulcer. When associated with shock, 80% of cases will continue to bleed or rebleed. **B** 'Visible vessel' (arrow). In reality, this is a pseudoaneurysm of the feeding artery seen here in a pre-pyloric peptic ulcer. It carries a 50% chance of rebleeding. **C** Haemostasis achieved after endoscopic clipping of bleeding vessel in duodenum.

3. Blood tests
- *Full blood count.* Chronic or subacute bleeding leads to anaemia, but the haemoglobin concentration may be normal after sudden, major bleeding until haemodilution occurs.
- *Urea and electrolytes.* This may show evidence of renal failure. The blood urea rises as the absorbed products of luminal blood are metabolised by the liver.
- *Liver function tests.*
- *Prothrombin time,* if there is clinical suggestion of liver disease or in anticoagulated patients.
- *Cross-matching* of at least 2 units of blood.

4. Resuscitation (p. 191)
Intravenous crystalloid fluids or colloid are given to restore the blood pressure. Blood is transfused when the patient is shocked or when the haemoglobin concentration is less than 100 g per litre.

Normal saline should be avoided in patients with liver disease because it can cause ascites.

Central venous pressure (CVP) monitoring is useful in severe bleeding, particularly in patients who have cardiac disease, to assist in defining the volume of fluid replacement and in identification of rebleeding.

5. Oxygen
This should be given by facemask to all patients in shock.

6. Endoscopy
This should be carried out after adequate resuscitation. A diagnosis will be achieved in 80% of cases. Patients who are found to have major endoscopic stigmata of recent haemorrhage (Fig. 22.18) can be treated endoscopically using a thermal modality such as a 'heater probe', by injection of dilute adrenaline (epinephrine) into the bleeding point, or by application of metallic clips. Endoscopic therapy may stop active bleeding and, combined with

---

22.14 ENDOSCOPIC THERAPY IN ACUTE UPPER GASTROINTESTINAL HAEMORRHAGE

'Injection of adrenaline (epinephrine) into the bleeding point, application of thermal energy or electrocoagulation reduces ulcer rebleeding rate, the need for urgent surgery, and hospital mortality rates.'

• British Society of Gastroenterology Endoscopy Committee. Gut 2002; 51(suppl IV):1–6.

For further information: 🖥 www.evidbasedgastro.com

22.15 ADJUNCTIVE DRUG THERAPY FOR BLEEDING ULCERS

'Intravenous proton pump inhibitor infusions reduce rebleeding ($NNT_B = 12$) and need for surgery ($NNT_B = 20$) but not mortality in patients who have been subjected to endoscopic therapy for major peptic ulcer haemorrhage.'

• Leontiadis GI, et al. BMJ 2005; 330:568–575.

For further information: 🖥 www.cochrane.org

---

intravenous PPI therapy, prevent rebleeding, thus avoiding the need for surgery (Boxes 22.14 and 22.15)

7. Monitoring

Patients should be closely observed, with hourly pulse, blood pressure and urine output measurements.

8. Surgical operation

An urgent surgical operation is indicated when:

• endoscopic haemostasis fails to stop active bleeding
• rebleeding occurs on one occasion in an elderly or frail patient, or twice in younger, fitter patients.

The choice of operation depends on the site and diagnosis of the bleeding lesion. Duodenal ulcers are treated by under-running with or without pyloroplasty. Under-running for gastric ulcers can also be carried out (a biopsy must be taken to exclude carcinoma). Local excision may also be performed, but when neither is possible, partial gastrectomy will be required. Following successful surgery for ulcer bleeding, all patients should be treated with *H. pylori* eradication therapy if positive and should avoid NSAIDs.

22.16 RISK FACTORS FOR DEATH IN PATIENTS WHO PRESENT WITH ACUTE UPPER GASTROINTESTINAL HAEMORRHAGE

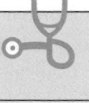

Factor	Comments
Increasing age	Risk increases over age 60 and especially in very elderly
Comorbidity	Advanced malignancy; renal and hepatic failure are associated with particularly high mortality
Shock	Defined as pulse > 100/min, BP < 100 mmHg
Diagnosis	Varices and cancer have the worst prognosis
Endoscopic findings	Active bleeding and a non-bleeding visible vessel at endoscopy are associated with a high risk of continuing bleeding
Rebleeding*	Associated with 10-fold rise in mortality

* Defined as fresh haematemesis or melaena associated with shock or a fall of Hb > 20 g/l over 24 hours.

Ulcer patients need confirmation of successful eradication by urea breath testing.

Prognosis

The mortality of patients admitted to hospital following a diagnosis of acute upper gastrointestinal bleeding is approximately 10%. Risk factors for death are shown in Box 22.16. Improved mortality can be achieved by specialised units in which joint management by physicians and surgeons and adherence to agreed protocols for transfusion and surgery are applied.

LOWER GASTROINTESTINAL BLEEDING

This may be due to haemorrhage from the small bowel, colon or anal canal. It is useful to distinguish those patients who present with profuse, acute bleeding from those who present with chronic or subacute bleeding of lesser severity (Box 22.17).

22.17 CAUSES OF LOWER GASTROINTESTINAL BLEEDING

Severe acute

• Diverticular disease
• Angiodysplasia
• Ischaemia
• Meckel's diverticulum

Moderate, chronic/subacute

• Anal disease, e.g. fissure, haemorrhoids
• Inflammatory bowel disease
• Carcinoma
• Large polyps
• Angiodysplasia
• Radiation enteritis
• Solitary rectal ulcer

Severe acute lower gastrointestinal bleeding

This is an unusual medical emergency. Patients present with profuse red or maroon diarrhoea and with shock.

Diverticular disease is the most common cause. Acute bleeding is due to erosion of an artery within the mouth of a diverticulum and bleeding almost always stops spontaneously. If bleeding continues, the diseased segment of colon will need to be resected after confirmation of the site (by angiography or colonoscopy).

Angiodysplasia is a disease of the elderly in which vascular malformations develop in the proximal colon. Bleeding can be acute and profuse; it usually stops spontaneously but commonly recurs. Diagnosis is often difficult. Colonoscopy reveals characteristic vascular spots which are reminiscent of spider naevi. In acute bleeding, visceral angiography shows bleeding into the intestinal lumen and an abnormal large, draining vein. In some patients diagnosis is only achieved by laparotomy with on-table colonoscopy. The treatment of choice is endoscopic thermal ablation, but resection of the affected bowel may be required if bleeding continues.

Ischaemia is due to occlusion of the inferior mesenteric artery and presents with abdominal colic and rectal bleeding. It should be considered in patients (particularly the elderly) who have evidence of generalised atherosclerosis. Diagnosis is made at colonoscopy. Resection is required only in the presence of peritonitis.

Meckel's diverticulum with ectopic gastric epithelium may ulcerate and erode into a major artery. The diagnosis should be considered in children or adolescents who present with profuse or recurrent lower gastrointestinal bleeding. A Meckel's ^{99m}Tc-pertechnate scan is sometimes positive but the diagnosis is commonly made only by laparotomy, at which time the diverticulum is excised.

Subacute or chronic lower gastrointestinal bleeding

This is extremely common at all ages and is usually due to haemorrhoids or anal fissure. Haemorrhoidal bleeding is bright red and occurs during or after defecation. Proctoscopy is used to make the diagnosis but in subjects who also have altered bowel habit and in all patients presenting at over 40 years of age, colonoscopy or barium enema is necessary to exclude coexisting colorectal cancer. Anal fissure should be suspected when fresh rectal bleeding and anal pain occur during defecation.

OBSCURE MAJOR GASTROINTESTINAL BLEEDING

In some patients who present with major gastrointestinal bleeding, upper endosopy and colonoscopy fail to reveal a diagnosis. When bleeding continues, urgent mesenteric angiography is indicated. This will usually identify the site if the bleeding rate exceeds 1 ml/min and embolisation can sometimes be used to stop the bleeding. If angiography is negative, enteroscopy can be used to visualise the proximal small intestine (Fig. 22.19) and treat the bleeding source. Wireless capsule endoscopy is also used to define a source of bleeding and, unlike push enteroscopy, the jejunum and ileum are visualised. When all else fails, laparotomy with on-table endoscopy is indicated.

OCCULT GASTROINTESTINAL BLEEDING

'Occult' means that blood or its breakdown products are present in the stool but cannot be seen. Occult bleeding may reach 200 ml per day, cause iron deficiency anaemia and signify serious gastrointestinal disease. Any cause of gastrointestinal bleeding may be responsible but the most important is colorectal cancer, particularly carcinoma of the caecum which may have no gastrointestinal symptoms.

In clinical practice, investigation of the gastrointestinal tract should be considered whenever a patient presents with unexplained iron deficiency anaemia. Testing the stool for the presence of blood is unnecessary and should not influence whether or not the gastrointestinal tract is imaged because bleeding from tumours is often intermittent and a negative faecal occult blood (FOB) test does not exclude important gastrointestinal disease. Many colorectal cancer patients are FOB-negative at presentation, and the only value of FOB testing is as a means of screening for colonic disease in asymptomatic populations (p. 928).

DIARRHOEA

The bowel frequency of the normal population ranges from three bowel movements per day to one bowel action every third day, and a normal stool consistency ranges from porridge-like to hard and pellety. The term 'diarrhoea' means different things to different people. Many patients and doctors think of diarrhoea in terms of increased stool frequency, and loose or watery stools. Gastroenterologists define diarrhoea as the passage of more than 200 g of stool daily, and measurement of stool volume is helpful. The most severe symptom in many patients is urgency of defecation, and faecal incontinence is a common event in acute and chronic diarrhoeal illnesses.

ACUTE DIARRHOEA

This is extremely common and usually due to faecal–oral transmission of bacteria, their toxins, viruses or parasites (Ch. 13). Infective diarrhoea is usually short-lived and patients who present with a history of diarrhoea lasting more than 10 days rarely have an infective cause. A variety of drugs, including antibiotics, cytotoxic drugs, proton pump inhibitors and NSAIDs, may be responsible for acute diarrhoea.

CHRONIC OR RELAPSING DIARRHOEA

The most common cause is irritable bowel syndrome (p. 920), which can present with increased frequency of defecation and loose, watery or pellety stools. Diarrhoea rarely occurs at night and is most severe before and after breakfast. At other times the patient is constipated and there are other characteristic symptoms of irritable bowel syndrome. The stool often contains mucus but never blood, and 24-hour stool volume is less than 200 g.

Chronic diarrhoea can be categorised as disease of the colon or small bowel, or malabsorption (Box 22.18). Clinical presentation, examination of the stool, routine blood tests and imaging reveal a diagnosis in many cases. A series of negative investigations usually implies irritable bowel syndrome but some patients clearly have organic disease and need more extensive investigations.

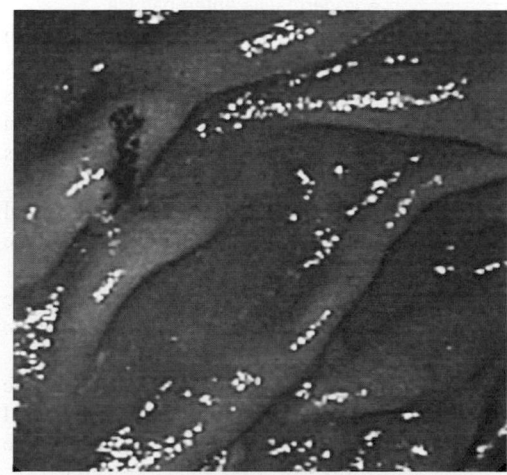

Fig. 22.19 **Jejunal angiodysplastic lesion seen at enteroscopy in a patient with recurrent obscure bleeding.**

22

22.18 CHRONIC OR RELAPSING DIARRHOEA

	Colonic	Malabsorption	Small bowel
Clinical features	Blood and mucus in stool Cramping lower abdominal pain	Steatorrhoea Undigested food in the stool Weight loss and nutritional disturbances	Large-volume, watery stool Abdominal bloating Cramping mid-abdominal pain

Some causes	Inflammatory bowel disease
	Neoplasia
	Ischaemia
	Irritable bowel syndrome
		Pancreatic
		  Chronic pancreatitis
		  Cancer of pancreas
		  Cystic fibrosis
		Enteropathy
		  Coeliac disease
		  Tropical sprue
		  Lymphoma
		  Lymphangiectasia
			VIPoma
			Drug-induced
			  NSAIDs
			  Aminosalicylates
			  Selective serotonin re-uptake
			  inhibitors (SSRIs)

Investigations	Colonoscopy with biopsies	Ultrasound, CT and MRCP Small bowel biopsy Barium follow-through	Stool volume Gut hormone profile Barium follow-through

MALABSORPTION

22

Digestion and absorption of nutrients is a complex, highly coordinated and extremely efficient process; normally, less than 5% of ingested carbohydrate, fat and protein is excreted in the faeces. Diarrhoea and weight loss in patients with a normal diet should always lead to the suspicion of malabsorption.

The symptoms of malabsorption are diverse in nature and

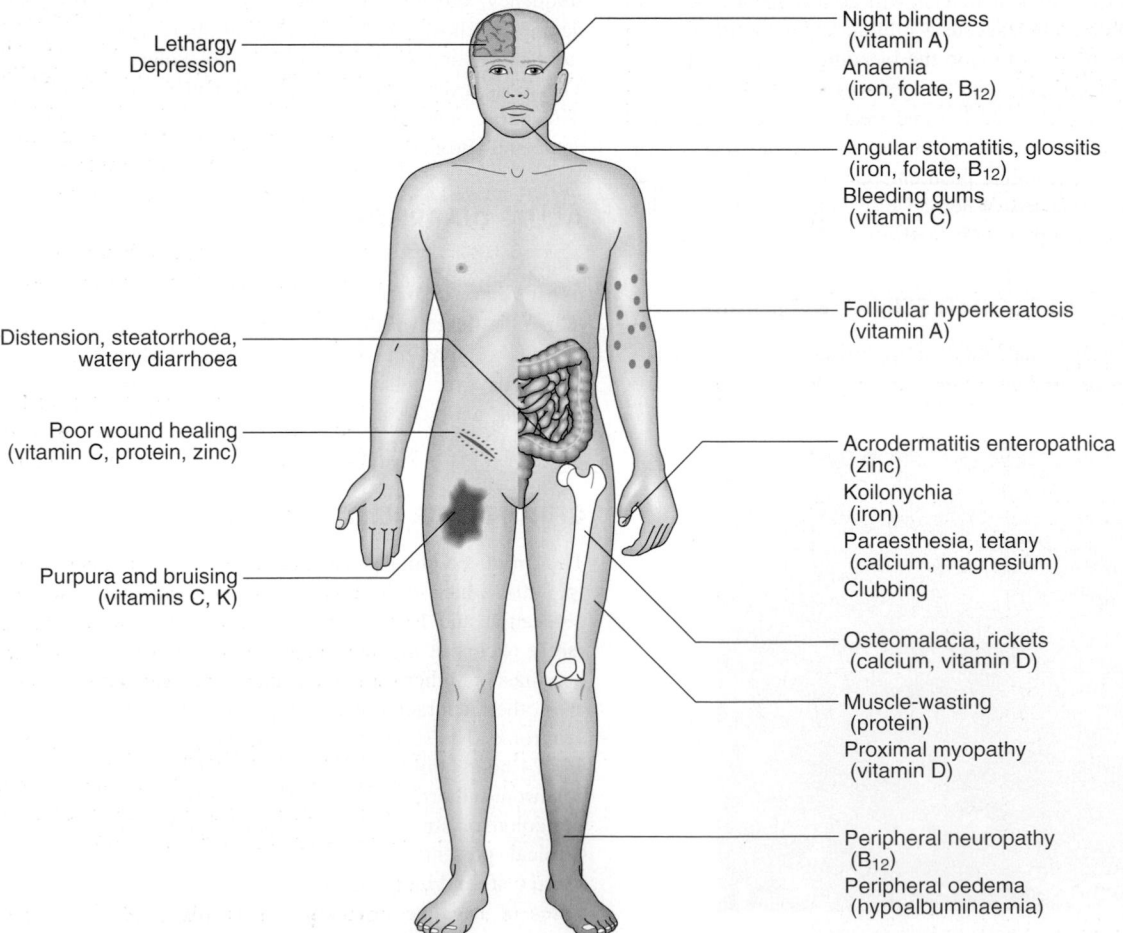

Lethargy
Depression

Distension, steatorrhoea,
watery diarrhoea

Poor wound healing
(vitamin C, protein, zinc)

Purpura and bruising
(vitamins C, K)

Night blindness
(vitamin A)
Anaemia
(iron, folate, B$_{12}$)

Angular stomatitis, glossitis
(iron, folate, B$_{12}$)
Bleeding gums
(vitamin C)

Follicular hyperkeratosis
(vitamin A)

Acrodermatitis enteropathica
(zinc)
Koilonychia
(iron)
Paraesthesia, tetany
(calcium, magnesium)
Clubbing

Osteomalacia, rickets
(calcium, vitamin D)

Muscle-wasting
(protein)
Proximal myopathy
(vitamin D)

Peripheral neuropathy
(B$_{12}$)
Peripheral oedema
(hypoalbuminaemia)

Fig. 22.20   Possible physical consequences of malabsorption.

variable in severity. A few patients have apparently normal bowel habit but diarrhoea is usual and may be watery and voluminous. Bulky, pale and offensive stools which float in the toilet (steatorrhoea) signify fat malabsorption. Abdominal distension, borborygmi, cramps, weight loss and undigested food in the stool may be present. Some patients complain only of malaise and lethargy. In others, symptoms related to deficiencies of specific vitamins, trace elements and minerals (e.g. calcium, iron, folic acid) may occur (Fig. 22.20).

Aetiology and pathogenesis

Malabsorption results from abnormalities of the three processes which are essential to normal digestion:

1. *Intraluminal maldigestion* occurs when deficiency of bile or pancreatic enzymes results in inadequate

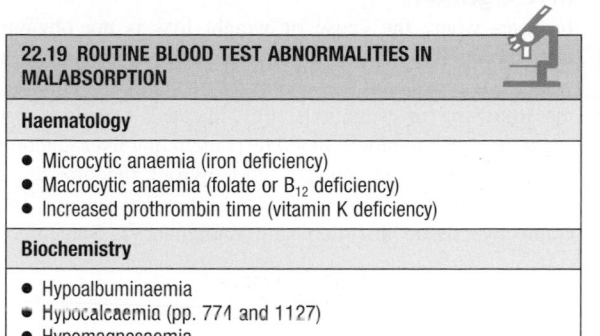

22.19 ROUTINE BLOOD TEST ABNORMALITIES IN MALABSORPTION

Haematology

- Microcytic anaemia (iron deficiency)
- Macrocytic anaemia (folate or B_{12} deficiency)
- Increased prothrombin time (vitamin K deficiency)

Biochemistry

- Hypoalbuminaemia
- Hypocalcaemia (pp. 774 and 1127)
- Hypomagnesaemia
- Deficiencies of phosphate, zinc

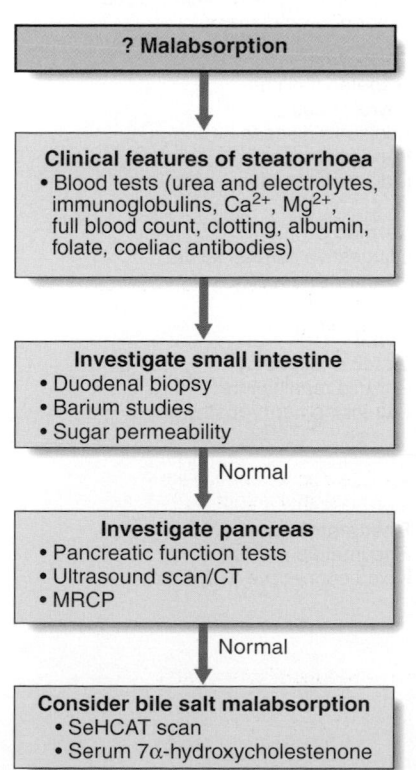

? Malabsorption

Clinical features of steatorrhoea
- Blood tests (urea and electrolytes, immunoglobulins, Ca^{2+}, Mg^{2+}, full blood count, clotting, albumin, folate, coeliac antibodies)

Investigate small intestine
- Duodenal biopsy
- Barium studies
- Sugar permeability

Normal

Investigate pancreas
- Pancreatic function tests
- Ultrasound scan/CT
- MRCP

Normal

Consider bile salt malabsorption
- SeHCAT scan
- Serum 7α-hydroxycholestenone

Fig. 22.21   Investigation for suspected malabsorption.

solubilisation and hydrolysis of nutrients. Fat and protein malabsorption results. This may also occur in the presence of small bowel bacterial overgrowth.

2. *Mucosal malabsorption* results from small bowel resection or conditions which damage the small intestinal epithelium, thereby diminishing the surface area for absorption and depleting brush border enzyme activity.

3. *'Postmucosal' lymphatic obstruction* prevents the uptake and transport of absorbed lipids into lymphatic vessels. Increased pressure in these vessels results in leakage into the intestinal lumen, leading to protein-losing enteropathy.

Diagnosis and investigations

Investigations are performed to confirm that malabsorption is present and then to determine the cause. Routine blood tests may show one or more of the abnormalities listed in Box 22.19. Tests to confirm fat and protein malabsorption are performed as described on page 863.

An approach to the investigation of malabsorption is shown in Figure 22.21.

WEIGHT LOSS

Weight loss may be 'physiological' due to dieting, exercise, starvation, or the decreased nutritional intake which accompanies old age. Alternatively, weight loss may signify disease; a loss of more than 3 kg over 6 months is significant. Hospital and general practice weight records may be valuable, as may reweighing patients at intervals, as sometimes weight is regained or stabilises in those with no obvious cause.

Pathological weight loss can be due to psychiatric illness, systemic disease, gastrointestinal causes or advanced disease of any specific organ system (Fig. 22.22).

History and examination

When weight loss is due to serious organic disease a careful history, physical examination and simple laboratory tests will usually define other features that lead to a specific diagnosis.

'Physiological' weight loss

This may be obvious in cases of young individuals who describe changes in physical activity or social circumstances. It may be more difficult to be sure in older patients when a history of nutritional intake may be unreliable; professional help from a dietitian is often valuable.

Psychiatric illness

Features of anorexia nervosa (p. 248), bulimia (p. 249) and affective disorders (p. 240) may only be apparent after formal psychiatric input. Alcoholic patients lose weight as a consequence of self-neglect and poor dietary intake.

Systemic diseases

Chronic infections including tuberculosis (p. 695), recurrent urinary or chest infections, and a range of parasitic and protozoan infections (Ch. 13) should be considered. A history of foreign travel, high-risk activities and specific features such as fever, night sweats, rigors, productive cough and dysuria must be sought. Sensitive, appropriate questions regarding lifestyle (promiscuous sexual activity and drug misuse) may suggest HIV-related illness (Ch. 14).

Weight loss is a late feature of disseminated malignancy (carcinoma, lymphoma or other haematological disorders). Specific symptoms, physical signs, relevant imaging, or biochemical or haematological abnormalities are almost invariable.

Gastrointestinal disease

Almost any disease of the gastrointestinal tract can cause weight loss. Dysphagia and gastric outflow obstruction (p. 889) cause defective dietary intake. Malignancy at any site may cause weight loss by mechanical obstruction, anorexia or cytokine-mediated systemic effects. Malabsorption from pancreatic diseases (p. 904) or small bowel causes may lead to profound weight loss with specific nutritional deficiencies (Ch. 5). Inflammatory diseases such as Crohn's disease or ulcerative colitis (p. 910) cause anorexia, fear of eating and loss of protein, blood and nutrients from the gut.

Specific diseases of any major organ system

These may be difficult to diagnose without a high index of suspicion. They may cause weight loss by a range of mechanisms, including altered metabolism in diabetes mellitus, Addison's disease and thyrotoxicosis (Chs 20 and 21).

Weight loss occurs as a consequence of increased metabolic demands in patients with end-stage respiratory and cardiac diseases. Multiple mechanisms are responsible in many cases: for example, patients with active or advanced rheumatological and collagen-vascular disorders (p. 1103) lose weight from a combination of anorexia, physical disability, altered metabolic demands and the systemic effects of their conditions.

In many diseases anorexia and weight loss may be compounded by the effects of drug therapies (e.g. digoxin) which may cause nausea, dyspepsia, constipation or depression.

Some easily overlooked causes of weight loss are listed in Box 22.20.

Investigations

In cases where the cause of weight loss is not obvious after thorough history-taking and physical examination, or where it is considered that an existing condition is unlikely, the following investigations are indicated: urinalysis for sugar, protein and blood; blood tests including liver function tests, random blood glucose, and thyroid function tests; ESR (may be raised in unsuspected infections such as TB, connective tissue disorders and malignancy). Sometimes

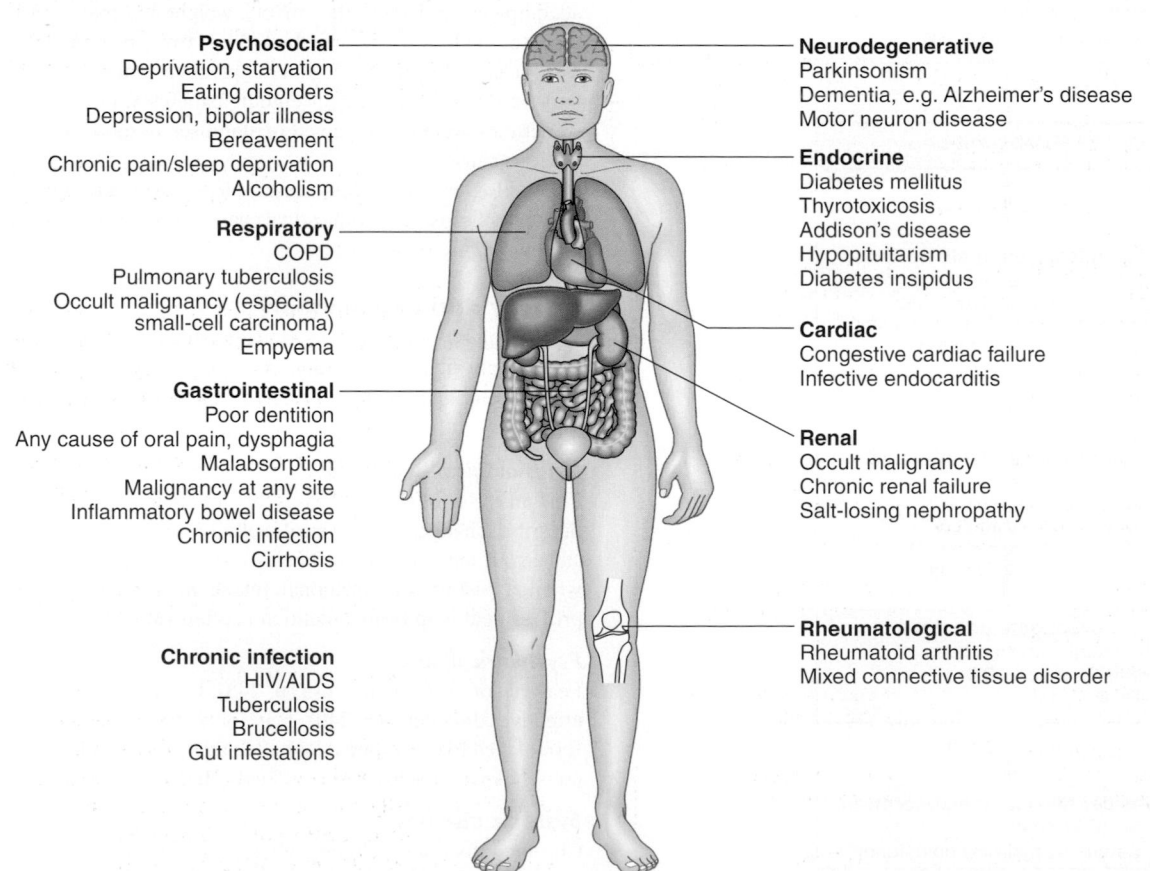

Psychosocial
Deprivation, starvation
Eating disorders
Depression, bipolar illness
Bereavement
Chronic pain/sleep deprivation
Alcoholism

Respiratory
COPD
Pulmonary tuberculosis
Occult malignancy (especially
small-cell carcinoma)
Empyema

Gastrointestinal
Poor dentition
Any cause of oral pain, dysphagia
Malabsorption
Malignancy at any site
Inflammatory bowel disease
Chronic infection
Cirrhosis

Chronic infection
HIV/AIDS
Tuberculosis
Brucellosis
Gut infestations

Neurodegenerative
Parkinsonism
Dementia, e.g. Alzheimer's disease
Motor neuron disease

Endocrine
Diabetes mellitus
Thyrotoxicosis
Addison's disease
Hypopituitarism
Diabetes insipidus

Cardiac
Congestive cardiac failure
Infective endocarditis

Renal
Occult malignancy
Chronic renal failure
Salt-losing nephropathy

Rheumatological
Rheumatoid arthritis
Mixed connective tissue disorder

Fig. 22.22 Some important causes of weight loss.

22.20 SOME EASILY OVERLOOKED CAUSES OF UNEXPLAINED WEIGHT LOSS

- Depression/anxiety
- Chronic pain or sleep deprivation
- Psychosocial deprivation/malnutrition in the elderly
- Existing conditions, e.g. severe chronic obstructive pulmonary disease (COPD), cardiac failure
- Diabetes mellitus/hyperthyroidism
- Occult malignancy (e.g. proximal colon, renal, lymphoma)
- Anorexia nervosa in atypical groups, e.g. young men
- Rare endocrine disorders, e.g. Addison's disease, panhypopituitarism

invasive tests such as bone marrow aspiration or liver biopsy may be necessary to identify conditions like cryptic miliary tuberculosis (p. 696). Rarely, abdominal and pelvic imaging by CT may be necessary, but before embarking on invasive or very costly investigations it is always worth revisiting the patient's history and reweighing patients at intervals.

CONSTIPATION

Constipation is defined as infrequent passage of hard stools. Patients may also complain of straining, a sensation of incomplete evacuation and either perianal or abdominal discomfort. Constipation may be the end result of many gastrointestinal and other medical disorders (Box 22.21).

22.21 CAUSES OF CONSTIPATION

Gastrointestinal disorders

Dietary
- Lack of fibre and/or fluid intake

Motility
- Slow-transit constipation (p. 930)
- Irritable bowel syndrome
- Drugs (see below)
- Chronic intestinal pseudo-obstruction

Structural
- Colonic carcinoma
- Diverticular disease
- Hirschsprung's disease

Defecation
- Obstructed defecation (p. 930)
- Anorectal disease (Crohn's, fissures, haemorrhoids)

Non-gastrointestinal disorders

Drugs
- Opiates
- Anticholinergics
- Calcium antagonists
- Iron supplements
- Aluminium-containing antacids

Neurological
- Multiple sclerosis
- Spinal cord lesions
- Cerebrovascular accidents
- Parkinsonism

Metabolic/endocrine
- Diabetes mellitus
- Hypercalcaemia
- Hypothyroidism
- Pregnancy

Others
- Any serious illness with immobility, especially in the elderly
- Depression

Clinical assessment and management

The onset, duration and characteristics are important; for example, a neonatal onset suggests Hirschsprung's disease, while a recent change in bowel activity in middle age should raise the suspicion of organic disorders such as colonic carcinoma. The presence of symptoms such as rectal bleeding, pain and weight loss is important, as are excessive straining, symptoms suggestive of irritable bowel syndrome, a history of childhood constipation and emotional distress.

Careful examination contributes more to the diagnosis than extensive investigation. A search should be made for general medical disorders as well as signs of intestinal obstruction. Neurological disorders, especially spinal cord lesions, should be sought. Perineal inspection and rectal examination are essential and may reveal abnormalities of the pelvic floor (e.g. abnormal descent, impaired sensation), anal canal or rectum (masses, faecal impaction, prolapse).

It is neither possible nor appropriate to investigate every person with this very common complaint. Most will respond to dietary fibre supplementation and the judicious use of laxatives. Middle-aged or elderly patients with a short history or worrying symptoms (rectal bleeding, pain or weight loss) must be investigated promptly, by either barium enema or colonoscopy. For those with simple constipation, investigation will usually proceed along the following lines.

Initial visit

Digital rectal examination, proctoscopy and sigmoidoscopy (to detect anorectal disease), routine biochemistry, including serum calcium and thyroid function tests, and a full blood count should be carried out. If these are normal, a 1-month trial of dietary fibre and/or laxatives is justified.

Next visit

If symptoms persist, then examination of the colon by barium enema or colonoscopy is indicated to look for structural disease.

Further investigation

If no cause is found and disabling symptoms are present, then specialist referral for investigation of possible dysmotility may be necessary. The problem may be one of infrequent desire to defecate ('slow transit') or else may result from excessive straining ('obstructed defecation', p. 930). Intestinal marker studies, anorectal manometry, electrophysiological studies and defecating proctography can all be used to define the problem.

ABDOMINAL PAIN

There are four types of abdominal pain:

- *Visceral.* Gut organs are insensitive to stimuli such as burning and cutting but are sensitive to distension, contraction, torsion and stretching. Pain from unpaired structures is usually but not always felt in the midline.
- *Parietal.* The parietal peritoneum is innervated by somatic nerves, and its involvement by disease processes, e.g. inflammation, infection or neoplasia, causes sharp, well-localised and lateralised pain.

22

22.22 CAUSES OF ACUTE ABDOMINAL PAIN ('SURGICAL')

Inflammation

- Appendicitis
- Diverticulitis
- Cholecystitis
- Pelvic inflammatory disease
- Pancreatitis
- Pyelonephritis
- Intra-abdominal abscess

Perforation/rupture

- Peptic ulcer
- Diverticular disease
- Ovarian cyst
- Aortic aneurysm

Obstruction

- Intestinal obstruction
- Biliary colic
- Ureteric colic

Other (rare)

- See 'extraintestinal' causes (Box 22.24)

- *Referred pain.* (For example, gallbladder pain is referred to the back or shoulder tip.)
- *Psychogenic.* Cultural, emotional and psychosocial factors influence everyone's experience of pain. In some patients, no organic cause can be found despite investigation, and psychogenic causes (depression or somatisation disorder) may be responsible (pp. 240 and 249).

THE ACUTE ABDOMEN

This accounts for approximately 50% of all urgent admissions to general surgical units. The acute abdomen is a consequence of one or more pathological processes (Box 22.22):

- *Inflammation.* Pain develops gradually, usually over several hours. It is initially rather diffuse until the parietal peritoneum is involved, when it becomes localised. Movement exacerbates the pain, and abdominal rigidity and guarding occur.
- *Perforation.* When a viscus perforates, pain starts abruptly; it is severe and leads to generalised peritonitis.
- *Obstruction.* Pain is colicky, with spasms which cause the patient to writhe around and double up. Colicky pain which does not disappear between spasms suggests complicating inflammation.

Initial clinical assessment

If there are signs of peritonitis (i.e. guarding and rebound tenderness with rigidity), adequate resuscitation should be arranged. In other circumstances further investigations are required (Fig. 22.23).

Investigations

In the majority of patients with acute abdominal pain full blood count (leucocytosis?), urea and electrolytes (dehydration?) and a serum amylase level (acute pancreatitis?) are measured. Further information can be obtained from an erect chest X-ray (air under the diaphragm?) and abdominal X-ray (obstruction?). An abdominal ultrasound may help

if acute gallstone disease (cholecystitis or cholangitis), ureteric colic or a soft tissue mass is suspected. Ultrasonography is also useful in the detection of free fluid and any possible intra-abdominal abscess. Contrast studies, by either mouth or anus, are useful in the further evaluation of intestinal obstruction, and essential in the differentiation of pseudo-obstruction from mechanical large bowel obstruction. Other investigations commonly used include CT (pancreatitis, retroperitoneal collections or masses, including an aortic aneurysm) and angiography (mesenteric ischaemia). Multi-slice CT angiography is now replacing angiography in many centres.

In those patients in whom the decision to operate remains in doubt and in whom the diagnosis has not been revealed by the appropriate investigations, diagnostic laparoscopy may be advised. All patients must be carefully and regularly reassessed (every 2–4 hours) so that any change in condition which might alter both the suspected diagnosis and clinical decision can be observed and acted upon early.

Management

In general, and depending on the organ affected, perforations are closed, inflammatory conditions are treated with antibiotics or resection, and obstructions are relieved. The speed of intervention and the necessity for surgery depend on a number of factors, of which the presence or absence of peritonitis is the most important. A treatment summary of some of the more common surgical conditions follows.

Acute appendicitis

Although non-operative treatment can be successful in some patients, the risk of perforation and subsequent recurrent attacks dictates that early surgery is undertaken. The appendix can be removed through a conventional right iliac fossa skin crease incision or by laparoscopic techniques.

Acute cholecystitis

This can be successfully treated non-operatively but the high risk of recurrent attacks and the low morbidity of surgery have made early laparoscopic cholecystectomy the treatment of choice.

Acute diverticulitis

Conservative therapy is usually recommended, but if perforation has occurred resection is advisable. Depending on peritoneal contamination and the state of the patient, primary anastomosis is preferable to a Hartmann's procedure (oversew of rectal stump and end colostomy).

Small bowel obstruction

If the cause is obvious and surgery inevitable (e.g. for an external hernia) an early operation is appropriate. If the suspected cause is adhesions from previous surgery, only those patients who do not resolve within the first 48 hours or who develop signs of strangulation (colicky pain becomes constant, peritonitis, tachycardia, fever, leucocytosis) will require surgery.

Large bowel obstruction

Pseudo-obstruction is treated non-operatively. Some patients benefit from colonoscopic decompression, but mechanical obstruction merits surgical resection, usually

22

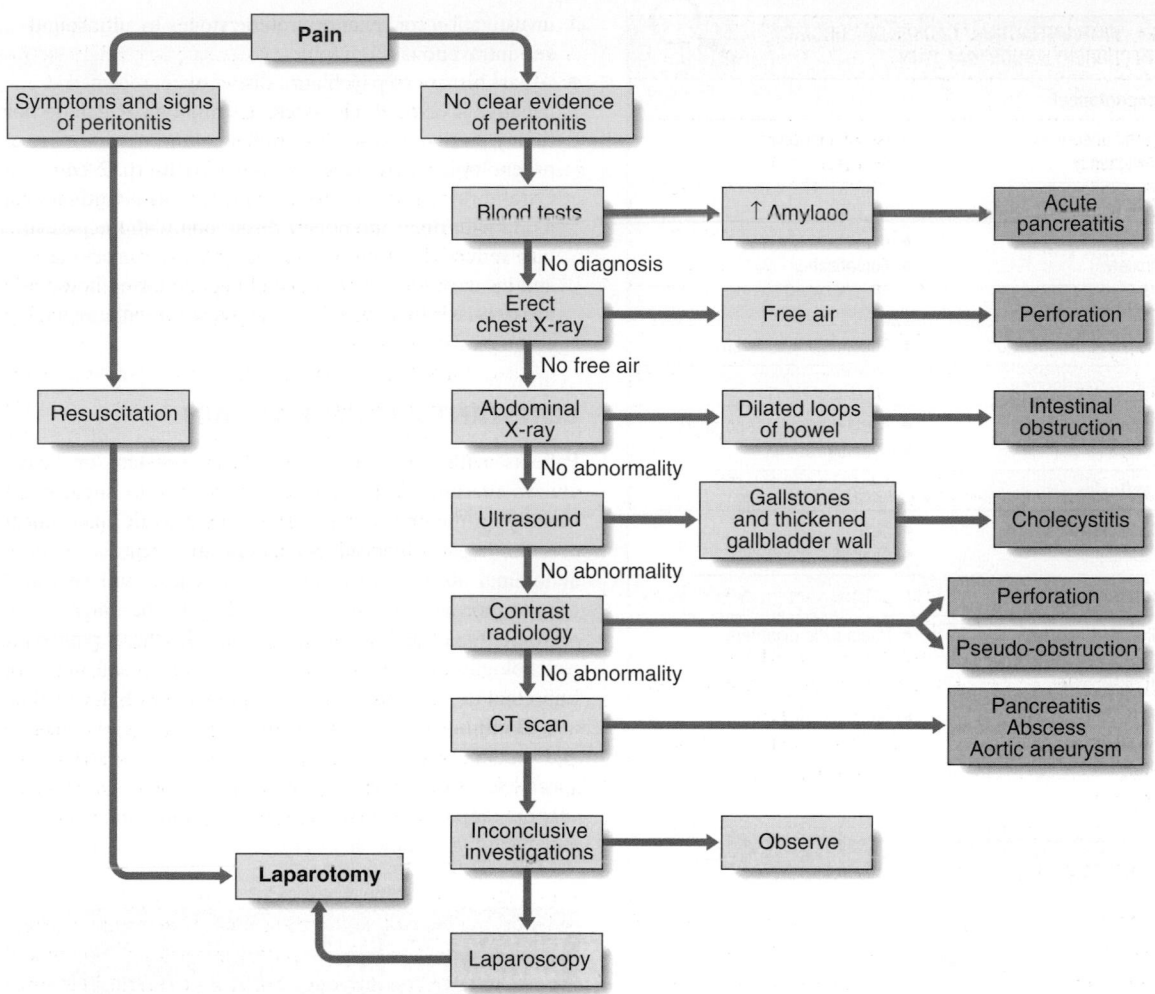

Fig. 22.23   Management of abdominal pain: an algorithm.

22.23 ACUTE ABDOMINAL PAIN IN OLD AGE

- **Presentation**: severity and localisation may blunt with age. Presentation may be atypical, even with perforation of a viscus.
- **Cancer**: a more common cause of acute pain in those over 70 years than in those under 50 years. Older people with vague abdominal symptoms should therefore be carefully assessed.
- **Non-specific symptoms**: intra-abdominal inflammatory conditions such as diverticulitis may present with non-specific symptoms such as acute confusion or anorexia and relatively little abdominal tenderness. The reasons for this are not clear but may result from altered sensory perception.
- **Outcome of abdominal surgery**: determined by the degree of comorbid disease and whether surgery is elective or emergency, rather than by chronological age.

---

with primary anastomosis. Differentiation between the two is made by a water-soluble contrast enema.

Perforated peptic ulcer

Although surgical closure of the perforation is standard practice, some patients without generalised peritonitis in whom a water-soluble contrast meal has confirmed spontaneous sealing of the perforation can be treated non-operatively. Adequate and aggressive resuscitation is mandatory before surgery.

For a more detailed discussion of acute abdominal pain the reader is referred to the sister volume of this text, *Principles and Practice of Surgery*.

CHRONIC OR RECURRENT ABDOMINAL PAIN

A detailed history, with particular attention to the features of the pain and any associated symptoms (Boxes 22.24 and 22.25), is essential.

Note should be made of the patient's general demeanour, mood and emotional state, signs of weight loss, fever, jaundice or anaemia. If a thorough abdominal and rectal examination is normal, a careful search should be made for evidence of disease affecting other structures, particularly the vertebral column, spinal cord, lungs and cardiovascular system.

The initial choice of investigations will obviously depend on the clinical features elicited during the history and examination:

22.24 'EXTRAINTESTINAL' CAUSES OF CHRONIC OR RECURRENT ABDOMINAL PAIN

Retroperitoneal

- Aortic aneurysm
- Malignancy
- Lymphadenopathy
- Abscess

Psychogenic

- Depression
- Anxiety
- Hypochondriasis
- Somatisation

Locomotor

- Vertebral compression
- Abdominal muscle strain

Metabolic/endocrine

- Diabetes mellitus
- Addison's disease
- Acute intermittent porphyria
- Hypercalcaemia

Drugs/toxins

- Corticosteroids
- Azathioprine
- Lead
- Alcohol

Haematological

- Sickle-cell disease
- Haemolytic disorders

Neurological

- Spinal cord lesions
- Tabes dorsalis
- Radiculopathy

22.25 IMPORTANT FACTORS IN THE ASSESSMENT OF ABDOMINAL PAIN

- Duration
- Site and radiation
- Severity
- Precipitating and relieving factors (food, drugs, alcohol, posture, movement, defaecation)
- Nature (colicky, constant, sharp or dull, wakes patient at night)
- Pattern (intermittent or continuous)
- Associated features (vomiting, dyspepsia, altered bowel habit)

- Epigastric pain, dyspepsia and relationship to food suggest gastroduodenal or biliary disease. Endoscopy and ultrasound are indicated.
- Altered bowel habit, rectal bleeding or features of obstruction suggest colonic disease. Barium enema and sigmoidoscopy, or colonoscopy are indicated.
- Pain provoked by food in a patient with widespread atherosclerosis may indicate mesenteric ischaemia. Mesenteric angiography may be necessary.
- Persistent symptoms require exclusion of colonic or small bowel disease. However, young patients with pain relieved by defecation, bloating and alternating bowel habit are likely to have irritable bowel syndrome (p. 920). Simple investigations (blood tests and sigmoidoscopy) may be sufficient.
- Upper abdominal pain radiating to the back, a history of alcohol misuse, weight loss and diarrhoea suggest chronic pancreatitis or pancreatic cancer. Ultrasound, CT and pancreatic function tests are required.
- Recurrent attacks of pain in the loins or radiating to the flanks with urinary symptoms should prompt

investigation for renal or ureteric stones by ultrasound and intravenous urography.

- A past history of psychiatric disturbance, repeated negative investigations or vague symptoms which do not fit any particular disease or organ pattern may point to a psychological origin for the patient's pain (p. 236). Careful review of case notes and previous investigations, along with open and honest discussion with the patient, may reduce the need for further cycles of unnecessary and invasive tests. Care must always be taken, however, not to miss rare pathology or atypical presentations of common diseases.

CONSTANT ABDOMINAL PAIN

Patients with chronic pain which is constant or nearly always present will usually have features to suggest the underlying diagnosis, e.g. malignancy (gastric, pancreatic, colonic, hepatic metastases), chronic pancreatitis or intra-abdominal abscess. In a minority no cause will be found despite thorough investigation, leading to the diagnosis of 'chronic functional abdominal pain'. In these patients a psychological cause is highly likely (p. 236) and the most important tasks are to provide symptom control, if not relief, and to minimise the effects of the pain on social, personal and occupational life. Patients are best managed in specialised pain clinics where, in addition to psychological support, appropriate use of drugs including amitriptyline, gabapentin, ketamine and opioids may be necessary.

DISEASES OF THE MOUTH AND SALIVARY GLANDS

APHTHOUS ULCERATION

Aphthous ulcers are superficial and painful; they occur in any part of the mouth. Recurrent ulcers afflict up to 30% of the population and are particularly common in women prior to menstruation. The cause is unknown, but in severe cases other causes of oral ulceration must be considered (Box 22.26). Occasionally, biopsy is necessary for diagnosis.

Topical corticosteroids (such as 0.1% triamcinolone in Orabase) or choline salicylate (8.7%) gel can effect healing. Symptomatic relief is achieved using local anaesthetic mouthwashes. Rare patients have very severe, recurrent aphthous ulcers and need oral corticosteroids.

ORAL CANCER

Squamous carcinoma of the oral cavity is common worldwide and the incidence has increased 19% since the mid-1990s in the UK. The mortality rate is around 50%, largely as a result of late diagnosis. Poor diet, alcohol excess and smoking or tobacco chewing are the main risk factors. In parts of Asia the disease is common among people who chew areca nuts wrapped in leaves of the betel plant ('betel nuts'). Oral cancer may present in many ways (Box 22.27) and a high index of suspicion is required. Patients with suspicious lesions should have all possible sources of local

22.26 CAUSES OF ORAL ULCERATION	

Aphthous

• Idiopathic	• Premenstrual

Infection

• Fungal, e.g. candidiasis • Viral, e.g. herpes simplex	• Bacterial, e.g. Vincent's angina, syphilis

Gastrointestinal diseases

• Crohn's disease	• Coeliac disease

Dermatological conditions

• Lichen planus • Pemphigoid	• Pemphigus

Drugs

• Hypersensitivity, e.g. Stevens–Johnson syndrome (p. 1308)	• Cytotoxics

Systemic diseases

• Systemic lupus erythematosus (SLE, p. 1132)	• Behçet's syndrome (p. 1142)

Neoplasia

• Carcinoma • Leukaemia	• Kaposi's sarcoma

22.27 SYMPTOMS AND SIGNS OF ORAL CANCER

- Solitary ulcer without precipitant, e.g. local trauma
- Solitary white patch ('leukoplakia') which fails to wipe off
- Solitary red patch
- Fixed lump
- Lip numbness in absence of trauma or infection
- Trismus (painful/difficult mouth opening)
- Cervical lymphadenopathy

trauma or infection treated and be reviewed after 2 weeks. If the lesion persists, biopsy is advisable. Small cancers can be resected but extensive surgery with neck dissection to remove involved lymph nodes may be necessary. Some patients can be treated with radical radiotherapy alone, and radiotherapy is sometimes also given after surgery to treat microscopic residual disease. Some tumours may be amenable to photodynamic therapy (PDT), avoiding the need for surgery.

VINCENT'S ANGINA

This is characterised by painful, deep, sloughing ulcers which principally affect the gums. It is due to invasion of the mucous membranes by organisms such as *Borrelia vincenti* and other commensals. Invasion occurs when host resistance is low and oral hygiene is poor. Malnutrition, general debility and the acquired immunodeficiency syndrome (AIDS) predispose. The illness is associated with halitosis, and many patients are feverish and systemically unwell.

Local treatment with hydrogen peroxide mouthwashes and broad-spectrum antibiotics is indicated.

CANDIDIASIS

The yeast *Candida albicans* is a normal mouth commensal but it may proliferate to cause thrush. This occurs in babies, debilitated patients, patients receiving corticosteroid or antibiotic therapy, diabetics and immunosuppressed patients, especially those receiving cytotoxic therapy and those with AIDS. White patches are seen on the tongue and buccal mucosa. Odynophagia or dysphagia suggests pharyngeal and oesophageal candidiasis. A clinical diagnosis is sufficient to instigate therapy, although brushings or biopsies can be obtained for mycological examination.

Oral thrush is treated using nystatin or amphotericin suspensions or lozenges. Resistant cases or immunosuppressed patients may require oral fluconazole.

PAROTITIS

Parotitis is due to viral or bacterial infection. Mumps causes a self-limiting acute parotitis (p. 302). Bacterial parotitis usually occurs as a complication of major surgery. It is a consequence of dehydration and poor oral hygiene and can be avoided by good post-operative care. Patients present with painful parotid swelling and this can be complicated by abscess formation. Broad-spectrum antibiotics are required, whilst surgical drainage is necessary for abscesses. Other causes of salivary gland enlargement are listed in Box 22.28.

22.28 CAUSES OF SALIVARY GLAND SWELLING	

• Infection
  Mumps
  Bacterial (post-operative)
• Calculi
• Sjögren's syndrome (p. 1137)
• Sarcoidosis
	• Tumours
	  Benign: pleomorphic adenoma (95% of cases)
	  Intermediate: mucoepidermoid tumour
	  Malignant: carcinoma

22.29 ORAL HEALTH IN OLD AGE

- **Dry mouth**: affects around 40% of healthy older people.
- **Gustatory and olfactory sensation**: declines and chewing power is diminished.
- **Salivation**: baseline salivary flow falls but stimulated salivation is unchanged.
- **Root caries and periodontal disease**: common partly because oral hygiene deteriorates with increasing frailty.
- **Bacteraemia and septicaemia**: may complicate Gram-negative anaerobic infection in the periodontal pockets of the very frail.

DISEASES OF THE OESOPHAGUS

GASTRO-OESOPHAGEAL REFLUX DISEASE

Gastro-oesophageal reflux resulting in heartburn affects approximately 30% of the general population.

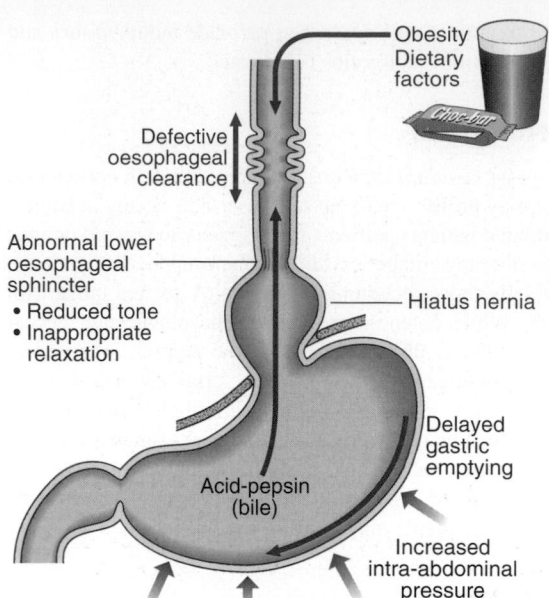

Obesity
Dietary factors

Defective oesophageal clearance

Abnormal lower oesophageal sphincter
• Reduced tone
• Inappropriate relaxation

Hiatus hernia

Acid-pepsin (bile)

Delayed gastric emptying

Increased intra-abdominal pressure

Fig. 22.24 Factors associated with the development of gastro-oesophageal reflux disease.

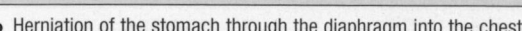

22.30 IMPORTANT FEATURES OF HIATUS HERNIA

- Herniation of the stomach through the diaphragm into the chest
- Occurs in 30% of the population over the age of 50 years
- Often asymptomatic
- Heartburn and regurgitation can occur
- Gastric volvulus may complicate large para-oesophageal hernias

Pathophysiology

Occasional episodes of gastro-oesophageal reflux are common in health. Reflux is normally followed by oesophageal peristaltic waves which efficiently clear the gullet, alkaline saliva neutralises residual acid, and symptoms do not occur. Gastro-oesophageal reflux disease develops when the oesophageal mucosa is exposed to gastric contents for prolonged periods of time, resulting in symptoms and, in a proportion of cases, oesophagitis. Several factors are known to be involved (Fig. 22.24).

Abnormalities of the lower oesophageal sphincter

In health, the lower oesophageal sphincter is tonically contracted, relaxing only during swallowing (p. 852).

Some patients with gastro-oesophageal reflux disease have reduced lower oesophageal sphincter tone, permitting reflux when intra-abdominal pressure rises. In others, basal sphincter tone is normal but reflux occurs in response to frequent episodes of inappropriate sphincter relaxation.

Hiatus hernia

Hiatus hernia (Box 22.30 and Fig. 22.25) causes reflux because the pressure gradient between the abdominal and thoracic cavities, which normally pinches the hiatus, is lost. In addition, the oblique angle between the cardia and oesophagus disappears. Many patients who have large hiatus hernias develop reflux symptoms, but the relationship between the presence of a hernia and symptoms is poor. Hiatus hernia is very common in individuals who have no symptoms, and some symptomatic patients have only a very small or no hernia. Nevertheless, almost all patients who develop oesophagitis, Barrett's oesophagus or peptic strictures have a hiatus hernia.

Delayed oesophageal clearance

Defective oesophageal peristaltic activity is commonly found in patients who have oesophagitis. It is a primary abnormality, since it persists after oesophagitis has been healed by acid-suppressing drug therapy. Poor oesophageal clearance leads to increased acid exposure time.

Gastric contents

Gastric acid is the most important oesophageal irritant and there is a close relationship between acid exposure time and symptoms.

Defective gastric emptying

Gastric emptying is delayed in patients with gastro-oesophageal reflux disease. The reason for this is unknown.

Increased intra-abdominal pressure

Pregnancy and obesity are established predisposing causes. Weight loss may improve symptoms.

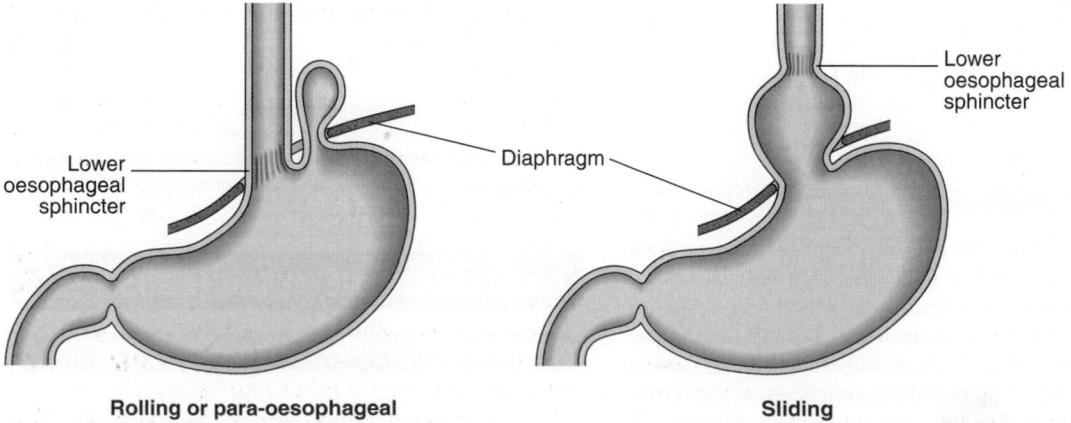

Lower oesophageal sphincter

Diaphragm

Lower oesophageal sphincter

Lower oesophageal sphincter

Rolling or para-oesophageal

Sliding

Fig. 22.25 Types of hiatus hernia.

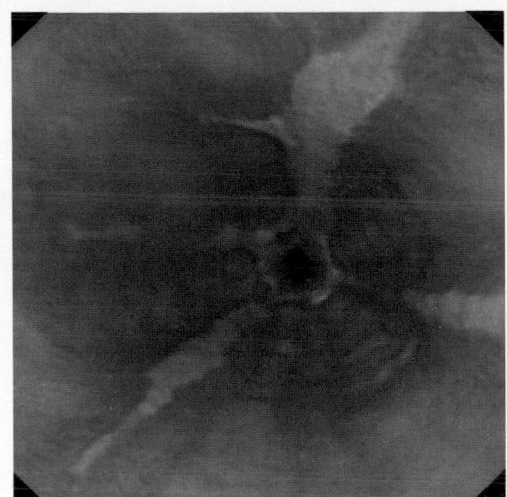

Fig. 22.26 **Reflux oesophagitis.** There are numerous linear streaks of superficial ulceration extending up the gullet.

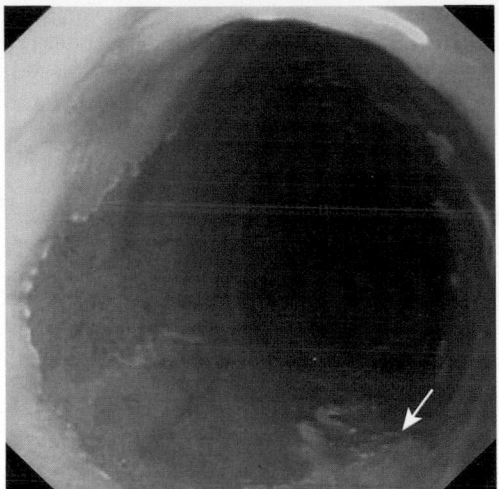

Fig. 22.27 **Barrett's oesophagus.** Pink columnar mucosa extends up the gullet. Small islands of squamous mucosa remain (arrow).

Dietary and environmental factors

Dietary fat, chocolate, alcohol and coffee relax the lower oesophageal sphincter and may provoke symptoms. There is little evidence to incriminate smoking or NSAIDs as causes of gastro-oesophageal reflux disease.

Clinical features

The major symptoms are heartburn and regurgitation, often provoked by bending, straining or lying down. 'Waterbrash', which is salivation due to reflex salivary gland stimulation as acid enters the gullet, is often present. A history of weight gain is common. Some patients are woken at night by choking as refluxed fluid irritates the larynx. Others develop odynophagia or dysphagia. A few present with atypical chest pain which may be severe, can mimic angina and is probably due to reflux-induced oesophageal spasm.

Complications

Oesophagitis

A range of endoscopic findings, from mild redness to severe, bleeding ulceration with stricture formation, are recognised (Fig. 22.26). There is a poor correlation between symptoms and histological and endoscopic findings. A normal endoscopy and normal oesophageal histology are perfectly compatible with significant gastro-oesophageal reflux disease.

Barrett's oesophagus

Background. Barrett's oesophagus ('columnar lined oesophagus'—CLO) is a pre-malignant glandular meta-plasia of the lower oesophagus, in which the normal squamous lining is replaced by columnar mucosa composed of a cellular mosaic containing areas of intestinal metaplasia (Fig. 22.27). It occurs as an adaptive response to chronic gastro-oesophageal reflux and is found in 10% of patients undergoing gastroscopy for reflux symptoms. Community-based epidemiological and autopsy studies suggest the true prevalence may be up to 20 times greater as the condition is often asymptomatic until first discovered when the patient presents with oesophageal cancer. CLO is the major risk factor for oesophageal adenocarcinoma, with a lifetime cancer risk of around 10%. The cancer incidence is estimated at 1 in 200 patient years (0.5% per year). The absolute risk is low, however, and more than 95% of patients with CLO die of causes other than oesophageal cancer. The epidemiology and aetiology of CLO are poorly understood. The prevalence is increasing, and it is more common in men (especially white) and those over 50 years of age. It is weakly associated with smoking but not alcohol. Cancer risk is more closely related to the severity and duration of reflux rather than the presence of CLO per se. Recent attention has focused on the importance of duodenogastro-oesophageal reflux, containing bile, pancreatic enzymes and pepsin in addition to acid. The molecular events underlying the progression of CLO from metaplasia to dysplasia to cancer are not well understood but E-cadherin polymorphisms, p53 mutations, transforming growth factor-β (TGF-β), epidermal growth factor (EGF) receptors, COX-2 and tumour necrosis factor-α (TNF-α) may play roles in neoplastic progression.

Diagnosis. This requires multiple systematic biopsies to maximise the chance of detecting intestinal metaplasia and/or dysplasia.

Management. Neither potent acid suppression nor antireflux surgery will stop progression or induce regression of CLO, and treatment is only indicated for symptoms of reflux or complications such as stricture. Endoscopic ablation therapy or photodynamic therapy can induce regression but 'buried islands' of glandular mucosa may persist underneath the squamous epithelium and cancer risk is not eliminated. At present these therapies remain experimental but show promise; they are also used in patients with high-grade dysplasia (HGD) or early malignancy who are not suitable for surgery.

Regular endoscopic surveillance can detect dysplasia and malignancy at an early stage and may improve 2-year survival but, because most CLO is undetected until cancer develops, surveillance strategies are unlikely to influence the overall mortality rate of oesophageal cancer. Surveillance is expensive and cost-effectiveness studies have been conflicting. Surveillance is currently recommended every 2–3 years for those without dysplasia and at 6–12-monthly intervals for those with low-grade dysplasia.

Oesophagectomy is widely recommended for those with HGD as the resected specimen harbours cancer in up to 40%. This may be an over-estimate and recent data suggest that HGD often remains stable and may not progress to cancer, at least in the medium term. Close follow-up with biopsies every 3 months is an alternative strategy for those with HGD.

Anaemia

Iron deficiency anaemia occurs as a consequence of chronic, insidious blood loss from long-standing oesophagitis. Almost all such patients have a large hiatus hernia and bleeding can occur from subtle erosions in the neck of the sac ('Cameron lesions'). Nevertheless, hiatus hernia is very common and other causes of blood loss, particularly colorectal cancer, must be considered in anaemic patients, even when endoscopy reveals oesophagitis and a hiatus hernia.

Benign oesophageal stricture

Fibrous strictures develop as a consequence of long-standing oesophagitis. Most patients are elderly and have poor oesophageal peristaltic activity. They present with dysphagia which is worse for solids than for liquids. Bolus obstruction following ingestion of meat causes absolute dysphagia. A history of heartburn is common but not invariable; many elderly patients presenting with strictures have no preceding heartburn.

Diagnosis is made by endoscopy, when biopsies of the stricture can be taken to exclude malignancy. Endoscopic balloon dilatation or bouginage is helpful. Subsequently, long-term therapy with a proton pump inhibitor drug at full dose should be started to reduce the risk of recurrent oesophagitis and stricture formation. The patient should be advised to chew food thoroughly, and it is important to ensure adequate dentition.

Gastric volvulus

Occasionally a massive intra-thoracic hiatus hernia may twist upon itself, either in the organoaxial or lateral axis, leading to a gastric volvulus. This leads to complete oesophageal or gastric obstruction and the patient presents with severe chest pain, vomiting and dysphagia. The diagnosis is made by chest X-ray (air bubble in the chest) and barium swallow. Most cases spontaneously resolve but tend to recur and surgery is usually advised after nasogastric decompression.

Investigations

Young patients who present with typical symptoms of gastro-oesophageal reflux, without worrying features such as dysphagia, weight loss or anaemia, can be treated empirically without investigation.

Investigation is advisable if patients present in middle or late age, if symptoms are atypical or if a complication is suspected. Endoscopy is the investigation of choice. This is performed to exclude other upper gastrointestinal diseases which can mimic gastro-oesophageal reflux, and to identify complications. A normal endoscopy in a patient with compatible symptoms should not preclude treatment for gastro-oesophageal reflux disease.

Twenty-four-hour pH monitoring is indicated if, despite endoscopy, the diagnosis is unclear or surgical intervention is under consideration. This involves tethering a slim catheter with a terminal radiotelemetry pH-sensitive probe above the gastro-oesophageal junction. The intraluminal pH is recorded whilst the patient undergoes normal activities, and episodes of pain are noted and related to pH. A pH of less than 4 for more than 6–7% of the study time is diagnostic of reflux disease.

Management

Lifestyle advice, including weight loss, avoidance of dietary items which the patient finds worsen symptoms, elevation of the bed head in those who experience nocturnal symptoms, avoidance of late meals and giving up smoking, are recommended but rarely heeded.

Proprietary antacids and alginates also provide symptomatic benefit. H_2-receptor antagonist drugs (p. 889) also help symptoms without healing oesophagitis.

Proton pump inhibitors (p. 887) are the treatment of choice for severe symptoms and for complicated reflux disease (Box 22.31). Symptoms almost invariably resolve and oesophagitis heals in the majority of patients. Recurrence of symptoms is common when therapy is stopped and some patients require life-long treatment at the lowest acceptable dose.

Patients who fail to respond to medical therapy, those who are unwilling to take long-term proton pump inhibitors and those whose major symptom is severe regurgitation should be considered for anti-reflux surgery. This can be undertaken by an open or laparoscopic operation. Although heartburn and regurgitation are alleviated in most patients, a small minority develop complications such as inability to vomit and abdominal bloating ('gas-bloat syndrome').

EBM

22.31 PHARMACOLOGICAL INTERVENTION IN GASTRO-OESOPHAGEAL REFLUX DISEASE

'Proton pump inhibitors are better than H_2-receptor antagonists in healing oesophagitis and relieving symptoms.'

- Bate CM, et al. Aliment Pharmacol Ther 1998; 12:41–47.

For further information: 🖥 www.evidbasedgastro.com

22.32 GASTRO-OESOPHAGEAL REFLUX DISEASE IN OLD AGE

- **Prevalence**: higher.
- **Severity of symptoms**: does not correlate with the degree of mucosal inflammation.
- **Complications**: late complications such as peptic strictures or bleeding from oesophagitis are more common.
- **Recurrent pneumonia**: consider aspiration from occult gastro-oesophageal reflux disease.

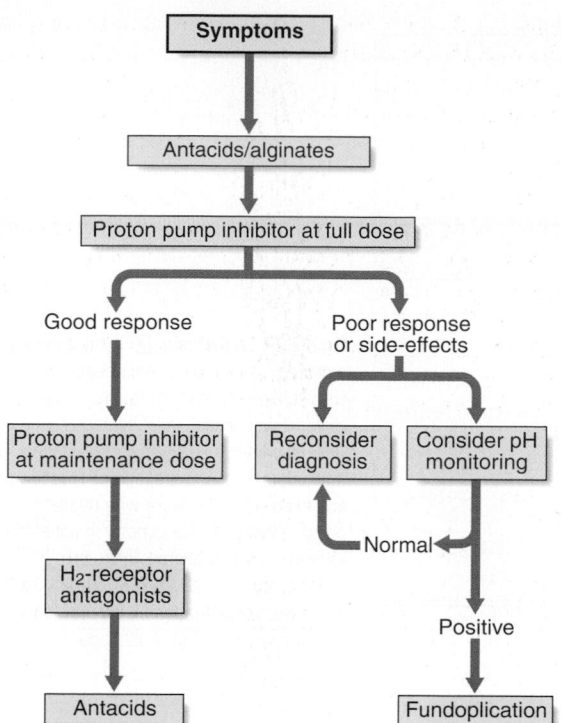

Fig. 22.28 Treatment of gastro-oesophageal reflux disease: a 'step-down' approach.

Recently, novel endoscopic methods of performing fundoplication or augmenting function of the lower oesophageal sphincter have been developed. A treatment algorithm is outlined in Figure 22.28.

OTHER CAUSES OF OESOPHAGITIS

Infection
Oesophageal candidiasis occurs in debilitated patients and those taking broad-spectrum antibiotics or cytotoxic drugs. It is a particular problem in AIDS patients, who are also susceptible to a spectrum of other oesophageal infections (p. 386).

Corrosives
Suicide attempt by strong household bleach or battery acid is followed by painful burns of the mouth and pharynx and by extensive erosive oesophagitis. This is complicated by oesophageal perforation with mediastinitis and by stricture formation. At the time of presentation treatment is conservative, based upon analgesia and nutritional support; vomiting and endoscopy should be avoided because of the high risk of oesophageal perforation. Following the acute phase, a barium swallow should be performed to demonstrate the extent of stricture formation. Endoscopic dilatation is usually necessary, although it is difficult and hazardous because strictures are often long, tortuous and easily perforated.

Drugs
Potassium supplements and NSAIDs may cause oesophageal ulcers when the tablets are trapped above an oesophageal stricture. Liquid preparations of these drugs should be used in such patients. Bisphosphonates, especially alendronate, cause oesophageal ulceration and should be used with caution in patients with known oesophageal disorders.

MOTILITY DISORDERS

PHARYNGEAL POUCH

Incoordination of swallowing within the pharynx leads to herniation through the cricopharyngeus muscle and formation of a pouch. Most patients are elderly and have no symptoms, although regurgitation, halitosis and dysphagia can occur. Some notice gurgling in the throat after swallowing. A barium swallow demonstrates the pouch and reveals incoordination of swallowing, often with pulmonary aspiration. Endoscopy may be hazardous since the instrument may enter and perforate the pouch. Surgical myotomy and resection of the pouch are indicated in symptomatic patients.

ACHALASIA OF THE OESOPHAGUS

Pathophysiology
Achalasia is characterised by:

- a hypertonic lower oesophageal sphincter which fails to relax in response to the swallowing wave
- failure of propagated oesophageal contraction, leading to progressive dilatation of the gullet.

The cause is unknown, although failure of non-adrenergic, non-cholinergic (NANC) innervation related to abnormal nitric oxide synthesis within the lower oesophageal sphincter has been found. Degeneration of ganglion cells within the sphincter and the body of the oesophagus occurs. Loss of the dorsal vagal nuclei within the brain stem can be demonstrated in later stages.

Chagas disease (p. 355) is endemic in South America; infestation with the protozoan organism *Trypanosoma cruzi* leads to myocarditis and a range of motility disorders of the gastrointestinal tract. Destruction of the myenteric plexus causes a syndrome which is clinically indistinguishable from achalasia.

Clinical features
Achalasia is an unusual disease affecting 1:100 000 people. It usually develops in middle life but can occur at any age. Dysphagia develops slowly, and is initially intermittent; it is worse for solids and is eased by drinking liquids, and by standing and moving around after eating. Heartburn does not occur because the closed oesophageal sphincter prevents gastro-oesophageal reflux. Some patients experience episodes of severe chest pain due to oesophageal spasm ('vigorous achalasia'). As the disease progresses dysphagia worsens, the oesophagus empties poorly and nocturnal pulmonary aspiration develops. Achalasia predisposes to squamous carcinoma of the oesophagus.

22

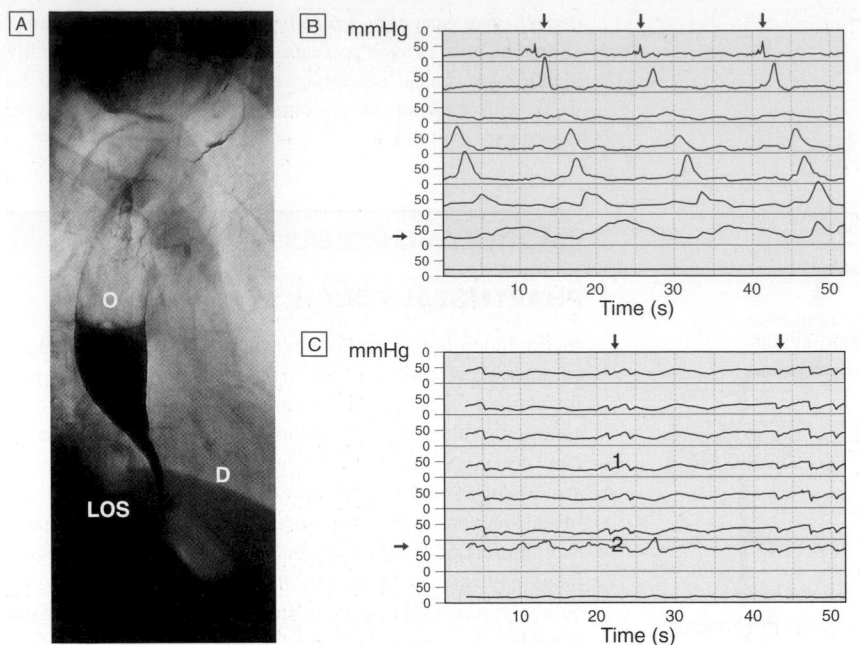

Fig. 22.29 Achalasia. A X-ray showing a dilated, barium-filled oesophagus (O) with fluid level and distal tapering, and a closed lower oesophageal sphincter (LOS). (D = diaphragm) B Normal oesophageal manometry showing propagated swallows and normal LOS pressure with relaxation on swallowing. C Manometry in achalasia showing non-propagated, ineffective contractions (1) and raised LOS pressure with failure of relaxation on swallowing (2). Compare with Figure 22.1, page 852.

Investigations

A chest X-ray may be abnormal in late disease, with widening of the mediastinum from gross oesophageal dilatation and features of aspiration pneumonia. A barium swallow shows tapered narrowing of the lower oesophagus. In late disease the oesophageal body is dilated, aperistaltic and food-filled (Fig. 22.29A). Endoscopy must always be carried out because carcinoma of the cardia can mimic the presentation and radiological and manometric features of achalasia ('pseudo-achalasia'). Manometry confirms the high-pressure, non-relaxing lower oesophageal sphincter with poor contractility of the oesophageal body (Fig. 22.29C).

Management

Endoscopic

Forceful pneumatic dilatation using a 30–35 mm diameter fluoroscopically positioned balloon disrupts the oesophageal sphincter and improves symptoms in 80% of patients. Some patients require more than one dilatation but those requiring frequent dilatation are best treated surgically. Endoscopically directed injection of botulinum toxin into the lower oesophageal sphincter induces clinical remission, but late relapse is common.

Surgical

Surgical myotomy ('Heller's operation'), performed either as an open operation or (increasingly) laparoscopically, is an extremely effective although more invasive option. Both pneumatic dilatation and myotomy may be complicated by gastro-oesophageal reflux, and this can lead to severe oesophagitis because oesophageal clearance is so poor in these patients. For this reason Heller's myotomy is accompanied by a partial fundoplication anti-reflux procedure. Proton pump inhibitor therapy is also often necessary.

OTHER OESOPHAGEAL MOTILITY DISORDERS

Diffuse oesophageal spasm presents in late middle age with episodic chest pain which may mimic angina, but is sometimes accompanied by transient dysphagia. Some cases occur in response to gastro-oesophageal reflux. Treatment is based upon the use of proton pump inhibitor drugs when gastro-oesophageal reflux is present. Oral or sublingual nitrates or nifedipine may relieve attacks of pain. Drug therapy is often disappointing and the alternatives, pneumatic dilatation and surgical myotomy, are also poor.

'Nutcracker' oesophagus is a condition in which extremely forceful peristaltic activity leads to episodic chest pain and dysphagia. Treatment is based upon the use of nitrates or nifedipine.

Non-specific motility disorders represent a collection of oesophageal motility disorders which do not fall into a specific disease entity. Patients are usually elderly and present with dysphagia and chest pain. Manometric abnormalities ranging from poor peristalsis to spasm occur.

SECONDARY CAUSES OF OESOPHAGEAL DYSMOTILITY

In systemic sclerosis the muscle of the oesophagus is replaced by fibrous tissue. Consequently, oesophageal peristalsis fails and this leads to heartburn and dysphagia. Oesophagitis is often severe, and benign fibrous strictures occur. Such patients require long-term therapy with proton pump inhibitor drugs. Dermatomyositis, rheumatoid arthritis and myasthenia gravis may also cause dysphagia.

22.33 CAUSES OF OESOPHAGEAL STRICTURE

- Gastro-oesophageal reflux disease
- Webs and rings
- Carcinoma of the oesophagus or cardia
- Extrinsic compression from bronchial carcinoma
- Corrosive ingestion
- Post-operative scarring following oesophageal resection
- Post-radiotherapy
- Following long-term nasogastric intubation

22.34 SQUAMOUS CARCINOMA: AETIOLOGICAL FACTORS

- Smoking
- Alcohol excess
- Chewing betel nuts or tobacco
- Coeliac disease
- Achalasia of the oesophagus
- Post-cricoid web
- Post-caustic stricture
- Tylosis (familial hyperkeratosis of palms and soles)

BENIGN OESOPHAGEAL STRICTURE

Benign oesophageal stricture is usually a consequence of gastro-oesophageal reflux disease (Box 22.33) and occurs most often in elderly patients who have poor oesophageal clearance. Rings, due to submucosal fibrosis, occur at the oesophago–gastric junction ('Schatzki ring') and cause intermittent dysphagia, often starting in middle age. A post-cricoid web is a rare complication of iron deficiency anaemia (Paterson–Kelly or Plummer–Vinson syndrome), and may be complicated by the development of squamous carcinoma.

Benign strictures are treated by endoscopic dilatation, in which wire-guided bougies or balloons are used to disrupt the fibrous tissue of the stricture.

TUMOURS OF THE OESOPHAGUS

BENIGN TUMOURS

The most common is a gastrointestinal stromal tumour (GIST). This is usually asymptomatic but may cause bleeding or dysphagia.

CARCINOMA OF THE OESOPHAGUS

Almost all are adenocarcinoma or squamous cancers. Small-cell cancer is a rare third type.

Squamous cancer

In Western populations squamous oesophageal cancer (Box 22.34) is relatively rare (approximately 4 cases per 100 000), whilst in Iran, parts of Africa and China it is common (200 per 100 000). Squamous cancer can arise in any part of the oesophagus from the post-cricoid region to the cardia. Almost all tumours above the lower third of the oesophagus are squamous cancers.

Adenocarcinoma

This arises in the lower third of the oesophagus from Barrett's oesophagus or from the cardia of the stomach. The incidence of this tumour is increasing and is now approximately 5:100 000 in the UK; this is possibly because of the high prevalence of gastro-oesophageal reflux and Barrett's oesophagus in Western populations.

Clinical features

Most patients have a history of progressive, painless dysphagia for solid foods. Others present acutely because of food bolus obstruction. In late stages weight loss is often

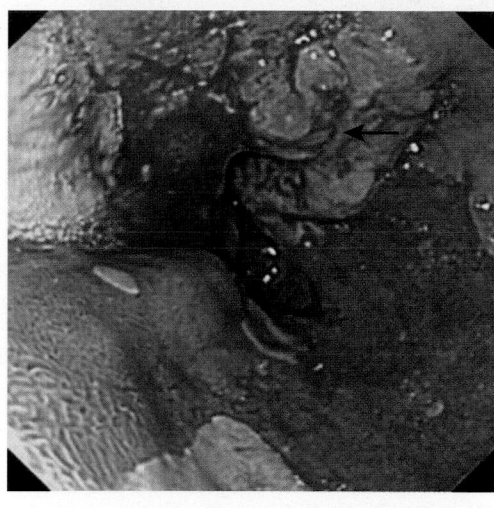

Fig. 22.30 Adenocarcinoma of the lower oesophagus. Adenocarcinoma in association with Barrett's oesophagus (arrow).

extreme; chest pain or hoarseness suggests mediastinal invasion. Fistulation between the oesophagus and the trachea or bronchial tree leads to coughing after swallowing, pneumonia and pleural effusion. Physical signs may be absent but even at initial presentation cachexia, cervical lymphadenopathy or other evidence of metastatic spread is common.

Investigations

The investigation of choice is upper gastrointestinal endoscopy (Fig. 22.30) with cytology and biopsy. A barium swallow demonstrates the site and length of the stricture but adds little useful information.

Once a diagnosis has been achieved, investigations are performed to stage the tumour and define operability. Thoracic and abdominal CT are carried out to identify metastatic spread and local invasion. Invasion of the aorta and other local structures may preclude surgery. Unfortunately, CT tends to understage tumours and the most sensitive modality is endoscopic ultrasound (EUS), in which an ultrasound transducer is incorporated into the tip of a modified endoscope (Fig. 22.31). These investigations will define the TNM stage of the disease (Ch. 11).

Management

Despite modern treatment, the overall 5-year survival of patients presenting with oesophageal cancer is 6–9%. Survival following oesophageal resection depends on stage. Tumours which have extended beyond the wall of the oesophagus and have lymph node involvement (T3, N1)

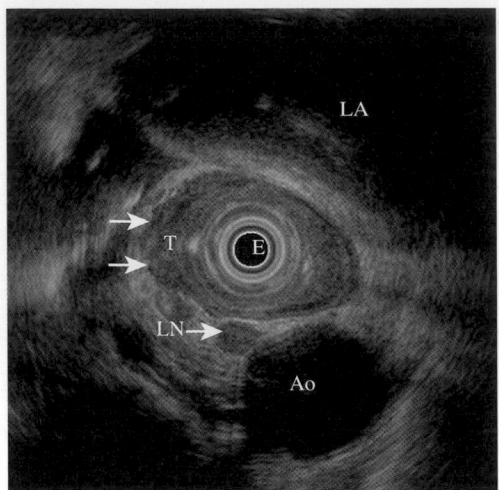

Fig. 22.31 Endoscopic ultrasound staging of oesophageal carcinoma. The tumour (T) has extended through the oesophageal wall (stage T3, arrows). A small peri-tumoral lymph node (LN) is also seen. (Ao = aorta; LA = left atrium; E = echoendoscope)

22

are associated with a 5-year survival of around 10% after surgery. However, this figure improves significantly if the tumour is confined to the oesophageal wall and there is no spread to lymph nodes. Overall survival following 'potentially curative' surgery (all macroscopic tumour removed) is about 30% at 5 years, but recent studies have suggested that this can be improved by neoadjuvant (pre-operative) chemotherapy with agents such as cisplatin and 5-fluorouracil. Although squamous carcinomas are radiosensitive, radiotherapy alone is associated with a 5-year survival of only 5%.

Approximately 70% of patients have extensive disease at presentation; in these, treatment is palliative and based upon relief of dysphagia and pain. Endoscopically directed tumour ablation using laser therapy or insertion of stents is the major method of improving swallowing. Palliative radiotherapy may induce shrinkage of both squamous cancers and adenocarcinomas but symptomatic response may be slow. Quality of life can be improved by nutritional support and appropriate analgesia.

PERFORATION OF THE OESOPHAGUS

The most common cause is endoscopic perforation complicating dilatation or intubation. Malignant, corrosive or post-radiotherapy strictures are more likely to be perforated than peptic strictures. A perforated peptic stricture is usually managed conservatively using broad-spectrum antibiotics and parenteral nutrition; most heal within days. Malignant, caustic and radiotherapy stricture perforations require surgical resection or intubation.

Spontaneous oesophageal perforation ('Boerhaave's syndrome') results from forceful vomiting and retching. Severe chest pain and shock occur as oesophago-gastric contents enter the mediastinum and thoracic cavity. Subcutaneous emphysema, pleural effusions and pneumothorax

develop. The diagnosis is made using a water-soluble contrast swallow, but in difficult cases both CT and careful endoscopy (usually in an intubated patient) may be required. Treatment is surgical. Delay in diagnosis is a key factor in the high mortality associated with this condition.

DISEASES OF THE STOMACH AND DUODENUM

GASTRITIS

Gastritis is a histological diagnosis, although it can sometimes be recognised at endoscopy.

ACUTE GASTRITIS

Acute gastritis is often erosive and haemorrhagic. Neutrophils are the predominant inflammatory cell in the superficial epithelium. Many cases result from aspirin or NSAID ingestion (Box 22.35). Acute gastritis often produces no symptoms but may cause dyspepsia, anorexia, nausea or vomiting, and haematemesis or melaena. Many cases resolve quickly and do not merit investigation; in others, endoscopy and biopsy may be necessary to exclude peptic ulcer or cancer. Treatment should be directed to the underlying cause. Short-term symptomatic therapy with antacids, and acid suppression using proton pump inhibitors or antiemetics (e.g. metoclopramide) may be necessary.

CHRONIC GASTRITIS DUE TO *HELICOBACTER PYLORI* INFECTION

This is the most common cause of chronic gastritis (Box 22.35). The predominant inflammatory cells are lymphocytes and plasma cells. Correlation between symptoms and

22.35 COMMON CAUSES OF GASTRITIS	

Acute gastritis (often erosive and haemorrhagic)

- Aspirin, NSAIDs
- *H. pylori* (initial infection)
- Alcohol
- Other drugs, e.g. iron preparations
- Severe physiological stress, e.g. burns, multi-organ failure, CNS trauma
- Bile reflux, e.g. following gastric surgery
- Viral infections, e.g. cytomegalovirus (CMV), herpes simplex virus in AIDS (pp. 384–385)

Chronic non-specific gastritis

- *H. pylori* infection
- Autoimmune (pernicious anaemia)
- Post-gastrectomy

Chronic 'specific' forms (rare)

- Infections, e.g. CMV, TB
- Gastrointestinal diseases, e.g. Crohn's disease
- Systemic diseases, e.g. sarcoidosis, graft-versus-host disease
- Idiopathic, e.g. granulomatous gastritis

endoscopic or pathological findings is poor. Most patients are asymptomatic and do not require any treatment but patients with dyspepsia may benefit from *H. pylori* eradication.

AUTOIMMUNE CHRONIC GASTRITIS

This involves the body of the stomach but spares the antrum; it results from autoimmune activity against parietal cells. The histological features are diffuse chronic inflammation, atrophy and loss of fundic glands, intestinal metaplasia and sometimes hyperplasia of enterochromaffin-like (ECL) cells. Circulating antibodies to parietal cell and intrinsic factor may be present. In some patients the degree of gastric atrophy is severe, and loss of intrinsic factor secretion leads to pernicious anaemia (p. 1028). The gastritis itself is usually asymptomatic. Some patients have evidence of other organ-specific autoimmunity, particularly thyroid disease. There is a fourfold increase in the risk of gastric cancer (see also p. 891).

MÉNÉTRIER'S DISEASE

In this rare condition the gastric pits are elongated and tortuous, with replacement of the parietal and chief cells by mucus-secreting cells. As a result, the mucosal folds of the body and fundus are greatly enlarged. Most patients are hypochlorhydric. Whilst some patients have upper gastro-intestinal symptoms, the majority present in middle or old age with protein-losing enteropathy (p. 900) due to exudation from the gastric mucosa. Barium meal shows enlarged, nodular and coarse folds which are also seen at endoscopy, although biopsies may not be deep enough to show all the histological features. Treatment with anti-secretory drugs may reduce protein loss but unresponsive patients require partial gastrectomy.

PEPTIC ULCER DISEASE

The term 'peptic ulcer' refers to an ulcer in the lower oesophagus, stomach or duodenum, in the jejunum after surgical anastomosis to the stomach or, rarely, in the ileum adjacent to a Meckel's diverticulum. Ulcers in the stomach or duodenum may be acute or chronic; both penetrate the muscularis mucosae but the acute ulcer shows no evidence of fibrosis. Erosions do not penetrate the muscularis mucosae.

GASTRIC AND DUODENAL ULCER

The prevalence of peptic ulcer is decreasing in many Western communities as a result of widespread use of *H. pylori* eradication therapy but it remains high in developing countries. The male to female ratio for duodenal ulcer varies from 5:1 to 2:1, whilst that for gastric ulcer is 2:1 or less.

Aetiology

Helicobacter pylori

In the industrialised world the prevalence of *H. pylori* infection in the general population rises steadily with age,

and in the UK approximately 50% of those over the age of 50 years are infected. In many parts of the developing world infection is much more common and is usually acquired in childhood. Up to 90% of the adult population are infected in some countries. The vast majority of colonised people remain healthy and asymptomatic and only a minority develop clinical disease. Around 90% of duodenal ulcer patients and 70% of gastric ulcer patients are infected with *H. pylori*; the remaining 30% of gastric ulcers are due to NSAIDs.

Pathogenesis and pathophysiology of infection. *H. pylori* is Gram-negative, spiral and has multiple flagella at one end which make it motile, allowing it to burrow and live deep beneath the mucus layer closely adherent to the epithelial surface. It uses an adhesin molecule (BabA) to bind to the Lewis b antigen on epithelial cells. Here the surface pH is close to neutral and any acidity is buffered by the organism's production of the enzyme urease. This produces ammonia from urea and raises the pH around the bacterium and between its two cell membrane layers. The bacteria spread by person-to-person contact via gastric refluxate or vomit. *H. pylori* exclusively colonises gastric-type epithelium and is only found in the duodenum in association with patches of gastric metaplasia.

The bacterium stimulates chronic gastritis by provoking a local inflammatory response in the underlying epithelium (Fig. 22.32). This depends on numerous factors, notably expression of bacterial cagA and vacA genes. The cagA gene is a marker for a segment of genome called the cag pathogenicity island (PaI), which encodes genes for a secretion system, comprising a syringe-like pilus through which the cagA product is injected into epithelial cells, ultimately interacting with numerous cell-signalling pathways involved in cell replication, apoptosis and morphology. *H. pylori* strains expressing cagA (cagA$^+$) are more often associated with disease than cagA$^-$ strains. Most strains also

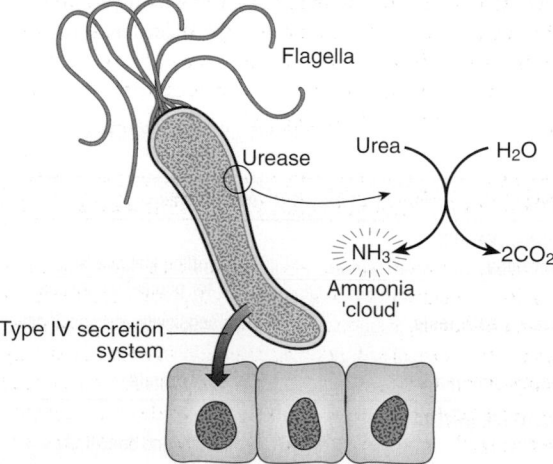

Other factors
- Vacuolating cytotoxin (vacA)
- Cytotoxin-associated gene (cagA)
- Adhesins (BabA)
- Outer inflammatory protein A (oipA)

Fig. 22.32 Factors which influence the virulence of *H. pylori*.

secrete a large pore-forming protein called vacA which causes large vacuoles to form in cells in vitro. In vivo, vacA has many effects including increased cell permeability, efflux of micronutrients from the epithelium, induction of apoptosis and suppression of local immune cell activity. Several forms of vacA exist and pathology is most strongly associated with the s1/m1 form of the toxin.

Host genetic polymorphisms are also important—for example, those that lead to greater levels of expression of the proinflammatory cytokine interleukin-1β (IL-1β) are associated with greater risk of gastric atrophy and subsequent carcinoma. Similar polymorphisms in other genes involved in the host inflammatory response to infection (e.g. IL-10 and TNF-α) may also be important.

In most people *H. pylori* causes antral gastritis associated with depletion of somatostatin (from D cells) and gastrin release from G cells. The subsequent hypergastrinaemia stimulates acid production by parietal cells, but in the majority of cases this has no clinical consequences. In a minority of patients (perhaps smokers) this effect is exaggerated, leading to duodenal ulceration (Fig. 22.33). The role of *H. pylori* in the pathogenesis of gastric ulcer is less clear but *H. pylori* probably acts by reducing gastric mucosal resistance to attack from acid and pepsin. In approximately 1% of infected people, *H. pylori* causes a pangastritis leading to gastric atrophy and hypochlorhydria. This allows bacteria to proliferate within the stomach; these may produce mutagenic nitrites from dietary nitrates, predisposing to the development of gastric cancer (Fig. 22.34).

Diagnosis. Many different diagnostic tests for *H. pylori* infection are available (Box 22.36). Some are invasive and require endoscopy; others are non-invasive. They vary in sensitivity and specificity. Overall, breath tests are best because of their accuracy, simplicity and non-invasiveness.

NSAIDs
See page 1090.

Smoking
Smoking confers an increased risk of gastric ulcer and, to a lesser extent, duodenal ulcer. Once the ulcer has formed, it

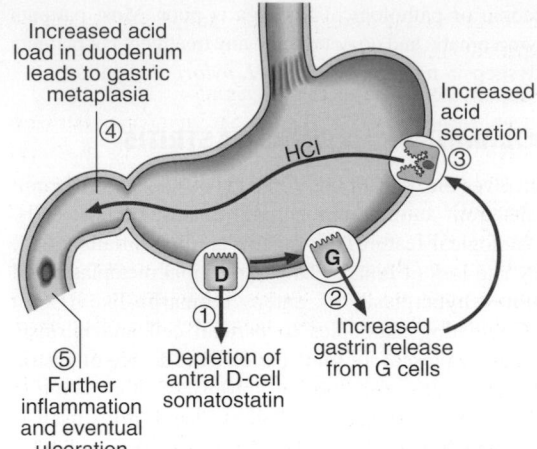

Fig. 22.33 Sequence of events in the pathophysiology of duodenal ulceration.

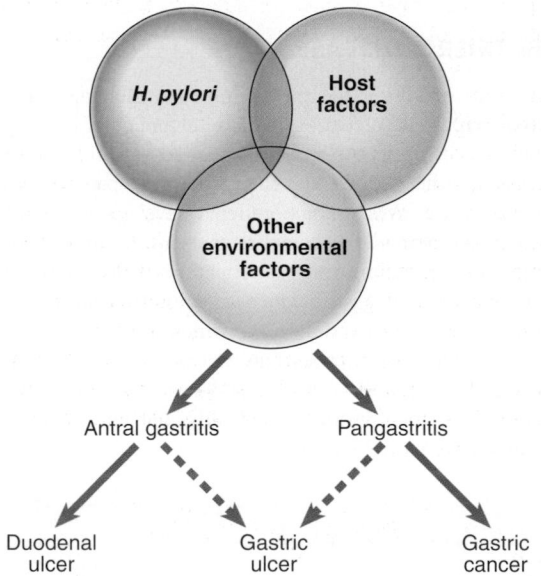

Fig. 22.34 Consequences of *H. pylori* infection.

22.36 METHODS FOR THE DIAGNOSIS OF *HELICOBACTER PYLORI* INFECTION		
Test	**Advantages**	**Disadvantages**
NON-INVASIVE		
Serology	Rapid office kits available Good for population studies	Lacks sensitivity and specificity Cannot differentiate current from past infection
Urea breath tests	High sensitivity and specificity	^{14}C uses radioactivity ^{13}C requires expensive mass spectrometer
Faecal antigen test	Cheap, accurate	Acceptability
INVASIVE (ANTRAL BIOPSY)		
Histology	Sensitivity and specificity	False negatives occur Takes several days to process
Rapid urease tests, e.g. CLO, Pyloritek	Cheap, quick Specificity	Lack sensitivity
Microbiological culture	'Gold standard' Defines antibiotic sensitivity	Slow and laborious Lacks sensitivity

is more likely to cause complications and less likely to heal if the patient continues to smoke.

Acid-pepsin versus mucosal resistance

An ulcer forms when there is an imbalance between aggressive factors, i.e. the digestive power of acid and pepsin, and defensive factors, i.e. the ability of the gastric and duodenal mucosa to resist this digestive power (Fig. 22.35). This mucosal resistance constitutes the gastric mucosal barrier. Ulcers occur only in the presence of acid and pepsin; they are never found in achlorhydric patients such as those with pernicious anaemia. On the other hand, severe intractable peptic ulceration nearly always occurs in patients with the Zollinger–Ellison syndrome (p. 890), which is characterised by very high acid secretion.

Most duodenal ulcer patients have markedly exaggerated acid secretion in response to stimulation by gastrin, and *H. pylori* (as already discussed) leads to hypergastrinaemia. In gastric ulcer patients the effects of *H. pylori* are more complex, and impaired mucosal defence resulting from a combination of *H. pylori* infection, NSAIDs and smoking may have a more important role.

Pathology

Chronic gastric ulcer is usually single; 90% are situated on the lesser curve within the antrum or at the junction between body and antral mucosa. Chronic duodenal ulcer usually occurs in the first part of the duodenum just distal to the junction of pyloric and duodenal mucosa; 50% are on the anterior wall. Gastric and duodenal ulcers coexist in 10% of patients and more than one peptic ulcer is found in 10–15% of patients. A chronic ulcer extends to below the muscularis mucosae and the histology shows four layers: surface debris, an infiltrate of neutrophils, granulation tissue and collagen.

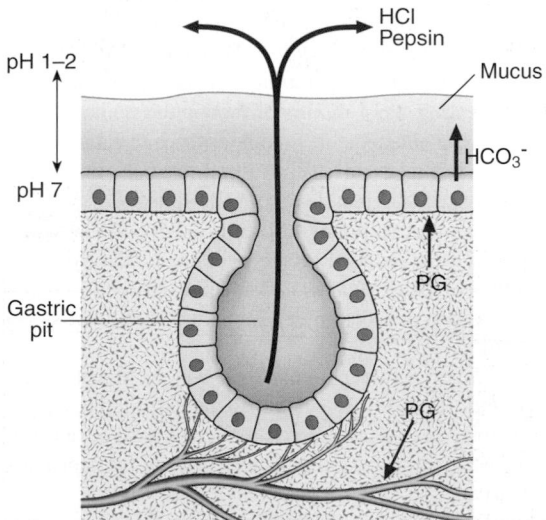

Fig. 22.35 Gastroduodenal mucosal protection. Prostaglandins (PG) stimulate bicarbonate and mucus secretion and increase mucosal blood flow. Bicarbonate ions are secreted into the unstirred mucus layer, neutralising hydrogen ions as they back-diffuse towards the epithelium. Rapid cell turnover and a rich mucosal blood supply are important protective elements.

Clinical features

Peptic ulcer disease is a chronic condition with a natural history of spontaneous relapse and remission lasting for decades, if not for life. Although they are different diseases, duodenal and gastric ulcers share common symptoms which will be considered together.

The most common presentation is that of recurrent abdominal pain which has three notable characteristics: localisation to the epigastrium, relationship to food and episodic occurrence. Occasional vomiting occurs in about 40% of ulcer subjects; persistent daily vomiting suggests gastric outlet obstruction.

In one-third of patients the history is less characteristic. This is especially true in elderly subjects under treatment with NSAIDs. In these patients pain may be absent or so slight that it is experienced only as a vague sense of epigastric unease. Occasionally, the only symptoms are anorexia and nausea, or a sense of undue repletion after meals. In some patients the ulcer is completely 'silent', presenting for the first time with anaemia from chronic undetected blood loss, as an abrupt haematemesis or as acute perforation; in others there is recurrent acute bleeding without ulcer pain between the attacks.

The diagnostic value of individual symptoms for peptic ulcer disease is poor; the history is therefore a poor predictor of the presence of an ulcer.

Investigations

Endoscopy is the preferred investigation. Gastric ulcers may occasionally be malignant and therefore must always be biopsied and followed up to ensure healing.

Management

The aims of management are to relieve symptoms, induce healing and prevent recurrence. *H. pylori* eradication is the cornerstone of therapy for peptic ulcers, as this will successfully prevent relapse and eliminate the need for long-term therapy in the majority of patients.

H. pylori eradication

All patients with proven acute or chronic duodenal ulcer disease and those with gastric ulcers who are *H. pylori*-positive should be offered eradication as primary therapy. Treatment is based upon a proton pump inhibitor taken simultaneously with two antibiotics (from amoxicillin, clarithromycin and metronidazole) for 7 days (Box 22.37). Success is achieved in over 90% of patients, although compliance, side-effects (Box 22.38) and metronidazole resistance influence the success of therapy.

Second-line therapy should be offered to those patients who remain infected after initial therapy once the reasons for failure of first-line therapy have been established. For those who are still colonised after two treatments, the choice lies between a third attempt with quadruple therapy (bismuth, proton pump inhibitor and two antibiotics) or long-term maintenance therapy with acid suppression.

H. pylori and NSAIDs are independent risk factors for ulcer disease but it is not clear whether patients requiring long-term NSAID therapy should first undergo eradication therapy to reduce ulcer risk. Current evidence suggests that this is not necessary in young, fit patients with no history of

22

22.37 ANTIBIOTIC REGIMENS FOR *H. PYLORI* ERADICATION

'First-line therapy is a proton pump inhibitor (12-hourly), clarithromycin 500 mg 12-hourly, and amoxicillin 1 g 12-hourly or metronidazole 400 mg 12-hourly, for 7 days. Second-line therapy is a proton pump inhibitor (12-hourly), bismuth 120 mg 6-hourly, metronidazole 400 mg 12-hourly, and tetracycline 500 mg 6-hourly, for 7 days.'

- Lind T, et al. Gastroenterology 1999; 116(2):248–253.

For further information: 💻 www.evidbasedgastro.com

22.38 COMMON SIDE-EFFECTS OF *H. PYLORI* ERADICATION THERAPY

- Diarrhoea
    30–50% of patients; usually mild but *Clostridium difficile*-associated colitis can occur
- Flushing and vomiting when taken with alcohol (metronizadole)
- Nausea, vomiting
- Abdominal cramp
- Headache
- Rash

22.39 INDICATIONS FOR *H. PYLORI* ERADICATION

Definite	
• Peptic ulcer • MALToma	• *H. pylori*-positive dyspepsia

Not indicated	
• Asymptomatic	• Gastro-oesophageal reflux disease

Uncertain	
• Family history of gastric cancer • Non-ulcer dyspepsia	• Long-term NSAID users

ulcer disease or dyspepsia but a 'test and treat' strategy for older patients with major comorbidity or a previous ulcer history is recommended. Subsequent co-prescription of a proton pump inhibitor along with the NSAID is advised but is not always necessary for patients being given low-dose aspirin in whom the risk of ulcer complications is lower.

Other indications for *H. pylori* eradication are shown in Box 22.39.

General measures

Cigarette smoking, aspirin and NSAIDs should be avoided. Alcohol in moderation is not harmful and no special dietary advice is required.

Short-term management

Many different drugs are available for the short-term management of acid peptic symptoms (Box 22.40).

Maintenance treatment

Continuous maintenance treatment should not be necessary after successful *H. pylori* eradication. For the minority who do require it, the lowest effective dose should be used.

Surgical treatment

The cure of most peptic ulcers by *H. pylori* eradication therapy and the availability of safe, potent acid-suppressing drugs have made elective surgery for peptic ulcer disease a rare event. Indications for surgery are listed in Box 22.41.

The operation of choice for a chronic non-healing gastric ulcer is partial gastrectomy, preferably with a Billroth I anastomosis, in which the ulcer itself and the ulcer-bearing area of the stomach are resected. The reason for this is to exclude an underlying cancer. Definitive anti-acid surgery in the form of vagotomy and drainage (pyloroplasty or gastroenterostomy) or highly selective vagotomy is no longer indicated for duodenal ulcer disease. In the emergency situation 'under-running' the ulcer for bleeding or 'oversewing' (patch repair) for perforation is all that is required, in addition to taking a biopsy. In the presence of giant duodenal ulcers partial gastrectomy using a 'Polya' or Billroth II reconstruction may be required.

Complications of gastric resection or vagotomy

Although gastric surgery is now rarely undertaken for benign disease, many patients underwent ulcer operations in the pre-*H. pylori* era and some degree of disability is seen in up to 50% of these. In most, the effects are minor but in 10% of cases they significantly impair quality of life.

Dumping. Rapid gastric emptying leads to distension of the proximal small intestine as the hypertonic contents draw fluid into the lumen. This leads to abdominal discomfort and diarrhoea after eating. Autonomic reflexes release a range of gastrointestinal hormones which lead to vasomotor features such as flushing, palpitations, sweating, tachycardia and hypotension. Patients should therefore avoid large meals with high carbohydrate content.

Bile reflux gastritis. Duodenogastric bile reflux leads to chronic gastritis. This is usually asymptomatic but dyspepsia can occur. Symptomatic treatment with aluminium-containing antacids or sucralfate may be effective. A few patients require revisional surgery with creation of a Roux en Y loop to prevent bile reflux into the stomach.

Diarrhoea and maldigestion. Diarrhoea may develop after any peptic ulcer operation and usually occurs 1–2 hours after eating. Poor mixing of food in the stomach, with rapid emptying, inadequate mixing with pancreatic biliary secretions, reduced small intestinal transit times and bacterial overgrowth, may lead to malabsorption.

Diarrhoea often responds to dietary advice to eat small, dry meals with a reduced intake of refined carbohydrates. Antidiarrhoeal drugs such as codeine phosphate (15–30 mg 4–6 times a day) or loperamide (2 mg after each loose stool) are helpful.

Weight loss. Most patients lose weight shortly after surgery and 30–40% are unable to regain all the weight which is lost. The usual cause is reduced intake because of a small gastric remnant, but diarrhoea and mild steatorrhoea also contribute.

Anaemia. Anaemia is common many years after subtotal gastrectomy. Iron deficiency is the most common cause; folic acid and B_{12} deficiency are much less frequent. Inadequate dietary intake of iron and folate, lack of acid and intrinsic factor secretion, mild chronic low-grade blood loss from the gastric remnant and recurrent ulceration are responsible.

22.40 DRUGS USED IN THE SHORT-TERM MANAGEMENT OF PEPTIC ULCERS

Group	Examples	Mechanism	Comments
Antacids and alginates	Aluminium hydroxide, magnesium trisilicate, alginic acid	Antacids; alginates form protective mucosal 'raft'	Aluminium salts block digoxin absorption and are constipating while magnesium salts can cause diarrhoea; some have high sodium content and can exacerbate cardiac failure
H$_2$-antagonists	Ranitidine, cimetidine, famotidine, nizatidine	Competitive inhibitors of H$_2$-receptors on parietal and ECL cells (Fig. 22.3)	Less potent than PPIs; good safety profile— some available without prescription; cimetidine may interfere with warfarin and phenytoin metabolism via cytochrome P450
Proton pump inhibitors (PPIs)	Omeprazole, esomeprazole, lansoprazole, pantoprazole, rabeprazole	Irreversible inhibitors of H$^+$/K$^+$ ATPase on parietal cell surface (Fig. 22.3)	Potent acid suppression and rapid ulcer healing; used in *H. pylori* therapy; superior to H$_2$ antagonists for healing ulcers and oesophagitis
Chelates	Tripotassium dicitratobismuthate	Ammoniacal suspension of complex bismuth salt; anti-*H. pylori* activity and enhances mucosal protection	May darken tongue and stools
Complex salts	Sucralfate	Aluminium salt of sucrose octasulphate; little effect on acid —may protect ulcer base from peptic activity and enhance epithelial cell turnover	Caution in renal impairment; reports of bezoar formation
Prostaglandin analogues	Misoprostol	Enhance mucosal blood flow, stimulate mucus and bicarbonate secretion; stimulate epithelial proliferation	Diarrhoea; abortifacient—contraindicated in women of child-bearing age

22

22.41 INDICATIONS FOR SURGERY IN PEPTIC ULCER

Emergency

- Perforation
- Haemorrhage

Elective

- Complications, e.g. gastric outflow obstruction
- Recurrent ulcer following gastric surgery

Metabolic bone disease. Both osteoporosis and osteo-malacia occur as a consequence of calcium and vitamin D malabsorption.

Gastric cancer. An increased risk of gastric cancer has been reported from several epidemiological studies. The risk is highest in those with hypochlorhydria, duodenogastric reflux of bile, smoking and *H. pylori* infection. Although the relative risk is increased, the absolute risk of cancer remains low and endoscopic surveillance is not indicated following gastric surgery.

Complications of peptic ulcer disease

These are perforation, gastric outlet obstruction and bleeding.

Perforation

When free perforation occurs, the contents of the stomach escape into the peritoneal cavity, leading to peritonitis. Perforation occurs more commonly in duodenal than in gastric ulcers, and is usually found with ulcers on the anterior wall. About one-quarter of all perforations occur in acute ulcers and NSAIDs are often incriminated.

Clinical features. Perforation is often the first sign of ulcer, and a history of recurrent epigastric pain is uncommon. The most striking symptom is sudden, severe pain; its distribution follows the spread of the gastric contents over the peritoneum. Pain initially develops in the upper abdomen and rapidly becomes generalised; shoulder tip pain is due to irritation of the diaphragm. The pain is accompanied by shallow respiration due to limitation of diaphragmatic movements, and by shock. The abdomen is held immobile and there is generalised 'board-like' rigidity. Bowel sounds are absent and liver dullness to percussion decreases due to the presence of gas under the diaphragm. After some hours symptoms may improve, although abdominal rigidity remains. Later the patient's condition deteriorates as general peritonitis develops.

In at least 50% of cases an erect chest X-ray shows free air beneath the diaphragm. If not, a water-soluble contrast swallow will confirm leakage of gastroduodenal contents.

Management and prognosis. After resuscitation, the acute perforation is treated surgically, either by simple closure, or by converting the perforation into a pyloroplasty if it is large. On rare occasions a 'Polya' partial gastrectomy is required. Following surgery *H. pylori* should be treated (if present) and NSAIDs avoided.

Perforation carries a mortality of 25%. This high figure reflects the advanced age and significant comorbidity of this population.

Gastric outlet obstruction

The causes are shown in Box 22.42. The most common is an ulcer in the region of the pylorus.

Clinical features. Nausea, vomiting and abdominal distension are the cardinal features of gastric outlet

22.42 DIFFERENTIAL DIAGNOSIS AND MANAGEMENT OF GASTRIC OUTLET OBSTRUCTION

Cause	Management
Fibrotic stricture from duodenal ulcer, i.e. 'pyloric stenosis'	Balloon dilatation or surgery
Oedema from pyloric channel or duodenal ulcer	Proton pump inhibitor therapy
Carcinoma of antrum	Surgery
Adult hypertrophic pyloric stenosis	Surgery

22.43 PEPTIC ULCER DISEASE IN OLD AGE

- **Gastroduodenal ulcers**: have a greater incidence, admission rate and mortality.
- **Causes**: high prevalence of *H. pylori* and NSAID use, and impaired defence mechanisms.
- **Atypical presentations**: pain and dyspepsia are frequently absent or atypical so older people develop complications such as bleeding or perforation more frequently.
- **Bleeding**: older patients require more intensive management (including central venous pressure measurement) than younger patients because they tolerate hypovolaemic shock poorly.

22

obstruction. Large quantities of gastric content are often vomited, and food eaten 24 hours or more previously may be recognised.

Physical examination frequently shows evidence of wasting and dehydration. A succussion splash may be elicited 4 hours or more after the last meal or drink. Visible gastric peristalsis is diagnostic of gastric outlet obstruction.

Investigations. Loss of gastric contents leads to dehydration with low serum chloride and potassium, and raised serum bicarbonate and urea concentrations. This results in enhanced renal absorption of Na^+ in exchange for H^+ and paradoxical aciduria. Nasogastric aspiration of at least 200 ml of fluid from the stomach after an overnight fast suggests the diagnosis.

Endoscopy should be performed after the stomach has been emptied by a wide-bore nasogastric tube. Endoscopic balloon dilatation of benign stenoses may be possible in some patients.

Barium studies are rarely advisable because they cannot usually distinguish between peptic ulcer and cancer. Moreover, barium remains in the stomach and is difficult to remove.

Management. Nasogastric suction and intravenous correction of dehydration are undertaken. In severe cases at least 4 litres of isotonic saline and 80 mmol of potassium may be necessary during the first 24 hours. Correction of metabolic alkalosis is not required. In some patients proton pump inhibitor drugs heal ulcers, relieve pyloric oedema and overcome the need for surgery. In others partial gastrectomy is necessary although this is best done after a 7-day period of nasogastric aspiration which enables the stomach to return to normal size. A gastroenterostomy is an alternative operation but, unless this is accompanied by vagotomy, patients will require long-term proton pump inhibitor therapy to prevent stomal ulceration.

Bleeding
See pages 866–868.

ZOLLINGER–ELLISON SYNDROME

This is a rare disorder characterised by the triad of severe peptic ulceration, gastric acid hypersecretion and a non-beta cell islet tumour of the pancreas ('gastrinoma'). It probably accounts for about 0.1% of all cases of duodenal ulceration. The syndrome occurs in either sex at any age, although it is most common between 30 and 50 years of age.

Pathophysiology
The gastrinoma secretes large amounts of gastrin, which stimulates the parietal cells of the stomach to secrete acid to their maximal capacity and increases the parietal cell mass three- to sixfold. The acid output may be so great that it reaches the upper small intestine, reducing the luminal pH to 2 or less. Pancreatic lipase is inactivated and bile acids are precipitated. Diarrhoea and steatorrhoea result.

Pathology
Around 90% of tumours occur in the pancreatic head or proximal duodenal wall, the latter site being more common. At least half are multiple, and tumour size can vary from 1 mm to 20 cm. Approximately one-half to two-thirds are malignant but are often slow-growing. Adenomas of the parathyroid and pituitary glands (multiple endocrine neoplasia, MEN type 1; p. 802) are present in 20–60% of patients.

Clinical features
Peptic ulcers are multiple, severe and may occur in unusual sites such as the post-bulbar duodenum, jejunum or oesophagus. There is a poor response to standard ulcer therapy. The history is usually short; bleeding and perforations are common. The syndrome may present as severe recurrent ulceration following a standard operation for peptic ulcer. Diarrhoea is seen in one-third or more of patients and can be the presenting feature. The diagnosis should be suspected in all patients with unusual or severe peptic ulceration, especially if a barium meal shows abnormally coarse gastric mucosal folds.

Investigations
Hypersecretion of acid under basal conditions with little increase following pentagastrin may be confirmed by gastric aspiration. Serum gastrin levels are grossly elevated (10- to 1000-fold). Injection of the hormone secretin normally causes no change or a slight decrease in circulating gastrin concentrations, but in Zollinger–Ellison syndrome produces a paradoxical and dramatic increase in gastrin. Tumour localisation is best achieved by endoscopic ultrasound and radio-labelled somatostatin receptor scintigraphy.

Management
Approximately 30% of small and single tumours can be localised and resected but many tumours are multifocal. Some patients present with metastatic disease and surgery is inappropriate. Proton pump inhibitors have made total gastrectomy unnecessary and in the majority of patients continuous therapy with omeprazole heals ulcers and

alleviates diarrhoea. Larger doses (60–80 mg daily) than those used to treat duodenal ulcer are required. The synthetic somatostatin analogue, octreotide, given by subcutaneous injection, reduces gastrin secretion and is sometimes of value. Overall 5-year survival is 60–75% and all patients should be monitored for the later development of other manifestations of MEN 1.

FUNCTIONAL DISORDERS

NON-ULCER DYSPEPSIA

This is defined as chronic dyspepsia (pain or upper abdominal discomfort) in the absence of organic disease. Other commonly reported symptoms include early satiety, fullness, bloating and nausea. 'Ulcer-like' and 'dysmotility-type' subgroups are reported, but there is great overlap between these and also with irritable bowel syndrome.

Aetiology
The condition of non-ulcer dyspepsia probably covers a spectrum of mucosal, motility and psychiatric disorders.

Clinical features
Patients are usually young (< 40 years) and women are affected twice as commonly as men. Abdominal pain is associated with a variable combination of other 'dyspeptic' symptoms, the most common being nausea and bloating after meals. Morning symptoms are characteristic and pain or nausea may occur on waking. Direct enquiry may elicit symptoms suggestive of irritable bowel syndrome. Peptic ulcer disease must be considered, whilst in older subjects intra-abdominal malignancy is a prime concern.

There are no diagnostic signs, apart perhaps from in-appropriate tenderness on abdominal palpation. Symptoms may appear disproportionate to clinical well-being and there is no weight loss. Patients often appear anxious.

A drug history should be taken and the possibility of a depressive illness should be considered. Pregnancy should be ruled out in young women before radiological studies are undertaken. Alcohol misuse should be suspected when early morning nausea and retching are prominent.

Investigations
The history will often suggest the diagnosis but in older subjects an endoscopy is necessary to exclude mucosal disease. While an ultrasound scan may detect gallstones, these are rarely responsible for dyspeptic symptoms.

Management
The most important elements are explanation and reassurance. Possible psychological factors should be explored and the concept of psychological influences on gut function should be explained. Idiosyncratic and restrictive diets are of little benefit, but fat restriction may help.

Drug treatment is not especially successful but merits trial. Antacids are sometimes helpful. Prokinetic drugs such as metoclopramide (10 mg 8-hourly) or domperidone (10–20 mg 8-hourly) may be given before meals if nausea, vomiting or bloating is prominent. Metoclopramide may induce extrapyramidal side-effects, including tardive dyskinesia in young subjects. H_2-receptor antagonist drugs may be tried if night pain or heartburn is troublesome. Low-dose amitriptyline is sometimes of value. The role of *H. pylori* eradication remains controversial, although up to 10% may benefit and a minority (5–15%) avoid ulcer development in the next 3 years. Eradication also removes a major risk factor for gastric cancer but at the cost of a small risk of side-effects and worsening symptoms of underlying gastro-oesophageal reflux disease.

Symptoms which can be associated with an identifiable cause of stress resolve with appropriate counselling. Some patients have major chronic psychological disorders resulting in persistent or recurrent symptoms and need behavioural or other formal psychotherapy (p. 238).

FUNCTIONAL CAUSES OF VOMITING

Psychogenic retching or vomiting may occur in anxiety. It typically occurs on wakening or immediately after breakfast and only rarely later in the day. The disorder is probably a reaction to facing up to the worries of everyday life; in the young it can be due to school phobia. Early morning vomiting also occurs in pregnancy, alcohol misuse and depression. Although functional vomiting may occur regularly over long periods, there is little or no weight loss. Children, and less often adults, sometimes suffer from acute and recurrent disabling bouts of vomiting for days at a time. The cause of this 'cyclical vomiting syndrome' is unknown.

In all patients it is essential to exclude other common causes (p. 866). Tranquillisers and antiemetic drugs (e.g. metoclopramide 10 mg 8-hourly, domperidone 10 mg 8-hourly, prochlorperazine 5–10 mg 8-hourly) have only a secondary place in management. Antidepressants in full dose may be effective (p. 237).

GASTROPARESIS

Defective gastric emptying without mechanical obstruction of the stomach or duodenum can occur as a primary event, due to inherited or acquired disorders of the gastric pacemaker, or can be secondary to disorders of autonomic nerves (particularly diabetic neuropathy) or the gastroduo-denal musculature (e.g. systemic sclerosis and amyloidosis). Early satiety and recurrent vomiting are the major symptoms; abdominal fullness and a succussion splash may be present on examination. Treatment is based upon the use of metoclopramide and domperidone. In severe cases nutritional failure can occur and long-term jejunostomy feeding or total parenteral nutrition is required. Surgical insertion of a gastric pacing device has been successful in some cases but remains experimental.

TUMOURS OF THE STOMACH

GASTRIC CARCINOMA

Although the incidence of gastric cancer in the UK has fallen markedly in recent years, it remains the leading cause of cancer death world-wide. There is marked geographical

22

variation in incidence. It is extremely common in China, Japan and parts of South America (mortality rate 30–40 per 100 000), less common in the UK (12–13 deaths per 100 000) and uncommon in the USA. Studies of Japanese migrants to the USA have revealed a much lower incidence in second-generation migrants, confirming the importance of environmental factors. Gastric cancer is more common in men and the incidence rises sharply after 50 years of age.

Aetiology

H. pylori is associated with chronic atrophic gastritis and gastric cancer (Fig. 22.36). *H. pylori* infection may be responsible for 60–70% of cases and acquisition of infection at an early age may be important. Although *H. pylori* infection is common in Africa, gastric cancer is uncommon and this 'enigma' may be explained by lower life expectancy in this part of the world. Although the majority of *H. pylori*-infected individuals have normal or increased acid secretion, a few become hypo- or achlorhydric and these people are thought to be at greatest risk. Chronic inflammation with generation of reactive oxygen species and depletion of the normally abundant antioxidant ascorbic acid are also important.

Diets rich in salted, smoked or pickled foods and the consumption of nitrites and nitrates may increase cancer risk. Carcinogenic N-nitroso-compounds are formed from nitrates by the action of nitrite-reducing bacteria which colonise the achlorhydric stomach. Diets lacking fresh fruit and vegetables as well as vitamins C and A may also contribute. Other risk factors are listed in Box 22.44.

No predominant genetic abnormality has been identified, although cancer risk is increased two- to threefold in first-degree relatives of patients, and links with blood group A

22.44 RISK FACTORS FOR GASTRIC CANCER
● *H. pylori*
● Smoking
● Alcohol
● Dietary associations (see text)
● Autoimmune gastritis (pernicious anaemia)
● Adenomatous gastric polyps
● Previous partial gastrectomy (> 20 years)
● Ménétrier's disease
● Hereditary diffuse gastric cancer families (HDC-1 mutations)
● Familial adenomatous polyposis (FAP, p. 924)

have been reported. Rare 'gastric cancer families' have also been described, in which diffuse gastric cancers occur in association with mutations of the *E-cadherin* gene. This is inherited as an autosomal dominant trait.

Pathology

Virtually all tumours are adenocarcinomas arising from mucus-secreting cells in the base of the gastric crypts. Most develop upon a background of chronic atrophic gastritis with intestinal metaplasia and dysplasia. Cancers are either 'intestinal', arising from areas of intestinal metaplasia with histological features reminiscent of intestinal epithelium, or 'diffuse', arising from normal gastric mucosa. Intestinal carcinomas are more common, and arise against a background of chronic mucosal injury. Diffuse cancers tend to be poorly differentiated and occur in younger patients.

In the developing world 50% of gastric cancers develop in the antrum, 20–30% occur in the gastric body, often on the greater curve, and 20% are found in the cardia. In Western populations, however, proximal gastric tumours are becoming more common than those arising in the body and distal stomach. This change in disease pattern may be a reflection of changes in lifestyle or the decreasing prevalence of *H. pylori* in the West. Diffuse submucosal infiltration by a scirrhous cancer (linitis plastica) is uncommon. Macroscopically, tumours may be classified as polypoid, ulcerating, fungating or diffuse.

Early gastric cancer is defined as cancer confined to the mucosa or submucosa, regardless of lymph node involvement (Fig. 22.37). It is often recognised in Japan, where widespread screening is practised. Over 80% of patients in the West present with advanced gastric cancer.

Clinical features

Early gastric cancer is usually asymptomatic but may occasionally be discovered during endoscopy for investigation of dyspepsia. Two-thirds of patients with advanced cancers have weight loss and 50% have ulcer-like pain. Anorexia and nausea occur in one-third, while early satiety, haematemesis, melaena and dyspepsia alone are less common features. Dysphagia occurs in tumours of the gastric cardia which obstruct the gastro-oesophageal junction. Anaemia from occult bleeding is also common.

Examination may reveal no abnormalities, but signs of weight loss, anaemia or a palpable epigastric mass are not infrequent. Jaundice or ascites may signify metastatic spread. Occasionally, tumour spread occurs to the supraclavicular

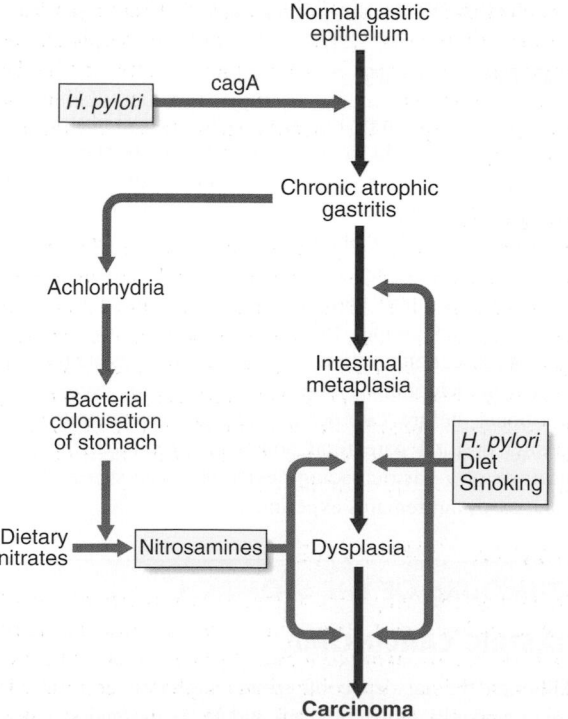

Fig. 22.36 Gastric carcinogenesis: a possible mechanism.

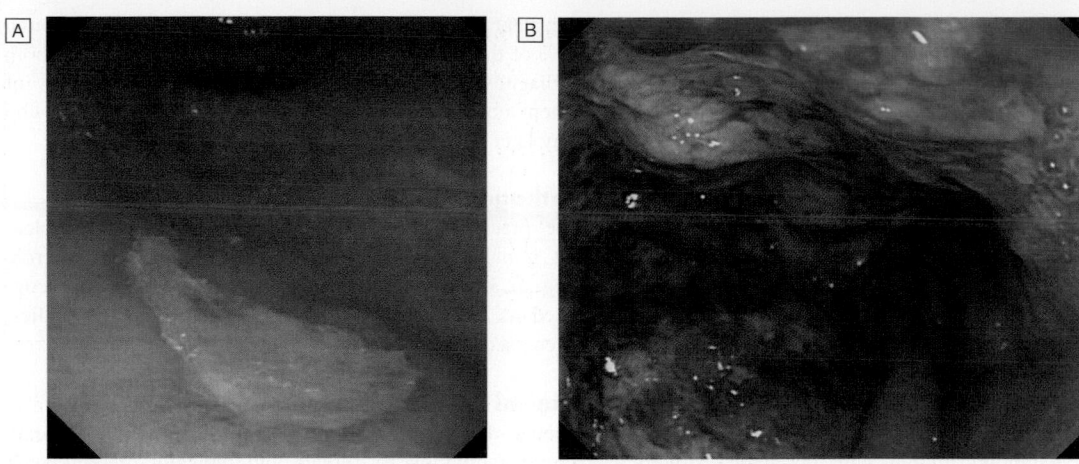

Fig. 22.37   Gastric carcinoma. A Endoscopic view of early cancer showing a shallow, depressed ulcer. B Advanced cancer seen as an infiltrating mass in the gastric body.

lymph nodes (Troisier's sign), umbilicus ('Sister Joseph's nodule') or ovaries (Krukenberg tumour). Paraneoplastic phenomena, such as acanthosis nigricans, thrombophlebitis (Trousseau's sign) and dermatomyositis, occur rarely. Metastases occur most commonly in the liver, lungs, peritoneum and bone marrow.

Diagnosis and staging

There are no laboratory markers of sufficient accuracy for the diagnosis of gastric cancer. Upper gastrointestinal endoscopy is the investigation of choice and should be performed promptly in any dyspeptic patient with 'alarm features' (p. 865). Multiple biopsies from the edge and base of a gastric ulcer are required and exfoliative brush cytology also improves the diagnostic yield. Barium meal is a poor alternative approach and any abnormalities must be followed by endoscopy to obtain biopsy. Once the diagnosis is made, further imaging is necessary for accurate staging and assessment of resectability. CT may not demonstrate small involved lymph nodes, but will show evidence of intra-abdominal spread or liver metastases. Even with these techniques, laparoscopy is required to determine whether the tumour is resectable as it is the only modality that will reliably detect peritoneal spread.

Management

Surgery

Resection offers the only hope of cure, which can be achieved in 90% of patients with early gastric cancer. For the majority who have locally advanced disease radical and total gastrectomy with lymphadenectomy is the operation of choice, preserving the spleen if possible. Proximal tumours involving the oesophago–gastric junction require an associated distal oesophagectomy. Small distally sited tumours can be managed by a partial gastrectomy with lymphadenectomy and either a Billroth I or Roux en Y reconstruction. More extensive lymph node resection may increase survival rates but carries greater morbidity. Even for those who cannot be cured, palliative resection may be necessary when patients present with bleeding or gastric

outflow obstruction. Following surgery, recurrence is much more likely if serosal penetration has occurred, although complete removal of all macroscopic tumour combined with lymphadenectomy will achieve a 50–60% 5-year survival. There is no current evidence to suggest that either neoadjuvant chemotherapy (before surgery and based on 5-fluorouracil) or adjuvant chemotherapy (after surgery) improves survival rates and post-operative radiotherapy has no value.

Unresectable tumours

The management of inoperable, locally advanced cancer is unsatisfactory. Modest palliation of symptoms can be achieved in some patients with chemotherapy using FAM (5-fluorouracil, doxorubicin and mitomycin C) or ECF (epirubicin, cisplatin and 5-fluorouracil). Endoscopic laser ablation of tumour tissue for control of dysphagia or recurrent bleeding benefits some patients. Carcinomas at the cardia may require endoscopic dilatation, laser therapy or insertion of expandable metallic stents to allow adequate swallowing.

Prognosis

With the exception of patients with early gastric cancer, overall prognosis remains very poor, with less than 30% surviving 5 years. Thus the best hope for improved survival lies in greater detection of tumours at an earlier stage. The low incidence of gastric carcinoma in many Western countries makes widespread endoscopic screening impractical but urgent referral and investigation of patients with new-onset dyspepsia over the age of 55, or those with 'alarm' features, are essential.

GASTRIC LYMPHOMA

Primary gastric lymphoma accounts for less than 5% of all gastric malignancies. The stomach is, however, the most common site for extranodal non-Hodgkin's lymphoma and 60% of all primary gastrointestinal lymphomas occur at this site. Lymphoid tissue is not found in the normal stomach but lymphoid aggregates develop in the presence of

H. pylori infection. Indeed, *H. pylori* infection is closely associated with the development of a low-grade lymphoma ('MALToma'). Superficial MALTomas may be cured by *H. pylori* eradication.

The clinical presentation is similar to that of gastric cancer and endoscopically the tumour appears as a polypoid or ulcerating mass. While initial treatment of low-grade MALTomas consists of *H. pylori* eradication and close observation, high-grade B-cell lymphomas are treated by a combination of chemotherapy, surgery and radiotherapy. The choice depends on the site and extent of tumour, the presence of comorbid illnesses, and other factors such as symptoms of bleeding and gastric outflow obstruction. The prognosis depends on the stage at diagnosis. Features predicting a favourable prognosis are stage I or II disease, small resectable tumours, tumours with low-grade histology, and age below 60 years.

OTHER TUMOURS OF THE STOMACH

Gastrointestinal stromal cell tumours (GIST) arising from the interstitial cells of Cajal are occasionally found at upper gastrointestinal endoscopy. They are differentiated from other mesenchymal tumours by expression of the c-kit proto-oncogene, which encodes a tyrosine kinase receptor. GISTs are usually benign and asymptomatic but may occasionally be responsible for dyspepsia; they can also ulcerate and cause gastrointestinal bleeding.

A variety of polyps occur. Hyperplastic polyps and fundic cystic gland polyps are common and of no consequence. Adenomatous polyps are rare; they have malignant potential and should be removed endoscopically.

Occasionally, gastric carcinoid tumours (p. 903) are seen in the fundus and body in patients with long-standing pernicious anaemia. These benign tumours arise from ECL or other endocrine cells, and are often multiple but rarely invasive. Unlike carcinoid tumours arising elsewhere in the gastrointestinal tract, they usually run a benign and favourable course. However, large (> 2 cm) carcinoids may metastasise and should be removed. Rarely, small nodules of ectopic pancreatic exocrine tissue are found. These 'pancreatic rests' may be mistaken for gastric neoplasms and usually cause no symptoms. Endoscopic ultrasound is the most useful investigation.

DISEASES OF THE SMALL INTESTINE

DISORDERS CAUSING MALABSORPTION

COELIAC DISEASE

Coeliac disease is an immunologically mediated inflammatory disorder of the small bowel occurring in genetically susceptible individuals and resulting from intolerance to wheat gluten and similar proteins found in rye, barley and, to a lesser extent, oats. It can result in malabsorption and responds to a gluten-free diet. The condition occurs worldwide but is more common in northern Europe. The true

prevalence in the UK is approximately 1 in 200, although 50% of these people are asymptomatic. These include both undiagnosed 'silent' cases of the disease and cases of 'latent' coeliac disease—genetically susceptible people who may later develop clinical coeliac disease.

Pathogenesis

The precise mechanism of mucosal damage is unclear but immunological responses to gluten play a key role (Fig. 22.38). Tissue transglutaminase (TTG) is now recognised as the autoantigen for anti-endomysial antibodies, often used in serological diagnosis.

Clinical features and associations

Coeliac disease presents at any age. In infancy it occurs after weaning on to cereals and typically presents with diarrhoea, malabsorption and failure to thrive. In older children it may present with non-specific features such as delayed growth. Features of malnutrition are often found on examination and mild abdominal distension may be present. Affected children have both growth and pubertal delay, leading to short stature in adulthood.

In adults peak onset is in the fifth decade and females are affected slightly more than males. The presentation is highly variable, depending on the severity and extent of small bowel involvement. Some patients have florid malabsorption while others develop non-specific symptoms such as tiredness, weight loss, folate deficiency or iron deficiency anaemia. Other recognised presentations include oral ulceration, dyspepsia and bloating.

Coeliac disease is associated with other human leucocyte antigen (HLA)-linked autoimmune disorders and with certain other diseases (Box 22.45).

Investigations

These are performed to confirm the diagnosis and to look for consequences of malabsorption.

Duodenal or jejunal biopsy

Endoscopic small bowel biopsy is the gold standard. The histological features are usually characteristic but other causes of villous atrophy should also be considered (Box 22.46 and Fig. 22.39). Sometimes the villi appear normal but there are excess numbers of intraepithelial lymphocytes present.

22.45 DISEASE ASSOCIATIONS OF COELIAC DISEASE

- Insulin-dependent diabetes mellitus (2–8%)
- Thyroid disease (5%)
- Primary biliary cirrhosis (3%)
- Sjögren's syndrome (3%)
- IgA deficiency (2%)
- Pernicious anaemia
- Inflammatory bowel disease
- Sarcoidosis
- Myasthenia gravis
- Neurological complications— encephalopathy, cerebellar atrophy, peripheral neuropathy, epilepsy

- Dermatitis herpetiformis
- Down's syndrome
- Enteropathy-associated T-cell lymphoma
- Small bowel carcinoma
- Squamous carcinoma of oesophagus
- Ulcerative jejunitis
- Pancreatic insufficiency
- Microscopic colitis
- Splenic atrophy

22

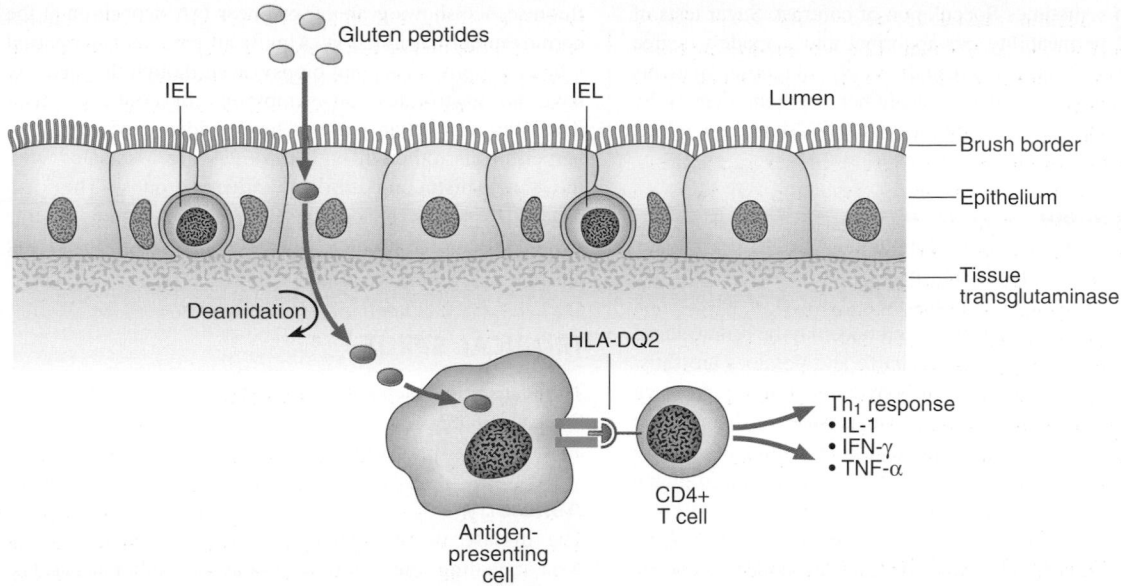

Fig. 22.38 Pathophysiology of coeliac disease. After being taken up by epithelial cells, gluten peptides are deamidated by the enzyme tissue transglutaminase in the subepithelial layer. They are then able to fit the antigen-binding motif on HLA-DQ2 positive antigen presenting cells. Recognition by CD4+ T cells triggers a Th₁ immune response with generation of pro-inflammatory cytokines (IL-1, IFN-γ and TNF-α). Lymphocytes infiltrate the lamina propria, and increased intraepithelial lymphocytes (IEL), crypt hyperplasia and villous atrophy ensue.

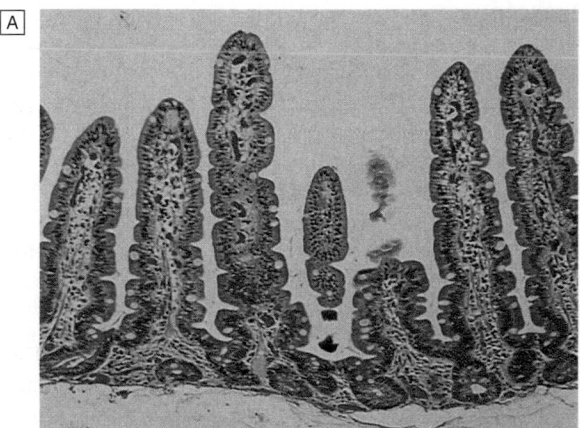

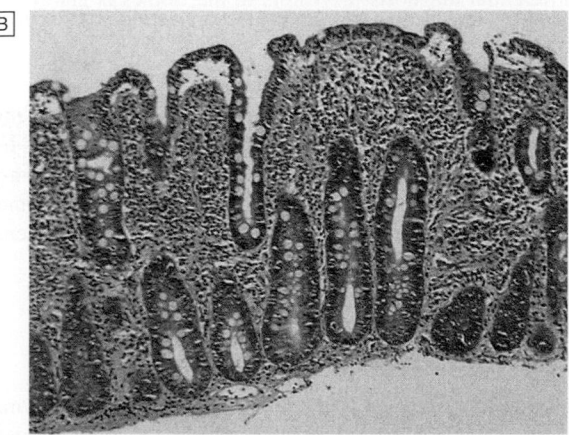

Fig. 22.39 Jejunal mucosa. A Normal. B Jejunum in coeliac disease showing subtotal villous atrophy and marked inflammatory infiltrate.

22.46 IMPORTANT CAUSES OF SUBTOTAL VILLOUS ATROPHY

- Coeliac disease
- Tropical sprue
- Dermatitis herpetiformis
- Lymphoma
- AIDS enteropathy
- Giardiasis
- Hypogammaglobulinaemia
- Radiation
- Whipple's disease
- Zollinger–Ellison syndrome

Antibodies

Serum antigliadin (especially IgA) and anti-endomysial antibodies are detectable in most untreated cases. IgA anti-endomysial antibodies are detected by immunofluorescence. They are not quantitative, but are sensitive (85–95%) and specific (approximately 99%) for the diagnosis, except in very young infants. IgG antibodies, however, must be analysed in patients with coexisting IgA deficiency. TTG assays have replaced other blood tests in many countries as they are easier to perform, semi-quantitative and more accurate in patients with IgA deficiency. These antibody tests constitute a valuable screening tool in patients with diarrhoea but are not a substitute for small bowel biopsy; they usually become negative with successful treatment.

Haematology and biochemistry

A full blood count may show microcytic or macrocytic anaemia from iron or folate deficiency and features of hyposplenism (target cells, spherocytes and Howell–Jolly bodies). Biochemical tests may reveal reduced concentrations of calcium, magnesium, total protein, albumin or vitamin D.

Other investigations

These are usually unnecessary. Barium follow-through X-rays may show dilated loops of bowel, coarse or diminished folds and sometimes flocculation of contrast. Sugar tests of intestinal permeability are abnormal and a modest degree of fat malabsorption is usual. Newly diagnosed patients should undergo baseline measurement of bone density by dual energy X-ray absorptiometry (DEXA scanning) to look for evidence of metabolic bone disease.

Management

The aims are to correct existing deficiencies of iron, folate, calcium and/or vitamin D, and to commence a life-long gluten-free diet. This requires the exclusion of wheat, rye, barley and initially oats, although oats may be reintroduced safely in most patients. Rice, maize and potatoes are satisfactory sources of complex carbohydrates. Initially, frequent dietary counselling is required to make sure the diet is being observed, as the most common reason for failure to improve with dietary treatment is accidental or unrecognised gluten ingestion. Mineral and vitamin supplements are also given when indicated but are seldom necessary when a strict gluten-free diet is adhered to. Booklets produced by coeliac societies in many countries, containing diet sheets and recipes for the use of gluten-free flour, are of great value. Regular monitoring of symptoms, weight and nutrition is essential. Patients who have an excellent clinical response, with disappearance of circulating anti-endomysial antibodies, probably do not need to undergo repeat jejunal biopsies. These should be reserved for patients who do not symptomatically improve or whose antibodies remain persistently positive.

Rarely, patients are 'refractory' and require treatment with corticosteroids or immunosuppressive drugs to induce remission. Dietary compliance should be carefully assessed in patients who fail to respond but if their diet is satisfactory, other conditions such as pancreatic insufficiency or microscopic colitis should be sought, as should complications of coeliac disease such as ulcerative jejunitis or enteropathy-associated T-cell lymphoma.

Prognosis and complications

There is an increased risk of malignancy, particularly of enteropathy-associated T-cell lymphoma, small bowel carcinoma and squamous carcinoma of the oesophagus. A few patients develop ulcerative jejunoileitis; fever, pain, obstruction or perforation may then supervene. The diagnosis of small bowel complications is rarely made by barium studies or enteroscopy, and laparotomy and full-thickness biopsy are usually necessary.

Treatment is difficult. Corticosteroids are used with mixed success and some patients require surgical resection and parenteral nutrition. The course is often progressive and relentless.

Metabolic bone disease is common in patients with long-standing, poorly controlled coeliac disease and is a source of considerable morbidity. This complication is less common in patients who adhere strictly to a gluten-free diet.

DERMATITIS HERPETIFORMIS

This is characterised by crops of intensely itchy blisters over the elbows, knees, back and buttocks (p. 1275). Immuno-

fluorescence shows granular or linear IgA deposition at the dermo–epidermal junction. Almost all patients have partial villous atrophy on jejunal biopsy, even though they usually have no gastrointestinal symptoms. In contrast, fewer than 10% of coeliac patients have evidence of dermatitis herpetiformis although both disorders are associated with the same histocompatibility antigen groups. The rash usually responds to a gluten-free diet but some patients require additional treatment with dapsone (100–150 mg daily).

TROPICAL SPRUE

Tropical sprue is defined as chronic, progressive malabsorption in a patient in or from the tropics, associated with abnormalities of small intestinal structure and function.

Aetiology

The disease occurs mainly in the West Indies and in Asia, including southern India, Malaysia and Indonesia. The epidemiological pattern and occasional epidemics suggest that an infective agent or agents may be involved. Although no single bacterium has been isolated, the condition often begins after an acute diarrhoeal illness. Small bowel bacterial overgrowth with *Escherichia coli*, *Enterobacter* and *Klebsiella* is frequently seen.

Pathology

The changes closely resemble those of coeliac disease. Partial villous atrophy is more common than subtotal villous atrophy.

Clinical features

There is diarrhoea, abdominal distension, anorexia, fatigue and weight loss. In visitors to the tropics the onset of severe diarrhoea may be sudden and accompanied by fever. When the disorder becomes chronic, the features of megaloblastic anaemia (folic acid malabsorption) and other deficiencies including ankle oedema, glossitis and stomatitis are common. Remissions and relapses may occur.

The differential diagnosis in the indigenous tropical population is an infective cause of diarrhoea. The important differential diagnosis in visitors to the tropics is giardiasis (p. 359).

Management

Tetracycline 250 mg 6-hourly for 28 days is the treatment of choice and brings about long-term remission or cure. In most patients pharmacological doses of folic acid (5 mg daily) improve symptoms and jejunal morphology. In some cases treatment must be prolonged before improvement occurs, and occasionally patients must leave the tropics.

SMALL BOWEL BACTERIAL OVERGROWTH ('BLIND LOOP SYNDROME')

The normal duodenum and jejunum contain less than 10^4/ml organisms which are usually derived from saliva. The count of coliform organisms never exceeds 10^3/ml. In bacterial overgrowth there may be 10^8–10^{10}/ml organisms, most of

22

22.47 CAUSES OF SMALL BOWEL BACTERIAL OVERGROWTH	
Mechanism	**Examples**
Hypo- or achlorhydria	Pernicious anaemia Partial gastrectomy Long-term proton pump inhibitor therapy
Impaired intestinal motility	Scleroderma Diabetic autonomic neuropathy Chronic intestinal pseudo-obstruction
Structural abnormalities	Gastric surgery (blind loop after Billroth II operation) Jejunal diverticulosis Enterocolic fistulae (e.g. Crohn's disease) Extensive small bowel resection Strictures (e.g. Crohn's disease)
Impaired immune function	Hypogammaglobulinaemia

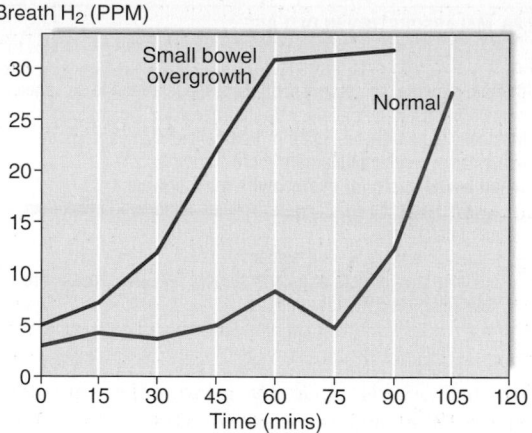

Fig. 22.40 **Early rise in breath hydrogen in small bowel bacterial overgrowth.**

which are normally found only in the colon. Disorders which impair the normal physiological mechanisms controlling bacterial proliferation in the intestine predispose to bacterial overgrowth (Box 22.47). The most important are loss of gastric acidity, impaired intestinal motility and structural abnormalities which allow colonic bacteria to gain access to the small intestine or provide a secluded haven from the peristaltic stream.

Clinical features

The patient presents with watery diarrhoea and/or steatorrhoea with anaemia due to B_{12} deficiency. These arise because of deconjugation of bile acids, which impairs micelle formation, and because of bacterial utilisation of vitamin B_{12}. There may also be symptoms from the underlying intestinal cause.

Investigations

Serum vitamin B_{12} concentration is low, whilst folate levels are normal or elevated because the bacteria produce folic acid. Barium follow-through or small bowel enema may reveal blind loops or fistulae. Endoscopic duodenal biopsies exclude mucosal disease such as coeliac disease. Jejunal contents for bacteriological examination can be aspirated at endoscopy; the laboratory analysis requires anaerobic and aerobic culture techniques. The diagnosis can often be made non-invasively using the glucose hydrogen or ^{14}C-glycocholic acid breath tests. In these tests breath samples are serially measured after oral ingestion of the test material. Bacteria within the small bowel cause an early rise in breath hydrogen from glucose (Fig. 22.40) or ^{14}C from ^{14}C-glycocholate.

Management

The underlying cause of small bowel bacterial overgrowth should be addressed. Tetracycline 250 mg 6-hourly for 7 days is then the treatment of choice, although up to 50% of patients do not respond adequately. Metronidazole 400 mg 8-hourly or ciprofloxacin 250 mg 12-hourly are alternatives. Some patients require up to 4 weeks of treatment and, in a few, continuous rotating courses of antibiotics are necessary.

Intramuscular vitamin B_{12} supplementation is needed in chronic cases.

Some specific causes of bacterial overgrowth

Jejunal diverticulosis

This is sometimes seen on barium follow-through examinations in patients over the age of 50 years. The diverticula are usually asymptomatic but predispose to bacterial overgrowth and subsequent malabsorption. Rarely, they may cause acute or chronic gastrointestinal bleeding, obstruction or perforation.

Diabetic diarrhoea

This results from diabetic autonomic neuropathy (p. 844), which reduces small bowel motility and affects enterocyte secretion. In some diabetic patients coexisting pancreatic insufficiency or coeliac disease may be responsible. The diarrhoea is watery and may be continuous or interrupted by bouts of constipation; it is often worse at night, frequently associated with faecal incontinence and may be refractory to antidiarrhoeal drugs. Treatment with antibiotics may be helpful but antidiarrhoeal drugs (diphenoxylate 5 mg 8-hourly orally or loperamide 2 mg 4–6-hourly orally) or opiates are usually needed. The α_2-adrenergic agonist clonidine (50–100 µg 8-hourly) or the somatostatin analogue octreotide may benefit some patients.

Progressive systemic sclerosis (scleroderma)

The circular and longitudinal layers of the intestinal muscle are fibrosed, motility is abnormal and malabsorption due to bacterial overgrowth is common. The patient may also have features of chronic intestinal pseudo-obstruction (p. 1135).

Hypogammaglobulinaemia

This rare disorder is characterised by a markedly reduced or absent IgA and IgM content in the serum and jejunal secretions. Chronic diarrhoea, malabsorption and respiratory infections are common. Diarrhoea is due to bacterial overgrowth and recurrent gastrointestinal infections (particularly giardiasis, p. 359).

22.48 MALABSORPTION IN OLD AGE

- **Coeliac disease**: symptoms such as dyspepsia tend to be vague; only 25% present classically with diarrhoea and weight loss. Metabolic bone disease, folate or iron deficiency, coagulopathy and small bowel lymphoma are more common.
- **Small bowel bacterial overgrowth**: more prevalent:
  — atrophic gastritis resulting in hypo- or achlorhydria becomes more common
  — jejunal diverticulosis is prevalent
  — the long-term effects of gastric surgery for ulcer disease are now being seen in older people.

The diagnosis is made by measurement of serum immunoglobulins and by intestinal biopsy which shows reduced or absent plasma cells and nodules of lymphoid tissue (nodular lymphoid hyperplasia). Some patients develop villous atrophy. Treatment involves control of giardiasis and, if necessary, regular parenteral replacement of immunoglobulins.

WHIPPLE'S DISEASE

This rare condition is characterised by infiltration of small intestinal mucosa by 'foamy' macrophages which stain positive with periodic acid–Schiff (PAS) reagent. The disease is a multisystem one and almost any organ can be affected, sometimes long before gastrointestinal involvement becomes apparent (Box 22.49).

Electron microscopy reveals small Gram-positive bacilli (*Tropheryma whipplei*) within the macrophages. Villi are widened and flattened; densely packed macrophages occur in the lamina propria. These may obstruct lymphatic drainage, causing fat malabsorption.

Clinical features

Middle-aged men are most commonly affected and the presentation depends on the pattern of organ involvement. Low-grade fever is common and most patients have joint symptoms to some degree, often as the first manifes-

---

22.49 CLINICAL FEATURES OF WHIPPLE'S DISEASE

Gastrointestinal
- Diarrhoea, steatorrhoea, weight loss, bloating, protein-losing enteropathy, ascites, hepatosplenomegaly (< 5%)

Musculoskeletal
- Seronegative large joint arthropathy, sacroiliitis

Cardiac
- Pericarditis (10%), myocarditis, endocarditis, coronary arteritis

Neurological
- Apathy, fits, dementia, myoclonus, meningitis, cranial nerve lesions

Pulmonary
- Chronic cough, pleurisy, pulmonary infiltrates

Haematological
- Anaemia, lymphadenopathy

Other
- Fever, pigmentation

---

tation. Occasionally, neurological manifestations may predominate.

Management

Whipple's disease is often fatal if untreated but responds well, at least initially, to co-trimoxazole and to a lesser degree, to tetracycline. Symptoms usually resolve quickly and biopsy changes revert to normal in a few weeks. Long-term follow-up is essential, as relapse occurs in up to one-third of patients. This often occurs within the CNS, in which case 2 weeks of parenteral ceftriaxone, followed by 6–12 months of oral co-trimoxazole, are necessary.

ILEAL RESECTION

The long-term effects of small bowel resection depend on the site and the amount of intestine resected, and vary from trivial to life-threatening.

Ileal resection usually occurs following surgery for Crohn's disease. Vitamin B_{12} and bile salt malabsorption develops (Fig. 22.41). Unabsorbed bile salts pass into the colon, stimulating water and electrolyte secretion and resulting in diarrhoea. If hepatic synthesis of new bile salts cannot keep pace with faecal losses, fat malabsorption occurs. Another consequence is the formation of lithogenic bile, leading to gallstones. Renal calculi, rich in oxalate, develop. Normally, oxalate in the colon is bound to and precipitated by calcium. Unabsorbed bile salts preferentially bind calcium, leaving free oxalate to be absorbed with subsequent development of urinary oxalate calculi.

Patients have urgent watery diarrhoea or mild steatorrhoea. Contrast studies of the small bowel and tests of B_{12} and bile acid absorption (pp. 863–864) are useful investigations. Parenteral vitamin B_{12} supplementation is necessary. Diarrhoea usually responds well to colestyramine, a resin which binds bile salts in the intestinal lumen. Aluminium hydroxide is an alternative therapy.

SHORT BOWEL SYNDROME

Short bowel syndrome is defined as malabsorption resulting from extensive small intestinal resection or disease.

Aetiology and pathogenesis

The syndrome has many causes (Box 22.50) but in adults it usually results from extensive surgery undertaken for Crohn's disease or mesenteric infarction.

Loss of surface area for digestion and absorption is the key problem. These processes are normally completed

---

22.50 AETIOLOGY OF SHORT BOWEL SYNDROME

Children	
• Congenital anomalies (e.g. mid-gut volvulus, atresia)	• Necrotising enterocolitis

Adults	
• Crohn's disease	• Radiation enteritis
• Mesenteric infarction	• Volvulus

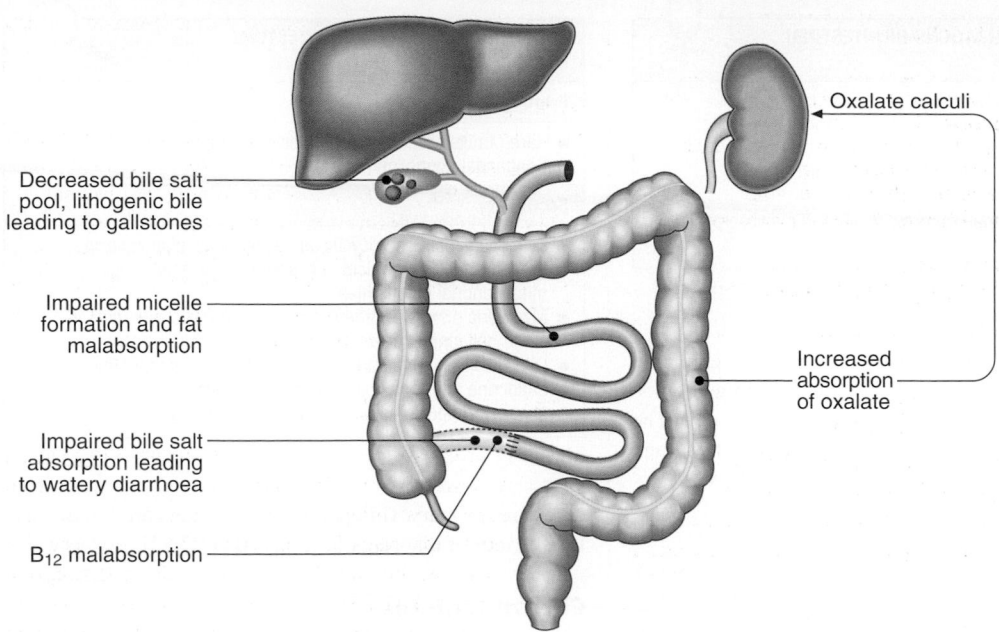

Oxalate calculi

Decreased bile salt pool, lithogenic bile leading to gallstones

Impaired micelle formation and fat malabsorption

Increased absorption of oxalate

Impaired bile salt absorption leading to watery diarrhoea

B_{12} malabsorption

Fig. 22.41 Consequences of ileal resection.

within the first 100 cm of jejunum, and enteral feeding is usually possible if this amount of small intestine remains. The proximal small bowel normally reabsorbs most of the 8 litres of fluid it receives daily, and patients with a high jejunostomy are at great risk of hypovolaemia, dehydration and electrolyte losses. The presence of some or all of the colon may markedly improve these losses by increased water reabsorption. The presence of an intact ileocaecal valve ameliorates the clinical picture by slowing small intestinal transit and reducing bacterial overgrowth. The remaining small bowel mucosa undergoes 'adaptation', whereby mucosal hyperplasia over months or years increases the effective surface area for absorption.

Clinical features
Severely affected patients have large volumes of jejuno-stomy fluid losses or, if the colon is preserved, diarrhoea and steatorrhoea. Dehydration and signs of hypovolaemia are common, as are weight loss, loss of muscle bulk and malnu-trition. Some patients remain in satisfactory but precarious fluid balance until a minor intercurrent illness or intestinal upset occurs, when they can rapidly become dehydrated.

Management
In the immediate post-operative period, total parenteral nutrition (TPN) should be started. Proton pump inhibitor therapy is given to reduce gastric secretions. Enteral feeding can be cautiously introduced after 1–2 weeks under careful supervision and slowly increased as tolerated.

The principles of long-term management are:

- Detailed nutritional assessments at regular intervals.
- Monitoring of fluid and electrolyte balance. Patients can usually be taught how to do this for themselves. A readily available supply of oral rehydration solution is useful for intercurrent illness.

- Adequate calorie and protein intake. Fats are a good energy source and should be taken as tolerated. Medium-chain triglyceride supplements are often given first because they are more easily absorbed.
- Replacement of B_{12}, calcium, vitamin D, magnesium, zinc and folic acid.
- Antidiarrhoeal agents, e.g. loperamide (2–4 mg 6-hourly) or codeine phosphate (30 mg 4–6-hourly).

Some patients are unable to maintain positive fluid balance. Octreotide (50–200 μg 8–12-hourly by subcutan-eous injection) reduces gastrointestinal secretions and is useful in such individuals. Despite these measures, some patients require long-term home TPN for survival and this is best managed in specialist centres. Small bowel trans-plantation is an option but rejection and 'graft-versus-host' disease (p. 1044) remain significant hurdles.

RADIATION ENTERITIS AND PROCTOCOLITIS

Intestinal damage occurs in 10–15% of patients undergoing radiotherapy for abdominal or pelvic malignancy. The risk varies with total dose, dosing schedule and the use of concomitant chemotherapy.

Pathology
The rectum, sigmoid colon and terminal ileum are most frequently involved. Radiation causes acute inflammation, shortening of villi, oedema and crypt abscess formation. These usually resolve completely but in some patients an obliterative endarteritis affecting the endothelium of sub-mucosal arterioles develops over 2–12 months. Fibroblastic proliferation produces progressive ischaemic fibrosis over years and may lead to adhesions, ulceration, strictures, obstruction or fistula to adjacent organs.

Clinical features

In the acute phase there is nausea, vomiting, cramping abdominal pain and diarrhoea. When the rectum and colon are involved, rectal mucus, bleeding and tenesmus occur. The chronic phase develops after 5–10 years in some patients and produces one or more of the problems listed in Box 22.51.

Investigations

In the acute phase the rectal changes at sigmoidoscopy resemble those of ulcerative proctitis (Fig. 22.54, p. 915). The extent of the lesion is determined by colonoscopy. Barium follow-through examination shows small bowel strictures, ulcers and fistulae.

Management

Diarrhoea in the acute phase is treated with codeine phosphate, diphenoxylate or loperamide in standard dosage. Local corticosteroid enemas help proctitis, and antibiotics may be required for bacterial overgrowth. Nutritional supplements are necessary when malabsorption is present. Colestyramine (4 g as a single sachet) is useful for bile salt malabsorption. Endoscopic laser or argon plasma coagulation therapy may reduce bleeding from proctitis. Surgery should be avoided, if possible, because the injured intestine is difficult to resect and anastomose, but it may be necessary for obstruction, perforation or fistula.

ABETALIPOPROTEINAEMIA

This rare autosomal recessive disorder results from deficiency of apolipoprotein B and subsequent failure of chylomicron formation. It leads to fat malabsorption and deficiency of fat-soluble vitamins. Jejunal biopsy reveals enterocytes distended with resynthesised triglyceride and normal villous morphology. Serum cholesterol and triglyceride levels are low. A number of other abnormalities occur in this syndrome, including acanthocytosis, retinitis pigmentosa and a progressive neurological disorder with cerebellar and dorsal column signs. Symptoms may be improved by a low-fat diet supplemented with medium-chain triglycerides and vitamins A, D, E and K.

MOTILITY DISORDERS

CHRONIC INTESTINAL PSEUDO-OBSTRUCTION

Small intestinal motility is disordered in conditions which affect the smooth muscle or nerves of the intestine. Many cases are 'primary' (idiopathic), while others are 'secondary' to a variety of disorders or drugs (Box 22.52).

Clinical features

There are recurrent episodes of nausea, vomiting, abdominal discomfort and distension, often worse after food. Alternating constipation and diarrhoea occur and weight loss results from malabsorption (due to bacterial overgrowth) and fear of eating. There may also be symptoms of dysmotility affecting other parts of the gastrointestinal tract, e.g. dysphagia, and, in primary cases, features of bladder dysfunction. Some patients have obscure but severe abdominal pain which is extremely difficult to manage.

Investigations

The diagnosis is often delayed and a high index of suspicion is needed. Plain X-rays show distended loops of bowel and air–fluid levels but barium studies demonstrate no mechanical obstruction. Laparotomy is sometimes performed to exclude obstruction and to obtain full-thickness biopsies of the intestine. Electron microscopy, histochemistry and special stains define rare, specific syndromes.

Management

This is often difficult. Underlying causes should be addressed and further surgery avoided if at all possible. Metoclopramide or domperidone may enhance motility, and antibiotics are given for bacterial overgrowth. Nutritional and psychological support is also necessary.

MISCELLANEOUS DISORDERS OF THE SMALL INTESTINE

PROTEIN-LOSING ENTEROPATHY

This term is used when there is excessive loss of protein into the gut lumen, sufficient to cause hypoproteinaemia. Protein-losing enteropathy occurs in many gut disorders but is most common in those where ulceration occurs (Box 22.53). In other disorders protein loss results from increased mucosal permeability or obstruction of intestinal lymphatic vessels.

22

22.53 CAUSES OF PROTEIN-LOSING ENTEROPATHY	
With mucosal erosions or ulceration	
• Crohn's disease • Ulcerative colitis • Radiation damage	• Oesophageal, gastric or colonic cancer • Lymphoma
Without mucosal erosions or ulceration	
• Ménétrier's disease • Bacterial overgrowth • Coeliac disease	• Tropical sprue • Eosinophilic gastroenteritis • SLE
With lymphatic obstruction	
• Intestinal lymphangiectasia • Constrictive pericarditis	• Lymphoma • Whipple's disease

Patients present with peripheral oedema and hypoproteinaemia in the presence of normal liver function and without proteinuria. There may also be features of the underlying cause.

The diagnosis is confirmed by measurement of faecal clearance of α_1-antitrypsin or ^{51}Cr-labelled albumin after intravenous injection. Other investigations are performed to determine the underlying cause. Treatment is that of the underlying disorder, with nutritional support and measures to control peripheral oedema.

INTESTINAL LYMPHANGIECTASIA

This may be primary, resulting from congenital malunion of lymphatics, or secondary to lymphatic obstruction due to lymphoma, filariasis or constrictive pericarditis. Impaired drainage of intestinal lymphatic vessels leads to discharge of protein and fat-rich lymph into the gastrointestinal lumen. The condition presents with peripheral lymphoedema, pleural effusions or chylous ascites, and steatorrhoea. Investigations reveal hypoalbuminaemia, lymphocytopenia and reduced serum immunoglobulin concentrations. Jejunal biopsies show greatly dilated lacteals, and lymphangiography shows lymphatic obstruction. Treatment consists of a low-fat diet with medium-chain triglyceride supplements.

ULCERATION OF THE SMALL INTESTINE

Small bowel ulcers are uncommon and are either idiopathic or secondary to underlying intestinal disorders (Box 22.54).

Ulcers are more common in the ileum, and cause

22.54 CAUSES OF SMALL INTESTINAL ULCERS
• Idiopathic   • Inflammatory bowel disease, e.g. Crohn's   • Drugs, e.g. NSAIDs, enteric-coated potassium tablets   • Ulcerative jejunoileitis   • Lymphoma and carcinoma   • Infections, e.g. TB, typhoid, *Yersinia*   • Others, e.g. radiation, vasculitis

bleeding, perforation, stricture formation or obstruction. Barium studies and enteroscopy confirm the diagnosis.

NSAID-ASSOCIATED SMALL INTESTINAL TOXICITY

These drugs cause a spectrum of small intestinal lesions ranging from erosions and ulcers to mucosal webs, strictures and, rarely, a condition known as 'diaphragm disease' in which intense submucosal fibrosis results in circumferential stricturing. The condition can present with pain, obstruction, bleeding or anaemia, and may mimic Crohn's disease, carcinoma or lymphoma. Enteroscopy or capsule endoscopy can reveal the diagnosis but sometimes this is only discovered at laparotomy.

EOSINOPHILIC GASTROENTERITIS

This disorder of unknown aetiology can affect any part of the gastrointestinal tract; it is characterised by eosinophil infiltration affecting the gut wall in the absence of parasitic infection or eosinophilia of other tissues. Peripheral blood eosinophilia is present in 80% of cases.

Inflammation and destruction affect mucosal, muscular and/or serosal layers.

Clinical features
There are features of obstruction and inflammation, such as colicky pain, nausea and vomiting, diarrhoea and weight loss. Protein-losing enteropathy occurs and up to 50% of patients have a history of other allergic disorders. Serosal involvement may produce eosinophilic ascites.

Diagnosis and management
The diagnosis is made by histological assessment of multiple endoscopic biopsies, although full-thickness biopsies are occasionally required. Other investigations are performed to exclude parasitic infection and other causes of eosinophilia. A raised serum IgE concentration is often seen.

Dietary manipulations are rarely effective although elimination diets, especially of milk, may benefit a few patients. Severe symptoms are treated with prednisolone 20–40 mg daily and/or sodium cromoglicate, which stabilises mast cell membranes. The prognosis is good in the majority of patients.

MECKEL'S DIVERTICULUM

This is the most common congenital anomaly of the gastrointestinal tract and occurs in 0.3–3% of people. Most patients are asymptomatic. The diverticulum results from failure of closure of the vitelline duct, with persistence of a blind-ending sac arising from the antimesenteric border of the ileum; it usually occurs within 100 cm of the ileocaecal valve, and is up to 5 cm long. Approximately 50% contain ectopic gastric mucosa; rarely, colonic, pancreatic or endometrial tissue is present.

Complications most commonly occur in the first 2 years of life but are occasionally seen in young adults. Bleeding results from ulceration of ileal mucosa adjacent to the ectopic parietal cells and presents as recurrent melaena or altered blood per rectum. Diagnosis can be made by scanning the abdomen using a gamma counter following an intravenous injection of ^{99m}Tc-pertechnate, which is concentrated by ectopic parietal cells. Other complications include intestinal obstruction, diverticulitis, intussusception and perforation. Intervention is unnecessary unless complications occur. The vast majority of patients remain asymptomatic throughout life.

ADVERSE FOOD REACTIONS

Adverse food reactions are common and are subdivided into food intolerance and food allergy, the former being much more common.

FOOD INTOLERANCE

This involves adverse reactions to food which are not immune-mediated and result from pharmacological (e.g histamine, tyramine or monosodium glutamate), metabolic (e.g. lactase deficiency) or other mechanisms (e.g. toxins or chemical contaminants in food).

Lactose intolerance

Human milk contains around 200 mmol/l of lactose which is normally digested to glucose and galactose by the brush border enzyme lactase prior to absorption. In most populations enterocyte lactase activity declines throughout childhood. The enzyme is deficient in up to 90% of adult Africans, Asians and South Americans, but only 5% of northern Europeans.

In cases of racially determined (primary) lactase deficiency, jejunal morphology is normal. 'Secondary' lactase deficiency occurs as a consequence of disorders which damage the jejunal mucosa, e.g. coeliac disease and viral gastroenteritis. Unhydrolysed lactose enters the colon, where bacterial fermentation produces volatile short-chain fatty acids, hydrogen and carbon dioxide.

Clinical features

In most people lactase deficiency is completely asymptomatic. However, some complain of colicky pain, abdominal distension, increased flatus, borborygmi and diarrhoea after ingesting milk or milk products. Irritable bowel syndrome is often suspected but the diagnosis is suggested by clinical improvement on lactose withdrawal. The lactose hydrogen breath test is a useful non-invasive confirmatory investigation.

Dietary exclusion of lactose is recommended, although most sufferers are able to tolerate small amounts of milk without symptoms. Addition of commercial lactase preparations to milk has been effective in some studies but is costly.

Diarrhoea due to other sugars

'Osmotic' diarrhoea can be caused by sorbitol, an unabsorbable carbohydrate which is used as an artificial sweetener. Fructose may also cause diarrhoea if consumed in greater quantities than can be absorbed (e.g. in fruit juices).

FOOD ALLERGY

Food allergies are immune-mediated disorders, most commonly due to IgE antibodies and type I hypersensitivity reactions, although type IV delayed reactions are also seen. Up to 20% of the population perceive themselves as suffering from food allergy but only 1–2% of adults and 5–7% of children have genuine food allergies. The most common culprits are peanuts, milk, eggs, soya and shellfish.

Clinical manifestations occur immediately on exposure and range from trivial to life-threatening or even fatal anaphylaxis. The common 'oral allergy syndrome' results from contact with benzoic acid in certain fresh fruit juices leading to urticaria and angioedema of the lips and oropharynx. This is, however, not an immune-mediated reaction. 'Allergic gastroenteropathy' has features similar to eosinophilic gastroenteritis, while 'gastrointestinal anaphylaxis' consists of nausea, vomiting, diarrhoea and sometimes cardiovascular and respiratory collapse. Fatal reactions to trace amounts of peanuts are well documented.

The diagnosis of food allergy is difficult to prove or refute. Skin prick tests and measurements of antigen-specific IgE antibodies in serum have limited predictive value. Double-blind placebo-controlled food challenges are the gold standard, but are laborious and are not readily available. In many cases clinical suspicion and trials of elimination diets are used.

Treatment of proven food allergy consists of detailed patient education and awareness, strict elimination of the offending antigen and in some cases antihistamines or sodium cromoglicate. Anaphylaxis should be treated as a medical emergency with resuscitation, airway support and intravenous adrenaline (epinephrine). Teachers and other carers of affected children should be trained to deal with this. Patients should wear an information bracelet and be taught to carry and use a preloaded adrenaline (epinephrine) syringe.

INFECTIONS OF THE SMALL INTESTINE

TRAVELLERS' DIARRHOEA, GIARDIASIS AND AMOEBIASIS

See pages 293, 359 and 358.

ABDOMINAL TUBERCULOSIS

Mycobacterium tuberculosis is a rare cause of abdominal disease in Caucasians but must be considered in people in and from the developing world and in AIDS patients. Gut infection usually results from human *M. tuberculosis* which is swallowed after coughing. Many patients have no pulmonary symptoms and a normal chest X-ray.

The area most commonly affected is the ileocaecal region; presentation and radiological findings may be very similar to those of Crohn's disease. Abdominal pain can be acute or of several months' duration, but diarrhoea is less common in TB than in Crohn's disease. Low-grade fever is common but not invariable. Like Crohn's disease, TB can affect any part of the gastrointestinal tract, and perianal disease with fistula is recognised. Peritoneal TB may result

22

in peritonitis with exudative ascites, associated with abdominal pain and fever. Granulomatous hepatitis occurs.

Diagnosis

Abdominal TB causes an elevated erythrocyte sedimentation rate (ESR); a raised serum alkaline phosphatase concentration suggests hepatic involvement. Histological confirmation is sought by endoscopy, laparoscopy or liver biopsy. Caseation of granulomas is not always seen and acid- and alcohol-fast bacteria are often scanty. Culture may be helpful but identification of the organism may take 6 weeks and diagnosis is now possible on biopsy specimens by rapid polymerase chain reaction techniques.

Management

When the presentation is very suggestive of abdominal TB, chemotherapy with four drugs—isoniazid, rifampicin, pyrazinamide and ethambutol (p. 701)—should be commenced even if bacteriological or histological proof is lacking.

CRYPTOSPORIDIOSIS

Cryptosporidiosis and other protozoal infections, including isosporiasis *(Isospora belli)* and microsporidiosis, are dealt with on pages 358–360.

TUMOURS OF THE SMALL INTESTINE

The small intestine is rarely affected by neoplasia, and fewer than 5% of all gastrointestinal tumours occur here.

Benign tumours

The most common are adenomas, GIST, lipomas and hamartomas. Adenomas are most often found in the peri-ampullary region and are usually asymptomatic, although occult bleeding or obstruction due to intussusception may occur. Transformation to adenocarcinoma is rare. Multiple adenomas are common in the duodenum of patients with familial adenomatous polyposis (FAP), who merit regular endoscopic surveillance. Hamartomatous polyps with almost no malignant potential occur in Peutz–Jeghers syndrome (p. 925).

Malignant tumours

These are rare and include, in decreasing order of frequency, adenocarcinoma, carcinoid tumour, malignant GIST and lymphoma. The majority occur in middle age or later. Kaposi's sarcoma is seen in patients with AIDS.

Adenocarcinomas occur with increased frequency in patients with FAP, coeliac disease and Peutz–Jeghers syndrome. The non-specific presentation and rarity of these lesions often lead to delay in diagnosis. Barium follow-through examination or small bowel enema studies will demonstrate most lesions of this type. Enteroscopy, capsule endoscopy, mesenteric angiography and CT also play a role in investigation. Treatment is by surgical resection.

CARCINOID TUMOURS

These are derived from enterochromaffin cells and are most common in the ileum. Localised spread and the potential for

22.55 CLINICAL FEATURES OF CARCINOID TUMOURS

- Small-bowel obstruction due to the tumour mass
- Intestinal ischaemia (due to mesenteric infiltration or vasospasm)
- Hepatic metastases causing pain, hepatomegaly and jaundice
- Flushing and wheezing
- Diarrhoea
- Cardiac involvement (tricuspid regurgitation, pulmonary stenosis, right ventricular endocardial plaques) leading to heart failure
- Facial telangiectasia

The diagnosis is made by detecting excess levels of the 5-HT metabolite, 5-HIAA, in a 24-hour urine collection.

metastasis to the liver increase with primary lesions over 2 cm in diameter. Carcinoid tumours also occur in the rectum and in the appendix; those in the latter are usually benign. Overall, these tumours are less aggressive than carcinomas and their growth is usually slow.

The term 'carcinoid syndrome' refers to the systemic symptoms produced when secretory products of the neoplastic enterochromaffin cells reach the systemic circulation (Box 22.55). When produced by the primary tumour they are usually metabolised in the liver and do not reach the systemic circulation. The syndrome is therefore only seen when 5-HT, bradykinin and other peptide hormones are released by hepatic metastases.

Management

The treatment of a carcinoid tumour is surgical resection. The treatment of carcinoid syndrome is palliative because hepatic metastases have occurred, although prolonged survival is common. Surgical removal of the primary tumour is usually attempted and the hepatic metastases can be excised as reduction of tumour mass improves symptoms. Hepatic artery embolisation retards growth of hepatic deposits. Octreotide 200 µg 8-hourly by subcutaneous injection is used to reduce tumour release of secretagogues. Cytotoxic chemotherapy has only a minor role.

LYMPHOMA

Non-Hodgkin lymphoma (p. 1049) may involve the gastrointestinal tract as part of more generalised disease or may rarely arise in the gut, with the small intestine being most commonly affected. Lymphomas occur with increased frequency in patients with coeliac disease, AIDS and other immunodeficiency states. Most are of B-cell origin, although lymphoma associated with coeliac disease is derived from T cells (enteropathy-associated T-cell lymphoma).

Colicky abdominal pain, obstruction and weight loss are the usual presenting features, and perforation is also occasionally seen. Malabsorption is only a feature of diffuse bowel involvement and hepatosplenomegaly is rare.

The diagnosis is made by small bowel biopsy, radiological contrast studies and CT. Staging investigations are performed. Surgical resection where possible is the treatment of choice, with radiotherapy and combination chemotherapy reserved for those with advanced disease. The

22

prognosis depends largely on the stage at diagnosis, cell type, patient age and the presence of 'B' symptoms.

IMMUNOPROLIFERATIVE SMALL INTESTINAL DISEASE (IPSID)

Also known as 'alpha heavy chain disease', this rare condition occurs mainly in the Mediterranean, Middle East, India and Pakistan, and North America. The aetiology is unknown but it may be a response to chronic stimulation by bacterial antigens. The condition varies in severity from relatively benign to frankly malignant.

The small intestinal mucosa is diffusely affected, especially proximally, by a dense lymphoplasmacytic infiltrate. Enlarged mesenteric lymph nodes are also common. Most patients are young adults who present with malabsorption, anorexia and fever. Serum electrophoresis confirms the presence of alpha heavy chains (from the F_c portion of IgA). Prolonged remissions can be obtained with long-term antibiotic therapy but chemotherapy is required for those who fail to respond or who have aggressive disease.

DISEASES OF THE PANCREAS

ACUTE PANCREATITIS

Acute pancreatitis accounts for 3% of all cases of abdominal pain admitted to hospital. It affects 2–28 per 100 000 of the population and may be increasing in incidence.

Pathophysiology

Acute pancreatitis occurs as a consequence of premature activation of zymogen granules, releasing proteases which digest the pancreas and surrounding tissue (Fig. 22.42). The normal pancreas has only a poorly developed capsule, and adjacent structures, including the common bile duct, duodenum, splenic vein and transverse colon, are commonly involved in the inflammatory process. The severity of acute pancreatitis is dependent upon the balance between activity of released proteolytic enzymes and antiproteolytic factors. The latter comprise an intracellular pancreatic trypsin inhibitor protein and circulating β_2-macroglobulin, α_1-antitrypsin and Cl-esterase inhibitors. Causes of acute pancreatitis are given in Box 22.56.

Acute pancreatitis is usually mild and self-limiting, with minimal organ dysfunction and uneventful recovery. In some patients, however, it is severe, with local complications such as necrosis, pseudocyst or abscess, and systemic complications leading to multi-organ failure. The mortality in this severe group is approximately 30%.

Clinical features

Severe, constant upper abdominal pain which radiates to the back in 65% of cases builds up over 15–60 minutes. Nausea and vomiting are common. There is marked epigastric tenderness, but in the early stages (and in contrast to a perforated peptic ulcer) guarding and rebound tenderness are absent because the inflammation is

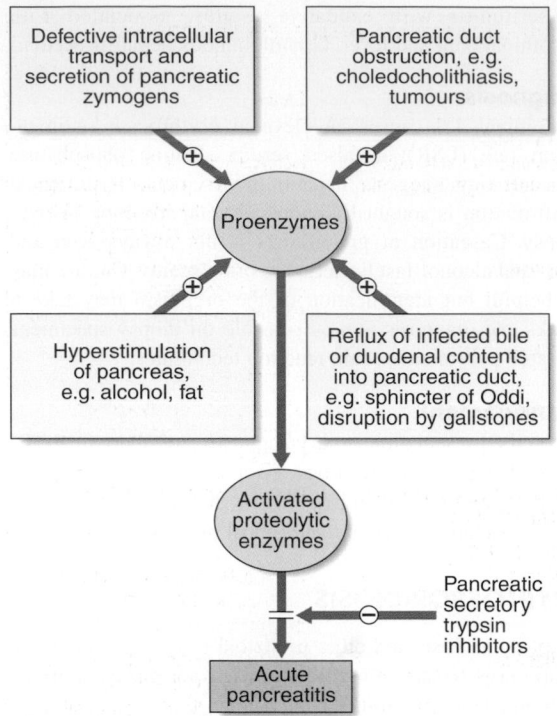

Fig. 22.42 Pathophysiology of acute pancreatitis.

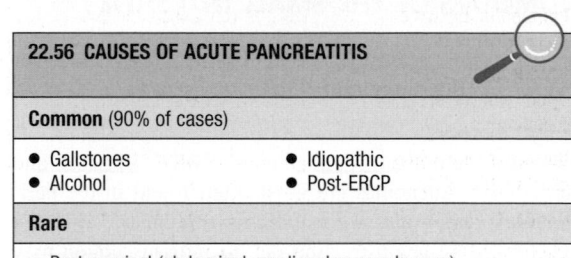

22.56 CAUSES OF ACUTE PANCREATITIS

Common (90% of cases)

- Gallstones
- Alcohol
- Idiopathic
- Post-ERCP

Rare

- Post-surgical (abdominal, cardiopulmonary bypass)
- Trauma
- Drugs (azathioprine, thiazide diuretics, sodium valproate)
- Metabolic (hypercalcaemia, hypertriglyceridaemia)
- Pancreas divisum (p. 908)
- Sphincter of Oddi dysfunction
- Infection (mumps, Coxsackie virus)
- Hereditary
- Renal failure
- Organ transplantation (kidney, liver)
- Severe hypothermia
- Petrochemical exposure

principally retroperitoneal. Bowel sounds become quiet or absent as paralytic ileus develops.

In severe cases the patient becomes hypoxic and develops hypovolaemic shock with oliguria. Discoloration of the flanks (Grey Turner's sign) or the periumbilical region (Cullen's sign) are features of severe pancreatitis with haemorrhage. The differential diagnosis includes a perforated viscus, acute cholecystitis and myocardial infarction.

Complications

These are listed in Box 22.57. An acute pancreatic pseudocyst is a localised peripancreatic collection of

22.57 COMPLICATIONS OF ACUTE PANCREATITIS

Complication	Cause
SYSTEMIC	
Systemic inflammatory response syndrome (SIRS)	Increased vascular permeability from cytokine, platelet aggregating factor and kinin release, paralytic ileus, vomiting, renal failure
Hypoxia	Acute respiratory distress syndrome (ARDS) due to microthrombi in pulmonary vessels
Hyperglycaemia	Disruption of islets of Langerhans with altered insulin/glucagon axis
Hypocalcaemia	Sequestration of calcium in fat necrosis, fall in ionised calcium (? cause)
Reduced serum albumin concentration	Increased capillary permeability
PANCREATIC	
Necrosis	Non-viable pancreatic tissue and peripancreatic tissue death; frequently infected
Abscess	Circumscribed collection of pus close to the pancreas and containing little or no pancreatic necrotic tissue
Pseudocyst	Disruption of pancreatic ducts
Pancreatic ascites or pleural effusion	Disruption of pancreatic ducts
GASTROINTESTINAL	
Upper gastrointestinal bleeding	Gastric or duodenal erosions
Variceal haemorrhage Erosion into colon	Splenic or portal vein thrombosis
Duodenal obstruction	Compression by pancreatic mass
Obstructive jaundice	Compression of common bile duct

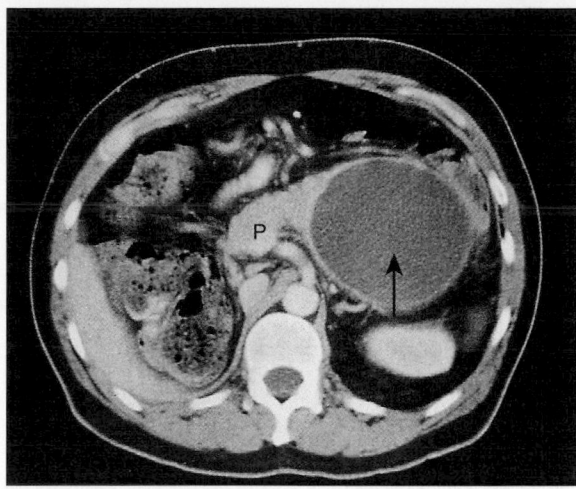

Fig. 22.43   CT showing large pancreatic pseudocyst (arrow) developing from the body of the pancreas (P).

22

pancreatic juice and debris which usually develops in the lesser sac following inflammatory rupture of the pancreatic duct. The pseudocyst is initially contained within a poorly defined, fragile wall of granulation tissue which matures over a 6-week period to form a fibrous capsule (Fig. 22.43). Small intrapancreatic cysts and pseudocysts are common features of both acute and chronic pancreatitis; they are usually asymptomatic and resolve as the pancreatitis recovers. Pseudocysts greater than 6 cm in diameter seldom disappear spontaneously. Large pseudocysts cause constant abdominal pain, can produce a palpable abdominal mass and may compress or erode surrounding structures including blood vessels to form pseudoaneurysms.

Pancreatic ascites occurs when fluid leaks from a disrupted pancreatic duct into the peritoneal cavity. Leakage into the thoracic cavity can result in a pleural effusion or a pleuro-pancreatic fistula.

Diagnosis

The diagnosis of acute pancreatitis is based upon elevation of serum amylase or lipase concentrations and ultrasound or CT evidence of pancreatic swelling. Plain X-rays are taken to exclude other diagnoses such as perforation or obstruction and to identify pulmonary complications.

Amylase is efficiently excreted by the kidneys, and concentrations may have returned to normal if measured 24–48 hours after the onset of pancreatitis. In this situation the diagnosis can be made by demonstrating an elevated urinary amylase:creatinine ratio. A persistently elevated serum amylase concentration suggests pseudocyst formation. Peritoneal amylase concentrations are massively elevated in pancreatic ascites. Serum amylase concentrations are also elevated (but less so) in intestinal ischaemia, perforated peptic ulcer and ruptured ovarian cyst, whilst the salivary isoenzyme of amylase is elevated in parotitis.

Ultrasound scanning confirms the diagnosis, although in the earlier stages the gland may not be grossly swollen. The ultrasound scan is also useful because it may show gallstones, biliary obstruction or pseudocyst formation.

CT between 3 and 10 days after admission is used to define the viability of the pancreas. Necrotising pancreatitis is associated with decreased pancreatic enhancement following intravenous injection of contrast material. The presence of gas within necrotic material (Fig. 22.44) suggests infection and impending abscess formation, in which case percutaneous aspiration of material for bacterial culture should be carried out and appropriate antibiotics prescribed. Involvement of the colon, blood vessels and other adjacent structures by the inflammatory process is best seen by CT.

Certain investigations stratify the severity of acute pancreatitis and have important prognostic value at the time of presentation (Box 22.58). In addition, serial assessment of C-reactive protein (CRP) is a useful indicator of progress. A peak CRP > 210 mg/l in the first 4 days predicts severe acute pancreatitis with 80% accuracy. It is worth noting that the serum amylase concentration has no prognostic value.

Management

Management of acute pancreatitis comprises several related steps:

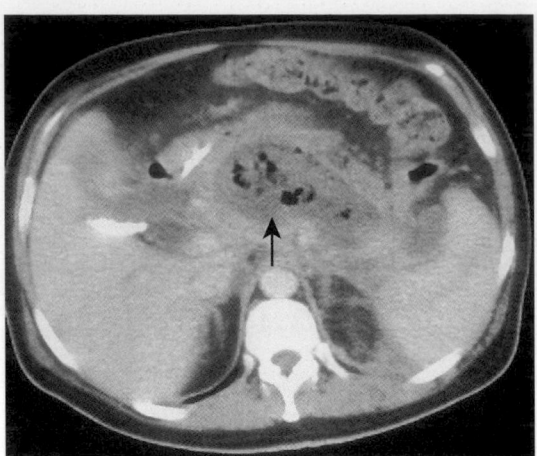

Fig. 22.44 Pancreatic necrosis. Lack of vascular enhancement of the pancreas during contrast-enhanced CT indicates necrosis (arrow). The presence of gas suggests infection has occurred.

EBM

22.58 ERCP IN ACUTE PANCREATITIS

'Emergency ERCP with biliary sphincterotomy and stone extraction when stones are identified in the common bile duct improves outcome in severe acute pancreatitis. Greatest benefit occurs in those patients who have ascending cholangitis.'

● Ayub K, et al. (Cochrane Review). Cochrane Library, issue 1, 2005. Oxford: Update Software.

For further information: 🖥 www.cochrane.org

● establishing the diagnosis and stratifying disease severity
● early treatment (resuscitation) according to whether the disease is mild or severe
● detection and treatment of complications
● treating the underlying cause—specifically gallstones.

The initial management is based upon analgesia using pethidine and correction of hypovolaemia using normal saline and/or colloids. All severe cases should be managed in a high-dependency or intensive care unit. A central venous line or Swan–Ganz catheter and urinary catheter are used to monitor patients with shock. Hypoxic patients need oxygen and patients who develop adult respiratory distress syndrome (ARDS) may require ventilatory support. Hyperglycaemia is corrected using insulin, but it is not necessary to correct hypocalcaemia by intravenous calcium injection unless tetany occurs.

Nasogastric aspiration is only necessary if paralytic ileus is present. Enteral feeding via a nasoenteral tube should be started at an early stage in patients with severe pancreatitis because they are in a severely catabolic state and need nutritional support (Box 22.59). In addition enteral feeding decreases endotoxaemia and thereby may reduce systemic complications. Prophylaxis of thromboembolism with low-dose subcutaneous heparin is also advisable. Prophylactic, broad-spectrum intravenous antibiotics such as imipenem or cefuroxime may improve outcome in severe cases.

Patients who present with cholangitis or jaundice in association with severe acute pancreatitis should undergo

---

EBM

22.59 NUTRITIONAL SUPPORT IN ACUTE PANCREATITIS

'Nasojejunal tube feeding is superior to total parenteral nutrition in acute pancreatitis.'

● Windsor AC, et al. Gut 1998; 42:431–435.

For further information: 🖥 www.bsg.org.uk

22.60 ADVERSE PROGNOSTIC FACTORS IN ACUTE PANCREATITIS (GLASGOW CRITERIA)*

● Age > 55 years
● PO_2 < 8 kPa (60 mmHg)
● White blood cell count (WBC) > 15×10^9/litre
● Albumin < 32 g/l
● Serum calcium < 2 mmol/l (8 mg/dl) (corrected)
● Glucose > 10 mmol/l (180 mg/dl)
● Urea > 16 mmol/l (45 mg/dl) (after rehydration)
● Alanine aminotransferase (ALT) > 200 U/l
● Lactate dehydrogenase (LDH) > 600 U/l

* Severity and prognosis worsen as the number of these factors increases. More than three implies severe disease.

---

urgent ERCP to diagnose and treat choledocholithiasis. In less severe cases of gallstone pancreatitis, biliary imaging (using MRCP) can be carried out after the acute phase has resolved. If the liver function tests return to normal and ultrasound has not demonstrated a dilated biliary tree, laparoscopic cholecystectomy with an on-table cholangiogram is appropriate because any common bile duct stones have probably passed. When the operative cholangiogram detects residual common bile duct stones, these are removed by laparoscopic exploration of the duct or by post-operative ERCP. Cholecystectomy should be undertaken within 2 weeks following resolution of pancreatitis to prevent further potentially fatal attacks of pancreatitis.

Management of complications
Patients who have developed necrotising pancreatitis or pancreatic abscess require urgent surgical débridement of the pancreas, followed by drainage of the pancreatic bed. Pancreatic pseudocysts are treated by drainage into the stomach, duodenum or jejunum (Roux en Y). This is usually performed after an interval of at least 6 weeks, once a pseudocapsule has matured, using open surgery or endoscopic methods.

Prognosis (Box 22.60)
Despite recent advances in management, mortality has remained unchanged at 10–15%. About 80% of all cases are mild with a mortality of less than 5%; 98% of deaths occur in the 20% of severe cases. One-third occur within the first week, usually from multi-organ failure. After this time the majority of deaths result from sepsis, especially that complicating infected necrosis.

CHRONIC PANCREATITIS

Chronic pancreatitis is a chronic inflammatory disease characterised by fibrosis and destruction of exocrine

22

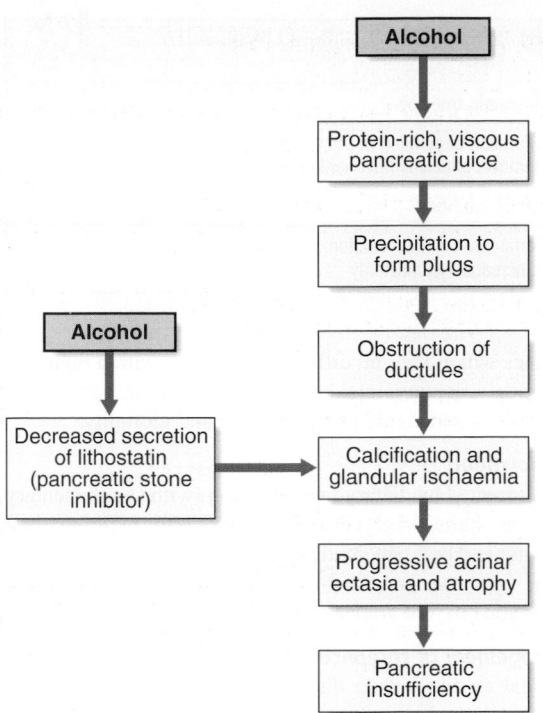

Fig. 22.45 Pathophysiology of chronic pancreatitis.

22.61 CAUSES OF CHRONIC PANCREATITIS

- Calcific
  Alcoholism
  Tropical (India)
- Obstructive
  Stenosis of the ampulla
  of Vater

- Pancreas divisum (p. 908)
- Cystic fibrosis
- Hereditary
- Idiopathic

N.B. Many patients have gallstones but these do not cause chronic pancreatitis.

22.62 COMPLICATIONS OF CHRONIC PANCREATITIS

- Pseudocysts and pancreatic ascites, which occur in both acute and chronic pancreatitis
- Extrahepatic obstructive jaundice due to a benign stricture of the common bile duct as it passes through the diseased pancreas
- Duodenal stenosis
- Portal or splenic vein thrombosis leading to segmental portal hypertension and gastric varices
- Peptic ulcer

22.63 INVESTIGATIONS IN CHRONIC PANCREATITIS

Tests to establish the diagnosis

- Ultrasound
- CT (may show atrophy, calcification or ductal dilatation)
- Abdominal X-ray (may show calcification)
- MRCP
- Endoscopic ultrasound

Tests of pancreatic function

- Collection of pure pancreatic juice after secretin injection (gold standard but invasive and seldom used)
- Pancreolauryl or PABA test (p. 863)
- Faecal pancreatic chymotrypsin or elastase
- Oral glucose tolerance test

Tests of anatomy prior to surgery

- MRCP

22

pancreatic tissue. Diabetes mellitus occurs in advanced cases because the islets of Langerhans are involved.

Pathophysiology

Around 80% of cases in Western countries result from alcohol misuse (Fig. 22.45). In southern India severe chronic calcific pancreatitis occurs in non-alcoholics, possibly as a result of malnutrition and cassava consumption. Other causes are listed in Box 22.61.

Clinical features

Chronic pancreatitis predominantly affects middle-aged alcoholic men. Almost all present with abdominal pain. In 50% this occurs as episodes of 'acute pancreatitis', although each attack results in a degree of permanent pancreatic damage. Relentless, slowly progressive chronic pain without acute exacerbations affects 35% of patients, whilst the remainder have no pain but present with diarrhoea. Pain is due to a combination of increased pressure within the pancreatic ducts and direct involvement of pancreatic and peripancreatic nerves by the inflammatory process. Pain may be relieved by leaning forwards or by drinking alcohol. Approximately one-fifth of patients chronically consume opiate analgesics.

Weight loss is common and results from a combination of anorexia, avoidance of food because of post-prandial pain, malabsorption and/or diabetes. Steatorrhoea occurs when more than 90% of the exocrine tissue has been destroyed; protein malabsorption only develops in the most advanced cases. Overall, 30% of patients are diabetic, but this figure rises to 70% in those with chronic calcific pancreatitis.

Physical examination reveals a thin, malnourished patient with epigastric tenderness. Skin pigmentation over the abdomen and back is common and results from chronic use of a hot water bottle (erythema ab igne). Many patients have features of other alcohol- and smoking-related diseases.

Complications are listed in Box 22.62.

Investigations

Investigations (Box 22.63 and Fig. 22.46) are carried out to:

- make a diagnosis of chronic pancreatitis
- define pancreatic function
- demonstrate anatomical abnormalities prior to surgical intervention.

Management

Alcohol misuse

Alcohol avoidance is crucial in halting the progression of the disease and reducing pain. Unfortunately, counselling

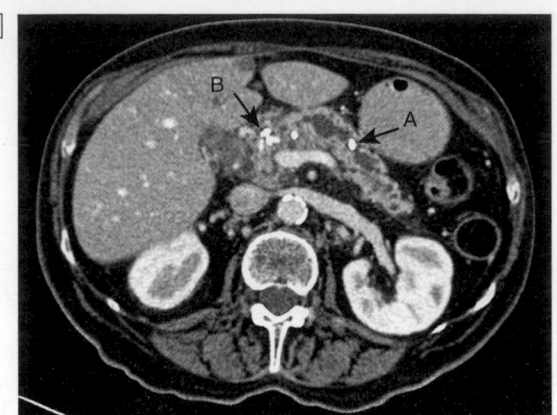

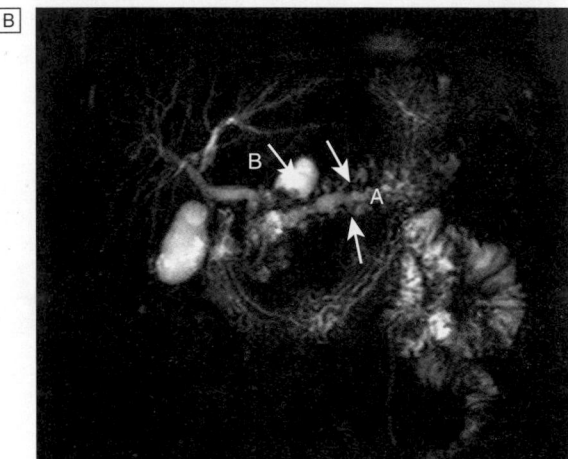

Fig. 22.46 Imaging in chronic pancreatitis. [A] CT scan showing a grossly dilated and irregular duct with a calcified stone (arrow A). Note the calcification in the head of the gland (arrow B). [B] MRCP of the same patient showing marked ductal dilatation with abnormal dilated side branches (arrows A). A small cyst is also present (arrow B).

and psychiatric intervention are rarely successful and the majority of patients continue to drink alcohol.

Pain relief

A range of analgesic drugs, particularly NSAIDs, are valuable, but the severe and unremitting nature of the pain often leads to opiate use with the risk of addiction. Oral pancreatic enzyme supplements suppress pancreatic secretion and their regular use reduces analgesic consumption in some patients.

Patients who are abstinent from alcohol and who have severe chronic pain which is resistant to conservative measures are considered for surgical or endoscopic pancreatic therapy (Box 22.64). Coeliac plexus neurolysis or minimally invasive thoracoscopic splanchnicectomy sometimes produces long-lasting pain relief although relapse eventually occurs in the majority of cases.

In some patients MRCP does not show a surgically or endoscopically correctable abnormality and in these patients the only surgical approach is total pancreatectomy. Unfortunately, even after this operation, some patients will continue to experience pain. Moreover, the procedure causes

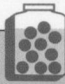

22.64 INTERVENTION IN CHRONIC PANCREATITIS

Endoscopic therapy

- Dilatation or stenting of pancreatic duct strictures
- Removal of calculi (mechanical or shock-wave lithotripsy)

Surgical methods

- Partial pancreatic resection, preserving the duodenum
- Pancreatico-jejunostomy

diabetes which may be difficult to control, with a high risk of hypoglycaemia (since both insulin and glucagon release are absent), and significant morbidity and mortality.

Steatorrhoea

This is treated by dietary fat restriction (with supplementary medium-chain triglyceride therapy in malnourished patients) and oral pancreatic enzyme supplements. A proton pump inhibitor is added to optimise duodenal pH for pancreatic enzyme activity.

Management of complications

Surgical or endoscopic therapy may be necessary for the management of pseudocysts, pancreatic ascites, common bile duct or duodenal stricture and the consequences of portal hypertension. Many patients with chronic pancreatitis also require treatment for other alcohol- and smoking-related diseases and for the consequences of self-neglect and malnutrition.

CONGENITAL ABNORMALITIES OF THE PANCREAS

PANCREAS DIVISUM

This is due to failure of the primitive dorsal and ventral ducts to fuse during embryonic development of the pancreas. As a consequence, most of the pancreatic drainage occurs through the smaller accessory ampulla rather than through the major ampulla.

Pancreas divisum occurs in 7–10% of the normal population and is usually asymptomatic. Some patients develop acute pancreatitis, chronic pancreatitis or atypical abdominal pain, possibly because drainage through the accessory papilla is restricted.

ANNULAR PANCREAS

In this congenital anomaly, the pancreas encircles the second/third part of the duodenum, leading to gastric outlet obstruction. Annular pancreas is associated with malrotation of the intestine, atresias and cardiac anomalies.

CYSTIC FIBROSIS

This disease is considered in detail on page 685. The major gastrointestinal manifestations of cystic fibrosis are pancreatic insufficiency and meconium ileus. Peptic ulcer, and hepatic and biliary disease also occur.

In cystic fibrosis pancreatic secretions are protein- and mucus-rich. The resultant viscous juice forms plugs which obstruct the pancreatic ductules, leading to progressive destruction of acinar cells. Steatorrhoea is universal and the large-volume bulky stools predispose to rectal prolapse. Malnutrition is compounded by the metabolic demands of respiratory failure and by diabetes which develops in 40% of patients by adolescence.

The majority of patients now survive well into adulthood and heart/lung transplantation can further prolong life. Optimal treatment of the cystic fibrosis patient depends upon an assiduous team approach to respiratory, nutritional and hepatobiliary complications. Nutritional counselling and supervision are important to ensure intake of high-energy foods, providing 120–150% of the recommended intake for normal subjects. Fats are an important calorie source and, despite the presence of steatorrhoea, fat intake should not be restricted. Supplementary fat-soluble vitamins are also necessary.

High-dose oral pancreatic enzymes are also required, in doses sufficient to control steatorrhoea and stool frequency. A proton pump inhibitor aids fat digestion by producing an optimal duodenal pH. Diabetic patients usually require insulin injections rather than oral hypoglycaemic agents.

Meconium ileus

Mucus-rich plugs within intestinal contents can obstruct the small or large intestine. Meconium ileus is treated by the mucolytic agent N-acetylcysteine given orally, by gastro-grafin enema or by gut lavage using polyethylene glycol. In resistant cases of meconium ileus surgical resection may be necessary.

TUMOURS OF THE PANCREAS

Pancreatic carcinoma affects 10–15 per 100 000 in Western populations, rising to 100 per 100 000 in those over the age of 70. Men are affected twice as often as women. The disease is associated with smoking and chronic pancreatitis. Between 5 and 10% of patients have a genetic predisposition (hereditary pancreatitis, MEN, hereditary non-polyposis colon cancer—HNPCC).

Pathology
Approximately 90% of pancreatic neoplasms are adeno-carcinomas which arise from the pancreatic ducts. These tumours involve local structures and metastasise to regional

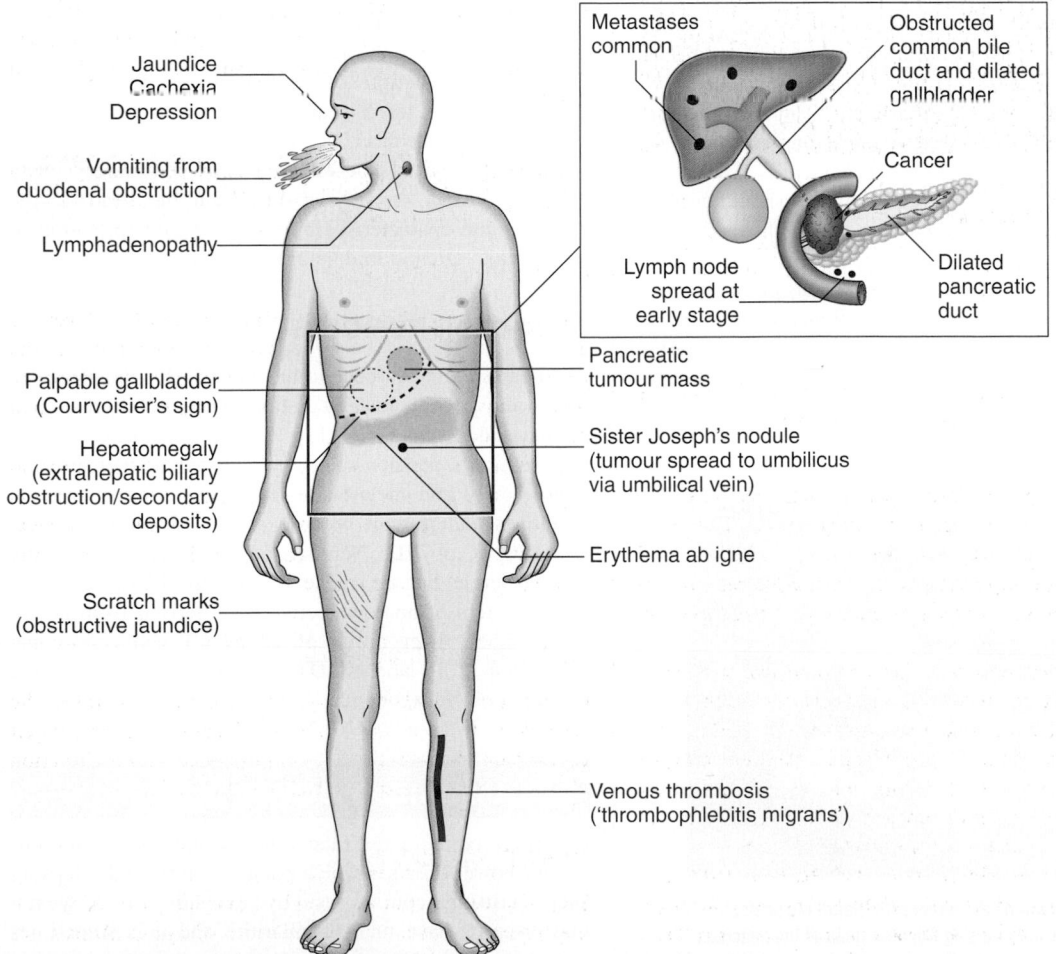

Fig. 22.47 Features of pancreatic cancer.

lymph nodes at an early stage. The majority of patients have advanced disease at the time of presentation.

Clinical features

The clinical features of pancreatic cancer are pain, weight loss and obstructive jaundice (Fig. 22.47). The pain results from invasion of the coeliac plexus and is characteristically incessant and boring. It often radiates from the upper abdomen through to the back and may be eased a little by bending forwards. Almost all patients lose weight and many are cachectic. Weight loss is the consequence of anorexia, steatorrhoea and metabolic effects of the tumour. Around 60% of tumours arise from the head of the pancreas, and involvement of the common bile duct results in the development of obstructive jaundice, often with severe pruritus.

A few patients present with diarrhoea, vomiting from duodenal obstruction, diabetes mellitus, recurrent venous thrombosis, acute pancreatitis or depression.

Physical examination reveals clear evidence of weight loss. An abdominal mass due to the tumour itself, a palpable gallbladder or hepatic metastasis is commonly found. A palpable gallbladder in a jaundiced patient is usually the consequence of distal biliary obstruction by a pancreatic cancer (Courvoisier's sign).

Investigations

When a patient presents with biochemically confirmed cholestatic jaundice the diagnosis is usually made by ultrasound and CT (Fig. 22.48). Diagnosis in non-jaundiced patients is often delayed because presenting symptoms are relatively non-specific.

Fit patients with small localised tumours should undergo staging to define operability. Laparoscopy with laparoscopic ultrasound will define tumour size, involvement of blood vessels and metastatic spread. In patients unsuitable for surgery because of advanced disease, frailty or comorbidity, ultrasound or CT-guided cytology or biopsy may be used to confirm the diagnosis. Endoscopic ultrasound with fine-needle aspiration is used to define vascular invasion and obtain cytological proof of diagnosis.

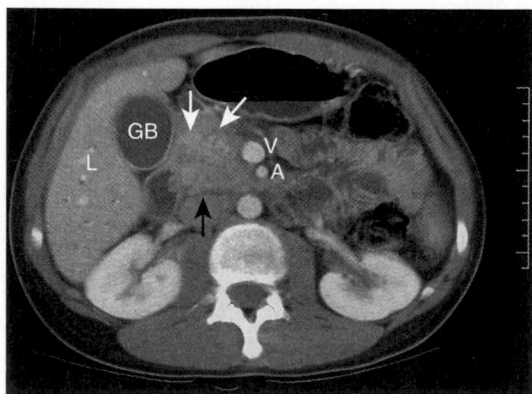

Fig. 22.48 Carcinoma of the pancreatic head. Multidetector CT showing an irregular mass arising from the head of the pancreas (arrows). (L = liver; GB = gallbladder; V = superior mesenteric vein; A = superior mesenteric artery)

MRCP and ERCP are sensitive methods of diagnosing pancreatic cancer and are valuable when the diagnosis is in doubt, although differentiation between cancer and localised chronic pancreatitis can be difficult. The main role of ERCP is to insert a stent into the common bile duct to relieve obstructive jaundice in inoperable patients.

Management

Surgical resection is the only method of effecting cure, and 5-year survival in patients undergoing a complete resection is around 20%. Recent trials have demonstrated improved survival with adjuvant chemotherapy using 5-fluorouracil. Unfortunately, a mere 15% of tumours are amenable to curative resection since most neoplasms are locally advanced at the time of diagnosis.

For the great majority of patients therapy is based on palliation of pain and obstructive jaundice. Pain relief is achieved using analgesic drugs and, in some patients, coeliac plexus neurolysis by a percutaneous or endoscopic ultrasound-guided alcohol injection. Jaundice is relieved by choledochojejunostomy in fit patients; percutaneous or endoscopic stenting is used in the elderly or in patients who have very advanced disease. Overall survival is only 3–5%.

Ampullary or periampullary adenocarcinomas are rare neoplasms which arise from the ampulla of Vater or adjacent duodenum. They are often polypoid and may ulcerate; they often infiltrate the duodenum but behave less aggressively than pancreatic adenocarcinoma. Around 25% of patients undergoing resection of ampullary or periampullary tumours survive for 5 years in contrast to patients with pancreatic ductal cancer.

Mucinous cystadenocarcinoma is a very rare, slowly growing tumour, usually arising from the head of the pancreas and characterised by mucinous cyst formation. It occurs most often in middle-aged women.

ENDOCRINE TUMOURS

These arise from neuroendocrine tissue within the pancreas. They may occur in association with parathyroid and pituitary adenomas (MEN 1, p. 802). The majority of endocrine tumours are non-secretory and, although malignant, grow slowly and metastasise late. Other tumours secrete hormones and present because of their endocrine effects (Box 20.50, p. 791). Neuroendocrine pancreatic tumours may be single, but are frequently multifocal and arise from other clusters of neuroendocrine cells derived from neural crest tissues. They are localised by CT and endoscopic ultrasound. ^{111}In-labelled DTPA is very sensitive in the diagnosis of glucagonoma.

INFLAMMATORY BOWEL DISEASE

Ulcerative colitis and Crohn's disease are chronic inflammatory bowel diseases which pursue a protracted relapsing and remitting course, usually extending over years. The diseases have many similarities and it is sometimes impossible to differentiate between them. A crucial distinction is that ulcerative colitis only involves the colon,

22

while Crohn's disease can involve any part of the gastrointestinal tract from mouth to anus.

The incidence of inflammatory bowel disease (IBD) varies widely between populations. Crohn's disease appears to be very rare in the developing world yet ulcerative colitis, although still unusual, is becoming more common. In the West, the incidence of ulcerative colitis is stable at 10–20 per 100 000, with a prevalence of 100–200 per 100 000, while the incidence of Crohn's disease is increasing and is now 5–10 per 100 000, with a prevalence of 50–100 per 100 000. Both diseases most commonly start in young adults, with a second incidence peak in the seventh decade. Approximately 240 000 people are affected by IBD in the UK.

Pathogenesis

IBD develops as a response to an environmental trigger in genetically susceptible individuals (Box 22.65). The cellular events involved in the pathogenesis of Crohn's disease and ulcerative colitis involve activation of macrophages, lymphocytes and polymorphonuclear cells with release of

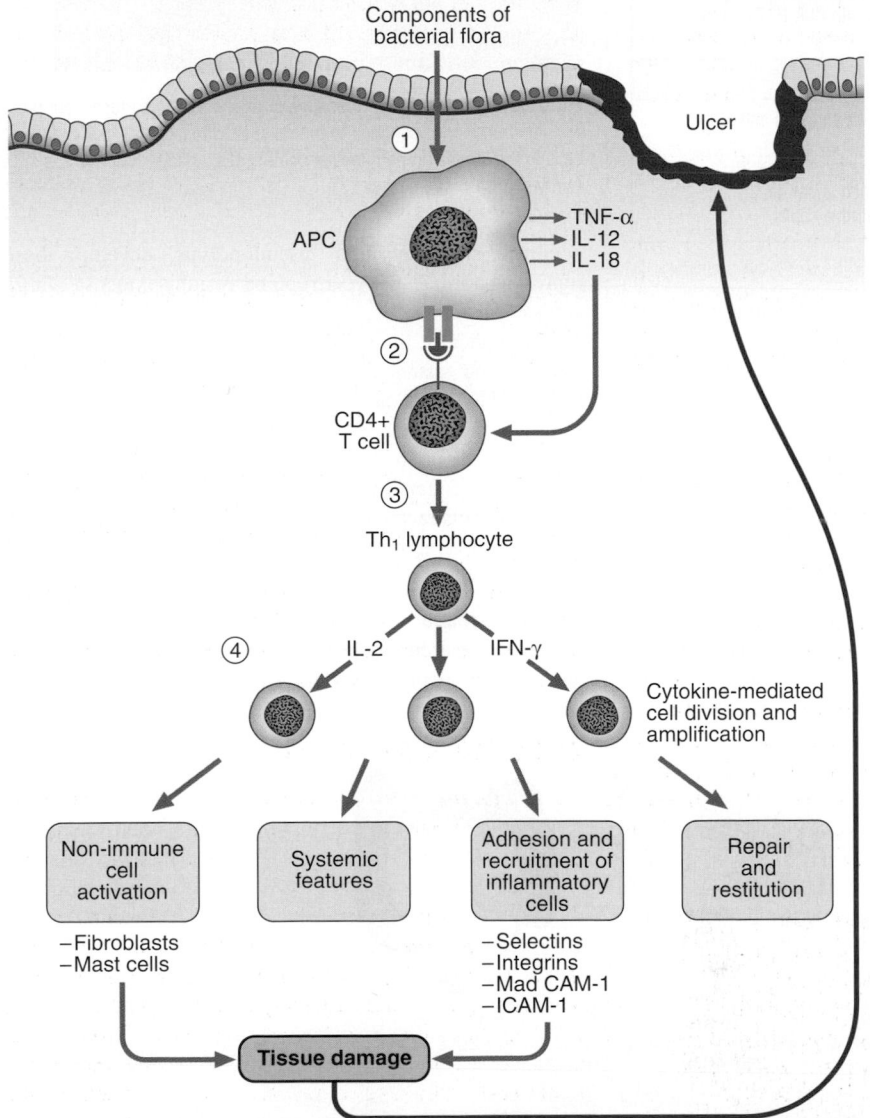

Fig. 22.49 Probable pathogenesis of inflammatory bowel disease. (1) Dietary or bacterial antigens either are taken up by specialised M cells, pass between leaky epithelial cells or enter the lamina propria through ulcerated mucosa. (2) After processing they are presented to CD4+ T cells by antigen-presenting cells (APC) in the lamina propria. APCs secrete pro-inflammatory cytokines such as tumour necrosis factor-α (TNF-α), interleukin 12 (IL-12) and interleukin-18 (IL-18). (3) T-cell activation and differentiation results in a Th$_1$ T cell-mediated cytokine response (4) with secretion of interleukin-2 (IL-2) and gamma interferon (IFN-γ). Further amplification of T cells perpetuates the inflammatory process with: activation of non-immune cells leading to tissue damage; expression of adhesion molecules on the vascular endothelium, leading to recruitment of inflammatory cells; systemic features such as fever, malaise and anorexia; and processes of tissue repair and restitution. Ulceration, inflammation and stricturing then ensue. These pathways occur in all normal individuals exposed to an inflammatory insult and this is self-limiting in healthy subjects. In genetically predisposed persons, dysregulation of these steps leads to chronic IBD, although evidence for this is stronger in Crohn's disease than ulcerative colitis. Mutations in the CARD 15/NOD-2 gene are prevalent in patients with Crohn's disease and may be involved in dysregulation of innate immunity: for example, abnormalities in NFκB responses to bacterial lipopolysaccharide.

22.65 FACTORS ASSOCIATED WITH THE DEVELOPMENT OF INFLAMMATORY BOWEL DISEASE

Genetic

- More common in Ashkenazi Jews
- 10% have a first-degree relative or at least one close relative with IBD
- High concordance between identical twins
- Associated with autoimmune thyroiditis and SLE
- Linkage with mutations in CARD 15/NOD-2 gene on chromosome 16 (IBD-1 locus)
- Other regions of linkage on chromosomes 12, 6 and 14 ('IBD 2–4')
- HLA-DR103 associated with severe ulcerative colitis
- Ulcerative colitis and Crohn's patients with HLA-B27 commonly develop ankylosing spondylitis

Environmental

- Ulcerative colitis—more common in non-smokers and ex-smokers
- Crohn's—most patients are smokers (relative risk = 3)
- Associated with low-residue, high refined sugar diet
- Appendicectomy protects against ulcerative colitis

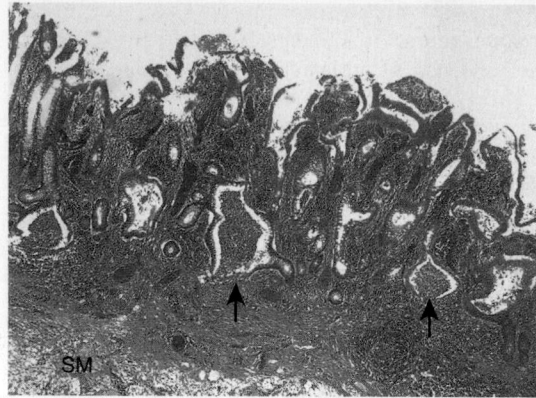

Fig. 22.51 Histology of ulcerative colitis. There is surface ulceration and inflammation is confined to the mucosa with excess inflammatory cells in the lamina propria, loss of goblet cells, and crypt abscesses (arrows). (SM = submucosa)

22

inflammatory mediators, and these events represent targets for future therapeutic intervention (Fig. 22.49).

Pathology

In both diseases the intestinal wall is infiltrated with acute and chronic inflammatory cells. There are important differences in the distribution of disease and in histological features (Fig. 22.50).

Ulcerative colitis

Inflammation invariably involves the rectum (proctitis). It may spread proximally to involve the sigmoid colon (proctosigmoiditis) and in a minority the whole colon is involved (pancolitis). Inflammation is confluent and is more severe distally. In long-standing pancolitis the bowel becomes shortened and 'pseudopolyps' develop; these represent normal or hypertrophied residual mucosa within areas of atrophy.

Histologically, the inflammatory process is limited to the mucosa and spares the deeper layers of the bowel wall (Fig. 22.51). Both acute and chronic inflammatory cells infiltrate the lamina propria and the crypts ('cryptitis'). Crypt abscesses are typical. Goblet cells lose their mucus and in long-standing cases glands become distorted. Dysplasia, characterised by heaping of cells within the crypts, nuclear atypia and increased mitotic rate may herald the development of colon cancer.

Crohn's disease

The sites most commonly involved, in order of frequency, are terminal ileum and right side of colon, colon alone, terminal ileum alone, ileum and jejunum. Characteristically,

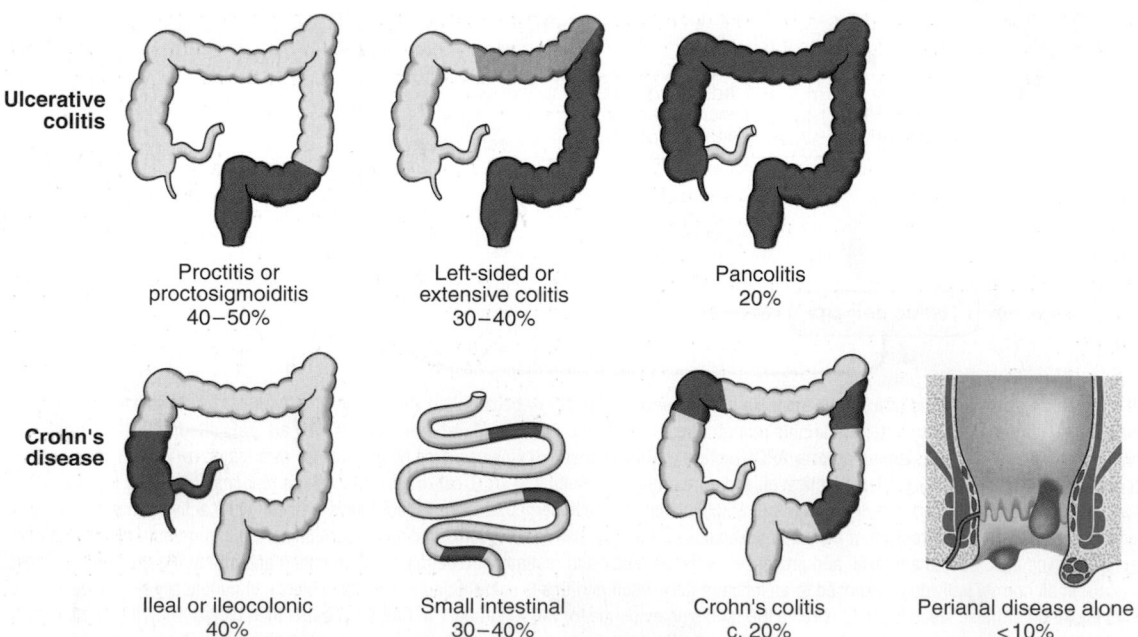

Ulcerative colitis

| Proctitis or proctosigmoiditis 40–50% | Left-sided or extensive colitis 30–40% | Pancolitis 20% |

Crohn's disease

| Ileal or ileocolonic 40% | Small intestinal 30–40% | Crohn's colitis c. 20% | Perianal disease alone <10% |

Fig. 22.50 Common patterns of disease distribution in inflammatory bowel disease.

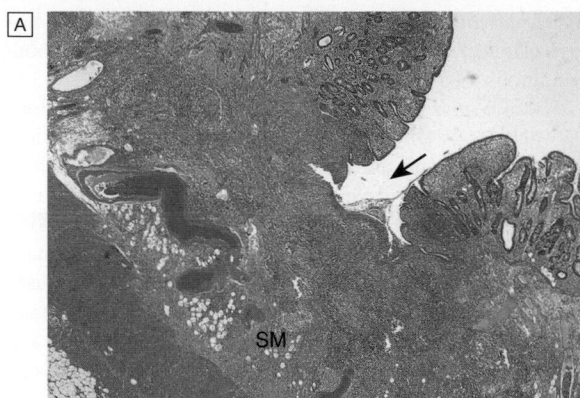

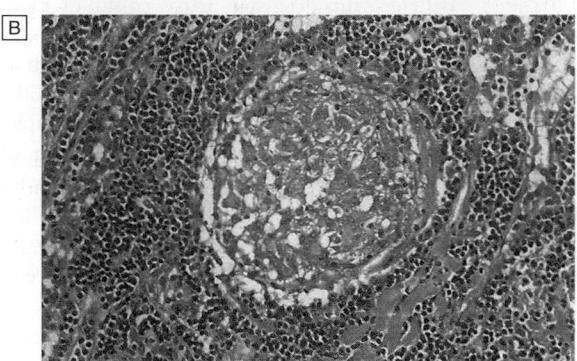

Fig. 22.52 Histology of Crohn's disease. Ⓐ Inflammation is 'transmural'; there is fissuring ulceration (arrow) with inflammation extending into the submucosa (SM). Ⓑ At higher power a characteristic non-caseating granuloma is seen.

the entire wall of the bowel is oedematous and thickened. There are deep ulcers which often appear as linear fissures; thus the mucosa between them is described as 'cobblestone'. Deep ulcers may penetrate through the bowel wall to initiate abscesses or fistulae. Fistulae may develop between adjacent loops of bowel or between affected segments of bowel and the bladder, uterus or vagina, and may appear in the perineum.

Characteristically, the changes are patchy. Even when a relatively short segment of bowel is affected, the inflammatory process is interrupted by islands of normal mucosa and the change from the affected part is abrupt. A small lesion separated in this way from a major area of involvement is referred to as a 'skip' lesion. The mesenteric lymph nodes are enlarged and the mesentery thickened.

Histologically, chronic inflammation is seen through all the layers of the bowel wall, which is thickened as a result (Fig. 22.52). There are focal aggregates of epithelioid histiocytes, which may be surrounded by lymphocytes and contain giant cells. Lymphoid aggregates or microgranulomas are also seen, and when these are near to the surface of the mucosa they often ulcerate to form tiny aphthous-like ulcers.

Clinical features

Ulcerative colitis
The major symptom is bloody diarrhoea. The first attack is usually the most severe and thereafter the disease is followed by relapses and remissions. Only a minority of patients have chronic, unremitting symptoms. Emotional stress, intercurrent infection, gastroenteritis, antibiotics or NSAID therapy may provoke a relapse. The clinical features depend upon the site and activity of the disease.

Proctitis causes rectal bleeding and mucus discharge, sometimes accompanied by tenesmus. Some patients pass frequent, small-volume fluid stools, while others are constipated and pass pellety stools. Constitutional symptoms do not occur.

Proctosigmoiditis causes bloody diarrhoea with mucus. Almost all patients are constitutionally well but a small minority who have very active, limited disease develop fever, lethargy and abdominal discomfort.

Extensive colitis causes bloody diarrhoea with passage of mucus. In severe cases anorexia, malaise, weight loss and abdominal pain occur, and the patient is toxic with fever, tachycardia and signs of peritoneal inflammation (Box 22.66).

Crohn's disease
The major symptoms are abdominal pain, diarrhoea and weight loss.

Ileal Crohn's disease causes abdominal pain, principally because of subacute intestinal obstruction, although an inflammatory mass, intra-abdominal abscess or acute obstruction may be responsible. Pain is often associated with diarrhoea which is watery and does not contain blood or mucus. Almost all patients lose weight. This is usually because they avoid food since eating provokes pain. Weight loss may also be due to malabsorption, and some patients present with features of fat, protein or vitamin deficiencies.

Crohn's colitis presents in an identical manner to ulcerative colitis, with bloody diarrhoea, passage of mucus and constitutional symptoms including lethargy, malaise, anorexia and weight loss. Rectal sparing and the presence of perianal disease are features which favour a diagnosis of Crohn's disease rather than ulcerative colitis.

Many patients present with symptoms of both small bowel and colonic disease. A few have isolated perianal

22.66 FACTORS CONSIDERED FOR DISEASE SEVERITY ASSESSMENT IN ULCERATIVE COLITIS		
	Mild	**Severe**
Daily bowel frequency	< 4	> 6
Blood in stools	+/−	+++
Stool volume (g/24 hrs)	< 200	> 400
Pulse (bpm)	< 90	> 90
Temperature (°C)	Normal	> 37.8, 2 days out of 4
Sigmoidoscopy	Normal or granular mucosa	Blood in lumen
Abdominal X-ray	Normal	Dilated bowel and/or mucosal islands
Haemoglobin (g/l)	Normal	< 100
ESR (mm/hr)	Normal	> 30
Serum albumin (g/l)	> 35	< 30

disease, vomiting from jejunal strictures or severe oral ulceration.

Physical examination often reveals evidence of weight loss, anaemia with glossitis and angular stomatitis. There is abdominal tenderness, most marked over the inflamed area. An abdominal mass due to matted loops of thickened bowel or an intra-abdominal abscess may occur. Perianal skin tags, fissures or fistulae are found in at least 50% of patients.

Complications

Intestinal

Severe, life-threatening inflammation of the colon. This occurs in both ulcerative colitis and Crohn's disease. In the most extreme cases the colon dilates (toxic megacolon) and bacterial toxins pass freely across the diseased mucosa into the portal then systemic circulation. This complication occurs most commonly during the first attack of colitis and is recognised by the features described in Box 22.66. An abdominal X-ray should be taken daily because when the transverse colon is dilated to more than 6 cm (Fig. 22.57, p. 916) there is a high risk of colonic perforation.

Perforation of the small intestine or colon. This can occur without the development of toxic megacolon.

Life-threatening acute haemorrhage. Haemorrhage due to erosion of a major artery is a rare complication of both conditions.

Fistulae and perianal disease. Fistulous connections between loops of affected bowel, or between bowel and bladder or vagina are specific complications of Crohn's disease and do not occur in ulcerative colitis. Enteroenteric fistulae cause diarrhoea and malabsorption due to blind loop syndrome. Enterovesical fistulation causes recurrent urinary infections and pneumaturia. An enterovaginal fistula causes a feculent vaginal discharge. Fistulation from the bowel may also cause perianal or ischiorectal abscesses, fissures and fistulae. These may sometimes be extremely severe and can be the source of great morbidity.

Cancer. Patients with extensive active colitis of more than 8 years' duration are at increased risk of colon cancer. The cumulative risk for ulcerative colitis may be as high as 20% after 30 years but is probably lower for Crohn's colitis. Tumours develop in areas of dysplasia and may be multiple. Small bowel adenocarcinoma is a rare complication of long-standing small bowel Crohn's disease. Patients with long-standing, extensive colitis are therefore entered into surveillance colonoscopy programmes beginning 8–10 years after diagnosis. Multiple random biopsies are taken

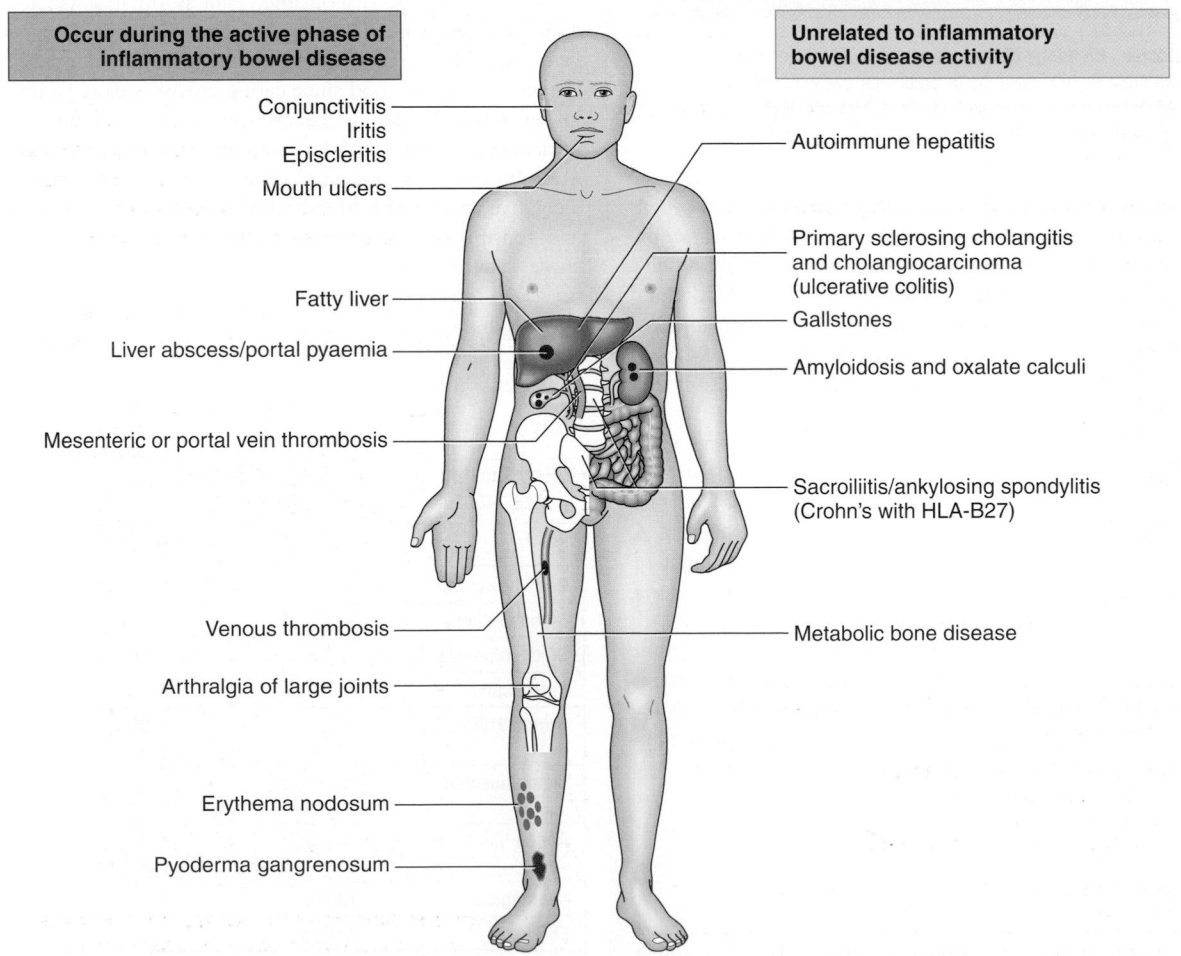

Occur during the active phase of inflammatory bowel disease

- Conjunctivitis
- Iritis
- Episcleritis
- Mouth ulcers
- Fatty liver
- Liver abscess/portal pyaemia
- Mesenteric or portal vein thrombosis
- Venous thrombosis
- Arthralgia of large joints
- Erythema nodosum
- Pyoderma gangrenosum

Unrelated to inflammatory bowel disease activity

- Autoimmune hepatitis
- Primary sclerosing cholangitis and cholangiocarcinoma (ulcerative colitis)
- Gallstones
- Amyloidosis and oxalate calculi
- Sacroiliitis/ankylosing spondylitis (Crohn's with HLA-B27)
- Metabolic bone disease

Fig. 22.53 Systemic complications of inflammatory bowel disease. (See also Chs 19 and 20.)

every 10 cm throughout the colon and additional biopsies are taken from raised or ulcerated areas. Dysplastic changes are graded by histopathologists as low-grade or high-grade. Assessment of biopsies is subjective and the presence of active inflammation makes analysis of dysplasia very difficult. Patients who have no evidence of dysplasia or only low-grade dysplasia are screened every 1–2 years, while those with high-grade dysplasia should be considered for panproctocolectomy because of the high risk of colon cancer development.

Extraintestinal

IBD can be considered as a systemic illness and in some patients extraintestinal complications dominate the clinical picture. Some of these occur during relapse of intestinal disease; others appear unrelated to intestinal disease activity (Fig. 22.53).

Differential diagnosis (Box 22.67)

Ulcerative colitis

The major diagnostic difficulty is to distinguish the first attack of acute colitis from infection. In general, diarrhoea

22.67 CONDITIONS WHICH CAN MIMIC ULCERATIVE OR CROHN'S COLITIS	
Infective	
Bacterial	
• *Salmonella*	• Gonococcal proctitis
• *Shigella*	• Pseudomembranous colitis
• *Campylobacter jejuni*	• *Chlamydia* proctitis
• *E. coli* O:157	
Viral	
• Herpes simplex proctitis	• Cytomegalovirus
Protozoal	
• Amoebiasis	
Non-infective	
Vascular	
• Ischaemic colitis	• Radiation proctitis
Idiopathic	
• Collagenous colitis	• Behçet's disease
Drugs	
• NSAIDs	
Neoplastic	
• Colonic carcinoma	
Other	
• Diverticulitis	

22.68 DIFFERENTIAL DIAGNOSIS OF SMALL BOWEL CROHN'S DISEASE 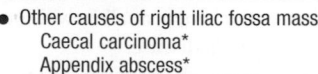
• Other causes of right iliac fossa mass 　Caecal carcinoma* 　Appendix abscess* 　Infection (TB, *Yersinia*, actinomycosis) • Mesenteric adenitis • Pelvic inflammatory disease • Lymphoma
* Common; other causes are rare.

lasting longer than 10 days in Western countries is unlikely to be the result of infection. A history of foreign travel, antibiotic exposure (pseudomembranous colitis) or homosexual contact suggests infection. Stool microscopy, culture and examination for *Clostridium difficile* toxin or for ova and cysts, sigmoidoscopy and rectal biopsy, blood cultures and serological tests for infection are useful.

Small bowel Crohn's disease

Crohn's disease can usually be diagnosed with confidence without histological confirmation in the appropriate clinical setting. Indium- or technetium-labelled white cell scanning may help identify inflamed intestinal segments. In atypical cases biopsy or surgical resection is necessary to exclude other diseases (Box 22.68). This can often be done endoscopically by ileal intubation at colonoscopy, but sometimes laparotomy or laparoscopy with resection or full-thickness biopsy is necessary.

Investigations

These confirm the diagnosis, define disease distribution and activity, and identify specific complications.

Full blood count may show anaemia resulting from bleeding or malabsorption of iron, folic acid or vitamin B_{12}. Serum albumin concentration falls as a consequence of protein-losing enteropathy, reflecting active and extensive disease, or because of poor nutrition. The ESR is raised in exacerbations or because of abscess. Elevation of CRP concentration is helpful in monitoring Crohn's disease activity.

Bacteriology

Stool cultures are performed to exclude superimposed enteric infection in patients who present with exacerbations of IBD. Blood cultures are also advisable in patients with known colitis or Crohn's disease who develop fever.

Endoscopy

Sigmoidoscopy (Fig. 22.54) with biopsies is a simple but essential investigation in all patients who present with

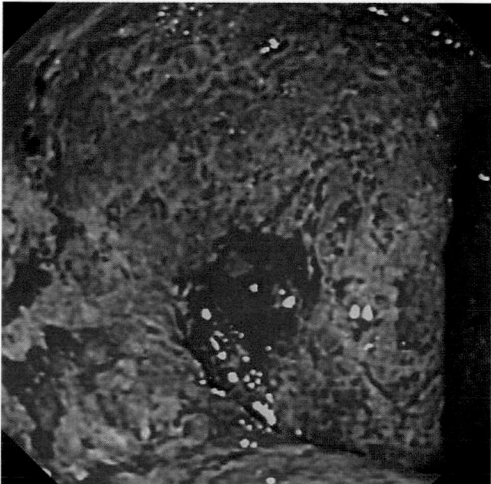

Fig. 22.54 Sigmoidoscopic view of moderately active ulcerative colitis. Mucosa is erythematous and friable with contact bleeding. Submucosal blood vessels are no longer visible.

22

22

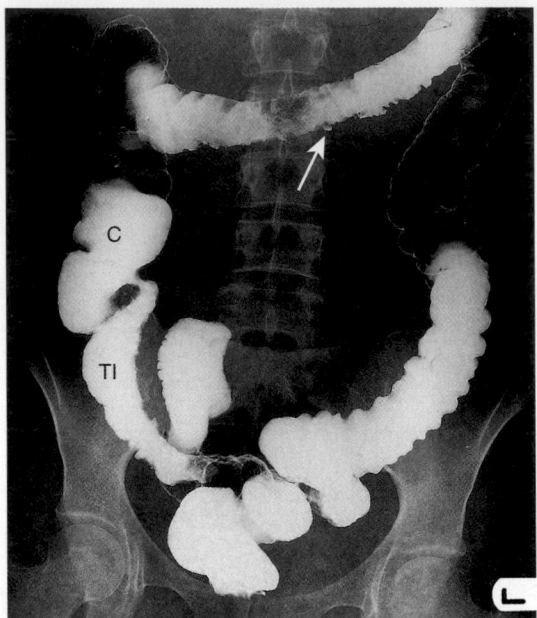

Fig. 22.55 Ileocolonic Crohn's disease. Barium enema showing normal rectum and sigmoid colon, typical aphthous ulceration in the descending colon, ulceration (arrow) and lack of haustra in the transverse colon. The ascending colon and caecum (C) are normal and there is typical Crohn's disease affecting the terminal ileum (TI), with coarse ulceration, rigidity and lack of mucosal folds.

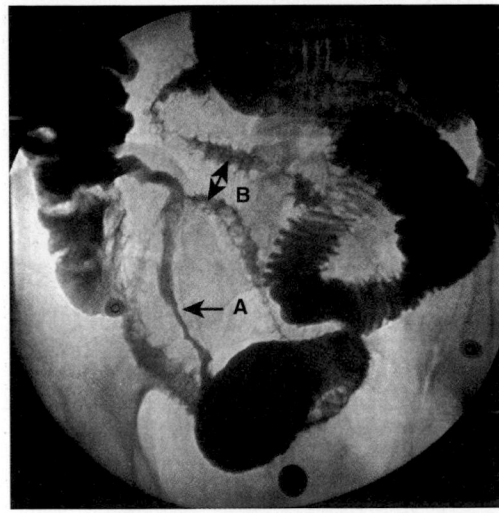

Fig. 22.56 Barium follow-through showing terminal ileal Crohn's disease. A long stricture is present (arrow A) and more proximally there is ulceration with characteristic 'rose thorn' ulcers (arrow B).

diarrhoea. In ulcerative colitis sigmoidoscopy is almost always abnormal with loss of vascular pattern, granularity, friability and ulceration. In Crohn's disease patchy inflammation with discrete, deep ulcers, perianal disease (fissures, fistulae and skin tags) or rectal sparing occurs.

Colonoscopy may show active inflammation with pseudopolyps or a complicating carcinoma. Biopsies are taken to define disease extent, as this is underestimated by endoscopic appearances alone, and to seek dysplasia in

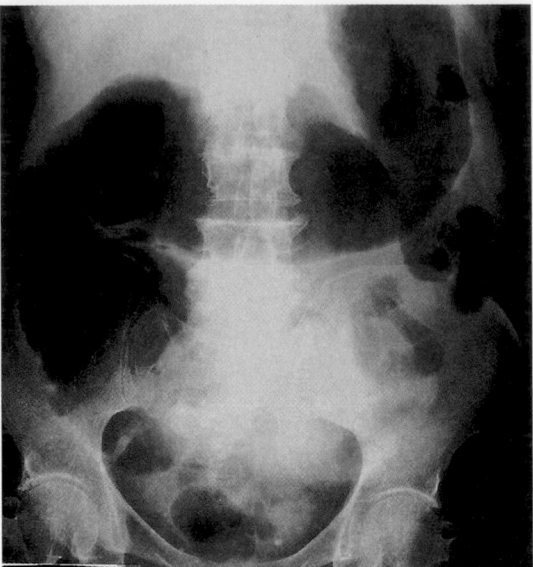

Fig. 22.57 Plain abdominal X-ray showing a grossly dilated colon due to severe ulcerative colitis.

patients with long-standing colitis. In ulcerative colitis the macroscopic and histological abnormalities are confluent and most severe in the distal colon and rectum. Stricture formation does not occur in the absence of a carcinoma. In Crohn's colitis the endoscopic abnormalities are patchy, with normal mucosa between the areas of abnormality. Aphthoid or deeper ulcers and strictures are common.

Barium studies

Barium enema is a less sensitive investigation than colonoscopy. In long-standing ulcerative colitis the colon is shortened and loses haustra to become tubular, and pseudopolyps are seen. In Crohn's colitis a range of abnormalities occur. The appearances may be identical to those of ulcerative colitis but skip lesions, strictures and deeper ulcers are characteristic (Fig. 22.55). Reflux into the terminal ileum may show stricture and ulcers.

Contrast studies of the small bowel are normal in ulcerative colitis, but in Crohn's disease affected areas are narrowed and ulcerated; multiple strictures are common (Fig. 22.56).

Other investigations

A straight abdominal X-ray is essential in the management of patients who present with severe active disease. Dilatation of the colon (Fig. 22.57), mucosal oedema ('thumb-printing') or evidence of perforation may be found. In small bowel Crohn's disease there may be evidence of intestinal obstruction or displacement of bowel loops by a mass. Ultrasound may identify thickened small bowel loops and abscess development in Crohn's disease.

Radio-labelled white cell scans show areas of active inflammation. They are less accurate than other imaging modalities with poor specificity but may be useful in severely ill patients in whom invasive tests are best avoided.

MRI scans are very accurate in delineating pelvic or perineal involvement by Crohn's disease.

Management

Best treatment depends upon a team approach involving physicians, surgeons, radiologists and dietitians. Both ulcerative colitis and Crohn's disease are life-long conditions and have psychosocial implications; counsellors and patient support groups have important roles in education, reassurance and coping. The key aims are to:

- treat acute attacks
- prevent relapses
- detect carcinoma at an early stage
- select patients for surgery.

Drugs used in the treatment of IBD are listed in Box 22.69.

Medical management of ulcerative colitis

Treatment depends upon the extent and activity of colitis.

Active proctitis

In mild to moderate disease mesalazine enemas or suppositories combined with oral mesalazine are effective first-line therapy. Topical corticosteroids are less effective and are reserved for patients who are intolerant of topical mesalazine. Patients who fail to respond are treated with oral prednisolone 40 mg daily.

Active left-sided or extensive ulcerative colitis

In mildly active cases, high-dose aminosalicylates combined with topical aminosalicylate and corticosteroids are effective. Oral prednisolone 40 mg daily is indicated for more active disease or when initial aminosalicylate therapy is ineffective.

Severe ulcerative colitis

Patients who fail to respond to maximal oral therapy and those who present with severe colitis are best managed in

22.69 DRUGS USED IN THE TREATMENT OF INFLAMMATORY BOWEL DISEASE		
Class	**Mechanism of action**	**Notes**
Aminosalicylates (mesalazine (Asacol, Salofalk, Pentasa), olsalazine, sulfasalazine, balsalazide)	Modulate cytokine release from mucosa Delivered to colon by one of three mechanisms: (1) pH-dependent (Asacol, Salofalk) (2) time-dependent (Pentasa) (3) bacterial breakdown by colonic bacteria from a carrier molecule (sulfasalazine, olsalazine, balsalazide)	Available as oral or topical (enema/suppository) preparation Sulfasalazine causes side-effects in 10–45%: headache, nausea, diarrhoea, blood dyscrasias Other aminosalicylates much better tolerated; diarrhoea, headache in 2–5% Rarely, renal impairment All safe during pregnancy
Corticosteroids (prednisolone, hydrocortisone, budesonide)	Anti-inflammatory Budesonide is a potent corticosteroid efficiently cleared from circulation by liver, thereby minimising adrenocortical suppression and steroid side-effects	Topical, oral or i.v. according to disease severity Bisphosphonates are co-prescribed to prevent osteopenia Budesonide considered for active ileitis and ileocolitis
Thiopurines (azathioprine, 6-mercaptopurine)	Immunomodulation by inducing T-cell apoptosis Azathioprine is metabolised in the liver to 6-mercaptopurine, then by thiopurine methyltransferase (TPMT) to thioguanine nucleotides	Effective 6–18 weeks after starting therapy. Complications in 20%. Flu-like syndrome with myalgia. Leucopenia in 3%, particularly in inherited TPMT deficiency No increased risk of cancer but probable increase in lymphoma Safe during pregnancy
Methotrexate	Anti-inflammatory	Intolerance in 10–18%. Nausea, stomatitis, diarrhoea, hepatotoxicity and pneumonitis
Ciclosporin	Suppresses T-cell expansion	'Rescue' therapy to prevent surgery in ulcerative colitis responding poorly to corticosteroids. No value in Crohn's disease Major side-effects in 0–17%: nephrotoxicity, infections, neurotoxicity (including fits) Minor complications in up to 50%: tremor, paraesthesiae, abnormal LFTs, hirsutism
Infliximab	Chimeric anti-TNF monoclonal antibody Given as i.v. infusion 4–8-weekly Induces apoptosis of inflammatory cells	Moderately to severely active Crohn's disease, especially fistulating Severe active ulcerative colitis Anaphylactic reactions after multiple infusions Contraindicated in the presence of infections; reactivation of TB Theoretical risk of lymphoma
Antibiotics	Antibacterial	Useful in perianal Crohn's disease Major concern is peripheral neuropathy with long-term metronidazole
Antidiarrhoeal agents (codeine phosphate, loperamide, lomotil)	Reduce gut motility and small bowel secretion Loperamide improves anal function	Avoided in moderately or severely active disease. May precipitate colonic dilatation

22

22.70 MEDICAL MANAGEMENT OF FULMINANT ULCERATIVE COLITIS

- Intravenous fluids
- Transfusion if Hb < 100 g/l
- I.v. methylprednisolone (60 mg daily) or hydrocortisone
- Antibiotics for proven infection
- Nutritional support
- Subcutaneous heparin for prophylaxis of venous thromboembolism
- Avoidance of opiates and antidiarrhoeal agents
- I.v. ciclosporin (2 mg/kg) or infliximab (5 mg/kg) in stable patients not responding to 3–5 days of corticosteroids

22.71 AMINOSALICYLATES AND REMISSION IN ULCERATIVE COLITIS **EBM**

'Six RCTs including a total of 485 5-ASA-treated patients and 401 placebo-treated patients indicate that active therapy is better than placebo (Chi Square 2.39).'

- Carter MJ, et al. Gut 2004; 53 (suppl. V):1–16.

For further information: 🖥 www.bsg.org.uk

22.72 INFLIXIMAB IN CROHN'S DISEASE **EBM**

'Anti-TNF antibody treatment (infliximab) improves remission rates in Crohn's disease refractory to conventional therapies including corticosteroids (NNT 4), heals enterocutaneous Crohn's fistulae and maintains longer remissions.'

- Akobeng AK, et al. (Cochrane Review). Cochrane Library, issue 1, 2005. Oxford: Update Software.

For further information: 🖥 www.cochrane.org

hospital and should be monitored jointly by a physician and surgeon:

- clinically— for the presence of abdominal pain, temperature, pulse rate, stool blood and frequency
- in the laboratory—haemoglobin, white cell count, albumin, electrolytes, ESR and CRP
- radiologically —for colonic dilatation on plain abdominal X-rays.

Supportive treatment includes intravenous fluids to correct dehydration along with nutritional support, usually as enteral rather than intravenous feeding, for malnourished patients (Box 22.70).

Intravenous corticosteroids (methylprednisolone 60 mg or hydrocortisone 400 mg/day) are given as a constant infusion. Topical and oral aminosalicylates are also used, although their value in severe disease is unclear.

Patients who do not promptly respond to corticosteroids are considered for intravenous ciclosporin or infliximab, which, in approximately 30% of cases, overcomes the need for urgent colectomy.

Patients who develop colonic dilatation (> 6 cm), those whose clinical and laboratory measurements deteriorate and those who do not respond after 7–10 days' maximal medical treatment usually proceed to urgent colectomy.

Maintenance of remission

Life-long maintenance therapy is recommended for all patients with extensive disease and patients with distal disease who relapse more than once a year.

Oral aminosalicylates—either mesalazine or balsalazide —are first-line agents (Box 22.71). Sulfasalazine has a higher incidence of side-effects, but should be considered in patients with co-existent arthropathy.

Patients who frequently relapse despite aminosalicylate drugs are treated with thiopurines.

Medical management of Crohn's disease

Active disease

Patients with active colitis or ileocolitis are initially treated in a similar manner to those with active ulcerative colitis. Aminosalicylates and corticosteroids are both effective and usually effect remission in active ileocolitis and colitis. In severe disease intravenous prednisolone is indicated, but abscess or fistulating disease should be excluded before instituting therapy with corticosteroids. In contrast to ulcerative colitis, nutritional therapy using polymeric or elemental diets induces remission. Possible mechanisms include

avoidance of dietary antigens, other ill-defined immunological effects and the non-specific effects of nutritional support. Prolonged nutritional therapy, which involves exclusion of a normal diet, is onerous for the patient; remission rates are comparable to those achieved by corticosteroids but relapse rates are higher and, except in paediatric practice, primary nutritional therapy is now seldom used.

Patients with isolated ileal disease are treated with corticosteroids. Budesonide is appropriate for treating moderately active disease, although it is marginally less effective than prednisolone. Aminosalicylates have little added value but there is some evidence to support the use of oral metronidazole. Poorly responding patients should, at an early stage, be considered for surgical resection since this is associated with prolonged remission in most cases.

Infliximab given as an intravenous infusion 4–8-weekly on three occasions induces remission in patients with active Crohn's disease at any site within the gastrointestinal tract (Box 22.72) and is also effective for the management of some extraintestinal complications including pyoderma gangrenosum and some forms of arthritis. Infliximab is contraindicated in the presence of infection, including TB, and may be complicated by allergic reactions. Relapse commonly occurs approximately 12 weeks after treatment and for this reason infliximab is combined with disease-modifying agents, either thiopurines or methotrexate, to maintain remission. Infliximab (in contrast to corticosteroids) causes remarkable mucosal healing, but this can lead to scarring and stricturing. It is therefore used with caution in patients with stenosing disease.

Patients with diffuse and extensive ileocolonic involvement present considerable therapeutic challenges. A combination of drug therapies, nutritional support which in the most severe cases involves prolonged parenteral nutrition, surgical intervention and endoscopic balloon dilatation of strictures may all be needed at different times.

Fistulating and perianal disease

Fistulae usually develop in association with active Crohn's disease and are often associated with sepsis. The first step in management is to define the site of fistulation; this may involve barium radiology, CT and MRI. Surgical intervention is then required, although treatment of underlying active disease with corticosteroids and nutritional support, usually by TPN, are required in many cases. For simple perianal disease metronidazole and/or ciprofloxacin are first-line therapies. Thiopurines are used in chronic disease. In many patients examination under anaesthetic is needed to determine the site of complicating abscess, fissure and fistula.

Infliximab, infused 4–8-weekly, has been shown to heal enterocutaneous fistulae and perianal disease.

Maintenance of remission

The most effective step, and one greater than any pharmacological intervention, is smoking cessation.

Aminosalicylates have minimal efficacy. Patients who relapse more than once a year are treated with thiopurines (Box 22.73). Those patients who are intolerant of, or resistant to azathioprine or 6-mercaptopurine are treated with once-weekly methotrexate combined with folic acid. Patients with aggressive disease are managed using a combination of immunomodulating agents and infliximab.

Chronic use of corticosteroids is avoided since this leads to osteopenia and other side-effects, without preventing relapse.

Surgical treatment

Ulcerative colitis

Up to 60% of patients with extensive ulcerative colitis eventually require surgery. The indications are listed in Box 22.74. Impaired quality of life, with impact upon occupation and on social and family life, is the most important of these.

Surgery involves removal of the entire colon and rectum and cures the patient. Before surgery, patients must be counselled by doctors, stoma nurses and patients who have undergone similar surgery. The choice of procedure is either panproctocolectomy with ileostomy, or proctocolectomy with ileal–anal pouch anastomosis. The sister surgical text to this book, *Principles and Practice of Surgery*, should be consulted for further details.

Crohn's disease

The indications for surgery are similar to those for ulcerative colitis. Operations are often necessary to deal with fistulae, abscesses and perianal disease, and may also be required to relieve small or large bowel obstruction.

In contrast to ulcerative colitis, surgery is not curative and disease recurrence is the rule. Surgical intervention should therefore be as conservative as possible in order to minimise loss of viable intestine and to avoid creation of a short bowel syndrome.

Obstructing or fistulating small bowel disease may require resection of affected tissue. Patients who have localised segments of Crohn's colitis may be managed by segmental resection and/or multiple stricturoplasties in which the stricture is not resected but instead incised in its longitudinal axis and sutured transversely. Others who have extensive colitis require total colectomy but ileal–anal pouch formation should be avoided because of the high risk of disease recurrence within the pouch and subsequent fistulae, abscess formation and pouch failure.

Patients who have perianal Crohn's disease are managed as conservatively as possible. Seton drainage, fistulectomy and use of advancement flaps are appropriate for complex fistulae in combination with medical therapies.

A summary of the main features of ulcerative colitis and Crohn's disease is provided in Box 22.75.

IBD in special circumstances

Childhood

Ulcerative colitis and Crohn's disease can develop before adolescence. Chronic ill health results in growth failure, metabolic bone disease and delayed puberty. Loss of schooling and social contact, as well as frequent hospitalisation, can have important psychosocial consequences. Treatment is similar to that described for adults and may require the use of corticosteroids, immunosuppressive drugs and surgery. Monitoring of height, weight and sexual development is important.

Pregnancy

The activity of IBD is not usually affected by pregnancy although relapse may be more common after parturition. Drug therapy, including aminosalicylates, corticosteroids and azathioprine, can be safely continued throughout the pregnancy.

Metabolic bone disease

Patients with IBD are prone to developing osteopenia, osteoporosis and fractures. This is partly a consequence of corticosteroid use and all patients treated with steroids for more than 3 months should also be given bisphosphonate therapy (p. 1124). Crohn's disease patients are particularly susceptible to metabolic bone disease, due to the combined effects of malnutrition, malabsorption,

---

22.73 AZATHIOPRINE (THIOPURINE) IN CROHN'S DISEASE   **EBM**

'Azathioprine is effective in preventing exacerbation of Crohn's disease.'

• Feagan BG, et al. In: McDonald J, et al., eds. Evidence-based gastroenterology and hepatology, 2nd edn. London: BMJ Books; 2003.

For further information: 💻 www.bsg.org.uk

22.74 INDICATIONS FOR SURGERY IN ULCERATIVE COLITIS

Impaired quality of life
• Loss of occupation or education
• Disruption of family life

Failure of medical therapy
• Dependence upon oral corticosteroids
• Complications of drug therapy

Fulminant colitis

Disease complications unresponsive to medical therapy
• Arthritis
• Pyoderma gangrenosum

Colon cancer or severe dysplasia

22.75 COMPARISON OF ULCERATIVE COLITIS AND CROHN'S DISEASE

	Ulcerative colitis	Crohn's disease
Age group	Any	Any
Gender	M = F	M = F
Ethnic group	Any	Any; more common in Ashkenazi Jews
Genetic factors	HLA-DR103 associated with severe disease	CARD 15/NOD-2 mutations predispose
Risk factors	More common in non-/ex-smokers Appendicectomy protects	More common in smokers
Anatomical distribution	Colon only; begins at anorectal margin with variable proximal extension	Any part of gastrointestinal tract; perianal disease common; patchy distribution—'skip lesions'
Extraintestinal manifestations	Common	Common
Presentation	Bloody diarrhoea	Variable; pain, diarrhoea, weight loss all common
Histology	Inflammation limited to mucosa; crypt distortion, cryptitis, crypt abscesses, loss of goblet cells	Submucosal or transmural inflammation common; deep fissuring ulcers, fistulae; patchy changes; granulomas
Management	5-ASA; corticosteroids; azathioprine; colectomy is curative	Corticosteroids; azathioprine; methotrexate; infliximab; nutritional therapy; surgery for complications is not curative

22

corticosteroid therapy and circulating cytokines. Regular assessment of bone density, with appropriate therapy (p. 1124), is indicated in all patients with ileocolonic Crohn's disease.

Prognosis

Life expectancy in patients with IBD is now similar to that of the general population. Although many patients require surgery and admission to hospital for other reasons, the majority have an excellent work record and pursue a normal life. Around 90% of ulcerative colitis patients have intermittent disease activity, whilst 10% have continuous symptoms. One-third of those with pancolitis undergo colectomy within 5 years of diagnosis.

Around 80% of Crohn's patients undergo surgery at some stage, and 70% of these require more than one operation during their lifetime. Clinical recurrence following resectional surgery is present in 50% of all cases at 10 years.

MICROSCOPIC COLITIS

Some patients experience watery diarrhoea as a consequence of microscopic ('lymphocytic') colitis. The colonoscopic appearances are normal but histological examination of biopsies shows a range of abnormalities.

Collagenous colitis is characterised by the presence of a thick submucosal band of collagen; a chronic inflammatory infiltrate is usually seen. The disease is more common in women and is associated with rheumatoid arthritis, diabetes and coeliac disease. Patients have a history of intermittent watery diarrhoea and treatment is based on antidiarrhoeal drugs, bismuth, aminosalicylates and topical corticosteroid enemas.

IRRITABLE BOWEL SYNDROME (IBS)

Functional gastrointestinal disorders are extremely common and are defined by the absence of structural pathology. Irritable bowel syndrome (IBS) is a functional bowel disorder in which abdominal pain is associated with defecation or a change in bowel habit.

Epidemiology

Approximately 20% of the general population fulfil diagnostic criteria for IBS but only 10% of these consult their doctors because of gastrointestinal symptoms. Nevertheless, IBS is the most common cause of gastrointestinal referral and accounts for frequent absenteeism from work and impaired quality of life. Young women are affected 2–3 times more often than men. There is wide overlap with non-ulcer dyspepsia, chronic fatigue syndrome, dysmenorrhoea and urinary frequency. A significant proportion of these patients have a history of physical or sexual abuse.

Aetiology

IBS encompasses a wide range of symptoms and a single cause is unlikely. It is generally believed that most patients develop symptoms in response to psychosocial factors, altered gastrointestinal motility, altered visceral sensation or luminal factors.

Psychosocial factors

Most patients seen in general practice do not have psychological problems but about 50% of patients referred to hospital meet criteria for a psychiatric diagnosis. A range of disturbances are identified, including anxiety, depression, somatisation and neurosis. Panic attacks are also common. Acute psychological stress and overt psychiatric disease are known to alter visceral perception and gastrointestinal motility in both irritable bowel patients and healthy people. There is an increased prevalence of abnormal illness behaviour with frequent consultations for minor symptoms and reduced coping ability (p. 236). These factors contribute to but do not cause IBS.

Altered gastrointestinal motility

A range of motility disorders are found but none is diagnostic. Patients with diarrhoea as a predominant symptom exhibit clusters of rapid jejunal contraction waves, rapid intestinal transit and an increased number of fast and propagated colonic contractions. Those who are predominantly constipated have decreased orocaecal transit and a reduced number of high-amplitude, propagated colonic contraction waves but there is no consistent evidence of abnormal motility.

Abnormal visceral perception ('visceral hypersensitivity')

IBS is associated with increased sensitivity to intestinal distension induced by inflation of balloons in the ileum, colon and rectum, a consequence of altered CNS processing of visceral sensation. This is more common in women and in diarrhoea-predominant IBS.

Luminal factors

Between 7 and 32% of patients develop IBS following an episode of gastroenteritis, more commonly young women and those with existing background psychological problems. Others may be intolerant of specific dietary components, particularly lactose and wheat. Abnormalities of gut microflora leading to increased fermentation and gas production and minimal inflammation have also been postulated.

Some patients have subtle, histologically undetectable mucosal inflammation, possibly leading to activation of inflammatory cells and release of cytokines, nitric oxide and histamine. These may trigger abnormal secretomotor function and sensitise enteric sensory nerve endings.

Clinical features

The most common presentation is that of recurrent abdominal pain (Box 22.76). This is usually colicky or 'cramping', is felt in the lower abdomen and relieved by defecation. Abdominal bloating worsens throughout the day; the cause is unknown but it is not due to excessive intestinal gas. The bowel habit is variable. Most patients alternate between episodes of diarrhoea and constipation but it is useful to classify patients as having predominantly constipation or predominantly diarrhoea. The constipated type tend to pass infrequent pellety stools, usually in association with abdominal pain or proctalgia. Those with diarrhoea have frequent defecation but produce low-volume stools and rarely have nocturnal symptoms. Passage of mucus is common but rectal bleeding does not occur.

Despite apparently severe symptoms, patients do not lose weight and are constitutionally well. Physical examination does not reveal any abnormalities, although abdominal bloating and variable tenderness to palpation are common.

Diagnosis

Investigations are normal. A positive diagnosis can confidently be made in patients under the age of 40 years without resorting to complicated tests. Full blood count, ESR and sigmoidoscopy are usually done routinely, but barium enema or colonoscopy should only be undertaken in older patients to exclude colorectal cancer. Those who present atypically require investigations to exclude organic gastrointestinal disease. Diarrhoea-predominant patients justify investigations to exclude microscopic colitis (p. 920), lactose intolerance (p. 902), bile acid malabsorption (p. 863), coeliac disease (p. 894), thyrotoxicosis and, in developing countries, parasitic infection. All patients who give a history of rectal bleeding should undergo colonoscopy to exclude colonic cancer or IBD.

Management

The most important steps are to make a positive diagnosis and reassure the patient. Many patients are concerned that they have developed cancer, and a cycle of anxiety leading to colonic symptoms, which further heighten anxiety, can be broken by explanation that symptoms are not due to organic disease but are the result of altered bowel motility and sensation. In patients who fail to respond to reassurance, treatment is tailored to the predominant symptoms (Fig. 22.58). Elimination diets are generally unhelpful but up to 20% may benefit from a wheat-free diet, some may respond to lactose exclusion, and excess intake of caffeine or artificial sweeteners such as sorbitol should be addressed. The role of probiotics has yet to be clearly established.

Patients with intractable symptoms sometimes benefit from several months of therapy with amitriptyline (Box 22.77). This is given in doses (10–25 mg at night) which are much lower than those used to treat depression. Side-effects include dry mouth and drowsiness but these are usually mild and the drug is generally well tolerated, although patients with features of somatisation tolerate the drug poorly and lower doses should be used. It may act by reducing visceral sensation and by altering gastrointestinal motility. Other drugs may overcome abnormalities of 5-HT signalling which have been identified in some IBS patients. These include 5-HT4 agonists. Active anxiety or affective disorders should be separately treated. Psychological interventions such as cognitive behavioural therapy, relaxation and gut-directed hypnotherapy are reserved for the most difficult cases.

Most patients have a relapsing and remitting course. Exacerbations often follow stressful life events, occupational dissatisfaction and difficulties with interpersonal relationships.

22

22.76 FEATURES OF IRRITABLE BOWEL SYNDROME

- Altered bowel habit
- Colicky abdominal pain
- Abdominal distension
- Rectal mucus
- Feeling of incomplete defecation

EBM

22.77 ANTIDEPRESSANTS IN IRRITABLE BOWEL SYNDROME

'Tricyclic antidepressant therapy improves symptoms in irritable bowel patients. Patients whose major symptoms are pain and diarrhoea benefit most; those with constipation as a predominant symptom benefit least.'

- Jackson JL, et al. Am J Med 2000;108:65–72.

For further information: 💻 www.evidbasedgastro.com

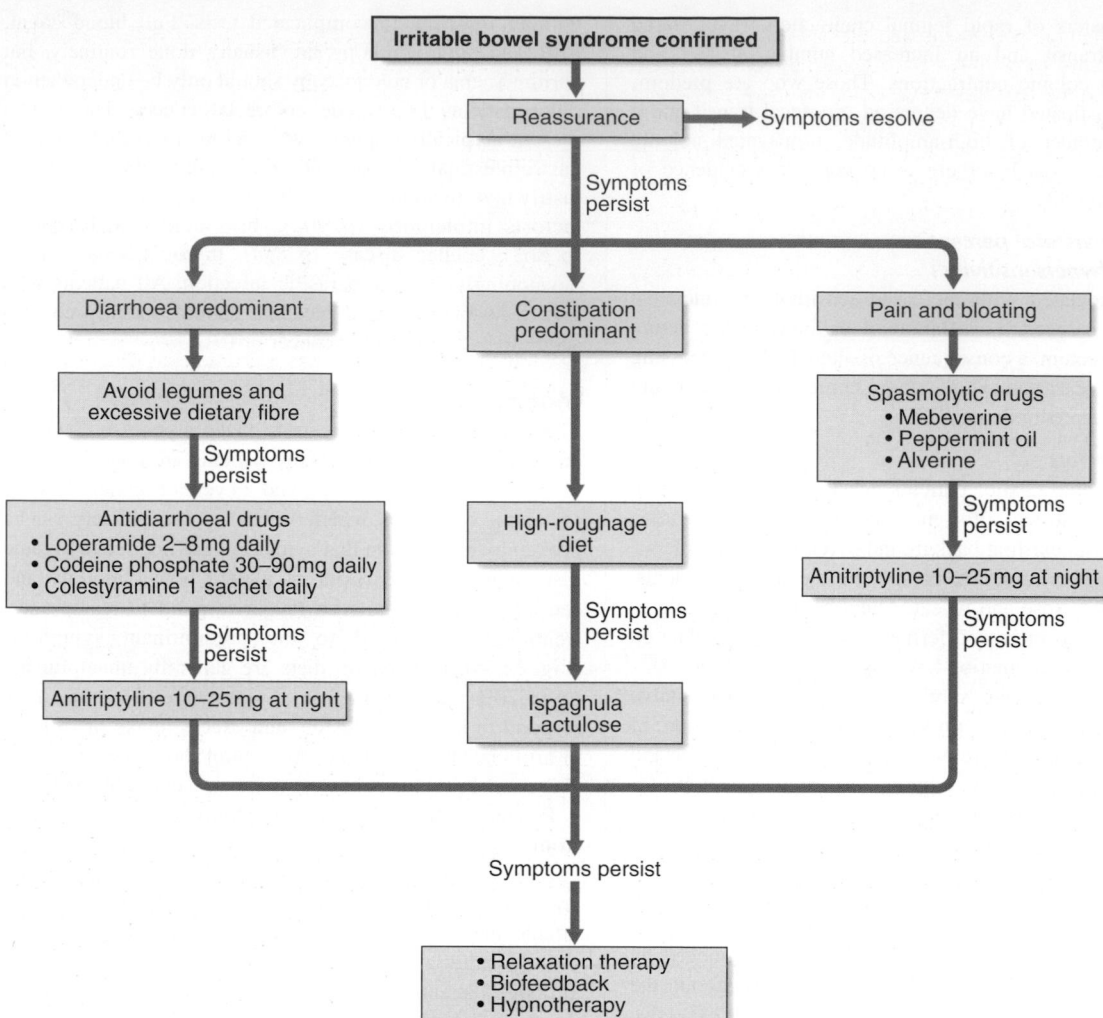

Fig. 22.58   Management of irritable bowel syndrome.

AIDS AND THE GASTROINTESTINAL TRACT

See page 386.

ISCHAEMIC GUT INJURY

Ischaemic gut injury is usually the result of arterial occlusion. Severe hypotension and venous insufficiency are less frequent causes (p. 197). The presentation is variable depending on the different vessels involved and the acuteness of the event. Diagnosis is often difficult.

ACUTE SMALL BOWEL ISCHAEMIA

An embolus from the heart or aorta to the superior mesenteric artery is responsible for 40–50% of cases, thrombosis of underlying atheromatous disease for ~25% and non-occlusive ischaemia due to hypotension complicating myocardial infarction, heart failure, arrhythmias or sudden blood loss for ~25%. Vasculitis or venous

occlusion are rare causes. The pathological spectrum ranges from transient alteration of bowel function to transmural haemorrhagic necrosis and gangrene. Patients usually have evidence of cardiac disease and arrhythmia. Almost all develop abdominal pain that is more impressive than the physical findings. In the early stages the only physical signs may be a silent, distended abdomen or diminished bowel sounds, peritonitis only developing later.

Leucocytosis, metabolic acidosis, hyperphosphataemia and hyperamylasaemia are typical. Plain abdominal X-rays show 'thumb-printing' due to mucosal oedema. Mesenteric or CT angiography reveals an occluded or narrowed major artery with spasm of arterial arcades, although most patients undergo laparotomy on the basis of a clinical diagnosis without angiography. Resuscitation, management of cardiac disease and intravenous antibiotic therapy, followed by laparotomy, are key steps. If treatment is instituted early, embolectomy and vascular reconstruction may salvage some small bowel. In these rare cases a 'second look' laparotomy is undertaken 24 hours later and further necrotic bowel resected. In patients at high surgical risk thrombolysis may sometimes be effective. The results of therapy depend on early intervention; patients treated late have a 75% mortality rate. Survivors often have nutritional failure from short bowel syndrome (p. 898) and require intensive nutritional support, sometimes including home parenteral nutrition, as well as anticoagulation. Small bowel transplantation is promising in selected patients. Patients with mesenteric venous thrombosis also require surgery if there are signs of peritonitis but are otherwise treated with anticoagulation. Investigations for underlying prothrombotic disorders should be performed (p. 1061).

ACUTE COLONIC ISCHAEMIA

The splenic flexure and descending colon have little collateral circulation and lie in 'watershed' areas of arterial supply. The spectrum of injury ranges from reversible colopathy to transient colitis, colonic stricture, gangrene and fulminant pancolitis. Arterial thromboembolism is usually responsible but colonic ischaemia can also follow severe hypotension, colonic volvulus, strangulated hernia, systemic vasculitis or hypercoagulable states. Ischaemia of the descending and sigmoid colon is also a complication of abdominal aortic aneurysm surgery (where the inferior mesenteric artery is ligated). The patient is usually elderly and presents with sudden onset of cramping left-sided lower abdominal pain and rectal bleeding. Symptoms usually resolve spontaneously over 24–48 hours and healing occurs within 2 weeks. Some have a residual fibrous stricture or segment of colitis. A minority develop gangrene and peritonitis. The diagnosis is established by colonoscopy or barium enema within 48 hours of presentation; otherwise, mucosal ulceration and oedema may have resolved. Resection is required for peritonitis.

CHRONIC MESENTERIC ISCHAEMIA

This results from atherosclerotic stenosis affecting at least two of the coeliac axis, superior mesenteric and inferior mesenteric arteries. Dull but severe mid- or upper abdominal pain develops about 30 minutes after eating. Patients lose weight because of reluctance to eat, and some experience diarrhoea. Physical examination invariably shows evidence of generalised arterial disease. An abdominal bruit is sometimes audible but is non-specific. Mesenteric angiography confirms at least two affected mesenteric arteries. Vascular reconstruction or percutaneous angioplasty is sometimes possible. Left untreated, many patients eventually develop intestinal infarction.

DISORDERS OF THE COLON AND RECTUM

TUMOURS OF THE COLON AND RECTUM

POLYPS AND POLYPOSIS SYNDROMES

Polyps may be neoplastic or non-neoplastic. The latter include hamartomas, metaplastic ('hyperplastic') polyps and inflammatory polyps. These have no malignant

22.78 RISK FACTORS FOR MALIGNANT CHANGE IN COLONIC POLYPS

- Large size (> 2 cm)
- Multiple polyps
- Villous architecture
- Dysplasia

22.79 COLONOSCOPIC POLYPECTOMY AND THE PREVENTION OF COLORECTAL CANCER | EBM

'In the US National Polyp Study, 1400 patients underwent follow-up for a mean of 5 years following colonoscopic polypectomy. The incidence of colorectal cancer was substantially less (75%) than expected. Although not a randomised study, these data support the view that colonoscopic polypectomy reduces the risk of subsequent colorectal cancer development.'

- Winawer SJ, et al. National Polyp Study Workgroup. N Engl J Med 1993; 329:1977–1981.

---

potential. Polyps may be single or multiple and vary from a few millimetres to several centimetres in size.

Colorectal adenomas are extremely common in the Western world and the prevalence rises with age; 50% of people over 60 years of age have adenomas, and in half of these the polyps are multiple. They are more common in the rectum and distal colon and are either pedunculated or sessile. Histologically, they are classified as either tubular, villous or tubulovillous, according to the glandular architecture. Nearly all forms of colorectal carcinoma develop from adenomatous polyps over 5–10 years, although not all polyps carry the same degree of risk. Features associated with a higher risk of subsequent malignancy in colonic polyps are listed in Box 22.78.

Adenomas are usually asymptomatic and discovered incidentally. Occasionally, they cause bleeding and anaemia. Villous adenomas sometimes secrete large amounts of mucus, causing diarrhoea and hypokalaemia.

Discovery of a polyp at sigmoidoscopy is an indication for colonoscopy because proximal polyps are present in 40–50% of such patients. Colonoscopic polypectomy should be carried out wherever possible, as this considerably reduces subsequent colorectal cancer risk (Fig. 22.59 and Box 22.79). Very large or sessile polyps can sometimes be removed safely by endoscopic mucosal resection (EMR) but will otherwise require surgery. Once all polyps have been removed, patients should undergo surveillance colonoscopy at 3–5-year intervals, as new polyps develop in 50% of patients. Patients over 75 years of age do not require repeated colonoscopies, as their subsequent lifetime cancer risk is low.

Between 10 and 20% of polyps show histological evidence of malignancy. When cancer cells are found within 2 mm of the resection margin of the polyp, when the polyp cancer is poorly differentiated or when lymphatic invasion is present, segmental colonic resection is recommended because residual tumour or lymphatic spread (in up to 10%) may be present. Malignant polyps without these features can be followed up by surveillance colonoscopy.

Polyposis syndromes are classified by histopathology (Box 22.80). It should be noted that, while the hamartoma-

22

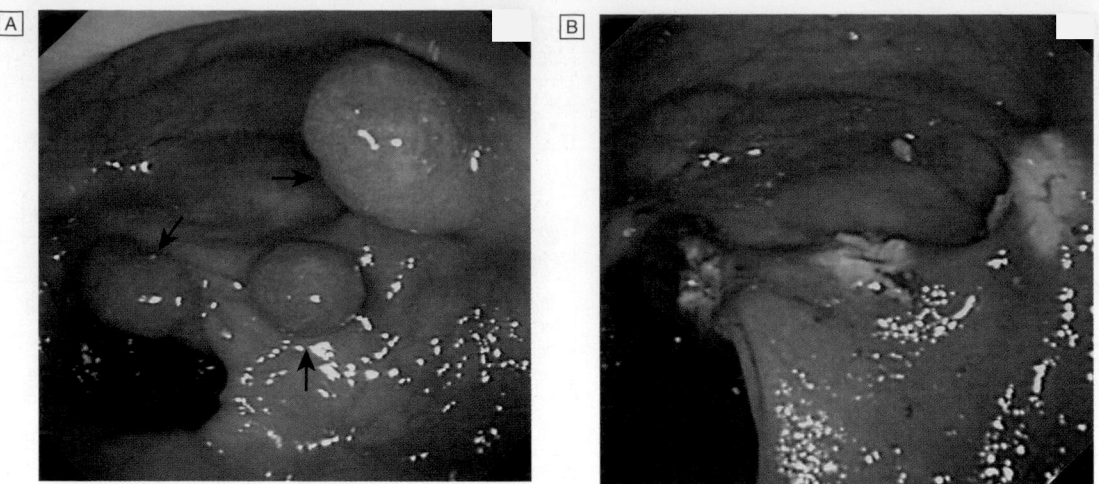

Fig. 22.59 Adenomatous colonic polyps. Ⓐ Before colonoscopic polypectomy (arrows show polyps). Ⓑ After polypectomy.

22

22.80 GASTROINTESTINAL POLYPOSIS SYNDROMES

	Neoplastic		Non-neoplastic		
	Familial adenomatous polyposis	Peutz–Jeghers syndrome	Juvenile polyposis	Cronkhite–Canada syndrome	Cowden's disease
Inheritance	Autosomal dominant	Autosomal dominant	Autosomal dominant in 1/3	None	Autosomal dominant
Oesophageal polyps	–	–	–	+	+
Gastric polyps	+	+	+	+++	+++
Small bowel polyps	++	+++	++	++	++
Colonic polyps	+++	++	++	+++	+
Other features	See text	See text	See text	Hair loss, pigmentation, nail dystrophy, malabsorption	Many congenital anomalies, oral and cutaneous hamartomas, thyroid and breast tumours

tous polyps in Peutz–Jeghers syndrome and juvenile polyposis are not themselves neoplastic, these disorders are associated with an increased risk of certain malignancies, e.g. breast, colon, ovary and thyroid.

Familial adenomatous polyposis (FAP)

This uncommon (1 in 13 000) autosomal dominant disorder accounts for 1% of all colorectal cancer. It results from germline mutation of the *APC* gene on the long arm of chromosome 5 followed by acquired mutation of the remaining allele ('chromosomal instability' pathway, p. 44). *APC* is a large gene and over 1400 different mutations have been reported but most result in a truncated APC protein. This protein has many functions in the regulation of colonic epithelial turnover. It normally binds to and sequesters β-catenin and is unable to do so when mutated, allowing β-catenin to translocate to the nucleus where it upregulates the expression of many genes.

Around 20% of cases arise as new mutations and have no family history. Hundreds to thousands of adenomatous colonic polyps will develop in 80% of patients by age 15 (Fig. 22.60), with symptoms such as rectal bleeding

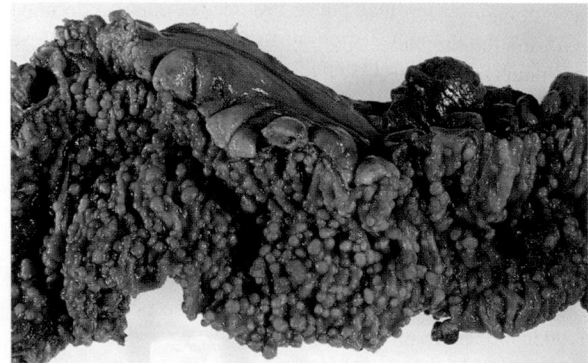

Fig. 22.60 Familial adenomatous polyposis. There are hundreds of adenomatous polyps throughout the colon.

beginning a few years later. In those affected, cancer will develop within 10–15 years of the appearance of adenomas and 90% will develop colorectal cancer by the age of 50 years. Despite surveillance approximately 1 in 4 patients with FAP has cancer by the time they undergo colectomy.

22.81 EXTRAINTESTINAL FEATURES OF FAMILIAL ADENOMATOUS POLYPOSIS

- Subcutaneous epidermoid cysts (extremities, face, scalp)*
- Benign osteomas, especially skull and angle of mandible*
- Dental abnormalities (15–20%)*
- Congenital hypertrophy of the retinal pigment epithelium (CHRPE)
- Desmoid tumours
- Lipomas

* Gardner's syndrome.

Non-neoplastic cystic fundic gland polyps occur in the stomach but adenomatous polyps also occur uncommonly. Duodenal adenomas occur in over 90% and are most common around the ampulla of Vater. Malignant transformation to adenocarcinoma occurs in 10% and is the leading cause of death in those who have had prophylactic colectomy. Many extraintestinal features are also seen in FAP and these are summarised in Box 22.81.

Desmoid tumours occur in up to one-third of patients and usually arise in the mesentery or abdominal wall. Although benign, they may become very large, causing compression of adjacent organs, intestinal obstruction or vascular compromise, and are difficult to remove. They sometimes respond to hormonal therapy with tamoxifen, and the non-steroidal drug sulindac may lead to regression in some, by unknown mechanisms. Congenital hypertrophy of the retinal pigment epithelium (CHRPE) occurs in some and is seen as dark, round, pigmented retinal lesions. When present in an at-risk individual, they are 100% predictive of the presence of FAP. A variant, Turcot's syndrome, is characterised by FAP with primary CNS tumours (astrocytoma or medulloblastoma).

Diagnosis and management

Early identification of affected individuals before symptoms develop is essential. The diagnosis can be excluded if sigmoidoscopy is normal. In newly diagnosed cases with new mutations, genetic testing by DNA linkage analysis confirms the diagnosis, and all first-degree relatives should also undergo testing (p. 51). In families with known FAP, at-risk family members should undergo direct mutation testing at 13–14 years of age. This is less invasive than regular sigmoidoscopy which is reserved for those known to have the mutation. Affected individuals should undergo colectomy after school or college education has been completed. The operation of choice is total proctocolectomy with ileal pouch–anal anastomosis. Periodic upper gastrointestinal endoscopy is recommended to detect duodenal adenomas.

Peutz–Jeghers syndrome

This is characterised by multiple hamartomatous polyps in the small intestine and colon, as well as melanin pigmentation of the lips, mouth and digits (Fig. 22.61). Most cases are asymptomatic, although chronic bleeding, anaemia or intussusception is seen. There is a small but significant risk of small bowel or colonic adenocarcinoma and of cancer of the pancreas, lung, ovary, breast and endometrium. The disorder is caused by truncating mutations in a serine-

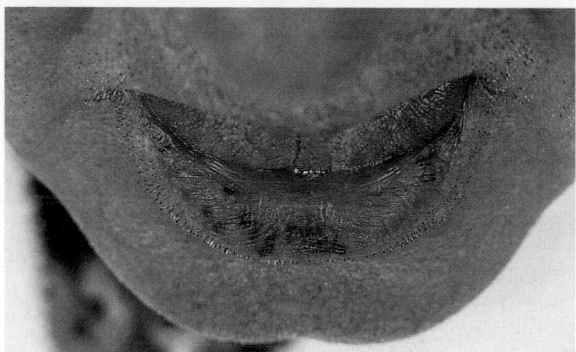

Fig. 22.61 Peutz–Jeghers syndrome. Typical lip pigmentation.

threonine kinase gene on chromosome 19p (STRK11-LKB1).

Tens to hundreds of mucus-filled hamartomatous polyps are found in the colon and rectum. One-third of cases are inherited in an autosomal dominant manner and up to 20% of patients develop colorectal cancer before the age of 40. Criteria for diagnosis are: 10 or more colonic juvenile polyps, juvenile polyps elsewhere in the gut or any number of polyps in those with a family history. Germline mutations in the tumour suppressor gene SMAD4 are often found, as are p53 and p21 mutations. Colonoscopy with biopsies should be performed every 1–3 years.

COLORECTAL CANCER

Although relatively rare in the developing world, colorectal cancer is the second most common internal malignancy and the second leading cause of cancer deaths in Western countries. In the UK the incidence is 50–60 per 100 000, equating to 30 000 cases per year. The condition becomes increasingly common over the age of 50.

Aetiology

Both environmental and genetic factors are important in colorectal carcinogenesis:

- 'sporadic' colorectal cancers: 80%
- hereditary non-polyposis colon cancer (HNPCC): 10%
- FAP: 1%
- other family history: 10%
- inflammatory bowel disease: 1%.

Environmental factors

Environmental factors probably account for over 80% of all 'sporadic' colorectal cancers. This figure is based on the wide geographic variation in incidence and the decrease in risk seen in migrants who move from high- to low-risk countries. Dietary factors are believed to be most important and these are summarised in Box 22.82; other recognised risk factors are listed in Box 22.83.

Genetic factors

Colorectal cancer development results from the accumulation of multiple genetic mutations arising from two major pathways: chromosomal instability and microsatellite instability (Fig. 22.62 and Box 22.84).

22

22.82 DIETARY RISK FACTORS FOR COLORECTAL CANCER DEVELOPMENT

Risk factor	Comments
INCREASED RISK	
Red meat*	High saturated fat and protein content Carcinogenic amines formed during cooking
Saturated animal fat*	High faecal bile acid and fatty acid levels May affect colonic prostaglandin turnover
DECREASED RISK	
Dietary fibre*	Effects vary with fibre type; shortened transit time, binding of bile acids and effects on bacterial flora proposed
Fruit and vegetables	Green vegetables contain anticarcinogens, e.g. glucosinolates and flavonoids. Little evidence for protection from vitamins A, C, E
Calcium	Binds and precipitates faecal bile acids
Folic acid	Reverses DNA hypomethylation

* Evidence is inconsistent and a clear relationship is unproven.

22.83 NON-DIETARY RISK FACTORS IN COLORECTAL CANCER

Medical conditions

- Colorectal adenomas (p. 923)
- Long-standing extensive ulcerative colitis or Crohn's colitis (p. 910)
- Ureterosigmoidostomy
- Acromegaly
- Pelvic radiotherapy

Others

- Obesity and sedentary lifestyle—may be related to dietary factors
- Smoking (relative risk 1.5–3.0)
- Alcohol (weak association)
- Regular aspirin use

Chromosomal instability. This involves mutations or deletions of portions of chromosomes with loss of heterozygosity (LOH) and inactivation of specific tumour suppressor genes. In LOH, one allele of a gene is deleted but gene inactivation only occurs when a subsequent unrelated mutation affects the other allele.

Microsatellite instability. This involves germline mutations in one of six genes encoding enzymes involved in repairing errors that occur normally during DNA replication

22.84 GENETIC FACTORS IN COLORECTAL CANCER DEVELOPMENT

	Chromosomal instability	Microsatellite instability
Inherited cancer type	FAP	HNPCC
Contribution to sporadic cancer	85%	15%
Mechanism	Loss of heterozygosity (LOH)	Germline mutations in DNA mismatch repair genes
Key genes involved	APC, K-ras, DCC, p53	Many, e.g. TGF-β receptor II

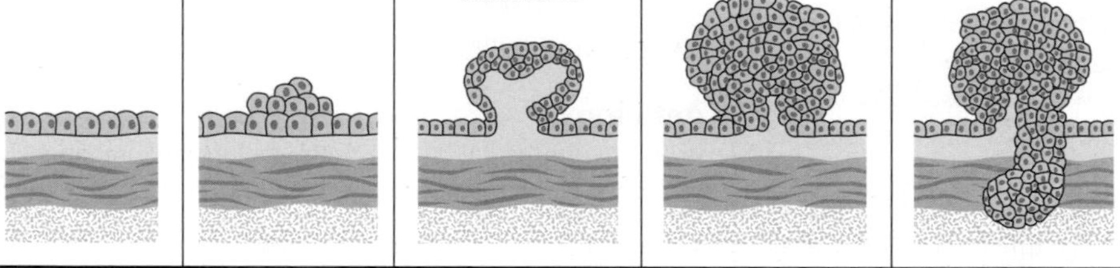

	Normal	Early adenoma	Intermediate adenoma	Late adenoma	Carcinoma	
						Further mutations
Key gene		APC (adenomatous polyposis coli)	K-ras	DCC (deleted in colon cancer)	p53	• Anchorage independence
Chromosome		5q	12p	18q	17p	• Protease synthesis
Normal function		'Gatekeeper'	Transmembrane GTP-binding protein mediating mitogenic signals (p21)	Multiple: role in apoptosis, tumour suppressor gene	Upregulated during cell damage to arrest cell cycle and allow DNA repair or apoptosis to occur	• Telomerase synthesis • Multidrug resistance
Alteration		Truncating mutations	Gain in function mutations	Allelic deletion	Allelic deletion; gain in function mutations	• Evasion of immune system
Effect		Progression to early adenoma development	Cell proliferation	? Role in invasion and metastasis	Cell proliferation; impaired apoptosis	

Fig. 22.62 The multistep origin of cancer: molecular events implicated in colorectal carcinogenesis. (GTP = guanine triphosphate)

(DNA mismatch repair); these genes are designated *hMSH*2, *hMSH*6, *hMLH*1, *hMLH*3, *hPMS*1 and *hPMS*2. Replication errors accumulate and can be detected in 'microsatellites' of repetitive DNA sequences. Replication errors also occur in important regulatory genes, resulting in a genetically unstable phenotype and accumulation of multiple somatic mutations throughout the genome that eventually lead to cancer formation. A minority of sporadic cancers develop this way and almost all cases of HNPCC.

HNPCC accounts for 10% of cancers; it occurs in those with a family history and often at a young age. Pedigrees of HNPCC families indicate an autosomal dominant pattern of inheritance. The criteria necessary for diagnosing this condition are given in Box 22.85. The lifetime risk of colorectal cancer in affected individuals is 80%. The mean age of cancer development is 45 years, and in contrast to sporadic colon cancer two-thirds of tumours occur proximally. In a subset of patients, there is also an increased incidence of cancers of the endometrium, ovary, urinary tract, stomach, pancreas, small intestine and CNS, related to inheritance of different mismatch repair gene mutations.

Those who fulfil the criteria for diagnosis should be referred for pedigree assessment, genetic testing and colonoscopy. These should begin around 25 years of age or 5–10 years earlier than the youngest case of cancer in the family. Colonoscopy needs to be repeated every 1–2 years but even then, interval cancers can still occur.

A further 10% of patients who do not have HNPCC still have a family history of colorectal cancer. The lifetime risk of developing cancer with one or two affected first-degree relatives is 1 in 12 and 1 in 6, respectively. The risk is even higher if relatives were affected at an early age. The genes mediating this increased risk are unknown.

Pathology

Most tumours arise from malignant transformation of a benign adenomatous polyp. Over 65% occur in the rectosigmoid and a further 15% recur in the caecum or ascending colon. Synchronous tumours are present in 2–5% of patients. Macroscopically, the majority of cancers are either polypoid and 'fungating', or annular and constricting. Spread occurs through the bowel wall. Rectal cancers may invade the pelvic viscera and side walls. Lymphatic invasion is common at presentation, as is spread through both portal and systemic circulations to reach the liver and, less commonly, the lungs. Tumour stage at diagnosis is the most important determinant of prognosis (p. 258).

Clinical features

Symptoms vary depending on the site of the carcinoma. In tumours of the left colon, fresh rectal bleeding is common and obstruction occurs early. Tumours of the right colon present with anaemia from occult bleeding, or altered bowel habit, but obstruction is a late feature. Colicky lower abdominal pain is present in two-thirds of patients and rectal bleeding occurs in 50%. A minority present with features of either obstruction or perforation, leading to peritonitis, localised abscess or fistula formation. Carcinoma of the rectum usually causes early bleeding, mucus discharge or a feeling of incomplete emptying. Between 10 and 20% of all patients present solely with iron deficiency anaemia or weight loss.

On examination there may be a palpable mass, signs of anaemia or hepatomegaly from metastases. Low rectal tumours may be palpable on digital examination.

Investigations

Rigid sigmoidoscopy will detect less than one-third of tumours. Colonoscopy (Fig. 22.63) is the investigation of choice because it is more sensitive and specific than barium enema. Furthermore, lesions can be biopsied and polyps removed. Endoanal ultrasound or pelvic MRI stages rectal cancers accurately. CT colography ('virtual colonoscopy') is a sensitive non-invasive technique for diagnosing tumours and polyps greater than 1 cm that can be used if colonoscopy is incomplete or high-risk. CT is valuable for detecting hepatic metastases, although intraoperative ultrasound is increasingly being used for this purpose. A proportion of patients have raised serum carcinoembryonic antigen (CEA) concentrations but this is variable and so of little use in diagnosis. Measurements of CEA are valuable, however, during follow-up and can help to detect early recurrence.

Management

Surgery

The tumour is removed, along with adequate resection margins and pericolic lymph nodes. Continuity is restored

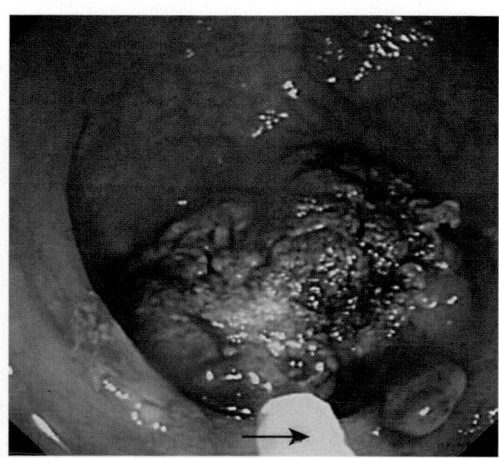

Fig. 22.63 Colonoscopic view of a polypoid rectal carcinoma undergoing laser therapy (arrow) in a patient unfit for surgery.

by direct anastomosis wherever possible. Carcinomas within 2 cm of the anal verge may require abdominoperineal resection and formation of a colostomy. All patients should be counselled pre-operatively about the possible need for a stoma. Total mesorectal excision (TME) reduces recurrence rates and increases survival in rectal cancer. Solitary hepatic or lung metastases are sometimes resected at a later stage.

Post-operatively, patients should undergo colonoscopy after 6–12 months and periodically thereafter to search for local recurrence or development of new 'metachronous' lesions, which occur in 6% of cases.

Adjuvant therapy

Two-thirds of patients have lymph node or distant spread (Dukes stage C, Fig. 22.64) at presentation and are, therefore, beyond cure with surgery alone. Most recurrences are within 3 years of diagnosis.

Colonic cancers recur locally at the site of resection, in lymph nodes, liver and peritoneum. Adjuvant chemotherapy with 5-fluorouracil and folinic acid (to reduce toxicity) for 6 months improves both disease-free and overall survival in patients with Dukes C colon cancer by around 4–13%. Pre-operative radiotherapy can be given to patients with large, fixed rectal cancers to 'down-stage' the tumour, making it resectable and reducing local recurrence. Dukes C and some Dukes B rectal cancers are given post-operative radiotherapy to reduce the risk of local recurrence if operative resection margins are involved.

Palliation

Surgical resection of the primary tumour is appropriate for some patients with metastases to treat obstruction, bleeding or pain. Palliative chemotherapy with 5-fluorouracil and folinic acid improves survival and second-line therapy with irinotecan is used when this fails. Pelvic radiotherapy is sometimes useful for distressing rectal symptoms such as pain, bleeding or severe tenesmus. Endoscopic laser therapy or insertion of an expandable metal stent can be used to relieve obstruction.

Prevention and screening

Evidence suggests that colorectal cancer is preventable. At present there are no guidelines in the UK for primary prevention by dietary or lifestyle changes.

Chemoprevention

No effective, safe, long-term agent yet exists. The most promising agents at present are aspirin, calcium and folic acid. COX-2 is over-expressed in many polyps and most colorectal cancers where it has anti-apoptotic actions. Lack of trial data and safety concerns over currently available selective COX-2 inhibitors have prevented their use as chemopreventive agents.

Secondary prevention (screening)

Secondary prevention aims to detect and remove lesions at an early or pre-malignant stage. Several potential methods exist:

- Widespread screening by regular *faecal occult blood (FOB) testing* reduces colorectal cancer mortality (Box 22.86) and increases the proportion of early cancers detected. These tests currently lack sensitivity and specificity and need to be improved. In the USA, annual FOB screening is recommended after the age of 50 years.
- *Colonoscopy* remains the gold standard but requires expertise, is expensive and carries risks; many countries lack the resources to offer this form of screening.
- *Flexible sigmoidoscopy* is an alternative option and has been shown to reduce overall colorectal cancer mortality

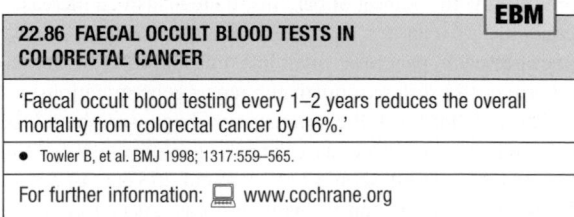

EBM

22.86 FAECAL OCCULT BLOOD TESTS IN COLORECTAL CANCER

'Faecal occult blood testing every 1–2 years reduces the overall mortality from colorectal cancer by 16%.'

- Towler B, et al. BMJ 1998; 1317:559–565.

For further information: 🖥 www.cochrane.org

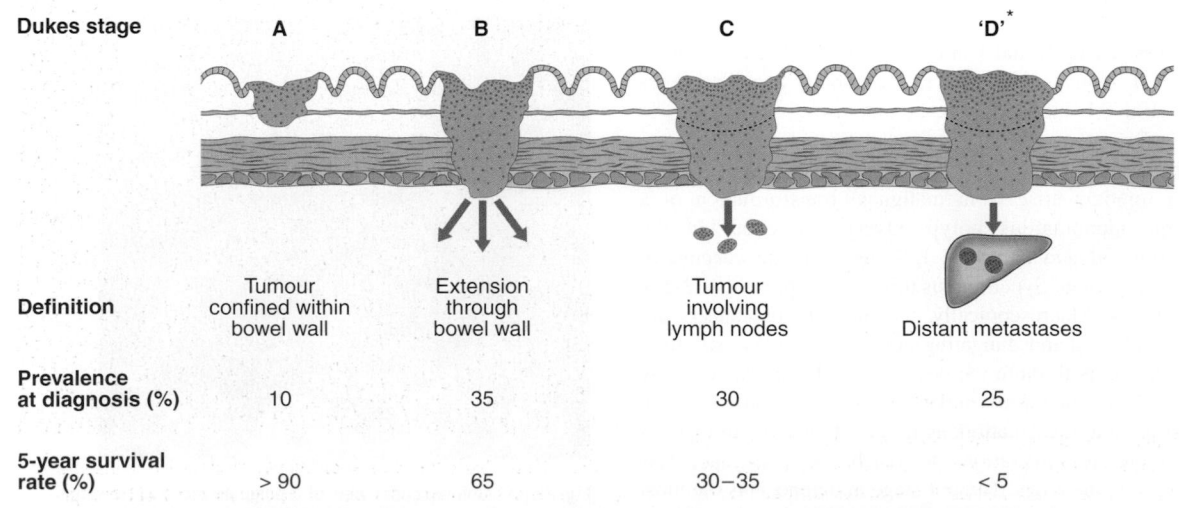

Dukes stage	A	B	C	'D'*
Definition	Tumour confined within bowel wall	Extension through bowel wall	Tumour involving lymph nodes	Distant metastases
Prevalence at diagnosis (%)	10	35	30	25
5-year survival rate (%)	> 90	65	30–35	< 5

Fig. 22.64 **Staging and survival in colorectal cancer.** (Modified Dukes classification. * Dukes' original staging only had stages A–C.)

by approximately 35% (70% for cases arising in the rectosigmoid). It is recommended in the USA every 5 years in all persons over the age of 50.

- Screening by *molecular genetic analysis* is an exciting prospect but is not yet available.

DIVERTICULOSIS

Diverticula are acquired and are most common in the sigmoid and descending colon of middle-aged people. Asymptomatic diverticula ('diverticulosis') are present in over 50% of people above the age of 70. Symptomatic ('diverticular disease') or complicated diverticulosis ('diverticulitis') is uncommon and supervenes in 10–25% of cases.

Aetiology
A life-long refined diet with a relative deficiency of fibre is widely thought to be responsible and the condition is rare in populations with a high dietary fibre intake, such as in Asia, where it more often affects the right side of the colon. It is postulated that small-volume stools require high intracolonic pressures for propulsion and this leads to herniation of mucosa between the taeniae coli (Fig. 22.65).

Pathology
Diverticula consist of protrusions of mucosa covered by peritoneum. There is commonly hypertrophy of the circular muscle coat. Inflammation is thought to result from impaction of diverticula with faecoliths. This may resolve spontaneously or progress to cause haemorrhage, perforation, local abscess formation, fistula and peritonitis. Repeated attacks of inflammation lead to thickening of

the bowel wall, narrowing of the lumen and eventual obstruction.

Clinical features
Symptoms are usually the result of associated constipation or spasm. Colicky pain is usually suprapubic or felt in the left iliac fossa. The sigmoid colon may be palpable and, in attacks of diverticulitis, there is local tenderness, guarding, rigidity ('left-sided appendicitis') and sometimes a palpable mass. During these episodes there may also be diarrhoea, rectal bleeding or fever. The differential diagnosis includes colorectal cancer, ischaemic colitis, inflammatory bowel disease and infection. Diverticular disease is complicated by perforation, pericolic abscess, fistula formation (usually colovesical) and acute rectal bleeding. These complications are more common in patients who take NSAIDs or aspirin. After one attack of diverticulitis, the recurrence rate is around 3% per year. Over 10–30 years, perforation, obstruction or bleeding will each affect around 5% of patients.

Investigations
These are usually performed to exclude colorectal neoplasia. Barium enema confirms the presence of diverticula (Fig. 22.66). Strictures and fistulae may also be seen. Flexible sigmoidoscopy is performed to exclude a coexisting neoplasm which is easily missed radiologically. Colonoscopy requires expertise and carries a risk of perforation. CT is used to assess complications.

Management
Diverticulosis which is asymptomatic and discovered coincidentally requires no treatment. Constipation can be relieved by a high-fibre diet with or without a bulking

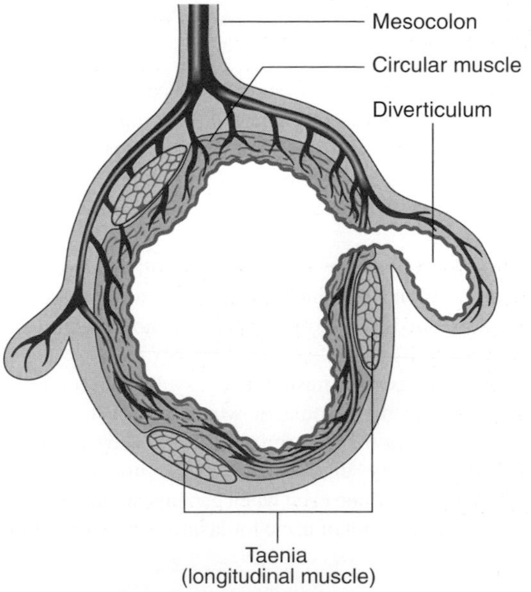

22

Mesocolon
Circular muscle
Diverticulum

Taenia
(longitudinal muscle)

Fig. 22.65 The human colon in diverticulosis. The colonic wall is weak between the taeniae. The blood vessels that supply the colon pierce the circular muscle and weaken it further by forming tunnels. Diverticula usually emerge through these points of least resistance.

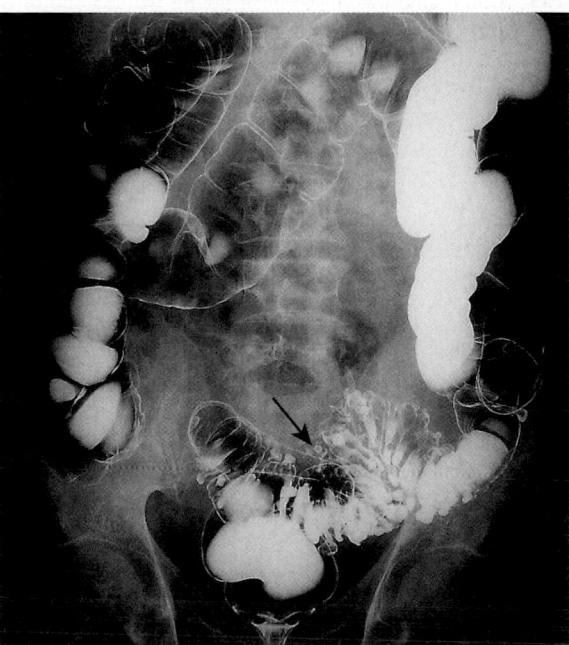

Fig. 22.66 Barium enema showing severe diverticular disease. There is tortuosity and narrowing of the sigmoid colon with multiple diverticula (arrow).

laxative (ispaghula husk, 1–2 sachets daily) taken with plenty of fluids. Stimulants should be avoided. Antispasmodics may sometimes help.

An acute attack of diverticulitis requires 7 days of metronidazole (400 mg 8-hourly orally), along with either a cephalosporin or ampicillin (500 mg 6-hourly orally). Severe cases require intravenous fluids, intravenous antibiotics, analgesia and nasogastric suction but randomised trials show no benefit from acute resection compared to conservative management, and emergency surgery is reserved for severe haemorrhage or perforation. Percutaneous drainage of acute paracolic abscesses can be effective and avoids the need for emergency surgery. Elective surgery is performed in patients after recovery from repeated acute attacks of obstruction, and resection of the affected segment with primary anastomosis is the procedure of choice.

CONSTIPATION AND DISORDERS OF DEFECATION

22

The clinical approach to patients with constipation and its aetiology have been described on page 873.

SIMPLE CONSTIPATION

This is extremely common and does not imply underlying organic disease. It usually responds to increased dietary fibre or the use of bulking agents; an adequate fluid intake is also essential. Many types of laxative are available, and these are listed in Box 22.87.

SEVERE IDIOPATHIC CONSTIPATION

This occurs almost exclusively in young women and often begins in childhood or adolescence. The cause is unknown but some have 'slow transit' with reduced motor activity in the colon. Others have 'obstructed defecation' resulting from inappropriate contraction of the external anal sphincter and puborectalis muscle (anismus).

22.87 LAXATIVES	
Class	**Examples**
Bulk-forming	Ispaghula husk Methylcellulose
Stimulants	Bisacodyl Dantron (only for terminally ill patients) Docusate Senna
Faecal softeners	Docusate Arachis oil enema
Osmotic laxatives	Lactulose Lactitol Magnesium salts
Others	Polyethylene glycol (PEG)* Phosphate enema*
* Used mainly for bowel preparation prior to investigation or surgery.	

22.88 CONSTIPATION IN OLD AGE	

- **Evaluation**: particular attention should be paid to immobility, dietary fluid and fibre intake, drugs and depression.
- **Immobility**: predisposes to constipation by increasing the colonic transit time; the longer this is, the greater the fluid absorption and the harder the stool.
- **Bulking agents**: can make matters worse in patients with slow transit times and should be avoided.
- **Overflow diarrhoea**: if faecal impaction develops, paradoxical overflow diarrhoea may occur. If antidiarrhoeal agents are given, the underlying impaction may worsen and result in serious complications such as stercoral ulceration and bleeding.

The condition is often resistant to treatment. Bulking agents may exacerbate symptoms but prokinetic agents or balanced solutions of polyethylene glycol '3350' benefit some patients with slow transit. Glycerol suppositories and biofeedback techniques are used for those with obstructed defaecation. Rarely, subtotal colectomy is necessary as a last resort.

FAECAL IMPACTION

In faecal impaction a large, hard mass of stool fills the rectum. This tends to occur in disabled, immobile or institutionalised patients, especially the frail elderly or those with dementia. Constipating drugs, autonomic neuropathy and painful anal conditions also contribute. Megacolon, intestinal obstruction and urinary tract infections may supervene. Perforation and bleeding from pressure-induced ulceration are occasionally seen. Treatment involves adequate hydration and careful digital disimpaction after softening the impacted stool with arachis oil enemas. Stimulants should be avoided.

MELANOSIS COLI AND LAXATIVE MISUSE SYNDROMES

Long-term consumption of stimulant laxatives leads to accumulation of lipofuscin pigment in macrophages in the lamina propria. This imparts a brown discoloration to the colonic mucosa, often described as resembling 'tiger skin'. The condition is benign and resolves when the laxatives are stopped.

Prolonged laxative use may rarely result in megacolon or 'cathartic colon', in which barium enema demonstrates a featureless mucosa, loss of haustra and shortening of the bowel.

Surreptitious laxative misuse is a psychiatric condition seen in young women, some of whom have a history of bulimia or anorexia nervosa (pp. 248–249). They complain of refractory watery diarrhoea. Laxative use is usually denied and may continue even when patients are undergoing investigation. Screening of urine for laxatives may reveal the diagnosis.

MEGACOLON

Megacolon is characterised by dilatation of the colon and refractory constipation. It may be congenital

(Hirschsprung's disease) or develop in later life (acquired megacolon).

Hirschsprung's disease

This is congenital aganglionosis of the large intestine, with an incidence of 1:5000. It may be local or diffuse and a family history is present in one-third of all cases. Mutations in the RET tyrosine kinase signalling system, important in enteric neurogenesis, are present in some hereditary cases and the condition results from failure of migration of neuroblasts into the gut wall during embryogenesis. Ganglion cells are absent from nerve plexuses, most commonly in a short segment of the rectum and/or sigmoid colon. As a result, the internal anal sphincter fails to relax. Constipation, abdominal distension and vomiting usually develop immediately after birth but a few cases do not present until childhood or adolescence. The rectum is empty on digital examination.

Barium enema shows a small rectum and colonic dilatation above the narrowed segment. Full-thickness biopsies are required to demonstrate nerve plexuses and confirm the absence of ganglion cells. Histochemical stains for acetylcholinesterase are also used. Anorectal manometry demonstrates failure of the rectum to relax with balloon distension. Treatment involves resection of the affected segment.

Acquired megacolon

This may develop in childhood as a result of voluntary withholding of stool during toilet training. In such cases it presents after the first year of life and is distinguished from Hirschsprung's disease by the urge to defecate and the presence of stool in the rectum. It usually responds to osmotic laxatives.

In adults, acquired megacolon has several causes. It is seen in depressed or demented patients, either as part of the condition or as a side-effect of antidepressant drugs. Prolonged misuse of stimulant laxatives may cause degeneration of the myenteric plexus, while interruption of sensory or motor innervation may be responsible in a number of neurological disorders. Scleroderma and hypothyroidism are other recognised causes.

Most patients can be managed conservatively by treatment of the underlying cause, high-residue diets, laxatives and the judicious use of enemas. Prokinetics are helpful in a minority of patients. Subtotal colectomy is a last resort for the most severely affected patients.

ACUTE COLONIC PSEUDO-OBSTRUCTION (OGILVIE'S SYNDROME)

This condition has many causes (Box 22.89) and is characterised by relatively sudden onset of painless, massive

22.89 CAUSES OF ACUTE COLONIC PSEUDO-OBSTRUCTION	
• Trauma, burns	• Respiratory failure
• Recent surgery	• Electrolyte and acid–base disorders
• Drugs, e.g. opiates, phenothiazines	• Diabetes mellitus
	• Uraemia

enlargement of the proximal colon accompanied by distension; there are no features of mechanical obstruction. Bowel sounds are normal or high-pitched rather than absent. Left untreated, it may progress to perforation, peritonitis and death.

Plain abdominal X-rays show colonic dilatation with air extending to the rectum. A caecal diameter greater than 10–12 cm is associated with a high risk of perforation. Single-contrast or water-soluble barium enemas demonstrate the absence of mechanical obstruction.

Management consists of treating the underlying disorder and correcting any biochemical abnormalities. The anticholinesterase, neostigmine, is often effective in enhancing parasympathetic activity and gut motility. Decompression either with a rectal tube or by careful colonoscopy may be effective but needs to be repeated until the condition resolves. In severe cases, surgical or fluoroscopic defunctioning caecostomy is necessary.

CLOSTRIDIUM DIFFICILE INFECTION

Antibiotic-associated diarrhoea, antibiotic-associated colitis and pseudomembranous colitis are part of the same disease spectrum which results from disturbance of the normal intestinal flora. *Cl. difficile* can be isolated from a variable proportion of patients and is thought to be the cause in most cases. The organism is a Gram-positive, anaerobic, spore-forming bacterium and is commonly found in hospital wards.

Pathogenesis

Around 5% of healthy adults and up to 20% of elderly patients in long-term care carry *Cl. difficile*. Infection is usually hospital-acquired and becomes established when the normal colonic bacterial flora is disrupted by antibiotic treatment. It can also occur, however, in debilitated patients who have not been exposed to antibiotics. Although almost any antibiotic may be responsible, the most commonly implicated are cephalosporins, ampicillin (± clavulanate), amoxicillin and clindamycin.

The organism produces two cytotoxic and inflammatory exotoxins (A and B), both of which contribute to virulence. It is not known why some people are asymptomatic carriers whilst others develop fulminant colitis. Host antibody responses to *Cl. difficile* toxin A may play a role in determining the clinical response to infection.

Pathology

Initially the mucosa shows focal areas of inflammation and ulceration. In severe cases the ulcers become covered by a creamy-white adherent 'pseudomembrane' composed of fibrin, debris and polymorphs.

Clinical features

Around 80% of cases occur in people over 65 years of age, many of whom are frail with comorbid diseases. Symptoms usually begin in the first week of antibiotic therapy but can occur at any time up to 6 weeks after treatment has finished. The onset is often insidious, with lower abdominal pain and diarrhoea which may become profuse and watery. The presentation may resemble acute ulcerative colitis with

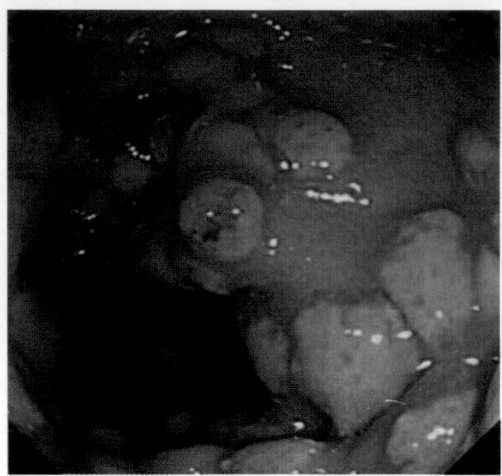

Fig. 22.67 *Clostridium difficile* infection. Colonoscopic view showing numerous adherent 'pseudomembranes' on the mucosa.

22

bloody diarrhoea, fever and even toxic dilatation and perforation. Ileus is also seen in pseudomembranous colitis.

Diagnosis

The diagnosis should be suspected in any patient who is currently taking or has recently taken antibiotics. The rectal appearances at sigmoidoscopy may be characteristic, with erythema, white plaques or an adherent pseudomembrane (Fig. 22.67). At other times the appearances resemble those of ulcerative colitis. In some cases the rectum is spared and the changes predominantly affect the proximal colon. Biopsies are carried out routinely.

Stool cultures isolate *Cl. difficile* in 30% of patients with antibiotic-associated diarrhoea and over 90% of those with pseudomembranous colitis. As some healthy people may harbour *Cl. difficile*, isolation of toxins A and B by cell cytotoxicity assays is required to prove the diagnosis. Culture and toxin isolation can be difficult and may take up to 72 hours.

Management

The offending antibiotic should be stopped and the patient should be isolated. Supportive therapy with intravenous fluids and bowel rest is often needed. Patients who are ill and those with evidence of ileus, dilatation or pseudo-membranous colitis should be treated with antibiotics. These are most effective when given orally and there is little to choose between metronidazole 400 mg 8-hourly and vancomycin 125 mg 6-hourly. Seven to ten days of therapy are usually effective, although relapses occur in 5–20% and require repeated treatment. Intravenous immunoglobulin is sometimes given in the most severe cases. Preventative measures include the responsible use of antibiotics and improved ward hygiene, hand-washing and disinfection policies.

ENDOMETRIOSIS

Ectopic endometrial tissue can become embedded on the serosal aspect of the intestine, most frequently in the sigmoid and rectum. The overlying mucosa is usually intact. Cyclical engorgement and inflammation result in pain, bleeding, diarrhoea, constipation and adhesions or obstruction. Low backache is frequent. The onset is usually between 20 and 45 years and is more common in nulliparous women. Bimanual examination may reveal tender nodules in the pouch of Douglas. Endoscopic studies only reveal the diagnosis if carried out during menstruation, when a bluish mass with intact overlying mucosa is apparent. In some patients laparoscopy is required. Treatment options include laparoscopic diathermy and hormonal therapy with progestagens (e.g. norethisterone), gonadotrophin-releasing hormone analogues or danazol.

PNEUMATOSIS CYSTOIDES INTESTINALIS

In this rare condition multiple gas-filled submucosal cysts line the colonic and small bowel walls. The cause is unknown but the condition may be seen in patients with chronic cardiac or pulmonary disease, pyloric obstruction, scleroderma or dermatomyositis. Most patients are asymp-tomatic, although there may be abdominal cramp, diarrhoea, tenesmus, rectal bleeding and mucus discharge. The cysts are recognised on sigmoidoscopy, plain abdominal X-rays or barium enema. Fasting breath hydrogen levels are elevated and fall with treatment. Therapies reported to be effective include prolonged high-flow oxygen, elemental diets and antibiotics.

ANORECTAL DISORDERS

FAECAL INCONTINENCE

The normal control of anal continence is described on page 857. Common causes of incontinence are listed in Box 22.90.

Patients are often embarrassed to admit incontinence and may complain only of 'diarrhoea'. A careful history and examination, especially of the anorectum and perineum, may help to establish the underlying cause. Endoanal ultrasound is valuable for defining the integrity of the anal sphincters, while anorectal manometry and electrophysio-logy are also useful investigations if available.

Management

This is often very difficult. Underlying disorders should be treated and diarrhoea managed with loperamide, diphenoxylate or codeine phosphate. Pelvic floor exercises and

22.90 CAUSES OF FAECAL INCONTINENCE
<ul><li>Obstetric trauma—childbirth, hysterectomy</li><li>Severe diarrhoea</li><li>Faecal impaction</li><li>Congenital anorectal anomalies</li><li>Anorectal disease—haemorrhoids, rectal prolapse, Crohn's disease</li><li>Neurological disorders—spinal cord or cauda equina lesions, dementia</li></ul>

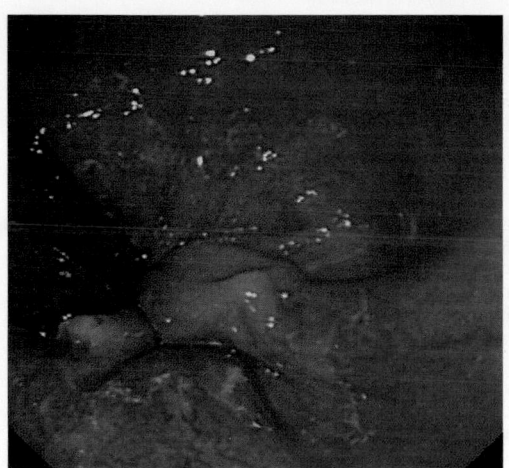

Fig. 22.68 Internal haemorrhoids seen as bluish cushions of prominent veins at sigmoidoscopy.

22.91 CAUSES OF PRURITUS ANI	
Local anorectal conditions	
• Haemorrhoids • Fistula, fissures	• Poor hygiene
Infections	
• Threadworms	• Candidiasis
Skin disorders	
• Contact dermatitis • Psoriasis	• Lichen planus
Other	
• Diarrhoea or incontinence of any cause	• Irritable bowel syndrome • Anxiety

biofeedback techniques help some patients, and those with confirmed anal sphincter defects may benefit from sphincter repair operations.

HAEMORRHOIDS ('PILES')

Haemorrhoids arise from congestion of the internal and/or external venous plexuses around the anal canal (Fig. 22.68). They are extremely common in adults. The aetiology is unknown, although they are associated with constipation and straining and may develop for the first time during pregnancy. First-degree piles bleed, while second-degree piles prolapse but retract spontaneously. Third-degree piles are those which require manual replacement after prolapsing. Bright red rectal bleeding occurs after defecation. Other symptoms include pain, pruritus ani and mucus discharge. Treatment involves measures to prevent constipation and straining. Injection sclerotherapy or band ligation is effective for most, but a minority of patients require haemorrhoidectomy, which is usually curative.

PRURITUS ANI

This is common and can result from many causes (Box 22.91), most of which result in contamination of the perianal skin with faecal contents.

Itching may be trivial or severe and results in an itch-scratch-itch cycle which exacerbates the problem. When no underlying cause is found, all local barrier ointments and creams must be stopped. Good personal hygiene is essential, with careful washing after defecation. The perineal area must be kept dry and clean. Bulk-forming laxatives may reduce faecal soiling.

SOLITARY RECTAL ULCER SYNDROME

This is most common in young adults and occurs on the anterior rectal wall. It is thought to result from localised chronic trauma and/or ischaemia associated with disordered puborectalis function and mucosal prolapse. The ulcer is seen at sigmoidoscopy and biopsies show a characteristic accumulation of collagen.

Symptoms include minor bleeding and mucus per rectum, tenesmus and perineal pain. Treatment is often difficult but avoidance of straining at defecation is important and treatment of constipation may help. Marked mucosal prolapse is treated surgically.

ANAL FISSURE

In this common problem traumatic or ischaemic damage to the anal mucosa results in a superficial mucosal tear, most commonly in the midline posteriorly. Spasm of the internal anal sphincter exacerbates the condition. Severe pain occurs on defecation and there may be minor bleeding, mucus discharge and pruritus. The skin may be indurated and an oedematous skin tag, or 'sentinel pile', adjacent to the fissure is common.

Avoidance of constipation with bulk-forming laxatives and increased fluid intake is important. Relaxation of the internal sphincter is normally mediated by nitric oxide, and 0.2% glyceryl trinitrate or diltiazem ointment, which donates nitric oxide and improves mucosal blood flow, is effective in 60–80% of patients. Resistant cases may respond to injection of botulinum toxin into the internal anal sphincter to induce sphincter relaxation. Manual dilatation under anaesthesia leads to long-term incontinence and should not be considered. The majority of cases can now be treated without surgery but where these measures fail, healing can usually be achieved surgically by lateral internal anal sphincterotomy or advancement anoplasty.

ANORECTAL ABSCESSES AND FISTULAE

Perianal abscesses develop between the internal and external anal sphincters and may point at the perianal skin. Ischiorectal abscesses occur lateral to the sphincters in the ischiorectal fossa. They usually result from infection of anal glands by normal intestinal bacteria. Crohn's disease (p. 910) is sometimes responsible.

Patients complain of extreme perianal pain, fever and/or discharge of pus. Spontaneous rupture may also lead to the development of fistulae. These may be superficial or may track through the anal sphincters to reach the rectum. Abscesses are drained surgically and superficial fistulae are laid open with care to avoid sphincter damage.

DISEASES OF THE PERITONEAL CAVITY

PERITONITIS

Surgical peritonitis occurs as the result of a ruptured viscus (see surgical textbooks). Peritonitis may also complicate ascites (spontaneous bacterial peritonitis) or may occur in children in the absence of ascites, due to infection with pneumococci or β-haemolytic streptococci.

Chlamydial peritonitis is a complication of pelvic inflammatory disease. The affected woman presents with right upper quadrant abdominal pain, pyrexia and a hepatic rub (the Fitz–Hugh–Curtis syndrome).

TB may cause peritonitis and ascites.

TUMOURS

The most common is secondary adenocarcinoma from the ovary or gastrointestinal tract.

Mesothelioma is a rare tumour complicating asbestos exposure. It presents as a diffuse abdominal mass, due to omental infiltration, and with ascites. The prognosis is extremely poor.

FURTHER INFORMATION

Books and journal articles

Cotton PB, Williams CB. Gastrointestinal endoscopy: the fundamentals. 5th edn. Oxford: Blackwell Science; 2003.

Feldman M, Friedman LS, Sleisenger M. Sleisenger and Fordtran's gastrointestinal and liver disease. 7th edn. Philadelphia: WB Saunders; 2002.

McDonald J, Burroughs A, Feagan B. Evidence-based gastro-enterology and hepatology. 2nd edn. London: BMJ Books; 2003.

Shearman DJC, Finlayson NDC, Camilleri M, et al. Diseases of the gastrointestinal tract and liver. 3rd edn. Edinburgh: Churchill Livingstone; 1997.

Websites

www.bsg.org.uk *British Society of Gastroenterology website. Contains Society guidelines for many gastrointestinal disorders and their management (downloadable via Adobe Acrobat).*

www.coeliac.co.uk *Website of the UK Coeliac Society with links to other websites of the Association of European Coeliac Societies.*

www.evidbasedgastro.com *Website of the textbook (see above).*

www.gastro.org *Website of the American Gastroenterological Association and the American Digestive Health Foundation. Useful site for information about many gastrointestinal disorders and sections for patient information and advice.*

www.gastrohep.com *Comprehensive resource with access and links to many textbooks, journals and relevant websites. Other features include abstracts of recent major journal articles, libraries of endoscopic images and case studies.*

www.ibsnetwork.org.uk *A site run by and for IBS sufferers, with input from leading medical experts.*

www.nacc.org.uk *The National Association for Colitis and Crohn's disease (NACC) is the UK's support, information and research-funding charity for people with Crohn's disease and colitis and their families.*

www.uegf.org *United European Gastroenterology Federation.*

22

23

R.W. CHAPMAN
J.D. COLLIER
P.C. HAYES

Liver and biliary tract disease

CLINICAL EXAMINATION OF THE ABDOMEN FOR LIVER AND BILIARY DISEASE

23

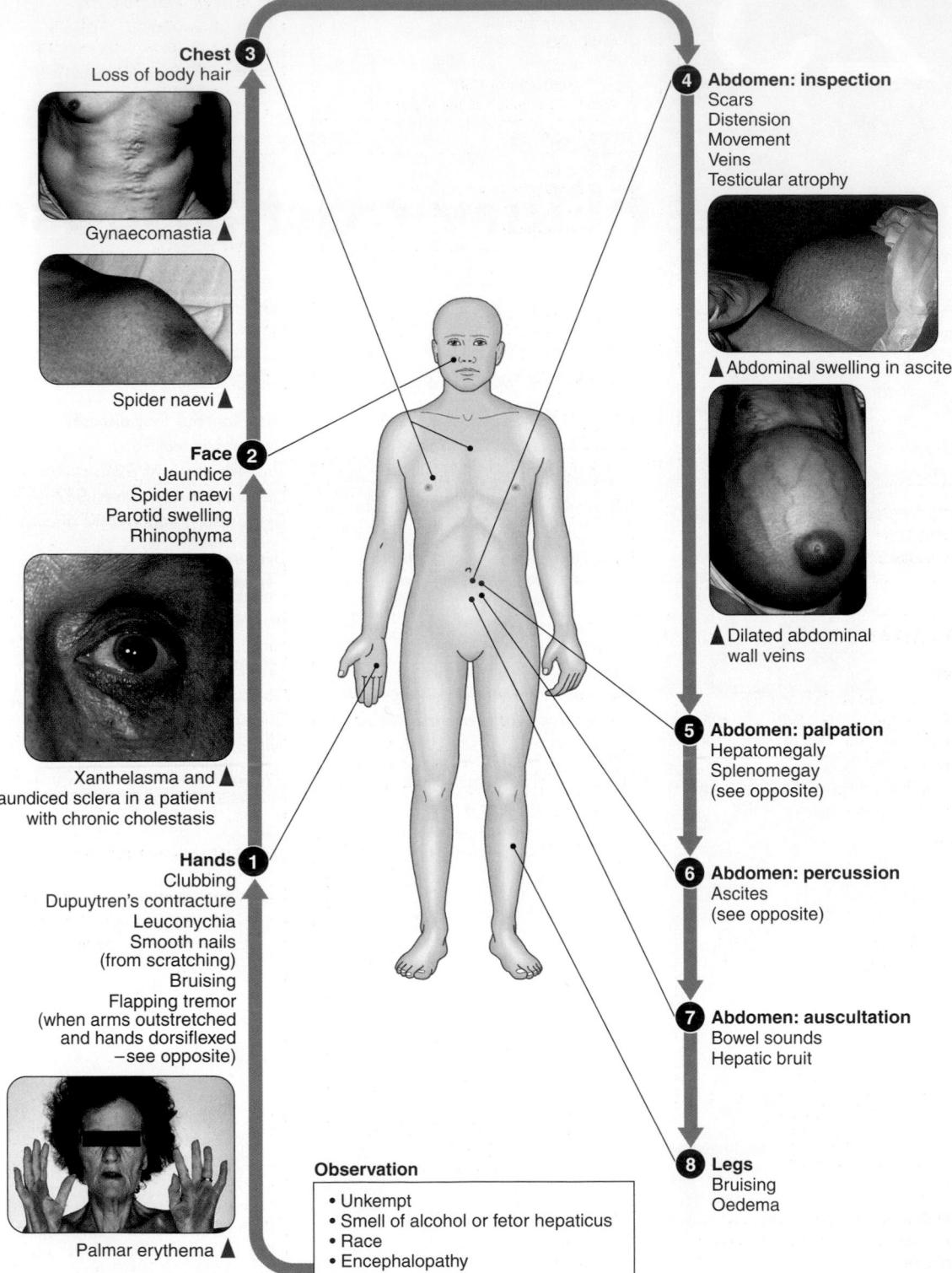

Chest 3
Loss of body hair

Gynaecomastia ▲

Spider naevi ▲

Face 2
Jaundice
Spider naevi
Parotid swelling
Rhinophyma

Xanthelasma and ▲
jaundiced sclera in a patient
with chronic cholestasis

Hands 1
Clubbing
Dupuytren's contracture
Leuconychia
Smooth nails
(from scratching)
Bruising
Flapping tremor
(when arms outstretched
and hands dorsiflexed
–see opposite)

Palmar erythema ▲

4 Abdomen: inspection
Scars
Distension
Movement
Veins
Testicular atrophy

▲ Abdominal swelling in ascites

▲ Dilated abdominal
wall veins

5 Abdomen: palpation
Hepatomegaly
Splenomegay
(see opposite)

6 Abdomen: percussion
Ascites
(see opposite)

7 Abdomen: auscultation
Bowel sounds
Hepatic bruit

8 Legs
Bruising
Oedema

Observation
• Unkempt
• Smell of alcohol or fetor hepaticus
• Race
• Encephalopathy

❶ FLAPPING TREMOR

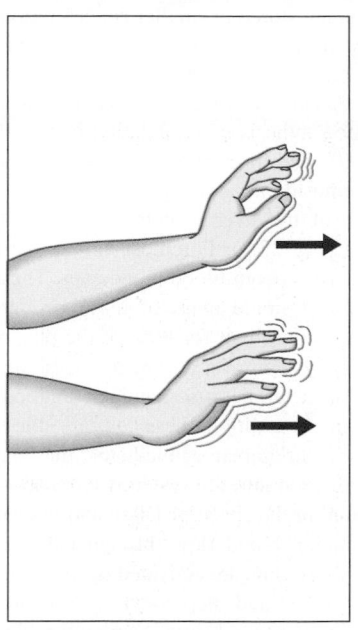

Jerky forward movements every 2–3 seconds when arms are outstretched and hands are dorsiflexed.

CAUSES OF ABNORMAL LIVER SIZE

Large liver (hepatomegaly)

- Liver metastases
- Cirrhosis
    Alcohol
    Haemochromatosis
- Hepatic venous outflow obstruction

Small liver

- Cirrhosis
    Autoimmune liver disease
    Alpha$_1$-antitrypsin deficiency
    Cryptogenic

CAUSES OF ASCITES

High protein (exudative)

- Carcinoma
- Tuberculosis

Low protein (transudative)

- Congestive heart failure
- Renal failure (including nephrotic syndrome)
- Cirrhosis

❻ PERCUSSION OF THE ABDOMEN

Liver

- Always start percussion from resonant to dull; i.e. percuss lower border from beneath and upper border from above.
- Percuss the abdomen gently, the chest more firmly.
- Once the upper border of the liver is identified, confirm its position by counting down the ribs from the sternal angle (second intercostal space).

Shifting dullness

- Start around the umbilicus (resonant).
- Percuss at 1 cm intervals around to the left flank.

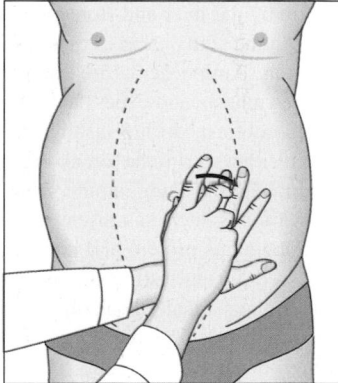

- Identify where dullness occurs.
- Roll the patient on to the left-hand side and note if the level of dullness moves towards the umbilicus.

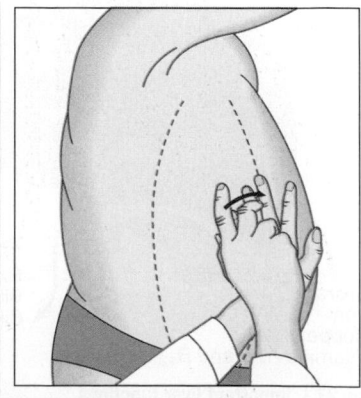

❺ PALPATION OF THE ABDOMEN

Liver

- Start in the right iliac fossa.
- Progress up the abdomen 2 cm with each breath (through open mouth)
- Confirm the lower border of the liver by percussion (see 6).

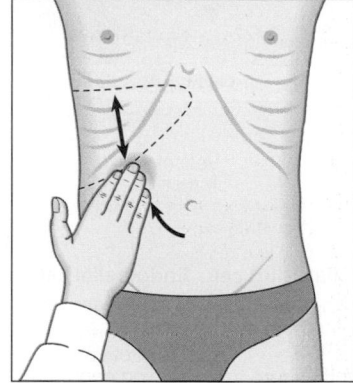

- Detect if smooth or irregular, tender or non-tender; ascertain shape.
- Identify the upper border by percussion (see 6).

Spleen

- Start again in the right iliac fossa.
- Progress towards the left upper quadrant at 2 cm intervals.
- Place the left hand around the lower lateral ribs as the costal margin is approached.

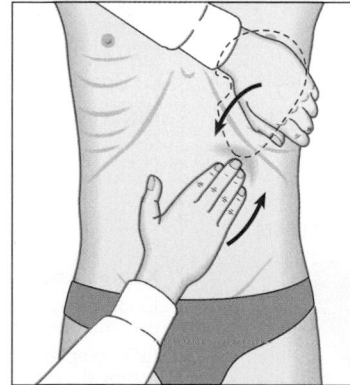

- Note the characteristics of the spleen
    – Notch
    – Superficial
    – Dull to percussion
    – Cannot get between ribs and spleen
    – Moves well with respiration.

23

The liver is the largest organ in the body and performs many important functions, so it is not surprising that diseases of the liver are a major cause of morbidity and mortality throughout the world. Cirrhosis, for example, was responsible for more than 25 000 deaths in the USA in 2003. In the developed world, the most common cause of liver disease is alcohol abuse, although in keeping with the rise in obesity rates, the incidence of non-alcoholic fatty liver disease (NAFLD) is rapidly increasing. In contrast, in the developing world, infections caused by hepatitis viruses and parasites are responsible for most chronic liver disease and hepatobiliary cancer.

FUNCTIONAL ANATOMY, PHYSIOLOGY AND INVESTIGATIONS

MAJOR HEPATIC FUNCTIONS

The liver performs a wide variety of functions (Fig. 23.1). Following a meal, more than half the glucose absorbed is taken up by the liver and stored as glycogen or converted to glycerol and fatty acids, thus avoiding marked hyperglycaemia. Amino acids are used for hepatic and plasma protein synthesis and excess amino acids are catabolised to urea. In contrast, during fasting the liver releases glucose, derived either from the breakdown of glycogen or from gluconeogenesis using amino acids released from extrahepatic tissues such as muscle (p. 808). Synthesis of urea, and endogenous protein and hepatic amino acid release are suppressed during fasting. In both the fed and fasting state the liver plays a central role in lipid metabolism, producing very low-density lipoproteins and further metabolising low- and high-density lipoproteins (p. 444).

The liver plays a central role in the metabolism of bilirubin, bile salts, drugs and alcohol (pp. 944, 990, 973 and 969 respectively). Some vitamins, such as A, D and B_{12}, are stored by the liver in large amounts, while others, such as vitamin K and folate, are stored in smaller concentrations and disappear rapidly if dietary intake is deficient. The liver is also able to metabolise vitamins to more active compounds, e.g. tryptophan and vitamin D. Vitamin K is essential for the hepatic synthesis of coagulation factors II, VII, IX and X (p. 1009). The liver stores minerals such as iron, in ferritin and haemosiderin, and copper.

Approximately 15% of the liver is composed of cells other than hepatocytes (Fig. 23.2). Foremost among these are the Kupffer cells, derived from blood monocytes. These cells constitute the largest single mass of tissue-resident monocytes in the body and account for 80% of the phagocytic capacity of this system. They remove aged and damaged red blood cells, bacteria, viruses, antigen–antibody complexes and endotoxin. In addition, these cells are able to produce a wide variety of inflammatory mediators that may act locally or may be released into the systemic circulation.

Stellate cells are found in the space of Disse and play an important role in regulating blood flow through the liver. Following liver injury, these cells are activated by cytokines produced by Kupffer cells and hepatocytes. Activated stellate cells become transformed into a myofibroblast phenotype and are an important source of extracellular matrix components such as collagen during the genesis of cirrhosis.

Endothelial cells line the hepatic sinusoids. These capillary vessels of the liver differ from other capillary beds in the body. No basement membrane is visible by electron microscopy and the endothelial cells have large fenestrae (0.1 microns), allowing free flow of fluid and particulate matter to the hepatocytes and other cells lining the space of Disse.

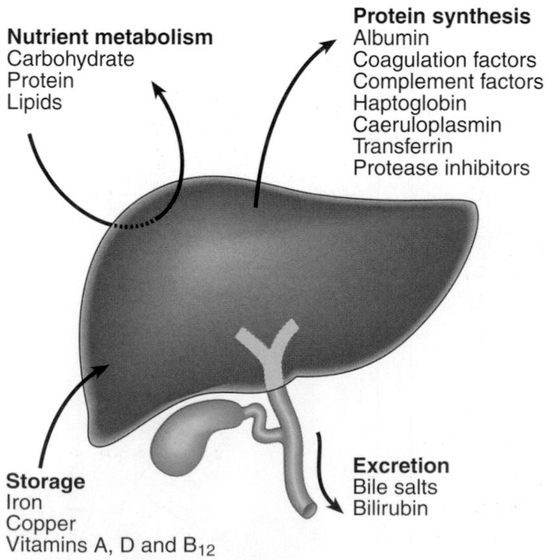

Nutrient metabolism
Carbohydrate
Protein
Lipids

Protein synthesis
Albumin
Coagulation factors
Complement factors
Haptoglobin
Caeruloplasmin
Transferrin
Protease inhibitors

Storage
Iron
Copper
Vitamins A, D and B_{12}

Excretion
Bile salts
Bilirubin

Fig. 23.1 Important liver functions.

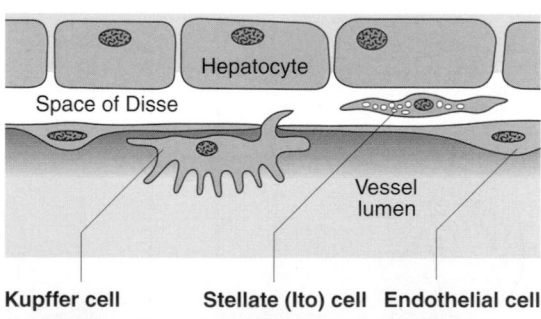

Kupffer cell	Stellate (Ito) cell	Endothelial cell
Lipoprotein uptake and metabolism	Uptake and storage of vitamin A	Hyaluronan uptake
IgG complex removal	Synthesis of extracellular matrix	Lipoprotein binding and uptake
Clearance of bacteria, viruses and erythrocytes	Synthesis and release of collagenase and metalloproteinase inhibitors	IgG complexes
Lipopolysaccharide binding and removal		Cytokine production
Cytokine production	Cytokine synthesis and release	

Fig. 23.2 Function of non-parenchymal liver cells.

FUNCTIONAL ANATOMY

The liver is one of the heaviest organs in the body, weighing 1.2–1.5 kg. It has traditionally been divided into the left and right lobes, by the falciform ligament, fissure of the ligamentum teres and fissure of the ligamentum venosum. Advances in hepatic surgery, however, have indicated a more useful division into right and left hemilivers based on the hepatic blood supply (Fig. 23.3). The right and left hemilivers are further divided into a total of eight segments in accordance with subdivisions of the hepatic and portal veins. The segments each have their own hepatic artery branch and biliary tree. Each segment is made up of multiple smaller units known as lobules, comprised of a central vein,

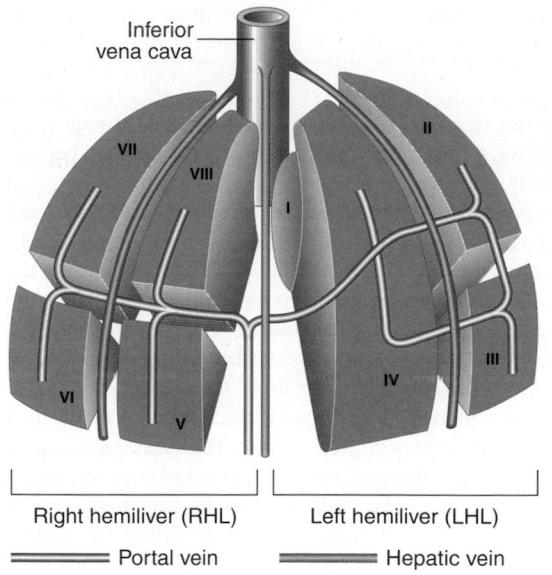

Fig. 23.3 **Schematic representation of the liver.**

radiating sinusoids separated from each other by single liver cell (hepatocyte) plates and peripheral portal tracts. However, the hepatic lobule has no functional significance. The functional unit of the liver is the hepatic acinus (Fig. 23.4), which anatomically is almost the reverse of the hepatic lobule. Blood flows into the hepatic acinus via the single terminal branches of the portal vein and hepatic artery located in the portal tracts, and along the hepatic sinusoids; it then drains into several hepatic venous tributaries at the periphery of the acinus. In contrast, the flow of bile is in the opposite direction along the biliary canaliculi into terminal bile ductules (cholangioles) and subsequently into the interlobular bile ducts located in the portal tracts. The hepatocytes in each acinus can be divided functionally into three different zones, in accordance with their position relative to the terminal portal tract. The hepatocytes in zone 1 are closest to the terminal branches of the portal vein and hepatic artery and therefore are supplied firstly with oxygenated blood, and secondly with blood containing the highest concentration of nutrients and toxins. The hepatocytes in zone 3 are furthest from the portal tracts and closest to the hepatic veins and are therefore relatively hypoxic compared with the hepatocytes in zone 1.

INVESTIGATION OF HEPATOBILIARY DISEASE

The aims of investigation in patients with suspected liver disease are shown in Box 23.1. When patients with suspected liver disease are being investigated, various testing modalities are integrated into batches (see below).

DETECTION OF HEPATIC ABNORMALITY

The clinical suspicion of liver disease usually leads to the measurement of the liver function tests or 'LFTs' (Box

23

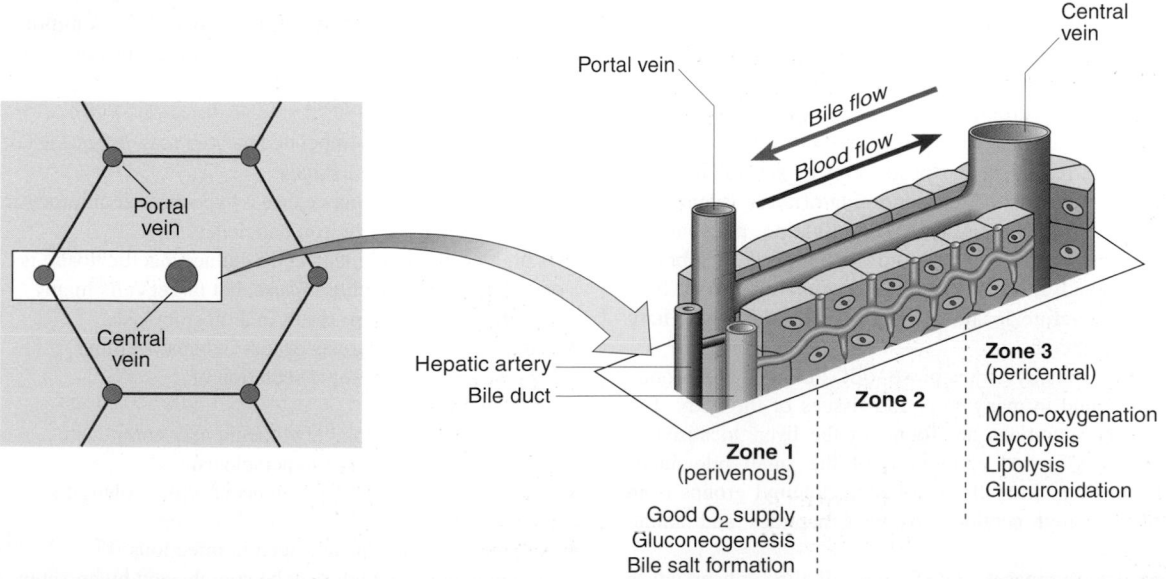

Fig. 23.4 **Hepatic acinus.** Functional unit of the liver.

23.1 AIMS OF INVESTIGATIONS IN PATIENTS WITH SUSPECTED LIVER DISEASE

- Detect hepatic abnormality
- Measure the severity of liver damage
- Define the structural effects on the liver
- Identify the specific cause
- Investigate possible complications

23.2 LIVER FUNCTION TESTS USED TO ASSESS LIVER DISEASE

- Bilirubin*
- Aminotransferases
- Alkaline phosphatase
- Gamma-glutamyl transferase
- Albumin

*Bilirubin detected in the urine identifies conjugated hyperbilirubinaemia and indicates hepatobiliary disease.

23.3 BIOCHEMICAL TESTS IN DIFFERENT CAUSES OF JAUNDICE

Enzyme combination		Diagnostic likelihood	
Amino-transferase	Alkaline phosphatase	Hepatocellular jaundice	Biliary obstruction
> × 6	< × 2.5	90%	10%
< × 6	> × 2.5	10%	80%
Other combinations		No clear separation	

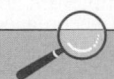

23.4 DRUGS INCREASING PLASMA GAMMA-GLUTAMYL TRANSFERASE

- Barbiturates
- Carbamazepine
- Ethanol
- Glucocorticoids
- Griseofulvin
- Isoniazid
- Meprobamate
- Phenytoin
- Primidone
- Rifampicin

23.2). The LFTs are not truly function tests, provide little prognostic information and do not indicate a specific diagnosis, although they may point to an underlying pathological process and direct further investigation. Several serum enzymes are measured in these widely available biochemical tests.

The activities of one or two transaminase enzymes, alanine aminotransferase (ALT) and aspartate aminotransferase (AST), are often measured. These enzymes function normally to transfer the amino group from an amino acid, alanine in the case of ALT and aspartate in the case of AST, to a ketoacid, producing pyruvate and oxaloacetate respectively. Both ALT and AST are located in the cytoplasm of the hepatocyte; an alternative form of AST is also located in the hepatocyte mitochondria. Although both transaminase enzymes are widely distributed in other tissues of the body, the activities of ALT outside the liver are low and therefore this enzyme is considered more specific for hepatocellular damage.

Alkaline phosphatase is a group of enzymes that are capable of hydrolysing phosphate esters at alkaline pH; they are widely distributed in the body, with significant activities in the liver, gastrointestinal tract, bone and placenta. Translational and post-translational modification of alkaline phosphatase results in the production of several different isoenzymes; the relative concentration of these isoenzymes differs in different tissues. The alkaline phosphatase enzymes are found in greatest concentration in membranes associated with absorptive or secretory functions; in the liver they are therefore localised in the sinusoidal and biliary canalicular membrane.

Gamma-glutamyl transferase (GGT) is a microsomal enzyme found in many cells and tissues of the body. The largest concentrations are found in the liver, localised in the hepatocytes and epithelium of the small bile ducts. GGT functions normally to transfer glutamyl groups from gamma-glutamyl peptides to other peptides and amino acids.

The transaminases, GGT and alkaline phosphatase concentrations should be considered together. Large increases of aminotransferase activity associated with small increases of alkaline phosphatase activity favour hepatocellular damage; small increases of aminotransferase activity and large increases of alkaline phosphatase and GGT activity favour biliary obstruction (Box 23.3). Unfortunately, these patterns do not absolutely separate the two diagnostic groups and further investigation with hepatic imaging is essential. Isolated elevation of the serum GGT is relatively common and may occur during ingestion of microsomal enzyme-inducing drugs (Box 23.4).

Other widely available biochemical tests may become altered in patients with liver disease. Hyponatraemia occurs in severe liver disease and is multifactorial in aetiology. Serum urea may be reduced due to impaired hepatic synthesis. Increased urea may occur following gastrointestinal haemorrhage but, when associated with a high serum creatinine and low urinary sodium excretion, is indicative of hepatorenal failure, which carries a grave prognosis.

Haematological investigations are also commonly abnormal in patients with liver disease and may suggest the underlying diagnosis:

- A normochromic normocytic anaemia may reflect recent gastrointestinal haemorrhage
- Chronic blood loss may cause a hypochromic microcytic anaemia secondary to iron deficiency.
- A high erythrocyte mean cell volume (macrocytosis) is associated with alcohol misuse, but target cells in any jaundiced patient also result in a macrocytosis.
- Rarely, an erythrocytosis occurs in hepatocellular carcinoma due to ectopic secretion of erythropoietin.
- Leucopenia and thrombocytopenia may complicate portal hypertension and hypersplenism.
- In contrast, leucocytosis may occur with cholangitis, alcoholic hepatitis and hepatic abscesses.
- Atypical lymphocytes are seen in infectious mononucleosis, which may be complicated by an acute hepatitis.

- Thrombocytosis may occur in those with active gastrointestinal haemorrhage and, rarely, in association with hepatocellular carcinoma.

TESTS TO DETERMINE THE SEVERITY AND ACTIVITY OF LIVER DISEASE

Simple and widely available biochemical and haematological investigations can give important information on the severity of both acute and chronic liver failure and provide prognostic information in these clinical situations.

Biochemical tests

Requesting the LFTs also routinely involves measurement of the serum bilirubin and albumin concentrations. These measurements are truly tests of liver function. Bilirubin metabolism is discussed on page 944. Albumin is one of the most important proteins involved in maintaining the normal colloidal oncotic pressure of the blood and is a major carrier of low molecular weight substances such as bilirubin, hormones and drugs. The liver normally produces 8–14 g of albumin per day. The reduction in serum albumin observed with liver diseases involves changes in the volume of distribution of albumin as well as a reduction in synthesis.

Coagulation tests

The liver synthesises most coagulation factors, and requires vitamin K to activate factors II, VII, IX and X. Severe liver damage and prolonged biliary obstruction, the latter reducing vitamin K absorption, are associated with a reduced plasma fibrinogen concentration and prolongation of the prothrombin time. The prothrombin time depends on factors I, II, V, VII and X, and is prolonged when the plasma concentration of any of these factors falls below 30% of normal. The normal half-lives of the vitamin K-dependent coagulation factors in the blood are short (5–72 hours). Therefore changes in the prothrombin time occur relatively quickly following liver damage, and provide valuable prognostic information in patients with both acute and chronic liver failure. An increased prothrombin time is evidence of severe liver damage in chronic liver disease, provided that vitamin K (10 mg by slow i.v. injection) is given to exclude deficiency.

RADIOLOGICAL IMAGING IN LIVER DISEASE

Several complementary imaging techniques can be used to determine the site and general nature of structural lesions in the liver and biliary tree.

Ultrasound requires a skilled operator but is safe and comfortable for the patient. It is most commonly used to identify gallstones (Fig. 23.5) and biliary obstruction. Ultrasound is also commonly used in the initial assessment of patients with liver disease to determine further investigation. However, it is often difficult to identify diffuse parenchymal diseases; moreover, focal lesions, such as tumours, may not be resolved unless they are more than about 2 cm in diameter and have echogenic characteristics sufficiently different from normal liver tissue. The advent of colour Doppler ultrasound has allowed blood flow in the

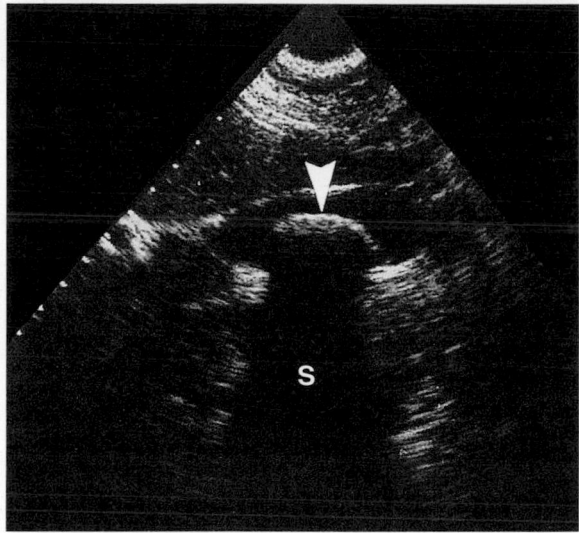

Fig. 23.5 Ultrasound showing stone in the gallbladder. Stone (arrow) with acoustic shadow (S).

hepatic artery, portal vein and hepatic veins to be investigated. Endoscopic and laparoscopic ultrasound provides high-resolution images of the pancreas, biliary tree and liver.

Computed tomography (CT) can be used for the same purposes as ultrasound, but detects smaller focal lesions in the liver, especially when combined with contrast injection. Magnetic resonance imaging (MRI) can also be used to localise and confirm the aetiology of focal liver lesions, particularly primary and secondary tumours.

Cholangiography can be undertaken by magnetic resonance cholangiopancreatography (MRCP, Fig. 23.6), endoscopy (endoscopic retrograde cholangiopancreatography, ERCP; Fig. 23.7) or the percutaneous approach (percutaneous transhepatic cholangiography, PTC). The

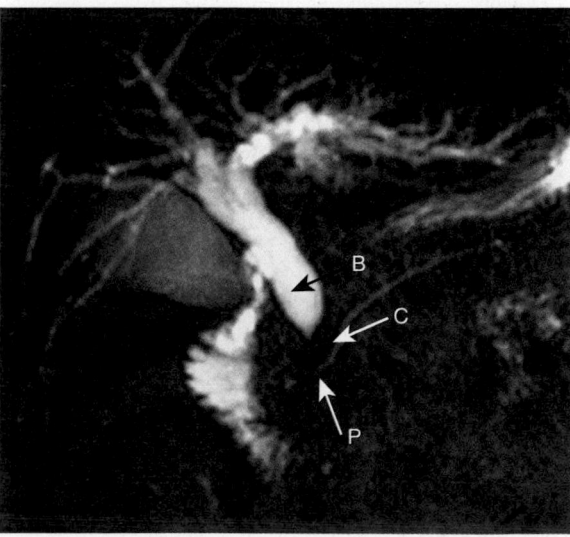

Fig. 23.6 A magnetic resonance cholangiopancreatogram (MRCP) showing a cholangiocarcinoma in the distal common bile duct (C). The proximal common bile duct (B) is dilated but the pancreatic duct (P) is normal.

23

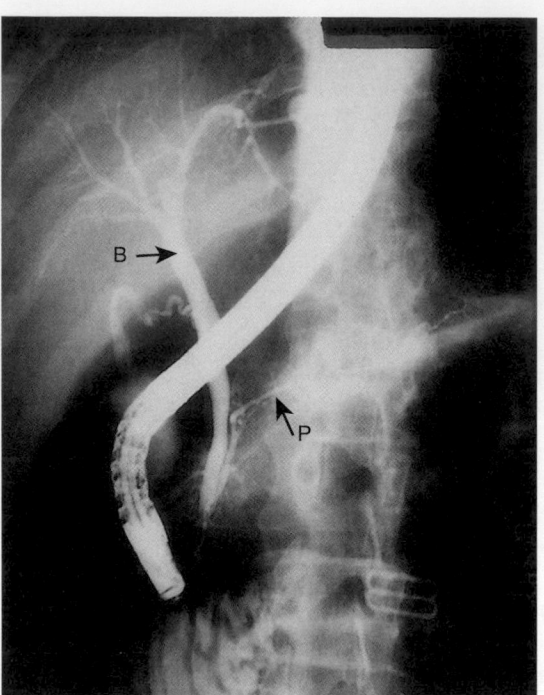

Fig. 23.7 ERCP showing normal biliary (B) and pancreatic (P) duct system.

23.5 CONDITIONS REQUIRED FOR SAFE LIVER BIOPSY

- Cooperative patient
- Prothrombin time < 4 seconds prolonged
- Platelet count > 100×10^9/l
- Exclusion of bile duct obstruction, localised skin infection, advanced chronic obstructive pulmonary disease, marked ascites and severe anaemia

latter does not allow the ampulla of Vater or pancreatic duct to be imaged. MRCP is as good as ERCP at imaging the biliary tree and does not have the same complications (pancreatitis in 5% and 1% bleeding if a sphincterotomy is performed); it is therefore the diagnostic test of choice. Both endoscopic and percutaneous approaches allow therapeutic interventions such as the insertion of biliary stents across malignant bile duct strictures. The percutaneous approach is therefore only used if it is not possible to access the bile duct endoscopically.

Hepatic angiography is now rarely needed, as both CT and MRI technology is able to characterise hepatic vasculature (arterial and venous). Hepatic portal venography is also rarely performed, but may be necessary to image the hepatic veins further in patients with suspected hepatic venous outflow obstruction (Budd–Chiari, p. 982).

Plain abdominal X-rays, oral cholecystography and radionucleotide liver scanning are now rarely employed to investigate liver diseases.

SPECIFIC AETIOLOGICAL INVESTIGATIONS

A variety of blood tests are available to determine the aetiology of hepatic disease, and are discussed under specific diseases. In certain clinical situations these blood tests may require further assessment by performing a liver biopsy.

LIVER BIOPSY

A liver biopsy can confirm the severity of liver damage and provide aetiological information; it is performed with a Trucut or Menghini needle, usually through an intercostal space, using local analgesia. Liver biopsy is a relatively safe procedure if the conditions detailed in Box 23.5 are met, but carries a mortality of about 0.5% and should never be undertaken lightly. The main complications are abdominal and/or shoulder pain, bleeding and biliary peritonitis, which is rare and usually occurs when a biopsy is performed in a patient with obstruction of a large bile duct. Liver biopsies can be carried out in patients with defective haemostasis if the defect is corrected with fresh frozen plasma and platelet transfusion, if the biopsy is obtained by the transjugular route, or if the procedure is conducted percutaneously under ultrasound control and the needle track is then plugged with procoagulant material. In patients with potentially resectable malignancy, biopsy should be avoided due to the potential risk of bleeding and tumour dissemination. Operative or laparoscopic liver biopsy may sometimes be valuable.

Histological assessment of hepatic biopsies

Histological assessment of liver biopsy tissue is enhanced by discussion between clinicians and pathologists. Although the pathological features of liver disease can be diverse and variable, with several features occurring together, liver disorders can be broadly classified histologically into fatty liver (steatosis), hepatitis and cirrhosis. The use of special histological stains can sometimes help in determining the aetiology of liver disorders. The clinical features and prognosis of these changes are dependent on the underlying aetiology, and are discussed in the relevant sections.

IDENTIFICATION OF POTENTIAL COMPLICATIONS OF LIVER DISEASE

Once the diagnosis of cirrhosis is made, endoscopy should be performed to look for oesophageal varices and ultrasound to check for hepatocellular carcinoma.

PRESENTING PROBLEMS IN LIVER DISEASE

'ASYMPTOMATIC' ABNORMAL LIVER FUNCTION TESTS

LFTs (Box 23.2) are frequently requested in patients who have no symptoms or signs of liver disease, e.g. in routine health checks, insurance medicals and drug monitoring. When abnormal results are found, it is important for the clinician to be able to interpret them and to investigate patients appropriately.

Why investigate?

Some, if not most, patients with chronic liver disease are asymptomatic or have only vague non-specific symptoms. Effective medical treatments for chronic liver disease (before cirrhosis is established) are becoming increasingly available and, since abnormal LFTs may be the only indication of these diseases, further evaluation is warranted. Indeed, when thorough investigations are performed, the majority of patients with abnormal LFTs will be found to have significant liver disease that merits treatment or follow-up. Moreover, those who do not have significant disease can safely be discharged.

How common are abnormal LFTs?

The prevalence of abnormal LFTs varies according to the population that is studied. When LFTs are measured routinely prior to elective surgery, 3.5% of patients will have some elevation of transaminase concentrations and 0.3% will have transaminase concentrations greater than twice normal. In other 'healthy' populations the prevalence of abnormal LFTs has been reported to be as high as 10%. The proportion of these individuals who have chronic liver disease is not clear; however, the majority of patients with persistently abnormal LFTs have significant liver disease (Box 23.6). The most common abnormality is alcoholic or non-alcoholic fatty liver disease (pp. 969–973).

Investigations

A thorough history should be taken to determine the patient's alcohol consumption, drug use (prescribed or otherwise), risk factors for viral hepatitis (e.g. blood transfusion, injection drug use), the presence of autoimmune diseases, family history, neurological symptoms, and the presence of diabetes and/or obesity.

23.6 COMMON CAUSES OF ELEVATED SERUM TRANSAMINASES	
Minor elevation (< 100 U/l)	
• Chronic hepatitis C	• Haemochromatosis
• Chronic hepatitis B	• Fatty liver disease
Moderate elevation (100–300 U/l)	
As above plus:	
• Alcoholic hepatitis	• Autoimmune hepatitis
• Non-alcoholic steatohepatitis (NASH)	• Wilson's disease
Major elevation (> 300 U/l)	
• Drug toxicity	• Ischaemic liver
• Paracetamol overdose	• Toxins, e.g. *Amanita phalloides* poisoning
• Acute viral hepatitis	
• Autoimmune liver disease	

Surprisingly, the presence or absence of stigmata of chronic liver disease (p. 954) does not reliably identify patients with significant chronic liver disease. The absence of these stigmata should not therefore preclude further investigation.

Most hepatologists investigate patients with LFTs that are greater than twice the normal range. The investigations that make up a standard liver screen and additional or confirmatory tests are shown in Box 23.7. An algorithm for investigating abnormal LFTs is illustrated in Figure 23.8.

It is important to realise that normal LFTs do not exclude the presence of significant chronic liver disease, which might progress to cirrhosis, e.g. primary sclerosing cholangitis, haemochromatosis and chronic hepatitis C.

23

23.7 TESTS TO IDENTIFY THE CAUSE OF LFT ABNORMALITY

Diagnosis	Clinical clue	Initial test	Additional tests
Alcoholic liver disease	AST > ALT; high MCV		Random blood alcohol
Non-alcoholic fatty liver disease (NAFLD)	Metabolic syndrome (central obesity, diabetes, hypertension)		
Chronic hepatitis B	Injection drug use, blood transfusion	HBsAg	HBeAg, HBeAb HBV-DNA
Chronic hepatitis C		HCV antibody	HCV-RNA
Primary biliary cirrhosis	Raised alkaline phosphatase	AMA	
Primary sclerosing cholangitis	Inflammatory bowel disease	MRCP	ANCA antibody
Autoimmune hepatitis	Other autoimmune diseases	ASMA, ANA, LKM, immunoglobulin	
Haemochromatosis	Diabetes/joint pain	Transferrin saturation, ferritin	HFE gene test
Wilson's disease	Neurological signs	Caeruloplasmin	24-hr urinary copper
Alpha$_1$-antitrypsin	Lung disease	α_1-antitrypsin level	α_1-antitrypsin phenotype
Drug-induced liver disease	Drug/herbal remedy history		
Coeliac disease	Malabsorption	Endomysial antibody	

(ALT = alanine aminotransferase; AMA = antimitochondrial antibody; ANA = antinuclear antibody; ANCA = antineutrophil cytoplasmic antibodies; ASMA = anti-smooth muscle antibody; AST = aspartate aminotransferase; HBeAg = hepatitis B e antigen; HBsAg = hepatitis B surface antigen; HBV = hepatitis B virus; HCV = hepatitis C virus; LKM = liver–kidney microsomal antibody; MCV = mean cell volume; MRCP = magnetic resonance cholangiopancreatography)

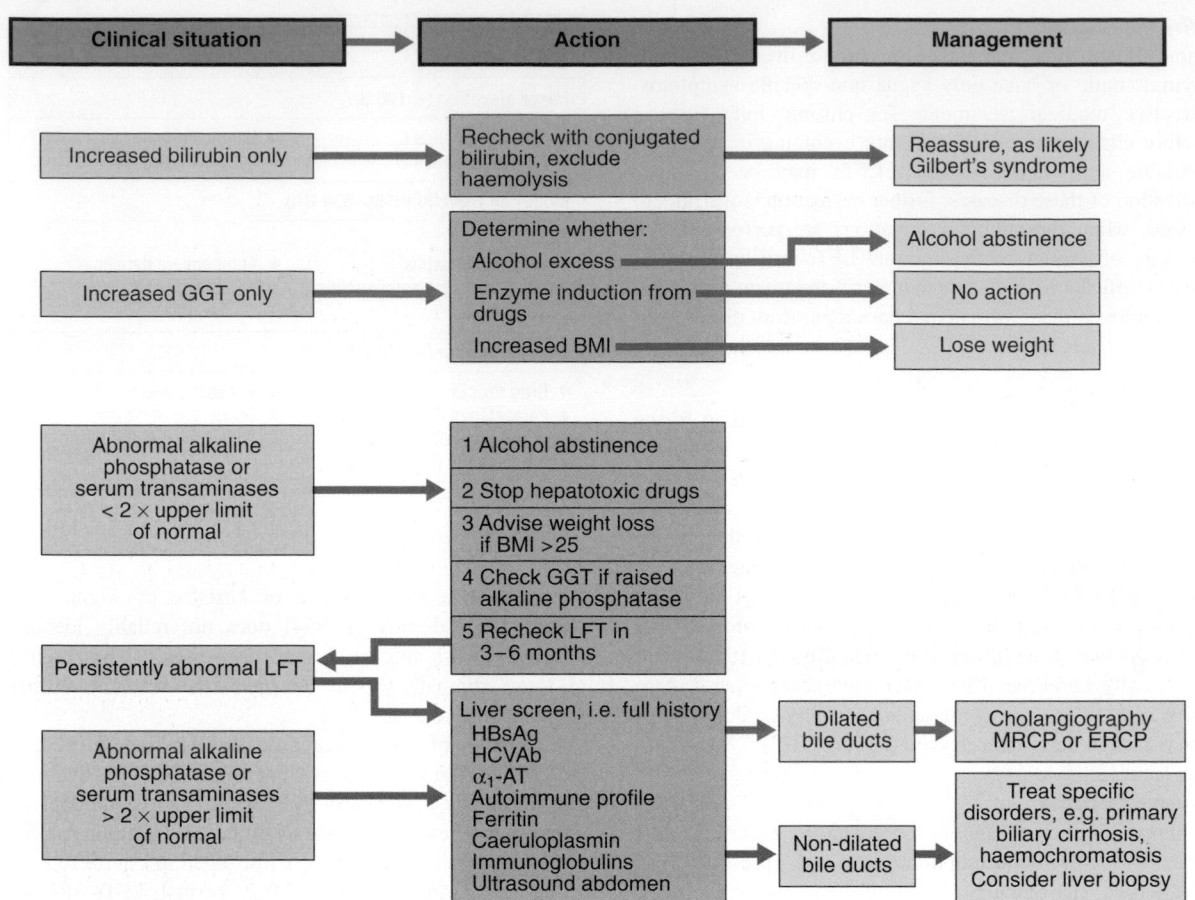

Clinical situation	Action	Management
Increased bilirubin only	Recheck with conjugated bilirubin, exclude haemolysis	Reassure, as likely Gilbert's syndrome
Increased GGT only	Determine whether: Alcohol excess Enzyme induction from drugs Increased BMI	Alcohol abstinence No action Lose weight
Abnormal alkaline phosphatase or serum transaminases < 2 × upper limit of normal	1 Alcohol abstinence 2 Stop hepatotoxic drugs 3 Advise weight loss if BMI >25 4 Check GGT if raised alkaline phosphatase 5 Recheck LFT in 3–6 months	
Persistently abnormal LFT		
Abnormal alkaline phosphatase or serum transaminases > 2 × upper limit of normal	Liver screen, i.e. full history HBsAg HCVAb α_1-AT Autoimmune profile Ferritin Caeruloplasmin Immunoglobulins Ultrasound abdomen	Dilated bile ducts → Cholangiography MRCP or ERCP Non-dilated bile ducts → Treat specific disorders, e.g. primary biliary cirrhosis, haemochromatosis Consider liver biopsy

Fig. 23.8 Suggested management of abnormal LFTs in asymptomatic patients.

JAUNDICE

Jaundice refers to the yellow appearance of the skin, sclerae and mucous membranes resulting from an increased bilirubin concentration in the body fluids. It is usually detectable clinically when the plasma bilirubin exceeds 50 µmol/l (~3 mg/dl) but recognition is often dependent on the ambient light available. The approach to investigating jaundice is shown in Figure 23.9.

Bilirubin metabolism

Between 425 and 510 mmol (250–300 mg) of unconjugated bilirubin is produced from the catabolism of haem every day. Bilirubin in the blood is normally almost all unconjugated and, because it is not water-soluble, is bound to albumin and does not pass into the urine. The metabolism of bilirubin is illustrated in Figure 23.10. Unconjugated bilirubin is conjugated by the endoplasmic reticulum enzyme, glucuronyl transferase, into bilirubin mono- and diglucuronide. These bilirubin conjugates are water-soluble and are exported into the bile via specific carriers on the hepatocyte membrane. Conjugated bilirubin is metabolised by colonic bacteria to form stercobilinogen, which may be further oxidised to stercobilin. Both stercobilinogen and stercobilin are then excreted in the stool. A small amount of stercobilinogen (4 mg/day) is absorbed from the bowel, passes through the liver and is excreted in the urine, where it is known as urobilinogen or, following further oxidisation, urobilin.

HAEMOLYTIC JAUNDICE

This results from increased destruction of red blood cells or their precursors in the marrow, causing increased bilirubin production. Jaundice due to haemolysis is usually mild because a healthy liver can excrete a bilirubin load six times greater than normal before unconjugated bilirubin accumulates in the plasma. However, this does not apply to the newborn.

There are no stigmata of chronic liver disease other than jaundice. Increased excretion of bilirubin and hence stercobilinogen leads to normal-coloured or dark stools, and increased urobilinogen excretion causes the urine to turn dark on standing as urobilin is formed. Pallor due to anaemia and splenomegaly due to excessive reticulo-endothelial activity are usually present.

The plasma bilirubin is usually less than 100 µmol/l (~6 mg/dl) and the LFTs are otherwise normal. There is no bilirubinuria because the hyperbilirubinaemia is predominantly unconjugated. The blood count and film may show evidence of haemolytic anaemia (p. 1030).

23

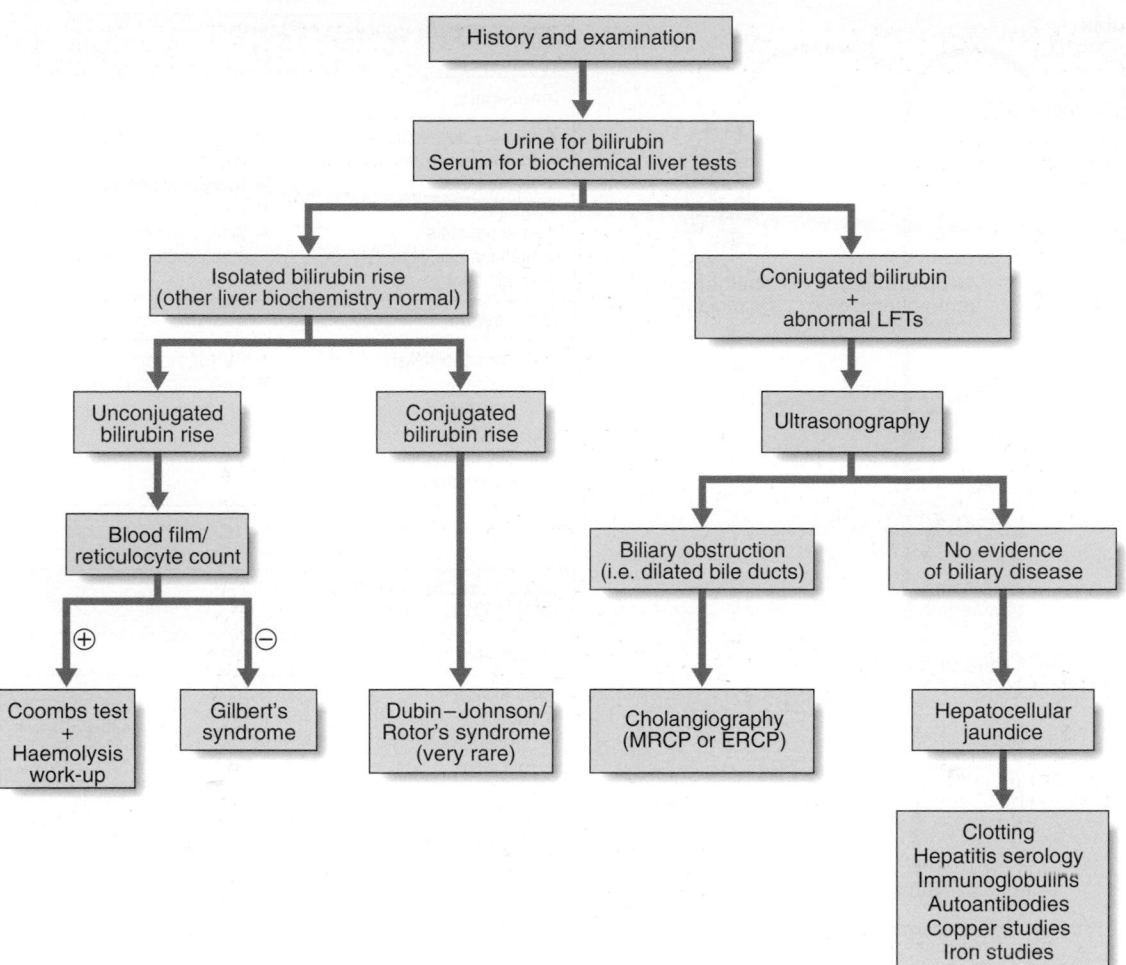

Fig. 23.9 Investigation of jaundice.

23.8 CONGENITAL NON-HAEMOLYTIC HYPERBILIRUBINAEMIA			
Syndrome	Inheritance	Abnormality	Clinical features/treatment
UNCONJUGATED HYPERBILIRUBINAEMIA			
Gilbert's	Autosomal dominant	↓ Glucuronyl transferase ↓ Bilirubin uptake	Mild jaundice, especially with fasting No treatment necessary
Crigler–Najjar			
Type I	Autosomal recessive	Absent glucuronyl transferase	Rapid death in neonate (kernicterus)
Type II	Autosomal dominant	↓↓ Glucuronyl transferase	Presents in neonate Phenobarbital, ultraviolet light or liver transplant as treatment
CONJUGATED HYPERBILIRUBINAEMIA			
Dubin–Johnson	Autosomal recessive	↓ Canalicular excretion of organic anions including bilirubin	Mild No treatment necessary
Rotor's	Autosomal dominant	↓ Bilirubin uptake ↓ Intrahepatic binding	Mild No treatment necessary

CONGENITAL NON-HAEMOLYTIC HYPERBILIRUBINAEMIA

Gilbert's syndrome is the only common form of congenital non-haemolytic hyperbilirubinaemia. All other forms are very rare (Box 23.8). Familial cases of Gilbert's syndrome have been linked to a mutation in the promoter region of the UDP-glucuronyl transferase enzyme, leading to reduced enzyme expression. This results in decreased conjugation of bilirubin, which accumulates as unconjugated bilirubin in the blood. The levels of unconjugated bilirubin increase during fasting and fall during treatment with phenobarbital (which can be used as confirmatory tests in difficult cases). The hyperbilirubinaemia is mild (< 100 μmol/l or

945

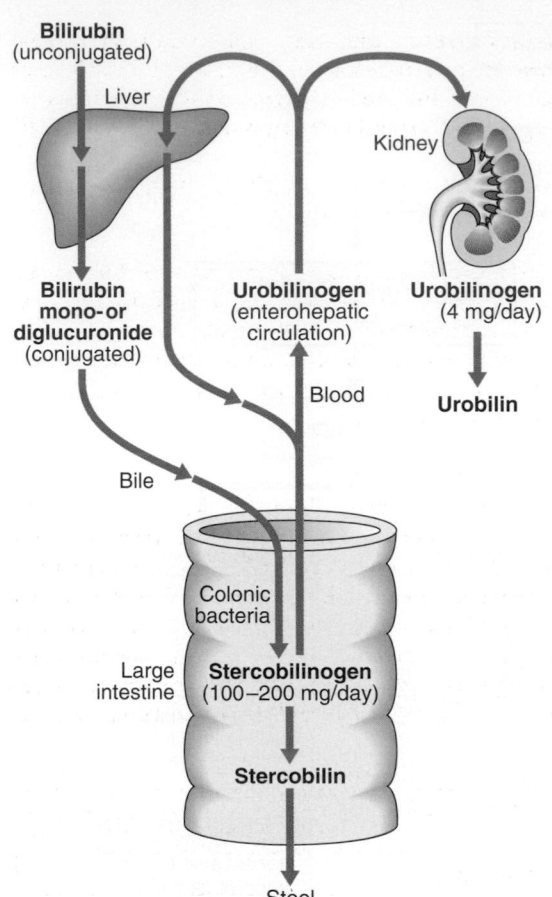

Fig. 23.10 Pathway of bilirubin excretion.

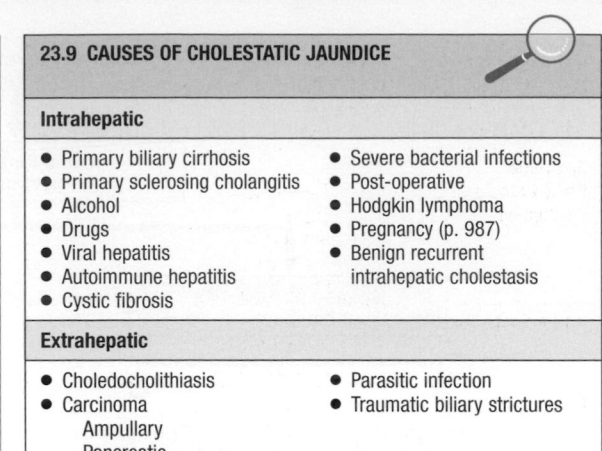

23.9 CAUSES OF CHOLESTATIC JAUNDICE

Intrahepatic

- Primary biliary cirrhosis
- Primary sclerosing cholangitis
- Alcohol
- Drugs
- Viral hepatitis
- Autoimmune hepatitis
- Cystic fibrosis
- Severe bacterial infections
- Post-operative
- Hodgkin lymphoma
- Pregnancy (p. 987)
- Benign recurrent intrahepatic cholestasis

Extrahepatic

- Choledocholithiasis
- Carcinoma
  Ampullary
  Pancreatic
  Bile duct (cholangiocarcinoma)
  Secondary
- Parasitic infection
- Traumatic biliary strictures

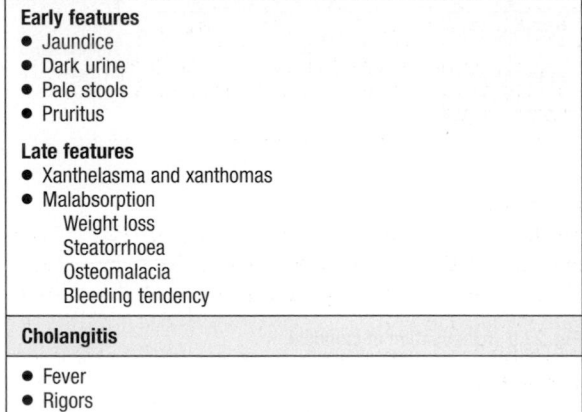

23.10 CLINICAL FEATURES IN CHOLESTATIC JAUNDICE

Cholestasis

Early features
- Jaundice
- Dark urine
- Pale stools
- Pruritus

Late features
- Xanthelasma and xanthomas
- Malabsorption
  Weight loss
  Steatorrhoea
  Osteomalacia
  Bleeding tendency

Cholangitis

- Fever
- Rigors
- Pain

< 6 mg/dl), and other LFTs and hepatic histology are normal. The condition has an excellent prognosis, needs no treatment, and is clinically important only because it may be mistaken for more serious liver disease.

HEPATOCELLULAR JAUNDICE

Hepatocellular jaundice results from an inability of the liver to transport bilirubin into the bile, occurring as a consequence of parenchymal liver disease. Bilirubin transport across the hepatocytes may be impaired at any point between uptake of unconjugated bilirubin into the cells and transport of conjugated bilirubin into the canaliculi. In addition, swelling of cells and oedema resulting from the disease itself may cause obstruction of the biliary canaliculi. In hepatocellular jaundice the concentrations of both unconjugated and conjugated bilirubin in the blood increase, perhaps because of the variable way in which bilirubin transport is disturbed. The severity of jaundice, the other clinical features, and the investigation and treatment vary with the underlying disease and are considered later in this chapter.

CHOLESTATIC JAUNDICE

In unrelieved cholestasis jaundice tends to become progressively more and more severe because conjugated bilirubin is unable to enter the bile canaliculi and passes back into the blood, and also because there is a failure of clearance of unconjugated bilirubin arriving at the liver cells.

Aetiology

The causes of cholestatic jaundice are listed in Box 23.9. Cholestasis may be due to failure of the hepatocytes to generate bile flow, to obstruction of bile flow in the bile ducts in the portal tracts, or to obstruction of bile flow in the extrahepatic bile ducts between the porta hepatis and the papilla of Vater. Causes of cholestasis can operate at more than one of these levels. Those confined to the extrahepatic bile ducts may be amenable to surgical correction.

Clinical assessment

Clinical features in cholestatic jaundice (Box 23.10) comprise those due to cholestasis itself, those due to secondary infection (cholangitis) and those of the underlying condition (Box 23.11).

23.11 CLINICAL FEATURES SUGGESTING AN UNDERLYING CAUSE OF CHOLESTATIC JAUNDICE*

Clinical feature	Causes
Jaundice Static or increasing Fluctuating	Carcinoma Stone Stricture Pancreatitis Choledochal cyst
Abdominal pain	Stone Pancreatitis Choledochal cyst
Cholangitis	Stone Stricture Choledochal cyst
Abdominal scar	Stone Stricture
Irregular hepatomegaly	Hepatic carcinoma
Palpable gallbladder	Carcinoma below cystic duct (usually pancreas)
Abdominal mass	Carcinoma Pancreatitis (cyst) Choledochal cyst
Occult blood in stools	Papillary tumour

* Each of the diseases listed here can give rise to almost any of the clinical features shown. The more likely causes of each clinical feature are given.

Investigations

The history and clinical findings determine investigations in individual patients. Usually, biochemical tests show greater elevation of the alkaline phosphatase and GGT compared with the aminotransferases, and an ultrasound is performed to identify any biliary dilatation. Subsequent investigation is shown in Figure 23.9.

Management

This depends on the underlying cause of the cholestasis and is discussed in detail in the relevant sections.

Benign recurrent intrahepatic cholestasis

This rare condition usually presents in adolescence and is characterised by recurrent episodes of cholestasis, lasting 1–6 months. It is mediated by the PFIC (progressive familial intrahepatic cholestasis) gene which lies on chromosome 18. The same gene is thought to be responsible for a cholestatic condition that causes cirrhosis in childhood (hence the name).

Episodes start with pruritus and painless jaundice develops later. LFTs show the pattern of cholestasis; liver biopsy shows cholestasis (bilirubin in hepatocytes) during an episode but is normal between episodes. Treatment is required to relieve pruritus and the long-term prognosis is good.

GASTROINTESTINAL BLEEDING

Acute upper gastrointestinal haemorrhage from oesophago-gastric varices or peptic ulcer disease (which is more common in patients with liver disease than in the general population) is a common manifestation of chronic liver disease and is discussed on pages 866–869. The specialist management of variceal bleeding is described on page 959.

ASCITES

Ascites refers to the accumulation of free fluid in the peritoneal cavity and is usually due to malignant disease, cirrhosis or heart failure; however, many primary disorders of the peritoneum and visceral organs can produce ascites, and these need to be considered even in a patient with chronic liver disease (Box 23.12).

Clinical features

Ascites causes abdominal distension with fullness in the flanks, shifting dullness on percussion and, when the ascites is marked, a fluid thrill (Fig. 23.11). These signs do not appear until the ascites volume exceeds 1 litre, even in thin patients, and much larger volumes can be hard to detect in the obese. Associated features of ascites include distortion or eversion of the umbilicus, herniae, abdominal striae, divarication of the recti and scrotal oedema. Pleural

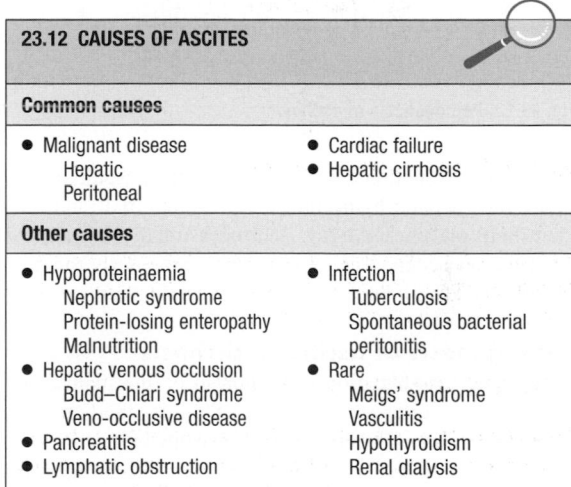

23.12 CAUSES OF ASCITES

Common causes	

● Malignant disease
    Hepatic
    Peritoneal
	● Cardiac failure
	● Hepatic cirrhosis

Other causes	

● Hypoproteinaemia
    Nephrotic syndrome
    Protein-losing enteropathy
    Malnutrition
● Hepatic venous occlusion
    Budd–Chiari syndrome
    Veno-occlusive disease
● Pancreatitis
● Lymphatic obstruction
	● Infection
	    Tuberculosis
	    Spontaneous bacterial
	    peritonitis
	● Rare
	    Meigs' syndrome
	    Vasculitis
	    Hypothyroidism
	    Renal dialysis

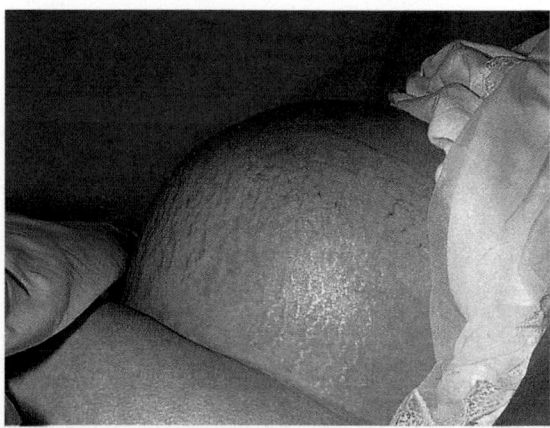

Fig. 23.11 Abdominal swelling in ascites.

23

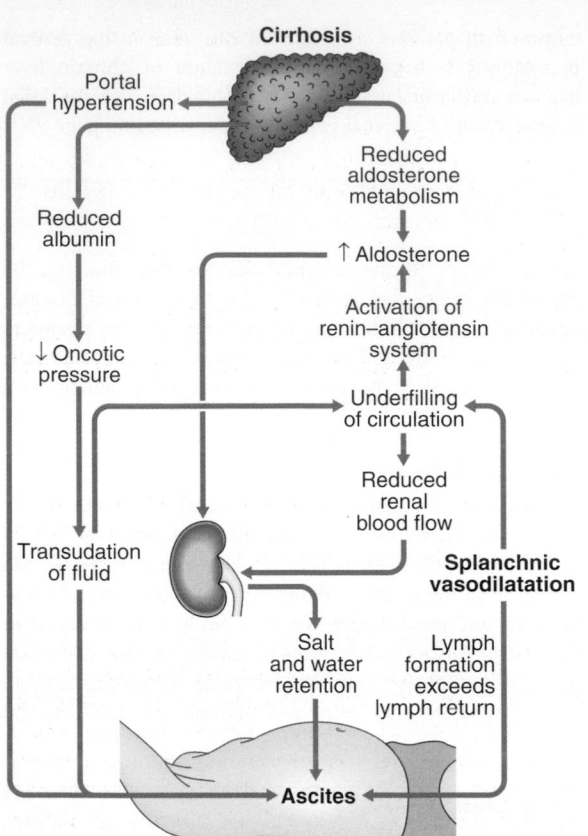

Fig. 23.12 Pathogenesis of ascites.

23.13 ASCITIC FLUID: APPEARANCE AND ANALYSIS
Cause/appearance
• Cirrhosis: clear, straw-coloured or light green • Malignant disease: bloody • Infection: cloudy • Biliary communication: heavy bile staining • Lymphatic obstruction: milky-white (chylous)
Useful investigations
• Total albumin (plus serum albumin) • Amylase • White cell count • Cytology • Microscopy and culture

effusions are found in about 10% of patients, usually on the right side (hepatic hydrothorax); most are small and only identified on chest X-ray, but occasionally a massive hydrothorax occurs. Pleural effusions, particularly those on the left side, should not be assumed to be due to the ascites.

Pathogenesis of ascites in cirrhosis

Splanchnic vasodilatation is thought to be the main factor leading to ascites in cirrhosis. This is mediated by vasodilators (mainly nitric oxide) that are released when portal hypertension causes shunting of blood into the systemic circulation. Systemic arterial pressure falls due to pronounced splanchnic vasodilatation as cirrhosis advances. This leads to activation of the renin–angiotensin system with secondary aldosteronism, increased sympathetic nervous activity, increased atrial natriuretic hormone secretion and altered activity of the kallikrein–kinin system (Fig. 23.12). These systems tend to normalise arterial pressure but produce salt and water retention. In this setting, the combination of splanchnic arterial vasodilatation and portal hypertension alter intestinal capillary permeability, promoting accumulation of fluid within the peritoneum.

Investigations

Ultrasonography is the best means of confirming ascites, particularly in the obese and those with small volumes of fluid. Paracentesis (if necessary under ultrasonic guidance) can also be used to confirm the presence of ascites but is most useful for obtaining ascitic fluid for analysis. The

appearance of the ascites may point to the underlying cause (Box 23.13). The ascites protein concentration and the serum-ascites albumin gradient are used to distinguish ascites due to transudation from ascites due to exudation.

Cirrhotic patients typically develop a transudate with a total protein concentration below 25 g/l and relatively few cells. However, in up to 30% of patients, the total protein concentration is more than 30 g/l. In these cases it is useful to calculate the serum-ascites albumin gradient by subtracting the concentration of the ascites fluid albumin from the serum albumin. A gradient of more than 11 g/l is strongly suggestive of portal hypertension and cirrhosis.

Exudative ascites (ascites protein concentration above 25 g/l or a serum-ascites albumin gradient of less than 11 g/l) raises the possibility of infection (especially tuberculosis), malignancy, hepatic venous obstruction, pancreatic ascites or, rarely, hypothyroidism. Ascites amylase activity above 1000 U/l identifies pancreatic ascites, and low ascites glucose concentrations suggest malignant disease or tuberculosis. Cytological examination may reveal malignant cells (one-third of cirrhotic patients with a bloody tap have a hepatoma). Polymorphonuclear leucocyte counts above 250×10^6/l strongly suggest infection (spontaneous bacterial peritonitis, see below). Laparoscopy can be valuable in detecting peritoneal disease.

Management

Successful treatment of ascites relieves discomfort but does not prolong life, and if over-vigorous, can produce serious disorders of fluid and electrolyte balance and precipitate hepatic encephalopathy (p. 950). Conventional treatment aims to reduce body sodium and water by restricting intake, promoting urine output and, if necessary, removing ascites directly by paracentesis. The rate of loss of sodium and water is most easily measured by regular weighing. No more than 900 ml can be mobilised from the peritoneum daily so the body weight should not fall by more than 1 kg daily if fluid depletion in the rest of the body is to be avoided.

Sodium and water restriction

Restriction of dietary sodium intake is essential to achieving negative sodium balance in patients with ascites. Restriction to 100 mmol/day ('no added salt diet') may be adequate, but restriction to 40 mmol/day (which requires close dietetic supervision) is necessary in more severe ascites. Drugs containing relatively large amounts of sodium and those promoting sodium retention, such as non-steroidal analgesic agents, must be avoided (Boxes 23.14 and 23.15). Restriction of water intake to 0.5–1.0 litre/day is necessary only if the plasma sodium falls below 125 mmol/l. A few patients can be managed satisfactorily on this treatment alone.

Diuretic drugs

Most patients require diuretic drugs in addition to sodium restriction. Spironolactone (100–400 mg/day) is the drug of choice for long-term therapy because it is a powerful aldosterone antagonist; unfortunately, it can cause painful gynaecomastia and hyperkalaemia. Some patients will also require powerful loop diuretics, e.g. furosemide, although these can cause fluid, electrolyte and renal function disorders. Diuresis is improved if patients are rested in bed while the diuretics are acting, perhaps because renal blood flow increases in the horizontal position. Patients who do not respond to doses of 400 mg spironolactone and 160 mg furosemide are considered to have refractory or diuretic-resistant ascites and should be treated by other therapeutic measures.

Paracentesis

The first-line treatment of refractory ascites is large-volume paracentesis with intravenous albumin. Paracentesis to dryness or the removal of 3–5 litres daily is safe, provided the circulation is supported by giving intravenous colloid such as human albumin (6–8 g per litre of ascites removed) or another plasma expander. Total paracentesis can therefore be used as an initial therapy or when other treatments fail.

Peritoneo-venous (LeVeen) shunt

The peritoneo-venous shunt is a long tube with a non-return valve running subcutaneously from the peritoneum to the internal jugular vein in the neck, which allows ascitic fluid to pass directly into the systemic circulation. It is effective in ascites resistant to conventional treatment but complications, including infection, superior vena caval thrombosis, pulmonary oedema, bleeding from oesophageal varices and disseminated intravascular coagulopathy, limit its use and insertion of these stents is now rare.

Transjugular intrahepatic portosystemic stent shunt (TIPSS)

TIPSS (p. 961) can relieve resistant ascites but does not prolong life. It can be used where liver function is reasonable or in patients awaiting liver transplantation, but should not be used in the terminally ill.

Prognosis

Ascites is a serious development in cirrhosis, as only 10–20% of patients survive 5 years from its appearance. The outlook is not universally poor, however, and is best in those with well-maintained liver function and where the response to therapy is good. The prognosis is also better when a treatable cause for the underlying cirrhosis is present (p. 954) or when a precipitating cause for ascites, such as excess salt intake, is found.

Complications

Ascites may be complicated by renal failure and also by infections which are spontaneous (see below) or, more commonly, precipitated by invasive investigations or treatment, such as upper gastrointestinal endoscopy and injection sclerotherapy. Both of these complications have adverse prognostic significance and may prompt referral for transplantation.

Hepatorenal syndrome

Ten per cent of patients with advanced cirrhosis and ascites develop the hepatorenal syndrome. There are two clinical types; both are mediated by severe renal vasoconstriction due to extreme underfilling of the arterial circulation.

Type 1 hepatorenal syndrome is characterised by progressive oliguria, a rapid rise of the serum creatinine and a very poor prognosis (without treatment median survival is less than 1 month). There is usually no proteinuria, a urine sodium excretion below 10 mmol/day and a urine/plasma osmolarity ratio of > 1.5. Other non-functional causes of renal failure must be excluded before the diagnosis is made. Treatment consists of albumin infusions in combination with terlipressin and is effective in about two-thirds of patients. Haemodialysis should not be used routinely because it does not improve the outcome. Patients who survive should be considered for liver transplantation.

Type 2 hepatorenal syndrome usually occurs in patients with refractory ascites, is characterised by a moderate and stable increase in serum creatinine, and has a better prognosis.

Spontaneous bacterial peritonitis (SBP)

Patients with cirrhosis are very susceptible to infection of ascitic fluid. SBP usually presents suddenly with abdominal pain, rebound tenderness, absent bowel sounds and fever in a patient with obvious features of cirrhosis and ascites. Abdominal signs are mild or absent in about one-third of patients, and in these patients hepatic encephalopathy and fever are the main features. Diagnostic paracentesis may show cloudy fluid, and an ascites neutrophil count above $250 \times 10^6/l$ almost invariably indicates infection. The source of infection cannot usually be determined, but most organisms isolated from ascitic fluid or blood cultures are of enteric origin and *Escherichia coli* is the organism most frequently found. Ascitic culture in blood culture bottles gives the highest yield of organisms. SBP needs to be differentiated from other intra-abdominal emergencies, and the finding of multiple organisms on culture should arouse suspicion of a perforated viscus.

Treatment should be started immediately with broad-spectrum antibiotics, such as cefotaxime. Recurrence of SBP is common and may be reduced by prophylactic quinolones such as norfloxacin (400 mg daily) or ciprofloxacin (250 mg daily) (Box 23.16).

23.16 ANTIBIOTICS AND SPONTANEOUS BACTERIAL PERITONITIS (SBP) | **EBM**

'In patients with a previous episode of SBP and continued ascites norfloxacin 400 mg/day prevents recurrence (NNT$_B$ 4.5).'

'In patients with cirrhosis who have had a gastrointestinal haemorrhage prophylactic antibiotics reduce the risk of bacterial peritonitis (NNT$_B$ 12.5) and improve survival (NNT$_B$ 11).'

- Gines P, et al. Hepatology 1990; 12:716.
- Bernard B, et al. Hepatology 1999; 29:1655–1661.

HEPATIC (PORTOSYSTEMIC) ENCEPHALOPATHY

Hepatic encephalopathy is a neuropsychiatric syndrome caused by liver disease. As encephalopathy progresses, confusion is followed by coma. Confusion needs to be differentiated from delirium tremens and Wernicke's encephalopathy, and coma from subdural haematoma which can occur in alcoholics after a fall (Box 23.17).

Aetiology

Hepatic encephalopathy is thought to be due to a biochemical disturbance of brain function because it is reversible and does not cause marked pathological changes in the brain. Liver failure and portosystemic shunting

---

23.17 DIFFERENTIAL DIAGNOSIS OF HEPATIC ENCEPHALOPATHY

- Subdural haematoma
- Drug or alcohol intoxication
- Delirium tremens
- Wernicke's encephalopathy
- Primary psychiatric disorders
- Hypoglycaemia
- Neurological Wilson's disease

---

of blood are two important factors underlying hepatic encephalopathy and the balance between these varies in different patients. Some degree of liver failure is a constant factor, as portosystemic shunting of blood hardly ever causes encephalopathy if liver function is normal. Little is known of the biochemical 'neurotoxins' causing the encephalopathy, but they are thought to be mainly nitrogenous substances produced in the gut, at least in part by bacterial action, which are normally metabolised by the healthy liver and therefore excluded from the systemic circulation. Ammonia has long been considered an important factor but much interest has centred recently on γ-aminobutyric acid. Additional putative culprit substances include other false neurotransmitters such as octopamine, amino acids, mercaptans and fatty acids. Ammonia-induced alteration in astrocyte glutamine and glutamate concentrations may be important. Some factors appear to precipitate hepatic encephalopathy by increasing the availability of these substances; in addition, the brain in cirrhosis may be sensitised to other factors such as drugs that are able to precipitate hepatic encephalopathy (Fig. 23.13). Disruption of the function of the blood–brain barrier is a feature of acute hepatic failure and may lead to cerebral oedema.

Clinical assessment

Features include changes of intellect, personality, emotions and consciousness, with or without neurological signs (Box 23.18). When an episode develops acutely, a precipitating factor may be found (Fig. 23.13). The earliest features are very mild and easily overlooked but, as the condition becomes more severe, apathy, inability to concentrate, confusion, disorientation, drowsiness, slurring of speech and eventually coma develop. Convulsions sometimes occur. Examination usually shows a flapping tremor (asterixis, p. 937), inability to perform simple mental arithmetic tasks (Fig. 23.14) or draw objects such as a star (constructional apraxia, Fig. 23.15), and, as the condition progresses, hyperreflexia and bilateral extensor plantar responses. Hepatic encephalopathy rarely causes focal neurological signs, and if these are present, other causes must be sought. Fetor hepaticus, a sweet musty odour to the breath, is usually present but is more a sign of liver failure and portosystemic shunting than of hepatic encephalopathy. Rarely, chronic hepatic encephalopathy (hepatocerebral degeneration) gives rise to variable combinations of cerebellar dysfunction, Parkinsonian syndromes, spastic paraplegia and dementia.

23.18 CLINICAL GRADING OF HEPATIC ENCEPHALOPATHY

Clinical grade	Clinical signs
Grade 1	Poor concentration, slurred speech, slow mentation, disordered sleep rhythm
Grade 2	Drowsy but easily rousable, occasional aggressive behaviour, lethargic
Grade 3	Marked confusion, drowsy, sleepy but responds to pain and voice, gross disorientation
Grade 4	Unresponsive to voice, may or may not respond to painful stimuli, unconscious

23

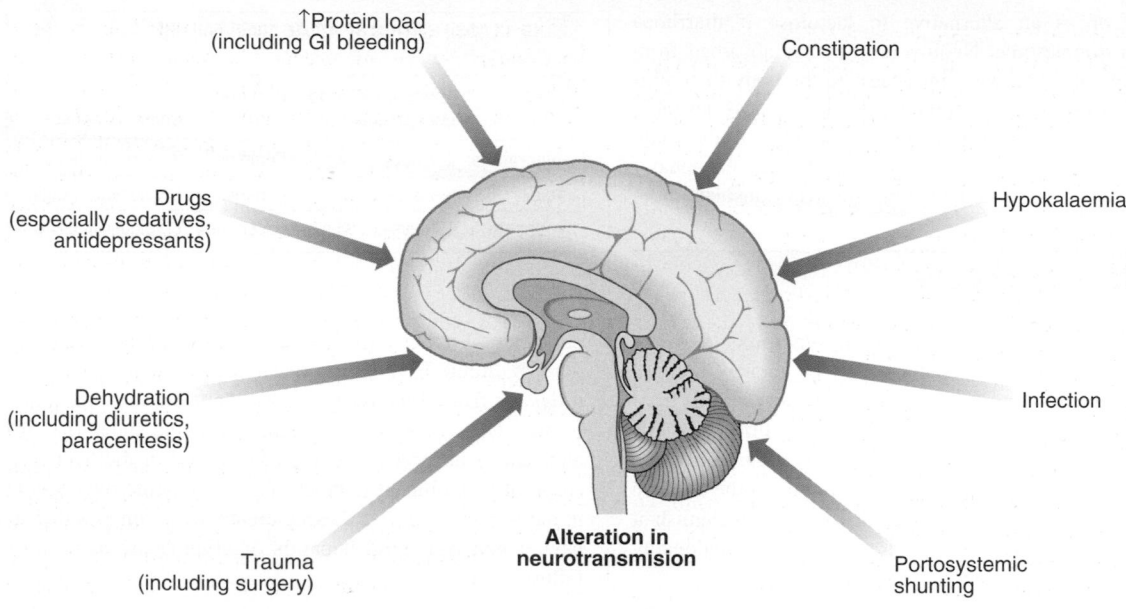

↑Protein load (including GI bleeding)

Constipation

Drugs (especially sedatives, antidepressants)

Hypokalaemia

Dehydration (including diuretics, paracentesis)

Infection

Trauma (including surgery)

Alteration in neurotransmision

Portosystemic shunting

Fig. 23.13 Factors precipitating hepatic encephalopathy.

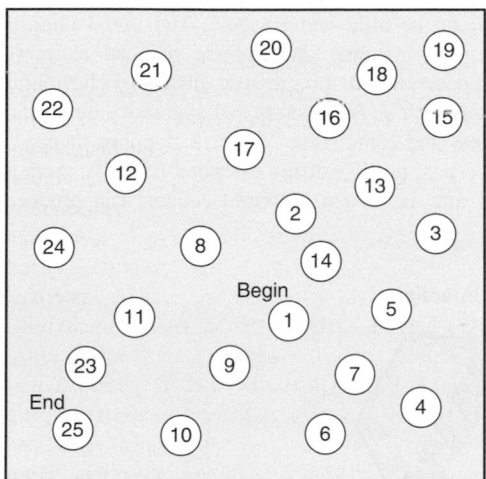

Fig. 23.14 Number connection test used in assessing encephalopathy. These 25 numbered circles can normally be joined together within 30 seconds. Serial observations may provide useful information as long as the position of the numbers is varied to avoid the patient learning their pattern.

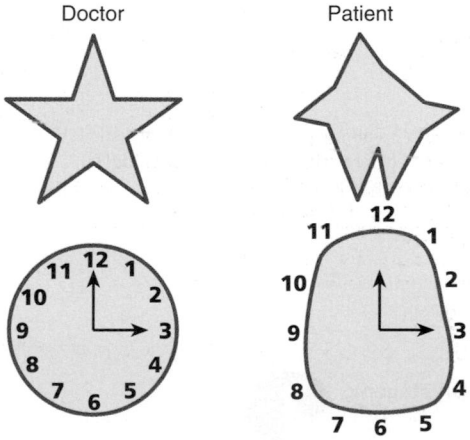

Doctor

Patient

Fig. 23.15 Constructional apraxia in encephalopathy. Drawing stars and clocks may reveal marked abnormality.

Investigations

The diagnosis can usually be made clinically, but when doubt exists, an electroencephalogram (EEG) shows diffuse slowing of the normal alpha waves with eventual development of delta waves. The arterial ammonia is usually increased in patients with hepatic encephalopathy. However, increased concentrations can occur in the absence of clinical encephalopathy so this investigation is of little or no diagnostic value.

Management

Episodes of encephalopathy are common in cirrhosis and are usually readily reversible until the terminal stages

occur. The principles of management are to treat or remove precipitating causes (Fig. 23.13) and to suppress production of neurotoxins by bacteria in the bowel. Dietary protein restriction is rarely needed and is no longer recommended as first-line treatment because it is unpalatable and can lead to worsening nutritional state in already malnourished patients. Lactulose (15–30 ml 8-hourly) is a disaccharide which is taken orally and reaches the colon intact, to be metabolised by colonic bacteria. The dose is increased gradually until the bowels are moving twice daily. It produces an osmotic laxative effect, reduces the pH of the colonic content, thereby limiting colonic ammonia absorption, and promotes the incorporation of nitrogen into bacteria. Lactitol is a rather more palatable alternative to lactulose, with a less explosive action on bowel function. Neomycin (1–4 g 4–6-hourly) is an antibiotic which acts by reducing the bacterial content of the bowel. It can be used in addition or as an alternative to lactulose if diarrhoea becomes troublesome. Neomycin is poorly absorbed from the bowel but sufficient gains access to the body to contra-indicate its use when uraemia is present. It is less desirable than lactulose for long-term use; ototoxicity is the main deleterious effect. Chronic or refractory hepatic encephalo-pathy is one of the main indications for liver transplantation.

ACUTE LIVER FAILURE

Acute liver failure is an uncommon syndrome in which hepatic encephalopathy, characterised by mental changes progressing from confusion to stupor and coma, results from a sudden severe impairment of hepatic function. The syndrome was originally defined further as occurring within 8 weeks of onset of the precipitating illness, in the absence of evidence of pre-existing liver disease, to distinguish it from those instances in which hepatic encephalopathy represents a deterioration in chronic liver disease.

Newer classifications have been developed to reflect differences in presentation and outcome of acute liver failure. One such classification divides acute liver failure into hyperacute, acute and subacute according to the interval between onset of jaundice and encephalopathy (Box 23.19).

Aetiology

Any cause of liver damage can produce acute liver failure, provided it is sufficiently severe (Fig. 23.16). Acute viral hepatitis is the most common cause world-wide; paracetamol toxicity (p. 208) is the most frequent cause in the UK. Acute liver failure occurs occasionally with other drugs, or from *Amanita phalloides* (mushroom) poisoning, in pregnancy, in Wilson's disease, following shock (p. 186) and, rarely, in extensive malignant disease of the liver. The cause of a significant number of cases of acute liver failure remains unknown and these patients are often labelled as having non-A–E viral hepatitis or cryptogenic acute liver failure.

Clinical assessment

Cerebral disturbance (hepatic encephalopathy) is the cardinal manifestation of acute liver failure, but in the early stages this can be mild and episodic. The initial clinical features are often subtle and include reduced alertness and poor concentration, progressing through behavioural abnormalities such as restlessness and aggressive outbursts, to drowsiness and coma (Box 23.18). A flapping 'hepatic' tremor (asterixis, p. 937) of the extended hands is charac-teristic but may be absent. Cerebral oedema can produce

23.19 CLASSIFICATION OF ACUTE LIVER FAILURE

Type	Time: jaundice to encephalopathy	Cerebral oedema	Common causes
Hyperacute	< 7 days	Common	Viral, paracetamol
Acute	8–28 days	Common	Cryptogenic, drugs
Subacute	29 days–12 weeks	Uncommon	Cryptogenic, drugs

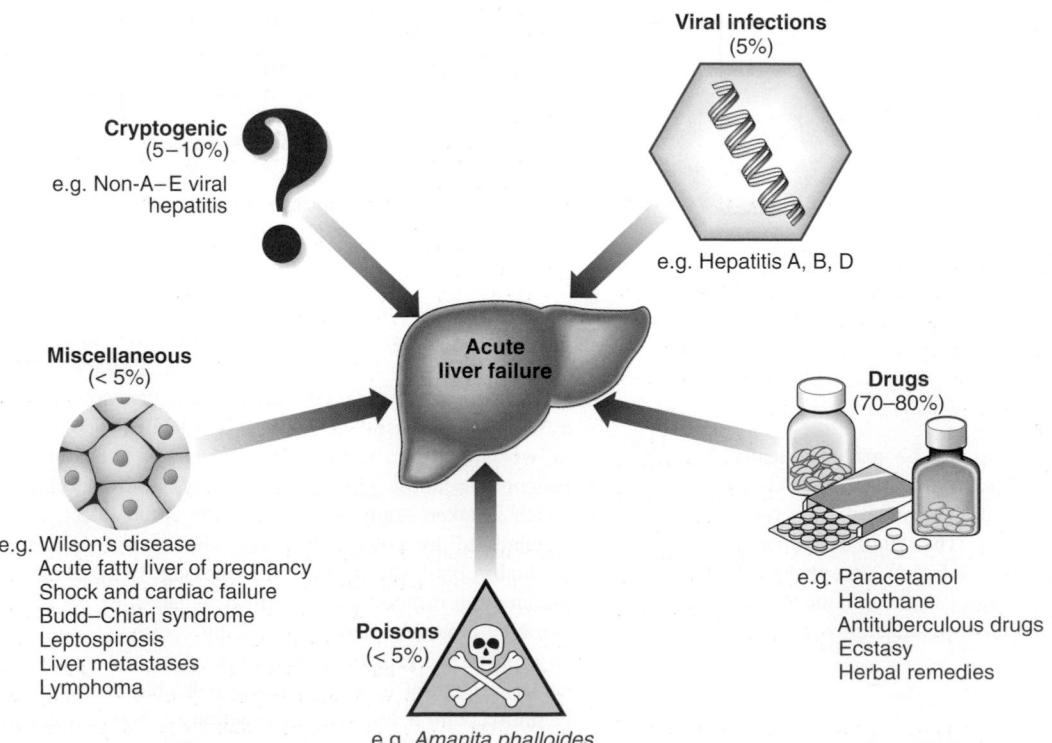

Viral infections
(5%)

e.g. Hepatitis A, B, D

Cryptogenic
(5–10%)

e.g. Non-A–E viral hepatitis

Acute liver failure

Miscellaneous
(< 5%)

e.g. Wilson's disease
Acute fatty liver of pregnancy
Shock and cardiac failure
Budd–Chiari syndrome
Leptospirosis
Liver metastases
Lymphoma

Drugs
(70–80%)

e.g. Paracetamol
Halothane
Antituberculous drugs
Ecstasy
Herbal remedies

Poisons
(< 5%)

e.g. *Amanita phalloides*

Fig. 23.16 Causes of acute liver failure in the UK. The relative frequency of the different causes varies according to geographical area.

23

23.20 INVESTIGATIONS TO DETERMINE THE CAUSE OF ACUTE LIVER FAILURE

- Toxicology screen of blood and urine
- IgM anti-HBc
- IgM anti-HAV
- Anti-HEV, HCV, cytomegalovirus, herpes simplex, Epstein–Barr virus
- Caeruloplasmin, serum copper, urinary copper, slit-lamp eye examination
- Autoantibodies: ANF, ASMA, LKM
- Immunoglobulins
- Ultrasound of liver and Doppler of hepatic veins

(ANF = antinuclear factor; ASMA = anti-smooth muscle antibody; LKM = liver–kidney microsomal antibody)

23.21 ADVERSE PROGNOSTIC CRITERIA IN ACUTE LIVER FAILURE*

Paracetamol overdose

- H^+ > 50 nmol/l (pH < 7.3) at or beyond 24 hours following the overdose

  or
- Serum creatinine > 300 μmol/l plus prothrombin time > 100 seconds plus encephalopathy grade 3 or 4

Non-paracetamol cases

- Prothrombin time > 100 seconds

  or
- Any three of the following:

  Jaundice to encephalopathy time > 7 days

  Age < 10 or > 40 years

  Indeterminate or drug-induced causes

  Bilirubin > 300 μmol/l

  Prothrombin time > 50 seconds

  or
- Factor V level of < 15% and encephalopathy grade 3 or 4

* Predict a mortality rate of ≥ 90%.
Creatinine of 300 μmol/l ≈ 3.38 mg/dl. Bilirubin of 300 μmol/l ≈ 17.6 mg/dl.

increased intracranial pressure causing unequal or abnormally reacting pupils, fixed pupils, hypertensive episodes, bradycardia, hyperventilation, profuse sweating, local or general myoclonus, focal fits or decerebrate posturing. Papilloedema occurs rarely and is a late sign. More general symptoms include weakness, nausea and vomiting. Right hypochondrial discomfort is an occasional feature.

Examination shows jaundice, which develops rapidly and is usually deep in subsequently fatal cases. Jaundice is not seen in Reye's syndrome, and death in other causes of acute liver failure occasionally occurs before jaundice develops. Fetor hepaticus can be present. The liver is usually of normal size but later becomes smaller. Hepatomegaly is unusual and, in the presence of a sudden onset of ascites, suggests venous outflow obstruction (Budd–Chiari). Splenomegaly is uncommon and never prominent. Ascites and oedema are late developments and may be a consequence of fluid therapy. Other features are related to the development of complications, which are considered below.

Investigations

Investigations are used to determine the cause of the liver failure and the prognosis (Boxes 23.20 and 23.21). Hepatitis B core IgM antibody is the best screening test for acute hepatitis B infection, as liver damage is due to the immunological response to the virus which has often been eliminated and HBsAg may be negative. The prothrombin time rapidly becomes prolonged as coagulation factor synthesis fails; this is the laboratory test of greatest prognostic value and should be carried out at least twice daily. Factor V levels can be used instead of the prothrombin time to assess the degree of liver impairment. The plasma bilirubin reflects the degree of jaundice. Plasma aminotransferase activity is particularly high after paracetamol overdose, reaching 100–500 times normal, but falls as liver damage progresses and is not helpful in determining prognosis. Plasma albumin concentration remains normal unless the course is prolonged. Percutaneous liver biopsy is contraindicated because of the severe coagulopathy, but biopsy can be undertaken by the transjugular route.

Management

A patient with acute hepatic damage should be observed in a high-dependency or intensive care unit as soon as a progressive prolongation of the prothrombin time or hepatic

23.22 OBSERVATIONS IN ACUTE LIVER FAILURE

Neurological

- Conscious level
- Intracranial pressure monitoring (specialist units, p. 197)

Cardiorespiratory

- Pulse
- Blood pressure
- Central venous pressure
- Respiratory rate

Fluid balance

- Input—oral, intravenous
- Hourly output (urine, vomiting, diarrhoea)

Blood analyses

- Arterial blood gases
- Peripheral blood count (including platelets)
- Creatinine, urea
- Sodium, potassium, HCO_3^-, calcium, magnesium
- Glucose (2-hourly in acute phase)
- Prothrombin time

Infection surveillance

- Cultures—blood, urine, throat, sputum, cannula sites
- Chest X-ray
- Temperature

encephalopathy is identified (Box 23.22) so that prompt treatment of complications can be initiated (Box 23.23). Conservative treatment aims to maintain life in the hope that hepatic regeneration will occur, but early transfer to a specialised transplant unit should always be considered. *N*-acetylcysteine therapy may improve outcome, particularly in patients with acute liver failure due to paracetamol poisoning. Liver transplantation is an increasingly important treatment option for acute liver failure, and criteria have

23

23.23 COMPLICATIONS OF ACUTE LIVER FAILURE

- Encephalopathy and cerebral oedema
- Hypoglycaemia
- Metabolic acidosis
- Infection (bacterial, fungal)
- Renal failure
- Multi-organ failure (hypotension and respiratory failure)

---

been developed to identify patients unlikely to survive without a transplant (Box 23.21). Patients should, wherever possible, be transferred to a transplant centre before these criteria are met to allow time for assessment and to maximise the time for a donor liver to become available. Survival following liver transplantation for acute liver failure is improving with increasing experience and 1-year survival rates of about 60% can be expected.

CHRONIC LIVER FAILURE

Chronic liver failure develops when the functional capacity of the liver can no longer maintain normal physiological conditions and is characterised by the presence of encephalopathy and/or ascites. The term 'hepatic decompensation' or 'decompensated liver disease' is often used when chronic liver failure occurs. The most common cause is cirrhosis, which is usually the result of chronic liver injury occurring over many years.

Chronic liver failure may occur as a consequence of insidious destruction of hepatocytes or acute on chronic injury such as may occur in viral or alcoholic hepatitis, and may also supervene when certain clinical situations lead to increased metabolic demands on the liver, e.g. infection or gastrointestinal haemorrhage.

A variety of clinical and laboratory features may be present (Box 23.24) in addition to encephalopathy and/or ascites; these include peripheral oedema, renal failure, jaundice, and hypoalbuminaemia and coagulation abnormalities due to defective protein synthesis.

23.24 FEATURES OF CHRONIC LIVER FAILURE

- Worsening synthetic liver function
  Prolonged prothrombin time
  Low albumin
- Jaundice
- Portal hypertension
  Variceal bleeding
- Hepatic encephalopathy
- Ascites
  Spontaneous bacterial peritonitis
  Hepatorenal failure

CHRONIC LIVER DISEASE

Chronic liver disease is defined as liver injury occurring over more than 6 months, in contrast to acute liver injury.

CIRRHOSIS

Hepatic cirrhosis can occur at any age and often causes prolonged morbidity. It frequently manifests itself in

---

23.25 CAUSES OF CIRRHOSIS

- Alcohol
- Chronic viral hepatitis (B or C)
- Non-alcoholic fatty liver disease
- Immune
  Primary sclerosing cholangitis
  Autoimmune liver disease
- Biliary
  Primary biliary cirrhosis
  Cystic fibrosis
- Genetic
  Haemochromatosis
  α_1-antitrypsin deficiency
  Wilson's disease
- Cryptogenic (unknown)

---

younger adults and is an important cause of premature death. Causes are listed in Box 23.25. Any condition leading to persistent or recurrent hepatocyte death may lead to hepatic cirrhosis. World-wide, the most common causes of cirrhosis are viral hepatitis and prolonged excessive alcohol consumption. Prolonged biliary damage or obstruction, as can occur in primary biliary cirrhosis, sclerosing cholangitis and post-surgical biliary strictures, will also result in cirrhosis. Persistent blockage of the venous return from the liver, e.g. veno-occlusive disease and Budd–Chiari syndrome, will eventually result in liver cirrhosis.

Common to all causes of liver cirrhosis is activation of the hepatic stellate cells. These cells are widely distributed throughout the liver in the perisinusoidal space of Disse. When activated, the quiescent fat-storing stellate cells become multifunctional cells, capable of collagen production, contraction and cytokine synthesis. This process is dependent on interaction with other cells in the liver, such as hepatocytes and Kupffer cells, and both paracrine and autocrine cytokine stimulation (Fig. 23.17).

Pathology

The changes in cirrhosis usually affect the whole liver; however, in biliary cirrhosis (e.g. primary biliary cirrhosis) they can be patchy (Fig. 23.18). They include progressive and widespread death of liver cells associated with inflammation and fibrosis, leading to loss of the normal liver architecture. Destruction of the liver architecture causes distortion and loss of the normal hepatic vasculature with the development of portosystemic vascular shunts and the formation of nodules rather than lobules due to the proliferation of surviving hepatocytes. The evolution of cirrhosis is gradual and progressive unless the aetiological agent is withdrawn: for example, by abstinence from alcohol (Fig. 23.18).

Cirrhosis can be classified histologically into two types.

- *Micronodular cirrhosis* is characterised by small nodules about 1 mm in diameter and is seen in alcoholic cirrhosis.
- *Macronodular cirrhosis* is characterised by larger nodules of various sizes. Areas of previous collapse of the liver architecture are evidenced by large fibrous scars.

Clinical features

These vary greatly and include any combination of the manifestations described below (Box 23.26). Cirrhosis may be entirely asymptomatic; in life it may be found

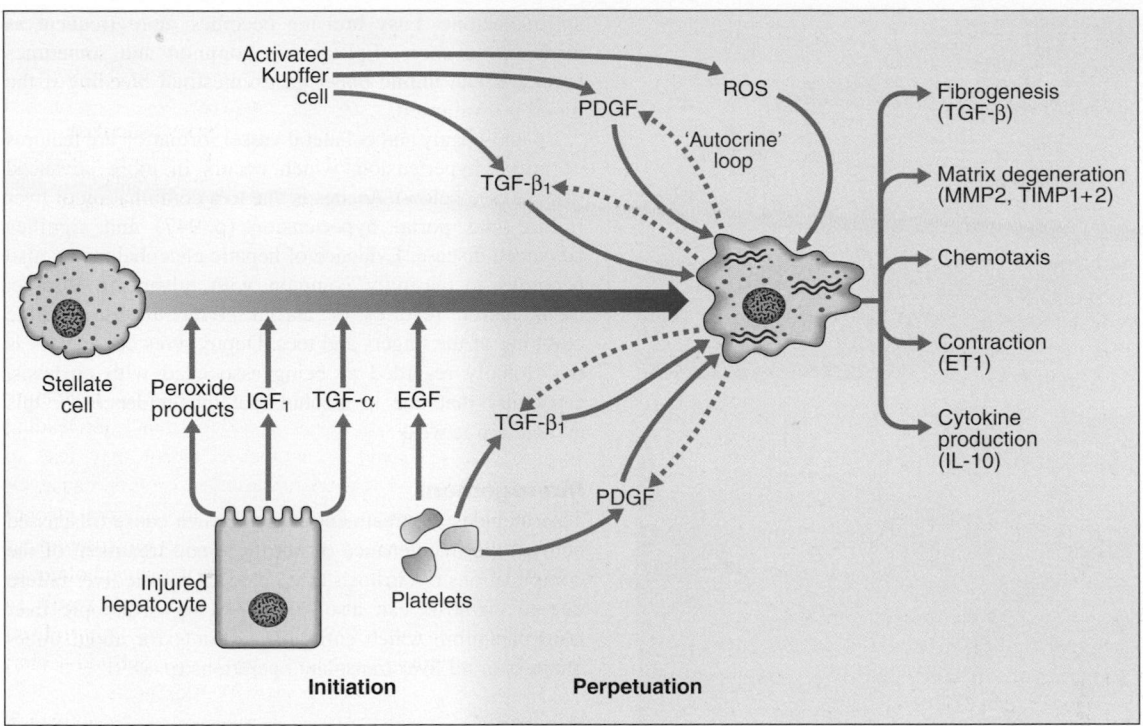

Figure 23.17 Pathogenic mechanisms in hepatic fibrosis. Stellate cell activation occurs under the influence of cytokines released by other cell types in the liver including hepatocytes, Kupffer cells (tissue macrophages), platelets and lymphocytes. Once stellate cells become activated, they can perpetuate their own activation by synthesis of transforming growth factor-beta (TGF-β_1) and platelet-derived growth factor (PDGF) through autocrine loops. Activated stellate cells produce TGF β_1, stimulating the production of collagen matrix as well as inhibitors of collagen breakdown. The inhibitors of collagen breakdown, matrix metalloproteinase 2 and 9 (MMP2 and MMP9), are inactivated in turn by tissue inhibitors TIMP1 and TIMP2 which are increased in fibrosis. Inflammation also contributes to fibrosis with the cytokine profile produced by Th2 lymphocytes, such as interleukin-6 and 13 (IL-6 and IL-13). Activated stellate cells also produce endothelin 1 (ET1), which may contribute to portal hypertension. (ROS = reactive oxygen species; IGF = insulin growth factor; EGF = epidermal growth factor)

23.26 CLINICAL FEATURES OF HEPATIC CIRRHOSIS

- Hepatomegaly (although liver may also be small)
- Jaundice
- Ascites
- Circulatory changes
    Spider telangiectasia, palmar erythema, cyanosis
- Endocrine changes
    Loss of libido, hair loss
    Men: gynaecomastia, testicular atrophy, impotence
    Women: breast atrophy, irregular menses, amenorrhoea
- Haemorrhagic tendency
    Bruises, purpura, epistaxis, menorrhagia
- Portal hypertension
    Splenomegaly, collateral vessels, variceal bleeding, fetor hepaticus
- Hepatic (portosystemic) encephalopathy
- Other features
    Pigmentation, digital clubbing

---

incidentally at surgery or may be associated with minimal features such as isolated hepatomegaly. Frequent complaints include weakness, fatigue, muscle cramps, weight loss and non-specific digestive symptoms such as anorexia, nausea, vomiting and upper abdominal discomfort. Otherwise, clinical features are due mainly to hepatic insufficiency and portal hypertension.

Hepatomegaly is common in alcoholic liver disease and haemochromatosis. Progressive hepatocyte destruction and fibrosis gradually reduce liver size as the disease progresses in other causes of cirrhosis. A reduction in liver size is especially common if the cause of cirrhosis is viral hepatitis or autoimmune liver disease. The liver is often hard, irregular and painless. Jaundice is usually mild when it first appears and is due primarily to a failure to excrete bilirubin. Mild haemolysis may occur due to hypersplenism but is not a major contributor to the jaundice. Palmar erythema can be seen early in the disease but is of limited diagnostic value as it occurs in many other conditions associated with a hyperdynamic circulation including normal pregnancy, as well as being found in some normal people. Spider telangiectasia are due to associated arteriolar changes and comprise a central arteriole (which occasionally raises the skin surface) from which small vessels radiate. They vary in size from 1–2 mm to 1–2 cm in diameter, are usually found only above the nipples, and can occur early in the disease. One or two small spider telangiectasia are found in about 2% of healthy people and can occur transiently in greater numbers in the third trimester of pregnancy, but otherwise they are a strong indicator of liver disease. Florid spider telangiectasia, gynaecomastia and parotid enlargement are most common in alcoholic cirrhosis. Pigmentation is most striking in haemochromatosis and in any cirrhosis

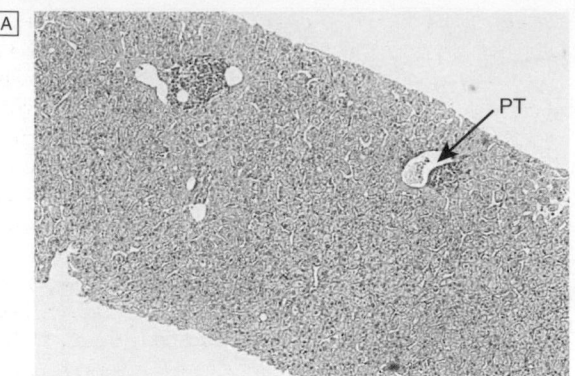

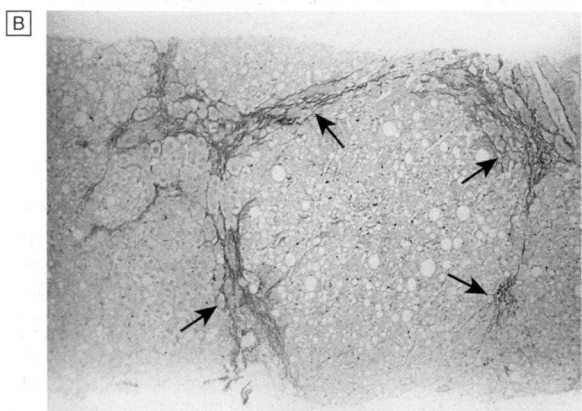

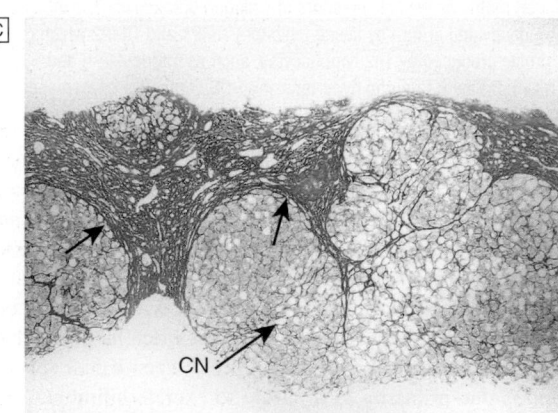

Fig. 23.18 Progressive liver fibrosis shown histologically.
A Normal liver. Columns of hepatocytes 1–2 cells thick radiate from the portal tracts to the central veins. The portal tract (PT) contains a normal intralobular bile duct branch of the hepatic artery and portal venous radical. B Fibrosis (stained pink, arrows) spreading out around the hepatic vein and single liver cells (pericellular). C A cirrhotic liver. The liver architecture is disrupted. The normal arrangement of portal tracts and hepatic veins is now lost and nodules of proliferating hepatocytes are broken up by strands of pink/orange-staining fibrous tissue (arrows) forming cirrhotic nodules (CN).

spironolactone. Easy bruising becomes more frequent as cirrhosis advances. Epistaxis is common and sometimes severe; it can mimic upper gastrointestinal bleeding if the blood is swallowed.

Splenomegaly and collateral vessel formation are features of portal hypertension, which occurs in more advanced disease (see below). Ascites is due to a combination of liver failure and portal hypertension (p. 947) and signifies advanced disease. Evidence of hepatic encephalopathy also becomes increasingly common with advancing disease. Non-specific features of chronic liver disease include clubbing of the fingers and toes. Dupuytren's contracture is traditionally regarded as being associated with cirrhosis, especially that due to alcohol, but the evidence for this association is weak.

Management

This includes the treatment of any known cause (discussed below), the maintenance of nutrition, and treatment of the complications of cirrhosis (see below). Chronic liver failure due to cirrhosis can also be treated by orthotopic liver transplantation, which currently accounts for about three-quarters of all liver transplant operations (p. 989).

Prognosis

The overall prognosis in cirrhosis is poor. Many patients present with advanced disease and/or serious complications that carry a high mortality. Overall, only 25% of patients

23.27 CHILD–PUGH CLASSIFICATION OF PROGNOSIS IN CIRRHOSIS

Score	1	2	3
Encephalopathy	None	Mild	Marked
Bilirubin (μmol/l)*	< 34	34–50	> 50
In primary biliary cirrhosis and sclerosing cholangitis	< 68	68–170	> 170
Albumin (g/l)	> 35	28–35	< 28
Prothrombin time (seconds prolonged)	< 4	4–6	> 6
Ascites	None	Mild	Marked

Add the individual scores: < 7 = Child's A
7–9 = Child's B
> 9 = Child's C

* To convert bilirubin in μmol/l to mg/dl, divide by 17.

23.28 SURVIVAL IN CIRRHOSIS

Child–Pugh grade	Survival (%)			Hepatic deaths* (%)
	1 year	5 years	10 years	
A	82	45	25	43
B	62	20	7	72
C	42	20	0	85

* Include hepatic failure, gastrointestinal bleeding and hepatocellular carcinoma.

associated with prolonged cholestasis. Pulmonary arterio-venous shunts also develop, leading to hypoxaemia and eventually to central cyanosis, but this is a late feature.

Endocrine changes are noticed more readily in men, who show loss of male hair distribution and testicular atrophy. Gynaecomastia is common and can be due to drugs such as

23.29 1-YEAR SURVIVAL RATE DEPENDING ON MELD SCORE

| MELD score | 1-year survival (%) | |
	No complications	Complications*
< 9	97	90
10–19	90	85
20–29	70	65
30–39	70	50

MELD = 3.8 [In serum bilirubin (mg/dl)] + 11.2 [In INR] + 9.6 [In serum creatinine (mg/dl)] + 6.4

In = natural log. To calculate on-line, go to www.unos.org/resources/meldpeldcalculator.

* Complications are the presence of ascites, encephalopathy or variceal bleeding.

survive 5 years from diagnosis but, where liver function is good, 50% survive for 5 years and 25% for up to 10 years. The prognosis is more favourable when the underlying cause of the cirrhosis can be corrected, as in alcohol misuse, haemochromatosis and Wilson's disease.

Laboratory tests give only a rough guide to prognosis in individual patients. Deteriorating liver function, as evidenced by jaundice, ascites or encephalopathy, indicates a poor prognosis unless a treatable cause such as infection is found. Increasing plasma bilirubin, falling plasma albumin or an albumin concentration < 30 g/l, marked hyponatraemia (< 120 mmol/l, not due to diuretic therapy) and a prolonged prothrombin time are all bad prognostic features (Boxes 23.27 and 23.28). The Child–Pugh score and, more recently, the MELD (Model for End-stage Liver Disease) score can be used to assess prognosis. The MELD is more difficult to calculate at the bedside but, unlike the Child–Pugh score, includes renal function; if this is impaired, it is known to be a poor prognostic feature in end-stage liver disease (Box 23.29). Despite the availability of these prognostic scores, the course of cirrhosis is uncertain, as unforeseen complications such as variceal bleeding may unexpectedly lead to death.

PORTAL HYPERTENSION

Portal hypertension is characterised by prolonged elevation of the portal venous pressure (normally 2–5 mmHg). Patients developing clinical features or complications of portal hypertension usually have portal venous pressures above 12 mmHg.

Aetiology and pathogenesis

Portal venous pressure is determined by the portal blood flow and portal vascular resistance. Increased vascular resistance is usually the main factor producing portal hypertension, irrespective of its cause, and consequently the causes of portal hypertension are classified in accordance with the main sites of obstruction to blood flow in the portal venous system (Fig. 23.19 and Box 23.30).

Extrahepatic portal vein obstruction is the usual cause of portal hypertension in childhood and adolescence, while cirrhosis causes 90% or more of portal hypertension in adults in developed countries. Schistosomiasis is the most common cause of portal hypertension world-wide but it is infrequent outside endemic areas. Increased portal vascular resistance leads to a gradual reduction in the flow of portal blood to the liver and simultaneously to the development of collateral vessels, allowing portal blood to bypass the liver and enter the systemic circulation directly. Increased portal blood flow contributes to portal hypertension but is not the dominant factor. Collateral vessel formation is widespread but occurs particularly in the gastrointestinal tract, especially the oesophagus, stomach and rectum, in the anterior abdominal wall, and in the renal, lumbar, ovarian and testicular vasculature. Normally, virtually all the portal blood flows through the liver but, as collateral vessel formation progresses, half or more (and occasionally almost all) of the portal blood flow can be shunted directly to the systemic circulation.

Clinical features

The clinical features of portal hypertension result principally from portal venous congestion and collateral vessel formation. Splenomegaly is a cardinal finding, and a diagnosis of portal hypertension is unlikely when splenomegaly cannot be detected clinically or by ultrasonography. The spleen is rarely enlarged more than 5 cm below the left costal margin in adults, but more marked splenomegaly can occur in childhood and adolescence. Hypersplenism is common and frequently results in thrombocytopenia. Platelet counts are usually around 100×10^9/l; values below 50×10^9/l are uncommon. Leucopenia occurs occasionally but anaemia can hardly ever be attributed directly to hypersplenism. Collateral vessels may be visible on the anterior abdominal wall and occasionally several radiate from the umbilicus to form a caput medusae. Rarely, a large umbilical collateral vessel has a blood flow sufficient to give a venous hum on auscultation (Cruveilhier–Baumgarten syndrome). The most important collateral vessels occur in the oesophagus and stomach, where they can cause severe bleeding. Rectal varices also cause bleeding and are often mistaken for haemorrhoids, which are no more common in portal hypertension than in the general population. Fetor hepaticus results from portosystemic shunting of blood, which allows mercaptans to pass directly to the lungs.

Investigations

Radiological and endoscopic examination of the upper gastrointestinal tract can show varices (Fig. 23.20). This establishes the presence of portal hypertension but not its cause. Imaging, particularly ultrasonography, can show features of portal hypertension, such as splenomegaly and collateral vessels, and can sometimes indicate the cause, such as liver disease or portal vein thrombosis. Portal venography demonstrates the site and often the cause of portal venous obstruction and is performed prior to surgical intervention.

Portal venous pressure measurements are rarely needed but can be used to confirm portal hypertension and to differentiate sinusoidal and pre-sinusoidal forms. They are usually made by using a balloon catheter to measure the wedged hepatic venous pressure (WHVP) and free hepatic

23

23.30 CAUSES OF PORTAL HYPERTENSION ACCORDING TO SITE OF ABNORMALITY

Extrahepatic post-sinusoidal ❶

• Budd–Chiari syndrome

Intrahepatic post-sinusoidal ❷

• Veno-occlusive disease

Sinusoidal ❸

• Cirrhosis*
• Cystic liver disease
• Partial nodular transformation of the liver
• Metastatic malignant disease

Intrahepatic pre-sinusoidal ❹

• Schistosomiasis*
• Sarcoidosis
• Congenital hepatic fibrosis
• Vinyl chloride
• Drugs

Extrahepatic pre-sinusoidal ❺

• Portal vein thrombosis due to sepsis* (umbilical, portal pyaemia) or procoagulopathy (thrombotic diseases, oral contraceptives, pregnancy), or secondary to cirrhosis
• Abdominal trauma, including surgery
• Malignant disease of pancreas or liver
• Pancreatitis
• Congenital

* Most common causes.
Numbers refer to Figure 23.19.

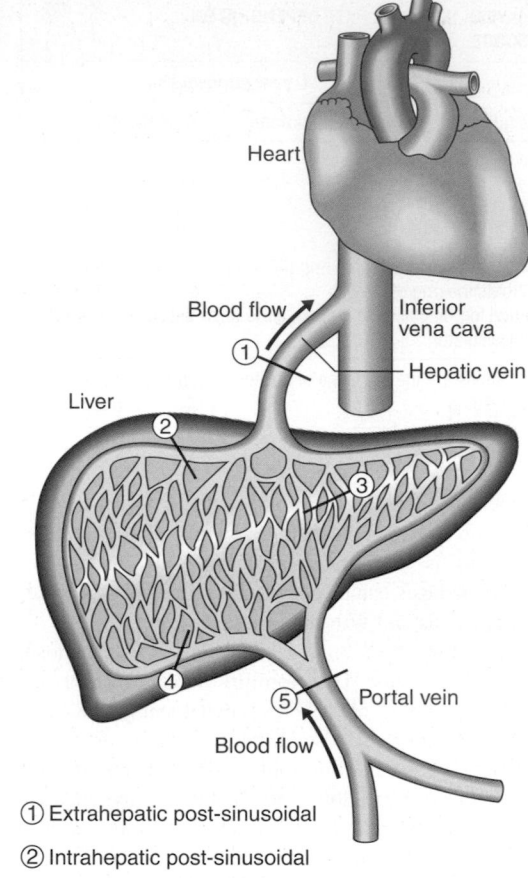

① Extrahepatic post-sinusoidal
② Intrahepatic post-sinusoidal
③ Sinusoidal
④ Intrahepatic pre-sinusoidal
⑤ Extrahepatic pre-sinusoidal

Fig. 23.19 Classification of portal hypertension according to site of vascular obstruction. See also Box 23.30.

venous pressure (FHVP). The WHVP minus the FHVP gives the hepatic venous pressure gradient (HVPG), which in cirrhosis reflects the portal pressure. The HVPG is low in pre-sinusoidal portal pressure, underestimating true portal pressure.

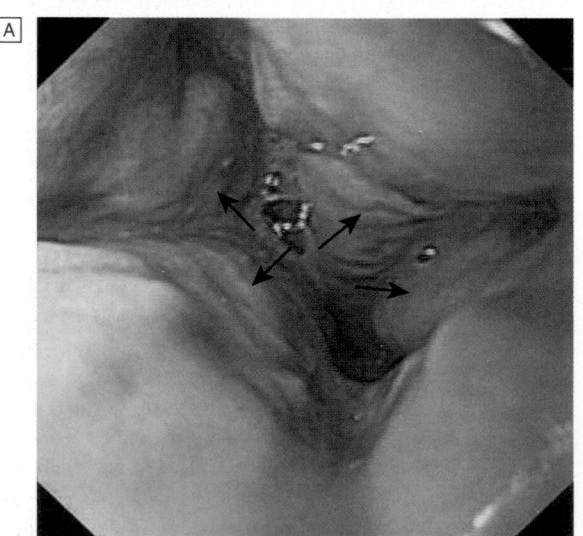

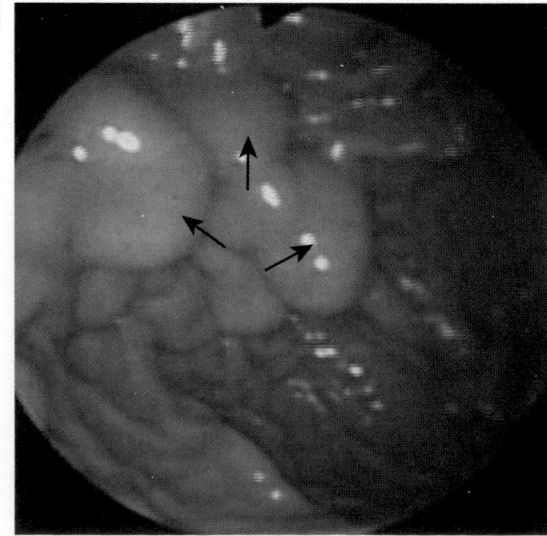

Fig. 23.20 Varices: endoscopic views. [A] Oesophageal varices (arrows) at the lower end of the oesophagus. [B] Gastric varices (arrows).

Complications

Gastrointestinal bleeding from varices or from congestive gastropathy is the main complication; others are listed in Box 23.31.

VARICEAL BLEEDING

Variceal bleeding occurs from oesophageal varices that are usually located within 3–5 cm of the oesophago-gastric junction, or from gastric varices. The size of the varices, endoscopic variceal features such as red spots and red stripes, high portal pressure and liver failure are all general factors that predispose to bleeding. Drugs capable of causing mucosal erosion, such as salicylates and other non-steroidal anti-inflammatory drugs (NSAIDs), can also precipitate bleeding. Variceal bleeding is often severe, and recurrent bleeding occurs if preventative treatment is not given. Bleeding from varices at other sites is comparatively uncommon but most often occurs from varices in the rectum or intestinal stomas. The mortality from bleeding oesophageal varices is high (up to 50% in those with advanced liver disease), and is largely dependent on the severity of liver dysfunction.

Management of acute variceal bleeding

The differential diagnosis and diagnostic approach in patients with acute upper gastrointestinal haemorrhage are detailed on pages 866–869.

The priority in acute bleeding from oesophageal varices is to restore the circulation with blood and plasma, not least because shock reduces liver blood flow and causes further deterioration of liver function. Even in patients with known varices, the source of bleeding should always be confirmed by endoscopy because about 20% of such patients are found to be bleeding from some other lesion, especially acute gastric erosions. Management of acute variceal bleeding is illustrated in Figure 23.21. All patients with cirrhosis and gastrointestinal bleeding should receive broad-spectrum antibiotics such as ciprofloxacin because sepsis is common and treatment with antibiotics has been shown to improve outcome.

Local measures

The measures used to control acute variceal bleeding include endoscopic therapy (banding or sclerotherapy), balloon tamponade and oesophageal transection.

Banding or sclerotherapy

This is the most widely used initial treatment and is undertaken if possible at the time of diagnostic endoscopy. It stops variceal bleeding in 80% of patients and can be repeated if bleeding recurs. Banding (Fig. 23.22) can be less easy to

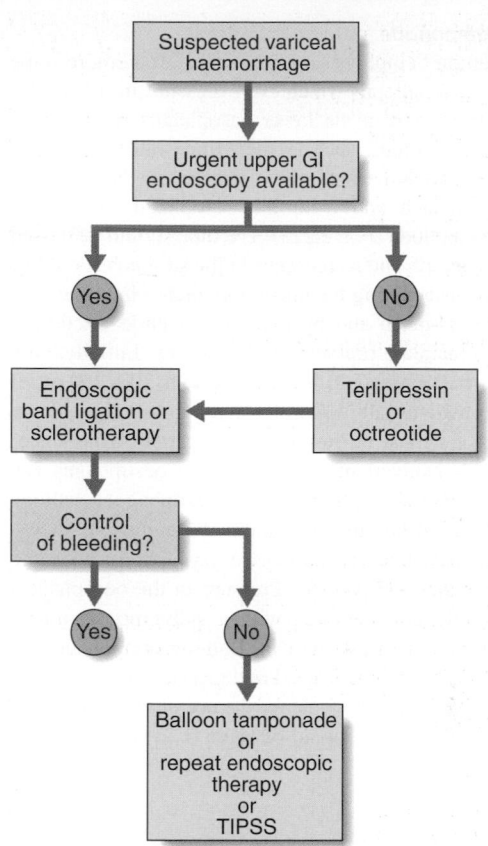

Fig. 23.21 **Management of acute bleeding from oesophageal varices.** (TIPSS = transjugular intrahepatic portosystemic stent shunt)

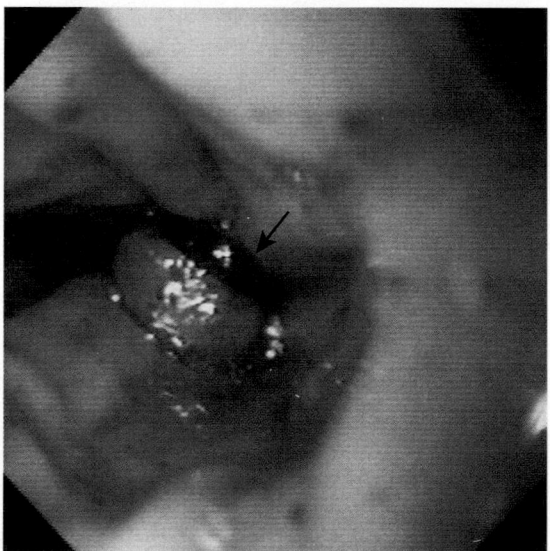

Fig. 23.22 **Appearances of oesophageal varices following application of strangulating bands (band ligation, arrow).**

apply than sclerotherapy. Active bleeding at endoscopy may make endoscopic therapy difficult; in such cases bleeding should be controlled by balloon tamponade prior to endoscopic therapy.

23

Balloon tamponade

This technique employs a Sengstaken–Blakemore tube possessing two balloons which exert pressure in the fundus of the stomach and in the lower oesophagus respectively. Current modifications, such as the Minnesota tube, incorporate sufficient lumens to allow material to be aspirated from the stomach and from the oesophagus above the oesophageal balloon (Fig. 23.23). The tube should be passed through the mouth and its presence in the stomach should be checked by auscultating the upper abdomen while injecting air into the stomach and by radiology. Gentle traction is essential to maintain pressure on the varices. Initially, only the gastric balloon should be inflated with 200–250 ml of air, as this will usually control bleeding. Inflation of the gastric balloon must be stopped if the patient experiences pain because inadvertent inflation in the oesophagus can cause oesophageal rupture. If the oesophageal balloon needs to be used because of continued bleeding, it should be deflated for about 10 minutes every 3 hours to avoid oesophageal mucosal damage. Pressure in the oesophageal balloon should be monitored with a sphygmomanometer and should not exceed 40 mmHg. Balloon tamponade will almost always stop oesophageal and gastric fundal variceal bleeding, but only creates time for the use of more definitive therapy. Particular care should be taken to avoid pulmonary aspiration whilst inserting the tube; patients unable to protect their airway should be intubated.

Oesophageal transection

Transection of the varices can be performed with a stapling gun, although it carries some risk of subsequent oesophageal stenosis, and is normally combined with splenectomy. The operation is used when transjugular intrahepatic portosystemic stent shunting (TIPSS) is not available and when bleeding cannot be controlled by the other therapies described. The operative morbidity and mortality are considerable.

Reduction of portal venous pressure

Pharmacological reduction of portal pressure is less important than sclerotherapy or banding, is expensive and is not always used. TIPSS is increasingly being used for reducing portal pressure (see below).

Pharmacological treatment

Terlipressin is the current drug of choice and releases the vasoconstrictor, vasopressin, over several hours in amounts sufficient to reduce the portal pressure without producing systemic effects. It is given in a dose of 2 mg i.v. 6-hourly until bleeding stops and then 1 mg 6-hourly for a further 24 hours.

Octreotide, the synthetic form of somatostatin, reduces the portal pressure and can stop variceal bleeding. It has few side-effects and is given in a dose of 50 μg intravenously, followed by an infusion of 50 μg hourly.

TIPSS and shunt surgery

TIPSS, described below, can be used for acute bleeding not responding to sclerotherapy or banding. Emergency portosystemic shunt surgery has a mortality of 50% or more and is now virtually never used for treating active variceal bleeding.

Prevention of recurrent bleeding

Recurrent bleeding is the rule rather than the exception in patients who have previously bled from oesophageal varices, and treatment to prevent this is needed.

Band ligation

This is a technique in which varices are sucked into an endoscope accessory, allowing them to be occluded with a tight rubber band. The occluded varix subsequently sloughs with variceal obliteration. Banding is repeated every 1–2 weeks until the varices are obliterated. Regular follow-up endoscopy is required to identify and treat any recurrence of varices. The technique is generally more effective than sclerotherapy, has fewer side-effects and is now the treatment of choice. Prophylactic acid suppression with proton pump inhibitors may reduce the risk of secondary bleeding from banding-induced ulceration.

Sclerotherapy

Sclerotherapy, a technique in which varices are injected with a sclerosing agent, has now been largely abandoned in preference to banding ligation. The treatment was not free of risk as injections could cause transient chest or abdominal pain, fever, transient dysphagia and occasionally oesophageal perforation. Oesophageal strictures may also develop.

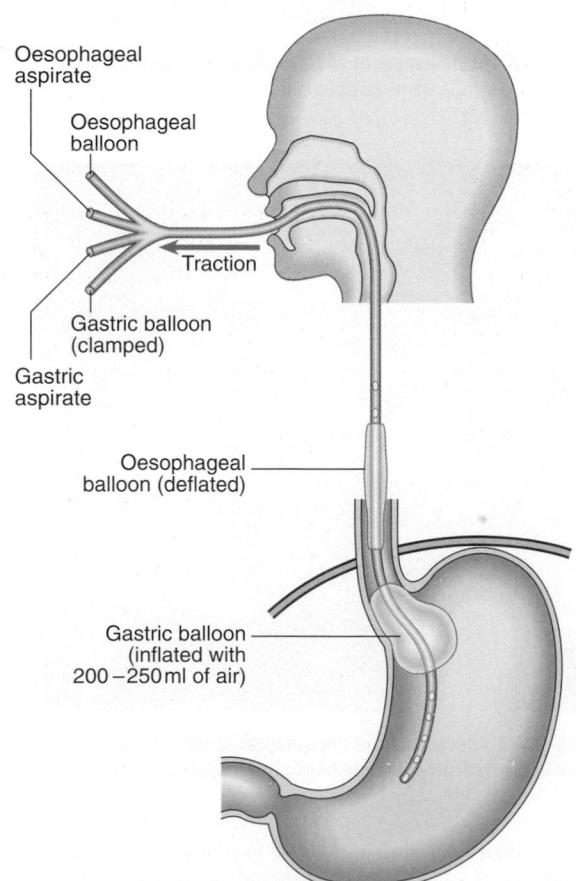

Oesophageal aspirate

Oesophageal balloon

Traction

Gastric balloon (clamped)

Gastric aspirate

Oesophageal balloon (deflated)

Gastric balloon (inflated with 200–250 ml of air)

Fig. 23.23 Sengstaken–Blakemore tube.

TIPSS

This technique uses a stent placed between the portal vein and the hepatic vein in the liver to provide a portosystemic shunt and therefore reduce portal pressure (Fig. 23.24). The procedure is carried out under radiological control via the internal jugular vein; prior patency of the portal vein must be determined angiographically, coagulation deficiencies may require correction with fresh frozen plasma, and antibiotic cover is provided. Successful shunt placement stops and prevents variceal bleeding. Further bleeding necessitates investigation and treatment (e.g. angioplasty) because it is usually associated with shunt narrowing or occlusion. Hepatic encephalopathy may occur following TIPSS and is managed by reducing the shunt diameter. Although TIPSS is associated with less rebleeding than endoscopic therapy, survival is not improved (Box 23.32).

Portosystemic shunt surgery

Although surgery prevents recurrent bleeding, it carries a high mortality and often leads to encephalopathy. Non-selective portacaval shunts can divert the majority of the portal blood away from the liver, rendering patients liable to post-operative liver failure and hepatic encephalopathy. This led to the development of more selective shunts (such as the distal splenorenal shunt); such shunts are associated with less post-operative encephalopathy, but with the passage of time liver portal blood flow falls and later encephalopathy may supervene. Furthermore, survival is not prolonged, as death from liver failure occurs. In practice, portosystemic shunts are now reserved for patients in whom other treatments have not been successful and are offered only to those with good liver function.

Beta-adrenoceptor antagonists (β-blockers)

Propranolol (80–160 mg/day) or nadolol reduces the portal venous pressure in portal hypertension and has been used to prevent recurrent variceal bleeding; however, it is not widely used in secondary prevention and compliance may be poor.

PRIMARY PROPHYLAXIS OF INITIAL VARICEAL BLEEDING

In view of the mortality and morbidity associated with variceal haemorrhage, portosystemic shunts, sclerotherapy and propranolol have all been used to try to prevent initial bleeding from varices. Propranolol or nadolol at a dose which reduces the heart rate by 25% has given beneficial results and should be used for primary prevention (Box 23.33). Prophylactic banding is probably as effective as a β-blocker.

CONGESTIVE GASTROPATHY

Long-standing portal hypertension causes chronic gastric congestion recognisable at endoscopy as multiple areas of punctate erythema. Rarely, similar lesions occur more

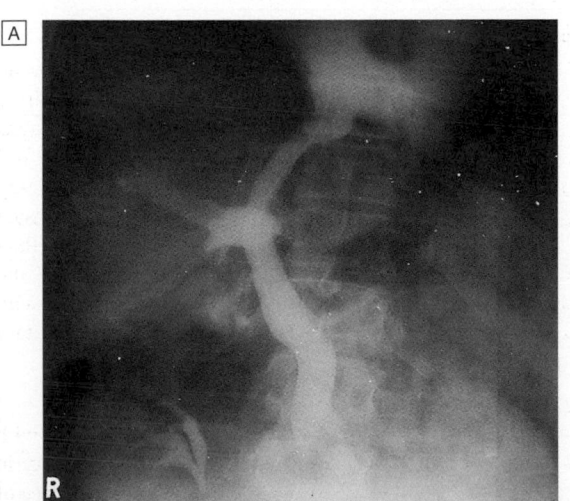
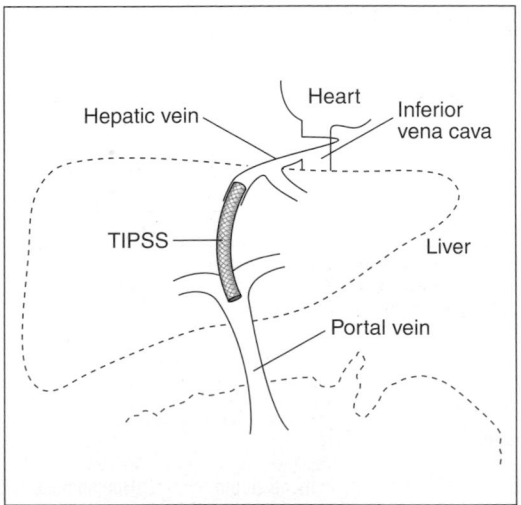

Fig. 23.24 Transjugular intrahepatic portosystemic stent shunt (TIPSS). A X-ray showing placement of TIPSS within the portal vein, allowing blood to flow from the portal vein into the hepatic vein and then the inferior vena cava. B Explanatory diagram.

distally in the gastrointestinal tract. These areas may become eroded, causing bleeding from multiple sites. Acute bleeding can occur, but repeated minor bleeding causing iron-deficiency anaemia is more common. Anaemia may be prevented by oral iron supplements but repeated blood transfusions can become necessary. Reduction of the portal pressure using propranolol 80–160 mg/day is the best initial treatment. If this is ineffective, a TIPSS procedure can be undertaken.

PULMONARY MANIFESTATIONS OF CHRONIC LIVER DISEASE

HEPATOPULMONARY SYNDROME

Many patients with cirrhosis are hypoxaemic due to a variety of factors, including pulmonary hypertension (see below), pleural effusions and the hepatopulmonary syndrome. The latter is characterised by resistant hypoxaemia (PaO_2 < 9.3 kPa or 70 mmHg), intrapulmonary vascular dilatation and chronic liver disease with portal hypertension. Clinical features include digital clubbing, cyanosis, spider naevi and a characteristic reduction in arterial oxygen saturation on standing. The hypoxia is due to intrapulmonary shunting through direct arteriovenous communications. It is believed that nitric oxide overproduction may be important, as exhaled NO correlates with the severity of hypoxia. The hepatopulmonary syndrome is now considered an indication for liver transplantation but, if severe (PaO_2 < 6.7 kPa or 50 mmHg), is associated with increased operative risk.

PORTOPULMONARY HYPERTENSION

This unusual complication of portal hypertension is similar to 'primary pulmonary hypertension' (p. 728) and is defined as pulmonary hypertension with increased pulmonary vascular resistance and a normal pulmonary artery wedge pressure in a patient with portal hypertension. It is caused by vasoconstriction and obliteration of the pulmonary arterial system and leads to breathlessness and fatigue.

VIRAL HEPATITIS

This is a common cause of jaundice and must be considered in anyone presenting with hepatitic liver blood tests (high transaminases). The causes are listed in Box 23.34.

All these viruses cause illnesses with similar clinical and pathological features and which are frequently anicteric or even asymptomatic. They differ in their tendency to cause acute and chronic infections. The features of the major hepatitis viruses are shown in Box 23.35.

Clinical features of acute infection

A non-specific prodromal illness characterised by headache, myalgia, arthralgia, nausea and anorexia usually precedes the development of jaundice by a few days to 2 weeks. Vomiting and diarrhoea may follow and abdominal discomfort is common. Dark urine and pale stools may precede jaundice. There are usually few physical signs. The liver is often tender but only minimally enlarged. Occa-

23.34 CAUSES OF VIRAL HEPATITIS	
Common	
● Hepatitis A	● Hepatitis C
● Hepatitis B ± hepatitis D	● Hepatitis E
Less common	
● Cytomegalovirus	● Epstein–Barr virus
Rare	
● Herpes simplex	● Yellow fever

23.35 FEATURES OF THE MAIN HEPATITIS VIRUSES					
	Hepatitis A	**Hepatitis B**	**Hepatitis C**	**Hepatitis D**	**Hepatitis E**
Virus					
Group	Enterovirus	Hepadna	Flavivirus	Incomplete virus	Calicivirus
Nucleic acid	RNA	DNA	RNA	RNA	RNA
Size (diameter)	27 nm	42 nm	30–38 nm	35 nm	27 nm
Incubation (weeks)	2–4	4–20	2–26	6–9	3–8
Spread					
Faeces	Yes	No	No	No	Yes
Blood	Uncommon	Yes	Yes	Yes	No
Saliva	Yes	Yes	Yes	?	?
Sexual	Uncommon	Yes	Uncommon	Yes	?
Vertical	No	Yes	Uncommon	Yes	No
Chronic infection	No	Yes	Yes	Yes	No
Prevention					
Active	Vaccine	Vaccine	No	Prevented by	No
Passive	Immune serum globulin	Hyperimmune serum globulin	No	hepatitis B vaccination	No

Note All body fluids are potentially infectious, although some (e.g. urine) are less infectious than others.

23

sionally, mild splenomegaly and cervical lymphadenopathy are seen. These are more frequent in children or those with Epstein–Barr virus infection.

Jaundice may be mild and the diagnosis may be suspected only after finding abnormal liver blood tests in the setting of non-specific symptoms. Symptoms rarely last longer than 3–6 weeks.

Investigations

A hepatitic pattern of LFTs develops, with serum transaminases typically between 200 and 2000 U/l. The plasma bilirubin reflects the degree of liver damage. The alkaline phosphatase rarely exceeds twice the upper limit of normal. Prolongation of the prothrombin time indicates the severity of the hepatitis but, except in rare cases of acute liver failure, rarely exceeds 25 sec. The white cell count is usually normal with a relative lymphocytosis. Serological tests confirm the aetiology of the infection.

Complications

Although recognised (Box 23.36), these are rare.

23.36 COMPLICATIONS OF ACUTE VIRAL HEPATITIS

- Acute liver failure
- Cholestatic hepatitis
- Aplastic anaemia
- Chronic liver disease and cirrhosis (hepatitis B and C)
- Relapsing hepatitis

Management

Most individuals do not need hospital care. Drugs such as sedatives and narcotics, which are metabolised in the liver, should be avoided. No specific dietary modifications are needed. Alcohol should be avoided during the acute illness. Elective surgery should be avoided in cases of acute viral hepatitis as there is a risk of post-operative liver failure.

Liver transplantation

This is very rarely indicated for acute viral hepatitis complicated by liver failure but is commonly performed for complications of cirrhosis resulting from chronic hepatitis B and C infection.

SPECIFIC VIRAL HEPATITIS

Although the hepatitis viruses all cause similar hepatic illnesses they belong to distinct viral groups.

HEPATITIS A

The hepatitis A virus (HAV) belongs to the picornavirus group of enteroviruses. HAV is highly infectious and is spread by the faecal–oral route. Infected individuals, who may be asymptomatic, excrete the virus in faeces for about 2–3 weeks before the onset of symptoms and then for a further 2 weeks or so. Infection is common in children but often asymptomatic, and so up to 30% of adults will have

serological evidence of past infection but give no history of jaundice. Infection is also more common in areas of overcrowding and poor sanitation. In occasional outbreaks water and shellfish have been the vehicles of transmission. In contrast to hepatitis B, a chronic carrier state does not occur.

Investigations

Only one HAV antigen has been found; individuals infected with HAV make an antibody to this antigen (anti-HAV). Anti-HAV is important in diagnosis as HAV is only present in the blood transiently during the incubation period. Excretion in the stools occurs for only 7–14 days after the onset of the clinical illness and the virus cannot be grown readily. Anti-HAV of IgM type, indicating a primary immune response, is already present in the blood at the onset of the clinical illness and is diagnostic of an acute HAV infection. Titres of this antibody fall to low levels within about 3 months of recovery. Anti-HAV of IgG type is of no diagnostic value as HAV infection is common and this antibody persists for years after infection, but it can be used to measure the prevalence of HAV infection. Its presence indicates immunity to HAV.

Prevention

Infection in the community is best prevented by improving social conditions, especially overcrowding and poor sanitation. Individuals can be given substantial protection from infection by active immunisation with an inactivated virus vaccine.

Immunisation should be considered for individuals with chronic hepatitis B or C infections. Immediate protection can be provided by immune serum globulin if this is given soon after exposure to the virus. The protective effect of immune serum globulin is attributed to its anti-HAV content. Immunisation should be considered for those at particular risk such as close contacts, the elderly, those with other major disease and perhaps pregnant women.

Immune serum globulin can be effective in an outbreak of hepatitis, in a school or nursery, as injection of those at risk prevents secondary spread to families. People travelling to endemic areas are best protected by vaccination.

Prognosis

Acute liver failure complicates acute hepatitis A in only 0.1% of cases and chronic infection does not occur. However, HAV infection in patients with chronic liver disease may cause serious or life-threatening disease. In adults a cholestatic phase with elevated alkaline phosphatase levels may complicate infection.

HEPATITIS B

The hepatitis B virus consists of a core containing DNA and a DNA polymerase enzyme needed for virus replication. The core of the virus is surrounded by surface protein (Fig. 23.25). The virus, also called a Dane particle, and an excess of its surface protein (known as hepatitis B surface antigen) circulate in the blood. Humans are the only source of infection.

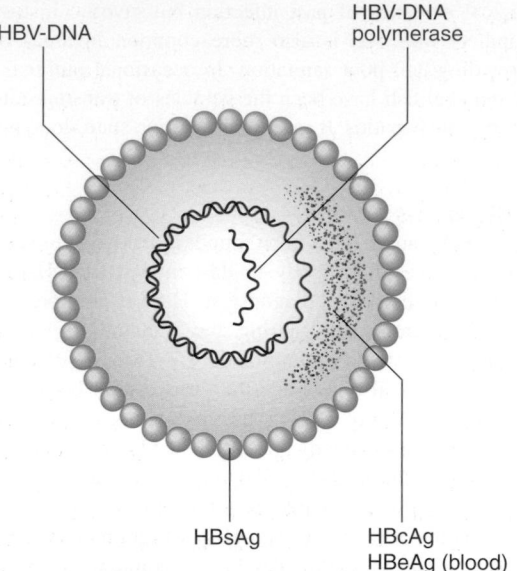

Fig. 23.25 Schematic diagram of hepatitis B virus. Hepatitis B surface antigen (HBsAg) is a protein which makes up part of the viral envelope. Hepatitis B core antigen (HBcAg) is a protein which makes up the capsid or core part of the virus (found in the liver but not in blood). Hepatitis B e antigen (HBeAg) is part of the HBcAg which can be found in the blood and indicates infectivity.

23

Hepatitis B infection affects 300 million people and is one of the most common causes of chronic liver disease and hepatocellular carcinoma world-wide.

Hepatitis B may cause an acute viral hepatitis; however, the acute infection is often asymptomatic, particularly when acquired at birth. Many individuals with chronic hepatitis B are also asymptomatic. Chronic hepatitis, associated with elevated serum transaminases, may occur and can lead to cirrhosis, usually after decades of infection (Fig. 23.26).

The risk of progression to chronic liver disease depends on the source of infection (Box 23.37). Vertical transmission, from mother to child in the perinatal period, is the most common cause of infection world-wide and carries the highest risk.

23.37 SOURCE OF HEPATITIS B INFECTION AND RISK OF CHRONIC INFECTION	
Route of transmission	Risk of chronic infection
Horizontal transmission Injection drug use Infected unscreened blood products Tattoos/acupuncture needles Sexual (homosexual and heterosexual)	10%
Vertical transmission HbsAg-positive mother	90%

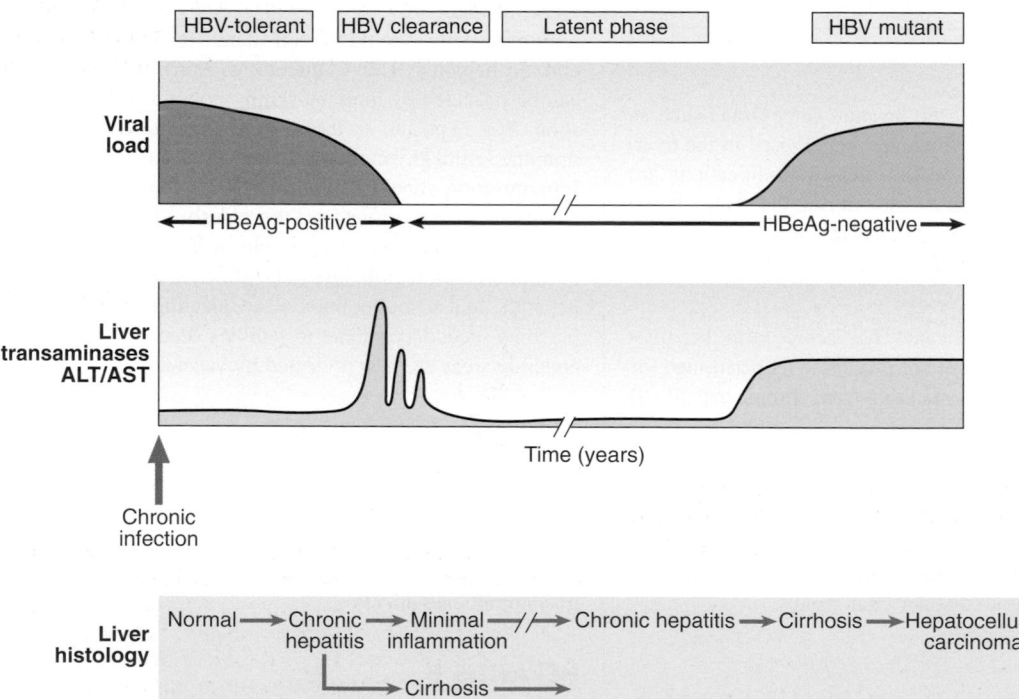

Fig. 23.26 Natural history of chronic hepatitis B infection. There is an initial immunotolerant phase with high levels of virus and normal liver biochemistry. An immunological response to the virus then occurs, with elevation in serum transaminases which causes liver damage: chronic hepatitis. If this response is sustained over many years and viral clearance does not occur promptly, chronic hepatitis may result in cirrhosis. In individuals where the immunological response is successful, viral load falls, HBe antibody develops and there is no further liver damage. Some individuals may subsequently develop HBV-DNA mutants, which escape from immune regulation, and viral load again rises with further chronic hepatitis. Mutations in the core protein result in the virus's inability to secrete HBe antigen despite high levels of viral replication; such individuals have HBeAg-negative chronic hepatitis. (ALT = alanine aminotransferase; AST = aspartate aminotransferase)

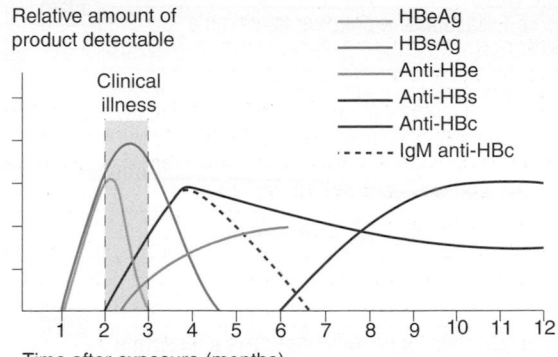

Fig. 23.27 Serological responses to hepatitis B virus infection.
(HBsAg = hepatitis B surface antigen; anti-HBs = antibody to HBsAg; HBeAg = hepatitis B e antigen; anti-HBe = antibody to HBeAg; anti-HBc = antibody to hepatitis B core antigen)

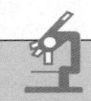

23.38 INTERPRETATION OF MAIN INVESTIGATIONS USED IN THE SEROLOGICAL DIAGNOSIS OF HEPATITIS B VIRUS INFECTION				
		Anti-HBc		
Interpretation	HBsAg	IgM	IgG	Anti-HBs
Incubation period	+	+	−	−
Acute hepatitis				
Early	+	+	−	−
Established	+	+	+	−
Established (occasional)	−	+	+	−
Convalescence				
(3–6 months)	−	±	+	±
(6–9 months)	−	−	+	+
Post-infection				
> 1 year	−	−	+	+
Uncertain	−	−	+	−
Chronic infection				
Usual	+	−	+	−
Occasional	−	−	+	−
Immunisation without infection	−	−	−	+
+ positive; − negative; ± present at low titre or absent.				

Investigations

Serology

HBV contains several antigens to which infected persons can make immune responses (Fig. 23.27); these antigens and their antibodies are important in identifying HBV infection (Box 23.38).

In acute infection the hepatitis B surface antigen (HBsAg) is a reliable marker of HBV infection, and a negative test for HBsAg makes HBV infection very unlikely but not impossible (Fig. 23.27). HBsAg appears in the blood late in the incubation period and before the prodromal phase of acute type B hepatitis; it may be present for only a few days, disappearing even before jaundice has developed, but usually lasts for 3–4 weeks and can persist for up to 5 months.

Antibody to HBsAg (anti-HBs) usually appears after about 3–6 months and persists for many years or perhaps permanently. Anti-HBs implies either a previous infection, in which case anti-HBc (see below) is usually also present, or previous vaccination when anti-HBc is not present.

The hepatitis B core antigen (HBcAg) is not found in the blood, but antibody to it (anti-HBc) appears early in the illness and rapidly reaches a high titre which then subsides gradually but persists. Anti-HBc is initially of IgM type with IgG antibody appearing later. Anti-HBc (IgM) can sometimes reveal an acute HBV infection when the HBsAg has disappeared and before anti-HBs has developed (Fig. 23.27 and Box 23.38).

The hepatitis B e antigen (HBeAg) appears only transiently at the outset of the illness and is followed by the production of antibody (anti-HBe). The HBeAg reflects active replication of the virus in the liver. The persistence of HBsAg for longer than 6 months indicates chronic infection.

Chronic HBV infection (see below) is marked by the presence of HBsAg and anti-HBc (IgG) in the blood. Usually, HBeAg or anti-HBe is also present; HBeAg indicates continued active replication of the virus in the liver while anti-HBe implies that replication is occurring at a much lower level or that HBV-DNA has become integrated into host hepatocyte DNA.

Viral load

HBV-DNA can be measured by polymerase chain reaction (PCR) in the blood. Viral loads are usually in excess of 10^5 copies/ml in the presence of active viral replication, as indicated by the presence of e antigen. In contrast, in those with low viral replication, HBsAg- and anti-HBe-positive, viral loads are less than 10^5 copies/ml. The exception is in patients who have a mutation in the pre-core protein, which

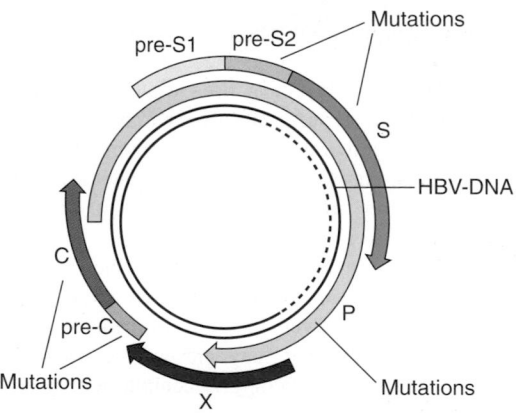

Fig. 23.28 The site of HBV-DNA mutations. HBV-DNA encodes four proteins: a DNA polymerase needed for viral replication (P), a surface protein (S), a core protein (C) and an X protein. The pre-C and C regions encode a core protein and an e antigen. Although mutations in the hepatitis B virus are frequent occurrences, certain mutations have important clinical effects. Pre-C encodes a signal sequence needed for the C protein to be secreted from the liver cell into serum as e antigen. A mutation in the pre-core region leads to a failure of secretion of e antigen into serum and so individuals have high levels of viral production but no detectable e antigen in the serum. Mutations can also occur in the surface protein and may lead to the failure of vaccination (surface antibodies produced against native S protein) to prevent infection. Mutations also occur in the DNA polymerase during antiviral treatment with lamivudine.

means they cannot secrete e antigen into serum (Fig. 23.28). Such individuals will be anti-HBe-positive but have a high viral load and often evidence of chronic hepatitis. These mutations are common in the Far East and those affected are classified as having e antigen-negative chronic hepatitis. They respond differently to antiviral drugs from those with classical e antigen-positive chronic hepatitis.

Measurement of viral load is important in monitoring antiviral therapy and identifying patients with pre-core mutants. Specific HBV genotypes can also be identified using PCR. Genotypes B and C appear to have more aggressive disease that responds less well to antiviral therapy.

Management

Acute hepatitis B

Treatment is supportive with monitoring for acute liver failure, which occurs in less than 1% of cases.

Chronic hepatitis B

Treatments are still limited, with no drug able to eradicate hepatitis B infection completely. The indication for treatment is a high viral load in the presence of active hepatitis, as demonstrated by elevated serum transaminases and/or histological evidence of inflammation.

Alfa-interferon. This is most effective in selected patients with a low viral load and serum transaminases greater than twice the upper limit of normal in whom it acts by augmenting a native immune response. In HBeAg-positive chronic hepatitis 33% lose e antigen after 4–6 months of treatment compared to 12% of controls. Response rates are lower in HBeAg-negative chronic hepatitis, even when patients are given longer courses of treatment. Interferon is contraindicated in the presence of cirrhosis as it may cause a flare in serum transaminases and precipitate liver failure. Longer-acting pegylated interferons which can be given once weekly have been evaluated in both HBeAg-positive and HBeAg-negative chronic hepatitis (Box 23.39). Other antiviral therapies are required because many patients with chronic hepatitis B have high levels of viraemia and/or low transaminase levels and are not therefore candidates for interferon.

Lamivudine. This is a nucleoside analogue which inhibits DNA polymerase and suppresses HBV-DNA levels. It is effective in improving liver function in patients with decompensated cirrhosis and may prevent the need for transplantation. Long-term therapy is complicated by the

---

23.39 PEGYLATED INTERFERONS IN CHRONIC HEPATITIS B INFECTION EBM

'In HBeAg-positive chronic hepatitis treatment with pegylated interferon for 6 months eliminates HBeAg in 35%, and normalises liver biochemistry in 25% of patients. In HBeAg-negative chronic hepatitis treatment with pegylated interferon for 12 months leads to normal liver biochemistry in 60%, and sustained suppression of hepatitis B virus load below 400 copies/ml in 20% of patients.'

● Cooksley WG, et al. J Viral Hep 2003; 10:298–302.
● Marcellin P. N Engl J Med 2004; 351:1206–1217.

For further information: 🖥 www.aasld.org

23.40 LAMIVUDINE IN CHRONIC HEPATITIS B INFECTION EBM

'48 weeks of treatment with lamivudine induces anti-HBe seroconversion in 27% of patients with HBeAg-positive chronic hepatitis, despite 38% developing HBV-DNA polymerase mutations. Treatment also improves histology and liver biochemistry.'

● Liaw YF, et al. Gastroenterology 2001; 121:1027–1028.

For further information: 🖥 www.aasld.org

23.41 ADEFOVIR IN CHRONIC HEPATITIS B INFECTION EBM

'In HBeAg-positive chronic hepatitis treatment with 10 mg of adefovir for 48 weeks produces normal liver biochemistry in 48% (NNT_B 3), suppresses serum HBV-DNA in 39% (NNT_B 5) and leads to e antigen seroconversion in 14% (NNT_B 16) of patients. In HBeAg-negative chronic hepatitis treatment with adefovir for 48 weeks reduces ALT to normal in 72% (NNT_B 2.3) and renders serum HBV-DNA undetectable in 55% (NNT_B 2) of patients.'

● Hadiziyannis SJ, et al. N Engl J Med 2003; 348:800–807.
● Marcellini P, et al. N Engl J Med 2003; 348:808–816.

For further information: 🖥 www.aasld.org

---

development of HBV-DNA polymerase mutants which may occur after 9 months of treatment and is characterised by a rise in viral load during treatment. These viral mutants are less hepatotoxic than native virus so the drug can often be continued (Box 23.40). Flares in transaminases occur when lamivudine is stopped if mutant virus is present, as native virus replaces mutant virus.

Adefovir. This is a nucleotide analogue that is phosphorylated to yield active drug which inhibits HBV-DNA polymerase. It reduces HBV-DNA levels by 3–4 logs, enhances the frequency of HBeAg seroconversion and leads to histological improvement, but is contraindicated in renal failure. The HBV-DNA mutants develop at a lower rate than with lamivudine, 2% being identified after 2 years of treatment (Box 23.41). Relapse occurs on stopping treatment and the optimum length of treatment remains unknown. Adefovir is effective in suppressing most of the lamivudine-induced DNA polymerase mutant viruses.

Other drugs. Other drugs which are currently been studied in chronic hepatitis B include tenofovir, which has anti-HIV efficacy, and L-deoxythymidine. The role of combination antiviral therapy, as used in HIV infection, is still unclear.

Liver transplantation. Historically, liver transplantation was contraindicated in the presence of hepatitis B because infection often recurred in the graft. However, the use of post-liver transplant prophylaxis with lamivudine and hepatitis B immunoglobulins has reduced the reinfection rate to 10% and increased 5-year survival to 80%, making transplantation an acceptable treatment option in selected cases.

Prevention

Individuals are most infectious when markers of continuing viral replication, such as HBeAg, and high levels of

HBV-DNA are present in the blood; they are least infectious when only anti-HBe is present with low levels of virus. HBV-DNA can be found in saliva, urine, semen and vaginal secretions. The virus is about ten times more infectious than hepatitis C, which in turn is about ten times more infectious than HIV.

A recombinant hepatitis B vaccine containing HBsAg is available (Engerix) and is capable of producing active immunisation in 95% of normal individuals. The vaccine gives a high degree of protection and should be offered to those at special risk of infection who are not already immune, as evidenced by anti-HBs in the blood (Box 23.42). The vaccine is ineffective in those already infected by HBV. Infection can also be prevented or minimised by the intramuscular injection of hyperimmune serum globulin prepared from blood containing anti-HBs. This should be given within 24 hours, or at most a week, of exposure to infected blood in circumstances likely to cause infection (e.g. needlestick injury, contamination of cuts or mucous membranes). Vaccine can be given together with hyper-immune globulin (active-passive immunisation).

Neonates born to hepatitis B-infected mothers should be immunised at birth and given immunoglobulin. Hepatitis B serology should then be checked at 12 months of age.

Prognosis

Acute hepatitis

Full recovery occurs in 90–95% of adults following acute HBV infection. The remaining 5–10% develop a chronic infection which usually continues for life, although later recovery occasionally occurs. Infection passing from mother to child at birth leads to chronic infection in the child in 90% of cases and recovery is rare. Chronic infection is also common in immunodeficient individuals such as those with Down's syndrome or HIV infection.

Recovery from acute HBV infection occurs within 6 months and is characterised by the appearance of antibody to viral antigens. Persistence of HBeAg beyond this time indicates chronic infection. Combined HBV and HDV infection causes more aggressive disease.

Chronic infection

Most patients with chronic hepatitis B are asymptomatic and develop complications such as cirrhosis and hepatocellular carcinoma only after many years (Fig. 23.26). Cirrhosis develops in 15–20% of patients with chronic HBV over 5–20 years. This proportion is higher in those who are e antigen-positive.

HEPATITIS D (DELTA VIRUS)

The hepatitis D virus (HDV) is an RNA-defective virus which has no independent existence; it requires HBV for replication and has the same sources and modes of spread. It can infect individuals simultaneously with HBV, or can superinfect those who are already chronic carriers of HBV. Simultaneous infections give rise to acute hepatitis which is often severe but is limited by recovery from the HBV infection. Infections in individuals who are chronic carriers of HBV can cause acute hepatitis with spontaneous recovery, and occasionally simultaneous cessation of the chronic HBV infection occurs. Chronic infection with HBV and HDV can also occur, and this frequently causes rapidly progressive chronic hepatitis and eventually cirrhosis.

HDV has a world-wide distribution. It is endemic in parts of the Mediterranean basin, Africa and South America, where transmission is mainly by close personal contact and occasionally by vertical transmission from mothers who also carry HBV. In non-endemic areas, transmission is mainly a consequence of parenteral drug misuse.

Investigations

HDV contains a single antigen to which infected individuals make an antibody (anti-HDV). Delta antigen appears in the blood only transiently, and in practice diagnosis depends on detecting anti-HDV. Simultaneous infection with HBV and HDV followed by full recovery is associated with the appearance of low titres of anti-HDV of IgM type within a few days of the onset of the illness. This antibody generally disappears within 2 months but persists in a few patients. Superinfection of patients with chronic HBV infection leads to the production of high titres of anti-HDV, initially IgM and later IgG. Such patients may then develop chronic infection with both viruses, in which case anti-HDV titres plateau at high levels.

Prevention

Preventing hepatitis B effectively prevents hepatitis D.

HEPATITIS C

This is caused by an RNA flavivirus. Primates have provided an animal model for infection as the virus has been difficult to grow in cell culture. Acute symptomatic infection with hepatitis C is rare. Most individuals will be unaware of when they became infected and are only identified when they develop chronic liver disease.

Eighty per cent of individuals exposed to the virus will become chronically infected and late spontaneous viral clearance is rare.

Hepatitis C is the cause of what used to be known as 'non-A, non-B hepatitis', a syndrome of acute hepatitis often with jaundice seen after a transfusion of blood or blood products. Following the identification of the virus in 1990, blood donors are now screened for infection in many parts of the world. New cases of post-transfusion hepatitis C no longer occur in the UK.

Hepatitis C infection is usually now identified in asymptomatic individuals screened because they have risk

23.43 RISK FACTORS FOR THE ACQUISITION OF CHRONIC HEPATITIS C INFECTION

- Intravenous drug misuse (95% of new cases in the UK)
- Unscreened blood products (before screening of donors, i.e. 1990 in UK)
- Vertical transmission (3% risk)
- Needlestick injury (3% risk)
- Iatrogenic parenteral transmission, i.e. unclean vaccination needles
- Sharing toothbrushes/razors

23.44 TREATMENT OF HEPATITIS C EBM

'The addition of ribavirin to pegylated α-interferon therapy improves the overall sustained virological response from 33% to 55%.'

- Manns MP, et al. Lancet 2001; 358:958–965.
- Hadziyannis SJ, et al. Ann Intern Med 2004; 140:346–553.

For further information: 🖥 www.nice.org.uk

factors for infection such as previous injection drug use (Box 23.43) or because they have incidentally been found to have abnormal liver blood tests. Although most individuals remain asymptomatic until progression to cirrhosis occurs, fatigue can complicate chronic infection and appears to be unrelated to the degree of liver damage.

Investigations

Serology and virology
HCV protein contains several antigens that give rise to antibodies in an infected person which are used in diagnosis. It may take 6–12 weeks for antibodies to appear in the blood following acute infection such as a needlestick injury. In these cases hepatitis C RNA can be identified in the blood as early as 2–4 weeks after infection. Active infection is confirmed by the presence of serum hepatitis C RNA in anyone who is antibody-positive.

Genotype
There are six common viral genotypes whose distribution varies world-wide. Genotype has no effect on progression of liver disease but does affect response to treatment. Genotype 1 is most common in northern Europe and is less easy to eradicate with current treatments.

Liver function tests
LFTs may be normal or show fluctuating serum transaminases with ALT between 50 and 200 U/l. Jaundice is rare and only usually appears in end-stage cirrhosis.

Liver histology
Serum transaminase levels in hepatitis C are a poor predictor of the degree of liver fibrosis which has developed as a result of chronic viral hepatitis, and so a liver biopsy is often required to stage the degree of liver damage. Non-invasive methods of assessing liver fibrosis in hepatitis C infection remain an area of active research. The degree of inflammation and fibrosis can be scored histologically. The most common scoring system used in hepatitis C is the Metavir system, which scores fibrosis from 1 to 4, the latter equating to cirrhosis.

Management
The aim of treatment is to eradicate infection. The treatment of choice is pegylated α-interferon given weekly subcutaneously, together with oral ribavirin, a synthetic nucleotide analogue (Box 23.44). The length of treatment and efficacy depend on viral genotype. The main side-effect of ribavirin is haemolytic anaemia. Side-effects of interferon are

significant and include flu-like symptoms, irritability and depression which can affect quality of life. Virological relapse can occur in the first 3 months after stopping treatment and cure is defined as loss of virus from serum 6 months after completing therapy (sustained virological response, or SVR).

Liver transplantation should be considered when complications of cirrhosis occur, such as diuretic-resistant ascites. Unfortunately, hepatitis C almost always recurs in the transplanted liver and up to 15% will develop cirrhosis in the liver graft within 5 years of transplantation.

Prevention and prognosis
There is no active or passive protection against HCV. Progression from chronic hepatitis to cirrhosis occurs over 20–40 years. Risk factors for progression include male gender, immunosuppression (such as co-infection with HIV) and heavy alcohol misuse. Not everyone with hepatitis C infection will necessarily develop cirrhosis but approximately 20% do so within 20 years. Once cirrhosis has developed, the 5- and 10-year survival rates are 95% and 81% respectively. One-quarter of cirrhotics will develop complications within 10 years and, once complications like ascites have arisen, the 5-year survival is around 50%. Once cirrhosis is present, 2–5% per year will develop primary hepatocellular carcinoma.

HEPATITIS E

Hepatitis E is caused by an RNA virus which is endemic in India and the Middle East. In northern Europe infection is usually seen in travellers from an endemic area.

The clinical presentation of hepatitis E is similar to hepatitis A. It is spread via the faecal–oral route; in most cases it presents as a self-limiting acute hepatitis and does not cause chronic liver disease.

It differs from hepatitis A in that infection during pregnancy is associated with the development of acute liver failure, which has a high mortality.

Investigations
In acute infection IgM antibodies to HEV are positive.

Prevention
There is no active or passive immunity to hepatitis E.

OTHER FORMS OF VIRAL HEPATITIS

Non-A, non-B, non-C (NANBNC) or non-A–E hepatitis is the term used to describe hepatitis thought to be due to a virus that is not HAV, HBV, HCV or HEV. Other viruses which affect the liver probably do exist, but the hepatitis viruses described above now account for the majority of hepatitis virus infections. Cytomegalovirus and Epstein–Barr virus infection causes abnormal LFTs in most patients, and occasionally icteric hepatitis occurs. Herpes simplex is a rare cause of hepatitis in adults, and most of these patients are immunocompromised. Abnormal LFTs are also common in chickenpox, measles, rubella and acute HIV infection.

ALCOHOLIC LIVER DISEASE

Alcohol remains one of the most common causes of chronic liver disease.

Epidemiology

The risk of alcoholic liver disease is variable and not everyone who drinks heavily will develop liver disease. Only 10% of alcoholics have evidence of cirrhosis at post-mortem. Alcoholic liver disease does not occur below a threshold of 21 units/week in women and 28 units/week in men (Box 23.45). Most individuals with liver disease will have drunk heavily for more than 5 years.

Although the average alcohol consumption of an individual with cirrhosis is 160 g/day for an average of 8 years, there is no clear linear relationship between dose and liver damage.

Some of the risk factors for alcoholic liver disease are:

23.45 AMOUNT OF ALCOHOL IN AN AVERAGE DRINK

Alcohol type	% Alcohol by volume	Amount	Units*
Beer	3.5%	440 ml (1 pint)	2
	9%	440 ml (1 pint)	4
Wine	10%	125 ml	1
Vodka/rum	37.5%	25 ml	1
'Alcopops'	6%	330 ml	2
*1 unit = 8 g.			

- *Drinking patterns.* Type of beverage drunk does not affect risk, but liver damage is more likely to occur in continuous rather than binge drinkers.
- *Gender.* The incidence of alcoholic liver disease is increasing in women, who often conceal alcohol misuse and have higher blood ethanol levels than men after drinking because their body mass is lower.
- *Genetics.* Alcoholism is more common in monozygotic than dizygotic twins. However, polymorphisms in the gene-coding enzymes involved in alcohol metabolism, tumour necrosis factor-alpha (TNF-α) and aldehyde dehydrogenase (ALD), have yet to be linked to alcoholic liver disease.
- *Nutrition.* Animals given a choline-deficient diet are more likely to develop alcoholic liver disease.

Aetiology

Alcohol is metabolised almost exclusively by the liver.

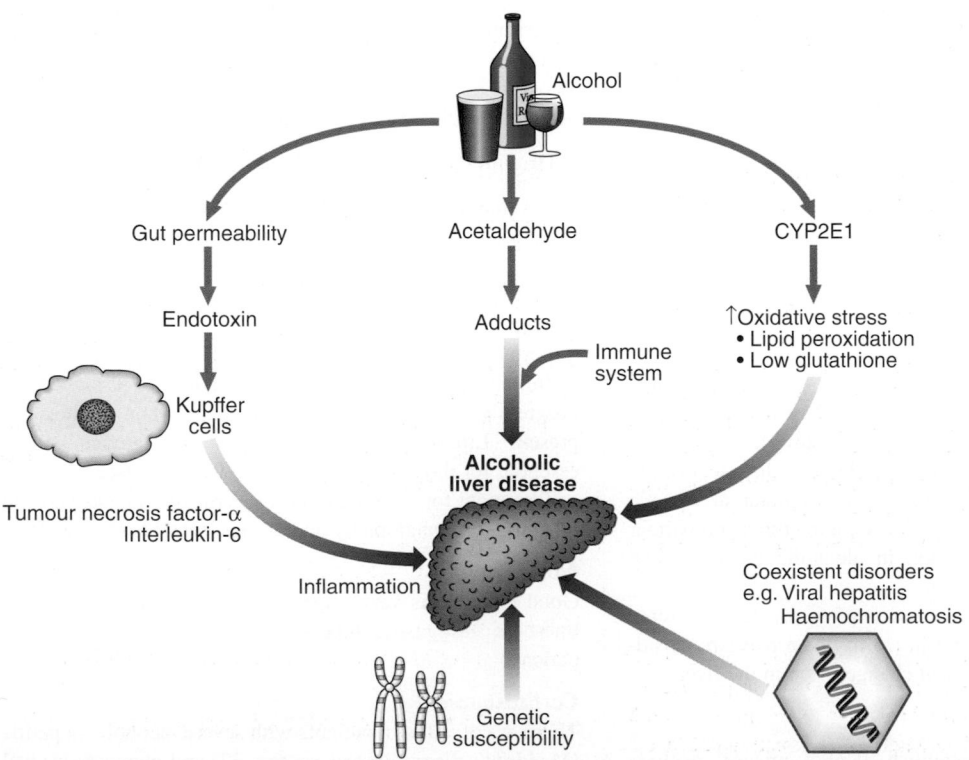

Fig. 23.29 Factors involved in the pathogenesis of alcoholic liver disease.

23.46 PATHOLOGICAL FEATURES OF ALCOHOLIC LIVER DISEASE	

• Alcoholic hepatitis
  Lipogranuloma
  Neutrophil infiltration
  Mallory's hyaline
  Pericellular fibrosis
	• Macrovesicular steatosis
	• Fibrosis and cirrhosis
	• Central hyaline sclerosis

Acetaldehyde

Eighty per cent of alcohol is metabolised to acetaldehyde by the mitochondrial enzyme, alcohol dehydrogenase (ADH). Acetaldehyde forms adducts with cellular proteins in hepatocytes which activate the immune system, leading to cell injury.

Acetaldehyde is then metabolised to acetyl coA and acetate by ALD. This generates NADH from NAD (nicotinamide adenine dinucleotide) which changes the redox potential of the cell.

Twenty per cent of alcohol is metabolised by the mixed function oxidase enzymes of the smooth endoplasmic reticulum. Cytochrome CYP2E1 is induced by alcohol, which increases oxygen consumption and lipid peroxidation. Microsomal peroxidation leads to oxygen free radicals which can induce mitochondrial damage.

The mechanisms leading to specific liver lesions of alcoholic liver disease are still poorly understood.

Cytokines

Increased endotoxin is released into the blood in alcoholic hepatitis via increased gut permeability. TNF-α production is increased from monocytes. Release of IL-1, 2 and 8 also occurs. These cytokines are also involved in fibrogenesis (Fig. 23.29).

Pathology

The pathological features of alcoholic liver disease are shown in Box 23.46. In about 80% of patients with severe alcoholic hepatitis, cirrhosis will coexist at presentation. Iron deposition is common and does not necessarily indicate haemochromatosis. Figure 23.31 (p. 972) shows the histological features of alcoholic liver disease, which are identical to those of non-alcoholic steatohepatitis.

Clinical features

Alcoholic liver disease manifests itself as a clinical spectrum ranging from incidental abnormal liver biochemistry with few physical signs to advanced cirrhosis. The liver is often enlarged in alcoholic liver disease, even in the presence of cirrhosis. Peripheral stigmata of chronic liver disease, including Dupytren's contractures and palmar erythema, are more common in alcoholic cirrhosis than cirrhosis of other aetiologies.

The spectrum of liver disease is often divided into three syndromes (Box 23.47) but in reality these overlap considerably, as do the pathological changes seen in the liver.

Investigations

Investigations aim to establish alcohol misuse, exclude alternative or coexistent causes of liver disease, such as

23.47 CLINICAL SYNDROMES OF ALCOHOLIC LIVER DISEASE	
Fatty liver	
• Asymptomatic abnormal liver biochemistry • Normal/large liver	
Alcoholic hepatitis	
• Jaundice • Malnutrition • Hepatomegaly • Features of portal hypertension (e.g. ascites, encephalopathy)	
Cirrhosis	
• Stigmata of chronic liver disease • Large, normal or small liver • Ascites/varices/encephalopathy • Hepatocellular carcinoma	

hepatitis C or haemochromatosis, and assess the severity of liver disease. The clinical history from patient, relatives and friends is most important in establishing alcohol misuse, duration and severity. Biological markers, particularly macrocytosis in the absence of anaemia, may suggest and support a history of alcohol misuse. A raised GGT is not specific for alcohol misuse and will be elevated in the presence of hepatic steatosis and fibrosis. The level may not therefore return to normal with abstinence if chronic liver disease is present. Unexplained rib fractures, particularly bilateral, on a chest X-ray are also suggestive of alcohol misuse.

The presence of jaundice suggests alcoholic hepatitis. Determining the extent of liver damage often requires a liver biopsy.

Prothrombin time and bilirubin can be used to give a 'discriminant function' (DF), also known as the Maddrey's score, which enables the clinician to assess prognosis in alcoholic hepatitis (PT = prothrombin time. Serum bilirubin in μmol/l is divided by 17 to convert to mg/dl):

$$DF = [4.6 \times \text{Increase in PT (sec)}] + \text{Bilirubin (mg/dl)}$$

A value over 32 implies severe liver disease with a poor prognosis.

Management

Cessation of alcohol consumption is the single most important treatment; without this all other therapies are of limited value. Abstinence is even effective at preventing progression of liver disease and death when cirrhosis is present. Life-long abstinence is the best advice and is essential for those with more severe liver disease.

Treatment for complications of cirrhosis, such as variceal bleeding, encephalopathy and ascites, may also be needed.

Nutrition

Good nutrition is very important and enteral feeding via a fine-bore nasogastric tube may be needed in severely ill patients.

Corticosteroids

These are of value in patients with severe alcoholic hepatitis (Maddrey's discriminative score > 32) and increase survival (Box 23.48). Sepsis is the main side-effect of steroids, and

23

23.48 CORTICOSTEROIDS IN ALCOHOLIC HEPATITIS	EBM

'In severe alcoholic hepatitis corticosteroids improve survival at 28 days from 65% to 85% (NNT_B 5).'

● Mathurin P, et al. J Hepatol 2002; 36:480–487.

For further information: 💻 www.aasld.org

23.49 PENTOXIFYLLINE IN ALCOHOLIC HEPATITIS	EBM

'In severe alcoholic hepatitis, oral pentoxifylline reduces inpatient mortality, particularly from hepatorenal failure, from 46% to 25% (NNT_B 5).'

● Akriviadis E, et al. Gastroenterology 2000; 119:1637–1648.

For further information: 💻 www.aasld.org

existing sepsis and variceal haemorrhage are the main contraindication to their use. If the bilirubin has not fallen 7 days after starting steroids, they are unlikely to reduce mortality and should be stopped.

Pentoxifylline

Pentoxifylline, which has a weak anti-TNF action, may be beneficial in severe alcoholic hepatitis. It appears to reduce the incidence of hepatorenal failure and its use is not complicated by sepsis (Box 23.49).

Liver transplantation

The role of liver transplantation in the management of alcoholic liver disease remains controversial. In many centres, however, alcoholic liver disease is a common indication for liver transplantation. The challenge is to identify patients with an unacceptable risk of returning to harmful alcohol consumption. Many programmes require a 6-month period of abstinence from alcohol before a patient is considered for transplantation. Although this relates poorly to the incidence of alcohol relapse after transplantation, liver function may improve to the extent that transplantation is no longer necessary. The outcome of transplantation for alcoholic liver disease is good (if the patient remains abstinent) because patients often require minimal immunosuppression and there is no risk of disease recurrence. Transplantation for alcoholic hepatitis has a poorer outcome than for complications of alcoholic cirrhosis.

Prognosis

The most important prognostic factor is the patient's ability to stop drinking alcohol. General health and life expectancy are improved when this occurs, irrespective of the form of alcoholic liver disease.

Alcoholic fatty liver disease

This has a good prognosis and steatosis usually disappears after 3 months of abstinence.

Alcoholic hepatitis

This has a significantly worse prognosis. About one-third of patients die in the acute episode, particularly those with hepatic encephalopathy or a prothrombin time sufficiently prolonged to exclude a percutaneous liver biopsy. Cirrhosis, if not already present, will occur if drinking continues. Patients with acute alcoholic hepatitis often deteriorate during the first 1–3 weeks in hospital. Even if they abstain, it may take up to 6 months for jaundice to resolve. In patients presenting with jaundice who subsequently abstain, the 3- and 5-year survival is 70%. In contrast, those who continue to drink have 3- and 5-year survival rates of 60% and 34% respectively.

Alcoholic cirrhosis

This often presents with a serious complication such as variceal haemorrhage or ascites, and only half of such patients will survive 5 years from presentation. However, most who survive the initial illness and who become abstinent will survive beyond 5 years.

NON-ALCOHOLIC FATTY LIVER DISEASE

Non-alcoholic fatty liver disease (NAFLD) is a disease of affluent societies and its prevalence is increasing in proportion to the rise in obesity. It has become the most common cause of chronic liver disease after hepatitis B, hepatitis C and alcohol. It can be classified into simple fatty liver disease (or non-alcoholic fatty liver, NAFL) and non-alcoholic steatohepatitis (NASH). The former has a benign prognosis but the latter is associated with fibrosis and progression to cirrhosis.

Epidemiology

NAFLD affects about 3% of the population in the USA. The prevalence is higher in those with diabetes and those with the metabolic syndrome (p. 1112). Rare causes of NAFLD include tamoxifen, amiodarone and exposure to certain petrochemicals. NAFLD has also been reported following weight-reducing jejenal bypass surgery. Many cases of cirrhosis that were previously labelled cryptogenic (i.e. cause unknown) are now thought to be due to NAFLD.

Aetiology and pathogenesis

Most individuals with NAFLD have insulin resistance but not necessarily overt glucose intolerance. The current two-hit hypothesis (Fig. 23.30) explains why not everyone with fatty liver disease develops hepatic fibrosis. The 'first hit' results in steatosis (fatty liver), which is only complicated by inflammation if a 'second hit occurs'. Leptin is probably then needed to cause hepatic fibrosis.

Clinical features

Most patients present with asymptomatic abnormal LFTs, particularly elevation of the transaminases or isolated elevation of the GGT. Occasionally, the condition presents with a complication of cirrhosis such as variceal haemorrhage or hepatocellular carcinoma. In contrast to alcoholic liver disease, jaundice only occurs when cirrhosis is established. NAFLD is the most likely diagnosis in a patient with elevated serum transaminases, no history of alcohol abuse and a negative chronic liver disease screen.

23

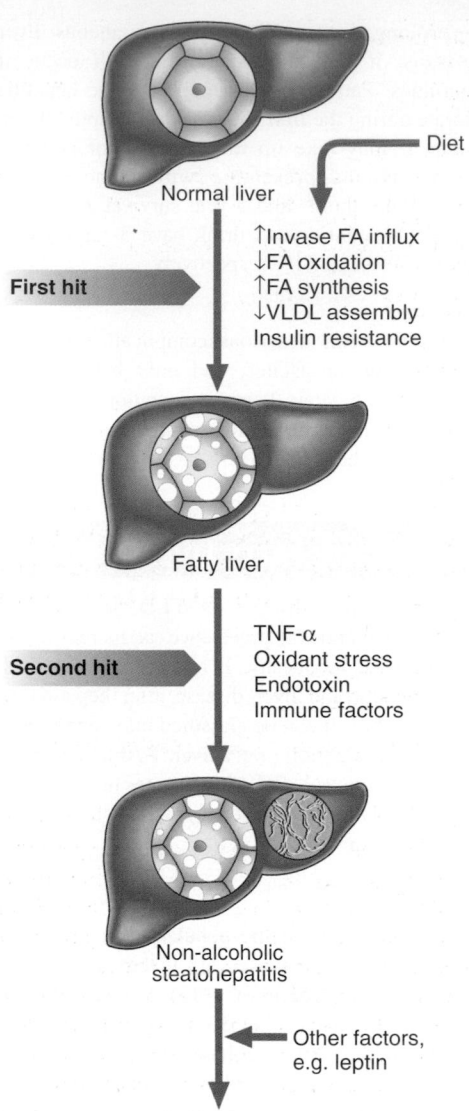

First hit

Diet

Normal liver

↑Invase FA influx
↓FA oxidation
↑FA synthesis
↓VLDL assembly
Insulin resistance

Fatty liver

Second hit

TNF-α
Oxidant stress
Endotoxin
Immune factors

Non-alcoholic
steatohepatitis

Other factors,
e.g. leptin

Fibrosis

Fig. 23.30 Pathogenesis of non-alcoholic fatty liver disease: the 'two-hit' hypothesis. Fatty liver occurs as a result of increased fat import into hepatocytes and reduced fat export. Insulin resistance causes hepatic steatosis, which also perpetuates insulin resistance. Subsequent activation of TNF-α, oxidant stress through the production of reactive oxygen species and production of endotoxin then results in inflammation and subsequently fibrosis. Factors including leptin are probably needed for fibrosis. (FA = fatty acids; VLDL = very low-density lipoproteins)

Investigations

Liver function tests

Unfortunately, there is no single diagnostic blood test; however, in contrast to alcoholic liver disease, the ALT is normally higher than the AST. Elevated alkaline phosphatase levels are seen in about 30% of cases. It is important to differentiate simple fatty liver disease (NAFL), which does not require follow-up, from NASH. Elevated serum transaminases greater than twice the upper limit of normal and the presence of the metabolic syndrome (hypertriglyceridaemia, hypertension, diabetes mellitus, an

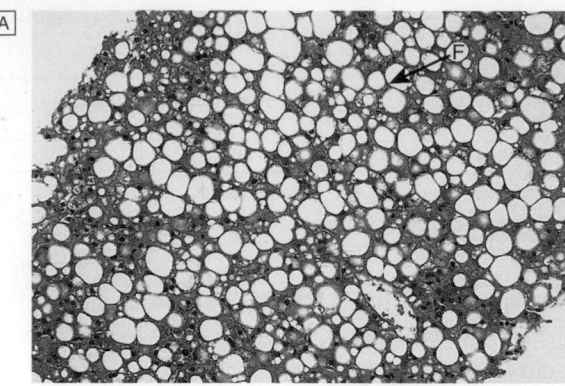

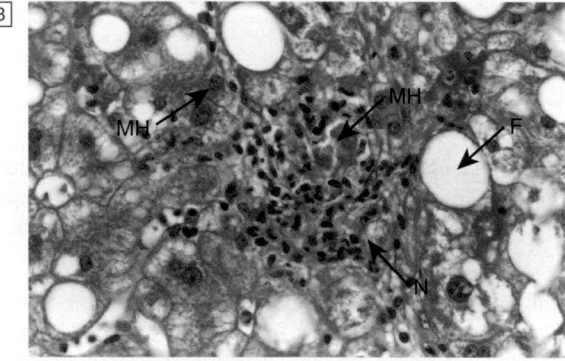

Fig. 23.31 Histology of non-alcoholic fatty liver disease.
Ⓐ Macroscopic steatosis (NAFL). Large fat droplets (F) fill hepatocytes but there is no inflammation. Ⓑ Non-alcoholic steatohepatitis at higher power. Fat (F) is associated with an inflammatory infiltrate of neutrophils (N) and dense pink Mallory's hyaline (MH).

elevated BMI > 25 and especially truncal obesity) are useful predictors of NASH.

Ultrasound

Ultrasound cannot differentiate simple fatty liver disease without fibrosis (NAFL) from NASH; in both cases the liver will appear bright on ultrasound.

Liver biopsy

Individuals with serum transaminases greater than twice the upper limit of normal and features of the metabolic syndrome should be offered a liver biopsy to determine whether inflammation and fibrosis are present. Histologically, fat deposition is usually macrovesicular (Fig. 23.31), in contrast to the microvesicular fat seen in acute fatty liver disease of pregnancy. NASH is characterised by fat, Mallory bodies, neutrophil infiltration and pericellular fibrosis. These features are indistinguishable histologically from alcoholic hepatitis, so a diagnosis of NASH relies on excluding alcohol misuse, the absence of jaundice, and the presence of risk factors such as obesity and diabetes. Fat often disappears by the time cirrhosis develops.

Management

Current treatments are aimed at reducing BMI and insulin resistance. Metformin has been shown to improve LFTs and should be the first-line treatment in type 2 diabetes with

23

NAFLD. Thiazolidinediones such as pioglitazone also improve LFTs in NAFLD and early data suggest they may improve inflammation and fibrosis. Weight loss will also reduce serum transaminase levels, improve liver fibrosis and reduce insulin resistance. Antioxidants such as vitamin E are not effective. There is no rationale for using HMG CoA reductase inhibitors (statins) in the treatment of NAFLD but they are not contraindicated for treatment of coexistent hyperlipidaemia.

Prognosis

Once cirrhosis has occurred, survival is similar to that in hepatitis C cirrhosis with 5- and 10-year survival rates of 90% and 84% respectively. Hepatocellular carcinoma frequently complicates NAFLD cirrhosis. Although less than 5% of liver transplants are currently performed for NAFLD, this is likely to increase. Unfortunately, the condition may recur in the graft.

DRUGS, TOXINS AND THE LIVER

The liver is the primary site of drug metabolism. Liver disease may affect the capacity of the liver to metabolise drugs and unexpected toxicity may occur when patients with liver disease are given drugs in normal doses (p. 26).

HEPATOTOXIC DRUG REACTIONS

Drug toxicity should be high in the differential diagnosis of acute liver failure, jaundice and abnormal liver biochemistry. Some typical patterns of drug toxicity are listed in Box 23.50; the most common picture is a mixed cholestatic hepatitis. The presence of jaundice indicates more severe liver damage. Although acute liver failure can occur, most drug reactions are acute and self-limiting; chronic liver damage is rare. LFTs often take weeks to return to normal following a drug-induced hepatitis and it may take months for them to normalise following a cholestatic hepatitis. Occasionally permanent bile duct loss (ductopenia) follows a cholestatic drug reaction, such as that due to co-amoxiclav, resulting in chronic cholestasis with persistent symptoms such as itching.

23.50 EXAMPLES OF COMMON CAUSES OF DRUG-INDUCED HEPATOTOXICITY	
Pattern	**Drug**
Cholestasis	Chlorpromazine High-dose oestrogens
Cholestatic hepatitis	NSAIDs Co-amoxiclav Statins
Acute hepatitis	Rifampicin Isoniazid
Non-alcoholic steatohepatitis	Amiodarone
Venous outflow obstruction	Busulfan Azathioprine
Fibrosis	Methotrexate

23.51 THE DIAGNOSIS OF ACUTE DRUG-INDUCED LIVER DISEASE

• Tabulate drugs taken
     Prescribed
     Self-administered
 • Establish if reported hepatoxicity in the literature
 • Relate time drugs taken to onset of illness
     4 days–8 weeks (usual)
 • Effect of stopping drugs on normalisation of liver biochemistry
     Hepatitic LFTs (2 months)
     Cholestatic/mixed LFTs (6 months)
 • Exclude other causes
     Viral hepatitis
     Biliary disease
 • Consider liver biopsy

N.B. Challenge tests with drugs should be avoided.

The key to diagnosing acute drug-induced liver disease is always to take a detailed drug history (Box 23.51). A liver biopsy should be considered if there is suspicion of pre-existing liver disease or if blood tests fail to improve when the suspect drug is withdrawn.

TYPES OF LIVER INJURY

Different histological patterns of liver injury may occur.

Cholestasis

Pure cholestasis (selective interference with bile flow in the absence of liver injury) can occur with oestrogens; this was seen quite frequently when higher concentrations of oestrogens (50 µg/day) were used as contraceptives. Both the current oral contraceptive pill and hormone replacement therapy can be safely used in chronic liver disease.

Chlorpromazine and antibiotics such as flucloxacillin are examples of drugs that cause cholestatic hepatitis, which is characterised by inflammation and canalicular injury. Co-amoxiclav is the most common antibiotic to cause abnormal LFTs but, unlike other antibiotics, it may not produce symptoms until 10–42 days after it is stopped. Anabolic steroids used by body-builders may also cause a cholestatic hepatitis. In some cases (e.g. NSAIDs and COX-2 inhibitors) there is overlap with acute hepatocellular injury.

Hepatocyte necrosis

Many drugs cause an acute hepatocellular necrosis with high serum transaminase concentrations; paracetamol (p. 208) is the best known. Inflammation is not always present but does accompany necrosis in liver injury due to diclofenac (an NSAID) and isoniazid (an anti-tuberculous drug). Granuloma may be seen in liver injury following the use of allopurinol. Acute hepatocellular necrosis has also been described following the use of several herbal remedies including germander, comfrey and jin bu huan. Recreational drugs, including cocaine and ecstasy, can also cause severe acute hepatitis.

Steatosis

Microvesicular hepatocyte fat deposition, due to direct effects on mitochondrial beta-oxidation, can follow exposure to tetracyclines and sodium valproate (Box 23.63, p. 988). Macrovesicular hepatocyte fat deposition has been

23

described with tamoxifen, and amiodarone toxicity can produce a similar histological picture to NASH (p. 971).

Vascular/sinusoidal lesions

Drugs such as alkylating agents used in oncology can damage the vascular endothelium and lead to hepatic venous outflow obstruction. Chronic overdose of vitamin A will also damage the sinusoids and trigger local fibrosis that can result in portal hypertension.

Hepatic fibrosis

Most drugs cause reversible liver injury and hepatic fibrosis is very uncommon. Methotrexate, however, as well as causing acute liver injury when it is started, can lead to cirrhosis when used in high doses over a long period of time. Risk factors for drug-induced hepatic fibrosis include pre-existing liver disease and a high alcohol intake.

DRUGS TO AVOID IN CIRRHOSIS

Most analgesics can precipitate complications and need to be used cautiously in cirrhosis (Box 23.52). NSAIDs are hepatotoxic and can potentiate hepatorenal failure; they should therefore be avoided in cirrhosis. Paracetamol up to a dose of 3 g/day can be used safely in chronic liver disease but higher doses may result in acute hepatic necrosis, particularly in patients with alcoholic liver disease.

23.52 DRUGS TO BE AVOIDED IN CIRRHOSIS		
Drug	**Problem**	**Toxicity**
NSAIDs	Reduced renal blood flow Ulceration	Hepatorenal failure Bleeding varices
ACE inhibitors	Reduced renal blood flow	Hepatorenal failure
Codeine	Constipation	Hepatic encephalopathy
Narcotics	Constipation Drug accumulation	Hepatic encephalopathy
Anxiolytics	Drug accumulation	Hepatic encephalopathy

INHERITED LIVER DISEASES

HAEMOCHROMATOSIS

Haemochromatosis is a condition in which the amount of total body iron is increased; the excess iron is deposited in and causes damage to several organs including the liver. It may be primary or secondary to other diseases (Box 23.53).

HEREDITARY (PRIMARY) HAEMOCHROMATOSIS

In this disease iron is deposited throughout the body and total body iron may reach 20–60 g (normally 4 g). The

23.53 CAUSES OF HAEMOCHROMATOSIS
Primary haemochromatosis
• Heriditary haemochromatosis • Congenital acaeruloplasminaemia • Congenital atransferrinaemia
Secondary iron overload
• Parenteral iron-loading (e.g. repeated blood transfusion) • Iron-loading anaemia (thalassaemia, sideroblastic anaemia, pyruvate kinase deficiency) • Liver disease • Dietary iron overload (prolonged oral iron therapy)
Complex iron overload
• Juvenile haemochromatosis • Neonatal haemochromatosis • Alcoholic liver disease • Porphyria cutanea tarda • African iron overload (Bantu siderosis)

important organs involved are the liver, pancreatic islets, endocrine glands and heart. In the liver, iron deposition occurs first in the periportal hepatocytes, extending later to all hepatocytes. The gradual development of fibrous septa leads to the formation of irregular nodules, and finally regeneration results in macronodular cirrhosis. An excess of liver iron can occur in alcoholic cirrhosis but this is mild by comparison with haemochromatosis.

Aetiology

Hereditary haemochromatosis (HHC) is caused by increased absorption of dietary iron and is inherited as an autosomal recessive gene located on chromosome 6. Approximately 90% of patients have a single-point mutation resulting in a cysteine to tyrosine substitution at position 282 (C282Y) in a protein (HFE) with structural and functional similarity to the human leucocyte antigen (HLA) proteins. The exact function of the HFE protein in regulating iron absorption is not known. However, it is believed that HFE is absent from the basolateral membrane of intestinal epithelial cells, where it normally interacts with the transferrin receptor. This defect in uptake of transferrin-associated iron may lead to up-regulation of enterocyte iron-specific divalent metal transporters and excessive iron absorption. A histidine to aspartic acid mutation at position 63 (H63D) in HFE causes a less severe form of haemochromatosis that is most commonly found in patients who are compound heterozygotes also carrying a C282Y mutated allele. Fewer than 50% of C282Y homozygotes will develop clinical features of haemochromatosis; therefore other factors must also be important. Iron loss in menstruation and pregnancy may protect females, as 90% of patients are male.

Clinical features

Symptomatic disease usually presents in men aged 40 years or over with features of hepatic cirrhosis (especially hepatomegaly), diabetes mellitus or heart failure. Tiredness, fatigue and arthropathy are early symptoms. Leaden-grey

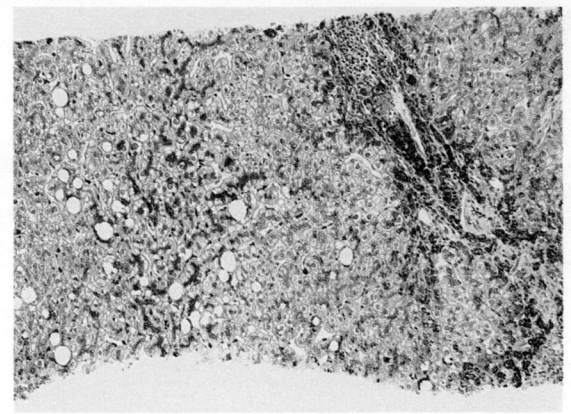

Fig. 23.32 Liver histology: haemochromatosis. This Perls stain shows accumulating iron within hepatocytes, which is stained blue. There is also accumulation of large fat globules in some hepatocytes (macrovesicular steatosis). Iron also accumulates in Kupffer cells and biliary epithelial cells.

skin pigmentation due to excess melanin occurs, especially in exposed parts, axillae, groins and genitalia; hence the term 'bronzed diabetes'. Impotence, loss of libido, testicular atrophy and arthritis with chondrocalcinosis secondary to calcium pyrophosphate deposition are also common. Cardiac failure or cardiac dysrhythmia may complicate heart muscle disease.

Investigations

The serum ferritin is greatly increased; the plasma iron is also increased, with a highly saturated plasma iron-binding capacity. CT may show features suggesting excess hepatic iron. The diagnosis is confirmed by liver biopsy, which shows heavy iron deposition and hepatic fibrosis which may have progressed to cirrhosis (Fig. 23.32). The iron content of the liver can be measured directly. Both the C282Y and H63D mutations can be identified by genetic testing.

Management

Treatment consists of weekly venesection of 500 ml blood (250 mg iron) until the serum iron is normal; this may take 2 years or more. Thereafter, venesection is continued as required to keep the serum ferritin normal. Liver and cardiac problems improve after iron removal, but joint pain is less predictable and can improve or worsen after iron removal. Diabetes mellitus does not resolve after venesection. Other therapy includes that for cirrhosis and diabetes mellitus. First-degree family members should be investigated, preferably by genetic screening and also by checking the plasma ferritin and iron-binding saturation. Liver biopsy is only indicated in asymptomatic relatives if the LFTs are abnormal and/or the serum ferritin is greater than 1000 μg/l because these features are associated with significant fibrosis or cirrhosis. Asymptomatic disease should also be treated by venesection until the serum ferritin is normal.

Prognosis

Pre-cirrhotic patients with HHC have a normal life expectancy; even cirrhotic patients have a relatively good prognosis, compared with other forms of cirrhosis (three-quarters of patients are alive 5 years after diagnosis). This is probably because liver function is usually well preserved at diagnosis and improves with therapy. Screening for hepatocellular carcinoma (p. 984) is mandatory because this is the main cause of death, affecting about one-third of patients with cirrhosis irrespective of therapy.

ACQUIRED IRON OVERLOAD (SECONDARY HAEMOCHROMATOSIS)

Many conditions, including chronic haemolytic disorders, sideroblastic anaemia, other conditions requiring multiple blood transfusion (generally over 50 litres), porphyria cutanea tarda, dietary iron overload and occasionally alcoholic cirrhosis, are associated with widespread secondary siderosis. The features are similar to primary haemochromatosis, but the history and clinical findings point to the true diagnosis. Some patients are heterozygotes for the primary haemochromatosis gene and this may contribute to the development of iron overload.

WILSON'S DISEASE (HEPATOLENTICULAR DEGENERATION)

Wilson's disease is a rare but important autosomal recessive disorder of copper metabolism that is caused by a variety of mutations in the gene ATP7B on chromosome 13. Total body copper is increased, with excess copper deposited in, and causing damage to, several organs.

Aetiology and pathology

Normally dietary copper is absorbed from the stomach and proximal small intestine and is rapidly taken into the liver, where it is stored and incorporated into caeruloplasmin, which is secreted into the blood. The accumulation of excessive copper in the body is ultimately prevented by its excretion, the most important route being via the bile. In Wilson's disease, there is almost always a failure of synthesis of caeruloplasmin; however, some 5% of patients have a normal circulating caeruloplasmin concentration and this is not the primary pathogenic defect. The amount of copper in the body at birth is normal, but thereafter it increases steadily; the organs most affected are the liver, basal ganglia of the brain, eyes, kidneys and skeleton.

The gene responsible for Wilson's disease (ATP7B, chromosome 13) encodes a member of the copper-transporting P-type adenosine triphosphatase family, which functions to export copper from the various cell types. At least 200 different mutations have been described. Although most of the mutations are rare, their relative frequency varies in different populations. The histidine to glucine single-base mutation at position 1069 is most common in Polish and Austrian patients, but rare in India, other Asian countries and Sardinia. In contrast, approximately 60% of Sardinian patients have a 15 nucleotide deletion in the 5' untranslated region of the Wilson's gene. Most cases are compound heterozygotes with two different mutations in the Wilson's gene. Attempts to correlate the genotype with the mode of presentation and clinical course have not shown any consistent patterns.

Clinical features

Symptoms usually arise between the ages of 5 and 45 years. Hepatic disease occurs predominantly in childhood and early adolescence, although it can present in adults in their fifties. Neurological damage causes basal ganglion syndromes and dementia which tends to present in later adolescence. These features can occur alone or simultaneously. Other manifestations include renal tubular damage and osteoporosis, but these are virtually never presenting features.

Liver disease

This can manifest in many ways which are not specific. Episodes of acute hepatitis, sometimes recurrent, can occur, especially in children, and may progress to acute fulminant liver failure. The latter is characterised by the liberation of free copper into the blood stream, causing massive haemolysis and renal tubulopathy. Chronic hepatitis can also develop insidiously and eventually present with established cirrhosis; liver failure and portal hypertension may supervene. Recurrent acute hepatitis of unknown cause, especially when accompanied by haemolysis, or chronic liver disease of unknown cause in a patient under 40 years old suggests Wilson's disease.

Neurological disease

Clinical features include a variety of extrapyramidal features, particularly tremor, choreoathetosis, dystonia, parkinsonism and dementia (p. 1216). Unusual clumsiness for age may be an early symptom.

Kayser–Fleischer rings

These are the most important single clinical clue to the diagnosis and can be seen in 60% of adults with Wilson's disease (less often in children but almost always in neurological Wilson's disease), albeit sometimes only by slit-lamp examination. Kayser–Fleischer rings are characterised by greenish-brown discoloration of the corneal margin appearing first at the upper periphery (Fig. 23.33). They eventually disappear with treatment.

Investigations

A low serum caeruloplasmin is the best single laboratory clue to the diagnosis. However, advanced liver failure from any cause can reduce the serum caeruloplasmin, and occasionally it is normal in Wilson's disease. Other features of disordered copper metabolism should therefore be sought; these include a high free serum copper concentration, a high urine copper excretion of greater than 0.6 µmol/24 hrs and a very high hepatic copper content. Measuring 24-hour urinary copper excretion whilst giving D-penicillamine is a useful confirmatory test; more than 25 µmol/24 hrs is considered diagnostic of Wilson's disease.

Genetic testing is limited by the existence of multiple genetic defects, but may be useful in screening families once the abnormality has been identified in an affected individual.

Management

The copper-binding agent penicillamine is the drug of choice. The dose given must be sufficient to produce

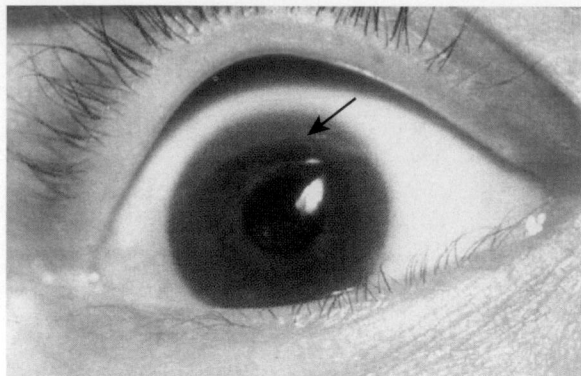

Fig. 23.33 Kayser–Fleischer rings at the junction of the cornea and sclera (arrow) in a patient with Wilson's disease.

cupriuresis and most patients require 1.5 g/day (range 1–4 g). The dose can be reduced once the disease is in remission but treatment must continue for life, even through pregnancy. Care must be taken to ensure that reaccumulation of copper does not occur. Abrupt discontinuation of treatment must be avoided because this may precipitate acute liver failure. Toxic effects of penicillamine occur in one-third of patients and include rashes, protein-losing nephropathy, lupus-like syndrome and bone marrow depression. If these do occur, trientine dihydrochloride (1.2–2.4 g/day) and zinc (50 mg 8-hourly) are alternative effective therapies.

Liver transplantation is indicated for fulminant liver failure or for advanced cirrhosis with liver failure. The value of liver transplantation in severe neurological Wilson's disease is highly controversial.

Prognosis

The prognosis is excellent, provided treatment is started before there is irreversible damage. Siblings and children of patients with Wilson's disease must be investigated and treatment should be given to all infected individuals, even if they are asymptomatic.

ALPHA₁-ANTITRYPSIN DEFICIENCY

Alpha₁-antitrypsin (α_1-AT) is a serine protease inhibitor (Pi) produced by the liver. The form of α_1-AT is genetically determined, and one of these forms (PiZ) cannot be secreted into the blood by liver cells because it is polymerised within the endoplasmic reticulum of the hepatocyte. Homozygous individuals (PiZZ) have low plasma α_1-AT concentrations, although globules containing α_1-AT are found in the liver, and they may develop hepatic and pulmonary disease (p. 678). Liver disease includes cholestatic jaundice in the neonatal period (neonatal hepatitis) which can resolve spontaneously, chronic hepatitis and cirrhosis in adults, and in the long term hepatocellular carcinoma. There are no clinical features distinguishing liver disease due to α_1-AT deficiency from other causes of liver disease, and the diagnosis is made from the low plasma α_1-AT concentration and the PiZZ genotype. Alpha₁-AT-containing globules can

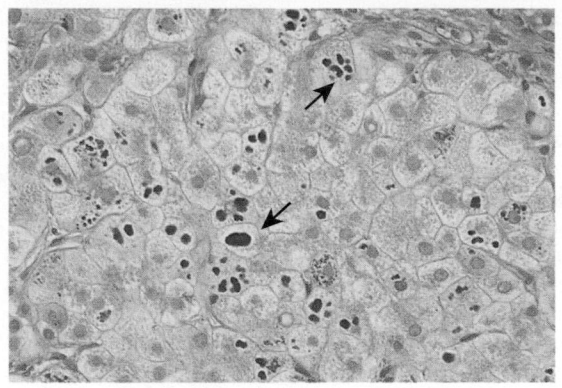

Fig. 23.34 Liver histology in α₁-antitrypsin deficiency. Accumulation of periodic acid–Schiff-positive granules (arrows) within individual hepatocytes is shown in this section from a patient with α₁-AT deficiency.

23.54 CONDITIONS ASSOCIATED WITH AUTOIMMUNE HEPATITIS

- Migrating polyarthritis
- Urticarial rashes
- Lymphadenopathy
- Hashimoto's thyroiditis
- Thyrotoxicosis
- Myxoedema
- Coombs-positive haemolytic anaemia
- Pleurisy
- Transient pulmonary infiltrates
- Ulcerative colitis
- Glomerulonephritis
- Nephrotic syndrome

23.55 FREQUENCY OF AUTOANTIBODIES IN CHRONIC NON-VIRAL LIVER DISEASES AND IN HEALTHY PEOPLE

Disease	Anti-nuclear antibody (%)	Anti-smooth muscle antibody (%)	Antimito-chondrial antibody* (%)
Healthy controls	5	1.5	0.01
Autoimmune hepatitis	80	70	15
Primary biliary cirrhosis	25	35	95
Cryptogenic cirrhosis	40	30	15

* Patients with antimitochondrial antibody frequently have cholestatic LFTs and may have primary biliary cirrhosis (see text).

be demonstrated in the liver (Fig. 23.34) but this is not necessary to make the diagnosis. Occasionally, patients with liver disease and minor reductions of plasma α₁-AT concentrations have α₁-AT phenotypes other than PiZZ, such as PiMZ or PiSZ, but the relationship of these genotypes to liver disease is uncertain. No specific treatment is available; the concurrent risk of severe and early-onset emphysema means that all patients should be advised to abandon cigarette smoking.

AUTOIMMUNE LIVER DISEASES

AUTOIMMUNE HEPATITIS

Autoimmune hepatitis is a liver disease of unknown aetiology characterised by a strong association with other autoimmune diseases (Box 23.54), high levels of serum immunoglobulins (hypergammaglobulinaemia) and auto-antibodies in the serum. It occurs most often in women, particularly in the second and third decades of life, but may develop in either sex at any age

Aetiology and pathology

Several subtypes of this disorder have been proposed which have differing immunological markers. Classical (type I) autoimmune hepatitis is characterised by a high frequency of other autoimmune disorders such as Graves' disease. Type I autoimmune hepatitis is associated with HLA-DR3 and DR4, particularly HLA-DRB3*0101 and HLA-DRB1*0401. These patients have high titres of antinuclear and anti-smooth muscle antibodies but none of these antibodies is cytotoxic. A suggested hypothesis for the development of type I autoimmune hepatitis is the aberrant expression on the hepatocyte of HLA antigen, influenced by viral, genetic and environmental factors. Type II auto-immune hepatitis is characterised by the presence of anti-LKM (liver–kidney microsomal) antibodies and lack of antinuclear and anti-smooth muscle antibodies. Anti-LKM antibodies recognise cytochrome P450-IID6, which is

expressed on the hepatocyte membrane. In Type III, serum immunoglobulin levels are elevated whilst the antibodies described above are absent, and antibodies against soluble liver antigen are present. The histopathological features of all forms of autoimmune hepatitis are similar.

Clinical features

The onset is usually insidious, with fatigue, anorexia and jaundice. In about one-quarter of patients the onset is acute, resembling viral hepatitis, but resolution does not occur. This acute presentation can lead to extensive liver necrosis and liver failure. Other features include fever, arthralgia, vitiligo and epistaxis. Amenorrhoea is the rule but general health may be good. Jaundice is mild to moderate or occasionally absent, but signs of chronic liver disease, especially spider naevi and hepatosplenomegaly, are usually present. Some patients have a 'Cushingoid' face with acne, hirsutism and pink cutaneous striae, especially on the thighs and abdomen.

Approximately two-thirds of patients have associated autoimmune disease such as Hashimoto's thyroiditis, renal tubular acidosis and rheumatoid arthritis.

Diagnosis and investigations

Serological testing for specific autoantibodies may suggest autoimmune hepatitis (Box 23.55). However, low titres of these antibodies occur in some healthy people. Antinuclear antibodies also occur in connective tissue diseases and other autoimmune diseases, including various thyroid disorders and pernicious anaemia, while anti-smooth muscle antibody has been reported in infectious mononucleosis and a variety of malignant diseases. Antimicrosomal antibodies (anti-LKM) occur particularly in children and adolescents. Elevated levels of serum IgG immunoglobulins are invariable and are an important diagnostic feature. Liver

23

EBM

23.56 IMMUNOSUPPRESSION IN AUTOIMMUNE HEPATITIS

'In autoimmune hepatitis treatment with prednisolone ± azathioprine improves serum biochemistry and hepatic histology. It also improves survival at 10 years from 27% to 63% (NNT_B 2.7).'

'In patients who have been in remission for more than 1 year, increasing the dose of azathioprine (from 1 to 2 mg/kg) and withdrawing prednisolone reduces steroid side-effects and does not increase the risk of relapse.'

- Kirk AP, et al. Gut 1980; 21:78–83.
- Johnson PJ, et al. N Engl J Med 1995; 333:958–963.

---

biopsy typically shows interface hepatitis, with or without cirrhosis.

Management

Treatment with corticosteroids is life-saving in autoimmune hepatitis, particularly during exacerbations of active and symptomatic disease. Initially, prednisolone 40 mg/day is given orally; the dose is then gradually reduced as the patient and LFTs improve. Maintenance therapy is required for at least 2 years after LFTs have returned to normal, and withdrawal of treatment should not be considered unless a liver biopsy is also normal. Azathioprine 1.0–1.5 mg/kg/day orally may allow the dose of prednisolone to be reduced (Box 23.56). Azathioprine can also be used as the sole maintenance immunosuppressive agent. Corticosteroids treat acute exacerbations and do not prevent cirrhosis; they are therefore less important in mild asymptomatic autoimmune hepatitis.

Prognosis

The disease is characterised by exacerbations and remissions, but most patients eventually develop cirrhosis and its complications. Hepatocellular carcinoma is uncommon. Approximately 50% of symptomatic patients will die of liver failure within 5 years if no treatment is given, but this falls to about 10% with therapy.

PRIMARY BILIARY CIRRHOSIS

Primary biliary cirrhosis (PBC) is a chronic, progressive cholestatic liver disease of unknown cause which predominantly affects middle-aged women. The condition is strongly associated with the presence of serum antibodies to mitochondria (AMA), which are diagnostic. It is characterised by a granulomatous inflammation of the portal tracts, leading to progressive damage and eventually loss of the small and middle-sized bile ducts. This in turn leads to fibrosis and cirrhosis of the liver. The condition typically presents with an insidious onset of itching and/or tiredness; it may also be found incidentally as the result of routine blood tests.

Epidemiology

The prevalence of PBC varies across the world. It is relatively common in northern Europe and North America (the prevalence in north-east England is 245/million) but is rare in Africa and Asia. There is a strong female to male

predominance of 9:1; it is also more common amongst cigarette smokers. Clustering of cases has been reported suggesting an infectious agent.

Aetiology and pathology

The cause of PBC is unknown but immune mechanisms are clearly involved in the pathogenesis of the bile duct damage. The condition is closely associated with other autoimmune non-hepatic diseases such as thyroid disease and there is a weak association with HLA-DR8. Antimitochondrial and antinuclear (nuclear pore antigens gp210) antibodies are found in the serum with elevations in serum immuno-globulin levels, particularly IgM; cellular immunity is impaired and abnormal cellular immune reactions have been described. Infectious agents, such as retroviruses, bacteria including *E. coli* and mycobacteria, have been suggested as the trigger for the disease process, but this hypothesis remains unproven.

The primary pathological lesion is a chronic granulomatous inflammation which damages and destroys the interlobular bile ducts; progressive lymphocyte-mediated inflammatory damage causes fibrosis which spreads from the portal tracts to the liver parenchyma and eventually leads to cirrhosis. A model of the natural history of the disease process is shown in Figure 23.35.

Clinical features

Non-specific symptoms, such as lethargy and arthralgia, are common and may precede diagnosis for years. Pruritus is the most common initial complaint, pointing to hepatobiliary disease, and may precede jaundice by months or years; jaundice is rarely a presenting feature. The itching is usually worse on the limbs. Although there may be right upper abdominal discomfort, fever and rigors (cholangitis), which are often features of large bile duct obstruction, do not occur. Bone pain or fractures can rarely result from osteomalacia (fat-soluble vitamin malabsorption) or more commonly, from accelerated osteoporosis (hepatic osteodystrophy).

Initially, patients are well nourished but considerable weight loss can occur as the disease progresses. Scratch marks may be found. Jaundice is only prominent late in the disease and can become intense. Xanthomatous deposits occur in a minority, especially around the eyes, in the hand creases and over the elbows, knees and buttocks. Hepatomegaly is virtually constant, and splenomegaly becomes increasingly common as portal hypertension develops. Liver failure may supervene.

Associated diseases

Autoimmune and connective tissue diseases occur with increased frequency in PBC, particularly the sicca syndrome (p. 1137), systemic sclerosis, coeliac disease (p. 894) and thyroid diseases. Hypothyroidism should always be considered in patients with fatigue.

Diagnosis and investigations

LFTs show the pattern of cholestasis (p. 943). Hyper-cholesterolaemia is common and worsens as disease progresses; however, it is of no diagnostic value. The anti-

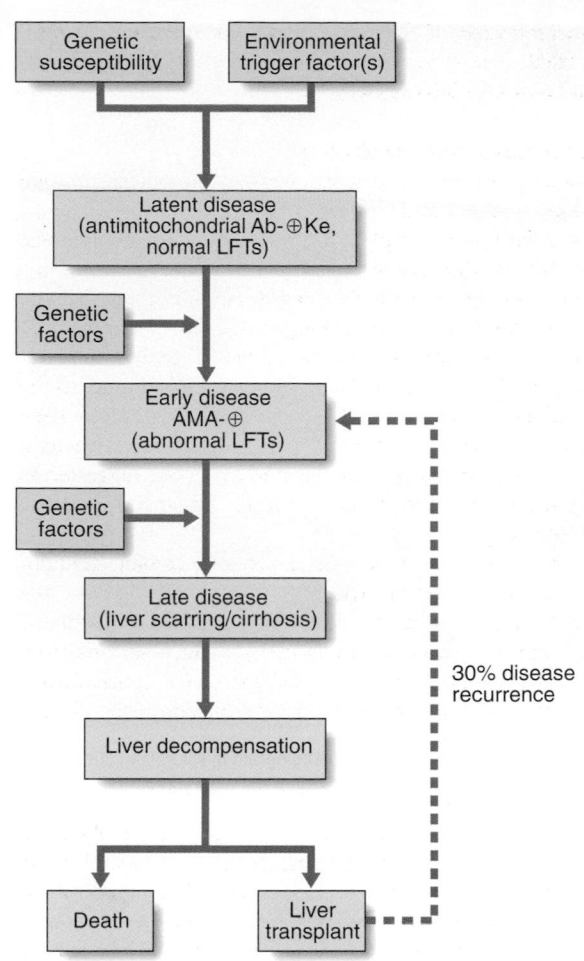

Fig. 23.35 Natural history of primary biliary cirrhosis.

23.57 URSODEOXYCHOLIC ACID (UDCA) IN PRIMARY BILIARY CIRRHOSIS (PBC)

EBM

'In PBC UDCA therapy (13–15 mg/kg/day) improves biochemical markers of cholestasis and jaundice. Some randomised trials have shown that UDCA treatment significantly slows disease progression but whether it affects mortality or transplantation rates remains controversial.'

- Poupon RE, et al. Gastroenterology 1997; 113:884–890.
- Corpechot C, et al. Hepatology 2000; 32:1196–1199.
- Goulis J, et al. Lancet 1999; 354:1053–1060.

down histological progression and has few side-effects (Box 23.57); it is therefore widely used in the treatment of PBC at a dose of 10–15 mg/kg/day.

Liver transplantation should be considered once liver failure has developed and may be indicated in patients with intractable pruritus. Prognostic models are available but serum bilirubin remains the most reliable marker of declining liver function. Transplantation is associated with an excellent 5-year survival of over 80%, although the disease will recur in over one-third of patients at 10 years.

Pruritus

This is the main symptom requiring treatment. The cause of itching is unknown but current research suggests that it is due to up-regulation of opioid receptors and increased levels of endogenous opioids. It is best treated with the anion-binding resin colestyramine, which probably acts by binding potential pruritogens in the intestine and increasing their excretion in the stool. A dose of 4–16 g/day orally is used. The powder is mixed in orange juice and the main dose (8 g) taken before and after breakfast when maximal duodenal bile acid concentrations occur. Colestyramine may bind other drugs in the gut (e.g. anticoagulants), which should therefore be taken 1 hour before the binding agent. Colestyramine is sometimes ineffective, especially in complete biliary obstruction. Alternative treatments include rifampicin 300 mg/day, naltrexone (an opioid antagonist) 25 mg/day initially increasing up to 300 mg/day, plasmapheresis and a liver support device (e.g. a molecular adsorbent recirculating system (MARS) machine).

Fatigue

Lethargy affects about one-third of patients with PBC. The cause is unknown but it may reflect intracerebral changes due to cholestasis. Unfortunately, once depression and hypothroidism have been excluded, there is no treatment.

Malabsorption

Prolonged cholestasis is associated with steatorrhoea and malabsorption of fat-soluble vitamins, which should be replaced as necessary. Associated coeliac disease requires exclusion.

Bone disease

Osteopenia and osteoporosis are common and normal post-menopausal bone loss is accelerated. Baseline bone density should be measured (p. 1122) and treatment started with replacement calcium and vitamin D_3. Bisphophonates such as risedronate should be used if there is evidence of osteopenia. Osteomalacia is rare.

mitochondrial antibody is present in over 95% of patients, and when it is absent the diagnosis should not be made without obtaining histological evidence and considering cholangiography (MRCP or ERCP) to exclude other biliary disease. Antinuclear and anti-smooth muscle antibodies are present in around 15% of patients (Box 23.55); autoantibodies found in associated diseases may also be present. Ultrasound examination shows no sign of biliary obstruction. Liver biopsy is only necessary if there is diagnostic uncertainty. The histological features of PBC correlate poorly with the clinical features; portal hypertension can develop before the histological onset of cirrhosis.

Management

Asymptomatic patients require monitoring on a yearly basis to assess the onset of symptoms and associated disease. Immunosuppressants such as corticosteroids, azathioprine, penicillamine and ciclosporin have all been tried in PBC but none is effective and all may have serious adverse effects. The hydrophilic bile acid, ursodeoxycholic acid (UDCA), improves bile flow, replaces toxic hydrophobic bile acids in the bile acid pool, and reduces apoptosis of the biliary epithelium. Clinically, UDCA improves LFTs, may slow

23

OVERLAP SYNDROMES

AMA-negative PBC ('autoimmune cholangitis')

A few patients demonstrate the clinical, biochemical and histological features of PBC but do not have detectable antimitochondrial antibodies in the serum. Serum transaminases, serum Ig levels and titres of antinuclear antibodies tend to be higher than in AMA-positive PBC. However, the clinical course mirrors classical PBC and these patients should be considered to have a variant of PBC.

PBC/autoimmune hepatitis overlap

A small minority of patients with AMA and cholestatic LFTs have elevated transaminases, high serum immuno-globulins and interface hepatitis on liver histology; in such patients a trial of corticosteroids may be beneficial.

SECONDARY BILIARY CIRRHOSIS

This develops after prolonged large duct biliary obstruction due to gallstones, benign bile duct strictures or sclerosing cholangitis (see below). Carcinomas rarely cause secondary biliary cirrhosis because few patients survive long enough. The clinical features are of chronic cholestasis with episodes of ascending cholangitis or even liver abscess (p. 986). Cirrhosis, ascites and portal hypertension are late features. Cholangitis requires treatment with antibiotics, which can be given continuously if attacks recur frequently.

PRIMARY SCLEROSING CHOLANGITIS

Primary sclerosing cholangitis is a cholestatic liver disease caused by diffuse inflammation and fibrosis that can involve the entire biliary tree and leads to the gradual obliteration of intrahepatic and extrahepatic bile ducts, and ultimately biliary cirrhosis, portal hypertension and hepatic failure. Cholangiocarcinoma develops in about 10–30% of patients during the course of the disease.

Primary sclerosing cholangitis occurs mainly in young men (male:female ratio 2:1). Most patients present at age 25–40 years, although the condition may be diagnosed at any age and is an important cause of chronic liver disease in children. The generally accepted diagnostic criteria are:

- generalised beading and stenosis of the biliary system on cholangiography (Fig. 23.36)
- absence of choledocholithiasis (or history of bile duct surgery)
- exclusion of bile duct cancer, usually by prolonged follow-up.

The term 'secondary sclerosing cholangitis' is used to describe the typical bile duct changes described above when a clear predisposing factor to duct fibrosis can be identified. The causes of secondary sclerosing cholangitis are shown in Box 23.58.

Aetiology

The cause of primary sclerosing cholangitis remains unknown. However, there is a close association with inflammatory bowel disease, particularly ulcerative colitis

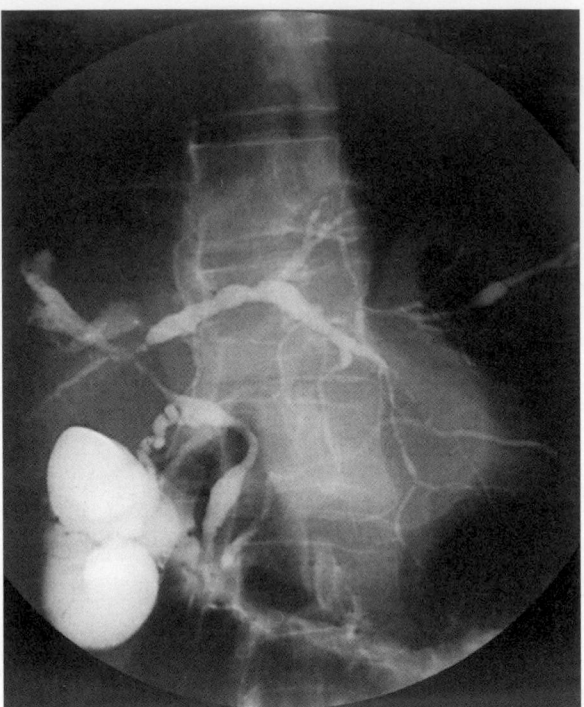

Fig. 23.36 A percutaneous cholangiogram in sclerosing cholangitis showing characteristic irregularity of the biliary tree.

23.58 CAUSES OF SECONDARY SCLEROSING CHOLANGITIS

- Previous bile duct surgery with stricturing and cholangitis
- Bile duct stones causing cholangitis
- Intrahepatic infusion of 5-fluorodeoxyuridine
- Insertion of formalin into hepatic hydatid cysts
- Insertion of alcohol into hepatic tumours
- AIDS (probably infective as a result of cytomegalovirus or *Cryptosporidium*)

23.59 DISEASES ASSOCIATED WITH PRIMARY SCLEROSING CHOLANGITIS

- Ulcerative colitis
- Crohn's colitis
- Chronic pancreatitis
- Retroperitoneal fibrosis
- Riedel's thyroditis
- Retro-orbital tumours
- Immune deficiency states
- Sjögren's syndrome
- Angio-immunoplastic lymphadenopathy
- Histiocytosis X
- Autoimmune haemolytic anaemia

(Box 23.59). About two-thirds of patients with primary sclerosing cholangitis have coexisting ulcerative colitis, and primary sclerosing cholangitis is the most common form of chronic liver disease found in ulcerative colitis. Between 3% and 10% of patients with ulcerative colitis develop primary sclerosing cholangitis, particularly those with substantial or total colitis. In a Swedish study, the prevalence of ulcerative colitis was 171/100 000 population and that of primary sclerosing cholangitis 6.3/100 000 population. The prevalence of primary sclerosing cholangitis is lower in patients with Crohn's colitis (about 1%). Patients with primary sclerosing cholangitis and ulcerative colitis are at greater risk of colorectal neoplasia than those with ulcerative colitis alone, and those who develop colorectal neoplasia are at greater risk of cholangiocarcinoma.

Any proposed aetiopathogenic factor must explain this close assocation with inflammatory bowel disease. Current evidence suggests that primary sclerosing cholangitis is an immunologically mediated disease, probably triggered in genetically susceptible individuals by acquired toxic or infectious agents, which may gain access through the leaky diseased colon.

Immunogenic factors

A close link with HLA haplotype A1 B8 DR3 DRW 52A has been identified. This haplotype is commonly found in association with other organ-specific autoimmune diseases (e.g. autoimmune hepatitis). The prevalence of HLA-DR2 and HLA-DR6 is greater in patients who are DR3-negative.

The importance of immunological factors has been emphasised by reports showing humoral and cellular abnormalities in primary sclerosing cholangitis. Perinuclear antineutrophil cytoplasmic antibodies (ANCA) have been detected in the sera of about 60–80% of patients with primary sclerosing cholangitis with or without ulcerative colitis, and in about 30–40% of patients with ulcerative colitis alone. The antibody is not specific for primary sclerosing cholangitis and is found in other chronic liver diseases (e.g. 50% of patients with autoimmune hepatitis).

Clinical features

The diagnosis is often made incidentally when persistently raised serum alkaline phosphatase is discovered in an individual with ulcerative colitis. Common symptoms include fatigue, intermittent jaundice, weight loss, right upper quadrant abdominal pain and pruritus. Attacks of acute cholangitis are uncommon and usually follow biliary instrumentation. Physical examination is abnormal in about 50% of symptomatic patients; the most common findings are jaundice and hepatomegaly/splenomegaly.

Investigations

Serum biochemical tests usually indicate cholestasis. However, alkaline phosphatase and bilirubin levels may vary widely in individual patients during the course of the disease (e.g. increasing during acute cholangitis, decreasing after therapy) and sometimes fluctuate for no apparent reason. Modest elevations in serum transaminases are usually seen, whereas hypoalbuminaemia and clotting abnormalities are found only at a late stage. In addition to ANCA, low titres of serum antinuclear and anti-smooth muscle antibodies have been found in primary sclerosing cholangitis but have no diagnostic significance; serum antimitochondrial antibody is absent. IgM concentrations are increased in about 50% of symptomatic patients and elevations of IgG are found in about one-third of adult patients tested.

Diagnosis

Radiological features

ERCP is usually diagnostic and may reveal multiple irregular stricturing and dilation (Fig. 23.36). MRCP is a

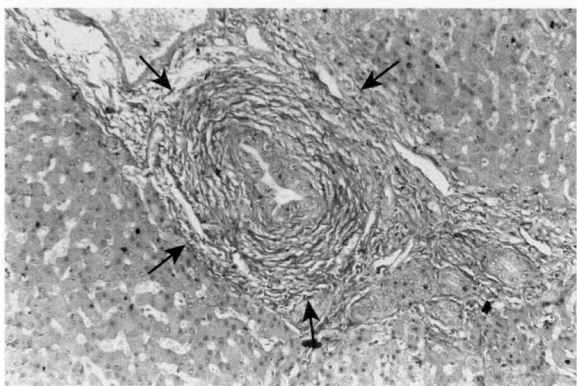

Fig. 23.37 Primary sclerosing cholangitis. Note onion-skin scarring (arrows) surrounding a bile duct.

non-invasive method of imaging the biliary tree; it is being assessed and will probably become the standard method of diagnosis.

Pathological features

Histological appearances are not usually diagnostic, although some form of biliary disease can usually be identified. The characteristic early features of primary sclerosing cholangitis are periductal 'onion-skin' fibrosis and inflammation, with portal oedema and bile ductular proliferation resulting in expansion of the portal tracts (Fig. 23.37). Later fibrosis spreads, leading inevitably to biliary cirrhosis; obliterative cholangitis leads to the so-called 'vanishing bile duct syndrome'.

Association with other diseases

Many diseases have been associated with primary sclerosing cholangitis (Box 23.59).

Management

Primary sclerosing cholangitis has no curative treatment but management of cholestasis and its complications and specific treatment of the disease process are required.

Management of cholestasis

Symptomatic patients often have pruritus, which is best managed initially with colestyramine; the dose should be increased until relief is obtained.

Management of complications

Broad-spectrum antibiotics (e.g. ciprofloxacin) should be given for acute attacks of cholangitis but have no proven prophylactic value. If cholangiography shows a well-defined obstruction to the extrahepatic bile ducts, mechanical relief can be obtained by placement of a prosthesis or by balloon dilatation performed at ERCP. Fat-soluble vitamin replacement is necessary in jaundiced patients. Metabolic bone disease (usually osteoporosis) is a common complication that requires treatment (p. 1121).

Specific treatment

UCDA is a non-hepatotoxic hydrophilic bile acid that has been used widely for treatment of cholestasis; it reduces levels of cholestatic liver enzymes, but controlled trials in conventional doses have shown no effect on symptoms,

23

histology or survival. Larger doses (20–25 mg/kg daily) have beneficial effects on liver histology and cholangiographic appearance. Immunosuppressive agents, including prednisolone, azathioprine, methotrexate and ciclosporin have been tried; generally, results have been disappointing but combination therapy with UDCA may be beneficial.

Surgical treatment

Orthotopic transplantation is the only option in young patients with primary sclerosing cholangitis and advanced liver disease; 5-year survival is 80–90% in most centres. Unfortunately, the condition may recur in the graft. Proven cholangiocarcinoma is a contraindication to transplantation.

Prognosis

The course of primary sclerosing cholangitis is variable. In symptomatic patients, median survival from presentation to death or liver transplantation is about 12 years. About 75% of asymptomatic patients survive 15 years or more. Most patients die in liver failure, about 30% die from bile duct carcinoma, and the remainder die from colonic cancer or complications of colitis.

VASCULAR LIVER DISEASES

HEPATIC ARTERIAL DISEASE

Hepatic arterial disease is rare and difficult to diagnose, but can cause serious liver damage. Hepatic artery occlusion may result from inadvertent injury during biliary surgery or may be caused by emboli, neoplasms, polyarteritis nodosa, blunt trauma or radiation. It usually causes severe upper abdominal pain with or without signs of circulatory shock. LFTs show a high transaminase activity, as in other causes of acute liver damage. Patients usually survive if the liver and portal blood supply are otherwise normal.

Hepatic artery aneurysms are extrahepatic in three-quarters of cases and intrahepatic in one-quarter. Atheroma, vasculitis, bacterial endocarditis, and surgical or biopsy trauma are the main causes. They usually cause bleeding into the biliary tree, peritoneum or intestine and are best diagnosed by arteriography. Treatment is radiological or surgical. Any of the vasculitides can affect the hepatic artery, but this rarely causes symptoms.

PORTAL VENOUS DISEASE

Portal venous thrombosis is rare but can occur in any condition predisposing to thrombosis. It may also complicate intra-abdominal inflammatory or neoplastic disease and is a recognised cause of portal hypertension. Acute portal venous thrombosis causes abdominal pain and diarrhoea, and may lead to bowel infarction. Treatment is surgical, although patients will require anticoagulation if an underlying thrombotic condition is diagnosed. Subacute thrombosis can be asymptomatic but may lead to extrahepatic portal hypertension (p. 957) later on.

HEPATIC VENOUS OUTFLOW OBSTRUCTION

Obstruction to hepatic venous blood flow can occur in the small central hepatic veins, the large hepatic veins, the inferior vena cava or the heart. The clinical features depend on the cause and on the speed with which obstruction develops, but congestive hepatomegaly and ascites are consistent features.

BUDD–CHIARI SYNDROME

Aetiology and pathology

This uncommon condition is characterised by thrombosis of the larger hepatic veins and sometimes the inferior vena cava. The cause cannot be found in about half of patients. Some have haematological disorders such as primary proliferative polycythaemia, paroxysmal nocturnal haemoglobinuria and antithrombin III, protein C or protein S deficiencies (pp. 1061–1062). Pregnancy and oral contraceptive use, obstruction due to tumours (particularly carcinomas of the liver, kidneys or adrenals), congenital venous webs and occasionally inferior vena caval stenosis are the other main causes. Hepatic congestion affecting the centrilobular areas is the initial consequence; centrilobular fibrosis develops later and eventually cirrhosis supervenes in those who survive long enough.

Clinical features

Sudden venous occlusion causes the rapid development of upper abdominal pain, marked ascites and occasionally acute liver failure. More gradual occlusion causes gross ascites and often upper abdominal discomfort. Hepatomegaly, often with tenderness over the liver, is almost always present. Peripheral oedema occurs only when there is inferior vena cava obstruction. Features of cirrhosis and portal hypertension develop in those who survive the acute event.

Investigations

LFTs vary considerably depending on the presentation and can show the features of acute hepatitis (p. 943) when the onset is rapid. Ascitic fluid analysis typically shows a protein concentration above 25 g/l (exudate) in the early stages; however, this often falls later in the disease. Doppler ultrasound examination may reveal obliteration of the hepatic veins and reversed flow or associated thrombosis in the portal vein. CT may show enlargement of the caudate lobe, as it often has a separate venous drainage system that is not involved in the disease. CT and MRI may also demonstrate occlusion of the hepatic veins and inferior vena cava. Liver biopsy demonstrates centrilobular congestion with fibrosis depending upon the duration of the illness. Venography is only needed if CT and MRI are unable to demonstrate the hepatic venous anatomy clearly.

Management

Predisposing causes should be treated as far as possible; where recent thrombosis is suspected, treatment with streptokinase followed by heparin and oral anticoagulation should be considered. Ascites is initially treated medically but often with limited success. Short hepatic venous strictures can be treated with angioplasty. In the case of more extensive hepatic vein occlusion many patients can be managed successfully by insertion of a covered TIPSS followed by anticoagulation. Surgical shunts, such as porta-caval shunts, are less commonly performed now that TIPPS is available. Occasionally, a web can be resected or an inferior vena caval stenosis dilated. Progressive liver failure is an indication for liver transplantation and life-long anticoagulation.

Prognosis

The prognosis without transplantation or shunting is poor, particularly following an acute presentation with liver failure. The 1- and 10-year survival following liver trans-plantation is 85% and 69% respectively, and this compares with a 5- and 10-year survival of 87% and 37% following surgical shunting.

VENO-OCCLUSIVE DISEASE

Widespread occlusion of central hepatic veins is the characteristic of this rare condition. Pyrrolizidine alkaloids in *Senecio* and *Heliotropium* plants used to make teas, cytotoxic drugs and hepatic irradiation are all recognised causes. In developed countries it is often seen a few months after bone marrow transplantation, due to pre-conditioning therapy with irradiation and cytotoxic chemotherapy. The clinical features are similar to those of the Budd–Chiari syndrome (see above). Investigations show evidence of venous outflow obstruction histologically but, in contrast to Budd–Chiari, the large hepatic veins appear patent radiologically.

CARDIAC DISEASE

Hepatic damage due primarily to congestion may develop in all forms of right heart failure (p. 542); the clinical features are usually dominated by the cardiac disease. Very rarely, long-standing cardiac failure and hepatic congestion cause cardiac cirrhosis.

Ischaemic hepatitis ('shock liver')

Acute heart failure sometimes causes a syndrome similar to acute hepatitis. This is usually mediated by a reduction in hepatic perfusion and is termed 'shock liver'. Pre-existing right heart dysfunction is often present. Common causes include heart surgery, myocardial infarction, decom-pensation of any chronic myocardial disease, respiratory conditions associated with cor pulmonale and tamponade. The patient is generally very ill with an enlarged tender liver, jaundice and LFTs showing very high serum transaminases (often over 2000 U/l). The correct diagnosis is made by recognising that the cardiac output is low, the jugular venous pressure is high and other signs of cardiac disease are present.

Ascites

Chronic congestive cardiac failure sometimes causes hepatomegaly and ascites disproportionate to the degree of peripheral oedema, and in the circumstances can mimic ascites due to liver disease. Constrictive pericarditis (p. 644) is particularly likely to mislead, as a normal heart size points away from heart disease. A raised jugular venous pressure is the most important single clue to the diagnosis.

Management

The treatment of these patients is that of the underlying heart disease.

NODULAR REGENERATIVE HYPERPLASIA OF THE LIVER

This disease is characterised by small hepatocyte nodules throughout the liver without fibrosis. It occurs in older people and has been associated with many conditions including connective tissue disease, haematological diseases and immunosuppressive and corticosteroid drugs. The condition usually presents as an abdominal mass or occasionally because of portal hypertension. Diagnosis is made by liver biopsy. Liver function is good and the prognosis is very favourable.

TUMOURS OF THE LIVER

HEPATOCELLULAR CARCINOMA

This is the most common primary liver tumour. Age-adjusted incidence rates vary in men from 28 per 100 000 in South-east Asia (reflecting the prevalence of hepatitis B) to 10 per 100 000 in southern Europe and 5 per 100 000 in northern Europe. The incidence in Europe and North America has risen recently; this is probably related to an increase in hepatitis C cirrhosis.

Aetiology

- *Chronic hepatitis B infection*. The major risk factor for hepatocellular carcinoma world-wide is chronic hepatitis B infection. The risk of hepatocellular carcinoma is 0.4%/year in the absence of cirrhosis and is four times higher in HBeAg-positive individuals than in those who have HBsAg alone.
- *Cirrhosis*. This is a an independent risk factor with an annual risk of 1–5% in hepatitis B and C cirrhosis. There is also an increased risk in cirrhosis due to haemochromatosis, alcohol, NASH and α_1-antitrypsin deficiency. In northern Europe 90% of those with hepatocellular carcinoma have underlying cirrhosis, compared to 30% in Taiwan where hepatitis B is the main risk factor.
- *Male gender and age*. The risk is higher in men and rises with age. Unlike their male counterparts, women with primary biliary cirrhosis do not require screening.

Pathology

Macroscopically, the tumour usually appears as a single mass in the absence of cirrhosis, or as a single or multiple nodules in the presence of cirrhosis. It takes its blood supply

23

from the hepatic artery and tends to spread by invasion into the portal vein and its radicles. Lymph node metastases are common but lung and bone metastases are rare.

Microscopically, the tumour resembles hepatocytes when well differentiated and can be difficult to distinguish from normal liver.

Clinical features

In patients with underlying cirrhosis there may be ascites, jaundice, worsening synthetic LFTs and variceal haemorrhage. Other symptoms include weight loss, anorexia and abdominal pain. Many tumours detected through screening programmes are asymptomatic. In patients without cirrhosis tumours are often much larger at presentation (usually > 5 cm), in which case abdominal pain and weight loss are more common.

Examination may reveal hepatomegaly or a right hypochondrial mass. Tumour vascularity can lead to an abdominal bruit, and hepatic rupture with intra-abdominal bleeding may occur.

Screening

Screening for hepatocellular carcinoma, by ultrasound scanning at 3–6-month intervals, is indicated in high-risk patients such as those with cirrhosis due to hepatitis B and C, haemochromatosis, alcohol and α_1-antitrypsin deficiency. Although no randomised controlled studies of outcome have been undertaken, screening has been shown to identify smaller tumours, often less than 3 cm, which are more likely to be cured by surgical resection, local ablative therapy or transplantation.

Investigations

Serum markers

Alpha-fetoprotein (AFP) is produced by 60% of hepatocellular carcinomas. Levels increase with the size of the tumour and are often normal in small tumours detected by ultrasound screening. Serum AFP also rises in the presence of active hepatitis B and C viral replication; very high levels are also seen in acute hepatic necrosis such as that following paracetamol toxicity. AFP is not therefore a useful screening tool for hepatocellular carcinoma.

Ultrasound

This will detect focal liver lesions as small as 2–3 cm. The use of ultrasound contrast agents has increased the sensitivity and specificity of the technique. Ultrasound may also show evidence of portal vein involvement and features to suggest coexistent cirrhosis.

CT

Helical CT, following intravenous contrast, identifies hepatocellular carcinoma by its classical hypervascular appearance (Fig. 23.38). Small lesions less than 2 cm can be difficult to differentiate from hyperplastic nodules in cirrhosis.

MRI

This can be used instead of helical CT. Hepatocellular cancers are characteristically hypointense on T1-weighted imaging and hyperintense on T2-weighted imaging.

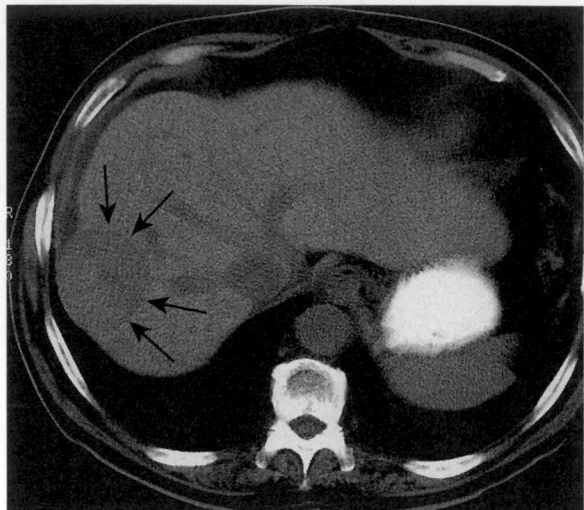

Fig. 23.38 CT showing a large hepatocellular carcinoma (arrows).

Imaging techniques tend to underestimate the multifocality of the tumour and combinations of ultrasound scanning and CT or MRI are often helpful.

Angiography

This has been superseded by helical CT and MRI, and is rarely required.

Liver biopsy

Histological confirmation is advisable in patients with large tumours who do not have cirrhosis or hepatitis B in order to confirm the diagnosis and exclude metastatic tumour. Biopsy is usually avoided in patients who may be eligible for transplantation or surgical resection because there is a small risk of tumour seeding along the needle tract.

Management

This differs between patients with and without cirrhosis.

Hepatic resection

This is the treatment of choice for non-cirrhotic patients. The 5-year survival in this group is about 50%. However, there is a 50% recurrence rate at 5 years; this may be due to a second de novo tumour or recurrence of the original tumour. Few patients with cirrhosis are amenable to hepatic resection because of the high risk of hepatic failure; nevertheless, surgery is offered, particularly in the Far East, to some cirrhotic patients with small tumours and good liver function (Child–Pugh A with no portal hypertension).

Liver transplantation

In the presence of cirrhosis transplantation has the benefit of curing the cirrhosis and removing the risk of a second de novo tumour. The 5-year survival following liver transplantation is 75% for single tumours less than 5 cm or three tumours less than 3 cm. Unfortunately, hepatitis B and C may recur in the transplanted liver.

Percutaneous ablation

Percutaneous ethanol injection into the tumour under ultrasound guidance is efficacious (80% cure rate) for tumours 3 cm or smaller. Recurrence rates (50% at 3 years) are similar to those following surgical resection. Radio-frequency ablation, using a single electrode inserted into the tumour under radiological guidance, is an alternative means of ablation that takes longer to perform but appears to cause more complete tumour necrosis.

Chemoembolisation

Hepatocellular cancers are not radiosensitive and the response rate to chemotherapy with drugs such as adriamycin is only around 30%. In contrast, hepatic artery embolisation with Gelfoam and adriamycin is more effective, with survival rates of 60% in cirrhotic patients with unresectable hepatocellular carcinoma and good liver function (compared with 20% in untreated patients) at 2 years. Unfortunately, any survival benefit is lost at 4 years.

Prevention

Hepatitis B vaccination has led to a fall in hepatocellular carcinoma in countries with a high prevalence of hepatitis B, such as Taiwan.

Prognosis

Prognosis depends on tumour size, the presence of vascular invasion, and liver function in those with cirrhosis. Screening has improved the outlook through early detection.

FIBROLAMELLAR HEPATOCELLULAR CARCINOMA

This rare variant differs from the more common hepato-cellular carcinoma in that it occurs in young adults, equally in males and females, in the absence of hepatitis B infection and cirrhosis. The tumours are often large at presentation and the AFP is usually normal. Histology of the tumour reveals malignant hepatocytes that are surrounded by a dense fibrous stroma. The treatment of choice is surgical resection. This variant of hepatocellular carcinoma has a better prognosis following surgery than an equivalent sized hepatocellular carcinoma, two-thirds of patients surviving beyond 5 years.

OTHER PRIMARY MALIGNANT TUMOURS

These are rare but include haemangio-endothelial sarcomas.

SECONDARY MALIGNANT TUMOURS

These are common and usually originate from carcinomas in the lung, breast, abdomen or pelvis. They may be single or multiple. Peritoneal dissemination frequently results in ascites.

Clinical features

The primary neoplasm is asymptomatic in about half of patients. There is usually liver enlargement and weight loss; jaundice may be present.

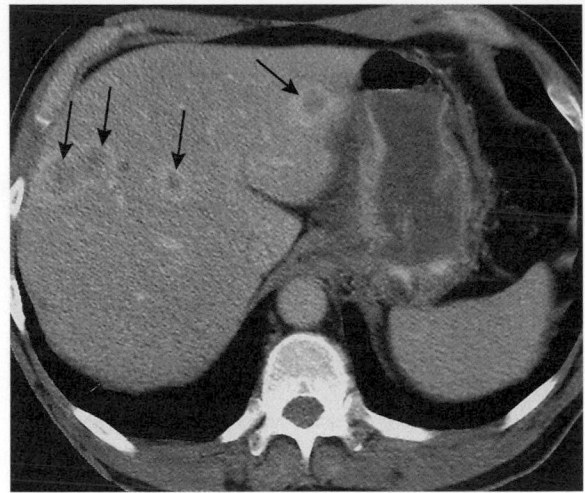

Fig. 23.39 CT showing multiple liver metastases (arrows).

Investigations

A raised alkaline phosphatase activity is the most common biochemical abnormality but LFTs may be normal. Ascitic fluid, if present, has a high protein content and may be blood-stained; cytology sometimes reveals malignant cells. Imaging (p. 941) usually reveals filling defects (Fig. 23.39); laparoscopy may reveal the tumour and facilitates liver aspiration or biopsy.

Management

Hepatic resection can improve survival for slow-growing tumours such as colonic carcinomas. Patients with hormone-producing tumours, such as gastrinomas, insulinomas and glucagonomas, and those with lymphomas may benefit from hormonal treatment or chemotherapy. Unfortunately, palliative treatment to relieve pain is all that is available for most patients; this may include arterial embolisation of the tumour masses.

BENIGN TUMOURS

The increasing use of ultrasound scanning has led to more frequent identification of incidental benign focal liver lesions.

HAEMANGIOMAS

These are the most common benign liver tumours; they are present in 5% of the population and rarely cause symptoms (Fig. 23.40).

HEPATIC ADENOMAS

These are rare vascular tumours which may present as an abdominal mass, or with abdominal pain or intraperitoneal bleeding. They are more common in women and may be caused by oral contraceptives, androgens and anabolic steroids. Resection is indicated for the relief of symptoms

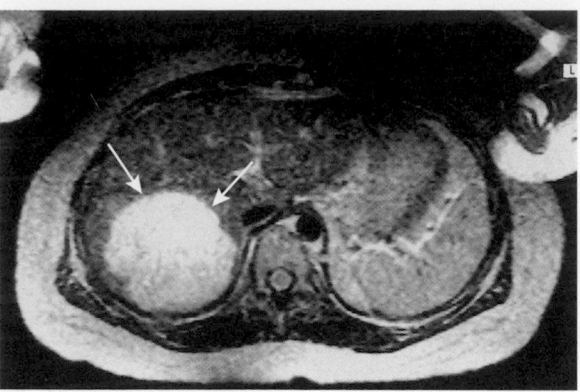

Fig. 23.40 MRI showing a haemangioma (arrows) in the liver.

and if pregnancy is contemplated, as they can increase in size during pregnancy.

FOCAL NODULAR HYPERPLASIA (FNH)

These lesions are asymptomatic but can be up to 10 cm in diameter; they can be differentiated from adenoma because of a focal central scar seen on CT or MRI. Histologically, they consist of nodular regeneration of hepatocytes but without fibrosis. They may be multiple and do not need to be resected.

23.60 LIVER DISEASE IN OLD AGE

- **Alcoholic liver disease:** 10% of cases present over the age of 70 years, when disease is more likely to be severe and has a worse prognosis.
- **Hepatitis A:** causes more severe illness and runs a more protracted course.
- **Primary biliary cirrhosis:** one-third of cases are over 65 years and age is an adverse prognostic factor.
- **Liver abscess:** more than 50% of all cases in the UK are over 60 years.
- **Hepatocellular carcinoma:** approximately 50% of cases present over the age of 65 years in the UK.
- **Surgery:** older people are less likely to survive liver surgery (including transplantation) because comorbidity is more prevalent.

MISCELLANEOUS LIVER DISEASES

LIVER ABSCESSES

Liver abscesses can be classified as pyogenic, hydatid or amoebic.

PYOGENIC LIVER ABSCESS

Pyogenic liver abscesses are uncommon but important because they are potentially curable, inevitably fatal if untreated, and readily overlooked.

23.61 CAUSES OF PYOGENIC LIVER ABSCESSES

- Biliary obstruction (cholangitis)
- Haematogenous
    Portal vein (mesenteric infections)
    Hepatic artery (bacteraemia)
- Direct extension
- Trauma
    Penetrating or non-penetrating
- Infection of liver tumour or cyst

Aetiology and pathology

Infection can reach the liver in several ways (Box 23.61). Abscesses are most common in older patients and usually result from ascending infection due to biliary obstruction (cholangitis) or contiguous spread from an empyema of the gallbladder. Abscesses complicating suppurative appendicitis used to be common in young adults but are now rare. Immunocompromised patients are particularly likely to develop liver abscesses. Single lesions are more common in the right liver; multiple abscesses are usually due to infection secondary to biliary obstruction. Abscesses vary greatly in size. *E. coli* and various streptococci, particularly *Strep. milleri*, are the most common organisms; anaerobes, including streptococci and *Bacteroides*, can often be found when infection has been transmitted from large bowel pathology via the portal vein, and multiple organisms are present in one-third of patients.

Clinical features

Patients are generally ill with fever, sometimes rigors and weight loss. Abdominal pain is the most common symptom and is usually in the right upper quadrant, sometimes with radiation to the right shoulder. The pain may be pleuritic in nature. Hepatomegaly is found in more than half of patients and tenderness can usually be elicited by gentle percussion over the organ. Mild jaundice may be present but is severe only when large abscesses cause biliary obstruction. Abnormalities are present at the base of the right lung in about one-quarter of patients. Atypical presentations are common and explain the frequency with which the diagnosis is made only at autopsy. This is a particular problem in patients with gradually developing illnesses or pyrexia of unknown origin without localising features. Necrotic colorectal metastases can be misdiagnosed as hepatic abscess.

Investigations

Liver imaging is the most revealing investigation and shows 90% or more of symptomatic abscesses. Needle aspiration under ultrasound guidance confirms the diagnosis and provides pus for culture. A leucocytosis is frequently found, plasma alkaline phosphatase activity is usually increased, and the serum albumin is often low. The chest X-ray may show a raised right diaphragm and lung collapse or an effusion at the base of the right lung. Blood culture should always be carried out as it may reveal the causative organism.

Management

This includes prolonged antibiotic therapy and drainage of the abscess. Pending the results of culture of blood and pus from the abscess, treatment should commence with a combination of antibiotics such as ampicillin, gentamicin and metronidazole. Aspiration or drainage with a catheter placed in the abscess under ultrasound guidance is required if the abscess is large or if it does not respond to antibiotics. Surgical drainage is rarely undertaken, although hepatic resection may be indicated for a chronic persistent abscess or 'pseudotumour'.

Prognosis

The mortality of liver abscesses is 20–40%; failure to make the diagnosis is the most common cause of death. Older patients and those with multiple abscesses also have a higher mortality.

HYDATID CYSTS

Hydatid cysts are caused by *Echinococcus granulosus* infection (p. 371). They have an outer layer derived from the host, an intermediate laminated layer and an inner germinal layer. They can be single (Fig. 23.41) or multiple. Chronic cysts become calcified. The cysts may be asymptomatic but may present with abdominal pain or a mass. There may be a peripheral blood eosinophilia, X-rays may show calcification, imaging shows the cyst(s), and serological tests are positive in 50% of cases. Rupture or secondary infection of cysts can occur, and a communication with the intrahepatic biliary tree can then result.

All patients are treated medically with albendazole or mebendazole prior to definitive therapy. In the absence of communications with the biliary tree, treatment consists of percutaneous aspiration of the cyst followed by the injection of 100% ethanol into the cysts and then re-aspiration of the cyst contents (PAIR). Where communication occurs between the cyst and biliary system, surgical removal of the intact cyst is the preferred treatment.

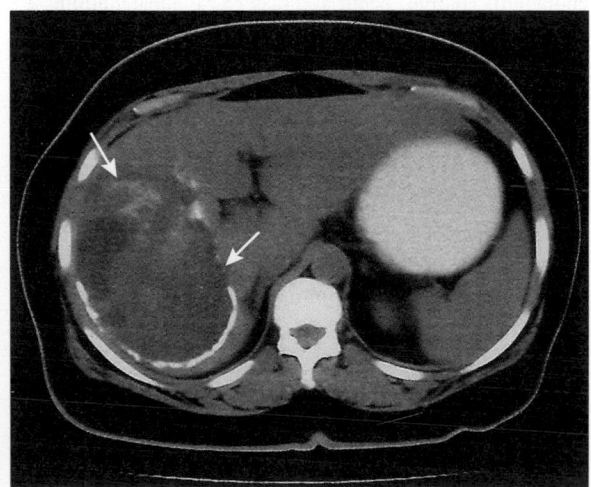

Fig. 23.41 Hydatid cyst of the liver on CT (arrows).

AMOEBIC LIVER ABSCESSES

Amoebic liver abscesses are caused by *Entamoeba histolytica* infection. Up to 50% of cases do not have a previous history of intestinal disease. Although amoebic liver abscesses are most often found in endemic areas, patients can present with no history of travel to these places. Abscesses are usually large, single and located in the right lobe; multiple abscesses may occur in advanced disease. Fever and abdominal pain or swelling are the most common symptoms. Diagnosis may depend on cyst aspiration revealing the classic anchovy sauce appearance of the cyst fluid. Treatment is described on page 359.

THE LIVER AND HIV

Some causes of abnormal LFTs in HIV infection are shown in Box 23.62. This topic is discussed in more detail on page 388.

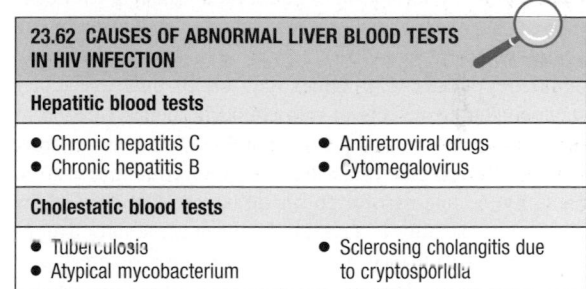

23.62 CAUSES OF ABNORMAL LIVER BLOOD TESTS IN HIV INFECTION	
Hepatitic blood tests	
• Chronic hepatitis C	• Antiretroviral drugs
• Chronic hepatitis B	• Cytomegalovirus
Cholestatic blood tests	
• Tuberculosis	• Sclerosing cholangitis due
• Atypical mycobacterium	to cryptosporidia

PREGNANCY AND THE LIVER

Liver disease in pregnancy may be intercurrent, pregnancy-associated or pre-existing.

INTERCURRENT LIVER DISEASE

When elevated serum transaminases are present, acute viral hepatitis and drug causes need to be excluded. Acute hepatitis A can occur during pregnancy but has no effect on the fetus. Gallstones (p. 991) are more common during pregnancy and may present with cholestatic LFTs and pain; they can be safely identified by ultrasound scanning.

PREGNANCY-ASSOCIATED LIVER DISEASE

These conditions only occur during pregnancy, may recur in subsequent pregnancies, and resolve after delivery of the baby.

Intrahepatic cholestasis of pregnancy

This usually occurs in the third trimester of pregnancy but can occur earlier; it is associated with intrauterine growth retardation and premature birth. There is a high prevalence in Chile. The condition characteristically presents with itching and cholestatic LFTs; however, the bilirubin may be normal and the liver biochemistry hepatitic. Bile salts are elevated in the serum. UDCA prevents premature birth and should be given at a daily dose of 15 mg/kg.

23

23.63 HEPATIC MITOCHONDRIAL CYTOPATHIES

- Acute fatty liver of pregnancy
- Reye's syndrome (aspirin toxicity in childhood)
- Toxins
    Bacillus cereus
- Drugs
    Sodium valproate
    Tetracyclines

Acute fatty liver of pregnancy

This is more common in twin and first pregnancies. It typically presents between 31 and 38 weeks of pregnancy with vomiting and abdominal pain followed by jaundice. In severe cases this may be followed by lactic acidosis, a coagulopathy, encephalopathy and renal failure. Hypoglycaemia can also occur. The features are characteristic of a defect in beta-oxidation of fatty acids in the mitochondria that leads to the formation of small fat droplets in liver cells (known as microvesicular fatty liver). Some women are heterozygous for long-chain 3-hydroxy-CoA dehydrogenase deficiency (LCHAD). Other causes of microvesicular steatosis due to defects in mitochondrial beta-oxidation of fatty acids are shown in Box 23.63. Differentiation from toxaemia of pregnancy (which is more common) can be made by the finding of high serum uric acid levels and the absence of haemolysis. Overlap between acute fatty liver of pregnancy, HELP (see below) and toxaemia of pregnancy can occur. Early diagnosis and delivery of the fetus has led to a fall in maternal mortality to 1–15%.

Toxaemia of pregnancy and HELP

The HELP syndrome is a variant of pre-eclampsia that tends to affect multiparous women and comprises **h**aemolysis, **e**levated **l**iver enzymes and thrombocyto**p**enia. Liver disease is associated with hypertension, proteinuria and fluid retention. Serum transaminases are high and the condition can be complicated by hepatic infarction and rupture.

PRE-EXISTING LIVER DISEASE

Pregnancy is uncommon in cirrhosis because of infertility. The risk of variceal bleeding increases during pregnancy and vaginal delivery is usually avoided if varices are present.

CYSTIC AND FIBROPOLYCYSTIC DISEASE

Fibropolycystic diseases of the liver and biliary system constitute a heterogeneous group of rare disorders, some of which are inherited. They are not distinct entities and combined lesions occur.

SOLITARY HEPATIC CYSTS

Isolated hepatic cysts may be discovered by chance; rarely, they give rise to complications, including pain or jaundice from cyst enlargement, haemorrhage or infection. Portal hypertension and bleeding from varices are exceptional.

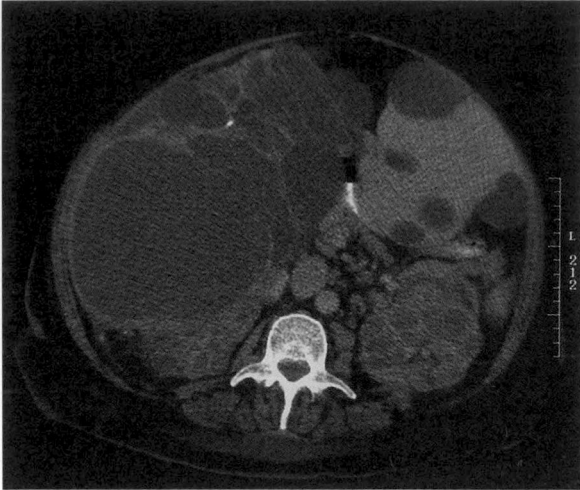

Fig. 23.42 CT showing multiple cysts in the liver and kidneys in polycystic disease.

Diagnosis is best made by ultrasonography. Resection of a large cyst or groups of cysts is only required if symptoms are troublesome. The prognosis is excellent.

ADULT HEPATORENAL POLYCYSTIC DISEASE

The kidneys are predominantly affected in this condition (Fig. 23.42), which is inherited as an autosomal dominant trait (p. 506). Hepatic cysts which do not communicate with the biliary system are present in over half of patients with renal cysts, and cysts can also be found in other organs. Cerebrovascular aneurysms may develop. Cysts restricted to the liver constitute a separate rare genetic disorder.

CAROLI'S SYNDROME

This is very rare and is characterised by segmental saccular dilatations of the intrahepatic biliary tree. The whole liver is usually affected, and extrahepatic biliary dilatation occurs in about one-quarter of patients. Recurrent attacks of cholangitis (p. 994) occur and may cause hepatic abscesses. Complications include biliary stones and cholangiocarcinoma. Antibiotics are required for episodes of cholangitis. Occasionally, localised disease can be treated by segmental liver resection.

CONGENITAL HEPATIC FIBROSIS

This is characterised by broad bands of fibrous tissue linking the portal tracts in the liver, abnormalities of the interlobular bile ducts, and sometimes a lack of portal venules. The renal tubules may show cystic dilatation (medullary sponge kidney, p. 507) and eventually renal cysts may develop. The condition can be inherited as an autosomal recessive trait. Liver involvement causes portal hypertension with splenomegaly and bleeding from oesophageal varices that usually presents in adolescence or in early adult life. The prognosis is good because liver function is preserved. Treatment may be required for variceal bleeding and occa-

23

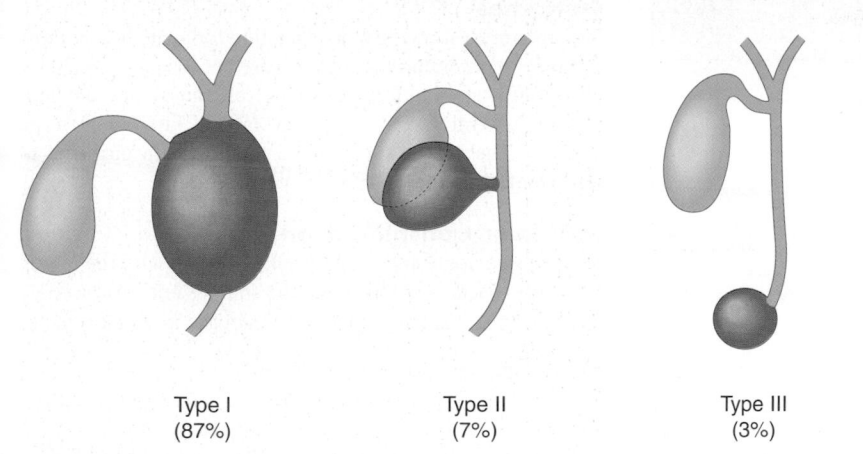
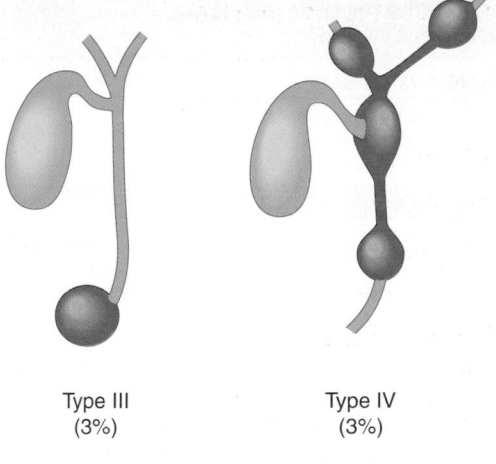

| Type I (87%) | Type II (7%) | Type III (3%) | Type IV (3%) |

Fig. 23.43 Classification and frequency of choledochal cysts.

sionally cholangitis. Patients can present during childhood with renal failure if the kidneys are severely affected.

CHOLEDOCHAL CYSTS

This term applies to cysts anywhere in the biliary tree (Fig. 23.43). The great majority cause diffuse dilatation of the common bile duct (type I), but others take the form of biliary diverticula (type II), dilatation of the intraduodenal bile duct (type III) and multiple biliary cysts (type IV). The last type merges with Caroli's syndrome (see above). In the neonate they may present with jaundice or biliary peritonitis. Recurrent jaundice, abdominal pain and cholangitis may arise in the adult. Liver abscess and biliary cirrhosis may develop, and there is an increased incidence of cholangiocarcinoma. Excision of the cyst with hepatico-jejunostomy is the treatment of choice.

CYSTIC FIBROSIS

Cystic fibrosis (p. 685) is associated with a biliary cirrhosis in about 5% of individuals. Splenomegaly and an elevated alkaline phosphatase are characteristic. Complications do not normally arise until late adolescence or early adulthood, when bleeding due to variceal haemorrhage may occur. UDCA improves liver blood tests but it is not known whether it can prevent progression of liver disease.

LIVER TRANSPLANTATION

The outcome following liver transplantation has improved significantly over the last decade and this is now an effective treatment for end-stage liver disease. The number of procedures is limited by cadaveric donor availability and in many parts of the world this had led to living donor transplant programmes. Despite this, 10% of those listed for liver transplantation will die while awaiting a donor liver. The main complications of liver transplantation relate to disease recurrence in the liver graft.

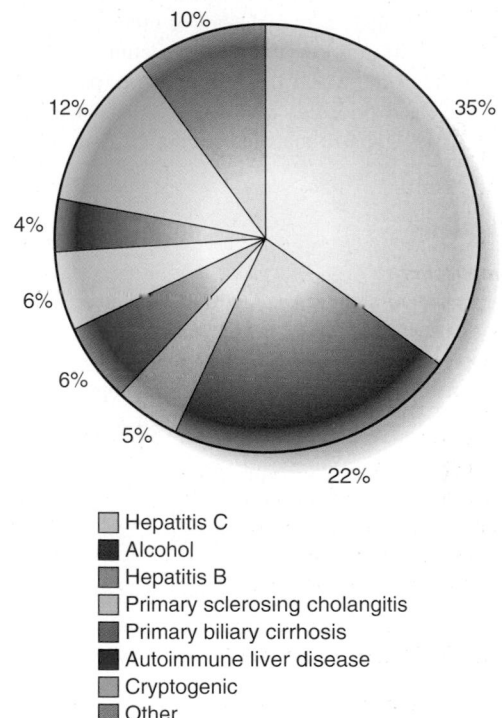

- ☐ Hepatitis C
- ■ Alcohol
- ☐ Hepatitis B
- ☐ Primary sclerosing cholangitis
- ■ Primary biliary cirrhosis
- ■ Autoimmune liver disease
- ☐ Cryptogenic
- ☐ Other

Fig. 23.44 Indications for liver transplantation for chronic liver disease in the USA in 2000. Many cases of cryptogenic liver disease are now considered to represent non-alcoholic fatty liver disease.

Indications

Currently around 9500 liver transplants per year are undertaken in Europe and the USA. About 10% are performed for acute liver failure, 6% for metabolic diseases, 71% for cirrhosis and 11% for hepatocellular carcinoma. Most patients are under 60 years of age and only 10% are aged between 60 and 70 years. The most common indication in North America is hepatitis C cirrhosis where about 10–20% of transplants are for alcoholic cirrhosis (Fig. 23.44). Patients with alcoholic liver disease need to show a capacity for abstinence.

23.64 INDICATIONS FOR LIVER TRANSPLANT ASSESSMENT FOR CIRRHOSIS

Complications

- First episode of bacterial peritonitis
- Diuretic-resistant ascites
- Recurrent variceal haemorrhage
- Hepatocellular carcinoma < 5 cm
- Persistent hepatic encephalopathy

Poor liver function

- Bilirubin > 100 μmol/l (5.8 mg/dl) in primary biliary cirrhosis
- MELD score > 12
- Child–Pugh C

Liver transplantation in cirrhosis is considered when the anticipated mortality without transplantation exceeds 50% at 1 year (Box 23.64).

The main contraindications to transplantation are sepsis, extrahepatic malignancy, active alcohol or other substance misuse, and marked cardiorespiratory dysfunction.

In many parts of the world the MELD score (p. 957) is used to identify and prioritise patients for transplantation. Patients are ABO- and size-matched but not HLA-matched with donors.

Complications

Early complications

Less immunosuppression is needed following liver transplantation than with kidney and heart/lung grafting. Initial immunosuppression is usually with tacrolimus or ciclosporin, prednisolone and azathioprine or mycophenolate. Some patients can eventually be maintained on a single agent.

Acute rejection. This occurs in up to 60% of patients, usually within the first 6 weeks after transplantation, and normally responds to 3 days of high-dose methylprednisolone.

Surgical complications. These include hepatic artery thrombosis which may necessitate retransplantation. Anastomotic biliary strictures can also occur and may respond to balloon dilatation or require surgical reconstruction. Portal vein thrombosis is rare.

Infections. Bacterial infections such as pneumonia and wound infections can occur in the first few weeks after transplantation. Cytomegalovirus (primary infection or reactivation) is a common infection in the 3 months after transplantation and can cause a hepatitis. Patients who have never had cytomegalovirus infection but who receive a liver from a donor who has been exposed are at greatest risk of infection and are usually given prophylactic antiviral therapy such as valciclovir. Tuberculous prophylaxis is given to recipients who have had previous exposure to tuberculosis for the first 6 months after transplantation to prevent reactivation.

Late complications

These include recurrence of the initial disease in the graft and complications due to the immunosuppressive therapy such as renal impairment from ciclosporin. Chronic vascular rejection is rare occurring in only 5% of cases.

Outcomes

The outcome following transplantation for acute liver failure is worse than for chronic liver disease because most patients have multi-organ failure at the time of transplantation. The 1-year survival is 65% but only falls a little to 59% at 5 years. The 1-year survival for patients with cirrhosis is 80–90% falling to 70–75% at 5 years.

Split liver transplantation

A cadaveric donor liver can be split into two with the larger right lobe used in an adult and the smaller left lobe used in a child. This practice has led to an increase in donor organs.

Living donor transplantation

This is normally performed using the left lateral segment or the right lobe. The donor mortality is significant at 0.5%–1%. Pre-operative assessment includes assessing donor liver size and psychological status.

GALLBLADDER AND EXTRAHEPATIC BILIARY DISEASE

FUNCTIONAL ANATOMY

The biliary tract begins in the biliary canaliculi, which are formed by the arrangement of hepatocytes, and the intrahepatic bile ducts derived from them join progressively to form the right and left hepatic ducts. These ducts join as they emerge from the liver to form the common hepatic duct, which becomes the common bile duct after joining the cystic duct (Fig. 23.45). The common bile duct is approximately 5 cm long; it has a thin-walled, wide-lumened proximal part and a thick-walled, narrow-lumened distal part surrounded by the choledochal sphincter. The distal common bile duct usually joins the pancreatic duct before it enters the duodenum. The gallbladder is a pear-shaped sac lying under the right hemiliver, with its fundus located anteriorly behind the tip of the 9th costal cartilage. Its body and neck pass posteromedially towards the porta hepatis, and the cystic duct then joins it to the common hepatic duct. The cystic duct mucosa has prominent crescentic folds (valves of Heister), giving it a beaded appearance on cholangiography.

BILE

The liver secretes 1–2 litres of bile daily. The hepatocytes provide the driving force for bile flow by creating osmotic gradients of bile acids, which form micelles in bile (bile acid-dependent bile flow), and of sodium (bile acid-independent bile flow). Common bile duct pressure is maintained by rhythmic contraction and relaxation of the ampullary sphincter; this pressure exceeds gallbladder pressure in the fasting state, so that bile normally flows into the gallbladder where it is concentrated some tenfold by resorption of water and electrolytes. Cholecystokinin released from the duodenal mucosa during feeding causes gallbladder contraction and reduces sphincter pressure, so that bile flows into the duodenum. Vagal activity maintains

23

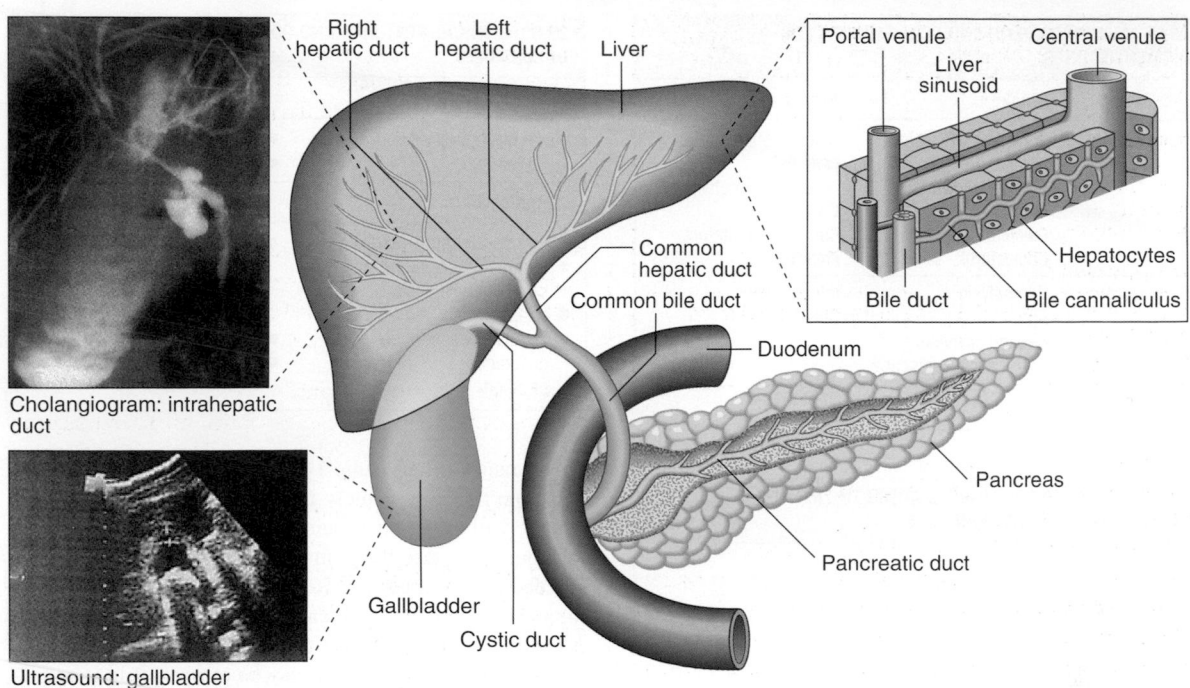

Right hepatic duct

Left hepatic duct

Liver

Portal venule

Central venule

Liver sinusoid

Common hepatic duct

Common bile duct

Hepatocytes

Bile duct

Bile cannaliculus

Duodenum

Cholangiogram: intrahepatic duct

Pancreas

Pancreatic duct

Gallbladder

Cystic duct

Ultrasound: gallbladder

Fig. 23.45 Functional anatomy of the biliary tree.

23

gallbladder tone, but sympathetic activity has little or no effect on the gallbladder.

GALLSTONES

Gallstone formation is the most common disorder of the biliary tree and it is unusual for the gallbladder to be diseased in the absence of gallstones.

Pathology

Gallstones are conveniently classified into cholesterol or pigment stones, although the majority are of mixed composition. Cholesterol stones are most common in developed countries, whereas pigment stones are more frequent in developing countries. Gallstones contain varying quantities of calcium salts, including calcium bilirubinate, carbonate, phosphate and palmitate, which are radio-opaque.

Epidemiology

In developed countries gallstones are common and occur in 7% of males and 15% of females aged 18–65 years, with an overall prevalence of 11%. In those under 40 years there is a 3:1 female preponderance, whereas in the elderly the sex ratio is about equal. In developed countries the incidence of symptomatic gallstones appears to be increasing and they occur at an earlier age. Gallstones are less frequent in India, the Far East and Africa.

There has been much debate over the role of diet in cholesterol gallstone disease; an increase in dietary cholesterol, fat, total calories and refined carbohydrate or lack of dietary fibre have all been implicated. At present the best data support an association between simple refined sugar in the diet and gallstones. There is a negative association between a moderate alcohol intake (2–3 units daily) and gallstones.

Aetiology

Gallstone formation is multifactorial, and the factors involved are related to the type of gallstone (Boxes 23.65 and 23.66).

Cholesterol gallstones

Cholesterol is held in solution in bile by its association with bile acids and phospholipids in the form of micelles and vesicles. Biliary lipoproteins may also have a role in solubilising cholesterol. In gallstone disease the liver produces bile which contains an excess of cholesterol, because there is either a relative deficiency of bile salts or a relative excess of cholesterol. Such bile, which is super-saturated with cholesterol, is termed 'lithogenic'. Disorders with the potential to induce the production of lithogenic bile

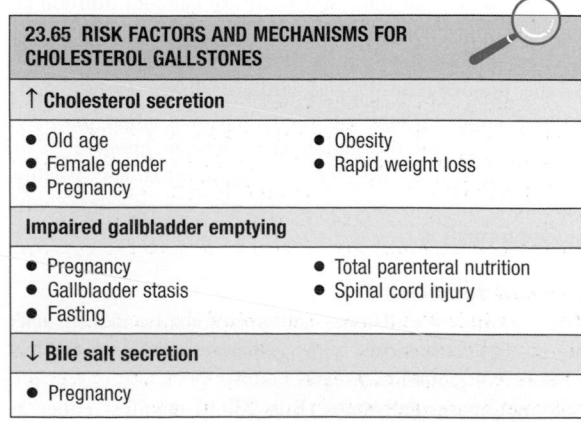

23.65 RISK FACTORS AND MECHANISMS FOR CHOLESTEROL GALLSTONES	
↑ **Cholesterol secretion**	
• Old age	• Obesity
• Female gender	• Rapid weight loss
• Pregnancy	
Impaired gallbladder emptying	
• Pregnancy	• Total parenteral nutrition
• Gallbladder stasis	• Spinal cord injury
• Fasting	
↓ **Bile salt secretion**	
• Pregnancy	

23.66 COMPOSITION OF AND RISK FACTORS FOR PIGMENT STONES

	Black	Brown
Composition	Polymerised calcium bilirubinates* Mucin glycoprotein Calcium phosphate Calcium carbonate Cholesterol	Calcium bilirubinate crystals* Mucin glycoprotein Cholesterol Calcium palmitate/ stearate
Risk factors	Haemolysis Age Hepatic cirrhosis Ileal resection/disease	Infected bile Stasis

* Major component.

23.67 PATHOGENIC FACTORS LEADING TO THE PRODUCTION OF LITHOGENIC BILE

- Defective bile salt synthesis
- Excessive intestinal loss of bile salts
- Over-sensitive bile salt feedback
- Excessive cholesterol secretion
- Abnormal gallbladder function

are shown in Box 23.67. Factors initiating crystallisation of cholesterol in lithogenic bile (nucleation factors) are also important; patients with cholesterol gallstones have gallbladder bile which forms cholesterol crystals more rapidly than equally saturated bile from patients who do not form gallstones. Factors favouring nucleation (mucus, calcium, fatty acids, other proteins) and antinucleating factors (apolipoproteins) have been described.

Pigment stones

Brown crumbly pigment stones are almost always the consequence of bacterial or parasitic infection in the biliary tree. They are found commonly in the Far East, where infection of the biliary tree allows bacterial β-glucuronidase to hydrolyse conjugated bilirubin to its free form, which then precipitates as calcium bilirubinate. The mechanism of black pigment gallstone formation in developed countries is not satisfactorily explained. Haemolysis is important, as these stones occur in chronic haemolytic disease.

Biliary sludge

The term 'biliary sludge' describes gelatinous bile that contains numerous microspheroliths of calcium bilirubinate granules and cholesterol crystals as well as glycoproteins; it is an important precursor to the formation of gallstones in the majority of patients. Biliary sludge is frequently formed under normal conditions, but then either dissolves or is cleared by the gallbladder; only in about 15% of patients does it persist to form cholesterol stones. Fasting, parenteral nutrition and pregnancy are also associated with sludge formation.

Clinical features

The majority of gallstones are asymptomatic; indeed, only about 10% of those with gallstones develop clinical evidence of gallstone disease.

Symptomatic gallstones (Box 23.68) manifest either as

23.68 CLINICAL FEATURES AND COMPLICATIONS OF GALLSTONES

Clinical features

- Asymptomatic
- Biliary colic
- Acute cholecystitis
- Chronic cholecystitis

Complications

- Empyema of the gallbladder
- Porcelain gallbladder
- Choledocholithiasis
- Pancreatitis
- Fistulae between the gallbladder and duodenum or colon
- Pressure on/inflammation of the common bile duct by a gallstone in the cystic duct (Mirizzi's syndrome)
- Gallstone ileus
- Cancer of the gallbladder

biliary pain ('biliary colic') or cholecystitis (see below). If a gallstone becomes acutely impacted in the cystic duct, the patient will experience pain. The term 'biliary colic' is a misnomer because the pain does not rhythmically increase and decrease in intensity like other forms of colic. Typically, the pain occurs suddenly and persists for about 2 hours; if it continues for more than 6 hours a complication such as cholecystitis or pancreatitis may be present. Pain is usually felt in the epigastrium (70% of patients) or right upper quadrant (20% of patients) and radiates to the interscapular region or the tip of the right scapula, but other sites include the left upper quadrant, the epigastrium and the lower chest. The pain can mimic intrathoracic disease, oesophagitis, myocardial infarction or dissecting aneurysm.

Combinations of fatty food intolerance, dyspepsia and flatulence not attributable to other causes have been referred to as 'gallstone dyspepsia'. These symptoms are not now recognised as being caused by gallstones and are best regarded as non-ulcer dyspepsia (p. 864).

Acute and chronic cholecystitis are described below.

Investigations

A plain abdominal X-ray will demonstrate calcified gallstones in less than 20% of patients. Ultrasonography is the method of choice for diagnosing gallstones (Fig. 23.5, p. 941) but oral cholecystography and CT can also be used (Fig. 23.46). MRCP is becoming increasingly available and can demonstrate gallstones and their complications.

Complications

A mucocele may develop if there is slow distension of the gallbladder from continuous secretion of mucus; if this material becomes infected, an empyema supervenes. Calcium may be secreted into the lumen of the hydropic gallbladder, causing limy bile, and if calcium salts are precipitated in the gallbladder wall the radiological appearance of 'porcelain' gallbladder results.

Gallstones in the gallbladder (cholecystolithiasis) migrate to the common bile duct (choledocholithiasis, p. 994) in approximately 15% of patients and cause biliary colic. Rarely, fistulae develop between the gallbladder and the duodenum, colon or stomach. Air will be seen in the biliary tree on plain abdominal X-rays. If a stone larger than 2.5 cm in diameter has migrated into the gut it may impact either at the terminal ileum or occasionally in the duodenum or

23

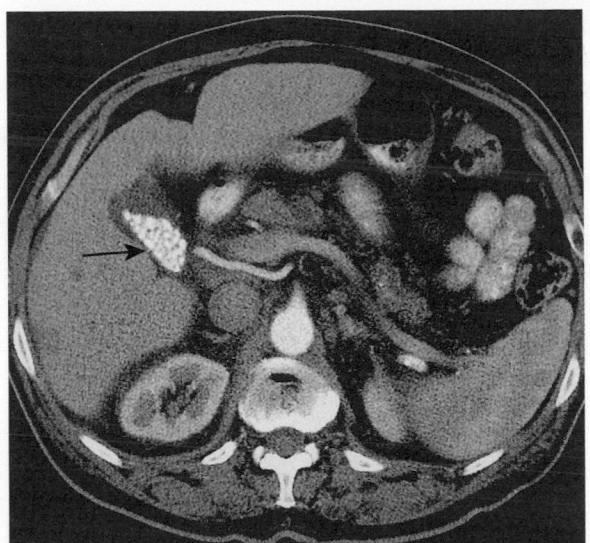

Fig. 23.46 CT showing a gallstone within the gallbladder (arrow).

sigmoid colon. The resultant intestinal obstruction may be followed by 'gallstone ileus'. Rarely, gallstones impacted in the cystic duct cause stricturing of the common hepatic duct (Mirizzi's syndrome) and obstructive jaundice.

Cancer of the gallbladder is uncommon (p. 995). In over 95% of patients with gallbladder cancer there are accompanying gallstones. Cancer is usually diagnosed as an incidental histological finding following cholecystectomy for gallstone disease.

Management
Asymptomatic gallstones found incidentally are not usually treated because the majority will never give symptoms. Symptomatic gallstones are best treated surgically using minimal access techniques. Gallstones can be dissolved and fragmented in the gallbladder or removed mechanically from the common bile duct (Box 23.69).

Medical dissolution of gallstones can be achieved by oral administration of the bile acid UDCA. Radiolucent gallstones, a gallbladder that opacifies on oral cholecysto-graphy, stones smaller than 15 mm in diameter, moderate obesity and no or at most mild symptoms are the features which suggest that drug therapy may be feasible. Success can be expected in approximately 75% of patients who fulfil these criteria. Extracorporeal shock-wave lithotripsy is expensive and not widely available. Bile salt therapy is necessary following lithotripsy to dissolve the gallstone fragments within the gallbladder. Only 30% of all patients with gallbladder disease are suitable for lithotripsy. All therapeutic regimens which retain the gallbladder have a 50% recurrence of stones after 5 years.

23.69 TREATMENT OF GALLSTONES

- Cholecystectomy—open or laparoscopic
- Oral bile acids—chenodeoxycholic or ursodeoxycholic
- Lithotripsy
- Endoscopic sphincterotomy

CHOLECYSTITIS

ACUTE CHOLECYSTITIS
Aetiology and pathology
Acute cholecystitis is almost always associated with obstruction of the gallbladder neck or cystic duct by a gallstone. Occasionally, obstruction may be by mucus, parasitic worms or a tumour. The pathogenesis is unclear, but the initial inflammation is possibly chemically induced. This leads to gallbladder mucosal damage which releases phospholipase, converting biliary lecithin to lysolecithin, a recognised mucosal toxin. At the time of surgery approx-imately 50% of cultures of the gallbladder contents are sterile. Infection occurs eventually and in elderly patients or those with diabetes mellitus a severe infection with gas-forming organisms can cause emphysematous cholecystitis. Acalculous cholecystitis can occur in the intensive care setting.

Clinical features
The cardinal feature is pain in the right upper quadrant but also in the epigastrium, the right shoulder tip or inter-scapular region. Differentiation between biliary colic (p. 992) and acute cholecystitis may be difficult; features suggesting cholecystitis include severe and prolonged pain, fever and leucocytosis.

Examination shows right hypochondrial tenderness, rigidity worse on inspiration (Murphy's sign) and occa-sionally a gallbladder mass. Fever is present but rigors are unusual. Jaundice occurs in less than 10% of patients and is usually due to the presence or recent passage of stones in the common bile duct.

Investigations
Peripheral blood leucocytosis is common, except in the elderly patient where the signs of inflammation may be minimal. Minor increases of plasma transaminases and plasma amylase concentration may be encountered. The plasma amylase should be measured to detect acute pancreatitis (p. 904), which may be a potentially serious complication of gallstones. Plain X-rays of the abdomen and chest may show radio-opaque gallstones, and rarely intrabiliary gas due to fistulation of a gallstone into the intestine, and are important in excluding lower lobe pneumonia and a perforated viscus. Ultrasonography detects gallstones and gallbladder thickening due to cholecystitis.

Management
Medical
This consists of bed rest, pain relief, antibiotics and maintenance of fluid balance. Moderate pain is relieved using diclofenac, and more severe pain should be relieved by pethidine. Antibiotics are required. A cephalosporin (such as cefuroxime) is the antibiotic of choice, and metronidazole is usually added in severely ill patients. Fluid balance is maintained by intravenous therapy, and naso-gastric aspiration is only needed for persistent vomiting. Cholecystitis usually resolves with medical treatment, but the inflammation may progress to an empyema or perforation and peritonitis.

23

Surgical

Urgent surgery is required when cholecystitis progresses in spite of medical therapy and when complications such as empyema or perforation develop. Operation should be carried out within 5 days of the onset of symptoms. Delayed surgery after 2–3 months is no longer favoured. Recurrent biliary colic or cholecystitis is frequent if the gallbladder is not removed.

CHRONIC CHOLECYSTITIS

Chronic inflammation of the gallbladder is almost invariably associated with gallstones. The usual symptoms are those of recurrent attacks of upper abdominal pain, often at night and following a heavy meal. The clinical features are similar to those of acute calculous cholecystitis but milder. The patient may recover spontaneously or following analgesia and antibiotics. Patients are usually advised to undergo elective laparoscopic cholecystectomy.

ACUTE CHOLANGITIS

Acute cholangitis is caused by bacterial infection of bile ducts and occurs in patients with other biliary problems such as choledocholithiasis (see below), biliary strictures or tumours, or after ERCP. Jaundice, rigors and abdominal pain are the cardinal presenting features. Treatment is with antibiotics and removal (if possible) of the underlying cause.

CHOLEDOCHOLITHIASIS

Stones in the common bile duct (choledocholithiasis) occur in 10–15% of patients with gallstones (Fig. 23.47) and have usually migrated from the gallbladder. Primary bile duct stones are rare but can develop within the common bile duct many years after a cholecystectomy and are sometimes related to biliary sludge arising from dysfunction of the sphincter of Oddi. In Far Eastern countries, where bile duct infection is common, primary common bile duct stones are thought to follow bacterial infection secondary to parasitic infections with *Clonorchis sinensis*, *Ascaris lumbricoides* or *Fasciola hepatica* (pp. 362 and 370) Common bile duct stones can cause partial or complete bile duct obstruction and may be complicated by cholangitis due to secondary bacterial infection, septicaemia, liver abscess and biliary stricture.

Clinical features

Choledocholithiasis may be asymptomatic, may be found incidentally by operative cholangiography at cholecystectomy, or may manifest as recurrent abdominal pain with or without jaundice. The pain is usually in the right upper quadrant and fever, pruritus and dark urine may be present. Rigors may be a feature; painless jaundice is uncommon. Physical examination may show the scar of a previous cholecystectomy; if the gallbladder is present, it is usually small, fibrotic and impalpable.

Investigations

LFTs show a cholestatic pattern and there is bilirubinuria. If cholangitis is present, the patient usually has a leucocytosis.

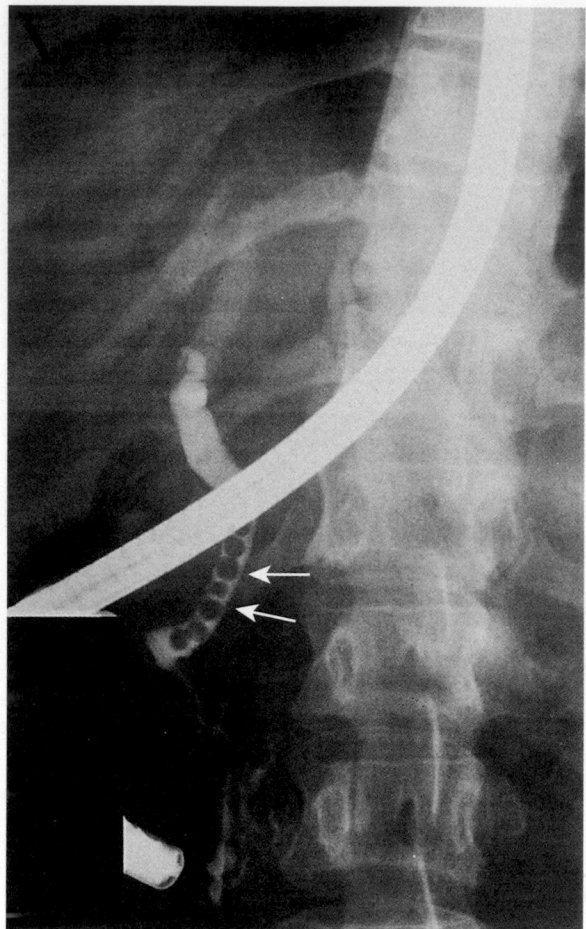

Fig. 23.47 ERCP showing common duct stones (arrows).

The most convenient method of demonstrating obstruction to the common bile duct is by ultrasonography; this shows dilated extrahepatic and intrahepatic bile ducts together with gallbladder stones, but does not always reveal the cause of the obstruction in the common bile duct (Fig. 23.48). ERCP can be used to diagnose obstruction and its cause, and to remove bile duct stones (Fig. 23.47). If ERCP fails, PTC may be undertaken.

Management

Cholangitis requires analgesia, intravenous fluids and broad-spectrum antibiotics such as cefuroxime and metronidazole. Blood cultures should be taken before the antibiotics are administered. Patients require urgent decompression of the biliary tree and stone removal. Endoscopic sphincterotomy and stone extraction is the treatment of choice, particularly in patients over the age of 60, and is successful in about 90% of patients. Less commonly used techniques include extracorporeal lithotripsy.

Surgical treatment of choledocholithiasis is performed less frequently than ERCP because it carries higher morbidity and mortality. Before the common bile duct is explored, an accurate diagnosis of choledocholithiasis should be confirmed by intraoperative cholangiography. If gallstones are found, the bile duct is explored, all stones are

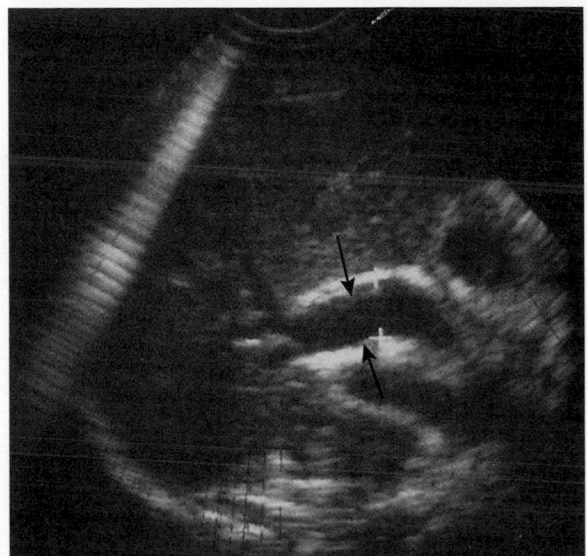

Fig. 23.48 Ultrasound showing dilated bile ducts (between arrows) in obstructive jaundice secondary to obstruction of the common bile duct.

removed, stone clearance is checked by cholangiography or choledochoscopy, and a T-tube is inserted into the common bile duct. It is now possible to achieve these goals in specialist centres by laparoscopic means.

RECURRENT PYOGENIC CHOLANGITIS

This disease occurs in South-east Asia. Biliary sludge, calcium bilirubinate concretions and stones accumulate in the intrahepatic bile ducts, with secondary bacterial infection. The patients present with recurrent attacks of upper abdominal pain, fever and cholestatic jaundice. Investigation of the biliary tree demonstrates that both the intrahepatic and extrahepatic portions are filled with soft biliary mud. Eventually, the liver becomes scarred and liver abscesses develop. The condition is difficult to manage and requires drainage of the biliary tract with extraction of stones, antibiotics and, in certain patients, partial resection of damaged areas of the liver.

TUMOURS OF THE GALLBLADDER AND BILE DUCT

CARCINOMA OF THE GALLBLADDER

This is an uncommon tumour, occurring more often in females and usually encountered above the age of 70 years. More than 90% of such tumours are adenocarcinomas; the remainder are anaplastic or, rarely, squamous tumours. Gallstones are usually present and are thought to be important in the aetiology of the tumour. Individuals with a 'porcelain gallbladder' (p. 992) are at high risk of malignant change.

The condition is usually diagnosed incidentally, following surgery for gallstone disease. Occasionally, it may manifest as repeated attacks of biliary pain and later persistent jaundice and weight loss. A gallbladder mass may be palpable in the right hypochondrium. LFTs show cholestasis, and gallbladder calcification (porcelain gallbladder) may be found on X-ray. The tumour may be diagnosed on ultrasonography and can be staged by CT. The treatment is surgical excision but local extension of the tumour beyond the wall of the gallbladder into the liver, lymph nodes and surrounding tissues is invariable and palliative management is usually all that can be offered. Survival is generally short, with death typically occurring within 1 year.

CHOLANGIOCARCINOMA

This uncommon tumour can arise anywhere in the biliary tree from the small intrahepatic bile ducts to the papilla of Vater, but it is the tumour involving the confluence of the right and left hepatic ducts (Klatskin tumour) which is the most challenging to manage. The cause is unknown but the tumour is associated with gallstones, primary and secondary sclerosing cholangitis, Caroli's disease and choledochal cysts (p. 989). In the Far East, particularly northern Thailand, chronic liver fluke infection is a major risk factor for the development of cholangiocarcinoma in men. Primary sclerosing cholangitis is associated with ulcerative colitis (p. 980), and cholangiocarcinoma may occur some years after proctocolectomy or as a presenting feature. Chronic biliary inflammation appears to be a common factor in the development of biliary dysplasia and cancer that is shared by all the predisposing causes.

Tumours typically invade the lymphatics and adjacent vessels, with a predilection for spread within perineural sheaths.

The patient presents with obstructive jaundice. Half the patients also have upper abdominal pain and weight loss. The diagnosis is made by a combination of ultrasound and cholangiography, but can be difficult to confirm in patients with sclerosing cholangitis. Cholangiocarcinomas can be treated surgically in about 20% of patients, which improves 5-year survival from less than 5% to 20–40%. Surgery involves excision of the extrahepatic biliary tree with or without a liver resection and a Roux loop reconstruction. However, most patients are treated by inserting drainage stents across the tumour, using endoscopic or transhepatic techniques (Fig. 23.49). Combination chemotherapy is increasingly used and palliation with photodynamic therapy has provided encouraging results.

CARCINOMA AT THE PAPILLA OF VATER

Nearly 40% of all adenocarcinomas of the small intestine arise in relationship to the papilla of Vater and present with pain, anaemia, vomiting and weight loss. Jaundice may be intermittent or persistent. Diagnosis is made by duodenal endoscopy and biopsy of the tumour. Ampullary carcinoma must be differentiated from carcinoma of the head of the pancreas and a cholangiocarcinoma because these latter conditions both have a worse prognosis.

Curative surgical treatment can be undertaken by pancreaticoduodenectomy and the 5-year survival may be as

23

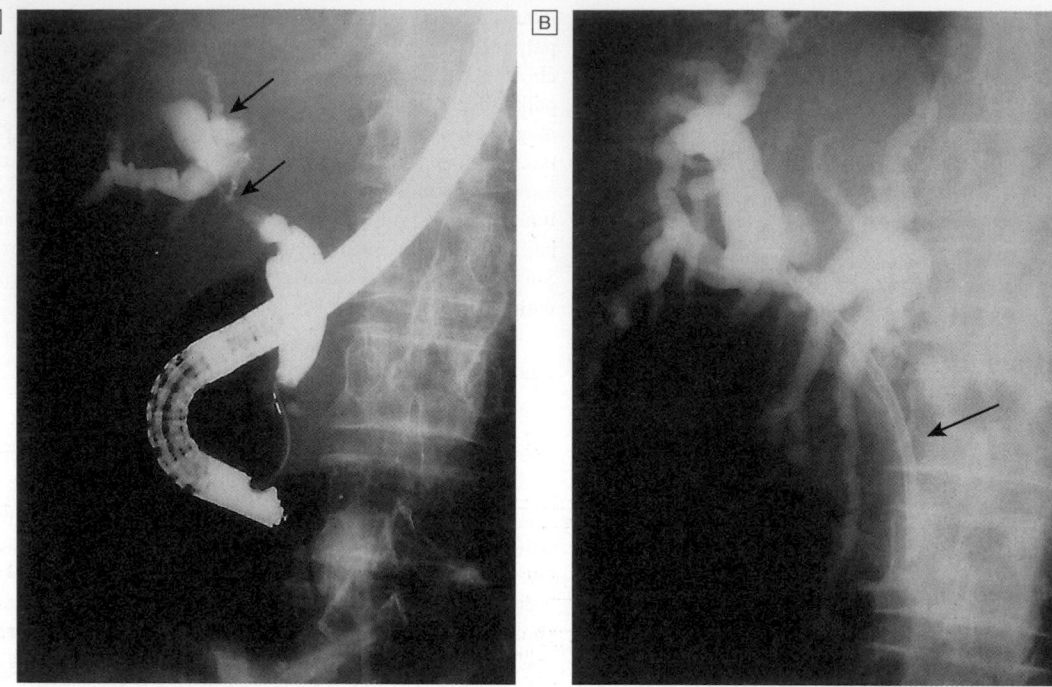

Fig. 23.49 Cholangiocarcinoma. A ERCP showing malignant biliary stricture (bottom arrow) and dilated intrahepatic bile ducts above (top arrow). B Post-ERCP stenting showing plastic endobiliary stent (arrow) which will draw bile from the dilated ducts above the stricture into the duodenum.

high as 50%. When this is impossible, a palliative bypass or insertion of a drainage stent is performed.

BENIGN GALLBLADDER TUMOURS

These are uncommon, often asymptomatic and usually found incidentally at operation or autopsy. Cholesterol polyps, sometimes associated with cholesterolosis, papillomas and adenomas, are the main types.

MISCELLANEOUS BILIARY DISORDERS

POST-CHOLECYSTECTOMY SYNDROME

Dyspeptic symptoms following cholecystectomy (post-cholecystectomy syndrome) occur in about 30% of patients depending on how the condition is defined, how actively symptoms are sought and the original indication for cholecystectomy. They occur most frequently in women, in patients who have had symptoms for more than 5 years before cholecystectomy, and in patients in whom the operation was undertaken for non-calculous gallbladder disease. An increase in bowel habit occurs in about 5–10% of patients after cholecystectomy, which often responds to colestyramine 4–8 g daily. Severe post-cholecystectomy syndrome occurs in only 2–5% of patients. The main causes are listed in Box 23.70.

The usual complaints include right upper quadrant abdominal pain, flatulence, fatty food intolerance, and occasionally jaundice and cholangitis. LFTs may be abnormal and sometimes show cholestasis. Ultrasonography

23.70 CAUSES OF POST-CHOLECYSTECTOMY SYMPTOMS	
Immediate post-surgical	
• Bleeding	• Abscess
• Biliary peritonitis	• Fistula
Biliary	
• Common bile duct stones	• Cystic duct stump syndrome
• Benign stricture	• Disorders of the ampulla of Vater
• Tumour	
Extrabiliary	
• Non-ulcer dyspepsia	• Gastro-oesophageal reflux
• Peptic ulcer	• Irritable bowel syndrome
• Pancreatic disease	• Functional abdominal pain

is used to detect biliary obstruction, and ERCP or MRCP is used to detect common bile duct stones. If retained bile duct stones are excluded, sphincter of Oddi dysfunction should be considered (see below). Other investigations which may be required include upper gastrointestinal endoscopy, barium examination of the small intestine, pancreatic function tests, cholescintigraphy and a liver biopsy. The possibility of a functional illness should also be considered (p. 236).

SPHINCTER OF ODDI DYSFUNCTION

The sphincter of Oddi (SO) is a small smooth muscle sphincter situated at the junction of the bile duct and pancreatic duct in the duodenum. Sphincter of Oddi dysfunction (SOD) is characterised by an increase in contractility that produces a benign non-calculus obstruction to the flow of bile or pancreatic juice. This may cause pancreatico-biliary pain, deranged LFTs or recurrent pancreatitis. A clinical classification system based on clinical history, laboratory results and ERCP findings is widely used (Boxes 23.71 and 23.72).

Clinical features

Patients with SOD who are predominantly female present with symptoms and signs suggestive of either biliary or pancreatic disease. Patients with biliary-type SOD experience recurrent episodic biliary-type pain. They have often had a cholecystectomy but the gallbladder may be intact. Patients with pancreatic SOD usually present with unexplained recurrent attacks of pancreatitis.

Investigations

The diagnosis is established by excluding gallstones and demonstrating a dilated or slowly draining bile duct. The gold standard for diagnosis is SO manometry. However, this is not widely available and is associated with a high rate of procedure-related pancreatitis.

Management

All biliary SOD patients with type I disease and the majority of those with type II are treated with endoscopic sphincterotomy. The results are good but patients should

23.73 GALLBLADDER DISEASE IN OLD AGE

- **Gallstones:** by the age of 70 years, prevalence is around 30% in women and 19% in men.
- **Acute cholecystitis:** tends to be severe, may have few localising signs, and is associated with a high frequency of empyema and perforation. If such complications supervene, mortality may reach 20%.
- **Cholecystectomy:** mortality after urgent cholecystectomy for acute uncomplicated cholecystitis is not significantly higher than in younger patients.
- **Endoscopic sphincterotomy and removal of common duct stones:** well tolerated by older patients and has a substantially lower mortality than surgical common bile duct exploration.
- **Cancer of the gallbladder:** a disease of old age, with a 1-year survival of 10%.

be warned that there is a high risk of complications, particularly acute pancreatitis. Type III patients with typical pain but normal cholangiography and laboratory tests should be offered medical therapy with nifedipine and/or low-dose tricyclic antidepressant drugs, such as amitriptyline.

Pancreatic SOD can be treated with pancreatic stenting followed by pancreatic sphincterotomy carried out in specialised units.

CHOLESTEROLOSIS OF THE GALLBLADDER

In this condition lipid deposits in the submucosa and epithelium appear as multiple yellow spots on the pink mucosa, giving rise to the description 'strawberry gallbladder'. The condition is usually asymptomatic but may occasionally present with right upper quadrant pain. Small, fixed filling defects may be visible on cholecystography or ultrasonography; the radiologist can usually differentiate between gallstones and cholesterolosis. The condition is usually diagnosed at cholecystectomy; if the diagnosis is made radiologically, cholecystectomy may be indicated, depending on symptoms.

ADENOMYOMATOSIS OF THE GALLBLADDER

In this condition there is hyperplasia of the muscle and mucosa of the gallbladder. The projection of pouches of mucous membrane through weak points in the muscle coat produces Rokitansky–Aschoff sinuses. There is much disagreement over whether adenomyomatosis is a cause of right upper quadrant pain or other gastrointestinal symptoms. It may be diagnosed by oral cholecystography when a halo or ring of opacified diverticula can be seen around the gallbladder. Other appearances include deformity of the body of the gallbladder or marked irregularity of the outline. Localised adenomyomatosis in the region of the gallbladder fundus causes the appearance of a 'Phrygian cap'. Most patients are treated by cholecystectomy but only after excluding other diseases in the upper gastrointestinal tract.

23.71 CLASSIFICATION OF BILIARY SPHINCTER OF ODDI DYSFUNCTION

Biliary type I

- Biliary-type pain
- Abnormal liver enzymes (ALT/AST > twice normal on two or more occasions)
- Dilated common bile duct (> 12 mm diameter)
- Delayed drainage of ERCP contrast beyond 45 minutes

Biliary type II

- Biliary-type pain with one or two of the above criteria

Biliary type III

- Biliary-type pain with no other abnormalities

23.72 CLASSIFICATION OF PANCREATIC SPHINCTER OF ODDI DYSFUNCTION

Pancreatic type I

- Pancreatic-type pain
- Twice normal amylase or lipase
- Pancreatic duct > 6 mm in the head or 5 mm in the body

Pancreatic type II

- Pancreatic-type pain with only one of the above criteria

Pancreatic type III

- Pancreatic-type pain with no other abnormalities

FURTHER INFORMATION

Books and journal articles

Bacon BR. Hemochromatosis: diagnosis and management. Gastroenterology 2001; 320:718–725.

Blei AT. Diagnosis and treatment of hepatic encephalopathy. Baillieres Best Pract Res Clin Gastroenterol 2000; 14(6):959–974.

EASL Conference on Hepatitis B. J Hepatol 2003; 39:suppl 1.

Fernandez J, Bauer TM, Navasa M, Rodes J. Diagnosis, treatment and prevention of spontaneous bacterial peritonitis. Baillieres Best Pract Res Clin Gastroenterol 2000; 14(6):975–990.

Friedman SL. Liver fibrosis—from bench to bedside. J Hepatol 2003; 38:S38–53.

Garcia-Tsao G. Current management of the complications of cirrhosis and portal hypertension: variceal haemorrhage, ascites, and spontaneous bacterial peritonitis. Gastroenterology 2001; 320:726–748.

Guruprasad P, et al. Clinical diagnostic scale: a useful tool in the evaluation of suspected hepatotoxic adverse drug reactions. J Hepatol 2000; 33:949–952.

Haydon GH, Neuberger J. Liver transplantation of patients in end-stage cirrhosis. Baillieres Best Pract Res Clin Gastroenterol 2000; 14(6):1049–1073.

Llovet JM, Bruix J. Early diagnosis and treatment of hepatocellular carcinoma. Baillieres Best Pract Res Clin Gastroenterol 2000; 14(6):991–1008.

National Institute of Health Consensus Development Conference. Management of hepatitis C. Hepatology 2002; 36:suppl 1.

Pratt DS, Kaplan MM. Evaluation of abnormal liver enzyme results in asymptomatic patients. New Engl J Med 2001; 342:1266–1271.

Torzilli G, Belghiti J, Makuuchi M. Third International Meeting Hepatocellular Carcinoma, Eastern and Western Experience. Hepatocellular Carcinoma. Liver Transplantation 2004; 10:suppl 1.

Websites

www.aasld.org *American Association for the Study of Liver Diseases.*

www.bsg.org.uk *British Society of Gastroenterology.*

www.easl.ch *European Association for the Study of the Liver.*

www.eltr.org *European Liver Transplant Registry.*

www.unos.org *American Transplant Register.*

23

J.I.O. CRAIG
D.B.L. McCLELLAND
C.A. LUDLAM

Blood disorders

CLINICAL EXAMINATION IN BLOOD DISORDERS

24

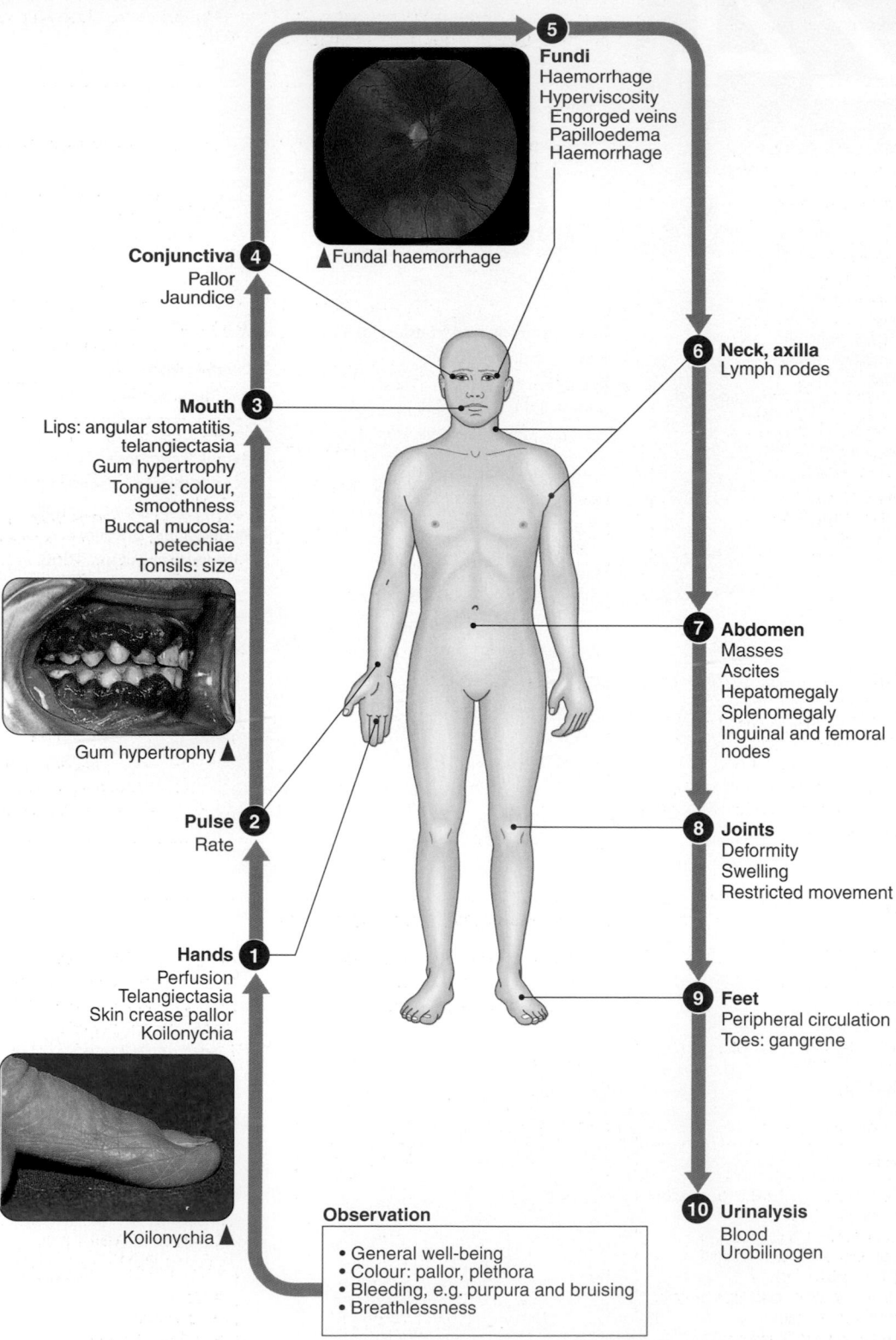

5 **Fundi**
Haemorrhage
Hyperviscosity
  Engorged veins
  Papilloedema
  Haemorrhage

▲ Fundal haemorrhage

Conjunctiva **4**
Pallor
Jaundice

6 **Neck, axilla**
Lymph nodes

Mouth **3**
Lips: angular stomatitis,
  telangiectasia
Gum hypertrophy
Tongue: colour,
  smoothness
Buccal mucosa:
  petechiae
Tonsils: size

Gum hypertrophy ▲

7 **Abdomen**
Masses
Ascites
Hepatomegaly
Splenomegaly
Inguinal and femoral
nodes

Pulse **2**
Rate

8 **Joints**
Deformity
Swelling
Restricted movement

Hands **1**
Perfusion
Telangiectasia
Skin crease pallor
Koilonychia

9 **Feet**
Peripheral circulation
Toes: gangrene

Koilonychia ▲

Observation

- General well-being
- Colour: pallor, plethora
- Bleeding, e.g. purpura and bruising
- Breathlessness

10 **Urinalysis**
Blood
Urobilinogen

❹ ANAEMIA

The box shows the symptoms and signs that will help to indicate the clinical severity of anaemia.

ANAEMIA 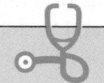
Search for symptoms and signs indicating the cause of anaemia
Non-specific symptoms
• Tiredness • Lightheadedness • Breathlessness • Ankle-swelling • Worsening of any previous coexisting disease such as angina
Non-specific signs
• Mucous membrane pallor • Tachypnoea • Raised jugular venous pressure • Flow murmurs • Ankle oedema • Postural hypotension • Tachycardia

BLEEDING

Bleeding can be due to congenital or acquired abnormalities in different components of the clotting system. The history and examination will help to clarify the severity and underlying cause of the bleeding problem.

BLEEDING
History
• Site of bleed • Duration of bleed • Precipitating causes including previous surgery • Family history • Drugs • Other medical conditions
Examination
There are two major patterns of bleeding: **1. Abnormal platelets** Abnormal function (e.g. aspirin) or reduced numbers (e.g. leukaemia) • Skin: petechiae, bruises • Gum and mucous membrane bleeding • Fundal haemorrhages **2. Abnormal coagulation cascade** (e.g. haemophilia) • Bleeding into joints (haemarthrosis) • Bleeding into soft tissues

Abnormalities in the blood are caused not only by primary diseases of the blood and lymphoreticular systems but also by diseases affecting other systems of the body. The clinical assessment of patients with haematological abnormalities must include a general history and examination as well as a search for symptoms and signs of abnormalities of red cells, white cells, platelets, bleeding and clotting systems, lymph nodes and lymphoreticular tissues.

❻ LYMPHADENOPATHY

Lymphadenopathy can be caused by benign or malignant disease. The clinical points to clarify are shown in the box.

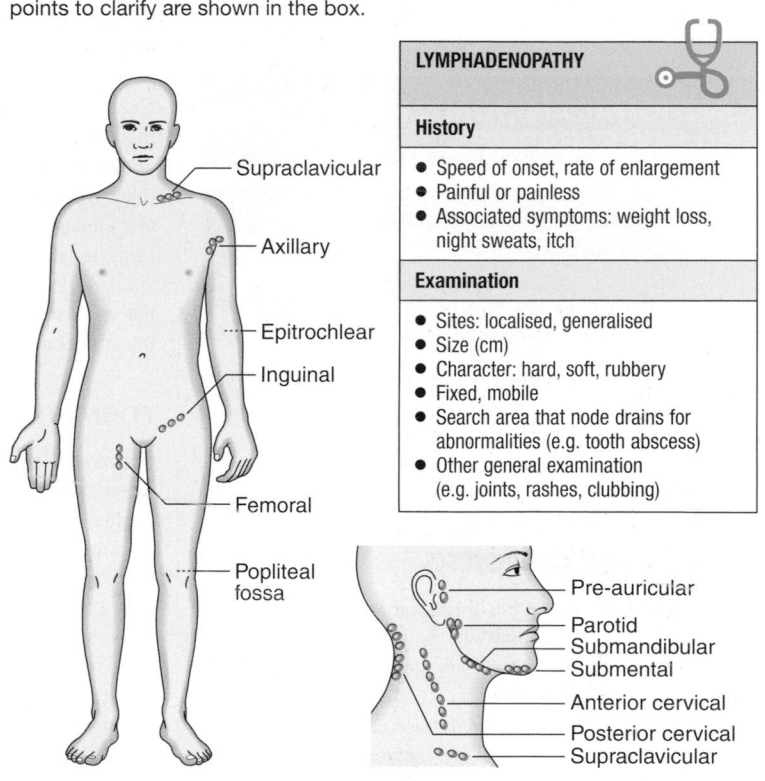

LYMPHADENOPATHY
History
• Speed of onset, rate of enlargement • Painful or painless • Associated symptoms: weight loss, night sweats, itch
Examination
• Sites: localised, generalised • Size (cm) • Character: hard, soft, rubbery • Fixed, mobile • Search area that node drains for abnormalities (e.g. tooth abscess) • Other general examination (e.g. joints, rashes, clubbing)

24

❼ EXAMINATION OF THE SPLEEN

• Move hand up from right iliac fossa, towards left upper quadrant on expiration.

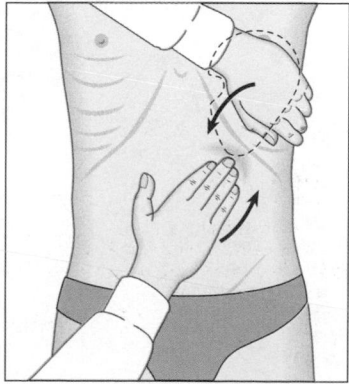

• Keep hand still and ask patient to take a deep breath through the mouth to feel spleen edge being displaced downwards.
• Place your left hand around patient's lower ribs and approach costal margin to pull spleen forward.
• To help palpate small spleens, roll patient on to the right side and examine as before.

CHARACTERISTICS OF THE SPLEEN
• Notch • Superficial • Dull to percussion • Cannot get between ribs and spleen • Moves well with respiration

Blood diseases cover a wide spectrum of illnesses, ranging from the anaemias that are amongst the most common disorders affecting mankind, to relatively rare conditions such as leukaemias and congenital coagulation disorders. Although the latter are uncommon, recent advances in understanding them at a cellular and molecular level are already impacting on diagnosis and treatment. Haematological change may occur as a consequence of disease affecting any system and measurement of haematological parameters is an important part of routine clinical assessment.

FUNCTIONAL ANATOMY, PHYSIOLOGY AND INVESTIGATIONS

FUNCTIONAL ANATOMY AND HAEMATOPOIESIS

Blood flows throughout the body in the vascular system, and consists of plasma and three cellular components:

- red cells, which transport oxygen from the lungs to the tissues
- white cells, which protect against infection
- platelets, which interact with blood vessels and clotting factors to maintain vascular integrity.

SITES OF HAEMATOPOIESIS

Haematopoiesis is the process of formation of blood cells. In the embryo this occurs initially in the yolk sac, followed by the liver and spleen; by 5 months in utero, haematopoiesis is established in the bone marrow. At birth, haematopoietic (red) marrow is found in the medullary cavity of all bones, but with age this is progressively replaced by fat (yellow marrow) so that by adulthood, haematopoiesis is restricted to the vertebrae, pelvis, sternum, ribs, clavicles, skull, upper humeri and proximal femora. Bone marrow usually accounts for 5% of an adult's weight but red marrow can expand in response to increased demands for blood cells.

Bone marrow occupies the intertrabecular spaces in trabecular bone and contains a range of immature haematopoietic precursor cells and a storage pool of mature cells for release at times of increased demand. Haematopoietic cells are set in and interact closely with a connective tissue stroma made of reticular cells, macrophages, fat cells, blood vessels and nerve fibres. This stroma provides the suitable microenvironment for blood cell growth and development. Normal marrow has a characteristic organisation (Fig. 24.1). Nests of red cell precursors cluster around a central macrophage which provides iron and phagocytoses extruded nuclei. Megakaryocytes are large cells which produce and release platelets into vascular sinuses. White cell precursors are clustered next to the bone trabeculae; maturing cells migrate into the marrow spaces towards the vascular sinuses. Plasma cells normally represent 5% or less of the marrow population and are scattered throughout the intertrabecular spaces.

FORMATION OF BLOOD CELLS

Stem cells

Haematopoiesis is an active process that must maintain normal numbers of circulating blood cells and be able to respond rapidly to increased demands such as bleeding or infection. All blood cells are derived from a pluripotent stem cell which has the ability to self-renew (make more stem cells) and to differentiate to form any of the blood elements. These comprise only 0.01% of the total marrow cells and produce a hierarchy of lineage-committed stem cells. As primitive progenitor cells cannot be distinguished morphologically, they are named according to the types of cell (or colony) they form during cell culture experiments. CFU–GM (colony-forming unit–granulocyte, monocyte) is

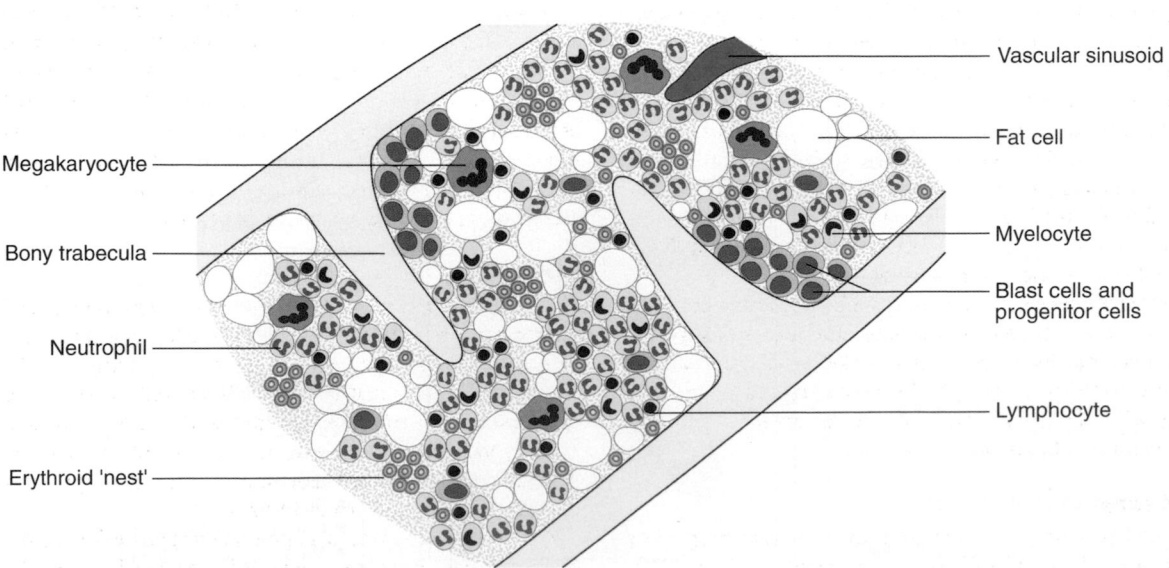

Megakaryocyte

Bony trabecula

Neutrophil

Erythroid 'nest'

Vascular sinusoid

Fat cell

Myelocyte

Blast cells and progenitor cells

Lymphocyte

Fig. 24.1 Structural organisation of normal bone marrow.

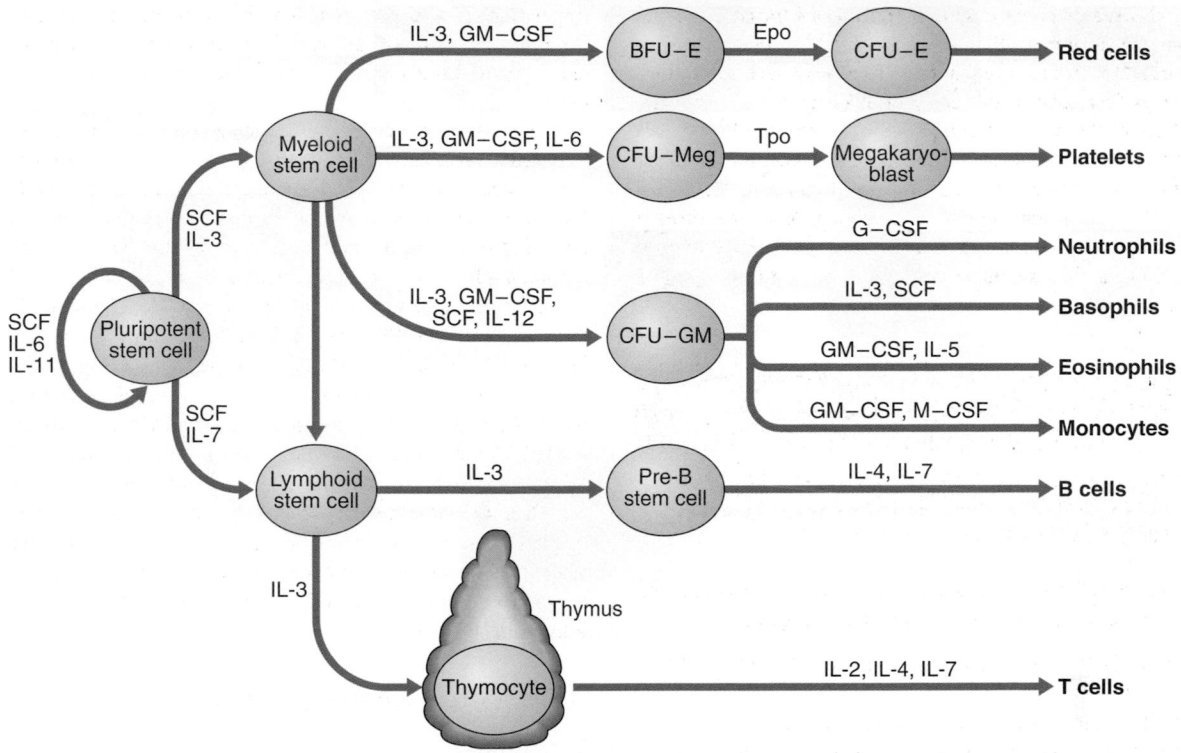

Fig. 24.2 **Stem cells and growth factors in haematopoietic cell development.** (BFU–E = blast-forming unit–erythroid; CFU–Meg = colony-forming unit–megakaryocyte; CFU–GM = colony-forming unit–granulocyte, monocyte; CFU–E = colony-forming unit–erythroid; IL = interleukin; SCF = stem cell factor; GM–CSF = granulocyte macrophage–colony stimulating factor; Epo = erythropoietin; Tpo = thrombopoietin; G-CSF = granulocyte–colony stimulating factor; M–CSF = macrophage–colony stimulating factor)

24

a stem cell that produces granulocytic and monocytic lines. CFU–E produces erythroid cells and CFU–Meg produces megakaryocytes and ultimately platelets (Fig. 24.2). The proliferation and differentiation of stem cells and their progeny are under the control of a range of growth factors produced by several cells, including stromal cells and lymphocytes. These growth factors bind to specific receptors on the cell surface and promote not only proliferation and differentiation but also survival and function of mature cells. Growth factors are often synergistic with other growth factors. Some, such as granulocyte macrophage–colony stimulating factor (GM–CSF), interleukin-3 (IL-3) and stem cell factor (SCF), act on a wide number of cell types at both early and late time points. Others, such as erythropoietin (Epo), granulocyte–colony stimulating factor (G–CSF) and thrombopoietin (Tpo), are lineage-specific. Many of these growth factors are now synthesised by recombinant DNA technology and used as treatments.

Recent evidence suggests that the bone marrow contains stem cells which can differentiate into cells from tissues other than the blood, such as nerve, skeletal muscle, cardiac muscle, liver and blood vessel endothelium. This is termed stem-cell plasticity and may have exciting clinical applications in the future.

Red cells

Red cell precursors formed from the erythroid progenitor cells are called erythroblasts or normoblasts (Fig. 24.3). These nucleated cells divide and acquire haemoglobin which turns the cytoplasm pink; the nucleus then condenses and is extruded from the cell. The first non-nucleated red cell is a reticulocyte which still contains ribosomal material in the cytoplasm. Under normal staining conditions reticulocytes are large cells with a faint blue tinge, termed polychromasia. Reticulocytes lose their ribosomal material and mature over 3 days, during which time they are released into the circulation. Increased numbers of circulating reticulocytes (reticulocytosis) reflect increased erythropoiesis. Red cell production is controlled by erythropoietin, a polypeptide hormone produced by renal tubular cells in response to hypoxia. Erythropoietin stimulates committed erythroid stem cells to proliferate and decreases maturation time. Patients with renal failure (p. 481) are anaemic due to failure of erythropoietin production, and exogenous recombinant hormone can be used to treat this.

White cells

Granulocytes (neutrophils, eosinophils, basophils) and monocytes are formed from the CFU–GM progenitor cell. The first recognisable granulocyte in the marrow is the myeloblast, a large cell with a small amount of basophilic cytoplasm and a primitive nucleus. As the cells divide and mature, the nucleus segments and the cytoplasm acquires specific neutrophilic, eosinophilic or basophilic granules (Fig. 24.3). This takes about 14 days.

A large storage pool of mature neutrophils exists in the bone marrow. Every day some 10^{14} neutrophils enter the circulation, where cells may be freely circulating or attached

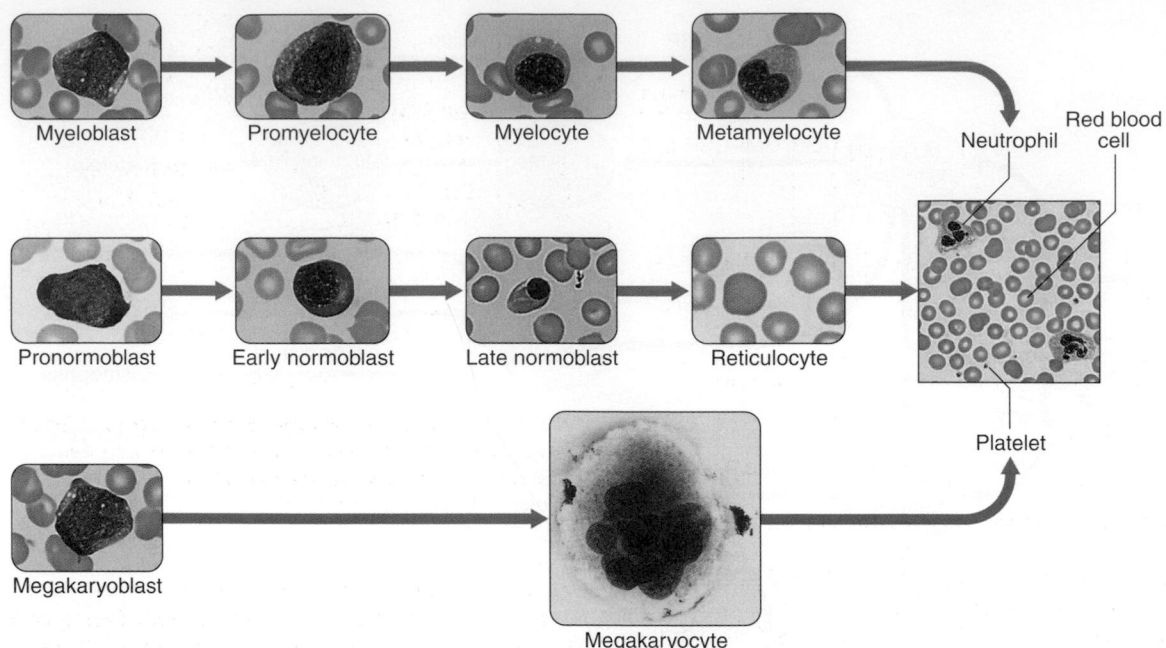

Fig. 24.3   Maturation pathway of red cells, granulocytes and platelets.

to endothelium in the marginating pool. These two pools are equal in size; factors such as exercise or catecholamines increase the cells flowing in the blood, so increasing the white cell count. Neutrophils spend 6–10 hours in the circulation before being removed, principally by the spleen. Alternatively, they pass into the tissues and either are consumed in the inflammatory process or undergo apoptotic cell death and phagocytosis by macrophages. Myelocytes or metamyelocytes are normally only found in the marrow but may appear in the circulation in infection or toxic states. The appearance of more primitive myeloid precursors in the blood is often associated with the presence of nucleated red cells and is termed a 'leucoerythroblastic' picture; this indicates a serious disturbance of marrow function. Monocytes are large cells derived from monoblasts. These cells circulate for a few hours and then migrate into the tissues where they can mature into macrophages which can proliferate for years. The cytokines G–CSF, GM–CSF and M–CSF are involved in the production of myeloid cells and can be used clinically, e.g. to hasten recovery of blood neutrophil counts after chemotherapy.

Lymphocytes are also derived from the pluripotent haematopoietic stem cell. There are two main types: T cells (80% of circulating lymphoid cells) and B cells. Lymphoid cells which migrate to the thymus develop into T cells, whereas B cells develop in the bone marrow.

Platelets

Platelets are derived from megakaryocytes. Megakaryocytic stem cells (CFU–Meg) divide to form a megakaryoblast; megakaryocytes are formed by endomitotic reduplication where the nucleus divides but not the cell. Thus mature megakaryocytes are large cells with several nuclei and cytoplasm containing platelet granules. Up to 3000 platelets

then fragment off from each megakaryocyte into the circulation in the marrow sinusoids. The formation and maturation of megakaryocytes are under the influence of Tpo, a recombinant form of which is in clinical use. Platelets circulate for 8–14 days before they are destroyed in the reticulo–endothelial system. Some 30% of peripheral platelets are normally pooled in the spleen and do not circulate.

MAJOR FUNCTIONS OF BLOOD CELLS

RED CELLS

The mature red cell is an 8 μm biconcave disc which delivers oxygen to the tissues from the lungs, and carbon dioxide in the reverse direction. It has no nucleus and no mitochondria; the normal red cell lifespan is about 120 days and in this time it will travel approximately 300 miles around the circulation. Red cells have to pass through the smallest capillaries in the circulation and their membrane structure is adapted to be deformable. The membrane has a lipid bilayer to which a 'skeleton' of filamentous proteins is attached via special linkage proteins (Fig. 24.4). Inherited abnormalities of any of these proteins result in loss of membrane as cells pass through the spleen, and the formation of abnormally shaped cells called spherocytes or elliptocytes (p. 1031). Red cells are exposed to osmotic stress in the pulmonary and renal circulation; to maintain normal homeostasis, the membrane contains ion pumps which control intracellular levels of sodium, potassium, chloride and bicarbonate. The energy for these functions is provided by the metabolic pathways of the cytosol; 90% of glucose metabolism occurs via anaerobic glycolysis which

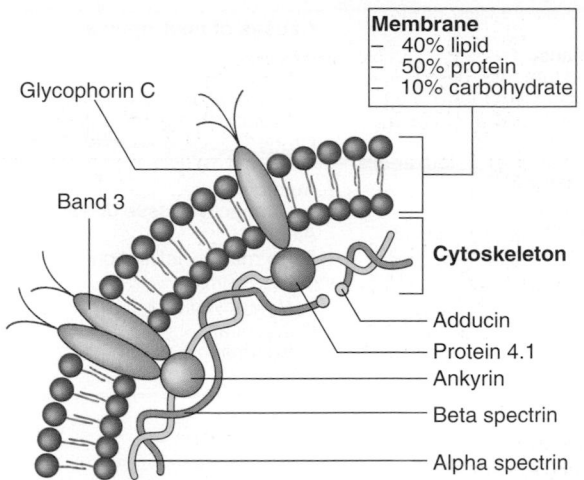

Membrane
- 40% lipid
- 50% protein
- 10% carbohydrate

Glycophorin C

Band 3

Cytoskeleton

Adducin
Protein 4.1
Ankyrin
Beta spectrin
Alpha spectrin

Fig. 24.4 Normal structure of red cell membrane.

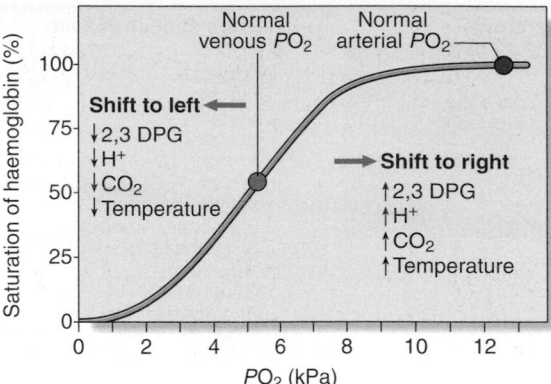

Fig. 24.5 The haemoglobin oxygen dissociation curve and factors which shift the curve to the right (more oxygen released from blood) and to the left (less oxygen released) at given PO_2. (To convert kPa to mmHg, multiply by 7.5.)

produces adenosine triphosphate (ATP), and 10% via the pentose phosphate pathway which produces nicotinamide adenine dinucleotide phosphate (reduced) (NADPH). Membrane proteins inserted into the lipid bilayer also form the antigens recognised by blood grouping. The ABO and Rhesus systems are the most commonly recognised (pp. 1020–1022) but over 400 blood group antigens have been described

Haemoglobin

Haemoglobin is a protein specially adapted for gas transport to and from the lungs. It is composed of four globin chains, each containing an iron-containing porphyrin pigment termed haem. Globin chains are a combination of two alpha and two non-alpha chains; haemoglobin A ($\alpha\alpha/\beta\beta$) represents over 90% of adult haemoglobin, whereas haemoglobin F ($\alpha\alpha/\gamma\gamma$) is the predominant type in the fetus. Each haem molecule contains a ferrous ion (Fe^{2+}) to which oxygen reversibly binds; the final oxygen to bind does so with 20 times the affinity of the first. When oxygen is bound, the beta chains 'swing' closer together; they move apart as oxygen is lost. In the 'open' deoxygenated state, 2,3 diphosphoglycerate (DPG), a product of red cell metabolism, binds to the haemoglobin molecule and lowers its oxygen affinity. These complex interactions produce the sigmoid shape of the oxygen dissociation curve (Fig. 24.5). The position of this curve depends upon the concentrations of 2,3 DPG, H^+ ions and CO_2; increased levels shift the curve to the right and cause oxygen to be released more readily. Tissue hypoxia increases all three and favours increased availability of oxygen from the red cell. Haemoglobin F is unable to bind 2,3 DPG and has a left-shifted oxygen dissociation curve; this increased affinity, together with the low pH of fetal blood, ensures fetal oxygenation. Amino acid mutations affecting the haem-binding pockets of globin chains or the 'hinge' interactions between globin chains result in haemoglobinopathies or unstable haemoglobins. Alpha globin chains are produced by two genes on chromosome 16 and beta globin chains by a single gene on chromosome 11; imbalance in the production of globin chains produces the thalassaemias (p. 1038).

Destruction

Red cells at the end of their lifespan are phagocytosed by the reticulo–endothelial system. Amino acids from globin chains are recycled and iron is removed from haem for reuse in haemoglobin synthesis. The remnant haem structure is degraded to bilirubin and conjugated to glucuronic acid before being excreted into bile. In the small bowel, bilirubin is converted to stercobilin; most of this is excreted, but a small amount is reabsorbed and excreted by the kidney as urobilinogen. Increased red cell destruction due to haemolysis or ineffective haematopoiesis will result in jaundice and increased urinary urobilinogen. Free intravascular haemoglobin is toxic and is normally bound by haptoglobins, which are plasma proteins produced by the liver.

WHITE CELLS

White cells or leucocytes in the blood consist of granulocytes (neutrophils, eosinophils and basophils), monocytes and lymphocytes (Fig. 24.6).

Neutrophils

Neutrophils, the most common white blood cells in the blood of adults, are 10–14 µm in diameter with a multilobular nucleus containing 2–5 segments and granules in their cytoplasm. Their main function is to recognise, ingest and destroy foreign particles and microorganisms. Two main types of granule are recognised: primary or azurophil granules, and the more numerous secondary or specific granules. Primary granules contain myeloperoxidase and other proteins important for killing ingested microbes. Secondary granules contain a number of membrane proteins including adhesion molecules, and components of the NADPH oxidase with which neutrophils produce superoxide anions for microbial killing. Granules fuse with the plasma membrane upon degranulation and their contents are released extracellularly. Granule staining becomes more intense in response to infection and is termed 'toxic granulation'.

Eosinophils

Eosinophils represent 1–6% of the circulating white cells. They are a similar size to neutrophils but have a bi-lobed

24

24

Neutrophil

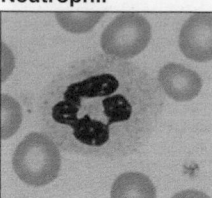

Causes of neutrophilia

Infection
    Bacterial
    Fungal
Trauma
    Surgery
    Burns
Infarction
    Myocardial infarct
    Pulmonary embolus
    Sickle-cell crisis
Inflammation
    Gout
    Rheumatoid arthritis
    Ulcerative colitis
    Crohn's disease

Malignancy
    Solid tumours
    Hodgkin lymphoma
Myeloproliferative disease
    Polycythaemia
    Chronic myeloid leukaemia
Physiological
    Exercise
    Pregnancy

Causes of neutropenia

Infection
    Viral
    Bacterial, e.g. *Salmonella*
    Protozoal, e.g. malaria
Drugs
    Box 24.10, p. 1014
Autoimmune
    Connective tissue disease
Alcohol
Bone marrow infiltration
    Leukaemia
    Myleodysplasia
Congenital
    Kostmann's syndrome

Eosinophil

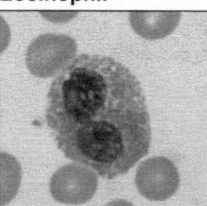

Causes of eosinophilia

Allergy
    Hay fever
    Asthma
    Eczema
Infection
    Parasitic
Drug hypersensitivity
    e.g. Gold, sulphonamides

Skin disease
Connective tissue disease
    Polyarteritis nodosa
Malignancy
    Solid tumours
    Lymphomas

Basophil

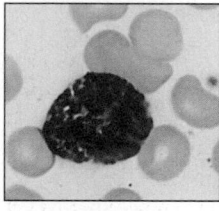

Causes of basophilia

Myeloproliferative disease
    Polycythaemia
    Chronic myeloid leukaemia
Inflammation
    Acute hypersensitivity
    Ulcerative colitis
    Crohn's disease
Iron deficiency

Monocyte

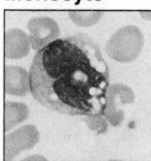

Causes of monocytosis

Infection
    Bacterial, eg tuberculosis
Inflammation
    Connective tissue disease
    Ulcerative colitis
    Crohn's disease
Malignancy
    Solid tumours

Lymphocyte

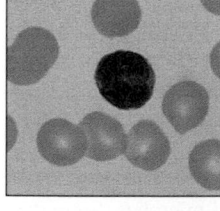

Causes of lymphocytosis

Infection
    Viral
    Bacterial, e.g. *Bordetella pertussis*
Lymphoproliferative disease
    Chronic lymphatic leukaemia
    Lymphoma
Post-splenectomy

Causes of lymphopenia

Inflammation
    Connective tissue disease
Lymphoma
Renal failure
Sarcoidosis
Drugs
    Corticosteroids
    Cytotoxics
Congenital
    Severe combined
    immunodeficiency

Fig. 24.6 Normal white blood cells.

nucleus and prominent orange granules on Romanowsky staining. Eosinophils are phagocytic and their granules contain a peroxidase capable of generating reactive oxygen species and proteins involved in the intracellular killing of protozoa and helminths (p. 296). They are also involved in allergic reactions (e.g. atopic asthma, p. 670; see also p. 83).

Basophils

These cells are less common than eosinophils, representing less than 1% of circulating white cells. They contain dense black granules which obscure the nucleus. Mast cells resemble basophils but are only found in the tissues. Basophils bind IgE antibody on their surface, and exposure to specific antigen results in degranulation with release of histamine, leukotrienes and heparin. These cells are involved in hypersensitivity reactions (p. 80).

Monocytes

Monocytes are the largest of the white cells, with a diameter of 12–20 μm and an irregular nucleus in abundant pale blue cytoplasm containing occasional cytoplasmic vacuoles. These cells migrate into the tissue where they become macrophages, Kupffer cells or antigen-presenting dendritic cells. The former phagocytose debris, apoptotic cells and microorganisms. They produce a variety of cytokines when activated, such as interleukin-1 (IL-1), tumour necrosis factor-α (TNF-α) and GM–CSF.

Lymphocytes

In children aged up to 7 years, lymphocytes are the most abundant white cell in the blood. They are heterogeneous, the smallest cells being the size of red cells and the largest being the size of neutrophils. Small lymphocytes are circular with scanty cytoplasm but the larger cells are more irregular with abundant blue cytoplasm. The majority of lymphocytes in the circulation are T cells (80%), which can be recognised by their expression of the CD antigens CD1, 2, 3, 4, 5, 7 and 8. The T cells mediate cellular immunity and two major types are recognised: CD4 positive helper cells and CD8 positive suppressor cells. The B cells mediate humoral immunity and can be recognised by their expression of immunoglobulin light chains (kappa or lambda in a ratio of 2:1). Lymphocyte subpopulations can be defined with specific functions and their lifespan can vary from several days to many years.

HAEMOSTASIS

Efficient mechanisms have evolved to maintain the circulation as a transport system, which both prevent blood loss from a damaged vessel by securing haemostasis, and also prevent the cessation of flow due to thrombosis. Haemostasis depends upon interactions between the vessel wall, platelets and clotting factors. There are two phases of haemostasis: primary and secondary. In the initial primary phase, the damaged vessel constricts and platelets aggregate at the site of damage to form a plug to arrest haemorrhage within a few minutes. This is followed by activation of the coagulation system with secondary deposition of a fibrin mesh to secure the platelet plug. These two phases are interlinked; damaged endothelium and the subendothelial matrix activate platelets, which then provide the optimal surface for the binding of the plasma clotting factors and the generation of insoluble fibrin.

PLATELETS

Under normal conditions platelets are discoid, with a diameter of 2–4 μm (Fig. 24.7). The surface membrane invaginates to form a tubular network, the canalicular system, which provides a conduit for the discharge of granule content. Three types of granule are present in the cytoplasm: alpha, delta and lysosomes. Their contents are shown in Figure 24.7.

When platelets are activated by ADP, thrombin or collagen they contract to become spherical and extend long pseudopodia which adhere to the subendothelium and other platelets. Upon activation, platelet granules discharge their contents, which encourages further platelet aggregation and fibrin formation. At the same time, arachidonic acid is released from the platelet membrane and converted by cyclo-oxygenase to endoperoxides and the powerful platelet aggregating agent, thromboxane A2. Aspirin and non-steroidal anti-inflammatory drugs (NSAIDs) inhibit platelet cyclo-oxygenase and impair platelet function. Platelet-binding to the subendothelium is dependent on high molecular weight von Willebrand factor released from endothelial cells and platelets, which bridges platelet

24

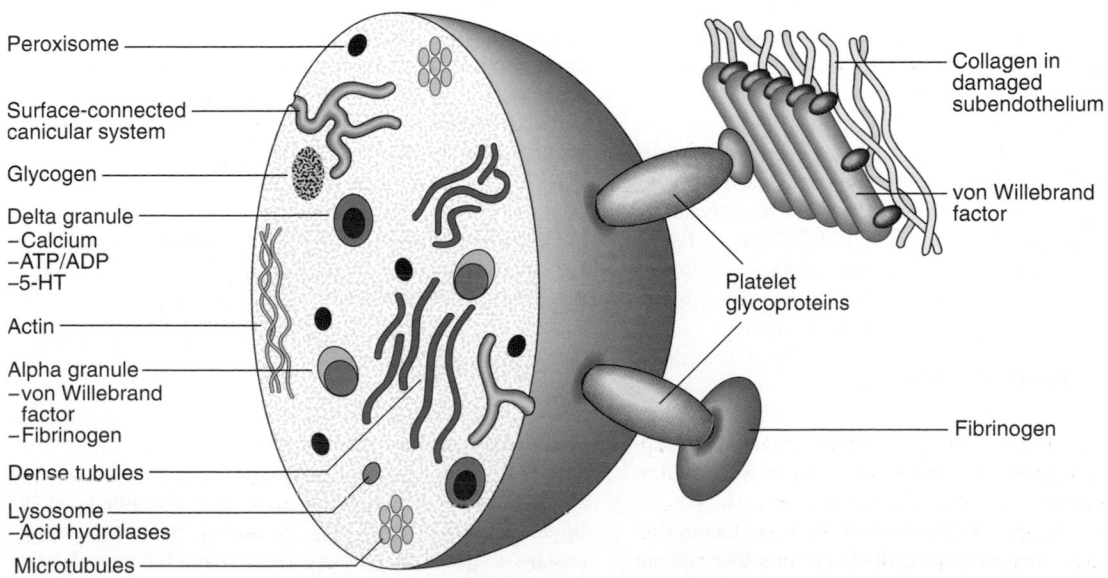

Fig. 24.7 Normal platelet structure. (ATP = adenosine triphosphate; ADP = adenosine diphosphate; 5-HT = 5-hydroxytryptamine, serotonin)

Peroxisome

Surface-connected canicular system

Glycogen

Delta granule
–Calcium
–ATP/ADP
–5-HT

Actin

Alpha granule
–von Willebrand factor
–Fibrinogen

Dense tubules

Lysosome
–Acid hydrolases

Microtubules

Collagen in damaged subendothelium

von Willebrand factor

Platelet glycoproteins

Fibrinogen

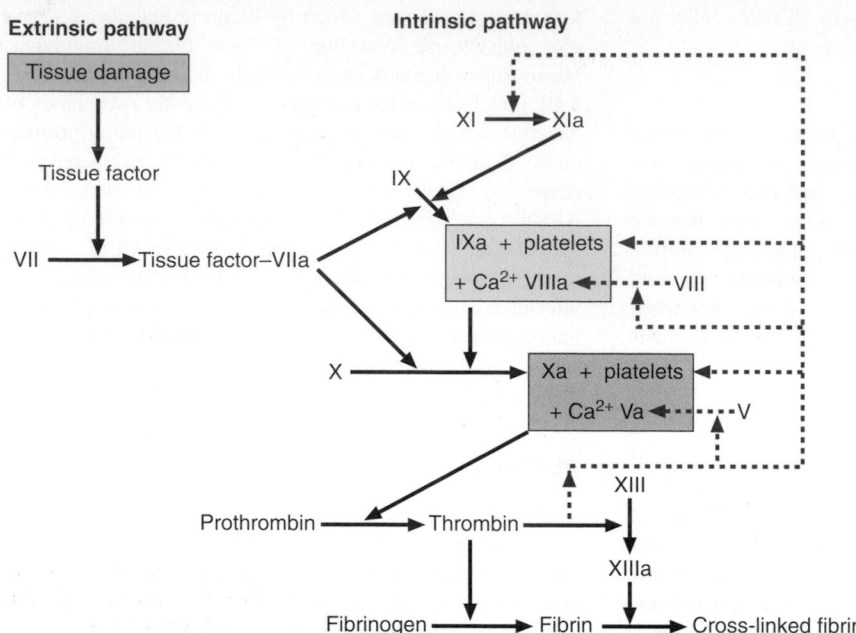

Extrinsic pathway

Intrinsic pathway

Fig. 24.8 Normal haemostatic mechanisms: clotting factors of the intrinsic and extrinsic pathways. The reactions of IXa/VIIIa and Xa/Va (in the boxes) take place on the platelet surface. The dotted lines represent positive feedback effects from small amounts of thrombin. This greatly enhances the activity of the coagulation network and results in large amounts of thrombin generation and thus fibrin formation in the clot.

membrane glycoproteins and subendothelial collagen. Interplatelet aggregation is dependent upon fibrinogen binding to platelet glycoproteins.

CLOTTING FACTORS

The coagulation system consists of a series of soluble inactive zymogen proteins designated by Roman numerals. When proteolytically cleaved and activated, each is capable of activating one or more components of the cascade. Activated factors are designated by the suffix 'a'. Some of these reactions require phospholipid and calcium. Two pathways of activation are recognised, named the 'extrinsic' and 'intrinsic' pathways. However, recent understanding has shown that the extrinsic pathway, where coagulation is initiated by factor VII interacting with tissue factor (TF), is the main physiological mechanism in vivo (Fig. 24.8). TF is a transmembrane protein expressed widely in the body, including the epidermis, monocytes, organ capsules, gastrointestinal and respiratory tracts, the brain and renal glomeruli. It is expressed during endothelial cell damage. Factor VII circulates in the plasma and can be activated to factor VIIa by TF, which in turn activates factor X. Factor Xa forms a complex with factor V on the surface of activated platelets which converts prothrombin to thrombin; this in turn converts fibrinogen to fibrin monomer, which polymerises and is cross-linked by factor XIII to form stable clot. Thrombin plays a crucial role in this 'final common pathway'; factors XI, VIII, V and platelets are activated by thrombin, which generates a positive feedback loop. Congenital deficiencies of any of these factors will result in a bleeding diathesis.

Clotting factors are synthesised by the liver; factor V is also produced by platelets and endothelial cells. The vitamin K-dependent factors II, VII, IX and X are produced as inactive proteins. These factors are rich in glutamic acid (Gla) residues, which must be further carboxylated to enable the proteins to maintain an active tertiary structure. The carboxylase enzyme responsible for this in the liver requires vitamin K as a co-factor (Fig. 24.9). Vitamin K is converted to an epoxide in this reaction and must be regenerated to its active form by a reductase enzyme. This reductase is inhibited by warfarin, which results in inhibition of the carboxylation cycle and is the basis of the anticoagulant effect of coumarins (p. 1009).

To prevent inappropriate over-activity of the clotting cascade, natural inhibitors of the clotting systems are present. The TF–VIIa complex, along with factor Xa, is rapidly inactivated by tissue factor pathway inhibitor (TFPI). Antithrombin is a protein produced by the liver which also has inhibitory activity, principally against thrombin and factor Xa. When heparin binds to antithrombin, however, its inhibitory activity is markedly accelerated and this forms the basis of the anticoagulant action of heparin. Protein C is a vitamin K-dependent factor produced by the liver; when activated by thrombin along with its co-factor, protein S, it degrades and inactivates factor Va and VIIIa. These natural inhibitors provide powerful mechanisms to prevent excessive coagulation in the circulation and any reduction in their functions result in a tendency to thrombus formation (pp. 1061–1062).

FIBRINOLYSIS

The excessive deposition of fibrin within the circulation is prevented in health by the fibrinolytic system (Fig. 24.10). This pathway is principally initiated by tissue plasminogen activator (tPA) which is released from endothelial cells. Some fibrinolysis is also promoted by the activator urokinase which is synthesised in the kidney and helps prevent obstruction of the urinary system by small clots of blood. These activators convert the circulating inactive

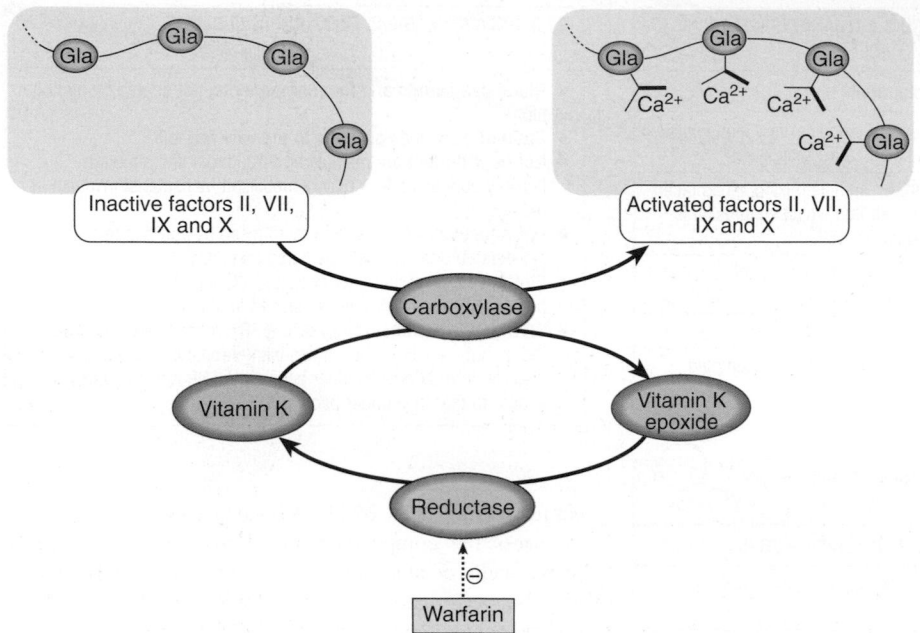

Fig. 24.9 The role of vitamin K in clotting and the mechanism of action of warfarin.

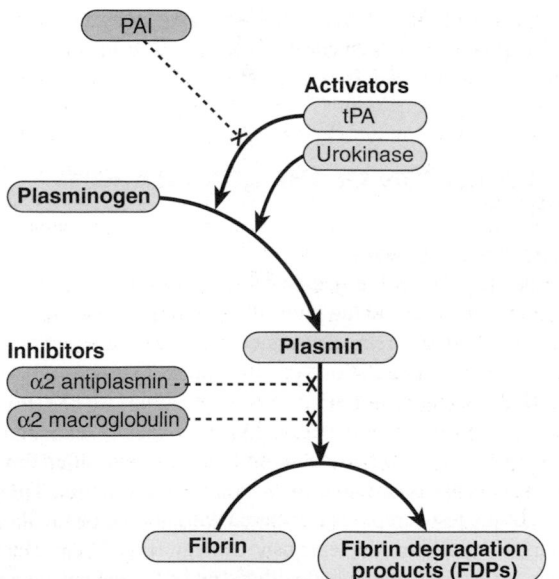

Fig. 24.10 Fibrinolysis. (tPA = tissue plasminogen activator; PAI = plasminogen activator inhibitor)

zymogen plasminogen to the active enzyme plasmin which hydrolyses fibrin. Within intravascular thrombi, both tPA and plasminogen bind to cross-linked fibrin, leading to the formation of plasmin which lyses the developing thrombus. The digested fibrin fragments, D-dimers, can be detected within the circulation and their concentration is raised in the presence of venous thrombosis.

Excessive tPA activity in the circulation is prevented by the presence of a further plasma component, plasminogen activator inhibitor (PAI), and plasmin is inactivated by α2 antiplasmin.

INVESTIGATION OF DISEASES OF THE BLOOD

24

THE FULL BLOOD COUNT

The full blood count (FBC) is the measurement of the number of circulating red cells (RBC), white cells (WBC) and platelets, the concentration of haemoglobin (Hb) and the characteristics of the red cells. Anticoagulated blood is processed through automatic blood analysers which use a variety of technologies (particle-sizing, radiofrequency and laser instrumentation) to measure the different haematological parameters. These include numbers of circulating cells, the proportion of red cells present in blood (the haematocrit, Hct), and the red cell indices which give information about the size of red cells (mean cell volume, MCV) and the amount of haemoglobin present in the red cells (mean cell haemoglobin, MCH). Modern blood analysers can detect the different types of white blood cell and give automated white cell differential counts including neutrophils, lymphocytes, monocytes, eosinophils and basophils. It is important to appreciate, however, that a number of conditions can lead to spurious results (Box 24.1). The reference values for a number of common haematological parameters in adults are given in the Appendix.

BLOOD FILM EXAMINATION

Although the technical advances of modern full blood count analysers have resulted in fewer blood films requiring examination, scrutiny of the blood film can often yield invaluable information (Box 24.2). Analysers cannot identify abnormalities of red cell shape and content (e.g. Howell–Jolly bodies, basophilic stippling, malarial parasites) or fully define abnormal white cells such as blasts.

24.1 SPURIOUS FBC RESULTS FROM AUTOANALYSERS

Result	Explanation
Increased haemoglobin	Lipaemia, jaundice, very high white cell count
Reduced haemoglobin	Improper sample mixing, blood taken from vein into which an infusion is flowing
Increased red cell volume (MCV)	Cold agglutinins, non-ketotic hyperosmolarity
Increased white cell count	Nucleated red cells present
Reduced platelet count	Clot in sample, platelet clumping

24.2 COMMON RED CELL APPEARANCES AND THEIR CAUSES

Microcytosis (reduced average cell size, MCV < 76 fl)

- Iron deficiency
- Thalassaemia
- Sideroblastic anaemia

Macrocytosis (increased average cell size, MCV > 100 fl)

- Vitamin B_{12}/folate deficiency
- Liver disease, alcohol
- Hypothyroidism
- Drugs (e.g. zidovudine)

Target cells (central area of haemoglobinisation)

- Liver disease
- Thalassaemia
- Post-splenectomy
- Haemoglobin C disease

Spherocytes (dense cells, no area of central pallor)

- Autoimmune haemolysis
- Post-splenectomy
- Hereditary spherocytosis

Red cell fragments (intravascular haemolysis)

- Disseminated intravascular coagulation (DIC)
- Haemolytic uraemic syndrome (HUS)/thrombotic thrombocytopenic purpura (TTP)

Nucleated red blood cells (normoblasts)

- Marrow infiltration
- Severe haemolysis
- Myelofibrosis
- Acute haemorrhage

Howell–Jolly bodies (small round nuclear remnants)

- Hyposplenism
- Post-splenectomy
- Dyshaemopoiesis

Polychromasia (young red cells—reticulocytes present)

- Haemolysis, acute haemorrhage
- Increased red cell turnover

Basophilic stippling (abnormal ribosomes appear as blue dots)

- Dyshaemopoiesis
- Lead poisoning

BONE MARROW EXAMINATION

In adults bone marrow examination is usually performed from the posterior iliac crest. After a local anaesthetic, marrow may be sucked out from the medullary space, stained and examined under the microscope (bone marrow aspirate). In addition, a core of bone may be removed (trephine biopsy), fixed and decalcified before sections are

24.3 HAEMATOLOGICAL FUNCTION IN OLD AGE

- **Blood cell counts and film components:** not altered by ageing alone.
- **Ratio of bone marrow cells to marrow fat:** falls.
- **Neutrophil function:** maintained throughout life, although leucocytes may be less readily mobilised by bacterial invasion in old age.
- **Lymphocytes:** functionally compromised by age due to a T cell-related defect in cell-mediated immunity.
- **Clotting factors:** no major changes, although mild congenital deficiencies may only be first noticed in old age.
- **Erythrocyte sedimentation rate (ESR):** raised above the normal range, but usually in association with chronic or subacute disease. In truly healthy older people the ESR range is very similar to that in younger people.

cut for staining (Fig. 24.11). A bone marrow aspirate is used to assess the composition and morphology of haemato-poietic cells or abnormal infiltrates. Further investigations may be performed such as cell surface marker analysis (immunophenotyping), chromosome and molecular studies to assess malignant disease, or marrow culture for suspected tuberculosis. A trephine biopsy is superior for assessing marrow cellularity, marrow fibrosis, and infiltration by abnormal cells such as metastatic carcinoma. Bone marrow aspiration can usually be safely performed in a thrombocytopenic patient.

INVESTIGATION OF THE COAGULATION SYSTEM

Bleeding disorders

The investigation of a patient with a possible bleeding disorder is directed by the clinical circumstances (p. 1055). The initial blood screening tests comprise a platelet count, blood film, and coagulation tests including the prothrombin time (PT), activated partial thromboplastin time (APTT) and fibrinogen (Box 24.4). Coagulation tests usually measure the length of time a plasma sample takes to clot after the clotting process is initiated by activators and calcium. The result of the test sample is compared with normal controls.

The PT assesses the extrinsic system (Fig. 24.8). The patient's plasma is incubated with tissue factor and calcium. The reaction proceeds with the activation of factor X by factor VIIa. The international normalised ratio (INR) is used only to assess the control of oral anticoagulant treatment. It is the ratio of the patient's PT to a normal control based on an international reference thromboplastin which ensures standardisation of anticoagulation between different centres.

The intrinsic system may be assessed by the APTT (sometimes known as the partial thromboplastin time with kaolin, PTTK). The APTT is determined by adding an activator to plasma—for instance, a suspension of kaolin—along with an extract of phospholipid (to mimic the platelet membrane). The normal ranges and causes of abnormalities are shown in Box 24.4. Special tests of coagulation including fibrinogen levels and individual clotting factor assays can be performed as indicated by the screening tests.

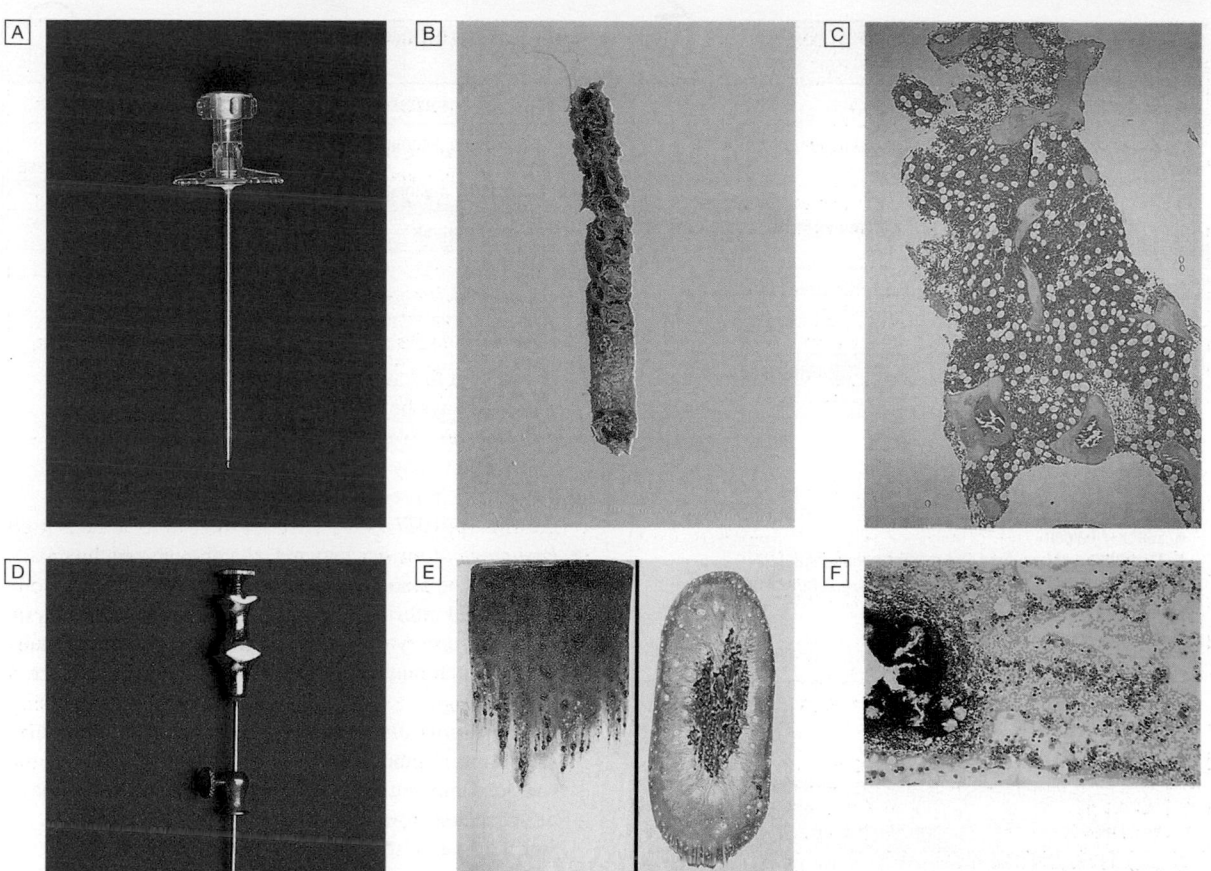

Fig. 24.11 Bone marrow aspirate and trephine. A Trephine biopsy needle. B Macroscopic appearance of a trephine biopsy. C Microscopic appearance of stained section of trephine. D Bone marrow aspirate needle. E Stained macroscopic appearance of marrow aspirate: smear (left) and squash (right). F Microscopic appearance of stained marrow particles and trails of haematopoietic cells.

24

24.4 COAGULATION SCREENING TESTS		
Investigation	**Normal range**	**Situations in which tests may be abnormal**
Platelet count	150–400 × 10⁹/l	Thrombocytopenia
Bleeding time	< 8 minutes	Thrombocytopenia Abnormal platelet function Deficiency of von Willebrand factor Vascular abnormalities
Prothrombin time (PT)	12–15 seconds	Deficiencies of factors II, V, VII or X
Activated partial thromboplastin time (APTT)	30–40 seconds	Deficiencies of factors II, V, VIII, IX, X, XI, XII Heparin Antibodies against clotting factors Lupus anticoagulant
Fibrinogen concentration	1.5–4.0 g/l	Hypofibrinogenaemia

N.B. International normalised ratio (INR) is not a coagulation screening test.

Platelet function may be assessed by performing a standardised template bleeding time test. A small standardised incision is made on the forearm below a sphygmomanometer cuff inflated to 40 mmHg. The bleeding time is prolonged in those with platelet functional defects, thrombocytopenia or von Willebrand disease. Platelet function can be further assessed by measuring aggregation in vitro in response to various agents, e.g. adrenaline (epinephrine) and collagen, or measuring the constituents of the intracellular granules, e.g. ATP/ADP.

Thrombotic disorders

The investigation of thrombosis depends upon the clinical situation (Box 24.5). The available investigations to assess thrombophilia, i.e. the propensity to thrombosis, are set out in Box 24.6. Anticoagulants can alter either the concentration or the activity of several of the plasma factors and, if possible, blood samples should therefore be collected before starting or after discontinuing anticoagulant therapy. On occasion this is not possible and the result has to be interpreted in the knowledge of the effect of the prevailing anticoagulant.

24.5 INDICATIONS FOR A THROMBOPHILIA SCREEN

- Venous thrombosis < 45 years
- Recurrent venous thrombosis
- Family history of venous thrombosis
- Venous thrombosis at an unusual site
  Cerebral venous thrombosis
  Hepatic vein (Budd–Chiari syndrome)
  Portal vein
- Arterial and venous thrombosis

24.6 LABORATORY INVESTIGATION OF THROMBOPHILIA

- Antithrombin
- Protein C
- Protein S
- Prothrombin G20210A
- Factor V Leiden
- Thrombin/reptilase time (for dysfibrinogenaemia)
- Antiphospholipid antibody/lupus anticoagulant/anticardiolipin antibody
- Homocysteine
- Factor VIII

24.7 CAUSES OF ANAEMIA

Decreased or ineffective marrow production

- Lack of iron, vitamin B_{12} or folate
- Hypoplasia
- Invasion by malignant cells
- Renal failure
- Anaemia of chronic disease

Peripheral causes

- Blood loss
- Haemolysis
- Hypersplenism

PRESENTING PROBLEMS IN BLOOD DISEASE

ANAEMIA

Anaemia refers to a state in which the level of haemoglobin in the blood is below the normal range appropriate for age and sex. Other factors, including pregnancy and altitude, also affect haemoglobin levels and must be taken into account when considering whether an individual is anaemic. The clinical features of anaemia reflect diminished oxygen supply to the tissue and depend upon the degree of anaemia, the rapidity of its development and the presence of cardiorespiratory disease. A rapid onset of anaemia (e.g. due to blood loss) will cause more profound symptoms than a gradually developing anaemia. Individuals with cardiorespiratory disease will have symptoms of anaemia at higher haemoglobin levels than those with normal cardiorespiratory function. The general symptoms and signs of anaemia are shown on page 1001.

The diagnosis of anaemia not only includes the assessment of its clinical severity but must also define the underlying cause. This rests on the clinical history and examination, assessment of the full blood count and blood film, and further appropriate investigations. Causes of anaemia are shown in Box 24.7.

History

- *Iron deficiency anaemia* (p. 1025) is the most common type of anaemia world-wide. A thorough gastrointestinal history is important, looking in particular for symptoms indicating blood loss. Menorrhagia is a common cause of anaemia in females still menstruating, so women should always be asked about their periods.
- *A dietary history* should assess the intake of iron and folate which may become deficient in comparison to needs (e.g. in pregnancy or during periods of rapid growth—p. 1027).
- *Past medical history* may reveal a disease which is known to be associated with anaemia, such as rheumatoid arthritis (the anaemia of chronic disease), or previous surgery (e.g. resection of the stomach or small bowel which may lead to malabsorption of iron and/or vitamin B_{12}).
- *Family history and ethnic background* of the patient are important. Haemolytic anaemias such as the haemoglobinopathies and hereditary spherocytosis may be suspected from the family history. Pernicious anaemia may also be familial.
- *A drug history* may reveal the ingestion of drugs which can be associated with blood loss (e.g. aspirin and anti-inflammatory drugs) or drugs that may cause haemolysis or aplasia.

Physical examination

As well as the general physical findings of anaemia shown on page 1001, there may be specific findings related to the aetiology of the anaemia; for example, a patient may be found to have a right iliac fossa mass due to an underlying caecal carcinoma. Haemolytic anaemias can cause jaundice. Vitamin B_{12} deficiency may be associated with neurological signs including peripheral neuropathy, dementia and signs of subacute combined degeneration of the cord (p. 1245). Sickle-cell anaemia (p. 1035) may result in leg ulcers. Anaemia may be multifactorial and the lack of specific symptoms and signs does not rule out silent pathology.

Schemes for the investigation of anaemias are often based on the size of the red cells, which is most accurately indicated by the mean cell volume (MCV) in the FBC. Commonly, in the presence of anaemia:

- A normal MCV (normocytic anaemia) suggests either acute blood loss or the anaemia of chronic disease (ACD) (Fig. 24.12).
- A low MCV (microcytic anaemia) suggests iron deficiency or thalassaemia (Fig. 24.12).
- A high MCV (macrocytic anaemia) suggests vitamin B_{12} or folate deficiency (Fig. 24.13).

Specific types of anaemia are dealt with separately later in this chapter (pp. 1023–1038).

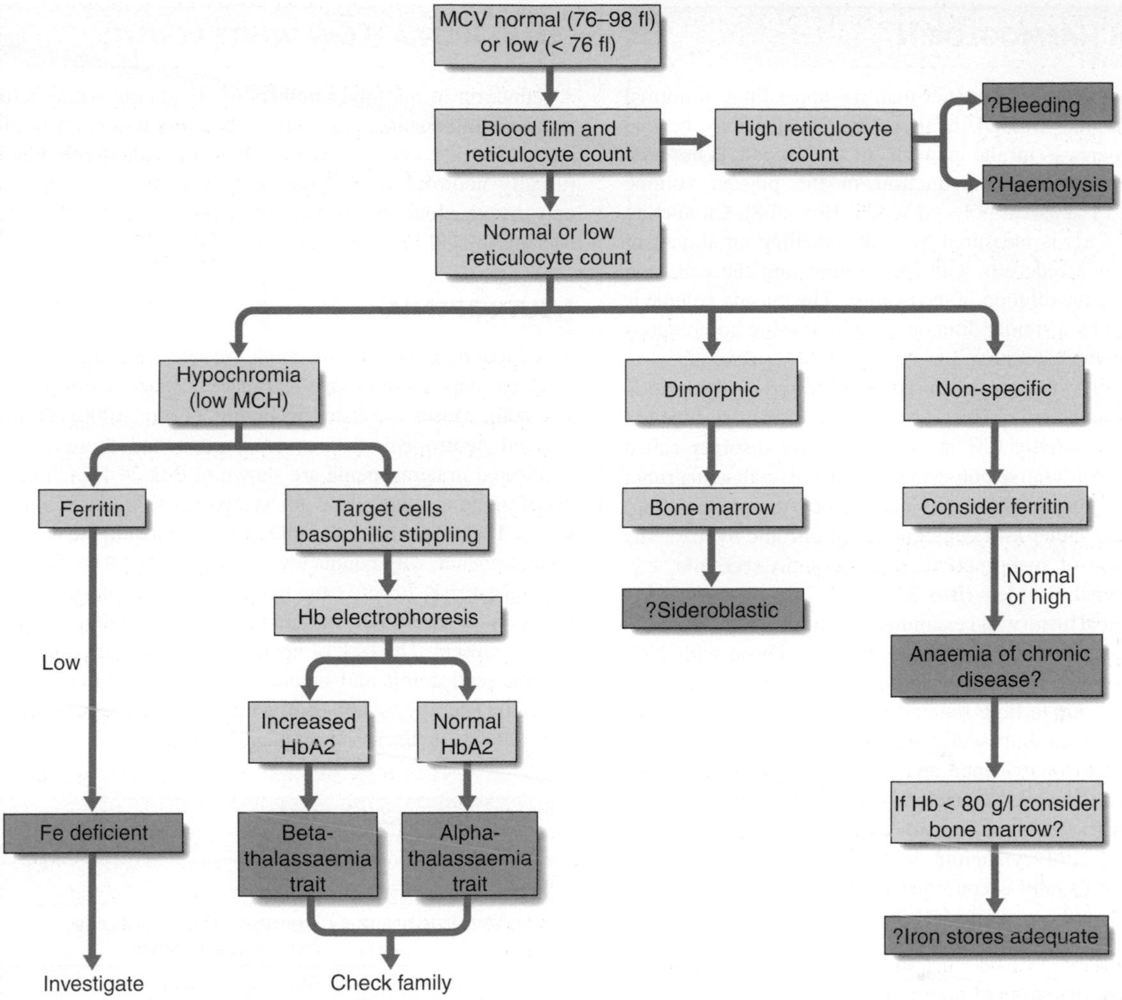

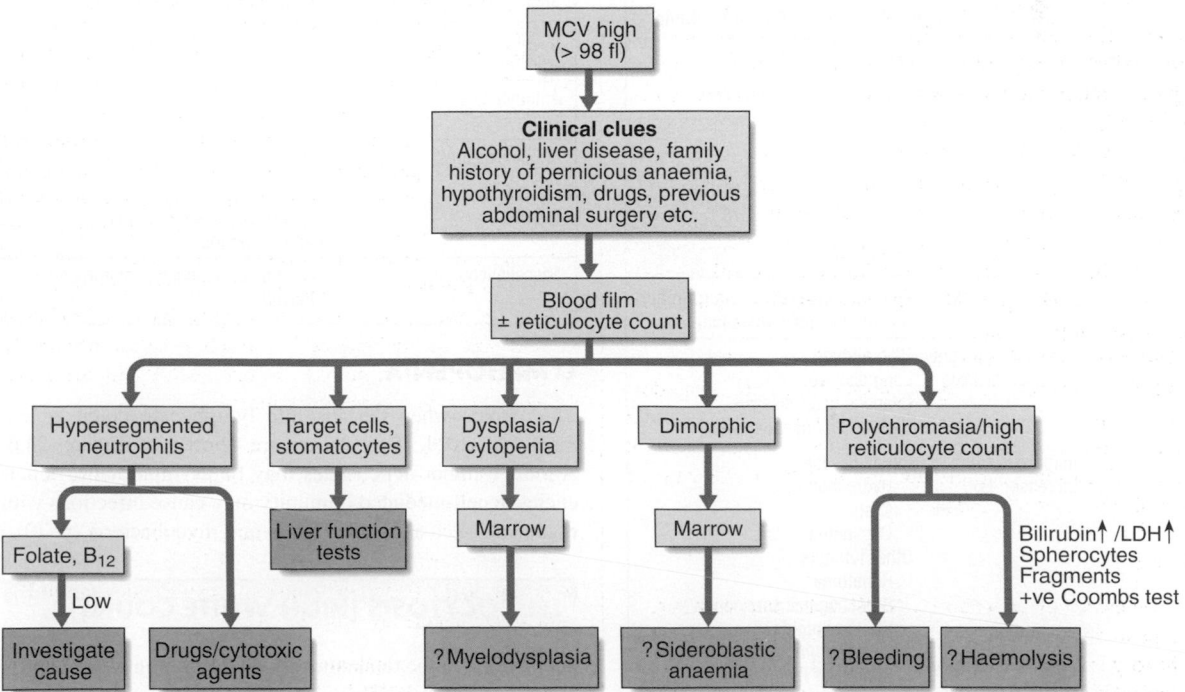

Fig. 24.12   Investigation of anaemia: normal or low MCV.

24

Fig. 24.13   Investigation of anaemia: high MCV. (LDH = lactate dehydrogenase)

24

HIGH HAEMOGLOBIN

A haemoglobin level greater than the upper limit of normal (adult females 165 g/l, adult males 180 g/l) may be due to an increase in the number of red blood cells (true polycythaemia) or a reduction in the plasma volume (relative or apparent polycythaemia, Box 24.8). Circulating red cell mass is measured by radio-labelling an aliquot of the patient's red cells with ^{51}Cr, reinjecting the cells and measuring the dilution of the isotope. The plasma volume is measured by a similar dilution technique using homologous albumin labelled with ^{125}I.

True polycythaemia is caused by increased erythropoiesis in the bone marrow. This occurs due to a primary increase in marrow activity (the myeloproliferative disorder called primary proliferative polycythaemia or polycythaemia rubra vera, PRV) or in response to increased erythropoietin (Epo) production either as a consequence of chronic hypoxaemia or because of inappropriate erythropoietin secretion, e.g. lung or renal disorders (Box 24.9).

A clinical history and examination will provide clues as to the aetiology of the true polycythaemia. Those with PRV may have arterial thromboses, pruritus worse after a hot bath, gout due to high red cell turnover and hepatosplenomegaly. The cardiovascular and respiratory systems should be assessed for evidence and causes of hypoxaemia, and further investigations to exclude inappropriate erythropoietin secretion should be performed.

Relative polycythaemia with a reduction in plasma volume is usually a consequence of dehydration, diuretic use or alcohol consumption.

24.8 CLASSIFICATION OF POLYCYTHAEMIA		
	Red cell mass	**Plasma volume**
True polycythaemia	Increased	Normal
Relative polycythaemia	Normal	Decreased

24.9 CAUSES OF TRUE POLYCYTHAEMIA		
	Aetiology	**Examples**
Primary	Myeloproliferative disorder	Polycythaemia rubra vera (primary proliferative polycythaemia)
Secondary	Increased Epo due to tissue hypoxia	High altitude Lung disease Cyanotic heart disease High-affinity haemoglobins

	Inappropriately increased Epo	Renal disease
		  Hydronephrosis
		  Cysts
		  Carcinoma
		Other tumours
		  Hepatoma
		  Bronchogenic carcinoma
		  Uterine fibroids
		  Phaeochromocytoma
		  Cerebellar haemangioblastoma

LEUCOPENIA (LOW WHITE COUNT)

A reduction in the total numbers of circulating white cells is called leucopenia. This may be due to a reduction in all types of white cell or a reduction in individual cell types (usually neutrophils or lymphocytes). In turn, leucopenia may occur alone or as part of a reduction in all three haematological lineages (pancytopenia, p. 1018).

NEUTROPENIA

A reduction in neutrophil count (usually less than $1.5 \times 10^9/l$, but dependent on age and race) is called neutropenia. The main causes are listed in Figure 24.6 (p. 1006). Drug-induced neutropenia is not uncommon and those drugs implicated in neutropenia are shown in Box 24.10. Clinical manifestations range from no symptoms to overwhelming sepsis. The risk of bacterial infection is related to the degree of neutropenia, with counts lower than $0.5 \times 10^9/l$ conferring the highest risk. Fever is the first and only manifestation of infection. A sore thoat, perianal pain or skin inflammation may be present. The lack of neutrophils allows the patient to become septicaemic and shocked within hours if immediate antibiotic therapy is not commenced. The management of such patients is discussed on page 1042.

24.10 DRUG-INDUCED NEUTROPENIA	
Group	**Examples**
Analgesics/anti-inflammatory agents	Phenylbutazone, gold, diflunisal, penicillamine, naproxen
Antithyroid drugs	Carbimazole, propylthiouracil
Anti-arrhythmics	Quinidine, procainamide
Antihypertensives	Captopril, enalapril, nifedipine
Antidepressants/ psychotropics	Amitriptyline, dosulepin, mianserin
Antimalarials	Pyrimethamine, dapsone, sulfadoxine, chloroquine
Anticonvulsants	Phenytoin, sodium valproate, carbamazepine
Antibiotics	Sulphonamides, penicillins, cephalosporins
Miscellaneous	Cimetidine, ranitidine, chlorpropamide, zidovudine

LYMPHOPENIA

This occurs when the absolute lymphocyte count is less than $1 \times 10^9/l$. The causes are shown in Figure 24.6. Although minor deficiencies may be asymptomatic, deficiencies in cell-mediated immunity may cause infections with organisms such as fungi, viruses and mycobacteria (p. 70).

LEUCOCYTOSIS (HIGH WHITE COUNT)

An increase in the total numbers of circulating white cells is called leucocytosis. This is usually due to an increase in a specific type of white blood cell (Fig. 24.6, p. 1006 for causes of a neutrophilia, eosinophilia, basophilia, monocytosis and lymphocytosis). It is important to realise that an increase in a single type of white cell (e.g. eosinophils or monocytes) may not increase the total WBC above the upper limit of normal and will only be apparent if the differential of the white count is examined.

NEUTROPHILIA

An increase in the number of circulating neutrophils is called a neutrophilia or a neutrophil leucocytosis. It can result from an increased production of cells from the bone marrow or redistribution from the marginated pool. The normal neutrophil count depends upon age, race and certain physiological parameters. In healthy neonates, the neutrophil count is higher than at other times of life. During pregnancy, not only is there an increase in neutrophils but also earlier forms such as promyelocytes can be found in the blood. The causes of a neutrophilia are shown in Figure 24.6.

LYMPHOCYTOSIS

A lymphocytosis is an increase in circulating lymphocytes above that expected for the patient's age. In adults this is $> 3.5 \times 10^9/l$. Infants and children have higher counts; age-related normal ranges should be consulted. Causes are shown in Figure 24.6; the most common is viral infection.

LYMPHADENOPATHY

Enlarged lymph glands may be an important indicator of haematological disease but they are not uncommon in

24.11 CAUSES OF LYMPHADENOPATHY
Infective
Bacterial   • Streptococcal, tuberculosis, brucellosis   **Viral**   • Epstein–Barr, HIV   **Protozoal**   • Toxoplasmosis   **Fungal**   • Histoplasmosis, coccidioidomycosis
Neoplastic
Primary   • Lymphomas, leukaemias   **Secondary**   • Lung, breast, thyroid, stomach   **Connective tissue disorders**   • Rheumatoid arthritis, systemic lupus erythematosus (SLE)
Sarcoidosis
Amyloidosis
Drugs
• Phenytoin

reaction to infection or inflammation (Box 24.11). The sites of lymph node groups, and symptoms and signs that may help elucidate the underlying cause are shown on page 1001. Reactive nodes usually expand rapidly and are painful, whereas those due to haematological disease are more frequently painless. Localised nodes should elicit a search for a source of inflammation in the appropriate drainage area: the scalp, ear, mouth, face or teeth for the neck; the breast for the axilla; and the perineum or external genitalia for inguinal nodes. Generalised lymphadenopathy may be secondary to infection, connective tissue disease or extensive skin disease but is more likely to signify underlying haematological malignancy. Weight loss and drenching night sweats which may require a change of night clothes are associated with haematological malignancies, particularly lymphoma.

Initial investigations in lymphadenopathy should include an FBC (to detect neutrophilia in infection or evidence of haematological disease), an ESR and a chest X-ray (to detect mediastinal lymphadenopathy). If the findings suggest malignancy, a formal cutting needle or excision biopsy of a representative node is indicated to confirm a histological diagnosis.

SPLENOMEGALY

The spleen may be enlarged due to involvement by lymphoproliferative disease, the resumption of extramedullary haematopoiesis in myeloproliferative disease, or enhanced reticulo-endothelial activity in autoimmune haemolysis. A list of the causes of splenomegaly is given in Box 24.12 overleaf. Massive splenomegaly occurs in chronic myeloid leukaemia, myelofibrosis, malaria or leishmaniasis. Hepatosplenomegaly is more suggestive of lympho- or myeloproliferative disease, liver disease or infiltration (e.g. with amyloid). The additional presence of lymphadenopathy makes a diagnosis of lymphoproliferative disease more likely. An enlarged spleen may cause abdominal discomfort, accompanied by back pain and abdominal bloating due to stomach compression. Splenic infarction may occur and produces severe abdominal pain radiating to the left shoulder tip, associated with a splenic rub on auscultation. Rarely, spontaneous or traumatic rupture may occur.

Investigation will centre on the suspected cause. Imaging of the spleen by ultrasound or computed tomography (CT) will detect variations in density in the spleen which may be a feature of lymphoproliferative disease; it also allows imaging of the liver or abdominal lymph nodes. Biopsy of the latter or of the superficial nodes may provide the diagnosis. A chest X-ray is required to exclude mediastinal nodes. An FBC may show pancytopenia secondary to hypersplenism and, if other abnormalities are present, such as abnormal lymphocytes or a leucoerythroblastic blood film, a bone marrow examination is indicated. Screening for infectious or liver disease (pp. 296 and 939) may be appropriate. If all investigations are unhelpful, splenectomy may be diagnostic.

24

24.12 CAUSES OF SPLENOMEGALY

Congestive

Intrahepatic portal hypertension
- Cirrhosis
- Hepatic vein occlusion

Extrahepatic portal hypertension
- Thrombosis, stenosis or malformation of the portal or splenic vein

Cardiac
- Chronic congestive cardiac failure
- Constrictive pericarditis

Infective

Bacterial
- Endocarditis
- Septicaemia
- Tuberculosis
- Brucellosis
- Salmonella

Viral
- Hepatitis
- Epstein–Barr
- Cytomegalovirus

Protozoal
- Malaria
- Leishmaniasis (kala-azar)
- Trypanosomiasis

Fungal
- Histoplasmosis

Inflammatory/granulomatous disorders

- Felty's syndrome, SLE
- Sarcoidosis

Haematological

Red cell disorders
- Megaloblastic anaemia
- Haemoglobinopathies

Autoimmune haemolytic anaemias

Myeloproliferative disorders
- Chronic myeloid leukaemia
- Myelofibrosis
- PRV
- Essential thrombocythaemia

Neoplastic
- Leukaemias
- Lymphomas

Other malignancies

- Metastatic cancer—rare

Storage diseases

- Gaucher's disease
- Niemann–Pick disease

Miscellaneous

- Cysts, amyloid, hyperthyroidism

BLEEDING

History

Bleeding results either from a breach of the vessel wall due to a specific insult (e.g. trauma) or from a defect in the haemostatic system. This may be due to a deficiency of one or more of the coagulation factors, thrombocytopenia, or occasionally excessive fibrinolysis which most commonly arises following therapeutic fibrinolytic therapy with tPA or streptokinase.

Prior to laboratory investigation it is important that a careful history is recorded of all bleeding episodes and a full clinical examination is performed. A history of bleeding is often remarkably reproducible, particularly after dental extraction; if a socket oozes for 2 days after removal of a tooth on one occasion, this is likely to recur following each subsequent extraction.

It is important to consider the following points:

- *Site of bleeds.* Muscle and joint bleeds indicate a coagulation defect, whereas purpura, prolonged bleeding from superficial cuts, epistaxis, gastrointestinal haemorrhage or menorrhagia indicates a platelet disorder, thrombocytopenia or von Willebrand disease. Recurrent bleeds at a single site suggest a local structural abnormality.
- *Duration of history.* It may be possible to assess whether the disorder is congenital or acquired.
- *Precipitating causes.* Bleeding arising spontaneously indicates a more severe defect than bleeding that occurs only after trauma.
- *Surgery.* Ask about all operations. Dental extractions, tonsillectomy and circumcision are particularly stressful tests of the haemostatic system. Bleeding that starts immediately after surgery indicates defective platelet plug formation and primary haemostasis, whereas that which comes on after several hours suggests a coagulation defect.
- *Family history.* Absence of relatives with clinically significant bleeding does not exclude a hereditary bleeding diathesis; about one-third of cases of haemophilia arise in individuals without a family history.
- *Systemic illnesses.* Many diseases (or their treatment) may be associated with bleeding but hepatic or renal failure, paraproteinaemia or a connective tissue disease in particular should be considered.
- *Drugs.* Almost any medicine can potentially cause bleeding, either by depressing marrow function with consequent thrombocytopenia or by interacting with warfarin. NSAIDs inhibit platelet function, and the effect of aspirin may last for up to 10 days after a single tablet.

Physical examination

Superficial examination may reveal bruises and purpura, or scars due to poor healing following prolonged superficial bleeding. Telangiectasia of lips and tongue points to hereditary haemorrhagic telangiectasia (p. 1055). Joints should be carefully scrutinised for evidence of haem-arthroses. A full general medical examination is important because it may give clues as to systemic illness—for example, stigmata of liver disease; splenomegaly may cause thrombocytopenia due to hypersplenism.

Investigations

Screening investigations and their interpretation are described on pages 1010–1011. If the patient has a history strongly suggestive of a bleeding disorder and all the preliminary screening tests give normal results, further investigations should be performed. The clinical history may be a useful guide as to whether attention should be directed to platelet function, e.g. von Willebrand disease, or a defect in coagulation, e.g. haemophilia.

24

THROMBOCYTOPENIA (LOW PLATELETS)

A reduced platelet count may arise by one of three mechanisms:

- failure of megakaryocyte maturation and hence platelet formation
- excessive platelet consumption after their release into the circulation
- platelet sequestration in an enlarged spleen.

The common causes of thrombocytopenia are listed in Box 24.13.

Spontaneous bleeding does not usually occur until the platelet count falls below about 30×10^9/l unless their function is also compromised. Purpura and spontaneous bruising are characteristic but there may also be oral, nasal, gastrointestinal or genitourinary bleeding. Severe thrombo-cytopenia results in optic fundal haemorrhage (Fig. 24.14), which may be a prelude to a rapidly fatal intracranial bleed.

Investigations are directed at the possible causes listed in Box 24.13. A blood film may give diagnostic information, e.g. acute leukaemia. Examination of the bone marrow may reveal an infiltrate such as carcinoma, a reduced number of megakaryocytes, e.g. hypoplastic anaemia, or an increased number of megakaryocytes indicating excessive peripheral destruction, e.g. idiopathic thrombocytopenic purpura (p. 1056).

THROMBOCYTOSIS (HIGH PLATELETS)

The platelet count is most commonly raised as part of the inflammatory response, as with infection, connective tissue disease, malignancy or gastrointestinal bleeding (Box 24.14), and the presenting clinical features are those of the underlying disorder. Thrombosis or bleeding secondary to a reactive increase in platelet count is rare.

In primary thrombocythaemia, there is primary proliferation of megakaryocytes in the marrow, and the patient may either have haemorrhagic features secondary to platelet dysfunction, e.g. gastrointestinal haemorrhage, or have hyperactive platelets and present with occlusion of a major artery, e.g. thrombotic stroke. Occlusion of smaller vessels may result in transient ischaemic attacks, amaurosis fugax, or distal ischaemia or gangrene (Fig. 24.15). A high platelet count is also a feature of other myeloproliferative disorders such as polycythaemia rubra vera or chronic myeloid leukaemia.

24.13 CAUSES OF THROMBOCYTOPENIA	
Marrow disorders	
Hypoplasia	
• Idiopathic	
• Drug-induced—cytotoxics, antimetabolites, thiazides	
Infiltration	
• Leukaemia	• Myelofibrosis
• Myeloma	• Osteopetrosis
• Carcinoma	
Vitamin B$_{12}$/folate deficiency	
Increased consumption of platelets	
• Disseminated intravascular coagulation (DIC)	
• Idiopathic thrombocytopenic purpura (ITP)	
• Viral infections, e.g. Epstein–Barr virus, human immunodeficiency virus (HIV)	
• Bacterial infections, e.g. Gram-negative septicaemia	
• Hypersplenism	
• Thrombotic thrombocytopenic purpura	
• Liver disease	
• Connective tissue diseases, e.g. SLE	

24.14 CAUSES OF A RAISED PLATELET COUNT	
Reactive thrombocytosis	
• Chronic inflammatory disorders	• Haemolytic anaemias
• Malignant disease	• Post-splenectomy
• Tissue damage	• Post-haemorrhage
Malignant thrombocytosis	
• Primary thrombocythaemia	• Myelofibrosis
• PRV	• Chronic myeloid leukaemia

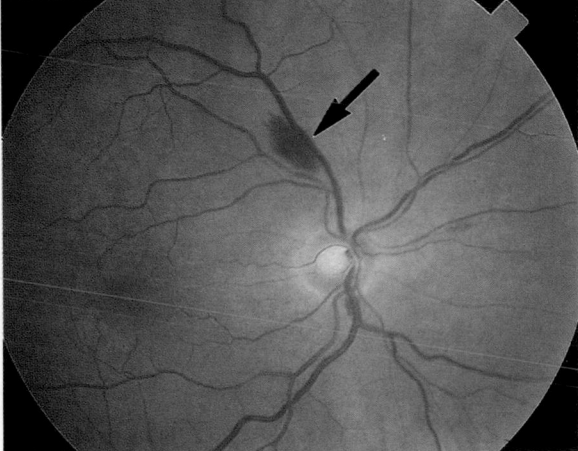

Fig. 24.14 Superficial fundal haemorrhage (arrow). The haemorrhage is in a patient with a platelet count of 5×10^9/l.

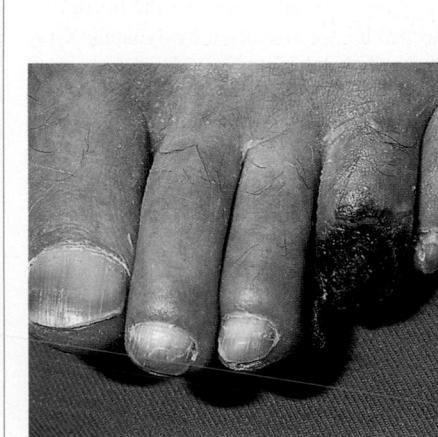

Fig. 24.15 Thrombocytosis causing vessel occlusion and gangrene.

24

VENOUS THROMBOSIS

Swelling of either one or both legs is a common presenting symptom. Deep venous thrombosis (DVT) is one possible cause; it characteristically causes pain, swelling, an increase in temperature and dilatation of the superficial veins. Often, however, there are only minimal symptoms and signs, and DVT cannot be excluded without appropriate investigations.

Unilateral leg-swelling may also result from a spontaneous or traumatic calf haematoma, cellulitis or a ruptured Baker's cyst (Box 24.15). The latter usually arises in individuals with pre-existing rheumatoid disease of the knee. The leak of synovial fluid into the calf is accompanied by a decrease in the size of the cyst in the popliteal fossa and an intense pain due to the irritant synovial fluid (p. 1103).

24.15 CAUSES OF A SWOLLEN LEG	
• Venous thrombosis	• Pelvic disease obstructing venous or lymphatic return
• Calf haematoma	
• Skin inflammation, including cellulitis	• Congestive cardiac failure/cor pulmonale
• Ruptured Baker's cyst	• Hypoalbuminaemia

Investigation of a swollen leg

For unilateral leg-swelling, it must be established whether or not a DVT is present. DVTs are usually unilateral but may be bilateral when they are extensive and extend into the pelvic veins and inferior vena cava (IVC). Other causes of bilateral leg-swelling, such as impaired venous or lymphatic return due to obstruction in the pelvis or above, right-sided heart failure and hypoalbuminaemia, should be excluded.

Using the patient's symptoms, a clinical risk of low, medium or high likelihood of DVT is established with Well's scoring system (Box 24.16). Those with a medium or high risk should undergo ultrasound or venography. For those with a low score, the plasma D-dimer level should be measured; if low, DVT is excluded, but if raised, further investigation with ultrasound or venography is required.

Venography remains the most accurate and reliable technique for assessing the presence of venous thrombosis. Radio-opaque dye is injected into a vein on the dorsum of the foot and the deep veins are visualised by dynamic X-ray imaging, with static films taken to provide a permanent record. Venography for thrombosis in the pelvic veins or IVC can be performed by femoral vein catheterisation.

Ultrasound is also a reliable, non-invasive method for detecting venous thrombosis. It depends upon demonstrating non-compressibility of the vein due to the presence of thrombus but can only detect thrombus in larger veins and is therefore only useful for assessing veins at or above the popliteal fossa as far as the inguinal ligament.

If a patient has a proven venous thrombosis, it may be necessary to consider whether s/he has a thrombophilic condition. Those fulfilling the clinical criteria set out in Box 24.5 (p. 1012) should be investigated, usually after anticoagulation has been discontinued, as in Box 24.6 (p. 1012).

24.16 PROCEDURE FOR PREDICTING THE PRE-TEST PROBABILITY OF DEEP VENOUS THROMBOSIS	
Clinical characteristic	**Score**
Active cancer (patient receiving treatment for cancer within the previous 6 months or currently receiving palliative treatment)	1
Paralysis, paresis or recent plaster immobilisation of the lower extremities	1
Recently bedridden for 3 days or more, or major surgery within the previous 12 weeks requiring general or regional anaesthesia	1
Localised tenderness along the distribution of the deep venous system	1
Entire leg swollen	1
Calf swelling at least 3 cm larger than that on the asymptomatic side (measured 10 cm below tibial tuberosity)	1
Pitting oedema confined to the symptomatic leg	1
Collateral superficial veins (non-varicose)	1
Previously documented DVT	1
Alternative diagnosis at least as likely as DVT	−2
Clinical probability	**Total score**
DVT unlikely	< 2
DVT likely	≥ 2

ABNORMAL COAGULATION SCREEN

A coagulation screen is undertaken when there is a history suggestive of a bleeding disorder (p. 1010), overt bleeding, or a clinical condition associated with a coagulation disorder, e.g. septicaemia. The prothrombin time is most sensitive to deficiencies of factors V, VII and X and may be prolonged in liver disease, DIC and patients on warfarin. The APTT is most sensitive to deficiencies in factors V, VIII, IX, X and XI and prolongation is seen in haemophilia A and B, DIC or those on standard or unfractionated heparin. The APTT is not prolonged by low molecular weight heparins. The most common cause of a low fibrinogen is DIC, although a reduced level in an otherwise well patient is seen in congenital hypofibrinogenaemia; this condition is uncommon. Fibrinogen is an acute phase reactant and is increased in patients with inflammatory conditions, e.g. infection.

PANCYTOPENIA

Pancytopenia refers to the combination of anaemia, leucopenia and thrombocytopenia. It may be due to reduced production of blood cells as a consequence of bone marrow suppression or infiltration, or there may be peripheral destruction or splenic pooling of mature cells. Causes are shown in Box 24.17. A bone marrow aspirate and trephine are usually required to establish the diagnosis.

INFECTION

Infection is a major complication of haematological disorders. The cause relates to the immune deficit caused by

24

24.17 CAUSES OF PANCYTOPENIA	
Bone marrow failure	
Hypoplastic/aplastic anaemia (p. 1054)	
• Inherited	• Viral
• Idiopathic	• Drugs
Bone marrow infiltration	
• Acute leukaemia	• Haemophagocytic syndrome
• Myeloma	• Myelodysplastic syndromes
• Lymphoma	• Acquired immunodeficiency
• Carcinoma	syndrome (AIDS)
Ineffective haematopoiesis	
• Megaloblastic anaemia	
Peripheral pooling/destruction	
Hypersplenism	
• Portal hypertension	• Malaria
• Felty's syndrome	• Myelofibrosis
SLE	

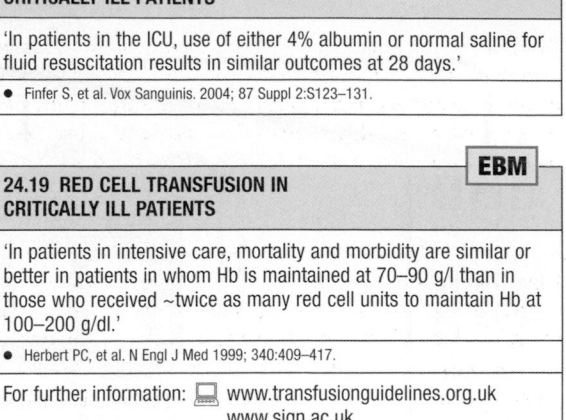

EBM

24.18 FLUID RESUSCITATION IN CRITICALLY ILL PATIENTS

'In patients in the ICU, use of either 4% albumin or normal saline for fluid resuscitation results in similar outcomes at 28 days.'

• Finfer S, et al. Vox Sanguinis. 2004; 87 Suppl 2:S123–131.

EBM

24.19 RED CELL TRANSFUSION IN CRITICALLY ILL PATIENTS

'In patients in intensive care, mortality and morbidity are similar or better in patients in whom Hb is maintained at 70–90 g/l than in those who received ~twice as many red cell units to maintain Hb at 100–200 g/dl.'

• Herbert PC, et al. N Engl J Med 1999; 340:409–417.

For further information: 💻 www.transfusionguidelines.org.uk
www.sign.ac.uk

the disease itself, to the treatment, e.g. chemotherapy, or commonly to a combination of both (p. 1014).

BLOOD PRODUCTS AND TRANSFUSION

A blood product is a therapeutic substance made from human blood. Transfusion may be needed when a patient has a deficiency or dysfunction of a blood constituent that causes symptoms or puts the patient at risk. It should only be prescribed if a useful improvement is likely to result. Patients who need transfusion require a safe and sufficient supply of blood. Transfusion from a donor is a form of allogeneic transplant and is never risk-free. Wherever possible, alternative treatments should be used (Boxes 24.18 and 24.19). For some patients, transfusion may be avoided by using strategies such as perioperative blood salvage or antifibrinolytic drugs.

A safe blood supply depends on a well-organised supply system that ensures regular donation by healthy individuals who have no excess risk of infections transmissible by blood. Every blood donation must be reliably tested to detect and exclude those containing transmissible agents. In the developed world, this includes hepatitis B, hepatitis C, HIV and human T lymphotropic virus (HTLV) which are detected with tests for antibody to the virus, viral antigen or nucleic acid. Platelet concentrates may be tested for bacterial contamination. The need for other microbiological tests depends on local epidemiology. For example, Chagas disease (p. 355) is transmissible by blood, and blood donations are tested for *Trypanosoma cruzi* in parts of South America where it is prevalent.

Effective control over the quality of safety testing, blood grouping, processing, storage and pre-transfusion testing of blood is also crucial. In the UK, blood services are licensed and regulated by the Pharmaceutical Regulatory Authority under European Union legislation. Figure 24.16 maps the main steps in blood collection, processing and storage.

Safe and effective clinical use of blood depends on:

• correct storage and handling throughout the life of the product right to the point of administration
• clinical protocols or guidelines for the management of patients at risk of transfusion
• a recorded assessment of the likely benefits and risks for each patient
• correct procedures for ordering and administration following the decision to transfuse.

BLOOD PRODUCTS

Blood products are subdivided as described below. In the UK, all blood components are processed to remove white cells. This is one of a number of precautions taken to minimise the risk of passing on the infective agent of variant Creutzfeldt–Jakob disease (vCJD, p. 1234) by transfusion, and blood donations are not accepted from individuals who have previously received a transfusion for the same reason.

Blood components are defined as whole blood or red cells, platelets, plasma or cryoprecipitate, prepared from single donations or by apheresis (Box 24.20).

Plasma derivatives are licensed pharmaceutical products produced from pooled human plasma obtained from many individuals. They are generally treated to remove or reduce virus contamination. Examples include the following:

• Coagulation factor concentrates factor VIII and IX for the treatment of conditions such as haemophilia and von Willebrand's disease. Coagulation factors made by recombinant DNA technology are preferred due to lack of infection risk.
• Intravenous immunoglobulin (IVIgG). This contains concentrated immunoglobulin and is used to replace IgG and reduce infective complications in hypogamma-globulinaemia. It also modulates the immune response and is sometimes effective in immune thrombocytopenia (p. 1056) and Guillain–Barré syndrome (p. 1249). At present, there is no alternative to the plasma derivative. IVIgG can cause acute renal failure, especially in the elderly. Specific immunoglobulins to, for example,

24

24

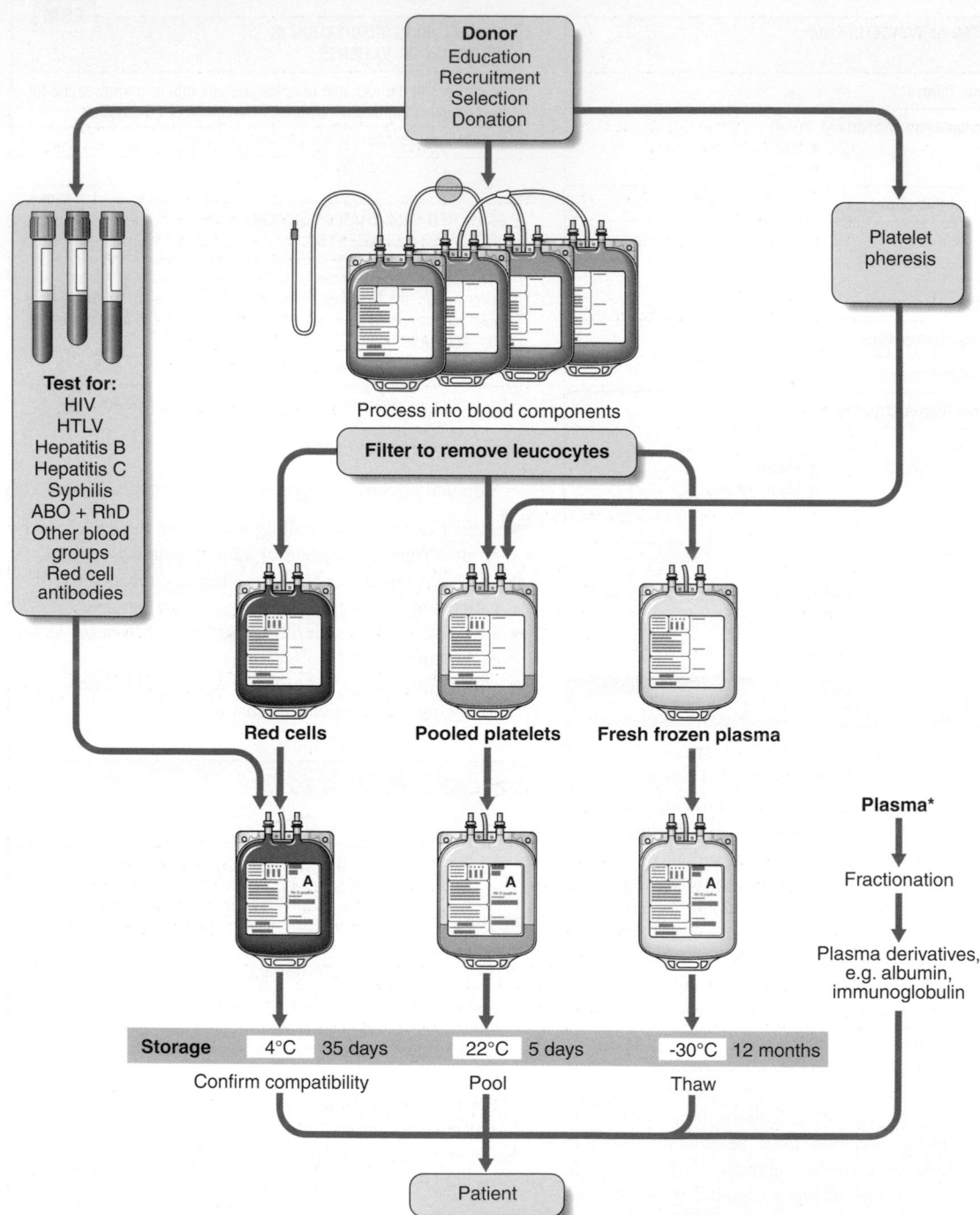

Test for:
HIV
HTLV
Hepatitis B
Hepatitis C
Syphilis
ABO + RhD
Other blood
groups
Red cell
antibodies

Donor
Education
Recruitment
Selection
Donation

Platelet
pheresis

Process into blood components

Filter to remove leucocytes

Red cells **Pooled platelets** **Fresh frozen plasma**

Plasma*

↓

Fractionation

↓

Plasma derivatives,
e.g. albumin,
immunoglobulin

| **Storage** | 4°C | 35 days | 22°C | 5 days | -30°C | 12 months |

Confirm compatibility   Pool   Thaw

Patient

Fig. 24.16 Blood donation, processing and storage. * In the UK, plasma for fractionation is imported as a precautionary measure against vCJD.

hepatitis B, tetanus and varicella zoster are made from donors with high titres of antibodies to these, and are used to prevent the development of infection in exposed non-immune people.

● Human albumin solution is available in two strengths. The 5% solution is indicated for replacement in plasma exchange. The 20% solution is used in the management of hypoproteinaemic oedema with nephrotic syndrome, and ascites in chronic liver disease. It is hyperoncotic and expands plasma volume by more than the amount infused.

RED CELL COMPATIBILITY

ABO RED CELL GROUPS

Transfusing red cells that have an ABO blood type that is incompatible with the recipient is the main cause of fatal, acute transfusion reaction.

There are four different ABO groups, determined by whether or not an individual's red cells express the A or B antigens. The frequency of ABO groups varies among

24.20 BLOOD COMPONENTS[1]

	Properties	Indications
Red cell components[2]	**N.B**. Red cell components *must* be compatible with the patient's ABO blood group	To increase circulating red cell mass to relieve clinical features caused by insufficient oxygen delivery in patients with low Hb levels
Whole blood	450 ml donor blood collected into 63 ml anticoagulant/preservative solution Stored at 2–6°C. Shelf life up to 5 weeks	Contains fibrinogen, other coagulation factors, and plasma as a colloid volume expander. Whole blood is suitable for replacement of acute blood loss but red cell concentrates plus colloid or crystalloid are acceptable alternatives
Red cell concentrate	Most of the plasma removed and replaced with a solution to optimise preservation of red cells	Most usual product in many countries, e.g. UK, US Some restrictions on use in infants; otherwise suitable for any patient requiring red cell replacement
Platelet concentrate[3]	One adult dose is made from four or five donations of whole blood, or from a single platelet apheresis procedure Stored at 20–24°C and must be agitated Shelf life up to 5 days from collection Platelets more effective if compatible with patient's ABO type Plasma in group O platelets can haemolyse red cells of group A patient	Treatment of bleeding due to thrombocytopenia and some forms of platelet dysfunction Prevention of bleeding due to thrombocytopenia in bone marrow failure
Plasma (Fresh frozen plasma, FFP)	150–300 ml plasma obtained from one donation of whole blood. Shelf life usually 1 year Should be compatible with patient's ABO type Group O plasma particularly is at risk of causing haemolysis in a group A patient	Replacement of coagulation factor deficiency if a suitable licensed virus-inactivated product is not available, e.g. multiple coagulation deficiencies in major haemorrhage Therapy of thrombotic thrombocytopenic purpura: by infusion or plasma exchange *Do not use* to replace circulatory fluid volume, to raise plasma albumin level or as an alternative to total parenteral nutrition
Virus-inactivated plasma	Plasma treated to remove or reduce infectivity of viruses from donor Obtained from a pool of donors' plasma treated with solvent and detergent, or from single donations treated with methylene blue and light	Indications as for FFP
Cryoprecipitate	High molecular weight proteins are modestly concentrated from plasma by precipitation near freezing point Each 10–20 ml pack of precipitate contains fibrinogen, factor VIII and von Willebrand factor	Replacement of fibrinogen if a suitable licensed virus-inactivated plasma derivative is not available Used for von Willebrand disease and haemophilia if virus-inactivated or recombinant products not available

[1] In the UK, all blood components are processed to reduce the leucocyte content to a level below 5×10^6 per pack.
[2] Alternative oxygen-delivering fluids: perfluorocarbon and haemoglobin solutions will NOT be licensed in the near future.
[3] Platelet preparations treated to inactivate microbial pathogens are in clinical trial and may become available.

populations. Normal healthy individuals have antibodies (mostly IgM), from early childhood, against the A or B antigens that are not expressed on their own cells (Box 24.21). These anti-A or anti-B antibodies in the recipient's plasma will bind to transfused red cells that express A or B antigen, as follows:

- Anti-A reacts with red cells of group A or AB.
- Anti-B reacts with red cells of group B or AB.

ABO-INCOMPATIBLE RED CELL TRANSFUSION

If red cells of an incompatible ABO group are transfused, the patient's IgM antibodies bind to the transfused cells as above. This activates complement which damages the red cell membranes and causes lysis of the red cells. Fragments of ruptured cell membrane may initiate DIC and released haemoglobin may cause renal failure. The risk of a severe or

24.21 THE ABO SYSTEM

Blood group	Red cell A or B antigens	Antibodies in plasma	UK frequency (%)
O	None	Anti-A and anti-B	46
A	A	Anti-B	42
B	B	Anti-A	9
AB	A and B	None	3

fatal reaction is greatest if group A red cells are infused to a group O recipient.

THE RHESUS D BLOOD GROUP AND HAEMOLYTIC DISEASE OF THE NEWBORN

About 15% of Caucasians are Rhesus-negative: that is, they lack the Rhesus D (RhD) red cell antigen. In other populations only 1–5% may be Rhesus-negative: for example, in Chinese and Bengalis. IgG antibodies to RhD-positive red cells are produced if such cells enter the circulation of an RhD-negative individual during pregnancy, via fetomaternal haemorrhage or transfusion. If a woman is so sensitised, during a subsequent pregnancy anti-RhD antibodies can cross the placenta and, if the fetus is RhD-positive, severe fetal anaemia and hyperbilirubinaemia can result. This may cause severe neurological damage or death due to haemolytic disease of the newborn (HDN). Therefore an RhD-negative female who may subsequently become pregnant, should never be transfused with RhD-positive blood.

Anti-RhD immunoglobulin (anti-D) is the only effective product for preventing the development of Rhesus antibodies in RhD-negative women who are at risk. It acts by blocking the immune response to the RhD antigen. Anti-D is given after delivery and other potentially sensitising events during pregnancy. In some countries, routine prophylactic anti-D is recommended for all Rh-negative women in later pregnancy. There is no alternative to the human plasma derivative, although monoclonal antibody products are in development.

Other red cell antigen groups also may stimulate the development of red cell antibodies with the potential to cause haemolytic transfusion reactions or to cross the placenta and cause HDN. These include the other Rhesus antigens (RhC, c, E, e) and the Kell, Duffy and Kidd blood group antigens.

SAFE TRANSFUSION PROCEDURES

It is essential to ensure that no ABO-incompatible red cell transfusion is ever given. Such an accident is likely to kill or harm the patient and is avoidable. Errors leading to patients receiving the wrong blood are one of the main causes of mortality and morbidity due to transfusion. The patient's safety depends not only on correct pre-transfusion testing in the laboratory but also on the use of standard procedures for taking correctly labelled blood samples from the patient and for making sure that blood is infused into the correct patient. The proposed transfusion and any alternatives should be discussed with the patient, or if that is not possible with a relative, and this should be documented. Some patients, e.g. Jehovah's Witnesses, may refuse transfusion and require specialised management to survive profound anaemia following blood loss.

PRE-TRANSFUSION TESTING

The red cells from the patient's blood sample are tested to determine the ABO and RhD type. The patient's plasma is tested to detect any red cell antibodies that could haemolyse transfused red cells. This is done by checking the patient's serum for reaction against two or three different red cell types, specially selected to express the most important antigens. If the patient's serum contains an antibody to one of these, the red cells will agglutinate. The antibody can then be identified by further testing so that red cell units that lack the corresponding antigen can be selected.

The transfusion laboratory will perform either a 'type and screen' or a cross-match. In the 'type and screen' (or 'group and hold' or 'group and save') procedure, after testing as above, the patient's sample is held in the laboratory for up to a week. During this period, provided no antibodies have been detected, the hospital blood bank can prepare compatible blood for collection within about 15 minutes. In a further development of this approach (often called 'electronic cross-match') blood can be issued for suitable patients with no red cell antibodies on the basis of blood group information held in the laboratory's computer.

In the cross-match (red cell compatibility testing) procedure, after pre-transfusion testing and a direct confirmation of compatibility ('cross-match'), red cell units are allocated to that patient for transfusion. Full cross-matching takes about 45 minutes if no red cell antibodies are present, but may require hours or days if a patient has multiple antibodies, which is usually due to previous transfusions or pregnancies.

STANDARD PROCEDURES FOR PRE-TRANSFUSION SAMPLING AND ADMINISTERING OF TRANSFUSIONS

Most incompatible transfusions result from mistakes in taking or labelling the blood sample for pre-transfusion testing, or from failure to carry out standard checks before infusion to make certain the correct pack has been selected for the patient. Every hospital where blood is transfused should have a written transfusion policy that is used by all staff ordering and administering blood products.

It should give clear instructions on the following:

- *Taking blood for pre-transfusion testing.* Positively identify the patient at the bedside. Label the sample tube and complete the request form clearly and accurately after identifying the patient. Do not write forms and labels in advance.
- *Administering blood.* Positively identify the patient at the bedside. Ensure that the identification of each blood pack matches the patient's identification. Check that the ABO and RhD groups of each pack are compatible with the patient's. Check each pack for evidence of damage. If in doubt, do not use and return to the blood bank. Complete the forms that document the transfusion of each pack.
- *Record-keeping and observations.* The reason for transfusion, the product given, any adverse effects and the clinical response should be recorded in the notes. Transfusions should only be given in a situation where the patient can be observed. Blood pressure, pulse and temperature should be monitored before and 15 minutes after starting each pack. If the patient is conscious, further observations are only needed if the patient has symptoms or signs of a reaction. An unconscious patient should have pulse and temperature checked at intervals during the transfusion. Signs of abnormal bleeding during the transfusion could be due to DIC resulting from an acute haemolytic reaction.

ADVERSE EFFECTS OF TRANSFUSION

The UK haemovigilance study, SHOT, has collated reports of Serious Hazards of Transfusion for the years 1996–2003, during which about 23 million units of blood components were supplied. The incidence of adverse events reported (expressed per unit of blood supplied) is shown in Boxes 24.22 and 24.23.

Fever and allergic symptoms or signs, such as itch or urticaria, occur during about 1% of transfusions, usually in patients who have had repeated transfusions. Usually these reactions are not serious but any new symptoms or signs that arise during a transfusion must be taken seriously as they may be the first warnings of a serious reaction. Infusion of fresh frozen plasma can rarely cause anaphylactic reactions.

Since it may be impossible to identify the cause of a severe reaction immediately, the initial supportive management should generally cover all the possible causes. Figure 24.17 overleaf outlines the symptoms and signs, management and investigation of reactions to blood products. Transfusion-associated graft-versus-host disease (TA GVHD) is a rare but always fatal complication. It occurs when there is sharing of an HLA haplotype between donor and recipient. Gamma irradiation of blood components prevents TA GVHD by preventing lymphocyte proliferation. Patients at risk of TA GVHD who must receive irradiated blood components include those with congenital T-cell immunodeficiencies, Hodgkin lymphoma, recipients of stem-cell transplants or blood from a family member, neonates and those treated with fludarabine (see www.transfusionguidelines.org.uk).

INFECTIONS TRANSMITTED BY TRANSFUSION

Over the past 30 years, the viruses that cause hepatitis B, AIDS and hepatitis C have been identified and effective tests introduced to detect and exclude infected blood units. Where blood is from 'safe' donors and correctly tested, the current risk of a donation being infectious is very small. In 2002–3 in the UK, the estimated chances that a unit of blood might transmit one of the viruses for which blood is tested, was 0.02 per 100 000 units for HIV, 0.005 for HCV and 0.24 for HBV. More patients are put at risk by receiving an unintended blood component (6 per 100 000), including ABO-incompatible blood (1 per 100 000).

However, some patients who received transfusions before these tests were available have suffered very serious consequences from these infections, and this is a reminder to avoid non-essential transfusions. Licensed plasma derivatives that have been virus-inactivated do not transmit HIV, human T lymphotrophic virus (HTLV), HBV, HCV, cytomegalovirus or other lipid-enveloped viruses.

Several viruses that are transmissible by transfusion have recently been described, but have not been shown to be pathogenic. These include GBV-C (wrongly referred to as 'hepatitis G'), TT virus and SEN-V. They may prove to be 'commensal' agents.

There is great concern in the UK about variant Creutzfeldt–Jakob disease (vCJD), a human prion disease linked to bovine spongiform encephalitis (BSE, p. 1234). The risk of a recipient acquiring the agent of vCJD from a transfusion is uncertain, but of 16 surviving recipients of blood from donors who later developed the disease, one has died with clinical vCJD and another has died of unrelated causes but was found to have immunohistological signs of infection.

Bacterial contamination of a blood component may rarely occur, causing very severe and often lethal transfusion reactions. In the UK, 16 incidents with 9 fatalities were identified during the 5 years to 1999; about 80% of these occurred with platelet transfusion. Tests for contamination of platelet units may reduce the risk.

Transfusion-transmitted malaria is extremely rare in the UK and US but may be more important where malaria is prevalent. Donor selection procedures are designed to exclude potentially infectious individuals from donating red cells for transfusion. Blood testing for *T. cruzi*, in parts of South America where Chagas disease is endemic (p. 355), can reduce the risk of transmitting infection.

ANAEMIAS

Around 30% of the total world population is anaemic and half of these, some 600 million people, have iron deficiency. The classification of anaemia by the size of the red cells (MCV) indicates the likely cause. Red cells in the bone marrow must acquire a minimum level of haemoglobin before being released into the blood stream (Fig. 24.18). Whilst in the marrow compartment red cell precursors undergo cell division driven by erythropoietin. If red cells cannot acquire haemoglobin at a normal rate they will undergo more divisions than normal and will have a low MCV when finally released into the blood. The MCV is low because component parts of the haemoglobin molecule are not fully available: that is, iron in iron deficiency, globin chains in thalassaemia, haem ring in congenital sideroblastic anaemia and, occasionally, poor iron utilisation in the

24.22 INCIDENCE OF ADVERSE EFFECTS FROM TRANSFUSION REPORTED TO SHOT	
• Wrong blood received	6.1 per 100 000
• ABO-incompatible blood received	1.0 per 100 000
• Transfusion-associated lung injury (TRALI)	0.6 per 100 000
• Transfusion-transmitted infections (mostly bacterial)	0.2 per 100 000
• Major morbidity	1.1 per 100 000
• Death probably due to transfusion	0.4 per 100 000

24.23 RISKS OF FATAL TRANSFUSION REACTIONS AS REPORTED TO SHOT — EBM

'Data from the UK SHOT scheme estimates the risk of death at ~ 0.4/100 000 blood component units supplied. The most common cause is transfusion of the wrong unit of blood leading to an incompatible red cell transfusion reaction and transfusion-associated acute lung injury.'

For further information: 💻 www.shotuk.org
www.transfusionguidelines.org.uk

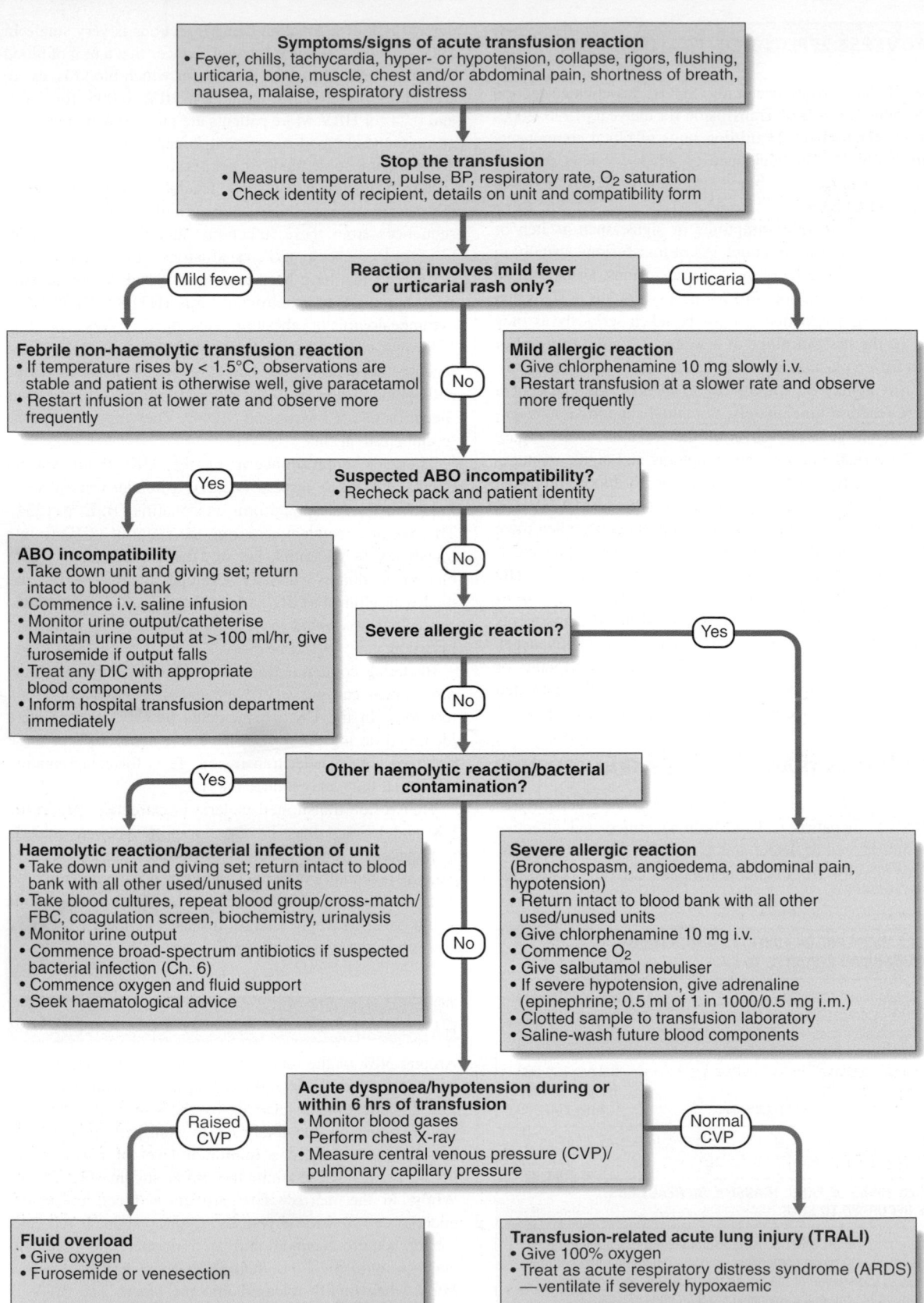

24

Fig. 24.17 Investigation and management of reactions to blood products.

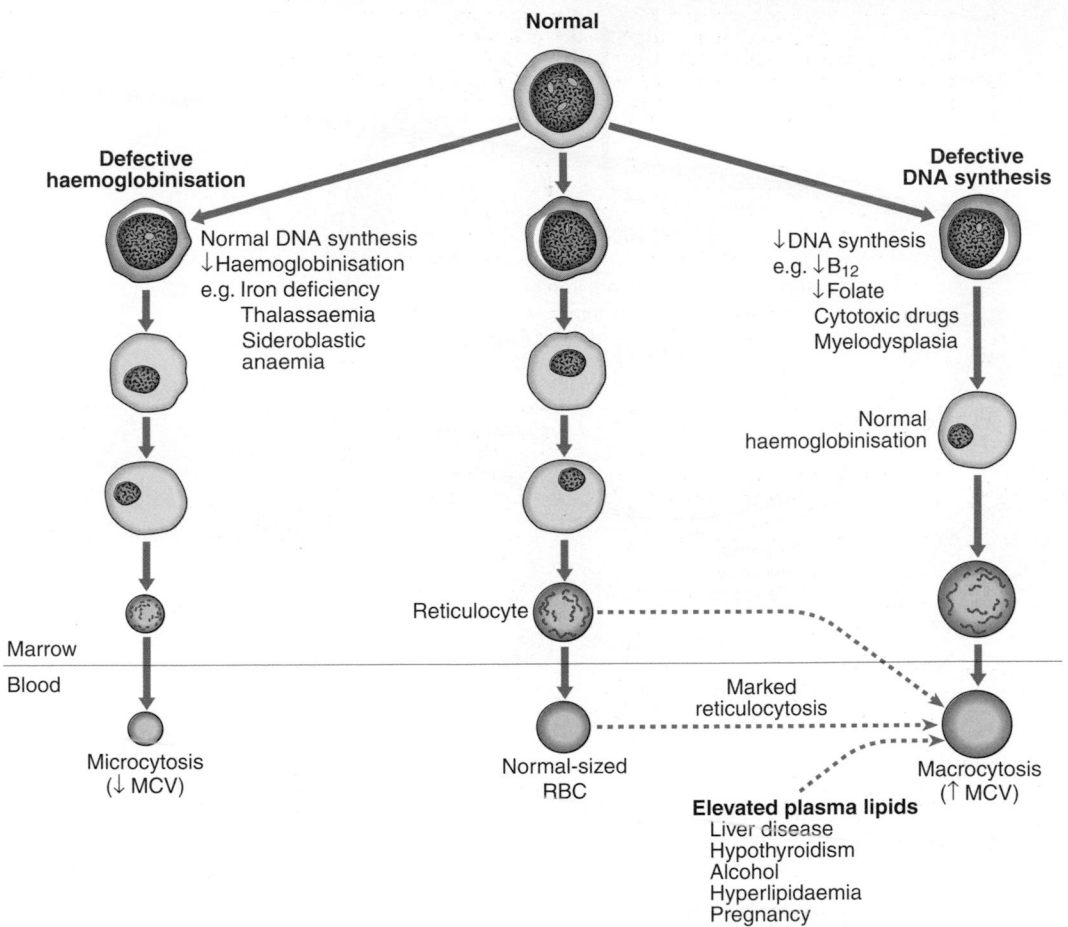

Fig. 24.18 **Factors which influence the size of red cells in anaemia.** ($\downarrow$ MCV is < 76 fl; $\uparrow$ MCV is > 100 fl)

anaemia of chronic disease. In megaloblastic anaemia the biochemical consequence of vitamin B_{12} or folate deficiency is an inability to synthesise new bases to make DNA. A similar defect of cell division is seen in the presence of cytotoxic drugs or haematological disease in the marrow such as myelodysplasia. In these states, cells haemoglobinise normally but undergo fewer cell divisions, resulting in circulating red cells with a raised MCV. The red cell membrane is composed of a lipid bilayer which will freely exchange with the plasma pool of lipid. Conditions such as liver disease, hypothyroidism, hyperlipidaemia and pregnancy are associated with raised lipids and may cause a raised MCV.

IRON DEFICIENCY ANAEMIA

This occurs when iron losses or physiological requirements exceed absorption.

Blood loss

The most common explanation in men and post-menopausal women is gastrointestinal blood loss (p. 866). This may result from occult gastric or colorectal malignancy, gastritis, peptic ulceration, inflammatory bowel disease, diverticulitis, polyps and angiodysplastic lesions. On a world-wide basis, hookworm and schistosomiasis are the most prevalent causes of gut blood loss (pp. 360 and 367). Gastrointestinal blood loss may be exacerbated by the chronic use of aspirin or NSAIDs, which cause intestinal erosions and impair platelet function. In women of child-bearing age, menstrual blood loss, pregnancy and breastfeeding contribute to iron deficiency by depleting iron stores; in developed countries one-third of women in this age bracket have low iron stores but only 3% display iron-deficient haematopoiesis. Rarely, chronic haemoptysis or haematuria may cause iron deficiency.

Malabsorption

A dietary assessment should be made in all patients to ascertain their iron intake. Gastric acid is required to release iron from food and helps to keep iron in the soluble ferrous state (Fig. 24.19). Hypochlorhydria in the elderly or that due to drugs such as proton pump inhibitors may contribute to the lack of iron availability from the diet, as may previous gastric surgery. Iron is absorbed actively in the upper small intestine and hence can be affected by coeliac disease (p. 894). Anyone with features of malabsorption or recurrent deficiency in the absence of other explanations, young men with normal diet or young women with normal menstruation and diet in association with iron deficiency, should be screened for coeliac disease.

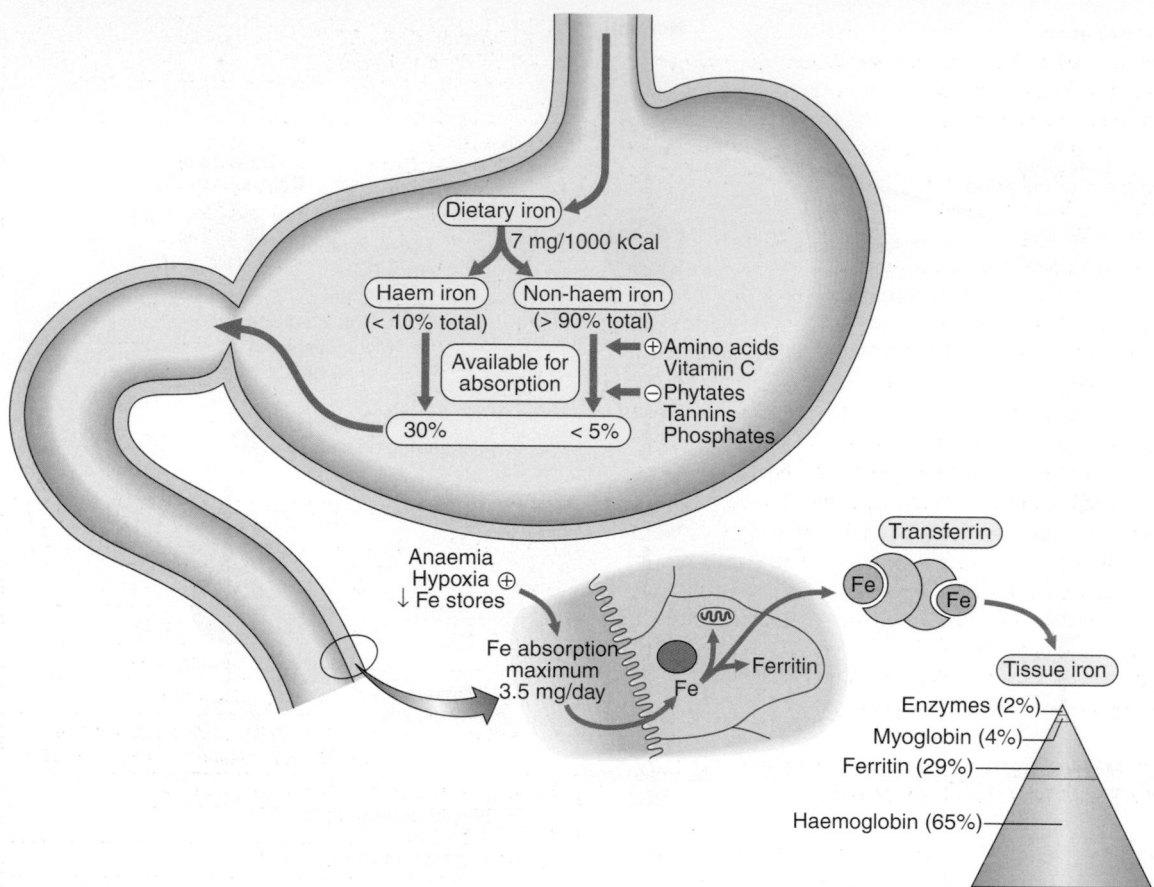

Fig. 24.19 Iron absorption, uptake and distribution in the body.

Physiological demands

At times of rapid growth such as infancy and puberty, iron demands increase and may outstrip absorption. This may be exacerbated by prematurity and breastfeeding in infants or menstruation in girls. In pregnancy, iron is diverted to the fetus, the placenta and the increased maternal red cell mass, and is lost with bleeding at parturition. There is no consensus about the routine use of iron supplementation in pregnancy but if women with a poor dietary history or previous heavy menstrual losses become pregnant and the side-effects are acceptable, it is a justifiable practice.

Investigations

Confirmation of iron deficiency

Plasma ferritin is a measure of iron stores and the best single test to confirm iron deficiency (Box 24.29, p. 1030). It is a very specific test; a subnormal level is due to iron deficiency, hypothyroidism or vitamin C deficiency. Levels can be raised by liver disease and in an acute phase response; in these conditions a ferritin level of up to 100 μg/l may still be associated with absent bone marrow iron stores. Plasma iron and total iron binding capacity (TIBC) are measures of iron availability, hence are affected by many factors besides iron stores. Plasma iron has a marked diurnal and day-to-day variation and becomes very low during an acute phase response but is raised in liver disease and haemolysis.

Transferrin levels are lowered by malnutrition, liver disease, an acute phase response and nephrotic syndrome but raised by pregnancy or the oral contraceptive pill. A transferrin saturation of less than 16% is consistent with iron deficiency but is less specific than a ferritin measurement.

All proliferating cells express membrane transferrin receptors to acquire iron; a small amount of this receptor is shed into blood and found in a free soluble form there. At times of poor iron stores, cells up-regulate transferrin receptor expression; hence the levels of soluble plasma transferrin receptor increase. This can now be measured by immunoassay and used to distinguish storage iron depletion in the presence of an acute phase response or liver disease where a raised level indicates iron deficiency. In difficult cases it may still be necessary to examine a bone marrow aspirate for iron stores.

Investigation of the cause

This will depend upon the age and sex of the patient as well as the history and clinical findings. In men over the age of 40 years and in post-menopausal women with a normal diet, the upper and lower gastrointestinal tract should be investigated by endoscopy or barium studies. If coeliac disease is suspected, serum antigliadin and anti-endomysium antibodies and duodenal biopsy are indicated (p. 894). In the tropics stool and urine should be examined for parasites (p. 297).

Management

Unless the patient has angina, heart failure or evidence of cerebral hypoxia, transfusion is not necessary and oral iron supplementation is appropriate. Ferrous sulphate 200 mg 8-hourly (120 mg of elemental iron per day) is more than adequate and should be continued for 3–6 months to replete iron stores. The occasional patient is intolerant of ferrous sulphate, with dyspepsia and altered bowel habit. In this case a reduction in dose to 200 mg 12-hourly or a switch to ferrous gluconate 300 mg 12-hourly (70 mg of elemental iron per day) should be made. Delayed-release preparations are not useful since they release iron beyond the upper small intestine where it cannot be absorbed.

The haemoglobin should rise by 10 g/l every 7–10 days and a reticulocyte response will be evident by 1 week. A failure to respond adequately may be due to non-compliance, continued blood loss, malabsorption or an incorrect diagnosis. The occasional patient with malabsorption or chronic gut disease may need parenteral iron with deep intramuscular injection of iron sorbitol (1.5 mg of iron per kg body weight). This will produce a haematological response and rapidly replete iron stores. Patients should be warned that a brown skin discoloration like a tattoo is likely to develop at the sites of administration.

MEGALOBLASTIC ANAEMIA

This results from a deficiency of vitamin B_{12} or folic acid, or from disturbances in folic acid metabolism. Folate is an important substrate of, and vitamin B_{12} a co-factor for, the generation of the essential amino acid methionine from homocysteine. This reaction produces tetrahydrofolate, which is converted to thymidine monophosphate for incorporation into DNA. Deficiency of either vitamin B_{12} or folate will therefore produce high plasma levels of homocysteine and impaired DNA synthesis.

The end result is cells with arrested nuclear maturation but normal cytoplasmic development: so-called nucleo-cytoplasmic asynchrony. All proliferating cells will exhibit megaloblastosis; hence changes are evident in the buccal mucosa, tongue, small intestine, cervix, vagina and uterus. The high proliferation rate of bone marrow results in striking changes in the haematopoietic system in megaloblastic anaemia. Cells become arrested in development and die within the marrow; this ineffective erythropoiesis results in an expanded hypercellular marrow. The megaloblastic changes are most evident in the early nucleated red cell precursors, and intramedullary haemolysis results in a raised bilirubin and lactate dehydrogenase (LDH) but no reticulocytosis. Iron stores are usually raised. The mature red cells are large and oval, and sometimes contain nuclear remnants. Nuclear changes are seen in the immature granulocyte precursors and a characteristic appearance is that of 'giant' metamyelocytes with a large 'sausage-shaped' nucleus. The mature neutrophils show hypersegmentation of their nuclei, with cells having six or more nuclear lobes. If severe, a pancytopenia may be present in the peripheral blood.

Vitamin B_{12} deficiency but not folate deficiency is associated with neurological disease in up to 40% of cases.

24.24 CLINICAL FEATURES OF MEGALOBLASTIC ANAEMIA

Symptoms

- Malaise (90%)
- Breathlessness (50%)
- Paraesthesiae (80%)
- Sore mouth (20%)
- Weight loss
- Altered skin pigmentation
- Grey hair
- Impotence
- Poor memory
- Depression
- Personality change
- Hallucinations
- Visual disturbance

Signs

- Smooth tongue
- Angular cheilosis
- Vitiligo
- Skin pigmentation
- Heart failure
- Pyrexia

24.25 DIAGNOSTIC FEATURES OF MEGALOBLASTIC ANAEMIA

Investigation	Result
Haemoglobin	Often reduced, may be very low
MCV	Usually raised, commonly > 120 fl
Erythrocyte count	Low for degree of anaemia
Blood film	Oval macrocytosis, poikilocytosis, red cell fragmentation, neutrophil hypersegmentation
Reticulocyte count	Low for degree of anaemia
Leucocyte count	Low or normal
Platelet count	Low or normal
Bone marrow	Increased cellularity, megaloblastic changes in erythroid series, giant metamyelocytes, dysplastic megakaryocytes, increased iron in stores, pathological non-ring sideroblasts
Serum ferritin	Elevated
Plasma LDH	Elevated, often markedly

24

The main pathological finding is focal demyelination affecting spinal cord, peripheral nerves, optic nerves and cerebrum. The most common manifestations are sensory with peripheral paraesthesia and ataxia of gait. The clinical and diagnostic features of megaloblastic anaemia are summarised in Boxes 24.24 and 24.25, the neurological findings of B_{12} deficiency in Box 24.26.

VITAMIN B_{12}

Vitamin B_{12} absorption

The average daily diet contains 5–30 µg of vitamin B_{12}, mainly in meat, fish, eggs and milk—well in excess of the 1 µg daily requirement. In the stomach, gastric enzymes release vitamin B_{12} from food and at gastric pH it binds to a carrier protein termed R protein. The gastric parietal cells produce intrinsic factor, a vitamin B_{12}-binding protein which optimally binds vitamin B_{12} at pH 8. As gastric emptying occurs, pancreatic secretion raises the pH and vitamin B_{12} released from the diet switches from the R protein to intrinsic factor. Bile also contains vitamin B_{12} which is available for reabsorption in the intestine. The vitamin B_{12} intrinsic factor complex binds to specific receptors in the

24.26 NEUROLOGICAL FINDINGS IN B₁₂ DEFICIENCY

Peripheral nerves

- Glove and stocking paraesthesiae

Spinal cord

- Subacute combined degeneration
- Posterior columns—diminished vibration and proprioception
- Corticospinal tracts—upper motor neuron signs

Cerebrum

- Dementia
- Optic atrophy

Autonomic neuropathy

terminal ileum and vitamin B_{12} is actively transported by the enterocytes to plasma, where it binds to transcobalamin II, a transport protein produced by the liver, which carries it to the tissues for utilisation. The liver stores enough vitamin B_{12} for 3 years and this, together with the entero-hepatic circulation, means that vitamin B_{12} deficiency takes years to become manifest even if all dietary intake is stopped.

Levels of cobalamins fall in normal pregnancy. Each laboratory must validate its own normal range but levels below 150 ng/l are common and in the last trimester 5–10% of women have levels below 100 ng/l. Similarly, paraproteins can interfere with vitamin B_{12} assays and so myeloma may be associated with a spurious low vitamin B_{12}.

Causes of vitamin B₁₂ deficiency

Dietary deficiency

This only occurs in strict vegans but the onset of clinical features can occur at any age between 10 and 80 years. The breastfed offspring of vegan mothers are at risk of developing nutritional vitamin B_{12} deficiency. Less strict vegetarians often have slightly low vitamin B_{12} levels but are not tissue vitamin B_{12}-deficient.

Gastric factors

Normal gastric acid and enzyme secretion is required for the release of vitamin B_{12} from the food. Hypochlorhydria in elderly patients or following gastric surgery can impair the release of vitamin B_{12} from food. Total gastrectomy invariably results in vitamin B_{12} deficiency within 5 years, often combined with iron deficiency. These patients need life-long 3-monthly vitamin B_{12} injections. After partial gastrectomy vitamin B_{12} deficiency only develops in 10–20% of patients by 5 years. An annual injection of vitamin B_{12} should prevent deficiency in this group.

Pernicious anaemia

This is an autoimmune disorder in which the gastric mucosa is atrophic with loss of parietal cells causing intrinsic factor deficiency. In the absence of intrinsic factor less than 1% of dietary vitamin B_{12} is absorbed. Pernicious anaemia has an incidence of 25/100 000 population over the age of 40 years in developed countries, but an average age of onset of 60 years. It is more common in individuals with other autoimmune disease (Hashimoto's thyroiditis, Graves'

disease, vitiligo, hypoparathyroidism or Addison's disease) or a family history of these or pernicious anaemia. Anti-parietal cell antibodies are present in over 90% of cases but are also present in 20% of normal females over the age of 60 years. A negative result makes pernicious anaemia less likely but a positive result is not diagnostic. Antibodies to intrinsic factor are found in the serum of 60% of patients with pernicious anaemia and, if present, are diagnostic.

Small bowel factors

One-third of all patients with pancreatic insufficiency fail to transfer dietary vitamin B_{12} from R protein to intrinsic factor. This usually results in slightly low vitamin B_{12} values but no tissue evidence of vitamin B_{12} deficiency.

Motility disorders or hypogammaglobulinaemia can result in bacterial overgrowth and the resulting competition for free vitamin B_{12} can result in deficiency. This will be corrected to some extent by a course of antibiotics.

A small number of people heavily infected with the fish tapeworm (p. 370) develop vitamin B_{12} deficiency.

Inflammatory disease of the terminal ileum, such as Crohn's disease, may impair the interaction of the vitamin B_{12}–intrinsic factor complex with its receptor, as will surgery on this part of the bowel. Both may result in vitamin B_{12} malabsorption.

It is possible to distinguish pernicious anaemia from intestinal problems with a two-part Schilling test (Fig. 24.20). The patient must be vitamin B_{12}-replete, have normal renal function and be able to comply with a 24-hour urine collection. This latter criterion is important as up to 25% of tests are invalidated by an incomplete urine collection. It is

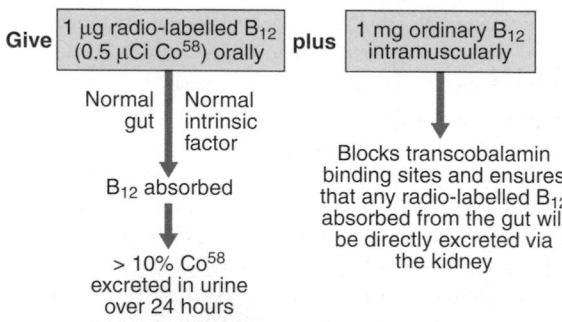

Part One

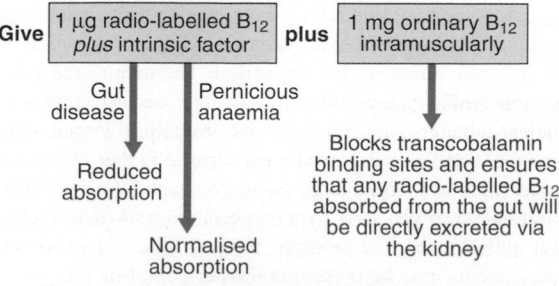

Part Two (if excretion ↓ in Part One)

Fig. 24.20 The two-part Schilling test in the diagnosis of the cause of vitamin B_{12} deficiency.

important to note that this is not a test of gut function, but simply distinguishes pernicious anaemia from the other causes of vitamin B_{12} deficiency.

FOLATE

Folate absorption

Folates are produced by plants and bacteria; hence dietary leafy vegetables (spinach, broccoli, lettuce), fruits (bananas, melons) and animal protein (liver, kidney) are a rich source. An average Western diet contains more than the minimum daily intake of 50 μg but excess cooking for longer than 15 minutes destroys folates. Most dietary folate is present as polyglutamates; these are converted to monoglutamate in the upper small bowel and actively transported into plasma. Plasma folate is loosely bound to plasma proteins such as albumin and there is an enterohepatic circulation. Total body stores of folate are small and deficiency can occur in a matter of weeks.

Folate deficiency

The causes and diagnostic features of folate deficiency are covered in Boxes 24.27 and 24.28. The edentulous elderly or psychiatric patient is particularly susceptible to dietary deficiency and this will be exacerbated in the presence of gut disease or malignancy. Pregnancy-induced folate deficiency is the most common cause of megaloblastosis world-wide and is more likely in the context of twin pregnancies, multiparity and hyperemesis gravidarum.

Serum folate is very sensitive to dietary intake; a single meal can normalise it in a patient with true folate deficiency, and anorexia, alcohol and anticonvulsant therapy can reduce it in the absence of megaloblastosis. For this reason red cell folate levels are a more accurate indicator of folate stores and tissue folate deficiency.

MANAGEMENT OF MEGALOBLASTIC ANAEMIA

Where a patient with a severe megaloblastic anaemia is very ill and treatment must be started before vitamin B_{12} and red cell folate results are available, always treat with both folic acid and vitamin B_{12}. The use of folic acid alone in the presence of vitamin B_{12} deficiency may result in worsening of neurological defects.

Vitamin B_{12} deficiency

Vitamin B_{12} deficiency is treated with hydroxycobalamin 1000 μg i.m. in five doses 2 or 3 days apart followed by maintenance therapy of 1000 μg every 3 months for life. The reticulocyte count will peak by the 5th–10th day after therapy and may be as high as 50%. The haemoglobin will rise by 10 g/l every week. The response of the marrow is associated with a fall in plasma potassium levels and rapid depletion of iron stores. If an initial response is not maintained and the blood film is dimorphic, the patient may need additional iron therapy. A sensory neuropathy may take 6–12 months to correct; long-standing neurological damage may not improve.

Folate deficiency

Oral folic acid 5 mg daily for 3 weeks will treat acute deficiency and 5 mg once weekly is adequate maintenance therapy. Prophylactic folic acid in pregnancy will prevent megaloblastosis in women at risk. Folic acid supplementation may reduce the risk of neural tube defects, and in some countries all pregnant women receive routine folic acid supplementation. Prophylactic supplementation is also given in chronic haematological disease associated with reduced red cell lifespan (e.g. autoimmune haemolytic anaemia or haemoglobinopathies). There is also evidence that supraphysiological supplementation (400 μg/day) can reduce the risk of coronary and cerebrovascular disease by reducing plasma homocysteine levels. This has led the US Food and Drug Administration to introduce fortification of bread, flour and rice with folic acid.

Rarely, if severe angina or heart failure is present, transfusion can be used in megaloblastic anaemia. The cardiovascular system is adapted to the chronic anaemia present in megaloblastosis, and the volume load imposed by transfusion may result in decompensation and severe cardiac failure. In such circumstances, exchange transfusion or slow administration of 1 unit each day with diuretic cover may be cautiously used.

ANAEMIA OF CHRONIC DISEASE

This is a common type of anaemia, particularly in hospital populations. It occurs in the setting of chronic infections,

24

chronic inflammation or neoplasia. The anaemia is not related to bleeding, haemolysis or marrow infiltration, is mild, in the range of 85–115 g/l, and is usually associated with a normal MCV (normocytic, normochromic), though this may be reduced in long-standing inflammation. The serum iron is low but iron stores are normal or increased, as indicated by the ferritin or stainable marrow iron.

Pathogenesis

The pathogenesis of this type of anaemia is thought to involve abnormalities of iron metabolism, including reduced release of iron to transferrin, and erythropoiesis. Recent interest has been centred on the role of erythropoietin and the inhibitory effect of various cytokines (e.g. IL-1 and TNF-α) on erythropoiesis. Erythropoietin levels appear to be lower than would be expected for the degree of anaemia, and administration of erythropoietin to patients with rheumatoid arthritis has a beneficial effect on the anaemia.

Diagnosis and management

It is often difficult to distinguish the anaemia of chronic disease (ACD) associated with a low MCV from iron deficiency. Box 24.29 summarises the investigations. Examination of the marrow may ultimately be required to assess iron

stores directly. A trial of oral iron can be given in difficult situations. A positive response occurs in true iron deficiency but not in ACD. Measures which reduce the severity of the underlying disorder generally help to improve the ACD.

HAEMOLYSIS

The normal red cell lifespan of 120 days may be shortened by a variety of abnormalities. The bone marrow may increase its output of red cells six- to eight-fold by increasing the proportion of red cells produced, expanding the volume of active marrow and releasing reticulocytes prematurely. If the rate of destruction exceeds this increased production rate, then anaemia will develop.

The basic laboratory diagnosis of haemolysis is outlined in Figure 24.21. The red cell destruction will overload pathways for haemoglobin breakdown, causing a modest rise in unconjugated bilirubin in the blood and mild jaundice. Increased reabsorption of urobilinogen from the gut results in an increase in urinary urobilinogen (pp. 1005 and 944). Red cell destruction releases LDH and increases serum levels. The bone marrow compensation results in a reticulocytosis, and nucleated red cell precursors may also appear in the blood. The expansion of the active bone marrow may result in a neutrophilia and immature granulocytes appearing in the blood to cause a leucoerythroblastic blood film. The appearances of the red cells may give an indication of the likely cause of the haemolysis. Spherocytes are small, dark-red cells and suggest autoimmune haemolysis or hereditary spherocytosis; sickle cells suggest haemoglobinopathy; and red cell fragments indicate microangiopathic haemolysis.

Intravascular haemolysis

When rapid red cell destruction occurs, free haemoglobin is released into the plasma. Free haemoglobin is toxic to cells and the body has evolved binding proteins to minimise this risk. Haptoglobin is an α_2-globulin produced by the liver which binds free haemoglobin, resulting in a fall in levels of haptoglobin. Once haptoglobins are saturated, free haemoglobin is oxidised to form methaemoglobin which binds to albumin, in turn forming methaemalbumin which can be detected by the Schumm's test. Methaemoglobin is degraded and any free haem is bound to a second binding protein termed haemopexin. If all the protective mechanisms are overloaded, free haemoglobin may appear in the urine. When fulminant, this gives rise to black urine as in severe *falciparum* malaria infection (p. 342). In smaller amounts renal tubular cells absorb the haemoglobin, degrade it and store the iron as haemosiderin. When the tubular cells are subsequently sloughed into the urine they give rise to haemosiderinuria, which is always indicative of intravascular haemolysis.

Extravascular haemolysis

Physiological red cell destruction occurs in the fixed reticulo–endothelial cells in the liver or spleen, so avoiding free haemoglobin in the plasma. In most haemolytic states, haemolysis is predominantly extravascular.

24

24.29 INVESTIGATIONS TO DIFFERENTIATE ANAEMIA OF CHRONIC DISEASE FROM IRON DEFICIENCY ANAEMIA					
	Ferritin	Iron	TIBC	Transferrin saturation	Soluble transferrin receptor
Iron deficiency anaemia	↓	↓	↑	↓	↑
Anaemia of chronic disease	↑/Normal	↓	↓	↓	↓/Normal
(TIBC = total iron binding capacity)					

24.30 ANAEMIA IN OLD AGE

- **Mean haemoglobin:** falls with age in both sexes, but remains well within the normal range. When a low haemoglobin does occur, it is generally due to disease.
- **Anaemia can never be considered 'normal' in old age.**
- **Symptoms:** may be subtle and insidious. Cardiovascular features such as dyspnoea and oedema, and cerebral features such as dizziness and apathy, tend to predominate.
- **Ferritin:** if less than 45 μg/l in older people is highly predictive of iron deficiency
- **Serum iron and transferrin:** fall with age because of the prevalence of other disorders, and are not reliable indicators of deficiency.
- **Most common cause of iron deficiency:** gastrointestinal blood loss.
- **Most common cause of vitamin B$_{12}$ deficiency:** pernicious anaemia, as the prevalence of chronic atrophic gastritis rises in old age.
- **Neuropsychiatric symptoms associated with vitamin B$_{12}$ deficiency:** well established but a causal relationship has not been clearly shown. Dementia associated with vitamin B$_{12}$ deficiency in the absence of haematological abnormalities is rare.
- **Anaemia of chronic disease:** frequent in old age because of the rising prevalence of diseases that reduce erythropoiesis.

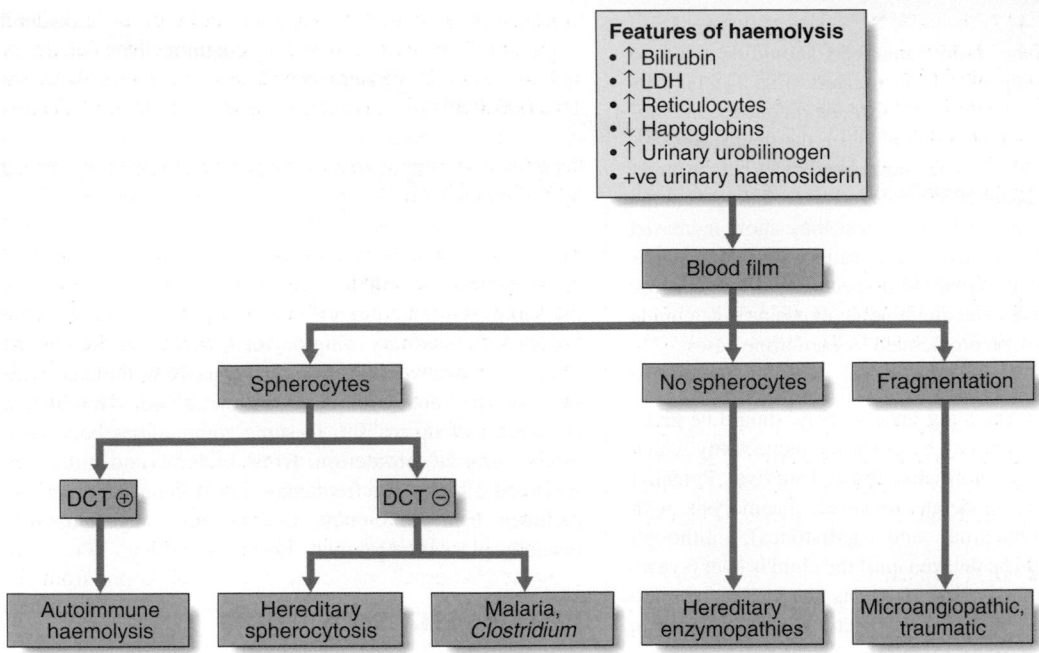

Fig. 24.21 **Laboratory features and classification of the causes of haemolysis.** (LDH = lactate dehydrogenase; DCT = direct Coombs test)

The compensatory erythroid hyperplasia may give rise to folate deficiency, when the blood findings will be complicated by the presence of megaloblastosis. Measurement of red cell folate is unreliable in the presence of haemolysis and serum folate will be elevated. Patients' red cells can be labelled with ^{51}chromium; when reinjected, they can be used to determine red cell survival, or when combined with surface counting may indicate whether the liver or the spleen is the main source of red cell destruction. This is seldom performed in clinical practice.

CONGENITAL HAEMOLYSIS

Inherited red cell defects of structure or metabolism may result in a chronic haemolytic state. The principal pathologies are red cell membrane defects (hereditary spherocytosis or elliptocytosis), glucose-6-phosphate dehydrogenase (G6PD) deficiency and the haemoglobinopathies (p. 1035).

RED CELL MEMBRANE DEFECTS

The structure of the red cell membrane is shown in Figure 24.4 (p. 1005). The basic structure is a cytoskeleton 'stapled' on to the lipid bilayer by special protein complexes. This structure ensures great deformability and elasticity; the red cell diameter is 8 μm but the narrowest point in the circulation is 2 μm in the spleen. When this normal structure is disturbed, usually by a quantitative or functional deficiency of one or more proteins in the cytoskeleton, cells lose their normal elasticity. Each time such cells pass through the spleen they lose membrane relative to their cell volume. This results in an increase in mean cell haemoglobin concentration (MCHC), abnormal cell shape and reduced red cell survival due to extravascular haemolysis.

Hereditary spherocytosis

This is usually inherited as an autosomal dominant condition, although 25% of cases have no family history and represent new mutations. The incidence is approximately 1:5000 in developed countries but this may be an underestimate since the disease may present de novo in patients over 65 years and is often discovered as a chance finding on a blood count. The pathogenesis varies between families; the most common abnormalities are deficiencies of beta spectrin or ankyrin (Fig. 24.4). The severity of spontaneous haemolysis varies. Most cases are associated with an asymptomatic compensated chronic haemolytic state with spherocytes present on the blood film and a reticulocytosis. Occasional cases are associated with more severe haemolysis; these may be due to co-incidental polymorphisms in alpha spectrin or co-inheritance of a second defect involving a different protein.

The clinical course may be complicated by crises:

- *A haemolytic crisis* occurs when the severity of haemolysis increases; this is rarely seen in association with infection.
- *A megaloblastic crisis* follows the development of folate deficiency; this may occur as a first presentation of the disease in association with pregnancy.
- *An aplastic crisis* occurs in association with erythrovirus infection. Erythrovirus causes a common exanthem in children but if individuals with chronic erythroid hyperplasia become infected, the virus directly invades red cell precursors and temporarily switches off red cell production. Patients present with severe anaemia and a low reticulocyte count.

Pigment gallstones are present in up to 50% of patients and may cause symptomatic cholecystitis.

Investigations

The patient and other family members should be screened for features of compensated haemolysis (Fig. 24.21). This may be all that is required to confirm the diagnosis. Haemoglobin levels are variable depending on the degree of compensation. The blood film will show spherocytes but the direct Coombs test (pp. 1033–1034) is negative excluding immune haemolysis. An osmotic fragility test may show increased sensitivity to lysis in hypotonic saline solutions but is limited by lack of sensitivity and specificity. More specific flow cytometric tests detecting binding of eosin-5-maleimide to red cells are now recommended in borderline cases.

Management

Folic acid prophylaxis, 5 mg once weekly, should be given for life. Consideration may be given to splenectomy which improves but does not normalise red cell survival. Potential indications include moderate to severe haemolysis with complications (anaemia and gallstones), although splenectomy should be delayed until the child is over 6 years of age in view of the risk of sepsis. Guidelines for the management of patients after splenectomy are presented in Box 24.31.

Acute, severe haemolytic crises require transfusion support but blood must be cross-matched carefully and transfused slowly as haemolytic transfusion reactions may occur. The typical blood film appearances are masked in the presence of iron deficiency or disorders which cause a raised MCV, such as jaundice; in these situations the red cell shape is normal but spherocytes will appear when the underlying abnormality is corrected.

Hereditary elliptocytosis

This term refers to a heterogeneous group of disorders that produce an increase in elliptocytic red cells on the blood film and a variable degree of haemolysis. Hereditary elliptocytosis is due to a functional abnormality of one or more anchor proteins in the red cell membrane, e.g. alpha spectrin or protein 4.1. Inheritance may be autosomal dominant or recessive. It is less common than hereditary spherocytosis in Western countries, with an incidence of 1/10 000, but is more common in equatorial Africa and parts of South-east Asia. The clinical course is variable and depends upon the degree of membrane dysfunction caused by the inherited molecular defect(s); most cases present as an asymptomatic blood film abnormality but occasional cases result in neonatal haemolysis or a chronic compensated haemolytic state. Management of the latter is the same as for hereditary spherocytosis. A characteristic variant of hereditary elliptocytosis occurs in South-east Asia, particularly Malaysia and Papua New Guinea, with stomatocytes and ovalocytes in the blood. This has a prevalence of up to 30% in some communities because it offers relative protection from malaria and thus has sustained a high gene frequency. The differential diagnosis includes iron deficiency, thalassaemia, myelofibrosis, myelodysplasia and pyruvate kinase deficiency.

RED CELL ENZYMOPATHIES

The mature red cell must produce energy via ATP to maintain a normal internal environment and cell volume whilst protecting itself from the oxidative stress presented from oxygen carriage. Anaerobic glycolysis via the Embden–Meyerhof pathway generates ATP, and the hexose monophosphate shunt produces NADPH and glutathione to protect against oxidative stress. The impact of functional or quantitative defects in the enzymes in these pathways will depend upon the importance of the steps affected and the presence of alternative pathways. In general, defects in the hexose monophosphate shunt result in periodic haemolysis induced by oxidative stress, whilst those in the Embden–Meyerhof pathway result in shortened red cell survival and chronic haemolysis.

Glucose-6-phosphate dehydrogenase deficiency

This enzyme is pivotal in the hexose monophosphate shunt and produces NADPH to protect the red cell against oxidative stress. Deficiencies of this enzyme are the most common human enzymopathy, affecting 10% of the world's population with a geographical distribution which parallels the malaria belt (pp. 1035–1036) because heterozygotes are protected from malarial parasitisation. The enzyme is a heteromeric structure made of catalytic subunits which are coded for by a gene on the X chromosome. The deficiency affects males but is carried by females, who are usually only affected in the neonatal period or in the presence of extreme lyonisation or homozygosity. There are over 400 subtypes of G6PD described. The most common types associated with normal activity are the B^+ enzyme present in most Caucasians and 70% of Afro-Caribbeans, and the A^+ variant present in 20% of Afro-Caribbeans. The two common variants associated with reduced activity are the A^- variety in approximately 10% of Afro-Caribbeans, and the Mediterranean or B^- variety in Caucasians. In East and West Africa up to 20% of males and 4% of females (homozygotes) are affected and have enzyme levels of approximately

---

24.31 MANAGEMENT OF THE SPLENECTOMISED PATIENT

- Vaccinate with pneumococcal, *Haemophilus influenzae* type B, meningococcal group C and influenza vaccines at least 2–3 weeks before elective splenectomy. Vaccination should be given after emergency surgery, but may be less effective. Pneumococcal re-immunisation should be given at least 5-yearly and influenza annually. Vaccination status must be documented
- Life-long prophylactic penicillin V 250 mg 12-hourly is recommended. In penicillin-allergic patients, consider erythromycin
- A card or bracelet should be carried by splenectomised patients to alert health professionals to the risk of overwhelming sepsis, wherever possible; it may be life-saving in unconscious patients by guiding the rapid administration of appropriate antibiotics
- In septicaemia, splenectomised patients should be resuscitated and given intravenous antibiotics to cover pneumococcus, *Haemophilus* and meningococcus
- The risk of malaria is increased
- Animal bites should be promptly treated with local disinfection and antibiotics, to prevent serious soft tissue infection and septicaemia

24.32 GLUCOSE-6-DEHYDROGENASE DEFICIENCY

Clinical features

Acute drug-induced haemolysis to (e.g.)
- Analgesics: aspirin, phenacetin
- Antimalarials: primaquine, quinine, chloroquine, pyrimethamine
- Antibiotics: sulphonamides, nitrofurantoin, ciprofloxacin
- Miscellaneous: quinidine, probenecid, vitamin K, dapsone

Chronic compensated haemolysis

Infection or acute illness

Neonatal jaundice
- May be a feature of the B⁻ enzyme

Favism or acute haemolysis after ingestion of the broad bean
Vicia faba

Laboratory features

Non-spherocytic intravascular haemolysis during an attack
The blood film will show:
- Bite cells (red cells with a 'bite' of membrane missing)
- Blister cells (red cells with surface blistering of the membrane)
- Irregularly shaped small cells
- Polychromasia reflecting the reticulocytosis
- Denatured haemoglobin visible as Heinz bodies within the red cell cytoplasm, if stained with a supravital stain such as methyl violet

G6PD level
- Can be indirectly assessed by screening methods which usually depend upon the decreased ability to reduce dyes
- Direct assessment of G6PD is made in those with low screening values
- Care must be taken close to an acute haemolytic episode because reticulocytes may have normal enzyme levels and give rise to a false normal result

---

15%. The deficiency in Caucasian and Oriental populations is more severe, with enzyme levels as low as 1%.

Clinical features and investigational findings are shown in Box 24.32.

Management aims to stop any precipitant drugs and treat any underlying infection. Acute transfusion support may be life-saving.

Pyruvate kinase deficiency

This is the second most common red cell enzyme defect and affects thousands of people world-wide. It results in deficiency of ATP production and a chronic haemolytic anaemia. It is inherited as an autosomal recessive trait. The extent of anaemia is variable; the blood film shows characteristic 'prickle cells' which resemble holly leaves. Enzyme activity is only 5–20% of normal. Transfusion support may be necessary.

Pyrimidine 5′ nucleotidase deficiency

This enzyme catalyses the dephosphorylation of nucleoside monophosphates and is important during the degradation of RNA in reticulocytes. It is inherited as an autosomal recessive trait and is as common as pyruvate kinase deficiency in Mediterranean, African and Jewish populations. The accumulation of excess ribonucleoprotein results in coarse basophilic stippling associated with a chronic haemolytic state. The enzyme is very sensitive to inhibition

by lead and this is the reason why basophilic stippling is a feature of lead poisoning.

ACQUIRED HAEMOLYTIC ANAEMIA

AUTOIMMUNE HAEMOLYTIC ANAEMIA

This results from increased red cell destruction due to red cell autoantibodies. The antibodies may be IgG or M, or more rarely IgE or A. If an antibody avidly fixes complement, it will result in intravascular haemolysis, but if complement activation is weak, the haemolysis will be extravascular. Antibody-coated red cells lose membrane to macrophages in the spleen and hence spherocytes are present in the blood. The optimum temperature at which the antibody is active (thermal specificity) is used to classify immune haemolysis:

- Warm antibodies bind best at 37°C and account for 80% of cases. The majority are IgG and usually react against Rhesus antigens.
- Cold antibodies bind best at 4°C but can bind up to 37°C in some cases. They are usually IgM and bind complement. They account for the other 20% of cases.

Warm autoimmune haemolysis

The incidence of warm autoimmune haemolysis is approximately 1/100 000 population per annum; it occurs at all ages but is more common in middle age and there is a female excess. No underlying cause is identified in up to 50% of cases. The remainder are secondary to a wide variety of other conditions:

- lymphoid neoplasms: lymphoma, chronic lymphocytic leukaemia, myeloma
- solid tumours: lung, colon, kidney, ovary, thymoma
- connective tissue disease: SLE, rheumatoid arthritis
- drugs: methyldopa, mefenamic acid, penicillin, quinine
- miscellaneous: ulcerative colitis, HIV.

Investigations

There is evidence of haemolysis and spherocytes on the blood film. The diagnosis is confirmed by the direct Coombs or antiglobulin test (Fig. 24.22). In this, red cells are mixed with Coombs reagent which contains antibodies against human IgG/M/complement. If the red cells have been coated by antibody in vivo, the Coombs reagent will induce their agglutination and this can be detected visually. The relevant antibody can be eluted from the red cell surface and tested against a panel of typed red cells to determine which red cell antigen it is directed against. The most common specificity is Rhesus and most often anti-e; this is helpful when choosing blood to cross-match. The direct Coombs test can be negative in the presence of brisk haemolysis; a positive test requires about 200 antibody molecules to attach to each red cell; with a very avid complement-fixing antibody, haemolysis may occur at lower levels of antibody-binding. The standard Coombs reagent will miss IgA or IgE antibodies.

24

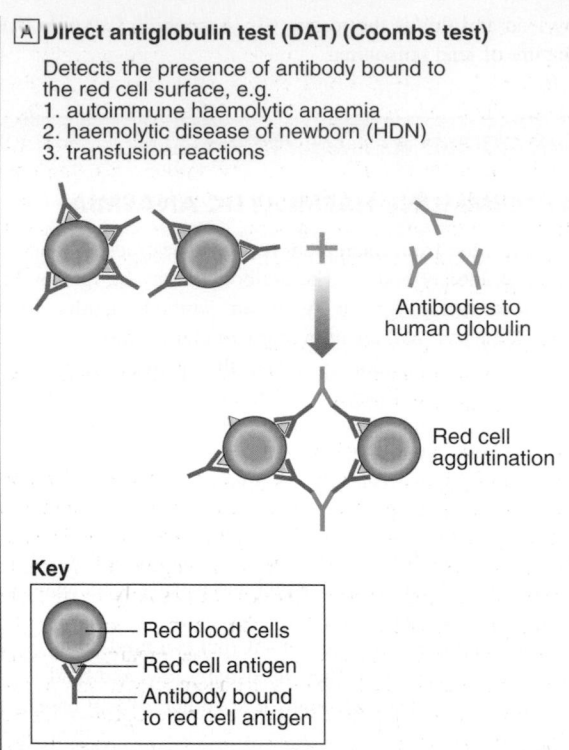

A Direct antiglobulin test (DAT) (Coombs test)

Detects the presence of antibody bound to the red cell surface, e.g.
1. autoimmune haemolytic anaemia
2. haemolytic disease of newborn (HDN)
3. transfusion reactions

Antibodies to human globulin

Red cell agglutination

Key

Red blood cells
Red cell antigen
Antibody bound to red cell antigen

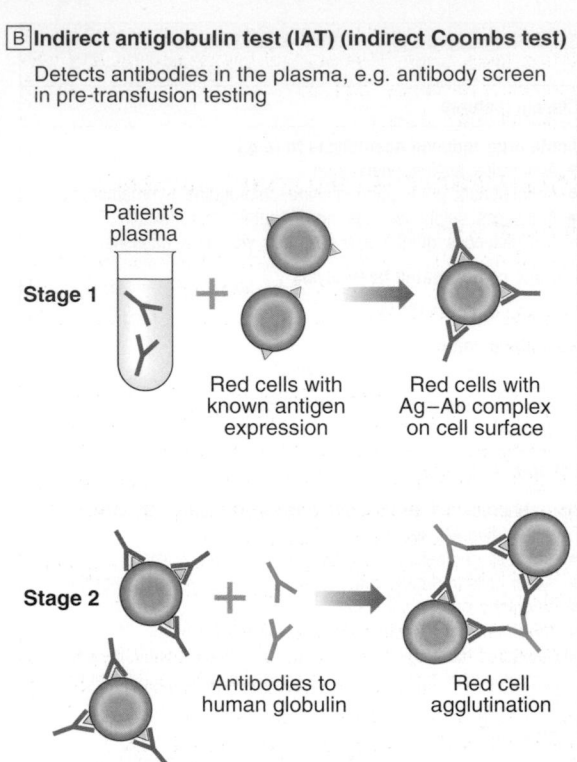

B Indirect antiglobulin test (IAT) (indirect Coombs test)

Detects antibodies in the plasma, e.g. antibody screen in pre-transfusion testing

Patient's plasma

Stage 1

Red cells with known antigen expression

Red cells with Ag–Ab complex on cell surface

Stage 2

Antibodies to human globulin

Red cell agglutination

Fig. 24.22   Direct and indirect antiglobulin tests.

Management

- If the haemolysis is secondary to an underlying cause, this must be treated and any offending drugs stopped.
- It is usual to treat patients initially with prednisolone 1 mg/kg orally. A response is seen in 70–80% of cases but this may take up to 3 weeks; a rise in haemoglobin will be matched by a fall in bilirubin and LDH levels. Once the haemoglobin has reached 100 g/l, the corticosteroid dose can be reduced by 5 mg per week to 10 mg daily, then reduced slowly to nothing over a further 10 weeks. Steroids work by decreasing macrophage destruction of antibody-coated red cells and reducing antibody production.
- Transfusion support may be required for life-threatening problems. The least incompatible blood should be used but may still give rise to transfusion reactions or the development of further alloantibodies.
- If the haemolysis fails to respond to corticosteroids or can only be stabilised by large doses, then splenectomy should be considered. This removes a main site of red cell destruction and antibody production with a good response in 50–60% of cases. The operation can be performed laparoscopically with reduced morbidity.
- For patients who fail to respond to corticosteroids or for whom splenectomy is not appropriate, alternative immunosuppressive therapy may be considered. This is least suitable for young patients, for whom long-term therapy may carry a risk of secondary neoplasms. The choice of drug is between azathioprine 1–2 mg/kg and cyclophosphamide 2 mg/kg, both orally; induction of a response usually takes 2–3 months.

Cold agglutinin disease

This is due to antibodies, usually IgM, which bind to the red cells at 4°C and cause them to agglutinate. It may cause intravascular haemolysis if complement fixation occurs. This can be chronic when the antibody is monoclonal, or acute or transient when the antibody is polyclonal.

Chronic cold agglutinin disease

This affects elderly patients and may be associated with an underlying low-grade B-cell lymphoma. It causes a low-grade intravascular haemolysis with cold, painful and often blue fingers, toes, ears or nose (so-called acrocyanosis). The latter is due to red cell agglutination in the small vessels in these exposed areas. The blood film shows red cell agglutination and the MCV may be spuriously raised because the automated analysers count aggregates as single cells. The monoclonal IgM usually has specificity against the I or, more rarely, i antigen and is present in a very high titre. Treatment is directed at any underlying lymphoma but if the disease is idiopathic, then patients must keep extremities warm, especially in winter. Some patients respond to corticosteroid therapy and blood transfusion may be considered, but the cross-match sample must be placed in a transport flask at a temperature of 37°C and blood administered via a blood-warmer.

Other causes of cold agglutination

Cold agglutination can occur in association with *Mycoplasma pneumoniae* or with infectious mononucleosis. Paroxysmal cold haemoglobinuria is a very rare cause seen in children in association with congenital syphilis. An IgG antibody binds to red cells in the peripheral circulation but lysis occurs in the central circulation when complement fixation takes place. This antibody is termed the Donath–Landsteiner antibody and has specificity against the P antigen on the red cells.

NON-IMMUNE HAEMOLYTIC ANAEMIA

Physical trauma

Physical disruption of red cells may occur in a number of conditions and is characterised by the presence of red cell fragments on the blood film and markers of intravascular haemolysis:

- *Mechanical heart valves*. High flow through incompetent valves or periprosthetic leaks through the suture ring holding a valve in place result in shear stress damage.
- *March haemoglobinuria*. Vigorous exercise such as prolonged marching or marathon running can cause red cell damage in the capillaries in the feet.
- *Thermal injury*. Severe burns cause thermal damage to red cells characterised by fragmentation and the presence of microspherocytes in the blood.
- *Microangiopathic haemolytic anaemia*. Fibrin deposition in capillaries can cause severe red cell disruption. It may occur in a wide variety of conditions: disseminated carcinomatosis, malignant or pregnancy-induced hypertension, haemolytic uraemic syndrome (p. 498), thrombotic thrombocytopenic purpura (p. 1057) and DIC (p. 1060).

Infection

Plasmodium falciparum malaria (p. 342) may be associated with intravascular haemolysis; when severe this is termed blackwater fever due to the associated haemoglobinuria. *Clostridium perfringens* septicaemia (p. 326), usually in the context of an ascending cholangitis, may cause severe intravascular haemolysis with marked spherocytosis due to bacterial production of a lecithinase which destroys the red cell's membrane.

Chemicals or drugs

These agents cause haemolysis by oxidant denaturation of haemoglobin. Dapsone and sulfasalazine can produce haemolysis associated with the presence of Heinz bodies in the red cells on supravital staining with brilliant cresyl blue. Heinz bodies contain denatured haemoglobin. Arsenic gas, copper, chlorates, nitrites and nitrobenzene derivatives may all cause haemolysis.

HAEMOGLOBINOPATHIES

Normal haemoglobin

The normal haemoglobin molecule is comprised of two alpha and two non-alpha globin chains (p. 1005). Alpha globin chains are produced from two genes present on each chromosome 16; these are active throughout embryonic, fetal, infant and adult life. Severe disorders of alpha globin chains may therefore cause intrauterine death. The non-alpha chains are produced by genes present in single copy on each chromosome 11. Production varies with age; fetal haemoglobin (HbF–$\alpha_2\gamma_2$) has two gamma chains but after the first trimester small amounts of haemoglobin A (HbA–$\alpha_2\beta_2$) with two beta chains are produced. At birth about 80% of haemoglobin is HbF and 20% HbA. Thereafter gamma chain production is suppressed, such that by 6 months of age HbA is the predominant haemoglobin with less than 1% HbF. Disorders affecting the beta chain do not present until after 6 months of age. A constant small amount of haemoglobin A_2 (HbA$_2$–$\alpha_2\delta_2$, usually < 2%) is made from birth.

Abnormal haemoglobins

The haemoglobinopathies can be classified into qualitative or quantitative abnormalities.

Qualitative abnormalities

In qualitative abnormalities (called the abnormal haemoglobins), there is an alteration in the amino acid structure of the polypeptide chains of the globin fraction of haemoglobin. The best-known example is haemoglobin S, found in sickle-cell anaemia. These abnormalities usually result from amino acid substitutions which change the function of the globin chain at critical sites. For example, mutations around the haem-binding pocket cause the haem ring to fall out of the structure and produce an unstable haemoglobin. These substitutions often change the charge of the globin chains, producing different electrophoretic mobility, and this forms the basis for the diagnostic use of electrophoresis to identify haemoglobinopathies. Several hundred such variants are known; they were originally designated by letters of the alphabet, e.g. S, C, D or E, but are now described by names usually taken from the town or district in which they were first described.

Quantitative abnormalities

In quantitative abnormalities (the thalassaemias), the amino acid sequence is normal but polypeptide chain production is impaired or absent for a variety of reasons. In these conditions the ratio of alpha to non-alpha chain production is disturbed. In alpha-thalassaemia excess beta chains are present, whilst in beta-thalassaemia excess alpha chains are present. The excess chains precipitate, causing red cell membrane damage and reduced red cell survival.

SICKLE-CELL ANAEMIA

Sickle-cell disease results from a single glutamic acid to valine substitution at position 6 of the beta globin polypeptide chain. It is inherited as an autosomal recessive trait. Homozygotes only produce abnormal beta chains that make haemoglobin S (HbS, termed SS), and this results in the clinical syndrome of sickle-cell disease. Heterozygotes produce a mixture of normal and abnormal beta chains that make normal HbA and HbS (termed AS), and this results in the clinically asymptomatic sickle trait. The inheritance of sickle-cell disease is shown in Figure 24.23.

Epidemiology

Individuals with sickle-cell trait are relatively resistant to the lethal effects of *falciparum* malaria in early childhood. The high incidence of this deleterious gene in equatorial

24

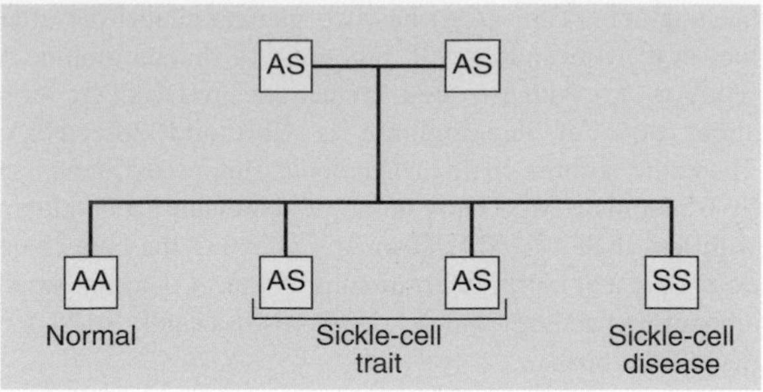

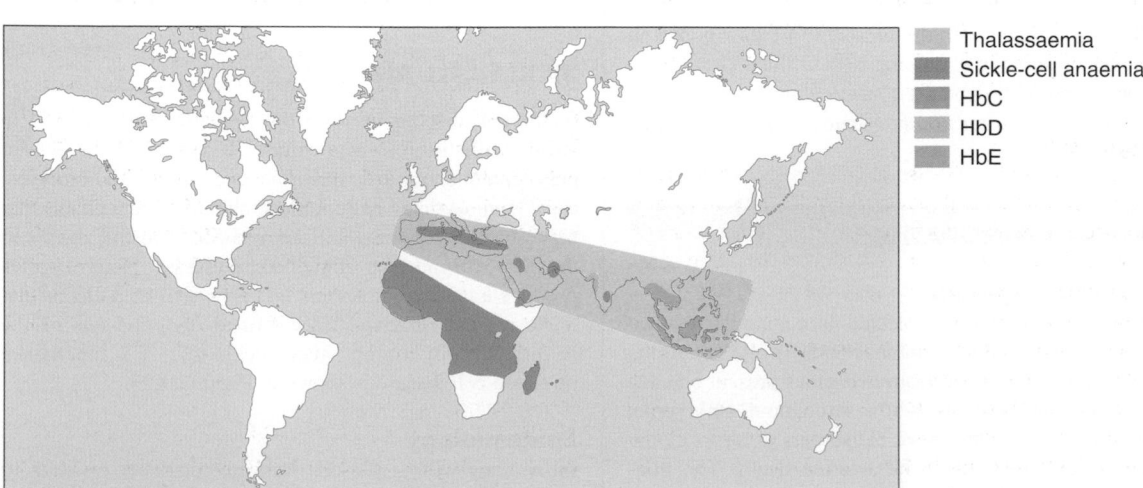

Fig. 24.23 **Possible genotype of offspring of parents with sickle-cell trait.**

Africa can be explained by the selective survival advantage it confers in areas where *falciparum* malaria is endemic. Patients with sickle-cell anaemia do not have correspondingly greater resistance to *falciparum* malaria. The geographical distribution of sickle-cell anaemia and the other common haemoglobinopathies is shown in Figure 24.24. The greatest prevalence of haemoglobinopathies occurs in tropical Africa, where the heterozygote frequency is over 20%. In black American populations, sickle-cell trait has a frequency of 8%.

Pathogenesis

When haemoglobin S is deoxygenated, the molecules of haemoglobin polymerise to form pseudocrystalline structures known as 'tactoids'. These distort the red cell membrane and produce characteristic sickle-shaped cells. The polymerisation is reversible when reoxygenation occurs. The distortion of the red cell membrane, however, may become permanent and the red cell 'irreversibly sickled'. The greater the concentration of sickle-cell haemoglobin in the individual cell, the more easily tactoids are formed, but this process may be enhanced or retarded by the presence of other haemoglobins. Thus haemoglobin C participates in the polymerisation more readily than haemoglobin A, whereas haemoglobin F strongly inhibits polymerisation.

Clinical features

Sickling is precipitated by hypoxia, acidosis, dehydration and infection. Irreversibly sickled cells have a shortened survival and plug vessels in the microcirculation. This results in a number of acute syndromes termed 'crises' and chronic organ damage as shown in Figure 24.25:

- *Vaso-occlusive crisis.* Plugging of small vessels in the bone produces acute severe bone pain. This affects areas of active marrow: the hands and feet in children (so-called dactylitis) or the femora, humeri, ribs, pelvis and vertebrae in adults. Patients usually have a systemic response with tachycardia, sweating and a fever. This is the most common crisis.
- *Sickle chest syndrome.* This may follow on from a vaso-occlusive crisis and is the most common cause of death in adult sickle disease. Bone marrow infarction results in fat emboli to the lungs which cause sickling and infarction, leading to ventilatory failure if not treated.
- *Sequestration crisis.* Thrombosis of the venous outflow from an organ causes loss of function and acute painful enlargement. In children the spleen is the most common site. Massive splenic enlargement may result in severe anaemia and circulatory collapse with death. Recurrent sickling in the spleen in childhood results in infarction and adults may have no functional spleen. In adults the liver may undergo sequestration with severe pain due to capsular stretching.
- *Aplastic crisis.* Infection of adult sicklers with human erythrovirus 19 results in a severe but self-limiting red cell aplasia. This produces a very low haemoglobin which may cause heart failure. Unlike in all other sickle crises, the reticulocyte count is low.

Investigations

Patients with sickle-cell disease have a compensated anaemia, usually around 60–80 g/l. The blood film shows sickle cells, target cells and features of hyposplenism. A reticulocytosis is present. The presence of HbS can be demonstrated by exposing red cells to a reducing agent such

Fig. 24.24 **The geographical distribution of the haemoglobinopathies.**

Thalassaemia
Sickle-cell anaemia
HbC
HbD
HbE

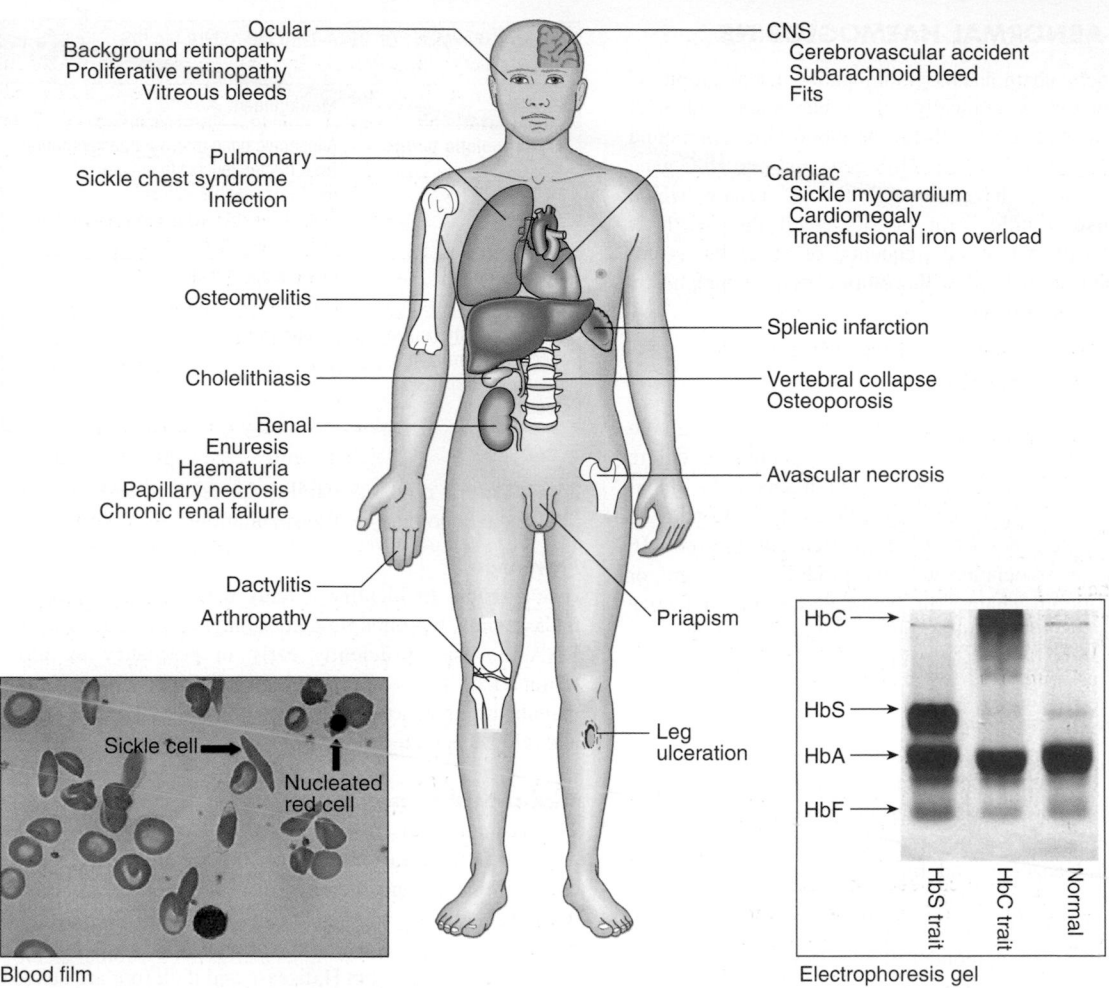

Ocular
Background retinopathy
Proliferative retinopathy
Vitreous bleeds

CNS
Cerebrovascular accident
Subarachnoid bleed
Fits

Pulmonary
Sickle chest syndrome
Infection

Cardiac
Sickle myocardium
Cardiomegaly
Transfusional iron overload

Osteomyelitis

Splenic infarction

Cholelithiasis

Vertebral collapse
Osteoporosis

Renal
Enuresis
Haematuria
Papillary necrosis
Chronic renal failure

Avascular necrosis

Dactylitis

Arthropathy

Priapism

Sickle cell

Nucleated red cell

Leg ulceration

Blood film

HbC
HbS
HbA
HbF

HbS trait   HbC trait   Normal

Electrophoresis gel

24

Fig. 24.25 Clinical manifestations of sickle-cell disease.

as sodium dithionite; HbA gives a clear solution, whereas HbS polymerises to produce a turbid solution. This forms the basis of emergency screening tests before surgery in appropriate ethnic groups but cannot distinguish between sickle trait and disease. The definitive diagnosis requires haemoglobin electrophoresis to demonstrate no HbA, 2–20% HbF and the predominance of HbS. Both parents of the affected individual will have sickle trait.

Management

All patients with sickle disease should receive prophylaxis with daily folic acid, and penicillin V to protect against pneumococcal infection which may be lethal in the presence of hyposplenism. These patients should be vaccinated against pneumococcus and, where available, *Haemophilus influenzae* B and hepatitis B.

Vaso-occlusive crises are managed by aggressive rehydration, oxygen therapy, adequate analgesia (which often requires opiates) and antibiotics. Transfusion should be with fully genotyped blood wherever possible. Simple top-up transfusion may be used in a sequestration or aplastic crisis. A regular transfusion programme to suppress HbS production and maintain the HbS level below 30% may be indicated in recurrent severe complications such as cerebrovascular accidents in children or chest syndromes in adults. Exchange transfusion, where a patient is simultaneously venesected and transfused to replace HbS with HbA, may be used in life-threatening crises or to prepare patients for surgery.

A high HbF level inhibits polymerisation of HbS and reduces sickling. Patients with sickle-cell disease and high HbF levels have a mild clinical course with few crises. Some agents are able to induce increased synthesis of HbF and this has been used to reduce the frequency of severe crises. The oral cytotoxic agent hydroxycarbamide has been shown to have clinical benefit with acceptable side-effects in children and adults who have recurrent severe crises. Relatively few allogeneic transplants from HLA-matched siblings have been performed but this procedure appears to be potentially curative.

Prognosis

In Africa few children with sickle-cell anaemia survive to adult life without medical attention. Even with standard medical care approximately 15% die by the age of 20 years and 50% by the age of 40 years.

OTHER ABNORMAL HAEMOGLOBINS

Another beta chain haemoglobinopathy, haemoglobin C (HbC) disease, is clinically silent but associated with microcytosis and target cells on the blood film. Compound heterozygotes inheriting one HbS gene and one HbC gene from their parents have haemoglobin SC disease, which behaves like a mild form of sickle-cell disease. It is associated with a reduced frequency of crises but is not uncommonly associated with complications in pregnancy and retinal vein thrombosis.

THE THALASSAEMIAS

Thalassaemia is an inherited impairment of haemoglobin production, in which there is partial or complete failure to synthesise a specific type of globin chain. In alpha-thalassaemia, the alpha genes are deleted; loss of one gene (α^-/α) or both genes (α^-/α^-) from each chromosome 16 may occur, in association with the production of some or no alpha globin chains. In beta-thalassaemia defective production usually results from disabling point mutations causing no (β^0) or reduced (β^-) beta chain production.

Beta-thalassaemia

Failure to synthesise beta chains (beta-thalassaemia) is the most common type of thalassaemia and is seen in highest frequency in the Mediterranean area. Heterozygotes have thalassaemia minor, a condition in which there is usually mild anaemia and little or no clinical disability. Homozygotes (thalassaemia major) either are unable to synthesise haemoglobin A or at best produce very little and, after the first 4 months of life, develop a profound hypochromic anaemia. The diagnostic features are listed in Box 24.33.

Beta-thalassaemia minor is often detected only when iron therapy for a mild microcytic anaemia fails. The diagnostic features are also summarised in Box 24.33. Symptoms are absent or mild. Intermediate grades of severity occur.

Management

The treatment of beta-thalassaemia major is given in Box

24.33 DIAGNOSTIC FEATURES OF BETA-THALASSAEMIA	
Major	
• Profound hypochromic anaemia	
• Evidence of severe red cell dysplasia	
• Erythroblastosis	
• Absence or gross reduction of the amount of haemoglobin A	
• Raised levels of haemoglobin F	
• Evidence that both parents have thalassaemia minor	
Minor	
• Mild anaemia	
• Microcytic hypochromic erythrocytes (not iron-deficient)	
• Some target cells	
• Punctate basophilia	
• Raised resistance of erythrocytes to osmotic lysis	
• Raised haemoglobin A_2 fraction	
• Evidence that one parent has thalassaemia minor	

24.34 TREATMENT OF BETA-THALASSAEMIA MAJOR	
Problem	**Management**
Erythropoietic failure	Allogeneic bone marrow transplantation from human leucocyte antigen (HLA)-compatible sibling Transfusion to maintain Hb > 100 g/l Folic acid 5 mg daily
Iron overload	Iron therapy forbidden Desferrioxamine therapy
Splenomegaly causing mechanical problems, excessive transfusion needs	Splenectomy

24.34. Cure is now a possibility for selected children, with allogeneic bone marrow transplantation.

Prevention

It is possible to identify a fetus with homozygous beta-thalassaemia by obtaining chorionic villous material for DNA analysis sufficiently early in pregnancy to allow termination. This examination is only appropriate if both parents are known to be carriers (beta-thalassaemia minor) and will accept a termination.

Alpha-thalassaemia

The reduction or absence of alpha-chain synthesis is common in Southeast Asia. There are two alpha gene loci on chromosome 16 and therefore four alpha genes. If one is deleted there is no clinical effect. If two are deleted there may be a mild hypochromic anaemia. If three are deleted the patient has haemoglobin H disease and if all four are deleted the baby is stillborn (hydrops fetalis). Haemoglobin H is a beta-chain tetramer formed from the excess of chains. It is functionally useless. Treatment of haemoglobin H disease is similar to that of beta-thalassaemia of intermediate severity. The combinations are shown in Box 24.35.

24.35 ALPHA-THALASSAEMIA
Cause
• Failure of production of haemoglobin alpha chains due to gene deletion
Age and sex incidence
• Both sexes from birth onward
Genetics
• Two alpha-chain genes from each parent
Presentation
• Hydrops fetalis if all genes deleted
• Haemoglobin H if three genes deleted
• Mild hypochromic microcytic anaemia if two genes deleted
Treatment
• Hydrops fetalis: none available
• Haemoglobin H: no specific therapy required; avoid iron therapy; folic acid if necessary

HAEMATOLOGICAL MALIGNANCIES

Haematological malignancies arise when the processes of proliferation or apoptosis are corrupted in blood cells. If mature differentiated cells are involved, the cells will have a low growth fraction and produce indolent neoplasms such as the low-grade lymphomas or chronic leukaemias, where patients have an expected survival of many years. In contrast, if more primitive stem cells are involved, the cells can have the highest growth fractions of all human neoplasms, producing rapidly progressive life-threatening illnesses such as the acute leukaemias or high-grade lymphomas. Involvement of the pluripotent stem cells produces the most aggressive acute leukaemias. In general, haematological neoplasms are diseases of elderly patients, the exceptions being acute lymphoblastic leukaemia which predominantly affects children, and Hodgkin lymphoma which affects young people in the 20–40-year age range (Fig. 24.26).

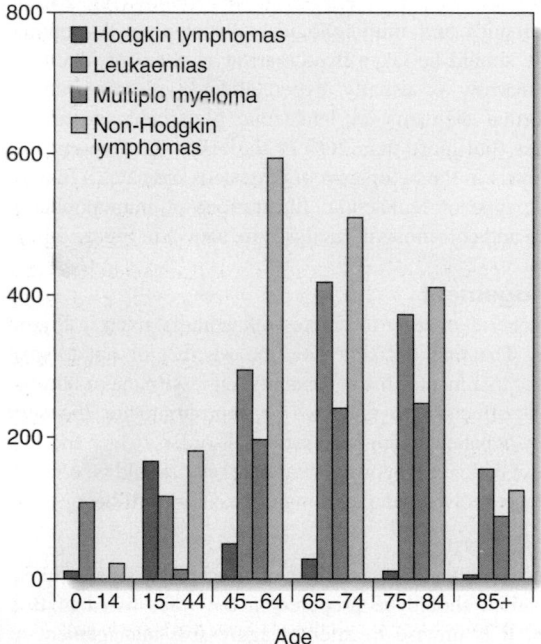

Fig. 24.26 **Variation in the incidence of different haematological malignancies in the UK by age.**

LEUKAEMIAS

Leukaemias are malignant disorders of the haematopoietic stem cell compartment, characteristically associated with increased numbers of white cells in the bone marrow and/or peripheral blood. The course of leukaemia may vary from a few days or weeks to many years, depending on the type.

Epidemiology

The incidence of leukaemia of all types in the population is approximately 10/100 000 per annum, of which just under half are acute leukaemia. Males are affected more frequently than females, the ratio being about 3:2 in acute leukaemia, 2:1 in chronic lymphocytic leukaemia and 1.3:1 in chronic myeloid leukaemia. Geographical variation in incidence does occur, the most striking being the rarity of chronic lymphocytic leukaemia in the Chinese and related races. Acute leukaemia occurs at all ages. Acute lymphoblastic leukaemia shows a peak of incidence in the 1–5 age group. All forms of acute myeloid leukaemia have their lowest incidence in young adult life and there is a striking rise over the age of 50. Chronic leukaemias occur mainly in middle and old age.

Aetiology

The cause of the leukaemia is unknown in the majority of patients. Several factors, however, are associated with the development of leukaemia and these are listed in Box 24.36.

Terminology and classification

In acute leukaemia there is proliferation of primitive stem cells leading to an accumulation of blasts, predominantly in the bone marrow, which causes bone marrow failure. In chronic leukaemia the malignant clone is able to differentiate, resulting in an accumulation of more mature cells.

Leukaemias are traditionally classified into four main groups:

- acute lymphoblastic leukaemia (ALL)
- acute myeloid leukaemia (AML)
- chronic lymphocytic leukaemia (CLL)
- chronic myeloid leukaemia (CML).

The diagnosis of leukaemia is usually suspected from an abnormal blood count, often a raised white count. The

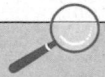

24.36 FACTORS ASSOCIATED WITH THE DEVELOPMENT OF LEUKAEMIA
Ionising radiation
• A significant increase in myeloid leukaemia followed the atomic bombing of Japanese cities • An increase in leukaemia was observed after the use of radiotherapy for ankylosing spondylitis and diagnostic X-rays of the fetus in pregnancy
Cytotoxic drugs
• These, particularly alkylating agents, may induce myeloid leukaemia, usually after a latent period of several years • Exposure to benzene in industry
Retroviruses
• One rare form of T-cell leukaemia/lymphoma appears to be associated with a retrovirus similar to the viruses causing leukaemia in cats and cattle
Genetic
• There is a greatly increased incidence of leukaemia in the identical twin of patients with leukaemia • Increased incidence occurs in Down's syndrome and certain other genetic disorders
Immunological
• Immune deficiency states (e.g. hypogammaglobulinaemia) are associated with an increase in haematological malignancy

24

24

diagnosis is made from examination of the bone marrow. This includes the morphology of the abnormal cells, analysis of cell surface markers (immunophenotyping), clone-specific chromosome abnormalities and molecular changes. Not only does this allow an accurate diagnosis but also gives valuable prognostic information, allowing therapy to be tailored to the patient's disease.

The World Health Organization (WHO) classification of tumours of haematopoietic and lymphoid tissues divides these diseases into lineages and incorporates results from immunophenotyping, genetic and molecular analysis. The subclassification of acute leukaemias is shown in Box 24.37.

ACUTE LEUKAEMIA

There is a failure of cell maturation in acute leukaemia. Proliferation of cells which do not mature leads to an accumulation of useless cells which take up more and more marrow space at the expense of the normal haematopoietic elements. Eventually, this proliferation spills into the blood. Acute myeloid leukaemia is about four times more common than acute lymphoblastic leukaemia in adults. In children the proportions are reversed, the lymphoblastic variety being more common. The clinical features are usually those of bone marrow failure (anaemia, bleeding or infection— pp. 1012, 1016 and 1018).

Investigations

Blood examination usually shows anaemia with a normal or raised MCV. The leucocyte count may vary from as low as $1 \times 10^9/l$ to as high as $500 \times 10^9/l$ or more. In the majority of patients the count is below $100 \times 10^9/l$. Severe thrombocytopenia is usual but not invariable. The appearance of blast cells in the blood film is usually diagnostic.

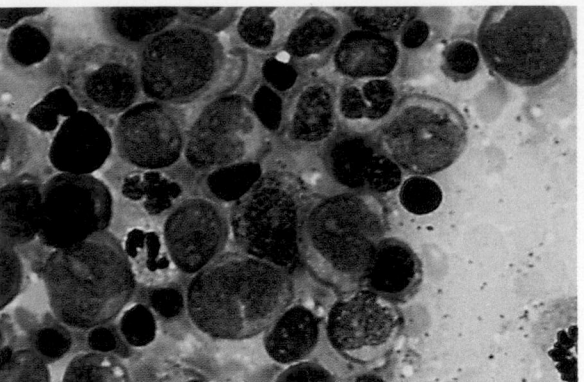

Fig. 24.27 Acute myeloid leukaemia. Bone marrow aspirate showing infiltration with large blast cells which display nuclear folding and prominent nucleoli.

Sometimes the blast cell count may be very low in the peripheral blood and a bone marrow examination is necessary to confirm the diagnosis.

The bone marrow is the most valuable diagnostic investigation and will provide material for cytology (Fig. 24.27), cytogenetics and immunological phenotyping. A trephine biopsy should be taken if no marrow is obtained (dry tap). The marrow is usually hypercellular, with replacement of normal elements by leukaemic blast cells in varying degrees (but more than 20% of the cells). The presence of Auer rods in the cytoplasm of blast cells indicates a myeloblastic type of leukaemia. Illustrations of immunophenotyping and chromosome analysis are shown in Figure 24.28.

Management

The general strategy for acute leukaemia is given in Figure 24.29. The first decision must be whether or not to give specific treatment. This is generally aggressive, has a number of side-effects, and may not be appropriate for the very elderly or patients with other serious disorders (Chs 7 and 11). In these patients supportive treatment only should be offered; this can effect considerable improvement in well-being.

Specific therapy

If a decision to embark on specific therapy has been taken, the patient should be prepared in the ways listed in Box 24.38. It is unwise to attempt aggressive management of acute leukaemia unless adequate services are available for the provision of supportive therapy.

The aim of treatment is to destroy the leukaemic clone of cells without destroying the residual normal stem cell compartment from which repopulation of the haematopoietic tissues will occur. There are three phases:

- *Remission induction.* In this phase, the bulk of the tumour is destroyed by combination chemotherapy. The patient goes through a period of severe bone marrow hypoplasia, requiring intensive support and inpatient care from specially trained medical and nursing staff.
- *Remission consolidation.* If remission has been achieved by induction therapy, residual disease is attacked by therapy during the consolidation phase. This consists of a number of courses of chemotherapy, again resulting in

24.37 WHO CLASSIFICATION OF ACUTE LEUKAEMIA
Acute myeloid leukaemia with recurrent genetic abnormalities
• AML with t(8;21) gene product AML/ETO • AML with eosinophilia inv(16) or t(16;16), gene product CBFβ/MYH11 • Acute promyelocytic leukaemia t(15;17), gene product PML/RARA • AML with 11q23 abnormalities (MLL)
Acute myeloid leukaemia with multilineage dysplasia
• e.g. Following a myelodysplastic syndrome
Acute myeloid leukaemia and myelodysplastic syndromes, therapy-related
• e.g. Alkylating agent or topoisomerase II inhibitor
Acute myeloid leukaemia not otherwise specified
• e.g. AML with or without differentiation, acute myelomonocytic leukaemia, erythroleukaemia, megakaryoblastic leukaemia, myeloid sarcoma
Acute lymphoblastic leukaemia
• Precursor B ALL • Precursor T ALL

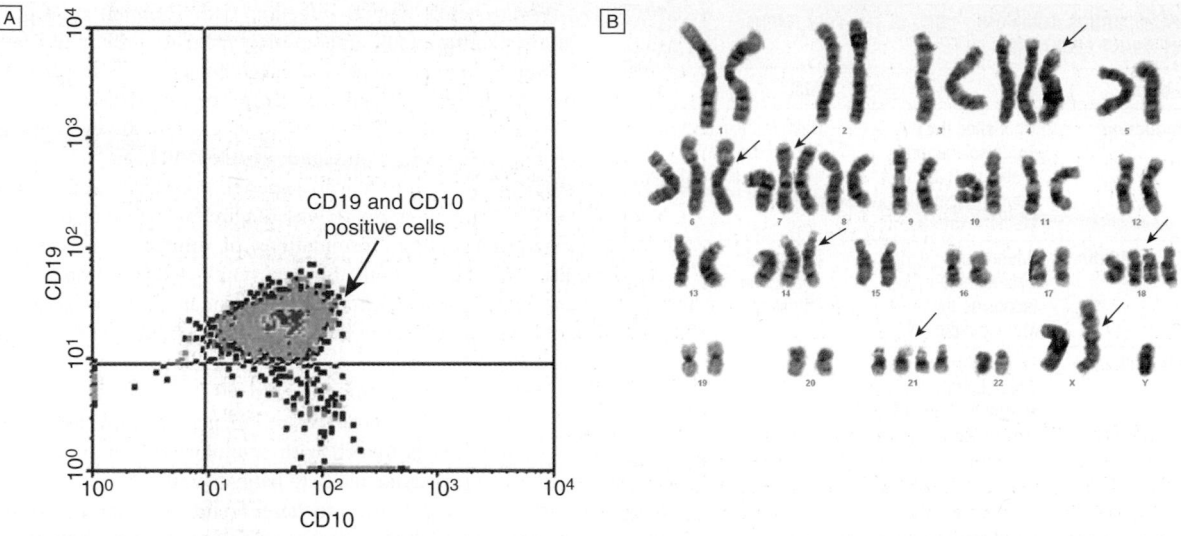

Fig. 24.28   Investigation of acute lymphoblastic leukaemia (ALL). Ⓐ Flow cytometric analysis of blasts labelled with the fluorescent antibodies anti-CD19 (y axis) and anti-CD10 (x axis). ALL blasts are positive for both CD19 and CD10 (arrow). Ⓑ Chromosome analysis (karyotype) of blasts showing additional chromosomes X, 4, 6, 7, 14, 18 and 21.

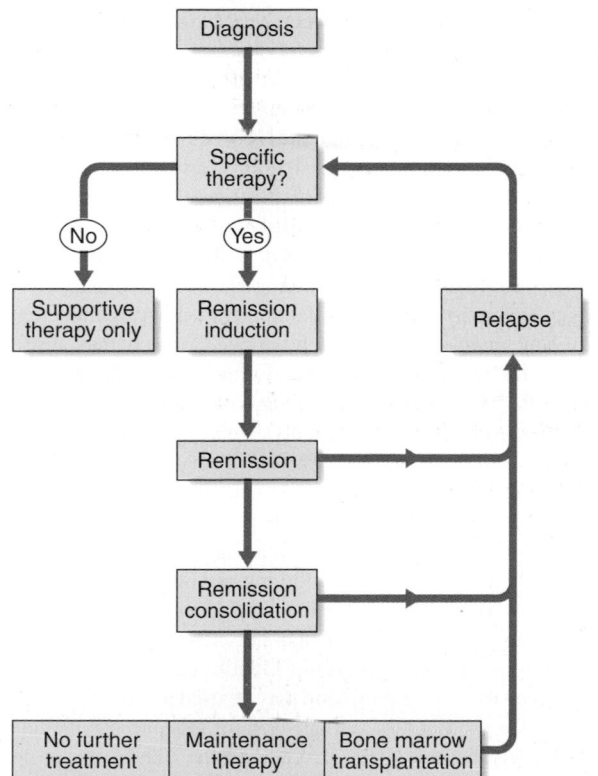

Fig. 24.29   Treatment strategy in acute leukaemia.

24.38 MANAGEMENT OF ACUTE LEUKAEMIA: SPECIFIC THERAPY

- Existing infections identified and treated (e.g. urinary tract infection, oral candidiasis, dental, gingival and skin infections)
- Anaemia corrected with red cell concentrate infusion
- Thrombocytopenic bleeding controlled with platelet transfusion
- If possible, central venous catheter (e.g. Hickman line) incerted to facilitate access to the circulation for delivery of chemotherapy
- Therapeutic regimen carefully explained to the patient and informed consent obtained

Thereafter, specific therapy is discontinued and the patient observed. (This maintenance phase is not thought to be of benefit in most patients with AML who have been brought into complete remission by induction and consolidation therapy.)

In patients with ALL it is necessary to give prophylactic treament to the central nervous system as this is a sanctuary site where standard therapy does not penetrate. This usually consists of a combination of cranial irradiation, intrathecal chemotherapy and high-dose methotrexate which crosses the blood–brain barrier.

The detail of the schedules for these treatments will be found in specialist texts. The drugs most commonly employed for the two main varieties of acute leukaemia are given in Box 24.39. Generally, if a patient fails to go into remission with induction treatment, alternative drug combinations may be tried but the outlook is poor unless remission can be achieved. Disease which relapses during treatment or soon after the end of treatment carries a poor prognosis and is difficult to treat. The longer after the end of treatment that relapse occurs, the more likely it is that further treatment will be effective.

Supportive therapy

Aggressive and potentially curative therapy which involves periods of severe bone marrow failure would not be possible

periods of marrow hypoplasia. In poor prognosis leukaemia this may include a stem cell transplant.

- *Remission maintenance.* If the patient is still in remission after the consolidation phase for acute lymphoblastic leukaemia, a period of maintenance therapy is given, consisting of a repeating cycle of drug administration. This may extend for up to 3 years if relapse does not occur and is usually given on an outpatient basis.

24

24.39 DRUGS COMMONLY USED IN THE TREATMENT OF ACUTE LEUKAEMIA		
Phase	**ALL**	**AML**
Induction	Vincristine (i.v.) Prednisolone (oral) L-asparaginase (i.m.) Daunorubicin (i.v.) Methotrexate (intrathecal)	Daunorubicin (i.v.) Cytarabine (i.v.) Etoposide (i.v. and oral)
Consolidation	Daunorubicin (i.v.) Cytarabine (i.v.) Etoposide (i.v.) Methotrexate (i.v.)	Cytarabine (i.v.) Amsacrine (i.v.) Mitoxantrone (i.v.)
Maintenance	Prednisolone (oral) Vincristine (i.v.) Mercaptopurine (oral) Methotrexate (oral)	

24

without adequate and skilled supportive care. The following problems commonly arise.

Anaemia. Anaemia is treated with red cell concentrate infusions to maintain a haemoglobin above 100 g/l.

Bleeding. Thrombocytopenic bleeding requires platelet transfusions unless the bleeding is trivial. Prophylactic platelet transfusion should be given to maintain the platelet count above 10×10^9/l. Coagulation abnormalities occur and need accurate diagnosis and treatment as appropriate, usually with fresh frozen plasma.

Infection. Fever (> 38°C) lasting over 1 hour in a neutropenic patient (absolute neutrophil count $< 1.0 \times 10^9$/l) indicates possible septicaemia. Parenteral broad-spectrum antibiotic therapy is essential. Empirical therapy is given with a combination of an aminoglycoside (e.g. gentamicin) and a broad-spectrum penicillin (e.g. piperacillin/tazobactam). This combination is synergistic and bactericidal and should be continued for at least 3 days after the fever has resolved. The organisms most commonly associated with severe neutropenia are Gram-positive bacteria such as *Staphylococcus aureus* and *Staph. epidermidis* which are present on the skin and gain entry via cannulae and central lines. Gram-negative infections often originate from the gastrointestinal tract, which is affected by chemotherapy-induced mucositis; organisms such as *Escherichia coli*, *Pseudomonas* and *Klebsiella* are more likely to cause rapid clinical deterioration and must be covered with the initial empirical therapy. Gram-positive infection may require vancomycin therapy.

Patients with lymphoblastic leukaemia are susceptible to infection with *Pneumocystis carinii* (now *jirovecii*, p. 389), which causes a severe pneumonia. Prophylaxis with co-trimoxazole is given during chemotherapy. Diagnosis may be difficult and may require either bronchoalveolar lavage or open lung biopsy. Treatment is with high-dose co-trimoxazole, initially intravenously, with change to oral treatment as soon as possible.

Oral and pharyngeal monilial infection is common. Fluconazole is effective for the treatment of established local infection. Prophylaxis against systemic fungal infections with either fluconazole or itraconazole is usual practice during intensive chemotherapy.

For systemic fungal infection with *Candida* or aspergillosis, intravenous amphotericin is required for at least 3 weeks, but is nephrotoxic and hepatotoxic. Renal and hepatic function should therefore be monitored closely, particularly if the patient is receiving antibiotics which are also nephrotoxic. Potassium supplementation is usually required. For patients who experience nephrotoxicity with standard amphotericin, or who require high-dose therapy for aspergillosis, lipid formulations of amphotericin can be administered without further renal deterioration. New antifungal agents such as caspofungin and voriconazole are now available in addition for treatment of fungal infection (p. 154).

Herpes simplex infection (p. 303) occurs frequently round the lips and nose during ablative therapy for acute leukaemia and is treated with aciclovir. This may also be prescribed prophylactically to patients with a history of cold sores or elevated titres to herpes simplex. Herpes zoster manifesting as chicken pox or, after reactivation, as shingles (p. 305) should be treated in the early stage with high-dose aciclovir as this can be fatal in immunocompromised patients.

The value of isolation facilities, such as laminar flow rooms, is debatable but may contribute to staff awareness of careful reverse barrier nursing practice. The isolation is often psychologically stressful for the patient.

Metabolic problems. Continuous monitoring of renal, hepatic and haemostatic function is necessary, together with fluid balance monitoring. Patients are often severely anorexic as a consequence of the side-effects of therapy; they may find drinking difficult and hence require intravenous fluids and electrolytes. Renal toxicity occurs with some antibiotics (e.g. aminoglycosides) and antifungal agents (amphotericin). Cellular breakdown during induction therapy increases uric acid production, which may cause renal failure. Allopurinol and intravenous hydration are given to try to prevent this, along with close monitoring of biochemistry. Occasionally dialysis may be required.

Psychological support. This is a key aspect of care. Patients should be kept informed, and their questions answered and fears allayed as far as possible. An optimistic attitude from the staff is vital. Delusions, hallucinations and paranoia are not uncommon during periods of severe bone marrow failure and septicaemic episodes, and should be met with patience and understanding.

Alternative chemotherapy. Gentle chemotherapy not designed to achieve remission may be used to curb excessive leucocyte proliferation. Drugs used for this purpose include hydroxycarbamide and mercaptopurine. The aim is to reduce the leucocyte count without inducing bone marrow failure.

Prognosis

Without treatment the median survival of patients with acute leukaemia is about 5 weeks. This may be extended to a number of months with supportive treatment. Patients who achieve remission with specific therapy have a better outlook. Around 80% of adult patients under 60 years of age with ALL or AML achive remission. Remission rates are lower for older patients. However, the relapse rate continues

24.40 OUTCOME IN ADULT ACUTE LEUKAEMIA		
Disease/risk	Risk factors	5-year overall survival
AML		
Good risk	Promyelocytic leukaemia: t(15;17) t(8;21) inv 16 or t(16;16)	76%
Poor risk	Cytogenetic abnormalities −5,−7,del 5q, abn(3q), complex (≥ 5)	21%
Intermediate risk	AML with none of the above	48%
ALL		
Poor risk	Philadelphia chromosome High white count > 100×10^9/l Abnormalities short arm of chromosome 11 t(1;19)	20%
Standard	ALL with none of the above	37%

to be high. Box 24.40 shows the survival in ALL and AML and the influence of prognostic features.

National and international studies have led to steady improvement in survival from leukaemia. Advances include the introduction of drugs such as ATRA (all transretinoic acid) in acute promyelocytic leukaemia; which has greatly reduced induction deaths from bleeding in this good-risk leukaemia. Current trials aim to improve survival, especially in standard and poor-risk disease, and also investigate the place of transplantation.

Bone marrow and peripheral blood stem cell transplantation

Traditionally, blood and marrow transplantation (BMT) has offered the only hope of 'cure' in a variety of haematological disorders. As standard treatment improves, the indications for BMT are being refined (Box 24.41). The type of transplant is defined according to donor and source of stem cell. In allogeneic BMT the stem cells come either from a related (usually an HLA-identical sibling) donor or from a closely HLA-matched volunteer unrelated donor (VUD). In an autologous transplant the stem cells are harvested from the patient and stored in the vapour phase of liquid nitrogen until required. Stem cells can be harvested from the bone marrow or from the blood.

Allogeneic BMT

Healthy marrow or blood stem cells from a donor are infused intravenously into the recipient who has been suitably 'conditioned'. The conditioning treatment (chemotherapy with or without radiotherapy) destroys malignant cells and immunosuppresses the recipient as well as ablating the recipient's haematopoietic tissues. The injected donor cells 'home' to the marrow, engraft and produce enough erythrocytes, granulocytes and platelets for the patient's needs after about 3–4 weeks. During this period of aplasia patients are at risk of infection and bleeding, and require intensive supportive care as described above. It may take

24.41 GENERAL INDICATIONS FOR ALLOGENEIC BONE MARROW TRANSPLANTATION
• Neoplastic disorders affecting the totipotent or pluripotent stem cell compartment (e.g. leukaemias)
• Those with a failure of haematopoiesis (e.g. aplastic anaemia)
• A major inherited defect in blood cell production (e.g. thalassaemia, immunodeficiency diseases)
• Inborn errors of metabolism with missing enzymes or cell lines

24.42 HAEMATOLOGICAL INDICATIONS FOR STEM CELL TRANSPLANTATION	
Allogeneic transplant	
• AML high-risk CR1, CR2	• Severe aplastic anaemia
• Adult ALL CR1, CR2	• Myelofibrosis
• CML chronic phase	• Severe immune deficiency
• Myelodysplastic syndrome	syndromes
Autologous transplant	
• AML CR2	• Mantle cell lymphoma
• Myeloma	• Poor-risk Hodgkin's lymphoma
• High-grade non-Hodgkin lymphoma second response	

24.43 COMPLICATIONS OF ALLOGENEIC BONE MARROW TRANSPLANTATION
• Mucositis   • Chronic graft-versus-host disease
• Infection   • Infertility
• Bleeding   • Acute graft-versus-host disease
• Cataract formation   • Secondary malignant disease
• Pneumonitis

several years to regain normal immunological function and patents remain at risk from opportunistic infections, in particular in the first year. An advantage of receiving donor stem cells is that the donor's immunological system can recognise residual malignant recipient cells and destroy them. This immunological 'graft versus disease' effect is a powerful tool against many haematological tumours and can be boosted in post-transplantation relapse by the infusion of T cells taken from the donor, so-called donor lymphocyte infusion (DLI).

The general indications for allogeneic transplantation are shown in Box 24.41 and specific haematological indications in Box 24.42. There is considerable morbidity and mortality associated with BMT. The best results are obtained in patients with minimal residual disease, and in those under 20 years of age who have an HLA-identical sibling donor. Older patients are routinely transplanted, but results become progressively worse with age and an upper age limit of 55 years is usually applied. The main complications of allogeneic BMT are outlined in Box 24.43. The risks and outcomes of transplant depend upon several patient- and disease-related factors. In general 25% die from procedure-related complications such as graft-versus-host disease (below), and there remains a significant risk of disease relapse. The long-term survival for patients undergoing allogeneic BMT in acute leukaemia is around 50%.

24

Graft-versus-host disease (GVHD)

GVHD is due to the cytotoxic activity of donor T lymphocytes which become sensitised to their new host, regarding it as foreign. This may cause either an acute or a chronic form of GVHD.

Acute GVHD. This occurs in the first 100 days after transplant in about one-third of patients. It can affect the skin causing rashes, the liver causing jaundice and the gut causing diarrhoea, and may vary from mild to lethal. Prevention includes HLA-matching of the donor, immunosuppressant drugs including methotrexate and ciclosporin, and antithymocyte globulin. The more severe forms prove very difficult to control and, despite high-dose corticosteroids, may result in death.

Chronic GVHD. This may follow acute GVHD or arise independently; it occurs later than acute GVHD. It often resembles a connective tissue disorder, although in mild cases a rash may be the only manifestation. Chronic GVHD is usually treated with corticosteroids and prolonged immunosuppression with, for example, ciclosporin. Associated with chronic GVHD is the graft-versus-leukaemia effect, which results in a lower relapse rate.

Infection

Infection is the other major problem encountered during recovery from BMT. Details are given in Box 24.44.

Reduced-intensity BMT

This concept has been developed in an attempt to reduce the mortality of allografting. Rather than use very intensive conditioning which causes morbidity from organ damage, relatively low doses of drugs such as fludarabine and cyclophosphamide are used simply to immunosuppress the recipient and allow donor stem cells to engraft. The emerging donor immune system then eliminates the malignant cells via the 'graft versus disease' effect, which may be boosted by the elective use of donor T-cell infusions post-transplant. This type of transplant is less toxic and allows BMT to be offered to an older group of patients. However, relapse and infections post-transplant remain a concern and the role of this type of transplant is still under investigation.

Autologous BMT

In this procedure the patient's own stem cells are first harvested and frozen. After conditioning therapy, the auto-

logous stem cells are reinfused in order to rescue the patient from the marrow damage and aplasia caused by the chemotherapy. Autologous BMT may be used for disorders which do not primarily involve the haematopoietic tissues, or in patients in whom very good remissions have been achieved. The preferred source of stem cells for autologous transplants is peripheral blood. These stem cells engraft more quickly, marrow recovery occurring within 2–3 weeks. There is no risk of GVHD and no immunosuppression is required. Thus autologous stem cell transplantation carries a lower procedure-related mortality rate than allogeneic BMT at around 5%, but there is a higher relapse rate. The issue of whether the stem cells should be treated (purged) in an attempt to remove any residual leukaemia cells is controversial.

CHRONIC MYELOID LEUKAEMIA (CML)

Chronic myeloid leukaemia is a myeloproliferative stem cell disorder resulting in proliferation of all haematopoietic lineages but manifesting predominantly in the granulocytic series. Maturation proceeds fairly normally. The disease occurs chiefly between the ages of 30 and 80 years, with a peak incidence at 55 years. It is rare, with an annual incidence in the UK of 1.8/100 000, and accounts for 20% of all leukaemias. The disease is found in all races. The aetiology is unknown.

Cytogenetic and molecular aspects

Approximately 95% of patients with CML have a chromosome abnormality known as the Philadelphia (Ph) chromosome. This is a shortened chromosome 22 and is the result of a reciprocal translocation of material with chromosome 9. The break on chromosome 22 occurs in the breakpoint cluster region (BCR). The fragment from chromosome 9 that joins the BCR carries the *abl* oncogene, which forms a chimeric gene with the remains of the BCR. This *BCR ABL* chimeric gene codes for a 210 kDa protein with tyrosine kinase activity, which plays a causative role in the disease, influencing cellular proliferation, differentiation and survival. In some apparently Ph chromosome-negative patients, the BCR ABL gene product is detectable by molecular techniques.

Natural history

The disease has three phases:

24.44 INFECTION DURING RECOVERY FROM BONE MARROW TRANSPLANTATION (BMT)		
Infection	**Time after BMT**	**Management**
Herpes simplex (p. 303)	0–4 weeks	Aciclovir
Bacterial, fungal	0–4 weeks	As for acute leukaemia (p. 1042)
Cytomegalovirus (p. 308)	7–21 weeks	If patient is CMV-negative, use CMV-negative blood products Hyperimmune immunoglobulin and ganciclovir for documented infections
Varicella zoster (p. 305)	After 13 weeks	Aciclovir i.v.
Pneumocystis jirovecii (p. 389)	8–26 weeks	Co-trimoxazole
Interstitial pneumonitis (non-infective)	6–18 weeks	No specific therapy Prednisolone may be tried

- *a chronic phase*, in which the disease is responsive to treatment and is easily controlled, typically lasting 3–5 years
- *an accelerated phase* (not always seen), in which disease control becomes more difficult
- *blast crisis*, in which the disease transforms into an acute leukaemia, either myeloid (70%) or lymphoblastic (30%), which is relatively refractory to treatment. Blast crisis occurs at a rate of 10% per year and is the cause of death in the majority of patients. Patient survival is therefore dictated by the timing of blast crisis, which cannot be predicted.

Patients who are Ph chromosome- and also BCR ABL-negative tend to be older, mostly male, with lower platelet counts and higher absolute monocyte counts, and respond poorly to treatment, with a median survival of less than 1 year.

Clinical features

The frequency of the more common symptoms at presentation is given in Box 24.45. About 25% of patients are asymptomatic at diagnosis. On examination the principal clinical finding is splenomegaly, which is present in 90% of patients. In about 10% the enlargement is massive, extending to over 15 cm below the costal margin. A friction rub may be heard in cases of splenic infarction. Hepatomegaly occurs in about 50% of patients. Lymphadenopathy is unusual.

Investigations

Examination of the blood usually shows a normocytic, normochromic anaemia. The mean haemoglobin is 105 g/l with a range of 70–150 g/l. The mean leucocyte count is 220×10^9/l with a range of 9.5–600. The mean platelet count is 445×10^9/l with a range of 162–2000. In the blood film the full range of granulocyte precursors from myeloblasts to mature neutrophils is seen but the predominant cells are neutrophils with a second peak at the myelocyte stage of maturation. Myeloblasts usually constitute less than 10% of all white cells. There is often an absolute increase in eosinophils and basophils, and nucleated red cells are common. If the disease progresses through an accelerated phase, the percentage of the more primitive cells increases. There is a dramatic increase in the number of circulating blasts as the disease enters blast transformation. In about one-third of patients very high platelet counts are seen during treatment, both in chronic and accelerated phases, but these usually drop dramatically at blast transformation. Basophilia tends to increase as the disease progresses.

The peripheral blood is useful diagnostically but bone marrow material should be obtained for chromosome analysis to demonstrate the presence of the Ph chromosome, and RNA analysis to demonstrate the presence of the BCR ABL gene product. Other characteristic findings on investigation include a very low neutrophil alkaline phosphatase score and very high vitamin B_{12} levels in the plasma. LDH levels are also elevated and the uric acid level may be high due to increased cell breakdown.

Management

Imatinib

This new agent specifically inhibits *BCR ABL* tyrosine kinase activity and reduces the uncontrolled proliferation of white cells. It is recommended as first-line therapy in chronic phase CML, producing complete cytogenetic response (disappearance of the Ph chromosome) in 76% at 18 months of therapy (Box 24.46). It is also recommended for those presenting in accelerated phase or blast crises and for those resistant to other therapies such as interferon.

The oral agent hydroxycarbamide was previously widely used for initial control of disease, and is still useful in this context or in palliative situations. It does not diminish the frequency of the Ph chromosome or affect the onset of blast cell transformation.

Alpha interferon was considered first-line treatment before imatinib was discovered. It is given alone or with the chemotherapy agent Ara-C, and can induce and maintain control of this disease in chronic phase in about 70% of patients. It causes reduction in the percentage of Ph-positive cells in about 20% of patients, and prolongs survival in those who achieve this. Interferon therapy causes 'flu-like' symptoms initially and although some of these may be controlled with paracetamol, others such as severe bone pain and severe weight loss are reasons for discontinuation.

Allogeneic or syngeneic bone marrow transplant from a matched sibling donor

In the imatinib era, the role of BMT in CML is less clear. It was previously considered the only cure for this disorder but long-term results with imatinib are awaited. A significant role for BMT remains in younger high-risk patients to effect a cure. The best results are obtained in patients in early chronic phase when about 80% can expect probable cure. Monitoring for relapse by detecting the presence of the *BCR ABL* protein and the use of donor T-cell infusion in such cases has proven very effective at returning patients to

24.45 SYMPTOMS AT PRESENTATION OF CHRONIC MYELOID LEUKAEMIA	
Symptom	**Present (%)**
Tiredness	37
Weight loss	26
Breathlessness	21
Abdominal pain and discomfort	21
Lethargy	13
Anorexia	12
Sweating	11
Abdominal fullness	10
Bruising	7
Vague ill health	7

24.46 IMATINIB AND CHRONIC MYELOID LEUKAEMIA | EBM

'As first-line therapy in CML, imatinib is better tolerated and induces a cytogenetic response in ~87% of cases at 18 months, compared with ~ 35% response to interferon + cytarabine.'

- O'Brien SG for the IRIS Investigators. N Engl J Med 2003; 348:994–1004.

24

durable complete remission. The results of transplantation in accelerated and blast transformation phases are significantly worse. Studies are under way to investigate the role of imatinib in transplantation for CML.

Treatment of the accelerated phase and blast crisis

This is more difficult. In accelerated phase, imatinib is indicated if the patient has not received it; hydroxycarbamide can be an effective single agent; and low-dose cytarabine can also be tried. When blast transformation occurs, the type of blast cell should be ascertained by cytochemical and immunological techniques. Response to appropriate treatment (Box 24.39, p. 1042) is better if lymphoblastic than if myeloblastic. Response to treatment for the latter is very poor. There is a strong case for supportive therapy only, particularly in older patients.

CHRONIC LYMPHOCYTIC LEUKAEMIA (CLL)

This is the most common variety of leukaemia, accounting for 30% of cases. The male to female ratio is 2:1 and the median age at presentation is between 65 and 70 years. In this disease B lymphocytes, which would normally respond to antigens by transformation and antibody formation, fail to do so. An ever-increasing mass of immuno-incompetent cells accumulate, to the detriment of immune function and normal bone marrow haematopoiesis.

Clinical features

The onset is very insidious. Indeed, in around 70% of patients the diagnosis is made incidentally on a routine full blood count. Presenting problems may be anaemia, infections, painless lymphadenopathy and systemic symptoms such as night sweats or weight loss. However, these more often occur later in the progress of the disease.

Investigations

The diagnosis is based on the peripheral blood findings of a mature lymphocytosis ($> 5 \times 10^9$/l) with characteristic morphology and cell surface markers. Immunophenotyping reveals the lymphocytes to be monoclonal B cells expressing the B-cell antigens CD19 and CD23 with either kappa or lambda immunoglobulin light chains and, characteristically, a T-cell antigen, CD5.

Other useful investigations in CLL include a reticulocyte count and a direct Coombs test as autoimmune haemolytic anaemia may occur (p. 1033). Serum immunoglobulin levels should be estimated to establish the degree of immunosuppression, which is common and progressive. Bone marrow examination by aspirate and trephine is not essential for the diagnosis of CLL, but may be helpful in difficult cases, for prognosis (patients with diffuse marrow involvement tend to do worse) and to monitor response to therapy. The main prognostic factor is stage of disease (Box 24.47); however, newer markers such as CD38 expression, mutations of IgVH genes, and cytogenetic abnormalities of chromosome 11 or 17 may also suggest a poorer prognosis.

Management

No specific treatment is required for most clinical stage A patients unless progression occurs. Life expectancy is

24.47 STAGING OF CHRONIC LYMPHOCYTIC LEUKAEMIA

Clinical stage A (60% patients)

- No anaemia or thrombocytopenia and less than three areas of lymphoid enlargement

Clinical stage B (30% patients)

- No anaemia or thrombocytopenia, with three or more involved areas of lymphoid enlargement

Clinical stage C (10% patients)

- Anaemia and/or thrombocytopenia, regardless of the number of areas of lymphoid enlargement

usually normal in older patients. The patient should be offered clear information about CLL, and reassured about the 'benign' nature of the disease, as the diagnosis of leukaemia inevitably causes anxiety.

Treatment is only required if there is evidence of bone marrow failure, massive or progressive lymphadenopathy or splenomegaly, systemic symptoms such as weight loss or night sweats, a rapidly increasing lymphocyte count or autoimmune cytopenias. Initial therapy for those requiring treatment (stages B and C) usually consists of oral chemotherapy with the alkylating agent chlorambucil. This will reduce the abnormal lymphocyte mass and produce symptomatic improvement in most patients. The median survival is 5–6 years. The purine analogue fludarabine is also useful, although it may lead to an increased risk of infection. Bone marrow failure or autoimmune cytopenias may respond to corticosteroid treatment.

Supportive care is increasingly required in progressive disease, e.g. transfusions for symptomatic anaemia or thrombocytopenia, prompt treatment of infections and for some patients with hypogammaglobulinaemia, immunoglobulin replacement. Radiotherapy may be used for lymph nodes causing discomfort or local obstruction, and for symptomatic splenomegaly. Splenectomy may be required to improve low blood counts due to autoimmune destruction or to hypersplenism, and can relieve massive splenomegaly.

Prognosis

The overall median survival for patients with CLL is about 6 years. The majority of clinical stage A patients have a normal life expectancy but stage C patients have a median survival of between 2 and 3 years. Approximately 50% of patients die of infection and 30% of causes unrelated to CLL. Unlike CML, CLL rarely transforms to an aggressive high-grade lymphoma, called Richter's transformation.

PROLYMPHOCYTIC LEUKAEMIA

This is a variant of chronic lymphatic leukaemia found mainly in males over the age of 60; 25% of cases are of the T-cell variety. There is massive splenomegaly with little lymphadenopathy and a very high leucocyte count, often in excess of 400×10^9/l; the characteristic cell is a large lymphocyte with a prominent nucleolus. Treatment is

24.48 HAEMATOLOGICAL MALIGNANCY IN OLD AGE

- **Median age:** approximately 70 years for most haematological malignancies.
- **Poor-risk biological features:** adverse cytogenetics or the presence of a multidrug resistance phenotype are more frequent.
- **Prognosis:** increasing age is an independent, adverse variable in myeloma, acute leukaemia and aggressive lymphoma.
- **Chemotherapy:** may be less well tolerated. Older people are more likely to have antecedent cardiac, pulmonary or metabolic problems, tolerate systemic infection less well and metabolise cytotoxic drugs differently.
- **Cure rates:** similar to those in younger patients, in those who do tolerate treatment well.
- **Decision to treat:** should be based on the individual's biological status, the level of social support available, and the patient's wishes and those of the immediate family, but not on chronological age.

24.49 WHO CLASSIFICATION OF MYELODYSPLASTIC SYNDROMES

Disease	Bone marrow findings
Refractory anaemia (RA)	Blasts < 5% Erythroid dysplasia only
Refractory anaemia with sideroblasts (RARS)	Blasts < 5% Ringed sideroblasts > 15%
Refractory cytopenias with multilineage dysplasia (RCMD)	Blasts < 5% 2–3 lineage dysplasia
Refractory anaemia with excess blasts (RAEB)	Blasts 5–20% 2–3 lineage dysplasia
Myelodysplastic syndrome with 5q–	Myelodysplastic syndrome associated with a del (5q) cytogenetic abnormality Blasts < 5% Often normal or increased blood platelet count
Myelodysplastic syndrome unclassified	None of the above or inadequate material

generally unsuccessful and the prognosis very poor. Leuka-pharesis, splenectomy and chemotherapy may be tried.

HAIRY CELL LEUKAEMIA

This is a rare chronic lymphoproliferative B-cell disorder. The male to female ratio is 6:1 and the median age at diagnosis is 50. Presenting symptoms are those of general ill health and recurrent infections. Splenomegaly occurs in 90% but lymph node enlargement is unusual.

Severe neutropenia, monocytopenia and the characteristic hairy cells in the blood and bone marrow are typical. These cells usually type as B lymphocytes and also characteristically express CD25 and CD103. A useful test is the demonstration that the acid phosphatase staining reaction in the cells is resistant to the action of tartrate.

Over recent years a number of treatments have been shown to produce long-lasting remissions. Cladribine and deoxycoformycin are effective in producing long periods of disease control.

MYELODYSPLASTIC SYNDROME (MDS)

This syndrome consists of a group of clonal haematopoietic disorders which represent steps in the progression to the development of leukaemia. It affects predominantly older people (median age 69 years); the overall incidence is 4/100 000 rising to more than 30/100 000 in the over-70s. It is characterised by blood cytopenias and abnormal-looking (dysplastic) blood cells, including macrocytic red cells and hypogranular neutrophils with nuclear hyper- or hypo-segmentation. The marrow is hypercellular with dysplastic changes in all three cell lines. Inevitably it progresses to acute myeloid leukaemia, although the time to progression varies with the subtype of MDS, being slowest in refractory anaemia and most rapid in refractory anaemia with excess of blasts. The WHO classification of MDS is shown in Box 24.49.

Clinical features and diagnosis

The most common presentation is due to the consequences of bone marrow failure: symptoms of anaemia, recurrent infections or bleeding. The blood film shows cytopenias and the dysplastic features indicated above. A bone marrow aspiration should be performed, which is usually hyper-cellular with evidence of dysplasia. Blast cells may be increased but do not reach the 20% level which indicates acute leukaemia. Chromosome analysis frequently reveals abnormalities, particularly of chromosomes 5 or 7.

Management

For the majority of patients the disease is incurable and supportive care with red-cell and platelet transfusions to maintain quality of life is the mainstay of treatment. A trial of erythropoietin and granulocyte–colony stimulating factor (G–CSF) is recommended in some patients with early disease to improve haemoglobin and white cell counts. Allogeneic stem cell transplants may afford a cure in younger patients. Transplantation should be preceded by intensive chemotherapy in those with more advanced disease.

Prognosis

The survival in MDS can vary from years in patients with RA and RARS to months in those with RAEB, who rapidly transform to acute myeloid leukaemia. Poor prognostic factors include blasts > 10% in the marrow, certain cyto-genetic abnormalities and more than one cytopenia in the blood.

LYMPHOMAS

These neoplasms arise from lymphoid tissues, and are diagnosed from the pathological findings on biopsy as Hodgkin or non-Hodgkin lymphoma. The majority are of B-cell origin. Non-Hodgkin lymphomas are classified as low- or high-grade tumours on the basis of their proliferation rate. High-grade tumours are dividing rapidly, have only been present for a matter of weeks before diagnosis and may be life-threatening. Low-grade tumours are dividing slowly,

24

may have been present for many months before diagnosis and behave in an indolent fashion.

HODGKIN LYMPHOMA (Box 24.50)

The histological hallmark of Hodgkin lymphoma (HL) is the presence of Reed–Sternberg cells, which are large malignant lymphoid cells of B-cell origin (Fig. 24.30). They are often only present in small numbers but are surrounded by large numbers of reactive normal T cells, plasma cells and eosinophils. The WHO classification is based on histology and is shown in Box 24.51. Nodular lymphocyte-predominant HL is slow-growing, localised and rarely fatal. Classical HL is divided into four histological subtypes from the appearance of the Reed–Sternberg cells and surrounding reactive cells. The nodular sclerosing type accounts for the initial peak in young patients and is more common in women. Mixed cellularity is more common in the elderly peak. Lymphocyte-rich HL usually presents in men. Lymphocyte-depleted HL is rare and probably represents large cell or anaplastic non-Hodgkin lymphoma.

Clinical features

There is painless rubbery lymphadenopathy, usually in the neck or supraclavicular fossae; the lymph nodes may fluctuate in size. Young patients with nodular sclerosing disease may have large mediastinal masses which are surprisingly asymptomatic but may cause dry cough and some breathlessness. Isolated subdiaphragmatic nodes occur in less than 10% at diagnosis. Hepatosplenomegaly may be present but does not always indicate disease. Spread is contiguous from one node to the next and extranodal disease, such as bone, brain or skin involvement, is rare.

Investigations

Treatment of HL depends upon the stage at presentation; therefore investigations aim not only to diagnose lymphoma but also to determine the extent of disease (Box 24.52).

- *Full blood count* may be completely normal. A normochromic, normocytic anaemia may be present and, together with lymphopenia, is a bad prognostic factor. An eosinophilia or a neutrophilia may be present.
- *ESR* may be raised.
- *Renal function tests* are required to ensure function is normal prior to treatment.
- *Liver function* may be abnormal in the absence of disease or reflect hepatic infiltration. An obstructive pattern may be caused by nodes at the porta hepatis.
- *LDH measurements*, as raised levels are an adverse prognostic factor.

24.50 EPIDEMIOLOGY AND AETIOLOGY OF HODGKIN LYMPHOMA	
Incidence	
• Approximately 4 new cases/100 000 population/year	
Sex ratio	
• Slight male excess (1.5:1)	
Age	
• Median age 31 years; first peak at 20–35 years and second at 50–70 years	
Aetiology	
• Unknown. More common in patients from well-educated backgrounds and small families. Three times more likely with a past history of infectious mononucleosis but no causal link to Epstein–Barr virus infection proven	

24

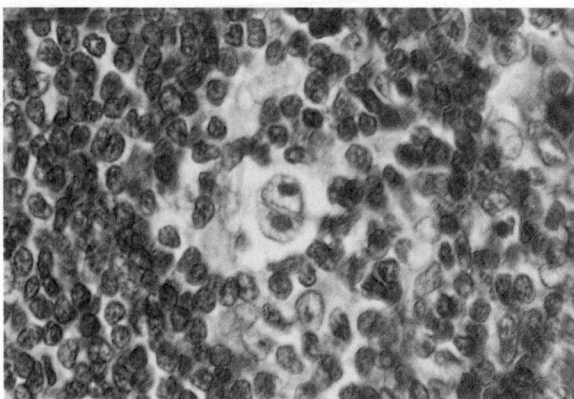

Fig. 24.30 Hodgkin lymphoma showing typical Reed–Sternberg cell.

24.51 WHO PATHOLOGICAL CLASSIFICATION AND INCIDENCE OF HODGKIN LYMPHOMA (HL)		
Type	**Histology**	**Incidence**
Nodular lymphocyte-predominant HL		5%
Classical HL	Nodular sclerosing	70%
	Mixed cellularity	20%
	Lymphocyte-rich	5%
	Lymphocyte-depleted	Rare

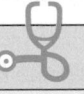

24.52 CLINICAL STAGES OF HODGKIN LYMPHOMA (ANN ARBOR CLASSIFICATION)	
Stage	**Definition**
I	Involvement of a single lymph node region (I) or extralymphatic site (IA$_E$)
II	Involvement of two or more lymph node regions (II) or an extralymphatic site and lymph node regions on the same side of (above or below) the diaphragm (II$_E$)
III	Involvement of lymph node regions on both sides of the diaphragm with (III$_E$) or without (III) localised extralymphatic involvement or involvement of the spleen (III$_S$) or both (III$_{SE}$)
IV	Diffuse involvement of one or more extralymphatic tissues, e.g. liver or bone marrow
A	No systemic symptoms
B	Weight loss, drenching sweats
The lymphatic structures are defined as the lymph nodes, spleen, thymus, Waldeyer's ring, appendix and Peyer's patches.	

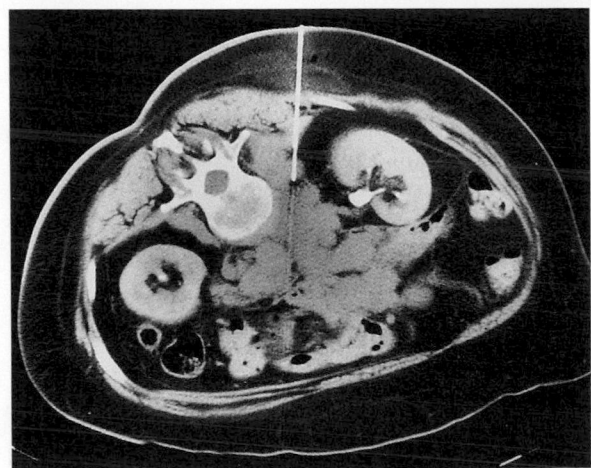

Fig. 24.31 CT-guided percutaneous needle biopsy of retroperitoneal nodes involved by lymphoma.

- *Chest X-ray* may show a mediastinal mass.
- *CT scan* of chest and abdomen to permit staging. Bulky disease (greater than 10 cm in a single node mass) is an adverse prognostic feature.
- *Lymph node biopsy* may be undertaken surgically or by percutaneous needle biopsy under radiological guidance (Fig. 24.31).

Management

Treatment options include radiotherapy, chemotherapy or a combination of the two (Box 24.53).

Radiotherapy

Good results are obtained in localised stage IA or stage IIA disease with no adverse prognostic features. Careful planning is required to limit the doses delivered to normal tissues. Fertility is usually preserved after radiotherapy. Women receiving breast irradiation during the treatment of chest disease have an increased risk of breast cancer and should be placed on a screening programme. Patients continuing to smoke after lung irradiation are at particular risk of lung cancer.

Chemotherapy

All other patients are treated initially with chemotherapy. The regimen in Box 24.54 is widely used in the UK. Over

24.53 THERAPEUTIC GUIDELINES FOR HODGKIN LYMPHOMA	

Indications for radiotherapy

- Stage I disease
- Stage IIA disease with three or fewer areas involved
- After chemotherapy to sites where there was originally bulk disease
- To lesions causing serious pressure problems

Indications for chemotherapy

- All patients with B symptoms
- Stage II disease with more than three areas involved
- Stages III and IV disease

24.54 THE ChIVPP REGIMEN FOR HODGKIN LYMPHOMA

Drug	Dose
Chlorambucil	6 mg/m² (up to 10 mg total) days 1–14 orally
Vinblastine	6 mg/m² (up to 10 mg total) days 1 and 8 i.v.
Procarbazine	100 mg/m² days 1–14 orally
Prednisolone	40 mg/m² days 1–14 orally

80% of patients will respond to this combination therapy, with drugs delivered on an outpatient basis every 3–4 weeks for a total of 6–8 cycles. Treatment response is assessed clinically and by repeat CT.

This type of chemotherapy carries a high risk of inducing permanent infertility in men; adequate counselling and sperm storage must be offered at diagnosis. The risk of infertility is lower for women but advice about obtaining ovarian tissue before starting treatment should be given as appropriate. Premature menopause may result from treatment and hormone replacement therapy should be discussed with the patient. Corticosteroids can cause avascular necrosis of bone, particularly the femoral head. Myelodysplasia and acute leukaemia can occur 5–10 years after alkylating therapy but the incidence is less than 5%.

Combined modality therapy

Radiotherapy may be given to the original sites of bulky disease after treatment by chemotherapy to reduce the risk of relapse. This form of treatment carries the greatest risk of long-term complications.

Prognosis

Over 90% of patients with stage IA disease are cured by radiotherapy alone. Patients with stage IIA disease have a reduced cure rate from radiotherapy. Approximately 70% of patients treated with chemotherapy are cured. The 15% of patients who fail to respond to initial chemotherapy have a poor prognosis but some may achieve long-term survival after high-dose chemotherapy and autologous stem cell rescue. Patients relapsing after local radiotherapy have a good cure rate after subsequent chemotherapy but with an increased risk of long-term toxicity. Those relapsing within a year of initial chemotherapy have a good salvage rate with high-dose therapy and autologous stem cell rescue. Patients relapsing after 1 year may obtain long-term survival with further chemotherapy.

NON-HODGKIN LYMPHOMA (Box 24.55)

Non-Hodgkin lymphoma (NHL) represents a monoclonal proliferation of lymphoid cells and may be of B-cell (70%) or T-cell (30%) origin. The incidence of these tumours increases with age, to 62.8/million population per year at age 75, and the overall rate is increasing at about 3% per year.

The difficulties of establishing a reproducible and clinically useful histological classification of NHL are reflected in the large number of classification systems to date. The current WHO classification stratifies according

24

24

24.55 EPIDEMIOLOGY AND AETIOLOGY OF NON-HODGKIN LYMPHOMA
Incidence
• 12 new cases/100 000 people/year
Sex ratio
• Slight male excess
Age
• Median age 65–70 years
Aetiology
• No single causative abnormality described
• Lymphoma is a late manifestation of HIV infection (p. 396)
• Specific lymphoma types are associated with EBV, human herpes virus 8 (HHV8) and HTLV infection
• The development of gastric lymphoma can be associated with *Helicobacter pylori* infection
• Some lymphomas are associated with specific chromosome lesions; the t(14:18) translocation in follicular lymphoma results in the dysregulated expression of the *BCL*-2 gene product which inhibits apoptotic cell death
• Lymphoma occurs in congenital immunodeficiency states and in immunosuppressed patients post-organ transplantation

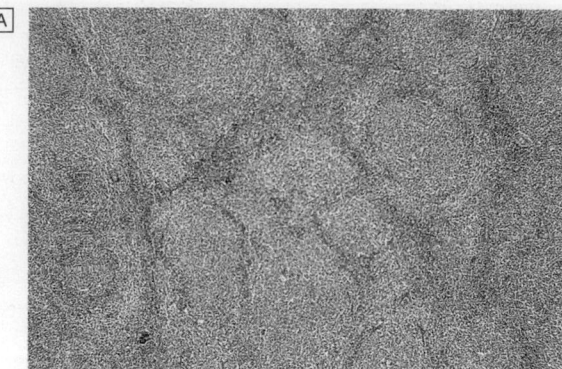

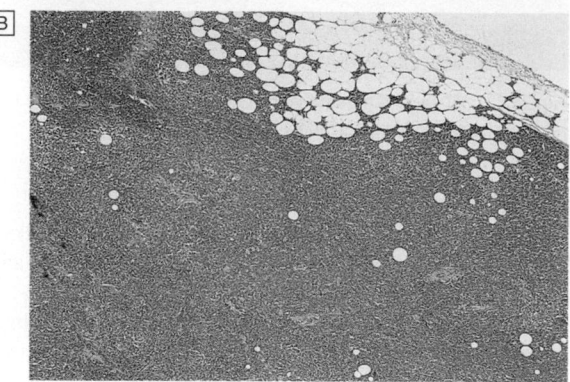

Fig. 24.32   Non-Hodgkin lymphoma. A (Low-grade) follicular or nodular pattern. B (High-grade) diffuse pattern of histology.

to cell lineage. Clinically, the most important factor is grade, which is a reflection of proliferation rate. High-grade NHL has high proliferation rates, rapidly produces symptoms, is fatal if untreated, but is potentially curable. Low-grade NHL has low proliferation rates, may be asymptomatic for many months before presentation, runs an indolent course, but is not curable by conventional therapy. Of all cases of NHL, 85% are either high-grade diffuse large-cell NHL or low-grade follicular NHL (Fig. 24.32). Other forms of NHL, including mantle cell lymphoma and malt lymphomas, are less common.

Clinical features

Compared to Hodgkin lymphoma, NHL is often widely disseminated at presentation. Patients present with lymph node enlargement which may be associated with systemic upset: weight loss, sweats, fever and itching. Hepatospleno-megaly may be present. Extranodal disease is more common in NHL, with involvement of the bone marrow, gut, thyroid, lung, skin, testis, brain and, more rarely, bone. Extranodal disease is more common in T-cell disease, whilst bone marrow involvement is more common in low-grade (50–60%) than high-grade (10%) disease. The same staging system (Box 24.52) is used for both HL and NHL but NHL is more likely to be stage III or IV at presentation. Compression syndromes may occur; gut obstruction, ascites, superior vena caval obstruction and spinal cord compression may all be presenting features.

Investigations

These are as for HL but in addition the following should be performed:

• *Routine bone marrow aspiration and trephine.*
• *Immunophenotyping of surface antigens to distinguish T- and B-cell tumours.* This may be done on blood, marrow or nodal material.

• *Immunoglobulin determination.* Some lymphomas are associated with IgG or IgM paraproteins which serve as markers for treatment response.
• *Measurement of uric acid levels.* Some very aggressive high-grade NHLs are associated with very high urate levels, which can precipitate renal failure when treatment is started.
• *HIV testing.* This may be appropriate if risk factors are present (p. 379).

Management

Low-grade NHL

Asymptomatic patients may not require therapy. Indications for treatment include marked systemic symptoms, lymph-adenopathy causing discomfort or disfigurement, bone marrow failure or compression syndromes. The options are:

• *Radiotherapy.* This can be used for localised stage I disease, which is rare.
• *Chemotherapy.* This is the mainstay of therapy. Most patients will respond to oral therapy with chlorambucil, which is well tolerated. More intensive intravenous chemotherapy in younger patients produces better quality of life but no survival benefit. Neither therapy will cure patients.
• *Monoclonal antibody therapy.* Humanised monoclonal antibodies can be used to target surface antigens on tumour cells, and induce tumour cell apoptosis directly. The anti-CD20 antibody rituximab has been shown to induce durable clinical responses in up to 60% of

patients. At present in England and Wales it is only recommended as last-line therapy for stage III and IV follicular lymphoma. Synergistic effects are seen when treatment is combined with standard chemotherapy, and trials are under way to define its optimal usage.

- *Transplantation.* Studies of autologous stem cell transplantation are in progress. Such high-dose therapy improves disease-free survival but longer follow-up is awaited before conclusions can be made about cure.

High-grade NHL

Patients with high-grade NHL need treatment at initial presentation:

- *Chemotherapy.* The majority (> 90%) will need intravenous combination chemotherapy. The CHOP regimen (cyclophosphamide, doxorubicin, vincristine and prednisolone) remains the mainstay of therapy.
- *Radiotherapy.* A few stage I patients without bulky disease may be suitable for radiotherapy. Radiotherapy is indicated for a residual localised site of bulk disease after chemotherapy, and for spinal cord and other compression syndromes.
- *Monoclonal antibody therapy.* When combined with CHOP chemotherapy, rituximab (R) increases the complete response rates and improves overall survival. The combination of R-CHOP is currently recommended for those with stage II or greater diffuse large-cell lymphoma as first-line therapy.
- *Transplantation.* Autologous stem cell transplantation benefits patients with relapsed chemosensitive disease (Box 24.56).

24.56 AUTOLOGOUS BONE MARROW TRANSPLANTATION IN NON-HODGKIN LYMPHOMA **EBM**

'The addition of autologous bone marrow transplantation to conventional salvage chemotherapy improves survival from 32% to 54% in relapsed high-grade NHL..'

- Philip T, et al. N Engl J Med 1995; 333:1540–1545.

For further information: 🖥 www.lymphoma.org.uk

Prognosis

Low-grade NHL runs an indolent remitting and relapsing course, with an overall median survival of 10 years. Transformation to a higher-grade NHL is associated with poor survival.

In high-grade NHL, some 80% of patients overall respond initially to therapy but only 35% will have disease-free survival at 5 years. The prognosis for patients with NHL is further refined according to the international prognostic index (IPI). For high-grade NHL, 5-year survival ranges from 75% in those with low-risk scores (age < 60, stage I or II, one or fewer extranodal sites, normal LDH and good performance status) to 25% in those with high-risk scores (increasing age, advanced stage, concomitant disease and a raised LDH).

Relapse is associated with a poor response to further chemotherapy (< 10% 5-year survival), but in patients under 65 years, stem cell transplantation improves survival.

PARAPROTEINAEMIAS

A gammopathy refers to over-production of one or more classes of immunoglobulin. It may be polyclonal in association with acute or chronic inflammation such as infection, sarcoidosis, autoimmune disorders or some malignancies. Alternatively, a monoclonal increase in a single immunoglobulin class may occur in association with normal or reduced levels of the other immunoglobulins. Gammopathies are detected by plasma immunoelectrophoresis. Such monoclonal proteins, also called M-proteins, paraproteins or monoclonal gammopathies, occur as a feature of myeloma, lymphoma and amyloidosis, in connective tissue disease such as rheumatoid arthritis or polymyalgia rheumatica, in infection such as HIV and in solid tumours. In addition, they may be present with no underlying disease.

MONOCLONAL GAMMOPATHY OF UNCERTAIN SIGNIFICANCE (MGUS)

In this condition (also known as benign monoclonal gammopathy or monoclonal gammopathy unclassified (MGu)), a paraprotein is present in the blood but with no other features of myeloma, Waldenström macroglobulinaemia (see below), lymphoma or related disease. It is a common condition associated with increasing age; a paraprotein can be found in 1% aged over 50 years increasing to 5% over 80 years.

Clinical features and investigations

Patients are usually asymptomatic, and the paraprotein is found on blood testing for other reasons. The routine blood count and biochemistry are normal, the paraprotein is usually present in small amounts with no associated immune paresis, and there are no lytic bone lesions. The bone marrow may have increased plasma cells but these usually constitute less than 10% of nucleated cells.

Prognosis

After follow-up of 20 years, only one-quarter will progress to myeloma or a related disorder. There is no way of predicting progression in an individual patient and if investigations remain stable, annual monitoring is all that is required.

WALDENSTRÖM MACROGLOBULINAEMIA

This is a low-grade lymphoplasmacytoid lymphoma associated with an IgM paraprotein causing clinical features of hyperviscosity syndrome. It is a rare tumour occurring in the elderly and affects a slight excess of males.

Patients classically present with features of hyperviscosity such as nosebleeds, bruising, confusion and visual disturbance. However, presentation may be with anaemia, systemic symptoms, splenomegaly or lymphadenopathy. Patients are found on investigation to have an IgM paraprotein associated with a raised plasma viscosity. The bone marrow has a characteristic appearance, with infiltration of lymphoid cells and prominent mast cells.

24

Management

Severe hyperviscosity and anaemia may necessitate plasmapheresis to remove IgM and make blood transfusion possible. Treatment with oral agents such as chlorambucil is effective but rather slow and fludarabine may be more active in this disease. The median survival is 5 years.

MULTIPLE MYELOMA

This is a malignant proliferation of plasma cells. Normal plasma cells are derived from B cells and produce immunoglobulins which contain heavy and light chains. Normal immunoglobulins are polyclonal, which means that a variety of heavy chains are produced and each may be of kappa or lambda light chain type. In myeloma plasma cells produce immunoglobulin of a single heavy and light chain, a monoclonal protein commonly referred to as a paraprotein. In some cases only light chain is produced and this appears in the urine as Bence Jones proteinuria. The frequency of different paraprotein types in myeloma is shown in Box 24.57.

24.57 CLASSIFICATION OF MULTIPLE MYELOMA

Type of paraprotein	Relative frequency (%)
IgG	55
IgA	21
Light chain only	22
Others (D, E, non-secretory)	2

Pathology

Although a small number of malignant plasma cells are present in the circulation, the majority are present in the bone marrow. The malignant plasma cells produce cytokines, which stimulate osteoclasts and result in net bone absorption. The resulting lytic lesions cause bone pain, fractures and hypercalcaemia. Marrow involvement can result in anaemia or pancytopenia. The aetiology of this condition is unknown.

Clinical features

The incidence of myeloma is 4/100 000 new cases per annum, with a male:female ratio of 2:1. The median age of diagnosis is 60–70 years and the disease is more common in Afro-Caribbeans. The clinical features are demonstrated in Figure 24.33.

Investigations

The diagnosis of myeloma requires two of the following criteria:

- increased malignant plasma cells in the bone marrow
- serum and/or urinary paraprotein
- skeletal lesions.

Bone marrow aspiration, plasma and urinary electrophoresis, and a skeletal survey are thus required. Other investigations are listed in Box 24.58, and their interpretation in Box 24.59.

24.58 RATIONALE FOR INVESTIGATIONS IN MULTIPLE MYELOMA

Problem	Investigations
Presence of lytic lesions, bone fractures	X-rays (skeletal survey)
Spinal cord compression	MRI spine
Presence of urine or plasma paraprotein	Blood and urine protein electrophoresis
Type of paraprotein	Blood and urine immunoelectrophoresis
Amount of paraprotein	Quantification of paraprotein
Degree of immune paresis	Plasma immunoglobulins
Presence of plasma cells in bone marrow	Bone marrow aspiration and trephine
Degree of bone marrow failure	Full blood count
Renal function	Urea and electrolytes, creatinine, urate
Presence of hypercalcaemia	Blood calcium Albumin
Degree of haemostasis	Bleeding time Coagulation screen

24.59 POINTS TO NOTE IN THE DIAGNOSIS OF MYELOMA

- Plasma alkaline phosphatase and the bone scan are normal in the absence of fractures or bone repair
- Serum β_2-microglobulin estimations may provide a useful assessment of prognosis
- Normal immunoglobulin levels, i.e. absence of immune paresis, should cast doubt on the diagnosis
- Only about 5% of patients with an ESR persistently above 100 mm/hr have myeloma

Management

If patients are asymptomatic, treatment may not be required. Otherwise, treatment consists of the measures described below.

Immediate support

- High fluid intake to treat renal impairment and hypercalcaemia.
- Analgesia for bone pain.
- Bisphosphonates for hypercalcaemia and to delay other skeletal related events (p. 1124).
- Allopurinol to prevent urate nephropathy.
- Plasmapheresis, as necessary, for hyperviscosity.

Chemotherapy

In frail older patients, melphalan is an effective oral therapy, whilst in younger patients treatment with intravenous agents may improve response. Higher doses of intravenous melphalan appear to be well tolerated even in patients over 65 years and may produce better clinical responses.

Treatment is administered until paraprotein levels have stopped falling. This is termed 'plateau phase' and may last for weeks or years. Successive relapses respond less well to treatment.

24

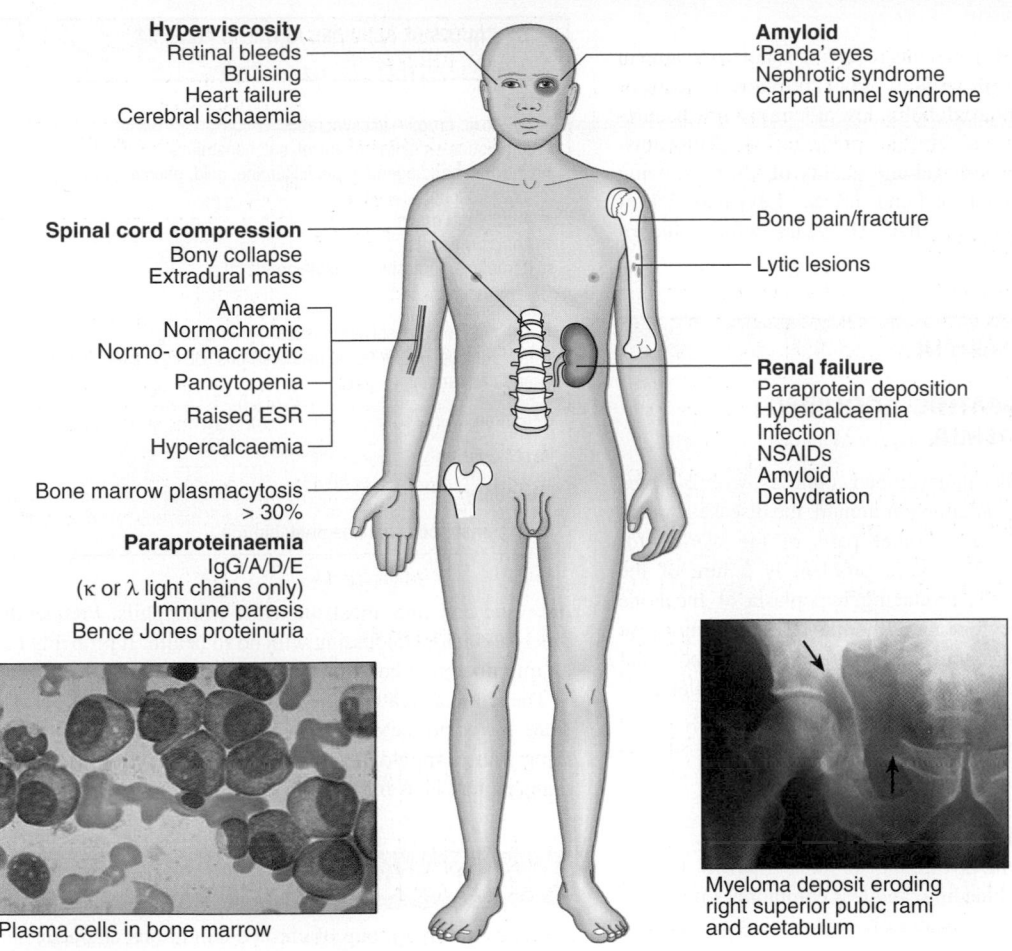

Hyperviscosity
Retinal bleeds
Bruising
Heart failure
Cerebral ischaemia

Amyloid
'Panda' eyes
Nephrotic syndrome
Carpal tunnel syndrome

Bone pain/fracture

Lytic lesions

Spinal cord compression
Bony collapse
Extradural mass

Anaemia
Normochromic
Normo- or macrocytic

Pancytopenia

Raised ESR

Hypercalcaemia

Bone marrow plasmacytosis
> 30%

Paraproteinaemia
IgG/A/D/E
(κ or λ light chains only)
Immune paresis
Bence Jones proteinuria

Renal failure
Paraprotein deposition
Hypercalcaemia
Infection
NSAIDs
Amyloid
Dehydration

Plasma cells in bone marrow

Myeloma deposit eroding
right superior pubic rami
and acetabulum

Fig. 24.33 Clinical manifestations of multiple myeloma.

Radiotherapy

This is effective for localised bone pain not responding to simple analgesia and for pathological fractures. It is also useful for the emergency treatment of spinal cord compression complicating extradural plasmacytomas.

Transplantation

Standard treatment does not cure myeloma. Autologous stem cell transplants improve quality of life and prolong survival (Box 24.60). All suitable patients under 65 years should be offered intravenous chemotherapy to maximum response and then an autologous stem cell transplant. Allogeneic bone marrow transplantation may cure some patients and should be considered in those under the age of 55 years with a sibling donor. Reduced-intensity allografting may improve outcomes by reducing transplant-related mortality and extending the upper age limit.

Bisphosphonates

Long-term bisphosphonate therapy reduces bone pain and skeletal events. These drugs protect bone and may cause apoptosis of malignant plasma cells.

Thalidomide

This drug has anti-angiogenic effects against tumour blood vessels and also immunomodulatory effects. At low doses it has been shown to be effective against refractory myeloma and when combined with dexamethasone, response rates over 50% are described. Trials are currently under way to investigate the use of thalidomide as an adjunct to other treatments earlier in the natural history of the disease. It can cause somnolence, constipation and a peripheral neuropathy. It is vital that females of child-bearing age use adequate contraception as it is teratogenic.

Other new agents include the proteasome inhibitor bortezomib which has also shown activity in advanced myeloma, and thalidomide derivatives which are currently being evaluated in clinical trials.

EBM

24.60 AUTOLOGOUS BONE MARROW TRANSPLANTATION IN MULTIPLE MYELOMA

'The addition of autologous bone marrow transplantation to conventional intravenous chemotherapy improves survival from 42 to 54 months.'

● Child JA, et al. N Engl J Med 2003; 348:1875–1883.

For further information: 💻 www.ukmf.org.uk

24

Prognosis

The median survival of patients receiving standard treatment is approximately 40 months. Poor prognostic features include a high β_2-microglobulin, low albumin, a low haemoglobin or a high calcium at presentation. Autotransplantation improves survival and quality of life by slowing the rate of progression of bone disease. Less than 5% of patients survive longer than 10 years with standard treatment.

APLASTIC ANAEMIA

PRIMARY IDIOPATHIC ACQUIRED APLASTIC ANAEMIA

This is a rare disorder in developed countries, with 2–4 new cases per million population per annum; the disease is much more common in certain other parts of the world—for example, east Asia. The basic problem is failure of the pluripotent stem cells, producing hypoplasia of the bone marrow with a pancytopenia in the blood. Usually no cause is found but careful enquiry should be made for potential causes such as exposure to drugs, chemicals and radiation, a history taken of viral illness, particularly hepatitis, and a search undertaken to exclude rare congenital causes such as Fanconi's anaemia.

Clinical features

Patients present with symptoms of bone marrow failure, usually anaemia or bleeding, and less commonly infections. A full blood count demonstrates pancytopenia, low reticulocytes and often macrocytosis. Bone marrow aspiration and trephine reveal hypocellularity.

Management

All patients will require blood product support and aggressive management of infection. The prognosis of severe aplastic anaemia managed with supportive therapy only is poor and more than 50% of patients die, usually in the first year. The curative treatment for patients under 30 years of age with severe idiopathic aplastic anaemia is allogeneic bone marrow transplantation if there is an available donor. Those with a compatible sibling donor should proceed to transplantation as soon as possible and have a 75–90% chance of long-term cure. In older patients, immunosuppressive therapy with ciclosporin and antithymocyte globulin gives 5-year survival rates of 75%. Such patients may relapse or evolve into other clonal disorders of haematopoiesis, such as paroxysmal nocturnal haemoglobinuria (PNH), MDS and even AML, and must be followed up long-term.

SECONDARY APLASIA

Causes of this condition are listed in Box 24.61. It is not practical to list all the drugs which have been suspected of causing aplasia. It is important to check the reported side-effects of all drugs taken over the preceding months. In some instances the cytopenia is more selective and affects

24.61 CAUSES OF ACQUIRED APLASTIC ANAEMIA

Drugs
- Cytotoxic drugs—idiosyncratic
- Antibiotics—chloramphenicol, sulphonamides
- Antirheumatic agents—penicillamine, gold, phenylbutazone, indometacin
- Antithyroid drugs
- Anticonvulsants
- Immunosuppressives—azathioprine

Chemicals
- Benzene toluene solvent misuse—glue-sniffing
- Insecticides—chlorinated hydrocarbons (DDT), organophosphates and carbamates (p. 216)

Radiation

Viral hepatitis

Pregnancy

Paroxysmal nocturnal haemoglobinuria

---

only one cell line, most often the neutrophils. Frequently, this is an incidental finding with no ill health. It probably has an immune basis but this is difficult to prove.

The clinical features and methods of diagnosis are the same as for primary idiopathic aplastic anaemia. An underlying cause should be treated or removed but otherwise management is as for the idiopathic form.

MYELOPROLIFERATIVE DISORDERS

These make up a group of chronic conditions characterised by clonal proliferation of marrow erythroid precursors (polycythaemia rubra vera, PRV), megakaryocytes (primary thrombocythaemia and myelofibrosis) or myeloid cells (chronic myeloid leukaemia). Although the majority of patients are classifiable as having one of these disorders, some have overlapping features. Furthermore, there is often progression from one to another, e.g. PRV to myelofibrosis.

CML is considered in detail above (p. 1044).

MYELOFIBROSIS

Myelofibrosis is characterised by bone marrow fibrosis, extramedullary haematopoiesis (blood cell formation outside the bone marrow) and a leucoerythroblastic blood picture. The marrow is initially hypercellular, with an excess of abnormal megakaryocytes which release growth factors, e.g. platelet-derived growth factor, to the marrow microenvironment, resulting in a reactive proliferation of fibroblasts. As the disease progresses, the marrow becomes fibrosed.

Most patients present over the age of 50 years with lassitude, weight loss and night sweats. The spleen can be massively enlarged due to extramedullary haematopoiesis, and painful splenic infarcts may occur.

The characteristic blood picture is a leucoerythroblastic anaemia, with circulating immature red blood cells (increased reticulocytes and nucleated red blood cells) and

24

granulocyte precursors (myelocytes). The red cells are shaped like teardrops (teardrop poikilocytes) and giant platelets may be seen in the blood. The white count varies from low to moderately high and the platelet count may be high, normal or low. Urate levels may be high due to increased cell breakdown, and folate deficiency is common. The marrow is often difficult to aspirate and a trephine biopsy shows an excess of megakaryocytes, increased reticulin and fibrous tissue replacement.

Median survival is 4 years from diagnosis but ranges from 1 year to over 20 years. Treatment is directed at control of symptoms, e.g. red cell transfusions for anaemia. Folic acid should be given to prevent deficiency. Cytotoxic therapy with hydroxycarbamide may help control spleen size, the white cell count or systemic symptoms. Splenectomy may be required for a grossly enlarged spleen or symptomatic pancytopenia secondary to splenic pooling of cells and hypersplenism. Bone marrow transplantation may be considered for younger patients.

PRIMARY THROMBOCYTHAEMIA

The malignant proliferation of megakaryocytes results in a raised level of circulating platelets that are often dysfunctional. Prior to making a diagnosis of essential thrombocythaemia it is essential to exclude reactive causes of increased platelets (p. 1017). Patients present at a median age of 60 years with vascular occlusion or bleeding events, or without symptoms and an isolated raised platelet count. In most individuals the condition is chronic, with the platelet count gradually increasing. A very small percentage may transform to acute leukaemia and others to myelofibrosis.

Low-risk patients (age less than 40 years, platelet count less than 1000×10^9/l and no bleeding or thrombosis) may require no treatment to reduce the platelet count. Aspirin therapy is often recommended. For those with a platelet count over 1000×10^9/l or those with symptoms, treatment to control platelets should be given. Agents include oral hydroxycarbamide or anagrelide, an inhibitor of mega-karyocyte maturation. Intravenous radioactive phosphorus (^{32}P) may be useful in old age. Aspirin should be considered for all patients to reduce the risk of thrombosis and is particularly useful therapy for those with digital ischaemia.

POLYCYTHAEMIA RUBRA VERA (PRV)

PRV occurs mainly in patients over the age of 40 years and presents either as an incidental finding of a high haemoglobin, or with symptoms of hyperviscosity such as lassitude, loss of concentration, headaches, dizziness, black-outs, pruritus and epistaxis. Some present with manifestations of peripheral arterial disease or a cerebrovascular accident. Patients are often plethoric and the majority have a palpable spleen at diagnosis. Thrombotic complications may occur and peptic ulceration is common, sometimes complicated by bleeding.

The diagnosis of polycythaemia is discussed on page 1014. It requires a raised red cell mass, the absence of causes of secondary erythrocytosis, and splenomegaly. The neutrophil and platelet counts are frequently raised, an abnormal karyotype may be found in the marrow, and in vitro culture of the marrow demonstrates autonomous growth in the absence of added growth factors.

Venesection gives prompt relief of hyperviscosity symptoms. Between 400 and 500 ml of blood (less if the patient is elderly) are removed and the venesection is repeated every 5–7 days until the haematocrit is reduced to below 45%. Less frequent but regular venesection will maintain this level until the haemoglobin remains reduced because of iron deficiency. The underlying myeloprolifera-tion can be suppressed by hydroxycarbamide or interferon. Radioactive phosphorus (5 mCi of ^{32}P i.v.) is reserved for older patients, as it increases the risk of transformation to acute leukaemia by six- to ten-fold. Treatment of marrow proliferation may reduce the risk of vascular occlusion, control spleen size and reduce transformation to myelo-fibrosis. Aspirin reduces the risk of thrombosis.

Median survival after diagnosis in treated patients exceeds 10 years. Some patients survive more than 20 years; however, cerebrovascular or coronary events occur in up to 60% of patients. The disease may convert to another myeloproliferative disorder, with about 15% developing myelofibrosis. Acute leukaemia develops principally in those patients who have been treated with radioactive phosphorus.

BLEEDING DISORDERS

DISORDERS OF PRIMARY HAEMOSTASIS

Platelet functional disorders, thrombocytopenia and von Willebrand disease, and diseases affecting the vessel wall, may all result in failure of the initial platelet plug formation in primary haemostasis. The causes of non-thrombocytopenic purpura are listed in Box 24.62.

24.62 CAUSES OF NON-THROMBOCYTOPENIC PURPURA

- Senile purpura
- Factitious purpura
- Henoch–Schönlein purpura (pp. 500 and 1141)
- Vasculitis (p. 1138)
- Paraproteinaemias
- Purpura fulminans

VESSEL WALL ABNORMALITIES

Vessel wall abnormalities may be congenital, such as heredi-tary haemophilia telangiectasis, or acquired as in a vasculitis.

Hereditary haemorrhagic telangiectasia

Hereditary haemorrhagic telangiectasia (HHT) is a dominantly inherited condition caused by mutations in the endothelial cell genes coding for endoglin and activator receptor-like kinase which are receptors for the transforming growth factor-beta (TGF-β), a potent angiogenic cytokine concerned with vascular modelling. Telangiectasia and small aneurysms are found on the fingertips, on the face, in the nasal passages, on the tongue, in the lung and in the gastrointestinal tract. A significant proportion of these patients develop larger pulmonary arteriovenous malformations (PAVMs) that cause arterial hypoxaemia due to a right-to-left shunt. These predispose to paradoxical embolism resulting in stroke or cerebral abscess. All patients with HHT should be screened for PAVMs which, if found, should be ablated by percutaneous embolisation.

Patients present either with recurrent bleeds, particularly epistaxis, or with iron deficiency due to occult gastrointestinal bleeding. Treatment can be difficult because of the multiple bleeding points but regular iron therapy often allows the marrow to compensate for blood loss. Local cautery or laser therapy may prevent single lesions from bleeding. A variety of medical therapies have been tried but none has been found to be universally effective.

Ehlers–Danlos disease

Ehlers–Danlos disease is a congenital disorder of collagen synthesis in which there is joint hyperextensibility, skin extensibility and tissue fragility such that capillaries are poorly supported by subcutaneous collagen and ecchymoses are commonly seen.

PLATELET FUNCTIONAL DISORDERS

Even in the presence of a normal platelet count, an individual may bleed if the function of the platelets is reduced. Congenital abnormalities include rare disorders of the membrane glycoproteins, e.g. thrombasthenia and Bernard–Soulier syndrome, or the presence of defective platelet granules, e.g. a deficiency of dense (delta) granules giving rise to storage pool disorders. Such patients exhibit bleeding of 'platelet type' (p. 1017) which varies in severity between patients, some presenting with frequent recurrent bleeds whilst others are only diagnosed because of excessive post-operative haemorrhage. Mild functional disorders, which only cause excessive bleeding after trauma or surgery, are often not diagnosed and are probably relatively common.

Many drugs inhibit platelets (Box 24.63). Aspirin and other NSAIDs inhibit platelet cyclo-oxygenase, preventing the conversion of arachidonic acid to the potent platelet aggregator thromboxane B_2.

24.63 DRUGS INHIBITING PLATELET FUNCTION

NSAIDs
- Aspirin
- Indometacin
- Phenylbutazone
- Sulfinpyrazone

Antibiotics
- Penicillins
- Cephalosporins

Dextran

Heparin

β-blockers

Thrombocytopenia

Thrombocytopenia causing bleeding constitutes a haematological emergency which should be promptly investigated and treated. Causes and investigations are described on page

1017. Treatment should be directed at the underlying condition as well as specific measures to raise the platelet count. Platelet transfusions should be given only if the platelet count is less than 10×10^9/l, to treat troublesome bleeding such as persistent epistaxis, or potentially life-threatening bleeding, e.g. gastrointestinal haemorrhage. Such transfusions provide only temporary relief because the survival of the platelets in the circulation is a few days at most, and only a matter of minutes or hours if the thrombocytopenia is due to increased platelet consumption, as in idiopathic thrombocytopenic purpura.

Idiopathic thrombocytopenic purpura

The presence of autoantibodies, often directed against platelet membrane glycoprotein IIb–IIIa, causes the premature removal of platelets by the monocyte–macrophage system. Occasionally, antigen–antibody immune complexes adhere to platelets at their F_c receptor, resulting in their premature removal from the circulation.

Clinical features and investigations

In children idiopathic thrombocytopenic purpura (ITP) often presents 2–3 weeks after a viral illness, with the sudden onset of purpura and sometimes oral and nasal bleeding. It is important to ascertain that the child does not have any other systemic illness, in particular DIC.

In adults ITP more commonly affects females and has an insidious onset. It is unusual for there to be a history of a preceding viral infection. At presentation some cases may be associated with symptoms or signs of a connective tissue disease, whilst in others these disorders may become apparent several years later. The condition is likely to become chronic, with remissions and relapses. The peripheral blood film is normal, apart from a greatly reduced platelet number, whilst the bone marrow reveals an obvious increase in megakaryocytes.

Management

Children. If the child has only mild bleeding symptoms, it is usual to withhold any specific treatment, as in the majority of instances the condition is self-limiting within a few weeks. The presence of moderate to severe purpura, bruising or epistaxis, and a platelet count less than 10×10^9/1 are indications for oral prednisolone 2 mg/kg daily. The platelet count usually rises promptly within 1–3 days. Persistent epistaxis, gastrointestinal bleeding, retinal haemorrhages or any suggestion of intracranial bleeding should be treated immediately by a platelet transfusion and intravenous immunoglobulin (IVIgG).

Adults. Treatment with prednisolone 1 mg/kg daily is often less rewarding than in children; the platelet count rises in response to therapy but may fall again when the dose is reduced or stopped. As with children, persistent or potentially life-threatening bleeding should be treated with platelet transfusion. Intravenous IgG (1 g/kg) should be given if the patient is very haemorrhagic or the bleeding is immediately life-threatening. IVIgG raises the platelet count by blocking the monocyte–macrophage F_c receptors, thus preventing the phagocytosis of antibody-coated platelets.

Relapses should be treated by increasing the dose of prednisolone. If a patient has two relapses, splenectomy is considered. This should be preceded by pneumococcal, meningococcal and *Haemophilus influenzae* vaccination and oral penicillin V daily for life (Box 24.31, p. 1032). As so many adults eventually require splenectomy, it is prudent to vaccinate all at presentation before they become immuno-suppressed with a prolonged course of corticosteroids. Vaccination should be performed by subcutaneous injection since, if given intramuscularly, it may result in a haematoma. Splenectomy is curative in about 70% of patients and, in the remainder, the aim should be to keep the patient free of symptoms rather than to treat the platelet count alone. Often patients have platelet counts of $20-30 \times 10^9/1$ without symptoms; some require long-term maintenance with prednisolone at 5 mg/day. If significant bleeding persists despite splenectomy and low-dose corticosteroid therapy, vincristine, immunosuppressive therapy—e.g. cyclophosphamide or rituximab, or repeated infusions of intravenous immunoglobulin should be considered.

Thrombotic thrombocytopenic purpura

This is a rare cause of thrombocytopenia that can present to a variety of specialties and requires urgent management. Platelet thrombi form in the microvasculature affecting in particular the renal (p. 498) and cerebral circulation. Excessive platelet aggregation is thought to occur because of the lack of a functioning protease enzyme which results in the presence of extra-large von Willebrand factor molecules. It can be associated with drugs, autoimmune disease and infection (e.g. *E. coli* O157). Clinically there is a pentad of diagnostic features: thrombocytopenia, micro-angiopathic haemolytic anaemia, fluctuating neurological signs, renal impairment and fever. Untreated mortality rates are 90%, this figure falling to 10–30% after treatment with fresh frozen plasma given during daily plasma exchange.

COAGULATION DISORDERS

Coagulation factor disorders can arise either from deficiency, usually congenital, of a single factor—e.g. factor VIII in haemophilia A—or from multiple factor deficiencies which are often acquired, e.g. secondary to liver disease. Of the single congenital deficiencies, haemophilia A and B are the most common although, rarely, any of the coagulation factors may be reduced. The congenital disorders almost exclusively arise as a result of an abnormality in the gene coding for the coagulation factor.

CONGENITAL BLEEDING DISORDERS

HAEMOPHILIA A

A reduction of factor VIII resulting in haemophilia A, which affects 1/10 000 individuals, is the most common congenital disorder of coagulation. Factor VIII is primarily synthesised by the liver and endothelial cells, but other organs such as the spleen, kidney and placenta may also contribute. Plasma factor VIII has a half-life of about 12 hours and is carried non-covalently bound to the von Willebrand factor (vWF).

Genetics

The factor VIII gene is located on the X chromosome and consists of 26 exons; many different defects in the gene have been identified, ranging from single-base changes to deletions and inversions. Major disruption of the gene, e.g a large deletion, results in severe haemophilia whereas a single base change will only cause a partial loss of function, with moderate or mild disease. As the factor VIII gene is on the X chromosome, haemophilia A is a sex-linked disorder. Thus all daughters of haemophiliacs are obligate carriers and sisters have a 50% chance of being a carrier. If a carrier has a son, he has a 50% chance of having haemophilia, and a daughter has a 50% chance of being a carrier. Haemophilia 'breeds true' within a family. All members will have the same abnormality of the factor VIII gene; thus if one individual has severe haemophilia, so will all others affected. Female carriers of haemophilia may have reduced factor VIII levels because of random inactivation of the X chromosome in the developing fetus (lyonisation). A reduced factor VIII level in a carrier will result in a mild bleeding disorder; thus all known or suspected carriers of haemophilia should have their factor VIII level measured.

The use of molecular genetic techniques has revolutionised the ability to identify carriers and make an antenatal diagnosis of haemophilia. If the factor VIII mutation causing the haemophilia in a particular family is known, antenatal diagnosis can be undertaken in a female who has a high probability of being a carrier. This is accomplished by chorionic villous sampling, usually around 11 weeks' gestation, sexing the fetus and using informative factor VIII probes.

Clinical features and investigations

Although haemophilia A is a congenital disorder, it is unusual for excessive bleeding to be noticed until about 6 months of age, when superficial bruising or a haemarthrosis may occur. This apparent delay in presentation is due to the relative inactivity of babies in the first few months of life and it is only when they begin to move about that the increase in trauma results in bleeding. It is not uncommon for children to be initially classified as having non-accidental injury.

The normal factor VIII level is 50–150% and is measured by a clotting assay. In haemophilia the propensity to bleeding is related to the plasma factor VIII level. The classification of severity of haemophilia is set out in Box 24.64.

24.64 SEVERITY OF HAEMOPHILIA (UK CRITERIA)

Degree of severity	Factor VIII or IX level	Clinical presentation
Severe	< 2%	Spontaneous haemarthroses and muscle haematomas
Moderate	2–10%	Mild trauma or surgery causes haematomas
Mild	10–50%	Major injury or surgery results in excess bleeding

24

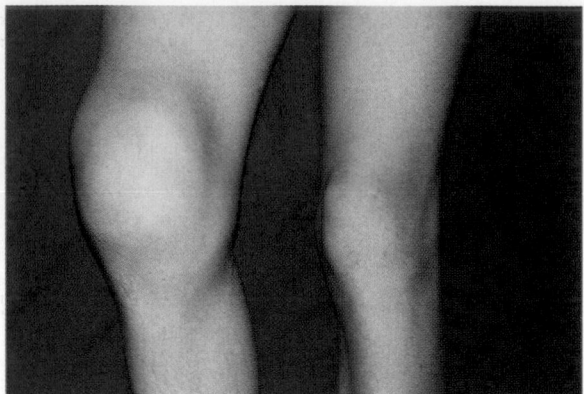

Fig. 24.34 Large haemarthrosis in the right knee of a boy with haemophilia A.

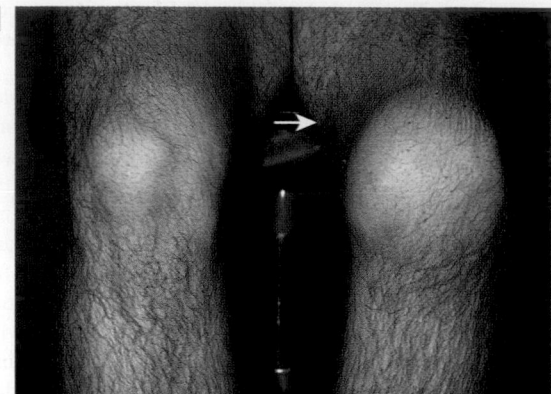

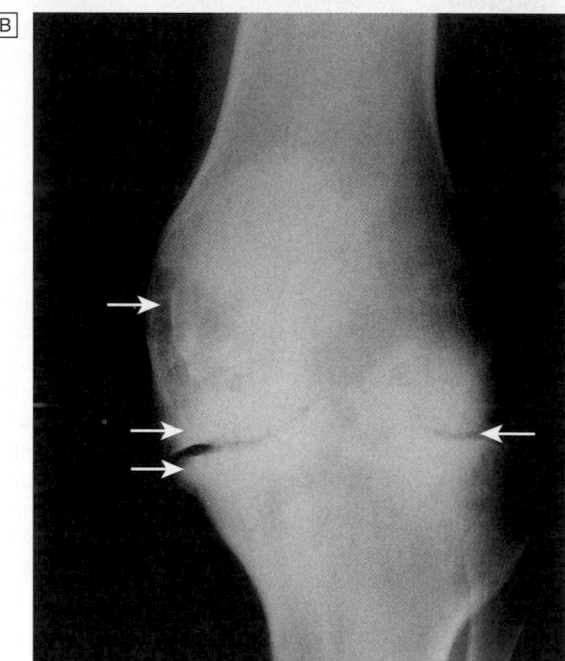

Fig. 24.35 Chronic haemophilic arthropathy of the left knee.
A Repeated bleeds have led to broadening of the femoral epicondyles. Unilateral atrophy of the quadriceps (A) is easily seen. **B** X-ray confirms broadening of femoral epicondyles. There is no cartilage present, as evidenced by the close proximity of the femur and tibia (B); sclerosis (C), osteophyte (D) and bony cysts (E) are present.

Individuals with severe haemophilia experience recurrent haemarthroses in large joints (Fig. 24.34). These usually begin spontaneously without apparent trauma and most commonly affect the knees, elbows, ankles and hips. A typical severe haemophiliac may have one or two bleeds each week. Patients are aware that bleeding has started because they experience an abnormal sensation in the joint. If treatment is not given at this stage, bleeding continues, resulting in a hot, swollen and very painful joint, which may persist for days before gradually subsiding. Recurrent bleeds into joints lead to synovial hypertrophy, destruction of the cartilage and secondary osteoarthrosis (Fig. 24.35). The resultant limitation of movement may greatly reduce the function of joints, making walking difficult.

Muscle haematomas are also characteristic of haemophilia. These occur most commonly in the calf and psoas muscles but they can arise in almost any muscle. Although less common than haemarthroses, a single episode can leave severe lasting damage if not effectively treated. A large psoas bleed, for example, may extend to compress the femoral nerve. Calf haematomas are also serious because of the inflexible fascial sheath surrounding the soleus and gastrocnemius muscles. Untreated haemorrhage causes a rise in pressure with eventual ischaemia, necrosis, fibrosis, and subsequent contraction and shortening of the Achilles tendon (Fig. 24.36).

Although joint and muscle bleeds are the most common sites for haemorrhage, bleeding can occur at almost any site. It is particularly serious if it takes place in a confined anatomical space associated with vital structures, such as the intracranial area where haemorrhage, unless treated very promptly, is often fatal (Fig. 24.37).

Individuals with moderate haemophilia usually only experience haemorrhage after minor trauma, and those with the mild form of the disorder, following more major trauma or surgery. Whereas severe haemophilia is usually diagnosed within the first 2 years of life, individuals with moderate and mild forms may escape diagnosis until adulthood.

Management
Bleeding episodes should be treated early by raising the factor VIII level. This is usually accomplished by intravenous infusion of factor VIII concentrate. Factor VIII concentrates are freeze-dried and stable at 4°C and can therefore be stored in domestic refrigerators. This allows many patients to treat themselves at home and has revolutionised haemophilia care. Factor VIII concentrates are prepared from blood donor plasma which has been screened for hepatitis B and C viruses and HIV, and has undergone a viral inactivation process during manufacture; they have a good safety record. However, factor VIII concentrates prepared by recombinant technology are now widely available and, although more expensive, are perceived as being safer than those derived from plasma.

In addition to factor VIII concentrate therapy, resting of the bleeding site by either bed rest or a splint reduces continuing haemorrhage. Once bleeding has settled, the

24

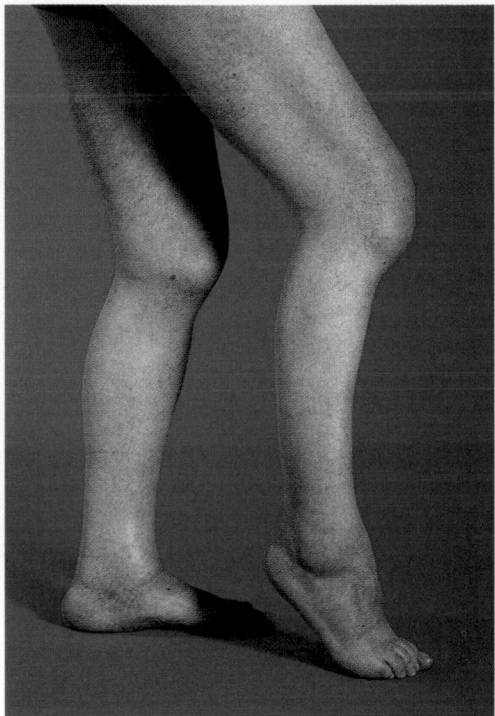

Fig. 24.36 Atrophy of the calf in an adult following an inadequately treated gastrocnemius haematoma as a child. The increased pressure of the haematoma caused ischaemia of the muscle, followed by necrosis, fibrosis and subsequent contraction to give the equinus deformity.

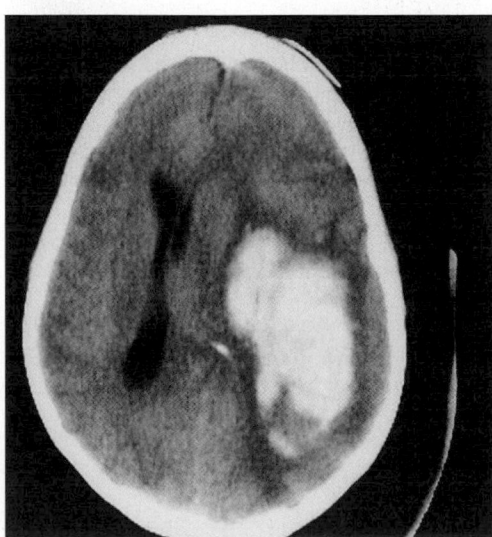

Fig. 24.37 CT revealing a major intracerebral haematoma. This arose spontaneously in a severe haemophiliac.

patient should be mobilised and physiotherapy used to restore strength to the surrounding muscles.

Complications of therapy

Although factor VIII concentrates have allowed many haemophiliacs to lead near-normal lives, this freedom has been bought at a cost (Box 24.65). Before 1985 concentrates

24.65 LONG-TERM SEQUELAE OF HAEMOPHILIA
Complications due to repeated haemorrhages
• Arthropathy of large joints, e.g. knees, elbows • Atrophy of muscles secondary to haematomas • Mononeuropathy resulting from pressure by haematomas
Complications due to therapy

• Anti-factor VIII antibody development
• Virus transmission
  Hepatitis A virus—acute self-limiting illness
  Hepatitis B virus—5–10% become chronic HBsAg carriers
  Hepatitis C virus—chronic progressive liver disease
  Hepatitis D virus—only arises in those with HBsAg
  Erythrovirus—acute systemic self-limiting illness

were not virally inactivated with heat or chemicals, and so many patients treated became infected with HIV and the hepatitis viruses. As a result, most adult severe haemophiliacs have been exposed to hepatitis B virus and have developed immunity, as evidenced by the development of anti-HBs (p. 963). A small number become chronic HBsAg carriers and may infect sexual partners, who should therefore be offered hepatitis B immunisation (p. 966). They are also at risk of delta virus infection. All potential recipients of pooled blood products should be offered hepatitis A and B immunisation because it will protect against hepatitis A, B and D infection. Hepatitis C virus was ubiquitously transmitted by concentrates prior to 1985, resulting in virtually all recipients becoming infected. It is clear that many of these patients have hepatitis, and a significant proportion progress to cirrhosis and hepatocellular carcinoma. Management of these is described in Chapter 23.

Prior to 1985, HIV was also transmitted to haemophiliacs by concentrates, with at least 60% of severe haemophiliacs becoming infected (p. 380). The clinical consequences are very similar to those for any individual infected with HIV, although their clinical course is perhaps more like those who become infected intravenously than those who become infected sexually. Kaposi's sarcoma is rare in haemophiliacs.

There is now concern that the infectious agent which causes variant CJD (p. 1234) might be transmissible by blood and blood products. Pooled plasma products, including factor VIII concentrate, are now manufactured from plasma collected in countries with a low incidence of BSE.

The other serious consequence of factor VIII infusion is the development of anti-factor VIII antibodies, which arises in about 20–30% of severe haemophiliacs. Such antibodies rapidly neutralise therapeutic infusions, making treatment relatively ineffective. Infusions of activated clotting factors, e.g. VIIa or FEIBA (factor eight inhibitor bypassing activity—an activated concentrate of factors II, IX and X), may stop bleeding.

In individuals with a basal factor VIII level of 10% or greater it may be possible to raise the level approximately three- to five-fold with desmopressin; this is best given intravenously but can be administered intranasally. This is often sufficient to treat a mild bleed or cover minor surgery such as dental extraction.

Surgery in haemophiliacs can be safely performed provided the patient does not have an inhibitor to factor VIII and receives appropriate doses of concentrate. A single infusion of factor VIII is usually adequate for simple dental extractions in an individual with severe haemophilia, along with a 10-day course of tranexamic acid (a fibrinolytic inhibitor) and an antibiotic. Major surgery, such as orthopaedic, requires twice-daily therapy for 14 days or longer.

HAEMOPHILIA B (CHRISTMAS DISEASE)

Aberrations of the factor IX gene, which is also present on the X chromosome, result in a reduction of the plasma factor IX level, giving rise to haemophilia B. This disorder is clinically indistinguishable from haemophilia A but is less common. The frequency of bleeding episodes is related to the severity of the deficiency of the plasma factor IX level.

Treatment is with a factor IX concentrate; it is used in much the same way as factor VIII for haemophilia A. Carrier identification and antenatal diagnosis can be accomplished if the specific mutation is known.

VON WILLEBRAND DISEASE

Von Willebrand disease is a common but usually mild bleeding disorder. The gene for von Willebrand factor (vWF) is located on chromosome 12 and therefore the disorder is inherited in an autosomal fashion. In most families it appears to be inherited dominantly; rarely, it appears in a clinically severe form with almost undetectable levels of vWF. In these circumstances the patient usually inherits a different abnormal vWF gene from each parent and is thus a compound heterozygote. Gene probes are available to trace the gene in a family and can be used to identify carriers and for antenatal diagnosis.

The vWF is a protein, synthesised by endothelial cells and megakaryocytes, that performs two principal functions. It acts as a carrier protein for factor VIII, to which it is non-covalently bound. A deficiency of vWF therefore results in a secondary reduction in the plasma factor VIII level. Its other function is to form bridges between platelets and sub-endothelial components (e.g. collagen), allowing platelets to adhere to damaged vessel walls (Fig. 24.7, p. 1007). A deficiency of vWF therefore also leads to prolonged primary haemorrhage after trauma.

Clinical features

As vWF participates along with platelets in primary haemostasis, patients present with haemorrhagic manifestations similar to those in individuals with reduced platelet function. Superficial bruising, epistaxis, and menorrhagic and gastrointestinal haemorrhage are common. Bleeding episodes are usually much less common than in severe haemophilia and excessive haemorrhage may only be observed after trauma or surgery. Within a single family the disease can be of very variable expression so that some members may have quite severe and frequent bleeds, whereas others are relatively little troubled.

Investigations

The disorder is characterised by a reduced level of vWF, which is often accompanied by a secondary reduction in factor VIII and a prolongation of the bleeding time.

Management

Many episodes of mild haemorrhage can be successfully treated with desmopressin, which raises the vWF level, resulting in a secondary increase in factor VIII. For more serious or persistent bleeds haemostasis can be achieved with selected factor VIII concentrates which contain considerable quantities of vWF in addition to factor VIII.

ACQUIRED BLEEDING DISORDERS

DISSEMINATED INTRAVASCULAR COAGULATION (DIC)

Clinical features

DIC can be initiated by a variety of different mechanisms in a number of diverse but distinct clinical situations (Box 24.66). Endothelial damage, due to many causes—e.g. endotoxaemia due to Gram-negative septicaemia—results in tissue factor expression, which leads to activation of the coagulation cascade through the extrinsic pathway (Fig. 24.8, p. 1008). Intravascular coagulation takes place with consumption of platelets, factors V and VIII, and fibrinogen. This results in a potential haemorrhagic state, due to the depletion of haemostatic components, which may be exacerbated by activation of the fibrinolytic system secondary to the deposition of fibrin.

Investigations

DIC should be suspected when any of the conditions in Box 24.66 are met. Definitive diagnosis depends on the finding of thrombocytopenia, prolongation of the prothrombin time (due to factor V and fibrinogen deficiency) and activated partial thromboplastin time (due to factors V, VIII and fibrinogen deficiency), a low fibrinogen concentration and increased levels of D-dimer (cleaved from fibrin by plasmin, establishing evidence of fibrin lysis).

Management

Therapy should be aimed at treating the underlying condition causing the DIC, e.g. intravenous antibiotics for

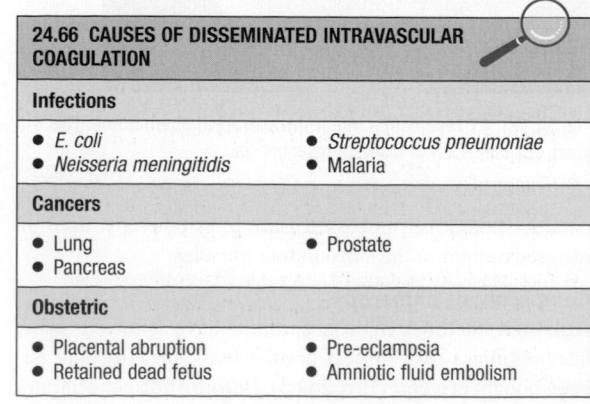

24.66 CAUSES OF DISSEMINATED INTRAVASCULAR COAGULATION	
Infections	
• E. coli	• Streptococcus pneumoniae
• Neisseria meningitidis	• Malaria
Cancers	
• Lung	• Prostate
• Pancreas	
Obstetric	
• Placental abruption	• Pre-eclampsia
• Retained dead fetus	• Amniotic fluid embolism

suspected septicaemia. Exacerbating factors such as acidosis, dehydration, renal failure and hypoxia should be corrected. If the patient is bleeding, blood products such as platelets and/or fresh frozen plasma should be given to correct identified abnormalities. It may also be reasonable to treat severe coagulation abnormalities in the absence of frank bleeding to prevent sudden catastrophic haemorrhage such as an intracranial bleed or massive gastrointestinal haemorrhage.

LIVER DISEASE

In severe parenchymal liver disease (Ch. 23), bleeding may arise from many different causes. Local anatomical abnormalities are often the site of major bleeding (such as oesophageal varices or peptic ulcer), and this may be difficult to arrest because of deficiencies in components of the haemostatic system. These may arise because of reduced hepatic synthesis, e.g. factors II, VII, IX, X and fibrinogen, DIC, reduced clearance of plasminogen activator, or thrombocytopenia secondary to hypersplenism. Treatment should be reserved for acute bleeds or to cover interventional procedures such as liver biopsy.

Cholestatic jaundice reduces vitamin K absorption and leads to a deficiency of function of factors II, VII, IX and X due to reduced gamma glutamate carboxylation. This deficiency can be readily and effectively treated with vitamin K_1 10 mg daily parenterally for several days.

RENAL FAILURE

The severity of the haemorrhagic state in renal failure is proportional to the plasma urea concentration (p. 481). Bleeding manifestations are of platelet type, with gastrointestinal haemorrhage being particularly common. The causes are multifactorial, including anaemia, mild thrombocytopenia and the accumulation of low molecular waste products, normally excreted by the kidney, that inhibit platelet function. Treatment is by dialysis to reduce the urea concentration, platelet concentrate infusions and red cell transfusions to raise the haemoglobin and decrease the propensity to bleed. Increasing the concentration of vWF, either by cryoprecipitate or by desmopressin (DDAVP), may promote haemostasis.

24.67 HAEMOSTASIS AND THROMBOSIS IN OLD AGE

- **Thrombocytopenia:** not uncommon because of the rising prevalence of disorders to which it may be secondary, and the greater use of drugs which can cause it.
- **'Senile' purpura:** thought to be due to age-associated loss of subcutaneous fat and the collagenous support of small blood vessels, making them more prone to damage from minor trauma.
- **Thrombosis-related events:** more frequent, possibly due to stasis to which older people are prone; possible increased platelet aggregation with age, or age-associated increase in levels of clotting factors which could cause a prothrombotic state.

VENOUS THROMBOSIS

Venous thrombosis may arise either because of damage to, or pressure on veins (e.g. varicose veins or pelvic tumour), or as a result of changes in the plasma or cellular elements of the blood. Predisposing conditions for venous thromboembolism are listed in Box 24.68. Its clinical features and investigation are described on page 1018.

HAEMATOLOGICAL DISORDERS PREDISPOSING TO VENOUS THROMBOEMBOLISM

When a thrombotic event arises in an individual under the age of 40 years, particularly if there is a family history of thrombosis, investigations for a predisposing blood abnormality should be undertaken (Box 24.68). Often several other risk factors are present when an acute deep venous thrombosis (DVT) occurs, e.g. obesity and surgery in a patient with factor V Leiden.

ANTITHROMBIN DEFICIENCY

Antithrombin is a protease inhibitor which inactivates factors IIa, IXa, Xa and XIa, especially in the presence of heparin (which greatly potentiates its activity). Familial deficiency of antithrombin is a dominantly inherited disorder and is associated with a marked predisposition to venous thromboembolism.

24

24.68 FACTORS PREDISPOSING TO VENOUS THROMBOSIS

Patient factors

- Age > 40 years
- Obesity
- Varicose veins
- Previous DVT
- Oral contraceptive
- Pregnancy/puerperium
- Dehydration
- Immobility

Surgical conditions

- Surgery, especially if > 30 minutes' duration
  Abdominal or pelvic
  Orthopaedic to lower limb

Medical conditions

- Myocardial infarction/heart failure
- Inflammatory bowel disease
- Malignancy
- Nephrotic syndrome
- Pneumonia
- Homocystinaemia

Haematological disorders

- Primary proliferative polycythaemia
- Essential thrombocythaemia
- Paroxysmal nocturnal haemoglobinuria
- Myelofibrosis

Deficiency of anticoagulants

- Antithrombin
- Protein C
- Prothrombin G20210A
- Protein S
- Factor V Leiden

Antiphospholipid antibody

- Lupus anticoagulant
- Anticardiolipin antibody

PROTEIN C AND S DEFICIENCIES

Protein C is a vitamin K-dependent plasma protein. When thrombin binds to thrombomodulin on the endothelial cell surface, it becomes an anticoagulant by activating protein C. In the presence of protein S, this inactivates factors Va and VIIIa. Thus a deficiency of either protein C or S results in a prothrombotic state due to reduced inhibition of activated factor V and VIII. A deficiency of either factor is usually inherited in an autosomal fashion.

FACTOR V LEIDEN

Factor V Leiden is associated with venous thrombosis. The abnormality resides with factor Va; a substitution of arginine by glutamine at position 506 prevents its cleavage and hence inactivation. Factor Va will therefore persist, resulting in a tendency to venous thrombosis.

The mutation has been identified in about 3–5% of healthy individuals in Western Europe and North America, and in about 20–40% of those with a history of venous thrombosis at a young age. The risk of venous thrombosis is substantially increased if the patient is homozygous for the mutation or has a second plasma abnormality, e.g. a lupus anticoagulant (see below).

PROTHROMBIN G20210A

This genetic polymorphism at the non-coding 3′ end of the prothrombin gene is associated with an increased plasma level of prothrombin and venous thromboembolism. It is present in about 2% of the normal population and about 6% of those with venous thrombus.

ANTIPHOSPHOLIPID ANTIBODY SYNDROME

In this syndrome an antibody in the patient's plasma has activity against enzymic reactions in the coagulation cascade that are dependent on platelet membranes (or in vitro by phospholipid). The antibody in vitro has the effect of prolonging the APTT because it interacts with phospholipid in the reaction tube and inhibits the binding or enzymic interactions of the coagulation components. It is most sensitively diagnosed by prolongation of the dilute Russell viper venom time (DRVVT) of plasma, an effect that can be neutralised by adding platelet membranes. When the antibody inhibits coagulation in these ways, it is known as the lupus anticoagulant. In some individuals the plasma protein β_2-glycoprotein-1 undergoes a conformational change after it has bound to anionic phospholipids, and is then recognised by the antibody. In vitro this is usually detected by its ability to bind to the β_2-glycoprotein-1 in an assay with cardiolipin, when it is known as an anticardiolipin antibody. The term antiphospholipid antibody encompasses both a lupus anticoagulant and an anticardiolipin antibody; some individuals are only positive for one of these activities, whereas in others both are present.

24.69 CLINICAL ASSOCIATIONS WITH ANTIPHOSPHOLIPID SYNDROME	
Primary antiphospholipid syndrome	
• Venous thromboembolic disease	
• Arterial thromboembolic disease	
• Sterile (Liebmann–Sachs) endocarditis with embolism	
• Recurrent pregnancy failure	
Secondary antiphospholipid syndrome	
• SLE	• Temporal arteritis
• Rheumatoid arthritis	• Sjögren's syndrome
• Systemic sclerosis	• Psoriatic arthropathy
• Behçet's syndrome	

Clinical features

The antiphospholipid antibody is associated with a constellation of clinical conditions (Box 24.69), found in association with a history of thromboembolism. The antibody has now been found in some individuals with a history of arterial or venous thromboembolism in one or several organs, often at a young age but without features of SLE; in this case it is known as the primary antiphospholipid antibody syndrome. In those with other conditions associated with thrombosis it is known as a secondary antiphospholipid antibody syndrome (Box 24.69). The antibody is also associated with recurrent spontaneous abortions and intrauterine fetal growth retardation. The mechanism by which the antibody predisposes to thrombosis is unclear but it may be related either to maintaining platelets in an activated state within the circulation, or to inhibiting the fibrinolytic activity of endothelial cells.

MANAGEMENT OF VENOUS THROMBOEMBOLISM

The treatment of a thrombosis depends on its site and extent and on the age of the thrombus. Prior to any antithrombotic therapy it is essential to consider whether the patient has a significant contraindication to anticoagulant therapy. On occasion therapy may have to be given to a patient who has a contraindication and in this instance the potential benefits have to be weighed against the risk of serious haemorrhage. Indications for and contraindications to anticoagulation are given in Boxes 24.70 and 24.71.

ANTICOAGULANT THERAPY

Heparin

Standard (unfractionated) heparin (SH) produces its anticoagulant effect by potentiating the activity of antithrombin which inhibits the procoagulant enzymic activity of factors IIa, VIIa, IXa, Xa and XIa (Fig. 24.8, p. 1008).

The more recently developed low molecular weight heparins (LMWHs) augment antithrombin activity preferentially against factor Xa. LMWH does not prolong the APTT, unlike SH, and if its plasma level needs to be measured this is accomplished using a specific anti-Xa-based assay. LMWH, because of its high bioavailability

24.70 INDICATIONS FOR ANTICOAGULATION

Heparin

- Treatment and prevention of DVT
- Pulmonary embolism
- Post-thrombolysis for myocardial infarction, to prevent coronary reocclusion
- Unstable angina pectoris
- Acute peripheral arterial occlusion

Warfarin

• Prophylaxis against DVT • Treatment of DVT and pulmonary embolism • Arterial embolism • Atrial fibrillation with specific stroke risk factors (p. 562) • Mobile mural thrombus on echo post-myocardial infarction • Extensive anterior myocardial infarction	Therapeutic corrected prothrombin ratio (INR) 2.5
• Recurrent DVT whilst on warfarin • Mechanical prosthetic cardiac valves	INR 3.5

(INR = international normalised ratio)

24.71 CONTRAINDICATIONS TO ANTICOAGULATION

- Recent surgery, especially to eye or CNS
- Pre-existing haemorrhagic state
  - e.g. Liver disease
  - Renal failure
  - Haemophilia
  - Thrombocytopenia

- Pre-existing structural lesions e.g. Peptic ulcer
- Recent cerebral haemorrhage
- Uncontrolled hypertension
- Cognitive impairment
- Frequent falls in old age

---

after subcutaneous injection, is given as either a standard or a weight-related dose. Normally, therefore, the plasma LMWH level does not need to be measured.

The therapeutic indications for heparin are listed in Box 24.70.

LMWHs are now widely used for the treatment of both DVT and pulmonary embolism and are replacing standard heparin as the initial treatment of choice for many patients. As injections of LMWH need only be given once daily subcutaneously and no monitoring is required, many patients can be treated at home. In patients who are elderly or who have low body weight or renal failure, there is an increased risk of bleeding. The LMWH dose should be reduced in these groups and in those with a creatinine clearance of less than 30 ml/min. If less than 10 ml/min, the use of standard heparin should be considered, especially where reversibility may be needed.

Standard heparin is often reserved for treating patients with very severe, life-threatening thromboembolism, e.g. major pulmonary embolism giving rise to significant hypoxaemia or hypotension. It should be started with a loading dose of 5000 U i.v., followed by a continuous infusion of 20 U/kg/hr initially. The level of anticoagulation should be assessed by the APTT after 6 hours and, if satisfactory, daily thereafter. It is usual to aim for a patient

EBM

24.72 ANTICOAGULATION IN VENOUS THROMBOEMBOLIC DISEASE

'Initial treatment with heparin before introducing warfarin reduces the risk of recurrent pulmonary emboli. Maintaining the INR at 2.0–3.0 has similar efficacy but induces fewer bleeds than maintaining the INR at 3.0–4.0.'

- Brandjes DP, et al. N Engl J Med 1992; 327:1485–1489.
- Hull R, et al. N Engl J Med 1982; 307:1676–1681.

---

time which is 1.5–2.5 times the control time of the test. The half-life of intravenous heparin is about 1 hour and if a patient bleeds, it is usually sufficient just to discontinue the infusion; however, if bleeding is severe, the excess can be neutralised with intravenous protamine. The short half-life of SH makes it useful for those with a predisposition to bleeding, e.g. who have peptic ulcer, or those who may require surgery. Treatment with either LMWH or SH should continue for 6–8 days, depending upon the extent of the thrombus. In most patients it is appropriate to start warfarin therapy at the same time as heparin, as it takes several days to decrease the concentration of the vitamin K-dependent clotting factors. Heparin should be continued until the INR is > 2.0 for 2 consecutive days (Box 24.72).

Heparin-induced thrombocytopenia (HIT)

In a small proportion of patients treated with heparin the platelet count declines after 5–7 days due to the development of an antibody to the heparin–platelet factor 4 on the platelet surface. HIT should be considered in all patients whose platelet count falls by more than 50% after starting heparin. It is a very serious complication because it is associated with a high incidence of arterial and venous thrombosis. The diagnosis is established by detecting the antibody to PF4–heparin complex. Heparin should be discontinued as soon as HIT is diagnosed and the direct thrombin inhibitor, hirudin, given instead.

Warfarin

Warfarin inhibits the vitamin K-dependent carboxylation of factors II, VII, IX and X in the liver (Fig. 24.9, p. 1009). Carboxylation of glutamyl residues of these coagulation factors increases their negative charge and allows them to maintain their active three-dimensional structure. The recognised indications for warfarin therapy are listed in Box 24.70.

Therapy with warfarin must be initiated with a loading dose—e.g. 10 mg orally—on the first day, and subsequent daily doses depending on the INR. The degree of anticoagulation depends on the clinical circumstances, and the appropriate target INRs are given in Box 24.70. Following a single episode of venous thromboembolism, it is usual to continue oral anticoagulation for 3–6 months. If a patient has had two episodes of venous thromboembolism, life-long warfarin is often considered appropriate. It is important to remember that nearly all drugs can potentially interact with warfarin, and therefore the INR should be checked 3–6 days after stopping or starting any other medicine.

Bleeding is the most common serious side-effect of warfarin and occurs in about 0.5–1.0% of patients each year.

24

The anticoagulant benefit of warfarin must therefore be demonstrably greater than the risk of serious bleeding. If the INR is above the desired therapeutic level, the warfarin dose should be reduced or withheld. If the patient is not bleeding, it may be appropriate to give a small dose of vitamin K, e.g. 5 mg orally or 2 mg by slow intravenous injection, especially if the INR is > 8. If the patient bleeds, the anticoagulant effect of warfarin may be reversed by vitamin K_1 1–5 mg slowly i.v. but this takes about 6 hours, and may not fully reverse anticoagulation for 1 or 2 days. The INR should be repeated after 6 hours and a further dose of vitamin K_1 given if appropriate. If the patient has a serious haemorrhage, reversal can be effected quickly by giving coagulation concentrate containing factors II, VII, IX and X (50 U/kg) or, if this is unavailable, fresh frozen plasma.

Other orally active anticoagulants are under development but not yet licensed for use, and include those which inhibit thrombin directly, e.g. ximelegatran. Their main potential advantage is that monitoring of the anticoagulant effect is not required. One of the disadvantages is that there is no specific antidote to reverse their effect in the event of bleeding.

PREVENTION OF VENOUS THROMBOSIS

All patients admitted to hospital should be assessed for their risk of developing venous thromboembolism. A summary of the risk categories is given in Box 24.73. Early mobilisation of all patients is important to prevent DVTs. Patients at medium or high risk may require additional antithrombotic measures. Full-length graduated compression stockings are effective in medium-risk individuals but SH or LMWH can also be used; it should be started pre-operatively and continued until the patient is fully mobile. High-risk individuals should receive anti-embolism stockings and LMWH at a higher prophylactic dose. Routine monitoring of SH or LMWH for prophylaxis is not necessary. Particular care should be taken with the use of heparin prophylaxis in any patient in whom intra- or post-operative bleeding could have serious consequences, e.g. following spinal anaesthesia, and it is usually contraindicated with neurosurgery. In individuals who have additional risk factors that increase the likelihood of thrombosis, care should be taken to ensure that the risk is lessened prior to surgery as far as possible—for instance, the haemoglobin reduced in polycythaemia. Over the next few years it is likely that other antithrombotic drugs will become available for prevention and treatment of venous thromboembolism including fondaparinux, a chemically synthesised penta-saccharide and oral thrombin inhibitor.

FURTHER INFORMATION

Books and journal articles

Bolton-Maggs PH, Pasi KJ. Haemophilias A and B. Lancet 2003; 361(9371):1801–1809.

Cines DB, Blanchette VS. Immune thrombocytopenic purpura. N Engl J Med 2002; 346(13):995–1008.

General Haematology Task Force of the British Committee for Standards in Haematology. Guidelines for the diagnosis and management of hereditary spherocytosis. Br J Haematol 2004; 126:455–474.

Guidelines Working Group of the UK CLL Forum. Guidelines on the diagnosis and management of chronic lymphocytic leukaemia. Br J Haematol 2004; 125:294–317.

Hirsh J, Guyatt G, Albers GW, Schunemann HJ. Seventh ACCP Conference on Antithrombotic and Thrombolytic Therapy: evidence-based guidelines. Chest 2004; 126(3 suppl.):172S–173S.

Jaffee ES, Harris NL, Stein H, Vardimann JW (eds). World Health Organization classification of tumours. Pathology and genetics of tumours of haematopoietic and lymphoid tissues. Lyons: IARC; 2001.

Lee AY, Hirsh J. Diagnosis and treatment of venous thromboembolism. Annu Rev Med 2002; 53:15–33.

Mannucci PM. Treatment of von Willebrand's disease. N Engl J Med 2004; 351(7):683–694.

Mannucci PM, Duga S, Peyvandi F. Recessively inherited coagulation disorders. Blood 2004; 104(5):1243–1252.

Murphy MF, Pamphilon DH. Practical transfusion medicine. Oxford: Blackwell Science; 2001.

Websites

www.bcshguidelines.com *British Committee for Standards in Haematology guidelines.*

www.ibmtr.org *International Bone Marrow Transplant Registry.*

www.show.scot.nhs.uk/sign/guidelines/fulltext/36/index.html *1999 SIGN guideline for antithrombotic therapy.*

www.transfusionguidelines.org.uk *Contains the UK Transfusion Services' Handbook of Transfusion Medicine and links to other relevant sites.*

24.73 ANTITHROMBOTIC PROPHYLAXIS	

Patients in the following categories should be considered for specific antithrombotic prophylaxis:

Moderate risk of DVT

- Major surgery in patients > 40 years or with other risk factor
- Major medical illness
  e.g. Heart failure
      Chest infection
      Malignancy
      Inflammatory bowel disease

High risk of DVT

- Hip or knee surgery
- Major abdominal or pelvic surgery for malignancy or with history of DVT or known thrombophilia (Box 24.4, p. 1011)

24

25

M. DOHERTY
P. LANYON
S.H. RALSTON

Musculoskeletal disorders

CLINICAL EXAMINATION OF THE MUSCULOSKELETAL SYSTEM

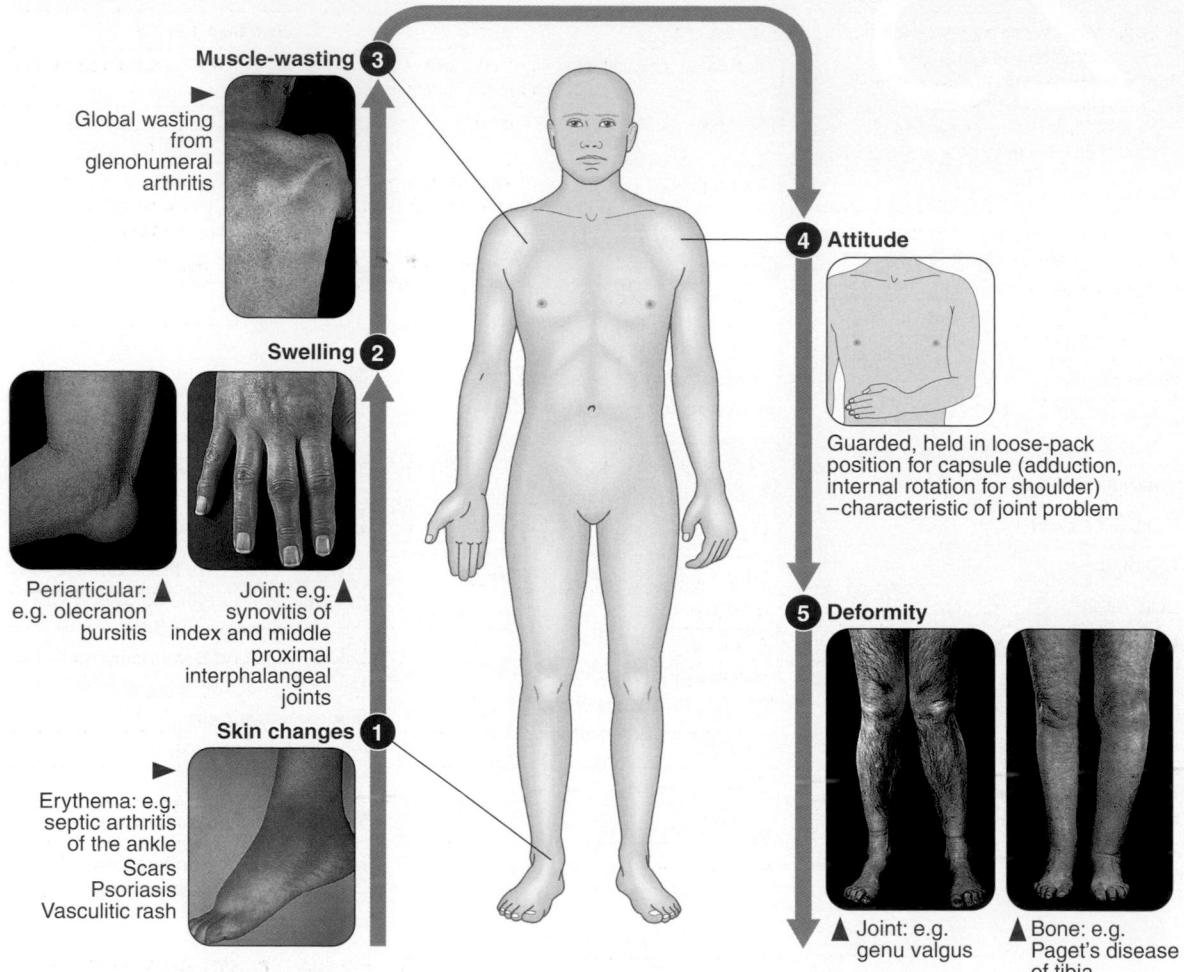

Muscle-wasting 3

► Global wasting from glenohumeral arthritis

Swelling 2

Periarticular: ▲ e.g. olecranon bursitis

Joint: e.g. ▲ synovitis of index and middle proximal interphalangeal joints

Skin changes 1

► Erythema: e.g. septic arthritis of the ankle
Scars
Psoriasis
Vasculitic rash

4 **Attitude**

Guarded, held in loose-pack position for capsule (adduction, internal rotation for shoulder) –characteristic of joint problem

5 **Deformity**

▲ Joint: e.g. genu valgus

▲ Bone: e.g. Paget's disease of tibia

Detailed regional examination involves 'look' (at rest and during movement), 'feel' and 'move'

A. Inspection at rest
(See figure above for examples)
• Skin changes
• Swelling
• Wasting of muscle
• Attitude
• Deformity

B. Inspection during movement
• Restriction
    Limited to one plane–periarticular lesion
    Affecting most or all movements–joint problem
• Increased range
    Hypermobility, instability
• Pain on usage
    Stress pain = increasing pain towards extremes of movement
    Universal stress pain (in most/all directions) –synovitis
    Selective stress pain (one plane only) –periarticular lesion

C. Palpation with movement
• Tenderness
    Joint line–intra-articular/joint problem
    Periarticular–periarticular lesion
• Increased warmth
    Inflammation (e.g. synovitis, bursitis)
• Swelling
    Fluid (fluctuant)
    Soft tissue (soft, non-fluctuant)
    Bone (hard)
• Crepitus
    Coarse, easily felt, may be readily audible–joint damage
    Fine, localised, heard with stethoscope–tendon sheath, bursa
• Stability
• Resisted active movements
    Reproduce pain from muscle, tendon, enthesis
• Stress tests
    Reproduce pain from ligament or tendon sheath

IMPORTANT MSK SYMPTOMS

Pain

- Usage pain—worse on use, relieved by rest (mechanical strain, damage)
- Rest pain—worse after rest, improved by movement (inflammation)
- Night or 'bone' pain—mostly at night, poorly related to movement (bone origin)

Stiffness

(Subjective feeling of inability to move freely)

- Duration and severity or early morning and inactivity stiffness that can be 'worn off' suggest degree of inflammation

Weakness

- Consider primary or secondary muscle abnormality

Swelling

(Fluid, soft tissue, bone)

Deformity

(Joint, bone)

Non-specific symptoms of systemic illness

(Reflecting acute phase response)

- Weight loss, ± reduction in appetite
- Fatigability, poor concentration
- Sweats and chills, particularly at night
- Feeling ill, low, irritable

REGIONAL EXAMINATION DIFFERENCES BETWEEN JOINT AND PERIARTICULAR LESIONS

Sign	Joint	Periarticular
Tenderness	Over joint line	Away from joint line
Restricted movement	Active and passive movement affected equally	Active more restricted than passive
Resisted active	Not painful	May reproduce muscle, tendon, ligament or enthesis pain
Stress pain	Present in all tight-pack positions (several directions)	Present in direction of use of ligament, tendon or enthesis (mainly one direction)
Swelling	Capsular pattern	Localised, periarticular
Crepitus ('crunching')	Coarse or fine	Fine

FEATURES THAT DIFFERENTIATE JOINT INFLAMMATION ('SYNOVITIS') FROM JOINT DAMAGE

Feature	Synovitis	Joint damage
Stiffness (early morning, inactivity)	+++	±
Increased warmth	+	−
Stress pain	+	−
Soft tissue swelling	+	−
Effusion	+++	±
Crepitus	−	+++
Deformity	−	+
Instability	−	+

25

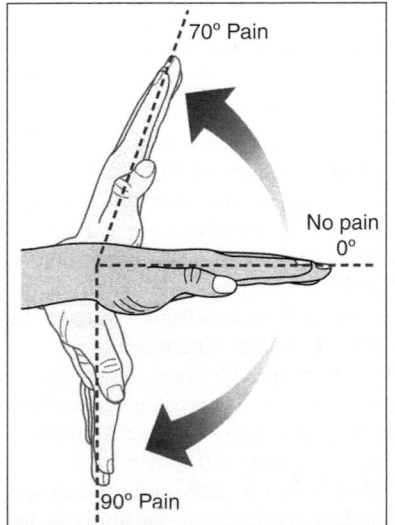

70° Pain

No pain 0°

90° Pain

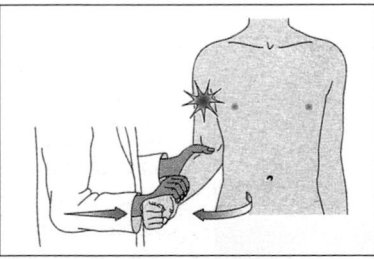

Example of resisted active movement. Attempted external rotation reproduces upper arm pain resulting from an infraspinatus/teres minor rotator cuff lesion.

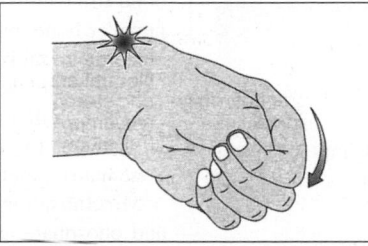

Example of a stress test. Passive ulnar flexion reproduces pain from de Quervain's tenosynovitis.

Example of 'stress pain' at the wrist. Pain worsens as the wrist moves towards the 'tight-pack' positions (flexion and extension) because of increased intracapsular pressure from inflammatory swelling and effusion. In the mid 'loose-pack' position, when the capsule is at its slackest, there is no pain. Stress pain is the earliest and most sensitive sign of synovitis, occurring before visible swelling or reduction of movement. With joint damage, pain is more evenly spread throughout the range.

Disorders of the musculoskeletal (MSK) system are prevalent throughout the world, affecting all ages and ethnic groups. The principal manifestations are pain and impairment of locomotor function.

Non-inflammatory conditions are far more prevalent than inflammatory disease (Box 25.1). Most MSK conditions predominate in women and show a strong association with ageing. In the UK up to 1 in 4 new consultations in general practice is for MSK symptoms and as many as 40% of those aged over 65 have a significant MSK disorder. Taken together, MSK disorders are the single most common cause of physical disability in the elderly, and around one-third of all people with physical disability have an MSK disorder as the primary cause.

Most regional MSK pain arises from muscles, tendons and periarticular structures. Osteoarthritis is the most common joint disorder, with knee involvement a major cause of disability in the community. Osteoporosis is the most prevalent bone disorder and constitutes a major public health problem. In developed countries about 1 in 3 women and 1 in 6 men sustain an osteoporotic fracture at some point during their lifetime.

25.1 RELATIVE PREVALENCE OF MUSCULOSKELETAL DISORDERS			
	Prevalence	Female: male	Age association
'Non-inflammatory' conditions			
Neck and back pain	20%	=	–
Osteoarthritis			
Knee	10%	F > M	++
Hip	4%	=	+
Osteoporosis	15%	F > M	++
Regional 'soft tissue' pain	10%	F > M	++
Fibromyalgia	3%	F > M	++
'Inflammatory' conditions			
Rheumatoid arthritis	1.5%	F > M	+
Gout	1.0%	M > F	–
Seronegative spondarthritis	0.8%	=	–
Polymyalgia rheumatica	0.04%	F > M	++
Connective tissue diseases (mainly lupus)	0.02%	F > M	–

FUNCTIONAL ANATOMY, PHYSIOLOGY AND INVESTIGATIONS

ANATOMY AND PHYSIOLOGY

The MSK system is responsible for body movements, providing a structural framework to protect internal organs and acting as a reservoir for storage of calcium and phosphate in the regulation of mineral homeostasis. Individual components are depicted in Figure 25.1.

BONE

Embryology

Bones are divisible into two main types on the basis of their embryonic development. Flat bones such as the skull develop by intramembranous ossification, in which embryonic mesenchymal fibroblasts differentiate directly into bone during early fetal life. Long bones such as the femur and radius develop by endochondral ossification from a cartilage template. The cartilage is gradually replaced by bone from centres of ossification situated in the middle and at the ends of the bone. A thin remnant of cartilage called the growth plate or epiphysis remains at each end of long bones, and chondrocyte proliferation in these regions is responsible for skeletal growth during childhood and adolescence. During puberty, the rise in circulating levels of sex hormones halts cell division in the growth plate. The cartilage remnant then disappears as the epiphysis fuses and longitudinal bone growth ceases.

Bone anatomy and microanatomy

Two types of bone are found in the normal skeleton (Fig. 25.1). Cortical bone is formed from Haversian systems, comprising concentric lamellae of bone tissue, surrounding a central canal that contains blood vessels. Cortical bone is dense and forms an envelope around the exterior of long bones, enclosing the marrow cavity. Trabecular or cancellous bone fills the centre of the bone and consists of an interconnecting meshwork of trabeculae, separated by spaces that are filled with bone marrow.

The three main cell types in bone are shown in Figure 25.1. Osteoclasts are multinucleated cells of haematopoietic origin, responsible for bone resorption. Osteoblasts are mononuclear cells of mesenchymal origin, responsible for bone formation. Osteocytes differentiate from osteoblasts during bone formation and become embedded in bone matrix. Osteocytes connect with one another by a series of cytoplasmic processes and are thought to be responsible for sensing and responding to mechanical loading.

The most important bone protein is type I collagen, which is formed from two α_1 peptide chains and one α_2 chain wound together in a triple helix. Type I collagen is proteolytically processed before being laid down in the extracellular space, releasing pro-peptide fragments that are used as biochemical markers of bone formation (p. 1076). After collagen is laid down the peptide chains are linked to one another by pyridinium cross-links which are important for bone strength. When bone is broken down by osteoclasts, these cross-links are degraded and released into the blood stream, thus providing biochemical markers of bone resorption (p. 1076). Under normal circumstances, bone collagen is laid down in an orderly fashion, producing lamellar bone, but in conditions such as Paget's disease, the collagen is laid down in a chaotic pattern, giving rise to 'woven bone' which is mechanically weak. Bone matrix contains small amounts of proteins and proteoglycans which are thought to be involved in helping bone cells attach to bone matrix, and in regulating bone cell activity.

Mineralisation of bone occurs by deposition of calcium and phosphate crystals between the collagen fibrils in the form of hydroxyapatite $[Ca_{10}(PO_4)_6(OH)_2]$. Normal mineralisation plays an important role in regulating bone strength and resistance to fracture, although overmineralisation can be detrimental by increasing brittleness, which contributes to bone fragility in diseases like osteogenesis imperfecta (p. 1131).

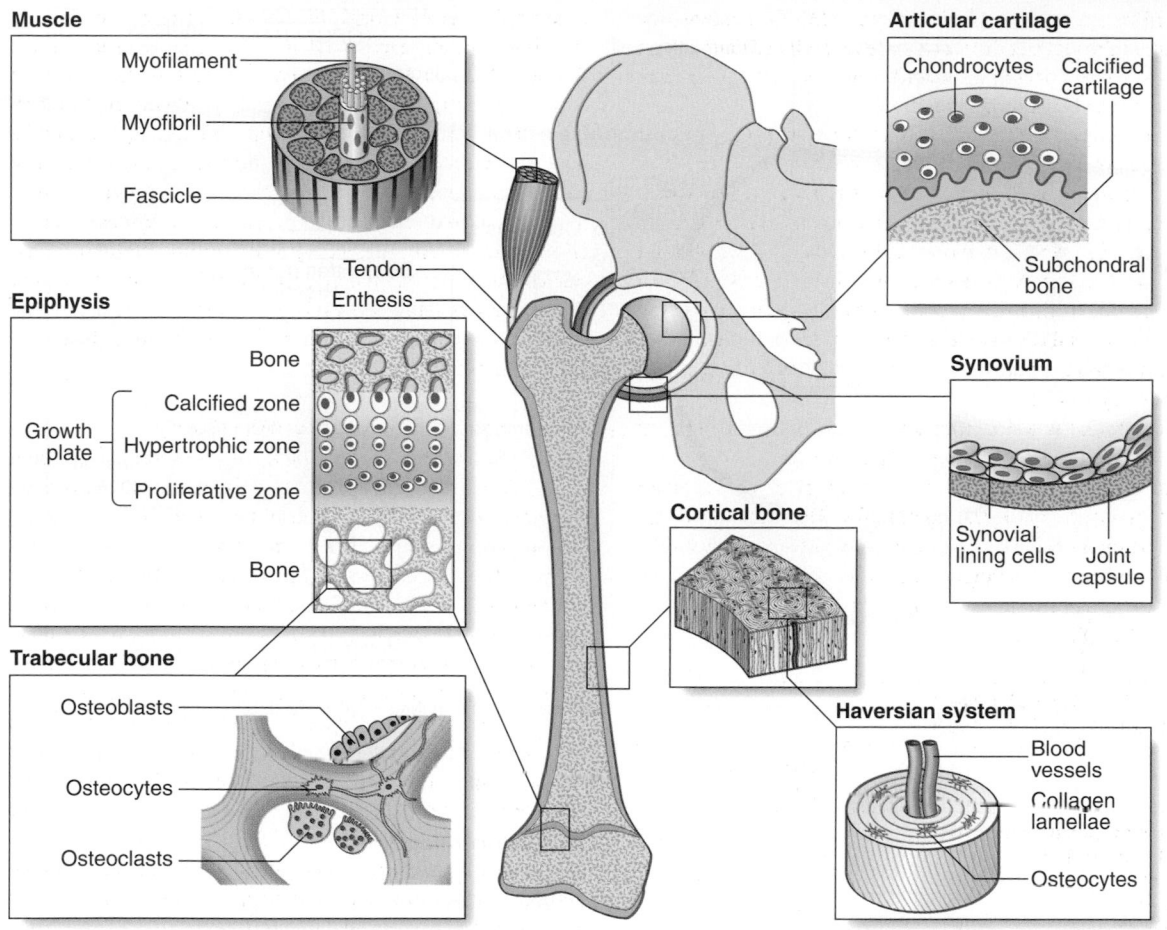

Fig. 25.1   Structure of major musculoskeletal tissues.

Bone remodelling

The skeleton is shaped during growth and repaired during adult life by the process of bone remodelling (Fig. 25.2). The remodelling cycle starts with attraction of osteoclast precursors in peripheral blood to the target site, probably by local release of chemotactic factors from areas of microdamage. The osteoclast precursors differentiate into mature osteoclasts in response to activation of the RANK receptor on their surface by a ligand called RANK ligand (RANKL) which is produced in osteoblasts and bone marrow cells. RANK activation is blocked by osteo-protegerin (OPG), a decoy receptor that inhibits osteoclast formation. Osteoclasts attach via a tight sealing zone to the bone surface and resorb bone by secreting hydrochloric acid and proteolytic enzymes into the space underneath, dissolving mineral and degrading bone matrix. When resorption is complete, osteoclasts undergo programmed cell death and bone formation begins with the attraction of osteoblast precursors to the resorption site. The osteoblast precursors differentiate into mature osteoblasts which deposit new bone matrix in the resorption lacuna, until the hole has been filled. Initially the matrix is uncalcified and is referred to as osteoid, but then becomes mineralised to form mature bone. Calcification of matrix is critically dependent on the enzyme alkaline phosphatase, which is produced by osteoblasts and degrades pyrophosphate—a natural inhibitor of mineralisation. The rate of bone remodelling is regulated by circulating hormones such as parathyroid hormone (PTH) and oestrogen as well as locally produced factors such as cytokines (Box 25.2). Most of these factors exert their effects by modulating local expression of RANK, RANKL or OPG (Fig. 25.2).

25.2 REGULATORS OF BONE REMODELLING			
Factor	Effect on osteoclasts	Effect on osteoblasts	Effect on bone mass
Parathyroid hormone (PTH) 1,25(OH)$_2$D	↑ ↑	↑ ↑	Variable
Interleukin-1 (IL-1) Tumour necrosis factor-α (TNF-α) Thyroid hormone Glucocorticoids	↑ ↑ ↑ ↑	↓ ↓ ↔ ↓	Bone loss
Calcitonin Oestrogen Testosterone Mechanical loading	↓ ↓ ↓ ↓	↔ ↑ ↑ ↑	Bone gain
↑ = stimulates; ↓ = inhibits; ↔ = neutral.			

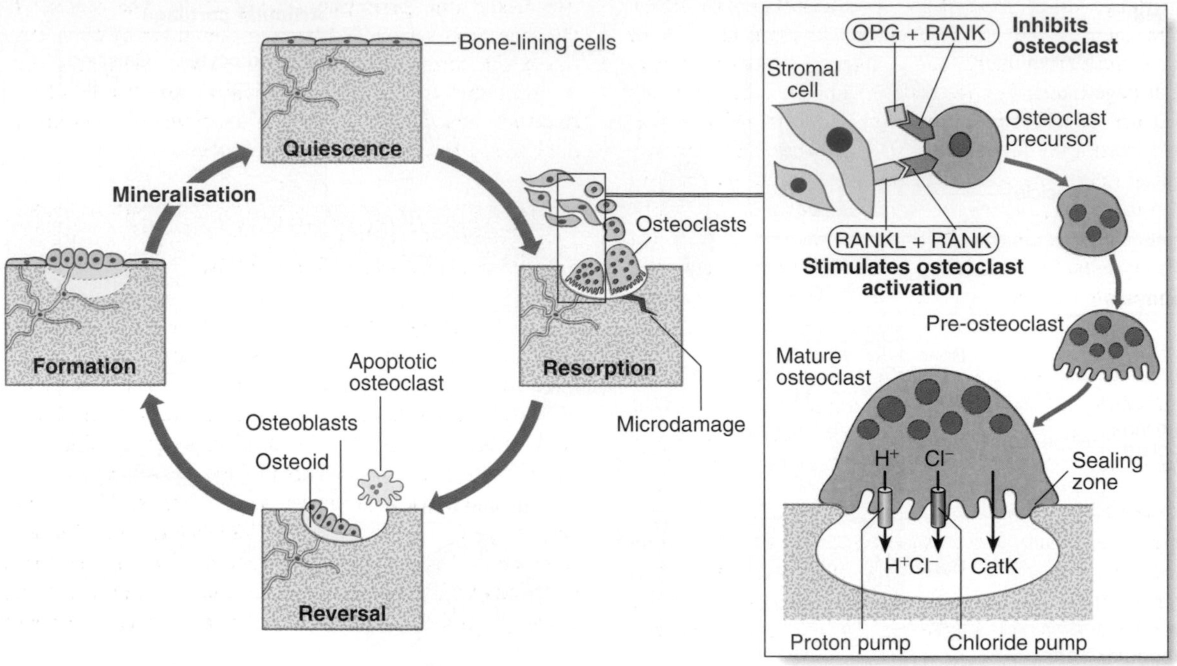

Fig. 25.2 **The bone remodelling cycle.** (RANK = receptor activator of nuclear factor kappa B; RANKL = RANK ligand; OPG = osteoprotegerin; CatK = cathepsin K)

25.3 TYPES OF JOINT		
Type	**Range of movement**	**Examples**
Fibrous	Minimal	Skull sutures
Fibrocartilaginous	Limited	Symphysis pubis Costochondral junctions Intervertebral discs
Synovial	Large	Most limb joints Temporomandibular Costovertebral

JOINTS

Bones are linked by joints. There are three main subtypes (Box 25.3).

Fibrous and fibrocartilaginous joints

These joints comprise a simple bridge of fibrous or fibrocartilaginous tissue joining two bones together where there is little requirement for movement. The intervertebral disc is a special type of fibrocartilaginous joint in which an amorphous area termed the nucleus pulposus lies in the centre of the fibrocartilaginous bridge. This structure has a high water content and acts as a cushion to provide the intervertebral disc with improved shock-absorbing properties.

Synovial joints

Synovial joints are more complex structures containing several cell types and are found where a wide range of movement is required.

Articular cartilage

In synovial joints the bone ends are covered by articular cartilage. This is an avascular tissue consisting of chondrocytes embedded in a meshwork of type II collagen fibrils that extend through a hydrated 'gel' of proteoglycan molecules (Fig. 25.3). The polysaccharide side-chains (keratan and chondroitin sulphates) on the proteoglycan molecules are negatively charged and avidly bind water molecules, so they occupy the maximum possible volume within the restrictive strength of the collagen meshwork, giving articular cartilage excellent shock-absorbing properties.

With ageing, the concentration of chondroitin sulphate decreases, whereas that of keratan sulphate increases, resulting in a reduction in water content and impairment of cartilage's shock-absorbing properties. Age-related changes

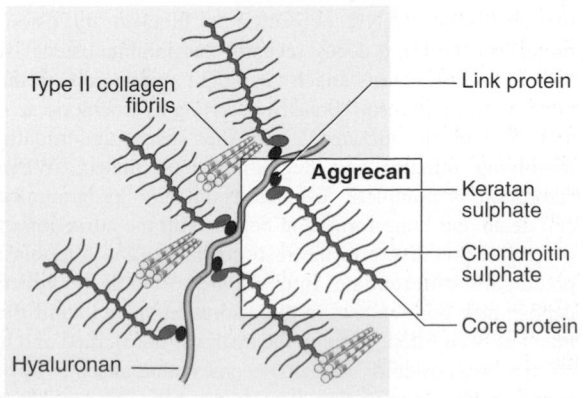

Fig. 25.3 **Ultrastructure of articular cartilage.**

in cartilage differ from those in osteoarthritis (p. 1096), where there is abnormal chondrocyte division, loss of proteoglycan from matrix and an increase in water content.

Cartilage matrix is constantly turning over, but in health a balance is maintained between synthesis and degradation. Cartilage degradation is mediated by enzymes such as matrix metalloproteinases and glycosidases. Pro-inflammatory cytokines such as interleukin-1 (IL-1) and tumour necrosis factor (TNF), which are released during joint inflammation, stimulate production of these enzymes and promote cartilage degradation.

Synovial fluid

The surfaces of articular cartilage are separated by a space filled with synovial fluid, a viscous liquid that lubricates the joint. Synovial fluid is an ultrafiltrate of plasma into which synovial cells secrete hyaluronan and proteoglycans.

Intra-articular discs

Some joints contain fibrocartilaginous discs within the joint space (for example, the menisci of the knee) that act as shock absorbers. Like articular cartilage, these structures are avascular and remain viable by diffusion of oxygen and nutrients from the synovial fluid.

The joint capsule and synovial membrane

The bones of synovial joints are connected by the joint capsule, a fibrous structure richly supplied with blood vessels, nerves and lymphatics that encompasses the joint cavity. Ligaments are discrete, regional thickenings of the joint capsule that act to stabilise joints. The inner surface of the joint capsule is lined by the synovial membrane, which comprises an outer vascular layer and a thin inner layer of synoviocytes. Type A synoviocytes are phagocytic and are responsible for removing particulate matter from the joint cavity; type B cells secrete synovial fluid. Most inflammatory and degenerative joint diseases are associated with thickening of the synovial membrane and infiltration by lymphocytes, polymorphs and macrophages.

Bursae are hollow sacs lined with synovium that contain a small amount of synovial fluid. They help tendons and muscles move smoothly in relation to the bones and other articular structures.

SKELETAL MUSCLE

Skeletal muscle consists of bundles of myocytes, embedded in a fine connective tissue containing nerves and blood vessels. Myocytes are large, elongated, multinucleated cells containing actin and myosin molecules that interdigitate with one another to form the myofibrils that are responsible for muscle contraction. The molecular mechanisms of skeletal muscle contraction are the same as for cardiac muscle (p. 524). Myocytes contain many mitochondria which provide the large amounts of adenosine triphosphate (ATP) necessary for muscle contraction and are rich in the protein myoglobin, which acts as a reservoir for oxygen during contraction, and glycogen, which provides glucose to fuel the mitochondria.

Individual myofibrils are organised into bundles (fasciculi) that are bound together by a thin layer of connec-

tive tissue (the perimysium) (Fig. 25.1). The surface of the muscle is surrounded by a thicker layer of connective tissue, the epimysium, which merges with the perimysium to form the muscle tendon. Tendons are tough, fibrous structures that attach muscles to the point of insertion on the bone surface that is called the enthesis.

INVESTIGATION OF MUSCULOSKELETAL DISEASE

For most MSK conditions clinical enquiry and examination alone give sufficient information for diagnosis and management. Investigations can be helpful in confirming the diagnosis and in assessing activity and progression of disease but few tests are specific. Investigations are an adjunct to, never a substitute for, competent clinical assessment.

The most valuable investigations are synovial fluid analysis and the plain X-ray. Confirmation of clinically assessed inflammatory disease activity and its response to treatment is mainly by the full blood count and either direct or indirect measures of the acute phase response (p. 75).

SYNOVIAL FLUID ANALYSIS

This is the pivotal investigation in patients suspected of having septic arthritis, crystal-associated arthritis and intra-articular bleeding, and it should be performed in all patients with acute monoarthritis, especially with overlying erythema.

Synovial fluid (SF) can readily be obtained from most peripheral joints and for diagnostic purposes only a small volume is required. Normal SF is present in small volume, contains very few cells, is clear and either colourless or pale yellow, and has high viscosity. With increasing joint inflammation the volume increases, the total cell count and proportion of neutrophils rise (causing turbidity), and the viscosity lowers (due to enzymatic degradation of hyaluronan and aggrecan). However, because of considerable variation and overlap between arthropathies these features have little diagnostic value. Frank pus or 'pyarthrosis' results from very high neutrophil counts and is not specific for sepsis. High concentrations of crystals, mainly urate or cholesterol, can make SF appear white.

Non-uniform blood-staining of SF is common, reflecting inconsequential needle trauma to the synovium. Uniform blood-staining—haemarthrosis—commonly accompanies florid synovitis but may also result from a bleeding diathesis, trauma or pigmented villonodular synovitis. A lipid layer floating above blood-stained fluid is diagnostic of intra-articular fracture with release of lipid from the bone marrow.

If sepsis is suspected, SF should be sent for urgent Gram stain and culture in a sterile universal container. If gonococcal sepsis or uncommon organisms are suspected, especially in immunocompromised patients, the microbiologist should be consulted to ensure that optimal cultures are established and that molecular techniques of antigen detection are used if appropriate.

25

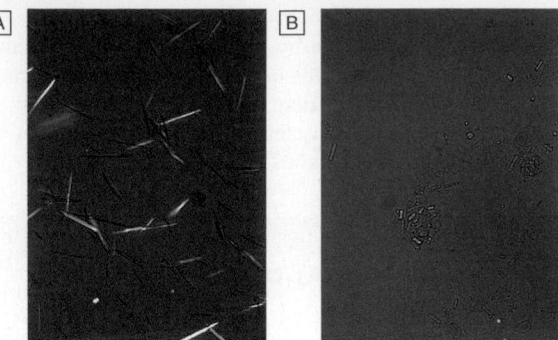

Fig. 25.4 Compensated polarised light microscopy of synovial fluids (× 400). [A] Monosodium urate crystals showing bright birefringence (negative sign) and needle-shaped morphology. [B] Calcium pyrophosphate crystals showing weak birefringence (positive sign), scant numbers and a predominantly rhomboid morphology. These are clearly more difficult to detect than urate crystals.

Identification of common SF crystals is by compensated polarised light microscopy of fresh unrefrigerated SF (to avoid problems of crystal dissolution and post-aspiration crystallisation). Urate crystals are long and needle-shaped and show a strong light intensity with a negative sign of birefringence (Fig. 25.4A). Calcium pyrophosphate crystals are smaller, rhomboid in shape, usually less numerous than urate and have weak intensity and positive birefringence (Fig. 25.4B).

PLAIN RADIOGRAPHY

X-rays can show anatomical changes that reflect important pathological processes, including:

- soft tissue swelling—seen as altered skin contours, displaced fat planes and intracapsular fat pads (fat appears dark on X-ray)
- decreased bone density (osteopenia) or increased bone density (osteosclerosis) which may be localised or generalised
- bone enlargement and deformity

- joint erosion (non-proliferative or proliferative marginal erosion, central erosion)
- joint-space narrowing (focal—osteoarthritis; generalised—inflammatory arthritis)
- new bone formation (osteophyte, enthesophyte, syndesmophyte) and periosteal reaction
- calcification (cartilage—chondrocalcinosis; synovium, capsule, ligament, tendon, muscle, fat, blood vessels, skin) and intra-articular osteochondral bodies.

Although most of these abnormalities have low individual specificity, various combinations of features, together with selective targeting of certain bones and joints (Fig. 25.5), result in characteristic patterns of abnormality and distribution that have high diagnostic specificity.

Choosing plain X-rays

Joints to be X-rayed are usually selected on the basis of localising symptoms and signs. An exception is seronegative spondarthritis where sacroiliac involvement is often asymptomatic and difficult to detect clinically; an antero-posterior (AP) view of the pelvis and a lateral thoracolumbar spine view (i.e. two films) are usually sufficient to show sacroiliitis or syndesmophytes. It is not always necessary to X-ray symptomatic joints. For example, to determine whether a patient with inflammatory polyarthritis has erosions typical of rheumatoid arthritis, postero-anterior (PA) views of hands and feet (i.e. two films), but not X-rays of all symptomatic joints, are appropriate, since rheumatoid erosions appear first in wrists and small joints of hands and feet and may appear first in metatarsophalangeal joints even if they are asymptomatic. However, if the degree of structural damage in one large joint is a cause for concern, an X-ray of that joint will be required.

Erosions

A hallmark of major inflammatory arthropathies is cartilage and bone erosion. Intracapsular bone erosion first occurs at the 'bare areas' of the joint margin ('marginal erosion') where bone is exposed directly to inflammatory synovium without the protection of overlying cartilage. Loss of the sharp cortical line is the first radiographic sign that precedes more definite scalloping of the bony contour (Fig. 25.6).

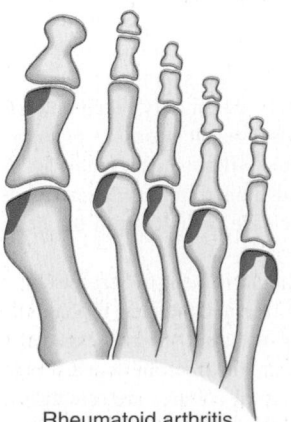
Rheumatoid arthritis

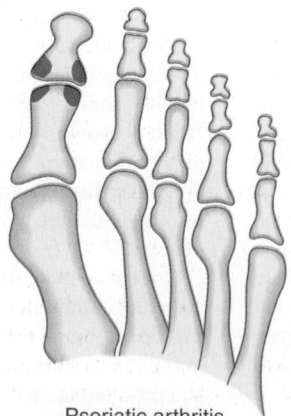
Psoriatic arthritis

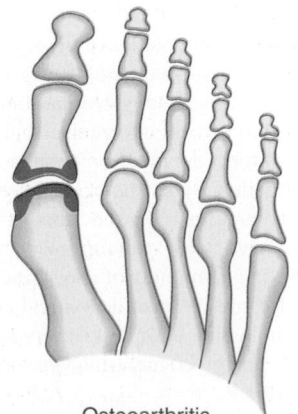
Osteoarthritis

Fig. 25.5 Examples of different target sites of involvement in the forefoot for arthritis.

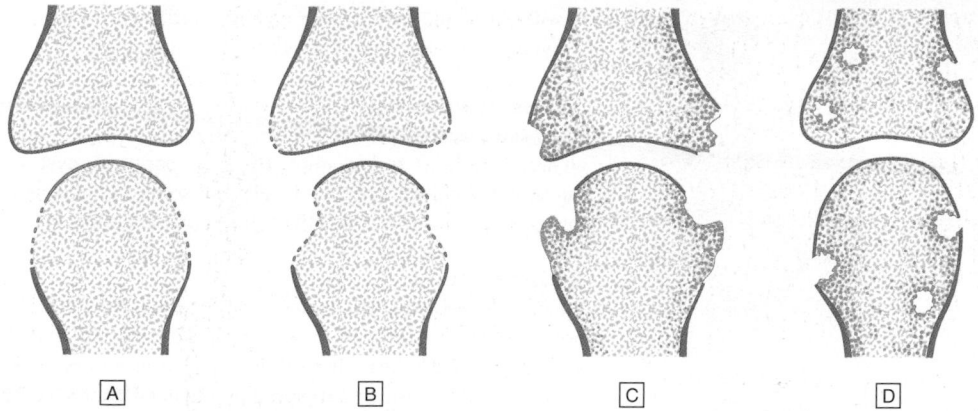

Fig. 25.6   Metacarpophalangeal joint. [A] Early dot-dash erosion of rheumatoid arthritis. [B] Later definite non-proliferative erosion of rheumatoid arthritis. [C] The proliferative erosion of psoriatic arthritis. [D] The intra- and extracapsular 'pressure erosions' of gout.

Cartilage erosion also starts at the margin and slowly works centrally, resulting in relatively late loss of 'joint space'. Both rheumatoid and seronegative spondarthritis (especially psoriatic arthritis) can cause marginal erosions. In rheumatoid arthritis the florid synovitis is not accompanied by any bone or periosteal reaction, resulting in atrophic 'non-proliferative' erosions (Fig. 25.6B), often with juxta-articular osteopenia and soft tissue swelling. By contrast, in seronegative spondarthritis there is often concomitant new bone formation and periosteal reaction with retained bone density, resulting in 'proliferative' erosions (Fig. 25.6C). Accompanying ossifying enthesopathy (enthesophytes) and the targeting of different joints further assist differentiation.

In the first 1–2 weeks of septic arthritis the X-ray is often normal, apart from osteopenia and soft tissue swelling. However, erosion proceeds rapidly and results in generalised loss of joint space with loss of cortical integrity centrally as well as marginally. In chronic gout bony defects develop slowly as massive crystal concretions ('tophi') cause pressure necrosis to surrounding bone. Such 'pressure erosions' (Fig. 25.6D) occur at extracapsular as well as intracapsular sites and are not accompanied by osteopenia.

Osteoarthritis

The two cardinal features of osteoarthritis (OA) are narrowing and osteophyte formation. In contrast to inflammatory arthritis, joint space narrowing in OA is focal not widespread (Fig. 25.7). Bony osteophytes are most noticeable at the joint margins. Subchondral sclerosis (focal increased density of bone), 'cysts' and osteochondral 'loose' bodies within the synovium are additional features, and there is an increased association with chondrocalcinosis. In contrast to inflammatory arthritis, bone density is normal or increased and marginal erosions are not a feature.

Calcification

Calcification of fibrocartilage and hyaline cartilage—chondrocalcinosis—is most commonly due to calcium pyrophosphate crystals or apatite. Calcification at other sites is mainly apatite. Spotty, multiple calcification of soft tissues—calcinosis—mainly targets peripheral and

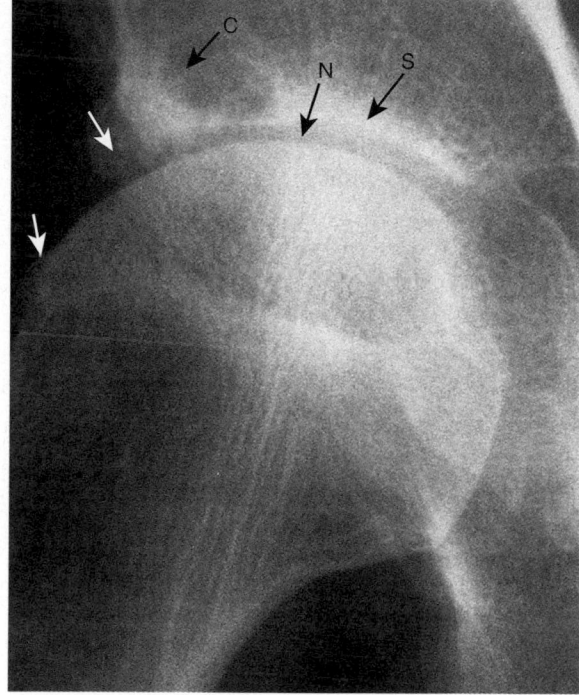

Fig. 25.7   X-ray of hip showing changes of osteoarthritis. Note the superior joint space narrowing (N), subchondral sclerosis (S), marginal osteophytes (O) and cysts (C).

intermediate sites such as finger pulps, wrists and forearms and is a feature of connective tissue disease.

OTHER IMAGING

Radionuclide bone scans

These involve gamma-camera imaging following an intravenous injection of ^{99m}Tc-bisphosphonate. Early post-injection images reflect vascularity and can show increased perfusion of inflamed synovium, Pagetic bone, or primary or secondary bone tumours (Fig. 25.8). Delayed images taken a few hours later reflect bone remodelling as the bisphosphonate localises to sites of active bone turnover.

25

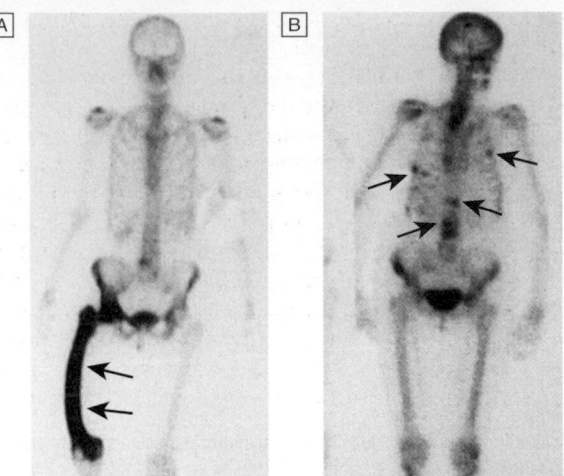

Fig. 25.8 Comparison of bone scan appearances in Paget's disease and metastatic bone disease. [A] Intense homogeneous uptake throughout the affected femur (arrows) in Paget's disease. [B] Patchy focal uptake affecting the spine, ribs (arrows) and skull in metastatic breast cancer.

Scintigraphy has a high sensitivity for detecting important bone and joint pathology that is not apparent on plain X-rays and may be clinically occult, including:

- the presence and extent of Paget's disease of bone
- bone metastases
- bone or joint sepsis
- early osteonecrosis
- bone fractures (including stress fractures)
- reflex sympathetic dystrophy (algodystrophy—p. 1131)
- hypertrophic osteoarthropathy (p. 1143).

Bone mineral density (BMD) measurements

Measurement of BMD plays a central role in the investigation and management of osteoporosis. Dual energy X-ray absorptiometry (DXA or DEXA) is the current method of choice because of its sensitivity and low radiation dose. Further details on the indications for, and interpretation of, BMD measurements are given in the section on osteoporosis (pp. 1122–1124).

Computerised tomography (CT) and magnetic resonance imaging (MRI)

These modalities allow detailed three-dimensional visualisation of anatomically complex structures, such as the spinal canal and facet joints, which may be inadequately assessed by plain X-rays. Drawbacks of CT include limited soft tissue resolution and a high radiation dose, and for many situations MRI is now preferred. MRI is particularly useful to detect and assess:

- early osteonecrosis
- intervertebral disc disease, root entrapment and spinal cord compression
- osteoarticular and soft tissue sepsis
- osteoarticular and soft tissue malignancy
- internal derangement of joints such as the knee

- soft tissue and periarticular pathology (e.g. early synovitis, rotator cuff tears, bursitis, tenosynovitis).

Ultrasonography

This safe, accessible technique can confirm soft tissue changes such as a hip joint effusion, popliteal cyst or thickened Achilles tendon. Limited resolution, however, makes it inferior to CT or MRI for defining anatomy.

Arthrography

Injection of positive (iodinated) or negative (air) contrast, or a combination of both, can help delineate the outline of a joint or bursa. The main use of plain film arthrography is at the knee to demonstrate a ruptured popliteal ('Baker's') cyst as the cause of calf pain and swelling. It may be combined with CT or MRI.

BLOOD TESTS IN RHEUMATIC DISEASES

C-reactive protein (CRP) and erythrocyte sedimentation rate (ESR)

Infections, inflammation and neoplasia all induce an acute phase response which is associated with changes in the full blood count, ESR and CRP (see p. 77 for fuller discussion of interpretation of these tests). Of the many acute phase proteins that react to inflammation and infection, CRP is the single most useful measure because it is the most sensitive and the quickest to respond. A notable exception is in connective tissue diseases such as lupus, systemic sclerosis and dermatomyositis where there is little elevation of CRP despite clear evidence of inflammation and tissue damage. Surprisingly, many patients with these diseases are capable of mounting an acute phase response to sepsis, and elevations of CRP in a patient with lupus or systemic sclerosis suggests an incidental cause such as sepsis rather than disease activation.

Full blood count (FBC)

The FBC may show non-specific changes in MSK diseases (Fig. 25.9). Furthermore, many slow-acting antirheumatic drugs have bone marrow toxicity requiring regular monitoring of the FBC.

Autoantibodies

Autoantibodies are described on page 81. They are important in several MSK disorders. Production of some autoantibodies is a common, age-related phenomenon that may be exaggerated by chronic inflammation. Their mere presence, therefore, often has low diagnostic specificity and little clinical relevance. If present in high concentrations, however, their disease specificity often increases. It is therefore important to know how much antibody is present (the titre or concentration in units) rather than just whether it is detectable, and to interpret the results of the tests in the light of the clinical picture.

Rheumatoid factor (RF)

A rheumatoid factor is an antibody, of any immunoglobulin class, directed against a specific region of the Fc fragment of human IgG. As described on page 81, RF was first identified in patients with rheumatoid arthritis but also

Increased		Decreased

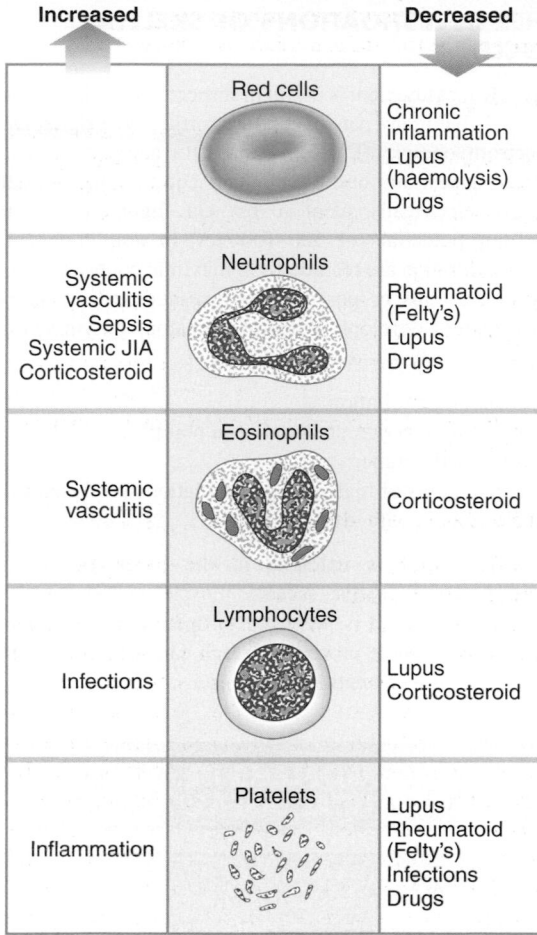

Increased		Decreased
	Red cells	Chronic inflammation Lupus (haemolysis) Drugs
Systemic vasculitis Sepsis Systemic JIA Corticosteroid	Neutrophils	Rheumatoid (Felty's) Lupus Drugs
Systemic vasculitis	Eosinophils	Corticosteroid
Infections	Lymphocytes	Lupus Corticosteroid
Inflammation	Platelets	Lupus Rheumatoid (Felty's) Infections Drugs

Fig. 25.9 Some of the non-specific changes that may occur in individual elements of the full blood count in patients with systemic rheumatic disease. (JIA = juvenile idiopathic arthritis)

occurs in a wide variety of other conditions and in some normal adults (Box 4.15, p. 81). Importantly, RF is not a 'test for rheumatoid arthritis'. Most patients with erosive rheumatoid disease have RF but this may only appear after months or years of disease, once the diagnosis is beyond dispute. It is therefore neither sufficient nor necessary for the diagnosis. Its principal use is as a prognostic marker; a high titre at presentation associates with a poorer prognosis. IgG RF has greater specificity for major rheumatic disease but the above caveats still remain.

Antinuclear antibodies

An antinuclear antibody (ANA) is any autoantibody directed against one or more components of the nucleus (p. 81). As with RF, the higher the titre of ANA, the greater its significance, although a high titre does not necessarily imply more severe disease. The specificity and sensitivity also vary according to the antigen preparation used in the test system and whether the ANA measured is IgG or IgM.

The many causes of a positive ANA are outlined in Box 4.16 (p. 82). The most common reason to test for ANA is if lupus is suspected. For lupus, ANA has high sensitivity (virtually 100%) so a negative ANA virtually excludes the

diagnosis. However, the specificity is low (10–40%) so a positive result does not make the diagnosis.

If a screening ANA test is positive, in most laboratories an attempt is made to establish the specific antigen, although in many cases this cannot be determined. Some antigens are soluble and can be extracted from the nucleus—'extractable nuclear antigens'. Compared to the ANA, antibodies against specific nuclear antigens may have higher specificity for certain diagnoses or for certain patterns of system involvement within the same disease. For example, ANA directed against double-stranded DNA (anti-dsDNA) is highly specific for lupus. Unfortunately, it is present in a minority of patients and those in whom it is positive often have classic severe lupus and a clear clinical diagnosis.

Antibodies to Sm occur in 10% of Caucasian and 30% of black and Chinese patients with lupus. They have high diagnostic specificity and associate with a greater likelihood of renal disease. Antibodies to Ro occur in both lupus and Sjögren's syndrome (in association with anti-La antibodies) and are associated with a high frequency of photosensitive rashes and risk of congenital heart block. Antibodies to ribonuclear protein (RNP) occur in lupus and also in overlap syndromes where features of lupus, myositis and scleroderma coexist (mixed connective tissue disease).

Anti-topoisomerase 1 (also termed Scl-70) is specific for diffuse systemic sclerosis and anti-centromere antibodies are reasonably specific for limited systemic sclerosis.

Antiphospholipid antibodies

These are part of the antiphospholipid syndrome (APS) which is characterised by arterial and venous thromboses, recurrent fetal losses and thrombocytopenia (p. 82). This condition may occur in lupus and other autoimmune diseases (secondary APS) or in isolation (primary APS). However, as described on page 82, antiphospholipid antibodies also occur in a wide variety of rheumatic, infectious (bacterial, viral, protozoal) and malignant conditions, and in these situations they are not usually associated with thromboses.

Biochemical tests

Biochemical tests are mainly of value in the assessment of patients with metabolic bone disease, but are also useful in the investigation of muscle diseases and gout.

Serum levels of uric acid are usually raised in patients with acute gout, but a normal level does not exclude the diagnosis. Moreover, a raised uric acid is not sufficient to make a diagnosis of gout since about 95% of subjects with hyperuricaemia never develop the condition.

Serum creatine kinase (CK) levels are an important investigation in patients suspected of having myopathy or myositis. The skeletal muscle isoform (CK–MM) is much more abundant in health than the cardiac muscle (CK–MB, p. 593) or brain (CK–BB) isoforms. Elevation of CK may result from a variety of causes (Box 25.4) and the specificity and sensitivity for muscle disease are poor. Patients who are clinically suspected of having muscle disease usually require additional investigations such as an electromyogram and muscle biopsy (see below). The normal range of CK in

25

25.4 CAUSES OF AN ELEVATED SERUM CREATINE KINASE

- Inflammatory myositis ± vasculitis
- Muscular dystrophy
- Motor neuron disease
- Alcohol, drugs
- Trauma, strenuous exercise
- Myocardial infarction*
- Hypothyroidism, metabolic myopathy

*In myocardial infarction, the CK-MB cardiac-specific isoform is disproportionately elevated compared with total CK.

some ethnic groups such as Afro-Caribbeans is higher than in Caucasians.

Biochemical investigation of bone metabolism

Several metabolic bone diseases, including Paget's disease, renal bone disease and osteomalacia, give a characteristic pattern of abnormalities on routine biochemical testing (Box 25.5). Other more specific biochemical markers reflect levels of bone resorption and bone formation. The best markers of bone resorption are N-telopeptide and C-telopeptide collagen cross-links (NTX and CTX) which can be measured in blood or urine samples. Bone formation can also be assessed by serum alkaline phosphatase (AP), but this marker is non-specific since elevations can also occur in patients with liver and kidney disease. The amino and carboxyl terminal fragments of procollagen (PINP and PICP), which are released during matrix deposition, are more specific markers of bone formation. These markers can be useful in monitoring the response of osteoporosis to treatment (p. 1126).

BONE BIOPSY

Bone biopsy is helpful in the differential diagnosis of metabolic bone diseases when other less invasive tests have proved inconclusive and is a key investigation in patients who are suspected of having osteomalacia. For systemic bone diseases, the biopsy should be taken using a large diameter (8 mm) trephine needle from the iliac crest under local anaesthesia. In patients with focal lesions, the biopsy should be taken under X-ray control or at open surgery from an affected site. If osteomalacia is suspected, the bone biopsy sample must be processed and examined without decalcification.

OTHER INVESTIGATIONS OF SKELETAL MUSCLE

Serum CK measurement is useful in suspected muscle disease (Box 25.4) but many patients require further investigations.

Electromyography (EMG) measures the action potentials produced at rest and during voluntary contraction. Normal muscle is electrically silent at rest. On slight contraction motor-unit potentials of 500–1000 μV in amplitude and 4–8 ms in duration are recorded. On maximal contraction, as many motor units as possible are recruited and an interference pattern develops. With inflammatory polymyositis the EMG may show a diagnostic triad of:

- spontaneous fibrillation
- short-duration action potentials in a polyphasic disorganised outline
- repetitive bouts of high-voltage oscillations produced by needle contact with diseased muscle.

Muscle biopsy is valuable in the investigation of myopathy and myositis. Needle muscle biopsy of the quadriceps or deltoid is preferred to open surgical biopsy because it is a simple procedure which can be repeated for serial monitoring of treatment response.

PRESENTING PROBLEMS IN MUSCULOSKELETAL DISEASE

JOINT PAIN

ACUTE MONOARTHRITIS

Causes of acute inflammation in a single previously healthy joint are listed in Box 25.6. Consideration of the following features usually suggests the most likely diagnosis:

- *Age and gender of the patient.* Reactive arthritis is the most common cause in young men; gout presents in middle-aged men; pseudogout mainly targets older women.
- *Joint involved.* Almost every joint disease can affect the knee, but classic target sites typical of certain conditions include the first metatarsophalangeal joint (gout); the big toe interphalangeal joint (reactive/ psoriatic arthritis); the elbow and ankle (haemarthrosis, seronegative spondarthrosis); the wrist and shoulder

25.5 BIOCHEMICAL ABNORMALITIES IN VARIOUS BONE DISEASES

	Serum calcium	Serum phosphate	Serum alkaline phosphatase	Serum PTH	Serum 25(OH)D
Osteoporosis	N	N	N	N	N or ↓
Paget's disease	N	N	↑↑	N or ↑	N
Renal osteodystrophy	↓	↑↑	↑	↑↑↑	N
Vitamin D-deficient osteomalacia	N or ↓	N or ↓	↑↑	↑↑	↓
Hypophosphataemic rickets	N	↓↓↓	↑↑	N	N

N = normal.

25

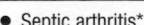

25.6 PRINCIPAL CAUSES OF ACUTE MONOARTHRITIS IN A PREVIOUSLY NORMAL JOINT

- Septic arthritis*
- Crystal synovitis—gout, pseudogout
- Monoarticular presentation of oligo- or polyarthritis
    Reactive, psoriatic or other seronegative spondarthritis
    Erythema nodosum
    Rheumatoid arthritis
    Juvenile idiopathic arthritis*
- Trauma—especially if associated with haemarthrosis
- Haemarthrosis associated with clotting abnormality
- Foreign body reaction (e.g. plant thorn)

* In children sepsis and juvenile idiopathic arthritis are the most common causes, but osteomyelitis and leukaemia may present in this way.

25.8 CAUSES OF CHRONIC SINGLE SITE SYNOVITIS

- Foreign body (e.g. plant thorn)
- Infection, including tuberculosis, fungi
- Chronic sarcoidosis
- Enteropathic arthritis (mainly Crohn's)
- Amyloidosis
- Pigmented villonodular synovitis
- Synovial chondromatosis
- Synovial sarcoma
- Monoarticular presentation of oligo-/polyarticular disease
    Rheumatoid arthritis
    Seronegative spondarthritis
    Juvenile idiopathic arthritis

(pseudogout); and finger joints (psoriasis, plant thorn synovitis).

- *Speed of onset.* Crystal synovitis develops very rapidly, often reaching maximum severity with extreme pain within just 2–12 hours, whereas sepsis is more subacute and continues to progress until treated.
- *Associated periarticular inflammation.* Acute synovitis with surrounding soft tissue swelling and overlying erythema is a classic feature of sepsis and crystals but may also occur with seronegative spondarthritis and erythema nodosum. Haemarthrosis can cause a very tense effusion, often splinting the joint in its loose-pack position, but there is no surrounding swelling or skin change. The combination of small joint synovitis and firm periarticular swelling in a digit—'dactylitis'—is characteristic of psoriasis (fingers, toes) or reactive arthritis (toes).
- *Additional circumstances surrounding the onset of pain.* These include dysentery or new sexual contact preceding reactive arthritis; intercurrent illness or surgery triggering crystal synovitis; clinical features or a family history of psoriasis; and streptococcal sore throat triggering erythema nodosum.

When acute monoarthritis occurs in a joint that is already abnormal the differential diagnosis is altered (Box 25.7). A common situation is an acute flare of inflammation in a single joint of a patient with known rheumatoid disease.

Rheumatoid has a strong negative association with crystal deposition, and disproportionate inflammation in one or even two joints in this situation, especially with overlying erythema, always suggests sepsis.

Investigation of acute monoarthritis varies according to the clinical situation, but aspiration of the joint is required if there is a possibility of sepsis or crystals.

CHRONIC INFLAMMATORY MONOARTHRITIS

Inflammatory monoarthritis that persists for more than 6 weeks may be due to a variety of causes (Box 25.8). The knee is the most common site but almost any joint may be involved. If no cause is apparent by 6 months, or if there are radiographic signs of osteopenia, erosion or periostitis, synovial biopsy is usually undertaken to exclude chronic infection or rare causes that have specific treatments. Retrospective studies suggest that about 25% of cases evolve to OA and about 25% to RA but that 30% remain undiagnosed, especially when the knee is involved.

OLIGOARTHRITIS

Oligo- or pauciarticular disease is arthritis affecting two, three or four joints or joint groups (for example, the wrist or midfoot, which have many joints but are counted as a single site). By far the most common cause is OA, which associates with non-inflammatory symptoms that usually affect just one or a few sites at any one time, even though

25

25.7 COMMON CAUSES OF ACUTE ARTHRITIS IN A PREVIOUSLY ABNORMAL JOINT

Damaged joint

- Pseudogout in association with osteoarthritis
- Bone problem
    Secondary avascular necrosis
    Subchondral collapse or fracture
- Cartilage problem
    Fibrocartilage tear, cartilage debris
- Haemarthrosis
- Septic arthritis

Existing inflammatory disease (with or without damage)

- Septic arthritis
- Exacerbation of underlying disease

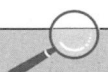

25.9 CAUSES OF INFLAMMATORY OLIGOARTHRITIS

- Seronegative spondarthritis
    Reactive arthritis
    Psoriatic arthritis
    Ankylosing spondylitis
    Enteropathic arthritis
- Erythema nodosum
- Juvenile idiopathic arthritis
- Oligoarticular presentation of polyarthritis
- Infection, including
    Bacterial endocarditis
    Neisseriae
    Mycobacteria

more asymptomatic multiple joint OA may be apparent on examination.

Acute or subacute inflammatory oligoarthritis mainly targets lower limb joints and is usually asymmetrical; it is a common presentation of seronegative spondarthritis (Box 25.9). Sequential joint involvement that ascends a limb—for example, a midfoot, followed by the ankle and then the knee on the same side — always suggests sepsis.

POLYARTHRITIS

Polyarthritis is involvement of five or more joints or joint groups. In determining the cause (Box 25.10) it is helpful to consider whether the polyarthritis:

- is symmetrical (approximately) or asymmetrical
- shows predominant or equal involvement of upper and lower limbs
- shows predominant or equal involvement of large and small joints
- has accompanying periarticular involvement
- has accompanying extra-articular features (Box 25.11).

A large number of viral infections may cause arthralgia (joint pain without abnormal examination findings) and rapid onset of an acute symmetrical inflammatory polyarthritis affecting small and large joints of upper and lower limbs that is usually self-limiting within 6 weeks. These include human erythrovirus 19, hepatitis B and C, mumps, rubella, chickenpox and infectious mononucleosis. The rapidity of onset, the presence of fever and the characteristic rash usually suggest the diagnosis. Arthritis usually

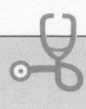

25.11 EXAMPLES OF EXTRA-ARTICULAR FEATURES THAT ASSOCIATE WITH INFLAMMATORY OLIGO- OR POLYARTHRITIS

Clinical feature	Disease association
Skin, nails and mucous membranes	
Psoriasis, nail pitting and dystrophy	Psoriatic arthritis
Raynaud's phenomenon	Lupus, systemic sclerosis
Photosensitivity	Lupus
Livedo reticularis	Lupus
Splinter haemorrhages, nail-fold infarcts	Vasculitis
Oral ulcers	Lupus, reactive arthritis, Behçet's syndrome
Large nodules (mainly extensor surfaces)	Rheumatoid arthritis, gout
Clubbing	Enteropathic arthritis, metastatic lung cancer, endocarditis
Eyes	
Uveitis	Seronegative spondarthritis
Conjunctivitis	Reactive arthritis
Episcleritis, scleritis	Rheumatoid arthritis, vasculitis
Heart, lungs	
Pleuro-pericarditis	Lupus, rheumatoid arthritis
Fibrosing alveolitis	Rheumatoid arthritis, lupus, other connective tissue disease
Abdominal organs	
Hepatosplenomegaly	Rheumatoid arthritis, lupus
Haematuria, proteinuria	Lupus, vasculitis, systemic sclerosis
Urethritis	Reactive arthritis
Fever, lymphadenopathy	Infection, systemic juvenile idiopathic arthritis

precedes jaundice from hepatitis B. Rubella arthritis mainly affects girls and women, occurring 1–7 days after the rash or 2–6 weeks after vaccination. Rubella is exceptional in that, although the symmetrical polyarthritis settles, oligoarthritis may persist for some months.

Polyarthritis that persists for more than 6 weeks is unlikely to be viral (Box 25.10). Certain presenting patterns are characteristic (Fig. 25.10), but a definitive diagnosis may only become apparent as more characteristic features develop with time. RA is by far the most common cause of chronic inflammatory, symmetrical polyarthritis affecting small and large joints of upper and lower limbs. Tenosynovitis and bursitis (i.e. synovial inflammation) are the main periarticular manifestations. Marked asymmetry, lower limb predominance and greater involvement of large joints than of small ones are all more characteristic of seronegative spondarthritis. Concurrence of enthesitis, associated diffuse periarticular swelling and inflammatory spondylitis may be further clinical markers of spondarthritis. Lupus usually causes more arthralgia and wrist extensor tenosynovitis than overt synovitis. Chronic polyarthritis due to gout is invariably preceded by a long history of acute attacks. Other causes of polyarthritis are rare.

A detailed history and examination often reveal the likely diagnosis and direct investigation. For inflammatory polyarthritis present for less than 6 weeks an FBC, liver function tests and viral serology are often appropriate. For early persistent polyarthritis of indeterminate cause appropriate initial investigation should include an FBC,

25.10 CAUSES OF POLYARTHRITIS

Cause	Characteristics
Non-inflammatory	
Generalised osteoarthritis	Very common, symmetrical, small and large joints, Heberden's nodes, only a few joints symptomatic at any one time
Haemochromatosis	Rare, small and large joints
Acromegaly	Rare, mainly large joints, spine
Inflammatory	
Viral arthritis	Very acute, self-limiting
Rheumatoid arthritis	Symmetrical, small and large joints, upper and lower limbs
Seronegative spondarthritis (psoriasis, reactive, ankylosing spondylitis, enteropathic arthropathy)	Asymmetrical, large > small joints, lower > upper limbs, spondylitis
Lupus	Symmetrical, small > large joints, joint damage uncommon
Chronic gout	Distal > proximal joints, preceded by acute attacks
Juvenile idiopathic arthritis	Symmetrical, small and large joints, upper and lower limbs
Chronic sarcoidosis	Symmetrical, small and large joints
Systemic sclerosis and polymyositis	Rare, small and large joints
Hypertrophic osteoarthropathy	Rare, large > small joints, clubbing

25

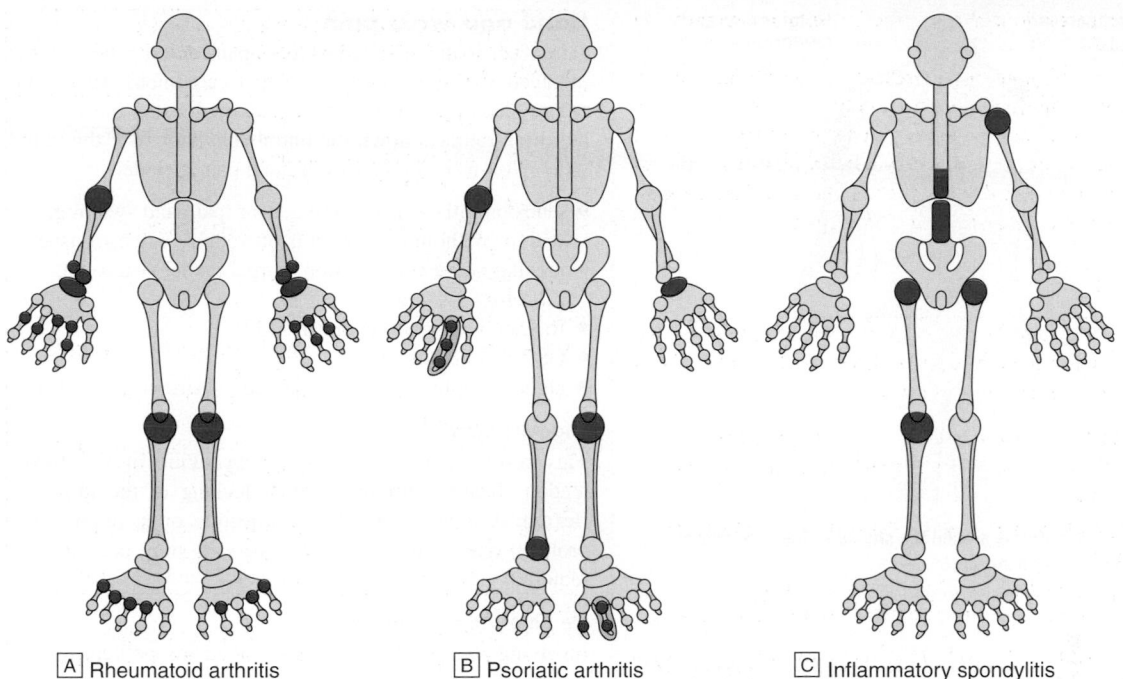

A Rheumatoid arthritis   B Psoriatic arthritis   C Inflammatory spondylitis

Fig. 25.10   Contrasting patterns of involvement in polyarthritis. A Rheumatoid arthritis (symmetrical, small and large joints, upper and lower limbs). B Seronegative psoriatic arthritis (asymmetrical, large > small joints, associated periarticular inflammation giving dactylitis). C Seronegative inflammatory spondylitis (axial involvement, large > small joints, asymmetrical).

ESR, CRP, tests of liver function, rheumatoid factor and antinuclear antibody, and X-rays of hands and feet.

REGIONAL PERIARTICULAR PAIN

SINGLE REGIONAL PAIN

This usually results from an over-usage strain or injury affecting a periarticular structure. The patient can often state the day or week that it started and may be able to name an obvious provoking event or injury. The pain is non-progressive and reproduced by just one or a few movements. Apart from the pain, the patient feels normal. Examination reveals localised periarticular tenderness and no sign or only mild signs of inflammation, and the pain may be reproduced by resisted active movement or by a stress test for the involved structure. Predisposing factors include increasing age, obesity, generalised hypermobility, and occupational and recreational usage.

Muscle injuries usually repair within days, whereas fibrous structures such as tendons and ligaments may take weeks or months to return to normal. The diagnosis is usually made clinically, although imaging, especially ultrasound and MRI, may be required to define the anatomy of more severe or resistant lesions. Management is aimed towards:

- identifying and avoiding, if possible, predisposing or adverse mechanical factors
- pain relief (topical and/or oral analgesics, local injection for severe pain)

25.12 EXAMINATION FINDINGS IN COMMON PERIARTICULAR LESIONS AT THE SHOULDER

Rotator cuff lesion

- Pain reproduced by resisted active movement
  Abduction—supraspinatus
  External rotation—infraspinatus, teres minor
  Internal rotation—subscapularis

Subacromial bursitis

- No pain on resisted active abduction (cf. supraspinatus lesion—the other cause of a painful middle arc)

Bicipital (long head) tendinitis

- Tender over bicipital groove
- Pain reproduced by resisted active wrist supination or elbow flexion

- appropriate exercise and rehabilitation to restore movement and function.

Surgery is only occasionally required for very resistant or disabling lesions.

Shoulder pain

Shoulder pain is a very common MSK complaint in men and women over the age of 40 years, principally due to rotator cuff lesions (Box 25.12). Varying pain patterns of common lesions are shown in Figure 25.11.

Adhesive capsulitis ('frozen shoulder')

This is an ill-understood condition which presents with upper arm pain that progresses over 4–10 weeks before

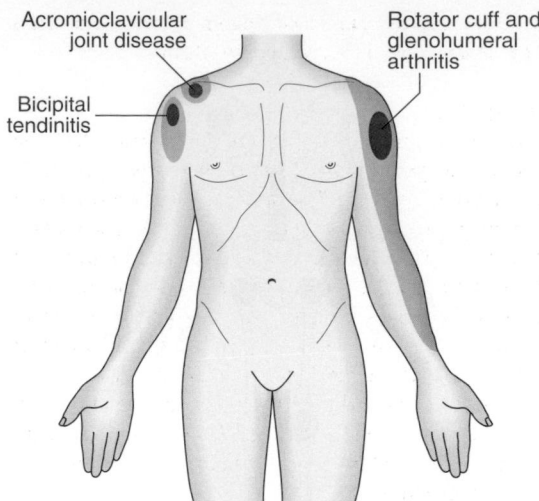

Acromioclavicular joint disease

Bicipital tendinitis

Rotator cuff and glenohumeral arthritis

Fig. 25.11 Pain patterns around the shoulder. The dark shading indicates sites of maximum pain.

receding over a similar time course. Glenohumeral restriction is present from the outset, but progresses and reaches its maximum as the pain is receding. In the early phase there is marked anterior joint/capsular tenderness and stress pain in a capsular pattern; later there is painless restriction, often of all movements. Frozen shoulder is more common in diabetics and may be triggered by a rotator cuff lesion, local trauma, myocardial infarction or hemiplegia. Treatment in the early stage is with analgesics, intra- and extracapsular corticosteroid injection and regular 'pendulum' exercises of the arm to prevent the capsule from over-tightening. Mobilising and strengthening exercises are the sole treatment in the painless 'frozen' stage. The natural history is for slow but complete recovery, the complete cycle sometimes taking as long as 2 years.

Elbow pain

Pain from the three joint compartments is felt maximally at the elbow, close to its origin, with occasional radiation down the forearm. Lateral epicondylitis is the most common periarticular lesion (Box 25.13). Olecranon bursitis can follow local repetitive trauma but infection, gout and RA also commonly affect this bursa.

25.13 PERIARTICULAR LESIONS PRESENTING AS ELBOW PAIN		
Lesion	**Pain**	**Examination findings, tests**
'Tennis elbow'	Lateral epicondyle Radiation to extensor forearm	Tender over epicondyle Pain reproduced by resisted active wrist extension
'Golfer's elbow'	Medial epicondyle Radiation to flexor forearm	Tender over epicondyle Pain reproduced by resisted active wrist flexion
Olecranon bursitis	Olecranon	Fluctuant tender swelling over olecranon

Hand and wrist pain

Joint disease in the hand produces pain well localised to the involved joints. Pain from the first carpometacarpal joint, commonly targeted by OA, is maximal at the thumb base but often radiates down the thumb and back over the radial wrist. Non-articular causes of hand pain include:

- tenosynovitis—flexor or extensor (pain and swelling, with or without fine crepitus on volar or extensor aspect)
- median nerve compression (carpal tunnel syndrome, p. 1248)
- Raynaud's phenomenon (p. 1132)
- C8/T1 radiculopathy
- algodystrophy (reflex sympathetic dystrophy, p. 1131).

Trigger finger

This results from stenosing tenosynovitis in the flexor tendon sheath, with intermittent locking of the finger in flexion. A local corticosteroid injection often relieves the problem and surgical decompression is only occasionally required.

De Quervain's tenosynovitis

Involving the tendon sheaths of abductor pollicis longus and extensor pollicis brevis, this produces pain maximal over the radial aspect of the distal forearm and wrist. There is tenderness (with or without warmth, linear swelling and fine crepitus) over the distal radius and marked pain on forced ulnar deviation of the wrist with the thumb held in the patient's palm (Finkelstein's sign). It is usually caused by repetitive over-usage, but bilateral symptoms may occur with gonococcal infection.

Dupuytren's contracture

This results from fibrosis and contracture of the superficial palmar fascia. Inability to extend the fingers fully is associated with puckering of the skin and the presence of palpable nodules. The ring and little fingers are usually the first and worst affected. It is usually painless and the main symptoms relate to the curled fingers becoming snagged in pockets or poking the eye during face-washing. It is age-related and usually bilateral, strongly predominates in men, and is often familial with a dominant inheritance. Occasional associations include plantar fibromatosis, Peyronie's disease, alcohol misuse and chronic vibration injury. It is very slowly progressive and fasciotomy is seldom necessary.

Hip pain

Hip joint pain is usually maximal deep in the anterior groin, with variable radiation to the buttock, anterolateral thigh, knee or shin (Fig. 25.12). Sacroiliac pain is maximal in the buttock, with radiation down the posterior thigh, worse on standing on that leg.

Trochanteric bursitis is the most common periarticular lesion (Box 25.14). It predominates in older, especially obese, women, occurring either in isolation or secondary to an abnormal gait, e.g. in hip or knee OA.

Hip pain may be referred from other structures. Back pain commonly radiates to the buttock and posterior thigh but the site of maximal pain is close to the spine or pelvic brim. Root entrapment can cause pain in the lateral thigh

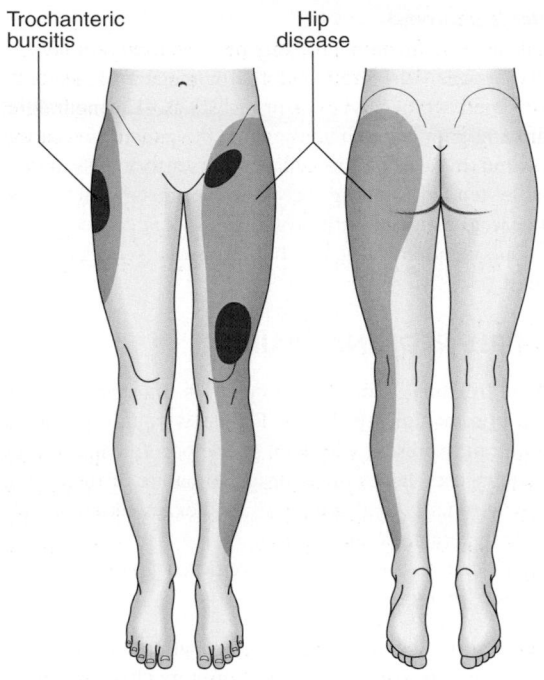

Trochanteric bursitis   Hip disease

Fig. 25.12 Pain patterns of hip disease and trochanteric bursitis. The dark shading indicates sites of maximum pain.

(T12–L1) or the inguinal region and lateral thigh (L2–4) but is worsened by coughing and straining more than by movement, and is often accompanied by sensory disturbance. A psoas abscess, retroperitoneal haemorrhage or pelvic inflammation can cause inguinal and lateral thigh pain that is aggravated by resisted hip flexion.

Knee pain

The knee is a common target site for arthritis but also for trauma and periarticular lesions. Pain arising from the patello-femoral or medial and lateral tibio-femoral compartments due to arthritis or internal derangement is anterior and well localised to the involved compartment. Patello-femoral pain is worse going down and up stairs or inclines. Locking—sudden painful inability to extend fully that often spontaneously unlocks and is followed by aching—reflects a mechanical derangement such as a meniscal tear or osteochondritis dissecans. Referred pain from the hip may present at the knee but is more diffuse and often relieved by rubbing; on examination hip not knee movement reproduces it.

Pain from periarticular lesions is well localised to the involved structure (Box 25.15). Inflammation of any of the three bursae around the patella usually results from repetitive occupational kneeling, but infection and gout may need consideration.

Anterior knee pain syndrome

This is a common problem, especially in adolescent girls. The pain has patello-femoral characteristics and is often aggravated by sports. In a small proportion there is evidence of non-progressive fibrillation of the retro-patellar cartilage ('chondromalacia patellae'). The condition is usually self-limiting and treatment should be conservative.

25

25.14 PERIARTICULAR LESIONS AT THE HIP		
Lesion	**Pain**	**Examination findings, tests**
Trochanteric bursitis	Upper lateral thigh, worse on lying on that side at night	Tender over greater trochanter
Gluteal enthesopathy	Upper lateral thigh, worse on lying on that side at night	Tender over greater trochanter Pain reproduced by resisted active hip abduction
Adductor tendinitis	Upper inner thigh Usually clearly sports-related	Tender over adductor origin/tendon/muscle Pain reproduced by resisted active hip adduction
Ischiogluteal bursitis	Buttock, worse on sitting	Tender over ischial prominence
Iliopectineal bursitis	Anterior groin	Tender (± fluctuant swelling) lateral to femoral pulse, not worsened by internal rotation of hip (cf. hip pain)

25.15 PERIARTICULAR LESIONS AT THE KNEE		
Lesion	**Pain**	**Examination findings, tests**
Pre-patellar bursitis	Anterior patella	Tender fluctuant swelling in front of patella
Superficial and deep infrapatellar bursitis	Anterior knee, inferior to patella	Tender fluctuant swelling in front of (superficial) or behind (deep) patella tendon
Anserine bursitis	Upper medial tibia	Tenderness (± warmth, swelling) over upper medial tibia
Inferior medial collateral ligament enthesopathy	Upper medial tibia	Localised tenderness of upper medial tibia Pain reproduced by valgus stress on mildly flexed knee
Popliteal ('Baker's') cyst	Popliteal fossa	Tender swelling of popliteal fossa, usually reducible by massage with knee in mid-flexion
Patella tendon enthesopathy (Osgood–Schlatter disease)	Anterior upper tibia Mainly energetic adolescents	Tenderness and firm swelling of tibial tubercle Pain on resisted active knee extension

Anterior tibial compartment syndrome

This is characterised by severe pain in the front of the lower leg, aggravated by exercise and relieved by rest. Symptoms result from fascial compression of the muscles in the anterior tibial compartment and may be associated with foot drop. Treatment is urgent surgical decompression.

Foot and ankle pain

Pain arising from articular and periarticular structures is usually well localised. Pain from the ankle joint is felt anteriorly between the two malleoli and is worse on standing or walking. Subtalar pain is mainly posterior between the malleoli and is particularly aggravated by walking on uneven surfaces, requiring eversion/inversion. Periarticular lesions that cause hindfoot pain are listed in Box 25.16.

Midtarsal disease causes pain in the 'bootlace' area, mainly during the late stance and toe-off phase of walking. Loss of the normal arches—pes planus ('flat foot')—may cause pain in the mid-sole. Pes planus is often congenital, but acquired causes include trauma, constitutional hypermobility, RA and neuropathic arthropathy. Medial arch supports in well-fitting shoes and/or intrinsic muscle-strengthening exercises usually relieve symptoms but rigid orthotics may be required for hyperpronated feet, provided the foot is not rigid from fusion of the tarsal bones (tarsal coalition).

Metatarsophalangeal (MTP) joint pain is felt below the metatarsal heads (metatarsalgia) and is often described as 'like walking on marbles'. Hallux valgus deformity with secondary bursitis (bunions) and OA of the first MTP joint often associates with flattening of the transverse metatarsal arch and is a common cause of forefoot pain. It predominates in women as a consequence of wearing narrow high-heeled shoes. Severe restriction of first MTP joint extension (hallux rigidus), usually due to OA, may cause marked pain during attempted toe-off. For both hallux problems, conservative treatment and appropriate footwear usually suffice, although surgery is required for a minority.

Pes cavus ('claw foot')

This is characterised by a high medial arch, secondary clawing of toes and metatarsal callosities. Rarely, it associates with neurological disorders such as Friedreich's ataxia, spina bifida or poliomyelitis. Associated pain is often helped by medial arch supports and metatarsal insoles, and fasciotomy or osteotomy is rarely indicated.

Morton's neuroma

This is an entrapment neuropathy of the interdigital nerves, mostly between the third and fourth metatarsal heads in middle-aged women with ill-fitting shoes. The neuralgic, lancinating pain occurs mainly when the patient is wearing shoes and may associate with local sensory loss and a palpable tender swelling between the metatarsal heads. Footwear adjustment, with or without a local corticosteroid injection, is often sufficient but excision is occasionally required.

MULTIPLE REGIONAL PAIN

Multiple regional 'soft tissue' pain is most commonly due to fibromyalgia (p. 1119). People with this prevalent condition may present with pain at one or a few index sites but enquiry establishes the widespread nature of their pain, often with other typical symptoms, and examination reveals multiple hyperalgesic tender sites.

Other causes of multiple regional pain without arthropathy include:

- *Seronegative spondarthritis.* Enthesopathy may affect several regions prior to the onset of more characteristic features. Chest wall pains, Achilles enthesopathy and plantar fasciitis are particularly common. Clues may lie in the inflammatory component (marked morning stiffness), coexistent back pain and stiffness, preceding uveitis or a strong family history.
- *Generalised hypermobility.* Joint mobility is variable but in general is greater in women than men and in Afro-Caribbeans than in whites, and declines with age. The 10% of adults at the lax end of the spectrum of joint mobility are predisposed to ligament strain, traumatic enthesopathy, mechanical back pain, arthralgia and dislocation (mainly glenohumeral). Such generalised hypermobility is recognised in adults by a modified Beighton score (Box 25.17). Within this 10% are individuals with disease-associated hypermobility such as in Marfan's syndrome, Ehlers–Danlos syndrome and acromegaly.
- *Endocrine disease.* Hyperparathyroidism, hypothyroidism and Addison's disease may all cause ill-defined, widespread pains.
- *Parkinsonism.* This may cause ill-defined regional pain, stiffness and disability. Rigidity, tremor,

25.16 PERIARTICULAR LESIONS CAUSING HINDFOOT PAIN		
Lesion	**Pain**	**Examination findings, tests**
Plantar fasciitis	Under heel, worse on standing and walking	Tender under distal calcaneus/plantar fascia insertion site
Subcalcaneal bursitis	Under heel, worse on standing and walking	Tender under middle of calcaneus
Achilles tendinitis	Localised to tendon	Tender on squeezing tendon, ± swelling of tendon Pain reproduced by standing on toes or resisted plantar flexion
Achilles enthesopathy	Localised to tendon insertion	Tender over insertion site, ± firm swelling Pain reproduced by standing on toes or resisted plantar flexion
Retro-Achilles bursitis	Posterior heel	Tenderness and soft swelling posterior to tendon
Pre-Achilles bursitis	Posterior heel	Tenderness and fluctuant swelling anterior to tendon

25

25.17 RECOGNITION OF GENERALISED HYPERMOBILITY IN ADULTS	
• Extend little finger > 90°	(1 point each side)
• Bring thumb back parallel to/touching forearm	(1 point each side)
• Extend elbow > 10°	(1 point each side)
• Extend knee > 10°	(1 point each side)
• Touch floor with flat of hands, legs straight	(1 point)
Hypermobile = 6 or more out of a possible 9 points.	

25.18 FEATURES OF SIMPLE MECHANICAL LOW BACK PAIN

- Pain varies with physical activity (improved with rest)
- Sudden onset, precipitated by lifting or bending
- Recurrent episodes
- Age 20–55
- Pain limited to back or upper leg
- No clear-cut nerve root distribution
- Systemically well
- Prognosis good (90% recovery at 6 weeks)

bradykinesia and other features are usually apparent (p. 1218).

- *Polymyalgia rheumatica* and *polymyositis*. These may both cause multiple regional symptoms with no clear examination findings. However, marked early morning stiffness and systemic upset are usually prominent.

BACK AND NECK PAIN

LOW BACK PAIN

Back pain is a 'human condition', with 60–80% of the world's population experiencing pain at some time in their lives. Although there is no evidence that back pain prevalence has increased, reported disability and absence from work due to back pain have increased significantly in the last 30 years. In the UK, 7% of the adult population consult their GP each year with back pain, at a cost of £500 million and 80 million working days lost.

Classification and clinical assessment

A minority of patients with back pain have a pathologically definable problem. The main role of history and examination is to identify the small number who have a serious or specific spinal disorder. Initial assessment should categorise the problem as in Figure 25.13.

Mechanical pain

This accounts for more than 90% of back pain episodes, usually affecting patients aged 20–55 years. Onset is often acute, associated with lifting or bending. Mechanical pain is related to activity and is generally relieved by rest (Box 25.18). It is usually confined to the lumbosacral region, buttock or thigh, is asymmetrical, and does not radiate beyond the knee (this implies nerve root irritation). On examination there may be asymmetric local paraspinal muscle spasm and tenderness, and painful restriction of some but not all movements. Back pain precipitated by extension may relate to facet joint hypertrophy or spinal stenosis. Low back pain is more common in heavy manual workers, particularly those in occupations that involve heavy lifting and twisting (e.g. construction, mining, agriculture and nursing). Psychological factors (e.g. job dissatisfaction, depression, anxiety) are important risk factors for both acute back pain and the transition to chronic pain and disability.

Non-mechanical pain

This is constant and has little variation in intensity or with activity. Anorexia, dyspepsia, change in bowel habit, prostatism or abnormal per vaginam bleeding may indicate gastric, pancreatic, colonic, prostatic or gynaecological malignancies respectively. Other 'red flags' for possible serious spinal pathology are indicated in Box 25.19. If there is evidence of a spinal cord or cauda equina lesion, this needs urgent neurosurgical assessment (Box 25.21 below).

Inflammatory pain

Pain due to spondylitis has a more gradual onset and often occurs before the age of 30. It is usually axial and symmetrical and spread over many segments which may include

25

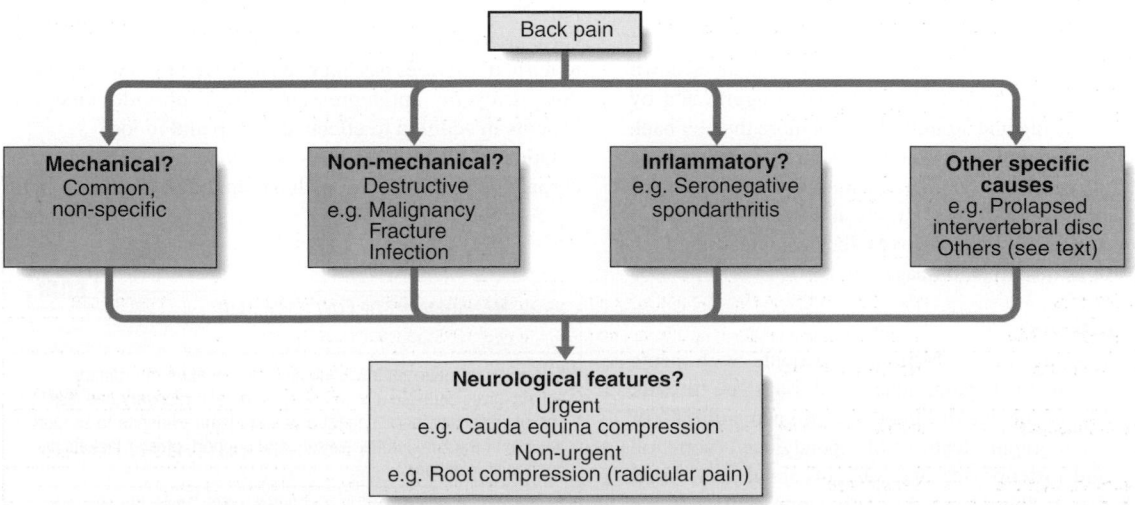

Fig. 25.13 Initial triage assessment of back pain.

25.19 RED FLAGS FOR POSSIBLE SPINAL PATHOLOGY

History

- Age—presentation under age 20 or over age 50
- Character—constant, progressive pain unrelieved by rest
- Location—thoracic pain
- Past medical history—carcinoma, tuberculosis, human immunodeficiency virus (HIV), systemic corticosteroid use
- Constitutional—sweats, malaise, weight loss
- Major trauma

Examination

- Painful spinal deformity
- Severe/symmetrical spinal deformity
- Saddle anaesthesia
- Progressive neurological signs/muscle-wasting
- Multiple levels of root signs

25.20 FEATURES OF NERVE ROOT PAIN

- Unilateral leg pain worse than low back pain
- Pain radiates beyond knee
- Paraesthesia in same distribution
- Nerve irritation signs (reduced straight leg raising which reproduces leg pain)
- Motor, sensory or reflex signs (limited to one nerve root)
- Prognosis reasonable (50% recovery at 6 weeks)

25.21 FEATURES OF CAUDA EQUINA SYNDROME

- Difficulty with micturition
- Loss of anal sphincter tone or faecal incontinence
- Saddle anaesthesia
- Progressive motor weakness/gait disturbance
- Sensory level

25

the thoracic region. Pain from sacroiliitis is maximal in the buttock, with radiation down the posterior thigh. Inflammatory pain associates with marked morning and inactivity stiffness and improves rather than worsens with activity.

Radicular (nerve root) pain

This has a severe, sharp, lancinating quality, radiates down the back of the leg beyond the knee and is aggravated by coughing, sneezing and straining at stool more than by back movement. On examination, there are signs of lumbar nerve root irritation (Box 25.20). Symptoms and signs of compression of multiple nerve roots in the cauda equina are shown in Box 25.21. It is vital to exclude compression of the spinal cord, as described on page 1243.

Investigations

Plain X-rays are rarely helpful in patients with acute mechanical low back pain, unless red flags are present (Box 25.19). By the age of 50, 60% of women and 80% of men have radiographic features of 'spondylosis' (vertebral sclerosis and osteophyte, and OA of apophyseal facet joints). However, there is no clear correlation between these universal degenerative changes and back pain. Similarly,

minor congenital abnormalities, such as spina bifida occulta and transitional vertebrae, are not specifically associated with low back pain.

Plain X-rays may be helpful in persistent pain in a young patient to help confirm a diagnosis of ankylosing spondylitis, and in an older patient to detect vertebral osteoporotic fracture, particularly if there is a history of trauma, prolonged corticosteroid use, height loss or clinical evidence of kyphosis.

If red flags are present, MRI should be undertaken even if plain X-rays are normal. CT is inferior to MRI for assessing soft tissue structures and nerves but is useful for detecting minor abnormalities of bone architecture and in cases where MRI is contraindicated (e.g. pacemaker or metallic clips).

A low haemoglobin and raised CRP or ESR may heighten the clinical suspicion of inflammation or malignancy. A raised acid phosphatase or prostate-specific antigen (PSA) is associated with metastatic carcinoma of the prostate, and raised alkaline phosphatase with other bone metastases and Paget's disease. Myeloma is associated with a monoclonal band on serum immunoelectrophoresis and the presence of urine light chains (Bence Jones proteinuria). EMG and nerve conduction studies, with or without measurement of somatosensory evoked responses, are occasionally required to confirm the localisation of nerve root lesions.

Management

Most episodes of mechanical low back pain settle spontaneously with explanation, reassurance and simple analgesics. After 2 days, 30% are better and at 6 weeks 90% have recovered. Recurrences of pain are common, however, and the 10–15% of patients with acute back pain who develop chronic pain consume 85% of back pain resources.

Patient education is paramount and should emphasise that hurt does not imply harm to the underlying structures and that exercise is helpful not damaging. Regular analgesia and/or non-steroidal anti-inflammatory drugs (NSAIDs) may be required to improve mobility and facilitate exercise. Return to work and normal activity should take place as soon as possible. Bed rest is not helpful and may increase the risk of chronic disability. Referral for physiotherapy (e.g. McKenzie technique of passive extension and postural correction) or manipulation should be considered if a return to normal activities has not been achieved by 6 weeks. Low-dose tricyclic antidepressant drugs provide analgesic benefits in addition to effects on sleep and mood.

Other treatment modalities occasionally used for acute or chronic low back pain include epidural and facet joint

25.22 MANAGEMENT OF LOW BACK PAIN   **EBM**

'For acute or recurrent low back pain continuation of ordinary activity gives equivalent or faster symptomatic recovery and less chronic disability than bed rest and there is no evidence to support the use of traction, lumbar corsets and support, plaster jackets or facet joint injections.'

- Waddell G, et al. Low back pain evidence review. London: Royal College of General Practitioners; 1996.

injection, spinal manipulation, traction and lumbar supports. There is currently no evidence from randomised controlled trials to support these interventions (Box 25.22). Surgery is required in fewer than 1% of patients with low back pain.

The management of serious spinal pathology is dictated by the cause.

SPECIFIC CAUSES OF LOW BACK PAIN

Spondylolysis and spondylolisthesis

Spondylolysis describes a break in the integrity of the neural arch. The principal cause is an acquired defect in pars interarticularis due to a fracture, mainly in gymnasts, dancers and long-distance runners in whom it is an important cause of back pain. Spondylolisthesis is where a defect causes slippage of a vertebra on the one below. This may be congenital, post-traumatic or degenerative. Rarely, it can result from metastatic destruction of the posterior elements.

Uncomplicated spondylolysis does not associate with symptoms but spondylolisthesis can variably associate with low back pain aggravated by standing and walking. More severe cases can result in nerve root compression or a lumbar stenosis syndrome and the vertebral slip is occasionally palpable. Spondylolysis and spondylolisthesis can usually be diagnosed from lateral X-rays of the lumbar spine. MRI may be required if there is nerve root involvement.

Advice on posture and muscle-strengthening exercises are required in mild cases. Surgical fusion is indicated for severe and recurrent low back pain, and surgical decompression is mandatory prior to fusion in patients with significant lumbar stenosis or symptoms of cauda equina compression.

Spinal stenosis

Symptoms of spinal stenosis occur due to limitation of space in the vertebral canal. The most common presentation is 'pseudoclaudication' with discomfort in the legs on walking that is relieved by rest, bending forwards or walking uphill. Patients may adopt a characteristic simian posture, with a forward stoop and slight flexion at the hips and knees. Diagnosis is confirmed by CT/MRI. Decompression is indicated if mobility or quality of life is significantly impaired.

Prolapsed intervertebral disc

Age-related reduction in proteoglycan size within the nucleus pulposus diminishes its viscoelasticity, leading to focal damage and disc herniation. These changes occur most frequently at L4 and L5 due to the increased mechanical forces across this area. Most patients have their first episode between the ages of 20 and 30 years. Presentation is with radicular pain (invariably felt below the knee) in combination with evidence of root involvement (sensory deficit, motor weakness, asymmetrical reflexes) and a positive sciatic or femoral stretch test. About 70% of patients improve by 4 weeks. Persistent neurological deficit at 6 weeks is an indication to consider surgery.

Arachnoiditis

Chronic inflammation of nerve root sheaths in the spinal canal can cause severe low back pain, sometimes combined with nerve root symptoms. Arachnoiditis can complicate meningitis or spinal surgery, but most frequently occurs as a late complication of myelography with oil-based contrast agents. MRI or radiculography can confirm the diagnosis but no satisfactory treatment is available.

Scheuermann's osteochondritis

This disorder predominates in adolescent boys who develop a painless dorsal kyphosis in association with irregular radiographic ossification of the vertebral end plates. Back pain, aggravated by exercise and relieved by rest, may occur if upper lumbar vertebrae are affected, and secondary spondylosis can follow in middle age. Excessive exercise and heavy manual labour before epiphyseal fusion has occurred may aggravate the symptoms. Treatment is avoidance of excessive activity and protective postural exercises. The deformity seldom warrants corrective surgery.

Diffuse idiopathic skeletal hyperostosis (DISH)

DISH ('Forrestier's disease') is a common disorder in the elderly, affecting 10% of men and 8% of women over the age of 65. It associates with obesity, hypertension and type 2 diabetes mellitus (Ch. 21). DISH is characterised by florid new bone formation along the antero-lateral aspect of at least four contiguous vertebral bodies (Fig 25.14). It is distinguished from lumbar spondylosis by the absence of disc space narrowing and marginal vertebral body sclerosis, and from spondylitis by the absence of sacroiliitis or apophyseal joint fusion. It rarely associates with pain and is usually an asymptomatic radiographic finding. Ossifying enthesopathy at peripheral sites may cause pain—for example, under the heel with calcaneal spur formation.

NECK PAIN

Neck pain is less common than back pain as a cause of disability in the working population but is a significant

25

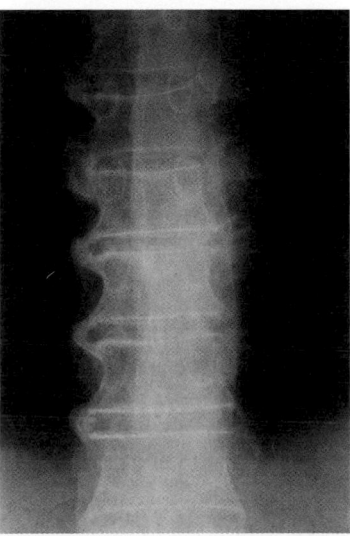

Fig. 25.14 Diffuse idiopathic skeletal hyperostosis (DISH). Antero-posterior X-ray of thoracic spine showing right-sided flowing new bone joining more than four contiguous vertebrae. The disc spaces are preserved.

25.23 CAUSES OF NECK PAIN	
Mechanical	
• Postural	• Disc prolapse
• Whiplash injury	• Cervical spondylosis
Inflammatory	
• Infections	• Rheumatoid arthritis
• Spondylitis	• Polymyalgia rheumatica
• Juvenile idiopathic arthritis	
Metabolic	
• Osteoporosis	• Paget's disease
• Osteomalacia	
Neoplasia	
• Metastases	• Reticuloses
• Myeloma	• Intrathecal tumours
Other	
• Fibromyalgia	• Torticollis
Referred pain	
• Pharynx	• Aortic aneurysm
• Cervical lymph nodes	• Pancoast tumour
• Teeth	• Diaphragm
• Angina pectoris	

problem in the elderly. Neck pain is usually due to mechanical or degenerative problems, although serious spinal disease needs to be excluded using the same principles as for back pain. Most episodes of transient mechanical neck pain are not associated with demonstrable spinal pathology. Other causes of neck pain are listed in Box 25.23.

Pain arising from neck structures is often poorly localised but maximal close to the neck. Pain from upper segments may radiate to the occiput, temple or face, and pain from lower segments to the scapula, shoulder, arm and occasionally chest wall. Mechanical neck pain is often acute in onset and associated with asymmetrical restriction of neck movements and a history of awkward posture or trauma. Radicular pain may arise from compression from osteophyte or disc prolapse. Most prolapse (70%) affects the C6 disc, compressing the C7 root; 20% affects C5. Massive cervical osteophytes or DISH occasionally cause dysphagia due to oesophageal indentation.

The principles of investigation and management are identical to those for low back pain. Surgery is only required when there are neurological signs of radiculopathy or progressive cervical myelopathy (p. 1241).

BONE PAIN

FRACTURE

This section focuses on the varieties of fracture which frequently involve medical as well as surgical management. Fracture is the major clinical manifestation of metabolic bone disease.

• *Fragility fractures* occur spontaneously or as the result of relatively minor trauma; they are typical of osteoporosis.
• *Pathological fractures* occur in bone that is structurally abnormal, such as in Paget's disease, osteomalacia, bone metastases and parathyroid bone disease. Like fragility fractures, they can occur spontaneously or follow minor trauma.
• *High-energy fractures* result from major trauma (e.g. car crash, falls from a height) and can affect normal bones. The same is true of stress (fatigue) fractures in healthy individuals, such as athletes and military recruits, who are exposed to repetitive trauma.

Clinical assessment

Long bone fractures present with acute pain and swelling following trauma. The main differential diagnosis is soft tissue injury, but fracture should be suspected when there is marked pain and swelling, abnormal movement of the affected limb, crepitus or deformity. Femoral neck fractures typically produce a shortened, externally rotated leg that is painful to move. Presentation of vertebral fractures is more variable. Some cause acute severe back pain with radiation to the anterior chest wall, mimicking acute myocardial infarction or pulmonary embolism. Others cause no symptoms or only minor ones, and present insidiously with intermittent back pain and height loss. The differential diagnosis for chronic back pain is potentially wide (pp. 1083–1084), but significant loss of height and acquired kyphosis suggests osteoporotic fracture. Rib fractures often cause pleuritic-type pain that may suggest intrathoracic disease, especially in patients with chronic respiratory disease and corticosteroid-induced osteoporosis. They are characterised by aggravation of the pain with movement, local tenderness and pain on springing the rib cage.

Investigations and management

X-rays of the affected bone should be taken in at least two perpendicular planes and examined for discontinuity of the cortical outline. If the X-rays are normal but clinical suspicion remains high, other imaging may be used—for example, radioisotope bone scans for fatigue fractures or scaphoid fractures, and CT or MRI for fractures of the pelvis or spine. CT or MRI can also help differentiate pathological fractures of the spine due to tumour from fractures due to osteoporosis.

Fractures should be treated by giving adequate pain relief, with opiates if necessary, by reducing the fracture to restore normal anatomy, and by immobilisation to promote healing, either by plaster cast or by fixation. Femoral neck fractures present a special management problem since non-union and avascular necrosis are common complications. This is especially true with intracapsular hip fractures, and in this situation, surgical treatment usually entails replacing the femoral head with a prosthesis. Rehabilitation is as important as reduction and fixation in determining outcome. A supervised exercise programme avoids muscle-wasting and joint stiffness, both of which impair long-term mobility, especially in the elderly. Older patients with hip fracture also benefit from nutritional supplementation during their hospital stay, and this should be instituted routinely.

25.24 CAUSES OF BONE PAIN

- Fracture
- Metastatic bone disease or primary bone tumour
- Paget's disease
- Osteomalacia
- Chronic infection (osteomyelitis)
- Osteonecrosis

Patients with high-energy and fatigue fractures generally require nothing further by way of investigation or treatment once the fracture has healed. Patients with fragility fractures or vertebral fractures should be screened to identify treatable secondary causes such as Paget's disease (p. 1129), osteomalacia (p. 1126), malignant disease and primary hyperparathyroidism (p. 775). Measurements of bone mineral density (BMD) should be undertaken to screen for the presence of osteoporosis (p. 1123).

BONE PAIN WITHOUT FRACTURE

Causes of bone pain are shown in Box 25.24. It is often difficult to differentiate bone pain from the regional pain syndromes associated with other rheumatic diseases. However, in the absence of fracture, bone pain has some characteristic features:

- localised to the affected bone, rather than the joint
- present at rest and worse at night-time
- not clearly worsened by movement or usage (unlike joint or periarticular pain)
- not readily reproduced by joint movement
- focal tenderness on local pressure.

Other features in the enquiry usually point to the most likely cause. For example, slowly but relentlessly progressive pain suggests a destructive disease like malignancy or chronic infection. Malignancy is usually associated with weight loss, fatigue and symptoms relating to the primary site. Pain that is experienced over a wider area of a bone and accompanied by deformity strongly suggests Paget's disease. Osteomalacia is associated with bone tenderness and limb girdle weakness. Pain from osteonecrosis is initially bony and progressive but then may develop superadded features of joint pain (worse on usage or weight-bearing, with or without radiation, reproduced by examination) as the adjacent joint cartilage collapses and the joint is involved (mainly hips, shoulders or elbows). Investigation of bone pain always includes plain X-rays of the symptomatic site and commonly a radioisotope bone scan, with other tests directed by the presumptive diagnosis.

MUSCLE PAIN AND WEAKNESS

Acute muscle weakness can arise from a variety of metabolic, endocrine, infective and neurological causes. It is important to distinguish between a subjective feeling of generalised weakness or fatigue and objective 'true' weakness with loss of muscle power and function. The former is a non-specific manifestation of many organic

25.25 CAUSES OF PROXIMAL MUSCLE PAIN AND WEAKNESS

Inflammatory	
- Polymyositis - Dermatomyositis	- Inclusion body myositis

Endocrine	
- Hypothyroidism - Hyperthyroidism - Osteomalacia	- Cushing's syndrome (usually iatrogenic) - Addison's disease

Metabolic	
- Myophosphorylase deficiency - Phosphofructokinase deficiency - Hypokalaemia	- Carnitine deficiency - Myoadenylate deaminase deficiency

Drugs/toxins	
- Alcohol - Cocaine - Fibrates	- Statins - Penicillamine - Zidovudine

Infections	
- Viral (HIV, cytomegalovirus, rubella, Epstein–Barr, echo) - Bacterial (*Clostridia*, staphylococci, tuberculosis, *Mycoplasma*)	- Parasitic (schistosomiasis, cysticercosis, toxoplasmosis)

diseases and also of psychological distress. Conversely, the diagnosis of muscle disease may be delayed because true weakness is misinterpreted as fatigue. It is also important to distinguish between muscle pain with weakness, and muscle pain with stiffness. The former is associated with intrinsic muscle diseases (Box 25.25). The latter is typical of polymyalgia rheumatica (p. 1139) and may be confused with the symptoms of large joint disease.

Proximal muscle weakness

This usually indicates a proximal myopathy which typically causes difficulty with standing from a seated position, squatting and lifting overhead. Distal power, such as grip, is usually preserved. The causes of proximal myopathy (Box 25.25) are either inflammatory (myositis) or non-inflammatory (due to endocrine or metabolic abnormalities, toxins or infections).

A history of exercise intolerance, with post-exertional cramps (with or without a family history), suggests a metabolic myopathy, the most common being the glycogen storage disorders (p. 442). A strong family history and onset in early adulthood suggest a muscular dystrophy. A drug history is important, notably alcohol, which can cause both an inflammatory myopathy and muscle atrophy. Myopathy can be associated with several viral infections, including HIV, due to either the virus itself or drug therapy with zidovudine.

Distal or generalised weakness

This usually indicates a neurological cause (e.g. motor neuron disease), which is even more likely if there are sensory abnormalities or if the weakness is unilateral or focal. The weakness of myasthenia gravis is characteristically worsened by repeated exertion (fatigability) and improved by rest, and usually involves the ocular muscles.

25

Clinical assessment and investigations

Physical examination should establish the presence, pattern and severity of muscle weakness, graded according to the Medical Research Council (MRC) 1–5 scale. General examination should assess for fasciculation, evidence of endocrine disease, malignancy, arthropathy and connective tissue disease.

The most sensitive biochemical test of muscle injury is CK (p. 1075). A raised level confirms the clinical suspicion of muscle inflammation or necrosis but does not establish the cause. Occasionally, the CK is normal, particularly if muscle changes are focal. Because the differential diagnosis of muscle pain and weakness and raised CK is wide, muscle biopsy and EMG are usually required for a precise diagnosis unless the cause is obvious. Using MRI to identify focal areas of muscle abnormality can increase the diagnostic yield from muscle biopsies. In inflammatory myositis, the typical features are muscle fibre necrosis and regeneration in the presence of focal lymphocytic infiltration. Atrophy of grouped fibres suggests a neuromyopathic cause such as denervation. Atrophy of type 2 fibres is a non-specific finding, and may occur with disuse and corticosteroid therapy as well as with a variety of connective tissue diseases.

Management

This is determined by the underlying cause, and is discussed further in other relevant sections. In all patients with muscle disease, physical therapy to maximise current muscle ability and to improve muscle conditioning may be helpful.

MSK DISEASE PRESENTING AS SYSTEMIC ILLNESS

Systemic illness may be the dominant presenting feature of multisystem MSK disease. The usual presentations are with arthralgia and myalgia in combination with weight loss, night sweats, fever, skin rashes, raised inflammatory markers and abnormal urinalysis.

The differential diagnosis is potentially wide but the most important possibility to consider is sepsis, particularly bacterial endocarditis and meningococcal infection. If the patient is febrile, unwell or hypotensive, empirical broad-spectrum antibiotics should be initiated after appropriate samples have been taken for culture.

The next important group of conditions to consider is systemic vasculitis (p. 1138). This may require urgent treatment prior to full diagnostic confirmation, particularly if there is evidence of critical organ inflammation. Additional symptoms suggesting vasculitis are shown in Box 25.26. Further investigation should include urine microscopy, antineutrophil cytoplasmic antibodies (ANCA, p. 1139) and biopsy of accessible affected organs. Immediate empirical management of vasculitis with critical organ involvement is with 1 g i.v. methylprednisolone on three consecutive days.

A number of other conditions may mimic both sepsis and vasculitis, including disseminated malignancy, lymphoma, atrial myxoma, cholesterol emboli and the antiphospholipid syndrome.

25.26 CLINICAL FEATURES THAT MAY ACCOMPANY MULTISYSTEM MSK DISEASE	
Systemic	
• Malaise • Fever • Night sweats	• Weight loss in combination with arthralgia and myalgia
Rashes	
• Palpable purpura • Pulp infarcts	• Ulceration • Livedo reticularis
Ear, nose and throat	
• Epistaxis • Recurrent sinusitis • Deafness	• Respiratory cough • Haemoptysis • Wheeze (uncontrolled asthma)
Gastrointestinal	
• Mouth ulcers • Diarrhoea	• Abdominal pain (due to mucosal inflammation or enteric ischaemia)
Neurological	
• Sensory or motor neuropathy	

PRINCIPLES OF MANAGEMENT OF MUSCULOSKELETAL DISORDERS

For the majority of MSK conditions the aims of management are to:

• educate the patient
• control pain
• optimise function
• beneficially modify the disease process.

These aims are interrelated and success in one area often benefits the others. Successful management inevitably requires careful assessment of the person as well as his or her MSK system. The management plan needs to be individualised according to:

• the person's daily activity requirements, and work and recreational aspirations
• the person's perceptions and knowledge of his or her condition
• medications and coping strategies already tried by the patient
• comorbid disease and its therapy
• risk factors and associations of the MSK condition (e.g. obesity, muscle weakness, non-restorative sleep).

The wide variety of treatment approaches may require the expertise of a number of health professionals, necessitating a coordinated multidisciplinary team approach for some patients. The patient's symptoms and signs will change with time, and require review and readjustment rather than rigid continuation of a single plan or algorithm.

The principal core interventions that should be considered for every patient with a painful MSK condition are listed in Box 25.27. In addition, there are other non-pharmacological and drug options from which to select, the choice depending largely on the nature and severity of the MSK diagnosis. Simple and safe interventions should be tried first.

25.27 INTERVENTIONS FOR PATIENTS WITH MUSCULOSKELETAL PAIN	
Core	

• Education
• Exercise
   Aerobic conditioning
   Strengthening
	• Reduction of adverse mechanical factors
	   Pacing of activities
	   Appropriate footwear
	• Weight reduction if obese
	• Simple analgesia

Other options	

• Other analgesic drugs
   Oral NSAIDs
   Topical creams
   Opioid analgesics
   Amitriptyline
• Slow-acting antirheumatic drugs
	• Corticosteroids
	• Local injections
	• Physical treatments
	   Heat, cold, aids, appliances
	• Surgery
	• Coping strategies

25.28 EDUCATION IN THE MANAGEMENT OF ARTHRITIS	EBM
'Education results in substantial and prolonged benefits in perceived ability to manage arthritis, pain and psychological well-being.' • Barlow JH, et al. Br J Rheumatol 1998; 37:1315–1319. • Fries JF, et al. J Rheumatol 1997; 24:1378–1383. • Mazzuca SA, et al. Arthritis Rheum 1999; 42:1267–1273.	

NON-PHARMACOLOGICAL INTERVENTIONS

Education

Education can reduce pain and disability, and reduce the health-care costs of many MSK conditions, including OA and RA (Box 25.28). Education of patients and their families/carers can be provided in various ways, including one-to-one discussion with health professionals, written literature, group education classes and interactive computer programs. The mechanisms of benefit are unknown but probably include improved adherence to the management plan.

Exercise

MSK tissues require regular movement for their health. If compromised by disease, it is even more important to maintain movement. Two types of exercise commonly require prescription:

- *Aerobic fitness training* can produce long-term reduction in MSK pain and disability. It improves well-being, encourages restorative sleep and benefits common comorbidity such as obesity, diabetes, chronic heart failure and hypertension.
- *Local strengthening exercise* for muscles that act over compromised joints also reduces pain and disability, with accompanying improvements in the reduced muscle strength, proprioception, coordination and balance that associate with chronic arthritis. 'Small amounts, often' of strengthening exercise are better than protracted episodes performed infrequently.

Reduction of adverse mechanical factors

Excessive impact-loading and adverse repetitive usage of a compromised joint or periarticular tissue can be reduced: for example, by cessation of contact sports or altered use of machinery or tools at the workplace. Simple 'pacing' of activities—dividing physically onerous tasks into shorter segments with brief breaks in between—is relevant to any patient with MSK pain. Use of shock-absorbing footwear with thick soft soles can reduce impact-loading through feet,

knees, hips and back, and improve symptoms at these sites. A walking-stick held on the contralateral side takes weight off a painful hip, knee or foot.

Advice on weight loss if obese

Obesity aggravates pain through increased mechanical strain, and is a risk factor for more rapid progression of joint damage in patients with arthritis. Obese subjects should receive an explanation of the mechanical effects and health implications of their weight and be offered advice on weight loss and maintenance of an appropriate weight (p. 113).

Physical treatments

Local heat, ice packs, wax baths and other local external applications can induce muscle relaxation and temporary relief of symptoms. Hydrotherapy permits muscle relaxation and enhanced movement in a warm, pain-relieving environment without the restraints of gravity and normal load-bearing. Various manipulative techniques may also help improve restricted movement. Such therapies are often combined with education and therapist contact, and this enhances their benefits.

Splints can give temporary rest and support for painful joints and periarticular tissues, and prevent disadvantageous involuntary postures during sleep. Prolonged rest, however, must be avoided. Orthoses are more permanent appliances used to reduce instability and excessive abnormal movement. Examples include working wrist splints, knee orthoses, and iron and T-straps to control ankle instability. Orthoses are particularly suited for severely disabled patients in whom a surgical option is inappropriate, and often need to be custom-made for the individual.

For those with severe disabilities it may be more appropriate to modify the environment around the patient than to try to restore irreversibly damaged joints to normal usage. A variety of simple aids and appliances may transform the lives of disabled patients, permitting dignity and independence in the activities of daily living. Common examples are a raised toilet seat, high rather than low chairs, extended handles on taps, a shower instead of a bath, thick-handled cutlery, and extended 'hands' to pull on tights and socks. Full assessment and advice from an occupational therapist can maximise the benefits from such adaptations.

Coping strategies

These are approaches that help patients to cope better with, and adjust to, their chronic pain and disability. They may be useful at any stage but should be considered particularly for patients with incurable problems who have received all other available treatment. The aim is to increase self-management through self-assessment, information and problem-solving. This involves patients recognising negative but potentially remediable aspects of their psyche (stress, frustration, anger, low self-esteem or prestige) and their situation (e.g. physical, social, financial). These may then be addressed by changes in attitude and behaviour. For example:

- learning yoga and relaxation techniques to reduce stress
- avoiding negative situations or activities that regularly produce stress, and increasing pleasant activities that give satisfaction
- altering beliefs about and perspectives on disease through information and discussion
- learning to reduce or avoid catastrophising and maladaptive pain behaviour
- learning imagery and distraction techniques for pain
- expanding social contact and better utilising social services.

PHARMACOLOGICAL OPTIONS FOR DIRECT SYMPTOM CONTROL

SIMPLE ANALGESIA

Paracetamol (1 g 6–8-hourly) is the oral analgesic of choice because of its efficacy, lack of contraindications or drug interactions, long-term safety, low cost and availability. Paracetamol inhibits prostaglandin synthesis centrally in the brain but has little effect on peripheral production of prostaglandins.

NON-STEROIDAL ANTI-INFLAMMATORY DRUGS (NSAIDS)

These are among the top five most prescribed drugs in many countries. Oral NSAIDs are often effective for the pain and stiffness of inflammatory disease. Long-acting NSAIDs given at night are particularly helpful for marked inflammatory early morning stiffness. NSAIDs may also reduce bone pain due to secondary malignant lesions. For chronic symptoms they may need to be taken for 2–3 weeks before their optimal effect is seen. Although NSAIDs show similar overall efficacy, there is marked variability in individual patient tolerance and response; patients who do not respond to one may still experience symptom relief from another.

Mechanism of action

As shown in Figure 25.15, NSAIDs reduce prostaglandin levels by inhibiting cyclo-oxygenases (COX). There are two isoforms of COX, encoded by distinct genes. COX-1 is constitutively expressed and functions largely as a 'house-keeping' enzyme in tissues such as the gastric mucosa, platelets and kidneys. In contrast, the 'inflammatory' enzyme COX-2, although constitutively expressed in some tissues (brain, ovary, uterus, cartilage, bone, kidney), is largely induced at sites of inflammation, producing prostaglandins that are involved in peripheral inflammation and pain. In response to inflammation COX-2 is also upregulated in the central nervous system, where it mediates

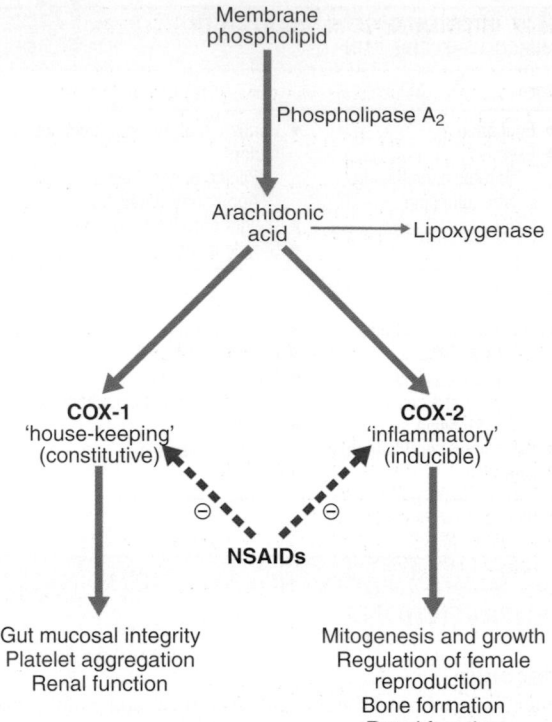

Fig. 25.15 COX-1 and COX-2 pathways.

pain and production of fever. Although NSAIDs inhibit both COX enzymes, COX-2 inhibition is largely responsible for their analgesic, anti-inflammatory and antipyretic effects. Whilst NSAIDs have 'anti-inflammatory' activity they do not reduce peripheral cytokine production, acute phase reactants or ESR.

Side-effects

Gastric ulceration and bleeding

The major drawback of NSAIDs is gastrointestinal toxicity. Prostaglandins of the E series play a major role in gastro-duodenal defence mechanisms. By depleting mucosal prostaglandin levels, aspirin and NSAIDs impair this 'cytoprotection', resulting in mucosal injury, erosions and ulceration. NSAIDs are an important aetiological factor in up to 30% of gastric ulcers. These drugs also reduce the integrity of the duodenal mucosa but are probably responsible for only a small proportion of duodenal ulcers. They greatly increase the risk of bleeding or perforation from pre-existing gastric and duodenal ulcers.

The magnitude of the risk is appreciable, as shown in Box 25.29. Dyspepsia is no guide to the presence of NSAID-associated ulceration or to the risk of complications. Principal risk factors for NSAID-associated bleeding and perforation are shown in Box 25.30, the most important being ageing and previous history of peptic ulceration. The main risk of dying from bleeding or perforation is in the elderly and in those with comorbidity, especially cardiovascular disease. Co-prescription of omeprazole (20 mg daily) or misoprostol (200 µg 8–12-hourly) can reduce the incidence of NSAID-associated ulceration and complications, but H_2-antagonists are ineffective in this respect (Box 25.31).

25.29 IMPACT OF NSAID-INDUCED GASTRIC BLEEDING

- Endoscopic evidence of peptic ulceration is found in 20% of NSAID users even in the absence of symptoms
- ~1% of patients with RA or OA are hospitalised each year with gastrointestinal bleeding
- Annual mortality ~16 000 people in the US and 2000 in the UK (i.e. higher than deaths from diseases such as myeloma, asthma, cervical cancer or Hodgkin lymphoma)

25.30 RISK FACTORS FOR NSAID-INDUCED ULCERS

- Age > 60 years
- Past history of peptic ulcer
- Past history of adverse event with NSAIDs
- Concomitant corticosteroid use
- High-dose or multiple NSAIDs
- Individual NSAID—highest with azapropazone, piroxicam, ketoprofen; lower with ibuprofen

25.31 TREATMENT OF NSAID-INDUCED PEPTIC ULCER
EBM

'Omeprazole is more effective than either misoprostol or ranitidine in healing peptic ulcers in patients taking NSAIDs. Omeprazole also prevents NSAID-induced ulcer formation.'

- Yeomans ND, et al. N Engl J Med 1998; 338:719–726.
- Hawkey CJ, et al. N Engl J Med 1998; 338:727–734.

Management of NSAID-induced ulcer. Where possible, the offending drug should be stopped. If an NSAID must be continued, then one with a lower risk of complications (Box 25.32), e.g. ibuprofen or diclofenac, should be used at the lowest effective dose. Co-prescription of a proton pump inhibitor (e.g. omeprazole 40 mg daily) will heal most, but not all, ulcers.

25.33 RECOMMENDATIONS FOR THE USE OF NSAIDs

- Current use of anticoagulants is a contraindication to NSAID use
- Avoid NSAIDs in the elderly and in those with important comorbidity including heart failure and hypertension
- Start with the lowest dose of one of the safer established NSAIDs (e.g. ibuprofen) and only increase the dose if required
- If an unsatisfactory result is obtained with one NSAID, a trial of another NSAID may be warranted
- Never prescribe more than one NSAID at a time
- Allow a 2–3-week trial to assess efficacy of any particular NSAID or dose
- For a patient with recognised risk factors for gastrointestinal ulceration (Box 25.30) consider co-prescription with omeprazole or misoprostol

Other side-effects of NSAIDs

These include fluid retention (reduced renal filtration rate and sodium excretion, and resistance to antihypertensives and diuretics), non-ulcer-associated dyspepsia, abdominal pain, altered bowel habit and rashes. Interstitial nephritis, asthma and anaphylaxis are rare. There are concerns that long-term NSAIDs may hasten cartilage and bone damage in OA, but human data on this are sparse. Aspirin is unusual amongst NSAIDs in causing irreversible inhibition of COX-1 at doses which are too low to inhibit most COX-2. Low-dose aspirin (75–300 mg daily) is therefore an effective antiplatelet agent. High-dose aspirin is an effective anti-inflammatory, but is poorly tolerated and has been superseded by other NSAIDs for relief of MSK symptoms.

Advice on NSAID prescribing is summarised in Box 25.33.

COX-2 INHIBITORS

Recently, highly selective COX-2 inhibitors without significant COX-1 inhibition have been developed ('coxibs'—e.g. celecoxib). These do not increase the risk of gastroduodenal ulceration. They do, however, have other

25

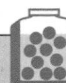

25.32 SOME COMMONLY USED NSAIDs AND THEIR RELATIVE RISK OF GASTRODUODENAL BLEEDING AND PERFORATION

Drug	Daily dose	Doses/day	Idiosyncratic side-effects, comments
Low risk			
Ibuprofen	< 1.6 g	3–4	Weak anti-inflammatory effect at this dose
Etodolac	600 mg	1	Partially selective COX-2 inhibitor
Meloxicam	7.5–15 mg	1	Partially selective COX-2 inhibitor
Nabumetone	500–1500 mg	1–2	Partially selective COX-2 inhibitor
Medium risk			
Ibuprofen	1600–2400 mg	3–4	–
Naproxen	500–1000 mg	1–2	–
Diclofenac	75–100 mg	2–3	Abnormal liver function tests
High risk			
Indometacin	50–200 mg	3–4	High incidence of dyspepsia and CNS side-effects (headache, dizziness, confusion)
Ketoprofen	100–200 mg	2–4	–
Highest risk			
Piroxicam	10–30 mg	1–2	Restricted use, especially in those over 60 years
Azapropazone	1200 mg	2–4	Marked uricosuric action Restricted use, especially in those over 60 years

25.34 USE OF ORAL NSAIDS IN OLD AGE

- **Gastrointestinal complications:** age is a strong risk factor for complications (bleeding, perforation) of NSAID-associated peptic ulceration.
- **Prognosis:** older people, especially those with cardiovascular comorbidity, are more likely to die if they suffer NSAID-associated bleeding or perforation.
- **Other side-effects:** older people are at greater risk of renal and cardiovascular side-effects of NSAIDs (peripheral oedema, cardiac failure).
- **Co-prescription of proton pump inhibitors or misoprostol:** reduces, but does not eliminate, the risk of life-threatening gastrointestinal complications, and is relatively expensive.
- **Paracetamol:** for many, oral paracetamol is as effective as oral NSAID for pain relief. Because of its greater safety and low expense, it remains the oral analgesic of choice.

NSAID side-effects, including cardio-renal effects, and theoretically may increase the risk of thromboembolic events compared to standard NSAIDs (due to inhibition of endothelial COX-2 generation of prostacyclin in the absence of inhibition of platelet COX-1 and aggregation). Indeed, one of the first coxibs, rofecoxib, was withdrawn in 2004 because of data showing increased risk of myocardial infarctions with chronic (2-year) usage, although it remains unclear as to whether this is a class- or drug-specific effect.

NUTRIPHARMACEUTICALS

A wide variety of compounds are available as food supplements and 'health foods' for relief of MSK symptoms. Their rationale for treatment is not always clear, although some, such as glucosamine sulphate and chondroitin sulphate, are normal constituents of cartilage, and others (e.g. selenium, zinc, manganese, copper, and vitamins C, D and E) are trace elements or vitamins required for normal health. Evidence from clinical trials is largely absent, although there are some data that glucosamine, chondroitin and avocado/soya bean may provide a slow onset (after several weeks) of modest pain relief in knee OA, and that regular glucosamine may slow further structural damage. Interest in such apparently safe compounds is growing and large independent clinical trials to determine their efficacy are in progress. Currently, however, these agents remain unlicensed and are available for self-medication only.

TOPICAL AGENTS

NSAID creams and gels and capsaicin (chilli extract; 0.025%) cream are safe and effective for pain relief from arthritis, especially OA, and superficial periarticular lesions affecting hands, elbows and knees. They may be used as monotherapy or as adjunctive treatment with oral analgesics. Topical NSAIDs can penetrate to superficial tissues and even to the joint capsule, though intrasynovial levels mainly reflect blood-borne drug delivery. Topical capsaicin causes pain fibres to discharge substance P. Initial application causes a burning sensation, but continued use 6-hourly reduces substance P activity, with subsequent

pain reduction that is optimal after 1–2 weeks. Topical rubefacients may act through counter-irritation. They often contain several compounds (e.g. nicotinates, camphor, diethylamine, chilli extract) and are mainly available over the counter for self-medication.

OTHER ANALGESICS

Stronger analgesics are sometimes required for moderate to severe pain which is unresponsive to other drug and non-pharmacological approaches. The non-opioid nefopam can help moderate MSK pain, although sympathomimetic and antimuscarinic side-effects (nausea, nervousness, dry mouth) often limit its use. The opioids codeine, dihydrocodeine and dextropropoxyphene are relatively mild analgesics, but when combined with paracetamol may give better analgesia than paracetamol alone. Any benefit, however, is often offset by side-effects such as constipation, headache and confusion, especially in the elderly. Because dependence and tolerance may develop with continuous use, such combinations are mainly reserved for intermittent control of painful 'flares'.

Patients whose pain is resistant to the measures above merit assessment by specialist teams. The centrally acting analgesics tramadol and meptazinol may be useful for temporary, but not long-term, control of severe pain. Both drugs have poor tolerability due to nausea, bowel upset, dizziness and somnolence, and withdrawal symptoms after chronic use. The tricyclic antidepressant amitriptyline can be an effective adjunctive treatment at lower doses (25–75 mg at night) than are used for depression. Amitriptyline is the primary drug treatment for fibromyalgia.

Pain management is discussed further in the palliative care chapter (p. 275).

SLOW-ACTING ANTIRHEUMATIC DRUGS

There are an increasing number of drugs that, like corticosteroids, non-specifically suppress chronic inflammatory disease. In contrast to corticosteroids, these drugs have a delayed action and must be taken for weeks or months before benefit occurs. Their precise mode of action is unclear. Nevertheless, such slow-acting drugs can reduce clinical signs of inflammation and improve or normalise objective parameters of the acute phase response. For some agents there is evidence that a successful response may reduce target tissue damage; hence the alternative name 'disease-modifying antirheumatic drug' (DMARD).

Slow-acting drugs are commonly indicated for rheumatoid arthritis, seronegative spondarthritis, juvenile idiopathic arthritis and connective tissue diseases (Box 25.35). The main indications for use are:

- persistent synovitis (> 6 weeks)
- severe extra-articular disease (e.g. vasculitis, scleritis, renal involvement)
- steroid-sparing effect (e.g. polymyalgia rheumatica resistant to low-dose corticosteroid)
- inflammatory myositis.

25.35 EXAMPLES OF MORE COMMONLY USED SLOW-ACTING ANTIRHEUMATIC DRUGS

Drug	Disease indications	Usual maintenance dose	Principal side-effects	Monitoring requirement	Frequency
Hydroxychloroquine	RA, lupus	200–400 mg/day	Rash, nausea, diarrhoea, headache, corneal deposits, retinopathy (rare)	Visual acuity, Amsler chart, fundoscopy	6–12-monthly
Sulfasalazine	RA, seroneg	2–3 g/day	Nausea, GI upset, rash, hepatitis, neutropenia, pancytopenia (rare)	FBC, LFTs	Monthly for 3 months, then 3-monthly
D-penicillamine	RA	250–750 mg/day	Rash, stomatitis, metallic taste, proteinuria, thrombocytopenia	FBC, urine (protein)	Initially 1–2-weekly; 4–6-weekly for maintenance
Gold	RA	50 mg/month by i.m. injection	Rash, stomatitis, alopecia, proteinuria, thrombocyto-penia, myelosuppression	FBC, urine (protein)	Each injection
Methotrexate	RA, seroneg, lupus, CTD, vasculitis, PMR	5–25 mg/week	GI upset, stomatitis, rash, alopecia, hepatotoxicity, acute pneumonitis	FBC, LFTs	Monthly
Azathioprine	RA, seroneg, lupus, CTD, vasculitis, PMR	50–150 mg/day	GI upset, stomatitis, hepatitis, myelosuppression	FBC, LFTs	Initially weekly, then monthly
Leflunomide	RA	20 mg/day	Nausea, GI upset, rash, alopecia, hepatitis, hypertension	FBC, LFTs, blood pressure	2–4-weekly
Cyclophosphamide	Vasculitis, lupus, myositis	0.5–1 g by i.v. injection, 1–4-weekly	Nausea, GI upset, alopecia, cystitis, myelosuppression, azoospermia, anovulation	FBC, urine (blood)	Each i.v. injection
Chlorambucil	RA	4–8 mg/day	Nausea, GI upset, hepato-toxicity, myelosuppression, azoospermia, anovulation	FBC, LFTs	Monthly
Ciclosporin	RA, psoriasis, lupus	150–300 mg/day	Nausea, GI upset, renal impairment, hypertension	FBC, LFTs, creatinine, blood pressure	2–4-weekly

(RA = rheumatoid arthritis; PMR = polymyalgia rheumatica; seroneg = peripheral arthritis due to seronegative spondarthritis; CTD = connective tissue disease; FBC = full blood count; LFTs = liver function tests)

25

All such drugs require regular monitoring for recognised side-effects and are contraindicated in pregnancy, especially the first trimester. They are mainly used as monotherapy, though certain combinations are increasingly used for RA. Slow-acting drugs are taken in addition to the patient's pain-relieving drugs but, if successful, may reduce analgesic and NSAID requirements.

Hydroxychloroquine

This antimalarial is often effective for mild to moderate lupus, especially when skin or locomotor involvement predominates. It is a relatively weak antirheumatic drug for RA, with a slower than usual onset of action (2–4 months). Despite a wide range of potential side-effects it is usually well tolerated.

Sulfasalazine

This compound has a good benefit-to-risk profile and is often a first-choice agent for RA and for the peripheral (not axial) arthritis of seronegative spondarthritis. Nausea and gastrointestinal intolerance are usually avoided by using enteric-coated tablets, always taken with food, starting with one tablet daily and building up to the full dose over 2 weeks. The patient should be warned of possible orange staining of urine and contact lenses.

D-penicillamine and intramuscular gold

These are no longer first-choice drugs for RA and require specialist supervision because of their high incidence of side-effects (Box 25.35).

Non-specific anti-inflammatory immunosuppressive drugs

Several cytotoxic and immunomodulatory drugs have slow-acting antirheumatic actions at low doses. Their use is mainly limited by toxicity. Because they are immuno-suppressive, they increase risks of bacterial and/or viral (e.g. herpes zoster) infections. Patients receiving such drugs should receive annual influenza vaccine, and pneumococcal vaccine every 5–10 years. In addition, these drugs may compromise immunosurveillance and increase the risk of neoplasia, especially solid tumours and lymphomas. The risk of drug-induced neoplasia appears to be lower in patients with rheumatic disease compared to organ transplant patients, possibly reflecting the lower doses used, and is mainly attributable to cyclophosphamide and chlorambucil.

Methotrexate

Methotrexate inhibits dihydrofolate reductase, interfering with DNA synthesis and cell division and causing cyto-toxicity at high doses. It is often the first-choice slow-acting drug (or second after sulfasalazine or hydroxychloroquine) for the indications shown in Box 25.35. It works relatively quickly, often within 1–2 months. It is usually given as a weekly oral dose starting at 5 mg and increasing in 2.5 mg increments every 3–4 weeks until benefit occurs (maximum 25 mg). It is usually well tolerated but can cause nausea and malaise for 24–48 hours after ingestion. Marrow suppression is rare but hepatotoxicity and hepatic fibrosis may occur, especially at higher doses. Folic acid (5 mg/day) reduces the incidence of adverse effects without reducing efficacy. Patients should be warned of drug interaction with sulphonamides and to avoid excess alcohol, which enhances methotrexate hepatotoxicity. Acute pulmonary toxicity (pneumonitis) is rare but can occur at any time during treatment. Patients should therefore be warned to seek early advice if they develop any new onset of unexplained dry cough, breathlessness or fever. Methotrexate should be stopped immediately and, if pneumonitis is suspected, intravenous high-dose corticosteroids are usually required.

Azathioprine

Following absorption, azathioprine is metabolised to 6-mercaptopurine (6-MP), which is then converted intra-cellularly to active purine thioanalogues which inhibit DNA and RNA biosynthesis. Common adverse effects are nausea, diarrhoea and mouth ulcers; hepatitis and marrow suppression are less common. Since 6-MP requires oxidation by xanthine oxidase before renal excretion, co-administration of allopurinol increases its toxicity; if both drugs are required, azathioprine should be reduced to 25% of the original dose.

Leflunomide

This novel isoxazole inhibits both uridine monophosphate production and tyrosine kinases and is an effective inhibitor of activated lymphocytes. It is currently only indicated for RA. It is given orally as a loading dose for 3 days (100 mg daily), followed by a daily dose of 20 mg. It is usually well tolerated, with low marrow toxicity.

Cyclophosphamide and chlorambucil

These alkylating agents directly bind DNA, RNA and proteins. Both are potentially mutagenic and teratogenic. Cyclophosphamide is the more commonly used. It is inactive until converted by the cytochrome P-450 oxidase system to phosphoramide mustard and acrolein. It may be given daily as tablets (1–2 mg/kg/day) or more commonly, for induction of remission, as 'pulse' intravenous injections (0.5–1.5 g/m^2) weekly or monthly. Common adverse effects include nausea, vomiting, reversible alopecia and suscept-ibility to infection. The incidence of acrolein-related haemorrhagic cystitis is reduced by good hydration and ingestion of mesna. Because of the high risk of azoospermia and anovulation, which may be permanent, pre-treatment sperm or ova collection and storage may need consideration.

Ciclosporin

This is a fungal cyclic polypeptide that blocks resting lymphocytes in the G0 or G1 phase of the cell cycle, inhibiting lymphokine production and release. It is toxic and expensive and usually reserved for patients resistant to other slow-acting agents.

OTHER TREATMENTS

TARGETED ANTICYTOKINE TREATMENT

The pro-inflammatory cytokines tumour necrosis factor alpha (TNF-α) and interleukin-1 (IL-1) play an important role in the pathogenesis of RA and are therefore prime therapeutic targets. Three anti-TNF biological agents are now commercially available. Infliximab is a chimeric human–murine anti-TNF-α monoclonal antibody which is administered by intravenous infusion every 1–2 months. Etanercept is a synthetic human TNF receptor–F$_c$ fusion protein, administered subcutaneously twice weekly. Adalimumab is a human monoclonal antibody to TNF-α administered subcutaneously every 2 weeks. Infliximab, but not etanercept or adalimumab, require co-prescription with methotrexate to reduce immunogenicity; however, all these agents are more effective in combination with methotrexate.

These drugs are more effective than standard DMARDs (with a faster onset of action, greater clinical efficacy and sustained benefit) but because of their cost many countries have set restrictive guidelines for their use. Current UK recommendations are that they should be initiated only in active RA when an adequate trial of at least two other DMARDs (including methotrexate) has failed.

The main potential side-effects are the risk of serious infection, particularly reactivation of latent tuberculosis, which appears to be more likely with infliximab than etanercept. There are theoretical risks of immuno-suppression-related malignancy, particularly lymphoma, but as yet no long-term studies have quantified this risk.

Anakinra is an IL-1 receptor antagonist also licensed for use in RA and is administered subcutaneously. This drug is effective in reducing the symptoms and radiographic damage of RA, but seems less efficacious than anti-TNF therapy. The combination of anti-TNF therapy and IL-1 receptor antagonist treatment has not demonstrated any greater benefit, but has shown an increased incidence of side-effects.

CORTICOSTEROIDS

Glucocorticoids have a rapid and dramatic anti-inflammatory action. However, the doses required to maintain adequate symptomatic relief are accompanied by an unacceptable level of side-effects (p. 784). Furthermore, whether glucocorticoids have any disease-modifying anti-rheumatic activity remains in question. Indications for their use are therefore restricted (Box 25.36). Since the incidence of steroid-related side-effects are largely dose- and duration-dependent, the aim is always to use the smallest amount for the shortest time possible to achieve the therapeutic goal.

In most cases corticosteroid therapy is initiated for rapid control of inflammatory disease at the same time as a slow-acting antirheumatic drug is commenced. After just a few months, when the slow-acting drug is exerting benefit, the steroid is withdrawn. It is usual to gain control with a high

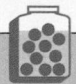

25.36 PRINCIPAL INDICATIONS FOR ORAL OR PARENTERAL CORTICOSTEROID

- For rapid, short-term (1–3 months) control of marked synovitis or systemic inflammation while awaiting efficacy from slow-acting antirheumatic agent
- For life-threatening (e.g. vasculitis) or organ-threatening (e.g. kidney, lung, eye) inflammatory multisystem disease
- For primary treatment of polymyalgia rheumatica
- For control of inflammatory disease during pregnancy

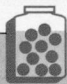

25.37 PRECAUTIONS FOR AVOIDING SEPSIS WITH INTRA-ARTICULAR CORTICOSTEROID INJECTION

- Never inject if the diagnosis is in doubt
- Do not inject if there is local or systemic infection
- Use an aseptic technique—single ampoules, sterile needle and syringe, clean hands, clean skin (alcohol/antiseptic)
- If aspirated fluid is turbid, send it for culture

initial dose of steroid that is then rapidly reduced to the lowest dose that will maintain control.

Prednisolone is the oral steroid of choice. It should be given as a single morning dose usually starting at 10–20 mg daily, although doses up to 60 mg daily may be used in severe disease. The dose can often be reduced after just a few days and the aim is for a maintenance dose of 7.5 mg daily or less, roughly equivalent to endogenous cortisol production. If higher maintenance doses are required, institution of a slow-acting antirheumatic drug should always be considered. Patients receiving oral corticosteroid should be given appropriate prophylaxis against osteoporosis (p. 1121) and should be alert to symptoms of infections or diabetes mellitus. Recommendations for withdrawal of glucocorticoids after long-term use are given on page 785.

Intramuscular injection of methylprednisolone (80–120 mg) may quickly and effectively control inflammation for variable periods (2–6 weeks). Such an approach, repeated if necessary at 3–6-week intervals, may provide equivalent short-term control whilst avoiding some of the problems of daily prednisolone.

LOCAL INJECTIONS

Intra-articular injections

Injection of a long-acting corticosteroid (e.g. triamcinolone acetonide or hexacetonide) may be useful adjunctive therapy for short-term pain relief (OA, inflammatory arthritis) and for temporary control of synovitis of just one or a few joints. The duration of benefit varies according to joint size and the nature and severity of the arthritis, but is in the order of 2–8 weeks. Frequently repeated injections may result in joint tissue atrophy and Cushing's syndrome, and some advise no more than four injections per year into a large joint such as the knee.

Iatrogenic infection is the most important adverse effect, but can be avoided with sensible precautions (Box 25.37). Other unwanted effects include facial flushing 24–72 hours post-injection, local skin atrophy, telangiectasia and permanent fat atrophy due to leakage along the needle track (especially with fluorinated triamcinolone preparations), and post-injection 'flare' with temporary (1–3 days) symptom exacerbation.

In knee OA intra-articular injection of one of several forms of hyaluronan (polymers of hyaluronate), usually given as a course of weekly injections for 3–5 weeks, can give modest pain relief that may be more prolonged (3–6 months) than following a single injection of corticosteroid. Intra-articular injection of radiocolloid (e.g. ^{90}yttrium

silicate for large to medium joints, ^{159}erbium for small joints) can give prolonged control of synovitis ('medical' or 'radiation' synovectomy) but should be avoided in patients under the age of 45. Joints are immobilised for 24–72 hours post-injection to reduce spread to regional lymph nodes. The synovium often recovers with return of synovitis after 1–3 years. Indications include inflammatory synovitis (e.g. rheumatoid) where just one or a few joints are resistant to other measures, synovitis of chronic haemophilic arthropathy, and pigmented villonodular synovitis.

Periarticular injections

Injection of local corticosteroid and/or anaesthetic may give rapid, effective control of pain from periarticular lesions (e.g. bursitis, tenosynovitis, enthesopathy). Such injection will not hasten healing (indeed, corticosteroids may retard healing) but its analgesic effect may extend beyond the natural history of the lesion. The rationale for injection is therefore relief of severe or resistant pain. A non-fluorinated steroid such as hydrocortisone should be used for superficial lesions (e.g. lateral epicondylitis, anserine bursitis) to avoid fat and skin atrophy. If anaesthetic is combined with the steroid, quick relief of pain confirms both the diagnosis and accurate placement of the injection. Injection of steroid into, or even adjacent to, certain tendons (e.g. long head of biceps tendon) can predispose to rupture and should be avoided. Steroid injection may also be used to confirm and give temporary benefit in peripheral nerve entrapment (e.g. carpal tunnel injection for median nerve entrapment at the wrist).

Nerve blocks

Nerve blocks using steroid and/or long-acting anaesthetics may be helpful for control of severe chronic arthritis or periarticular pain resistant to other means (e.g. suprascapular nerve block for severe glenohumeral arthritis or chronic rotator cuff pain). Epidural injections of corticosteroid may also give temporary relief of troublesome root entrapment symptoms.

SURGERY

There are a variety of surgical interventions that may relieve pain and conserve or restore function in patients with joint and periarticular disease (Box 25.38).

Soft tissue release and tenosynovectomy may reduce inflammatory symptoms, improve function, and prevent or retard tendon damage for variable periods, sometimes indefinitely. Synovectomy of joints does not prevent disease progression but may be indicated for pain relief when drugs, physical therapy and intra-articular injections have been

25

25.38 EXAMPLES OF COMMON USEFUL SURGICAL PROCEDURES FOR MSK DISORDERS

Procedure	Indication
Soft tissue release (decompression)	
Carpal tunnel	Median nerve compression
Tarsal tunnel	Posterior tibial nerve entrapment
Flexor tenosynovectomy	Relief of 'trigger' fingers
Ulnar nerve transposition	Ulnar nerve entrapment at elbow
Fasciotomy	Severe Dupuytren's contracture
Tendon repairs and transfers	
Hand extensor tendons	Extensor tendon rupture
Thumb and finger flexor tendons	Flexor tendon rupture
Synovectomy	
Wrist and extensor tendon sheath (+ excision of radial head)	Pain relief and prevention of extensor tendon rupture in RA
Knee synovectomy	Resistant inflammatory synovitis
Osteotomy	
Femoral osteotomy	Early OA of hip
Tibial osteotomy	Unicompartmental knee OA
Deformed tibia in OA	Paget's disease
Excision arthroplasty	
First metatarsophalangeal joint (Keller's procedure)	Painful hallux valgus
Radial head	Painful distal radio-ulnar joint
Lateral end of clavicle	Painful acromioclavicular joint
Metatarsal head	Painful subluxed metatarsophalangeal joints
Joint replacement arthroplasty	
Knee, hip, shoulder, elbow	Painful damaged joints (mainly OA)
	Fractured neck of femur (hemiarthroplasty)
Arthrodesis	
Wrist	Damaged joint—pain relief, improvement of grip
Ankle/subtalar joints	Damaged joint—pain relief, stabilisation of hindfoot

insufficient. Tendon repairs and transfers may also prove useful. The main approaches for damaged joints are osteotomy (cutting bone to alter joint mechanics and load transmission), excision arthroplasty (removing part or all of the joint), joint replacement (insertion of prosthesis in place of the excised joint) and arthrodesis (joint fusion).

The main aims of such operations are pain relief and improvements in function and quality of life. Patient expectations need to be realistic. If surgery is to be successful, the aims and consequences of each operation should be carefully explained and considered as part of an integrated programme of management and rehabilitation. This is often best achieved by multidisciplinary teams of surgeons, allied health professionals and physicians. Assessment of motivation, social support and environment are no less important than careful consideration of patients' general health, their risks for major surgery, the extent of disease in other joints and their ability to mobilise following the operation. In particular, it must be appreciated that for some severely compromised people pain relief and functional independence are better served by provision of a suitable wheelchair, home adjustments, physical aids and social services than by surgery that is technically successful but from which the patient cannot mobilise.

OSTEOARTHRITIS

Osteoarthritis (OA, osteoarthrosis) is by far the most common form of arthritis. It shows a strong association with ageing and is a major cause of pain and disability in the elderly. Pathologically, it may be defined as a condition of synovial joints characterised by focal loss of articular hyaline cartilage with proliferation of new bone and remodelling of joint contour. Inflammation is not a prominent feature. OA preferentially targets only certain small and large joints (Fig. 25.16) but is not a disease or a single condition. It is best viewed as the dynamic repair process of synovial joints that may be triggered by a variety of insults, some but not all of which result in symptomatic 'joint failure'.

Epidemiology

There is a steady rise in prevalence from age 30 such that by 65, 80% of people have radiographic evidence of OA, though only 25–30% are symptomatic. The knee and hip are the principal large joints involved, affecting 10–25% of those aged over 65 years. Even in joints less frequently targeted by OA, such as the elbow, glenohumeral joint or ankle, OA remains the most common cause of arthritis because it is far more prevalent than inflammatory arthropathies.

Risk factors for OA are shown in Figure 25.17. Twin and family studies show that inheritance is a major factor, particularly for hand and generalised OA but also for hip and knee OA, although the responsible genes have yet to be determined. Knee OA is prevalent in all racial groups but hip, hand and generalised OA are only prevalent in Caucasians. OA is more prevalent and more commonly symptomatic in women, except at the hip where men are equally affected. Although overt trauma is a commonly recognised predisposing factor, more subtle repetitive

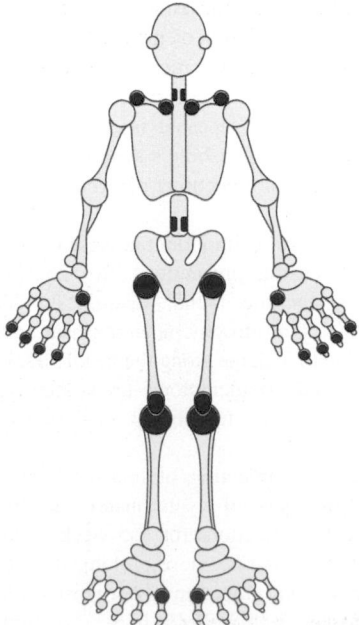

Fig. 25.16 The distribution of osteoarthritis. Although OA can affect any synovial joint, those shown in red are the most commonly targeted.

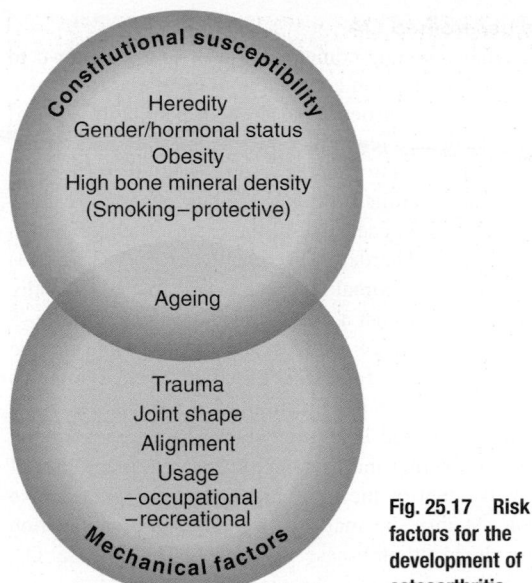

Fig. 25.17 Risk factors for the development of osteoarthritis.

adverse loading of joints during occupation or competitive sports also appears important: for example, in farmers (hip OA), miners (knee OA) and professional footballers (knee OA).

Aetiology and pathogenesis

A variety of mechanical, metabolic, genetic or constitutional insults may damage a synovial joint and trigger the need for repair. Most often the insult remains unclear ('primary' OA) but sometimes there is an obvious cause such as trauma or ligament rupture ('secondary' OA). All the joint tissues (cartilage, bone, synovium, capsule, ligament, muscle) depend on each other for health and function. Insult to any one tissue impacts on the others, resulting in a common OA phenotype affecting the whole joint. The OA process involves dynamic new tissue production and remodelling of joint shape. Often the slow but efficient OA process compensates for the insults, resulting in an anatomically altered but pain-free functioning joint ('compensated' OA). Sometimes, however, because of either overwhelming or chronic insult or an inherently poor repair response, it fails, resulting in progressive tissue damage, more frequent association with symptoms, and presentation as 'joint failure'. Such a perspective readily explains the clinical heterogeneity of OA.

Cartilage changes

These are highly characteristic. There is enzymatic degradation of the major structural components aggrecan and collagen (Fig. 25.3, p. 1070). The chondrocytes increase their production of matrix components and divide to produce nests of metabolically active cells. Although the turnover of aggrecan components is increased, the concentration of aggrecan eventually falls. The decrease in size of the hydrophilic aggrecan molecules increases the water concentration and swelling pressure in cartilage, further disrupting the retaining scaffolding of type II collagen and making the cartilage vulnerable to load-bearing injury. There is eventual fissuring of the cartilage surface ('fibrillation'), development of deep vertical clefts, localised chondrocyte death and decrease in cartilage thickness. Cartilage loss is focal rather than widespread and usually restricted to the maximum load-bearing part of the joint (Fig. 25.18). The changes in OA cartilage encourage deposition of calcium pyrophosphate and apatite crystals.

Bone changes

The bone response immediately below the compromised cartilage increases its trabecular thickness. In some cases this reflects healed trabecular microfractures. Holes ('cysts') often develop, possibly the result of small areas of osteonecrosis caused by the increased pressure in bone as the cartilage fails in its load-transmitting function. At the margins of the joint there is production of new fibrocartilage which then undergoes endochondral ossification to form osteophyte. Despite central and marginal new bone formation, with severe cartilage loss there may be attrition of bone as the two unprotected bone ends wear on each other. Such wear may ablate the trabeculae and lead to a smooth, shiny surface ('eburnation'), often with deep linear grooves. Bone remodelling and cartilage thinning slowly alter the shape of the OA joint, increasing its surface.

25

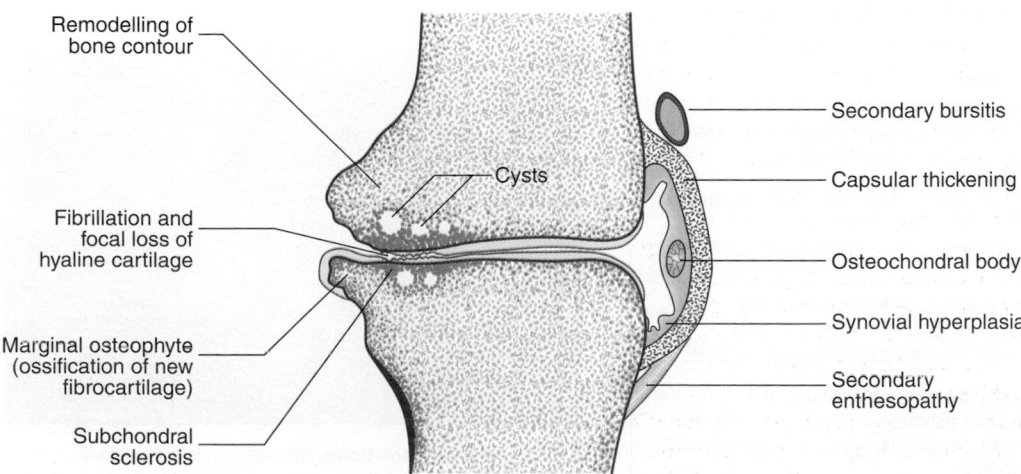

Fig. 25.18 Pathological changes in osteoarthritis.

Other changes

The synovium undergoes variable degrees of hyperplasia. Sometimes histological changes are as florid, though less widespread, as those of RA. Osteochondral bodies commonly occur within the synovium, reflecting chondroid metaplasia or secondary uptake and growth of damaged cartilage fragments. The outer capsule also thickens and contracts, usually retaining the stability of the remodelling joint. The muscles that act over the joint commonly show non-specific type II fibre atrophy.

Clinical features

The main presenting symptoms of OA are pain and functional restriction. Pain may directly relate to the OA process through increased pressure in subchondral bone (mainly causing night pain), trabecular microfractures, capsular distension and low-grade synovitis, or may result from bursitis and enthesopathy secondary to the altered joint mechanics. OA pain typically has the characteristics listed in Box 25.39. For many people functional restriction of the hands, knees or hips is an equal, if not greater, problem than pain. The clinical findings vary according to severity but are principally those of joint damage (Box 25.39).

The correlation between the presence of structural OA (clinical signs, radiographic changes) and pain and disability varies according to site. Correlation is stronger at the hip than the knee, and poor at most small joints. Risk factors for pain and disability may differ from those for structural change. At the knee, for example, reduced quadriceps muscle strength and adverse psychosocial factors (anxiety, depression) correlate more strongly with pain and disability than the degree of radiographic change.

It should be remembered that OA is prevalent in middle-aged and elderly subjects, and commonly asymptomatic. Therefore the presence of OA cannot necessarily be taken as an explanation of the patient's problem.

Nodal generalised OA

Characteristics of this common form of OA are shown in Box 25.40. Presentation is typically in middle-aged women (in their forties or fifties) who develop pain, stiffness and swelling of one or a few finger interphalangeal joints (IPJs). Gradually, over many months, more finger IPJs (distal > proximal) are recruited. Affected joints develop postero-lateral swellings on each side of the extensor tendon which slowly enlarge and harden to become Heberden's (distal IPJ) and Bouchard's (proximal IPJ) nodes (Fig. 25.19). Typically each joint goes through a phase of episodic symptoms (1–5 years) while the node evolves and OA develops in the underlying IPJ. Once fully established, however, symptoms usually subside and hand function often remains relatively unimpaired. Affected IPJs often show characteristic lateral deviation, reflecting the asymmetric focal cartilage loss of OA. Involvement of the first carpometacarpal joint is also common. At this site marked osteophyte and subluxation may result in 'thumb-base squaring'. Thumb-base OA occasionally causes more chronic symptoms and functional impairment than IPJ OA.

Some patients with otherwise typical nodal OA have a more prolonged symptom phase and more overt IPJ inflammation, and subsequently develop IPJ instability in some fingers, with subchondral erosions on X-rays. Such 'erosive' OA is rare and is probably part of the spectrum of nodal OA rather than a distinct subset.

People with nodal OA are at increased risk of OA at other sites ('generalised OA'), especially the knee. Nodal generalised OA has a very strong genetic predisposition, probably the strongest of all major rheumatic conditions.

25.40 CHARACTERISTICS OF NODAL GENERALISED OSTEOARTHRITIS

- Polyarticular finger interphalangeal joint OA
- Heberden's (± Bouchard's) nodes
- Marked female preponderance
- Peak onset in middle age
- Good functional outcome for hands
- Predisposition to OA at other joints, especially knees
- Strong genetic predisposition

25.39 TYPICAL CHARACTERISTICS OF PAIN AND CLINICAL SIGNS OF OSTEOARTHRITIS

Pain

- Patient over age 45 (often over age 60)
- Insidious onset over months or years
- Variable or intermittent over time ('good days, bad days')
- Mainly related to movement and weight-bearing, relieved by rest
- Only brief (< 15 minutes) morning stiffness and brief (< 1 minute) 'gelling' after rest
- Usually only one or a few joints painful (not multiple regional pain)

Clinical signs

- Restricted movement (capsular thickening, blocking by osteophyte)
- Palpable, sometimes audible, coarse crepitus (rough articular surfaces)
- Bony swelling (osteophyte) around joint margins
- Deformity, usually without instability
- Joint-line or periarticular tenderness
- Muscle weakness, wasting
- No or only mild synovitis (effusion, increased warmth)

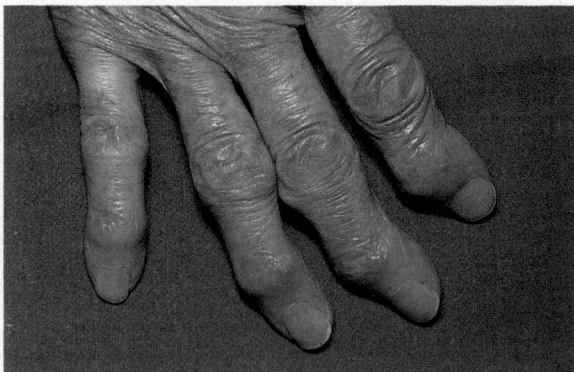

Fig. 25.19 Nodal osteoarthritis. Heberden's nodes and lateral deviation of distal interphalangeal joints, with mild Bouchard's nodes at the proximal interphalangeal joints.

The daughter of an affected mother has approximately a 1 in 3 chance of developing nodal OA herself. Nodal OA with multiple nodes and symptom onset in middle age should not be confused with just one or two asymptomatic nodes related to past trauma, a common finding, particularly in the elderly.

Knee OA

OA principally targets the patello-femoral and medial tibio-femoral compartments of the knee. It may be isolated or occur as part of nodal generalised OA. Trauma is a more important risk factor in men and may result in unilateral OA. Most knee OA, particularly in women, is bilateral and symmetrical.

OA knee pain is usually localised to the anterior or medial aspect of the knee and upper tibia. Patello-femoral pain is usually worse going up and down stairs or inclines. Posterior knee pain suggests a complicating popliteal 'cyst'. Common functional difficulties are prolonged walking, rising from a chair, getting in or out of a car, or bending to put on shoes and socks. Local examination findings may include:

- a jerky, asymmetric 'antalgic' gait—less time weight-bearing on the painful side
- a varus (Fig. 25.20), less commonly valgus, and/or fixed flexion deformity
- joint-line and/or periarticular tenderness (secondary anserine bursitis (Box 25.15, p. 1081) and medial ligament enthesopathy are common, giving tenderness of the upper medial tibia)
- weakness and wasting of the quadriceps muscle
- restricted flexion/extension with coarse crepitus
- bony swelling around the joint line.

Calcium pyrophosphate dihydrate (CPPD) crystal deposition in association with OA is most common at the knee. This may result in a more overt inflammatory component (stiffness, effusions) and superadded acute attacks of synovitis ('pseudogout'—p. 1115), which predicts more rapid radiographic and clinical progression.

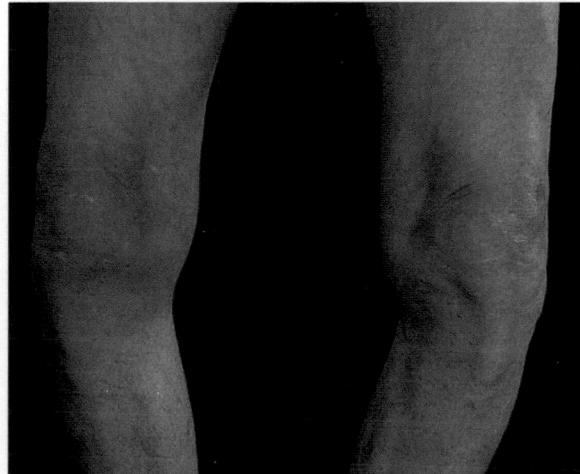

Fig. 25.20 **Typical varus deformity resulting from marked medial tibio-femoral osteoarthritis.**

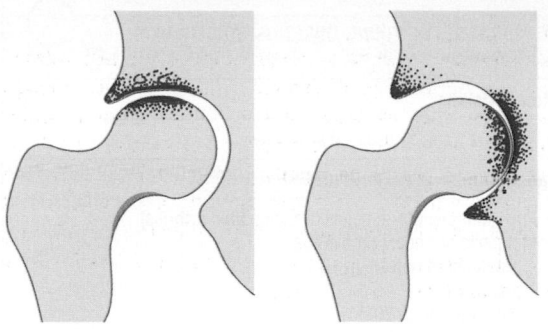

Superior pole osteoarthritis   Medial osteoarthritis

Fig. 25.21 **Patterns of hip osteoarthritis.**

Hip OA

Hip OA most commonly targets the superior aspect of the joint (Fig. 25.21). Such 'superior pole' OA is often unilateral at presentation, often progresses with superolateral migration of the femoral head, and has a poor prognosis. The less common central (medial) OA shows more central cartilage loss and is largely confined to women. It is often bilateral at presentation, may associate with nodal generalised OA, uncommonly progresses with axial femoral migration, and has a better prognosis.

The hip shows the best correlation between symptoms and radiographic change. Hip pain is usually maximal deep in the anterior groin, with variable radiation to the buttock, antero-lateral thigh, knee or shin. Lateral hip pain, worse on lying on that side with tenderness over the greater trochanter, suggests secondary trochanteric bursitis. Common functional difficulties are the same as for knee OA; in addition, restricted hip abduction in women may cause pain on intercourse.

Examination may reveal:

- an antalgic gait
- weakness and wasting of quadriceps and gluteal muscles
- pain and restriction of internal rotation with the hip flexed—the earliest and most sensitive sign of hip OA; other movements may subsequently be restricted and painful
- anterior groin tenderness just lateral to the femoral pulse
- fixed flexion, external rotation deformity of the hip
- ipsilateral leg shortening with severe joint attrition and superior femoral migration.

Although obesity is not a major risk factor for development of hip OA, it is a risk factor for its more rapid progression.

Young-onset OA

Unusually, patients present with typical symptoms and clinical signs of OA before the age of 45. In most cases they have OA at a single joint such as the knee and a clear explanation of previous overt trauma. However, in people with apparently young-onset OA affecting several or many joints, especially those not normally targeted by OA, rare causes need to be considered (Box 20.41). Patients with endemic OA, due to unknown environmental cartilage toxins, will have grown up in just a few specific areas of the

25.41 CAUSES OF YOUNG-ONSET OSTEOARTHRITIS (< 45 YEARS)
Monoarticular
• Previous trauma, localised instability
Pauciarticular or polyarticular

• Prior joint disease (e.g. juvenile idiopathic arthritis)
• Metabolic or endocrine disease
    Haemochromatosis (p. 974)
    Ochronosis
    Acromegaly (p. 801)
• (Spondylo-)epiphyseal dysplasia
• Late avascular necrosis
• Neuropathic joint
• Endemic OA

world: for example, eastern Russia and northern China ('Kashin–Beck disease').

Investigations
A plain X-ray is usually the only useful investigation. This may show one or more of the typical features of OA described on page 1073 (Fig. 25.7). The main use of an X-ray is to assess severity of structural change, an issue if surgery is being considered. Although a non-weight-bearing PA view of the pelvis is adequate for assessment of hip OA, standing (stressed) AP X-rays are needed to assess tibio-femoral cartilage loss, and a flexed skyline view is best for patello-femoral OA.

OA does not trigger the acute phase response and therefore has no impact on the FBC, ESR or CRP. Synovial fluid aspirated from OA knees shows variable characteristics but is predominantly viscous with low turbidity; CPPD crystals may be identified in up to 50% of knee OA fluids. Radioisotope bone scans performed for other reasons often show, as an incidental finding, discrete increased uptake in OA joints due to bone remodelling.

Unexplained young-onset OA requires additional investigation. X-rays are often helpful—for example, in showing typical features of dysplasia or avascular necrosis, widening of joint spaces in acromegaly (p. 801), multiple cysts and chondrocalcinosis in haemochromatosis (p. 974), or disorganised architecture in neuropathic joints. Other tests are guided by the suspected underlying condition.

Management
Treatment follows the principles on pages 1088–1092 and 1095–1096 and always requires:

- *Full explanation of the nature of OA* (with or without support literature). This should include relevant risk factors (e.g. obesity, heredity, trauma); the fact that established structural changes are permanent but that pain and function can improve; discussion of prognosis (good for hand OA, more optimistic for knee than hip OA); and the fact that appropriate action can improve the prognosis of large joint OA.
- *Advice and instruction on appropriate exercise*. This should cover both strengthening and aerobic exercise, preferably with reinforcement by a physiotherapist (Box 25.42).

25.42 EXERCISE IN KNEE OR HIP OSTEOARTHRITIS   **EBM**
'Both aerobic and strengthening exercise produce modest but long-term improvements in pain, disability and physical performance in people with knee or hip OA.'
• FAST (Fitness Arthritis and Seniors Trial). Ettinger WH, et al. JAMA 1997; 277:25–31. • Van Baar ME, et al. J Rheumatol 1998; 25:2432–2439.

- *Reduction of any adverse mechanical factors*. These could include weight loss if obese, shock-absorbing footwear, pacing of activities, use of a walking-stick for painful knee or hip OA, or provision of built-up shoes to equalise leg lengths.
- *Initial trial of paracetamol*. Consider the addition of a topical NSAID, and then capsaicin, for knee and hand OA. If required, consider the ascending use of opioid (including combined) analgesics and oral NSAIDs (pp. 1090–1092).

For temporary benefit of moderate to severe pain consider intra-articular injection of corticosteroid (particularly for knee and thumb-base OA) and hyaluronan (knee OA), and local physical therapies such as heat or cold.

At present there are no disease-modifying drugs for OA. However, the measures above may reduce structural progression as well as benefit symptoms.

25.43 CRITERIA FOR JOINT REPLACEMENT IN OSTEOARTHRITIS
• Pain severity (walking limited to 10 minutes, severe rest/night pain) • Age (the older the patient, the better, since prostheses have a limited lifespan of approximately 15 years) • Fitness for surgery and anaesthesia (especially lung and heart disease), although surgery can be performed under regional anaesthesia • Exclusion of patients with an unacceptable risk of complications (e.g. active sepsis, leg ulcers or severe peripheral vascular disease)

25.44 OSTEOARTHRITIS IN OLD AGE
• **OA:** the major MSK cause of pain and disability in older people. • **Functional impact:** the reduced muscle strength, reduced proprioception and impaired balance that accompany ageing all associate with and contribute to pain and disability from knee and hip OA. • **Coexistent calcium pyrophosphate crystal deposition:** an age-associated phenomenon that may result in superimposed acute attacks of synovitis ('pseudogout'). • **Regular strengthening exercise:** can safely reduce the pain and disability of knee OA with accompanying improvements in lower limb muscle strength, proprioception and balance. • **Oral paracetamol and topical NSAIDs:** safe in the older people, with no important drug interactions or contraindications, and often effective for pain relief. • **Total joint replacement:** with appropriate rehabilitation, an excellent cost-effective treatment for severe disabling knee or hip OA in old age.

Surgery

Surgery should be considered if conservative measures fail, the main indications being uncontrolled pain and progressive immobility and functional impairment. Osteotomy may prolong the life of malaligned joints and relieve pain by reducing intra-osseous pressure. Joint replacement can, however, effectively transform the quality of life of people with severe knee or hip OA. Factors that influence patient selection for joint replacement are shown in Box 25.43.

Contrary to popular opinion, total joint replacements are required for the minority of people with large joint OA. The failure rate for replacements (mainly loosening) is about 15% at 15 years for hip replacements, and 10% at 15 years for knee replacements.

INFLAMMATORY JOINT DISEASE

RHEUMATOID ARTHRITIS

Rheumatoid arthritis (RA) is the most common inflammatory arthritis in women and hence an important cause of potentially preventable disability. Many of the clinical features and management strategies in RA are relevant across the spectrum of inflammatory joint disease. The typical clinical phenotype of RA is a symmetrical, deforming, small and large joint polyarthritis, often associated with systemic disturbance and extra-articular disease. The clinical course is usually life-long, with intermittent exacerbations and remissions and highly variable severity.

RA occurs throughout the world and in all ethnic groups. The prevalence is lowest in black Africans and Chinese, and highest in the Pima Indians of Arizona. In Caucasians it is around 1.0–1.5% with a female:male ratio of 3:1. Before the age of 45, the female:male ratio is 6:1. Prevalence increases with age, with 5% of women and 2% of men over 55 years being affected.

Aetiology

RA is an autoimmune disease (p. 80). Concordance rates are higher in monozygotic twins (12–15%) than in dizygotic twins (3%) and frequency of disease is increased in first-degree relatives of patients with RA. Up to 50% of the genetic contribution to susceptibility is due to genes in the HLA region. HLA–DR4 is the major susceptibility haplotype in most ethnic groups, occurring, for example, in 50–75% of Caucasian patients with RA compared to 20–25% of the normal population. However, DR1 is more important in Indians and Israelis and DW15 in Japanese. It is likely that genetic factors influence both susceptibility and severity, with DR4 positivity more common in those with severe erosive disease.

Female gender is a risk factor and this susceptibility is increased post-partum and by breastfeeding. No infectious agents have been consistently isolated and there is no evidence of disease clustering. Cigarette smoking is a risk factor for RA and for positivity for rheumatoid factor in non-RA subjects.

Pathology

RA is characterised by persistent cellular activation, autoimmunity and the presence of immune complexes at sites of articular and extra-articular lesions (Fig. 25.22). This leads to chronic inflammation, granuloma formation and joint destruction. The earliest change is swelling and congestion of the synovial membrane and the underlying connective tissues, which become infiltrated with lymphocytes (especially CD4 T cells), plasma cells and macrophages. Effusion of synovial fluid into the joint space takes place during active phases of the disease. Hypertrophy of the synovial membrane occurs, with the formation of lymphoid follicles resembling an immunologically active lymph node. Inflammatory granulation tissue (pannus) spreads over and under the articular cartilage, which is progressively eroded and destroyed. Later, fibrous or bony ankylosis may occur. Muscles adjacent to inflamed joints atrophy and there may be focal infiltration with lymphocytes.

Subcutaneous nodules consist of a central area of fibrinoid material surrounded by a palisade of proliferating mononuclear cells. Similar granulomatous lesions may occur in the pleura, lung, pericardium and sclera. Lymph nodes are often hyperplastic, showing many lymphoid follicles with large germinal centres and numerous plasma cells in the sinuses and medullary cords. Immunofluorescence confirms 'rheumatoid factor' autoantibody synthesis by plasma cells in synovium and lymph nodes.

Clinical features

The diagnosis of RA can only be established by an accurate and careful history and physical examination. Only limited help is provided by laboratory tests. The clinical hallmark of inflammatory joint disease is persistent synovitis. A set of classification criteria is shown in Box 25.45 but note that these were designed to distinguish patients with RA from those with other arthropathies in epidemiological studies rather than in individual cases; their sensitivity for diagnosing early inflammatory disease in a primary care setting is unknown, so they cannot be applied dogmatically. The requirement for symptoms to persist beyond 6 weeks is a useful cutoff to ensure that self-limiting or viral arthritis is not labelled prematurely as RA. However, irreversible damage occurs early in RA and diagnosis and treatment should not be delayed.

Patterns of presentation

The most common presentation is with a gradual onset of symmetrical arthralgia and synovitis of small joints of the

---

25.45 CRITERIA FOR DIAGNOSIS OF RHEUMATOID ARTHRITIS*

Diagnosis of RA is made with four or more of the following:
- Morning stiffness (> 1 hour)
- Arthritis of three or more joint areas
- Arthritis of hand joints
- Symmetrical arthritis
- Rheumatoid nodules
- Rheumatoid factor
- Radiological changes
- Duration of 6 weeks or more

* American Rheumatism Association 1988 revision.

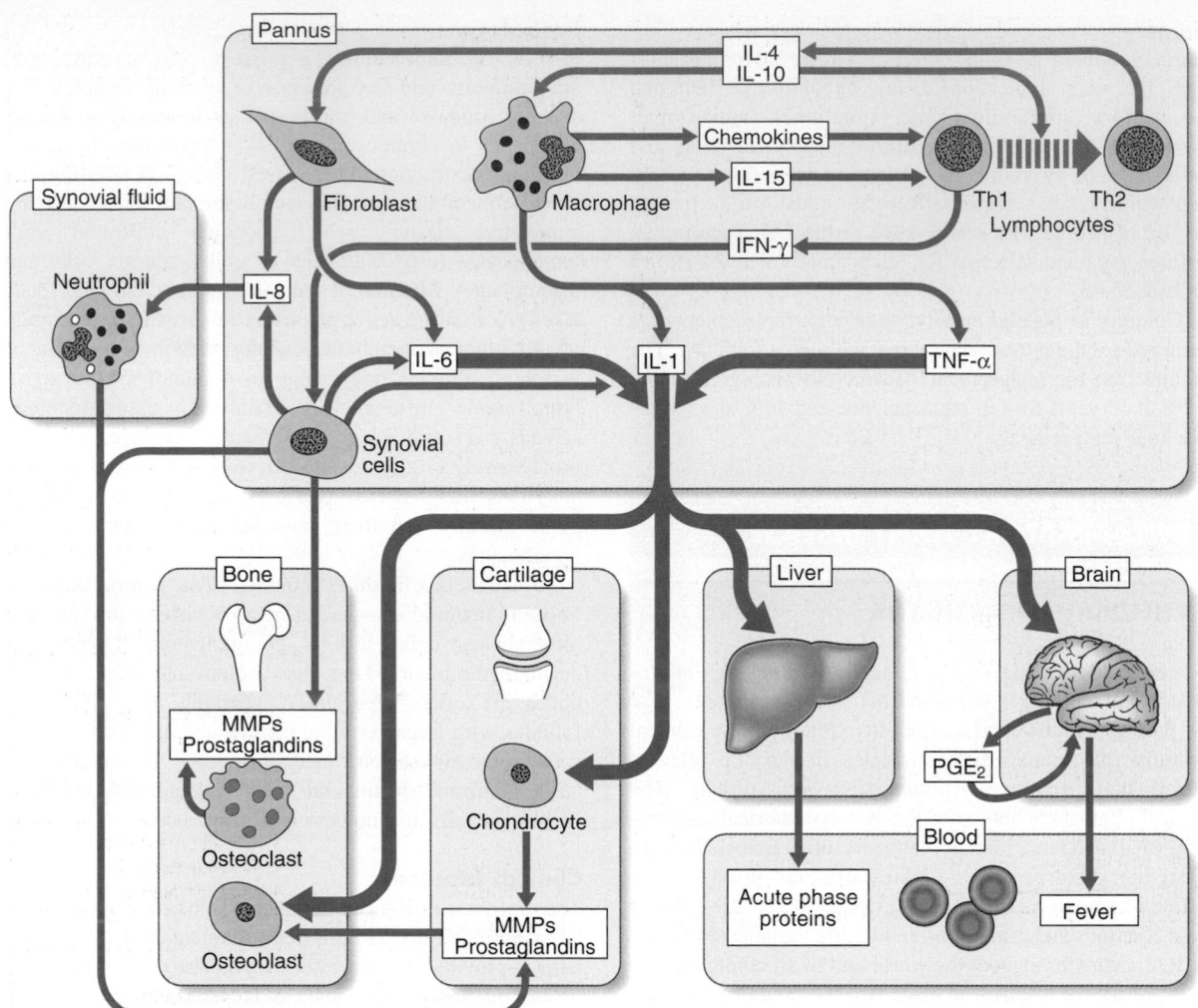

Fig. 25.22 Pathogenesis of rheumatoid arthritis. Possible sequence of events with network of cells, cytokines and mediators. (IL = interleukin; TNF-α = tumour necrosis factor-α; Th1 and Th2 = Th1 and Th2 lymphocyte subsets; IFN = interferon; MMPs = matrix metalloproteinases; PGE$_2$ = prostaglandin E$_2$)

hands, feet and wrists. This insidious onset has traditionally been considered to imply a poor prognosis, possibly because of the delay in presenting for medical advice. A dramatic acute onset, sometimes over just a few days, with florid morning stiffness, polyarthritis and pitting oedema, occurs more commonly, but not exclusively, in the elderly. Some elderly patients present acutely with an initial polymyalgic illness with marked proximal muscle stiffness, the synovitis appearing only after several months as initial corticosteroid therapy is withdrawn. Occasionally the onset is palindromic, with recurrent symmetrical acute episodes of joint pain and swelling which last only for a few hours or days. Whatever the pattern, most patients have evidence of morning and inactivity stiffness and stress pain (p. 1067). Involvement of other synovial structures (tenosynovium, bursae) is common but, unlike in seronegative spondarthritis, the entheses are not targeted.

Specific joints

The hand is crucial to overall patient function and provides a good reflection of overall disease activity. The typical features are symmetrical swelling of the metacarpophalangeal (MCP) and proximal interphalangeal (PIP) joints. These and other joints are considered to be actively inflamed if they are tender on pressure, and have stress pain on passive movement or non-bony effusion/swelling. Note that erythema is not a feature of RA and usually implies coexistent sepsis. Specific hand abnormalities (usually seen with long-standing active disease) include 'swan neck' deformity, the boutonnière or 'button hole deformity', and a Z deformity of the thumb (Fig. 25.23). Dorsal subluxation of the ulnar styloid of the wrist is common and may contribute to rupture of the fourth and fifth extensor tendons. Triggering of fingers may occur due to nodules in the flexor tendon sheath.

In the forefoot dorsal subluxation of the metatarsophalangeal (MTP) joints results in 'cock-up' toe deformities. This causes pain on weight-bearing on the exposed metatarsal heads and development of secondary adventitious bursae and callosities. In the hindfoot, calcaneovalgus (eversion) is the most common deformity, reflecting damage to the ankle and subtalar joint. This is often associated with

25

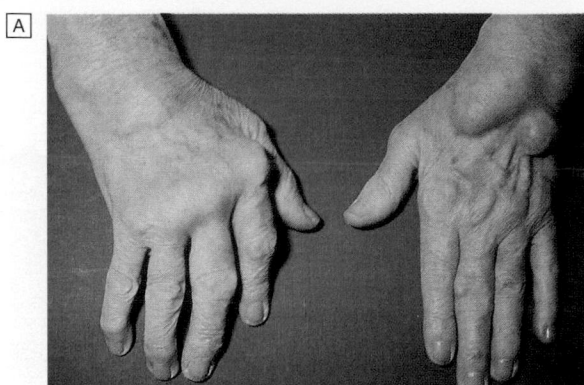

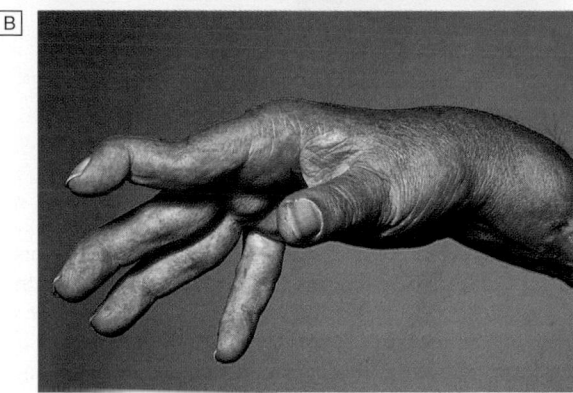

Fig. 25.23 The hand in rheumatoid arthritis. [A] Ulnar deviation of the fingers with wasting of the small muscles of the hands and synovial swelling at the wrists, the extensor tendon sheaths, the metacarpophalangeal and proximal interphalangeal joints. [B] 'Swan neck' deformity of the fingers.

25.46 EXTRA-ARTICULAR MANIFESTATIONS OF RHEUMATOID DISEASE	
Systemic	
• Fever	• Fatigue
• Weight loss	• Susceptibility to infection
Musculoskeletal	
• Muscle-wasting	• Bursitis
• Tenosynovitis	• Osteoporosis
Haematological	
• Anaemia	• Eosinophilia
• Thrombocytosis	
Lymphatic	
• Splenomegaly	• Felty's syndrome
Nodules	
• Sinuses	• Fistulae
Ocular	
• Episcleritis	• Scleromalacia
• Scleritis	• Keratoconjunctivitis sicca
Vasculitis	
• Digital arteritis	• Mononeuritis multiplex
• Ulcers	• Visceral arteritis
• Pyoderma gangrenosum	
Cardiac	
• Pericarditis	• Conduction defects
• Myocarditis	• Coronary vasculitis
• Endocarditis	• Granulomatous aortitis
Pulmonary	
• Nodules	• Bronchiolitis
• Pleural effusions	• Caplan's syndrome
• Fibrosing alveolitis	
Neurological	
• Cervical cord compression	• Peripheral neuropathy
• Compression neuropathies	• Mononeuritis multiplex
Amyloidosis	

25

loss of the longitudinal arch (flat foot) due to rupture of the tibialis posterior tendon.

Popliteal ('Baker's') cysts usually occur in combination with knee synovitis, with synovial fluid communicating with the cyst but being prevented from returning to the joint by a valve-like mechanism. Rupture, often induced by knee flexion in the presence of a large effusion, leads to calf pain and swelling. Differentiation from a deep venous thrombosis (DVT) can usually be made on the presence of pre-existing joint problems, but a Doppler ultrasound or arthrogram is required to establish the correct diagnosis, since DVT and Baker's cyst may coexist. It is important to be aware of this differential diagnosis, as anticoagulating a patient with Baker's cyst can cause further leg swelling and lead to a compartment syndrome.

Extra-articular features

RA is a systemic disease. Anorexia, weight loss and fatigue are common and may occur throughout the disease course. Generalised osteoporosis and muscle-wasting (sarcopenia) result from systemic inflammation. Extra-articular features are more common in patients with long-standing seropositive erosive disease but may occasionally occur at presentation, especially in men. Most features are due to serositis, granuloma/nodule formation or vasculitis (Box 25.46).

Cutaneous features

Subcutaneous rheumatoid nodules occur almost exclusively in seropositive patients, usually at sites of pressure or friction such as the extensor surfaces of the forearm, sacrum, Achilles tendon and toes (Fig. 25.24). They may be complicated by ulceration and secondary infection. Systemic rheumatoid vasculitis usually occurs in elderly seropositive patients in the context of systemic symptoms and multiple extra-articular features. The cutaneous clinical manifestations vary from relatively benign nail-fold infarcts to widespread cutaneous ulceration with skin necrosis.

Ocular features

The most common symptom is dry eyes (keratoconjunctivitis sicca) due to secondary Sjögren's syndrome. Painless episcleritis frequently accompanies nodular seropositive disease; it may cause intense redness but the conjunctival vessels remain normal. It is not usually associated with

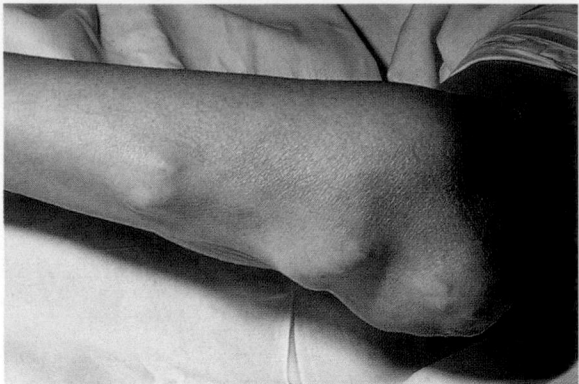

Fig. 25.24 Rheumatoid nodules and olecranon bursitis. Nodules were palpable within as well as outside the bursa.

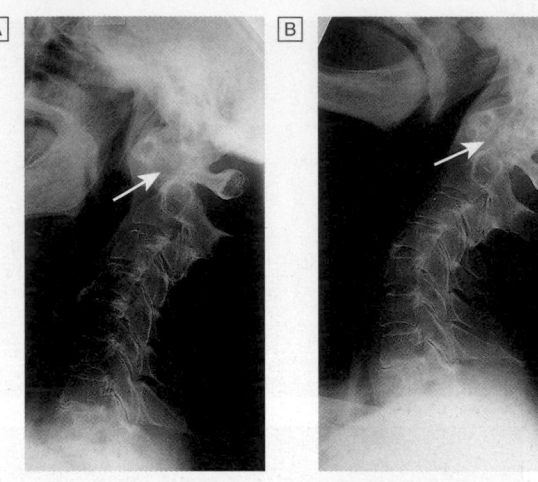

Fig. 25.25 Subluxation of cervical spine. Ⓐ Flexion, showing widening of the space (arrow) between the odontoid peg of the axis (behind) and the anterior arch of the atlas (in front). Ⓑ Extension, showing reduction in this space.

visual disturbance. If treatment is required, local corticosteroids or systemic NSAIDs are usually effective.

Scleritis is more serious and potentially sight-threatening; the eye is red and painful, with inflammatory changes throughout the sclera and uveal tract. The pupil may appear irregular due to adhesions (synechiae) that can lead to secondary glaucoma and visual impairment. NSAIDs may be effective but if no response is obtained, oral corticosteroids are required.

Scleromalacia is painless bilateral thinning of the sclera, with the affected area appearing blue or grey (the colour of the underlying choroid). No specific treatment is required.

Corneal melting is a rare but devastating manifestation. It usually occurs in long-standing disease and is associated with systemic vasculitis. The clinical features are pain, redness and blurred vision with corneal thinning. If untreated, progression to perforation is common. Immunosuppression with corticosteroids and ciclosporin or cyclophosphamide is usually required.

Cardiovascular features
Asymptomatic pericarditis occurs in approximately 30% of patients with seropositive RA, with pericardial effusions and constrictive pericarditis being rare complications. Occasionally, granulomatous lesions result in heart block, cardiomyopathy, coronary artery occlusion or aortic regurgitation. Vasculitis of medium-sized arteries may lead to mesenteric, renal or coronary artery occlusion.

Pulmonary features
These are listed in Box 25.46 and described further on page 722.

Neurological features
Entrapment neuropathies result from compression of peripheral nerves due to hypertrophied synovium or joint subluxation. Median nerve compression in the carpal tunnel is the most common, and bilateral compression may be an early clinical manifestation of RA. Other common features include ulnar nerve compression at the elbow, compression of the lateral popliteal nerve at the head of the fibula, and tarsal tunnel syndrome (entrapment of the posterior tibial nerve in the flexor retinaculum) which causes burning, tingling and numbness in the distal sole and toes.

Diffuse symmetrical peripheral neuropathy and mononeuritis multiplex may occur due to a vasculitic neuropathy.

Cervical cord compression can result from subluxation of the cervical spine at the atlantoaxial joint or at a subaxial level (Fig. 25.25). Atlantoaxial subluxation is a common finding in long-standing RA and is due to erosion of the transverse ligament around the posterior aspect of the odontoid peg. On neck flexion, this leads to the peg moving posteriorly and indenting the cord. If unrecognised, it can lead to cord compression or sudden death following minor trauma or manipulation. Atlantoaxial subluxation should be suspected in any RA patient who describes new onset of occipital headache, particularly if symptoms of paraesthesia or 'electric shock' are present in the arms. Alternatively, onset may be insidious, with subtle loss of function that is initially attributed to active disease. Reflexes and power can be very difficult to assess in the presence of marked joint damage, and therefore sensory or upper motor signs are the most important to elicit. Lateral X-rays should be taken in flexion and extension, and the degree of compression established with MRI. Operative stabilisation and fixation may be required, though the outcome is poor if the patient already has tetraparesis.

Haematological features
Microcytic iron deficiency anaemia due to NSAID-induced gastrointestinal blood loss and normochromic, normocytic anaemia (with or without thrombocytosis) due to active disease may both occur, the latter being unresponsive to oral iron. Felty's syndrome is the association of splenomegaly and neutropenia with RA which occurs in < 1% of RA patients (Box 20.47). Lymphadenopathy may be found in nodes draining actively inflamed joints, but generalised lymphadenopathy should be investigated by biopsy since there is an increased risk of lymphoma in patients with long-standing disease. Amyloidosis (p. 79) is a rare complication of prolonged active disease and usually presents with nephrotic syndrome.

25

<table>
<tr><td colspan="2">

25.47 FELTY'S SYNDROME   ⓘ

Risk factors

</td></tr>
</table>

25.47 FELTY'S SYNDROME

Risk factors

- Age of onset 50–70
- F > M
- Caucasians > blacks
- Long-standing RA

- Deforming but inactive disease
- Seropositive for rheumatoid factor

Common clinical features

- Splenomegaly
- Lymphadenopathy
- Weight loss
- Skin pigmentation

- Keratoconjunctivitis sicca
- Nodules
- Vasculitis, leg ulcers
- Recurrent infections

Laboratory findings

- Anaemia (normochromic, normocytic)
- Neutropenia
- Abnormal liver function

- Thrombocytopenia
- Impaired T- and B-cell immunity

25.48 INVESTIGATIONS AND MONITORING OF RHEUMATOID ARTHRITIS

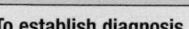

To establish diagnosis

- Clinical criteria
- Acute phase response

- Serological tests
- X-rays

To monitor disease activity and drug efficacy

- Pain (visual analogue scale)
- Early morning stiffness (minutes)

- Joint tenderness (number of inflamed joints, articular index)
- Acute phase response

To monitor disease damage

- X-rays

- Functional assessment

To monitor drug safety

- Urinalysis
- Biochemistry

- Haematology

Investigations

The diagnosis should be confirmed according to clinical criteria (Box 25.48). The acute phase response is usually elevated in patients with widespread disease, but may be normal in isolated small joint synovitis. Rheumatoid factor has low specificity and sensitivity (pp. 1074 and 81).

The typical radiographic appearances of RA are periarticular osteopenia and marginal non-proliferative erosions (p. 1072). Although osteopenia may be present within the first 6 months, erosions are uncommon within the first year. Therefore it is not appropriate to await radiographic changes before making the diagnosis.

Management

This follows the principles outlined on pages 1088–1096.

Physical rest, targeted anti-inflammatory therapy and passive exercises are the mainstay of treatment for acute RA. Hospital admission in order for the patient to undergo multiple intra-articular injections, joint splinting, regular hydrotherapy, physiotherapy and education may be beneficial. However, most flares can be managed out of hospital

---

by judicious use of either intramuscular or intra-articular corticosteroids, oral analgesics and NSAIDs, and adjustment of DMARDs. Periodic assessment of disease activity, progression (damage) and disability is required. Patient education, counselling and a coordinated multidisciplinary approach are required for successful management.

Drug therapy

Prompt introduction of DMARDs (p. 1092), either singly or in combination, is central to the modern management of RA. These drugs do not have immediate anti-inflammatory or analgesic effects but will improve symptoms and acute phase response, and reduce radiographic progression, at least in the medium term (Box 25.49). They are likely to be most useful when started early in disease before irreversible damage has occurred. Methotrexate and sulfasalazine are currently first-choice DMARDs for RA. If they fail to control disease or are not tolerated, other DMARDs (or anti-TNF therapy) should be used, either sequentially or in combination. The addition of a fixed dose of 7.5 mg prednisolone daily to NSAID and DMARD therapy may slow the rate of radiological progression over 2 years in patients with early RA. Symptomatic management with continued use of NSAIDs and analgesics may also be required.

Surgery

Synovectomy of the wrist or finger tendon sheaths of the hands may be required for pain relief or to prevent tendon rupture when other medical interventions have failed. In later stages of the disease osteotomy, arthrodesis or arthroplasties play a major part in patient rehabilitation (Box 25.38, p. 1096).

Progression and prognosis

Past views about the treatment of RA were based on the concept that it was a benign, non-fatal and slowly evolving disease, often responsive to simple therapy. This led to a conservative management approach, predominantly based on the use of NSAIDs, that has been challenged by the following findings:

- There is increased mortality in RA patients, highest in those with the most severe disease. Average lifespan is reduced by 8–15 years by RA and the 5-year survival for patients with severe disease is only 50%.
- Around 40% of patients will be registered disabled within 3 years.
- Around 80% will be moderately to severely disabled within 20 years and 25% will have required a large joint replacement.

Functional capacity decreases most rapidly at the beginning of disease and it is therefore essential to control

25.50 RHEUMATOID ARTHRITIS IN OLD AGE

- **Presentation:** may be atypical—for example, with an initial polymyalgic picture or with synovitis and marked peripheral oedema.
- **Increasing age and comorbidity** (e.g. cardiac, renal, gastrointestinal tract disease): increase the risks of NSAID gastrotoxicity; comorbidity can also make overall management more difficult.
- **Steroid-induced osteoporosis:** patients aged over 65 years are at increased risk. Prophylaxis should be co-prescribed in those on corticosteroid therapy for > 3 months (bisphosphonates).
- **Slow-acting antirheumatic drug therapy:** age alone is not a contraindication.

25.51 SERONEGATIVE SPONDARTHRITIDES

- Ankylosing spondylitis
- Reactive arthritis, including Reiter's syndrome
- Psoriatic arthropathy
- Arthritis associated with inflammatory bowel disease (Crohn's disease, ulcerative colitis)

25.52 CLINICAL FEATURES COMMON TO SERONEGATIVE SPONDARTHRITIS

- Asymmetrical inflammatory oligoarthritis (lower > upper limb)
- Sacroiliitis and inflammatory spondylitis
- Inflammatory enthesitis
- Tendency for familial aggregation
- No association with seropositivity for rheumatoid factor
- Absence of nodules and other extra-articular features of RA
- Overlapping extra-articular features typical of the group:
    Mucosal surface inflammation—conjunctivitis, buccal ulceration, urethritis, prostatitis, bowel ulceration
    Pustular skin lesions, nail dystrophy
    Anterior uveitis
    Aortic root fibrosis (aortic incompetence, conduction defects)
    Erythema nodosum

disease as soon as possible. Joint damage and erosions occur early, and the functional status of patients after only 1 year of RA correlates with long-term outcome. However, it is not possible to predict the outcome accurately at the time of diagnosis, so caution and careful follow-up are needed in all patients. The following factors at presentation are associated with a poor prognosis:

- higher baseline disability
- female gender
- involvement of MTP joints
- positive rheumatoid factor
- disease duration of over 3 months.

SERONEGATIVE SPONDARTHRITIS

This term is applied to a group of inflammatory joint diseases (Box 25.51), distinct from RA, that are thought to share a similar pathogenesis. They show considerable overlap and similarity of articular and extra-articular clinical features (Box 25.52) and a striking genetic association with the histocompatibility antigen HLA–B27.

Pathology

The synovitis is non-specific and, apart from the absence of granulomas, is often indistinguishable from rheumatoid synovitis. However, a distinctive feature is the marked degree of extrasynovial inflammation, especially of the enthesis but also affecting capsule, periarticular periosteum, cartilage and subchondral bone. The inflammation tends to resolve with extensive fibrosis and the resulting scar tissue is prone to calcify and ossify. This may characteristically lead to joint fusion. The periarticular osteitis and periostitis may result in bony spurs that bridge adjacent vertebral bodies (syndesmophytes) or protrude at sites of ligament attachment (e.g. calcaneal or olecranon 'spurs'). Large central cartilaginous joints (sacroiliac, intervertebral, symphysis pubis) are particularly involved, but even when synovial joints are affected (often spinal apophyseal joints, hips, knees, shoulders), extrasynovial inflammation is still prominent.

Aetiology

An association with HLA–B27 occurs in all seronegative spondarthritides but is particularly strong for ankylosing

spondylitis (> 95%) and Reiter's disease (90%), and when there is sacroiliitis, uveitis or balanitis. The suggested pathogenesis is an aberrant response to infection in genetically predisposed persons—the 'reactive' concept. In some situations a triggering organism can be identified, as in Reiter's disease following bacterial dysentery or chlamydial urethritis, but in others the environmental trigger remains obscure.

There is a strong aggregation of seronegative spondarthritis conditions within families, each syndrome showing an increased familial incidence of the other conditions. It is tempting to speculate that such families share an inherited 'reactive' potential but the phenotypic expression is modified according to the inciting trigger and other genetic and constitutional features of the individual.

ANKYLOSING SPONDYLITIS

This prototype of the seronegative spondarthritis group is a chronic inflammatory arthritis with a predilection for the sacroiliac joints and spine. It is characterised by progressive stiffening and fusion of the axial skeleton.

Epidemiology

The disease has a peak onset in the second and third decades, with a male:female ratio of about 3:1. The overall prevalence is around 0.5% in most communities, but is much greater in the Pima and Haida Indians who have a high prevalence of HLA–B27.

Infective triggers have not been identified conclusively. Chronic prostatitis is more common than expected but appears non-infective. Increased faecal carriage of *Klebsiella* aerogenes occurs in patients with established ankylosing spondylitis and may relate to exacerbation of both joint and eye disease.

Clinical features

Spinal features

The onset is usually insidious, over months or years, with recurring episodes of low back pain and marked stiffness. Radiation to the buttocks or posterior thighs may be misdiagnosed as sciatica. Unlike mechanical back pain (p. 1083), symptoms extend over many segments and are axial and symmetrical in distribution. Symptoms are most marked in the early morning and after inactivity and are relieved by movement. Although the lumbosacral area is usually the first and worst affected region, some patients present with mainly thoracic or neck symptoms. The disease tends to ascend the spine slowly and eventually, after several years, the whole spine may be affected. As the spine becomes progressively ankylosed, spinal rigidity and secondary osteoporosis predispose to spinal fracture, presenting as acute, severe, well-localised pain. Secondary spinal cord compression is a rare complication.

Early physical signs include failure to obliterate the lumbar lordosis on forward flexion, pain on sacroiliac compression, and restriction of movements of the lumbar spine in all directions. As the disease progresses, stiffness increases throughout the spine, and chest expansion frequently becomes restricted. Spinal fusion varies in its extent but in a few patients results in marked kyphosis of the dorsal and cervical spine that can interfere with forward vision. This may prove incapacitating, especially when associated with fixed flexion contractures of hips or knees.

Extraspinal features

Most patients have additional locomotor symptoms reflecting the widespread nature of the condition. 'Pleuritic' chest pain aggravated by breathing results from involvement of the costovertebral joints. Plantar fasciitis, Achilles tendinitis and tenderness over bony prominences such as the iliac crest and greater trochanter result from inflammatory enthesopathy. Fatigue is often a major complaint and may

---

25.53 EXTRA-ARTICULAR FEATURES OF ANKYLOSING SPONDYLITIS

- Anterior uveitis (25%) and conjunctivitis (20%)
- Prostatitis (80% men)—usually asymptomatic
- Cardiovascular disease
    - Aortic incompetence
    - Mitral incompetence
    - Cardiac conduction defects
    - Pericarditis
- Amyloidosis
- Atypical upper lobe pulmonary fibrosis

---

result from chronic interruption of sleep due to pain and from chronic systemic inflammation.

Up to 40% of patients have extraspinal synovial joint involvement. This is usually asymmetrical at first and may cause inflammatory symptoms mainly affecting hips, knees, ankles or shoulders. Involvement of a peripheral joint (mainly ankle, knee or elbow) precedes the development of spinal symptoms in around 10% of cases. In a further 10% symptoms begin in childhood as one variety of pauciarticular juvenile idiopathic arthritis.

Most extra-articular features are rare (Box 25.53), except ocular involvement which occasionally precedes joint disease.

Investigations

The ESR and CRP are usually raised. Serum rheumatoid factor is negative or present in low titre.

Radiographic signs provide the strongest investigational evidence but may take years to develop. Sacroiliitis is often the first abnormality, beginning in the lower synovial parts of the joints with irregularity and loss of cortical margins, widening of the joint space and subsequently sclerosis, narrowing and fusion. Lateral thoracolumbar spine X-rays may show anterior 'squaring' of vertebrae due to erosion

25

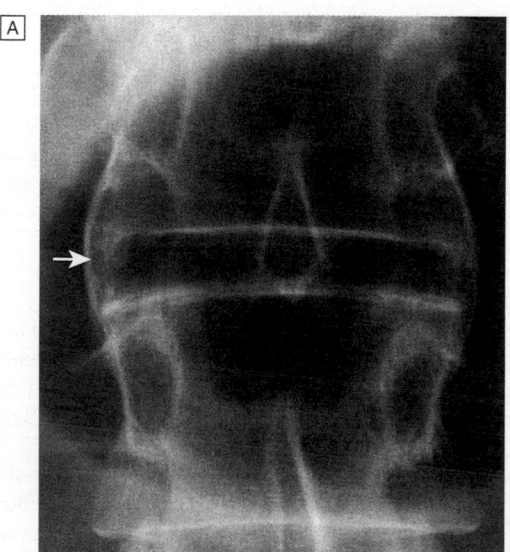

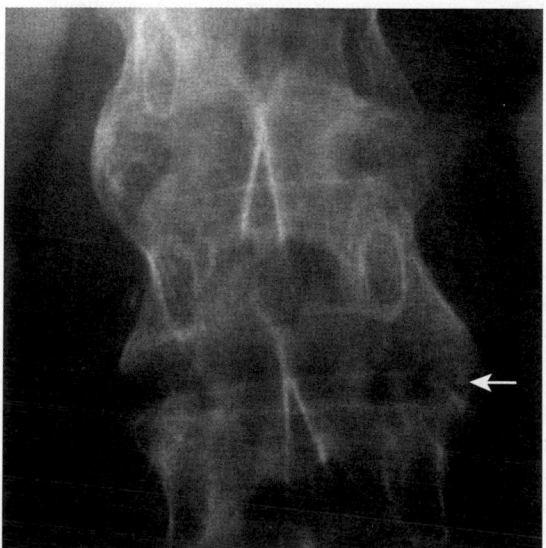

Fig. 25.26   Radiographic syndesmophyte (arrows). A Fine symmetrical marginal syndesmophytes typical of ankylosing spondylitis. B Coarse, asymmetrical non-marginal syndesmophytes typical of psoriatic/Reiter's spondylitis.

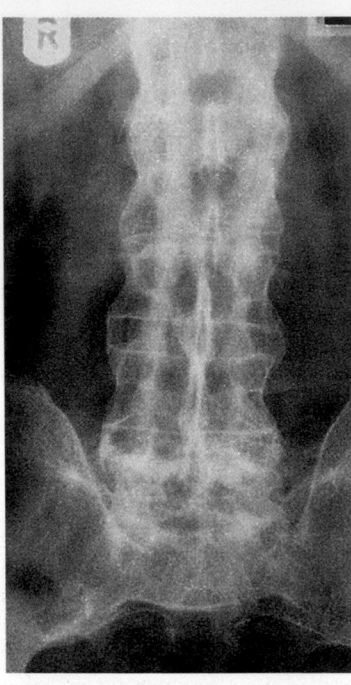

Fig. 25.27 'Bamboo' spine of severe late ankylosing spondylitis. Note the symmetrical marginal syndesmophytes, sacroiliac joint fusion and generalised osteopenia.

and sclerosis of the anterior corners and periostitis of the waist. Bridging syndesmophytes are fine and symmetrical and follow the outermost fibres of the annulus (Fig. 25.26). Ossification of the anterior longitudinal ligament and facet joint fusion may also be visible. The combination of all these features results in the typical 'bamboo' spine (Fig. 25.27). Erosive changes may be seen in the symphysis pubis, the ischial tuberosities and peripheral joints. Osteoporosis and atlantoaxial dislocation can occur.

Management

The aims are to relieve pain and stiffness, maintain a maximal range of skeletal mobility and avoid deformity. Education and appropriate physical activity are the cornerstones of management. Early in the disease patients should be taught to perform regular daily back extension exercises, including a morning 'warm-up' routine, and to punctuate prolonged periods of inactivity (e.g. driving, computer work) with regular breaks. Swimming is ideal exercise. Poor bed and chair posture must be avoided.

NSAIDs are effective in relieving symptoms but do not alter the course of the disease. A long-acting NSAID at night is particularly helpful for marked morning stiffness. The slow-acting antirheumatic drugs sulfasalazine, methotrexate or azathioprine may control persistent peripheral joint synovitis but appear to have little or no impact in suppressing axial disease. However, recent studies have shown that anti-TNF therapy may improve the symptoms and signs of ankylosing spondylitis, including spinal mobility.

Local corticosteroid injections can be useful for persistent plantar fasciitis and other enthesopathies. Oral steroid may occasionally be required for acute uveitis but should otherwise be avoided. Severe hip, knee or shoulder restriction may require surgery. Total hip arthroplasty has largely obviated the need for difficult spinal surgery in those with advanced deformity.

Around 75% of patients with ankylosing spondylitis are able to remain in employment and enjoy a good quality of life. Even if severe ankylosis develops, functional limitation may not be marked as long as the spine is fused in an erect posture. Severe hip, knee or shoulder disease carries a worse prognosis.

REACTIVE ARTHRITIS

Characteristics of Reiter's disease are shown in Box 25.54.

Epidemiology

Reactive arthritis is predominantly a disease of young men with a sex ratio of 15:1 and is possibly the most common cause of inflammatory arthritis in men aged 16–35; however, it may occur at any age. Between 1% and 2% of patients with non-specific urethritis seen at clinics for sexually acquired diseases (p. 406) have reactive arthritis. Following an epidemic of *Shigella* dysentery, 20% of HLA–B27-positive men develop reactive arthritis.

Clinical features

The onset is typically acute, with development of urethritis, conjunctivitis (in about 50%) and an inflammatory oligoarthritis affecting the large and small joints of the lower limbs 1–3 weeks following sexual exposure or an attack of dysentery. There may be considerable systemic disturbance with fever, weight loss and vasomotor changes in the feet.

Less classic attacks may be subacute or insidious. Many patients present with single joint involvement that turns into an asymmetric oligoarthritis over several days. Symptoms and signs of urethritis or conjunctivitis may be minimal or absent and there may be no clear history of prior dysentery. In such cases the coexistence of both synovitis and periarticular inflammation, marked asymmetry and lower limb predominance all suggest seronegative spondarthritis. Achilles tendinitis or plantar fasciitis may be present as further clues.

Extra-articular features (Box 25.54)

Circinate balanitis starts as vesicles on the coronal margin of the prepuce and glans, later rupturing to form superficial

25.54 REITER'S DISEASE	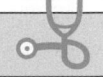

Classic triad*

- Non-specific urethritis
- Conjunctivitis (~50%)
- Reactive arthritis

Additional extra-articular features

- Circinate balanitis (20–50%)
- Keratoderma blennorrhagica (15%)
- Nail dystrophy
- Buccal erosions (10%)

Precipitated by

- Bacterial dysentery—mainly *Salmonella*, *Shigella*, *Campylobacter* or *Yersinia*, or
- Sexually acquired infection with *Chlamydia*

* Incomplete forms with just one or two of the classic triad are more frequent than the full syndrome.

25

erosions with minimal surrounding erythema, some coalescing to give the circular pattern. Lesions are often painless and may escape notice. Buccal erosions are painless shallow red patches on tongue, palate, buccal mucosa and lips which last only a few days. Keratoderma blennorrhagica skin lesions appear as discrete waxy yellow-brown vesico-papules with desquamating margins, occasionally coalescing to form large crusty plaques. Palms and soles are particularly affected but spread may occur to the scrotum, scalp and trunk. Clinically and histologically, these lesions are indistinguishable from pustular psoriasis (p. 1287). The nail dystrophy with subungual hyperkeratosis is indistinguishable from psoriatic nail dystrophy.

Chronic features

The first attack of arthritis is usually self-limiting, with spontaneous remission of symptoms within 2–4 months of onset. However, recurrent or chronic arthritis develops in more than 60% of patients and is not necessarily related to further infection. In chronic arthropathy low back pain and stiffness from sacroiliitis are common and 15–20% of patients develop spondylitis. Ankles, midtarsal joints, metatarsophalangeal joints and knees are usually the other target sites. Uveitis is rare with the first attack but occurs in 30% of patients with recurring arthritis. Other uncommon features include cardiac abnormalities (aortic incompetence, conduction defects, pleuro-pericarditis), peripheral neuropathy (foot drop, ulnar neuritis) and CNS disease (seizures, meningoencephalitis).

Around 10% of patients have evidence of active disease 20 years after the onset. Spondylitis, chronic erosive arthritis, recurrent acute arthritis and uveitis are the major causes of long-term morbidity.

Investigations

The acute phase response is usually evident from a raised ESR and CRP and subsequently from a normochromic, normocytic anaemia. Aspirated synovial fluid is inflammatory (low viscosity, turbid) and often contains giant macrophages (Reiter's cells). Urethritis may be confirmed in the 'two-glass test' by demonstration of mucoid threads in the first void specimen that clear in the second. High vaginal swabs may reveal *Chlamydia* on culture. Except for post-*Salmonella* arthritis, stool cultures are usually negative by the time the arthritis presents; serum agglutinin tests, however, may help confirm previous dysentery. Serum tests for rheumatoid factor and antinuclear factor are negative.

In most cases there are no radiographic changes in the acute attack other than soft tissue swelling. However, mild periarticular osteopenia, joint space narrowing and marginal proliferative erosions may develop with chronic or recurrent disease. There may also be periostitis, especially of metatarsals, phalanges and pelvis, and large 'fluffy' calcaneal spurs. In contrast to changes in ankylosing spondylitis, radiographic sacroiliitis is often asymmetrical and sometimes unilateral, and syndesmophytes are predominantly coarse, asymmetrical and beyond the contours of the annulus fibres (i.e. 'non-marginal', Fig. 25.26). The radiographic changes in the peripheral joints and spine are identical to those seen in psoriasis.

Management

In the first attack this is mainly symptomatic and supportive. NSAIDs are helpful during the acute phase, together with judicious aspiration of joints and intra-articular or other local corticosteroid injections. Systemic steroids are rarely required. Severe progressive arthritis and intractable keratoderma blennorrhagica occasionally warrant anti-rheumatic therapy with azathioprine or methotrexate. Non-specific chlamydial urethritis is usually treated with a short course of tetracycline and this may reduce the frequency of arthritis in sexually acquired cases. Anterior uveitis is a medical emergency requiring topical, subconjunctival or systemic corticosteroids.

PSORIATIC ARTHROPATHY

Approximately 20% of all patients with seronegative polyarthritis have psoriasis. The onset is usually between 25 and 40 years of age, most commonly in patients with current or previous skin psoriasis (70%) (p. 1287), but in some cases (20%) it predates the onset of psoriasis. A small minority of patients have synchronous onset of skin and joint features (5%) or have arthritis but never develop skin lesions (5%). The association with nail dystrophy is stronger than with skin plaques.

Psoriatic arthritis occurs in about 1 in 1000 of the population and in 7% of patients with psoriasis.

Clinical features

A wide spectrum of joint disease is seen but five major presentations are recognised:

1. *Asymmetrical inflammatory oligoarthritis* (40%). This may affect lower and upper limb joints, often with the combination of synovitis and periarticular inflammation. It is most characteristic when a finger or toe is involved by synovitis of its joints and tenosynovitis, enthesitis and inflammation of intervening tissue to give a 'sausage digit' or dactylitis (Fig. 25.28A). Usually only one or two large joints are involved, mainly knees, with often very large effusions. Onset is often abrupt but with mild symptoms and no systemic features. Dactylitis typically settles, with a good outcome after several months.
2. *Symmetrical polyarthritis* (25%). This predominates in women and may strongly resemble RA, with symmetrical involvement of small and large joints in both upper and lower limbs. However, nodules and other extra-articular features of RA are absent and joint disease is generally less extensive and more benign. Much of the hand deformity often results from tenosynovitis and soft tissue contractures.
3. *Predominant distal interphalangeal joint (DIPJ) arthritis* (15%). This is a very characteristic form that mainly affects men and predominantly targets finger DIPJs and surrounding periarticular tissues, almost invariably with accompanying nail dystrophy (Fig. 25.28B).
4. *Psoriatic spondylitis* (15%). This presents a similar clinical picture to ankylosing spondylitis but tends to be

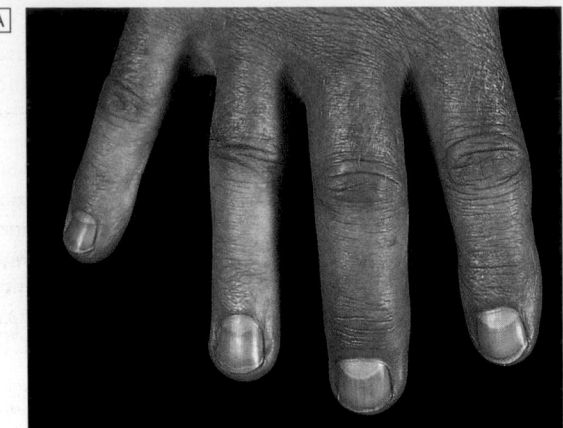

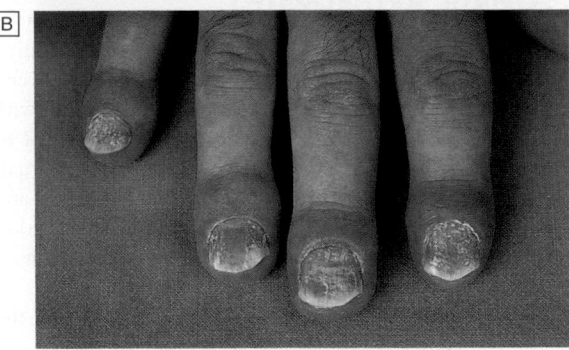

Fig. 25.28 Psoriatic arthropathy. A 'Sausage' middle finger of a patient with psoriatic arthritis. B Typical distal interphalangeal joint pattern with accompanying nail dystrophy (pitting and onycholysis).

less severe. It may occur alone or with any of the other clinical patterns of peripheral arthritis.

5. *Arthritis mutilans* (5%). This deforming erosive arthritis targets fingers and toes. Marked cartilage and bone attrition results in loss of the joint and instability. The encasing skin appears invaginated and 'telescoped' ('main en lorgnette') and traction can pull the finger back to its original length. Other joints in the hand or foot may show ankylosis.

The general pattern of psoriatic arthritis is one of intermittent exacerbation followed by varying periods of complete or near-complete remission. Residual damage and disability in many cases, except arthritis mutilans, are relatively mild.

Extra-articular features are limited to:

- *Skin lesions* (p. 1288).
- *Nail changes* (p. 1288). These may be present in the absence of skin lesions and are more common in psoriatic arthritis (85%) than in uncomplicated psoriasis (30%).
- *Conjunctivitis and uveitis.* Conjunctivitis is most common. Uveitis is mainly in HLA–B27-positive individuals with sacroiliitis and spondylitis.

Investigations

The ESR and CRP may be raised, especially with poly-articular disease, but are often unimpressive. Tests for rheumatoid factor and antinuclear antibody are generally negative. X-rays may be normal or show erosive change with joint space narrowing. Features that permit distinction from RA include marginal proliferative erosions, retained bone density and increased sclerosis of small bones ('ivory phalanx'). Arthritis mutilans and peripheral joint ankylosis can occur in both conditions. The changes in the axial skeleton resemble those of chronic reactive arthritis (coarse, asymmetrical, non-marginal syndesmophytes (Fig. 25.26) and asymmetrical sacroiliitis).

Management

The prognosis is better than for RA, except in arthritis mutilans. Symptomatic agents such as simple analgesics, and topical or oral NSAIDs are usually all that is required. Intra-articular injections may help to control florid synovitis temporarily. In general, splints and prolonged rest are avoided because of the increased tendency to fibrous and bony ankylosis. The same regime of regular exercise and attention to posture should be prescribed as in those with spondylitis (p. 1108).

For persistent peripheral arthritis sulfasalazine, metho-trexate or azathioprine may be required but these have little or no benefit for axial disease. Methotrexate and azathio-prine may also help severe skin psoriasis. Antimalarials should be avoided since they can give exfoliative reactions. The retinoid acitretin (p. 1292) is effective in treating the arthritis as well as the skin lesions but must be avoided in young women because of its teratogenicity. Its use is com-plicated by mucocutaneous side-effects, hyperlipidaemia, myalgias and extraspinal calcification. Photochemotherapy with methoxypsoralen and long-wave ultraviolet light (PUVA, p. 1291) is primarily used for patients with severe skin lesions but can also help some patients with synchronous exacerbations of inflammatory arthritis.

ARTHRITIS ASSOCIATED WITH INFLAMMATORY BOWEL DISEASE

Two patterns of seronegative inflammatory arthritis are associated with ulcerative colitis and Crohn's disease:

- Enteropathic arthritis is an acute inflammatory oligoarthritis that occurs in 12% of patients with ulcerative colitis and 20% of those with Crohn's disease. Large lower limb joints (knees, ankles, hips) are most commonly affected but the wrists and small joints of the fingers and toes can also be involved. The arthritis coincides with exacerbations of the underlying bowel disease, sometimes in association with aphthous mouth ulcers, iritis and erythema nodosum. It ceases to be a problem following total colectomy for ulcerative colitis. The higher prevalence of arthritis in Crohn's disease may reflect the greater difficulty in eradicating the bowel problem.
- Sacroiliitis (16%) and ankylosing spondylitis (6%) are not correlated with the activity of the bowel disease. Clinically and radiologically, such axial disease is indistinguishable from classic ankylosing spondylitis.

25

CRYSTAL-ASSOCIATED DISEASE

A variety of crystals can deposit in and around joints and associate with both acute inflammatory and chronic syndromes (Box 25.55). In some instances crystals are the primary pathogenic agents—true 'crystal deposition disease' (e.g. gout). In other situations MSK disease predisposes to secondary crystal formation (e.g. predisposition to calcium pyrophosphate and apatite crystal formation in OA). Such crystals may subsequently amplify symptoms and damage, or be an incidental epiphenomenon of no clinical consequence.

Several factors influence crystal formation (Fig. 25.29). Firstly, there must be sufficient concentration of the chemical components (ionic product). Whether a crystal then forms, however, depends on the balance of tissue factors that promote or inhibit crystal nucleation and growth. Many tissues are supersaturated for various products but depend on natural inhibitors to prevent crystallisation. Alteration in the balance of inhibitors and promoters may allow crystallisation. Crystals can also dissolve and the yield of crystals at any one time will depend on the relative rates of crystallisation, growth and dissolution.

The inflammatory potential of crystals resides in the physical irregularity and high negative charge of their surface which can induce inflammation and damage cell membranes. Crystals can also cause mechanical damage to the tissues in which they lie and act as wear particles at the joint surface. Crystals forming deep within cartilage or tendon are prevented from interaction with proteins and cells and can paradoxically reside in MSK tissues for years without causing inflammation or symptoms. It is only when they are released from their protected sites of origin ('crystal shedding') that they trigger acute attacks of inflammation. Such attacks may occur spontaneously, result from mechanical loosening (local trauma), partial dissolution and reduced crystal size (e.g. initiation of hypouricaemic

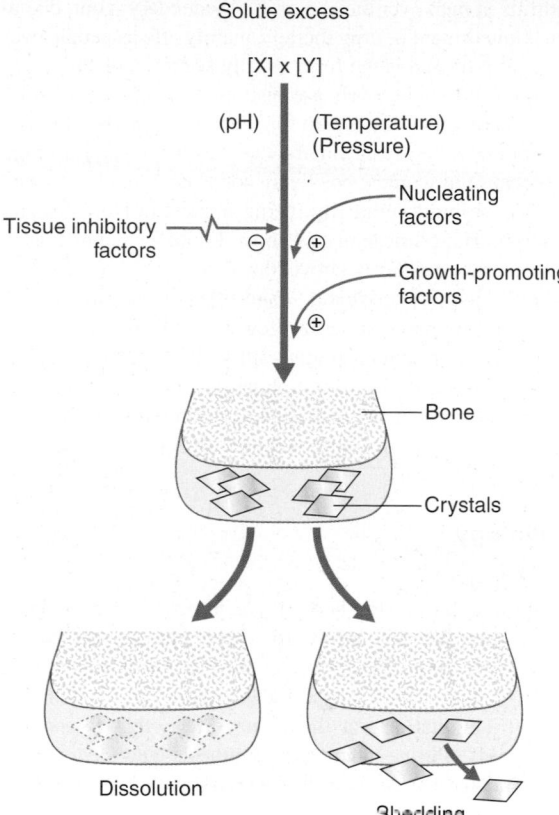

Fig. 25.29 Factors relating to crystal formation and tissue concentration at any one time.

treatment), or occur in association with an acute phase response due to intercurrent illness or surgery (mechanism unknown).

GOUT

Gout is a true crystal deposition disease. It can be defined as the pathological reaction of the joint or periarticular tissues to the presence of monosodium urate monohydrate (MSUM) crystals. MSUM crystals preferentially deposit in peripheral connective tissues in and around synovial joints, initially favouring lower rather than upper limbs and especially targeting the first metatarsophalangeal and small joints of feet and hands. As the crystal deposits slowly increase and enlarge there is progressive involvement of more proximal sites and the potential for cartilage and bone damage, and development of 'secondary' OA. MSUM crystals take months or years to grow to a detectable size, implying a long asymptomatic phase.

Prolonged hyperuricaemia is necessary, but not sufficient, for development of gout.

Epidemiology

The prevalence of gout varies between populations but is around 1% with a strong male predominance (> 10:1). Prevalence increases with age and increasing serum uric acid concentration. 'Primary' gout is almost exclusively a male disease and the most common cause of inflammatory

25.55 CRYSTAL-ASSOCIATED ARTHRITIS AND DEPOSITION IN CONNECTIVE TISSUE	
Crystal	**Associations**
Common	
Monosodium urate monohydrate	Acute gout Chronic tophaceous gout
Calcium pyrophosphate dihydrate	Acute 'pseudogout' Chronic (pyrophosphate) arthropathy Chondrocalcinosis
Basic calcium phosphates	Calcific periarthritis Calcinosis
Uncommon	
Cholesterol	Chronic effusions in RA
Calcium oxalate	Acute arthritis in dialysis patients
Extrinsic crystals/ semi-crystalline particles	
Synthetic crystals	Acute synovitis
Plant thorns/sea urchin spines	Chronic monoarthritis, tenosynovitis

25

arthritis in men over the age of 40. 'Secondary' gout, due to renal impairment or drug therapy, mainly affects people over the age of 65 and is the form usually seen in women.

Serum uric acid levels are distributed in the community as a continuous variable (p. 7). Levels are higher in men than women; they rise from the twenties in men and after the menopause in women, positively correlate with obesity, and vary according to ethnicity (being highest in New Zealand Maoris). Hyperuricaemia is most logically defined as a serum uric acid level above the theoretical solubility of MSUM in physiological conditions (0.42 mmol/l or 7.1 mg/dl). In practical terms, however, it is usually defined as a serum uric acid level greater than 2 standard deviations above the mean for the population (c. 0.40 mmol/l or 6.7 mg/dl for men, 0.35 mmol/l or 5.9 mg/dl for women). Probably 95% of hyperuricaemic subjects never develop gout.

Aetiology

Primary gout

About one-third of the body uric acid pool is derived from dietary sources and two-thirds from endogenous purine metabolism (Fig. 25.30). The concentration of uric acid in body fluids depends on the balance between its synthesis and its elimination via the kidneys (two-thirds) and gut (one-third). Purine nucleotide synthesis and degradation are regulated by a network of enzyme pathways; xanthine

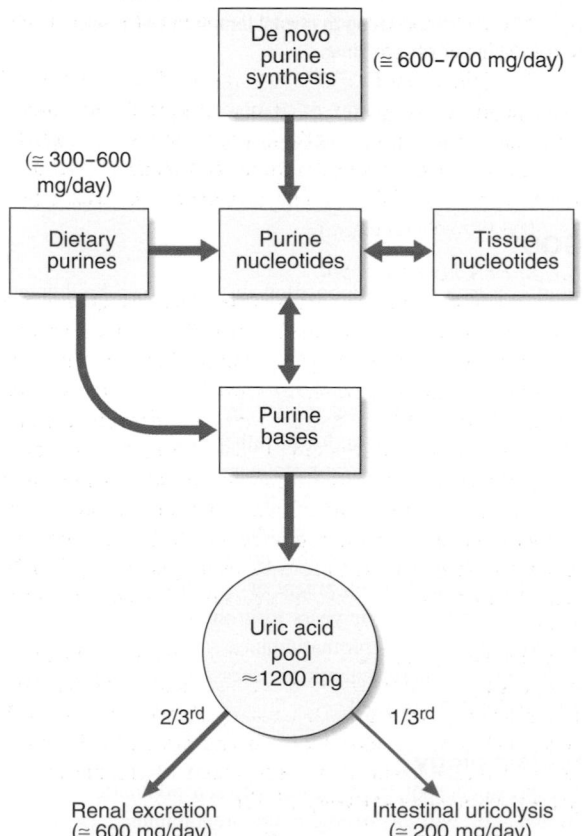

Fig. 25.30 The uric acid pool. Origins and disposal of uric acid in normal humans.

25.56 FACTORS THAT PREDISPOSE TO CHRONIC HYPERURICAEMIA AND GOUT
Diminished renal excretion—common
● Inherited isolated renal tubular defect ('under-excretors')
● Renal failure
● Chronic drug therapy
Thiazide and loop diuretics
Low-dose aspirin
Ciclosporin
Pyrazinamide
● Lead toxicity (e.g. in 'moonshine' drinkers)
● Lactic acidosis (alcohol)
Increased production of uric acid—uncommon
● Increased purine turnover
Chronic myeloproliferative or lymphoproliferative disorders
(e.g. polycythaemia, chronic lymphatic leukaemia)
● Increased de novo synthesis ('over-producers')
Unidentified abnormality (most common)
Specific enzyme defect (rare)
Hypoxanthine-guanine phosphoribosyl transferase deficiency
Phosphoribosyl pyrophosphate synthetase over-activity
Glucose-6-phosphatase deficiency

oxidase catalyses the end conversion of hypoxanthine to xanthine and then xanthine to uric acid.

Causes of hyperuricaemia are shown in Box 25.56. In over 90% of patients with primary gout, hyperuricaemia results from an inherited isolated renal defect in fractional uric acid excretion which impairs their ability to increase renal excretion in response to a purine load ('under-excretors'). Some primary gout patients are intrinsic 'over-producers' of uric acid through no identifiable cause. Rare individuals (< 1% primary gout patients) have a specific inherited enzyme defect of purine synthesis which should be suspected if gout develops under the age of 25 years, in patients presenting with uric acid stones in the urinary tract, or if there is a strong family history of early-onset gout.

Apart from hyperuricaemia, other risk factors and interrelated associations for primary gout include metabolic syndrome (insulin resistance, dyslipidaemia and hypertension which independently reduce renal uric acid clearance) and high alcohol intake (predominantly beer which contains guanosine).

Secondary gout

Secondary gout results from chronic hyperuricaemia due to renal impairment or chronic diuretic use. In diuretic-induced gout nodal generalised OA is a further risk factor, especially in women. This presumably relates to a non-specific predisposition to crystallisation in osteoarthritic cartilage, possibly due to reduced levels of proteoglycan and other inhibitors of crystal formation.

Clinical features

Acute gout

In almost all first attacks a single distal joint is affected. The first metatarsophalangeal joint is affected in over 50% of cases—'podagra' (Fig. 25.31). Other common sites (in order of decreasing frequency) are the ankle, midfoot, knee, small joints of hands, wrist and elbow. The axial skeleton and

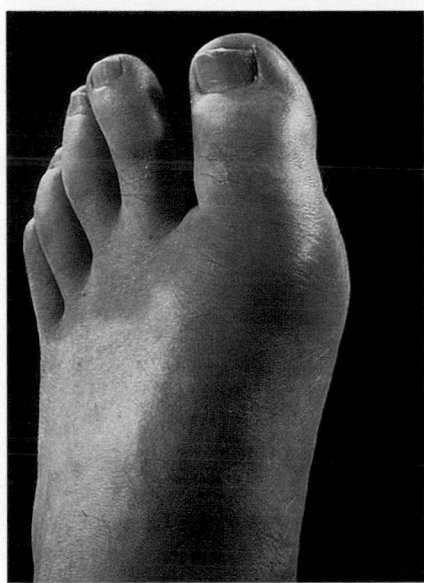

Fig. 25.31 Podagra. Acute gout causing swelling, erythema and extreme pain and tenderness of the first metatarsophalangeal joint.

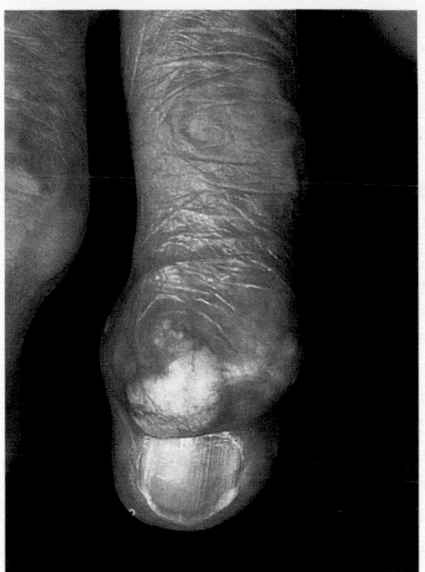

Fig. 25.32 Tophus with white MSUM crystals visible beneath the skin. This was diuretic-induced gout in a patient with pre-existing nodal OA.

large proximal joints are rarely involved and never as the first site. Typical attacks have the following characteristics:

- extremely rapid onset, reaching maximum severity in just 2–6 hours, often waking the patient in the early morning
- severe pain, often described as the 'worst pain ever'
- extreme tenderness—the patient is unable to wear a sock or to let bedding rest on the joint
- marked swelling with overlying red, shiny skin
- self-limiting over 5–14 days, with complete return to normality.

During the attack the joint shows signs of marked synovitis but also periarticular swelling and erythema. There may be accompanying fever, malaise and even confusion, especially if a large joint such as the knee is involved. As the attack subsides, pruritus and desquamation of overlying skin are common. The main differential diagnosis is septic arthritis, infective cellulitis or another crystal disease. Sepsis, however, is usually more subacute in onset and progresses in severity until treated.

Acute attacks may also manifest as bursitis, tenosynovitis or cellulitis. These attacks have the same characteristics— rapid onset, severe pain, florid inflammation and erythema. Many patients describe milder episodes lasting just a few days ('petite attacks'). Some have attacks in more than one joint; sometimes one attack, by triggering the acute phase response, triggers attacks in other joints a few days later ('cluster attacks'). Polyarticular attacks are rare.

Recurrent and chronic gout

After an acute attack some people never have a second episode; in others the next episode occurs after years. In most, however, a second attack occurs within 1 year and the frequency of attacks gradually increases with time. Later attacks are more likely to involve several joints and to be

more severe. Eventually, continued MSUM deposition causes joint damage and chronic pain. The interval between the first attack and the development of chronic symptoms is variable, but averages around 10 years. The main determinant is the serum uric acid level—the higher it is, the earlier and more extensive the development of joint damage and MSUM deposits.

The joints most commonly involved with signs of damage and varying degrees of synovitis are the first metatarsophalangeal joint, midfoot, finger joints and wrists, occasionally with severe deformity and marked functional impairment, especially of feet and hands. As with tophi, asymmetry is characteristic.

Chronic tophaceous gout

Large MSUM crystal deposits produce irregular firm nodules ('tophi') at the usual sites for nodules around extensor surfaces of fingers, hands, forearm, elbows, Achilles tendons and sometimes the helix of the ear. The white colour of MSUM crystals may be evident and permits distinction from rheumatoid nodules (Fig. 25.32). Large nodules may ulcerate, discharging white gritty material and associating with local inflammation (erythema, pus), even in the absence of secondary infection. Although tophi are usually a very late feature, they may appear surprisingly rapidly, in under 1 year, in patients with chronic renal failure.

Secondary gout may present with painful, sometimes discharging tophi without preceding acute attacks. This is particularly seen in older, mainly female patients with nodal OA who develop tophi in and around their osteoarthritic finger joints as a consequence of chronic (> 1–2 years) diuretic therapy (Fig. 25.32).

Renal and urinary tract manifestations

Uric acid (not MSUM) stones cause renal colic (p. 471) in around 10% of gout patients in Europe. The incidence is

25

higher in hot climates and is favoured by purine over-production, uricosuric drugs, defects in tubular reabsorption of uric acid, dehydration and lowering of urine pH (e.g. chronic diarrhoea or ileostomy).

Progressive renal disease is an important complication confined to untreated severe chronic tophaceous gout. This results from MSUM crystal deposition in the interstitium of the medulla and pyramids with consequent chronic inflammation, giant-cell reaction, fibrosis, glomerulo-sclerosis and secondary pyelonephritis.

Investigations

Definitive diagnosis requires identification of MSUM crystals in the aspirate from a joint, bursa or tophus. In acute gout synovial fluid shows increased turbidity due to the greatly elevated cell count (> 90% neutrophils); chronic gouty fluid is more variable but occasionally appears white due to the high crystal load. During remission aspiration of an asymptomatic first metatarsophalangeal joint or knee may still permit crystal identification.

Although hyperuricaemia is usually consistently present, it does not confirm gout. Equally, a normal uric acid level, especially during an attack, does not exclude gout (uric acid falls as part of the acute phase reaction). Measurement of 24-hour urinary uric acid excretion on a low purine diet will identify an over-producer. Assessment of renal function (serum creatinine, urine testing), hypertension, blood glucose and serum lipid profile should be undertaken. An FBC and ESR should detect myeloproliferative disorders during remission of acute gout. During an attack a marked acute phase response (elevated CRP, neutrophilia) is usual; the ESR is often modestly raised in tophaceous gout.

X-rays can assess the degree of joint damage. In early disease they are usually normal, but narrowing of joint space, sclerosis, cysts and osteophyte (changes of OA) may develop in affected joints with time, or be present as a predisposing factor in secondary gout. Gouty 'erosions' (bony tophi) are a less common but more specific feature occurring as para-articular 'punched-out' defects with well-delineated borders and retained bone density. Tophi may also be visible as eccentric soft tissue swellings. In late disease changes may be hard to distinguish from other forms of inflammatory polyarthritis.

25.57 GOUT IN OLD AGE

- **Aetiology:** gout is usually secondary to chronic (>18 months) diuretic therapy (thiazides, loop diuretics) or chronic renal failure.
- **Nodal generalised osteoarthritis:** an important additional risk factor for gout.
- **Presentation:** in contrast to primary gout, secondary gout in older people often presents as painful tophi rather than as acute attacks. Hands, not feet, are the target site.
- **Treatment of acute attacks:** best treated by aspiration and intra-articular injection of long-acting corticosteroid followed by early mobilisation. Oral NSAID and colchicine are best avoided because of increased toxicity.
- **Allopurinol:** because of increased toxicity, should be started at the low dose of 100 mg/day.

Management

The acute attack

A fast-acting oral NSAID (e.g. naproxen, diclofenac, indometacin) can give effective pain relief and is the standard treatment. Patients can keep a supply of an NSAID with which they are familiar and take it as soon as the first symptoms are noticed, continuing for the duration of the attack. Oral colchicine (a potent inhibitor of neutrophil microtubular assembly) can be very effective, but unfortunately often causes vomiting and severe diarrhoea at the doses needed for rapid relief (1 mg loading dose, then 0.5 mg 6-hourly until symptoms abate). The compromise is to try lower doses (0.5 mg 8–12-hourly) for a slower onset of benefit. Aspiration of the joint will give instant relief and, when combined with an intra-articular corticosteroid injection to prevent fluid reaccumulation, often effectively aborts the attack.

Long-term management

Correction of any predisposing factors should always be attempted. Lifestyle alteration to correct obesity and reduce excess beer consumption may significantly reduce hyper-uricaemia. Diuretics should be stopped if possible. Although a very high purine diet (large amounts of seafood, red meat and offal) should be tempered, there is no need for a specific highly restrictive diet.

Indications for hypouricaemic drugs are shown in Box 25.58. Allopurinol is the usual drug of choice because of its once-daily convenience and low incidence of side-effects. It inhibits xanthine oxidase and reduces conversion of hypoxanthine and xanthine to uric acid. The usual starting dose is 100–300 mg daily but lower doses (100 mg or less) should be used in older patients or if renal function is impaired. The sharp reduction in tissue uric acid levels that follows initiation of treatment can partially dissolve MSUM crystals and trigger acute attacks. The patient should be warned of this and told to continue treatment even if an attack occurs. This risk can be minimised by using a lower starting dose (100 mg) or by concurrent administration of oral colchicine (0.5 mg 12-hourly) or an NSAID for the first few weeks. Initiation of treatment during an attack can exacerbate and prolong the episode so it is prudent to wait until the attack settles.

The aim of treatment is to bring the serum uric acid level into the lower half of the normal range to ensure dissolution of crystals and to prevent new ones forming. The serum uric acid should therefore be measured every 3–4 weeks and the dose of allopurinol increased in 100 mg increments until this is achieved (maximum 900 mg daily). Infrequent (e.g. yearly) monitoring is advised to ensure

---

25.58 INDICATIONS FOR HYPOURICAEMIC DRUGS

- Recurrent attacks of acute gout
- Tophi
- Evidence of bone or joint damage
- Associated renal disease
- Gout with greatly elevated serum uric acid

25

maintenance of effective treatment. In most cases allopurinol will need to be continued indefinitely.

Uricosuric drugs such as probenecid or sulfinpyrazone can achieve equivalent reductions in serum uric acid to allopurinol but require several doses each day and maintenance of a high urine flow (to avoid uric acid crystallisation in renal tubules). Salicylates antagonise the uricosuric action of these drugs and should be avoided. Uricosurics are contraindicated in over-producers (they already have gross uricosuria), those with renal impairment (ineffective), and in patients with urolithiasis (increased stone formation). The uricosuric benzbromarone is effective in patients with mild to moderate renal impairment but can cause hepatotoxicity and has limited availability in most countries.

Asymptomatic hyperuricaemia

There is no evidence that hyperuricaemia itself is damaging. Treatment is therefore unnecessary unless there is a strong family history of gout, urolithiasis or persistently very high levels (> 0.6 mmol/l or 10.1 mg/dl). Causes of secondary hyperuricaemia should be considered.

CALCIUM PYROPHOSPHATE DIHYDRATE (CPPD) CRYSTAL DEPOSITION

CPPD crystal deposition in hyaline and fibrocartilage of joints causes chondrocalcinosis. Sporadic, familial and metabolic disease-associated forms are recognised (Box 25.59). Radiographic chondrocalcinosis is rare under the age of 55, but rises from 10–15% in those aged 65–75 to 30–60% in those over 85. The knee (hyaline cartilage and menisci) is by far the most prevalent site, followed by the wrist (triangular fibrocartilage) and pelvis (symphysis pubis). It is often clinically occult, but can cause acute self-limiting synovitis ('pseudogout') or occur as a chronic arthritis showing a strong association/overlap with OA, especially at the knee (Fig. 25.33).

Aetiology

In OA, CPPD crystal deposition may be favoured by a reduction in concentration of proteoglycan and other natural inhibitors of crystal formation, and increased extracellular pyrophosphate levels due to up-regulated chondrocyte metabolism.

The rare autosomal dominant syndrome of CPPD deposition in some cases results from mutations in the ANKH gene which regulates extracellular pyrophosphate metabolism. Other metabolic diseases are associated with CPPD deposition, but of these only haemochromatosis also predisposes to OA-like structural change. All of these conditions are characterised by elevated levels of extracellular pyrophosphate in joint tissues, mainly through reduced concentrations or activity of alkaline phosphatase and other pyrophosphatases, resulting in ectopic mineralisation.

Clinical features

Acute synovitis: 'pseudogout'

This is the most common cause of acute monoarthritis in the elderly. The knee is by far the most common site, followed by the wrist, shoulder, ankle and elbow. It may be the first presentation of disease in the joint, or occur on a background of chronic symptomatic arthritis. Triggering factors include direct trauma and intercurrent illness or surgery.

The typical attack resembles acute gout and develops rapidly, with severe pain, stiffness and swelling, maximal within 6–24 hours of onset. Overlying erythema is common and examination reveals a very tender joint held in the flexed 'loose-pack' position with signs of marked synovitis (large/tense effusion, warmth, restricted movement with stress pain). Fever is common and the patient may appear confused and ill. The attack is self-limiting but may take 1–3 weeks to resolve.

25

25.59 ASSOCIATIONS OF CPPD CRYSTAL DEPOSITION		
	Chondro-calcinosis	Structural arthritis
Ageing (sporadic) (Most common)	+	–
Osteoarthritis, joint damage (Common)	+	+
Familial predisposition (Rare)	+	Variable
Metabolic disease (Rare)		
Haemochromatosis	+	+
Hyperparathyroidism	+	–
Hypophosphatasia	+	–
Hypomagnesaemia	+	–
Wilson's disease	+	–

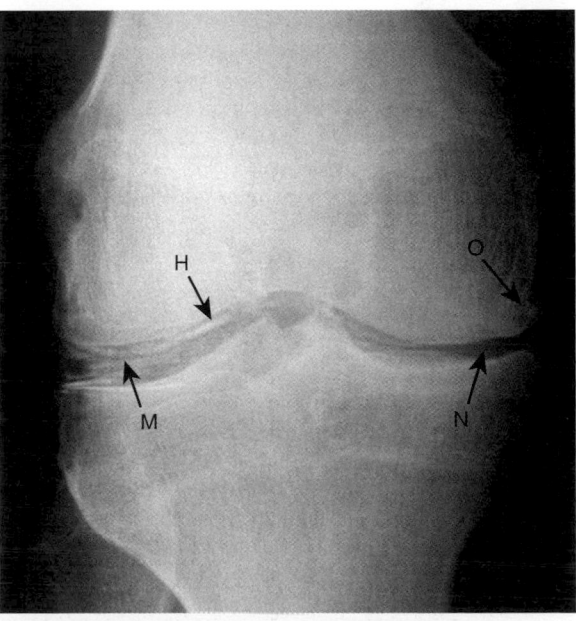

Fig. 25.33 Knee X-ray showing chondrocalcinosis of the fibrocartilaginous menisci (M) and articular hyaline cartilage (H). There is also narrowing (N) and osteophyte (O) of the medial tibio-femoral compartment.

Sepsis and gout are the main differential diagnoses. Although sepsis is often more subacute in onset and progressive, it often needs to be considered, especially when pseudogout has been triggered by chest infection or surgery and if the patient is unwell. It is noteworthy, however, that sepsis and pseudogout can coexist (infection 'strip-mining' CPPD crystals from cartilage). Gout is unlikely in patients over the age of 65 without a preceding history of primary gout or chronic diuretic therapy and seldom involves the knee in a first attack.

Chronic ('pyrophosphate') arthritis

Most patients with chronic symptoms are elderly women. The distribution is similar to that of pseudogout, with knees being the worst affected, then wrists, shoulders, elbows, hips and midtarsals. In the hand the second and third meta-carpophalangeal joints are most affected. Symptoms are chronic pain, variable early morning and inactivity stiffness, and functional impairment. Acute attacks may be super-imposed on this chronic history. Affected joints show features of OA (bony swelling, crepitus, restriction) with varying degrees of synovitis. Effusion and synovial thickening are usually most apparent at knees and wrists; wrist involvement may result in carpal tunnel syndrome. Examination often reveals more widespread but asympto-matic signs of OA, and Heberden's nodes and generalised OA commonly coexist.

Inflammatory features may be sufficiently pronounced to suggest RA. However, tenosynovitis and extra-articular involvement are absent, and large and medium rather than small joints are targeted. Severe damage and instability of knees or shoulders may occasionally lead to consideration of a neuropathic joint, though neurological findings are normal.

Incidental findings

Due to its high age-associated prevalence radiographic chondrocalcinosis often occurs as an incidental finding in older subjects. As with uncomplicated OA, asymptomatic clinical and radiographic features of 'pyrophosphate' arthritis are not uncommon in the elderly. Thorough history and examination are always required to determine the relevance of such findings to symptom causation.

Investigations

In acute pseudogout examination of synovial fluid using compensated polarised microscopy will demonstrate CPPD crystals (Fig. 25.4B, p. 1072) and permit distinction from urate gout. The aspirated fluid is often turbid and may be uniformly blood-stained, reflecting the severity of inflammation. Gram stain and culture of the fluid will exclude sepsis. CPPD crystals may also be identified in the less inflamed fluids aspirated from chronic pyrophosphate arthritis.

X-rays may show chondrocalcinosis in hyaline cartilage and/or fibrocartilage (occasionally capsule or ligament) with or without associated structural changes of OA (Fig. 25.33). Chondrocalcinosis is not always evident, especially in joints showing some degree of cartilage loss, and its absence does not exclude the diagnosis of pseudogout.

Screening for metabolic or familial predisposition (Box 25.59) should be undertaken in patients who show CPPD deposition aged < 55; florid polyarticular, as opposed to pauciarticular, chondrocalcinosis; recurrent acute attacks without chronic arthropathy; or additional clinical or radiographic features of predisposing disease.

Management

For acute pseudogout, aspiration quickly reduces pain and may alone be sufficient. Fluid reaccumulation, however, is common, particularly early in an attack, and additional intra-articular injection of corticosteroid is usually required. Oral NSAIDs and colchicine are also effective, as in gout, but should be avoided if possible in older people. Early active mobilisation is also important in this age group. For chronic arthropathy management is the same as for OA (p. 1100).

BASIC CALCIUM PHOSPHATE (BCP) DEPOSITION

Hydroxyapatite (apatite) is the principal mineral in bone and teeth. Apatite and other basic, as opposed to acidic, calcium phosphates (octacalcium phosphate, tricalcium phosphate) are also the usual minerals to deposit in extraskeletal tissues. In MSK tissues abnormal deposition may occur in:

- periarticular tissues, particularly tendon
- hyaline cartilage in association with OA
- subcutaneous tissue and muscle, principally in connective tissue diseases.

Aetiology

Under normal circumstances mineralisation of soft tissues is prevented by inhibitors such as pyrophosphate and proteoglycans. When these protective mechanisms break down, abnormal calcification due to BCP occurs. There are many causes, some of which are shown in Box 25.60.

In most situations such calcification is of no consequence, possibly because of encasement by protein and surrounding fibrous tissue. However, BCP crystals have inflammatory

---

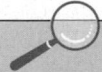

25.60 SOME CAUSES OF ECTOPIC CALCIFICATION

Elevated $[Ca^{2+}] \times [PO_4^{2-}]$ product (metastatic calcification)

- Hyperparathyroidism (especially tertiary, p. 775)
- Renal dialysis
- Vitamin D intoxication
- Basal ganglia in pseudohypoparathyroidism

Altered tissue balance of inhibitors and promoters of crystal formation (dystrophic calcification)

- Calcific periarthritis
- Atherosclerotic arteries
- Fibrotic lymph nodes
- Scarred lung parenchyma
- Scarred adrenal glands (tuberculosis)
- Polymyositis
- Systemic sclerosis (calcinosis)
- Tumours (e.g. craniopharyngioma)

25

potential and in some MSK situations their deposition associates with clinical problems.

Individual apatite crystals are too small to be viewed by light microscopy but their aggregated spherulites can be seen using calcium stains. Sophisticated analytical techniques are required to identify individual BCPs but for clinical purposes presumptive diagnosis based on radiographic calcification or non-specific calcium staining of synovial fluid or histological tissue is sufficient.

Calcific periarthritis

Deposition of apatite in the supraspinatus tendon (Fig. 25.34) is an incidental radiographic finding in around 7% of adults. It occasionally results in severe acute inflammation of the subacromial bursa and periarticular tissues through crystal shedding from the tendon into and around the bursa. Periarticular sites around the greater trochanter of the hip, foot or hand are less commonly affected.

The acute episode may occur spontaneously or follow local trauma. Within just a few hours shoulder pain and tenderness are extreme and the area appears swollen, hot and sometimes red. Modest systemic upset and fever are common. X-rays confirm the diagnosis by showing tendon calcification. If the subacromial bursa is aspirated, thick white fluid containing many calcium-staining (alizarin red S) aggregates may be obtained.

The condition usually resolves spontaneously over 1–3 weeks, often accompanied by radiographic dispersal and disappearance of small to modest-sized deposits (i.e. complete crystal shedding). Calcific periarthritis may result from metabolic abnormality (renal failure, hyperparathyroidism, hypophosphatasia) but measurements of serum creatinine, calcium and alkaline phosphatase are usually normal. The CRP is elevated during the episode.

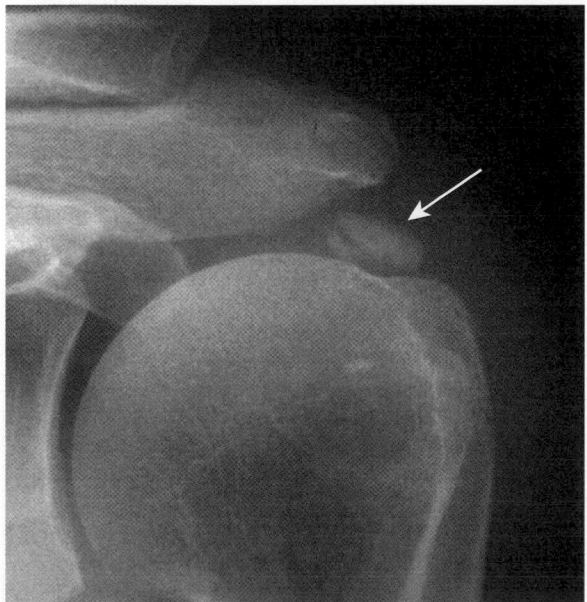

Fig. 25.34 Shoulder X-ray showing supraspinatus tendon calcification (arrow).

Oral analgesics and NSAIDs ameliorate symptoms and the attack may be abbreviated by aspiration and injection of corticosteroid. Exceptionally large deposits may cause mechanical blocking and painful impingement on abduction rather than acute periarthritis, and require surgical removal.

Osteoarthritis and BCP crystal deposition

Modest amounts of BCP aggregates are commonly found in synovial fluid from osteoarthritic joints, either alone or with CPPD crystals ('mixed crystal deposition'). Whether they contribute to joint damage or cause minor inflammatory episodes remains unclear. Large amounts of BCP, however, have been associated with an uncommon but distinctive form of OA characterised by:

- presence in elderly people (> 75), predominantly women
- involvement of knee, hip or shoulder (large joints) only
- rapid progression, often leading to severe pain and disability in just a few months
- development of marked instability and large effusions of knees or shoulders
- an atrophic radiographic appearance with marked loss of cartilage and bone, and minimal osteophyte.

Aspiration yields large volumes of relatively non-inflammatory fluid containing abundant BCP aggregates and often cartilage fragments. The differential diagnosis of such rapidly destructive arthropathy is end-stage avascular necrosis, chronic sepsis or neuropathic joint. Unlike in sepsis, the acute phase response is not triggered and synovial fluid cultures are negative.

Treatment is with analgesics, intra-articular injection of corticosteroids, local physical treatments and physiotherapy. The clinical outcome, however, is poor and most patients require joint replacement. It is most likely that the BCP aggregates, rather than being causal pathogenic agents, are a marker of the speed of joint damage in such 'apatite-associated destructive arthritis', which represents the most severe end of the spectrum of OA.

25

BONE AND JOINT INFECTION

SEPTIC ARTHRITIS

Septic arthritis is a medical emergency. It is the most rapid and destructive joint disease and has a significant morbidity and a mortality of 10%. This has not improved over the last 20 years despite advances in antimicrobial therapy. The incidence is 2–10 per 100 000 in the general population and 30–70 per 100 000 in those with pre-existing joint disease or joint replacement.

Patients with septic arthritis inevitably have a bacteraemia. Haematogenous spread from either skin or upper respiratory tract is the most common source; infection from direct puncture wounds or secondary to joint aspiration is uncommon. Risk factors for septic arthritis include increasing age, pre-existing joint disease (principally RA), diabetes mellitus and immunosuppression (through drugs or disease). In patients with RA the skin is a frequent portal of bacterial entry, especially because of maceration of skin between the toes due to joint deformity, compounded by difficulties in washing and drying the feet due to hand deformities.

Lyme disease (p. 319) may present with monoarthritis, often with other features including headaches, neurological signs and fatigue. There is usually a history of rash (erythema migrans) occurring 7–10 days after tick bite. Diagnosis is confirmed by *Borrelia* serology, although false positives may occur.

Clinical features

The usual presentation is with acute or subacute mono-arthritis. The joint is usually swollen, hot and red and is held in the 'loose-pack' position, with rest pain and stress pain on movement. Although any joint can be affected, the lower limb, particularly knee and hip, is the most common site. In patients with pre-existing arthritis involvement of one or more joints is not uncommon and a full MSK examination should be undertaken.

In adults the most likely organism is *Staphylococcus aureus*, particularly in patients with RA and diabetes. In young, sexually active adults disseminated gonococcal infection is an important cause (p. 413). This occurs in up to 3% of untreated gonorrhoea, usually presenting with migratory arthralgia, low-grade fever and tenosynovitis, which may precede the development of oligo- or mono-arthritis. Painful pustular skin lesions may also be present. Amongst the elderly or those who misuse intravenous drugs, Gram-negative bacilli or group B, C and G streptococci are important causes. Other organisms that are occasionally isolated include group A streptococci, pneumococci, meningococci and *Haemophilus influenzae*.

Investigations

Joint aspiration is essential whenever septic arthritis is suspected. Synovial fluid should be sent for Gram stain and culture. Aspirated fluid often looks turbid or blood-stained but may appear more normal. Blood cultures should also be taken. If the joint is not readily accessible (e.g. hip, spine, sacroiliac joint), aspiration should be performed under image guidance or in theatre. Prosthetic joints should only be aspirated in theatre.

Synovial fluid culture is positive in around 90% of cases of septic arthritis, though the initial Gram stain is positive in only 50% of these. By contrast, synovial fluid culture is positive in only 30% of gonococcal infections, making it important to obtain concurrent cultures from the genital tract (positive in 70–90% of cases). Although fever with peripheral leucocytosis and raised ESR occur in most patients, these may be absent in elderly or immuno-compromised patients or early in the disease course.

Management

Hospitalisation is essential. The principles of management are:

- pain relief
- parenteral antibiotics
- adequate drainage
- early active rehabilitation.

The recommended first-line antibiotic regime in adults is flucloxacillin (2 g i.v. 6-hourly), which will cover both staphylococcal and streptococcal infection until identification of the organism and its antibiotic sensitivities is possible. Intravenous treatment is usually continued for 2–3 weeks followed by oral treatment for 6 weeks in total. Initially, the joint should be aspirated daily to minimise the effusion. If this proves unsuccessful or the joint is inaccessible, surgical drainage may be required. Regular passive movement should be undertaken from the outset, and active movements encouraged once the condition has stabilised.

VIRAL ARTHRITIS

Most forms of viral arthritis are self-limiting. The usual presentation is with acute polyarthritis, fever or viral prodrome and rash. Erythrovirus arthropathy is the most common and, unlike children, adults may not have the characteristic facial rash. Diagnosis is confirmed by a rise in specific IgM. Polyarthritis may also rarely occur with hepatitis B and C, rubella and HIV infection.

OSTEOMYELITIS

Some degree of adjacent bone infection is usual with septic arthritis. In some cases, however, the primary site of infection is bone or bone marrow (osteomyelitis). Any part of a bone may be involved but there is preferential targeting of the juxta-epiphyseal regions of long bones adjacent to joints. The usual source of infection is haematogenous spread (septicaemia), although directly introduced infection may complicate a compound fracture, penetrating injury or orthopaedic surgery. Organisms most frequently implicated are staphylococci, *Pseudomonas* and *Mycobacterium tuberculosis*. Risk factors include childhood and adolescence, diabetes mellitus (especially involving the foot), compromised immunity (including AIDS) and sickle-cell disease (the latter particularly increasing the risk of *Salmonella* infection). Pathologically, the infection often results in a florid inflammatory response, greatly increased intra-osseous pressure and localised areas of osteonecrosis (bone death). A separated shard of dead bone in this context is called a 'sequestrum'. Eventual perforation of the cortex by pus stimulates local new bone formation ('involucrum') by the subperiosteum and periosteum, often with sinuses that discharge through the skin.

25.61 BONE INFECTION IN OLD AGE

- **Vertebral infection:** more common. Recognition is often delayed as symptoms may be attributed to compression fractures caused by osteoporosis.
- **Peripheral vascular disease:** leads to more frequent involvement of the bones of the feet, and diabetic foot ulcers are also commonly complicated by osteomyelitis.
- **Prosthetic joint infections:** now more common because of the increased frequency of prosthetic joint insertion in older people.
- **Gram-negative bacilli:** more frequent pathogens than in youth.

25

Clinical features and investigations

Presentation is with localised bone pain and tenderness, often with malaise, night sweats and pyrexia. The adjacent joint may be painful to move and may develop a sterile ('sympathetic') effusion or secondary septic arthritis. The earliest radiographic abnormality is localised osteopenia adjacent to an epiphysis; this may be followed by more obvious areas of bone lucency mixed with patchy sclerosis (osteonecrosis) and adjacent periosteal new bone formation. X-rays may be normal for the first few weeks, but bone technetium scans, labelled white cell scans and MRI are much more sensitive and show clear abnormalities at presentation. Confirmation of the diagnosis may be obtained by blood culture and/or culture of a bone aspirate or biopsy.

Management

Management of acute osteomyelitis is similar to that for septic arthritis, requiring:

- pain relief
- parenteral antibiotics for at least 2 weeks, followed by oral antibiotics for at least 4 weeks
- surgical decompression and removal of any dead bone
- rehabilitation.

Early recognition and management is critical. Once osteomyelitis becomes established and chronic it may prove very hard to eradicate the infection with antibiotics alone. Many patients require resection of the infected bone and subsequent reconstruction: for example, with callus distraction and external fixators. Complications of chronic osteomyelitis include secondary amyloidosis (p. 79) and skin malignancy at the margin of a discharging sinus (Marjolin's ulcer).

TUBERCULOSIS OF BONE AND JOINTS

This is usually secondary to an established focus in the lung (p. 695) or kidney. Although any joint or bone may be involved, the hip, knee and vertebrae are key target sites. Presentation is extremely variable. Tuberculous arthritis usually presents as a chronic mildly inflammatory monoarthritis or oligoarthritis with pain, swelling and eventual deformity, usually over several years. Spinal involvement may result in contiguous involvement of several vertebrae as infection spreads under the anterior longitudinal ligament. This classically results in anterior wedging of one or more adjacent vertebrae and an angular kyphosis ('gibbus') with possible paraplegia from spinal cord compression. Radiographic changes include bone destruction, joint narrowing and soft tissue calcification, and MRI typically confirms extensive involvement of adjacent soft tissues. There may be evidence of active or inactive tuberculosis on the chest X-ray and Mantoux skin-testing may be useful. However, definite diagnosis requires biopsy and appropriate PCR and culture of synovium (peripheral joint) or bone (spinal involvement). It is uncommon to grow mycobacteria from aspirated synovial fluid.

Management is with appropriate combination chemotherapy for several months, as for pulmonary tuberculosis (p. 701). Additional surgical débridement may be required for extensive peripheral joint or bone disease, and spinal involvement may require surgical stabilisation and decompression.

FIBROMYALGIA

This is a very common cause of multiple regional MSK pain and disability. It commonly associates with medically unexplained symptoms in other systems (p. 236).

The crude prevalence in UK and US communities is 2–3%. Although fibromyalgia can occur at any age, including in teenagers, it shows a progressive increase with age, reaching a maximum prevalence of 7% in women aged over 70. There is a strong female predominance of around 10:1. Other risk factors include a wide variety of life events that associate with psychosocial distress: for example, divorce, marital disharmony, alcoholism in the family, traumatic injury or assault, low income and self-reported childhood abuse (Box 25.62). The condition is reported in a wide variety of racial groups and cultural settings.

Aetiology

The condition is poorly understood. Despite intensive and invasive investigation, no structural, inflammatory, metabolic or endocrine abnormality has been identified. Two abnormalities, however, have consistently been reported:

- *Sleep abnormality.* Delta waves are characteristic of the deep stages of non-rapid eye movement (non-REM) sleep, which usually occurs in the first few hours and is thought to have primarily a restorative function. People with fibromyalgia have reduced delta sleep in a pattern distinct from the sleep abnormalities associated with depression. Furthermore, deprivation of delta but not REM sleep in normal volunteers produces the symptoms and signs of fibromyalgia, supporting the concept of fibromyalgia as a non-restorative sleep disorder.
- *Abnormal pain processing.* A reduced threshold to pain perception and tolerance at characteristic sites throughout the body is a central feature of fibromyalgia. Affected people also have spinal cord 'wind-up' (pain amplification), as evidenced by the exaggerated skin flare response to topically applied capsaicin and frequent occurrence of dermatographism and allodynia (when normally non-noxious stimuli become painful). Other observations to support abnormal pain processing include altered cerebrospinal fluid levels of substance P (increased) and 5-HT (5-hydroxytryptamine or serotonin—reduced), and reduced regional cerebral blood flow in the caudate and thalamus.

EBM
25.62 ASSOCIATIONS OF FIBROMYALGIA
'Epidemiological studies show that widespread body pain, fatigue, psychological distress and multiple hyperalgesic tender sites cluster together and associate with stressful life events.'
• Wolfe F, et al. Arthritis Rheum 1995; 38:19–28.
• Croft P, et al. BMJ 1994; 309:696–699.

25

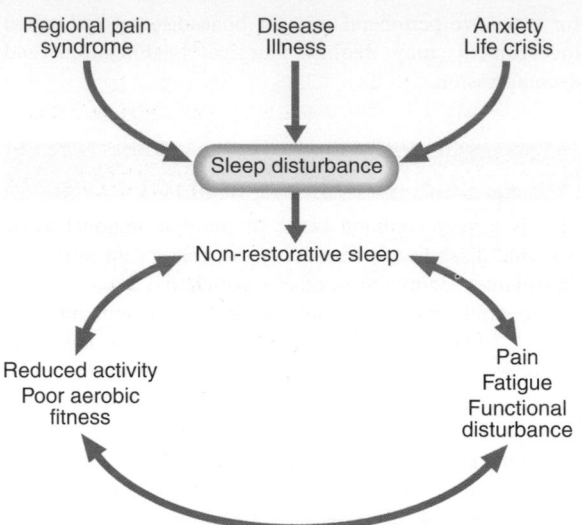

Fig. 25.35 Possible mechanisms involved in fibromyalgia.

25.63 SYMPTOMS OF FIBROMYALGIA

Usual symptoms

- Multiple regional pain
- Marked fatigability
- Marked disability
- Broken non-restorative sleep
- Low affect, irritability, weepiness
- Poor concentration, forgetfulness

Variable locomotor symptoms

- Early morning stiffness
- Swelling of hands, fingers
- Numbness, tingling of all fingers

Additional, variable, non-locomotor symptoms

- Non-throbbing bifrontal headache ('tension headache')
- Colicky abdominal pain, bloating, variable bowel habit ('irritable bowel syndrome')
- Bladder fullness, nocturnal frequency ('irritable bladder')
- Hyperacusis, dyspareunia, discomfort when touched (allodynia)
- Common side-effects with drugs ('chemical sensitivity')

These abnormalities may interrelate. Poor sleep may impair normal descending inhibition to the spinal cord centres that gate pain and, equally, chronic pain may interrupt sleep. The strong association with distressing life events might also explain initial disruption of normal sleep and restoration. A current hypothesis to explain these interrelations is outlined in Figure 25.35.

Clinical features

The main presenting feature is multiple regional pain, often focusing on the neck and back (Box 25.63). At presentation just one or a few regions may dominate the picture, but over the preceding months pain will have affected all body quadrants—both arms, both legs, neck and back. The pain is characteristically unresponsive to traditional measures (analgesics, NSAIDs) and physiotherapy often makes it worse. Fatigability, most prominent in the morning, is the second major problem. Reported disability is often marked. Although people can usually dress, feed and groom themselves, they may be unable to perform daily tasks such as shopping, housework or gardening. They may have experienced major difficulties at work or even given up employment because of pain and fatigue.

Examination usually reveals no abnormality of the MSK system in terms of joint synovitis or damage, and no overt neurological defect or wasting. Depending on their age, people may have signs of OA or other prevalent MSK conditions, but of insufficient severity to explain such widespread symptoms and severe disability. The principal finding is hyperalgesia at tender sites (Fig. 25.36). Moderate digital pressure at each site may be uncomfortable in a normal subject but in fibromyalgia it produces a wince/ withdrawal response. Metered dolorimeters are available for research purposes but moderate digital pressure, strong enough just to whiten the nail, is sufficient for clinical diagnosis. Crucially, tenderness should also be tested at negative control sites (pressure on forehead, squeezing across the distal radius and ulna, pressure over the proximal

fibular head). If a person exhibits hyperalgesia wherever pressure is applied, he or she is likely to have severe psychological disturbance or to be malingering.

People with recognised MSK or other disease (e.g. RA, lupus, cancer) are not exempt from developing fibromyalgia. Assessment may prove challenging since many of the symptoms could relate to activity of their multisystem disease. Marked discordance between the severity of reported and observed abnormality, however, is an important feature that suggests fibromyalgia, and widespread hyperalgesic tender sites are not explained by polyarticular disease.

Investigations

Fibromyalgia does not associate with any abnormality of routine testing. However, it is important to screen for alternative conditions that may account for some of the symptoms without producing overt clinical signs (Box 25.64).

Management

The aims of management are education concerning the nature of the problem, pain control and improvement of sleep. Principles of management of medically unexplained symptoms are outlined on pages 250–251.

Education is central. Wherever possible, discussion should include the spouse, family or carer. The fact that

25.64 A MINIMUM INVESTIGATION SCREEN IN PEOPLE WITH FIBROMYALGIA

Test	Condition screened
FBC	Anaemia, lymphopenia of lupus
ESR, CRP	Inflammatory disease
Thyroid function	Hypothyroidism
Calcium, alkaline phosphatase	Hyperparathyroidism, osteomalacia
Antinuclear antibody	Lupus

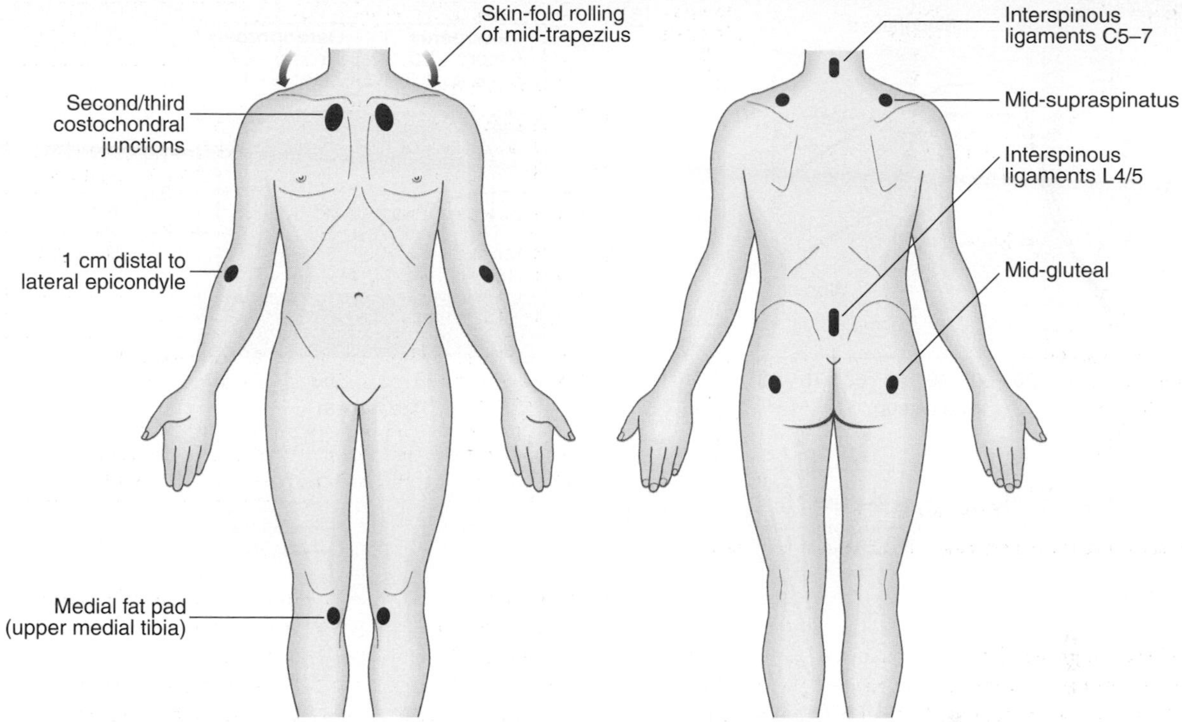
Skin-fold rolling of mid-trapezius
Second/third costochondral junctions
1 cm distal to lateral epicondyle
Medial fat pad (upper medial tibia)
Interspinous ligaments C5–7
Mid-supraspinatus
Interspinous ligaments L4/5
Mid-gluteal

Fig. 25.36 Major tender sites that become hyperalgesic with fibromyalgia.

we recognise the condition but have no clear medical explanation for it should be acknowledged. It is important to explain that the person's chronic pain does not reflect inflammation, damage or disease. The model of a self-perpetuating cycle of loss of sleep and pain in Figure 25.35 is often readily accepted and is a useful framework for problem-based management. Ascribing the symptoms to a cause for which the patient cannot be blamed, and knowing that it is very common often help. Repeat or drawn-out investigation may reinforce beliefs in occult serious pathology and should be avoided.

Low-dose amitriptyline (10–75 mg nocte) with or without fluoxetine may be useful. Many people with fibromyalgia, however, are intolerant of even small doses of amitriptyline. A graded increase in aerobic exercise can improve well-being and sleep quality. The use of self-help strategies and a cognitive behavioural approach, with relaxation techniques and other coping strategies, should be encouraged. Many people with chronic pain 'for no obvious cause' adopt maladaptive illness behaviour which can sometimes be modified to improve coping. Sublimated anxiety relating to distressing life events should be specifically explored with appropriate counselling. There are patient organisations from which to obtain additional information and support.

The prognosis for hospital-diagnosed fibromyalgia is poor. Although treatment may improve quality of life and ability to cope, most people do not lose their symptoms or diagnostic criteria over 5 years. Subjects diagnosed in primary care, or who have sublimated anxiety that can be successfully addressed, may fare better.

DISEASES OF BONE

OSTEOPOROSIS

Osteoporosis is by far the most common bone disease. It is characterised by reduced bone mineral density (BMD), micro-architectural deterioration of bone tissue and an increased risk of fracture. The prevalence of osteoporosis and osteoporosis-related fractures increases markedly with age, reflecting the age-related decline in bone mass and the increased risk of falling in the elderly (Fig. 25.37). Fractures related to osteoporosis are a major public health problem in all developed countries, affecting up to 30% of women and 12% of men at some time in their life. In the UK alone, fractures affect over 250 000 individuals annually with treatment costs of about £1.4 million.

Pathogenesis

Post-menopausal osteoporosis

Post-menopausal osteoporosis occurs because of:

- low peak bone mass
- accelerated bone loss after the menopause and with ageing
- a combination of both factors.

In normal individuals, bone mass increases during skeletal growth to reach a peak between age 20–40 but falls thereafter. There is an accelerated phase of bone loss in women after the menopause (Fig. 25.37) as a result of oestrogen

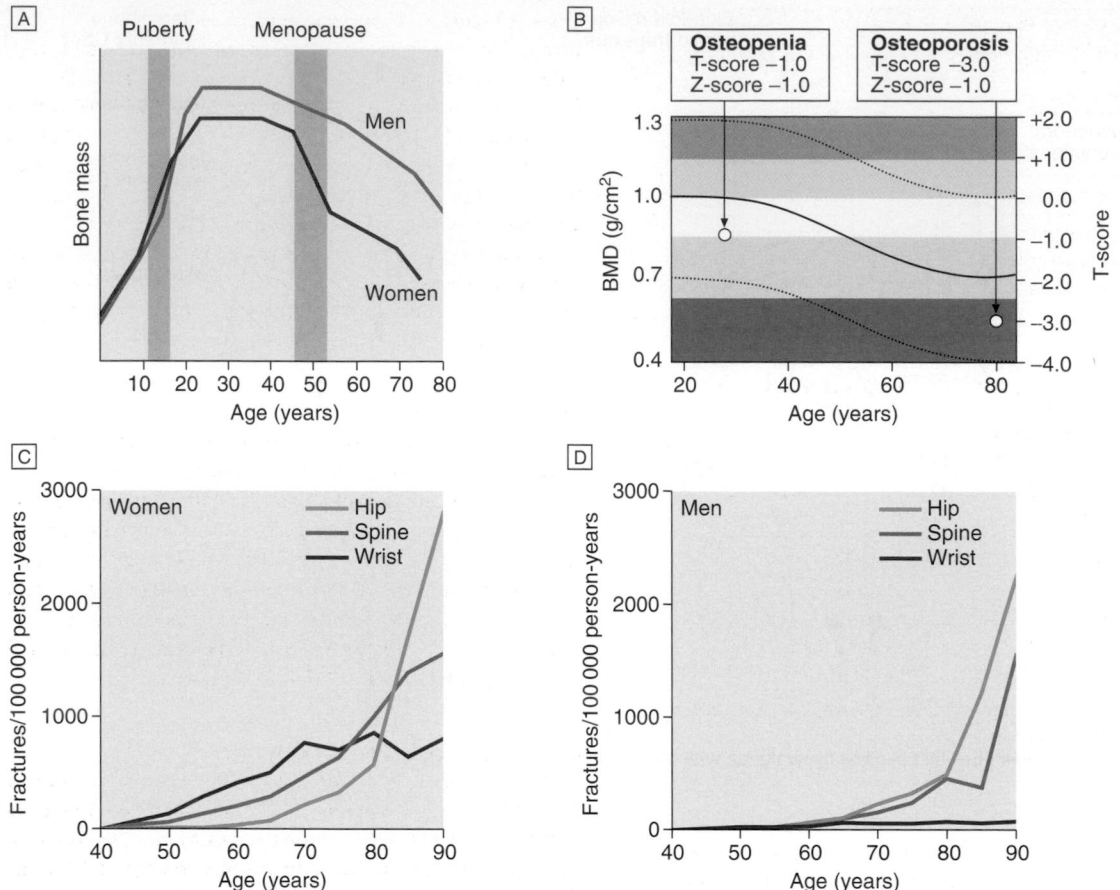

Fig. 25.37   Bone mineral density. ⒶChanges in bone mass with age in men and women. ⒷOutput from DXA scan of the femoral neck comparing BMD values (left axis), T-score values (right axis) and Z-score values (arrows) in patients of different ages. The solid line represents the population average plotted against age, whereas the interrupted lines are ± 2 standard deviations from the average. Patient A, aged 30, has a T-score value of –1.0 and a Z-score value of –1.0, both of which are within the normal range. Patient B, aged 80, also has a Z-score of –1.0 but a T-score of –3.0, reflecting bone loss with age. Patient B therefore has osteoporosis, even though the BMD value is in the 'normal range' for someone of that age. ⒸChanges in fracture incidence with age in women. ⒹChanges in fracture incidence with age in men.

deficiency which causes uncoupling of bone resorption and bone formation, such that the amount of bone removed during the bone remodelling cycle slightly exceeds that which is replaced (Fig. 25.2, p. 1070).

Bone mass and bone loss are regulated by a combination of genetic and environmental factors. Genetic factors play an important role, accounting for up to 80% of the population variance in peak bone mass and other determinants of fracture risk such as bone turnover and bone size. Polymorphisms have been identified in several genes that contribute to the pathogenesis of osteoporosis, including the oestrogen receptor, vitamin D receptor and collagen type I, though most of the genes responsible remain unidentified. Environmental factors such as exercise and calcium intake during growth and adolescence are important in maximising peak bone mass and in regulating rates of post-menopausal bone loss. Smoking has a detrimental effect on BMD and also associates with increased fracture risk, partly because female smokers have an earlier menopause than non-smokers. Moderate amounts of alcohol do not appreciably influence the risk of osteoporosis, although alcoholism is a recognised cause of secondary osteoporosis.

Osteoporosis in men

Osteoporosis is less common in men than in women, and a secondary cause can be identified in about 50% of cases, most notably hypogonadism, corticosteroid use or alcoholism. The pathogenesis of osteoporosis secondary to hypogonadism in men is similar to that in post-menopausal osteoporosis, in that testosterone deficiency results in an increase in bone turnover and uncoupling of bone resorption from bone formation. No obvious cause can be identified in 50% of men with osteoporosis and it is likely that genetic factors play an important role in these cases.

Secondary osteoporosis

Osteoporosis can occur as a complication of many diseases and drug treatments (Box 25.65). In primary hyperparathyroidism, osteoporosis mainly occurs in post-menopausal women and here it appears that the high levels of PTH increase bone turnover and aggravate the uncoupling of bone resorption and bone formation which already occurs due to oestrogen deficiency. A similar mechanism operates in thyrotoxicosis, driven by raised levels of thyroid hormones. The mechanism in Cushing's disease is as

25.65 CAUSES OF OSTEOPOROSIS AND OSTEOPOROTIC FRACTURES	
Endocrine disease	
• Hypogonadism* • Hyperthyroidism	• Hyperparathyroidism • Cushing's syndrome
Inflammatory disease	
• Inflammatory bowel disease • Ankylosing spondylitis	• Rheumatoid arthritis
Drugs	
• Corticosteroids • Gonadotrophin-releasing hormone (GnRH) agonists* • Aromatase inhibitors • Thyroxine over-replacement	• Sedatives • Anticonvulsants • Alcohol excess • Heparin
Gastrointestinal disease	
• Malabsorption	• Chronic liver disease
Miscellaneous	
• Myeloma • Homocystinuria • Anorexia nervosa* • Highly trained athletes*	• Gaucher's disease • Systemic mastocytosis • Immobilisation • Poor diet/low body weight

* Hypogonadism plays an important role in osteoporosis associated with these conditions.

described below for corticosteroid induced osteoporosis. Anorexia nervosa causes osteoporosis through several mechanisms including calcium deficiency, weight loss and hypogonadism, whereas malabsorption predisposes to osteoporosis through calcium deficiency and secondary hyperparathyroidism. Inflammatory diseases cause osteoporosis by increasing bone resorption and suppressing bone formation through release of pro-inflammatory cytokines such as IL-1 and TNF, and similar mechanisms operate in certain types of cancer where a variety of bone-resorbing factors are released by the tumour, including TNF, lymphotoxin and parathyroid hormone-related protein (PTHrP). Release of bone resorbing factors is also thought to underlie the pathogenesis of osteoporosis in Gaucher's disease and mastocytosis.

Corticosteroid-induced osteoporosis

Corticosteroid treatment is an important cause of osteoporosis, the risk of which is directly related to dose and duration of therapy. Although there is no 'safe' dose of corticosteroid, osteoporosis is less likely to occur in patients who are receiving inhaled glucocorticoids, short-term courses of steroids or prednisolone doses of less than 5 mg daily. The risk becomes substantial when the dose of prednisolone exceeds 7.5 mg daily and is continued for more than 3 months. Corticosteroids have adverse effects on several aspects of calcium metabolism. Intestinal calcium absorption is decreased and renal calcium excretion increased, leading to secondary hyperparathyroidism and increased bone turnover. This is combined with inhibition of bone formation due to a direct inhibitory effect on osteoblast activity and stimulation of osteoblast death through apoptosis. The combination of all of these factors leads to rapid bone loss and a greatly increased risk of fracture.

Unusual causes of osteoporosis

Juvenile osteoporosis is a rare condition associated with reduced BMD and bone fractures in children. Genetic factors are important and one syndrome, termed osteoporosis–pseudoglioma syndrome, is caused by mutations in the lipoprotein receptor-related protein-5 gene, which is important in regulating bone formation. Pregnancy-associated osteoporosis is a rare condition that presents with back pain and multiple vertebral fractures during the second or third trimester. The cause is unknown but may relate to an exaggerated bone loss that occurs in normal pregnancy in patients with pre-existing low peak bone mass.

Clinical features

The clinical presentation of osteoporosis is with fragility fractures, back pain, height loss and kyphosis, although many patients are asymptomatic. A common presentation is with radiological osteopenia in otherwise asymptomatic patients who are undergoing X-ray examination for trauma or another condition. Osteoporotic fractures can affect virtually any bone, but the most common sites are the forearm (Colles fracture), spine (vertebral fracture) and femur (hip fracture) (Fig. 25.38).

Investigations and diagnosis

Measurements of BMD are necessary to make or exclude the diagnosis of osteoporosis. The preferred technology is dual energy X-ray absorptiometry (DXA) and the preferred measurement sites are the lumbar spine and hip. Indications for bone densitometry are shown in Box 25.66. Bone densitometers work on the principle that the calcium in bone attenuates passage of X-ray beams in proportion to the amount of mineral present. By comparing the degree of attenuation with known standards, BMD values can be estimated for various skeletal sites and the values are expressed in grams of hydroxyapatite per cm^2 of the area scanned. In addition to giving absolute BMD values, DXA machines give results as 'T-scores' and 'Z-scores'. The T-score measures by how many standard deviations the patient's BMD value differs from that of a young healthy control, whereas the Z-score measures by how many standard deviations the BMD deviates from that of an aged-matched control (Fig. 25.37B). Osteoporosis is diagnosed when the T-score value falls to −2.5 or below (shaded orange in the figure), whereas T-score values that lie between −1.0

25

25.66 INDICATIONS FOR BONE DENSITOMETRY
• Low trauma fracture (fall from standing height or less)   • Clinical features of osteoporosis (height loss, kyphosis)   • Osteopenia on plain X-ray   • Corticosteroid therapy (> 7.5 mg prednisolone daily for > 3 months)   • Family history of osteoporotic fracture   • Low body weight (body mass index < 19)   • Early menopause (< 45 years)   • Diseases associated with osteoporosis   • Assessing response of osteoporosis to treatment

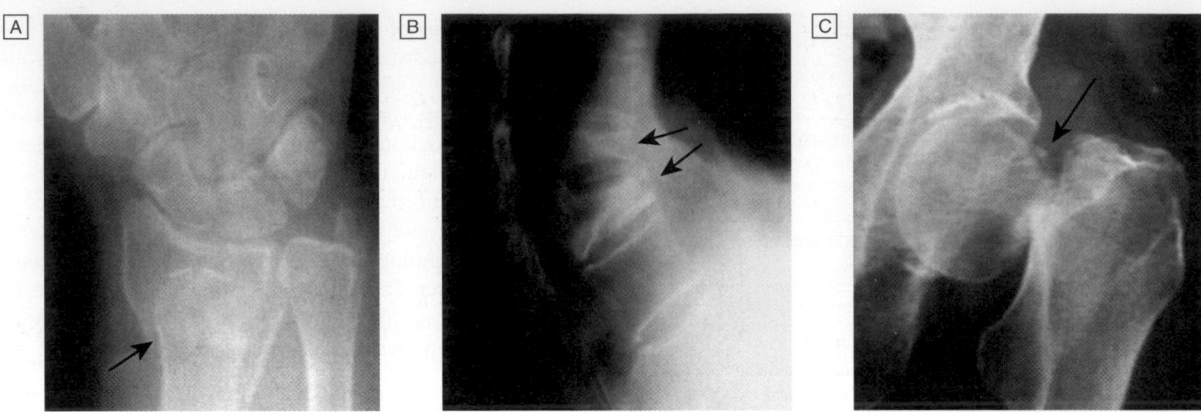

Fig. 25.38 **Common osteoporotic fractures (arrows).** A Colles fracture. B Vertebral fractures. C Neck of femur fracture.

and −2.5 are defined as being in the osteopenic range (shaded beige in the figure). Values of BMD above −1.0 are regarded as normal. The importance of age-related bone loss to the pathogenesis of osteoporosis is reflected by the fact that about 50% of all Caucasian women will be osteoporotic on the basis of BMD T-score values by the age of 80 years.

If the diagnosis of osteoporosis is confirmed by bone densitometry, a history should be taken to identify predisposing causes such as early menopause, excessive alcohol intake, smoking and corticosteroid therapy. Physical examination should include a search for endocrine disease (thyrotoxicosis, Cushing's disease, hypogonadism), neoplasia (evidence of weight loss, lymphadenopathy) and inflammatory disease. Routine biochemical and haematological screens should include serum calcium and phosphate, thyroid function tests, immunoglobulins and ESR. Additional investigations such as serum 25(OH)D and PTH measurement may be required if there is reason to suspect vitamin D deficiency or primary hyperparathyroidism. Levels of sex hormones and gonadotrophins should be measured in men with osteoporosis and in amenorrhoeic women below 50. Transiliac bone biopsy is only required in patients with early-onset osteoporosis of unknown cause or when coexisting osteomalacia is suspected.

Management

An algorithm for the management of patients with suspected osteoporosis is shown in Figure 25.39. Individuals with normal BMD can be reassured, whereas patients with osteopenia should be given advice on lifestyle factors such as smoking (stop), alcohol (limit to < 20 U/week), dietary calcium (aim for 1500 mg daily) and exercise (encourage). Osteopenic patients with BMD values between −2.0 and −2.5 should be offered a repeat BMD measurement in 2–3 years. Specific anti-osteoporosis treatment should be considered in patients with BMD values in the osteoporotic range, especially those who have a previous history of fragility fractures (Box 25.67). Treatment options are discussed in more detail below.

Bisphosphonates

Bisphosphonates are currently the market-leading drugs for osteoporosis. They are synthetic analogues of pyrophosphate that adsorb on to bone surfaces and become incorporated within bone matrix. When osteoclasts resorb bone that contains bisphosphonate, the drug is released within the cell, where it inhibits signalling pathways that are essential for osteoclast function. Bisphosphonate therapy results in a decrease in bone resorption, but bone formation is also suppressed because of coupling between these

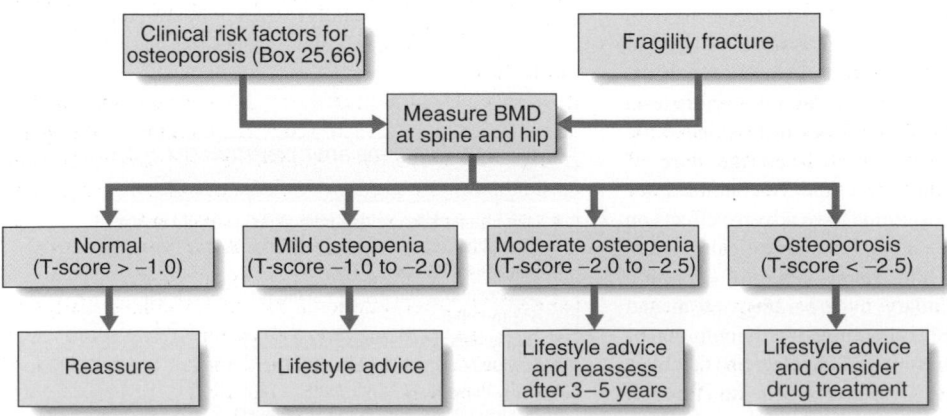

Fig. 25.39 Diagnosis and management of suspected osteoporosis. See page 1086 for fragility fractures.

25.67 RELATIVE EFFICACY OF DRUG TREATMENTS FOR OSTEOPOROSIS

Drug	↑ BMD	↓ Vertebral fracture	↓ Non-vertebral fracture
Alendronate and risedronate	+++	++	++
Etidronate	+	+	–
HRT	++	++	++
Raloxifene	+	++	–
Calcitonin	+	+/–	–
Strontium	+++	++	+
Calcium and vitamin D	+	–	–
Teriparatide	+++	++	++

(+++ most effective; ++ highly effective; + effective; +/– mixed results; – ineffective)

25.68 BMD AND TREATMENT RESPONSE IN OSTEOPOROSIS

'The beneficial effects of bisphosphonates in preventing fractures are restricted to patients with low BMD.'

- Cummings SR, et al. JAMA 1998; 280:2077–2082.
- McClung MR, et al. N Engl J Med 2001; 344:333–340.

25.69 BISPHOSPHONATES PREVENT OSTEOPOROTIC FRACTURES

'The aminobisphosphonates aledronate and residronate reduce the risk of osteoporotic fractures by about 50% in post-menopausal osteoporosis.'

- Black DM, et al. Lancet 1996; 348:1535–1541.
- Harris ST, et al. JAMA 1999; 282:1344–1352.

Hormone replacement therapy (HRT)

HRT with oestrogen and progestagens prevents post-menopausal bone loss and reduces the risk of osteoporotic fractures. The use of HRT as a treatment for osteoporosis has diminished in recent years following publication of the large Women's Health Initiative study which showed that long-term HRT increased the risk of breast cancer, thromboembolic disease, stroke and cardiovascular disease (Box 20.23, p. 766). These risks are lower with oestrogen-only HRT in women who have had a hysterectomy, but even in this group HRT is regarded as second-line treatment because safer alternatives are available. Testosterone is indicated for men with osteoporosis who have hypogonadism (p. 766).

Calcium and vitamin D supplements

These are generally used as an adjunct to other treatments. Calcium is typically given in doses of 500–1000 mg daily, and vitamin D supplements in doses of 400–800 U daily. When given as monotherapy, calcium and vitamin D supplements have been shown to prevent fragility fractures in elderly institutionalised patients with vitamin D deficiency, but they do not seem to be effective at preventing fractures in other patient groups.

Calcitonin

Calcitonin is an osteoclast inhibitor which is effective in preventing post-menopausal bone loss and in the secondary prevention of vertebral fractures in patients with established osteoporosis. However, the effects are not as robust as those of the aminobisphosphonates and there is doubt concerning calcitonin's effectiveness in preventing non-vertebral fractures. There is evidence that calcitonin has analgesic properties and may be helpful in reducing the pain of acute vertebral fracture when given by subcutaneous or intramuscular injection (100–200 U daily). An intranasal spray of calcitonin is also available in some countries.

Raloxifene

Raloxifene binds to the oestrogen receptor and inhibits osteoclastic bone resorption in patients with post-menopausal osteoporosis. Raloxifene has differential effects on the oestrogen receptor in different tissues, acting as an agonist in some tissues such as bone and liver, but as an antagonist in the breast and endometrium. Therefore it is classified as a selective oestrogen receptor modulator (SERM). Administration of raloxifene (60 mg daily) to women with post-menopausal osteoporosis results in a modest increase in BMD (2%) and a reduction in the risk of vertebral fractures. It can provoke muscle cramps and hot flushes and increases the risk of venous thromboembolism to a similar extent to HRT, but reduces the risk of breast

processes in the bone remodelling cycle (Fig. 25.2, p. 1070). The suppression of bone resorption acts to prevent bone loss, however, and allows mineralisation of existing bone to increase. Patients who are treated with bisphosphonates usually experience a gradual increase in BMD of about 5–8% with a plateau about 2 years after commencing therapy (Box 25.68).

The bisphosphonate etidronate is given cyclically in a daily dose of 400 mg for 2 weeks, every 3 months, with administration of calcium supplements during the intervening period. Etidronate slows post-menopausal bone loss and reduces the risk of osteoporotic vertebral fractures, and has been found to be effective in the prevention and treatment of corticosteroid-induced osteoporosis. Etidronate does not prevent non-vertebral fracture. Nitrogen-containing (amino) bisphosphonates such as alendronate (10 mg daily, or 70 mg once weekly) and risedronate (5 mg daily, or 35 mg once weekly) are considerably more potent than etidronate and are generally considered to be more effective. Alendronate and risedronate have similar therapeutic profiles and have both been shown to prevent post-menopausal bone loss and reduce the risk of vertebral and non-vertebral fractures (Box 25.69). They are also effective in the prevention and treatment of corticosteroid-induced osteoporosis and alendronate has been found to be of benefit in male osteoporosis.

Bisphosphonates are poorly absorbed from the gastro-intestinal tract and should be taken on an empty stomach with plain water only, avoiding food for 45–60 minutes after administration. Upper gastrointestinal upset can occur, especially with aminobisphosphonates such as alendronate and risedronate. These drugs should be used with caution in patients with gastro-oesophageal reflux disease, and avoided in patients with oesophageal stricture or achalasia.

cancer and does not have the adverse cardiovascular or cerebrovascular side-effects of HRT. Raloxifene is not generally considered as first-line treatment for osteoporosis because it does not reduce the risk of non-vertebral fractures, but it can be useful in patients with vertebral osteoporosis who are intolerant of bisphosphonates.

Parathyroid hormone (PTH)

PTH is an effective treatment for osteoporosis and works by stimulating bone formation. The beneficial effects of PTH on the skeleton are thought to depend on its intermittent mode of administration which results in peaks and troughs of circulating hormone. This contrasts with the situation in primary hyperparathyroidism (p. 775) where there is a sustained elevation in PTH which causes bone loss and can result in an increased risk of osteoporosis.

The formulation currently available is the 1–34 fragment amino acid (teriparatide), given by single daily subcutaneous injection of 20 μg over a 12–18-month period. Teriparatide increases BMD by 10% or more in osteoporotic subjects and reduces the risk of both vertebral and non-vertebral fractures. It is also effective in male osteoporosis and corticosteroid-induced osteoporosis. Teriparatide has been successfully combined with HRT but administration of bisphosphonate therapy prior to or during teriparatide treatment has been shown to blunt the anabolic effect. Because of its high cost, teriparatide is currently reserved for patients with severe osteoporosis or those who have not responded adequately to other therapies.

Strontium ranelate

Strontium ranelate is an effective agent for secondary prevention of vertebral and non-vertebral fractures in post-menopausal osteoporosis. Strontium incorporates within bone mineral and inhibits bone resorption by mechanisms that are poorly understood. Strontium treatment is accompanied by large changes in BMD, although this is partly arte-factual due to substitution of heavier strontium atoms for calcium atoms. Adverse effects include lower gastrointestinal upset and an increased risk of venous thromboembolism.

Other treatments

The anabolic steroids stanozolol and nandrolone decanoate have been used to treat osteoporosis but there are no data on fracture prevention, and adherence is poor due to side-effects such as hirsutism, weight gain, fluid retention and disturbance of liver function. Tibolone is a steroid hormone receptor modulator that acts as a partial agonist at oestrogen, progestagen and androgen receptors. It increases BMD in post-menopausal osteoporosis but there are no data on fracture prevention. Calcitriol (1,25(OH)$_2$D), the active metabolite of vitamin D, is licensed for treatment of osteoporosis, but the data on fracture prevention are less robust than for other agents.

Monitoring response to treatment

Response to treatment can be monitored either by repeated BMD measurement or by measuring biochemical markers of bone turnover. If BMD measurements are to be used, the preferred site is the lumbar spine because precision here is greater than at the hip. Since treatment changes in BMD

25.70 OSTEOPOROSIS IN OLD AGE

- **Bone loss:** due to an age-associated increase in PTH secretion which leads to increased bone turnover, and an age-related defect in osteoblast function.
- **Fractures due to osteoporosis:** a common cause of morbidity and mortality, although fracture healing is not delayed by age.
- **Recurrent fractures:** elderly patients who suffer fragility fractures are at increased risk for further fracture. They should be investigated for osteoporosis and treated if the diagnosis is confirmed.
- **Falls:** risk factors for falls (such as visual and neuromuscular impairments) are independent risk factors for hip fracture in elderly women, so intervention to prevent falls is as important as treatment of osteoporosis (p. 166).
- **Bisphosphonates:** the most effective agents currently available for the prevention of osteoporotic fractures, but their use should be restricted to patients in whom BMD is low (T-score below −2.5).
- **Calcium and vitamin D supplements:** a safe and effective way of preventing hip and other non-vertebral fractures in elderly housebound or institutionalised individuals, irrespective of BMD values.

occur slowly and are relatively modest, it is advisable to wait 18–24 months between starting therapy and repeating BMD. Biochemical markers of bone turnover such as NTX (p. 1076) respond more quickly than BMD and have been shown to correlate with antifracture efficacy of antiresorptive therapy. If neither BMD nor biochemical markers are available, treatment response can be assessed by monitoring changes in height and the occurrence of clinical fractures. It should be noted, however, that even if patients develop fractures, this does not necessarily indicate treatment failure since even the best treatments reduce fracture risk by only 50–65%.

Duration of treatment

Antiresorptive therapy should be continued long-term in patients with established osteoporosis. With teriparatide the duration of treatment is limited to 18 months, because of concerns over osteosarcoma with long-term treatment. Courses of teriparatide should be followed up with long-term antiresorptive treatment (e.g. bisphosphonates) in order to maintain the increase in BMD.

OSTEOMALACIA AND RICKETS

Osteomalacia is characterised by defective bone mineral-isation, bone pain, increased bone fragility and fractures. Rickets is the clinical syndrome that results when osteo-malacia occurs in the growing skeleton and these patients develop bone deformity in addition to the above features. Full-blown osteomalacia is now relatively rare in developed countries, but subclinical disease is still quite common, especially in people who have a poor diet or limited sunlight exposure such as elderly housebound individuals and Muslim women who live in northern latitudes. Four broad categories of osteomalacia and rickets can be identified based on the underlying cause, specifically:

- deficiency of vitamin D or defects in vitamin D metabolism

25

- hypophosphataemia
- drug-induced inhibition of bone mineralisation
- defects in pyrophosphate metabolism.

Pathogenesis

The role of vitamin D in calcium metabolism is shown in Figure 20.16 (p. 772). Vitamin D occurs in only small quantities in most foods except oily fish, so the amount in the diet is generally insufficient to meet requirements. Maintenance of normal levels of vitamin D therefore depends on ultraviolet sunlight exposure which permits formation of cholecalciferol (D) in the skin from 7-dehydrocholesterol. Lack of cholecalciferol due to inadequate sunlight exposure, dietary deficiency, malabsorption or a combination of these factors is accompanied by a reduction in 25(OH)D3 synthesis in the liver. This causes reduced production of the biologically active metabolite 1,25(OH)$_2$D3 in the kidneys, reduced intestinal calcium absorption and low serum calcium. The low serum calcium level stimulates PTH secretion, resulting in secondary hyperparathyroidism and subsequent increased osteoclastic bone resorption, reduced renal calcium excretion and increased renal phosphate excretion. This sequence of events represents an attempt by the parathyroid glands to restore serum calcium levels to normal; however, this cannot be achieved with continuing vitamin D deficiency so there is progressive loss of both calcium and phosphate from bone and defective mineralisation.

Osteomalacia also occurs in association with inherited and acquired metabolic defects of vitamin D metabolism and function. Patients with chronic renal failure cannot synthesise the active metabolite of vitamin D (1,25(OH)$_2$D) due to renal damage and this causes secondary hyperparathyroidism and, in some cases, osteomalacia. Osteomalacia also occurs in the inherited disorder vitamin D-resistant rickets type I, which is caused by inactivating mutations in the renal α-hydroxylase enzyme, rendering the enzyme unable to convert 25(OH)D to 1,25(OH)$_2$D. In type II vitamin D-resistant rickets, mutations in the vitamin D receptor occur, rendering it resistant to activation by 1,25(OH)$_2$ D.

Clinical features

Rickets in children has many manifestations, including enlargement of epiphyses at the lower end of the radius, and swelling of the costochondral junctions ('rickety rosary'). Osteomalacia in adults presents much more insidiously and, when mild, can be relatively asymptomatic or mimic osteoporosis. With further progression, however, features of bone pain, pathological fractures and general malaise occur. Proximal muscle weakness is prominent and the patient may walk with a waddling gait and experience difficulty in climbing stairs or getting out of a chair. Bone and muscle tenderness on pressure is common and focal bone pain may occur in association with fissure fractures of the ribs and pelvis.

Investigations and diagnosis

Patients suspected of having osteomalacia should have a routine biochemical screen (renal function, serum calcium, phosphate, albumin and alkaline phosphatase), along with serum 25(OH)D and PTH levels (Box 25.5, p. 1076). A diagnosis of vitamin D-deficient osteomalacia should be suspected by the presence of low or low-normal calcium and phosphate, raised alkaline phosphatase, low 25(OH)D and raised PTH. Radiological examination is of limited value in diagnosis, except in advanced cases where focal radiolucent areas (pseudofractures or Looser's zones) may be seen in the ribs, pelvis and long bones (Fig. 25.40A). Radiological osteopenia is common and the presence of vertebral crush fractures may cause confusion with osteoporosis. In children, the pathognomonic feature is thickening and widening of the epiphyseal plate. The diagnosis of osteomalacia can be confirmed by bone biopsy, which shows the pathognomonic features of increased thickness and extent of osteoid seams (Fig. 25.40B).

The clinical features of vitamin D-resistant rickets (VDRR) are similar to those of vitamin D-deficient rickets and the diagnosis is usually first suspected when patients fail to respond to vitamin D supplementation. Biochemical features of type I VDRR are similar to vitamin D deficiency except that levels of 25(OH)D are normal and 1,25(OH)$_2$D is undetectable (reflecting failure of 1-α-hydroxylation of vitamin D). In VDRR type II, 25(OH)D is normal but PTH and 1,25(OH)$_2$D values are raised.

Management

Rickets and osteomalacia caused by vitamin D deficiency respond rapidly to treatment with 25(OH) (50 µg daily) or active vitamin D metabolites (1-α-(OH)D 1–2 µg daily or

25

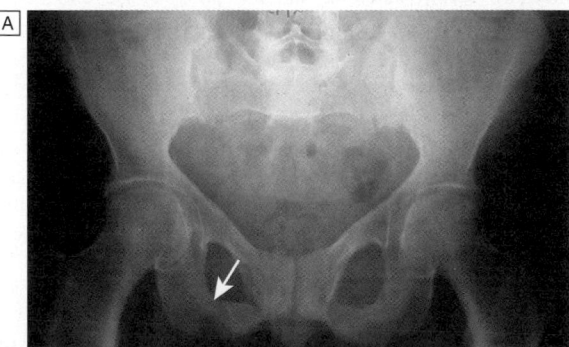

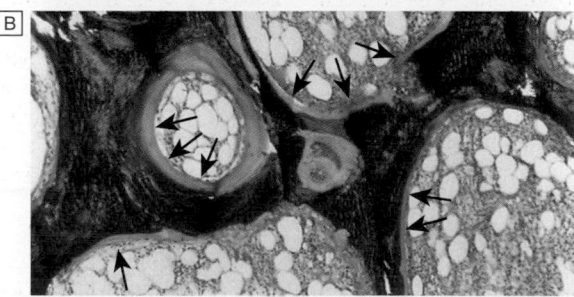

Fig. 25.40   Osteomalacia. [A] X-ray of the pelvis showing Looser's zones (arrow). [B] Photomicrograph of bone biopsy from osteomalacic patient showing thick osteoid seams (stained light blue) which cover almost all of the bone surface. Calcified bone is stained dark blue.

1,25(OH)$_2$D 0.25–1.5 µg daily) and calcium supplementation (500–1000 mg daily). Higher doses or systemic administration may be required in patients with malabsorption. Healing of the bone disease is accompanied by rapid clinical improvement, normalisation of biochemical abnormalities and radiographic improvement. After 3–4 months, treatment can generally be stopped or the dose of vitamin D reduced to a maintenance level of 10–20 µg cholecalciferol for those in whom underlying disease or lifestyle factors put them at risk of recurrence.

Osteomalacia secondary to chronic renal failure and VDRR type I require treatment with active vitamin D metabolites (1-α-(OH)D or 1,25 (OH)$_2$D) since these bypass the metabolic defect in 1-α-hydroxylation of 25(OH)D. Management of VDRR type II is difficult as the defect is at the receptor level, but a partial response to high doses of vitamin D metabolites and parenteral calcium and phosphate may be observed.

During treatment of osteomalacia it is important to measure serum calcium, alkaline phosphatase and renal function on a regular basis to screen for development of hypercalcaemia. Healing of osteomalacia is reflected by a return of alkaline phosphatase values to normal.

HYPOPHOSPHATAEMIC RICKETS

Osteomalacia and rickets can occur as the result of renal phosphate wasting in the absence of vitamin D deficiency. Hypophosphataemic rickets is most often caused by inherited defects in key genes that regulate phosphate metabolism but can also arise in patients who develop tumours that secrete phosphaturic substances.

Pathogenesis

Serum phosphate levels in normal individuals are primarily regulated by modulation of phosphate reabsorption in the renal tubules. One of the most important regulators is the circulating phosphaturic hormone, fibroblast growth factor 23 (FGF23), the levels of which, in turn, are regulated by the enzyme PHEX which degrades FGF23 (Fig. 25.41). Most inherited cases of hypophosphataemic rickets are due to mutations in the FGF23 or PHEX genes. The condition of X-linked hypophosphataemic rickets (XLH) is caused by inactivating mutations in the PHEX gene, which prevent PHEX from degrading FGF23. Autosomal dominant hypophosphataemic rickets (ADHR) is caused by mis-sense mutations in the FGF23 gene that render the FGF23 hormone resistant to PHEX-mediated inactivation, thus raising levels of bioactive FGF23 in the circulation. Most cases of tumour-induced osteomalacia appear to be due to 'ectopic' production of FGF23 by mesenchymal tumours, sometimes in combination with other phosphaturic factors.

Investigations and diagnosis

The diagnosis of XLH and ADHR is often made on the basis of the family history. In XLH, female carriers are clinically unaffected but pass the condition to 50% of their male offspring. Male-to-male transmission is never observed. In ADHR, an autosomal dominant pattern of inheritance is observed, and affected individuals pass the condition on to 50% of their offspring. Both conditions are characterised by severe hypophosphataemia, phosphaturia, raised alkaline phosphatase levels, normal or low-normal serum calcium levels and normal 25(OH)D and 1,25(OH)D levels. Patients with tumour-induced osteomalacia present with a similar biochemical picture, but with a later age at onset and no family history. In most cases, the causal tumour is clinically occult and whole-body MRI or CT may be required for localisation.

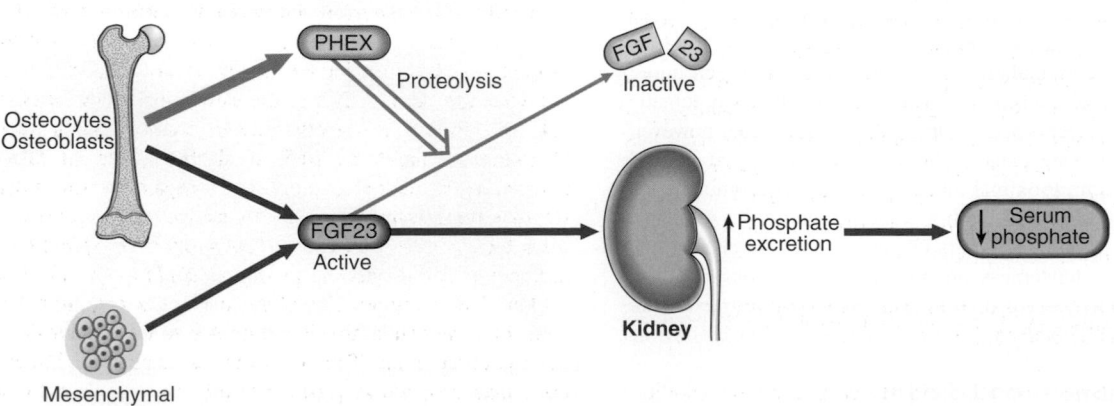

Fig. 25.41 **Regulation of phosphate metabolism.**

Management

Treatment of hypophosphataemic rickets is with phosphate supplements (1–4 g daily), combined with active metabolites of vitamin D to promote intestinal calcium and phosphate absorption (1-α-(OH)D 1–2 µg daily or 1,25(OH)$_2$D 0.25–1.5 µg daily). The aim is to ameliorate symptoms, restore normal growth, maintain serum phosphate levels within the normal range and normalise alkaline phosphatase levels. Levels of calcium, phosphate, alkaline phosphatase and renal function should be monitored during treatment. Whilst tumour-induced osteomalacia can also be managed medically, it is best treated by localisation and removal of the causal tumour.

OTHER CAUSES OF OSTEOMALACIA

Aluminium intoxication

This can cause osteomalacia due to direct inhibition of mineralisation. The most common scenario is patients with chronic renal failure who are undergoing dialysis and taking aluminium-containing phosphate binders. Aluminium-induced osteomalacia presents clinically with symptoms of osteomalacia and fragility fractures. Serum calcium levels are high-normal or raised, whereas alkaline phosphatase and PTH values are normal or only slightly elevated. The diagnosis can be confirmed by demonstration of aluminium at the calcification front in a bone biopsy.

Bisphosphonates

These can cause osteomalacia due to direct inhibition of mineralisation. This has been described mostly in patients with Paget's disease receiving etidronate, but it can occur with high doses of other bisphosphonates. The osteomalacia is usually asymptomatic and spontaneous healing occurs when treatment is stopped.

Fluoride

Excessive intake of fluoride causes osteomalacia due to direct inhibition of mineralisation. Fluoride-induced osteomalacia can result from fluoride treatment for osteoporosis, or can be endemic due to high fluoride content in drinking water.

Hypophosphatasia

This is an autosomal recessive disorder in which osteomalacia occurs as the result of inactivating mutations in the alkaline phosphatase gene. The causal mutations impair alkaline phosphatase function, resulting in accumulation of pyrophosphate, subsequent inhibition of mineralisation and, in adults, chondrocalcinosis. On investigation, the pathognomonic feature is reduced serum alkaline phosphatase with normal levels of calcium, phosphate and vitamin D metabolites. There is no effective medical treatment but bone marrow transplantation has been used successfully in severe cases.

PAGET'S DISEASE

Paget's disease of bone (PDB) is a common condition characterised by focal areas of increased and disorganised bone remodelling, most commonly affecting the axial skeleton in sites such as the pelvis, femur, tibia, lumbar spine, skull and scapula. Paget's disease is seldom diagnosed before the age of 40 but gradually increases in prevalence thereafter to affect up to 10% of the UK population by the age of 85. The disease is common in Caucasians from north-west and southern Europe but is rare in Scandinavians, Asians, Chinese and Japanese. These ethnic differences in susceptibility persist after migration, illustrating the importance of genetic factors in aetiology, but the incidence of PDB has also been found to be decreasing in some countries over the past 25 years, suggesting that environmental factors also play a role.

Pathogenesis

The primary abnormality in PDB is increased osteoclastic bone resorption, which is accompanied by marrow fibrosis, increased vascularity of bone and increased osteoblast activity. The bone in PDB is architecturally abnormal and has reduced mechanical strength. Osteoclasts in PDB are increased in number, are unusually large, and contain characteristic inclusion bodies. Inclusion bodies in osteoclast nuclei have led to speculation that PDB might be caused by a slow virus infection with measles or distemper but the evidence is conflicting. Biomechanical factors may be important in determining the pattern of involvement, since PDB tends to start at the site of muscle insertions to bone and, in some cases, localises to bones or limbs that have been subjected to repetitive trauma or over-use.

Genetic factors are important in PDB. Between 15 and 40% of patients have a positive family history with autosomal dominant inheritance and a high degree of penetrance by the age of 65. Several rare inherited syndromes have also been described which are similar to PDB but have an earlier age of onset. These include the dominantly inherited conditions familial expansile osteolysis, expansile skeletal hyperphosphatasia and early-onset PDB, and the recessively inherited idiopathic hyperphosphatasia.

Clinical features

The classic presentation of PDB is with bone pain, deformity, deafness and pathological fractures, but many patients are discovered to have asymptomatic disease as the result of an incidental finding on biochemical testing or X-ray examination. Clinical signs of PDB include bone deformity and expansion, increased warmth over affected bones and pathological fracture. Bone deformity is most evident in weight-bearing bones such as the femur and tibia, but when the skull is affected the patient may complain that hats no longer fit properly due to cranial enlargement. Neurological problems such as deafness, cranial nerve defects, nerve root pain, spinal cord compression and spinal stenosis are recognised complications due to enlargement of the affected bones and encroachment upon the spinal cord and nerve foraminae. Surprisingly, deafness in PDB is seldom due to compression of the auditory nerve, but rather appears to be conductive in nature due to osteosclerosis of the temporal bone. The increased vascularity of Pagetic bone makes operative procedures difficult and, in extreme cases, the high bone blood flow can precipitate cardiac failure in elderly patients with limited cardiac reserve.

25

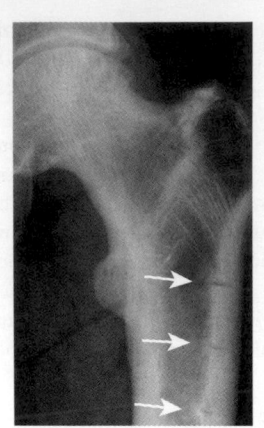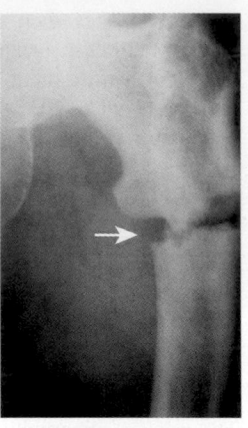

Fig. 25.42 Paget's disease. A Radiographic features, illustrating bone expansion and osteosclerosis with pseudofractures breaching the bone cortex (arrows). B X-ray some weeks later from the same patient who developed a pathological fracture (arrow) at the site of a pre-existing pseudofracture while walking down the street.

Osteosarcoma is a rare but serious complication of Paget's disease that has a poor prognosis. It should be suspected in a patient with Paget's who suffers a sudden increase in pain or swelling of an affected bone.

Investigations and diagnosis

A routine biochemistry screen is helpful in diagnosis, giving the characteristic picture of an 'isolated' elevation in alkaline phosphatase in over 90% of cases. However, the alkaline phosphatase can be normal in PDB, especially when only a single bone is affected. A radionuclide bone scan is a useful way of screening for the presence of PDB and documenting its extent (Fig. 25.8, p. 1074). If the bone scan is positive, X-rays should be taken of an affected bone to confirm the diagnosis. Typical features on X-ray are osteosclerosis alternating with osteolysis, bone expansion and bone deformity (Fig. 25.42). Bone biopsy is not usually required to make the diagnosis of PDB, but it can be helpful in differentiation from osteosclerotic metastases (for example, from adenocarcinoma of breast or prostate).

Management

Treatment of PDB is primarily indicated for the control of bone pain. In many cases, pain can be adequately controlled by administration of painkillers such as paracetamol or NSAIDs, but if these measures are ineffective, then bisphosphonates should be tried (Box 25.72). Aminobisphosphonates such as pamidronate, risedronate and zoledronate are more effective than older bisphosphonates such as etidronate and tiludronate at suppressing biochemical markers of bone turnover in PDB, but they have not, as yet, been shown to offer any significant advantage in terms of pain control. Calcitonin can be used as an alternative to bisphosphonate therapy in PDB, but is less convenient to administer and significantly more expensive. Repeated courses of bisphosphonates or calcitonin can be given to patients whose symptoms recur.

The long-term effects of antiresorptive therapy with bisphosphonates and calcitonin on complications such as deafness, bone deformity and fracture are unknown. Currently, there is no evidence to show that prophylactic therapy with bisphosphonates in asymptomatic patients is effective in preventing complications.

25.73 PAGET'S DISEASE OF BONE IN OLD AGE
• **Prevalence:** affects about 3% of individuals over the age of 55 in the UK.
• **Symptoms:** usually asymptomatic and often discovered by finding an elevated serum alkaline phosphatase in patients with otherwise normal biochemistry.
• **Investigation:** the diagnosis is usually obvious on X-ray but can be confirmed by radionuclide bone scan, which also gives information on the extent of the disease.
• **Treatment:** none required in those who are asymptomatic. Anti-Pagetic therapy with bisphosphonates is the treatment of choice in patients with bone pain that does not respond to analgesics.

PRIMARY BONE TUMOURS

Primary bone tumours are less common than secondary bone tumours but have a peak incidence in childhood and adolescence. An exception is in patients with Paget's disease of bone, which accounts for most cases of osteosarcoma occurring above the age of 40. The presentation of primary bone tumours is with local pain and swelling. Plain X-rays show expansion of the bone with a surrounding soft tissue mass, often containing islands of calcification. The diagnosis is confirmed by biopsy. Treatment depends on

25.72 MEDICAL MANAGEMENT OF PAGET'S DISEASE			
Drug	**Route of administration**	**Dose**	**Inhibitory effect on bone turnover**
Etidronate	Oral	400 mg daily for 3–6 months	+
Tiludronate	Oral	400 mg daily for 3–6 months	++
Risedronate	Oral	30 mg daily for 2 months	+++
Pamidronate	Intravenous	1–3 × 60 mg	+++
Zoledronate	Intravenous	1 × 5 mg	+++
Calcitonin	Subcutaneous	100–200 U 3 times weekly for 2–3 months	+
(+ moderately effective; ++ effective; +++ highly effective)			

histological type but generally involves surgical removal of the tumour followed by chemotherapy and radiotherapy. The prognosis is generally good in cases that present in childhood and adolescence, but poor in elderly patients with osteosarcomas related to Paget's disease.

OTHER DISEASES OF BONE

ALGODYSTROPHY (REFLEX SYMPATHETIC DYSTROPHY SYNDROME)

Algodystrophy is characterised by gradual onset of pain, swelling and local tenderness, usually of a limb extremity, accompanied by localised osteoporosis, abnormal sweating, and colour and temperature change. Algodystrophy is commonly triggered by a fracture or other trauma, but can also occur in association with pregnancy, as the result of an intercurrent illness, or may arise spontaneously. The cause is unknown but local over-activity of the sympathetic nervous system is thought to be responsible for many of its features. Diagnosis is based upon the clinical picture, coupled with patchy local osteoporosis of the affected region on X-ray, and a local increase in isotope uptake on bone scan examination.

The differential diagnosis includes infection, inflammation and malignancy. Algodystrophy can usually be distinguished from infection and inflammation by the absence of an acute phase response and lack of synovitis. The X-ray appearances in algodystrophy are also usually quite distinct from those of focal osteolytic lesions in

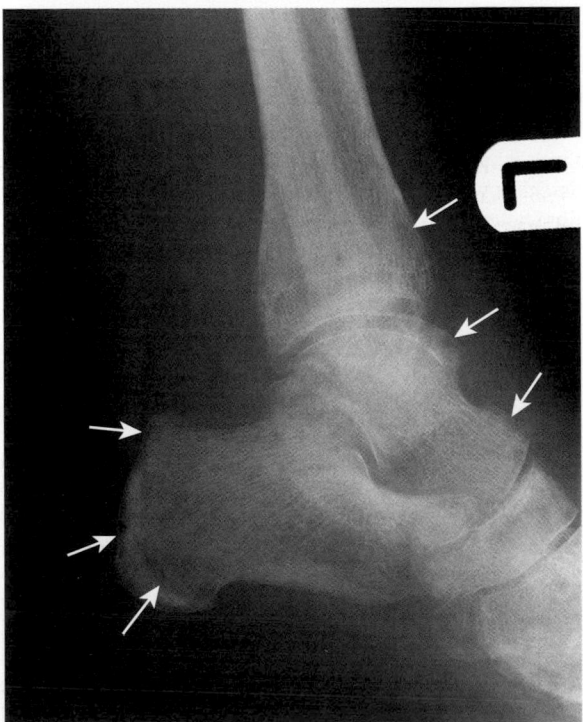

Fig. 25.43 Lateral X-ray of the foot in a patient with algodystrophy. There is generalised osteopenia and also some more focal areas of patchy osteolysis (arrows).

malignant disease (Fig. 25.43), but in cases of doubt, biopsy of the affected site can be performed. In algodystrophy the appearances are non-specific, showing osteopenia and evidence of increased bone turnover.

Management of algodystrophy is difficult. Several treatments have been tried with varying levels of success, including calcitonin, corticosteroids, sympathetic blockade and bisphosphonates. The best results have been obtained with intravenous aminobisphosphonates which may improve pain, swelling and BMD values. Nevertheless, many patients have persisting symptoms despite therapy and the overall prognosis for return of normal function is poor.

OSTEOGENESIS IMPERFECTA (OI)

OI is a rare disease that typically presents with multiple fractures in infancy and childhood. BMD values are often reduced but not invariably so, and the bone fragility is out of proportion to the reduction in BMD. Other common features include blue sclerae and abnormal dentition. Most cases are due to mutations in the type I collagen genes (*COLIA1*, *COLIA2*), causing either reduced collagen production or formation of abnormal collagen molecules that are rapidly degraded. The disease is inherited in a dominant manner, but most cases represent new mutations and often there is no positive family history. The severity varies from neonatal lethal (type II), through very severe with multiple fractures in infancy and childhood (types III and IV), to mild (type I) which is classically accompanied by blue sclerae and in which bone deformity is less marked. Severe OI can usually be diagnosed on clinical grounds, but in milder cases, osteoporosis enters into the differential diagnosis. In these cases, molecular diagnosis by mutation screening of the *COLIA1* and *COLIA2* genes can be performed, but this is not widely available.

Treatment of OI is multidisciplinary in nature. Orthopaedic surgery is required for the treatment of fractures and correction of limb deformities while physiotherapists and occupational therapists play an important role in rehabilitation of patients and in managing the consequences of bone deformity. Encouraging but uncontrolled results have been obtained using intravenous pamidronate in the treatment of children with OI.

OSTEOPETROSIS

Osteopetrosis describes a group of rare inherited diseases characterised by increased bone density due to defective osteoclast function. The presentation is highly variable, ranging from a lethal disorder that presents with bone marrow failure in infancy to a milder and sometimes asymptomatic form that presents in adulthood. Severe osteopetrosis is inherited in an autosomal recessive manner and presents with failure to thrive, delayed dentition, cranial nerve palsies (due to absent cranial foramina), blindness, anaemia and recurrent infections due to bone marrow failure. The adult-onset type (Albers–Schönberg disease) shows autosomal dominant inheritance and presents either with bone pain, cranial nerve palsies, osteomyelitis and OA, or as an incidental radiographic finding (Fig. 25.2, p. 1070).

Most cases of osteopetrosis are caused by mutations in genes that are responsible for acidification of the resorption lacuna or for matrix degradation. Many cases of recessive osteopetrosis are caused by mutations in *TCIRG1*, which encodes a component of the osteoclast proton pump, whereas mutations in the *CLCN7* gene, which encodes the osteoclast chloride pump, are responsible for most cases of autosomal dominant osteopetrosis. Mutations in the carbonic anhydrase II gene are responsible for a syndrome of osteopetrosis and renal tubular acidosis (p. 438) due to failure of acid production within the osteoclast and renal tubules. Another recessive type of osteopetrosis, termed pyknodysostosis, is caused by mutations in cathepsin K, which is essential for degradation of bone matrix.

The treatment of osteopetrosis is difficult. Interferon-gamma treatment can improve blood counts and reduce frequency of infections, but in severe cases bone marrow transplantation may be required to provide a source of normal osteoclasts that resorb bone normally.

SCLEROSING BONE DYSPLASIAS

Sclerosing bone dysplasias are a rare heterogeneous group of diseases characterised by osteosclerosis due to increased bone formation. Van Buchem's disease and sclerosteosis are recessive disorders characterised by enlargement of the cranium and jaw, tall stature and cranial nerve palsies. They are caused by mutations of the *SOST* gene which normally suppresses bone formation. Treatment is symptomatic. Camurati–Engelmann disease is an autosomal dominant condition characterised by bone pain, muscle weakness and osteosclerosis predominantly affecting the diaphysis of the long bones and caused by activating mutations in the *TGF beta 1* gene. Corticosteroid treatment can help the bone pain, but often the doses required for symptom control are unacceptably high.

POLYOSTOTIC FIBROUS DYSPLASIA

This condition is characterised by bone pain, bone deformity, and expansion and pathological fractures on a focal or multifocal basis through the skeleton. Associated features include endocrine dysfunction, especially precocious puberty, and café-au-lait skin pigmentation (McCune–Albright syndrome). It is caused by mutations in the *GNAS1* gene which encodes the stimulatory G-protein Gsα. Imaging shows focal osteolytic lesions on X-ray and focal increases on bone scan. The condition can resemble PDB but the earlier age of onset and pattern of involvement is usually distinctive. Management is symptomatic with orthopaedic treatment of fracture and deformity. Intravenous pamidronate has been reported to help bone pain and healing of lytic lesions, but studies performed so far are not blinded or placebo-controlled.

SYSTEMIC CONNECTIVE TISSUE DISEASE

The connective tissue diseases are a group of chronic inflammatory disorders that involve multiple body systems and therefore exhibit a wide spectrum of clinical manifestations. Their aetiology is multifactorial and involves genetic, immunological (especially autoantibody production) and environmental factors. Although each disease displays different clinical and pathological features, the group shares enough characteristics to be considered a family of overlapping conditions. They were initially grouped as 'collagen disease' because of common pathological changes (especially fibrinoid changes in the connective tissues) but the term connective tissue disease is now preferred as it avoids confusion with unrelated monogenic disorders of collagen such as Marfan's syndrome.

SYSTEMIC LUPUS ERYTHEMATOSUS (SLE)

SLE is the most common multisystem connective tissue disease. It is characterised by a wide variety of clinical features and a diverse spectrum of autoantibody production. The prevalence varies according to geographical and racial background, from 30/100 000 in Caucasians to 200/100 000 in Afro-Caribbeans. Around 90% of affected individuals are women, with peak onset in the second and third decades.

Aetiology and pathogenesis

At least 50 antigen targets for autoantibody production are described in SLE. However, none of the diverse manifestations of SLE can be attributed to a single antigenic stimulus, and it is likely that this wide spectrum of auto-antibody production results from polyclonal B- and T-cell activation. Many autoantigens in SLE are components of the intracellular and intranuclear machinery. In normal health these antigens are 'hidden' from the immune system and do not provoke an immune response. Although the triggers that lead to autoantibody production in SLE are unknown, one mechanism may be exposure of intracellular antigens on the cell surface during apoptosis. This hypothesis is supported by the fact that environmental factors that associate with flares of lupus—such as sunlight and artificial ultraviolet (UV) light, pregnancy and infection—increase oxidative stress and subsequent apoptosis.

Few of the autoantibodies found in SLE have been ascribed a specific pathological role. An exception is in the anti-phospholipid syndrome (p. 1062), in which antibodies against components of the coagulation cascade are responsible for the predisposition to thromboembolic disease.

Diagnosis

Diagnosis depends on the recognition of specific symptoms and identification of autoantibodies (Box 25.74). Patients who are antinuclear antibody (ANA)-negative are very unlikely to have SLE unless they are extractable nuclear antigen (Ro)-positive; most Ro-positive patients also have rashes. Anti-dsDNA antibodies occur in only 30–50% of patients.

Clinical features

Raynaud's phenomenon

Arthralgia or arthritis in combination with Raynaud's phenomenon (p. 604) is the most common presentation

25

25.74 REVISED AMERICAN RHEUMATISM ASSOCIATION CRITERIA FOR SYSTEMIC LUPUS ERYTHEMATOSUS[1]	
Features	**Characteristics**
Malar rash	Fixed erythema, flat or raised, sparing the nasolabial folds
Discoid rash	Erythematous raised patches with adherent keratotic scarring and follicular plugging
Photosensitivity	Rash as a result of unusual reaction to sunlight
Oral ulcers	Oral or nasopharyngeal ulceration, which may be painless
Arthritis	Non-erosive, involving two or more peripheral joints
Serositis	Pleuritis (convincing history of pleuritic pain or rub, or pleural effusion) *or* Pericarditis (rub, ECG evidence or effusion)
Renal disorder	Persistent proteinuria > 0.5 g/day *or* Cellular casts (red cell, granular or tubular)
Neurological disorder	Seizures or psychosis, in the absence of offending drugs or metabolic derangement
Haematological disorder	Haemolytic anaemia *or* Leucopenia[2] ($< 4 \times 10^9$/l), *or* Lymphopenia[2] ($< 1 \times 10^9$/l), *or* Thrombocytopenia[2] ($< 100 \times 10^9$/l) in the absence of offending drugs
Immunological disorder	Anti-DNA antibodies in abnormal titre *or* Presence of antibody to Sm antigen *or* Positive antiphospholipid antibodies
Antinuclear antibody (ANA) disorder	Abnormal titre of ANA by immunofluorescence

[1] For the purpose of identifying patients for clinical studies, a person has SLE if any 4 out of 11 features are present serially or simultaneously.
[2] On two separate occasions.

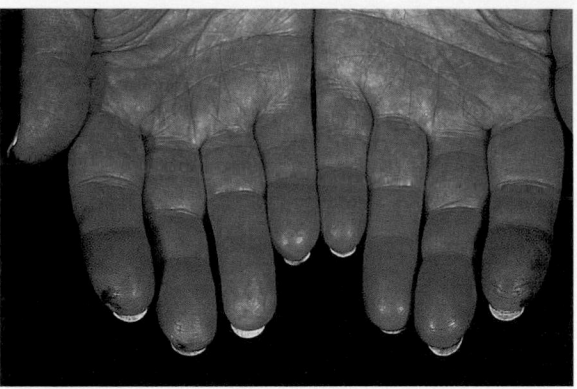

Fig. 25.44   Severe secondary Raynaud's phenomenon leading to digital ulceration.

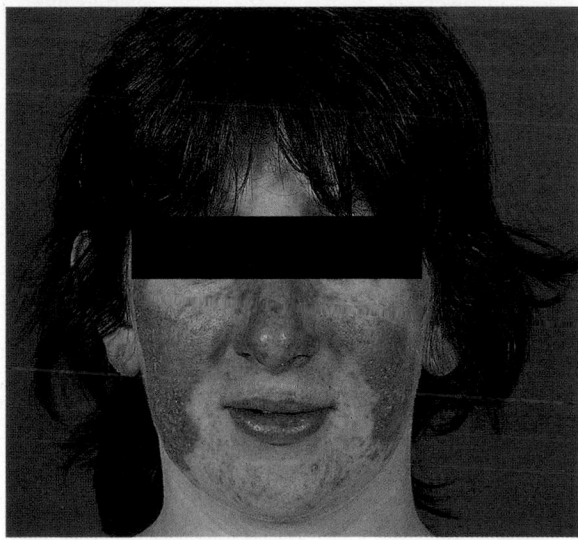

Fig. 25.45 Butterfly (malar) rash of systemic lupus erythematosus, sparing the nasolabial folds.

25

(Fig. 25.44). It is important to elicit a history of Raynaud's since it is very uncommon for this to associate with other arthropathies such as RA. Raynaud's phenomenon in a teenage girl, with no other associated symptoms and especially if there is a family history, is likely to be idiopathic 'primary' Raynaud's. By contrast, onset in a male, or in a woman over the age of 30 years suggests a secondary cause, usually underlying connective tissue disease. Examination of capillary nail-fold loops using an ophthalmoscope may help distinguish primary from secondary Raynaud's. Loss of the normal loop pattern and capillary 'fallout' with haemorrhage and dots indicate underlying disease.

Musculoskeletal features

A variety of joint problems may occur, including migratory arthralgia with mild morning stiffness, tenosynovitis and small joint synovitis that may mimic RA. In contrast to RA, joint deformities are rare. Deformities that do occur result from tendon inflammation and damage rather than from bone erosion ('Jaccoud's arthropathy').

Mucocutaneous features

Painful oral ulcers are common in SLE. In comparison with aphthous ulceration, they usually last longer and may scar. Diffuse, usually non-scarring, alopecia may occur with active disease. There are three main types of rash in SLE:

● *The classic butterfly facial rash* (20–30% of patients) is raised and painful or pruritic and occurs in a photosensitive distribution that spares the nasolabial folds (Fig. 25.45).
● *Subacute cutaneous lupus erythematosus* (SCLE) rashes are migratory, non-scarring and either papulosquamous (psoriaform) or annular.
● *Discoid lupus* lesions are characterised by hyperkeratosis and follicular plugging and may cause scarring alopecia if present on the scalp.

Other skin manifestations include periungual erythema, vasculitis and livedo reticularis, the latter also being a common feature of the antiphospholipid antibody syndrome (Fig. 25.46).

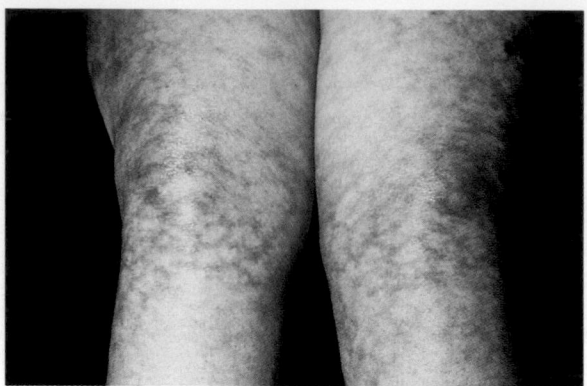

Fig. 25.46 Livedo reticularis in systemic lupus erythematosus.

Renal features

Renal involvement is one of the main determinants of prognosis, and regular monitoring of urinalysis and blood pressure is essential. The typical renal lesion is a proliferative glomerulonephritis (p. 499), characterised by heavy haematuria, proteinuria and casts on urine microscopy.

Cardiopulmonary features

The most common manifestation is chest pain from pleurisy or pericarditis. Myocarditis and sterile Libman–Sacks endocarditis may also occur, the latter being due to non-infectious vegetations, usually seen as a manifestation of procoagulability in association with antiphospholipid antibodies. SLE patients with antiphospholipid antibodies are at increased risk of venous thromboembolism, which should always be considered in the presence of chest pain or dyspnoea. Alveolitis and lung fibrosis occur, particularly in overlap connective tissue diseases.

Central nervous system features

Fatigue, headache, poor concentration and other non-specific features similar to fibromyalgia are common accompaniments of SLE and often occur in the absence of active disease. Specific features of cerebral lupus include visual hallucinations, chorea (also associated with antiphospholipid antibody syndrome), organic psychosis, transverse myelitis and lymphocytic meningitis.

Haematological features

Antibody-mediated destruction of peripheral blood cells may cause neutropenia, lymphopenia, thrombocytopenia or haemolytic anaemia. The degree of leucopenia, most commonly lymphopenia, is often a good guide to disease activity. Although the ESR is usually elevated, CRP is often normal unless there is serositis or infection.

Other manifestations

Fever, weight loss and mild lymphadenopathy commonly accompany active disease. Gastrointestinal involvement is rare and other causes of abdominal pain should always be considered, e.g. appendicitis, perforation secondary to drugs, or infection.

There is also significant morbidity from chronic fatigue and other features of fibromyalgia, which affect up to 80% of patients. These symptoms are typically unresponsive to corticosteroids and should be managed according to standard fibromyalgia protocols, e.g. low-dose amitriptyline, graded exercise therapy and cognitive behavioural interventions if appropriate (p. 238).

25.75 MANAGEMENT OF LUPUS NEPHRITIS   **EBM**

'In SLE nephritis pulse i.v. cyclophosphamide is more effective than pulse i.v. methylprednisolone alone and combination therapy is more effective still. Continuing quarterly i.v. treatment for 1 year after renal remission decreases the risk of renal flares.'

- Boumpas DT, et al. Lancet 1992; 340:741–745.
- Gourley MF, et al. Ann Intern Med 1996; 125:549–557.

Management

All patients require education on the importance of avoiding sun and UV light exposure, and the use of high-factor sun blocks (sun protection factor 25–50). Many patients have mild disease requiring only intermittent analgesics or NSAIDs. Hydroxychloroquine (200–400 mg daily) is often effective for more troublesome cutaneous and joint symptoms. Short courses of oral corticosteroids may be required for mild to moderate disease activity (e.g. rashes, synovitis, pleuro-pericarditis).

Acute or life-threatening disease (i.e. renal, cerebral) requires high-dose corticosteroids (e.g. oral prednisolone 40–60 mg daily or i.v. methylprednisolone 500 mg–1 g) in combination with pulse i.v. cyclophosphamide (Box 25.75). Other immunosuppressive drugs (azathioprine, methotrexate, ciclosporin, tacrolimus, mycophenolate mofetil) are useful either alone or in combination with corticosteroids for severe but non-life-threatening manifestations or as step-down therapy after cyclophosphamide. Lupus patients with the antiphospholipid antibody syndrome who have had previous thrombosis will require life-long warfarin. If repeated thromboses occur despite warfarin, the INR target range is usually increased to 2.5–3.5.

Prognosis

Overall 5-year survival is greater than 90%. Early mortality within 5 years of diagnosis is usually due to organ failure or overwhelming sepsis, both of which are modifiable by early intervention. However, compared to the normal population, the late mortality of patients with lupus is increased five-fold. This mainly results from premature cardiovascular disease to which chronic corticosteroid therapy contributes. To reduce this, steroids should be used at the lowest effective dose and for the shortest period possible; combination therapy with immunosuppressive drugs may help to achieve this. It is also important to control other cardiovascular risk factors.

SYSTEMIC SCLEROSIS

Systemic sclerosis (previously called 'scleroderma') is a generalised disorder of connective tissue affecting the skin, internal organs and vasculature. The clinical hallmark is the presence of sclerodactyly in combination with Raynaud's phenomenon or digital ischaemia. The peak age of onset

25

is in the fourth and fifth decades, and overall prevalence is 10–20 per 100 000 with a 4:1 female:male ratio. It is sub-divided into diffuse cutaneous systemic sclerosis (DCSS) and limited cutaneous systemic sclerosis (LCSS). Many patients with LCSS have features which are phenotypically grouped into the 'CREST' syndrome (**c**alcinosis, **R**aynaud's, **o**esophageal involvement, **s**clerodactyly, **t**elangiectasia).

Aetiology and pathogenesis

The aetiology is unknown, with no consistent genetic, geographical or racial associations. Environmental factors are important in isolated cases that result from exposure to silica dust, vinyl chloride, hypoxy resins and trichloroethylene.

Early in the disease there is skin infiltration by T lymphocytes and abnormal fibroblast activation that leads to increased production of extracellular matrix in the dermis, primarily type I collagen. This results in symmetrical thickening, tightening and induration of the skin (sclerodactyly). In addition to skin changes there is arterial and arteriolar narrowing due to intimal proliferation and vessel wall inflammation. Endothelial injury causes release of vasoconstrictors and platelet activation, resulting in further ischaemia.

Clinical features and diagnosis

Systemic sclerosis is predominantly a clinical diagnosis based on the presence of sclerodactyly (Fig. 25.47). Most patients are ANA-positive, and approximately 30% of patients with diffuse disease and 60% with limited disease have antibodies to topoisomerase 1 and centromere respectively.

Cutaneous changes

Raynaud's phenomenon is universal and may precede other clinical features.

The initial phase of skin disease is characterised by non-pitting oedema of the fingers and flexor tendon sheaths. Subsequently, the skin becomes shiny and taut, and distal skin creases disappear. There is usually erythema and tortuous dilatation of capillary loops in the nail-fold bed, readily visible with an ophthalmoscope set to +20. The face and neck are usually involved next, with thinning of the lips and radial furrowing. In some patients skin thickening

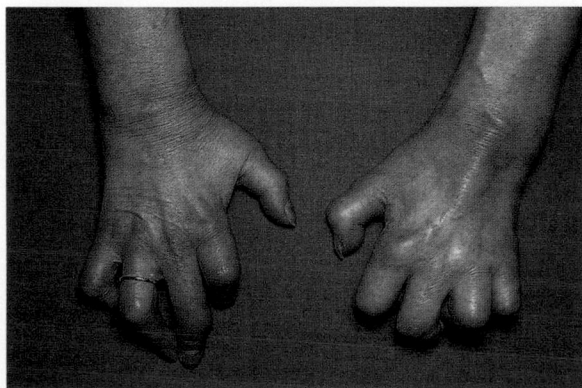

Fig. 25.47 Systemic sclerosis. Hands showing tight shiny skin, sclerodactyly, flexion contractures of the fingers and thickening of the left middle finger extensor tendon sheath.

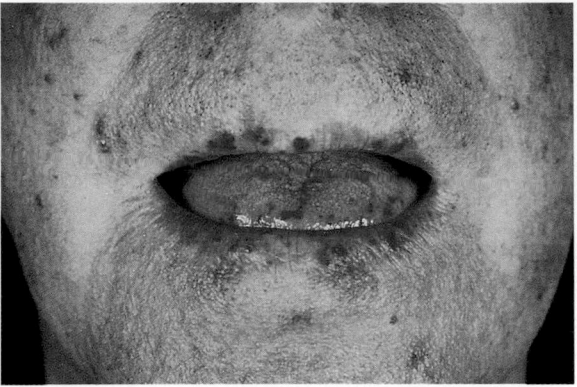

Fig. 25.48 Typical facial appearance in the CREST syndrome.

stops at this stage. Skin involvement restricted to sites distal to the elbow or knee (apart from the face) is classified as 'limited cutaneous disease' or CREST syndrome (Fig. 25.48). Involvement proximal to the knee and elbow and on the trunk is classified as 'diffuse cutaneous disease'. In the distal extremities, the combination of intimal fibrosis and vessel wall inflammation may cause critical tissue ischaemia, leading to skin ulceration over pressure areas, localised areas of infarction and pulp atrophy at the fingertips.

Musculoskeletal features

Arthralgia, morning stiffness and flexor tenosynovitis are common. Restricted hand function is due to skin rather than joint disease and erosive arthropathy is uncommon. Muscle weakness and wasting are usually due to myositis.

Gastrointestinal features

Gut involvement is common. Smooth muscle atrophy and fibrosis in the lower two-thirds of the oesophagus lead to acid reflux with erosive oesophagitis. Since this may progress to further fibrosis, adequate treatment of reflux (usually with proton pump inhibitors) is important. Dysphagia and odynophagia (painful dysphagia) may also occur. Involvement of the stomach causes early satiety and occasionally outlet obstruction. Recurrent occult upper gastrointestinal bleeding may indicate a 'watermelon stomach' (antral vascular ectasia), which occurs in up to 20% of patients. Small intestine involvement may lead to malabsorption due to bacterial overgrowth and intermittent bloating, pain or constipation. Dilatation of large or small bowel due to autonomic neuropathy may cause pseudo-obstruction.

Cardiorespiratory features

Pulmonary involvement is a major cause of morbidity and mortality. Fibrosing alveolitis mainly affects patients with diffuse disease, particularly those with antibodies to topoisomerase 1. Pulmonary hypertension is a complication of long-standing disease and is six times more prevalent in limited than in diffuse disease. The clinical features are rapidly progressive dyspnoea (more rapid than interstitial lung disease), right heart failure and angina, often in association with rapidly progressing digital ischaemia. Treatment strategies include vasodilators, continuous

25

infusions of epoprostenol, the oral endothelin 1 antagonist bosentan and heart–lung transplantation.

Renal features

One of the main causes of death is hypertensive renal crisis characterised by rapidly developing malignant hypertension and renal failure. Treatment is by angiotensin-converting enzyme (ACE) inhibition even if renal impairment is present. Hypertensive renal crisis is much more likely to occur in patients with diffuse rather than limited disease. It is also more prevalent in patients with topoisomerase 1 antibodies, and many clinicians use prophylactic ACE inhibitors in patients with diffuse disease to prevent this manifestation.

Management and prognosis

Five-year survival is approximately 70%. Risk factors at presentation that associate with a poor prognosis include older age, diffuse skin disease, proteinuria, high ESR, a low gas transfer factor for carbon monoxide (TLCO) and pulmonary hypertension.

Self-management to maintain core body temperature and avoid peripheral cold exposure is important. Infection of ulcerated skin should be treated with prompt antibiotic therapy. Antibiotics penetrate poorly into the skin lesions of systemic sclerosis and therefore need to be given at higher dose for longer periods (e.g. flucloxacillin 500 mg 6-hourly for 14 days). Calcium antagonists (e.g. nifedipine, amlodipine) or angiotensin II receptor antagonists (e.g. valsartan) may be effective for Raynaud's symptoms. For severe digital ischaemia, intermittent infusions of epoprostenol may be helpful.

Corticosteroids and cytotoxic drugs are indicated in patients with myositis or alveolitis. No agent has been shown to arrest or improve skin changes.

POLYMYOSITIS AND DERMATOMYOSITIS

The idiopathic inflammatory myopathies (IIMs) are rare connective tissue disorders defined by the presence of muscle weakness and inflammation. The incidence is 2–10 per million/year with no significant world-wide variation. The aetiology is unknown and genetic associations differ amongst ethnic groups. The most common clinical forms of IIM are polymyositis, dermatomyositis and inclusion body myositis. Other systemic autoimmune diseases such as SLE or vasculitis can also cause myositis. Usually only skeletal muscle is affected. Occasionally, the distribution is focal (e.g. orbital myositis).

There is an increased risk of malignancy in patients with dermatomyositis (about a threefold increase) and polymyositis (an increase of about 30%). Malignancy may be apparent at the time of diagnosis or manifest itself later.

Polymyositis

The typical presentation is with symmetrical proximal muscle weakness, usually affecting the lower extremities first. Patients report difficulty rising from a chair, climbing stairs and lifting, sometimes in combination with muscle pain. The onset is usually between 40 and 60 years of age

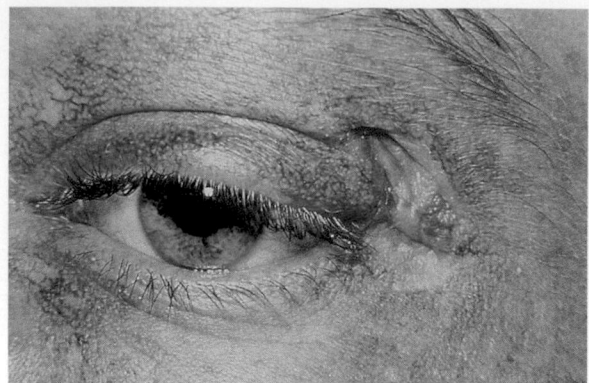

Fig. 25.49 Typical eyelid appearance in dermatomyositis. Note the oedema and telangiectasia.

and is typically gradual, over a few weeks, although both more explosive and more insidious onsets may occur. Systemic features of fever, weight loss and fatigue are common. Respiratory or pharyngeal muscle involvement leading to ventilatory failure/aspiration is ominous and requires urgent treatment. Interstitial lung disease occurs in up to 30% of patients and is strongly associated with the presence of antisynthetase (e.g. Jo1) antibodies.

Dermatomyositis

The muscle manifestations are identical to polymyositis, but occur in combination with characteristic cutaneous manifestations. Gottron's papules are scaly erythematous/violaceous plaques or papules occurring over the extensor surfaces of the proximal and distal interphalangeal joints. The heliotrope rash is a violaceous discoloration of the eyelid in combination with periorbital oedema (Fig. 25.49). Similar rashes occur on the upper back, chest and shoulders ('shawl' distribution). Periungual nail-fold capillaries are often abnormal. Other systemic manifestations include arthralgia, weight loss and fever.

Investigations

These conditions should be suspected in anyone who presents with proximal muscle weakness without evidence of neuropathy, particularly if there is evidence of systemic disease. Creatine kinase (CK) is usually raised and is a guide to disease activity. However, a normal CK does not exclude the diagnosis, particularly in juvenile myositis where only 70% of patients have a raised CK at the time of diagnosis. Electromyography (EMG) may confirm the presence of myopathy and exclude neuropathy. Most patients will then need a muscle biopsy to look for the typical features of fibre necrosis, regeneration and inflammatory cell infiltrate (Fig. 25.50). Occasionally, a biopsy may be normal, particularly if myositis is patchy. MRI is a useful means of identifying areas of abnormal muscle that are amenable to biopsy. When underlying malignancy is suspected screening investigations should include chest/abdomen/pelvis CT, gastrointestinal tract imaging and mammography.

Management

Oral corticosteroids (e.g. prednisolone 40–60 mg daily) are the mainstay of initial treatment. Patients with severe

25

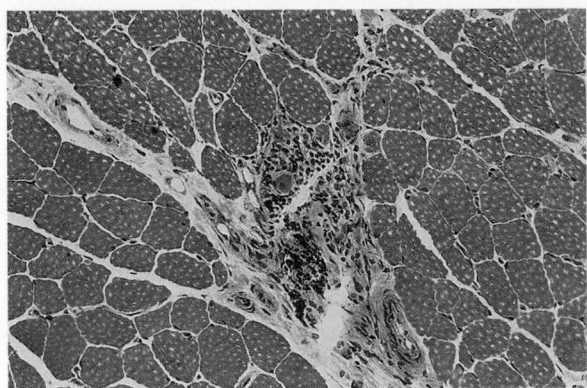

Fig. 25.50 Muscle biopsy from a patient with inflammatory myositis. The sample shows an intense inflammatory cell infiltrate in an area of degenerating and regenerating muscle fibres.

weakness or evidence of respiratory or pharyngeal weakness may need methylprednisolone 1 g daily for 3 days. If there is a good response, the prednisolone dose should be reduced by approximately 25% per month to a maintenance dose of 5–7.5 mg. Although most patients have an initial response to steroids, many will need additional immunosuppressive therapy, especially if the disease relapses. Azathioprine and methotrexate are the initial agents of choice. If these are ineffective or not tolerated, then ciclosporin, cyclophosphamide, tacrolimus and intravenous immunoglobulin are alternatives. If the patient fails to respond clinically to treatment, this may be due to steroid-induced myopathy or the development of inclusion body myositis. Further biopsy is indicated at this stage. If active necrosis and regeneration are present, then the disease is still active, whereas the presence of type 2 fibre atrophy suggests steroid myopathy.

INCLUSION BODY MYOSITIS

This is the most common disease of muscle in patients over the age of 50 and predominates in men. Although proximal weakness does occur, distal involvement is more common and may be asymmetrical. Evaluation is along the same lines as for IIM. CK may be marginally elevated and both myopathic and neurogenic abnormalities may be present on EMG. The characteristic findings on muscle biopsy are abnormal fibres containing rimmed vacuoles and filamentous inclusions in the nucleus and cytoplasm. These inclusions contain paired helical filaments that resemble those seen in the brain in Alzheimer's disease. Treatment is controversial and not as successful as in IIM. Some patients do have an inflammatory component and are corticosteroid-responsive; a trial of steroids is therefore warranted, and if a response occurs then immunosuppressive therapy should be substituted.

MIXED CONNECTIVE TISSUE DISEASE

This is an overlap connective tissue disease with features of SLE, systemic sclerosis and myositis. The usual clinical features include synovitis and oedema of the hands in combination with Raynaud's phenomenon and muscle pain/weakness. Most patients have anti-ribonucleoprotein (RNP) antibodies, although these also occur in SLE without overlap features.

SJÖGREN'S SYNDROME

This is an autoimmune disorder of unknown aetiology characterised by lymphocytic infiltration of salivary and lachrymal glands, leading to glandular fibrosis and exocrine failure. Age of onset is usually in the fourth and fifth decades with a female:male ratio of 9:1. The disease may be primary or secondary in association with other autoimmune disease such as RA, SLE, thyroiditis or primary biliary cirrhosis.

Clinical features

The eye symptoms, termed keratoconjunctivitis sicca, are due to a lack of tears and lubrication. Conjunctivitis and blepharitis are frequent manifestations, and may lead to filamentary keratitis due to tenacious mucous filaments binding to the cornea and conjunctiva. Oral involvement typically leads to the patient needing water to swallow food, and there is a high incidence of dental caries. Other sites of extraglandular involvement are listed in Box 25.76.

The disease is associated with a 40-fold increased lifetime risk of lymphoma and can be viewed as being at the crossroads between an exaggerated autoimmune response and malignancy.

25

25.76 FEATURES OF SJÖGREN'S SYNDROME	
Risk markers	
• Age of onset 40–60	• HLA–B8/DR3
• F > M	
Common clinical features	
• Keratoconjunctivitis sicca	• Non-erosive arthritis
• Xerostomia	• Raynaud's phenomenon
• Salivary gland enlargement	• Fatigue
Less common features	
• Low-grade fever	• Peripheral neuropathy
• Interstitial lung disease	• Lymphadenopathy
• Anaemia, leucopenia	• Lymphoreticular malignancy
• Thrombocytopenia	• Glomerulonephritis
• Cryoglobulinaemia	• Renal tubular acidosis
• Vasculitis	
Autoantibodies frequently detected	
• Rheumatoid factor	• SS-B (anti-La)
• ANA	• Gastric parietal cell
• SS-A (anti-Ro)	• Thyroid
Associated autoimmune disorders	
• SLE	• Chronic active hepatitis
• Progressive systemic sclerosis	• Myasthenia gravis
• Primary biliary cirrhosis	

Investigations

Most patients will have an elevated ESR secondary to hypergammaglobulinaemia and one or more autoantibodies, of which antinuclear antibody (ANA) and rheumatoid factor are the most common. Sicca can be established by the Schirmer tear test, which measures flow of tears over 5 minutes using absorbent paper strips placed in the lower lachrymal sac; a normal result is greater than 6 mm of wetting. If the diagnosis is still in doubt, it can be confirmed by finding focal lymphocytic infiltrate in the minor salivary glands on lip biopsy.

Management

Artificial lubrication is the mainstay of symptomatic treatment. Lachrymal substitutes such as hypromellose should be used during the day in combination with more viscous lubricating ointment at night. Soft contact lenses can be useful for corneal protection in patients with filamentary keratitis, and occlusion of the lachrymal ducts is occasionally needed. Artificial saliva and oral gels can be tried for xerostomia, but are often not effective. Stimulation of saliva flow by sugar-free chewing gum or lozenges may be helpful. Adequate post-prandial oral hygiene and prompt treatment of oral candidiasis are essential. Vaginal dryness is treated with lubricants such as K-Y jelly.

Extraglandular and MSK manifestations may respond to corticosteroids and, if so, other immunosuppressive drugs such as azathioprine can be added for steroid-sparing effect. One of the most difficult symptoms to treat is fatigue; this is usually due to non-restorative sleep (often because of xerostomia) and is unresponsive to steroids. Immunosuppression does not improve sicca symptoms. If massive lymphadenopathy or salivary gland enlargement develops during the disease course, biopsy should be performed to detect malignancy.

INHERITED DISEASES OF CONNECTIVE TISSUE

Marfan's syndrome is characterised by skeletal disproportion (arm span greater than height), arachnodactyly (long, thin, 'spider' fingers), sternal depression, generalised hypermobility of joints, lens dislocation and a high arched palate. It results from mutations of the fibrillin gene, a component of extracellular matrix. The most serious complications are in the cardiovascular system, with mitral valve prolapse, aortic incompetence and aortic dissection (Ch. 18).

Ehlers–Danlos syndrome is characterised by generalised hypermobility, skin laxity and easy bruising, with scoliosis, short stature, ocular fragility and visceral vascular catastrophes. It may result from mutations in several genes including *COLIA2*, lysyl oxidase, fibronectin and elastin.

Osteoporosis and a Marfanoid appearance occur in homocystinuria, which is due to deficiency of the enzyme cystathionine synthetase. Other features include mental retardation, and venous and arterial thrombosis. The diagnosis is confirmed by finding homocystine in the urine, and patients respond to treatment with pyridoxine.

SYSTEMIC VASCULITIS

The vasculitides are a heterogeneous group of diseases characterised by inflammation and necrosis of blood vessel walls (Box 25.77). The spectrum of disease ranges from benign and self-limiting (e.g. cutaneous leucocytoclastic vasculitis limited to skin) to life-threatening (e.g. fulminant Wegener's granulomatosis with renal failure and pulmonary haemorrhage).

Vasculitis may occur in many types of inflammatory or infectious diseases, such as SLE, RA, endocarditis and hepatitis B and C. Primary systemic vasculitis is less common, with an annual incidence of approximately 18–40 new cases per million, which peaks in the 65–74-year age group. The aetiology remains unclear, although geographic, environmental and genetic factors are important.

Clinical features

These are due to a combination of local tissue ischaemia (caused by vessel inflammation and narrowing) and the systemic effects of widespread inflammation. Typical features are shown in Box 25.26 (p. 1088). Systemic vasculitis should be considered in any patient with fever, weight loss, fatigue, evidence of multisystem involvement, rashes, raised inflammatory markers and abnormal urinalysis. Early diagnosis and management are essential to prevent irreversible organ damage. Vasculitis may be difficult to distinguish from widespread malignancy, occult sepsis (particularly subacute bacterial endocarditis and meningococcal septicaemia), cholesterol emboli, atrial myxoma and the antiphospholipid syndrome. The key to recognition is the presence of multisystem involvement.

Investigations

If vasculitis is suspected, the diagnosis should ideally be confirmed by tissue biopsy, in order to determine the vessel size involved and guide therapy. Skin biopsies are easily obtained. Nasal septal tissue can be taken from areas of ulceration or granulation. Muscle biopsy is positive in about 50% of patients with muscle pain. The most important bedside test is the urine dip test for protein and blood, and subsequent microscopy, since the prognosis of vasculitis is often determined by the degree of renal involvement. In patients with abnormal renal function and active urinary

25.77 SIZE OF VESSEL INVOLVEMENT IN VASCULITIS	
Large vessel	
• Giant cell arteritis	• Takayasu's arteritis
Medium vessel	
• Classical polyarteritis nodosa	• Kawasaki disease (in childhood)
Small vessel	
• Microscopic polyangiitis	• Henoch–Schönlein purpura
• Wegener's granulomatosis	• Mixed essential
• Churg–Strauss syndrome	cryoglobulinaemia

25

sediment, renal biopsy should be considered. Visceral angiography to detect microaneurysms (e.g. classical polyarteritis nodosa) is most useful where involved tissue is not available to biopsy.

Antineutrophil cytoplasmic antibodies (ANCA) are directed against enzymes present in neutrophil granules. Two main patterns of immunofluorescence are distinguished: cytoplasmic (c-ANCA) and perinuclear (p-ANCA). c-ANCA are usually directed against proteinase 3 and are particularly associated with Wegener's granulomatosis and Churg–Strauss syndrome. p-ANCA are usually directed against myeloperoxidase and associate with microscopic polyangiitis. However, positive ANCAs occur in many other diseases, including malignancy, infection (bacterial and HIV), inflammatory bowel disease, RA, lupus and pulmonary fibrosis. Therefore, the diagnosis of these conditions cannot be made or refuted on the ANCA test alone.

POLYMYALGIA RHEUMATICA (PMR)

PMR is a clinical syndrome of muscle pain and stiffness and, classically, an increased ESR. It is not a true vasculitis but there is a close association with giant cell arteritis. The prevalence is approximately 20 per 100 000 over the age of 50. The mean age of onset is 70, and diagnosis is rarely made in patients under 60. Women are affected more often than men in a ratio of 3:1.

Clinical features

The cardinal features are muscle stiffness and pain, symmetrically affecting the proximal muscles of the neck, upper arms and, less commonly, the buttocks and thighs. There is marked early morning stiffness, often with night pain. Constitutional features of weight loss, fatigue, depression and night sweats also occur. Most patients have a rapid onset of symptoms, sometimes overnight, although occasionally the onset is more insidious. On examination there may be stiffness and painful restriction of active shoulder movement but passive movements are preserved. Muscles may be tender to palpation but there should not be muscle-wasting; if there is, then primary muscle or neurological disease is more likely.

Investigations

In the majority of patients the ESR is elevated above 40 mm/hour and there may be a normochromic, normocytic anaemia. Very occasionally the ESR is low, usually in the acute situation where there has not been sufficient time for it to rise. In this situation the CRP may be elevated prior to the ESR.

Management

The only effective treatment is corticosteroids, and prednisolone should be started at a dose of 15 mg daily. The majority of patients should have a dramatic response within 72 hours. If there is no response by 72 hours or an incomplete response by 7 days, then the diagnosis is not PMR. Other conditions that may mimic PMR are shown in Box 25.78.

If there has been a good response to prednisolone, the daily dose should be reduced to 10 mg after 4 weeks and

25.78 CONDITIONS THAT MAY MIMIC POLYMYALGIA RHEUMATICA

- Fibromyalgia
- Hypothyroidism
- Cervical spondylosis
- Rheumatoid arthritis
- Inflammatory myopathy (particularly inclusion body myositis)
- Systemic vasculitis
- Malignancy

then by 1 mg per month, assuming that symptoms remain controlled. If symptoms recur, the dose should be increased to that which previously controlled the symptoms, and reduction attempted in another few months. Most patients need steroids for an average of 12–18 months and osteoporosis prophylaxis with bisphosphonates should be considered. Some patients require steroid-sparing agents such as methotrexate or azathioprine, particularly if prednisolone cannot be withdrawn at 2 years or is needed at doses greater than 7.5 mg daily.

Occasionally, RA presents with a polymyalgic illness (Box 20.78). This is more common in men and the diagnosis is usually revealed by the appearance of peripheral synovitis when prednisolone doses are reduced below 10 mg/day.

Approximately 15–20% of patients develop features of giant cell arteritis at some point in the course of their disease. All patients should therefore be instructed to seek prompt medical advice if such symptoms occur.

GIANT CELL ARTERITIS (GCA)

GCA is a large vessel vasculitis predominately affecting branches of the temporal and ophthalmic arteries. The mean age of onset is 70 years with a 4:1 female:male ratio.

Clinical features

As with PMR, onset of symptoms may be abrupt but is often insidious over the course of several weeks or months. The most important clinical features are:

- *Headache*. This is usually the first symptom and is often localised to the temporal or occipital region, with scalp tenderness.
- *Jaw pain*. This is brought on by chewing or talking and is due to ischaemia of the masseters.
- *Visual disturbance*. The optic nerve head is supplied by the posterior ciliary artery, vasculitis of which leads to occlusion and acute anterior ischaemic optic neuropathy. Damage to the optic nerve results in loss of visual acuity and field, reduced colour perception and pupillary defects. Sudden visual symptoms in one eye, leading rapidly to blindness, constitute the most common pattern. On fundoscopy the optic disc may appear pale and swollen with haemorrhages, but these changes may take 24–36 hours to develop. Once blindness has occurred corticosteroids have a negligible effect but are indicated to prevent blindness in the other eye.

There may be associated constitutional symptoms of anorexia, fatigue, weight loss, fever, depression and general malaise. Occasionally presentation is with neurological complications that include transient ischaemic attacks, brain-stem infarcts and hemiparesis.

25

Investigations

The ESR and CRP are elevated as for PMR (see above). Ideally, a temporal artery biopsy should also be obtained. However, corticosteroid treatment should not be delayed whilst this is organised; diagnostic information will still be present on biopsies taken a week later. Characteristic biopsy findings are fragmentation of the internal elastic lamina with necrosis of the media in combination with a mixed inflammatory cell infiltrate (lymphocytes, plasma cells and eosinophils). However, 'skip' lesions are common and a negative biopsy does not exclude the diagnosis.

Management

If GCA is suspected, systemic corticosteroid (prednisolone 60 mg daily) should be started immediately to prevent visual loss. Steroid reduction should be guided by symptoms and ESR, aiming for approximately 10 mg daily by 6 weeks. Thereafter, doses should be reduced by 1 mg per month. Patients with known GCA should be advised to take 60 mg prednisolone and seek prompt medical advice should they experience any recurrence of headache or visual disturbance. Maintenance therapy is required for at least 1 year, and occasionally for the rest of the patient's life. Relapse occurs in 30%, and is an indication to restart high-dose steroids with additional immunosuppressive agents, typically azathioprine or methotrexate.

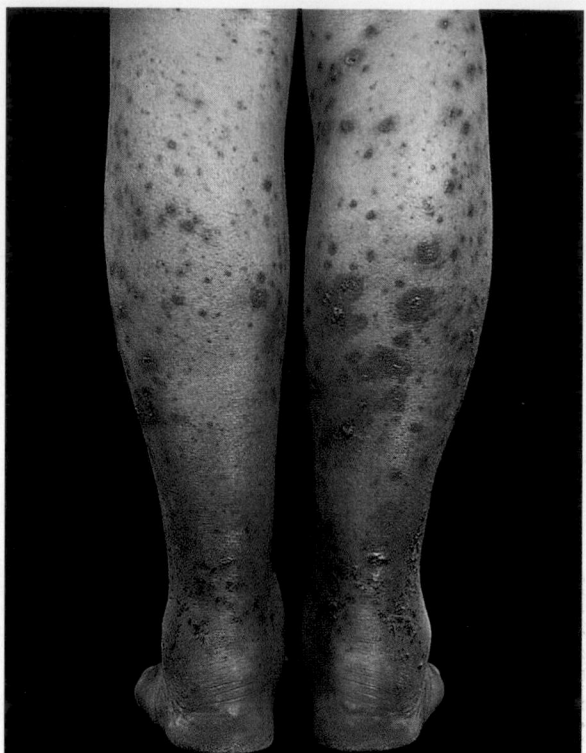

Fig. 25.51 Rash of systemic vasculitis (palpable purpura).

TAKAYASU'S ARTERITIS

Takayasu's disease is a chronic inflammatory granulomatous panarteritis of elastic arteries. The vessels most commonly involved are the aorta and its branches, and the carotid, ulnar, brachial, radial and axillary arteries. Pulmonary arteries are occasionally affected. It is more common in women (female:male ratio 8:1) with a typical onset at the age of 25–30 years. It has a world-wide distribution but is most common in Asia. The aetiology is unknown. In contrast to other vasculitides Takayasu's arteritis is characterised by thickened and inflamed intima without fibrinoid degeneration.

The usual presentation is with claudication and systemic symptoms of fever, arthralgia and weight loss. Clinical examination may reveal loss of pulses, bruits, hypertension and aortic incompetence.

Laboratory investigations are usually non-specific, with high ESR and normocytic, normochromic anaemia. Diagnosis is usually based on angiographic findings of coarctation, occlusion and aneurysmal dilatation.

The 5-year survival rate is ~80%. Most patients respond to initial high-dose oral prednisolone (1–2 mg/kg daily). Additional therapy with methotrexate or cyclophosphamide is usually required. Reconstructive vascular surgery should be avoided during periods of active inflammation but may benefit selected patients, especially those with hypertension secondary to aortic or renal lesions.

CLASSICAL POLYARTERITIS NODOSA (PAN)

Classical PAN is a necrotising vasculitis characterised by transmural inflammation of medium-sized to small arteries.

PAN is a rare disorder with an annual incidence of 2 per million in most populations. All age groups can be affected, with a peak incidence in the fourth and fifth decades, and a male:female ratio of 2:1. Hepatitis B is a risk factor, and the incidence of PAN is 10 times higher in the Inuit population of Alaska, where hepatitis B infection is endemic.

Clinical presentation is with myalgia, arthralgia, fever and weight loss in combination with manifestations of multisystem disease. The most common skin lesions are palpable purpura, ulceration, infarction and livedo reticularis (Figs 25.46 and 25.51). In 70% of patients arteritis of the vasa nervorum leads to neuropathy which is typically symmetrical and affects both sensory and motor function. Severe hypertension and/or renal impairment may occur due to multiple renal infarctions; glomerulonephritis is rare (in contrast to microscopic polyangiitis). Diagnosis is confirmed by finding multiple aneurysms and smooth narrowing of either the mesenteric, hepatic or renal systems on angiography. Tissue biopsy may be definitive (muscle or sural nerve), even in the absence of angiographic abnormality.

Treatment for hepatitis B-related disease is to remove the source of the antigen, i.e. antiviral therapy (p. 966). Corticosteroids and cyclophosphamide are the treatment of choice for idiopathic disease. Mortality is less than 20%, although relapse occurs in up to 50% of patients.

ANCA-ASSOCIATED VASCULITIS

Microscopic polyangiitis, Wegener's granulomatosis and Churg–Strauss syndrome can be grouped together as

'ANCA-associated vasculitis', although not all patients are ANCA-positive at diagnosis. All patients may present similarly with arthralgia, myalgia and evidence of multi-system disease, the precise 'subtype' being determined by other specific clinical features.

Microscopic polyangiitis (MPA)

MPA is more common than PAN, with an annual incidence of 8 per million in the UK. Classic presentation is with rapidly progressive glomerulonephritis (p. 499), often associated with pulmonary alveolar haemorrhage. Cutaneous and gastrointestinal involvement, similar to PAN, is common. Other features include neuropathy (15%) and pleural effusions (15%). Patients are usually p-ANCA-positive.

Wegener's granulomatosis (WG)

The annual incidence of WG is 5–10 per million. The most common presentation is with upper airway involvement (typically epistaxis, nasal crusting and sinusitis), haemoptysis, mucosal ulceration and deafness due to serous otitis media. Symptoms may have been present for several months and erroneously attributed to infection or allergy. The most common ocular abnormality is proptosis, due to inflammation of the retro-orbital tissue. This may cause diplopia due to entrapment of the extraocular muscles, or loss of vision due to optic nerve compression (Fig. 25.52). Untreated nasal disease ultimately leads to destruction of bone and cartilage. Migratory pulmonary infiltrates and nodules occur in 50% of patients. A minority of patients present with glomerulonephritis. Patients are usually c-ANCA-positive.

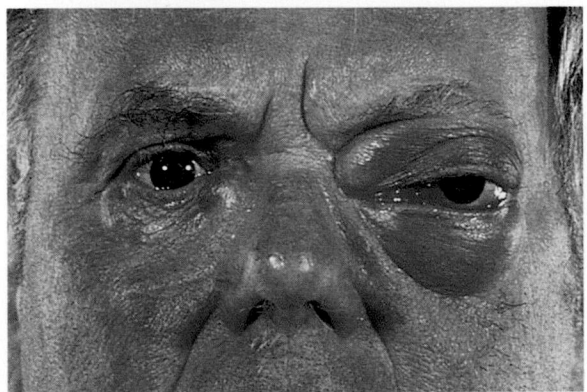

Fig. 25.52 Eye involvement in Wegener's granulomatosis.

Churg–Strauss syndrome (CSS)

The annual incidence is 1–3 per million in the UK. Most patients have a prodromal period for many years, characterised by allergic rhinitis, nasal polyposis and late-onset asthma that is often difficult to control. The typical acute presentation is with a triad comprising skin lesions (purpura or nodules), asymmetric mononeuritis multiplex and eosinophilia on a background of resistant asthma. Pulmonary infiltrates and pleural or pericardial effusions due to serositis may be present. Up to 50% of patients have abdominal symptoms due to mesenteric vasculitis. Either c-ANCA or p-ANCA is present in around 40% of cases.

Management of MPA, WG and CSS

Treatment should be instituted as early as possible to prevent irreversible damage, even in advance of biopsy confirmation if there is life-threatening or critical organ involvement. Remission can be induced either with oral high-dose prednisolone (1 mg/kg daily) and continuous oral cyclophosphamide (2 mg/kg daily) or with bolus i.v. methylprednisolone (10 mg/kg) and cyclophosphamide (15 mg/kg), initially fortnightly and subsequently monthly. Doses of cyclophosphamide should be reduced in the elderly and those with renal impairment. Once remission has been induced (3–6 months) the dose of oral prednisolone is rapidly reduced and cyclophosphamide is usually replaced with azathioprine. Co-trimoxazole is usually given at a prophylactic dose (960 mg thrice weekly) in conjunction with cyclophosphamide to prevent *Pneumocystis* pneumonia, unless there is a history of drug allergy. Mesna is used with bolus cyclophosphamide to reduce the risks of haemorrhagic cystitis. Occasionally, cyclophosphamide fails to induce a remission, in which case the diagnosis should be reconsidered. Patients who have ANCA-positive vasculitis with acute renal failure (creatinine > 500 µmol/l or 5.66 mg/dl) have a better outcome when also treated with adjunctive plasma exchange.

OTHER FORMS OF VASCULITIS

Henoch–Schönlein purpura

This small vessel vasculitis usually occurs in children and young adults and has a good prognosis. Typical presentation is with purpura over the buttocks and lower legs, abdominal symptoms (pain and bleeding) and arthritis (knee or ankle) following an upper respiratory tract infection. Nephritis occurs in 40% of patients and may occur up to 4 weeks after the onset of other symptoms (pp. 500 and 515). The diagnosis can only be confirmed by demonstrating IgA deposition within and around blood vessel walls. Prognosis is determined by the degree and severity of renal involvement. Although only 1% of patients develop end-stage renal failure, adverse features at presentation in adults include hypertension, abnormal renal function and proteinuria > 1.5 g/day. Corticosteroids alone are effective for gastrointestinal and joint involvement but nephritis usually requires treatment with both pulse i.v. steroids and immunosuppression.

Cryoglobulinaemic vasculitis

Cryoglobulins are circulating immunoglobulins that precipitate out in the cold. They are classified into three types (Box 25.79); types II and III are associated with cryoglobulinaemic vasculitis. The typical clinical features are palpable purpura over the lower extremities, arthralgia, Raynaud's phenomenon and neuropathy. Type II cryoglobulinaemia is secondary to hepatitis C virus (HCV) infection in most patients, the virus being present in the vasculitic lesions complexed with IgG and IgM. For HCV-positive patients, interferon-alpha is currently the treatment of choice; for high HCV loads, combination with ribavirin may be more effective (p. 968).

25.79 CLASSIFICATION OF CRYOGLOBULINS

Type	Antibody type	Associations
I	Monoclonal IgM	Malignant B-cell disease, e.g. Waldenström's macroglobulinaemia, lymphoma, myeloma
II ('mixed essential')	Monoclonal IgM and anti-IgG antibody (RhF)	Hepatitis C, SLE, B-cell malignancy
III	Polyclonal IgM and anti-IgG antibody (RhF)	RA, SLE, chronic infections

Behçet's syndrome

This is a vasculitis of unknown aetiology that characteristically targets venules. It is rare in Western Europe but more common in 'Silk Route' countries around the Mediterranean and in Japan where there is a strong association with HLA–B51.

There is a wide range of clinical features, and the disease is characterised by unpredictable exacerbations. There are no defining investigations and the diagnosis is made using clinical criteria (Box 25.80). Oral ulcers are universal (Fig. 25.53). Unlike aphthous ulcers they are usually deep

25.80 CRITERIA FOR THE DIAGNOSIS OF BEHÇET'S SYNDROME

- Recurrent oral ulceration—minor aphthous, major aphthous or herpetiform ulceration at least three times in a 12-month period

Plus two of:
- Recurrent genital ulceration
- Eye lesions—anterior uveitis, posterior uveitis, cells in vitreous on slit-lamp examination, retinal vasculitis
- Skin lesions—erythema nodosum, pseudofolliculitis, papulopustular lesions, acneiform nodules
- Positive pathergy test

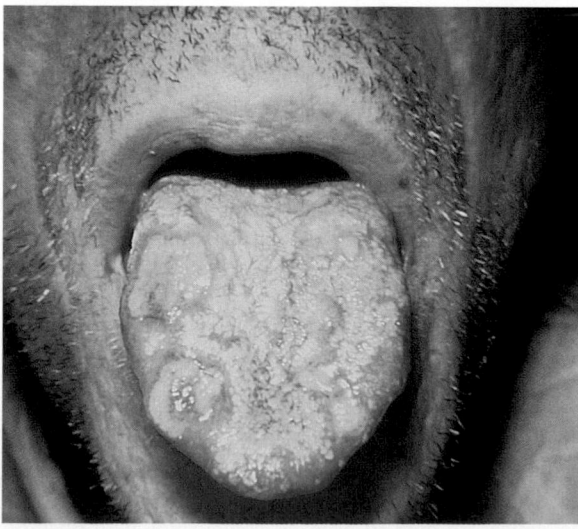

Fig. 25.53 Oral ulceration in Behçet's syndrome.

and multiple, and last for 10–30 days. Genital ulcers are less common (60–80%). The usual skin lesions are erythema nodosum or acneiform lesions but migratory thrombophlebitis and vasculitis also occur. The pathergy reaction is hyper-reactivity at the site of minor trauma. A formal pathergy test involves intradermal skin pricking with a needle, and is positive if a pustule develops within 48 hours. Ocular involvement is usually bilateral and may include anterior or posterior uveitis or retinal vasculitis. Neurological involvement occurs in 5% and mainly involves the brain stem, although the meninges, hemispheres and spinal cord can also be involved to cause pyramidal signs, cranial nerve lesions, brain-stem symptoms or hemiparesis. Recurrent thromboses also occur. Renal involvement is extremely rare.

Treatment of oral ulceration is with topical corticosteroid preparations (e.g. soluble prednisolone mouthwashes, corticosteroid pastes). Colchicine is sometimes effective for erythema nodosum and arthralgia. Thalidomide (100–300 mg daily for 28 days initially) is very effective for resistant oral and genital ulceration but is teratogenic and neurotoxic. Systemic disease is more problematic and usually requires oral corticosteroids in combination with other immunosuppressive drugs.

MUSCULOSKELETAL MANIFESTATIONS OF DISEASE IN OTHER SYSTEMS

Many systemic diseases result in MSK symptoms and signs and in some cases this may be the presentation of the disease. Furthermore, drugs used for other system disease may result in MSK complications (Box 25.81). The following examples illustrate the variety of conditions that may be encountered but the list is not exhaustive.

25.81 EXAMPLES OF DRUG-INDUCED EFFECTS ON THE MUSCULOSKELETAL SYSTEM

Musculoskeletal problem	Principal drug
Secondary gout	Diuretic—thiazide, loop diuretic
Osteoporosis	Corticosteroids, heparin
Osteomalacia	Anticonvulsants
Osteonecrosis	Corticosteroids
Drug-induced lupus syndrome	Procainamide, hydralazine, isoniazid, chlorpromazine
Arthralgias or arthritis	Corticosteroid withdrawal, glibenclamide, methyldopa, ciclosporin, isoniazid, barbiturates
Myalgias	Corticosteroid withdrawal, L-tryptophan, fibrates, statins
Myopathy	Corticosteroid, chloroquine
Myositis, myasthenia	Penicillamine
Cramps	Corticosteroid, adrenocorticotrophic hormone (ACTH), diuretics, carbenoxolone
Vasculitis	Amphetamines, thiazides

MALIGNANT DISEASE

Malignancy can present with polyarthritis (e.g. in acute leukaemia, p. 1039), dermatomyositis/polymyositis (p. 1136) and, rarely, polymyalgia rheumatica (but not giant cell arteritis). Bone involvement in cancer presents in several ways:

- hypercalcaemia
- metastatic bone disease
- osteoporosis
- hypophosphataemic osteomalacia (p. 1126).

Hypercalcaemia is one of the most common metabolic complications of cancer. In most cases, it is due to excessive release of parathyroid hormone-related protein (PTHrP) by the tumour, which causes hypercalcaemia by stimulating osteoclastic bone resorption and increasing renal tubular calcium reabsorption. The mechanisms are different in haematological tumours. In myeloma, hypercalcaemia occurs as the result of local bone destruction by metastases, mediated by the release of factors which stimulate bone resorption and suppress bone formation; these include TNF, lymphotoxin, MIP-1α and sFRP. Hypercalcaemia in lymphoma is most often due to increased production of $1,25(OH)_2D$ by the tumour, due to expression of 1-α hydroxylase in tumour cells. Treatment of hypercalcaemia is with intravenous saline and intravenous bisphosphonates (p. 776).

Metastatic bone disease

Bone metastases are a common and serious complication of cancer, occurring particularly in patients with tumours of the breast, prostate or lung and in multiple myeloma. The clinical presentation of metastatic bone disease is with bone pain, pathological fracture and neurological symptoms due to nerve root or spinal cord compression. Most bone metastases are osteolytic, but osteosclerotic metastases can also occur and are characteristic of prostate carcinoma. Radionuclide bone scan is the most sensitive investigation for documenting the presence and extent of bone metastases, but false negative results can occur in myeloma. If this diagnosis is suspected, a radiological skeletal survey should be performed.

The treatment of metastatic bone disease is interdisciplinary, involving four broad strategies (Box 25.82).

25.82 MANAGEMENT OF METASTATIC BONE DISEASE	
Treatment of the primary tumour	
• Chemotherapy	• Radiotherapy
• Hormone therapy	
Treatment of local lesions	
• Fixation of fractures	• Radiotherapy
• Spinal cord decompression	
Inhibition of osteoclastic bone resorption	
• Bisphosphonates	
Treatment of pain	
• Analgesics/NSAIDs	• Radiotherapy
• Nerve blocks	

25.83 BISPHOSPHONATES IN BONE METASTASES	EBM

'Bisphosphonates can prevent skeletal morbidity and improve bone pain in patients with breast cancer and myeloma who have metastatic bone disease.'

- Berenson JR, et al. N Engl J Med 1996; 334:488–493.
- Lipton A, et al. Cancer 2000; 88:1082–1090.

If antitumour therapy is not possible, efforts should focus on controlling pain with analgesics, NSAIDs, nerve blockade or local radiotherapy. Orthopaedic surgery may be required for the treatment of pathological fractures and to stabilise local osteolytic lesions that might progress to fracture. Surgical decompression can be of value as a palliative manoeuvre in the treatment of metastases that are encroaching on the spinal cord. Bisphosphonates such as clodronate, pamidronate and zoledronate have been shown to be of value in the secondary prevention of skeletal complications in patients with metastatic bone disease secondary to breast carcinoma and multiple myeloma. Zoledronate has also been found to be effective at reducing skeletal events in prostate carcinoma and other tumours (Box 25.83).

Primary bone tumours are far less common than metastases. They present with local pain and swelling. Treatment depends on histological tumour type, but often involves surgical removal of the tumour followed by chemotherapy and radiotherapy.

Hypertrophic osteoarthropathy

This poorly understood condition comprises clubbing, painful swelling of distal limbs (usually symmetrical), periosteal new bone formation and arthralgia/arthritis. Many causes of clubbing can result in this uncommon syndrome but it mainly occurs with bronchial carcinoma (5%—the most common cause, p. 705) and mesothelioma (40%, p. 736). The pain is characteristically worsened by dependency and relieved by elevation. Bone scans show increased periosteal activity before new bone is apparent on X-ray. The course follows that of the underlying malignancy.

ENDOCRINE DISEASE

Hypothyroidism (p. 750) may present with carpal tunnel syndrome and, occasionally, a severely painful, symmetrical proximal myopathy with muscle hypertrophy. All MSK lesions show excellent recovery following thyroxine replacement.

The MSK manifestations of hyperparathyroidism are described on page 775. There is predisposition to radiographic chondrocalcinosis, pseudogout attacks due to calcium pyrophosphate crystals and, especially with disease secondary to renal failure, calcific periarthritis.

Diabetes mellitus (Ch. 21) commonly causes diabetic 'stiff hands' (cheiroarthropathy) due to tightening of skin and periarticular structures, giving flexion deformities of many fingers which is sometimes painful. Diabetic osteopathy presents as forefoot pain and shows radiographic progression from osteopenia to complete osteolysis of the

25

phalanges and metatarsals. There is also predisposition to 'frozen shoulder', Dupuytren's contracture, septic arthritis and neuropathic joints.

Acromegaly (p. 801) commonly causes MSK symptoms, which are occasionally the presenting complaint. These include low mechanical back pain, carpal tunnel syndrome and late-onset Raynaud's phenomenon (25%). Acromegalic arthropathy (50%) mainly affects knees, hips and shoulders. Radiographic signs include widening of joint spaces, squaring of bone ends, generalised osteopenia and tufting of terminal phalanges. Unfortunately, the arthropathy persists after cure of growth hormone excess.

METABOLIC DISEASE

Approximately 50% of people with haemochromatosis (p. 974) develop arthropathy, usually in their forties or fifties, and this may predate other classic features. Presentation is usually with pain and stiffness of wrists, fingers and metacarpophalangeal joints, though hips, shoulders and knees are also commonly affected. Radiographic changes resemble OA with narrowing, sclerosis and cysts, but cysts are often multiple and prominent. There is little osteophyte, and atypical sites for OA (e.g. radiocarpal joint, metacarpophalangeal joints) are targeted. About 30% have superimposed pseudogout attacks and radiographic chondrocalcinosis as additional clues to the diagnosis. Treatment of the haemochromatosis does not influence the arthropathy.

SARCOIDOSIS

Acute self-limiting arthritis, presenting as polyarthralgia and erythema nodosum, may accompany the onset of acute sarcoidosis (p. 715). Chronic sarcoidosis may associate with a more persistent arthritis that targets the same joints.

NEUROPATHIC (CHARCOT) JOINTS

Neurological disease (Ch. 26) may result in rapidly destructive arthritis of joints, first described by Charcot in association with syphilis. Common causes and the joints affected are shown in Box 25.84. Although repetitive microtrauma following sensory loss was one popular explanation, the more likely pathogenesis is altered blood flow secondary to impaired sympathetic nervous system control.

Presentation is usually with chronic monoarthritis or dislocation. Pain can occur, especially at the onset, but the

25.84 NEUROPATHIC (CHARCOT) JOINTS

Causes	Joints affected
Diabetic neuropathy	Hindfoot
Syringomyelia	Shoulder, elbow, wrist
Leprosy	Hands, feet
Tabes dorsalis	Knees, spine

striking clinical feature is that signs are disproportionately greater than symptoms would suggest. The joint is often grossly swollen, with effusion, crepitus, marked instability and deformity, though usually no increased warmth. It may eventually become flail and be complicated by peripheral nerve entrapment or spinal cord compression. Radiographic features are gross loss of cartilage and bone, with disorganisation of normal architecture and often multiple loose bodies, and either no (atrophic) or gross (hypertrophic) new bone formation. Management principally involves orthoses and occasionally arthrodesis.

FURTHER INFORMATION

Books and journal articles

Bone health in the balance. Science 2000; 289:1497–1514. *A series of reviews on basic aspects of bone cell biology and bone turnover.*

Brandt KD, Doherty M, Lohmander LS, eds. Osteoarthritis. 2nd edn. Oxford: Oxford University Press; 2003.

Coleman RE. Metastatic bone disease: clinical features, pathophysiology and treatment strategies. Cancer Treat Rev 2001; 27:165–176.

Cush JJ, Kavanaugh AF, Olsen N, et al. Rheumatology diagnosis and therapeutics. Baltimore: Williams & Wilkins; 1999.

Doherty M, Hazleman BL, Huttin CW, et al. Rheumatology examination and injection techniques. London: WB Saunders; 1999.

Eastell R. Treatment of postmenopausal osteoporosis. N Engl J Med 1998; 33(8):736–746.

Firestein GS, Panayi GS, Wollheim FA, eds. Rheumatoid arthritis: new frontiers in pathogenesis and treatment. Oxford: Oxford University Press; 2000.

Langston AL, Ralston SH. Management of Paget's disease of bone. Rheumatology 2004; 43:955–959.

Maddison PJ, Isenberg DA, Woo P, Glass DN, eds. Oxford textbook of rheumatology. 2nd edn. Oxford: Oxford University Press; 1998.

Websites

www.eBandolier.com *Updates on management.*
www.rheumatology.com *Updates on management.*

26

C.M.C. ALLEN
C.J. LUECK
M. DENNIS

Neurological disease

CLINICAL EXAMINATION OF THE NERVOUS SYSTEM

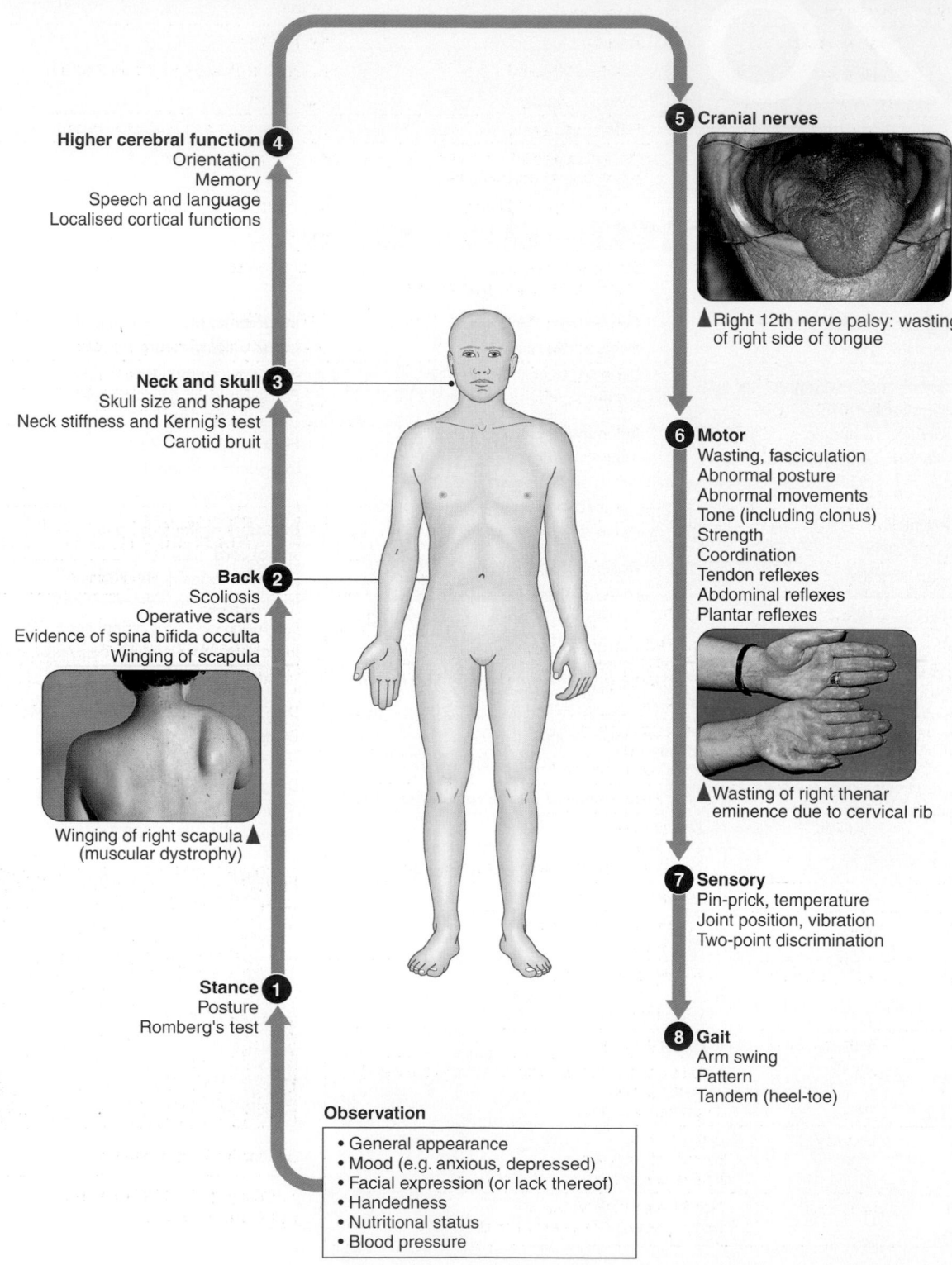

Higher cerebral function ❹
Orientation
Memory
Speech and language
Localised cortical functions

Neck and skull ❸
Skull size and shape
Neck stiffness and Kernig's test
Carotid bruit

Back ❷
Scoliosis
Operative scars
Evidence of spina bifida occulta
Winging of scapula

▲ Winging of right scapula
(muscular dystrophy)

Stance ❶
Posture
Romberg's test

Observation
- General appearance
- Mood (e.g. anxious, depressed)
- Facial expression (or lack thereof)
- Handedness
- Nutritional status
- Blood pressure

❺ **Cranial nerves**

▲ Right 12th nerve palsy: wasting
of right side of tongue

❻ **Motor**
Wasting, fasciculation
Abnormal posture
Abnormal movements
Tone (including clonus)
Strength
Coordination
Tendon reflexes
Abdominal reflexes
Plantar reflexes

▲ Wasting of right thenar
eminence due to cervical rib

❼ **Sensory**
Pin-prick, temperature
Joint position, vibration
Two-point discrimination

❽ **Gait**
Arm swing
Pattern
Tandem (heel-toe)

26

❶ + ❽ EXAMINATION OF GAIT AND POSTURE

Step	Procedure	Abnormality	Disease
1	Examine posture	Stooped	Parkinsonism
	Axial tone	Axial tone increased	Parkinsonism (Parkinson's plus syndrome)
	Retropulsion/anteropulsion	Postural instability	Parkinsonism
2	Examine arms during walking	Reduced arm swing	Parkinsonism, upper motor neuron lesion
3	Examine routine walking	Circumduction (stiff leg moves outwards in 'circular' manner)	Upper motor neuron lesion
		'Slapping' due to foot drop	Lower motor neuron lesion
		Narrow-based, short strides	Parkinsonism
		Wide-based, short strides (marche à petits pas, magnetic gait)	Frontal lobe lesion
		Wide-based, irregular strides	Cerebellar lesion
		High-stepping gait	Dorsal column lesion/sensory neuropathy
4	Examine tandem gait	Inability to perform task	Cerebellar lesion, dorsal column lesion
5	Perform Romberg test	Patient falls with eyes shut	Loss of joint position sense at ankles

❺ EXAMINATION OF CRANIAL NERVES

Nerve	Name	Tests
I	Olfactory	Ask patient
II	Optic	Visual acuity Visual fields 'Swinging' torch test for relative afferent pupillary defect Ophthalmoscopy
III	Oculomotor	Eye movements (nystagmus) Eyelid movement Pupil size, symmetry, reactions
IV	Trochlear	Eye movements (nystagmus)
V	Trigeminal	Sensation to face Corneal reflex Jaw movements (deviates on opening to side of lesion)
VI	Abducens	Eye movements (nystagmus)
VII	Facial	Facial symmetry and movements Ask patient about taste
VIII	Vestibulocochlear	Hearing (whisper to each ear) Tuning fork tests (Rinne and Weber) Look for nystagmus
IX	Glossopharyngeal	Gag reflex (sensory)
X	Vagus	Palatal elevation (uvula deviates to side opposite lesion) Gag reflex (motor) Cough (bovine cough)
XI	Accessory	Look for wasting Elevation of shoulders Turning head to right and left
XII	Hypoglossal	Look for wasting/fasciculation Tongue protrusion (deviates to side of lesion)

❻ ROOT VALUES OF TENDON REFLEXES

Reflex	Root value
Upper limb	
Biceps jerk	C5/C6
Supinator jerk	C5/C6
Triceps jerk	C7
Finger jerk	C8
Lower limb	
Knee jerk	L3/L4
Ankle jerk	S1/S2

26

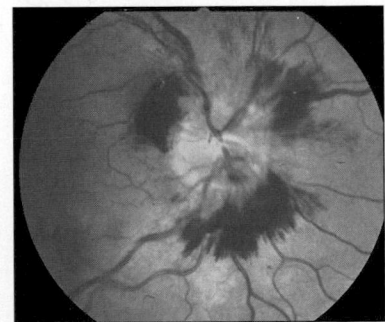

Haemorrhagic papilloedema.

See also page 1149 for neurological examination in old age.

The brain, spinal cord and peripheral nerves constitute an organ responsible for perception of the environment, a person's behaviour within it, and the maintenance of the body's internal milieu in readiness for this behaviour. Some 10% of the population in the United Kingdom consult their general practitioner each year with a neurological symptom, and neurological disorders account for about one-fifth of acute medical admissions and a large proportion of chronic physical disability in the UK. However, neurological symptoms are often not associated with disease, and considerable clinical skill is needed to distinguish those with significant disease from those who need sympathetic reassurance.

A carefully taken history of the pattern of presenting neurological symptoms should suggest a short list of diagnoses that can then be tested on examination. During the neurological examination, knowledge of the relevant anatomy and physiology of the nervous system helps to determine the site of the lesion. The underlying pathology is often suggested by the time course of the symptoms and the epidemiological context. Increasingly sophisticated investigations, particularly imaging, are available to refine this clinical diagnosis.

Once the patient's neurological lesion (the deficit) is identified, the clinician needs to assess what impact this has had on the patient's functioning (the disability) and, in turn, how this is affecting his or her life (the handicap). Even when a complete cure cannot be effected, much can be done to improve the disability by pharmacological correction of the pathophysiology and through rehabilitation (p. 169).

FUNCTIONAL ANATOMY, PHYSIOLOGY AND INVESTIGATIONS

ANATOMY AND PHYSIOLOGY

CELLS OF THE NERVOUS SYSTEM

In addition to a variety of neurons, the nervous system includes specialised blood vessels, ependymal cells lining the cerebral ventricles and glial cells, of which there are three types. Astrocytes form the structural framework for the neurons and control their biochemical environment. Astrocyte foot processes are closely associated with the blood vessels to form the blood–brain barrier (Fig. 26.1). Oligodendrocytes are responsible for the formation and maintenance of the myelin sheath, which surrounds axons and is essential for the rapid transmission of action potentials by saltatory conduction. Microglia are blood-derived mononuclear macrophages. Peripheral neurons have axons invested in myelin made by Schwann cells.

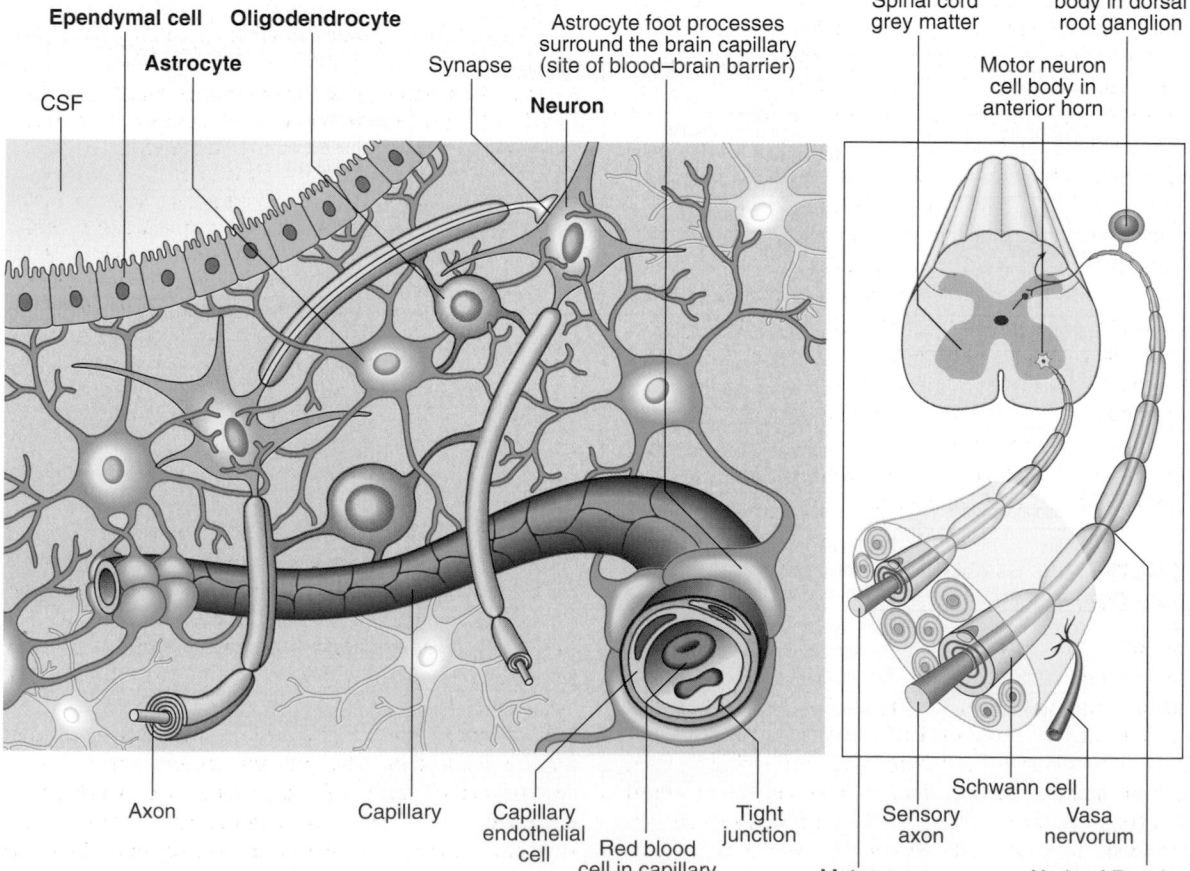

26

Fig. 26.1 Cells of the nervous system.

THE GENERATION AND TRANSMISSION OF THE NERVOUS IMPULSE

The functioning of the nervous system rests upon two physiological processes: the generation of an action potential with its conduction down axons, and the synaptic transmission of impulses between neurons and/or muscle cells. These processes depend upon the energy-demanding maintenance of an electrochemical gradient across neuron cell membranes, and alterations in this are effected by specialised ion channels in the membrane. Synaptic transmission involves the release from a neuron of neurotransmitter molecules that bind to specific receptors on the membrane of the receptor cell. These molecules alter either that cell's membrane potential via effects upon ion channel permeability, or its metabolic function (Fig. 26.2). There are over 20 different neurotransmitters known to act at different sites in the nervous system, all potentially amenable to pharmacological manipulation (Box 26.2).

The neuronal cell bodies are acted upon by synapses with large numbers of other neurons. Each neuron therefore acts as a microprocessor, reacting to the influences upon it by changes to its cell membrane potential, causing it to be more or less ready to discharge an impulse down its axon(s). The synapsing neuron terminals are also subject to regulation by receptor sites on their pre-synaptic membrane, which modify the release of transmitter across the synaptic cleft. The effect of some neurotransmitters is to produce long-term modulation of metabolic function or gene expression rather than simply to change the membrane potential. This effect probably underlies more complex processes in cognition, such as long-term memory.

FUNCTIONAL ANATOMY OF THE NERVOUS SYSTEM (Fig. 26.3)

Cerebral hemispheres

The cerebral cortex constitutes the highest level of nervous function, the anterior half dealing with executive ('doing') functions and the posterior half constructing a perception of the environment ('receiving and perceiving'). Each cerebral hemisphere has four functionally specialised lobes (Fig. 26.4 and Box 26.3). Many of the functions are lateralised. To which side depends on which of the two hemispheres is 'dominant', i.e. where language function is represented. In right-handed individuals this is almost

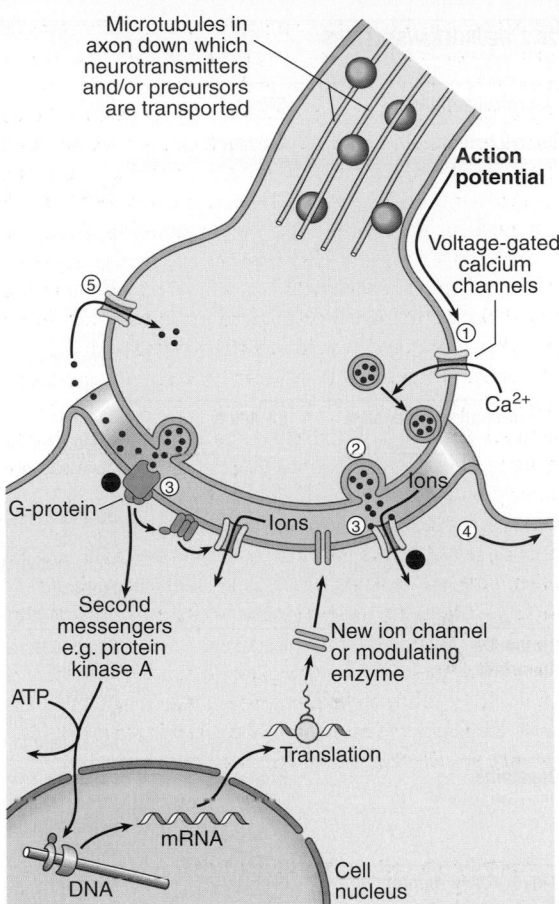

Fig. 26.2 Neurotransmission and neurotransmitters. (1) An action potential arriving at the nerve terminal depolarises the membrane and this opens voltage-gated calcium channels. (2) Entry of calcium causes the fusion of synaptic vesicles containing neurotransmitters with the pre-synaptic membrane and release of the neurotransmitter across the synaptic cleft. (3) The neurotransmitter binds to receptors on the post-synaptic membrane to either (A) open ligand-gated ion channels which, by allowing ion entry, depolarise the membrane and initiate an action potential (4), or (B) bind to metabotrophic receptors, which activate an effector enzyme (e.g. adenylyl cyclase) and thus via the intracellular second messenger system modulate gene transcription, leading to changes in synthesis of ion channels or modulating enzymes. (5) Neurotransmitters are taken up at the pre-synaptic membrane and/or metabolised.

always the left hemisphere while in left-handers either hemisphere may be dominant with about equal frequency.

The frontal lobes are concerned with executive function, movement and behaviour. In addition to the primary and supplementary motor cortex, there are specialised areas for the control of eye movements, speech (Broca's area) and micturition control.

The parietal lobes are concerned with the integration of sensory perception. The primary sensory cortex lies in the post-central gyrus of the parietal lobe. Much of the remainder is devoted to 'association' cortex, which integrates the input from the various sensory modalities. The supramarginal and angular gyri of the dominant parietal lobe form part of the language area (p. 1190). Close to these

26.2 NEUROTRANSMITTERS

Neurotransmitter	Effect	Clinical relevance	Pharmacology
Acetylcholine	Excitatory	Alzheimer's disease	Central acetylcholinesterase inhibitors, e.g. donepezil, rivastigmine
		Myasthenia gravis	Peripheral acetylcholinesterase inhibitors, e.g. edrophonium, pyridostigmine
		Parkinson's disease	Anticholinergics, e.g. benztropine, orphenadrine, procyclidine
		Huntington's chorea	
		Motion sickness	Anticholinergics, e.g. hyoscine
		Bladder control	Anticholinergics, e.g. oxybutinin
		Cataplexy	
		Botulinum toxicity	Used therapeutically as i.m. botulinum toxin injections
		Pesticide toxicity	
Noradrenaline/adrenaline	Excitatory	Migraine	β-adrenoceptor antagonists (β-blockers)
		Mood disorders	Antidepressants
		Cardiovascular control	β-adrenoceptor antagonists (β -blockers), α-adrenergic antagonists (α-blockers)
		Bladder control	α-adrenoreceptor antagonists (α-blockers)
		Appetite	Amphetamines, sibutramine
		Multi-system atrophy	
		Spasticity	Tizanidine
		Sleep disorders	Dexamfetamine
Glutamate	Excitatory	Cerebral ischaemia	
Aspartate		Epilepsy	Lamotrigine, topiramate
		Memory	
		Alzheimer's disease	Memantine
		Motor neuron disease	Riluzole
Dopamine	Excitatory	Parkinson's disease	Levodopa, dopamine agonists
		Alzheimer's disease	
		Schizophrenia	Antipsychotics
		Vomiting	Metoclopramide
5-hydroxytryptamine (5-HT, serotonin)	Excitatory	Migraine	Pizotifen, triptans
		Depression	Selective serotonin re-uptake inhibitor (SSRI) antidepressants
		Pain	
		Vomiting	Ondansetron
		Sleep	
Gamma-aminobutyric acid (GABA)	Inhibitory	Epilepsy	Phenobarbital, vigabatrin
		Anxiety	Benzodiazepines
		Spasticity	Baclofen, benzodiazepines
Glycine	Inhibitory	Startle syndromes	
Histamine	Inhibitory	Uncertain	
Neuropeptides	Excitatory and inhibitory		
Vasopressin		Memory	
Adrenocorticotrophic hormone (ACTH)		Uncertain	
Melanocyte-stimulating hormone (MSH)			
Substance P		Pain	
Opioid peptides (> 20)			
Endorphins			Morphine
Enkephalins			Morphine
Dynorphins			Morphine
Purines	Excitatory and modulation of neurotransmission	Uncertain	
Adenosine triphosphate/ diphosphate (ATP/ADP)			
Adenosine monophosphate (AMP)			
Adenosine			
Nitric oxide	Modulation of neurotransmission	Penile erection	Sildenafil
		Memory	
		Cerebral ischaemia	
Endocannabinoids	Modulation of neurotransmission	Pain	Nabilone
		Motor control	

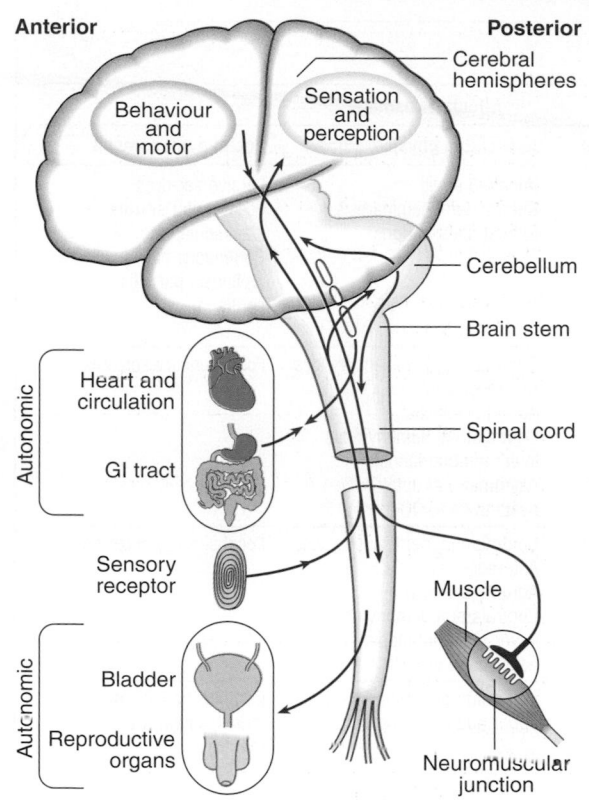

Fig. 26.3 The major anatomical components of the nervous system.

are regions dealing with numerical function. The non-dominant parietal lobe houses areas concerned with spatial awareness and orientation.

In the temporal lobes are the primary auditory cortex and primary vestibular cortex. On the medial side lie the olfactory cortex and the parahippocampal cortex which is involved in memory function. The temporal lobes also contain many structures associated with the limbic system, including the hippocampus and the amygdala, which are involved in the processing of memory and emotions. The dominant temporal lobe also participates in language functions, particularly verbal comprehension (Wernicke's area). Music processing occurs in both temporal lobes, rhythm being processed on the dominant side and melody/pitch more on the non-dominant side.

The occipital lobes are principally concerned with visual processing. The contralateral visual hemifield is represented in the primary visual (striate) cortex, and areas immediately surrounding this are involved in the processing of specific visual submodalities such as colour, movement or depth, and the analysis of more complex visual patterns such as faces.

Collections of cells in the depths of the hemispheres deal with motor control (the basal ganglia), the appropriate attention to sensory perception (the thalamus), emotion and memory (the limbic system), and control over internal bodily functions (the hypothalamus). The cerebral ventricles contain the choroid plexus; this produces the cerebrospinal fluid (CSF), which cushions the brain within the cranium. From the fourth ventricle the CSF leaves through foramina

26

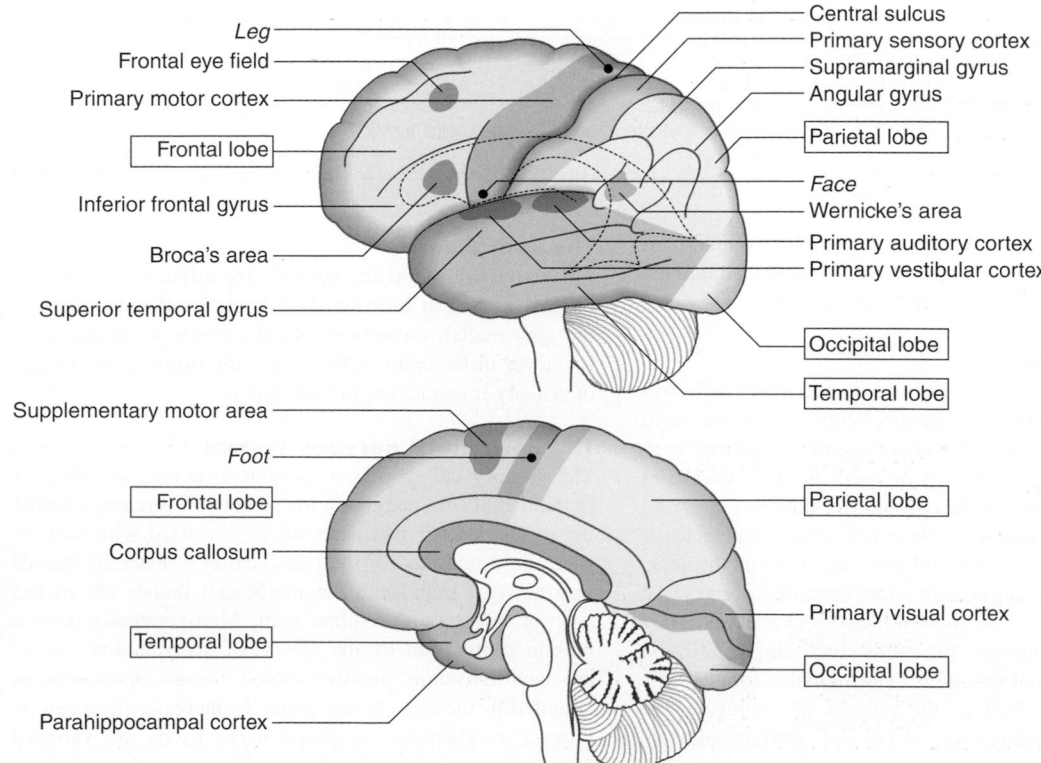

Fig. 26.4 The anatomy of the cerebral cortex.

26.3 CORTICAL LOBAR FUNCTIONS

Lobe	Function	Effects of damage		
		Cognitive/behavioural	Associated physical signs	Positive phenomena
Frontal	Personality Emotional control Social behaviour Contralateral motor control Language Micturition	Disinhibition Lack of initiation Antisocial behaviour Impaired memory Expressive dysphasia Incontinence	Impaired smell Contralateral hemiparesis Frontal release signs[1]	Versive seizures Focal motor seizures (Jacksonian march) Continuous partial seizures (epilepsia partialis continua)
Parietal: dominant	Language Calculation	Dysphasia Dyscalculia Dyslexia Apraxia[4] Agnosia[5]	Contralateral hemisensory loss Astereognosis[2] Agraphaesthesia[3] Contralateral homonymous lower quadrantanopia Asymmetry of optokinetic nystagmus (OKN)	Focal sensory seizures
Parietal: non-dominant	Spatial orientation Constructional skills	Neglect of contralateral side Spatial disorientation Constructional apraxia Dressing apraxia	Contralateral hemisensory loss Astereognosis Agraphaesthesia Contralateral homonymous lower quadrantanopia Asymmetry of OKN	Focal sensory seizures
Temporal: dominant	Auditory perception Language Verbal memory Smell Balance	Receptive aphasia Dyslexia Impaired verbal memory	Contralateral homonymous upper quadrantanopia	Complex hallucinations (smell, sound, vision, memory)
Temporal: non-dominant	Auditory perception Melody/pitch perception Non-verbal memory Smell Balance	Impaired non-verbal memory Impaired musical skills (tonal perception)	Contralateral homonymous upper quadrantanopia	Complex hallucinations (smell, sound, vision, memory)
Occipital	Visual processing	Visual inattention Visual loss Visual agnosia	Homonymous hemianopia (macular sparing)	Simple visual hallucinations (e.g. phosphenes, zigzag lines)

[1] Grasp reflex, palmomental response, rooting reflex.
[2] Inability to determine 3-D shape by touch.
[3] Inability to 'read' numbers or letters drawn on hand, with eyes shut.
[4] Inability to perform complex movements in the presence of normal motor, sensory and cerebellar function.
[5] Inability to recognise or discriminate.

in the brain stem to circulate down around the spinal cord and over the surface of brain, where it is reabsorbed into the cerebral venous system (Fig. 26.51, p. 1240).

The brain stem

In addition to containing all the sensory and motor pathways entering and leaving the hemispheres, the brain stem houses the nuclei of the cranial nerves, nuclei projecting to the cerebrum and cerebellum as well as other important collections of neurons in the reticular formation (Fig. 26.5). The cranial nerve nuclei provide motor control to muscles of the head (including the face and eyes) and some in the neck, along with coordinating sensory input from the special sense organs and the face, nose, mouth, larynx and pharynx. They also control autonomic functions including pupillary, salivary and lacrimal functions. The reticular formation is predominantly involved in the control of conjugate eye movements, the maintenance of balance, cardiorespiratory control and the maintenance of arousal.

The spinal cord

The spinal cord contains not only the afferent and efferent fibres arranged in functionally discrete bundles but also, in the grey matter, collections of cells which are responsible for lower-order motor reflexes and the primary processing of sensory information, including pain.

The peripheral nervous system

The sensory cell bodies of peripheral nerves are situated in the dorsal root ganglia in the spinal exit foramina, whilst the distal ends of their neurons are invested with various specialised endings for the transduction of external stimuli into nervous impulses. The motor cell bodies are in the anterior horns of the spinal cord. Motor neurons initiate muscle contraction by the release of acetylcholine across the neuromuscular junction which results in change in potential in the muscle end plate. To increase the speed of impulse conduction, peripheral nerve axons are variably invested in myelin sheaths consisting of the wrapped

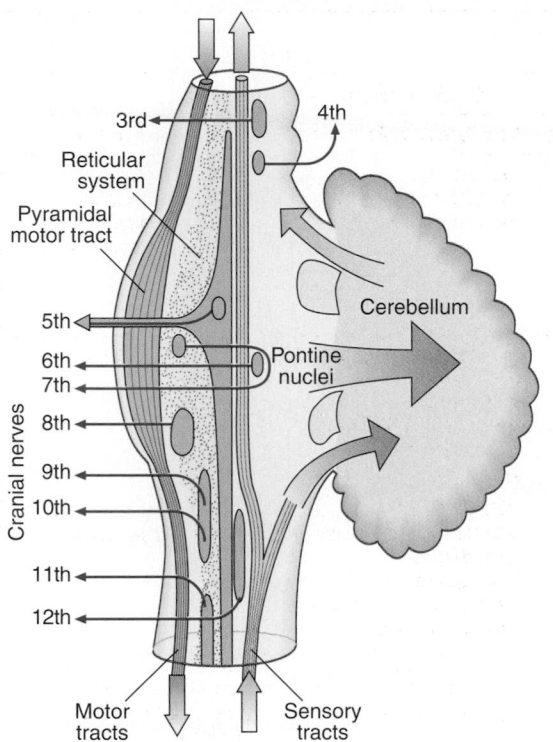

Fig. 26.5   Anatomy of the brain stem.

membranes of Schwann cells. Thus, any peripheral nerve is made up of a combination of large, fast, myelinated axons (which carry information about joint position sense and commands to muscles), and smaller, slower, unmyelinated axons (which carry information about pain and temperature, as well autonomic function).

The autonomic system

The unconscious neural control of the body's physiology is effected through the autonomic system. This innervates the cardiovascular and respiratory systems, smooth muscle of the gastrointestinal tract, and glands throughout the body. The autonomic system is controlled centrally by diffuse modulatory systems in the brain stem, limbic system and frontal lobes, which are concerned with arousal and background behavioural responses to threat. The output of the autonomic system is divided functionally and pharmacologically into two divisions: the parasympathetic and sympathetic systems.

INVESTIGATION OF NEUROLOGICAL DISEASE

TESTS OF FUNCTION (CLINICAL NEUROPHYSIOLOGY)

In the investigation of neurological disease, tests of function have a somewhat more restricted application than tests of structure (i.e. imaging). Nevertheless, recording of electrical activity over the brain and assessment of nerve and muscle

function are essential in certain conditions. The major tests are electroencephalography (EEG), evoked potentials (EPs) and nerve conduction studies/electromyography (NCS/EMG).

Electroencephalography

Electrical activity arising in the cerebral cortex can be detected using electrodes placed on the scalp, although this is estimated to detect only 0.1–1% of the brain's electrical activity at any one time. An array of electrodes provides spatial information. Rhythmical waveforms can be detected and are distinguished by their frequency. When the eyes are shut, the most obvious frequency over the occipital cortex is 8–13/s; this is known as alpha rhythm, and disappears when the eyes are opened. Other frequency bands seen over different parts of the brain in different circumstances are beta (faster than 13/s), theta (4–8/s) and delta (slower than 4/s). Lower frequencies predominate in the very young and during sleep.

Various diseases result in abnormalities of the EEG. These may be continuous or episodic, focal or diffuse. Examples of continuous abnormalities include a global increase in fast frequencies (beta) seen with sedating drugs (e.g. benzodiazepines), or marked slowing seen over a structural lesion such as a tumour or an infarct. With the advent of modern neuro-imaging, EEG has lost its use in localising lesions, except in the management of epilepsy (see below and Fig. 26.6). However, it is still useful in the management of patients who have disturbance of consciousness or disorders of sleep, in the diagnosis of cerebral diseases such as encephalitis, and in certain dementias (e.g. sporadic Creutzfeldt–Jakob disease).

The most important use of EEG is in the management of epilepsy. It must be stressed, however, that only in rare circumstances will an EEG provide unequivocal evidence of epilepsy, and it is therefore not useful as a diagnostic test for the presence of epilepsy. Its use is predominantly to distinguish the type of epilepsy present, and whether there is an epileptic focus, particularly if surgery for epilepsy is contemplated.

During an epileptic seizure, high-voltage disturbances of the background activity ('transients') can be recorded. These may be generalised, as in the 3 cycle/s 'spike and wave' of childhood absence epilepsy (petit mal), or more focal, as in partial epilepsies (Fig. 26.6). However, it is unusual to record a seizure itself, except in the case of childhood absence epilepsy. Nevertheless, it is often possible to detect 'epileptiform' abnormalities in between seizures in the form of 'spikes' and 'sharp waves' that lend support to a clinical diagnosis. The likelihood of detecting these abnormalities is enhanced by hyperventilation, photic flicker, sleep and some drugs. Even so, some 50% of patients with proven epilepsy will have a normal 'routine' EEG, and conversely, the presence of features often seen in association with epilepsy does not of itself make a diagnosis (although the false positive rate for clear-cut epileptiform features is < 1/1000).

It is possible to enhance the information provided by a variety of means. For example, the usual 30-minute recording session can be lengthened to 24 hours by the use of a

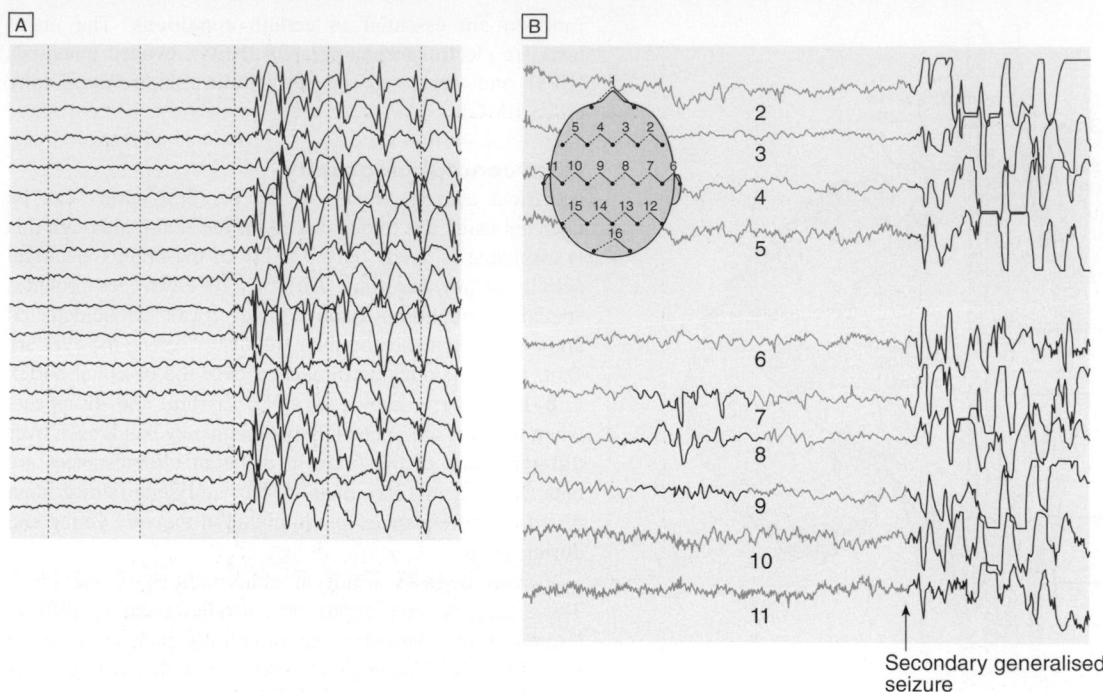

Fig. 26.6 EEGs in epilepsy. A Primary generalised epileptic discharge. B Focal sharp waves over the right parietal region (between electrodes 7 and 8—shown in purple) with secondary generalised discharge.

lightweight tape recorder. The addition of video information to the EEG allows comparison of behaviour with cerebral activity. In special circumstances, electrodes can be surgically positioned, e.g. through the foramen ovale, to record from the inferior temporal surface.

Evoked potentials

If a stimulus is provided—for example, to the eye—it would normally be impossible to detect the small EEG response evoked over the occipital cortex as the signal would be lost in background noise. However, if the EEG data from 100–1000 repeated stimuli are averaged electronically, this noise is removed and an evoked potential recorded whose latency (the time interval between stimulus onset and the maximum positive value of the evoked potential, P_{100}) and amplitude can be measured.

Evoked potentials can be measured following visual, auditory or somatosensory stimuli if electrodes are appropriately positioned, although visual evoked potentials are by far the most commonly used (Fig. 26.7). Abnormalities of the evoked potential indicate damage to the relevant pathway, either in the form of a conduction delay (increased latency) or reduced amplitude, or both.

With the advent of magnetic resonance imaging (MRI), the use of evoked potentials is becoming restricted to specialised indications, such as providing a semi-objective measure of visual function.

Nerve conduction studies and electromyography

Using surface or needle electrodes, it is possible to record action potentials from nerves which lie close to the skin

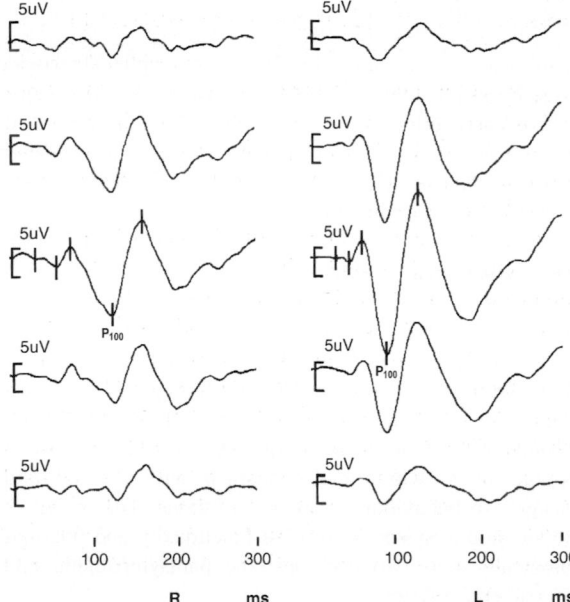

Fig. 26.7 Visual evoked responses (VER) recording showing abnormal delay on right. The latency of the P_{100} (the point of maximum positivity) on the left is 90 ms, that on the right 115 ms.

surface as well as from muscles. If a nerve trunk is stimulated with a small electric potential, it is possible to record the resulting compound action potential (the sum of all the individual nerves' action potentials) as it travels down the nerve. A normal compound action potential would have an amplitude of 5–30 microvolts, depending upon the nerve. If the recorded potential is smaller than expected,

26

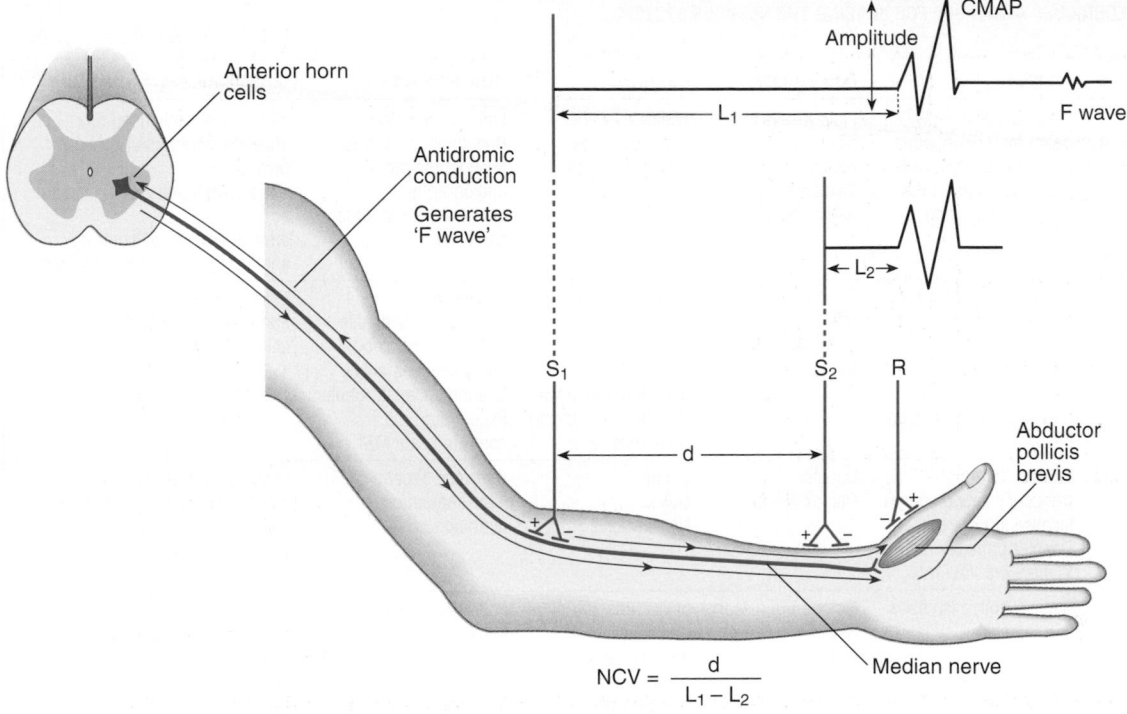

$$NCV = \frac{d}{L_1 - L_2}$$

Fig. 26.8 **Motor nerve conduction tests.** Dipolar electrodes (R) on the muscle (abductor pollicis brevis here) record the compound motor action potential (CMAP) from stimulation at the median nerve at the elbow (S_1) and from the wrist (S_2). The CMAP amplitude is related to the number of axons, and the velocity can be determined if the distance between the two stimulating electrodes (d) is known. The latency (L) of the F wave is a measure of the conduction time in the nerve proximal to the elbow (see text). (NCV = nerve conduction velocity)

26

this provides evidence of a reduction in the overall number of functioning axons. Central conduction times can be measured using electromagnetic induction of action potentials in the cortex or spinal cord by the local application of specialised coils.

Compound motor action potentials (CMAPs) can also be recorded over muscles in response to motor nerve stimulation (Fig. 26.8). These are easier to record because the muscle amplifies the response, typical amplitudes being 1–20 millivolts. By measuring the response latency to stimulation of a nerve at two different points along its length, it is possible to calculate nerve conduction velocities (NCVs). This can be done for both sensory and motor nerves; typical values are 50–60 m/s. Slowing of conduction velocity is suggestive of peripheral nerve demyelination which may be either diffuse (as in a demyelinating peripheral neuropathy) or focal (as in pressure palsies or conduction block).

The principal use of nerve conduction studies is to identify damage to peripheral nerves, and to determine whether the pathological process is focal or diffuse, and whether the damage is principally axonal or demyelinating. It is also possible to obtain some information about nerve roots by more sophisticated analysis of responses to impulses initially conducted antidromically (i.e. the 'wrong' way) back up to the spinal cord, and then returning orthodromically (the 'right' way) down to the stimulation point ('F waves').

Fine concentric needle electrodes can be inserted into muscle bellies themselves and the potentials from individual motor units recorded. It is possible to record abnormal spontaneous activity arising from muscles at rest, such as fibrillations (a sign of denervation) or myotonic discharges. Abnormalities in the shape and size of muscle potentials can help in the differential diagnosis of denervation and structural muscle diseases. Myopathies caused by metabolic abnormalities (causing electromechanical dissociation rather than loss of fibre structure) show no changes on needle EMG.

Electromyography can also be used to investigate the neuromuscular junction. Repetitive stimulation of a nerve with trains of electrical impulses at 3–15/s does not normally result in a significant fall-off in the amplitude of the resulting muscle action potential. However, such a decrement is seen in myasthenia gravis (p. 1252) and provides one of the key diagnostic features. Augmentation of the response to repetitive stimulation is seen in the Lambert–Eaton myasthenic syndrome, though usually at higher stimulation frequencies.

IMAGING

Imaging is crucial to the identification of lesions of the nervous system in disease. There are various techniques, based on the use of X-rays (plain X-rays, computed tomography (CT), myelography and angiography), magnetic resonance (MR imaging—MRI, or MR angiography—MRA), ultrasound (Doppler imaging of blood vessels), and radio-isotopes (single photon emission computed tomography —SPECT, and positron emission tomography—PET). The

26.4 TECHNIQUES AVAILABLE FOR IMAGING THE NERVOUS SYSTEM

Technique	Principle	Applications	Advantages	Disadvantages	Comments
X-ray	Attenuation of X-ray beam by radio-opaque tissues and substances (bone, calcium, metal, iodinated contrast)	Plain X-rays CT Radiculography Myelography Angiography	Widely available Relatively cheap Relatively quick	Ionising radiation Reactions to contrast Myelography and angiography are invasive and thus carry risk	Plain X-rays only used for showing fractures or foreign bodies CT is investigation of choice for stroke Intra-arterial X-ray contrast angiography still 'gold standard'
Magnetic resonance imaging (MRI)	Magnetic resonance of different tissues depends on free hydrogen/water content; signals changed by movement (e.g. flowing blood)	Structural imaging MRA Functional MRI MR spectroscopy	High-quality soft tissue imaging Good views of posterior fossa and temporal lobes No ionising radiation Non-invasive	Expensive Less widely available MRA looks at blood flow not vessel anatomy Scanners claustrophobic Pacemakers contraindicate MRI	Increasing application Functional MR and spectroscopy still mainly research tools
Ultrasound	Echoes from high-frequency sound source localise structure; Doppler principle used to measure flow rate	Doppler Duplex scans	Cheap Quick Non-invasive	Operator-dependent Poor anatomical definition	Useful as screening tool Increasingly used as basis for carotid endarterectomy
Radio-isotope	Radio-labelled isotopes	Isotope brain scan SPECT PET	In vivo imaging of functional anatomy (e.g. ligand binding, blood flow)	Poor spatial resolution Ionising radiation Expensive (especially PET) Not widely available	Isotope scans now obsolete SPECT and PET largely research tools but used increasingly in management of epilepsy and dementia

(CT = computed tomography; MRA = magnetic resonance angiography; MRI = magnetic resonance imaging; PET = positron emission tomography; SPECT = single photon emission computed tomography)

indications, usefulness and limits of each technique are listed in Box 26.4. The choice of technique depends upon the area of the neuraxis that is being investigated.

Head and orbit

The use of plain skull X-rays is largely restricted to the diagnosis of fractures and sinus disease. CT or MRI is needed to image pathology inside the skull. Which is used depends on what information is being sought and, to some extent, how urgently it is required, as CT is often more easily available than MRI. CT will show bone and calcium well, and will easily image collections of blood. It will also detect abnormalities of the brain and ventricles, such as atrophy, tumours, cysts, abscesses, vascular lesions and hydrocephalus. Diagnostic yield is often improved by the use of intravenous contrast and spiral CT methods. It is, however, limited in its ability to image the posterior fossa (because of the surrounding bone density), and it is poor at detecting abnormalities of white matter and at allowing detailed analysis of grey matter.

MRI is much more useful in the investigation of posterior fossa disease as it is not affected by the surrounding bone. It is much more sensitive than CT to abnormalities of white and grey matter and is therefore useful in the investigation of inflammatory conditions such as multiple sclerosis, and in investigating epilepsy. MRI can also provide additional information about structural brain lesions, which may complement that available from CT. It is also useful in imaging the orbits, where special imaging sequences can be used to compensate for orbital fat and thereby allow clear views of extraocular muscles, optic nerve and other orbital structures.

Standard isotope brain scans are of little value in assessing structure if other imaging facilities are available. However, the blood flow and function of the cerebral hemispheres can be assessed by using either SPECT or PET. Examples of brain imaged by the various techniques are shown in Figure 26.9.

Neck

Plain X-rays of the neck are useful in the investigation of structural damage to vertebrae, such as that resulting from trauma or inflammatory damage (e.g. rheumatoid arthritis). They can also provide implicit information about intervertebral disc disease, but not detailed information about the cervical cord or nerve roots, for which myelography or MRI is needed.

Myelography is invasive. Potential complications include headache, seizures and meningitis. With the advent of MRI its use is declining. Nevertheless, it is still of value if MRI is not available or the patient cannot tolerate lying within an MRI scanner. Radio-opaque contrast is injected into the lumbar theca and then moved up to the cervical region by tilting the patient. The contrast outlines the nerve roots and spinal cord, thereby providing information about abnormal structure. Examples of the neck imaged by plain X-rays, myelography and MRI are shown in Figure 26.10.

Lumbo-sacral region

Imaging of this region is similar to imaging the neck, and plain X-rays are of limited use. Contrast can be injected into the lumbar thecal space and used to outline the lower nerve roots only (radiculography), or it can be run up to outline the conus and spinal cord (myelography). The information

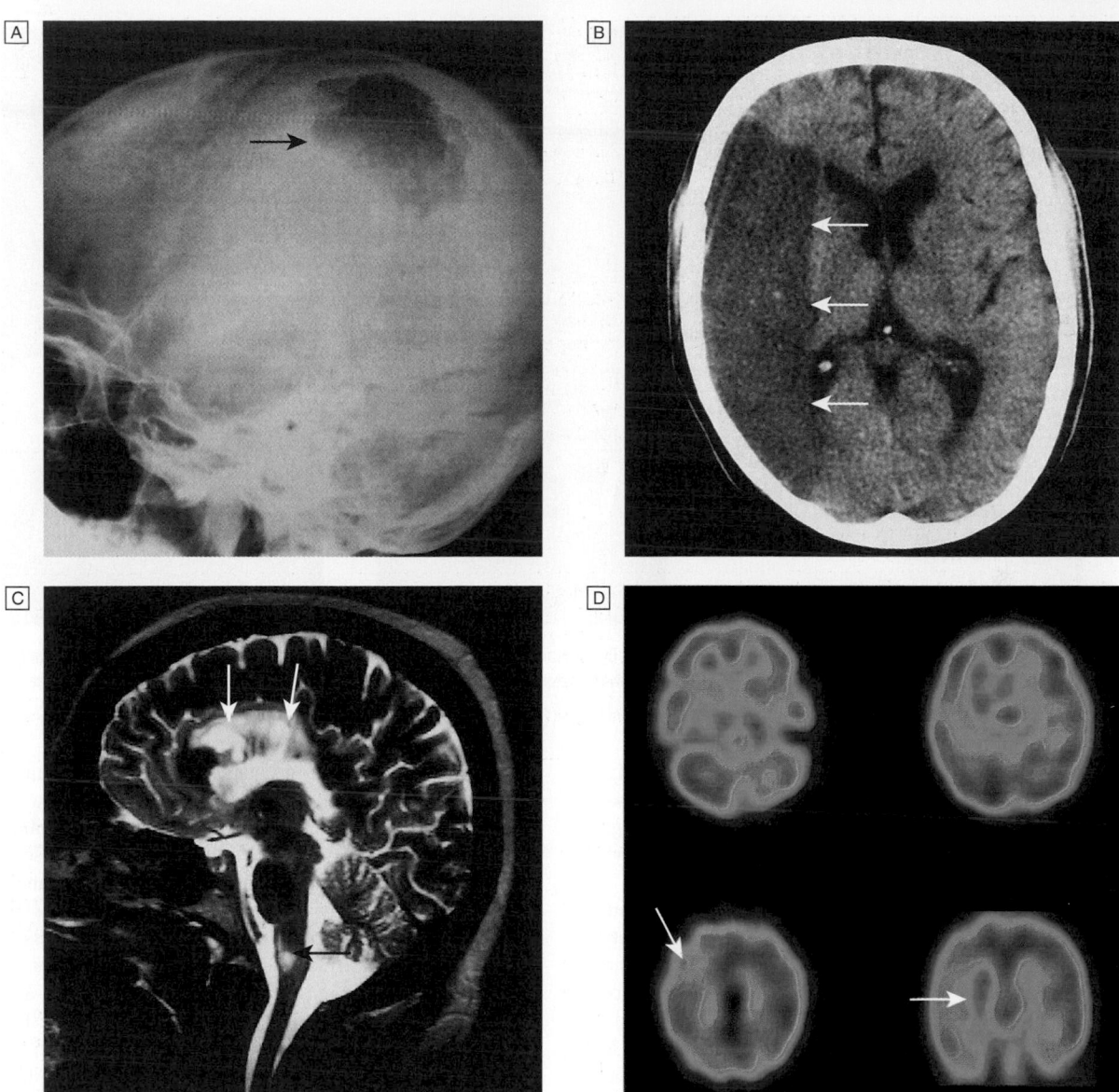

Fig. 26.9 Different techniques of imaging the head and brain. [A] Skull X-ray showing lytic vault lesion (eosinophilic granuloma—arrow).
[B] CT showing complete middle cerebral artery infarct (arrows). [C] MRI showing widespread areas of high signal in multiple sclerosis (arrows).
[D] SPECT after caudate infarct shows relative hypoperfusion of overlying right cerebral cortex (arrows).

26

obtained may be enhanced by the additional use of CT following myelography (contrast CT). Non-contrast CT of the lumbar spine can only be used to image the vertebrae and discs. As with the cervical spine, MRI provides a non-invasive way of obtaining high-resolution images of both the vertebral column and the relevant neural structures.

Blood vessels

Various techniques are available to investigate extracranial and intracranial blood vessels. The least invasive is ultra-sound (Doppler or duplex scanning), which is used to investigate the carotid and the vertebral arteries in the neck, usually as part of the investigation of stroke. In skilled hands, reliable information can be provided about the degree of arterial stenosis, and the technique often gives

useful anatomical information, e.g. whether there is an ulcerated plaque. Information concerning the blood flow in the intracerebral vessels is also becoming increasingly possible to obtain using transcranial Doppler. While the anatomical resolution of Doppler imaging is limited, this is improving with increased experience and many centres no longer require formal angiography before performing carotid endarterectomy (pp. 1204–1206). This has the advantage of eliminating the small but significant risk of stroke or even death associated with catheter angiography.

Blood vessels can be outlined by the injection of radio-opaque contrast. The X-ray images obtained can be enhanced by the use of computer-assisted digital subtrac-tion, or by the use of spiral CT. Contrast may be injected intravenously or intra-arterially. The former requires a much

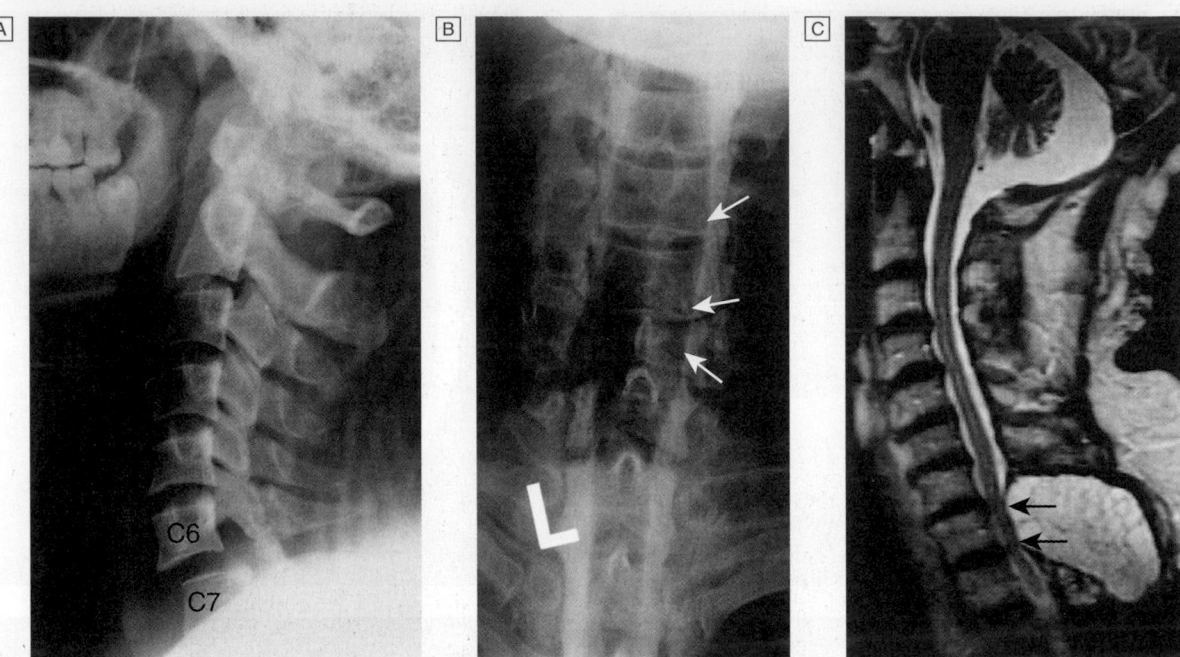

Fig. 26.10 Different techniques of imaging the cervical spine. [A] Lateral X-ray showing bilateral C6/7 facet dislocation. [B] Myelogram showing widening of cervical cord due to astrocytoma (arrows). [C] MRI showing posterior epidural compression from adenocarcinomatous metastasis to the posterior arch of T1 (arrows).

higher total dose of contrast, and the images obtained are not as good, but the latter involves feeding catheters up through the arterial tree and is thus associated with a higher complication rate. Formal intra-arterial angiography is still required in many centres to delineate lesions of the extracranial carotid artery prior to endarterectomy, and is also used to investigate abnormalities of intracerebral vessels such as arterial (berry) aneurysms or arteriovenous malformations, or to delineate the blood supply of tumours prior to surgery.

Flowing blood can be detected by specialised MR sequences in MR angiography. The anatomical resolution is still not comparable to that of intra-arterial angiography, but the investigation is non-invasive. Examples of these different techniques are given in Figure 26.11.

SPECIAL TESTS

Blood tests

Many systemic conditions affect the nervous system and these can often be diagnosed with the help of blood tests: for example, confusion due to hypothyroidism, a stroke due to systemic lupus erythematosus, ataxia due to vitamin B_{12} deficiency, or myelopathy due to syphilis. The blood tests relating to general medical conditions which affect the nervous system are dealt with in the sections dealing with the conditions themselves.

There are, however, a number of blood tests which are used in investigating specific neurological diseases. These include haematological tests (e.g. looking for acanthocytes to diagnose neuroacanthocytosis), biochemical tests (e.g. creatine kinase in muscle diseases, copper studies to diagnose Wilson's disease) or tests to help diagnose

innumerable infections of the nervous system. In addition, there are a number of specific antibodies that are useful diagnostically. These include antibodies to acetylcholine receptors and muscle-specific tyrosine kinase (MuSK), seen in myasthenia gravis, and to voltage-gated calcium channels in Lambert–Eaton myasthenic syndrome. Antibodies to different types of ganglioside (glycoproteins expressed on nerve membranes) can be seen in various types of neuropathy including multifocal motor neuronopathy, and the Guillain–Barré syndrome (particularly the Miller–Fisher variant). Also, antineuronal antibodies provide markers of paraneoplastic cerebellar or neuropathic syndromes. Antibodies to basal ganglia neurons are found in Sydenham's chorea and encephalitis lethargica.

An increasing number of inherited neurological conditions can now be diagnosed by DNA analysis (p. 50). These include diseases caused by increased numbers of trinucleotide repeats, such as Huntington's disease, myotonic dystrophy and some types of spinocerebellar ataxia. Also, defects of mitochondrial DNA can be detected in many conditions including Leber's hereditary optic neuropathy, and some syndromes causing epilepsy or stroke-like syndromes.

Lumbar puncture

This involves the insertion of a needle between lumbar spinous processes, through the dura and into the CSF under local anaesthetic. Intracranial pressure can be measured and CSF removed for analysis. CSF is normally clear and colourless. Tests usually performed on CSF include centrifuging to determine the colour of the supernatant (yellow, or xanthochromic, some hours after subarachnoid haemorrhage), biochemistry (glucose, total protein, and protein electrophoresis to detect oligoclonal bands),

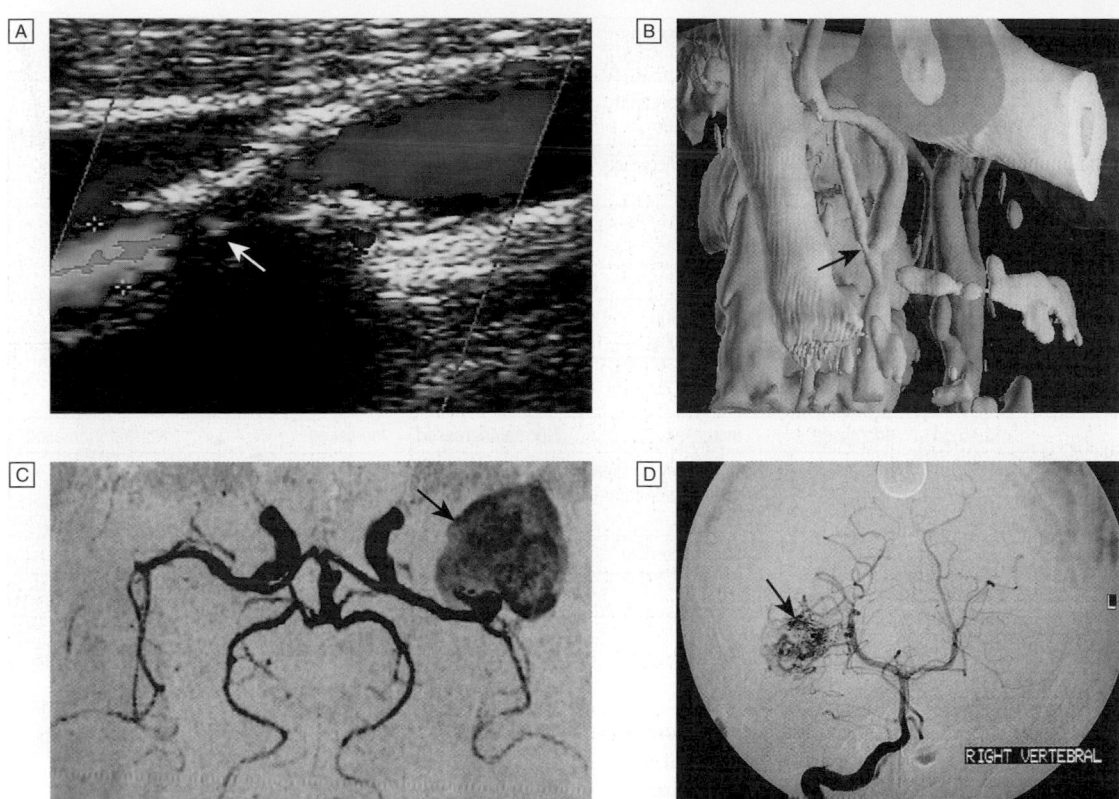

Fig. 26.11 **Different techniques of imaging blood vessels.** [A] Doppler scan showing 80% stenosis of internal carotid artery (arrow). [B] 3-D reconstruction of CT angiogram showing stenosis at the carotid bifurcation (arrow). [C] MR angiogram showing giant aneurysm at the middle cerebral artery bifurcation (arrow). [D] Intra-arterial angiography showing arteriovenous malformation (arrow).

26

microbiology (e.g. polymerase chain reaction (PCR) for herpes simplex or tuberculosis), immunology (e.g. paraneoplastic antibodies) and cytology (to detect malignant cells). Normal values and various abnormalities found in diseases are shown in Box 26.5.

Lumbar puncture is indicated in the investigation of infections (e.g. meningitis or encephalitis), subarachnoid haemorrhage, inflammatory conditions (e.g. multiple sclerosis, sarcoidosis and cerebral lupus) and some neurological malignancies (e.g. carcinomatous meningitis, lymphoma and leukaemia), and to measure CSF pressure (e.g. in idiopathic intracranial hypertension). It is, of course, part of the procedure of myelography, and can be used in therapeutic procedures, either to lower CSF pressure or to administer drugs.

If there is a space-occupying lesion in the head, lumbar puncture can result in a shift of intracerebral contents downwards, towards and into the spinal canal. This process is known as coning, and is potentially fatal (p. 1235). Consequently, lumbar puncture is contraindicated if there is any suggestion of raised intracranial pressure (e.g. papilloedema), depressed level of consciousness, or focal neurological signs suggesting a cerebral lesion, until imaging of the head (by CT or MRI) has excluded a space-occupying lesion or hydrocephalus. It is also contraindicated if the patient is likely to bleed, as in thrombocytopenia, disseminated intravascular coagulation or warfarin therapy, unless

specific measures are taken to compensate for the clotting deficit on a temporary basis. Lumbar puncture is not contraindicated in those on aspirin.

About 30% of lumbar punctures are followed by low-pressure headache, which can be severe. Other minor complications involve transient radicular pain during the procedure, and pain over the lumbar region. Provided the test is performed under sterile conditions, infections such as meningitis are extremely rare.

Biopsies
Nerve and muscle are occasionally biopsied to assist in the diagnosis and management of a number of neurological conditions. Likewise, it is occasionally necessary to biopsy brain or meninges.

Nerve is sometimes biopsied as part of the investigation of peripheral neuropathies. Usually, the sural nerve is sampled at the ankle or the radial nerve at the wrist. Histology can help identify underlying causes in demyelinating neuropathies (e.g. vasculitic) or, occasionally, infiltration with abnormal substances such as amyloid. However, nerve biopsy is not performed unless it is reasonably likely to diagnose a potentially treatable condition such as an inflammatory neuropathy, since there is an appreciable morbidity.

Skeletal muscle biopsy is performed more frequently. The quadriceps muscle is often sampled, although this depends somewhat on which muscles are affected. Indications

26.5 CSF PARAMETERS IN HEALTH AND SOME COMMON DISORDERS*

	Normal	Subarachnoid haemorrhage	Acute bacterial meningitis	Viral meningitis	Tuberculous meningitis	Multiple sclerosis
Pressure	50–180 mm of water	Increased	Normal/increased	Normal	Normal/increased	Normal
Colour	Clear	Blood-stained Xanthochromic	Cloudy	Clear	Clear/cloudy	Clear
Red cell count	$0-4 \times 10^6$/l	Raised	Normal	Normal	Normal	Normal
White cell count	$0-4 \times 10^6$/l	Normal/slightly raised	1000–5000 polymorphs	10–2000 lymphocytes	50–5000 lymphocytes	0–50 lymphocytes
Glucose	> 60% of blood level	Normal	Decreased	Normal	Decreased	Normal
Protein	< 0.45 g/l	Increased	Increased	Normal/increased	Increased	Normal/increased
Microbiology	Sterile	Sterile	Organisms on Gram stain and/or culture	Sterile/virus detected	Ziehl–Nielson/auramine stain or tuberculosis culture positive	Sterile
Oligoclonal bands	Negative	Negative	Can be positive	Can be positive	Can be positive	Often positive

* See also Box 26.94, page 1225.

include the investigation of primary muscle disease, as muscle histology can be used to distinguish neurogenic wasting, myositis and myopathy, which may be difficult to distinguish clinically. Histology and enzyme histochemistry can also be helpful in the diagnosis of more widespread metabolic disorders, such as mitochondrial and some storage diseases. Although pain and infection can follow the procedure, these are much less of a problem than after nerve biopsy.

The nature of lesions demonstrated by brain imaging can often be inferred from the appearances as well as the history, examination and other, less invasive, investigations. However, there are situations in which the nature of lesions is not clear, and it is important to obtain tissue for histological examination. Likewise, it is sometimes necessary to biopsy the brain parenchyma itself in unexplained degenerative diseases (e.g. unusual dementias) so as not to miss potentially treatable disease.

Brain biopsy used to require full craniotomy. However, owing to the increased availability and sophistication of cerebral imaging, it is now possible to biopsy most lesions stereotactically through a burrhole in the skull. The complication rate of such stereotactic biopsies is much lower than that of open craniotomy, but haemorrhage, infection and death still occur. Hence, brain biopsy is only considered if a diagnosis cannot be reached in any other way.

PRESENTING PROBLEMS IN NERVOUS SYSTEM DISEASE

HEADACHE AND FACIAL PAIN

Headache is a frequently encountered neurological symptom but is seldom associated with significant neurological disease unless accompanied by other symptoms or

26.6 COMMON AND IMPORTANT HEADACHE AND FACIAL PAIN SYNDROMES

- Tension-type headache (persistent daily headache)
- Migraine
- Cluster headache
- Raised intracranial pressure
- Benign paroxysmal headaches (Box 26.11, p. 1163)
- Trigeminal neuralgia
- Atypical facial pain
- Post-herpetic neuralgia

neurological signs. Nevertheless, patients suffering from headaches usually fear serious brain disease. In order to manage them effectively, it is important to be aware of this mismatch between fear of disease and its actual likelihood. Careful clinical assessment usually identifies one of a limited number of headache or facial pain syndromes (Box 26.6). After taking a careful history and performing the appropriate neurological examination, it is often not necessary to perform further investigations. The patient can be reassured and provided with symptomatic treatment.

Pathophysiology

It is often difficult to explain the pain of headaches by reference to current neurobiological understanding of the mechanisms of pain, especially in those not caused by serious disease. Within the skull, the dura (including the dural sinuses and falx cerebri) and the proximal parts of the large pial blood vessels are the main structures sensitive to pain. The brain parenchyma, pial arteries over the convexities, and the cerebral ventricles and choroid plexus are known to be insensitive to pain. The pain-sensitive intracranial structures are mostly innervated by branches of the trigeminal nerve and some by branches of the upper cervical nerves. This probably accounts for the patterns of pain referral seen in intracranial disease when these pain-

26

26.7 IMPORTANT POINTS IN THE HEADACHE HISTORY

- The overall pattern (intermittent or continuous)
- The tempo of onset
- The time of day of onset of maximal pain
- The effect of posture, coughing and straining
- The location of the pain
- Any associated symptoms

26.8 HEADACHE OF RAISED INTRACRANIAL PRESSURE

- Worse in morning, improves through the day
- Associated with morning vomiting
- Worse bending forward
- Worse with cough and straining
- Relieved by analgesia
- Dull ache, often mild

26.9 HEADACHES IN OLD AGE

- **Prevalence:** less common in those aged over 60 years than in younger people.
- **Common causes:** trigeminal neuralgia, temporal arteritis and post-herpetic neuralgia, which occur rarely in younger patients.
- **Migraine and tension headache:** less common than in younger people.
- **Raised intracranial pressure:** not always associated with headache, vomiting or papilloedema because intracranial mass lesions can reach larger sizes before presentation, as the involutional process that occurs in ageing brains allows the accommodation of an expanding lesion more easily than in younger patients.

sensitive parts of the intracranial contents are stretched, distended or otherwise irritated.

A DIAGNOSTIC APPROACH TO THE PATIENT WITH HEADACHE

Unless the history is suggestive of structural disease, patients with headache who are normal on neurological examination are unlikely to have a serious disorder, however distressing their symptoms. The features of a patient's history that are helpful in making a clear diagnosis of the cause of a headache are shown in Box 26.7.

Patients can be divided into those with chronic headache (a duration of several weeks or more) and those with more acute headache. Serious acute neurological disease should always be considered in patients with headaches of very sudden onset. Subarachnoid haemorrhage (p. 1210) causes a very sudden headache which may or may not be localised, although only one person in eight who has such a 'thunderclap' headache will have had a subarachnoid haemorrhage. A patient with subarachnoid haemorrhage almost invariably develops other symptoms including vomiting and neck stiffness, although the latter may take some hours to develop. The main differential diagnosis in a patient with a sudden severe headache is between subarachnoid haemorrhage and a migraine variant (Fig. 26.35, p. 1211). Meningitis occasionally presents apoplectically, but the headache is usually less dramatic in onset.

Headache coming on over a matter of hours is less likely to be associated with structural disease and more likely to be due to migraine, unless accompanied by other significant symptoms or signs. Patients with bacterial meningitis are usually generally ill and pyrexial, and exhibit meningism (p. 1224). Patients with viral meningitis may present with a pyrexia and quite sudden and severe headache coming on over an hour or so, but are less likely to have neck stiffness or other signs of meningism. Migraine headaches (see below) may be accompanied or preceded by vomiting and focal neurological symptoms (usually in the form of zigzag 'fortification spectra' or tingling moving slowly over part of the body).

When headaches are intermittent rather than continuous over a period of days or weeks, they are most likely to be migrainous but it is worthwhile paying attention to the time of day they occur and to the presence or absence of precipitating factors. The headache of raised intracranial pressure is present on waking and often resolves or improves as the patient becomes upright (reducing the intracranial pressure) or takes simple analgesia (Box 26.8). It is unusual for a patient to present with such a headache alone since it is usually not sufficiently severe to cause

alarm, the presentation of the causative mass lesion more often being provoked by a seizure or by focal neurological dysfunction (aphasia, hemiplegia etc.). The exceptions to this are patients with acute hydrocephalus who present with a more severe headache. As with other causes of raised intracranial pressure, this is worse when lying, bending forward or coughing, and frequently causes vomiting in the morning (especially in children). Hydrocephalus may cause no other symptoms except gait ataxia, although examination may reveal papilloedema.

Headaches that persist for weeks, are present all day and are poorly responsive to simple analgesia are very likely to be tension-type headaches, whatever their other characteristics. Headaches so well localised by the patient that a finger is used to locate the exact spot on the skull are never associated with significant disease.

In a patient over 60 years with head pain localised to one or both temples, giant cell arteritis (p. 1139) should be considered, especially if the temporal pulses are not palpable and/or the arteries are enlarged and tender.

TENSION-TYPE HEADACHE

Clinical assessment

This is the most common type of headache and is experienced at some time by the majority of the population in some form. The pain is usually constant and generalised but often radiates forward from the occipital region. It is described as 'dull', 'tight' or like a 'pressure', and there may be a sensation of a band round the head or pressure at the vertex. In contrast to migraine, the pain may continue for weeks or months without interruption, although the severity may vary, and there is no associated vomiting or photophobia. The patient can usually continue normal activities, and the pain may be less noticeable when the patient is occupied. The pain is characteristically less severe in the

26

early part of the day and becomes more troublesome as the day goes on. Local tenderness may be present over the skull vault or in the occiput but this should be distinguished from the acute pain precipitated by skin contact in trigeminal neuralgia and the exquisite tenderness of temporal arteritis. Typically, the headache is reported to be poorly responsive to ordinary analgesia.

Pathogenesis

The cause of tension-type headaches is obscure. There is little evidence for the hypothesis that they are caused by excessive contraction of the muscles of the head and neck. Emotional strain or anxiety is a common precipitant to tension-type headache and there is sometimes an associated depressive illness. Anxiety about the headache itself may lead to continuation of symptoms, and patients often become convinced of a serious underlying condition.

Management

Careful assessment followed by discussion of likely precipitants and explanation of the fact that the symptoms are not due to any sinister underlying pathology is more likely to be beneficial than analgesics. Excessive use of analgesics, particularly of codeine, may actually worsen the headache (analgesic headache). Physiotherapy (with muscle relaxation and stress management) is usually beneficial, but low-dose amitriptyline (10 mg nocte increased gradually to 30–50 mg) may be necessary. There is evidence that patients benefit from a perception that their problem has been taken seriously and rigorously assessed, but over-investigation can worsen a patient's anxiety.

MIGRAINE

Clinical assessment

Patients may refer to any episodic paroxysmal headache as migraine. However, it is best to look upon migraine as a triad of paroxysmal headache, nausea and/or vomiting, and an 'aura' of focal neurological events (usually visual). Patients with all three of these features are said to have migraine with aura ('classical' migraine). Those with paroxysmal headache (with or without vomiting) but no 'aura' are said to have migraine without aura ('common' migraine). It has been estimated that the lifetime prevalence of migraine is about 20% in females and 6% in males. Over 90% of migraine sufferers will have their first attack by the time they are 40 years old. Typically, a classical migraine attack starts with a non-specific prodrome of malaise and irritability followed by the 'aura' of a focal neurological event, and then a severe, throbbing, hemicranial headache with photophobia and vomiting. During the headache phase, patients prefer to be in a quiet, darkened room and to sleep. The headache may persist for several days.

The 'aura' most often takes the form of 'fortification spectra': shimmering, silvery zigzag lines which march across the visual fields over 20 minutes, sometimes leaving a trail of temporary visual field loss. In some patients there is a sensory aura: a spreading front of tingling followed by numbness which moves, over 20–30 minutes, from one part of the body to another. If the dominant hemisphere is involved, the patient may also experience transient aphasia. True weakness is distinctly unusual in migraine, so 'hemiplegic migraine' should be diagnosed with extreme caution. In some patients the focal events may occur by themselves ('migraine equivalent'), but in this case other structural disorders of the brain, or even focal epilepsy, need to be considered in the differential diagnosis. In a smaller number of patients, the symptoms of the aura do not resolve, leaving more permanent neurological disturbance ('complicated migraine').

Aetiology and pathogenesis

The aetiology of migraine is largely unknown. There is often a family history, suggesting a genetic predisposition. The great female preponderance and the tendency for some women to have migraine attacks at certain points in their menstrual cycle hint at hormonal influences. The relevance of the contraceptive pill in this context is difficult to establish, but it does appear to exacerbate migraine in many patients, and to increase the small risk of stroke in patients who suffer from migraine with aura (Box 26.10). In some patients there are identifiable dietary precipitants such as cheese, chocolate or red wine. When psychological stress is involved, the migraine attack often occurs after the period of strain so that some patients tend to have attacks at weekends or at the beginning of a holiday.

The 'aura' of classical migraine probably represents a spreading front of electrical excitation followed by depression of activity of cortical cells. The cause of this is not understood but it probably represents a paroxysmal alteration in cortical modulation pathways from the brain stem (especially serotoninergic projections). The observation that migraine-like phenomena occur in rare genetic disorders associated with mutations in calcium channel genes, suggests the possibility that the aura may be due to paroxysmal changes in the function of neuronal ion channels. The headache is thought to be caused by vasodilatation of extracranial vessels and may, like the headache following an epileptic seizure, be a non-specific effect of the disturbance of neuronal function.

Management

Identification and avoidance of precipitants or exacerbating factors (such as the contraceptive pill) may prevent attacks. Treatment of an acute attack consists of simple analgesia with aspirin or paracetamol, often combined with an antiemetic such as metoclopramide or domperidone. Long-term use of codeine-containing analgesic preparations should be

---

EBM

26.10 MIGRAINE AND STROKE RISK

'There is a slight increase in the risk of thromboembolic stroke in patients who suffer from migraine, particularly migraine with aura. This risk is considerably elevated by concomitant use of oestrogen-based contraception.'

- Buring JE, et al. Arch Neurol 1995; 52:129–134.
- Chang CL, et al. World Health Organization Collaborative Study of Cardiovascular Disease and Steroid Hormone Contraception. BMJ 1999; 318:13–18.

For further information: 💻 www.cochrane.org

avoided. Severe attacks can be treated with one of the 'triptans' (e.g. sumatriptan), 5-HT agonists that are potent vasoconstrictors of the extracranial arteries. These can be administered orally, sublingually, by subcutaneous injection or by nasal spray. Ergotamine preparations should be avoided since they easily lead to dependence. This is less likely to happen with the triptans, but it can occur. If attacks are frequent, they can often be prevented with propranolol (80–160 mg daily, in a sustained-release preparation), a tricyclic such as amitriptyline (10–50 mg at night) or sodium valproate (300–600 mg/day), or pizotifen (1.5–3.0 mg daily). Women should be warned that the small risk of ischaemic stroke attributable to taking oral contraception is increased if they have migraine (see above), especially if they also smoke.

CLUSTER HEADACHE (MIGRAINOUS NEURALGIA)

Clinical assessment

This is some 10–50 times less common than migraine. There is a 5:1 predominance of males and onset is usually in the third decade. The characteristic syndrome comprises periodic, severe, unilateral periorbital pain accompanied by unilateral lacrimation, nasal congestion and conjunctival injection, often with the other features of Horner's syndrome. The pain, whilst being very severe, is characteristically brief (30–90 minutes). Typically, the patient develops these symptoms at a particular time of day (often in the early hours of the morning). The syndrome may occur repeatedly for a number of weeks, followed by a respite for a number of months before another cluster occurs.

Pathogenesis

There is little genetic predisposition, no provoking dietary factors and a male predominance, which suggest a different aetiology from that of migraine, but this remains unknown. Patients are usually heavy smokers with a higher than average alcohol consumption.

Management

Acute attacks are usually halted by subcutaneous injections of sumatriptan or by inhalation of 100% oxygen; other migraine therapies are ineffective, probably because of the brevity of the individual attacks. Preventative therapy with the agents used for migraine is often ineffective but attacks can be prevented in some patients by verapamil (80–120 mg 8-hourly), methysergide (4–10 mg daily, for a maximum of 3 months only) or short courses of corticosteroids. Patients with severe and debilitating clusters can be helped with lithium therapy, although the usual precautions concerning the use of this drug should be observed (p. 237).

LESS COMMON NEURALGIC HEADACHES

There are a number of rare headache syndromes which produce pains about the eye similar to cluster headaches (Box 26.11). These include chronic and episodic paroxysmal hemicrania, and SUNCT (Short-lasting Unilateral Neuralgiform headaches with Conjunctival injection and Tearing). The recognition of these syndromes is useful since they often respond to specific treatments such as indometacin

COITAL AND EXERCISE-INDUCED CEPHALGIA

Clinical assessment

Patients are almost exclusively middle-aged men who develop a sudden, severe headache at the climax of sexual intercourse. There is usually no vomiting and no neck stiffness, and it does not persist for more than 10–15 minutes, though a less severe, dull headache may persist for

26

26.11 BENIGN PAROXYSMAL HEADACHES				
	Character of pain	Duration	Location	Comment
Ice pick	Stabbing	Very brief (split-second)	Variable, usually temporal or parietal	Benign, more common in migraine
Ice cream	Sharp, severe	30–120 seconds	Bitemporal/occipital	Obvious trigger by cold stimuli
Exertional/coital	Bursting, thunderclap	Severe for minutes then less severe for hours	Generalised	Subarachnoid haemorrhage needs exclusion
Cough	Bursting	Seconds to minutes	Occipital or generalised	Intracranial pathology needs exclusion (especially craniocervical junction)
Cluster headache (migrainous neuralgia)	Severe unilateral, with ptosis, tearing, conjunctival injection, unilateral nasal congestion	30–90 minutes 1–3 times per day	Periorbital	Usually men, occurring in clusters over weeks/months
Chronic paroxysmal hemicrania	Severe unilateral with cluster headache-like autonomic features (above)	5–20 minutes, frequently through day	Periorbital/temporal	Usually women, responds to indometacin
SUNCT*	Severe, sharp, triggered by touch or neck movements	15–120 seconds, repetitive through day	Periorbital	May respond to carbamazepine

* Short-lasting, Unilateral, Neuralgiform headache with Conjunctival injection, Tearing, rhinorrhoea and forehead sweating.

some hours. This type of paroxysmal headache often needs to be distinguished, by CT and/or CSF examination, from the thunderclap headache of a subarachnoid haemorrhage (Fig. 26.35, p. 1121). A very similar headache may occur during physical exertion, especially if this is attempted with unaccustomed vigour in an unfit person. The pathogenesis is unknown.

Management

Coital or exertional cephalgia is usually brief though frightening and may not need more than ordinary analgesia for the residual headache. The syndrome may not recur but prevention with propranolol or indometacin (75 mg daily) may be necessary.

Other paroxysmal headaches are described in Box 26.11.

A DIAGNOSTIC APPROACH TO THE PATIENT WITH FACIAL PAIN

Pain in and around the eye, when not caused by ocular disease, should be considered as a headache (above). This includes the dramatic pain of cluster headache and rarer variants. Rarely, inflammatory or infiltrative lesions at the apex of the orbit or the cavernous sinus may cause pain in or around the eye, but tell-tale signs from involvement of the ocular motor nerves usually accompany this. Pain in the eye may accompany disorders of the carotid artery, particularly dissections, and may then be accompanied by a Horner's syndrome.

Pain in other parts of the face can be due to problems with the teeth or the temporo-mandibular joint. Inflamed nasal sinuses are seldom the cause of lasting facial pain in the absence of obvious nasal congestion. The very rare but serious condition of subdural empyema (p. 1231) needs to be considered if 'sinusitis' is followed by very severe unilateral facial pain and signs of cerebral irritation (seizures and/or obtundation). Destructive lesions of the trigeminal nerve causing pain are extremely rare since such lesions usually cause loss of sensation in the nerve's territory rather than pain.

Most patients with persisting pain in the face have trigeminal neuralgia, atypical facial pain or post-herpetic neuralgia. The main distinction between these is in the nature of the pain. In trigeminal neuralgia, the pain is very brief, though severe and recurrent, described as 'like lightning' and is most frequently felt in the second and third divisions of the nerve. Atypical facial pain, on the other hand, is continuous and unremitting, and is centred over the maxilla, usually on the left side. It occurs most frequently in middle-aged women. Post-herpetic neuralgia is continuous and is felt as a burning pain throughout the affected territory, which is often very sensitive to light touch. The cause is usually obvious from a history of 'shingles' in the ophthalmic division of the trigeminal nerve.

TRIGEMINAL NEURALGIA

Clinical assessment

This condition causes lancinating pains in the second and third divisions of the trigeminal nerve territory, usually in patients over age 50 years. The pain is severe and very brief but repetitive, causing the patient to flinch as if with a motor tic; hence the French term for the condition, 'tic douloureux'. The pain may be precipitated by touching trigger zones within the trigeminal territory or by eating. Usually there are no other signs, although similar symptoms may occur in multiple sclerosis or rarely with other lesions, in which case there may be sensory changes in the trigeminal nerve territory or other brain-stem symptoms and signs. There is a tendency for the condition to remit and relapse over many years.

Pathogenesis

The current aetiological hypothesis suggests that the neuralgia is most commonly caused by compression of the trigeminal nerve rootlets at their entry to the brain stem by aberrant loops of the cerebellar arteries. Other compressive lesions, usually benign, are occasionally found in the site. When trigeminal neuralgia occurs in multiple sclerosis, there is a plaque of demyelination in the trigeminal root entry zone.

Management

The pain usually responds to carbamazepine, in doses of up to 1200 mg daily. It is wise to start with much lower doses and escalate the dose according to effect, as when used for epilepsy. In patients who cannot tolerate carbamazepine, gabapentin or phenytoin may be effective, but other anticonvulsants are not. Various surgical treatments are available; the simplest is the injection of alcohol or phenol into a peripheral branch of the nerve. Probably more effective is the percutaneous placing of a radiofrequency lesion in the nerve near the Gasserian ganglion. Care has to be taken not to cause excessive damage to sensation in the face to prevent the complication of neurogenic pain ('anaesthesia dolorosa') which is worse than the neuralgia. Alternatively, the vascular compression of the trigeminal nerve can be relieved through a small posterior craniotomy, often with substantial success. This latter approach is usually favoured in younger patients in whom the other injection treatments may have to be repeated and become less effective.

DIZZINESS, BLACKOUTS AND 'FUNNY TURNS'

Episodes of lost or altered consciousness are a frequent symptom in primary care and in hospital practice, especially in the elderly. A patient may complain of 'blacking out', 'going dizzy', 'coming over queer', 'having a funny turn' or other local variants. The first task is to discover exactly what the patient means by the terms used. Some patients, for example, mean by 'blackout' that their vision darkens without alteration in consciousness (defined here as an awareness of the environment and ability to respond to it). More often 'blackout' is used to describe an episode of lost consciousness with or without falling down. The terms 'blackout' and 'funny turn' can also be used to refer to transient periods of amnesia, when the patient loses memory

26

consciousness, vertigo, transient amnesia or something else. The former two symptoms suggest a problem in mechanisms maintaining normal awareness. Vertigo is caused by an alteration in function of the peripheral vestibular organs or the central control mechanisms of balance and posture.

A DIAGNOSTIC APPROACH TO THE PATIENT WITH VERTIGO (Fig. 26.12)

Abnormal perception of movement of the environment occurs as a result of a mismatch between the information about a person's position reaching the brain from the eyes, limb proprioception and the vestibular system. Vertigo arising from inappropriate input from the labyrinthine apparatus is within the experience of most people, since this is the 'dizziness' which occurs after someone has spun round vigorously and then stops. Vertigo caused by labyrinthine disorders is usually short-lived, though it may recur, whilst vertigo arising from central (brain-stem) disorders is often persistent and accompanied by other signs of brain-stem dysfunction. A careful analysis of the history will reveal the likely cause in most patients.

for a period of time. 'Dizziness' is used frequently to describe an abnormal perception of movement of the environment (vertigo), but may be used to mean a feeling of faintness, some other alteration of consciousness, or unsteadiness (p. 1193).

After a careful history from the patient, supplemented by a witness account, it should be clear whether the patient is describing an episode of loss of consciousness, altered

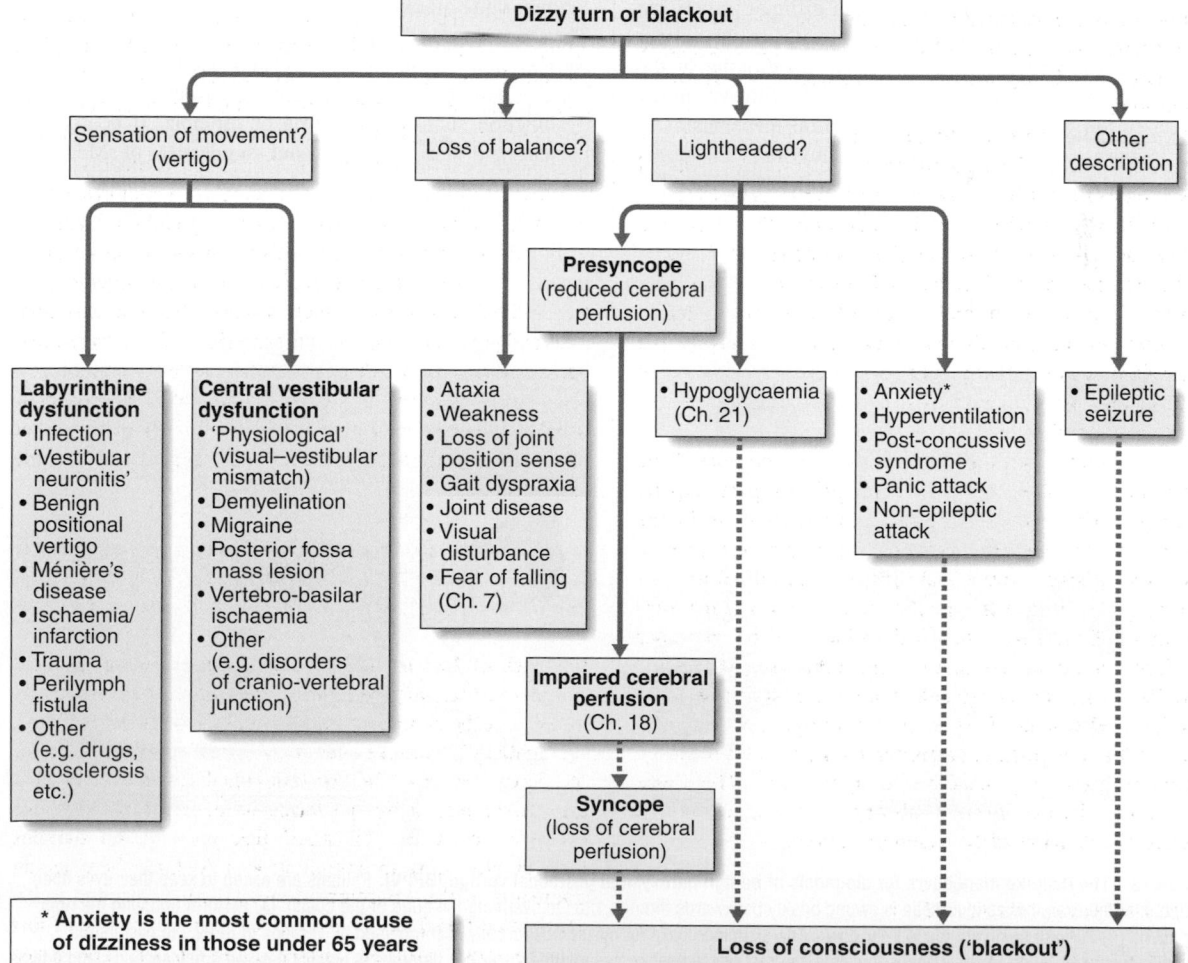

Fig. 26.12 **A diagnostic approach to the patient with dizziness, funny turns or blackouts.**

VERTIGO CAUSED BY LABYRINTHINE DISTURBANCES

Labyrinthitis ('vestibular neuronitis')

This is the most common cause of severe vertigo, but the cause of the labyrinthitis is unknown; it usually presents in the third or fourth decade as severe vertigo, with vomiting and ataxia but no tinnitus or deafness, often coming on when waking. The vertigo is most severe at onset and settles down over the next few days, though afterwards head movement may provoke vertigo (positional vertigo) for some time. During the attack, nystagmus (p. 1196) will be present but does not persist for long.

Benign paroxysmal positional vertigo

Especially in older patients, paroxysms of vertigo occurring with certain head movements may be due to the presence of degenerative material affecting the free flow of endolymph in the labyrinth (cupulolithiasis). Each attack of vertigo lasts seconds but patients often become very distressed and reluctant to move their head, which can in turn produce a muscle tension-type of headache. Secondary hyperventilation attacks and associated depressive features are also common. The diagnosis can be confirmed by using the 'Hallpike manoeuvre' to demonstrate positional nystagmus (Fig. 26.13). Although this test is often difficult to perform adequately, it is useful since it demonstrates to the patient that the vertigo fatigues with repetitive positioning of the head. The vertigo can then be treated with vestibular exercises designed to habituate the central mechanisms to the inappropriate signals from the labyrinth. Positional vertigo may also occur after concussive head injuries but this usually resolves after a period of weeks.

Ménière's disease

This is a cause of labyrinthine vertigo that is probably diagnosed too readily. Patients usually present first with tinnitus and distorted hearing, and then develop paroxysmal attacks of vertigo preceded by a sense of fullness in the ear. Examination in this circumstance shows sensorineural hearing loss on the affected side.

Drug treatment of labyrinthine vertigo

Symptomatic relief of labyrinthine causes of vertigo can be achieved with 'vestibular sedatives' (e.g. cinnarizine, prochlorperazine, betahistine). Patients with intractable symptoms should be referred to an ENT specialist for assessment.

CENTRAL CAUSES OF VERTIGO

Any disease that affects the vestibular nucleus in the brain stem or its connections can cause vertigo. This can be distinguished from peripheral causes of vertigo by its persistence and the usual association of other signs, especially persistent nystagmus. Positionally induced central vertigo persists for as long as the position is maintained, unlike the common peripheral positional vertigo that fatigues quite quickly if the inducing position is maintained. The same is true of any accompanying nystagmus. Transient causes such as brain-stem ischaemia can be recognised by the association with other symptoms of brain-stem dysfunction such as dysarthria or diplopia. If deafness is present and the history is not suggestive of Ménière's disease, extra-axial compression of the 8th cranial nerve by a lesion such as an acoustic neuroma (p. 1238) should be

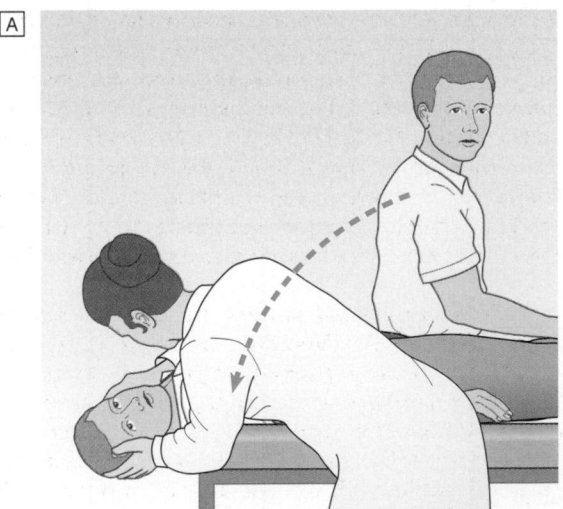
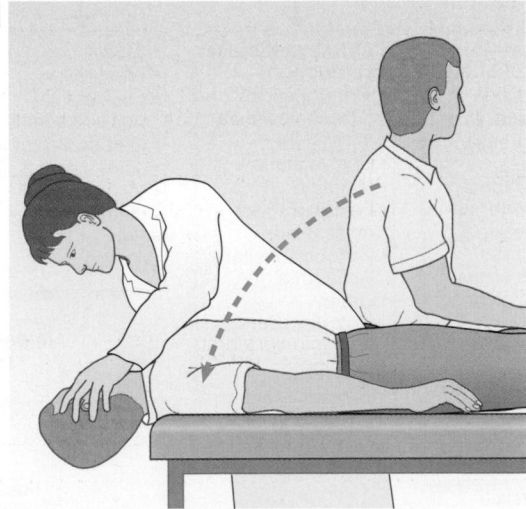

Fig 26.13 **The Hallpike manoeuvre for diagnosis of benign paroxysmal positional vertigo (BPPV).** Patients are asked to keep their eyes open and look at the examiner as their head is swung briskly backwards through 120° to overhang the edge of the couch. [A] Perform first with the right ear down. [B] Perform next with the left ear down. The examiner looks for nystagmus (usually accompanied by vertigo). In BPPV, the nystagmus typically occurs in [A] or [B] only and is torsional, the fast phase beating towards the lower ear. Its onset is usually delayed a few seconds, and it lasts 10–20 seconds. As the patient is returned to the upright position, transient nystagmus may occur in the opposite direction. Both nystagmus and vertigo typically decrease (fatigue) on repeat testing.

26

suspected. Rarely, vertigo originating from the cerebral cortex may be a manifestation of a partial seizure in the temporal lobe.

A DIAGNOSTIC APPROACH TO THE PATIENT WITH EPISODIC LOSS OF CONSCIOUSNESS

Loss of consciousness, other than in sleep, suggests a global dysfunction of the brain. As a transient phenomenon, this most commonly occurs because of a recoverable loss of adequate blood supply to the brain, i.e. syncope (see below). Alternatively, loss of consciousness occurs from sudden electrical dysfunction of the brain during a seizure (epileptic fit). Episodes of loss of consciousness are therefore either fits or faints, though many patients who have various types of psychogenic blackout or non-epileptic seizure confuse this clear distinction.

The distinction of a seizure from a faint can only be made from the patient's history, with help from a witness to the attack. No amount of investigation can replace a clear history in these circumstances. Features in the history useful in distinguishing a seizure from a faint are shown in Box 26.13.

SYNCOPE

A brief feeling of 'lightheadedness' often precedes a faint; vision then darkens and there may be a ringing in the ears. Vasovagal syncope (p. 553) may be provoked by some emotionally charged event (e.g. venepuncture) and usually occurs from the standing position. Cardiac syncope (p. 551), caused by a sudden decline in cardiac output and hence cerebral perfusion, may be provoked by exertion (e.g. with severe aortic stenosis) or may occur completely 'out of the blue' (as in heart block).

In vasovagal syncope, the loss of consciousness is gradual and brief, and the patient recovers quickly without confusion as long as he or she has assumed the horizontal position. It is rare for the syncope to cause injury and there is no amnesia for events that occur after regaining awareness. During a syncopal attack, incontinence of urine can occur and there is often stiffening and brief twitching of the limbs, but tongue-biting never occurs.

26.13 FEATURES HELPFUL IN DISTINGUISHING SEIZURES FROM FAINTS		
	Seizure	Faint
Aura (e.g. olfactory)	+	−
Cyanosis	+	−
Tongue-biting	+	−
Post-ictal confusion	+	−
Post-ictal amnesia	+	−
Post-ictal headache	+	−
Rapid recovery	−	+

SEIZURES

A seizure is any clinical event caused by an abnormal electrical discharge in the brain, whilst epilepsy is the tendency to have recurrent seizures (p. 1169). Major seizures cause loss of consciousness, with the patient falling to the ground and presenting with a history of 'blackouts'. Minor seizures causing alteration of consciousness, without the patient falling to the ground, may also be described by patients as 'blackouts'.

Pathophysiology

In the normally functioning cortex, recurrent and collateral inhibitory circuits limit synchronous discharge amongst neighbouring groups of neurons. The inhibitory transmitter gamma-aminobutyric acid (GABA) is particularly important in this role, and drugs that block GABA receptors provoke seizures. There is also a large number of excitatory neurotransmitters, of which acetylcholine and the amino acids glutamate and aspartate are examples (Box 26.2, p. 1150). 'Epileptic' cerebral cortex exhibits hypersynchronous repetitive discharges involving large groups of neurons. Intracellular recordings show bursts of rapid action potential firing, with reduction of the transmembrane potential (paroxysmal depolarisation shift). It is likely that both reduction in inhibitory systems and excessive excitation play a part in the genesis of seizure activity. Cells undergoing repetitive 'epileptic' discharges undergo morphological and physiological changes which make them more likely to produce subsequent abnormal discharges ('kindling').

The chief division of seizure types on physiological grounds is between partial (focal) seizures in which paroxysmal neuronal activity is limited to one part of the cortex, and generalised seizures where the electrophysiological abnormality involves both hemispheres simultaneously and synchronously (Fig. 26.14). If partial seizures remain localised, the symptomatology depends on the cortical area affected. If consciousness (the awareness of and ability to respond to the environment) is preserved, the attack is termed a 'simple partial seizure'. However, if the activity involves parts of the brain concerned with awareness (such as the temporal or frontal lobes), then consciousness is affected and a 'complex partial seizure' results. Further spread into the diencephalon and thence throughout the remainder of the cortex leads to a secondarily generalised seizure.

In primary generalised seizures, the abnormal activity begins synchronously throughout the cortex without an initial partial onset. It probably originates in the central diencephalic mechanisms controlling cortical activation (Fig. 26.14). This is recognisable on an EEG as spike and wave discharges (Fig. 26.6, p. 1154) and quite often hyperventilation and/or photic stimulation provoke such discharges. This may cause a major seizure identical to a secondarily generalised seizure, or a more restricted clinical manifestation if the abnormal electrical activity fails to affect muscle tone. In the latter case there is an 'absence', in which consciousness is lost but the patient remains standing or sitting. Such attacks may be difficult to distinguish clinically from a complex partial seizure in the temporal lobe.

26

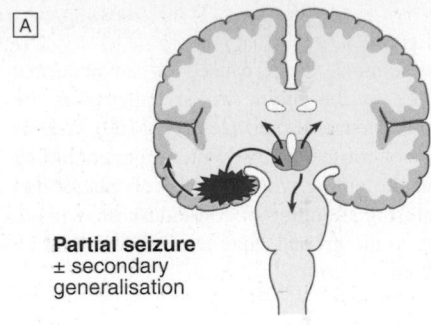

Partial seizure
± secondary
generalisation

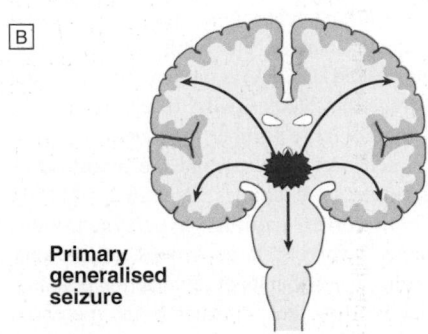

**Primary
generalised
seizure**

Fig. 26.14   The pathophysiological classification of seizures. [A] A partial seizure originates from a paroxysmal discharge in a focal area of the cerebral cortex (often the temporal lobe); the seizure may subsequently spread to the rest of the brain (secondary generalisation) via diencephalic activating pathways. [B] In primary generalised seizures the abnormal electrical discharges originate from the diencephalic activating system and spread simultaneously to all areas of the cortex.

Clinical assessment

Tonic clonic seizures

A tonic clonic seizure may be preceded by a partial seizure (the 'aura') which can take various forms, described below. However, a history of such an 'aura' is commonly not obtained, probably because the subsequent generalised seizure causes some retrograde amnesia for immediately preceding events. The patient then goes rigid and becomes unconscious, falling down heavily if standing and often sustaining injury. During this phase, respiration is arrested and central cyanosis may be witnessed. After a few moments, the rigidity is periodically relaxed, producing clonic jerks. Some patients do not have a clonic phase and the rigidity is replaced by a flaccid state of deep coma which can persist for some minutes. The patient then gradually regains consciousness, but is in a confused and disorientated state for half an hour or more after regaining consciousness. Full memory function may not be recovered for some hours. During the attack, urinary incontinence may occur, as may tongue-biting. A severely bitten, bleeding tongue after an attack of loss of consciousness is pathognomonic of a generalised seizure. After a generalised seizure the patient usually feels terrible, may have a headache and will want to sleep. Witnesses of a seizure are usually frightened by the events, often believing the person to be dying, and may not give a clear account; this is in itself a helpful diagnostic

pointer since syncope seldom produces such fear in onlookers. Patients may have no tonic or clonic phase, and may not become cyanosed or bite their tongue. However, post-ictal confusion or headache and a period of subsequent malaise and/or confusion are usually seen, and this is useful in differentiating seizures from faints. Psychogenic non-epileptic attacks ('pseudo-seizures') may be accompanied by dramatic flailing of the limbs and arching of the back; however, these are not usually followed by the same degree of post-ictal confusion and do not cause cyanosis.

Complex partial seizures

Partial seizures may cause episodes of altered consciousness without the patient collapsing to the ground, especially if arising from the temporal or, less frequently, the frontal lobe. These may be referred to as 'blackouts'. The patient stops what he or she is doing and stares blankly, often making rhythmic smacking movements of the lips or displaying other automatisms, such as picking at their clothes. After a few minutes the patient returns to consciousness but may be initially muddled and feel drowsy. Immediately before such an attack the patient may report alterations of mood, memory and perception such as undue familiarity (déjà vu) or unreality (jamais vu), complex hallucinations of sound, smell, taste, vision, emotional changes (fear, sexual arousal) or visceral sensations (nausea, epigastric discomfort). If these changes of memory or perception occur without subsequent alteration in awareness, the seizure is said to be a simple partial seizure.

Complex partial seizures arising from the anterior parts of the frontal lobe may produce bizarre behaviour patterns including frenetic ill-directed motor activity and incoherent screaming. These can be very difficult to distinguish from psychogenic attacks (which are more common). However, the abruptness of their onset and relative brevity may help distinguish frontal seizures, as may their tendency to occur out of sleep.

Absence seizures

A type of minor seizure that resembles a complex partial seizure occurs in some generalised epilepsies, including the generalised absence epilepsy of childhood known as 'petit mal'. In petit mal epilepsy, which always starts in childhood, the attacks are usually briefer and very much more frequent (up to 20 or 30 a day) than complex partial seizures and are not associated with post-ictal confusion. Absence attacks are caused by a generalised discharge that does not spread out of the hemispheres and so does not cause loss of posture.

Atonic seizures

These are seizures involving brief loss of muscle tone, usually resulting in heavy falls with or without loss of consciousness. They only occur in the context of epilepsy syndromes with other forms of seizure. They should not be considered in the differential diagnosis of collapse in patients not known to have epilepsy.

Partial motor seizures

Epileptic activity arising in the pre-central gyrus causes partial motor seizures affecting the contralateral face, arm, trunk or leg. Seizures are characterised by rhythmical jerking or sustained spasm of the affected parts. They

26

may remain localised to one part, or may spread to involve the whole side. Some attacks begin in one part (e.g. mouth, thumb, great toe etc.) and spread gradually; this is 'Jacksonian epilepsy'. Attacks vary in duration from a few seconds to several hours. More prolonged episodes may leave paresis of the involved limb lasting for several hours after the seizure ceases (Todd's palsy).

Partial sensory seizures

Seizures arising in the sensory cortex cause unpleasant tingling or 'electric' sensations in the contralateral face and limbs. A spreading pattern like a Jacksonian seizure may occur, the abnormal sensation spreading much faster over the body (in seconds) than the 'march' of a migrainous focal sensory attack, which spreads over 10–15 minutes.

Versive seizures

A frontal epileptic focus may involve the frontal eye field, causing forced deviation of the eyes and sometimes turning of the head to the opposite side. This type of attack often becomes generalised to a tonic clonic seizure.

Partial visual seizures

Occipital epileptic foci cause simple visual hallucinations such as balls of light or patterns of colour. Formed visual hallucinations of faces or scenes arise more anteriorly in the temporal lobes.

Factors precipitating seizures

Sometimes specific trigger factors can be identified. Some are listed in Box 26.14.

EPILEPSY

Epilepsy means a tendency to have seizures and is a symptom of brain disease rather than a disease itself. A single seizure is not epilepsy but an indication for investigation. Medication should await evidence of a tendency to recurrent seizures. However, the recurrence rate after a first seizure approaches 70% during the first year, most recurrent attacks occurring within a month or two of the first. Further seizures are less likely if a trigger factor is definable and avoidable (Box 26.14). There is a group of disorders whose only or main symptom is epilepsy, whilst in other disorders, epilepsy is just one of the manifestations. The annual incidence of new cases of epilepsy after infancy is 20–70/100 000. The lifetime risk of having a single seizure is about 5%, whilst the prevalence of epilepsy in European countries is about 0.5%. Prevalence in developing countries

is up to five times higher than in developed countries; incidence is double.

Types of epilepsy

The classification of epilepsy is best achieved by considering the clinical events (the seizures), the abnormal electrophysiology, the anatomical site of seizure genesis and the pathological cause of the problem (Box 26.15).

Primary generalised epilepsy

The primary or idiopathic epilepsies make up some 10% of all epilepsies, including some 40% of those with tonic clonic seizures. Onset is almost always in childhood or adolescence. No structural abnormality is present and there is often a substantial genetic predisposition. Some, like childhood absence epilepsy, are relatively uncommon, whilst others, like juvenile myoclonic epilepsy, are common (5–10% of all patients with epilepsy). The more common varieties of primary generalised epilepsy are listed in Box 26.16, along with their clinical features and management.

Secondary generalised epilepsy

Generalised epilepsy may arise from spread of partial seizures due to structural disease, or may be secondary to drugs or metabolic disorders (Box 26.17). Epilepsy presenting in adult life is almost always secondary generalised, even if there is no clear history of a partial seizure before the onset of a major attack (an 'aura').

Partial epilepsy

Partial seizures may arise from any disease of the cerebral cortex, congenital or acquired, and frequently generalise. With the exception of a few idiopathic partial epilepsies of benign outcome in childhood, the presence of partial seizures signifies the presence of focal cerebral pathology. Common causes are listed in Box 26.18.

26.14 TRIGGER FACTORS FOR SEIZURES
• Sleep deprivation
• Alcohol (particularly withdrawal)
• Recreational drug misuse
• Physical and mental exhaustion
• Flickering lights, including TV and computer screens (primary generalised epilepsies only)
• Intercurrent infections and metabolic disturbances
• Uncommonly: loud noises, music, reading, hot baths

26.15 CLASSIFICATION OF EPILEPSY	
Seizure type	
• Simple partial	• Tonic
• Complex partial	• Atonic
• Absence	• Myoclonic
• Tonic clonic	
Physiology (EEG)	
• Focal spikes/sharp waves	• Generalised spike and wave
Anatomical site	
• Cortex 　Temporal 　Frontal 　Parietal 　Occipital	• Generalised (diencephalon) • Multifocal
Pathological cause	
• Genetic	• Infections
• Developmental	• Inflammation
• Tumours	• Metabolic
• Trauma	• Drugs, alcohol and toxins
• Vascular	• Degenerative

26

26.16 PRIMARY GENERALISED EPILEPSIES

	Incidence	Age of onset	Type of seizure	EEG features	Provoking factors	Treatment	Prognosis
Childhood absence epilepsy	6–8/100 000	4–8 yrs	Frequent brief absences	3/s spike and wave	Hyperventilation, fatigue	Ethosuximide Sodium valproate	40% develop tonic clonic seizures, 80% remit in adulthood
Juvenile absence epilepsy	1–2/100 000	10–15 yrs	Less frequent absences than childhood absence	Poly-spike and wave	Hyperventilation, sleep deprivation	Sodium valproate	80% develop tonic clonic seizures, 80% seizure-free in adulthood
Juvenile myoclonic epilepsy	25–50/100 000	15–20 yrs	GTCS, absences, morning myoclonus	Poly-spike and wave, photosensitivity	Sleep deprivation, alcohol withdrawal	Sodium valproate	90% remit with sodium valproate but relapse on AED withdrawal
GTCS on awakening	Common	10–25 yrs	GTCS, sometimes myoclonus	Spike and wave on waking and sleep onset	Sleep deprivation	Sodium valproate	65% controlled with AEDs but relapse off treatment

(GTCS = generalised tonic clonic seizure; AED = anti-epilepsy drug)

26.17 CAUSES OF SECONDARY GENERALISED EPILEPSY

Secondary generalisation from partial seizures
- See Box 26.18 for causes of partial seizures

Genetic
- Inborn errors of metabolism
- Storage diseases

Cerebral birth injury

Hydrocephalus

Cerebral anoxia

Drugs
- Antibiotics: penicillin, isoniazid, metronidazole
- Antimalarials: chloroquine, mefloquine
- Ciclosporin
- Cardiac anti-arrhythmics: lidocaine; disopyramide
- Psychotropic agents: phenothiazines, tricyclic antidepressants, lithium
- Amphetamines (withdrawal)

Alcohol (especially withdrawal)

Toxins
- Heavy metals (lead, tin)
- Organophosphates (sarin)

Metabolic disease
- Hypocalcaemia
- Hyponatraemia
- Hypomagnesaemia
- Hypoglycaemia
- Renal failure
- Liver failure

Infective
- Meningitis
- Post-infectious encephalopathy

Inflammatory
- Multiple sclerosis (uncommon)
- SLE

Diffuse degenerative diseases
- Alzheimer's disease (uncommonly)
- Creutzfeldt–Jakob disease (rarely)

26.18 CAUSES OF PARTIAL SEIZURES

Idiopathic
- Benign Rolandic epilepsy of childhood
- Benign occipital epilepsy of childhood

Focal structural lesions

Genetic
- Tuberous sclerosis
- Neurofibromatosis
- von Hippel–Lindau disease
- Cerebral migration abnormalities

Infantile hemiplegia

Dysembryonic
- Cortical dysgenesis
- Sturge–Weber syndrome

Mesial temporal sclerosis (associated with febrile convulsions)

Cerebrovascular disease
- Intracerebral haemorrhage
- Cerebral infarction
- Arteriovenous malformation
- Cavernous haemangioma

Tumours (primary and secondary)

Trauma (including neurosurgery)

Infective
- Cerebral abscess (pyogenic)
- Toxoplasmosis
- Cysticercosis
- Tuberculoma
- Subdural empyema
- Encephalitis
- Human immunodeficiency virus (HIV)

Inflammatory
- Sarcoidosis
- Vasculitis

Investigations

After a single seizure, cerebral imaging with CT or MRI is advisable, although the yield of structural lesions is low unless there are focal features to the seizure or there are focal signs. Similarly, toxic and metabolic causes (Box 26.17) should be considered. An EEG performed very soon after a seizure may be more helpful in showing focal

26.19 INVESTIGATION OF SUSPECTED EPILEPSY	
Epileptic nature of attacks?	
• Ambulatory EEG	• Videotelemetry
Type of epilepsy?	
• Standard EEG • Sleep EEG	• EEG with special electrodes (foramen ovale, subdural)
Structural lesion?	
• CT	• MRI
Metabolic disorder?	
• Urea and electrolytes • Liver function tests	• Blood glucose • Serum calcium, magnesium
Inflammatory or infective disorder?	
• Full blood count, erythrocyte sedimentation rate (ESR), C-reactive protein (CRP) • Chest X-ray • Serology for syphilis, HIV, collagen disease • CSF examination	

26.20 INDICATIONS FOR BRAIN IMAGING IN EPILEPSY
• Epilepsy starts after the age of 20 years • Seizures have focal features clinically • EEG shows a focal seizure source • Control of seizures is difficult or deteriorates

26.21 IMMEDIATE CARE OF SEIZURES
First aid (by relatives and witnesses)
• Move person away from danger (fire, water, machinery, furniture) • After convulsions cease, turn into 'recovery' position (semi-prone) • Ensure airway is clear • Do **NOT** insert anything in mouth (tongue-biting occurs at seizure onset and cannot be prevented by observers) • If convulsions continue for more than 5 minutes or recur without person regaining consciousness, summon urgent medical attention • Person may be drowsy and confused for some 30–60 minutes and should not be left alone until fully recovered
Immediate medical attention
• Ensure airway is patent • Give oxygen to offset cerebral hypoxia • Give intravenous anticonvulsant (e.g. diazepam 10 mg) **ONLY IF** convulsions are continuous or repeated (if so, manage as for status epilepticus) • Consider taking blood for anticonvulsant levels (if known epileptic) • Investigate cause

features than if performed after an interval. An EEG is certainly useful when more than one seizure has occurred, in order to establish the type of epilepsy and guide therapy. The increasing sophistication of imaging techniques now allows the identification of the cause of epilepsy in an increasing number of patients, especially those with partial seizures. These patients warrant intensive investigation, especially if seizures arise for the first time in adult life. Investigations should be pursued more vigorously if the epilepsy is intractable to treatment. The investigations that may be undertaken in a patient with suspected epilepsy are shown in Box 26.19.

Electroencephalography (EEG)

The EEG (p. 1153) may help to establish a diagnosis and characterise the type of epilepsy (i.e. primary generalised or partial with or without secondary generalisation). Inter-ictal records are abnormal in only about 50% of patients so the EEG is not a sensitive test for the presence or absence of epilepsy. However, 'epileptiform changes' (sharp waves or spikes) are fairly specific (falsely positive in 1/1000). The sensitivity can be increased to about 85% by prolonging recording time and including a period of natural or drug-induced sleep. Ambulatory EEG recording or video/EEG monitoring may provide helpful information when attacks are frequent.

Brain imaging

Imaging can never establish a diagnosis of epilepsy but is useful in defining or excluding a structural cause; indications are summarised in Box 26.20. Imaging is not required if a confident diagnosis of primary generalised epilepsy can be made with an EEG. CT is often sufficient to exclude a major structural cause of epilepsy. MRI of the brain may be indicated if CT shows no abnormality but a subtle structural change is still suspected, as in the case of patients with partial seizures (with or without secondary generalisation) which are resistant to therapy.

Management

It is important to explain the nature and cause of seizures to patients and their relatives, and to instruct relatives in the first aid management of major seizures (Box 26.21). Many people with epilepsy feel stigmatised by society and may become unnecessarily isolated from work and social life. It should be emphasised that any brain can develop a seizure, that epilepsy is a common disorder which affects about 1% of the population, and that good control of seizures can be expected in more than 80% of patients.

Immediate care of seizures

Little can or need be done for a person whilst a major seizure is occurring except first aid and common-sense manoeuvres to limit damage or secondary complications (Box 26.21).

Restrictions

Patients should be made aware of the riskiness of any activity where loss of awareness would be dangerous, until good control of seizures has been established. This includes work or recreational activities involving exposure to heights, dangerous machinery, open fires or water. Only shallow baths or showers should be taken, and then with someone else in the house and with the bathroom door unlocked. Cycling should be discouraged until at least 6 months' freedom from seizures has been achieved. Activities requiring prolonged proximity to water (e.g. swimming, fishing or boating) should always be in the company of someone who is aware of the risk of a seizure and able to rescue the

26

26.22 UK DRIVING REGULATIONS

Private use

Single seizure
- Cease driving for 1 year free of recurrence, then Driver and Vehicle Licensing Authority (DVLA) will restore a full licence (i.e. until age of 70 years)

Epilepsy
- Licence restored when patient is free from all types of seizure for 1 year *or* seizures exclusively during sleep for a period of 3 years (licence will require renewal every 3 years thereafter until 10 seizure-free years)

Withdrawal of anticonvulsants
- Cease driving during withdrawal and for 6 months thereafter

Vocational drivers (heavy goods and public service vehicles)

- No licence permitted if any seizure occurs after the age of 5 years until off medication and seizure-free for more than 10 years, and no potentially epileptogenic brain lesion

26.23 ANTI-EPILEPTIC DRUGS (AEDs) AFTER A SINGLE SEIZURE

EBM

'After a single seizure there is a 40% risk of subsequent seizures. The use of AEDs after a single seizure reduces the frequency of second seizures by half over 2 years but does not alter the long-term prognosis.'

- Berg AT, Shinnar S. Neurology 1991; 41:965–972.
- Musicco M, et al. for the FIRST group. Neurology 1997; 49:991–998.

For further information: 💻 www.clinicalevidence.org

26.24 GUIDELINES FOR ANTICONVULSANT THERAPY

- Start with one first-line drug (Box 26.26)
- Start with low dose; gradually increase to effective control of seizures or until side-effects (drug levels occasionally helpful)
- Check compliance (use minimum division of doses)
- If first drug fails (seizures continue or side-effects), start second-line drug whilst gradually withdrawing first
- Try three agents singly before using combinations (beware interactions)
- Do not use more than two drugs in combination at any one time
- If above fails, consider occult structural or metabolic lesion and whether seizures are truly epileptic

26.25 RELATIVE EFFICACY OF THE MAIN AEDs IN GENERALISED TONIC CLONIC SEIZURES

EBM

'The main AEDs as monotherapy for generalised tonic clonic seizures have similar efficacy but different side-effects.'

- Heller AJ, et al. J Neurol Neurosurg Psychiatry 1995; 8:44–50.
- Richens A, et al. J Neurol Neurosurg Psychiatry 1994; 57:682–687.

For further information: 💻 www.clinicalevidence.org

patient if necessary. In the UK and many other countries, legal restrictions regarding vehicle driving apply to patients with epilepsy, defined as more than one seizure over the age of 5 years (Box 26.22). The patient should inform the licensing authorities about the onset of seizures. It is also wise for patients to notify their motor insurance company. Certain occupations, such as airline pilot, are not open to anyone who has ever had an epileptic seizure; further information is often available from epilepsy support organisations.

Anticonvulsant drug therapy

Drug treatment should certainly be considered after more than one seizure has occurred and the patient agrees that seizure control is worthwhile; the use of anti-epilepsy drugs (AEDs) is more controversial after a first seizure (Box 26.23). Quite a range of anti-epilepsy drugs is available (Box 26.30, pp. 1174–1175). The mode of action is either to increase inhibitory neurotransmission in the brain or to alter neuronal sodium channels in such a way as to prevent abnormally rapid transmission of impulses. Of patients whose epilepsy is controllable, only a single drug is necessary in 80%, providing the choice of agent is appropriate and the dosage correct. The combination of more than two drugs is seldom necessary. Dose regimens should be kept as simple as possible to promote compliance. Some useful guidelines are listed in Box 26.24.

Choice of drug. With the exception of absence attacks and juvenile myoclonic epilepsy, there is no hard evidence indicating that one drug is superior to another in the treatment of epilepsy (Box 26.25). The first line of treatment should be one of the established first-line drugs (Box 26.26), with the more recently introduced drugs as second choice. Phenytoin and carbamazepine are not ideal agents for a young woman wishing to use oral contraception, because the drugs induce liver enzymes. Carbamazepine, lamotrigine and sodium valproate are preferable to phenytoin as first-line drugs because of the side-effect profile of the latter and its complicated pharmacokinetics.

Anticonvulsant drug blood levels. With some AEDs, such as phenytoin and carbamazepine, occasional measurement of the blood level can be a guide to whether the patient is on

26.26 GUIDELINES FOR CHOICE OF AED

Epilepsy type	First-line	Second-line	Third-line
Partial and/or secondary GTCS	Carbamazepine	Lamotrigine Sodium valproate Topiramate Tiagabine Gabapentin	Clobazam Phenytoin Primidone Phenobarbital Oxcarbazepine Levetiracetam Vigabatrin Acetazolamide
Primary GTCS	Sodium valproate	Lamotrigine Topiramate Carbamazepine	Phenytoin Gabapentin Primidone Phenobarbital Tiagabine Acetazolamide
Absence	Ethosuximide	Sodium valproate	Lamotrigine Clonazepam Acetazolamide
Myoclonic	Sodium valproate	Clonazepam	Piracetam Lamotrigine Phenobarbital

N.B. Preferably one and no more than two drugs should be used at one time.

26

a useful dose and is complying with the medication, but blood levels need to be interpreted intelligently. With other AEDs, such as sodium valproate, there is no relationship between drug levels and anticonvulsant efficacy. Repeated measurement of plasma levels of AEDs is not generally useful since the dose used in any individual patient will be determined by the efficacy of seizure control and the development of side-effects, whatever the plasma level happens to be. Plasma level monitoring is especially useful in dealing with suspected toxicity (particularly if more than one drug is being taken), dealing with the pharmacokinetic effects of pregnancy, or in suspected non-compliance.

Prognosis

Overall, generalised seizures are more readily controlled than partial seizures. The presence of a structural lesion makes complete control of the epilepsy less likely. The overall prognosis for epilepsy is shown in Box 26.27. There is a forty-fold increased risk of sudden unexplained death in epilepsy (SUDEP) and patients may need to be made aware of this in order to help them rearrange their lifestyle and comply with treatment.

Withdrawal of anticonvulsant therapy

After complete control of seizures for 2–4 years, withdrawal of medication may be considered. Childhood-onset epilepsy, particularly classical absence seizures, carries the best prognosis for successful drug withdrawal. Other primary generalised epilepsies, such as juvenile myoclonic epilepsy, have a marked liability to recur after AED withdrawal. Seizures that begin in adult life, particularly those with partial features, are also likely to recur, especially if there is an identified structural lesion. Overall, the recurrence rate of seizures after drug withdrawal is about 40% (Box 26.28). Some adult patients tend to opt for continuation of therapy because they feel that the threat of further attacks (especially regarding driving) outweighs the complications of continuing with medication. The EEG is generally a poor predictor of seizure recurrence but if the record is still very abnormal, drug withdrawal is unwise. Withdrawal should be undertaken slowly, reducing the drug dose gradually over 6–12 months. In the UK, patients must stop driving whilst withdrawing from their anti-epileptic medication and not drive for 6 months after full withdrawal of the drugs.

Status epilepticus

Status epilepticus exists when a series of seizures occurs without the patient regaining awareness between attacks over a period of 30 minutes. Most commonly, this refers to recurrent tonic clonic seizures (major status) and is a life-threatening medical emergency. Partial motor status is obvious clinically, but complex partial status and absence status may be difficult to diagnose because the patient may

merely present in a dazed, confused state. Status is never the presenting feature of idiopathic epilepsy but may be precipitated by abrupt withdrawal of anticonvulsant drugs, the presence of a major structural lesion or acute metabolic disturbance, and tends to be more common with frontal epileptic foci. Management is summarised in Box 26.29. It should be remembered that psychogenic or non-epileptic attacks commonly masquerade as 'status epilepticus', so electrophysiological confirmation of the seizures should be obtained as early as possible.

Epilepsy, pregnancy and oral contraception

Hepatic enzyme induction caused by carbamazepine, phenytoin, topiramate and barbiturates accelerates

26

26

26.30 ANTICONVULSANT DRUGS

Drug	Seizure types	Dose range (mg/day)	Doses per day	Therapeutic range (µmol/l)	Dose-related side-effects	Idiosyncratic side-effects	Long-term side-effects	Interactions
Acetazolamide	Primary and secondary GTCS, absences, partial	250–1000	2–3	Not applicable	Paraesthesia, anorexia, headache, nausea, diarrhoea, visual changes	Rashes, agranulocytosis, thrombocytopenia, photosensitivity, liver damage	Renal calculi	Aspirin, quinidine, phenytoin, carbamazepine, digoxin, ulcer-healing drugs
Carbamazepine	Partial, secondary GTCS	200–2000	2–3	30–50	Drowsiness, ataxia, nystagmus, diplopia, hyponatraemia	Rashes, thrombocytopenia, other blood dyscrasias	None	Other AEDs, warfarin, OCP, corticosteroids, antimalarials, cimetidine
Clobazam	Partial (adjunctive)	20–30	1	Not applicable	Sedation, irritability		Anticonvulsant effect wears off after a few weeks	Other AEDs
Clonazepam	Partial (adjunctive), myoclonus	1–8	2–4	Not applicable	Sedation, irritability	Blood dyscrasias	Anticonvulsant effect wears off after a few weeks	Other AEDs
Ethosuximide	Childhood absence	500–1500	2	200–700	Dizziness, insomnia, ataxia	Rashes, blood dyscrasias		Other AEDs, antidepressants
Gabapentin	Partial	300–2400	3	Not applicable	Drowsiness, ataxia		Not yet known	Antacids
Lamotrigine	Partial, secondary GTCS	25–500	1–2	Not applicable	Drowsiness, ataxia, diplopia, confusion	Rashes, blood dyscrasias	Not yet known	Carbamazepine
Levetiracetam	Partial, secondary GTCS	1000–3000	2	Not applicable	Somnolence, tiredness, dizziness, headache	None recorded	Not yet known	Phenytoin
Lorazepam	Status epilepticus	4 mg (intravenous)		Not applicable	Sedation, hypotension, apnoea		None known	Other AEDs
Oxcarbazepine	Partial, secondary GTCS	600–2400	2	50–125	Drowsiness, ataxia, nystagmus, diplopia, hyponatraemia	Rash	None known	Fewer than carbamazepine, but equally problematic for OCP
Paraldehyde	Status epilepticus	5–10 ml diluted (intravenous or rectally)		Not applicable	Respiratory depression, lactic acidosis		None known	Other AEDs
Phenobarbital	Partial, secondary GTCS	60–180	1	50–150	Drowsiness, ataxia, nystagmus, diplopia	Rashes, depression (adults), excitement (children), megaloblastic anaemia, SLE	Folate deficiency, osteomalacia, neuropathy	Other AEDs, anticoagulants, calcium channel blockers, digoxin, corticosteroids, OCP, theophylline, levothyroxine sodium (thyroxine sodium), antidepressants, antimalarials

PRESENTING PROBLEMS IN NERVOUS SYSTEM DISEASE

26.30 ANTICONVULSANT DRUGS—cont'd

Drug	Seizure types	Dose range (mg/day)	Doses per day	Therapeutic range (μmol/l)	Dose-related side-effects	Idiosyncratic side-effects	Long-term side-effects	Interactions
Phenytoin	Partial, secondary GTCS	150–350	1	40–80	Drowsiness, ataxia, nystagmus, diplopia, tremor, dystonia, asterixis	Rashes, blood dyscrasias, liver damage, SLE	Gum hypertrophy, facial dysmorphism, hirsutism, folate deficiency, osteomalacia, neuropathy	Other AEDs, warfarin, amiodarone and other anti-arrhythmics, antimalarials, corticosteroids, OCP, cimetidine, oral hypoglycaemics, theophylline, thyroxine
Piracetam	Myoclonus	7200–20 000	2–3	Not applicable	Dizziness, insomnia, nausea, weight gain, drowsiness, tremor, agitation	Rash	None known	None known
Primidone	Partial, secondary GTCS	250–1000	1–2	50–150	Drowsiness, ataxia, nystagmus, diplopia	Rashes, depression (adults), excitement (children), megaloblastic anaemia, SLE	As for phenobarbital*	As for phenobarbital*
Sodium valproate	Primary and secondary GTCS, absences, myoclonus	400–2500	1–2	Not applicable	Drowsiness, nausea, ataxia, nystagmus, diplopia, tremor	Alopecia, rashes, blood dyscrasias, liver damage, pancreatitis	Weight gain	Other AEDs, antimalarials, cimetidine
Tiagabine	Partial, secondary GTCS	15–30	2–3	Not applicable	Drowsiness, nausea, ataxia, tremor	Headache, psychosis, depression	Reduced peripheral vision	Other AEDs
Topiramate	Partial, secondary GTCS	200–600	1–2	Not applicable	Drowsiness, nausea, ataxia, confusion	Nephrolithiasis, depression, taste alteration, diarrhoea, weight loss	Not yet known	Other AEDs, OCP
Vigabatrin	Partial, secondary GTCS, infantile spasms	2000–6000	1–2	Not applicable	Drowsiness, nausea, ataxia, confusion	Aggression, alopecia, skin rash, increase in seizures, retinal atrophy	Reduced peripheral vision	

(GTCS = generalised tonic clonic seizures; AEDs = anti-epileptic drugs; OCP = oral contraceptive pill; SLE = systemic Lupus erythematosus)
* Primidone is converted in the liver to phenobarbital.
N.B. Doses of all drugs should be adjusted for patient age and body mass.

26

metabolism of oestrogen, causing breakthrough bleeding and contraceptive failure. The safest policy is to use an alternative contraceptive method, but it is sometimes possible to overcome the problem by giving a higher oestrogen dose preparation. Sodium valproate has little interaction with oral contraception.

Epilepsy may worsen during pregnancy, particularly during the third trimester when plasma anticonvulsant levels tend to fall. Therefore, monitoring of blood levels (in those drugs in which levels are relevant) during pregnancy may be helpful. Almost all the major anticonvulsant drugs have been associated with an increased incidence of fetal congenital abnormalities (e.g. cleft lip, spina bifida and cardiac defects), but this has not yet been demonstrated for gabapentin. The risk of fetal abnormality, which is greatest if the exposure is in the first trimester, rises from the background risk of 1–3% to about 7% with one anti-epileptic drug and to about 15% with two or more drugs. Folic acid (5 mg daily) taken 2 months before conception may reduce the risk of some fetal abnormalities. Occasionally, in a well-controlled patient, anticonvulsants can be withdrawn before conception, but if major seizures have occurred in the preceding year this is unwise as the risk to the fetus from uncontrolled maternal major seizures is probably greater than the teratogenic effects. Partial seizures probably carry little risk to the fetus.

The incidence of haemorrhagic disease of the newborn due to vitamin K deficiency may be increased by maternal use of hepatic enzyme-inducing anticonvulsants. Therefore, maternal vitamin K supplements (20 mg orally per day) in the last month of pregnancy and intramuscular vitamin K (1 mg) at birth for the infant are widely advised.

Non-epileptic attack disorder ('psychogenic attacks', 'pseudo-seizures')

Patients may present with attacks that superficially resemble epileptic seizures but which are caused by psychological phenomena and not associated with abnormal epileptic discharges in the brain. Such patients may present in apparent status epilepticus. People with epilepsy may have non-epileptic attacks as well, and this diagnosis should be considered if a patient fails to respond to anti-epileptic therapy, especially in the absence of a structural abnormality. Non-epileptic attacks may be quite difficult to distinguish from truly epileptic attacks. Clues pointing towards non-epileptic attacks include elaborate arching of the back in an attack, pelvic thrusting and/or wild flailing of limbs. Cyanosis and severe biting of the tongue are rare in non-epileptic attacks, but urinary incontinence can occur. The distinction between epileptic attacks originating in the frontal lobes and non-epileptic attacks may be especially difficult, and may require videotelemetry with prolonged EEG recordings. Non-epileptic attacks are three times more common in women than in men and have been associated with a history of sexual abuse in childhood. They are not necessarily associated with formal psychiatric illness. Treatment is often difficult and usually requires psychotherapy and/or counselling rather than drug therapy (p. 238).

26.31 EPILEPSY IN OLD AGE
• **Incidence and prevalence:** late-onset epilepsy is very common and the annual incidence in those over 60 years is rising.
• **Fits and faints:** the features that usually differentiate these may be less definitive than in younger patients.
• **Complex partial status epilepticus:** should be considered as a cause of confusion in the frail older patient.
• **Cerebrovascular disease** accounts for 30–50% of cases in people over the age of 50 years. A seizure may occur with an overt stroke or with otherwise occult vascular disease (e.g. identified on CT). Secondary prevention with aspirin and appropriate cardiovascular risk factor reduction is required.
• **Anti-epileptic drug regimens:** as simple as possible, and care should be taken to avoid potential interactions with other drugs being prescribed.
• **Carbamazepine-induced hyponatraemia:** increases significantly with age; particularly important in patients on diuretics or who have heart failure.
• **Withdrawal of anticonvulsant therapy:** late-onset epilepsy is associated with an increased relapse rate, so this should not be attempted where it was commenced appropriately.

A DIAGNOSTIC APPROACH TO THE PATIENT WITH TRANSIENT AMNESIA

Loss of memory for a period of time may be due to a transient toxic confusional state, a psychological fugue state, the post-ictal period after seizure or the syndrome known as transient global amnesia. These are usually distinguished on the basis of the history. A period of amnesia often follows either a complex partial or generalised seizure, and this may cause diagnostic confusion if the seizure was not witnessed—for example, if it occurred in sleep.

TRANSIENT GLOBAL AMNESIA

This is a syndrome affecting predominantly middle-aged patients in which there is an abrupt, discrete and reversible loss of short-term memory function for a period of some hours. During this time patients know who they are and can perform motor acts normally, but act in a bemused way, repeatedly asking the same questions. During the attack there is retrograde amnesia for the events of the past few weeks. After 4–6 hours, memory functions and behaviour return to normal but the patient is left with a period of time for which he or she has complete amnesia. There are none of the phenomena associated with seizures and, unlike epileptic amnesia, transient global amnesia tends not to recur. There are no associated cerebrovascular risk factors, making a vascular aetiology unlikely. Transient global amnesia is thought to be due to a benign process similar to that causing a migraine aura, occurring in the hippocampus. The patient has no physical signs and further investigation may not be needed if epilepsy can be excluded.

SLEEP DISORDERS

Disturbances of sleep are common. Apart from insomnia, patients may complain of excessive daytime sleepiness, disturbed behaviour during night-time sleep, the parasomnias (sleep walking and talking, or night terrors) or disturbing subjective experiences during sleep and/or its onset (nightmares, hypnagogic hallucinations, sleep paralysis). A careful history will allow certain patterns of sleep disturbance to be identified.

Normal sleep is controlled by the reticular activating system in the upper brain stem and diencephalon. During overnight sleep, a series of repeated cycles of EEG patterns can be recorded. As drowsiness occurs, alpha rhythm disappears and the EEG gradually becomes dominated by deepening slow-wave activity. After 60–80 minutes this slow-wave pattern is replaced by a short spell of low-amplitude EEG background on which are superimposed rapid eye movements (REM). After a few minutes of REM sleep, another slow-wave spell starts and the cycle repeats several times throughout the night. The REM periods tend to become longer as the sleep period progresses. Dreaming takes place during REM sleep. This is accompanied by muscle relaxation, penile erection and loss of tendon reflexes. REM sleep seems to be the most important part of the sleep cycle for refreshing cognitive processes. Deprivation of REM sleep causes tiredness, irritability and impaired judgement.

PARASOMNIAS

Automatic behaviour that is not recalled may take place during light sleep. Sleep talking and sleep walking are innocuous and common in normal children. Sleep walking is uncommon in adults and has no pathological significance. Nightmares are frightening dreams from which the sufferer wakes in a state of fear or agitation. Most normal people have experienced such phenomena and they are not of any significance in terms of organic disease.

Night terrors occur as sudden arousals from deep slow-wave sleep. They are more common in children but may affect adults. The sufferer wakes in a state of agitation, screaming and fearful. Occasionally, violent behaviour occurs. The agitation may last many minutes. Such events may be confused with nocturnal seizures, particularly those arising from the frontal lobe, or their post-ictal effects.

DAYTIME SOMNOLENCE

Excessive sleepiness in the day is most commonly due to inadequate night-time sleep related to fatigue and poor sleep hygiene, including the excessive use of caffeine and/or alcohol in the evening. Night-time sleep may also be disturbed by sleep apnoea (p. 666), periodic limb movements and the restless leg syndrome. Somnolence due to disturbed night-time sleep particularly occurs after meals and during dull monotonous activities, such as long car journeys. Such causes of daytime sleepiness need to be distinguished from narcolepsy.

NARCOLEPSY

This disorder has a prevalence of about 1 in 4000 and is associated with HLA (human leucocyte antigen) DR-1501 and DQB1-0602 in 85% of cases. There is a familial

26.32 THE NARCOLEPSY TETRAD
Sleep attacks
● Brief, frequent and unlike normal somnolence
Cataplexy
● Sudden loss of muscle tone set off by surprise, laughter, strong emotion etc.
Hypnagogic hallucinations
● Frightening hallucinations experienced during sleep onset or waking (can occur in normal people)
Sleep paralysis
● Brief paralysis on waking (can occur in normal people)

tendency suggesting an autosomal dominant inheritance with low penetrance. Recurrent bouts of irresistible sleep are experienced, during which the EEG often shows direct entry into REM sleep. Sufferers tend to fall asleep when eating or talking, not just when under-stimulated. The periods of sleep are usually short and the person can be woken relatively easily. He or she usually feels refreshed after waking. In addition, patients with narcolepsy will report at least one other of the 'narcolepsy tetrad' (Box 26.32). These four symptoms may occur together or in combinations in the same patient; most often, sleep attacks and cataplexy occur together.

Narcoleptic attacks can be treated with CNS stimulants such as dexamfetamine (5–10 mg 8-hourly) or methylphenidate (10–60 mg per day) but fewer side-effects occur with modafinil (200–400 mg per day). Cataplexy responds to clomipramine (25–50 mg 8-hourly) or fluoxetine (20 mg per day).

OTHER DISORDERS OF SLEEP

Restless leg syndrome

This is a common syndrome, also known as Ekbom's syndrome, affecting up to 2% of the population. Unpleasant sensations in the legs that are ameliorated by moving the legs occur when the patient is tired in the evenings and at the onset of sleep. This condition has a strong familial tendency and can present with daytime somnolence due to disturbed night-time sleep. It needs to be distinguished from the daytime sense of restlessness of the limbs known as akathisia that is a side-effect of major tranquillisers, and the related condition of periodic limb movements during sleep. Restless legs can be symptomatic of an underlying peripheral neuropathy or iron deficiency, or general medical conditions (e.g. uraemia).

Treatment is with clonazepam (0.5–2.0 mg), small doses of levodopa (100–200 mg) or dopamine agonists (p. 1221) at night.

Periodic limb movements

In this syndrome, sleep is disturbed by repetitive jerky flexion movements of the limbs which occur in the early stages of sleep. The history of abnormal limb movements

26

during sleep may need to be obtained from the patient's bed partner, since the patient may not be aware of the arousals that are occurring as a result of the movements, even though they may be sufficient to cause daytime somnolence. Treatment may be effected with small doses of levodopa (100–200 mg at night) or a dopamine agonist (p. 1219).

DISORDERS OF MOVEMENT

Lesions in various parts of the motor system produce distinctive patterns of motor deficit. These can take the form of negative symptoms of weakness, lack of coordination, lack of stability and stiffness, or positive symptoms such as tremor, dystonia, chorea, athetosis, hemiballismus, tics and myoclonus. When the lower limbs are affected, characteristic patterns of gait disorder may result.

THE MOTOR SYSTEM

A programme of movement formulated by the pre-motor cortex is converted into a series of muscle movements in the motor cortex and then transmitted to the spinal cord in the pyramidal tract (Fig. 26.15). This passes through the

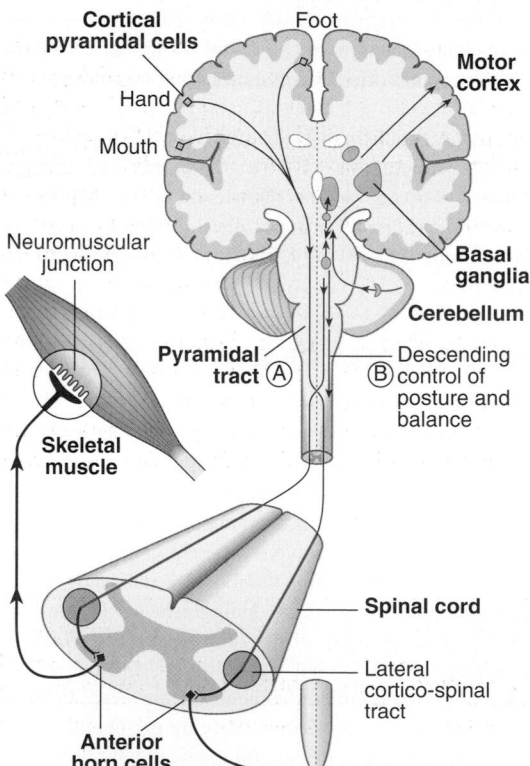

Fig. 26.15 The motor system. Neurons from the motor cortex descend as the pyramidal tract in the internal capsule and cerebral peduncle to the ventral brain stem, where most cross low in the medulla (A). In the spinal cord the upper motor neurons form the cortico-spinal tract in the lateral column before synapsing with the lower motor neurons in the anterior horns. The activity in the motor cortex is modulated by influences from the basal ganglia and cerebellum. Pathways descending from these structures control posture and balance (B).

internal capsule and the ventral brain stem before decussating in the medulla to enter the lateral columns of the spinal cord. The pyramidal tract 'upper motor neurons' end by synapsing with the anterior horn cells of the spinal cord grey matter, which form the 'lower motor neurons'.

Movement of a body part necessitates changes in posture and alteration in the tone of many muscles, some quite distant from the part being moved. The motor system consists of a hierarchy of control mechanisms that maintain body posture and baseline muscle tone upon which a specific movement is superimposed. The lowest order of this hierarchy comprises the mechanisms in the grey matter of the spinal cord which control the muscle tone response to stretch, and the reflex withdrawal response to noxious stimuli. The afferent side of the stretch reflex consists of the muscle spindles that detect lengthening of the muscle and initiate a monosynaptic reflex leading to muscle contraction. The predominantly inhibitory descending input from the brain stem and cerebral hemispheres modulates the sensitivity of the stretch reflex. It is the state of this stretch reflex that is tested clinically when a patient's tendon reflexes are elicited.

Polysynaptic connections in the spinal cord grey matter control more complex reflex actions of flexion and extension of the limbs that form the basic building blocks of coordinated actions, but these require control from above to function usefully. Above the spinal cord, circuits between the basal ganglia and the motor cortex constitute the extrapyramidal system which controls background muscle tone and body posture, and gates the initiation of movement (Fig. 26.15).

Accurately targeted and coordinated movements require the functioning of the cerebellum, which fine-tunes goal-directed movements initiated by the motor cortex. In addition, the cerebellum, through its reciprocal connections with the thalamus and cortex, participates in the planning and learning of skilled movements.

Lower motor neuron lesions

A group of muscle fibres innervated by a single anterior horn cell (lower motor neuron) form a 'motor unit'. Loss of function of lower motor neurons will cause the loss of contraction in their units' muscle fibres and the muscle will be weak and flaccid. Denervated muscle fibres atrophy in time, causing wasting of the muscle, and depolarise spontaneously, causing fibrillations which, except in the tongue, are only perceptible on an EMG. Re-innervation from neighbouring intact motor neurons occur with time but the neuromuscular junctions of the enlarged motor units are unstable and depolarise spontaneously, causing fasciculations (which are visible to the naked eye because the motor units are larger than normal). Thus fasciculations imply chronic partial denervation with re-innervation.

Upper motor neuron (pyramidal) lesions

When the spinal cord is disconnected from the modulating influence of the higher motor hierarchies, the anterior horn motor neurons are under the uninhibited influence of the spinal reflex mechanisms. Their motor units have an exaggerated response to stretch. The limbs show reflex patterns of movement, like flexion withdrawal to noxious stimuli and spasms of extension. An upper motor neuron lesion therefore manifests clinically with brisk tendon stretch reflexes, 'spastic' increase in tone greater in the extensors of the lower limbs and the flexors of the upper limbs, and extensor plantar responses. Spastic increase in tone can be seen on clinical examination to vary with both the degree and speed of stretch. The increased tone is more obvious with rapid stretch, the 'clasp-knife' phenomenon. Spasticity takes time to develop and may not be present for weeks after the onset of an upper motor neuron lesion. Spasticity will be exacerbated by increased sensory input into the reflex arc, as may be caused by a pressure sore or urinary tract infection in a patient with a spinal cord lesion. The weakness found in upper motor neuron lesions is more pronounced in the extensors of the upper limbs and the flexors of the lower limbs.

Extrapyramidal lesions

Lesions of the extrapyramidal system produce an increase in tone, which is not an exaggerated response to stretch but is continuous throughout the range of movement at any speed of stretch ('lead pipe' rigidity). Involuntary movements are also a feature of extrapyramidal lesions (see below), and a tremor combined with rigidity produces typical 'cogwheel' rigidity. Rapid movements are slowed and clumsy (bradykinesia). Extrapyramidal lesions also cause postural instability, precipitating falls.

Cerebellar lesions

A lesion in a cerebellar hemisphere causes lack of coordination on the same side of the body. The initial part of movement is normal but as the target is approached, the accuracy of the movement deteriorates, producing an 'intention tremor'. The distances of targets are misjudged (dysmetria), resulting in 'past-pointing'. The ability to produce rapid, accurate, regularly alternating movements is impaired (dysdiadochokinesis).

The central vermis of the cerebellum is concerned with the coordination of gait and posture. Disorders of this part therefore produce a characteristic ataxic gait (see below).

'MEDICALLY UNEXPLAINED' ('PSYCHOGENIC'/'NON-ORGANIC'/ 'FUNCTIONAL') WEAKNESS

Patients may present with limb weakness which is not due to organic (structural, physiological or biochemical) disease but which is caused by psychological phenomena: for example, a conversion disorder (p. 236). This weakness does not conform to known pathophysiological patterns (reflexes are normal) and the deficit cannot be attributed to a lesion in a specific anatomical site in the nervous system. During formal testing of power, a patient's strength may appear to 'give way', yet demonstrate bursts of full power at other times. Alternatively, if a 'weak' limb is held up and then suddenly allowed to drop, the limb may be momentarily held up, something which does not happen in organic weakness. Apparently 'non-organic' weakness may occur as elaboration upon a 'genuine' organic weakness, and physical signs such as 'give-way weakness' therefore do not necessarily imply absence of pathology. Great care should be exercised in making the diagnosis of a functional disorder, and all unusual manifestations of nervous system disease should be considered before such a diagnosis is made.

A DIAGNOSTIC APPROACH TO THE PATIENT WITH LIMB WEAKNESS

Establishing the diagnosis in a patient with weakness requires the application of basic anatomy, physiology and some pathology to the interpretation of the history and clinical findings (Box 26.33 and Fig. 26.16). Points to consider are shown in Box 26.34.

Weakness in only some muscles in a limb suggests a problem in the peripheral nerve(s) or motor root(s). Weakness of the whole of one limb may be due to problems in the brachial or lumbosacral plexuses, or to a central lesion. Weakness in both lower limbs (paraparesis) or all four limbs (tetraparesis) suggests either a spinal cord lesion or a diffuse peripheral nerve problem such as Guillain–Barré syndrome (p. 1249). In such cases the condition of the reflexes is the most discriminating sign. The reflexes are absent in the Guillain–Barré syndrome (or other lower

26

26.33 PHYSICAL SIGNS IN DIFFERENT TYPES OF MOTOR DEFICIT					
Clinical sign	Upper motor (pyramidal) lesion	Lower motor lesion	Extrapyramidal lesion	Cerebellar lesion	Functional
Power	Weak Upper limbs: extensors weaker Lower limbs: flexors weaker	Weak	No weakness	No weakness	Give-way weakness
Wasting	None	Yes, after interval	None	None	None
Fasciculation	None	Yes, after interval	None	None	None
Tone	Spastic increase (after interval)	Flaccid from onset	Rigidity (cogwheel)	Normal/reduced	Normal
Reflexes	Increased	Reduced/absent	Normal	Normal	Normal
Plantar response	Extensor	Flexor	Flexor	Flexor	Normal
Coordination	Reduced by weakness	Reduced by weakness	Normal (but slowed)	Impaired	Normal (may be laborious)

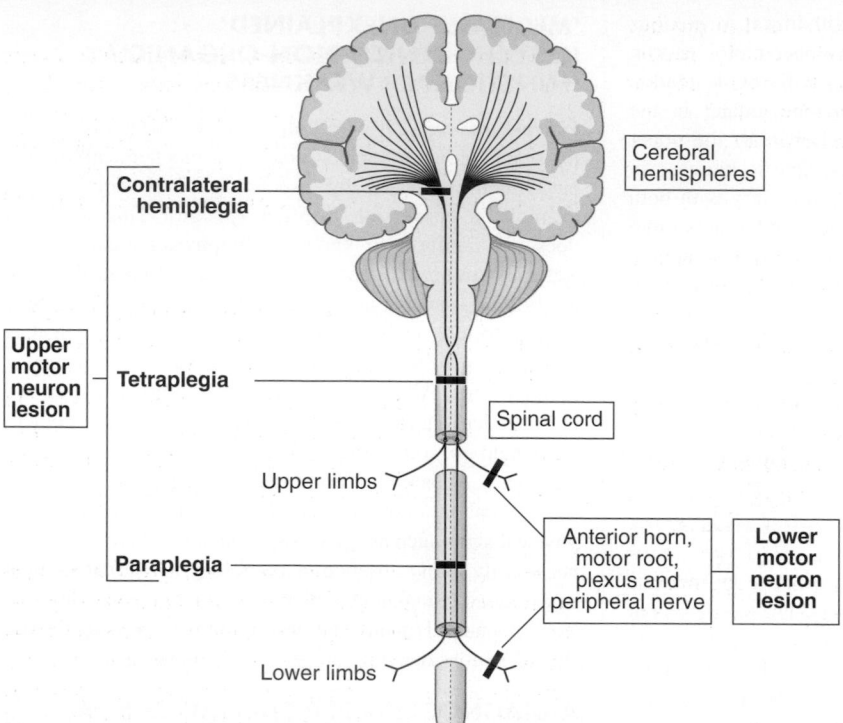

Fig. 26.16 Patterns of motor loss according to the anatomical site of the lesion.

26.34 ASSESSMENT OF WEAKNESS
Distribution
• A few muscles • A limb • Both lower limbs (paraparesis) • Both limbs on one side (hemiparesis)
Type of weakness
• Upper motor neuron lesion • Lower motor neuron lesion
Evolution of the weakness
• Sudden and improving • Gradually worsening over days or weeks • Evolving over months or years

26.35 LIMB WEAKNESS—ASSESSING THE CAUSE
Vascular (stroke) lesions
• Sudden onset (over minutes) followed by a stable period and gradual recovery
Neoplastic lesions
• Deficit is gradual in onset and progressive over weeks or months • There may be signs caused by the mass effect of the lesion
Inflammatory lesions
• May be fairly acute in onset (over a few days), persist for a time and then improve (e.g. in multiple sclerosis)
Degenerative disorders
• May evolve over months or years (e.g. motor neuron disease or cervical spondylotic myelopathy)

motor nerve lesions) and brisk in spinal cord (upper motor neuron) lesions. The paraparesis or tetraparesis of spinal cord lesions may be associated with a specific pattern of sensory loss (p. 1183) which gives a clue to the site of the cord lesion.

Patients with a bradykinetic limb often complain of weakness. Therefore if there are no reflex, wasting or sensory changes when a patient is complaining of weakness in a limb, extrapyramidal signs of rigidity (cogwheel or leadpipe) and bradykinesia should be sought. Patients with Parkinson's disease usually present with symptoms in one limb that may be described as weak and clumsy, especially for fine manipulations. Often the typical rest tremor is a clue to the diagnosis.

Weakness down one side of the body (hemiparesis) is almost always due to a cerebral hemisphere lesion, although it can be caused by spinal cord or brain-stem lesions. The lesion is of upper motor neuron type, and the site and often the size of the lesion can be deduced by the concurrence of other signs and symptoms, such as higher cerebral function abnormalities or sensory change.

The evolution of a motor deficit over time suggests the likely underlying pathology (Box 26.35).

GAIT DISORDERS

Seeing a patient walk can be very revealing for neurological diagnosis and is an important element of assessing disability. Patterns of weakness, loss of coordination and proprioceptive sensory loss produce a range of abnormal

26

gaits. Neurogenic gait disorders need to be distinguished from those due to skeletal abnormalities, usually characterised by pain producing an antalgic gait, or limp. Gaits that do not fit either pattern may be due to 'functional' or non-organic disorders and are usually incompatible with any anatomical or physiological deficit.

Pyramidal gait

Upper motor neuron (pyramidal) lesions cause a gait in which the upper limb is held in flexion and the lower limb kept relatively extended. The pyramidal tract lesion slows the normally rapid ankle dorsiflexion necessary to keep the toes from striking the ground as the leg swings through. In an attempt to overcome this, the leg is swung out at the hip (circumduction), but the affected foot still scuffs along the ground at the toes. The shoe on the affected side may be worn at the toes as evidence of this type of gait. In a hemiplegia, the asymmetry between the affected and normal sides is obvious in walking. In a paraparesis, both lower limbs move slowly, swung from the hips and dragged stiffly on the ground in extension, an effect that can often be heard as well as seen.

Foot drop

In normal walking, toe strike follows heel strike during the gait cycle. Weakness of ankle dorsiflexion disrupts this pattern. The result is a less controlled descent of the foot making a slapping noise. If the distal weakness is more severe, the foot will have to be lifted higher at the knee to allow room for the inadequately dorsiflexed foot to swing through, producing a high stepping gait.

Waddling gait of proximal muscle weakness

During walking, alternate placement of the body's weight through each leg requires careful control of the hips by the gluteal muscles. In proximal muscle weakness, usually caused by muscle disease, the hips are not properly fixed by these muscles and trunk movements are exaggerated, producing a rolling or waddling gait.

Cerebellar ataxia

Patients with lesions of the central parts of the cerebellum (the vermis) walk with a characteristic broad-based gait, 'like a drunken sailor' (cerebellar function is particularly sensitive to alcohol). Patients with acute vestibular disturbances walk in a similar broad-based fashion, though the accompanying vertigo distinguishes them from those with cerebellar lesions. Less severe degrees of cerebellar ataxia can be detected by asking the patient to walk heel to toe; patients with vermis lesions are unable to do this.

Gait apraxia

In an apraxic gait, there is normal power in the legs and no abnormal cerebellar signs or proprioception loss, yet the patient cannot formulate the motor act of walking. This is a higher cerebral dysfunction in which the feet appear stuck to the floor and the patient cannot walk, even though movement is normal on the examination couch. Gait apraxia occurs in bilateral hemisphere disease such as normal pressure hydrocephalus and diffuse frontal lobe disease.

Marche à petits pas

Patients with multiple small-vessel cerebrovascular disease walk with small slow steps with instability. This looks different from the festinant gait of Parkinson's disease (see below) in that it does not have the variable pace and freezing. There are usually signs of bilateral upper motor neuron disease (bilateral extensor plantar responses and brisk jaw jerk).

Sensory ataxia

Loss of joint position sense makes walking unreliable, especially in poor light. The feet tend to be placed on the ground with greater emphasis, presumably in an attempt to increase what proprioceptive input is available. This results in a 'stamping' gait which is often combined with foot drop when caused by a peripheral neuropathy, but it can occur in disorders of the dorsal columns in the spinal cord.

Extrapyramidal gait

Patients with Parkinson's disease (p. 1218) and other extrapyramidal diseases have difficulty initiating walking and difficulty controlling the pace of their gait. The patient may get stuck whilst trying to start walking or when walking through doorways ('freezing') but, once started, may shuffle and then have problems with controlling the speed of walking and with stopping. This produces the festinant gait: initial stuttering steps that quickly increase in frequency while decreasing in length.

INVOLUNTARY MOVEMENTS

Abnormal movements usually imply a disorder in the basal ganglia, in which there is disinhibition of the activity of intrinsic rhythm generators or a disorder of postural control. Some, like tremor, are commonplace. Others, like chorea, athetosis and dystonia, have become more common as a result of adverse effects from drugs used in the treatment of Parkinson's disease and psychiatric disease.

Tremor

A tremor is a rhythmic oscillating movement of a limb or part of a limb, or of the head. Tremors are usefully divided into those occurring at rest and those seen only when a limb is in action. The other characteristic by which tremors can be classified is their frequency.

Rest tremor

This is pathognomonic of Parkinson's disease (p. 1218). The tremor is characteristically 'pill-rolling' and usually presents asymmetrically. However, patients with Parkinson's disease may have an abnormal action tremor as well. Tremor of the head in the upright position ('titubation') is not a rest tremor since this is a postural tremor, disappearing when the head is supported.

Action tremor

This is more frequently seen than rest tremor and potential causes are more numerous (Box 26.36). A physiological tremor (frequency between 8 and 12 Hz) can be identified in the limbs of normal subjects; exaggeration of this physiological tremor occurs in anxiety and other situations, listed in Box 26.37.

26

26.36 CAUSES OF TREMOR ON ACTION

- Exaggerated physiological tremor (Box 26.37)
- Essential tremor (may be familial)
- Parkinson's disease (rest tremor more usual)
- Wilson's disease
- Postural ('Holmes', 'rubral') tremor
  Multiple sclerosis
  Other lesions in cerebellar outflow/red nucleus
- Intention tremor
  Cerebellar hemisphere disease

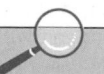

26.37 CAUSES OF EXAGGERATED PHYSIOLOGICAL TREMOR

Anxiety

Fatigue

Endocrine
- Thyrotoxicosis
- Cushing's disease
- Phaeochromocytoma
- Hypoglycaemia

Drugs
- β-agonists (e.g. salbutamol)
- Theophylline
- Caffeine
- Lithium
- Dopamine agonists
- Sodium valproate
- Tricyclics
- Phenothiazines
- Amphetamines

Toxins
- Mercury
- Lead
- Arsenic

Alcohol withdrawal

26

26.38 CAUSES OF ASTERIXIS

- Renal failure
- Liver failure
- Hypercapnia
- Drug toxicity (e.g. phenytoin)
- Acute focal parietal or thalamic lesions

26.39 CAUSES OF CHOREA

Hereditary
- Huntington's disease
- Wilson's disease
- Neuroacanthocytosis
- Porphyria
- Paroxysmal choreoathetosis

Cerebral birth injury (including kernicterus)

Cerebral trauma

Drugs
- Levodopa
- Dopamine agonists
- Phenothiazines
- Tricyclics
- Oral contraceptive

Endocrine
- Pregnancy
- Oral contraceptive
- Thyrotoxicosis
- Hypoparathyroidism
- Hypoglycaemia

Infective/inflammatory
- Post-streptococcal (Sydenham's chorea)
- Henoch–Schönlein purpura
- Creutzfeldt–Jakob disease
- Antiphospholipid antibody syndrome
- SLE

Vascular
- Lacunar infarction
- Arteriovenous malformation

Essential tremor is distinct from a physiological tremor, although resembling it superficially. It is slower than a physiological action tremor and may become quite disabling. The condition is often familial, and in some families the tremor is most obvious during certain specific actions such as writing; here there is an overlap with focal dystonias (see below). Characteristic of essential tremor is that alcohol suppresses it, sometimes to the extent that the patient becomes addicted. Centrally acting β-adrenoceptor antagonists (β-blockers) such as propranolol are often effective in treatment.

An 'intention tremor' is the characteristic oscillation at the end of a movement which occurs in cerebellar disease, due to the breakdown of feedback control of targeted movements. Asterixis, the 'flapping' tremor seen in metabolic disturbances (Box 26.38), is the result of intermittent failure of the parietal mechanisms required to maintain a posture. Thus, when a patient is asked to hold out the arms with the hands extended at the wrists, this posture is periodically dropped, allowing the hands to drop transiently before the posture is taken up again. Occasionally, unilateral asterixis can be seen in an acute parietal lesion, usually vascular.

A more dramatic action tremor occurs with lesions in the superior cerebellar peduncle (the site of the cerebellar outflow towards the red nucleus). Known variously as a 'peduncular', 'rubral' or 'Holmes' tremor, this is a violent, large-amplitude postural tremor that worsens as a target is approached. It is common in advanced multiple sclerosis and may be a source of considerable disability. Stereotactic

thalamotomy can reduce the tremor, although the overall functional result is often disappointing.

Chorea, athetosis, ballism and dystonia

Non-rhythmic involuntary movements may be combinations of fragments of purposeful movements and abnormal postures. All of these abnormal movements represent disorders of the balance of activity in the complex basal ganglia circuitry. Jerky, small-amplitude, purposeless involuntary movements are termed 'chorea' (the Greek for 'dance'). In the limbs they resemble fidgety movements, and in the face, grimaces; they suggest disease in the caudate nucleus (as in Huntington's disease, pp. 52–54) or excessive activity in the striatum due to dopaminergic drugs used to treat Parkinson's disease. There is a range of other causes (Box 26.39). More dramatic ballistic movements of the limbs usually occur unilaterally (hemiballismus) in vascular lesions of the subthalamic structures. Slower writhing movements of the limbs are called athetosis. These are often combined with chorea (and have a similar list of causes) and are then termed 'choreo-athetoid' movements.

The term 'dystonia' is used to describe the movement disorder in which a limb (or the head) involuntarily takes up an abnormal posture. This may be generalised in various diseases of the basal ganglia or may be focal or segmental, as in spasmodic torticollis when the head involuntarily turns to one side. Other segmental dystonias may cause abnormal disabling postures of a limb to be taken up during certain specific actions, such as in writer's cramp or numerous other occupational 'cramps'. These segmental dystonias can be treated by the administration of botulinum toxin to a few of the responsible muscles, which seems to overcome the abnormal distribution of muscle activity for a period of time.

Myoclonus

Myoclonus refers to brief, isolated, random, non-purposeful jerks of muscle groups in the limbs. Myoclonic jerks occur normally at the onset of sleep (hypnic jerks). Similarly, a myoclonic jerk is a component of the normal startle response which may be exaggerated in some rare (mostly genetic) disorders. Unlike the movement disorders discussed so far, myoclonus may occur in disorders of the cerebral cortex, when groups of pyramidal cells fire spontaneously. Such myoclonus occurs in some forms of epilepsy in which the jerks are fragments of seizure activity. Alternatively, myoclonus can arise from subcortical structures or, more rarely, from diseased segments of the spinal cord. Myoclonus, especially of cortical origin, often responds to clonazepam, sodium valproate or piracetam.

Tics

Tics are repetitive semi-purposeful movements such as blinking, winking, grimacing or screwing up of the eyes. They are distinguished from other involuntary movements by the ability of the patient to suppress their occurrence, at least for a short time. An isolated tic may be no more than a mild embarrassment, but may become frequent at certain times in childhood and then disappear. The uncommon syndrome of Gilles de la Tourette consists of a tendency to multiple tics and odd vocalisations, with obsessive behavioural abnormalities. The pathogenic basis is not understood, but there may be some response to major tranquillisers.

SENSORY DISTURBANCE

Sensory symptoms are very common but do not always denote nervous system disorder. For example, tingling in the fingers of both hands and around the mouth commonly suggests hyperventilation (p. 660) or, very rarely, hypocalcaemia (p. 774). The accuracy of patients in describing sensory disturbances is very variable and skill is needed in sifting through the history to make anatomical and pathophysiological sense of the complaints. Damage to the afferent nervous pathways conveying sensations of touch and pain produces either the negative sensation of numbness or positive symptoms, such as paraesthesia and pain. When there is dysfunction of the cerebral mechanisms of somatic sensation there may be distortion of the patient's perception of the wholeness or actual presence of the relevant part of the body.

A DIAGNOSTIC APPROACH TO THE PATIENT WITH SENSORY SYMPTOMS

In the history, the most useful features are the anatomical distribution and mode of onset of numbness, paraesthesia or pain. Certain patterns of onset of sensory symptoms can be recognised. For example, in a migraine attack the aura may consist of a front of tingling paraesthesia followed by numbness which takes 20–30 minutes to spread over one half of the body, splitting the tongue. Sensory loss due to a vascular lesion, on the other hand, will occur over the whole territory of the lesion more or less instantaneously, and at onset is not associated with positive sensory phenomena like tingling. The rare, unpleasant paraesthesia of sensory epilepsy 'shoots' down one side of the body in seconds. The numbness and paraesthesia of spinal cord lesions often ascend one or both lower limbs to a level on the trunk over hours or days. Sensory symptoms of tingling and numbness can be of 'functional' or non-organic origin, as a manifestation of anxiety or as part of a conversion disorder (p. 236). In these circumstances the pattern of sensory symptoms does not conform to known anatomical distribution or fit with any known pattern of sensory involvement in organic disease. As with weakness (see above), care should be taken to avoid misdiagnosing an unusual organic sensory impairment as a functional disorder.

Examination of the sensory system needs to be approached with care since it is easy to produce confusing false positive results because of the inescapably subjective nature of sensory testing. However, the distribution of sensory loss and associated deficits in motor and/or cranial nerve function may enable a diagnostically helpful pattern of sensory loss to be identified.

PATTERNS OF SENSORY DISTURBANCE
(Fig. 26.17)

Peripheral nerve lesions

In peripheral nerve lesions, the symptoms are usually of sensory loss and simple paraesthesia (pins and needles). Single peripheral nerve lesions will, as expected, cause disturbance in the sensory distribution of that nerve. In diffuse neuropathies the longest neurons are affected first, giving the characteristic 'glove and stocking' distribution. If the smaller nerve fibres are preferentially affected (e.g. in alcoholic neuropathy), temperature and pin-prick (pain) are lost, whilst modalities served by the larger well myelinated sensory nerves may be spared. On the other hand, the latter are particularly affected if the neuropathy is demyelinating in character (p. 1250), producing symptoms of tightness and swelling with impairment of proprioception and vibration sensation.

Nerve root lesions

Pain is more often a feature of lesions of nerve roots, within the spine or of the limb plexuses. It is often felt in the muscles innervated by a root, i.e. the myotome rather than the dermatome. The site of nerve root lesions may be deduced from the dermatomal pattern of sensory loss, although this is often smaller than would be expected because of the overlap of sensory 'territories'.

Spinal cord lesions

Somatic sensory information from the limbs ascends the nervous system in two anatomically discrete systems, differential involvement of which is often of diagnostic

26

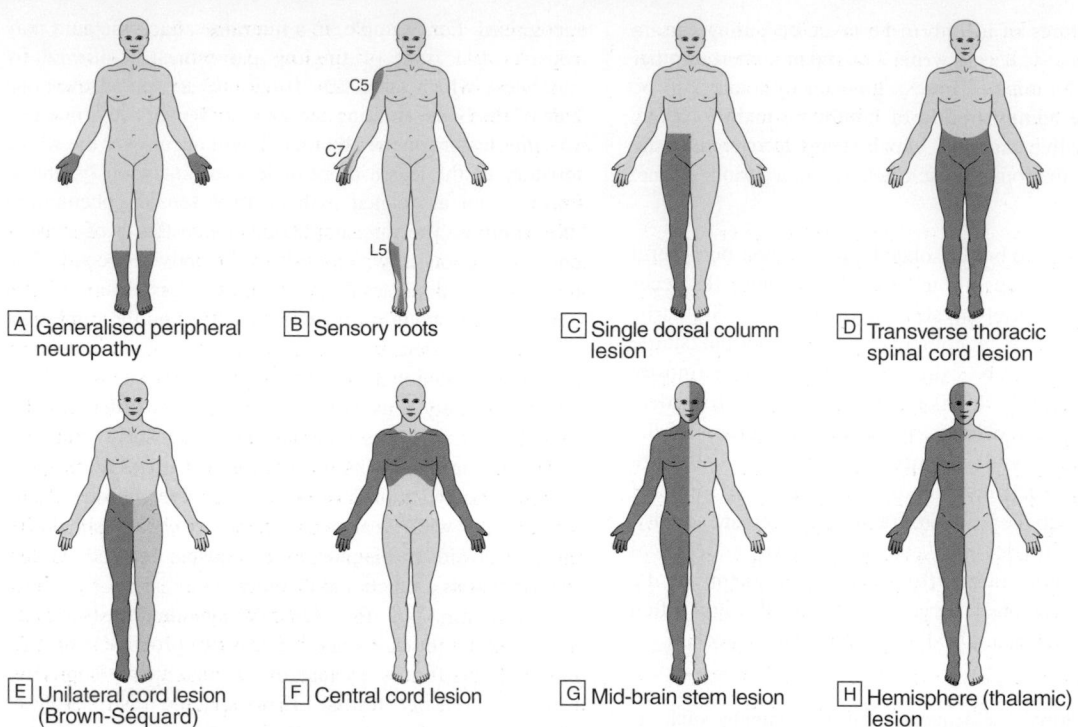

A Generalised peripheral neuropathy	B Sensory roots	C Single dorsal column lesion	D Transverse thoracic spinal cord lesion
E Unilateral cord lesion (Brown–Séquard)	F Central cord lesion	G Mid-brain stem lesion	H Hemisphere (thalamic) lesion

Fig. 26.17 Patterns of sensory loss. A Generalised peripheral neuropathy. B Sensory roots. C Single dorsal column lesion (proprioception and some touch loss). D Transverse thoracic spinal cord lesion. E Unilateral cord lesion (Brown–Séquard): ipsilateral dorsal column (and motor) deficit and contralateral spinothalamic deficit. F Central cord lesion: 'cape' distribution of spinothalamic loss. G Mid brain stem lesion: ipsilateral facial sensory loss and contralateral loss on body below the vertex. H Hemisphere (thalamic) lesion: contralateral loss on one side of face and body.

26

assistance (Fig. 26.18). Fibres from proprioceptive organs and those mediating well-localised touch (including vibration) enter the spinal cord at the posterior horn and pass without synapsing into the ipsilateral posterior columns. Fibres conveying pain and temperature sensory information synapse with second-order neurons which cross the midline in the spinal cord before ascending in the contralateral anterolateral spinothalamic tract to the brain stem.

Transverse lesions of the spinal cord produce loss of all modalities below that segmental level, although the level obtained clinically may vary by two or three segments. Very often, at the top of the area of sensory loss, there is a band of paraesthesia or hyperaesthesia. If the transverse lesion is vascular in origin (e.g. due to anterior spinal artery thrombosis), the posterior one-third of the spinal cord (and therefore the dorsal column modalities) may be spared.

Lesions damaging one side of the spinal cord will produce sensory loss for spinothalamic modalities (pain and temperature) on the opposite side and for dorsal column modalities (joint position and vibration) on the same side as the lesion. This is the pattern seen in the Brown–Séquard syndrome (p. 1243).

Lesions in the centre of the spinal cord (e.g. syringomyelia, Box 26.118, p. 1245) spare the dorsal columns but affect the spinothalamic fibres crossing the cord from both sides over the length of the lesion. The sensory loss is therefore dissociated (in terms of the modalities affected) and suspended (in the sense that segments above and below the lesion are spared), often with reflex loss if afferent fibres of the reflex arc within the cord are affected.

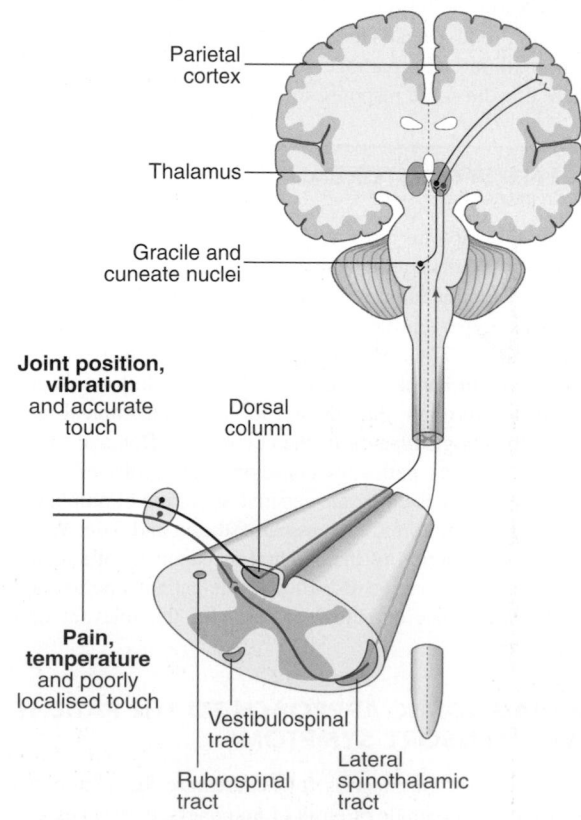

Fig. 26.18 The main somatic sensory pathways.

There may be a lesion in the dorsal column alone, particularly in multiple sclerosis. This produces a characteristic unpleasant tight feeling over the limb involved and loss of proprioception that may severely affect the function of the limb without any loss of pin-prick or temperature sensation.

Brain-stem lesions

The second-order neurons of the dorsal column sensory system cross the midline in the upper medulla to ascend through the brain stem. Here they lie just medial to the (already crossed) spinothalamic pathway. Brain-stem lesions can therefore cause sensory loss affecting all modalities of the contralateral side of the body. Sensory loss on the face due to brain-stem lesions is dependent upon the anatomy of the trigeminal fibres within the brain stem. Fibres from the back of the face (near the ears) descend within the brain stem to the upper part of the spinal cord before synapsing, the second-order neurons crossing the midline and then ascending with the spinothalamic fibres. Fibres conveying sensation from progressively more forward areas of the face descend a shorter distance in the brain stem. Thus, sensory loss in the face from low brain-stem lesions is in a 'balaclava helmet' distribution, as the longer descending trigeminal fibres are affected.

Hemisphere lesions

Both the dorsal column and spinothalamic tracts end in the thalamus, relaying from there to the parietal cortex. Lesions in the hemispheres can therefore affect all modalities of sensation. In the thalamus, discrete lesions (as may occur in small lacunar strokes) can cause loss of sensation over the whole contralateral half of the body. Lesions in the sensory cortex have to be very small (and therefore affect only a restricted area of the body) to avoid affecting the motor tracts deeper in the hemispheres. With substantial lesions of the parietal cortex (as with large strokes) there is severe loss of proprioception and even conscious awareness of the existence of the affected limb(s). The resulting loss of function in the limb may be impossible to distinguish from paralysis.

Pain

Pain is a complex percept that is only partly related to activity in nociceptor neurons (Fig. 26.19). In the posterior horn of the spinal cord, the second-order neuron of the spinothalamic tract is subject to modulation by a number of influences in addition to its synapse with the fibres from nociceptors. Branches from the larger mechanoceptor fibres destined for the posterior column also synapse with the second-order spinothalamic neurons and with interneurons of the grey matter of the posterior horn. The nociceptor neurons release neurotransmitters (such as substance P), in addition to excitatory transmitters, which influence the excitability of the spinothalamic neurons. Neurons in the posterior horn are also subject to modulation by fibres descending from the peri-aqueductal grey matter of the mid-brain and raphe nuclei of the medulla. Neurons of this 'descending analgesia system' are activated by endogenous opiate (endorphin) peptides. The spinal cord's posterior horn is therefore much more than a way-station in the transmission of nociceptive sensory information; it is a complex organ for gating and modulating information about painful stimuli before this ascends in the spinothalamic tract. In the diencephalon the perception of pain is further influenced by the rich interconnections of the thalamus with the limbic system.

Neuropathic pain

Pain is of two main types: nociceptive pain, arising from a pathological process in a body part, and neuropathic pain,

26

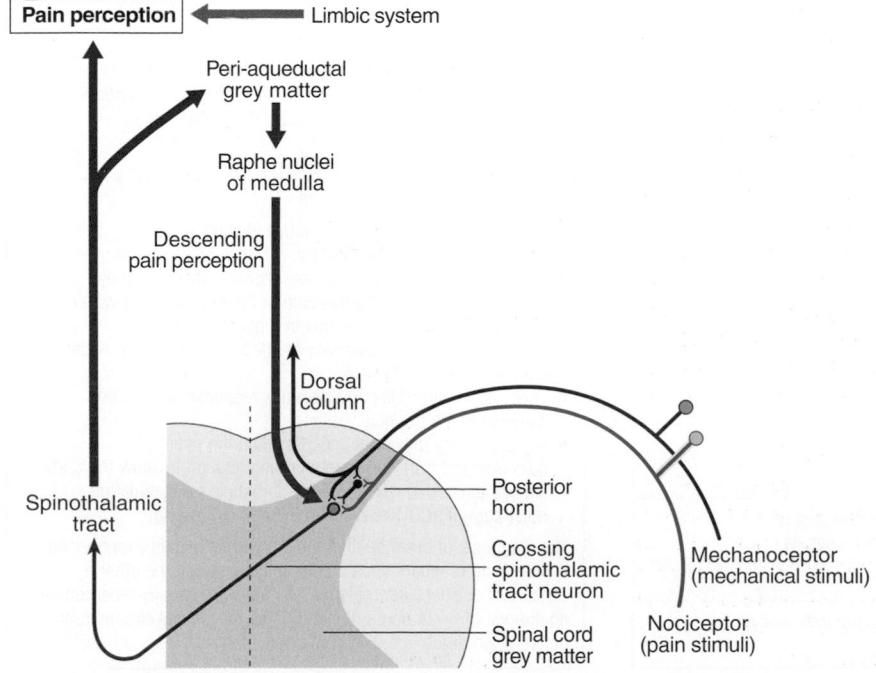

Fig. 26.19 The pain perception system.

caused by dysfunction of the pain perception apparatus itself. Neuropathic pain has distinctive features and is described as a very unpleasant persistent burning sensation. There is often increased sensitivity to touch, so that light brushing touches cause exquisite pain (hyperpathia). Painful stimuli appear to come from a larger area than that touched and spontaneous bursts of pain may occur. The perception of pain may be elicited by stimuli from other modalities such as loud sounds (allodynia) and is considerably affected by emotional influences. The most common syndromes of neuropathic pain are seen where there is partial damage to peripheral nerves ('causalgia'), to the trigeminal nerve (post-herpetic neuralgia) or to the thalamus. Treatment of these syndromes is very difficult. Drugs which modulate various parts of the nociceptive system, such as carbamazepine, tricyclics or phenothiazines, may help but usually only do so partially. Neurosurgical attempts to interrupt various pain pathways sometimes succeed but often increase the sensory deficit and may worsen the situation. Implantation of electrical stimulators has occasionally proved successful. For further information, see Chapter 12.

COMA AND BRAIN DEATH

COMA

Persistent loss of consciousness or coma indicates disorder of the arousal mechanisms in the brain stem and diencephalon, and indicates bilateral hemisphere or brain-stem disease. There are many causes of coma (Box 26.40). The history of the mode of onset of coma and of any

26.40 CAUSES OF COMA

Metabolic disturbance

- Drug overdose
- Diabetes mellitus
  Hypoglycaemia
  Ketoacidosis
  Hyperosmolar coma
- Hyponatraemia
- Uraemia
- Hepatic failure
- Respiratory failure
- Hypothermia
- Hypothyroidism

Trauma

- Cerebral contusion
- Extradural haematoma
- Subdural haematoma

Cerebrovascular disease

- Subarachnoid haemorrhage
- Intracerebral haemorrhage
- Brain-stem infarction/ haemorrhage
- Cerebral venous sinus thrombosis

Infections

- Meningitis
- Encephalitis
- Cerebral abscess
- General sepsis

Others

- Epilepsy
- Brain tumour
- Thiamin deficiency

26.41 GLASGOW COMA SCALE

Eye-opening (E)

• Spontaneous	4
• To speech	3
• To pain	2
• Nil	1

Best motor response (M)

• Obeys	6
• Localises	5
• Withdraws	4
• Abnormal flexion	3
• Extensor response	2
• Nil	1

Verbal response (V)

• Orientated	5
• Confused conversation	4
• Inappropriate words	3
• Incomprehensible sounds	2
• Nil	1

Coma score = E + M + V

• Minimum	3
• Maximum	15

26.42 UK CRITERIA FOR THE DIAGNOSIS OF BRAIN DEATH

Preconditions for considering a diagnosis of brain death

- The patient is deeply comatose
  (a) There must be no suspicion that coma is due to depressant drugs, e.g. narcotics, hypnotics, tranquillisers
  (b) Hypothermia has been excluded—rectal temperature must exceed 35°C
  (c) There is no profound abnormality of serum electrolytes, acid–base balance or blood glucose concentrations, and any metabolic or endocrine cause of coma has been excluded
- The patient is maintained on a ventilator because spontaneous respiration had been inadequate or had ceased. Drugs, including neuromuscular blocking agents, must have been excluded as a cause of the respiratory failure
- The diagnosis of the disorder leading to brain death has been firmly established. There must be no doubt that the patient is suffering from irremediable structural brain damage

Tests for confirming brain death

All brain-stem reflexes are absent

- The pupils are fixed and unreactive to light
- The corneal reflexes are absent
- The vestibulo-ocular reflexes are absent—there is no eye movement following the injection of 20 ml of ice-cold water into each external auditory meatus in turn
- There are no motor responses to adequate stimulation within the cranial nerve distribution
- There is no gag reflex and no reflex response to a suction catheter in the trachea
- No respiratory movement occurs when the patient is disconnected from the ventilator long enough to allow the carbon dioxide tension to rise above the threshold for stimulating respiration ($PaCO_2$ must reach 6.7 kPa (50 mmHg))

The diagnosis of brain death should be made by two experienced doctors, one of whom should be a consultant and the other a consultant or specialist registrar. The tests are usually repeated after an interval of 6–24 hours, depending on the clinical circumstances, before brain death is finally confirmed

precipitating event is crucial to establishing the cause, and this should be obtained from family or other witnesses. As with any medical emergency, the top priority is assessment and stabilisation of the vital functions. Neurological examination may reveal important findings, e.g. evidence of head injury, papilloedema, meningism or eye movement disorder. In the majority of cases, however, there are no focal neurological signs since drug overdose and metabolic disturbance are the most common causes of unexplained coma requiring hospital admission. Some patients will require intensive care unit (ICU) support.

Assessment of conscious level

This is an essential component of the neurological examination. Terms such as 'stuporose', 'semiconscious' and 'obtunded' are ill defined, and a clear description of the patient's level of arousal and response to stimuli is more helpful. Systematic assessment of the unconscious patient by the application of the Glasgow Coma Scale provides a grading of coma by using a numerical scale which allows serial comparison and may provide prognostic information, particularly in traumatic coma (Box 26.41).

BRAIN DEATH

The widespread availability of mechanical ventilators has resulted in the survival of patients with severe and irreversible brain damage but functioning cardiovascular systems. Diagnostic criteria for brain death have been established in order that those patients without functioning brains who have no chance of recovery may be identified and ventilation discontinued.

The diagnosis of brain death depends on meeting a set of preconditions, all of which must coexist, and then applying a series of clinical tests (Box 26.42), all of which must be fulfilled.

ACUTE CONFUSIONAL STATE

This is also known as delirium, and is seen much more commonly than dementia. Unlike dementia, there is a disturbance of arousal that accompanies the global impairment of mental function. This usually takes the form of drowsiness with disorientation, perceptual disturbances and muddled thinking. Patients typically fluctuate, confusion being worse at night, and there may be associated emotional disturbance (e.g. anxiety, irritability or depression) or psychomotor changes (e.g. agitation, restlessness or retardation).

There are many possible causes of acute confusion (Box 26.43), including acute decompensation of a more chronic dementia. (See also Ch. 7.)

Diagnosis

The diagnosis of an acute confusional state involves careful history taking. Patients are usually disorientated, often in both time and place, and therefore their account may not be helpful. As with dementia, it is vital to take a history from a witness (either a relative or a carer). Examination may yield

26

26.43 CAUSES OF ACUTE CONFUSIONAL STATE

Type	Common	Unusual
Infective	Chest infection Urinary infection Septicaemia Viral illness Meningitis Encephalitis	Cerebral abscess Subdural empyema AIDS
Metabolic/endocrine	Hypoxia (respiratory failure) Cardiac failure Acute (internal) haemorrhage Hyper-/hypoglycaemia Hyper-/hypocalcaemia Hyponatraemia Liver failure, renal failure	Hypo-/hyperthyroidism Adrenal disease Porphyria
Vascular	Acute cerebral haemorrhage/infarction Subarachnoid haemorrhage	Vasculitis (e.g. SLE) Cerebral venous thrombosis Hyperviscosity
Toxic	Alcohol intoxication/withdrawal Drugs (therapeutic/illicit)	Carbon monoxide poisoning Industrial exposure (e.g. heavy metals)
Neoplastic	Secondary deposits	Primary cerebral tumour Paraneoplastic syndrome
Trauma	Head injury (cerebral contusions) Subdural haematoma	
Other	Post-ictal state Perioperative Acute decompensation of dementia (Box 26.46)	Acute hydrocephalus Complex partial status epilepticus Hashimoto's encephalopathy Altitude sickness Migraine

26.44 INVESTIGATION OF ACUTE CONFUSIONAL STATE

	First-line	Other useful tests
Blood tests	Full blood count, ESR Urea and electrolytes Glucose Calcium, magnesium Liver function tests Thyroid function tests	Cardiac enzymes Protein electrophoresis Vitamin B_{12} Copper studies Syphilis serology Antinuclear antibody (ANA), anti-double-stranded DNA (anti-dsDNA), antithyroid antibodies Tumour markers, prostate-specific antigen
CNS investigations	Head imaging (CT and/or MRI)	Lumbar puncture EEG
Other	Arterial blood gases ECG Infection screen (blood cultures, chest X-ray, urine culture)	Viral screen, as appropriate (e.g. consider HIV) Urinary porphyrins

26.45 ACUTE CONFUSIONAL STATE IN OLD AGE

- **Increased risk:** in the context of relatively minor systemic disturbances.
- **Predisposing factors:**
  - *dementia:* conversely, an acute confusional state may herald the onset of dementia
  - *malnutrition*
  - *visual and/or auditory impairments*
  - *infections:* chest or urinary tract infections are the most common causes of confusion in old age, and a low threshold of suspicion is essential. Typical symptoms including pyrexia may not be present, so if there is no other obvious cause, it may be appropriate to treat with antibiotics 'blind' once cultures have been taken
  - *surgery:* very common after emergency surgery, and only slightly less so after elective surgery
  - *drugs:* because of polypharmacy and changes in the response to and elimination of drugs in old age.
- See also Chapter 7.

other clues to the cause (e.g. pyrexia, or focal chest or neurological signs). It is important to distinguish confusion from a fluent aphasia, since patients with this speech disorder may appear confused. Often, however, the cause is not immediately obvious, and a wide screen of tests must be performed (Box 26.44).

Management

The management of acute confusional states involves identifying the cause and correcting it if possible. Confused patients should be nursed in a well-lit room. During the period of confusion, sedative drugs are best avoided, as they may exacerbate the confusion, although occasionally drugs such as haloperidol (1–10 mg 8-hourly) may be required. In delirium tremens (alcohol withdrawal), the treatment is a tapered course of diazepam with high-dose intravenous thiamin (p. 246).

DISTURBANCE OF MEMORY

Patients with memory disorders are assessed and investigated with a view to placing them in one of three categories. These are mild or subjective disorders which simply require reassurance, treatable disorders, and disorders which are due to progressive, irreversible memory decline, i.e. dementia (see below). It is important to find out exactly what the patient has noticed wrong. In general, memory problems which have been observed by relatives or colleagues are likely to be more significant than those of which only the patient is aware. Problems of concentration must be distinguished from true problems with memory, as concentration difficulties are much more likely to be due to underlying depressive or anxiety disorders.

It is important to determine for how long the problem has existed, and exactly which aspects of memory are affected. Complaints of getting lost or of forgetting about burners on the kitchen stove are more likely to be significant than simply forgetting names. Disturbance of episodic memory (previously called 'short-term memory') must be distinguished from semantic memory. The former can be selectively impaired in Korsakoff's syndrome (often secondary to alcohol) or bilateral temporal lobe damage, but is seen in conjunction with other disturbance of cortical function in different types of dementia. Progressive deterioration over many months suggests the possibility of an underlying dementia, but it is important to take a full medical history to detect any underlying medical problem which could be responsible (see below). A family history of a memory disorder such as dementia is clearly important.

It is worth stressing that it is important to look for features suggesting depression for two reasons. First, depression can present as a 'pseudo-dementia' with concentration and memory impairment as a dominant feature, and this is often reversible with antidepressant medication. Second, many patients with dementia may develop depression in the early stages of their illness, and this is potentially treatable.

DEMENTIA

Dementia is a clinical syndrome characterised by a loss of previously acquired intellectual function in the absence of impairment of arousal. There are many potential causes of dementia (Box 26.46) but Alzheimer's disease and diffuse vascular disease are the most common. The distinction of senile from pre-senile dementia is unhelpful. However, rarer causes of dementia should be more actively sought in younger patients and those with short histories.

When a patient presents with disturbance of personality or memory dysfunction, the first step is to exclude a focal lesion by determining that there is cognitive disturbance in more than one area. A careful history is, of course, essential and it is important to interview not just the patient but a close family member too. Simple bedside tests such as the Mini-Mental State Examination (MMSE; p. 230) are useful in assessing the cognitive deficit, but more formal help from clinical psychology may be required. General history and

26

26.46 CAUSES OF DEMENTIA

Type	Common	Unusual	Rare
Vascular	Diffuse small-vessel disease	Amyloid angiopathy Multiple emboli	Cerebral vasculitis
Degenerative/inherited (p. 1217)	Alzheimer's disease	Leucodystrophies Huntington's disease Wilson's disease Pick's disease Dystrophia myotonica Cortical Lewy body disease Progressive supranuclear palsy Others (e.g. cortico-basal degeneration)	Mitochondrial encephalopathies
Neoplastic (p. 1236)	Secondary deposits	Primary cerebral tumour	Paraneoplastic syndrome (limbic encephalitis)
Inflammatory		Multiple sclerosis	Sarcoidosis
Traumatic	Chronic subdural haematoma Post-head injury	Punch-drunk syndrome	
Hydrocephalus (p. 1239)		Communicating/non-communicating 'Normal pressure' hydrocephalus	
Toxic/nutritional	Alcohol	Thiamin deficiency B_{12} deficiency	Anoxia/carbon monoxide poisoning Heavy metal poisoning
Infective		Syphilis HIV	Post-encephalitic Whipple's disease Subacute sclerosing panencephalitis
Prion diseases (p 1234)		Sporadic Creutzfeldt–Jakob disease (CJD)	Variant CJD Kuru Gerstmann–Sträussler–Scheinker disease

26

examination may give further clues to aetiology.

Dementias are broadly divided into 'cortical' and 'sub-cortical' types, depending upon their clinical features. Many of the primary degenerative diseases that cause dementia have characteristic features that may allow a specific diagnosis during life. Creutzfeldt–Jakob disease is usually relatively rapidly progressive (over months), is associated with myoclonus, and there may be characteristic abnormalities on EEG. Of the more slowly progressive dementias, Pick's disease presents with rather focal (temporal or frontal lobe) dysfunction often affecting language function early, and Lewy body dementia may present with visual hallucinations. However, it is often difficult to distinguish these dementias from each other or from Alzheimer's disease during life.

Investigations

The aim is to discover a treatable cause, if present, and to try to give an idea of prognosis, using a standard set of investigations (Box 26.47). Imaging of the brain is important to exclude potentially treatable structural lesions such as hydrocephalus, cerebral tumour or chronic subdural haematoma, though often the only abnormality seen is generalised atrophy. If the initial tests fail to yield an answer, more invasive tests such as lumbar puncture or, rarely, brain biopsy may be indicated. If there is concern that the memory disturbance may be a manifestation of depressive illness, formal neuropsychological evaluation is helpful.

26.47 INITIAL INVESTIGATION OF DEMENTIA

In most patients

- Imaging of head (CT and/or MRI)
- Blood tests
    Full blood count, ESR
    Urea and electrolytes, glucose
    Calcium, liver function tests
    Thyroid function tests
    Vitamin B_{12}
    Venereal Diseases Reasearch Laboratory (VDRL) test
    ANA, anti-dsDNA
- Chest X-ray
- EEG

In selected patients

- Lumbar puncture
- HIV serology
- Brain biopsy

Management

This is directed at removing correctable causes, and providing support for patient and carers (p. 237) if no specific treatment exists. Anticholinesterases, such as donepezil, rivastigmine and galantamine, or NMDA (N-methyl-D-aspartate receptor antagonists (memantine) appear to improve cognitive function to some extent in Alzheimer's disease (pp. 247 and 1217).

CHANGES IN PERSONALITY AND BEHAVIOUR

While this is generally considered the province of the psychiatrist (p. 233), there are a number of ways in which organic conditions can result in altered personality and behaviour. This particularly applies to conditions which alter the function of the frontal lobes which are involved in the control of executive function, movement and behaviour (Box 26.3, p. 1152). The frontal lobes may be damaged structurally (e.g. trauma, strokes, hydrocephalus or tumour) or functionally (e.g. metabolic disturbances). It is therefore always worth considering these possibilities, as correct diagnosis will allow appropriate treatment.

Personality can be affected in three broad directions as a result of frontal lobe damage. Patients with mesial frontal lesions become increasingly withdrawn, unresponsive and mute (abulic), and this is often associated with urinary incontinence, gait apraxia and an increase in tone known as gegenhalten, in which the patient varies the resistance to movement in proportion to the force exerted by the examiner. Patients with lesions of the dorsolateral prefrontal cortex develop difficulties with speech and motor planning and organisation (dysexecutive syndrome). Those with orbitofrontal lesions of the frontal lobes become disinhibited, sometimes to the point of grandiosity, or exhibit irresponsible behaviour (e.g. with financial affairs). Memory is substantially intact, and there may be focal physical signs such as a grasp reflex, palmo-mental response or pout. As the frontal lobe overlies the olfactory bulb and tracts, structural lesions such as tumours in the inferior frontal lobes may be associated with anosmia.

Personality can also be affected by damage to the temporal lobes, usually as a result of memory impairment. Disturbance to the cortical areas responsible for speech can result in speech difficulties which may be interpreted as changes in personality.

SPEECH AND LANGUAGE DISTURBANCE

Speech is the process whereby vocal sounds are used to convey meaning between individuals. A large volume of the cerebral cortex is involved in this complex process, mostly in the dominant hemisphere (Box 26.3, p. 1152). The decoding of speech sounds (phonemes) is a function of the upper part of the posterior temporal lobe. The perception of these sounds as meaningful language, as well as the formulation of the language required for the expression of ideas and concepts, occurs predominantly in the lower parts of the anterior parietal lobe (the angular and supramarginal gyri). The temporal speech comprehension region is referred to as Wernicke's area. Other parts of the temporal lobe contribute to language processing in areas specialising in verbal memory, where lexicons of meaningful words are 'stored'. The language information so generated then passes anteriorly via the arcuate fasciculus to Broca's area in the posterior end of the inferior frontal gyrus on the dominant side. The motor commands generated in Broca's area pass to

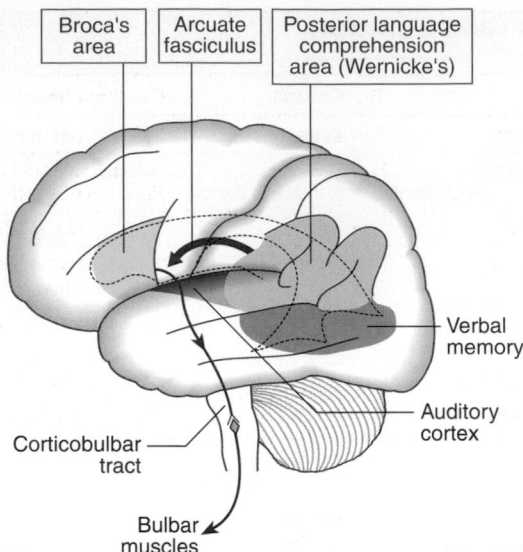

Fig. 26.20 Areas of the cerebral cortex involved in the generation of spoken language.

the cranial nerve nuclei in the pons and medulla, as well as to the anterior horn cells in the spinal cord. The cerebellum has an important coordinating function. Nerve impulses then travel to the lips, tongue, palate, pharynx, larynx and respiratory muscles via the facial nerve and cranial nerves 9, 10 and 12, and result in the series of ordered sounds known as speech (Fig. 26.20).

These ordered sounds are detected by a listener in whom nerve impulses are passed from the ears to the auditory cortex in the temporal lobe and hence to the speech comprehension areas. Parts of the non-dominant parietal lobe appear to contribute to non-verbal aspects of language in the recognition of meaningful intonation patterns of spoken words.

DYSPHONIA AND DYSARTHRIA

At a simple level, the vocal cords may fail to generate sounds properly in speech, and this results in hoarse or whispered speech (dysphonia). This may be due to a local problem affecting the proper functioning of the cords or a higher-level problem (dystonia) of vocal cord operation. If the muscles or nerves controlling the mouth, tongue, pharynx and lips are not functioning correctly, poorly articulated speech will result (dysarthria). There is no problem with choice of words, but the speech may or may not be intelligible, depending on severity. Cerebellar or brain-stem disease, lower cranial nerve lesions, myasthenia or muscle disease may all result in dysarthria. The quality of the speech tends to differ somewhat depending on the cause but it can be very difficult to distinguish the different types clinically (Box 26.48).

APHASIA

Aphasia (or dysphasia) is a disorder of the language content of speech. It can occur with lesions over a wide area of the

26

26.48 CAUSES OF DYSARTHRIA

Type	Site	Characteristics	Associated features
Myopathic	Muscles of speech	Indistinct, poor articulation	Weakness of face, tongue and neck
Myasthenic	Motor end plate	Indistinct with fatigue and dysphonia. Fluctuating severity	Ptosis, diplopia, facial and neck weakness
Bulbar	Brain stem	Indistinct, slurred, often nasal	Dysphagia, diplopia, ataxia
'Scanning'	Cerebellum	Slurring, impaired timing and cadence, 'sing-song' quality	Ataxia of limbs and gait, tremor of head/limbs. Nystagmus
Spastic	Pyramidal tracts	Indistinct, breathy, mumbling	Poor rapid tongue movements, increased reflexes and jaw jerk
Parkinsonian	Basal ganglia	Indistinct, rapid, stammering, quiet	Tremor, rigidity, slow shuffling gait
Dystonic	Basal ganglia	Strained, slow, high-pitched	Dystonia, athetosis

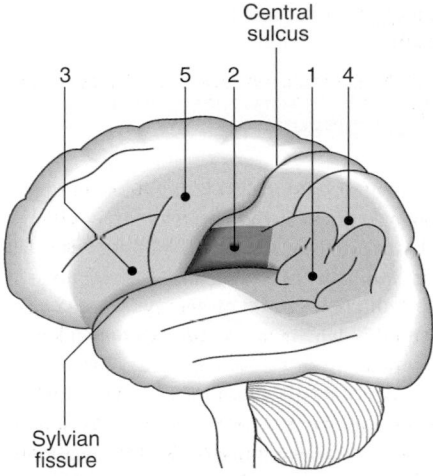

Central sulcus

3 5 2 1 4

Sylvian fissure

Fig. 26.21 Classification of aphasia, according to the site of the lesion and type of language deficit. All have naming difficulty (anomia). Fluent aphasias arise from lesions posterior to the central fissure; repetition is affected by lesions around the Sylvian fissure. (1) Wernicke aphasia: fluent aphasia with poor comprehension and poor repetition. (2) Conduction aphasia: fluent aphasia with good comprehension and poor repetition. (3) Broca aphasia: non-fluent aphasia with good comprehension and poor repetition. (4) Transcortical sensory aphasia: fluent aphasia with poor comprehension and good repetition. (5) Transcortical motor aphasia: non-fluent aphasia with good comprehension and good repetition. **N.B.** Large lesions affecting all of regions 1–5 cause global aphasia.

dominant hemisphere. Aphasia is detected by the patient's inability to produce the correct word (anomia). When patients are asked to name objects or parts of objects, if anomia is present either no word will be produced or the wrong word or a nonsense word produced (paraphasia). Aphasia can be classified according to whether the speech output is 'fluent', in which a normal or increased number of (the wrong) words is produced, or 'non-fluent' if the verbal output is reduced. Patients with lesions anterior to the central (Rolandic) fissure have non-fluent aphasia whilst those with lesions posterior to the central fissure in the speech areas have a fluent aphasia (and are often mistakenly thought to be 'confused'). By testing patients for the comprehension of words and their ability to repeat, their aphasia can be further classified into distinct syndromes of aphasia which have localising and prognostic implications (Fig. 26.21).

If a patient is found to have difficulty with speech comprehension there is likely to be a lesion in the superior part of the posterior temporal lobe and/or the adjoining part of the parietal lobe (Wernicke's area). Patients with lesions around the lateral (Sylvian) fissure will have difficulty with repetition, whilst those with lesions away from the Sylvian fissure can repeat and may do so compulsively. Patients with large lesions over much of the speech area are not testable in such a refined manner, having no language production, and are said to have 'global aphasia'. Some patients with patchy lesions in the speech areas may not be easily classified according to the above scheme and are said to have anomic aphasia. Patients with fluent aphasia tend not to have an associated hemiparesis since the pyramidal tract is not involved, whilst those with the more anteriorly placed lesions causing non-fluent aphasia often do have a hemiparesis.

DISORDERS OF PERCEPTION

The temporal, parietal and occipital lobes receive a variety of sensory information including the various different modalities of touch, vision, hearing and balance (Box 26.3, p. 1152). The initial points of entry into the cortex are the respective primary cortical areas (Fig. 26.4, p. 1151). Damage to any of these areas will result in reduction or loss of the ability to perceive that particular modality. This is referred to as 'negative' symptomatology. Abnormal excitation of these areas (e.g. by epilepsy or migraine) will result in an apparent perception which is not based in physical reality (i.e. a hallucination). Such 'positive' stimuli can be visual (flashing lights or formed images), somatosensory (tingling, burning or pain), auditory (noises) or vestibular (vertigo).

The parietal lobes are also involved in the higher processing and integration of the primary sensory information. This occurs in areas which may be highly specialised (e.g. the areas involved in the production and understanding of speech; see above) or less specialised. Less specialised

26

areas are referred to as 'association' cortex. Damage to association cortex gives rise to sensory (including visual) inattention and disorders of spatial perception and hence the disruption of spatially orientated behaviour leading to apraxia. Apraxia is the inability to perform complex, organised activity in the presence of a normal basic motor, sensory and cerebellar system (i.e. after weakness, numbness and ataxia have been excluded as causes). Such complex activities include dressing, using cutlery and finding one's way around geographically. Other abnormalities which may result from damage to association cortex involve difficulty reading (dyslexia) or writing (dysgraphia), or the inability to detect that something is wrong (agnosia). The results of damage to particular lobes of the brain are given in Box 26.3 on page 1152.

PROBLEMS WITH BRAIN-STEM FUNCTION

Many different functional areas are tightly packed into the brain stem (p. 1152 and Fig. 26.5, p. 1153). Thus, damage to even a small area of the brain stem potentially causes major disturbance of several systems. As the anatomy of the brain stem is very precisely organised, it is usually possible to localise the site of a lesion on the basis of careful history and examination to determine exactly which tracts/nuclei are affected. Lesions can occur singly, multiply or diffusely, but the standard neurological approach is to try to explain all of a patient's problems in the minimum number of lesions (ideally just one).

An example would be a patient presenting with sudden onset of upper motor neuron features affecting the right face, arm and leg in association with a left 3rd nerve palsy. The lesion would have to be in the left cerebral peduncle in the brain stem where the pathology is likely to have been a small stroke, as the onset was sudden. This combination of signs is known as Weber's syndrome, and this is one of several well-described brain-stem syndromes which are listed in Box 26.49. These are often, but not always, caused by vascular lesions.

The effects of damage to the individual cranial nerves which arise in the brain stem, or to their nuclei, are discussed in the sections on eye movements (p. 1195) and on nerve and muscle, below (p. 1246). The lower cranial nerves, 9, 10, 11 and 12, are frequently affected bilaterally, producing dysphagia (see below) and dysarthria (see above). The term 'bulbar palsy' is used if this results from lower motor neuron lesions, either at nuclear or fascicular level within the medulla, or from bilateral lesions of the lower cranial nerves outside the brain stem. The tongue is wasted and fasciculating and the palate moves very little. A 'pseudobulbar palsy' arises from an upper motor neuron lesion of the bulbar muscles from lesions of the corticobulbar pathways in the pyramidal tracts. Here the tongue is small and contracted, and moves slowly; the jaw jerk is brisk. Causes of bulbar and pseudobulbar palsies are shown in Box 26.50.

SWALLOWING DIFFICULTIES

Swallowing is a complex activity involving the coordinated action of lips, tongue, soft palate, pharynx and larynx, which are innervated by the facial nerve and cranial nerves 9, 10, 11 and 12. This mechanism is potentially vulnerable to damage to many different areas of the nervous system, resulting in dysphagia which is usually accompanied by dysarthria. Structural causes of dysphagia are considered on page 864. Acute onset of dysphagia may occur as a result of brain-stem stroke, a rapidly developing neuropathy such as the Guillain–Barré syndrome or diphtheria. The upper motor neuron innervation of the cranial nerves responsible for swallowing is bilateral, so persistent dysphagia is unusual with a unilateral upper motor lesion. However, dysphagia may occur in the early stages of such a lesion if it is very acute, such as a hemisphere stroke. Dysphagia developing

26.49 MAJOR FOCAL BRAIN-STEM SYNDROMES		
Name of syndrome	**Site of lesions**	**Clinical features**
Weber	Anterior cerebral peduncle (mid-brain)	Ipsilateral 3rd palsy Contralateral upper motor neuron 7th palsy Contralateral hemiplegia
Claude	Cerebral peduncle involving red nucleus	Ipsilateral 3rd palsy Contralateral cerebellar signs
Parinaud	Dorsal mid-brain (tectum)	Vertical gaze palsy Convergence disorders Convergence retraction nystagmus Pupillary and lid disorders
Millard–Gubler	Ponto-medullary junction	Ipsilateral 6th palsy Ipsilateral lower motor neuron 7th palsy Contralateral hemiplegia
Wallenberg	Lateral medulla	Ipsilateral 5th, 9th, 10th, 11th palsy Ipsilateral Horner's syndrome Ipsilateral cerebellar signs Contralateral spinothalamic sensory loss Vestibular disturbance

26

26.50 CAUSES OF BULBAR AND PSEUDOBULBAR PALSY

	Pseudobulbar	Bulbar
Genetic		Kennedy's disease (X-linked bulbo-spinal neuronopathy)
Vascular	Bilateral hemisphere (lacunar) infarction	Medullary infarction
Degenerative	Motor neuron disease (p. 1223)	Motor neuron disease Syringobulbia
Inflammatory/infective	Multiple sclerosis (p. 1212) Cerebral vasculitis	Myasthenia (p. 1252) Guillain–Barré (p. 1249) Poliomyelitis (p. 1230) Lyme disease (p. 319) Vasculitis
Neoplastic	High brain-stem tumours	Brain-stem glioma Malignant meningitis

subacutely may be seen in myasthenia gravis, motor neuron disease, polymyositis, basal meningitis and inflammatory brain-stem disease. More slowly developing dysphagia suggests a myopathy or possibly a brain-stem or skull-base tumour.

DISORDERS OF BALANCE

Balance is a complicated process which involves modification of both axial and limb muscle function to compensate for the effects of gravity and alterations in body position and load (and hence centre of gravity) in order to prevent the person from falling. This process involves input from a variety of sensory modalities (visual, vestibular, proprioceptive), processing by the cerebellum and brain stem, and output via a number of descending pathways (e.g. vestibulospinal, rubrospinal and reticulospinal tracts). The process also results in a cognitive perception of 'vertical' which is mediated through the cerebral cortex.

Disorders of balance can therefore arise from a number of different abnormalities which may affect input (loss of vision, vestibular disorders or lack of joint position sense), processing (damage to vestibular nuclei or cerebellum) or motor function (spinal cord lesions, leg weakness of any cause). The patient may complain of different symptoms depending on what is actually wrong. For example, loss of joint position sense or cerebellar function may result in a sensation of 'unsteadiness', while damage to the vestibular nuclei or labyrinth may result in an illusory sensation of movement, i.e. 'vertigo' (p. 1165). A careful history is vital. Patients may well have other associated symptoms, depending on the site of damage (e.g. dysarthria in a cerebellar lesion). As vision can often compensate for lack of joint position sense, patients with peripheral neuropathies or dorsal column loss will often find their problem more noticeable in the dark.

Examination of such patients may yield physical signs that depend on the site of the problem. Sensory abnormalities may be manifest as altered visual acuities or visual fields, possibly with abnormalities on fundoscopy, altered eye movements (including nystagmus), impaired vestibular function (p. 1166) or lack of joint position sense.

Disturbance of cerebellar function may be manifest as nystagmus (p. 1196), dysarthria or incoordination of limb movements (ataxia), demonstrated as abnormalities of finger-nose testing, heel-shin testing, inability to perform alternating movements (dysdiadochokinesis) or difficulty with gait (unsteadiness or inability to perform tandem gait, p. 1181). Leg weakness will be detectable on examination of the limbs.

VISUAL DISTURBANCE

Disturbances of vision are common and often related to problems with the eye rather than disorders of the nervous system. A common reason for presentation is loss of vision, but patients may also present with positive visual symptoms, e.g. hallucinations. The movements of the two eyes may be disturbed and give rise to double vision (diplopia) or blurred vision. Alternatively, patients may present with disordered appearance of their visual apparatus, which includes the eyelids, the globe, the eye movements, the pupils or the appearance of the optic disc on fundoscopy (e.g. papilloedema).

VISUAL LOSS

The visual pathway from the retina to the occipital cortex is topographically organised, so the pattern of visual field loss allows precise localisation of the site of the lesion. Fibres from ganglion cells in the retina pass to the optic disc and then backwards through the lamina cribrosa to the optic nerve. Nasal optic nerve fibres (subserving the temporal visual field because the image on the retina is inverted) cross at the chiasm, but temporal fibres do not. Hence, all fibres in the optic tract and further posteriorly subserve both eyes' representation of contralateral visual space. From the lateral geniculate nucleus, lower fibres pass through the temporal lobes on their way to the primary visual area in the occipital cortex, while the upper fibres pass through the parietal lobe. Patterns of visual field loss are explained by this anatomy, as seen in Figure 26.22, and associated clinical manifestations are described in Box 26.51.

26

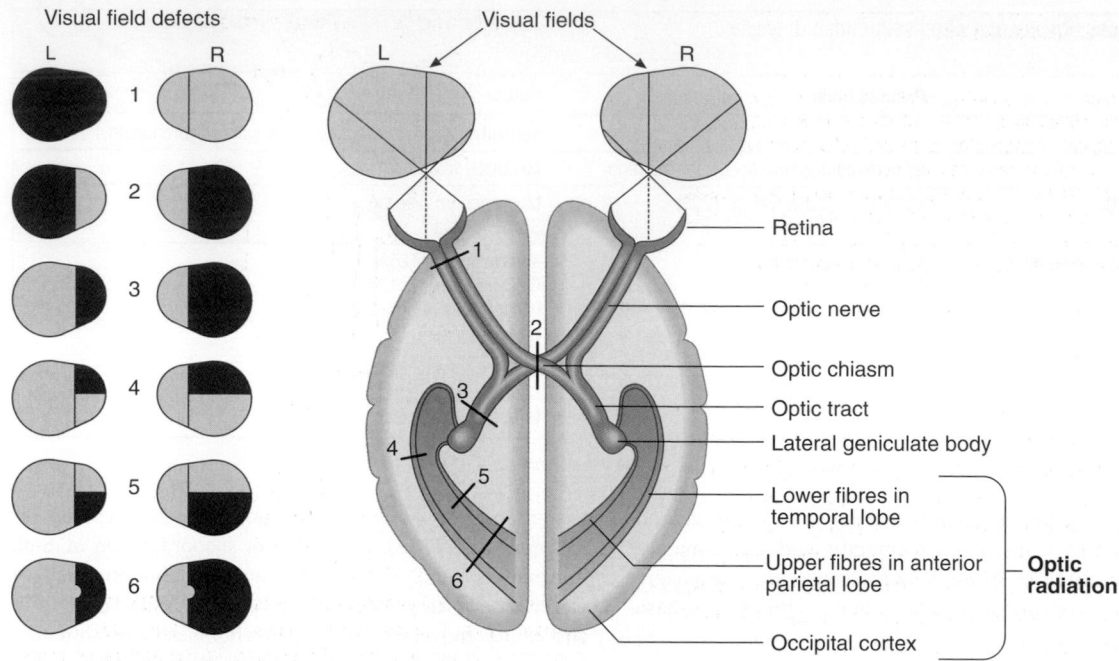

Fig. 26.22 **Visual pathways and visual field defects.** Schematic representation of eyes and brain in transverse section.

26.51 CLINICAL MANIFESTATIONS OF VISUAL FIELD LOSS

Site	Common causes	Complaint	Visual field loss	Associated physical signs
Retina/optic disc	Vascular disease (including vasculitis) Glaucoma Inflammation	Partial/complete visual loss depending on site	Altitudinal field defect Arcuate scotoma	Reduced acuity Visual distortion (macula) Abnormal retinal appearance
Optic nerve	Optic neuritis Sarcoidosis Tumour Leber's hereditary optic neuropathy	Partial/complete loss of vision in one eye Often painful Central vision particularly affected	Central scotoma Paracentral scotoma Monocular blindness	Reduced acuity Reduced colour vision Relative afferent pupillary defect Optic atrophy (late)
Optic chiasm	Pituitary tumours Craniopharyngioma Sarcoidosis	May be none Rarely diplopia ('hemifield slide')	Bitemporal hemianopia	Pituitary function abnormalities
Optic tract	Tumour Inflammatory disease	Disturbed vision to one side of midline	Incongruous contralateral homonymous hemianopia	
Temporal lobe	Stroke Tumour Inflammatory disease	Disturbed vision to one side of midline	Contralateral homonymous upper quadrantanopia	Memory/language disorders
Parietal lobe	Stroke Tumour Inflammatory disease	Disturbed vision to one side of midline Bumping into things	Contralateral homonymous lower quadrantanopia	Contralateral sensory disturbance Asymmetry of optokinetic nystagmus
Occipital lobe	Stroke Tumour Inflammatory disease	Disturbed vision to one side of midline Difficulty reading Bumping into things	Homonymous hemianopia (may be macula-sparing)	Damage to other structures supplied by posterior cerebral circulation

It is not uncommon for patients to present with transient visual loss. Visual loss lasting from 1–20 minutes is likely to have a vascular cause. This can affect one eye (amaurosis fugax) or one visual field. Whether the field loss was monocular (carotid circulation) or a homonymous hemianopia (vertebro-basilar circulation) is crucial to further management, and this must be distinguished by careful history (e.g. did the patient try shutting each eye in turn?). Transient visual loss lasting 20–30 minutes suggests migraine, especially if accompanied by headache and/or positive visual phenomena.

26

POSITIVE VISUAL SYMPTOMS

The most common cause of a positive visual disturbance is migraine, in which patients may see silvery zigzag lines (fortification spectra) or flashing coloured lights (teichopsia) which precede the headache. Simple flashes of light (phosphenes) can also be seen as a result of damage to the retina (e.g. detachment) or damage to the primary visual cortex. Visual hallucinations may be caused by drugs, or may be due to structural damage resulting in epilepsy or 'release phenomena', i.e. hallucinations which occur in a blind visual field.

EYE MOVEMENT DISORDERS

Under normal circumstances, the eyes move conjugately, though horizontal vergence allows visual fusion of objects at different distances. The control of eye movements begins in the cerebral hemispheres, particularly within the frontal eye fields, and the pathway then descends to the brain stem with input from the visual cortex, superior colliculus and cerebellum. Horizontal and vertical gaze centres in the pons and mid-brain, respectively, coordinate output to the ocular motor nerve nuclei (3, 4 and 6), which are connected to each other by the medial longitudinal fasciculus (MLF) (Fig. 26.23). The MLF is particularly important in yoking the horizontal movements of the two eyes. The extraocular muscles are then supplied by the oculomotor (3rd), trochlear (4th) and abducens (6th) nerves.

Diplopia

This arises when eye movement is impaired so that the image of an object is not projected to homologous points on the two retinae. This may result from central disorders or from disturbance of the ocular motor nerves, muscles or the neuromuscular junction. The pattern of double vision, along with any associated features, usually allows localisation of the lesion, whilst the mode of onset and subsequent behaviour (e.g. fatigability in myasthenia) suggest the aetiology.

The trochlear (4th) nerve innervates the superior oblique muscle, and the abducens (6th) nerve innervates the lateral rectus. The oculomotor (3rd) nerve innervates the remainder of the extraocular muscles along with the levator palpebrae superioris and the ciliary body (pupil constriction and accommodation). Causes of ocular motor nerve palsies are given in Box 26.53.

Complete oculomotor (3rd) nerve lesions cause ptosis and a dilated pupil, and the eye tends to rest in a 'down and out'

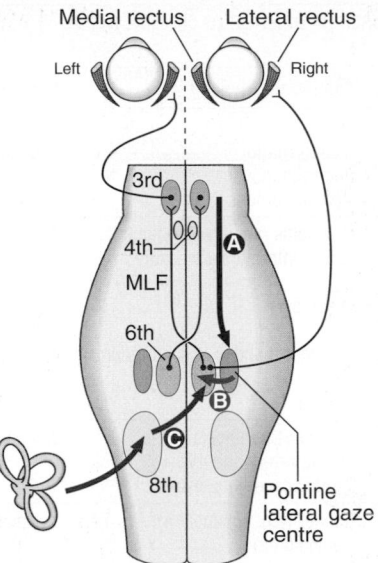

Fig. 26.23 Control of conjugate eye movements. Downward projections pass from the cortex to pontine lateral gaze centre (A). Pontine gaze centre projects to the 6th cranial nerve nucleus (B), which innervates the ipsilateral lateral rectus and projects to the contralateral 3rd nerve nucleus (and hence medial rectus) via the medial longitudinal fasciculus (MLF). Tonic inputs from the vestibular apparatus (C) project to the contralateral 6th nerve nucleus via the vestibular nuclei.

position due to unopposed tonic activity of the unaffected lateral rectus and superior oblique muscles. The pupil is often spared in ischaemic lesions (e.g. in diabetes), and its involvement requires that compressive lesions such as aneurysm be excluded. Trochlear (4th) nerve palsy presents with vertical diplopia (especially noticeable going downstairs), and the patient may have a head tilt to the contralateral side and double vision when looking down to the side opposite the lesion. Abducens (6th) nerve palsy causes horizontal double vision when trying to look towards the side of the lesion. In diplopia of any cause, the image projected furthest away from primary position arises from the paretic eye, and covering each eye in turn can often determine this. Note that this image is not necessarily any less clear than the image from the non-paretic eye—it is the relative position, not the clarity, of the images which is important in determining which muscle is weak.

Myasthenia gravis (p. 1252) can cause diplopia by affecting any or all of the extraocular muscles. It is often associated with ptosis, and the hallmark is fatiguability. Similarly, diseases of the extraocular muscles themselves can cause diplopia. These include thyroid eye disease, myopathies and orbital myositis.

Central lesions can also give rise to diplopia. Brain-stem lesions affecting the 3rd, 4th or 6th nerves or nuclei will cause diplopia, as will lesions of the MLF. The hallmark of an MLF lesion is an internuclear ophthalmoplegia (INO), most commonly seen in multiple sclerosis (p. 1212). The lateral gaze centre in the pons sends fibres to the ipsilateral 6th nerve nucleus. The nucleus contains two populations of neurons. Half the cells send their axons directly into the 6th nerve to supply the lateral rectus, while the remaining

26

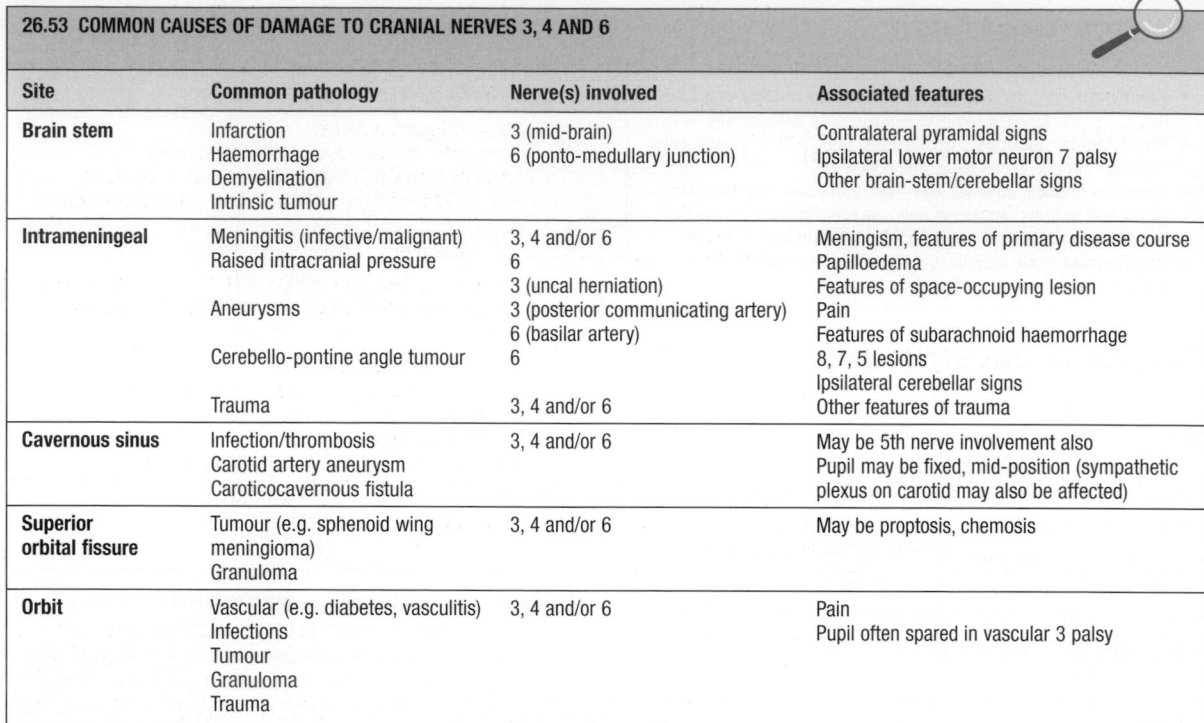

26.53 COMMON CAUSES OF DAMAGE TO CRANIAL NERVES 3, 4 AND 6

Site	Common pathology	Nerve(s) involved	Associated features
Brain stem	Infarction Haemorrhage Demyelination Intrinsic tumour	3 (mid-brain) 6 (ponto-medullary junction)	Contralateral pyramidal signs Ipsilateral lower motor neuron 7 palsy Other brain-stem/cerebellar signs
Intrameningeal	Meningitis (infective/malignant) Raised intracranial pressure Aneurysms Cerebello-pontine angle tumour Trauma	3, 4 and/or 6 6 3 (uncal herniation) 3 (posterior communicating artery) 6 (basilar artery) 6 3, 4 and/or 6	Meningism, features of primary disease course Papilloedema Features of space-occupying lesion Pain Features of subarachnoid haemorrhage 8, 7, 5 lesions Ipsilateral cerebellar signs Other features of trauma
Cavernous sinus	Infection/thrombosis Carotid artery aneurysm Caroticocavernous fistula	3, 4 and/or 6	May be 5th nerve involvement also Pupil may be fixed, mid-position (sympathetic plexus on carotid may also be affected)
Superior orbital fissure	Tumour (e.g. sphenoid wing meningioma) Granuloma	3, 4 and/or 6	May be proptosis, chemosis
Orbit	Vascular (e.g. diabetes, vasculitis) Infections Tumour Granuloma Trauma	3, 4 and/or 6	Pain Pupil often spared in vascular 3 palsy

half send their fibres into the contralateral MLF and up to the contralateral 3rd nerve nucleus, where they synapse with neurons destined for the medial rectus (Fig. 26.23). Hence, damage to the 6th nerve nucleus itself will prevent both eyes from moving ipsilaterally (gaze palsy), and a lesion of the MLF will interfere with adduction of the ipsilateral eye (INO). In this situation, the ipsilateral eye will either fail to adduct past midline if the lesion is complete, or adduct very slowly if it is partial. Nystagmus may sometimes be seen in the other (abducting) eye, giving rise to the archaic term 'ataxic nystagmus'.

Nystagmus

If the eye movement control systems are defective, the eyes may drift off target and recurrent corrections become necessary to return fixation to the object of interest. This results in a repetitive to-and-fro movement (drift-correction-drift etc.) which is known as nystagmus. Usually the drifts are slower than the corrections (slow and fast phases, respectively). The direction of the fast phase is usually designated as the direction of the nystagmus because it is easier to see, although the abnormality is the slower drift of the eyes off target. Nystagmus may be horizontal, vertical or torsional, and is usually conjugate, i.e. the two eyes usually move together. Nystagmus is seen as a physiological phenomenon in response to sustained vestibular stimulation or movement of the visual world (optokinetic nystagmus). There are, however, many different causes of pathological nystagmus, the most common being disorders of the vestibular system (peripheral and central components) and brain-stem/cerebellar lesions.

In lesions of the vestibular system (most commonly peripheral labyrinthine lesions), damage to the horizontal canal or its connections on one side will allow the tonic output from the healthy, contralateral side to cause the eyes to drift towards the side of the lesion. This causes recurrent compensatory fast movements away from the side of the lesion; hence unidirectional horizontal nystagmus to the opposite side is seen. Vertical and torsional components can be seen with damage to other parts of the vestibular apparatus. The nystagmus of peripheral labyrinthine lesions disappears (fatigues) quite quickly and is always accompanied by vertigo and quite often nausea and vomiting. Central vestibular nystagmus is more persistent.

The brain stem and the cerebellum are involved in maintaining eccentric positions of gaze. Lesions will therefore allow the eyes to drift back in towards primary position. This produces nystagmus whose fast component beats in the direction of gaze (gaze-evoked nystagmus). This is the most common type of 'central' nystagmus and is most commonly bi-directional and not usually accompanied by vertigo, but there may be other signs of brain-stem dysfunction. Brain-stem disease may also cause vertical nystagmus.

Unilateral cerebellar lesions may result in gaze-evoked nystagmus when looking in the direction of the lesion, where the fast phases are directed towards the side of the lesion. Cerebellar hemisphere lesions also cause 'ocular dysmetria', an overshoot of target-directed, fast eye movements (saccades) resembling 'past-pointing' in limbs.

Nystagmus also occurs as a result of toxicity (especially drugs) and nutritional (thiamin) deficiency. The severity is variable, and it may or may not result in visual degradation, though it may be associated with a sensation of movement of the visual world (oscillopsia). Nystagmus may occur as a congenital phenomenon, in which case the nystagmus is

26

26.54 COMMON CAUSES OF PTOSIS

Mechanism	Causes	Associated clinical features
3rd nerve palsy	Isolated palsy (Box 26.53) Central/supranuclear lesion	Ptosis is usually complete Extraocular muscle palsy (eye 'down and out') Depending on site of lesion, other cranial nerve palsies (e.g. 4, 5 and 6) or contralateral upper motor neuron signs
Sympathetic lesion (Horner's syndrome) (Fig. 26.24)	Central (hypothalamus/brain stem) Peripheral (lung apex, carotid artery pathology) Idiopathic	Ptosis is partial Lack of sweating on affected side Depending on site of lesion, brain-stem signs, signs of apical lung/brachial plexus disease, or ipsilateral carotid artery stroke
Myopathic	Myasthenia gravis Dystrophia myotonica	Extraocular muscle palsies More widespread muscle weakness, with fatigability in myasthenia Progressive external ophthalmoplegia Other characteristic features of individual causes
Other	Pseudo-ptosis (e.g. blepharospasm) Local orbital/lid disease Age-related levator dehiscence	Eyebrows depressed rather than raised May be local orbital abnormality

26.55 PUPILLARY DISORDERS

Disorder	Cause	Ophthalmological features	Associated features
3rd nerve palsy	Box 26.53	Dilated pupil Extraocular muscle palsy (eye is typically 'down and out') Complete ptosis	Other features of 3rd nerve palsy (Box 26.54)
Horner's syndrome (Fig. 26.24)	Lesion to sympathetic supply	Small pupil Partial ptosis Iris heterochromia (if congenital)	Ipsilateral failure of sweating (anhidrosis)
Holmes–Adie syndrome (tonic pupil)	Lesion of ciliary ganglion (usually idiopathic)	Dilated pupil Light-near dissociation (accommodate but do not react to light) Vermiform movement of iris during contraction Disturbance of accommodation	Generalised areflexia
Argyll Robertson pupil	Dorsal mid-brain lesion (syphilis or diabetes)	Small, irregular pupils Light-near dissociation	Other features of tabes dorsalis (p. 1233)
Local pupillary damage	Trauma/inflammatory disease	Irregular pupils, often with adhesions to lens (synechiae) Variable degree of reactivity	Other features of trauma/ underlying inflammatory disease (e.g. cataract, blindness etc.)
Relative afferent pupillary defect (Marcus Gunn pupil)	Damage to optic nerve (Box 26.51, p. 1194)	Pupils symmetrical, but degree of dilatation depends on which eye stimulated	Decreased visual acuity/ colour vision Central scotoma Papilloedema/optic disc pallor

26

often quasi-sinusoidal ('pendular') rather than having alternating fast and slow phases ('jerk').

EYELID, GLOBE AND PUPIL DISORDERS

Various disorders may cause drooping or ptosis of the eyelid, and these are listed in Box 26.54.

In some circumstances the globe is pushed forward in the orbit, either unilaterally (proptosis) or bilaterally (exophthalmos). By far the most common cause of both is thyroid eye disease (p. 756), but other causes include orbital tumours or granulomas, cavernous sinus disease and inflammatory orbital disease ('pseudotumour').

Disorders of the pupil

Pupillary response to light is due to a combination of parasympathetic and sympathetic activity. Parasympathetic fibres originate in the Edinger–Westphal subnucleus of the 3rd nerve, and pass with the 3rd nerve to synapse in the ciliary ganglion before supplying the constrictor pupillae of the iris. Sympathetic fibres originate in the hypothalamus, pass down the brain stem and cervical spinal cord to emerge at T1, return up to the eye in association with the internal carotid artery and supply the dilator pupillae. Lesions in the sympathetic pathway cause Horner's syndrome (Fig. 26.24). The pupils also constrict as part of the near reflex (in association with accommodation and convergence).

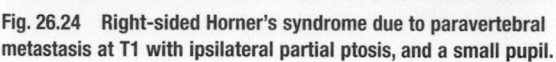

Fig. 26.24 **Right-sided Horner's syndrome due to paravertebral metastasis at T1 with ipsilateral partial ptosis, and a small pupil.**

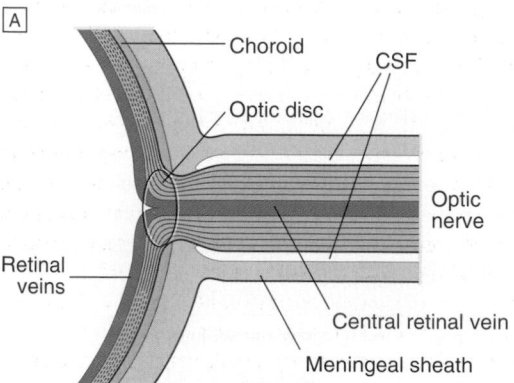

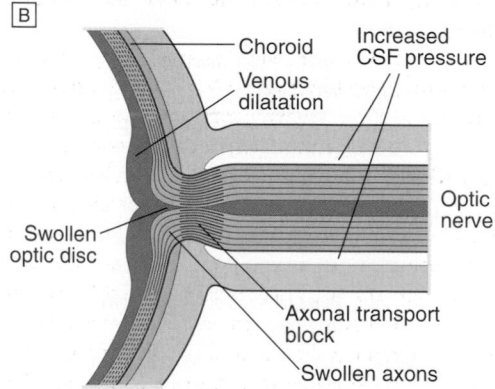

26

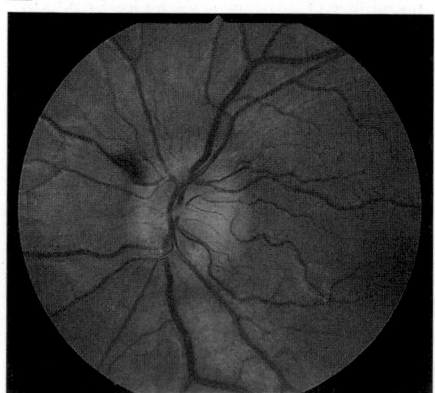

Fig. 26.25 **Mechanism of optic disc oedema (papilloedema).**
Ⓐ Normal. Ⓑ Disc oedema (e.g. due to cerebral tumour). Ⓒ Fundus photograph of the left eye showing optic disc oedema with a small haemorrhage on the nasal side of the disc.

26.56 COMMON CAUSES OF OPTIC DISC SWELLING
Raised intracranial pressure
• Cerebral mass lesion (tumour, abscess)   • Hydrocephalus, haemorrhage, haematoma   • Idiopathic intracranial hypertension
Obstruction of ocular venous drainage
• Central retinal vein occlusion   • Cavernous sinus thrombosis
Systemic disorders affecting retinal vessels
• Hypertension   • Vasculitis   • Hypercapnia
Optic nerve damage
• Demyelination (optic neuritis/papillitis)   • Leber's hereditary optic neuropathy   • Ischaemia   • Toxins (e.g. methanol)   • Infiltration of optic disc   • Sarcoidosis   • Glioma   • Lymphoma

Lesions of the oculomotor nerve, ciliary ganglion and sympathetic supply produce characteristic 'efferent' disorders of pupillary function. 'Afferent' defects occur as a result of damage to an optic nerve, impairing the direct response of a pupil to light, although leaving the consensual response from stimulation of the normal eye intact. Structural damage to the iris itself can also result in pupillary abnormalities. A summary is given in Box 26.55.

Optic disc disorders

Optic disc swelling

There are several causes of swelling of the optic disc, but the term 'papilloedema' is reserved for swelling in association with raised intracranial pressure. In raised intracranial pressure from any cause, axoplasmic flow from retinal ganglion cells is held up at the cribriform plate. This results in swollen nerve fibres, which in turn cause capillary and venous congestion, producing papilloedema. The first sign is the cessation of normal venous pulsation seen at the disc, and the disc margins then become red (hyperaemic). The margins become indistinct and the whole disc is raised up, often with haemorrhages in the retina (Fig. 26.25).

Other causes of optic disc swelling are listed in Box 26.56. Some normal variations of disc appearance can look like pathological disc swelling (pseudo-papilloedema).

Optic atrophy

Loss of nerve fibres causes the optic disc to appear pale, as the choroid becomes visible (Fig. 26.26). A pale disc (optic atrophy) follows optic nerve damage, and causes include previous optic neuritis or ischaemic damage, long-standing papilloedema, optic nerve compression, trauma and degenerative conditions (e.g. Friedreich's ataxia, Box 26.88, p. 1222).

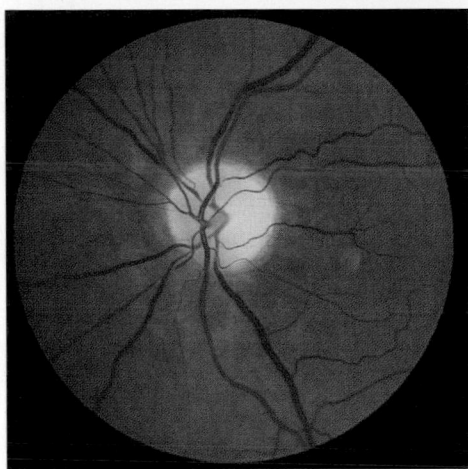

Fig. 26.26 Fundus photograph of the left eye of a patient with familial optic atrophy. Note marked pallor of optic disc.

SPHINCTER DISTURBANCE

Incontinence and its management are discussed on pages 167 and 474. However, many different symptoms of bladder and bowel disturbance can arise as a result of nervous system dysfunction.

BLADDER

The bladder is analogous to skeletal muscle in that neural control can be divided into upper and lower 'motor neuron' components. Conscious control of micturition resides within the pre-frontal cortex. Connections pass from here to the main controlling and coordinating centre in the pons, the pontine micturition centre, and from here down into the spinal cord, where they are found in the lateral columns bilaterally. The sympathetic supply to the bladder leaves from T10–L2 to synapse in the inferior hypogastric plexus, while the parasympathetic supply leaves from S2–4. In addition, a further somatic supply to the distal (voluntary) sphincter arises from S2–4, traveling via the pudendal nerves. Stimulation of sympathetic fibres causes relaxation of the detrusor muscle and contraction of the bladder neck, while stimulation of the parasympathetic fibres causes the reverse effects.

Afferent fibres from the bladder wall pass via the pelvic and hypogastric nerves. In the absence of conscious control (stroke, dementia), distension of the bladder to near-capacity evokes reflex detrusor contraction (analogous to the muscle stretch reflex). Reciprocal changes in sympathetic activation and relaxation of the distal sphincter result in coordinated bladder emptying. Normally, however, conscious control from the medial pre-frontal cortex inhibits bladder emptying until it is socially acceptable.

Damage to the 'lower motor neuron' component, i.e. the pelvic and pudendal nerves, gives rise to a flaccid bladder and sphincter with overflow incontinence, often accompanied by loss of pudendal sensation. Such damage may be due to disease of the conus medullaris or sacral nerve roots, either within the dura (as in inflammatory or carcinomatous

meningitis), or as they pass through the sacrum (trauma or malignancy), or due to damage to the nerves themselves in the pelvis (infection, haematoma, trauma or malignancy).

Damage to the pons or spinal cord results in an 'upper motor neuron' pattern of bladder dysfunction due to uncontrolled overactivity of the parasympathetic supply. The bladder is small and highly sensitive to being stretched (analogous to spasticity). This results in frequency, urgency and urge incontinence. The loss of the coordinating control of the pontine micturition centre will also result in the phenomenon of detrusor–sphincter dyssynergia, where detrusor contraction and sphincter relaxation are not coordinated; hence the spastic bladder will often try to empty against a closed sphincter. This manifests as both urgency and an inability to pass urine, which is distressing and painful, and may last some minutes before partial emptying of the bladder is achieved. There is often a post-micturition residuum of urine which is prone to infection, and the prolonged high bladder pressure may result in renal failure. More severe lesions of the spinal cord, as in spinal cord compression or trauma, can result in urinary retention; this will be painless as bladder sensation, normally carried in the lateral spinothalamic tracts, will be cut off.

Damage to the mesial frontal lobes gives rise to loss of awareness of bladder fullness and consequent incontinence. Coexisting cognitive impairment may result in inappropriate micturition. These features are seen typically in hydrocephalus, frontal tumours, dementia and bifrontal subdural haematomas.

When faced with a patient who has bladder symptoms, it is important to try to localise the lesion on the basis of history and examination, remembering that most bladder problems are not neurological unless there are overt neurological signs. Clinical features are summarised in Box 26.57.

Management of bladder disturbance involves identifying the cause and correcting it if possible. Overactive (spastic) bladders are common in neurological disease, and the unwanted detrusor activity (and hence urgency) can be lessened by anticholinergic drugs such as oxybutynin, tolterodine or imipramine. However, this will not solve the problem of detrusor–sphincter dyssynergia, and it may be necessary to teach the patient how to perform intermittent clean self-catheterisation (ISC); by emptying the bladder regularly, urinary frequency is reduced, as is the likelihood of infection. Bladder ultrasound is often helpful in this regard; a large (> 100 ml) post-micturition residual volume suggests that ISC will be necessary. Flaccid bladders are less common and unfortunately there is no effective drug treatment. These patients therefore need to perform ISC. Long-term catheterisation (urethral or suprapubic) may be necessary in either spastic or flaccid bladders, but this is avoided if at all possible as it is associated with increased infection as well as blockage.

RECTUM

The rectum has an excitatory cholinergic input from the parasympathetic sacral outflow, and inhibitory sympathetic supply similar to the bladder. Continence depends largely on skeletal muscle contraction in the puborectalis and pelvic

26.57 NEUROGENIC BLADDER: CLINICAL FEATURES AND TREATMENT

	Site of lesion	Result	Treatment
Atonic ('lower motor neuron')	Lesions of sacral segments of cord (conus medullaris) Lesions of sacral roots and nerves	Loss of detrusor contraction Difficulty initiating micturition Bladder distension with overflow	Intermittent self-catheterisation In-dwelling catheterisation

Hypertonic ('upper motor neuron')	Pyramidal tract lesion in spinal cord or brain stem	Urgency with urge incontinence
		Bladder sphincter incoordination (dyssynergia)
		Incomplete bladder emptying
			Anticholinergics
			  Oxybutynin (5 mg 8–12-hourly)
			  Imipramine (25 mg 12-hourly)
			  Tolterodine (2 mg 12-hourly)
			Intermittent self-catheterisation

Cortical	Post-central Pre-central Frontal	Loss of awareness of bladder fullness Difficulty initiating micturition Inappropriate micturition Loss of social control	Intermittent catheterisation

floor muscles supplied by the pudendal nerves, as well as the internal and external anal sphincters. Damage to the autonomic components usually causes constipation but diabetic neuropathy can be associated with diarrhoea. Lesions affecting the conus medullaris, the somatic S2–4 roots and the pudendal nerves cause faecal incontinence.

PENILE ERECTION AND EJACULATION

These related functions are under autonomic control via the pelvic nerves (parasympathetic, S2–4) and hypogastric nerves (sympathetic, L1–2). Descending influences from the cerebrum are important for psychogenic erection, but erection can occur as a purely reflex phenomenon in response to genital stimulation. Erection is largely parasympathetic, mediated by nitric oxide, and is impaired by drugs which have anticholinergic effects and also by some antihypertensive and antidepressant agents. Sympathetic activity is important for ejaculation, and may be inhibited by α-adrenoceptor antagonists (α-blockers). For further information on erectile impotence, see page 476.

CEREBROVASCULAR DISEASE

Stroke is the third most common cause of death in the developed world after cancer and ischaemic heart disease, and is the most common cause of severe physical disability. It is the most frequent clinical manifestation of diseases of the cerebral blood vessels, although cerebrovascular disease may present, particularly in the elderly, as a dementia (p. 1188). Traditionally, the term 'stroke' has been used to include episodes of focal brain dysfunction due to focal ischaemia or haemorrhage as well as subarachnoid haemorrhage (SAH). However, because SAH has rather different clinical manifestations, underlying pathology and management, it is dealt with separately (p. 1210).

Stroke is a common medical emergency with an annual incidence of between 180 and 300 per 100 000. The incidence rises steeply with age, and in many developing countries, the incidence is rising because of the adoption of less healthy lifestyles. About one-fifth of patients with an acute stroke will die within a month of the event, and at least half of those who survive will be left with physical disability.

ACUTE STROKE

Acute stroke is characterised by the rapid appearance (usually over minutes) of a focal deficit of brain function, most commonly a hemiplegia with or without signs of focal higher cerebral dysfunction (such as aphasia), hemisensory loss, visual field defect or brain-stem deficit. Provided that there is a clear history of a rapid-onset focal deficit, the chance of the brain lesion being anything other than vascular is 5% or less. However, care needs to be taken to exclude other differential diagnoses if the symptoms progress over hours or days, and could be explained by causes other than focal cerebral dysfunction. Confusion, memory or balance disturbance may reflect focal deficits but are more often due to other causes.

Clinical classification of stroke

Several terms have been used to classify strokes, often based on duration and evolution of symptoms.

- *Transient ischaemic attack (TIA).* This describes strokes in which symptoms resolve within 24 hours—an arbitrary cut off which has little value in practice apart from perhaps indicating that underlying cerebral haemorrhage or extensive cerebral infarction is extremely unlikely. The term TIA traditionally also includes patients with transient monocular blindness (also known as amaurosis fugax), usually due to a vascular occlusion in the retina. Transient symptoms, such as syncope, amnesia, confusion and dizziness, which do not reflect focal cerebral dysfunction, are often mistakenly attributed to TIA (Fig. 26.12, p. 1165, and Box 26.58).
- In epidemiological studies, the term *stroke* is reserved for those events in which symptoms last more than 24 hours. The differential diagnosis of patients with symptoms lasting a few minutes or hours is similar to those with persisting symptoms (Box 26.58).
- *Progressing stroke (or stroke in evolution).* This describes a stroke in which the focal neurological deficit

worsens after the patient first presents. Such worsening may be due to increasing volume of infarction, haemorrhage or related oedema.

- *Completed stroke.* This describes a stroke in which the focal deficit persists and is not progressing.

In clinical practice, it is probably most important to distinguish those patients with strokes who, when seen, have persisting focal neurological symptoms, from those whose symptoms have resolved. When assessing a patient within hours of symptom onset, it is not possible to distinguish stroke from TIA unless the symptoms have already resolved. In patients with persisting symptoms, it is necessary to confirm the diagnosis and then consider treatments to reverse the underlying pathology, prevent complications, alleviate the functional consequences of any persisting neurological impairments and reduce the risks of further stroke or other vascular events. In those patients without persisting symptoms, the emphasis should be on confirming the diagnosis and preventing further vascular events.

Clinical features

The clinical assessment provides an estimate of the site of the lesion (i.e. which arterial territory is involved) and its size, both of which will have a bearing on management, such as suitability for carotid endarterectomy. The neurological deficits can be identified from the patient's history and, if these are persistent, from the neurological examination. The presence of a unilateral motor deficit, higher cerebral function deficit (e.g. aphasia or neglect) or a visual field defect usually places the lesion in the cerebral hemisphere. Ataxia, diplopia, vertigo and/or bilateral weakness usually indicate a lesion in the brain stem or cerebellum. Different combinations of these deficits can define several stroke syndromes (Fig. 26.27) which reflect the site and size of the lesion and may provide clues to underlying pathology.

Reduced conscious level usually indicates a large-volume lesion in the cerebral hemisphere but may result from a lesion in the brain stem or complications such as obstructive hydrocephalus, hypoxia or severe systemic infection.

Clinical assessment of the patient with a stroke should also include a general examination (Box 26.59) since this may provide clues to the cause of the stroke, and identify important comorbidities and complications of the stroke.

Pathology

Of patients presenting with a stroke, 85% will have sustained a cerebral infarction due to inadequate blood flow to part of the brain. The remainder will have had an intracerebral haemorrhage. Brain imaging is required to

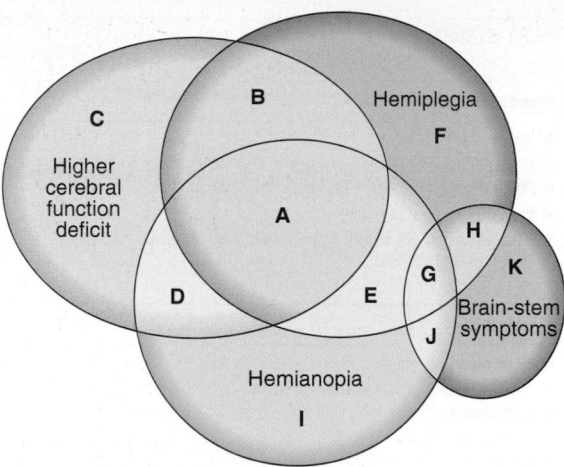

Fig. 26.27 Syndromes of acute stroke. Total anterior circulation syndrome—TACS (A). Partial anterior circulation syndromes—PACS (B, C, D and E). Pure motor stroke—lacunar syndrome (F). Posterior circulation syndromes—POCS (G, H, I, J and K).

distinguish these pathologies and to guide management. The combination of severe headache and vomiting at the onset of the focal neurological deficits increases the likelihood of a haemorrhagic stroke.

CEREBRAL INFARCTION

Cerebral infarction is mostly due to thromboembolic disease secondary to atherosclerosis in the major extracranial

26.60 STROKE RISK FACTORS

Fixed

- Age
- Gender (male > female, except in the very young and very old)
- Race (Afro-Caribbean > Asian > European)
- Heredity
- Previous vascular event, e.g. myocardial infarction, stroke or peripheral embolism
- High fibrinogen

Modifiable

- High blood pressure
- Heart disease (atrial fibrillation, heart failure, endocarditis)
- Diabetes mellitus
- Hyperlipidaemia
- Smoking
- Excess alcohol consumption
- Polycythaemia
- Oral contraceptives
- Social deprivation

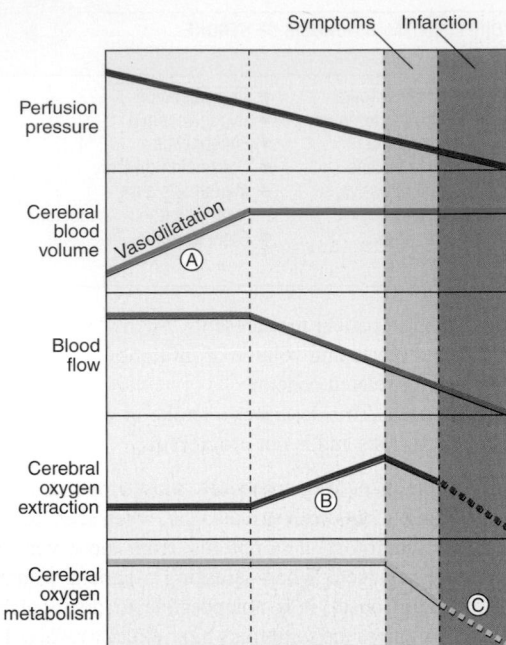

Fig. 26.28 Homeostatic responses to falling perfusion pressure in the brain following arterial occlusion. Vasodilatation initially maintains cerebral blood flow (A), but after maximal vasodilatation further falls in perfusion pressure lead to a decline in blood flow. An increase in tissue oxygen extraction, however, maintains the cerebral metabolic rate for oxygen (B). Still further falls in perfusion, and therefore blood flow, cannot be compensated; cerebral oxygen availability falls and symptoms appear, then infarction (C).

arteries (carotid artery and aortic arch). About 20% of infarctions are due to embolism from the heart, and a further 20% are due to intrinsic disease of small perforating vessels (lenticulostriate arteries), producing so-called 'lacunar' infarctions. The risk factors for ischaemic stroke reflect the risk factors for the underlying vascular disease (Box 26.60). Perhaps 5% are due to rare causes, including vasculitis (p. 1138), endocarditis (p. 629) and cerebral venous disease (p. 1211).

Pathophysiology

Cerebral infarction is a process which takes some hours to complete, even though the patient's deficit may be maximal close to the onset of the causative vascular occlusion. After the occlusion of a cerebral artery, the opening of anastomotic channels from other arterial territories may restore perfusion to its territory. Similarly, a reduction in perfusion pressure leads to compensatory homeostatic changes to maintain oxygenation (Fig. 26.28). These changes can sometimes prevent even occlusion of a carotid artery from having any clinically apparent effect.

However, if and when these homeostatic mechanisms fail, the process of ischaemia starts and ultimately leads to infarction. As the cerebral blood flow declines, different neuronal functions fail at various thresholds (Fig. 26.29). Once blood flow falls below the threshold for the maintenance of electrical activity, neurological deficit appears. At this level of blood flow, the neurons are still viable; if the blood flow increases again, function returns and the patient will have had a transient ischaemic attack. However, if the blood flow falls further, a level is reached at which the process of cell death starts. Hypoxia leads to an inadequate supply of adenosine triphosphate (ATP), which in turn leads to failure of membrane pumps, thereby allowing influx of sodium and water into the cell (cytotoxic oedema) and the release of the excitatory neurotransmitter glutamate into the extracellular fluid. Glutamate opens membrane channels, allowing the influx of calcium and more sodium into the neurons. Calcium entering the neurons

activates intracellular enzymes that complete the destructive process. The release of inflammatory mediators by microglia and astrocytes produces death of all cell types in the area of maximum ischaemia. The infarction process is worsened by the anaerobic production of lactic acid (Fig. 26.30) and consequent fall in tissue pH. Attempts to produce 'neuroprotective drugs' to slow down the processes leading to irreversible cell death have so far been largely disappointing (p. 1208).

The final result of the occlusion of a cerebral blood vessel therefore depends upon the competence of the circulatory homeostatic mechanisms, and the severity and duration of the reduction in blood flow. Higher brain temperature, as might occur in fever, and higher blood sugar have both been associated with a greater volume of infarction for a given reduction in cerebral blood flow. If ischaemic damage has occurred to the vascular endothelium, subsequent restoration of blood flow may cause haemorrhage into the infarcted area (so-called haemorrhagic transformation). This is particularly likely to occur in larger infarcts, in patients given antithrombotic and thrombolytic drugs, and possibly following embolic occlusion when the embolus is lysed by the blood's intrinsic thrombolytic mechanisms.

Radiologically, a cerebral infarct can be seen as a lesion which comprises brain tissue that is ischaemic and swollen but recoverable (the ischaemic penumbra), as well as dead brain tissue that is already undergoing autolysis. The infarct swells with time and is at its maximal size a couple of days

26

Cerebral blood flow
ml/100 g/min

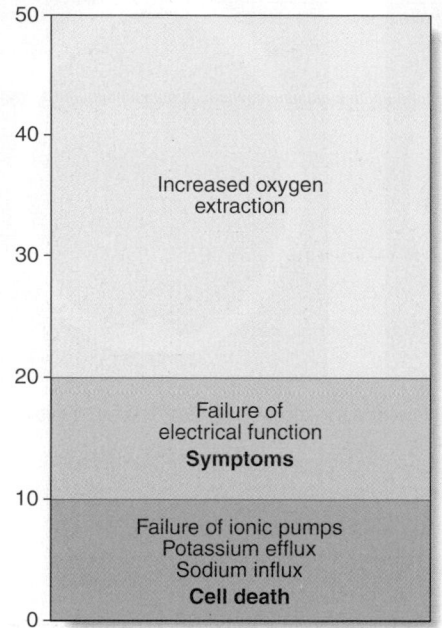

Fig. 26.29   **Thresholds of cerebral ischaemia.** Symptoms of cerebral ischaemia appear when the blood flow has fallen to less than half of normal and energy supply is insufficient to sustain neuronal electrical function. Full recovery can occur unless this level of flow is sustained for long periods. Further blood flow reduction below the next threshold causes failure of cell ionic pumps and starts the ischaemic cascade, leading to cell death. Brain tissue can sustain such depths of blood flow reduction only for brief periods without infarction.

after the stroke onset. At this stage it may be big enough to exert some mass effect both clinically and radiologically. As the weeks go by, the oedema subsides and the infarcted area is replaced by a sharply defined fluid-filled cavity.

INTRACEREBRAL HAEMORRHAGE

This usually results from rupture of a blood vessel within the brain parenchyma: a primary intracerebral haemorrhage. It may also occur in a patient with a subarachnoid haemorrhage if the artery ruptures into the brain substance as well as into the subarachnoid space (p. 1210). Haemorrhage frequently occurs into an area of brain infarction; if the volume of haemorrhage is large, this may be difficult to distinguish from primary intracerebral haemorrhage both

26.61 CAUSES OF INTRACEREBRAL HAEMORRHAGE AND ASSOCIATED RISK FACTORS	
Disease	**Risk factors**
Complex small vessel disease with disruption of vessel wall	Age Hypertension
Amyloid angiopathy	Familial (rare) Age
Impaired blood clotting	Anticoagulant therapy Blood dyscrasia Thrombolytic therapy
Vascular anomaly	Arteriovenous malformation Cavernous haemangioma
Substance misuse	Alcohol Amphetamines Cocaine

26

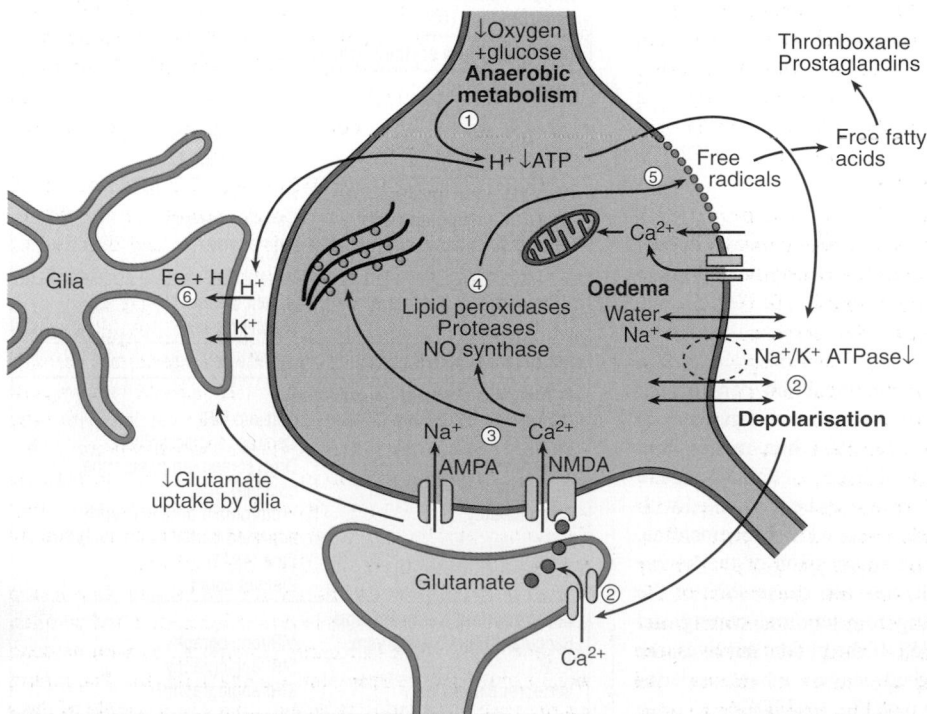

Fig. 26.30   **The process of neuronal ischaemia and infarction.** (1) Reduction of blood flow reduces supply of oxygen and hence ATP. H^+ is produced by anaerobic metabolism of available glucose. (2) Energy-dependent membrane ionic pumps fail, leading to cytotoxic oedema and membrane depolarisation, allowing calcium entry and releasing glutamate. (3) Calcium enters cells via glutamate-gated channels and (4) activates destructive intracellular enzymes, (5) destroying intracellular organelles and cell membrane, with release of free radicals. Free fatty acid release activates pro-coagulant pathways which exacerbate local ischaemia. (6) Glial cells take up H^+, can no longer take up extracellular glutamate and also suffer cell death, leading to liquefactive necrosis of whole arterial territory.

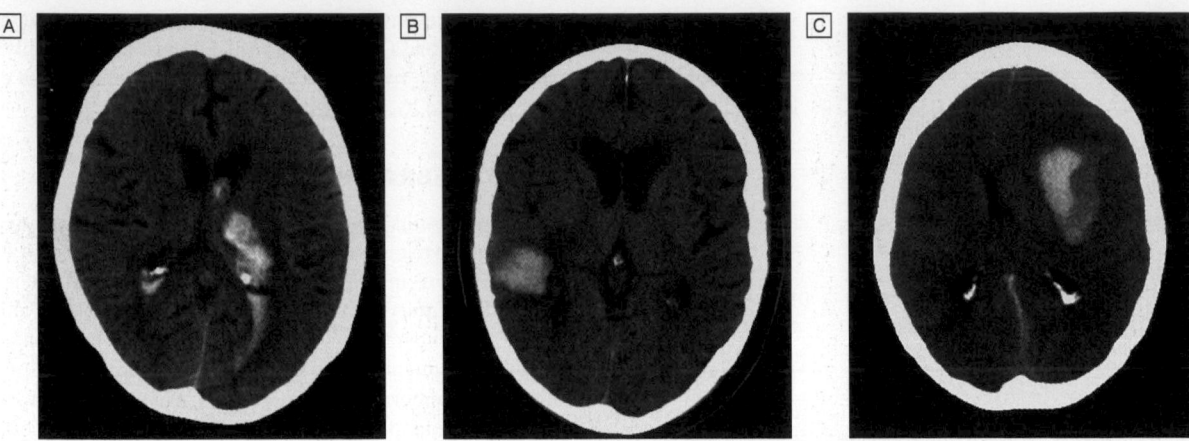

Fig. 26.31   CT scans of intracerebral haemorrhage. Ⓐ Basal ganglia haemorrhage with intraventricular extension. Ⓑ Small cortical haemorrhage. Ⓒ Large haemorrhage with mass effects.

26

26.62 INVESTIGATION OF A PATIENT WITH AN ACUTE STROKE	
Diagnostic question	**Investigation**
Is it a vascular lesion?	CT/MRI
Is it ischaemic or haemorrhagic?	CT/MRI
Is it a subarachnoid haemorrhage?	CT Lumbar puncture
Is there any cardiac source of embolism?	Electrocardiogram (ECG) Echocardiogram
What is the underlying vascular disease?	Duplex ultrasound of carotids Magnetic resonance angiography (MRA) CT angiography (CTA) Contrast angiography
What are the risk factors?	Full blood count Cholesterol Blood glucose
Is there an unusual cause?	ESR Clotting/thrombophilia screen

26.63 CAUSES AND INVESTIGATION OF ACUTE STROKE IN YOUNG PATIENTS	
Cause	**Investigation**
Cardiac embolism	Echocardiography (including transoesophageal)
Premature atherosclerosis	Serum lipids
Arterial dissection	MRI Angiography
Thrombophilia	Protein C Protein S Antithrombin III
Homocystinuria (p. 442)	Urinary amino acids Methionine loading test
Antiphospolipid antibody syndrome (p. 1062)	Anticardiolipin antibodies/lupus anticoagulant
Systemic lupus erythematosus	Antinuclear antibodies
Vasculitis	ESR CRP Antineutrophil cytoplasmic antibody (ANCA)
CADASIL (Cerebral Autosomal Dominant Ateriopathy with Subcortical Infarcts and Leucoencephalopathy)	MRI brain Genetic analysis Skin biopsy
Mitochondrial cytopathy	Serum lactate Muscle biopsy
Neurovascular syphilis	Syphilis serology
Primary intracerebral haemorrhage Arteriovenous malformation (AVM) Drug misuse Coagulopathy	Delayed MRI Contrast angiography Drug screen (amphetamine, cocaine) Prothrombin time (PT) and activated partial thromboplastin time (APTT) Platelet count
Subarachnoid haemorrhage Saccular ('berry') aneurysm AVM Vertebral dissection	MRI/angiography MRI/angiography MRI/angiography

clinically and radiologically (Fig. 26.33C, p. 1206). The risk factors and underlying causes of intracerebral haemorrhage are listed in Box 26.61.

Pathophysiology

The explosive entry of blood into the brain parenchyma causes immediate cessation of function in that area as neurons are structurally disrupted and white matter fibre tracts are split apart. The haemorrhage itself may expand over the first minutes or hours or it may be associated with a rim of cerebral oedema, which, along with the haematoma, acts like a mass lesion to cause progression of the neurological deficits. If big enough, this can cause shift of the intracranial contents, producing transtentorial coning and sometimes rapid death (p. 1235). If the patient survives, the haematoma is gradually absorbed, leaving a haemosiderin-lined slit in the brain parenchyma (Fig. 26.32D).

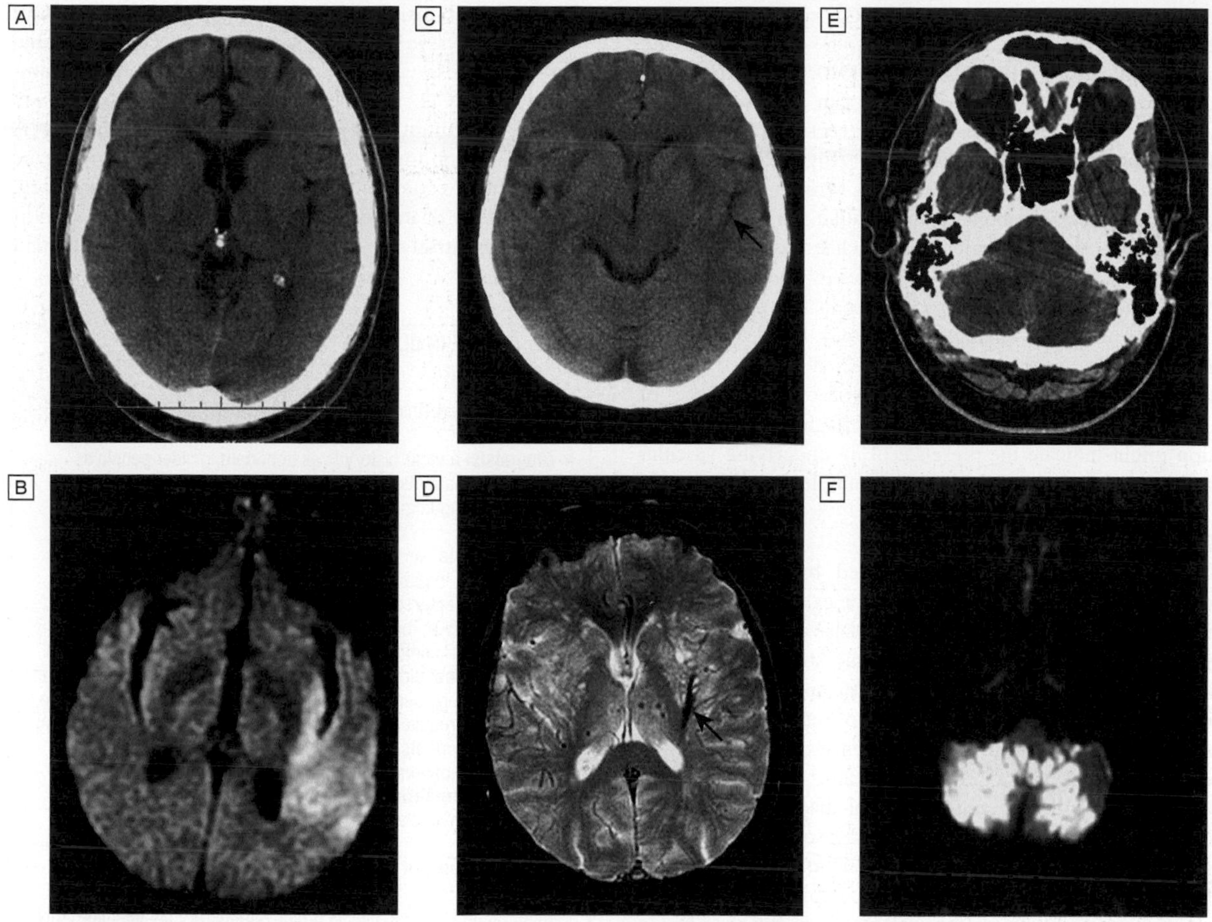

Fig 26.32 Acute stroke seen in CT scans with corresponding MRI appearances. A CT may show no evidence of early infarction. B Corresponding image seen on MRI diffusion weighted imaging (DWI) with changes in MCA territory. C Late appearance of haemorrhage on CT (arrow). D Corresponding appearance on gradient echo MRI (arrow). E Subtle appearance of massive cerebellar infarction on CT. F Corresponding appearance more obvious on DWI MRI.

INVESTIGATION OF ACUTE STROKE

Investigation of a patient presenting with an acute stroke aims to confirm the vascular nature of the lesion, distinguish cerebral infarction from haemorrhage and identify the underlying vascular disease and risk factors (Box 26.62).

Initial investigation of all patients with stroke includes a range of simple blood tests to detect common vascular risk factors and markers of rarer causes, an electrocardiogram and brain imaging. Where there is uncertainty about the nature of the stroke, further investigations are usually indicated. This especially applies to younger patients who are less likely to have atherosclerotic disease (Box 26.63).

Imaging the brain

Brain imaging with either CT or MRI should be performed in all patients with stroke. Exceptions to this include patients in whom the brain scan results would not influence management, such as the patient who has a stroke in the latter stages of a terminal illness.

CT is the most practical and widely available method of imaging the brain. It will usually exclude non-stroke lesions,

> **26.64 INDICATIONS FOR AN IMMEDIATE CT/MRI IN ACUTE STROKE**
>
> - Patient on anticoagulants or with abnormal coagulation
> - Plan to give thrombolysis or immediate anticoagulants
> - Deteriorating conscious level or rapidly progressing deficits
> - Suspected cerebellar haematoma, to exclude hydrocephalus

including subdural haematomas and brain tumours. It will demonstrate intracerebral haemorrhage within minutes of stroke onset (Fig. 26.31). However, especially within the first few hours after symptom onset, CT changes in cerebral infarction may be completely absent or very subtle, though changes usually evolve over time (Fig. 26.32). For most purposes, a CT scan performed within the first day or so is adequate for clinical care but there are certain circumstances in which an immediate CT scan is essential (Box 26.64). Even in the absence of changes suggesting infarction, abnormal perfusion of brain tissue can be imaged with CT after injection of contrast media (i.e. perfusion scanning). This can be useful in guiding hyper-acute treatment of ischaemic stroke.

26

MRI is not as widely available as CT, scanning times are longer and it cannot be used in some individuals with contraindications (Box 26.4, p. 1156). However, MRI diffusion weighted imaging (DWI) can detect ischaemia earlier than CT, and other MRI sequences can also be used to demonstrate abnormal perfusion (Fig. 26.32). MRI is more sensitive than CT in detecting strokes affecting the brain stem and cerebellum, and unlike CT, can reliably distinguish haemorrhagic from ischaemic stroke even several weeks after the onset (Fig. 26.32C and D).

CT and MRI may reveal clues as to the nature of the arterial lesion. For example, there may be a small, deep lacunar infarct indicating small vessel disease, or a more peripheral infarct suggesting an extracranial source of embolism (Fig. 26.33B). In a haemorrhagic lesion, the location might indicate the presence of an underlying vascular malformation, saccular aneurysm or amyloid angiopathy.

Imaging blood vessels

Many ischaemic strokes are caused by atherosclerotic thromboembolic disease of the major extracranial vessels. Detection of extracranial vascular disease can help establish why the patient has had an ischaemic stroke and may, in highly selected patients, lead on to specific treatments including carotid endarterectomy to reduce the risk of further stroke (p. 1210). The presence or absence of a carotid bruit is not a reliable indicator of the degree of carotid stenosis. Extracranial arterial disease can be non-invasively identified with duplex ultrasound, MR angiography (MRA) or CT angiography (Fig. 26.11, p. 1159). Because of the significant risk of complications, intra-arterial contrast angiography is reserved for patients in whom non-invasive methods have provided contradictory or incomplete information, or in whom it is necessary to image the intracranial circulation in detail: for example, to delineate a saccular aneurysm, an arteriovenous malformation or vasculitis.

Detecting a cardiac source of embolism

Approximately 20% of ischaemic strokes are thought to be due to embolism from the heart. The most common causes of cardiac embolism are atrial fibrillation, prosthetic heart valves, other valvular abnormalities and recent myocardial infarction. These can often be identified by clinical examination and ECG. However, cardiac sources of embolism can exist without obvious clinical or ECG signs. A transthoracic or transoesophageal echocardiogram can be useful, either to confirm the presence of a clinically apparent cardiac source or to identify an unsuspected source such as endocarditis, atrial myxoma, intracardiac thrombus or patent

26.65 STROKE IN OLD AGE

- **Incidence:** two-thirds of stroke patients are aged over 60 years.
- **Diagnosis:** a clear history is as important in older people as in younger patients, but will be more difficult to obtain if there is pre-existing cognitive impairment or communication difficulties.
- **Thrombolysis:** very few data are available concerning the risk and benefits in patients over 80 years.
- **Carotid endarterectomy:** the benefits accrue quickly after transient stroke; therefore, when it is indicated, advanced age alone is not a contraindication to surgery.
- **Comorbidities:** older patients with stroke are more likely to have other pathology such as ischaemic heart disease, cardiac failure, chronic obstructive pulmonary disease (COPD), osteoarthritis and visual impairments. All will have to be addressed as part of overall management.
- **Cognitive impairment:** adversely affects outcome, as much of rehabilitation involves the learning and retention of new skills (p. 169).
- **Over-diagnosis of recurrent stroke:** the reappearance of neurological signs from a previous stroke in a patient who has other acute systemic illness or is hypotensive may be incorrectly attributed to a new event.
- **Diffuse small-vessel cerebrovascular disease:** very common, and may present insidiously with gait abnormalities and/or significant memory impairment. It also predisposes to confusional states when intercurrent infection or metabolic disturbance supervenes.
- **Anticoagulation for secondary prevention after stroke:** may be indicated in certain circumstances, but must be used with caution because the associated risks in frail older patients are higher due to comorbidity, falls, cognitive impairment and interaction with other medication.

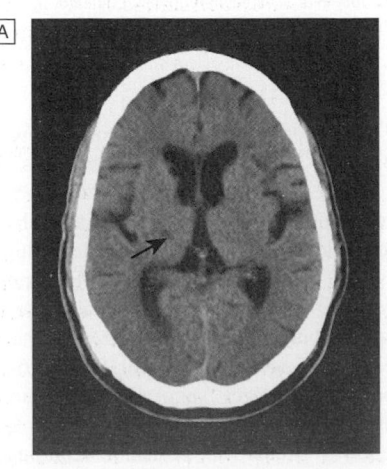
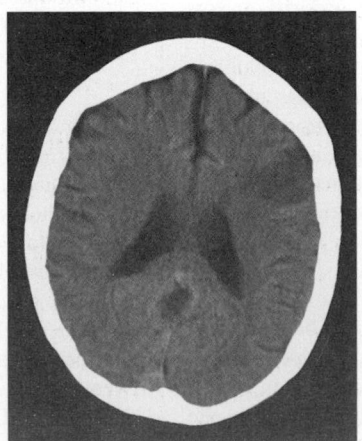
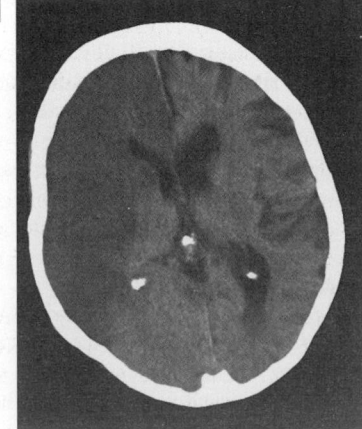

Fig 26.33 CT scans in ischaemic stroke. A Typical appearance of a lacunar infarct in the basal ganglia (arrow). B Small cortical infarct. C Large middle and anterior cerebral artery territory infarct with mass effect.

26.66 COMPLICATIONS OF ACUTE STROKE

Complication	Prevention	Treatment
Chest infection	Nurse semi-erect Avoid aspiration	Antibiotics Physiotherapy
Epileptic seizures	Maintain cerebral oxygenation Avoid metabolic disturbance	Anticonvulsants
Deep venous thrombosis/pulmonary embolism	Maintain hydration Early mobilisation Anti-embolism stockings Heparin (for high-risk patients only)	Anticoagulation (exclude haemorrhagic stroke first)
Painful shoulder	Avoid traction injury Shoulder/arm supports Physiotherapy	Physiotherapy Local corticosteroid injections
Pressure sores	Frequent turning Monitor pressure areas Avoid urinary damage to skin	Nursing care Pressure-relieving mattress
Urinary infection	Avoid catheterisation if possible Use penile sheath	Antibiotics
Constipation	Appropriate aperients and diet	Appropriate aperients
Depression and anxiety	Maintain positive attitude and provide information	Antidepressants

26.67 SPECIALIST STROKE UNITS

EBM

'Admitting 1000 patients to a stroke unit prevents about 50 patients from being dead or dependent at 6 months.'

- Langhorne P, Pollock A in conjunction with the Stroke Unit Trialists Collaboration. Age Ageing 2002; 31:365–371.

For further information: 🖥 www.cochrane.org

foramen ovale. Such findings may lead on to specific treatment (Ch. 18).

GENERAL MANAGEMENT OF PATIENTS WITH ACUTE STROKE

Management is aimed at minimising the volume of brain that is irreversibly damaged, preventing complications (Box 26.66), reducing the patient's disability and handicap through rehabilitation, and reducing the risk of recurrent episodes. Early admission of patients to a specialised stroke unit facilitates coordinated care from a specialised multi-disciplinary team (Ch. 7) and has been shown to reduce both mortality and residual disability amongst survivors (Box 26.67). Consideration of a patient's rehabilitation needs should commence at the same time as acute medical management.

Dysphagia is common after stroke and can be detected by an early bedside test of swallowing, which allows hydration, feeding and medication to be given safely, if necessary by nasogastric tube or intravenously. In the acute phase it may be useful to refer to a checklist (Box 26.68) to ensure that all the factors which might influence the patient's outcome have been addressed.

The deteriorating stroke patient

The patient's neurological deficits may worsen during the hours or days after their onset. This is probably most common amongst those with lacunar infarction but may occur in other patients, due to extension of the area of infarction, haemorrhage into it or the development of oedema with consequent mass effect. It is important to distinguish such patients from those who are deteriorating as a result of complications such as hypoxia, sepsis, epileptic seizures or metabolic abnormalities which may be more easily reversed. Patients with cerebellar haematomas or infarcts with mass effect may develop obstructive hydrocephalus and some will benefit from insertion of a ventricular drain and/or decompressive surgery. Some patients with large haematomas or infarction with massive oedema in the cerebral hemispheres may benefit from anti-oedema agents, such as mannitol, artificial ventilation and/or surgical decompression to reduce intracranial pressure, although evidence for the effectiveness of these interventions is still incomplete.

Specific medical treatment for ischaemic stroke

Thrombolysis and other revascularisation treatments

Intravenous thrombolysis with recombinant tissue plasminogen activator (rt-PA) increases the risk of haemorrhagic transformation of the cerebral infarct with potentially fatal results. However, if given within 3 hours of symptom onset to highly selected patients, the haemorrhagic risk may be offset by an improvement in overall outcome (Box 26.69). Alternative methods of revascularisation, including intra-arterial thrombolysis, mechanical dissolution or removal of the thrombus, are used but little evidence is available concerning the balance of risks and benefits.

26

26.68 ACUTE STROKE MANAGEMENT: ADMISSION CHECKLIST

Airway

- Is the patient able to protect his/her airway?
- Can the patient swallow without evidence of aspiration?
- Perform a swallow screen and keep patient nil by mouth if swallowing unsafe

Breathing

- Is the patient breathing adequately?
- Check oxygen saturation and give supplementary oxygen if oxygen saturation < 95%

Circulation

- Are peripheral perfusion, pulse and blood pressure adequate?
- Treat with fluid replacement, anti-arrhythmics and inotropic drugs as appropriate

Hydration

- Is the patient dehydrated or unable to swallow?
- Give fluids parenterally or by nasogastric tube if swallow is unsafe

Nutrition

- Assess nutritional status
- Consider nutritional supplements
- If dysphagia persists for a day or two, start feeding via a nasogastric tube

Medication

- If the patient is dysphagic, consider alternative routes for essential medications

Blood pressure

- Unless there is heart failure or renal failure, evidence of hypertensive encephalopathy or aortic dissection, do not lower the blood pressure in the first week since it will often return towards the patient's normal level within the first few days
- Early blood pressure reduction may decrease cerebral perfusion and increase infarction to offset potential benefits. Trials of early blood pressure lowering are ongoing

Blood glucose

- Is the blood glucose ≥ 11.1 mmol/l (200 mg/dl)?
- Hyperglycaemia may increase infarct volume, therefore use insulin (via infusion or glucose/potassium/insulin (GKI)) to normalise levels but monitor closely to avoid hypoglycaemia
- Trials of more rigorous glycaemic control are ongoing

Temperature

- Is the patient pyrexial?
- Raised brain temperature may increase infarct volume
- Investigate and treat any cause but give antipyretics early

Pressure areas

- These should be formally assessed and measures taken to reduce the risk
- Treat infection, maintain nutrition, provide a pressure-relieving mattress and turn immobile patients regularly

Incontinence

- Ensure the patient is not constipated or in urinary retention
- Avoid urinary catheterisation unless the patient is in acute urinary retention or incontinence is threatening pressure areas

---

26.69 THROMBOLYSIS IN ACUTE ISCHAEMIC STROKE — EBM

'rt-PA increases the risk of fatal intracranial haemorrhage, but this risk is offset by an improvement in longer-term outcome amongst survivors. The maximum benefit appears to be when thrombolysis is given within 3 hours of onset. Treating 1000 patients within 3 hours prevents about 60 patients from being dead or dependent at 3 months.'

- Wardlaw JM, et al. (Cochrane Review). Cochrane Library, issue 4, 2005. Oxford: Update Software.
- Mielke O, Wardlaw JM, Liu M (Cochrane Review). Cochrane Library, issue 4, 2005. Oxford: Update Software.

For further information: 💻 www.cochrane.org

26.70 ASPIRIN IN ACUTE ISCHAEMIC STROKE — EBM

'After an acute persistent stroke, aspirin started within 48 hours of onset improves long-term outcome. Treating 1000 patients for 2 weeks prevents 13 being dead or dependent by 6 months.'

- Gubitz G, et al. (Cochrane Review). Cochrane Library, issue 3, 2004. Oxford: Update Software.
- Chen ZM, et al. on behalf of the CAST and IST Collaborative Groups. Stroke 2000; 31:1240–1249.

For further information: 💻 www.cochrane.org

Aspirin

Aspirin (300 mg daily) should be started immediately after an ischaemic stroke unless rt-PA has been given, in which case it should be withheld for at least 24 hours. Aspirin reduces the risk of early recurrence and has a small but clinically worthwhile effect on long-term outcome (Box 26.70); it may be given by rectal suppository or by nasogastric tube in dysphagic patients.

Heparin

Formal anticoagulation with heparin has been widely used in treating acute ischaemic stroke in the past. Whilst this does reduce the risk of early ischaemic recurrence and venous thromboembolism, these benefits are offset by a definite increase in the risk of both intracranial and extracranial haemorrhage. Furthermore, routine use of heparin does not result in better long-term outcomes, and therefore it should not be used in the routine management of acute stroke. It is unclear whether anticoagulation with heparin might provide benefit in selected patients, such as those with recent myocardial infarction, arterial dissection or progressing strokes. Intracranial haemorrhage must be excluded on brain imaging before considering anticoagulation.

Corticosteroids, haemodilution, vasodilators and 'neuroprotective' agents

Routine use of these agents should be avoided since they may all have adverse effects and none has been shown to improve patient outcomes.

Specific treatment for haemorrhagic stroke

Coagulation abnormalities, most commonly due to oral anticoagulants, should be reversed as quickly as possible to reduce the likelihood of the haematoma enlarging. Promising research suggests that, in highly selected patients,

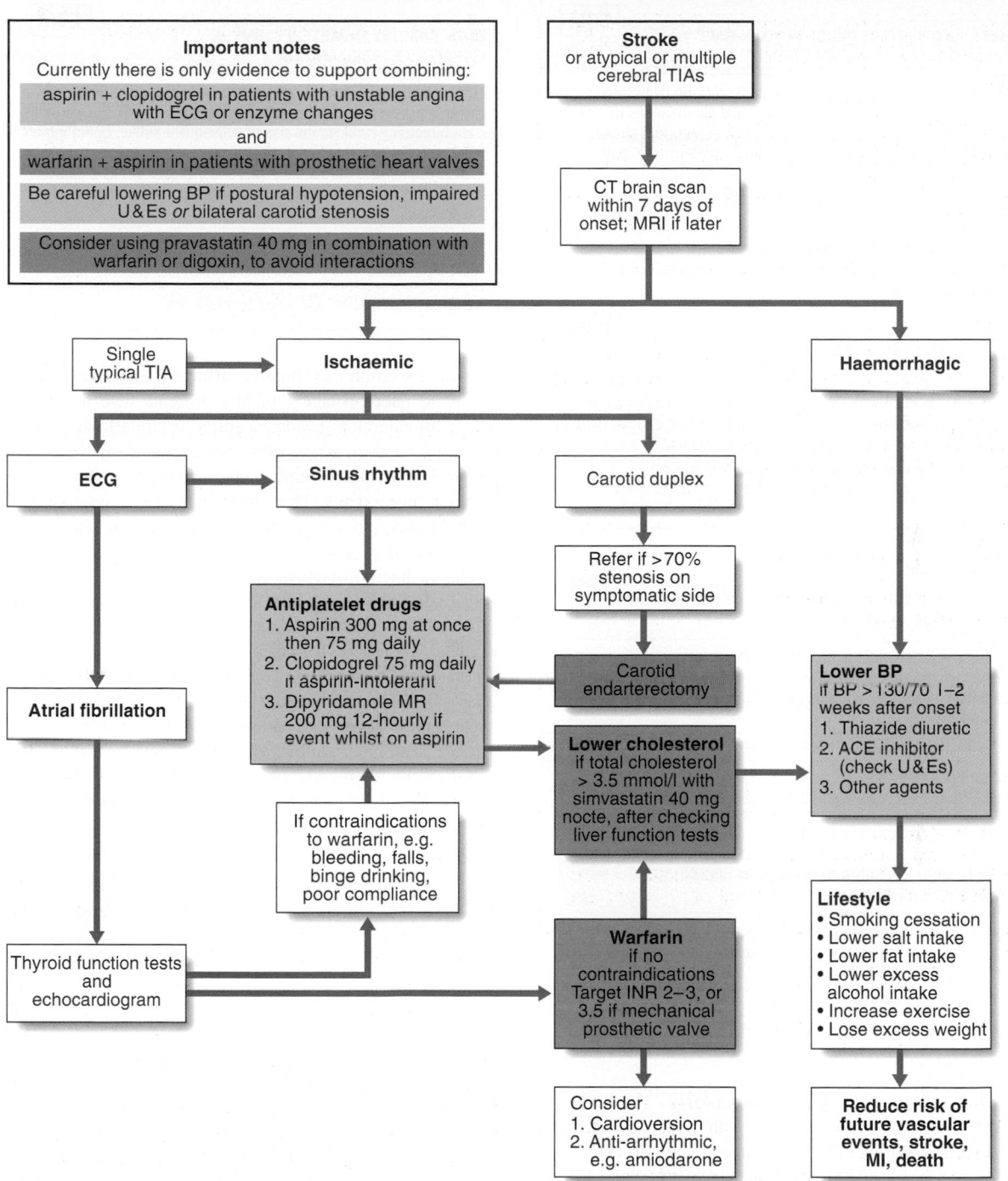

Important notes
Currently there is only evidence to support combining:

aspirin + clopidogrel in patients with unstable angina with ECG or enzyme changes

and

warfarin + aspirin in patients with prosthetic heart valves

Be careful lowering BP if postural hypotension, impaired U&Es *or* bilateral carotid stenosis

Consider using pravastatin 40 mg in combination with warfarin or digoxin, to avoid interactions

Stroke
or atypical or multiple cerebral TIAs

CT brain scan within 7 days of onset; MRI if later

Ischaemic

Haemorrhagic

Single typical TIA

ECG

Sinus rhythm

Carotid duplex

Refer if >70% stenosis on symptomatic side

Antiplatelet drugs
1. Aspirin 300 mg at once then 75 mg daily
2. Clopidogrel 75 mg daily if aspirin-intolerant
3. Dipyridamole MR 200 mg 12-hourly if event whilst on aspirin

Carotid endarterectomy

Lower BP
if BP > 130/70 1–2 weeks after onset
1. Thiazide diuretic
2. ACE inhibitor (check U&Es)
3. Other agents

Atrial fibrillation

If contraindications to warfarin, e.g. bleeding, falls, binge drinking, poor compliance

Lower cholesterol
if total cholesterol > 3.5 mmol/l with simvastatin 40 mg nocte, after checking liver function tests

Lifestyle
• Smoking cessation
• Lower salt intake
• Lower fat intake
• Lower excess alcohol intake
• Increase exercise
• Lose excess weight

Thyroid function tests and echocardiogram

Warfarin
if no contraindications
Target INR 2–3, or 3.5 if mechanical prosthetic valve

Consider
1. Cardioversion
2. Anti-arrhythmic, e.g. amiodarone

Reduce risk of future vascular events, stroke, MI, death

26

Fig 26.34 Secondary prevention strategy for stroke.

haematoma enlargement may be reduced by the early administration of recombinant factor VII even in patients without a clotting problem.

Reducing the risk of further strokes and other vascular problems (Fig. 26.34)

The average risk of a further stroke is 5–10% within the first week of a stroke or TIA, perhaps 15% in the first year and 5% per year thereafter. The risks are not clearly different for intracerebral haemorrhage. Patients with ischaemic events should be put on long-term antiplatelet drugs (Box 26.71) and statins to lower cholesterol (Box 26.72). For patients in atrial fibrillation the risk can be reduced by about 60% by oral anticoagulation to achieve an INR of 2–3 (Box 26.73). The risk of recurrence after both ischaemic and haemorrhagic strokes can be reduced by blood pressure reduction, even for those with blood pressures in the normal range (Box 26.74).

26.71 ANTIPLATELET DRUGS IN SECONDARY PREVENTION OF ISCHAEMIC STROKE `EBM`

'Ongoing treatment with either aspirin 75–300 mg daily, clopidogrel 75 mg daily or a combination of aspirin and dipyridamole modified release 200 mg 12-hourly reduces the risk of recurrent stroke, myocardial infarction and vascular deaths. Treating 1000 patients for a year prevents about 10 strokes.'

- Antithrombotic Trialists' Collaboration. BMJ 2002; 324:71–86.
- Hankey GJ, et al. Stroke 2000; 31:1779–1784.

For further information: 💻 www.cochrane.org

26.72 STATINS IN SECONDARY PREVENTION OF ISCHAEMIC STROKE `EBM`

'Ongoing treatment with simvastatin 40 mg daily reduces the risk of recurrent stroke, myocardial infarction and vascular deaths. Treating 1000 patients for a year prevents about 17 strokes.'

- Heart Protection Study Collaborative Group. Lancet 2002; 360:7–22.

For further information: 💻 www.cochrane.org

26.73 ANTICOAGULANTS IN SECONDARY PREVENTION OF ISCHAEMIC STROKE `EBM`

'There is no net benefit to be gained in the routine use of anticoagulants after acute stroke except in the presence of atrial fibrillation, when treating 1000 patients for a year prevents about 80 strokes.'

- Hart RG, et al. Ann Intern Med 1999; 131:492–501.

For further information: 💻 www.cochrane.org

26.74 BLOOD PRESSURE LOWERING IN SECONDARY PREVENTION OF STROKE `EBM`

'Lowering blood pressure even in the 'normal range' reduces the risk of recurrent stroke, myocardial infarction and vascular deaths. Treating 1000 patients for a year prevents about 22 strokes.'

- PROGRESS Collaborative Group. Lancet 2001; 358:1033–1041.

For further information: 💻 www.cochrane.org

Carotid endarterectomy and angioplasty

A small proportion of patients with a carotid territory ischaemic stroke or TIA will have a greater than 70% stenosis of the carotid artery on the side of the brain lesion. Such patients have a greater than average risk of stroke recurrence. For those without major residual disability, removal of the stenosis has been shown to reduce the overall risk of recurrence, although the operation itself carries a 5% risk of stroke (Box 26.75). Carotid angioplasty and stenting are technically feasible but the long-term effects on the risk of stroke are unclear.

SUBARACHNOID HAEMORRHAGE

About three-quarters of those presenting with a subarachnoid haemorrhage (SAH) are under 65 years, and

26.75 CAROTID ENDARTERECTOMY IN ISCHAEMIC STROKE AND TIA `EBM`

'After a stroke with good functional recovery in the carotid territory and in the presence of an ipsilateral severe stenosis (70%), carotid endarterectomy reduces the risk of subsequent stroke. Operating on 1000 patients prevents about 40 strokes over the next year.

In asymptomatic carotid stenosis, endarterectomy has a smaller benefit. Operating on 1000 patients prevents about 13 strokes over the next year.'

- Rothwell PM, et al. Lancet 2003; 361:107–16.
- Executive Committee for the Asymptomatic Carotid Atherosclerosis Study. JAMA 1995; 273:1421–1428.

For further information: 💻 www.cochrane.org

women are more frequently affected than men. Subarachnoid haemorrhage typically presents with a sudden, severe 'thunderclap' headache (often occipital) which lasts for hours or even days, often accompanied by vomiting. Physical exertion, straining and sexual excitement are common antecedents. There may be loss of consciousness at the onset, so subarachnoid haemorrhage should be considered if a patient is found comatose. Since subarachnoid haemorrhage is rare (incidence 6/100 000) and only 1 patient in 8 with a sudden severe headache has had a subarachnoid haemorrhage, clinical vigilance is necessary to avoid a missed diagnosis. All patients with a sudden severe headache require investigation to exclude a subarachnoid haemorrhage (Fig. 26.35).

On examination the patient is usually distressed and irritable, with photophobia. There may be neck stiffness due to subarachnoid blood but this may take some hours to develop. Focal hemisphere signs (hemiparesis, aphasia etc.) may be present at onset if there is an associated intracerebral haematoma. A 3rd nerve palsy may be present due to local pressure from an aneurysm of the posterior communicating artery, though this is rare. Fundoscopy may reveal a subhyaloid haemorrhage, which represents blood tracking along the subarachnoid space around the optic nerve.

Pathology

Of all subarachnoid haemorrhages, 85% are caused by saccular ('berry') aneurysms bulging out from the bifurcations of the cerebral arteries, particularly in the region of the circle of Willis. These rarely present before the age of 20 years. There is an increased risk in first-degree relatives of those with saccular aneurysms, and with polycystic kidney disease and congenital collagen defects, e.g. Ehlers–Danlos syndrome. Of the remainder, 10% are non-aneurysmal haemorrhages (so called peri-mesencephalic haemorrhages), which have a very characteristic appearance on CT and a benign outcome in terms of mortality and recurrence. Some 5% of SAHs are due to rarities including arteriovenous malformations and vertebral artery dissection.

Management and prognosis

The immediate mortality of aneurysmal subarachnoid haemorrhage is about 30%. Survivors have a recurrence, or re-bleed, rate of about 40% in the first 4 weeks and 3% annually thereafter. Insertion of platinum coils into an aneurysm (via an endovascular procedure) or surgical

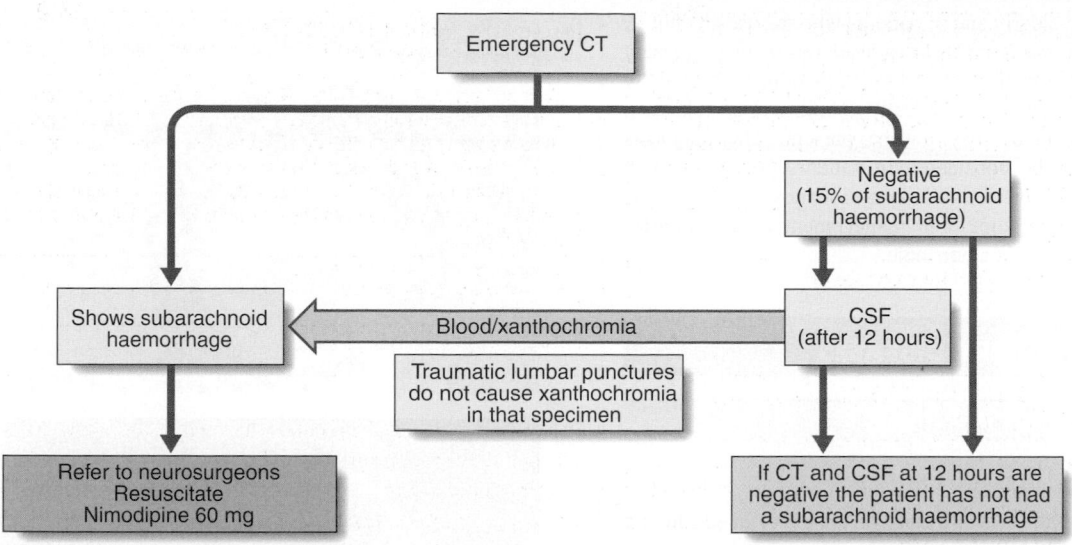

Fig. 26.35   The investigation of sudden severe headache.

clipping of the aneurysm neck reduces the risk of both early and late recurrence. Coiling may be associated with fewer perioperative complications and better outcomes.

A re-bleed is not the only cause of early deterioration. The clinician should also consider obstructive hydrocephalus, delayed cerebral ischaemia due to vasospasm, hyponatraemia and systemic complications associated with immobility, e.g. chest infection or pulmonary embolism. Nimodipine (60 mg) is given to prevent vasospasm in the acute phase.

CEREBRAL VENOUS DISEASE

Thrombosis of cerebral veins and venous sinuses is relatively uncommon, although probably more so than previously thought. The causes are listed in Box 26.76.

Cerebral venous sinus occlusion causes raised intracranial pressure and patchy ischaemia, which is often haemorrhagic. The clinical features vary according to the part of the cerebral venous system involved (see below). Anticoagulation is usually given, though the evidence for this is scanty; similarly, in selected patients, the use of endovascular thrombolysis has been advocated. Management of underlying causes and complications, such as persistently raised intracranial pressure, is also important.

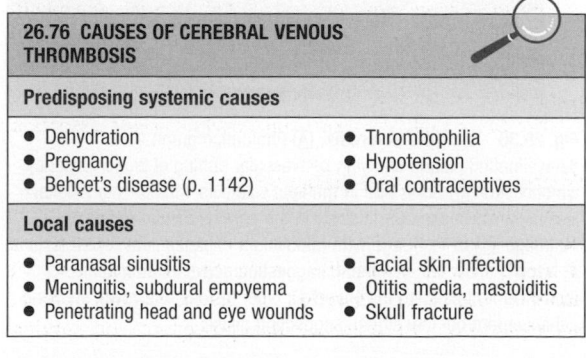

26.76 CAUSES OF CEREBRAL VENOUS THROMBOSIS	
Predisposing systemic causes	
• Dehydration	• Thrombophilia
• Pregnancy	• Hypotension
• Behçet's disease (p. 1142)	• Oral contraceptives
Local causes	
• Paranasal sinusitis	• Facial skin infection
• Meningitis, subdural empyema	• Otitis media, mastoiditis
• Penetrating head and eye wounds	• Skull fracture

26.77 CLINICAL FEATURES OF CEREBRAL VENOUS THROMBOSIS	
Cavernous sinus	
• Proptosis, ptosis, headache, external and internal ophthalmoplegia, papilloedema, reduced sensation in trigeminal first division	
• Often bilateral, patient ill and febrile	
Superior sagittal sinus	
• Headache, papilloedema, seizures	
• May involve veins of both hemispheres, causing advancing motor and sensory focal deficits	
Transverse sinus	
• Hemiparesis, seizures, papilloedema	
• May spread to jugular foramen to involve cranial nerves 9, 10, 11	

CORTICAL VEIN THROMBOSIS

This may present with focal cortical deficits, such as aphasia and hemiparesis, and epilepsy (focal or generalised), according to the area involved. The deficit may enlarge if spreading thrombophlebitis occurs.

CEREBRAL VENOUS SINUS THROMBOSIS

The clinical features of cerebral venous sinus thrombosis depend on the sinus involved (Box 26.77). About 10% of cerebral venous sinus thrombosis is associated with infection, particularly thrombosis of the cavernous sinus. Antibiotics are obviously indicated in this situation. Otherwise, the treatment of choice is anticoagulation, as above.

SUBDURAL HAEMATOMA

This is a collection of blood which forms between the dura and the surface of the brain, due to rupture of veins on the surface of the brain. It usually follows trauma but may occur spontaneously, particularly in patients on anticoagulants. It

26

is common in elderly and in patients who misuse alcohol. A history of trauma is not always available. Patients present with subacute impairment of brain function, both globally (obtundation, coma) and focally (hemiparesis, seizures). Headaches may or may not be present. The diagnosis should always be considered in patients presenting with unexplained reduction of consciousness. CT is the investigation of choice, and management entails surgical drainage, usually via a burr hole.

INFLAMMATORY DISEASES

MULTIPLE SCLEROSIS

In multiple sclerosis, one of the most common neurological causes of long-term disability, the myelin-producing oligodendrocytes of the central nervous system are the target of recurrent cell-mediated autoimmune attack. In the UK the prevalence is 120 per 100 000 of the population, with an annual incidence of around 7 per 100 000. The lifetime risk of developing multiple sclerosis is about 1 in 400. The incidence is higher in temperate climates and in Northern Europeans, and the disease is about twice as common in women as men.

Aetiology

Epidemiological and genetic evidence suggests that multiple sclerosis is caused by an interplay of multiple genetic and environmental factors. The incidence varies with latitude, being low in equatorial areas and higher in the temperate zones of both hemispheres, with people retaining the risk of the zone in which they grew up. However, no specific environmental factors such as exposure to viral infections have so far been correlated with an increased risk. The risk of familial recurrence is 15%, with highest being for first-degree relatives (age-adjusted risk: 2–3%) and a monozygotic twin concordance of 35%. The heritability is polygenic, with associations with various class II MHC alleles and the gene for TNF-α, as well as HLA haplotypes, although the latter vary between countries. An immune mechanism is suggested by increased levels of activated T lymphocytes in the CSF, and increased immunoglobulin synthesis within the central nervous system.

Pathology

An attack of central nervous system inflammation in multiple sclerosis starts with the entry of activated T lymphocytes through the blood–brain barrier. These recognise myelin-derived antigens on the surface of the nervous system's antigen-presenting cells, the microglia, and undergo clonal proliferation. The resulting inflammatory cascade releases cytokines and initiates destruction of the oligodendrocyte–myelin unit by macrophages. Histologically, the characteristic lesion is a plaque of inflammatory demyelination occurring most commonly in the periventricular regions of the brain, the optic nerves and the subpial regions of the spinal cord (Fig. 26.36). Initially, this is a circumscribed area of disintegration of the myelin

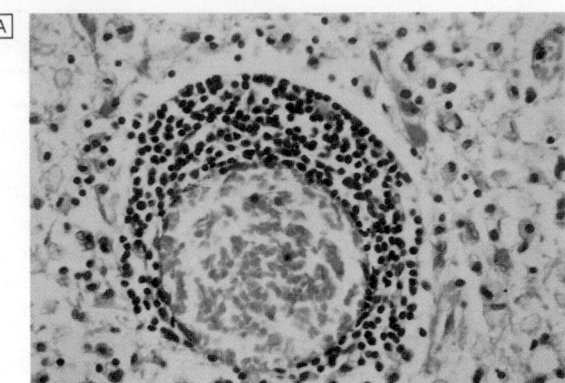

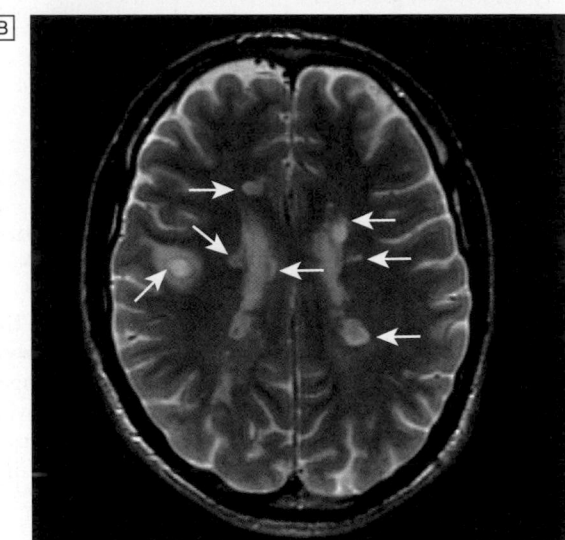

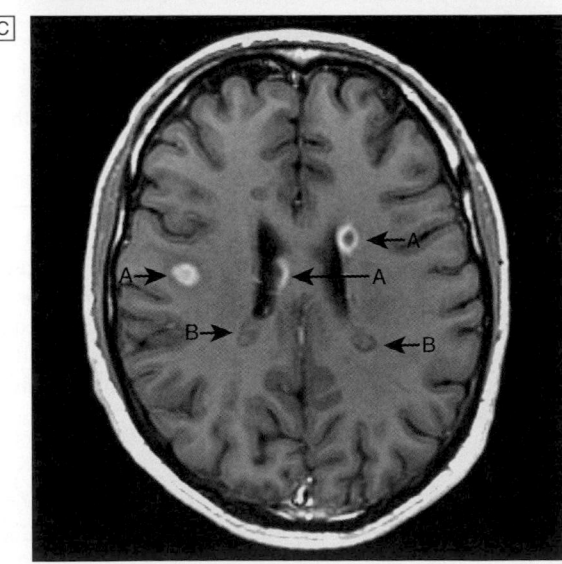

Fig. 26.36   Multiple sclerosis. Ⓐ Photomicrograph from demyelinating plaque showing perivascular cuffing of blood vessel by lymphocytes. Ⓑ Brain MRI in multiple sclerosis. Multiple high-signal lesions (arrows) seen particularly in the paraventricular region on T2 image. Ⓒ In T1 image with gadolinium enhancement recent lesions (A arrows) show enhancement, suggesting active inflammation (enhancement persists for 4 weeks); older lesions (B arrows) show no enhancement but low signal, suggesting gliosis.

26

sheath, accompanied by infiltration by activated lymphocytes and macrophages, often with conspicuous perivascular inflammation. After an acute attack, gliosis follows, leaving a shrunken grey scar.

Much of the initial acute clinical deficit is caused by the effect of inflammatory cytokines upon transmission of the nervous impulse rather than structural disruption of the myelin, which explains the rapid recovery of some deficits and probably the efficacy of corticosteroids in ameliorating the acute deficit. However, the myelin loss that results from an attack reduces the safety factor for impulse propagation or causes complete conduction block, which lowers the efficiency of central nervous system functions. Inflammatory mediators released during the acute attack (particularly nitrous oxide) probably also initiate axonal damage, which is a feature of the latter stages of the disease. In established multiple sclerosis there is progressive axonal loss, probably due to direct damage to axonal integrity by the inflammatory mediators released in acute attacks and subsequently the loss of neurotrophic factors from oligodendrocytes. This axonal loss is the cause of the phase of the disease where there is progressive and persistent disability (Fig. 26.37).

Clinical features

A diagnosis of multiple sclerosis requires the demonstration of lesions in more than one anatomical site at more than one time for which there is no other explanation (Box 26.78).

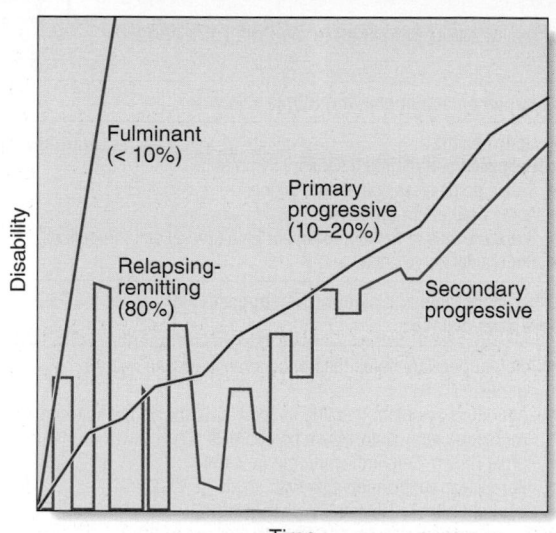

Fig. 26.37 **The progression of disability in fulminant, relapsing-remitting and progressive multiple sclerosis.**

Around 80% of patients have a relapsing and remitting clinical course of episodic dysfunction of the central nervous system with variable recovery. Of the remaining 20%, most follow a slowly progressive clinical course, with a tiny minority who have a fulminant variety leading to early

26.78 THE MACDONALD CRITERIA FOR THE DIAGNOSIS OF MULTIPLE SCLEROSIS[1]	
Clinical presentation[2]	**Additional evidence required for diagnosis of MS**
Two or more attacks separated in 'time' (at least 3 months apart) and 'space' (involving different parts of the CNS) with objective clinical evidence of two or more lesions	None
Two or more attacks separated in 'time' and 'space', but with objective clinical evidence for only one lesion	MRI demonstrates dissemination in 'space' (multiple lesions in several different sites) *or* Two or more MRI-detected lesions consistent with MS *and* oligoclonal bands in CSF *or* Await further clinical attack at different anatomical site
One attack with objective clinical evidence of two or more lesions in different parts of the CNS (i.e. dissemination in 'space')	Dissemination in 'time', demonstrated by serial MRI scans (looking for a new lesion developing at least 3 months after the inital presentation) *or* Await further (second) clinical attack at different anatomical site
One attack with clinical evidence of only one lesion (clinically isolated syndrome)	MRI demonstration of dissemination in 'space' and 'time' (as above) *or* Two or more MRI-detected lesions with CSF showing oligoclonal bands *and* dissemination in time, demonstrated by MRI *or* Await further (second) clinical attack at different anatomical site
Insidious neurological progression suggestive of MS	CSF positive for oligoclonal bands *and* Dissemination in 'space' and 'time' on MRI and/or abnormal VER[3] *or* Continued progression for a year

[1]Published by the International Panel on MS Diagnosis (Ann Neurol 2001; 50:121–127.) Starting from the clinical presentation in the left-hand column, if the evidence available fulfils the criteria in the right-hand column, the diagnosis is MS. If the criteria are not completely met, the diagnosis is 'possible MS'. If the criteria are fully explored but not met, then the patient does not have MS.
[2]Assumes other possible causes for CNS inflammation (e.g. sarcoidosis, SLE) have been excluded.
[3]VER = visual evoked response.

26.79 CLINICAL FEATURES OF MULTIPLE SCLEROSIS

Common presentations of multiple sclerosis

- Optic neuritis
- Relapsing and remitting sensory symptoms
- Subacute painless spinal cord lesion
- Acute brain-stem syndrome
- Subacute loss of function of upper limb (dorsal column deficit)
- 6th cranial nerve palsy

Other symptoms and syndromes suggestive of CNS demyelination

- Afferent pupillary defect and optic atrophy (previous optic neuritis)
- Lhermitte's symptom (tingling in spine or limbs on neck flexion)
- Progressive non-compressive paraparesis
- Partial Brown–Séquard syndrome (p. 1184)
- Internuclear ophthalmoplegia with ataxia (p. 1195)
- Postural ('rubral', 'Holmes') tremor (p. 1182)
- Trigeminal neuralgia (p. 1164) under the age of 50
- Recurrent facial palsy

26.80 INVESTIGATIONS IN A PATIENT SUSPECTED OF HAVING MULTIPLE SCLEROSIS

Exclude other structural disease and identify plaques of demyelination

- Image area of clinical involvement (MRI, myelography)

Demonstrate other sites of involvement

- Imaging (MRI)
- Visual evoked potentials
- Other evoked potentials

Demonstrate inflammatory nature of lesion(s)

- CSF examination
  Cell count
  Protein electrophoresis (oligoclonal bands)

Exclude other conditions

- Chest X-ray
- Serum angiotensin-converting enzyme (ACE)—sarcoidosis
- Serum B_{12}
- Antinuclear antibodies—SLE
- Antiphospholipid antibodies

death (Fig. 26.37). The peak age of onset is in the fourth decade, with onset before puberty or after the age of 60 years being rare. There are a number of clinical symptoms and syndromes suggestive of multiple sclerosis, some of which may occur at presentation while others may develop in the course of the illness (Box 26.79).

Demyelinating lesions cause symptoms and signs that usually come on subacutely over days or weeks and resolve over weeks or months, although rarely a stroke-like presentation may occur. After a variable interval there may be a recurrence, often within 2 years. Frequent relapses with incomplete recovery indicate a poor prognosis, and in many patients a phase of secondary progression, caused by secondary axonal degeneration, supersedes the phase of relapse and remission. In a minority of patients, there may be an interval of years or even decades between attacks, and in some, particularly if optic neuritis is the initial manifestation, there is no recurrence. Some presentations, such as optic neuritis with purely sensory relapses, have a good prognosis.

The physical signs observed in multiple sclerosis depend on the anatomical site of demyelination. Combinations of spinal cord and brain-stem signs are common, maybe with evidence of previous optic neuritis in the form of an afferent pupillary deficit. Significant intellectual impairment is unusual until late in the disease, when loss of frontal functions and impairment of memory are common.

Investigations

There is no specific test for multiple sclerosis, and the results of investigation are taken in conjunction with the clinical picture in making a diagnosis of varying probability (Box 26.78). The clinical diagnosis of multiple sclerosis should be supported by investigations to exclude other conditions, provide evidence for an inflammatory disorder and identify multiple sites of neurological involvement (Box 26.80).

Following the first clinical event, investigations may help prognostically in confirming the disseminated nature of the disease. Visual evoked potentials (p. 1154) can detect

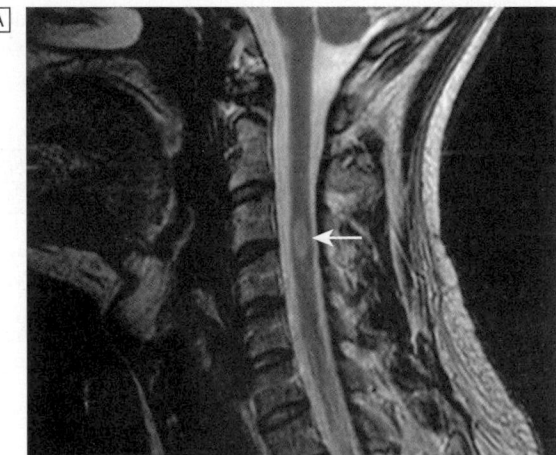

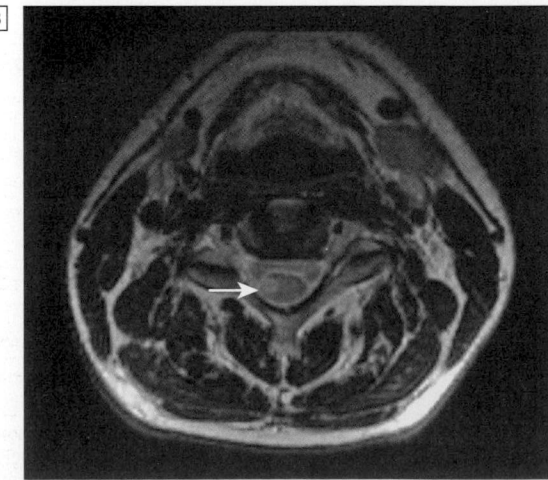

Fig. 26.38 Multiple sclerosis: demyelinating lesion in cervical spinal cord, high-signal T2 images (arrows). A Sagittal plane. B Axial plane.

26

clinically silent lesions in up to 70% of patients, but auditory and somatosensory evoked potentials are seldom of diagnostic value. The CSF may show a lymphocytic pleocytosis in the acute phase and oligoclonal bands of IgG in 70–90% of patients between attacks. Oligoclonal bands are not specific to multiple sclerosis but denote intrathecal inflammation and occur in a range of other disorders. MRI is the most sensitive technique for imaging lesions in both brain and spinal cord (Fig. 26.38) and in excluding other causes of the neurological deficit. However, the MRI appearances in multiple sclerosis may be confused with those of cerebrovascular disease or cerebral vasculitis. Diagnosis depends on the clinical history and examination, taken in combination with the investigative findings. It is important to exclude other potentially treatable conditions such as infection, vitamin B_{12} deficiency and spinal cord compression.

Management

The management of multiple sclerosis involves treatment of the acute relapse, prevention of future relapses, treatment of complications and management of the patient's disability.

Acute relapse

In a function-threatening relapse, pulses of high-dose methylprednisolone, either intravenously (1 g daily for 3 days) or orally (500 mg daily for 5 days), shorten the duration of the relapse but do not affect long-term outcome (Box 26.81). Pulsed steroids also have some effect in reducing spasticity. Prolonged administration of steroids does not alter the long-term outcome and is therefore avoided. Pulses of steroids can be given up to three times in a year but their administration should be restricted to those with significant function-threatening deficits.

Preventing relapses

Immunosuppressive agents including azathioprine have some effect in reducing relapses and improving long-term outcome. In relapsing and remitting multiple sclerosis, subcutaneous or intramuscular interferon beta-1a/b reduces the number of relapses by some 30%, with a small effect on long-term disability (Boxes 26.82 and 26.83); glatiramer acetate has similar effects. The effects of other immune modulation therapies (Box 26.83) may be of some use in severely affected patients. Special diets including gluten-free, linoleic acid supplements or hyperbaric oxygen therapy are popular with patients, but are of no proven benefit.

Complications

The treatment of the complications of multiple sclerosis is summarised in Box 26.84. Of prime importance is a careful explanation of the nature of the disease and its outcome, along with support of patients and their relatives when disability occurs. Specialist nurses working in a multi-disciplinary team of health-care professionals are of great value in managing the chronic phase of the disease. Periods

---

26.81 PULSED CORTICOSTEROIDS IN MULTIPLE SCLEROSIS **EBM**

'In people with multiple sclerosis with acute exacerbations, corticosteroids (methylprednisolone or corticotrophin) improve symptoms compared with placebo within 5 weeks of treatment. The optimal dose, route and duration of treatment are unclear.'

- Filippini G, et al. (Cochrane Review). Cochrane Library, issue 4, 2000. Oxford: Update Software.
- Barnes D, et al. Lancet 1997; 349:902–906.

For further information: ▢ www.clinicalevidence.org

26.82 INTERFERON BETA-1a/b IN MULTIPLE SCLEROSIS **EBM**

'In people experiencing a first demyelinating event, interferon beta-1a decreases the risk of conversion to clinically definite multiple sclerosis over 2–3 years compared with placebo. In people with active relapsing-remitting multiple sclerosis, there is limited evidence that, compared with placebo, interferon beta-1a/b reduces exacerbations and disease progression over 2 years.'

- PRISMS Study Group. Lancet 1998; 352:1498–1504.
- IFNB Multiple Sclerosis Study Group. Neurology 1993; 43:655–661.

For further information: ▢ www.clinicalevidence.org

26

26.83 DISEASE-MODIFYING TREATMENTS IN MS

Treatment	Mode of action	Comment
Interferon beta	Immune modulation	In widespread use for reducing relapse rate (RCT evidence)
Glatiramer acetate	Immune modulation	Similar efficacy to interferon beta (RCT evidence)
Azathioprine	Immune suppression	Similar efficacy to interferon beta (RCT evidence)
Cyclophosphamide	Immune suppression (cytotoxic)	Occasionally used in aggressive disease. Not recommended for widespread use (no proven benefit in RCTs)
Mitoxantrone	Immune suppression (cytotoxic)	Early trials in aggressive disease (no proven benefit in RCTs)
Plasmapheresis	Immune modulation	Occasionally used in aggressive disease (no proven efficacy in RCTs)
Intravenous immunoglobulin	Immune modulation	Occasionally used in aggressive disease
Monoclonal antibodies to beta-integrins (e.g. natalizumab)	Immune modulation (lymphocyte entry into CNS)	Encouraging experimental results (no proven efficacy in RCTs)
Monoclonal antibodies to lymphocyte epitopes (e.g. campath1-H)	Immune suppression (lymphocyte depletion)	Encouraging experimental results (no proven efficacy in RCTs)

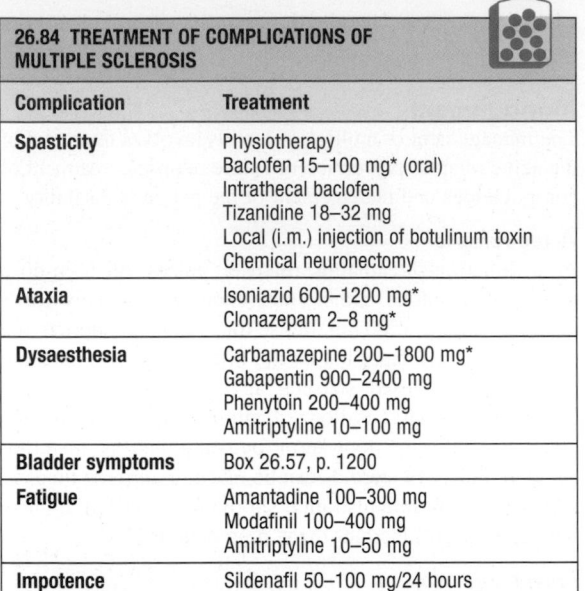

26.84 TREATMENT OF COMPLICATIONS OF MULTIPLE SCLEROSIS

Complication	Treatment
Spasticity	Physiotherapy Baclofen 15–100 mg* (oral) Intrathecal baclofen Tizanidine 18–32 mg Local (i.m.) injection of botulinum toxin Chemical neuronectomy
Ataxia	Isoniazid 600–1200 mg* Clonazepam 2–8 mg*
Dysaesthesia	Carbamazepine 200–1800 mg* Gabapentin 900–2400 mg Phenytoin 200–400 mg Amitriptyline 10–100 mg
Bladder symptoms	Box 26.57, p. 1200
Fatigue	Amantadine 100–300 mg Modafinil 100–400 mg Amitriptyline 10–50 mg
Impotence	Sildenafil 50–100 mg/24 hours

* In divided doses.

of physiotherapy and occupational therapy may improve functional capacity in those patients who become disabled, and can provide guidance in the provision of aids at home, reducing handicap.

Care of the bladder is particularly important. Urgency and frequency may be treated pharmacologically (Box 26.57, p. 1200), but this may lead to a degree of retention that promotes the development of infection; this needs appropriate treatment. Retention can be managed initially by intermittent urinary catheterisation (by the patient, if possible), but an in-dwelling catheter may become necessary.

Sexual dysfunction is a frequent source of distress. Sildenafil helps impotence in men, and skilled counselling and prosthetic aids are often useful.

Prognosis

The outlook is difficult to predict with confidence in any individual patient, especially early in the disease. Furthermore, the ability to diagnose disease at an earlier stage means that older studies may not reliably reflect the outcome of those diagnosed with modern techniques. About 15% of those having one attack of demyelination do not suffer any more events, whilst those with relapsing and remitting multiple sclerosis have, on average, 1–2 relapses every 2 years. Approximately 5% of patients die within 5 years of onset, whilst others have a very benign outcome. Overall, after 10 years about one-third of patients are disabled to the point of needing help with walking, rising to about 50% after 15 years.

ACUTE DISSEMINATED ENCEPHALOMYELITIS

This is an acute, usually monophasic, demyelinating condition in which there are areas of perivenous demye-

lination widely disseminated throughout the brain and spinal cord. The illness may apparently occur spontaneously but often occurs a week or so after a viral infection, especially measles and chickenpox, or following vaccination, suggesting that it is immunologically mediated.

Clinical features

Headache, vomiting, pyrexia, confusion and meningism may be presenting features, often with focal or multifocal brain and spinal cord signs. Seizures or coma may occur. A minority of patients who recover have further episodes.

Investigations

MRI shows multiple high-signal areas in a pattern similar to that of multiple sclerosis, although often with larger areas of abnormality. The CSF may be normal or show an increase in protein and lymphocytes (occasionally over 100×10^6 cells/l); oligoclonal bands may be found in the acute episode but do not persist upon recovery, unlike in multiple sclerosis. The differential diagnosis from a first severe attack of multiple sclerosis may be difficult.

Management

The disease may be fatal in the acute stages but is otherwise self-limiting. Treatment with high-dose intravenous methylprednisolone, using the same regimen as for a relapse of multiple sclerosis, is recommended.

ACUTE TRANSVERSE MYELITIS

Transverse myelitis is an acute, often monophasic, inflammatory demyelinating disorder affecting the spinal cord over a variable number of segments. Patients may be of any age and present with a subacute paraparesis with a sensory level, often with severe pain in the neck or back at the onset. MRI is needed to distinguish this from a compressive lesion of the spinal cord. CSF examination shows cellular pleocytosis, often with polymorphs at the onset, and oligoclonal bands are usually absent. Treatment is with high-dose intravenous methylprednisolone. The outcome is variable; in some cases, near-complete recovery occurs despite a severe initial deficit. Some patients who present with acute transverse myelitis go on to develop multiple sclerosis in later years.

The concurrence of transverse myelitis with bilateral optic neuritis—neuromyelitis optica (Devic's disease)—is a more common cause of central nervous demyelination in Africa and Asia than multiple sclerosis.

DEGENERATIVE DISEASES

Many diseases cause degeneration in different parts of the nervous system without an identifiable external cause. Genetic factors are known to be involved in several, but the cause is still unknown for the majority. Clinical features depend on which structures are affected. Degeneration of the cerebral cortex causes dementia, the most common type

26

being Alzheimer's disease. Degeneration of the basal ganglia results in movement disorder, which may manifest as either too little or too much movement, depending on the structures involved. Examples of these conditions are Parkinson's disease and Huntington's disease. Cerebellar degeneration usually causes ataxia. Degeneration can also occur in the spinal cord or peripheral nerves, giving rise to motor, sensory or autonomic disturbance.

DEGENERATIVE CAUSES OF DEMENTIA

As many as 5% of the population over 65 years of age suffer from a dementing illness. Over the age of 80, this rises to over 20%. Dementia therefore has major implications for health resources.

ALZHEIMER'S DISEASE

This is the most common cause of dementia, occurring mostly in patients over 45 years. About 15% of cases are familial, and these cases fall into two main groups: an early-onset, autosomal dominant pattern, and a later-onset group whose inheritance is not so clear. Genetic abnormalities on several different chromosomes have been described. The inheritance of one of the alleles of apolipoprotein ε, apo ε4, is associated with an increased risk of developing the disease (2–4 times in heterozygotes and 6–8 times in homozygotes). However, its presence is neither necessary nor sufficient for the development of the disease, so screening for its presence is not clinically useful.

Pathology

Macroscopically, the brain is atrophic, particularly the cerebral cortex and hippocampus. Histology reveals the presence of senile plaques and neurofibrillary tangles in the cerebral cortex. Histochemical staining demonstrates significant quantities of amyloid in plaques (Fig. 26.39). Many different neurotransmitter abnormalities have been described, in particular impairment of cholinergic transmission, although noradrenaline, 5-HT, glutamate and substance P are also involved (Box 26.2, p. 1150).

Clinical features

The key clinical feature is impairment of delayed recall, i.e. the inability to retrieve (remember) information acquired in the past. Hence, patients present with gradual impairment of memory, usually in association with disorders of other cortical functions. Both short-term and long-term memory are affected, but defects in the former are usually more obvious. Later in the course of the disease, typical features are apraxia, visuo-spatial impairment and aphasia. In the early stages, patients themselves may complain of difficulties, but as the disease progresses, it is common for patients to deny that there is anything wrong (anosognosia). In this situation, patients are often brought to medical attention by their carers. Depression is common. Occasionally, patients become aggressive, and the clinical features are made acutely worse by coexistent intercurrent illness.

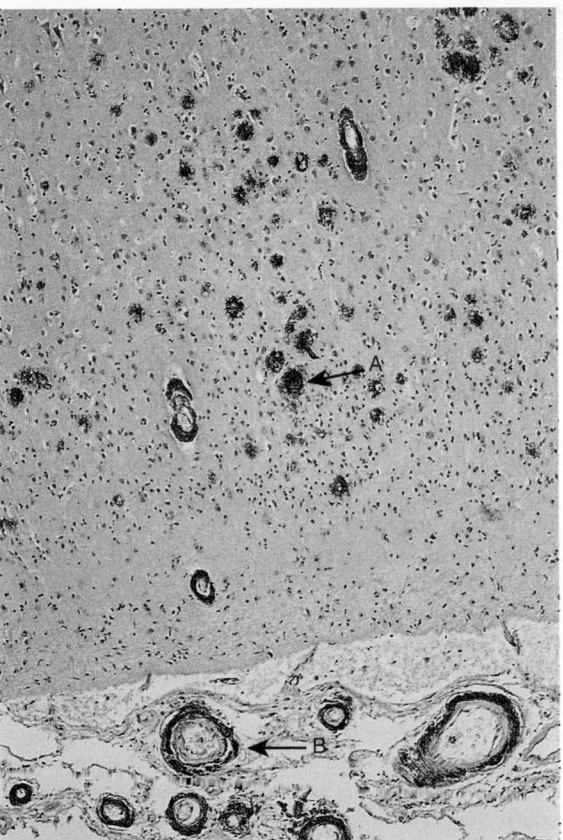

Fig. 26.39 Alzheimer's disease. Section of neocortex stained with polyclonal antibody against βA4 peptide showing amyloid deposits in plaques in brain substance (arrow A) and in blood vessel walls (arrow B).

26

Investigations and management

Investigation is aimed at excluding other treatable causes of dementia (Box 26.47, p. 1189), as histological confirmation of the diagnosis usually occurs only after death. There is no known treatment, though recently anticholinesterases such as donepezil, rivastigmine and galantamine, and the NMDA receptor antagonist, memantine, have been shown to be of some benefit (Box 26.85). Management consists largely

---

EBM

26.85 DONEPEZIL, GALANTAMINE, MEMANTINE, RIVASTIGMINE AND ALZHEIMER'S DISEASE

'In selected patients with mild or moderate Alzheimer's disease treated for periods of up to a year, donepezil, galantamine, memantine and rivastigmine produce modest improvements in cognitive function. However, the effects on quality of life of both patient and carer are still not clear, and hence the practical importance of these drugs has not been established.'

- Areosa Sastre A, Sherriff F (Cochrane Review). Cochrane Library, issue 2, 2004. Chichester: John Wiley.
- Birks JS, Harvey R (Cochrane Review). Cochrane Library, issue 2, 2004. Chichester: John Wiley.
- Birks J, et al. (Cochrane Review). Cochrane Library, issue 2, 2004. Chichester: John Wiley.
- Olin J, Schneider L (Cochrane Review). Cochrane Library, issue 2, 2004. Chichester: John Wiley.

For further information: 💻 www.cochrane.org

of providing a familiar environment for the patient, and providing support for the carers (p. 169). However, many patients are depressed, and treatment with antidepressant medication may be helpful.

OTHER DEGENERATIVE CAUSES OF DEMENTIA

Wernicke–Korsakoff disease

Deficiency of thiamin (vitamin B_1) usually presents with an acute confusional state (Wernicke's encephalopathy) and brain-stem abnormalities such as ataxia, nystagmus and extraocular muscle weakness, particularly lateral rectus weakness. If inadequately treated, this results in a dementia characterised by a profound disturbance of short-term memory associated with a tendency to confabulate, called Korsakoff's syndrome (p. 245). The deficiency can arise as a result of malnutrition (particularly when due to chronic alcohol misuse), malabsorption or even protracted vomiting (as in hyperemesis gravidarum). The diagnosis can be made biochemically by the finding of a reduced red cell transketolase, but this test is often difficult to obtain and so the diagnosis is usually made clinically. Because it is potentially treatable, the condition must be considered in any confused or demented patient; if there is any doubt, it is usually better to treat anyway. Treatment consists of intravenous thiamin (in the form of Pabrinex, 2 vials 8-hourly for 48 hours) initially, followed by oral (100 mg 8-hourly), in addition to treating the underlying cause.

Pick's disease

In this condition, much rarer than Alzheimer's, degeneration predominantly affects frontal and temporal lobes. The histology is characterised by the presence of argyrophilic cytoplasmic inclusion bodies (Pick bodies) and chromatolytic ballooned neurons (Pick cells) (Fig. 26.40). Patients may present with personality change due to frontal lobe involvement or with progressive aphasia. Memory is relatively preserved in the early stages. There is no specific treatment for Pick's disease.

Lewy body dementia

In diffuse Lewy body disease, pathology similar to that found in the substantia nigra in Parkinson's disease is found in the cerebral cortex. This condition usually presents as cognitive impairment in the context of an extrapyramidal syndrome, and the cognitive features may be indistinguishable from those of Alzheimer's disease. Patients' cognitive state often fluctuates; they have a high incidence of visual hallucinations, and are particularly sensitive to the side-effects of anti-parkinsonian medication and also to neuroleptic medication. There is no specific treatment for this condition, although there may be clinical benefit with anticholinesterase agents such as rivastigmine.

PARKINSON'S DISEASE AND AKINETIC-RIGID SYNDROMES

There are a number of degenerative diseases affecting the basal ganglia, which present with differing combinations of slowness of movement (bradykinesia), increased tone (rigidity), tremor and loss of postural reflexes. The most common cause of these parkinsonian or akinetic-rigid syndromes is idiopathic Parkinson's disease.

IDIOPATHIC PARKINSON'S DISEASE

This condition has an annual incidence of about 0.2/1000 and a prevalence of 1.5/1000 in the UK. Prevalence rates are similar throughout the world, though lower rates have been reported for China and West Africa. Whilst 10% of the patients are under 45 years at presentation, the incidence and prevalence both increase with age, the latter rising to over 1% in those over 60. Sex incidence is about equal. It is less common in cigarette smokers.

Aetiology

The cause is unknown, and no strong genetic factors have been identified, though recent work on twins has suggested that the genetic influence may be greater than previously thought. The discovery that methyl-phenyl-tetrahydro-

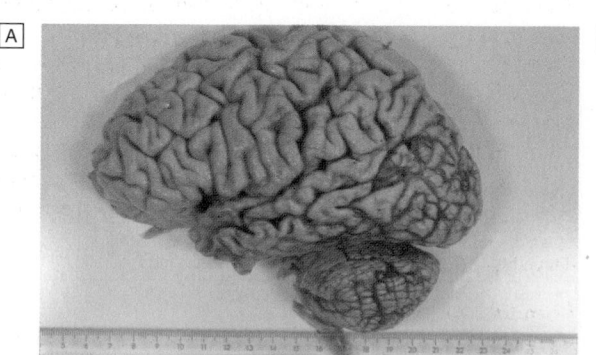
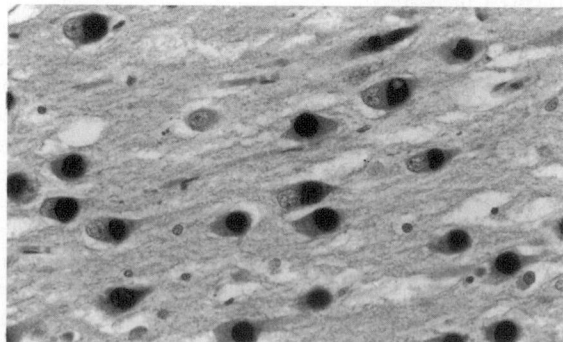

Fig. 26.40 Pick's disease. **A** Lateral view of formalin-fixed brain from a patient who died of Pick's disease, showing gyral atrophy of frontal and parietal lobes and a more severe degree of atrophy affecting the anterior half of the temporal lobe. **B** High power (× 200) of hippocampal pyramidal layer, prepared with monoclonal anti-tau antibody. Many neuronal cell bodies contain sharply circumscribed, spherical cytoplasmic inclusion bodies (Pick bodies).

26

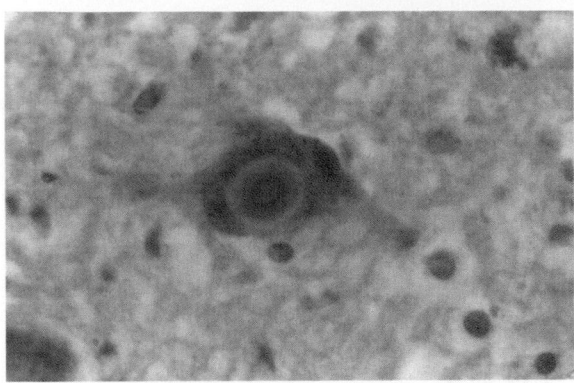

Fig. 26.41 Parkinson's disease. High power (× 400) of substantia nigra of a patient with Parkinson's disease to show classical Lewy body (haematoxylin and eosin).

pyridine (MPTP) caused severe parkinsonism in young drug users suggests that the idiopathic disease might be due to an environmental toxin; many candidate toxins have been studied, but there is no strong evidence in favour of any of them.

Pathology

There is depletion of the pigmented dopaminergic neurons in the substantia nigra, hyaline inclusions in nigral cells (Lewy bodies—Fig. 26.41), atrophic changes in the substantia nigra and depletion of neurons in the locus coeruleus. Reduced dopaminergic output from the substantia nigra to the globus pallidus leads to reduced inhibitory effects on the subthalamic nucleus, neurons of which become more active than usual in inhibiting activation of the cortex. This in turn results in bradykinesia.

Clinical features

The classical syndrome of tremor, rigidity and bradykinesia may be absent initially, when non-specific symptoms of tiredness, aching limbs, mental slowness, depression and small handwriting (micrographia) may be noticed.

The presentation is almost always unilateral, a resting tremor in an upper limb being a common presenting feature. The tremor may also affect the legs, mouth and tongue. It may remain the predominant symptom for some years. Bradykinesia may develop gradually. Most patients have difficulty with rapid fine movements, and this manifests itself as slowness of gait and difficulty with tasks such as fastening buttons, shaving or writing. Rigidity, or increased muscular tone, causes stiffness and a flexed posture. Postural righting reflexes are impaired early on in the disease, but falls tend not to occur until later. As the disease advances, speech becomes softer and indistinct. There are a number of abnormalities on neurological examination, and these are listed in Box 26.86.

Although parkinsonian features are initially unilateral, gradual bilateral involvement is the rule. Muscle strength and reflexes remain normal, and plantar responses are flexor. There is a paucity of facial expression (hypomimia) and the blink reflex may be exaggerated and fail to habituate (glabellar tap sign). Eye movements are normal to standard

26.86 PHYSICAL ABNORMALITIES IN PARKINSONISM

General
- Expressionless face
- Greasy skin
- Soft, rapid, indistinct speech
- Flexed posture
- Impaired postural reflexes

Gait
- Slow to start walking
- Shortened stride
- Rapid, small steps, tendency to run (festination)
- Reduced arm swing
- Impaired balance on turning

Tremor

Resting 4–6 Hz
- Usually first in fingers/thumb
- Coarse, complex movements, flexion/extension of fingers
- Abduction/adduction of thumb
- Supination/pronation of forearm
- May affect arms, legs, feet, jaw, tongue
- Intermittent, present at rest and when distracted
- Diminished on action

Postural 8–10 Hz
- Less obvious, faster, finer amplitude
- Present on action or posture, persists with movement

Rigidity
- Cogwheel type, mostly upper limbs
- Plastic (leadpipe) type, mostly legs

Bradykinesia
- Slowness in initiating or repeating movements
- Impaired fine movements, especially of fingers

26

clinical testing, provided allowance is made for the normal limitation of upward gaze with age. Sensation is normal and intellectual faculties are not affected initially. As the disease progresses, about one-third of patients develop cognitive impairment.

Investigations

The diagnosis is made clinically, as there is no diagnostic test for Parkinson's disease. Sometimes it is necessary to investigate patients to exclude other causes of parkinsonism if there are any unusual features. Patients presenting before the age of 50 are usually tested for Wilson's disease, and imaging (CT or MRI) of the head may be needed if there are any features suggestive of pyramidal, cerebellar or autonomic involvement, or the diagnosis is otherwise in doubt.

Management

Drug therapy

Levodopa combined with a peripheral-acting dopa-decarboxylase inhibitor provides the mainstay of treatment in Parkinson's disease but should only be started to help overcome significant disability. Other agents include anticholinergic drugs, dopamine receptor agonists, selegiline, COMT inhibitors and amantadine (Fig. 26.42).

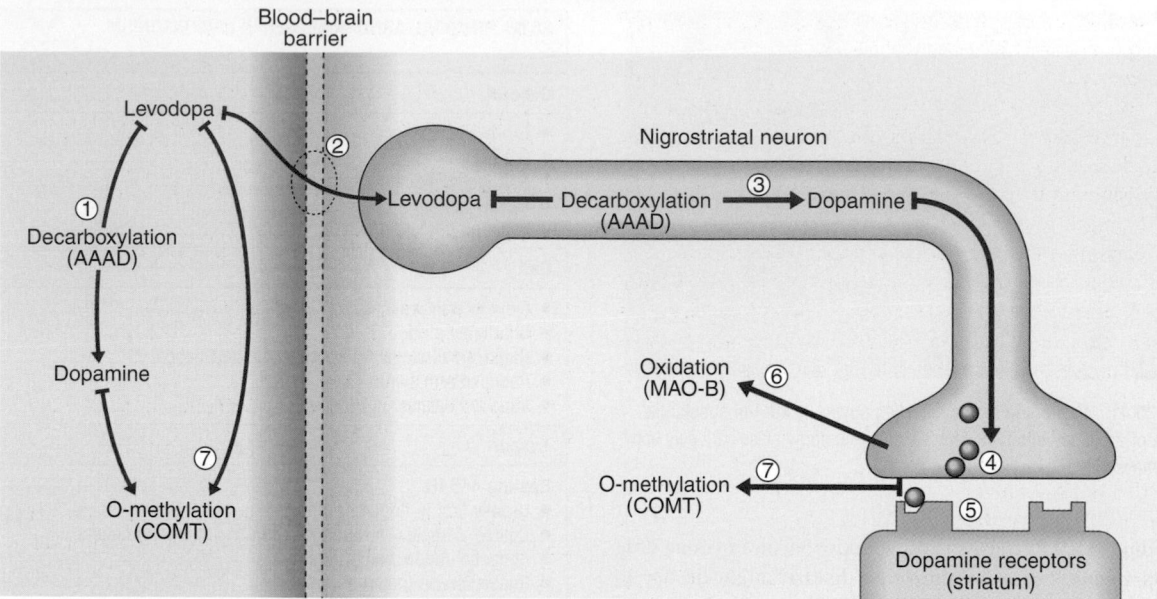

Fig. 26.42 Mechanisms of drug action in Parkinson's disease. (1) Decarboxylase inhibitors (carbidopa and benserazide) decrease side-effects by reducing peripheral conversion of levodopa to dopamine by aromatic amino acid decarboxylase (AAAD). (2) Active transport of levodopa into the brain may be inhibited by competition from dietary amino acids after a high-protein meal. (3) In the nigrostriatal neurons, levodopa is converted into dopamine. (4) Amantadine enhances the release of dopamine at the nerve terminal. (5) Dopamine agonists act directly on striatal receptors. (6) The monoamine oxidase type B (MAO-B) inhibitor selegiline increases the availability of neuronal dopamine by reducing its metabolism outside the neuron. (7) The catechol-O-methyl-transferase (COMT) inhibitor entacapone prolongs the availability of dopamine by inhibiting the metabolism of dopamine and levodopa outside the neuron.

Levodopa. Although the number of dopamine-releasing terminals in the striatum is diminished in Parkinson's disease, remaining neurons can be driven to produce more dopamine by administering its precursor, levodopa. If levodopa is administered orally, more than 90% is decarboxylated to dopamine peripherally in the gastrointestinal tract and blood vessels, and only a small proportion reaches the brain. This peripheral conversion of levodopa is responsible for the high incidence of side-effects if used alone. The problem is largely overcome by giving a decarboxylase inhibitor that does not cross the blood–brain barrier along with the levodopa. Two peripheral decarboxylase inhibitors, carbidopa and benserazide, are available as combination preparations with levodopa, as Sinemet and Madopar.

The initiation of levodopa therapy should be delayed until there is significant disability, since there is concern regarding long-term side-effects. With this in mind, some authorities suggest that it is advisable to initiate treatment with a dopamine agonist (see below) or a slow-release preparation of levodopa in order to minimise or delay the onset of long-term side-effects, particularly in patients who develop the disease before age 70. Levodopa is particularly effective at improving bradykinesia and rigidity. Tremor is also helped but rather unpredictably. The initial dose is 50 mg 8- or 12-hourly, increased if necessary. The total levodopa dose may be increased to over 1000 mg/day, but should be kept as low as possible. Side-effects include postural hypotension, nausea and vomiting, which may be offset by the use of a peripheral dopamine antagonist such as domperidone. Other dose-related side-effects are involuntary movements, particularly orofacial dyskinesias,

limb and axial dystonias, and occasionally depression, hallucinations and delusions.

Late deterioration despite levodopa therapy occurs after 3–5 years in one-third to one-half of patients. Usually this manifests as fluctuation in response. The simplest form of this is end-of-dose deterioration due to progression of the disease and loss of capacity to store dopamine. More complex fluctuations present as sudden, unpredictable changes in response, in which periods of severe parkinsonism alternate with dyskinesia and agitation (the 'on-off' phenomenon). End-of-dose deterioration can often be improved by dividing the levodopa into smaller but more frequent doses, or by converting to a slow-release preparation. The 'on-off' phenomenon is difficult to treat, but sometimes subcutaneous injections of apomorphine (a dopamine agonist) are helpful to 'rescue' the patient rapidly from an 'off' period.

Involuntary movements (dyskinesia) may occur as a peak-dose phenomenon, or as a biphasic phenomenon (occurring during both the build-up and wearing-off phases). Management is difficult, but again involves modifying the way levodopa is administered to obtain constant levels in the brain, and the use of alternative drugs, particularly dopamine agonists.

Anticholinergic agents. These have a useful effect on tremor and rigidity, but do not help bradykinesia. They can be prescribed early in the disease before bradykinesia is a problem, but should be avoided in elderly patients in whom they cause confusion and hallucinations. Other side-effects include dry mouth, blurred vision, difficulty with micturition and constipation. Many anticholinergics are available—

for example, trihexyphenidyl (benzhexol; 1–4 mg 8-hourly) and orphenadrine (50–100 mg 8-hourly).

Amantadine. This has a mild, usually short-lived effect on bradykinesia, but may be used early in the disease before more potent treatment is needed. Amantadine can be particularly useful in controlling the dyskinesias produced by dopaminergic treatment later in the disease. The dose is 100 mg 8- or 12-hourly. Side-effects include livedo reticularis, peripheral oedema, confusion and seizures.

Selegiline. Selegiline has a mild therapeutic effect in its own right. Evidence that it slows the progression of the disease is highly controversial. There has been some doubt as to its safety, but this is also controversial and the subject of ongoing research. The usual dose is 5–10 mg in the morning.

COMT (catechol-O-methyl-transferase) inhibitors. Entacapone (200 mg with each dose of levodopa) prolongs the effects of each dose and reduces motor fluctuations when used with levodopa. This allows the levodopa dose to be reduced and given less frequently.

Dopamine receptor agonists. An increasing number of these drugs are becoming available. They all have slightly different activity at the various dopamine receptors in the brain. Apomorphine given alone causes marked vomiting and has to be administered parenterally. The vomiting can be overcome by the concomitant use of domperidone, and parenteral administration achieved through continuous subcutaneous infusion from a portable pump, or direct injection as needed. This requires considerable nursing support but, used correctly, can be very useful.

More easily administered drugs include bromocriptine, lisuride, pergolide, cabergoline, ropinirole and pramipexole, which can all be taken orally. These drugs are less powerful than levodopa in controlling features of parkinsonism, but they are much less likely to cause dose fluctuations or dyskinesia, though they will certainly exacerbate the latter once these have developed. Side-effects include nausea, vomiting, confusion and hallucinations. The dose of bromocriptine is 1 mg initially, increased to 2.5 mg 8-hourly, and thereafter up to 30 mg/day. Pergolide dose starts at 50 µg, increased to 250 µg 8-hourly, and possibly to 3000 µg/day. Dopamine agonists derived from ergot (e.g. pergolide and cabergoline) have recently been associated with the development of fibrotic reactions and thickening of heart valves. For this reason, most patients are screened with echocardiogram, chest X-ray and renal function tests before commencing therapy. The optimal frequency of screening by repeating these tests has not been determined, but many neurologists screen their patients every 6 months.

Surgery

Stereotactic thalamotomy can be used to treat tremor, though this is needed relatively infrequently because of the medical treatments available. Other stereotactic lesions are currently undergoing evaluation, in particular pallidotomy to help in the management of drug-induced dyskinesia. The implantation of fetal mid-brain cells into the basal ganglia to enhance dopaminergic activity remains experimental.

Physiotherapy and speech therapy

Patients at all stages of Parkinson's disease benefit from physiotherapy, which helps reduce rigidity and corrects

---

26.87 PARKINSON'S DISEASE IN OLD AGE

- **Incidence:** increasingly common with age.
- **Drug therapy:** the long-term side-effects of levodopa, such as dyskinesia, are less of a problem in patients whose disease starts after age 70, so it is reasonable to prescribe levodopa as the first-line agent, as opposed to a dopamine agonist in a younger patient.
- **Side-effects of medication:** much more common, particularly confusion and hallucinations, particularly with anticholinergic drugs.
- **Autonomic disturbances:** more likely, especially medication-induced postural hypotension and bladder instability.
- **Cognitive changes and dementia:** more common than in younger people with Parkinson's disease.
- **Prognosis:** better in those developing the disease over the age of 70.

---

abnormal posture. Speech therapy may help in cases where dysarthria and dysphonia interfere with communication.

Prognosis

The outlook for patients with Parkinson's disease is variable, and depends partly on the age of onset. If symptoms start in middle life, the disease is usually slowly progressive and likely to shorten lifespan because of the complications of immobility and tendency to fall. Onset after 70 is unlikely to shorten life or become severe.

OTHER AKINETIC-RIGID SYNDROMES

There are many conditions which can rarely manifest as parkinsonian syndromes, including other degenerative diseases (e.g. Huntington's disease, Wilson's disease) and infective diseases (e.g. syphilis). Drug-induced parkinsonism is much more common (particularly with neuroleptic agents and anti-emetics). These conditions should always be borne in mind in the differential diagnosis. In particular there are several specific degenerative conditions that can mimic idiopathic Parkinson's disease, particularly in the early stages. These conditions are relatively uncommon, but about 10% of those thought to have idiopathic Parkinson's disease have one of these variants. The variants are notable in causing a more rapid clinical deterioration than idiopathic Parkinson's disease and in being more resistant to treatment with dopaminergic medication.

Multiple systems atrophy (MSA)

This is a sporadic condition seen in middle-aged and elderly patients. Features of parkinsonism, often without tremor, are combined with varying degrees of autonomic failure, cerebellar involvement and pyramidal tract dysfunction. The combination of parkinsonism with autonomic failure was called the Shy–Drager syndrome, but this term is declining in use. Degeneration is more widespread than in idiopathic Parkinson's disease, and the disappointing response to levodopa and other anti-parkinsonian drugs is probably because of degeneration of post-synaptic neurons in the basal ganglia. Autonomic features include postural hypotension, sphincter disturbance and sometimes respiratory stridor; diagnosis is often assisted by performing tests of

26

autonomic function. Management of postural hypotension includes physical measures such as head-up sleeping position and compression stockings, and drugs such as fludrocortisone and midodrine (p. 554). Falls are much more common than in idiopathic Parkinson's disease, and life expectancy is considerably reduced.

Progressive supranuclear palsy

Like MSA, this sporadic condition presents in middle-aged patients, and is due to more widespread degeneration in the brain than is seen in idiopathic Parkinson's disease. The clinical features include parkinsonism, though with rigidity in extension rather than flexion, and tremor is usually minimal. In addition, there must be a supranuclear paralysis of eye movements, usually downgaze, for the diagnosis to be made. Other features include pyramidal signs and cognitive impairment.

WILSON'S DISEASE

This is an inherited disorder transmitted in an autosomal recessive manner, involving a defect of copper metabolism. It is discussed on page 975. It is a treatable cause of various movement disorders, including ataxia and akinetic rigid syndromes, and so must always be considered in the differential diagnosis of these disorders.

HUNTINGTON'S DISEASE

This is an inherited disorder with autosomal dominant transmission, affecting both males and females, and usually starting in adult life. It is due to expansion of a trinucleotide repeat on chromosome 4 (p. 45) and frequently demonstrates anticipation, i.e. a younger age of onset in subsequent generations. Slightly different features of the disease occur, depending on whether the abnormal gene is inherited from father or mother.

Clinical features

Symptoms usually begin in middle adult life with the development of chorea, which gradually worsens. This is accompanied by cognitive impairment which often manifests initially as psychiatric symptoms, but later becomes frank dementia. In juvenile-onset disease, there may be parkinsonian features with rigidity. Seizures may occur late in the disease.

Investigations

The diagnosis is made clinically but is supported by the finding of atrophy of the caudate nucleus on CT or MRI. DNA analysis can be used to confirm the diagnosis and provide pre-symptomatic testing for other family members after appropriate counselling (p. 57).

Management

At present this is symptomatic only. The chorea may respond to tetrabenazine or dopamine antagonists such as sulpiride. Long-term psychological support and eventually institutional care are often needed as dementia progresses. Depressive symptoms are common, and may be helped by antidepressant medication. Genetic counselling of relatives is important.

HEREDITARY ATAXIAS

This is a group of inherited disorders in which degenerative changes occur to varying extents in the cerebellum, brain stem, pyramidal tracts, spinocerebellar tracts, optic and peripheral nerves. Onset may be in childhood or adulthood, and different disorders demonstrate recessive, sex-linked or dominant inheritance. Recently, the genetic abnormalities responsible for some types of spinocerebellar ataxia have been shown to be due to abnormal numbers of trinucleotide repeats in various genes, and these can now be detected by DNA analysis, allowing diagnostic confirmation, pre-diagnostic testing and genetic counselling. Other conditions

26.88 HEREDITARY ATAXIAS			
Type	**Inheritance**	**Onset**	**Clinical features**
Friedreich's ataxia	Autosomal recessive	8–16 years	Ataxia, nystagmus, dysarthria, spasticity, areflexia, proprioceptive impairment, diabetes mellitus, optic atrophy, cardiac abnormalities. Usually chairbound by age 20
Ataxia telangiectasia	Autosomal recessive	Childhood	Progressive ataxia, athetosis, telangiectasia on conjunctivae, impaired DNA repair, immune deficiency, tendency to malignancies
Abetalipoproteinaemia	Autosomal recessive	Childhood	Steatorrhoea, sensorimotor neuropathy, retinitis pigmentosa, malabsorption of vitamins A, D, E, K, cardiomyopathy
Spinocerebellar ataxia types 1–21	Autosomal dominant	Childhood to middle age	Progressive ataxia, some types have associated retinitis pigmentosa, pyramidal tract abnormalities, peripheral neuropathy and cognitive deficits
Dentato-rubro-pallido-luysian atrophy (DRPLA)	Autosomal dominant	Childhood to middle age	Children present with myoclonic epilepsy and progressive ataxia; adults have progressive ataxia with psychiatric features, dementia and choreoathetosis
Episodic ataxias (types 1–4)	Autosomal dominant	Childhood and early adulthood	Brief episodes of ataxia, sometimes induced by stress or startle. Some develop progressive fixed ataxia

26

which may manifest as progressive ataxia, including Friedreich's ataxia, are shown in Box 26.88.

MOTOR NEURON DISEASE

This is a progressive disorder of unknown cause, in which there is degeneration of motor neurons in the spinal cord and cranial nerve nuclei, and of pyramidal neurons in the motor cortex. About 5% of cases are familial, showing autosomal dominant inheritance. In many such families, the genetic defect lies on chromosome 21, the enzyme involved being a superoxide dismutase (SOD1). For the remaining 95%, possible causes include viral infection, trauma, exposure to toxins and electric shock, but no sound evidence exists to support any of these. The prevalence of the disease is about 5/100 000.

Clinical features

Patients present with a combination of lower and upper motor neuron signs without sensory involvement. The presence of brisk reflexes in wasted fasciculating limb muscles is typical. Common presenting features are listed in Boxes 26.89 and 26.90.

Investigations

In many patients the clinical features are highly suggestive but alternative diagnoses need to be carefully excluded. In particular, potentially treatable disorders such as diabetic amyotrophy, spinal disorders and multifocal motor neuronopathy should be excluded. Electromyography helps to confirm the presence of fasciculation and denervation, and is particularly helpful when pyramidal features predominate. Sensory nerve conduction and motor conduction studies are normal but there may be some reduction in amplitude of action potentials due to loss of axons. Spinal imaging and brain scanning may be necessary to exclude focal spinal or

26.89 CLINICAL FEATURES OF MOTOR NEURON DISEASE	

Onset

- Usually after the age of 50 years
- Very uncommon before the age of 30 years
- Affects males more commonly than females

Symptoms

- Limb muscle weakness, cramps, occasionally fasciculation
- Disturbance of speech/swallowing (dysarthria/dysphagia)

Signs

- Wasting and fasciculation of muscles
- Weakness of muscles of limbs, tongue, face and palate
- Pyramidal tract involvement causes spasticity, exaggerated tendon reflexes, extensor plantar responses
- External ocular muscles and sphincters usually remain intact
- No objective sensory deficit
- No intellectual impairment in most cases

Course

- Symptoms often begin focally in one part and spread gradually but relentlessly to become widespread

26.90 PATTERNS OF INVOLVEMENT OF MOTOR NEURON DISEASE	

Progressive muscular atrophy

- Predominantly spinal motor neurons affected
- Weakness and wasting of distal limb muscles at first
- Fasciculation in muscles
- Tendon reflexes may be absent

Progressive bulbar palsy

- Early involvement of tongue, palate and pharyngeal muscles
- Dysarthria/dysphagia
- Wasting and fasciculation of tongue
- May be pyramidal signs as well

Amyotrophic lateral sclerosis

- Combination of distal and proximal muscle-wasting and weakness, fasciculation
- Spasticity, exaggerated reflexes, extensor plantars
- Bulbar and pseudobulbar palsy follow eventually
- Pyramidal tract features may predominate

26.91 RILUZOLE AND MOTOR NEURON DISEASE | **EBM**

'Riluzole 100 mg per day appears to be modestly effective in prolonging survival for patients with motor neuron disease by about 2 months. However, the economics of its use have yet to be fully assessed.'

- Miller RG, et al. (Cochrane Review). Cochrane Library, issue 2, 2004. Chichester: John Wiley.

For further information: 💻 www.cochrane.org

cerebral disease. CSF examination is usually normal, though a slight elevation in protein concentration may be found.

Management

The glutamate antagonist, riluzole, has recently been shown to have a small effect in prolonging life expectancy by about two months (Box 26.91). It is not clear at which stage of the illness this prolongation occurs, and therefore it may not be particularly helpful. Other agents such as nerve growth factor show promise. Psychological and physical support, with help from occupational and speech therapists and physiotherapists, are essential to maintain the patient's quality of life. Mechanical aids such as splints, walking aids, wheelchairs and communication devices all help to reduce handicap. Feeding by percutaneous gastrostomy may be necessary if bulbar palsy is marked. Sometimes non-invasive ventilatory support may help distress from weak respiratory muscles although maintenance ventilation is usually not requested. Relief of distress in the terminal stages usually requires the use of opiates and sedative drugs (p. 275).

Prognosis

Motor neuron disease is progressive; the mean time from diagnosis to death is 1 year, with most patients dying within 3–5 years of the onset of symptoms. Younger patients and those with early bulbar symptoms tend to show a more rapid course. Death is usually from respiratory infection and failure, and the complications of immobility.

26.92 TYPES OF SPINAL MUSCULAR ATROPHY				
Type	**Onset**	**Inheritance**	**Features**	**Prognosis**
Werdnig–Hoffmann	Infancy	Autosomal recessive	Severe muscle-wasting/weakness	Poor
Kugelberg–Welander	Childhood, adolescence	Autosomal recessive	Proximal weakness and wasting, EMG shows denervation	Slowly progressive disability
Distal forms	Early adult life	Autosomal dominant	Distal weakness and wasting of hands and feet	Good, seldom disabling
Bulbospinal	Adult life, males only	X-linked	Facial and bulbar weakness, proximal limb weakness, gynaecomastia	Good

SPINAL MUSCULAR ATROPHIES

This is a group of genetically determined disorders affecting spinal motor and cranial motor neurons, characterised by proximal and distal wasting, fasciculation and weakness of muscles. Involvement is usually symmetrical but occasional localised forms occur. With the exception of the infantile form, progression is slow and the prognosis better than for motor neuron disease (Box 26.92).

INFECTIONS OF THE NERVOUS SYSTEM

The clinical features of nervous system infections depend upon the location of the infection (the meninges or in the parenchyma of the brain and spinal cord), the causative organism (virus, bacterium or parasite), and whether the infection is acute or chronic. The major infections of the nervous system are listed in Box 26.93. The frequency of these varies geographically. Helminthic infections such as cysticercosis and hydatid disease, and protozoal infections are described in Chapter 13.

MENINGITIS

Acute infection of the meninges presents with a characteristic combination of pyrexia, headache and meningism. Meningism, which can occur in other situations (e.g. subarachnoid haemorrhage), consists of stiffness of the neck, often with other signs of meningeal irritation: Kernig's sign (with the hip joint flexed, extension at the knee causes spasm in the hamstring muscles) and Brudzinski's sign (passive flexion of the neck causes flexion of the thighs and knees). The severity of these features varies somewhat according to the causative organism, as does the presence of other features such as a rash. Abnormalities in the CSF (Box 26.94) are very helpful in distinguishing the cause of meningitis. Causes of meningitis are listed in Box 26.95.

VIRAL MENINGITIS

Viral infection is the most common cause of meningitis, and usually results in a benign and self-limiting illness

26.93 INFECTIONS OF THE NERVOUS SYSTEM	
Bacterial infections	
• Meningitis	• Neurosyphilis
• Suppurative encephalitis	• Leprosy (peripheral nerves)
• Brain abscess	• Diphtheria (peripheral nerves)
• Tuberculosis	• Tetanus (motor cells)
• Paravertebral (epidural) abscess	
Viral infections	
• Meningitis	• Subacute sclerosing
• Encephalitis	panencephalitis (late sequel)
• Transverse myelitis	• Poliomyelitis
• Progressive multifocal	• Rabies
leucoencephalopathy	• HIV infection (Ch. 14)
Prion diseases	
• Creutzfeldt–Jakob disease	• Kuru
Protozoal infections	
• Malaria*	• Trypanosomiasis*
• Toxoplasmosis (in	• Amoebic abscess*
immunosuppressed)*	
Helminthic infections	
• Schistosomiasis (spinal cord)*	• Hydatid disease*
• Cysticercosis*	• Strongyloidiasis*
Fungal infections	
• Cryptococcal meningitis	• Candida meningitis or brain abscess
*These infections are not detailed in this chapter. They can be found in Chapter 13.	

requiring no specific therapy. It is a much less serious illness than bacterial meningitis unless there is associated encephalitis, which is rare. A number of viruses can cause meningitis (Box 26.95), the most common being echoviruses and, where specific immunisation is not employed, the mumps virus.

Clinical features

The condition occurs mainly in children or young adults, with acute onset of headache and irritability and the rapid development of meningism. In viral meningitis, the headache is usually the more severe feature. There may be a high pyrexia, but focal neurological signs rarely occur.

26

26.94 CEREBROSPINAL FLUID INDICES IN MENINGITIS*

Condition	Cell type	Cell count	Glucose	Protein	Gram stain
Normal	Lymphocytes	$0–4 \times 10^6/l$	> 60% of blood glucose	Up to 0.45 g/l	–
Viral	Lymphocytes	10–2000	Normal	Normal	–
Bacterial	Polymorphs	1000–5000	Low	Normal/elevated	+
Tuberculous	Polymorphs/lymphocytes/mixed	50–5000	Low	Elevated	Often –
Fungal	Lymphocytes	50–500	Low	Elevated	±
Malignant	Lymphocytes	0–100	Low	Normal/elevated	–

* See also Box 26.5, page 1160.

26.95 CAUSES OF MENINGITIS

Infective

Bacteria (Box 26.96)
- *Brucella*

Viruses
- Enteroviruses (echo, Coxsackie, polio)
- Mumps
- Influenza
- Herpes simplex
- Varicella zoster
- Epstein–Barr
- HIV
- Lymphocytic choriomeningitis
- Mollaret's meningitis (HSV type 2)

Protozoa and parasites
- *Toxoplasma*
- Amoeba
- *Cysticercus*

Fungi
- *Cryptococcus neoformans*
- *Candida*
- *Histoplasma*
- *Blastomyces*
- *Coccidioides*
- *Sporothrix*

Non-infective ('sterile')

Malignant disease
- Breast cancer
- Bronchial cancer
- Leukaemia
- Lymphoma

Inflammatory disease (may be recurrent)
- Sarcoidosis
- SLE
- Behçet's disease

Investigations

The CSF usually contains an excess of lymphocytes, but glucose and protein levels are commonly normal or the protein level may be raised. It is extremely important to verify that the patient has not received antibiotics (for whatever cause) prior to the lumbar puncture, as this picture can also be found in partially treated bacterial meningitis.

Management

There is no specific treatment and the condition is usually benign and self-limiting. The patient should be treated symptomatically in a quiet environment. Recovery usually occurs within days, although a lymphocytic pleocytosis may persist in the CSF.

Meningitis may also occur as a complication of a viral infection primarily involving other organs: for example, in mumps, measles, infectious mononucleosis, herpes zoster and hepatitis. Complete recovery without specific therapy is the rule.

PYOGENIC BACTERIAL MENINGITIS

Many bacteria can cause meningitis. Certain organisms are particularly common at different age ranges (Box 26.96). Bacterial meningitis is usually secondary to a bacteraemic illness, although infection may result from direct spread from an adjacent focus of infection in the ear, skull fracture or sinus. Bacterial meningitis has become less common but the mortality and morbidity remain significant despite the availability of an increasing range of antibiotics. An important factor in determining prognosis is early diagnosis and the prompt initiation of appropriate therapy.

The meningococcus *(Neisseria meningitidis)* is now second to *Streptococcus pneumoniae* as the most common cause of bacterial meningitis in Western Europe, whilst in the USA, *Haemophilus influenzae* remains common. In India, *Haemophilus influenzae* B and *Streptococcus pneumoniae* are probably the most common causes of bacterial meningitis, at least in children.

The meningococcus and other common causes of meningitis are normal commensals of the upper respiratory tract. New and potentially pathogenic strains are acquired by the air-borne route, but close contact is necessary. Epidemics of meningococcal meningitis occur, particularly in cramped living conditions or where the climate is hot and dry, e.g. areas of Africa. The organism invades through the nasopharynx, producing septicaemia that is usually associated with pyogenic meningitis. Complications of meningococcal septicaemia are listed in Box 26.97. Chronic meningococcaemia is a rare condition in which the patient can be unwell for weeks or even months with recurrent fever, sweating, joint pains and transient rash. It usually occurs in the middle-aged and elderly and those who have previously had a splenectomy.

In pneumococcal and *Haemophilus* infections there may be an associated otitis media. Pneumococcal meningitis may be associated with pneumonia and occurs especially in older patients and alcoholics, as well as those without functioning spleens. *Listeria monocytogenes* has recently emerged as an increasing cause of meningitis and rhombencephalitis

26

26.96 BACTERIAL CAUSES OF MENINGITIS

Age of onset	Common	Less common
Neonate	Gram-negative bacilli (*Escherichia coli*, *Proteus* etc.) Group B streptococci	*Listeria monocytogenes*
Pre-school child	*Haemophilus influenzae* *Neisseria meningitidis* *Streptococcus pneumoniae*	*Mycobacterium tuberculosis*
Older child and adult	*Neisseria meningitidis* *Streptococcus pneumoniae*	*Listeria monocytogenes* *Mycobacterium tuberculosis* *Staphylococcus aureus* (skull fracture) *Haemophilus influenzae*

26.97 COMPLICATIONS OF MENINGOCOCCAL SEPTICAEMIA

- Meningitis
- Rash (morbilliform, petechial or purpuric)
- Shock
- Intravascular coagulation
- Renal failure
- Peripheral gangrene
- Arthritis (septic or reactive)
- Pericarditis (septic or reactive)

(brain-stem encephalitis) in the immunosuppressed, diabetics, alcoholics and pregnant women (p. 323). It can also cause meningitis in the neonatal period.

Pathology

The pia-arachnoid is congested and infiltrated with inflammatory cells. A thin layer of pus forms and this may later organise to form adhesions. These may cause obstruction to the free flow of CSF leading to hydrocephalus, or they may damage the cranial nerves at the base of the brain. The CSF pressure rises rapidly, the protein content increases, and there is a cellular reaction that varies in type and severity according to the nature of the inflammation and the causative organism. An obliterative endarteritis of the leptomeningeal arteries passing through the meningeal exudate may produce secondary cerebral infarction. Pneumococcal meningitis is often associated with a very purulent CSF and a high mortality, especially in older adults.

Clinical features

Headache, drowsiness, fever and neck stiffness are the usual presenting features. In severe bacterial meningitis the patient may be comatose and later there may be focal neurological signs. Meningococcal meningitis is associated with a purpuric rash in 70% of cases. When accompanied by septicaemia, it may present very rapidly, with abrupt onset of obtundation due to cerebral oedema, probably as a result of endotoxin and/or cytokine release, and circulatory collapse.

Investigations

Lumbar puncture is mandatory unless there are contraindications (p. 1158). Particularly if the patient is drowsy with focal neurological signs or seizures, it is wise to obtain

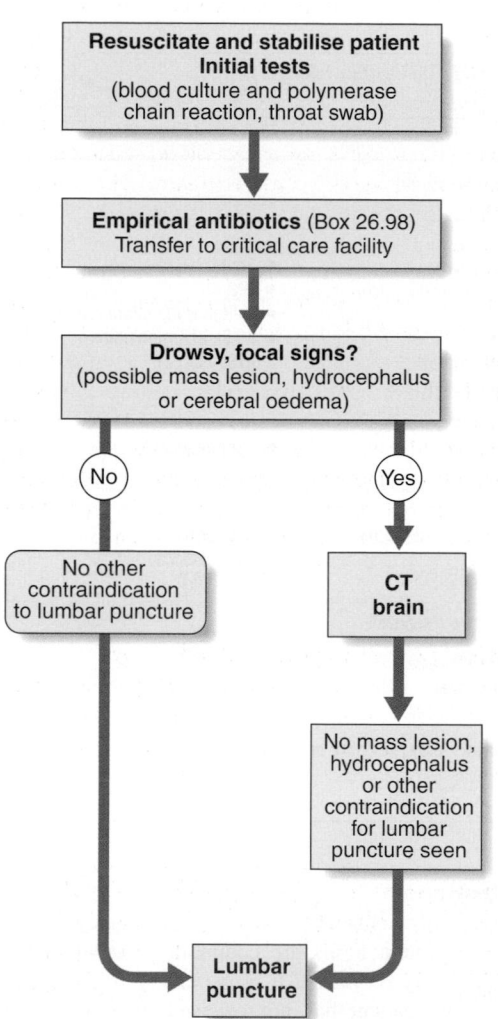

Fig. 26.43 **The investigation of meningitis.**

a CT to exclude a mass lesion (such as a cerebral abscess) before lumbar puncture because of the risk of coning, but this should not delay treatment of a presumptive meningitis. If lumbar puncture is deferred or omitted, it is essential to take diagnostic specimens and to start empirical treatment (Fig. 26.43).

In bacterial meningitis the CSF is cloudy (turbid) due to the presence of many neutrophils (often $> 10^9$ cells/litre),

26

the protein content is significantly elevated and the glucose reduced. Gram film and culture may allow identification of the organism. Blood cultures may be positive. Polymerase chain reaction (PCR) techniques can be used on both blood and CSF to identify bacterial DNA. These methods are useful in detecting meningococcal infection and in typing the organism.

Management

If meningococcal or other bacterial meningitis is suspected, the patient should be given parenteral benzylpenicillin immediately (intravenous is preferable to intramuscular) and prompt admission to hospital should be arranged. The only contraindication is a history of penicillin anaphylaxis. Recommended empirical therapy before the cause of meningitis is known is given in Box 26.98. The antibiotic regimen may be modified after CSF examination, depending on the infecting organism. Guidance as to the preferred antibiotic is given in Box 26.99 (for when the organism is known) and in Box 26.98 (for when the organism has not been identified). Adjunctive corticosteroid therapy is useful in both children (Box 26.100) and, as demonstrated more recently, adults.

In meningococcal disease, mortality is doubled if the patient presents with features of septicaemia rather than meningitis. Patients likely to require intensive care facilities and expertise include those with cardiac, respiratory or renal involvement, and those with CNS depression prejudicing the airway. Early endotracheal intubation and mechanical ventilation protect the airway and may prevent the development of the acute respiratory distress syndrome (ARDS, p. 187). Adverse prognostic features include hypotensive shock, a rapidly developing rash, a haemorrhagic diathesis, multisystem failure and an age of more than 60 years.

Prevention of meningococcal infection

Household and other close contacts of patients with meningococcal infections, especially children, should be given 2 days of oral rifampicin (age 3–12 months 5 mg/kg 12-hourly, > 1 year 10 mg/kg 12-hourly, adults 600 mg 12-hourly). In adults, a single dose of 500 mg of

26.98 TREATMENT OF PYOGENIC MENINGITIS OF UNKNOWN CAUSE

1. Patients with a typical meningococcal rash

- Benzylpenicillin 2.4 g i.v. 6-hourly

2. Adults aged 18–50 years without a typical meningococcal rash

- Cefotaxime 2 g i.v. 6-hourly
  or
- Ceftriaxone 2 g i.v. 12-hourly

3. Patients in whom penicillin-resistant pneumococcal infection is suspected

- As for (2) but add:
  Vancomycin 1 g i.v. 12-hourly
  or
  Rifampicin 600 mg i.v. 12-hourly

4. Adults aged over 50 years and those in whom *Listeria monocytogenes* infection is suspected (e.g. brain-stem signs, immunosuppression, diabetic, alcoholic)

- As for (2) but add:
  Ampicillin 2 g i.v. 4-hourly
  or
  Co-trimoxazole 50 mg/kg i.v. daily in two divided doses

5. Patients with a clear history of anaphylaxis to β-lactams

- Chloramphenicol 25 mg/kg i.v. 6-hourly
  plus
  Vancomycin 1 g i.v. 12-hourly

EBM

26.100 ADJUNCTIVE DEXAMETHASONE FOR BACTERIAL MENINGITIS IN CHILDREN

'Adjunctive dexamethasone therapy prevents severe deafness following *H. influenzae* type B meningitis and, if commenced with or before parenteral antibiotics, in pneumococcal meningitis in childhood. Limiting dexamethasone therapy to 2 days may be optimal.'

- McIntyre PB, et al. JAMA 1997; 278:925–931.
- Coyle PK. Arch Neurol 1999; 56:796–801.

For further information: 💻 www.clinicalevidence.org

26

26.99 CHEMOTHERAPY OF BACTERIAL MENINGITIS WHEN THE CAUSE IS KNOWN

Pathogen	Regimen of choice	Alternative agent(s)
N. meningitidis	Benzylpenicillin 2.4 g i.v. 4-hourly for 5–7 days	Cefuroxime, ampicillin Chloramphenicol*
Strep. pneumoniae (sensitive to β-lactams, minimum inhibitory concentration (MIC) < 1 mg/l)	Cefotaxime 2 g i.v. 6-hourly *or* ceftriaxone 2 g i.v. 12-hourly for 10–14 days	Chloramphenicol*
Strep. pneumoniae (resistant to β-lactams)	As for sensitive strains but add vancomycin 1 g i.v. 12-hourly *or* rifampicin 600 mg i.v. 12-hourly	Vancomycin *plus* rifampicin*
H. influenzae	Cefotaxime 2 g i.v. 6-hourly *or* ceftriaxone 2 g i.v. 12-hourly for 10–14 days	Chloramphenicol*
Listeria monocytogenes	Ampicillin 2 g i.v. 4-hourly *plus* gentamicin 5 mg/kg i.v. daily	Ampicillin 2 g i.v. 4-hourly *plus* co-trimoxazole 50 mg/kg daily in two divided doses

*For patients with a history of anaphylaxis to β-lactam antibiotics.

ciprofloxacin is an alternative. If not treated with ceftriaxone, the index case should be given similar treatment to clear infection from the nasopharynx before hospital discharge. Vaccines are available for the prevention of disease caused by meningococci of groups A and C, but not group B which is the most common serogroup isolated in many countries, including the UK.

TUBERCULOUS MENINGITIS

Now rare in developed countries in previously healthy individuals, tuberculous meningitis remains common in developing countries and is seen more frequently as a secondary infection in patients with AIDS.

Pathology

Tuberculous meningitis occurs most commonly shortly after a primary infection in childhood or as part of miliary tuberculosis. The usual local source of infection is a caseous focus in the meninges or brain substance adjacent to the CSF pathway. The brain is covered by a greenish, gelatinous exudate, especially around the base, and numerous scattered tubercles are found on the meninges.

Clinical features

The clinical features are listed in Box 26.101.

Investigations

The CSF is under increased pressure. It is usually clear but, when allowed to stand, a fine clot ('spider web') may form. The fluid contains up to 5×10^8 cells/litre, predominantly lymphocytes. There is a rise in protein and a marked fall in glucose. Detection of the tubercle bacillus in a smear of the centrifuged deposit from the CSF may be difficult. The CSF should be cultured but as this result will not be known for up to 6 weeks, treatment must be started without waiting for confirmation. Brain imaging may show hydrocephalus, brisk meningeal enhancement on enhanced CT and/or an intracranial tuberculoma.

Management

As soon as the diagnosis is made or strongly suspected, chemotherapy should be started using one of the regimens including pyrazinamide described on page 701. The use of corticosteroids in addition to antituberculous therapy has been controversial. Recent evidence suggests that it

improves mortality but not focal neurological damage, especially if given early. Surgical ventricular drainage may be needed if obstructive hydrocephalus develops. Skilled nursing is essential during the acute phase of the illness, and measures should be put in place to maintain adequate hydration and nutrition.

Prognosis

Untreated tuberculous meningitis is fatal in a few weeks but complete recovery is the rule if treatment is started before the appearance of focal signs or stupor. When treatment is started at a later stage, the recovery rate is 60% or less and the survivors show permanent neurological deficit.

OTHER FORMS OF MENINGITIS

Fungal meningitis (especially cryptococcosis—p. 375) usually occurs in patients who are immunosuppressed and is a recognised complication of HIV infection (p. 394). The CSF findings are similar to those of tuberculous meningitis, but the diagnosis can be confirmed by microscopy or specific serological tests.

In some areas, meningitis may be caused by spirochaetes (leptospirosis, Lyme disease and syphilis—pp. 321, 319 and 411), rickettsiae (typhus fever—p. 338) or protozoa (amoebiasis—p. 358).

Meningitis can also be due to non-infective pathologies. This is seen in recurrent aseptic meningitis due to SLE, Behçet's disease or sarcoidosis, as well as a condition of previously unknown origin known as Mollaret's syndrome in which the recurrent meningitis is associated with epithelioid cells in the spinal fluid ('Mollaret' cells). Recent evidence suggests that this condition may be due to human herpes virus type 2, and therefore infective after all. Meningitis can also be seen due to direct invasion of the meninges by neoplasm ('malignant meningitis'—Box 26.95, p. 1225).

PARENCHYMAL VIRAL INFECTIONS

Infection of the substance of the nervous system will produce symptoms of focal dysfunction (focal deficits and/or seizures) with general signs of infection depending upon the acuteness of the infection and the type of organism.

VIRAL ENCEPHALITIS

A range of viruses can cause encephalitis but only a minority of patients have a history of recent viral infection. In Europe, the most serious cause of viral encephalitis is herpes simplex (p. 303), which probably reaches the brain via the olfactory nerves. The development of effective therapy for some forms of encephalitis has increased the importance of clinical diagnosis and virological examination of the CSF. In some parts of the world, viruses transmitted by mosquitoes and ticks (arboviruses) are an important cause of encephalitis. The epidemiology of some of these infections is changing. Japanese encephalitis (p. 312) has spread relentlessly across Asia to Australia, and

26.101 CLINICAL FEATURES OF TUBERCULOUS MENINGITIS	
Symptoms	
• Headache	• Depression
• Vomiting	• Confusion
• Low-grade fever	• Behaviour changes
• Lassitude	
Signs	
• Meningism (may be absent)	• Depression of conscious level
• Oculomotor palsies	• Focal hemisphere signs
• Papilloedema	

26

there have been outbreaks of West Nile encephalitis in Romania, Israel and New York. Acute encephalitis may occur in HIV infection, occasionally at the time of infection, but more commonly as a manifestation of AIDS (p. 391).

Pathology

Inflammation can occur in the cortex, white matter, basal ganglia and brain stem, and the distribution of lesions varies with the type of virus. In herpes simplex encephalitis, the temporal lobes are usually primarily affected. Inclusion bodies may be present in the neurons and glial cells and there is an infiltration of polymorphonuclear cells in the perivascular space. There is neuronal degeneration and diffuse glial proliferation, often associated with cerebral oedema.

Clinical features

Viral encephalitis presents with acute onset of headache, fever, focal neurological signs (aphasia and/or hemiplegia) and seizures. Disturbance of consciousness ranging from drowsiness to deep coma supervenes early and may advance dramatically. Meningism occurs in many patients. Rabies presents a distinct clinical picture and is described below.

Investigations

CT of the head, which should precede lumbar puncture, may show low-density lesions in the temporal lobes. MRI is more sensitive in detecting early abnormalities The CSF usually contains excess lymphocytes, but polymorphonuclear cells may predominate in the early stages. Occasionally, the CSF is normal. The protein content may be elevated but the glucose is normal. The EEG is usually abnormal in the early stages, especially in herpes simplex encephalitis, with characteristic periodic slow-wave activity in the temporal lobes. Virological investigations of the CSF, including PCR for viral DNA, may reveal the causative organism but the initiation of treatment should not await this.

Management

Anticonvulsant treatment is often necessary (p. 1172) and raised intracranial pressure is treated with dexamethasone 8 mg 12-hourly. Herpes simplex encephalitis responds to aciclovir 10 mg/kg i.v. 8-hourly for 2–3 weeks. This should be given early to all patients suspected of suffering from viral encephalitis.

Even with optimum treatment, mortality is 10–30% and significant proportions of survivors have residual epilepsy or cognitive impairment. For details of post-infectious encephalomyelitis, see page 1216.

BRAIN-STEM ENCEPHALITIS

This presents with ataxia, dysarthria, diplopia or other cranial nerve palsies. The CSF is lymphocytic, with a normal glucose. The causative agent is presumed to be viral. However, *Listeria monocytogenes* may cause a similar syndrome with meningitis (and often a polymorphonuclear CSF pleocytosis) and requires specific treatment with ampicillin 500 mg 6-hourly (Box 26.99).

RABIES

Rabies is caused by a rhabdovirus which infects the central nervous tissue and salivary glands of a wide range of mammals, and is usually conveyed by saliva through bites or licks on abrasions or on intact mucous membranes. Humans are most frequently infected from dogs. In Europe, the maintenance host is the fox.

The incubation period varies in humans from a minimum of 9 days to many months but is usually between 4 and 8 weeks. Severe bites, especially if on the head or neck, are associated with shorter incubation periods.

Clinical features

At the onset there may be fever, and paraesthesia at the site of the bite. A prodromal period of 1–10 days, during which the patient is increasingly anxious, leads to the characteristic 'hydrophobia'. Although the patient is thirsty, attempts at drinking provoke violent contractions of the diaphragm and other inspiratory muscles. Delusions and hallucinations may develop, accompanied by spitting, biting and mania, with lucid intervals in which the patient is markedly anxious. Cranial nerve lesions develop and terminal hyperpyrexia is common. Death ensues, usually within a week of the onset of symptoms.

Investigations

During life, the diagnosis is usually made on clinical grounds but rapid immunofluorescent techniques can detect antigen in corneal impression smears or skin biopsies.

Management

A few patients with rabies have survived. All received some post-exposure prophylaxis, and needed intensive care facilities to control cardiac and respiratory failure. Otherwise, only palliative treatment is possible once symptoms have appeared. The patient should be heavily sedated with diazepam 10 mg 4–6-hourly, supplemented by chlorpromazine 50–100 mg if necessary. Nutrition and fluids should be given intravenously or through a gastrostomy.

Prevention

Pre-exposure prophylaxis

Pre-exposure prophylaxis is required by those who professionally handle potentially infected animals, those who work with rabies virus in laboratories and those who live at special risk in rabies-endemic areas. Protection is afforded by two intradermal injections of 0.1 ml human diploid cell strain vaccine, or two intramuscular injections of 1 ml, given 4 weeks apart, followed by yearly boosters.

Post-exposure prophylaxis

The wounds should be thoroughly cleaned, preferably with a quaternary ammonium detergent or soap; damaged tissues should be excised and the wound left unsutured. Rabies can usually be prevented if treatment is started within a day or two of biting. Delayed treatment may still be of value. For maximum protection, hyperimmune serum and vaccine are required.

26

The safest antirabies antiserum is human rabies immune globulin; the dose is 20 U/kg body weight. Half is infiltrated around the bite and half is given intramuscularly at a different site from the vaccine. The dose of hyperimmune animal serum is 40 U/kg; hypersensitivity reactions, including anaphylaxis, are common.

The safest vaccine, free of complications, is human diploid cell strain vaccine; 1.0 ml is given intramuscularly on days 0, 3, 7, 14, 30 and 90. In developing countries, where human rabies globulin may not be obtainable, 0.1 ml of vaccine should be given intradermally into eight sites on day 1, with single boosters on days 7 and 28. Where human products are not available and when risk of rabies is slight (licks on the skin, or minor bites of covered arms or legs), it may be justifiable to delay starting treatment for up to 5 days while observing the biting animal or awaiting examination of its brain, rather than use the older vaccine.

Control of spread

Human rabies is a rare disease, even in endemic areas. However, because it is usually fatal, major efforts are directed to limiting its spread and preventing its importation into uninfected countries such as the UK.

POLIOMYELITIS

Aetiology and pathology

The disease is caused by one of three polioviruses, which are a subgroup of the enteroviruses. It is much less common in developed countries following the widespread use of oral vaccines but is still a problem in the developing world, especially parts of Africa. Infection usually occurs through the nasopharynx.

The virus causes a lymphocytic meningitis and infects the grey matter of the spinal cord, brain stem and cortex. There is a particular propensity to damage anterior horn cells, especially in the lumbar segments.

Clinical features

The incubation period is 7–14 days. Figure 26.44 illustrates the various features of the infection. Many patients recover fully after the initial phase of a few days of mild fever and headache. In others, after a week of well-being, there is recurrence of pyrexia, headache and meningism. Weakness may start later in one muscle group and can progress to widespread paresis. Respiratory failure may supervene if intercostal muscles are paralysed or the medullary motor nuclei are involved.

Investigations

The CSF shows a lymphocytic pleocytosis, a rise in protein and a normal sugar content. Poliomyelitis virus may be cultured from CSF and stool.

Management

In the early stages, bed rest is imperative because exercise appears to worsen the paralysis or precipitate it. At the onset of respiratory difficulties, a tracheostomy and ventilation are required. Subsequent treatment is by physiotherapy and orthopaedic measures.

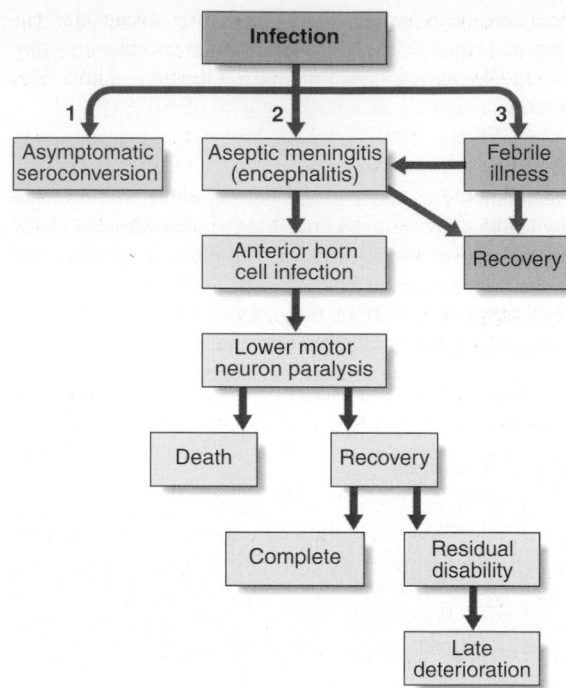

Fig. 26.44 Poliomyelitis. Possible consequences of infection.

Prognosis

Epidemics vary widely in their incidence of non-paralytic cases and in mortality rate. Death occurs from respiratory paralysis. Muscle weakness is maximal at the end of the first week and gradual recovery may then take place for several months. Muscles showing no signs of recovery by the end of a month will probably not regain useful function. Second attacks are very rare but occasionally patients show late deterioration in muscle bulk and power many years after the initial infection.

Prevention

Prevention of poliomyelitis is by immunisation with live (Sabin) vaccine. In developed countries where polio is now very rare, the live vaccine has been replaced by the killed vaccine in childhood immunisation schedules.

HERPES ZOSTER (SHINGLES)

Herpes zoster is the result of reactivation of the varicella zoster virus that has lain dormant in a nerve root ganglion following chickenpox earlier in life. Reactivation may be spontaneous (as usually occurs in the middle-aged or elderly) or due to immunosuppression (as in patients with diabetes, malignant disease or AIDS). Full details are given on page 305.

SUBACUTE SCLEROSING PANENCEPHALITIS

This is a rare, chronic, progressive and eventually fatal neurological disease caused by the measles virus, presumably as a result of an inability of the nervous system to eradicate the virus. It occurs in children and adolescents, usually many years after the primary virus infection. The onset is insidious, with intellectual deterioration, apathy and clumsiness followed by myoclonic jerks, rigidity and dementia.

The CSF may show a mild lymphocytic pleocytosis and the EEG is distinctive, with periodic bursts of triphasic waves. Although there is persistent measles-specific IgG in serum and CSF, antiviral therapy is ineffective and death ensues within years.

PROGRESSIVE MULTIFOCAL LEUCOENCEPHALOPATHY

This was originally described as a rare complication of lymphoma, leukaemia or carcinomatosis. Nowadays it occurs more frequently as a feature of AIDS (p. 393). It is an infection of oligodendrocytes by human polyomavirus JC, which causes widespread demyelination of the white matter of the cerebral hemispheres. Clinical signs include dementia, hemiparesis and aphasia which progress rapidly, usually leading to death within weeks or months. Areas of low density in the white matter are seen on CT but MRI is more sensitive, showing diffuse high signal in the cerebral white matter on T2-weighted images.

PARENCHYMAL BACTERIAL INFECTIONS

CEREBRAL ABSCESS

Bacteria may enter the cerebral substance through penetrating injury, by direct spread from paranasal sinuses or the middle ear, or by haematogenous spread from septicaemia. The site of abscess formation and the likely causative organism are both related to the source of infection (Box 26.102). Initial infection leads to local suppuration followed by loculation of pus within a surrounding wall of gliosis, which in a chronic abscess may form a tough capsule. Multiple abscesses may occur, particularly with haematogenous spread.

Clinical features

A cerebral abscess may present acutely with fever, headache, meningism and drowsiness, but more commonly

presents over days or weeks as a cerebral mass lesion with little or no evidence of infection. Seizures, raised intracranial pressure and focal hemisphere signs occur alone or in combination. Distinction from a cerebral tumour may be impossible on clinical grounds.

Investigations

Lumbar puncture is potentially hazardous in the presence of raised intracranial pressure, and CT should always precede it. CT reveals single or multiple low-density areas, which show ring enhancement with contrast and surrounding cerebral oedema (Fig. 26.45). There may be an elevated white blood cell count and ESR in patients with active local infection. The possibility of cerebral toxoplasmosis or tuberculous disease secondary to HIV infection should always be considered.

Management and prognosis

Antimicrobial therapy is indicated once the diagnosis is made. The likely source of infection should guide the choice of antibiotic (Box 26.102). Surgical treatment by burr-hole aspiration or excision may be necessary, especially where the presence of a capsule may lead to a persistent focus of infection. Anticonvulsants are often necessary, as epilepsy frequently develops acutely or in the recovery phase.

The mortality rate remains at 10–20% despite an improvement in available surgical and medical treatments, and in some patients this is related to delay in diagnosis and initiation of treatment.

SUBDURAL EMPYEMA

This is a rare complication of frontal sinusitis, osteomyelitis of the skull vault, or middle ear disease. A collection of pus in the subdural space spreads over the surface of the hemisphere, causing underlying cortical oedema or thrombophlebitis. Patients present with severe pain in the face or head and pyrexia, often with a history of preceding paranasal sinus or ear infection. The patient then becomes drowsy with seizures and focal signs such as a progressive hemiparesis.

The diagnosis rests on a strong clinical suspicion in patients with a local focus of infection. Careful assessment of a head CT (with contrast) or MRI may show a subdural

26.102 AETIOLOGY AND TREATMENT OF BACTERIAL CEREBRAL ABSCESS

Site of abscess	Source of infection	Likely organisms	Recommended treatment
Frontal lobe	Paranasal sinuses / Teeth	Streptococci / Anaerobes	Cefuroxime 1.5 g i.v. 8-hourly *plus* metronidazole 500 mg i.v. 8-hourly
Temporal lobe	Middle ear	Streptococci / Enterobacteriaceae	Ampicillin 2–3 g i.v. 8-hourly *plus* metronidazole 500 mg i.v. 8-hourly *plus* either ceftazidime 2 g i.v. 8-hourly *or* gentamicin* 5 mg/kg i.v. daily
Cerebellum	Sphenoid sinus / Mastoid/middle ear	*Pseudomonas* spp. / Anaerobes	
Any site	Penetrating trauma	Staphylococci	Flucloxacillin 2–3 g i.v. 6-hourly *or* cefuroxime 1.5 g i.v. 8-hourly
Multiple	Metastatic and cryptogenic	Streptococci / Anaerobes	Benzylpenicillin 1.8–2.4 g i.v. 6-hourly if endocarditis or cyanotic heart disease / Otherwise cefuroxime 1.5 g i.v. 8-hourly *plus* metronidazole 500 mg i.v. 8-hourly

*Monitor gentamicin levels.

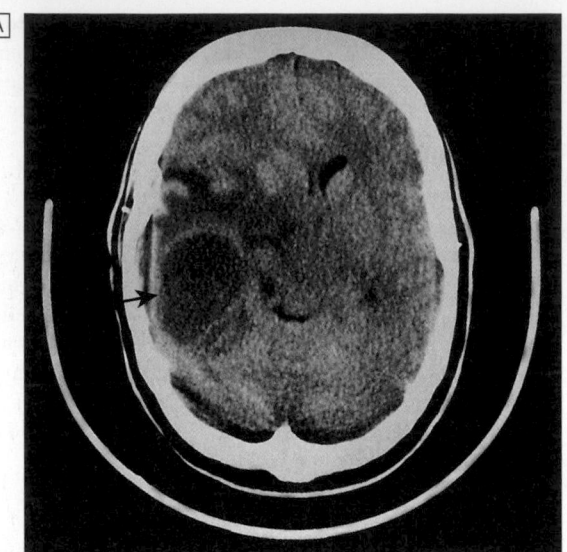 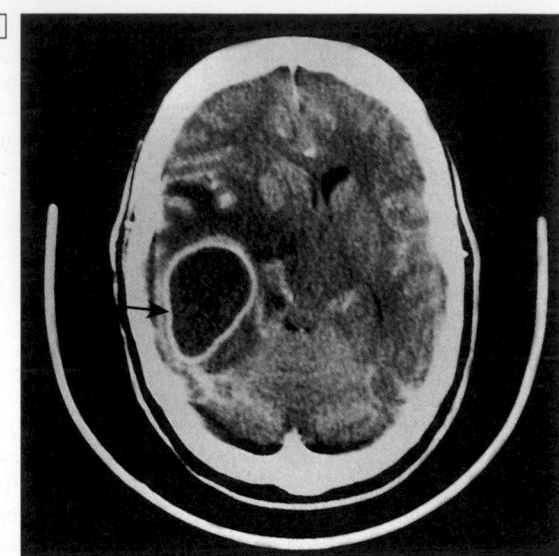

Fig. 26.45 **Right temporal cerebral abscess (arrows), with surrounding oedema and midline shift to the left.** Ⓐ Unenhanced CT image. Ⓑ Contrast-enhanced CT image.

collection with underlying cerebral oedema. Management requires aspiration of pus via a burr hole and appropriate parenteral antibiotics. Any local source of infection must be treated to prevent re-infection.

SPINAL EPIDURAL ABSCESS

The characteristic clinical features are pain in a root distribution and progressive transverse spinal cord syndrome with paraparesis, sensory impairment and sphincter dysfunction. Infection is usually haematogenous but a primary source of infection is easily overlooked. The resurgence of staphylococcal infection, often linked to intravenous drug misuse has contributed to a marked rise in incidence in recent years.

Plain X-rays of the spine may show osteomyelitis but such changes are often late. MRI or myelography should precede urgent neurosurgical intervention. Decompressive laminectomy with draining of the abscess relieves the pressure on the dura. This, together with appropriate anti-biotics, may prevent complete and irreversible paraplegia. Organisms may be cultured from the pus or blood.

TETANUS

This disease results from infection with *Clostridium tetani*, a commensal in the gut of humans and domestic animals which is found in soil. Infection enters the body through wounds, often trivial. It is rare in the UK, occurring mostly in gardeners and farmers but with a recent increase in intravenous drug misusers. By contrast, the disease is common in many developing countries, where dust contains spores derived from animal and human excreta. If childbirth takes place in an unhygienic environment, *Tetanus neonatorum* may result from infection of the umbilical stump, or the mother may develop the disease. Tetanus is still one of the major killers of adults, children and neonates

in developing countries, where the mortality rate can be nearly 100% in the newborn and around 40% in others.

In circumstances unfavourable to the growth of the organism, spores are formed and these may remain dormant for years in the soil. Spores germinate and bacilli multiply only in the anaerobic conditions which occur in areas of tissue necrosis or if the oxygen tension is low as a result of the presence of other organisms, particularly aerobic ones. The bacilli remain localised but produce an exotoxin with an affinity for motor nerve endings and motor nerve cells.

The anterior horn cells are affected after the exotoxin has passed into the blood stream and their involvement results in rigidity and convulsions. Symptoms first appear from 2 days to several weeks after injury—the shorter the incubation period, the more severe the attack and the worse the prognosis.

Clinical features

By far the most important early symptom is trismus— spasm of the masseter muscles, which causes difficulty in opening the mouth and in masticating; hence the name 'lockjaw'. Lockjaw in tetanus is painless, unlike the spasm of the masseters due to dental abscess, septic throat or other causes. Conditions that can mimic tetanus include hysteria and phenothiazine overdosage, or overdose in intravenous drug misusers.

In tetanus, the tonic rigidity spreads to involve the muscles of the face, neck and trunk. Contraction of the frontalis and the muscles at the angles of the mouth leads to the so-called 'risus sardonicus'. There is rigidity of the muscles at the neck and trunk of varying degree. The back is usually slightly arched ('opisthotonus') and there is a board-like abdominal wall.

In the more severe cases, violent spasms lasting for a few seconds to 3–4 minutes occur spontaneously, or may be induced by stimuli such as moving the patient or noise. These convulsions are painful, exhausting and of very serious significance, especially if they appear soon after the onset of symptoms. They gradually increase in frequency and severity for about 1 week and the patient may die from exhaustion, asphyxia or aspiration pneumonia. In less severe illness, convulsions may not commence for about a week after the first sign of rigidity, and in very mild infections they may never appear. Autonomic involvement may cause cardiovascular complications such as hypertension.

Rarely, the only manifestation of the disease may be 'local tetanus'—stiffness or spasm of the muscles near the infected wound—and the prognosis is good if treatment is commenced at this stage.

Investigations

The diagnosis is made on clinical grounds. It is rarely possible to isolate the infecting organism from the original locus of entry.

Management

This should be begun as soon as possible, as shown in Box 26.103.

26.103 TREATMENT OF TETANUS
Neutralise absorbed toxin
• I.v. injection of 3000 U of human tetanus antitoxin
Prevent further toxin production
• Débridement of wound • Benzylpenicillin 600 mg i.v. 6-hourly (metronidazole if allergic to penicillin)
Control spasms
• Nurse in a quiet room • Avoid unnecessary stimuli • I.v. diazepam—if spasms continue, paralyse patient and ventilate
General measures
• Maintain hydration and nutrition • Treat secondary infections

Prevention

Active immunisation must be given. Contaminated injuries are treated by débridement. The immediate danger of tetanus can be greatly reduced by the injection of 1200 mg of penicillin followed by a 7-day course of oral penicillin. For those who are allergic to penicillin, erythromycin should be used. When the risk of tetanus is judged to be present, an intramuscular injection of 250 U of human tetanus antitoxin should be given, along with toxoid which should be repeated 1 month and 6 months later. For those already immunised, only a booster dose of toxoid is required.

LYME DISEASE

See page 319.

NEUROSYPHILIS

Neurosyphilis may present as an acute or chronic process and may involve the meninges, blood vessels and/or parenchyma of the brain and spinal cord. In developed countries, syphilis is now most commonly seen in patients with AIDS. The clinical manifestations are diverse and, although the condition is now rare, early diagnosis and treatment remain important.

Clinical features

The clinical and pathological features of the three most common presentations are summarised in Box 26.104.

Neurological examination reveals signs appropriate to the anatomical localisation of lesions. Delusions of grandeur suggest general paresis of the insane, but more commonly there is simply progressive dementia. The pupillary abnormality described by Argyll Robertson may accompany any neurosyphilitic syndrome, but most commonly tabes dorsalis; the pupils are small and irregular, and react to convergence but not directly to light.

Investigations

Routine screening for syphilis is warranted in the great majority of neurological patients. Serological tests (p. 412) are positive in the serum in most patients, but CSF

26

26.104 CLINICAL AND PATHOLOGICAL FEATURES OF NEUROSYPHILIS		
Type	**Pathology**	**Clinical features**
Meningovascular (5 years)*	Endarteritis obliterans Meningeal exudate Granuloma (gumma)	Stroke Cranial nerve palsies Seizures/mass lesion
General paralysis of the insane (5–15 years)*	Degeneration in cerebral cortex/cerebral atrophy Thickened meninges	Dementia Tremor Bilateral upper motor signs
Tabes dorsalis (5–20 years)*	Degeneration of sensory neurons Wasting of dorsal columns Optic atrophy	Lightning pains Sensory ataxia Visual failure Abdominal crises Incontinence Trophic changes
* Interval from primary infection.		

examination is essential if neurological involvement is suspected. Active disease is suggested by an elevated cell count, usually lymphocytic, and the protein content may be elevated to 0.5–1.0 g/l with an increased gamma globulin fraction. Serological tests in the CSF are usually positive, but progressive disease can occur with negative CSF serology.

Management

The injection of procaine benzylpenicillin (procaine penicillin) and probenecid for 17 days is essential in the treatment of neurosyphilis of all types (p. 413). Further courses of penicillin must be given if symptoms are not relieved, if the condition continues to advance or if the CSF continues to show signs of active disease. The cell count returns to normal within 3 months of completion of treatment, but the elevated protein takes longer to subside and some serological tests may never revert to normal. Evidence of clinical progression at any time is an indication for renewed treatment.

PRION DISEASES: TRANSMISSIBLE SPONGIFORM ENCEPHALOPATHIES

Transmissible spongiform encephalopathies (TSEs) include a number of conditions affecting both animals and humans which are characterised by the histopathological triad of spongiform change, neuronal cell loss and gliosis in the grey matter of the brain. Associated with these changes, there is deposition of amyloid made up of an altered form of a normally occurring protein, the prion protein. These diseases can be transmitted by inoculation; the precise nature of the infective agent is not yet clear but almost certainly involves the abnormal prion protein. They may also occur spontaneously or as an inherited disorder. Diseases affecting animals include bovine and feline spongiform encephalopathies (BSE and FSE). In humans, the most common TSE is Creutzfeldt–Jakob disease (CJD). This occurs sporadically, with a world-wide incidence of approximately 1/1 000 000, but can also be transmitted by inoculation (e.g. via depth EEG electrodes, corneal grafts, neurosurgery, especially when cadaveric dura mater grafts were used, and by the use of pooled cadaveric growth hormone). Some 10% of cases arise due to a mutation in the gene coding for the prion protein. A variant form of CJD has recently been described which is probably due to the same agent which causes BSE. Other extremely rare inherited human TSEs include Gerstmann–Sträussler–Scheinker disease, fatal familial insomnia and kuru. Kuru occurred only in members of a cannibalistic New Guinea tribe and was probably transmitted by people eating the brains of dead tribal members. Clinical features involved progressive ataxia and dementia.

CREUTZFELDT–JAKOB DISEASE (CJD)

Sporadic CJD usually occurs in middle-aged to elderly patients. Clinical features usually involve a rapidly progressive dementia, with myoclonus and a characteristic EEG pattern (repetitive slow wave complexes), although a number of other features such as visual disturbance or ataxia may also be seen. These are particularly common in CJD transmitted by inoculation. Death occurs after a mean of 4–6 months. There is as yet no known treatment.

Variant CJD

A variant of CJD (vCJD) has been described in a small number of patients, mostly in the UK. The causative agent appears to be identical to that causing BSE in cows, and it has been suggested that the disease appeared in humans as a result of the epidemic of BSE in the UK which started in the late 1980s. Patients affected by vCJD are typically younger than those with sporadic CJD and present with neuro-psychiatric changes and sensory symptoms in the limbs, followed by ataxia, dementia and death, progressing at a slightly slower rate than patients with sporadic CJD (mean time to death is over a year). Characteristic EEG changes are not present but MRI scans of the head show characteristic high signal changes in the pulvinar in a high proportion of cases. The brain pathology is distinct, with very florid plaques containing the prion proteins. Abnormal prion protein has been identified in tonsil specimens from sufferers of vCJD, leading to the suggestion that the disease could be transmitted by reticulo-endothelial tissue (like TSEs in animals but unlike sporadic CJD in humans). This has caused great concern in the UK, leading to precautionary measures such as leucodepletion of all blood used for transfusion, and the mandatory use of disposable surgical instruments wherever possible for tonsillectomy, appendicectomy and ophthalmological procedures.

INTRACRANIAL MASS LESIONS AND RAISED INTRACRANIAL PRESSURE

There are many different types of mass lesion in the head (Box 26.105). In developing countries, tuberculoma is a very common cause, but in developed countries cerebral neoplasms are the most frequent. The clinical features relate to the site of the mass, its nature and its rate of expansion. Symptoms and signs are produced by a number of mechanisms (Box 26.106).

RAISED INTRACRANIAL PRESSURE

Raised intracranial pressure may be caused by mass lesions (especially tumours), cerebral oedema, obstruction to CSF circulation (causing hydrocephalus) or impaired CSF absorption, as in idiopathic intracranial hypertension and cerebral venous obstruction.

Clinical features

The major features of raised intracranial pressure are listed in Box 26.106. Impairment of conscious level is related to the level of intracranial pressure. Cerebral mass lesions will tend to increase intracerebral pressure, but the amount by which the pressure is raised depends on the rate of growth of the mass. If it is slow, various compensatory mechanisms

26.105 INTRACRANIAL MASS LESIONS

Traumatic

- Subdural haematoma
- Extradural haematoma

Vascular

- Intracerebral haematoma

Infective

- Cerebral abscess (pyogenic, *Toxoplasma* etc.)
- Tuberculoma
- Cysticercosis (p. 371)
- Echinococcosis (as hydatid cysts, p. 371)
- Schistosomiasis (p. 367)

Inflammatory

- Sarcoid mass

Neoplastic

- Cerebral neoplasm (benign and malignant)

Other

- Embryonic dysplastic lesions (e.g. craniopharyngiomas, hamartomas)
- Arachnoid cyst
- Colloid cyst (in the ventricles)

26.106 CLINICAL FEATURES OF INTRACRANIAL MASS LESIONS

Local effects on adjacent brain tissue (e.g. seizures, focal signs)

- Depends on the site of the lesion (Box 26.3, p. 1152)

Raised intracranial pressure

- Headache (p. 1160)
- Impairment of conscious level
- Papilloedema
- Vomiting, bradycardia, arterial hypertension

False localising signs

- Pupillary dilatation (ipsilateral to lesion)
- 6th cranial nerve lesion (unilateral or bilateral)
- Hemiparesis (ipsilateral to lesion)
- Bilateral extensor plantar responses

may occur, including alteration in the volume of fluid in CSF spaces and venous sinuses, thereby allowing some tumours to achieve considerable size. More rapid growth (as in highly malignant tumours or abscesses) does not allow the compensatory mechanisms to take place, so raised intracranial pressure develops early, especially if the CSF circulation is also obstructed. Papilloedema is not always present, either because raised intracranial pressure has developed too recently, or because of anatomic anomalies of the meningeal sheath of the optic nerve. Vomiting, bradycardia and arterial hypertension develop as late features of raised intracranial pressure and usually parallel the other clinical signs; sudden vomiting may be an early feature of tumours of the cerebellum, especially in children.

Management

The management of raised intracranial pressure is largely dictated by its specific cause (see below). ICU support may be required (p. 198).

'CONING' AND FALSE LOCALISING SIGNS

The rise in intracranial pressure from a mass lesion is not usually uniform within the cerebral substance and alterations in pressure relationships within the skull may lead to displacement of parts of the brain between its various compartments. Downward displacement of the temporal lobes through the tentorium due to a large hemisphere mass may cause 'temporal coning' (Fig. 26.46). This may stretch the 3rd and/or 6th cranial nerves, or cause pressure on the contralateral cerebral peduncle (causing ipsilateral upper motor neuron signs). Downward movement of the cerebellar tonsils through the foramen magnum may compress the medulla—'tonsillar coning' (Fig. 26.47). This coning may result in brain-stem haemorrhage and/or acute obstruction of the CSF pathways. As coning progresses, the patient may adopt a decerebrate posture and, unless rapidly treated, death almost invariably ensues. The process may be acutely accelerated if the pressure dynamics are suddenly disturbed by lumbar puncture.

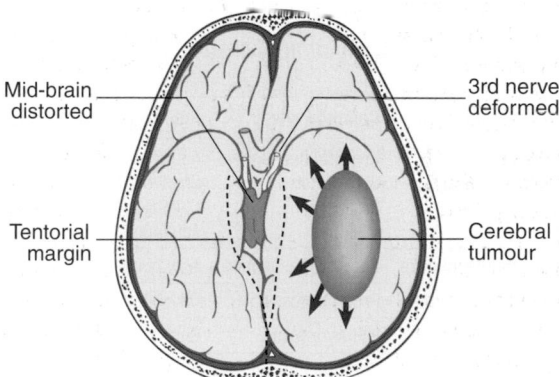

Fig. 26.46 Cerebral tumour displacing medial temporal lobe and causing pressure on the mid-brain and 3rd cranial nerve.

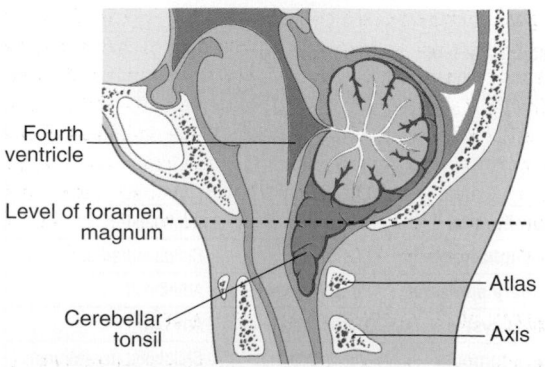

Fig. 26.47 Tonsillar cone. Downward displacement of the cerebellar tonsils below the level of the foramen magnum.

26

INTRACRANIAL NEOPLASMS

In the developed world, cerebral tumours account for 2% of deaths at all ages. The majority are metastatic from malignancies outside the nervous system. Meningiomas account for about one-fifth of intracranial tumours. Benign or malignant neoplasms of central nervous system tissue account for the remainder.

PRIMARY AND SECONDARY BRAIN TUMOURS

Pathology

Metastases from extracranial primary tumours are usually located in the white matter of the cerebral or cerebellar hemispheres, and common sources are bronchus, breast and gastrointestinal tract. Primary intracerebral tumours are classified by their cell of origin and degree of malignancy, and vary in incidence by age and localisation (Boxes 26.107 and 26.108). Even when malignant they do not metastasise outside the nervous system.

Clinical features

- *Headache* is not an invariable manifestation of cerebral tumour. If present, it may have characteristics suggesting raised intracranial pressure, or be caused by traction on the pain-sensitive intracranial structures (p. 1161). The site of the headache often does not correlate with the site of the tumour, although posterior fossa tumours often cause pain in the occiput or neck.
- *The focal deficits* produced by a cerebral tumour are of slow onset and progressive. Tumours may present at an early stage in some areas, such as the brain stem where structural disturbance quickly results in a neurological deficit. In other regions, especially the frontal lobe, a tumour may be quite large before symptoms occur. The clinical features of dysfunction in the various lobes of the brain are outlined in Box 26.3, page 1152. Occasionally, localised oedema in the brain tissue surrounding a tumour will cause a rapid progression of symptoms. Rarely, haemorrhage into a tumour presents like an acute stroke.
- *Seizures* are caused by infiltration by tumour cells of an area of cerebral cortex which excites seizure activity. The resulting seizures may be generalised or partial in nature, and the development of focal seizures in adult life should always suggest the possibility of a tumour.

Investigations

CT or MRI of the head allows accurate localisation of the tumour and provides some guidance as to the likely histological type (Fig. 26.48). MRI is of particular value in the investigation of tumours of the posterior fossa and brain stem (Fig. 26.49) and in delineating the nature and extent of tumours prior to surgery. Distortion of intracranial structures and the size of the ventricular system can be assessed and

26.107 PRIMARY MALIGNANT INTRACRANIAL TUMOURS

Histological type	Common site	Age
Glioma (astrocytoma)	Cerebral hemisphere	Adulthood
	Cerebellum	Childhood/adulthood
	Brain stem	Childhood/young adulthood
Oligodendroglioma	Cerebral hemisphere	Adulthood
Medulloblastoma	Posterior fossa	Childhood
Ependymoma	Posterior fossa	Childhood/adolescence
Cerebral lymphoma (microglioma)	Cerebral hemisphere	Adulthood

26.108 PRIMARY BENIGN INTRACRANIAL TUMOURS

Histological type	Common site	Age
Meningioma	Cortical dura	Adulthood
	Parasagittal	
	Sphenoid ridge	
	Suprasellar	
	Olfactory groove	
Neurofibroma	Acoustic neuroma	Adulthood
Craniopharyngioma	Suprasellar	Childhood/adolescence
Pituitary adenoma	Pituitary fossa	Adulthood
Colloid cyst	Third ventricle	Any age
Pineal tumours	Quadrigeminal cistern	Childhood (teratomas) Young adulthood (germ cell)

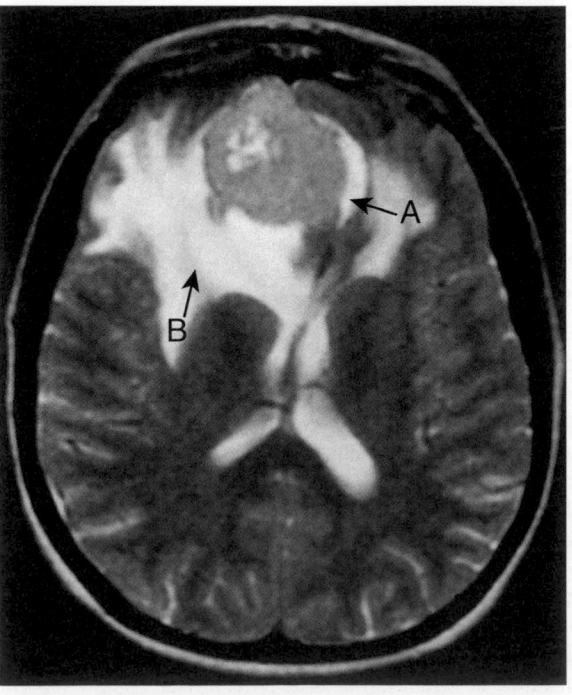

Fig. 26.48 MRI showing meningioma in frontal lobe (arrow A) with associated oedema (arrow B).

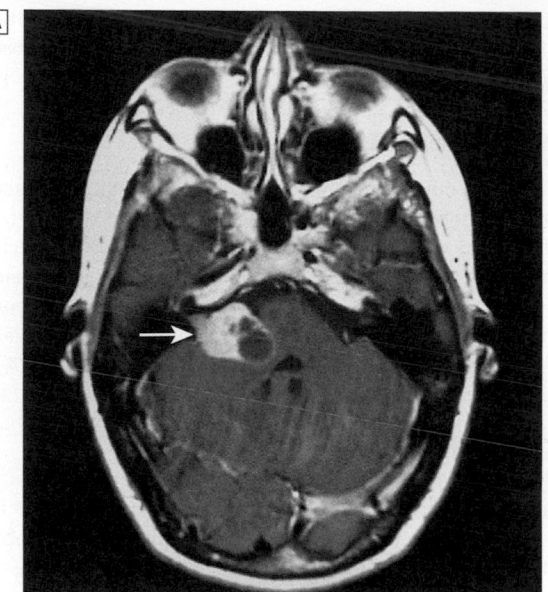
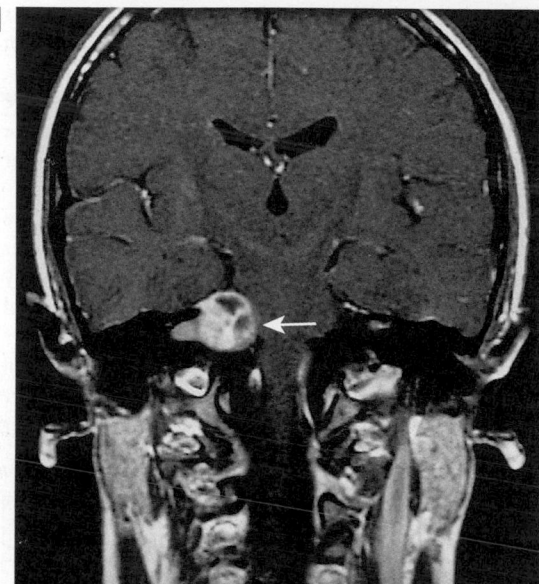

Fig. 26.49 MRI of an acoustic neuroma (arrows) in the posterior fossa compressing the brain stem. A Axial image. B Coronal image.

may provide accurate evaluation of the extent of the tumour. Plain skull X-rays are rarely of diagnostic value except in pituitary tumours. Chest radiography is an important investigation and may provide evidence of a primary pulmonary tumour or other systemic malignancy.

Management

Medical

Relief of raised intracranial pressure is often required when surgery is not possible or when life is threatened before investigation has revealed the diagnosis. Dexamethasone, 8 mg 12-hourly either orally or by injection, is used to lower intracranial pressure by resolving the reactive oedema around a tumour. A striking improvement in conscious level is often produced and focal disabilities may regress. In severe and acutely raised intracranial pressure, 16–20 mg of dexamethasone may be given intravenously or 200 ml of a 20% solution of mannitol may be infused.

Prolactin- or growth hormone-secreting pituitary tumours (p. 797) may respond to treatment with the dopamine agonists bromocriptine, cabergoline or quinagolide.

Surgical

Surgery is the mainstay of treatment, although only partial excision may be possible if the tumour is inaccessible or if its removal is likely to cause unacceptable brain damage. Biopsy by a direct or stereotactic technique should be considered even if the tumour cannot be removed, since the histological diagnosis has important implications for management and prognosis.

Meningiomas and acoustic neuromas offer the best prospects for complete removal without unacceptable damage to surrounding structures. Meningiomas can recur, particularly those of the sphenoid ridge when partial excision is often all that is possible. Pituitary adenomas can often be removed by a trans-sphenoidal route, thereby avoiding the need for a craniotomy.

Radiotherapy and chemotherapy

Radiotherapy and chemotherapy have only a marginal effect on survival in cerebral metastases and malignant gliomas in adults, but their combination has greatly improved the prognosis in medulloblastoma in children. Radiotherapy reduces the risk of recurrence of pituitary adenoma after surgery and may also be helpful as an adjunct to operative treatment in those meningiomas whose anatomical site precludes complete excision or whose histology suggests an increased tendency to recurrence. Ependymomas, some pineal tumours and low-grade gliomas in children and young adults are often radiosensitive.

Prognosis

Gliomas are rarely completely excised, as infiltration spreads beyond the radiologically evident boundaries of the tumour. Recurrence is therefore common, even if the mass of the tumour is apparently removed completely. Partial excision ('debulking') may be useful in alleviating raised intracranial pressure, but survival in highly malignant gliomas is poor even if such a decompressive procedure is attempted. Prognosis is related to histological grade; patients with better grades (I–II) may survive many years, whilst only 20% of patients with grade IV gliomas (glioblastoma multiforme) survive 1 year.

The prognosis for benign tumours is good, provided complete surgical excision can be achieved. Ependymomas and medulloblastomas can often be excised with minimal residual disability, but may recur with seeding of the tumour via the CSF. Oligodendrogliomas are often slow-growing and relatively benign in the early stages, but may transform to a more malignant form and behave as gliomas.

NEUROFIBROMATOSIS

This is a disorder of autosomal dominant inheritance due to an abnormal gene on chromosome 17 (q11.2, type 1

26

neurofibromatosis, NF1) or 22 (q12.2, type 2 neurofibromatosis, NF2). Multiple fibromatous tumours develop from the neurilemmal sheaths of peripheral and cranial nerves. Most of the lesions are benign but sarcomatous change may occur. In NF1 (von Recklinghausen's disease) there are characteristic cutaneous manifestations and other extracranial manifestations (Box 26.109).

Patients with NF1 are easily recognised because of the cutaneous lesions (Fig. 26.50), which increase in number throughout life. Investigation and treatment are only indicated if there are symptoms of cerebral or spinal involvement, or if malignant change is suspected.

Patients with NF2 present with acoustic neuromas, often bilateral, and/or other central neoplasms, and have fewer if any cutaneous lesions. A family history of cerebral or

spinal tumours should be noted with care, since relatives of patients with NF2 may require screening for acoustic neuromas.

ACOUSTIC NEUROMA

This is a benign tumour of Schwann cells of the 8th cranial nerve, which may arise in isolation or as part of NF2 (see above). As an isolated finding, an acoustic neuroma occurs after the third decade and is more frequent in females. The tumour commonly arises near the nerve's entry point into the medulla or in the internal auditory meatus, usually on the vestibular division. Such lesions make up 80–90% of tumours at the cerebello–pontine angle.

Clinical features

These depend on the site of the tumour along the acoustic or vestibular nerve. Similar tumours arise rarely from the trigeminal nerve. Hearing loss is almost invariable, although it may not be the presenting feature. Sensory symptoms in the face and vertigo are also common at presentation. Distortion of the brain stem and/or cerebellar peduncle may cause ataxia and/or cerebellar signs in the limbs. Distortion of the fourth ventricle and cerebral aqueduct may cause hydrocephalus, which may be the presenting feature (see below). Facial weakness is unusual at presentation, but facial palsy may follow surgical removal of the tumour.

Investigations

MRI is the investigation of choice (Fig. 26.49), CT being less useful in this region of the posterior fossa.

Management

This involves surgical removal. If this is complete, the prognosis is excellent. Deafness and facial weakness, if not present before surgery, usually result from the operation.

VON HIPPEL–LINDAU DISEASE

This is a dominantly inherited disease due to a defective gene on chromosome 3p25–26, characterised by the combination of retinal and intracranial (typically cerebellar) haemangiomas and haemangioblastomas. There may be associated extracranial hamartomatous lesions, which may undergo malignant change. About 10% of posterior fossa tumours are cerebellar haemangioblastomas. Von Hippel–Lindau disease needs to be considered in patients with such lesions, so that screening for other lesions and, if necessary, of family members can be instituted.

PARANEOPLASTIC NEUROLOGICAL DISEASE

Neurological disease may occur with systemic malignant tumours in the absence of metastases. Mild degrees of myopathy and neuropathy are quite frequent with the common malignancies. Much rarer are certain disabling, and often fatal, paraneoplastic syndromes which often have an inflammatory basis, with associated autoantibodies

26.109 TYPES OF NEUROFIBROMATOSIS
Type 1 Peripheral form (> 70% of cases)
• Multiple cutaneous neurofibromas • 'Soft' papillomas • Café au lait patches • Axillary freckling • Iris fibromas   • Plexiform neurofibromas • Spinal neurofibromas • Aqueduct stenosis • Scoliosis • Endocrine tumours
Type 2 Central form
• Few or no cutaneous lesions • Bilateral acoustic neuromas • Cerebral and optic nerve gliomas   • Meningiomas • Spinal neurofibromas

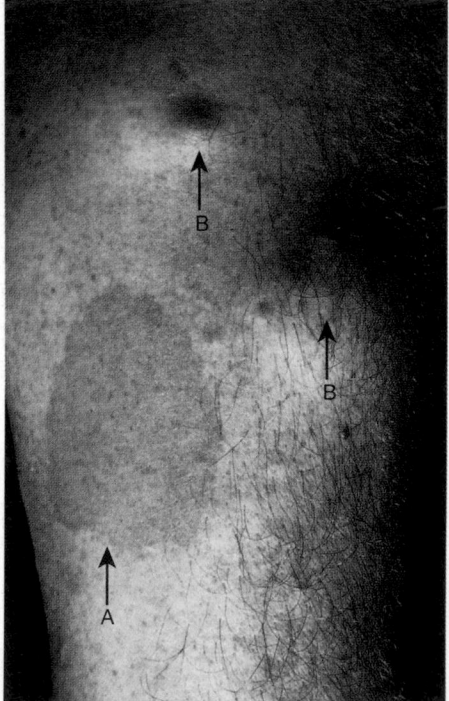

Fig. 26.50   A café au lait spot (arrow A) and subcutaneous nodules (arrows B) on the forearm of a patient with neurofibromatosis type 1.

26

which cross-react with neural and tumour antigens (Box 26.110). In the case of the Lambert–Eaton myasthenic syndrome the autoantibodies have a functional effect on neuromuscular transmission (p. 1253).

These syndromes are particularly associated with small-cell carcinoma of the lung, ovarian tumours, and lymphomas. In addition to the presence of autoantibodies in the serum and/or CSF, there is usually a lymphocytic infiltrate of the neural tissue affected.

Clinical features

These are summarised in Box 26.110. In most instances the neurological disease progresses quite rapidly over a few months. In 50% of patients with a paraneoplastic syndrome, the neurological disease precedes clinical presentation of the primary neoplasm. Paraneoplastic disease should be considered in the diagnosis of any unusual progressive neurological syndrome.

Investigations

See Box 26.110. The presence of characteristic autoantibodies in the context of a suspicious clinical picture may be diagnostic. The causative tumour may be very small and therefore CT of the chest or abdomen is often necessary to find it. The CSF often shows an increased protein and lymphocyte count with oligoclonal bands.

Management

This is directed at the primary tumour. Occasionally, successful therapy of the tumour is associated with improvement of the paraneoplastic syndrome. Some improvement may occur following administration of intravenous immunoglobulin.

HYDROCEPHALUS

COMMUNICATING AND OBSTRUCTIVE HYDROCEPHALUS

Hydrocephalus (dilatation of the ventricular system) may be due to obstruction of the CSF circulation (Fig. 26.51). Hydrocephalus is said to be 'communicating' if the obstruction is outside the ventricular system (usually in the basal cisterns). Obstruction within the ventricles is most common in the narrow channels of the third ventricle and aqueduct, and may be caused by tumour or a congenital anomaly such as aqueduct stenosis (Fig. 26.52). Causes of hydrocephalus are given in Box 26.111.

Diversion of the CSF by means of a shunt procedure between the ventricular system and the peritoneal cavity or right atrium may result in prompt relief of symptoms in obstructive or communicating hydrocephalus.

26.110 PARANEOPLASTIC SYNDROMES				
Syndrome	**Clinical features**	**Antibody**	**Associated tumours**	**Investigations**
Retinal degeneration	Painless progressive visual loss	Antiretinal	Small-cell carcinoma of lung Melanoma	Chest X-ray, CT chest Electroretinogram
Opsoclonus-myoclonus	Arrhythmic chaotic rapid eye movements	Anti-Ri	Ovarian, lung Neuroblastoma (in children)	Chest X-ray, CT chest Pelvic ultrasound or CT
Sensory neuropathy	Limb pain, paraesthesia Distal numbness	Anti-Hu	Small-cell carcinoma of lung Hodgkin lymphoma	Chest X-ray, CT chest Nerve conduction studies
Limbic encephalitis	Memory loss, progressive dementia Seizures	Anti-Hu	Small-cell carcinoma of lung Hodgkin lymphoma	Chest X-ray, CT chest MRI (head) CSF (pleocytosis, raised protein)
Myelitis	Progressive spinal cord lesion (usually cervical cord)	Anti-Hu	Small-cell carcinoma of lung	Chest X-ray, CT chest MRI (cord, head)
Cerebellar degeneration	Progressive ataxia, nystagmus (down-beating), vertigo	Anti-Yo Anti-Hu	Small-cell carcinoma of lung Ovarian Hodgkin lymphoma	Chest X-ray, CT chest Pelvic ultrasound or CT CSF (raised protein, oligoclonal bands)
Subacute motor neuropathy	Subacute, patchy progressive, usually lower limb, weakness and wasting	Anti-Hu	Hodgkin lymphoma Small-cell carcinoma of lung	Chest X-ray, CT chest Nerve conduction studies/EMG
Sensorimotor peripheral neuropathy	Mild, non-disabling peripheral limb numbness and paraesthesia	Not known	Small-cell carcinoma of lung Breast Other carcinoma	Chest X-ray, CT chest Nerve conduction studies/EMG
Lambert–Eaton myasthenic syndrome	Weakness of proximal limb muscles, fatigue with exertion after initial improvement, areflexia	Anti-Ca^{2+} channel	Small-cell carcinoma of lung	Chest X-ray, CT chest EMG
Dermatomyositis/ polymyositis	Proximal limb weakness and pain, heliotrope skin rash, Gottron's papules on knuckles	Anti-Jo-1	Lung, breast, ovary	Chest X-ray, CT chest Creatine kinase EMG, muscle biopsy
Guillain–Barré	Ascending weakness, distal paraesthesia	Not known	Hodgkin lymphoma	Nerve conduction studies/EMG

26

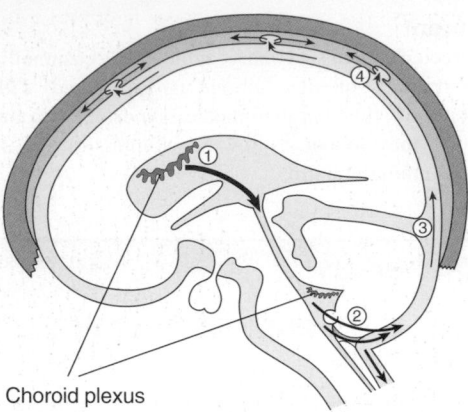

Choroid plexus

Fig. 26.51 The circulation of cerebrospinal fluid. (1) CSF is synthesised in the choroid plexus of the ventricles, and flows from the lateral and third ventricles through the aqueduct to the fourth ventricle. (2) At the foramina of Luschka and Magendie it exits the brain, flowing over the hemispheres (3) and down around the spinal cord and roots in the subarachnoid space. (4) It is then absorbed into the dural venous sinuses via the arachnoid villi.

NORMAL PRESSURE HYDROCEPHALUS

In this condition the dilatation of the ventricular system is caused by intermittent rises in CSF pressure, which occur particularly at night. It occurs predominantly in old age and is suggested by the combination of gait apraxia (p. 1181) and dementia, often with urinary incontinence as an early feature. This cause of dilatation of the ventricles can be very difficult to distinguish from that occurring due to cerebral atrophy, where the cortical sulci are also dilated. The result of shunting procedures for normal pressure hydrocephalus is unpredictable.

26.111 CAUSES OF HYDROCEPHALUS

Communicating (obstruction outside ventricular system)

- Bacterial meningitis (especially tuberculous)
- Sarcoidosis
- Subarachnoid haemorrhage
- Head injury
- Idiopathic ('normal pressure')

Non-communicating (obstruction within ventricular system)

- Tumours
- Colloid cyst
- Arnold–Chiari malformation
- Aqueduct stenosis
- Cerebellar abscess
- Cerebellar or brain-stem haematoma

IDIOPATHIC INTRACRANIAL HYPERTENSION

This condition, previously known as 'benign intracranial hypertension' and 'pseudotumour cerebri', usually occurs in obese young women. Raised intracranial pressure develops without a space-occupying lesion, ventricular dilatation or impairment of consciousness. The aetiology is uncertain but there may be a diffuse defect of CSF reabsorption by the arachnoid villi. The condition can be precipitated by drugs, including tetracycline, and rarely vitamin A, retinoids, Addison's disease (p. 782) and withdrawal of corticosteroid therapy.

Clinical features

Characteristically, there is a headache, sometimes with transient diplopia and visual obscurations, but few other symptoms. There are usually no signs other than papill-

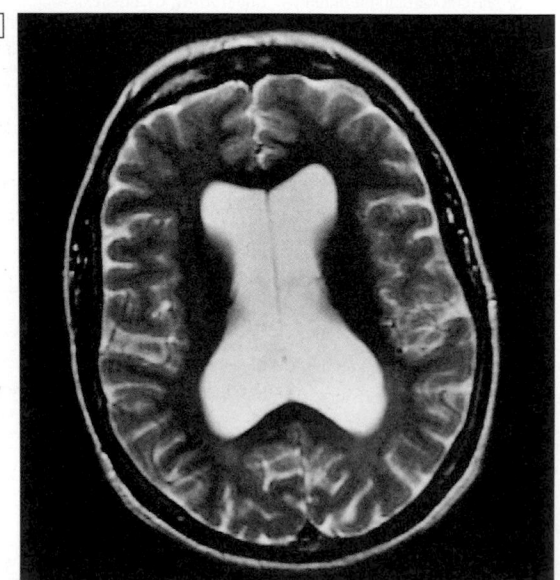

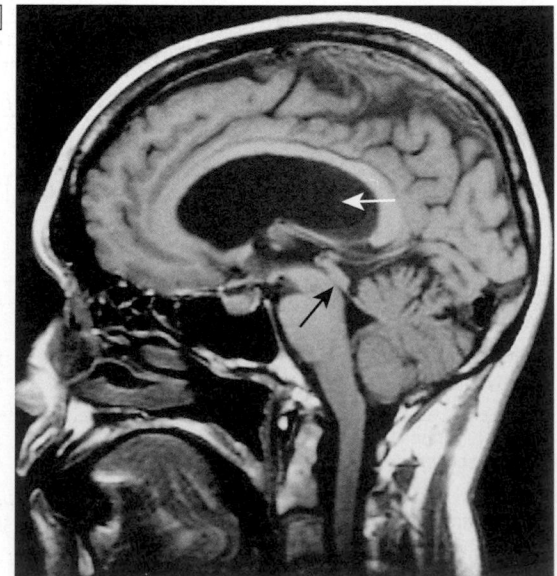

Fig. 26.52 MRI of hydrocephalus due to aqueduct stenosis. A Axial image: note the dilated lateral ventricles. B Sagittal image: note the dilated ventricles (top arrow) and narrowed aqueduct (bottom arrow).

26

oedema, which may be discovered incidentally at a routine visit to an optician, but a 6th nerve palsy may be present.

Investigations

The CT is normal, with normal-sized or small ventricles. Once this has been demonstrated, a lumbar puncture is safe and will allow confirmation of the raised CSF pressure and form part of treatment. MR angiography or cerebral venography will exclude cerebral venous sinus thrombosis or stenosis of other cause. True papilloedema may need to be distinguished from other causes of disc swelling by fluorescein angiography.

Management

Any precipitating condition should be sought, relevant medication should be withdrawn and a weight-reducing diet instigated, if indicated. The carbonic anhydrase inhibitor, acetazolamide, may help to lower intracranial pressure. Repeated lumbar puncture can be considered, but is often unacceptable to the patient. Patients failing to respond, in whom chronic papilloedema threatens vision, may require optic nerve sheath fenestration or a lumbo-peritoneal shunt.

DISORDERS OF THE SPINE AND SPINAL CORD

The spinal cord and spinal roots may be affected by intrinsic disease or by disorders of the surrounding meninges and bones. The clinical presentation of these conditions depends on the anatomical level at which the cord or roots are affected, as well as the nature of the pathological process involved. It is important to recognise when emergency surgical intervention is necessary and to plan investigations to identify such patients.

CERVICAL SPONDYLOSIS

In the cervical spine, some degree of osteoarthritic degenerative change is a normal radiological finding in the middle-aged and elderly. Degeneration of the intervertebral discs and secondary osteoarthrosis (cervical spondylosis) is often asymptomatic, but may be associated with neurological dysfunction. The C5/6, C6/7 and C4/5 vertebral levels and C6, C7 and C5 roots, respectively, are most commonly affected (Fig. 26.53).

CERVICAL SPONDYLOTIC RADICULOPATHY

Compression of a nerve root occurs when a disc prolapses laterally, which may develop acutely or more gradually due to osteophytic encroachment of the intervertebral foramina.

Clinical features

The patient complains of pain in the neck that may radiate in the distribution of the affected nerve root. The neck is held rigidly and neck movements may exacerbate pain. Paraesthesia and sensory loss may be found in the affected segment and there may be lower motor neuron signs, including weakness, wasting and reflex impairment (Box 26.112).

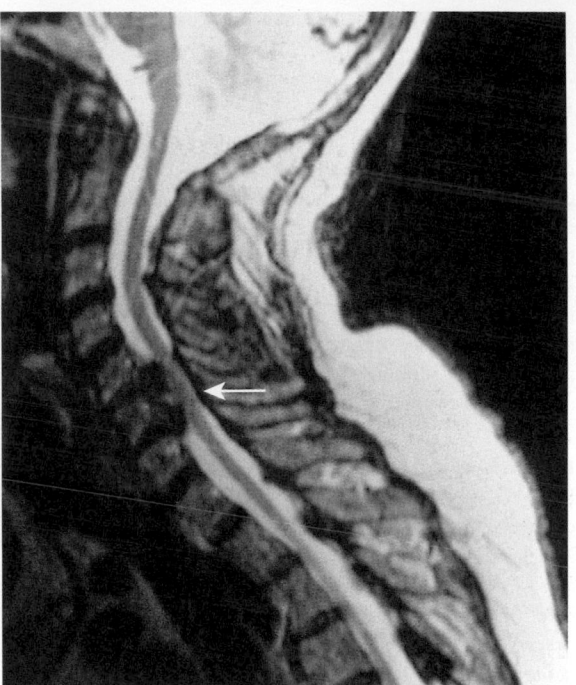

Fig. 26.53 MRI showing cervical cord compression (arrow) in cervical spondylosis.

26.112 PHYSICAL SIGNS IN CERVICAL ROOT COMPRESSION			
Root	Muscle weakness	Sensory loss	Reflex loss
C5	Biceps, deltoid, spinati	Upper lateral arm	Biceps
C6	Brachioradialis	Lower lateral arm, thumb, index finger	Supinator
C7	Triceps, finger and wrist extensors	Middle finger	Triceps

Investigations

Plain X-rays, including lateral and oblique views, should be obtained to confirm the presence of degenerative changes and to exclude other conditions, including destructive lesions. If surgery is contemplated, MRI is required. Electrophysiological studies rarely add to the clinical examination, but may be necessary if there is doubt about the differential diagnosis between root and peripheral nerve lesions.

Management

Conservative treatment with analgesics and physiotherapy results in resolution of symptoms in the great majority of patients, but a few require surgery in the form of foraminotomy or disc excision.

CERVICAL SPONDYLOTIC MYELOPATHY

Dorsomedial herniation of a disc and the development of transverse bony bars or posterior osteophytes may result in pressure on the spinal cord or the anterior spinal artery which supplies the anterior two-thirds of the cord (Fig. 26.53).

Clinical features

The onset is usually insidious and painless, but acute deterioration may occur after trauma, especially hyper-extension injury. Upper motor neuron signs develop in the limbs, with spasticity of the legs usually appearing before the arms are involved. Sensory loss in the upper limbs is common, producing tingling, numbness and proprioception loss in the hands, with progressive clumsiness. Sensory manifestations in the legs are much less common. The neurological deficit usually progresses gradually and disturbance of micturition is a very late feature.

Investigations

Plain X-rays confirm the presence of degenerative changes, and MRI (Fig. 26.53) or myelography may be indicated if surgical treatment is being considered. MRI may also show areas of high signal within the spinal cord at the level of compression. Imaging of the cervical spine should be considered if there is diagnostic doubt or if surgery is contemplated.

Management

Surgical procedures, including laminectomy and anterior discectomy, may arrest progression of disability but may not result in neurological improvement. The judgement on whether surgery should be undertaken may be difficult. Manipulation of the cervical spine is of no proven benefit and may precipitate acute neurological deterioration.

Prognosis

The prognosis of cervical myelopathy is variable. In many patients the condition stabilises or even improves without intervention, but if progressive disability does develop, surgical decompression should be considered.

LUMBO-SACRAL SPONDYLOSIS

In developed countries, low back pain ('lumbago') is the most common medical cause of inability to work. In the great majority of patients it is due to abnormalities of joints and ligaments in the lumbar spine rather than herniation of an intervertebral disc. Pain in the distribution of the lumbar or sacral roots ('sciatica') is often due to disc protrusion, but can be a feature of other rare but important disorders including spinal tumour, malignant disease in the pelvis and tuberculosis of the vertebral bodies.

LUMBAR DISC HERNIATION

Acute lumbar disc herniation is often precipitated by trauma, usually by lifting heavy weights while the spine is flexed. The nucleus pulposus may bulge or rupture through the annulus fibrosus, giving rise to pressure on nerve endings in the spinal ligaments, changes in the vertebral joints or pressure on nerve roots.

26.113 PHYSICAL SIGNS IN LUMBAR ROOT COMPRESSION				
Disc level	Root	Sensory loss	Weakness	Reflex loss
L3/L4	L4	Inner calf	Inversion of foot	Knee
L4/L5	L5	Outer calf and dorsum of foot	Dorsiflexion of hallux/toes	
L5/S1	S1	Sole and lateral foot	Plantar flexion	Ankle

Clinical features

The onset may be sudden or gradual. Alternatively, repeated episodes of low back pain may precede sciatica by months or years. Constant aching pain is felt in the lumbar region and may radiate to the buttock, thigh, calf and foot. Pain is exacerbated by coughing or straining but may be relieved by lying flat.

The altered mechanics of the lumbar spine result in loss of lumbar lordosis and there may be spasm of the paraspinal musculature. Root pressure is suggested by limitation of flexion of the hip on the affected side if the straight leg is raised (Lasègue's sign). If the third or fourth lumbar roots are involved, Lasègue's sign may be negative, but pain in the back may be induced by hyperextension of the hip (femoral nerve stretch test). The roots most frequently affected are S1, L5 and L4; the signs of root pressure at these levels are summarised in Box 26.113.

Investigations

Plain X-rays of the lumbar spine are of little value in the diagnosis of lumbar disc disease, although they may show other conditions such as malignant infiltration of a vertebral body. CT, especially using spiral scanning techniques, can provide helpful images of the disc protrusion and/or narrowing of the exit foramina. MRI is the investigation of choice if available, since soft tissues are well imaged.

Management

Some 90% of patients with sciatica recover with conservative treatment with analgesia and early mobilisation; bed rest does not help recovery. The patient should be instructed in back-strengthening exercises and advised to avoid physical manoeuvres likely to strain the lumbar spine. Injections of local anaesthetic or corticosteroids may be useful adjunctive treatment if symptoms are due to ligamentous injury or joint dysfunction. Surgery may have to be considered if there is no response to conservative treatment or if progressive neurological deficits develop. Central disc prolapse with bilateral symptoms and signs and disturbance of sphincter function requires urgent surgical decompression.

LUMBAR CANAL STENOSIS

This is due to a congenital narrowing of the lumbar spinal canal, exacerbated by the degenerative changes that commonly occur with age.

Clinical features

The patients, who are usually elderly, develop exercise-induced weakness and paraesthesia in the legs (cauda equina claudication). These symptoms progress with continued exertion, often to the point that the patient can no longer walk, but are quickly relieved by a short period of rest. Physical examination at rest shows preservation of peripheral pulses with absent ankle reflexes. Weakness or sensory loss may only be apparent if the patient is examined immediately after exercise.

Investigations

Myelography, CT or MRI will demonstrate narrowing of the lumbar canal.

Management

Extensive lumbar laminectomy often results in complete relief of symptoms and recovery of normal exercise tolerance.

COMPRESSION OF THE SPINAL CORD

Acute spinal cord compression is one of the most common neurological emergencies encountered in clinical practice and the common causes are listed in Box 26.114. A space-occupying lesion within the spinal canal may damage nerve tissue either directly by pressure or indirectly by interfering with blood supply. Oedema from venous obstruction impairs neuronal function, and ischaemia from arterial obstruction may lead to necrosis of the spinal cord. The early stages of damage are reversible but severely damaged neurons do not recover; hence the importance of early diagnosis and treatment.

Clinical features

The onset of symptoms of spinal cord compression is usually slow (over weeks), but can be acute as a result of trauma or metastases, especially if there is associated arterial occlusion. The symptoms are shown in Box 26.115.

Pain and sensory symptoms occur early, while weakness and sphincter dysfunction are usually late manifestations. The signs vary according to the level of the cord compression and the structures involved. There may be tenderness to percussion over the spine if there is vertebral disease, and this may be associated with a local kyphosis. Involvement of the roots at the level of the compression may cause dermatomal sensory impairment and corresponding lower motor signs. Interruption of fibres in the spinal cord causes sensory loss (p. 1183) and upper motor neuron signs below the level of the lesion, and there is often disturbance of sphincter function. The distribution of these signs varies with the level of the lesion, as shown in Box 26.116.

The Brown–Séquard syndrome (Fig. 26.17E, p. 1184) results if damage is confined to one side of the cord; the findings are explained by the anatomy of the sensory tracts (Fig. 26.18, p. 1184). On the side of the lesion there is a band of hyperaesthesia with loss of proprioception and

26.115 SYMPTOMS OF SPINAL CORD COMPRESSION
Pain
• Localised over the spine or in a root distribution, which may be aggravated by coughing, sneezing or straining
Sensory
• Paraesthesia, numbness or cold sensations, especially in the lower limbs, which spread proximally, often to a level on the trunk
Motor
• Weakness, heaviness or stiffness of the limbs, most commonly the legs
Sphincters
• Urgency or hesitancy of micturition, leading eventually to urinary retention

26

26.116 SIGNS OF SPINAL CORD COMPRESSION
Cervical, above C5
• Upper motor neuron signs and sensory loss in all four limbs • Diaphragm weakness (phrenic nerve)
Cervical, C5 to T1
• Lower motor neuron signs and segmental sensory loss in the arms; upper motor neuron signs in the legs • Respiratory (intercostal) muscle weakness
Thoracic cord
• Spastic paraplegia with a sensory level on the trunk
Conus medullaris
• Lesions at the end of the spinal cord cause sacral loss of sensation and extensor plantar responses
Cauda equina
• Spinal cord ends at approximately the T12/L1 spinal level and spinal lesions below this level can only cause lower motor neuron signs by affecting the cauda equina

26.114 CAUSES OF SPINAL CORD COMPRESSION		
Site	**Frequency**	**Causes**
Vertebral	80%	Trauma (extradural) Intervertebral disc prolapse Metastatic carcinoma (e.g. breast, prostate, bronchus) Myeloma Tuberculosis
Meninges (intradural extramedullary)	15%	Tumours (e.g. meningioma, neurofibroma, ependymoma, metastasis, lymphoma, leukaemia) Epidural abscess
Spinal cord (intradural intramedullary)	5%	Tumours (e.g. glioma, ependymoma, metastasis)

upper motor neuron signs below it. On the other side there is loss of spinothalamic sensation (pain and temperature). With compressive lesions there is usually a band of pain at the level of the lesion in the distribution of the nerve roots subject to compression.

Investigations

Patients with a short history of a progressive spinal cord syndrome should be investigated urgently. Investigations necessary are listed in Box 26.117.

Plain X-rays may show bony destruction and soft-tissue abnormalities and are an essential initial investigation (Fig. 26.54). Routine investigations, including chest X-ray, may provide evidence of systemic disease. MRI of the spine is the investigation of choice (Fig. 26.55); myelography also localises the lesion and, with CT in suitable cases, defines

26.117 INVESTIGATION OF ACUTE SPINAL CORD SYNDROME
• Plain X-rays of spine
• Chest X-rays
• MRI of spine or myelography
• CSF
• Serum B$_{12}$

the extent of compression and associated soft-tissue abnormality (Fig. 26.56). CSF should be taken for analysis at the time of myelography. In cases of complete spinal block this shows a normal cell count with a very elevated protein causing yellow discoloration of the fluid (Froin's syndrome). Acute deterioration may develop after myelography and the neurosurgeons should be alerted before it is

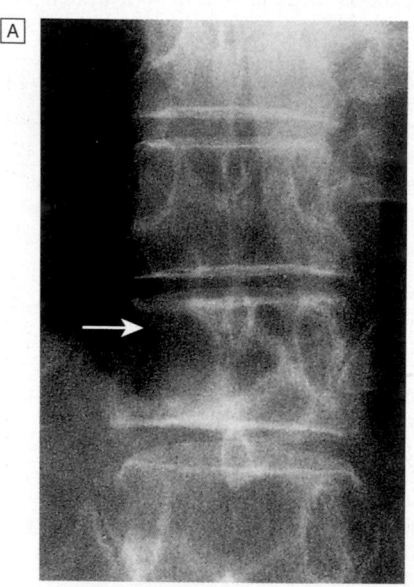

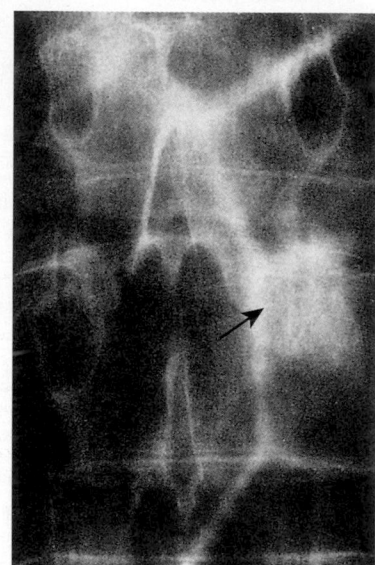

Fig. 26.54 Plain X-rays of the spine. A Loss of vertebral pedicle (arrow) by bony erosion of an osteolytic metastasis. B An osteosclerotic metastasis (arrow).

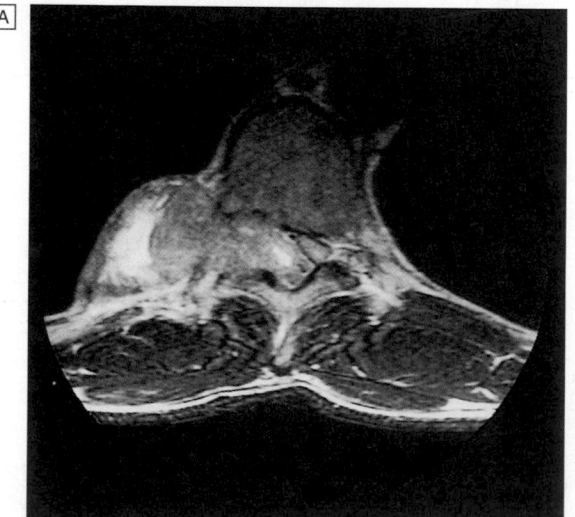

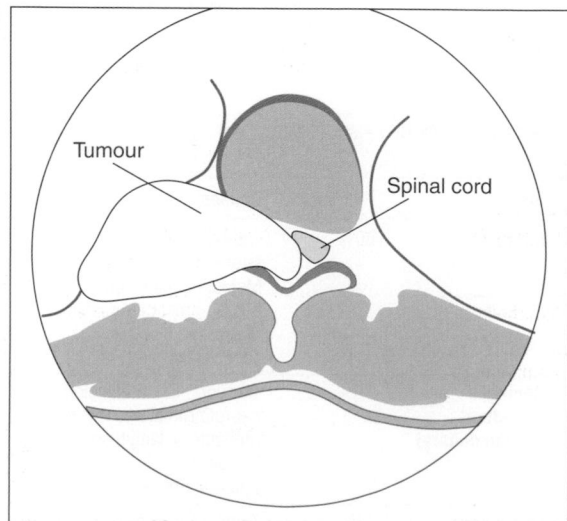

Fig. 26.55 Axial MRI of thoracic spine. A A neurofibroma is compressing the spinal cord and emerging in a 'dumbbell' fashion through the vertebral foramen into the paraspinal space. B Line diagram illustrating major structures.

26

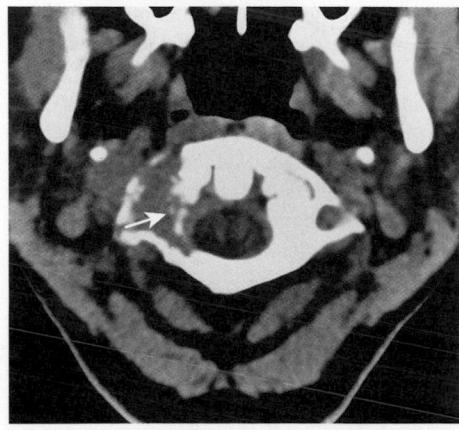

Fig. 26.56 CT myelogram of cervical spine at the level of C2 showing bony erosion of vertebra by a metastasis (arrow).

undertaken. Needle biopsy is required prior to radiotherapy to establish the histological nature of the tumour.

Management
Treatment and prognosis depend on the nature of the underlying lesion. Benign tumours should be surgically

excised, and a good functional recovery can be expected unless a marked neurological deficit has developed before diagnosis. Extradural compression due to malignancy is the most common cause of spinal cord compression in developed countries and has a poor prognosis, although useful function can be regained if treatment is initiated within 24 hours of the onset of severe weakness or sphincter dysfunction. Surgical decompression may be appropriate in some patients, but has a similar outcome to radiotherapy. Spinal cord compression due to tuberculosis is common in some areas of the world, and requires surgical treatment if seen early. This should be followed by appropriate anti-tuberculous chemotherapy (p. 701) for an extended period. Traumatic lesions of the vertebral column require specialised neurosurgical treatment.

INTRINSIC DISEASES OF THE SPINAL CORD

There are many disorders which interfere with spinal cord function due to non-compressive involvement of the spinal cord itself. A list of such disorders is given in Box 26.118. The symptoms and signs are generally similar to those

26.118 INTRINSIC DISEASES OF THE SPINAL CORD

Type of disorder	Condition	Clinical features
Congenital	Diastematomyelia (spina bifida)	Features variably present at birth and deteriorate thereafter LMN features, deformity and sensory loss of legs Impaired sphincter function Hairy patch or pit over low back Incidence reduced by increased maternal intake of folic acid during pregnancy
	Hereditary spastic paraplegia	Onset usually in adult life Autosomal dominant inheritance usual Slowly progressive UMN features affecting legs > arms Little, if any, sensory loss
Infective/inflammatory	Transverse myelitis due to viruses (HZV), schistosomiasis, HIV, MS, sarcoidosis	Weakness and sensory loss, often with pain, developing over hours to days UMN features below lesion Impaired sphincter function
Vascular	Anterior spinal artery infarct Intervertebral disc embolus	Abrupt onset Anterior horn cell loss (LMN) at level of lesion UMN features below it Spinothalamic sensory loss below lesion but spared dorsal column sensation
	Spinal AVM/dural fistula	Onset variable (acute to slowly progressive) Variable LMN, UMN, sensory and sphincter disturbance Symptoms and signs often not well localised to site of AVM
Neoplastic	Glioma, ependymoma	Weakness and sensory loss, often with pain, developing over months to years UMN features below lesion in cord; additional LMN features in conus Impaired sphincter function
Metabolic	Vitamin B$_{12}$ deficiency (subacute combined degeneration)	Progressive spastic paraparesis with proprioception loss, absent reflexes due to peripheral neuropathy ± optic nerve and cerebral involvement (p. 1027)
Degenerative	Motor neuron disease	Relentlessly progressive LMN and UMN features, associated bulbar weakness, no sensory involvement. See page 1222
	Syringomyelia	Gradual onset over months or years, pain in cervical segments Anterior horn cell loss (LMN) at level of lesion, UMN features below it Suspended spinothalamic sensory loss at level of lesion, dorsal columns preserved. See Figures 26.17 (p. 1184) and 26.57

(AVM = arteriovenous malformation; HIV = human immunodeficiency virus; HZV = herpes zoster virus; LMN = lower motor neuron; MS = multiple sclerosis; UMN = upper motor neuron)

26

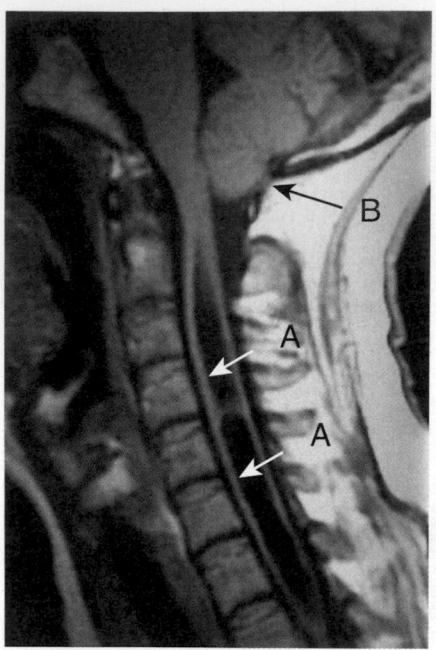

Fig. 26.57 MRI scan showing syrinx (arrows A), with herniation of cerebellar tonsils (arrow B).

Investigation of intrinsic disease starts with imaging, importantly to exclude a compressive lesion. If available, MRI provides the most information about structural lesions such as diastematomyelia, syringomyelia (Fig. 26.57), or intrinsic tumours. Non-specific signal change may be seen in the spinal cord in inflammatory (Fig. 26.38, p. 1214) or infective conditions and others such as B12 deficiency. Other investigations such as lumbar puncture or blood tests are required to make a specific diagnosis.

DISEASES OF NERVE AND MUSCLE

DISEASES OF THE PERIPHERAL NERVOUS SYSTEM

Numerous inherited and acquired pathological processes may affect the nerve roots (radiculopathy), the nerve plexuses (plexopathy) and/or the individual nerves (neuropathy). Cranial nerves 3–12 share the same tissue characteristics as peripheral nerves elsewhere and are subject to the same range of diseases. Nerve fibres of different types (motor, sensory or autonomic) and of different sizes may be variably involved. Disorders may be primarily directed at the axon, the myelin sheath (Schwann cells) or both (Fig. 26.1, p. 1148).

An acute or chronic peripheral nerve disorder may be focal (affecting a single nerve: mononeuropathy), multifocal (several nerves: mononeuropathy multiplex) or generalised (polyneuropathy). Neurophysiological tests (p. 1154), and sometimes nerve biopsy, will help determine whether the pathology is primarily affecting the nerve axon (axonal

which would occur with extrinsic compression (Boxes 26.115 and 26.116), although a suspended sensory loss (Fig. 26.17F, p. 1184) can only occur with intrinsic disease such as syringomyelia. Urinary symptoms usually occur earlier in the course of an intrinsic cord disorder than with compressive disorders.

		Multifocal (mononeuropathy multiplex)		Generalised (polyneuropathy)	
Neurophysiology	Focal (mononeuropathy)	Acute	Chronic	Acute	Chronic
Demyelinating on NCS; slowed conduction ± conduction block	Entrapment*	Diphtheria	Leprosy* Paraproteinaemia MMN HNPP	Guillain-Barré* Suramin toxicity	Hereditary* CIDP Lymphoma Osteoclastic myeloma IgM paraproteinaemia Arsenic toxicity Amiodarone toxicity Diphtheria
Axonal on NCS; reduced or absent action potentials, normal conduction velocities	Severe entrapment*	Diabetes* Vasculitis Lyme disease Cryoglobulinaemia	Diabetes* Neoplastic infiltration HIV Sarcoidosis Amyloid	Alcohol* Guillain–Barré variants Toxins Critical illness Porphyria Paraneoplastic Tick paralysis	Metabolic/endocrine diseases (including diabetes)* Alcohol* Drugs and toxins (Boxes 26.120 and 26.121)* Vitamin deficiency* (Box 26.120) Hereditary* IgG paraproteinaemia Paraneoplastic Primary amyloidosis

26.119 TYPES AND CAUSES OF PERIPHERAL NEUROPATHY

*Common and/or important causes.
(CIDP = chronic inflammatory demyelinating peripheral neuropathy; MMN = multifocal motor neuropathy with conduction block; HNPP = hereditary neuropathy with tendency to pressure palsies; NCS = nerve conduction studies)

26.120 SYSTEMIC DISORDERS AND TOXINS ASSOCIATED WITH NEUROPATHY

	Common	Unusual	Rare
Metabolic/endocrine	Diabetes mellitus Chronic renal failure	Hypothyroidism	Porphyria (p. 451) Acromegaly
Toxic	Alcoholism Chronic liver disease Drugs (Box 26.121)	Lead Radiation	Arsenic (p. 226) Mercury Thallium Organophosphates (p. 216) Acrylamide Hexacarbons (glue)
Immune-mediated/ inflammatory		Polyarteritis nodosa Churg–Strauss disease SLE Rheumatoid arthritis Sjögren's disease Cryoglobulinaemia Paraproteinaemia	Coeliac disease Sarcoidosis Primary amyloidosis
Infective		HIV/AIDS	Lyme disease
Neoplastic		Lymphoma Carcinoma (infiltration and paraneoplastic) Myeloma	
Vitamin deficiencies		Vitamin B_{12} Thiamin Pyridoxine Folic acid Vitamin E Pantothenic acid	

26

26.121 DRUGS CAUSING PERIPHERAL NEUROPATHY

Cardiovascular agents

- Amiodarone
- Statins
- Hydralazine

Chemotherapy agents

- Cisplatin
- Thalidomide
- Vincristine
- Paclitaxel

Anti-infective agents

- Chloramphenicol
- Isoniazid
- Nitrofurantoin
- Ethambutol
- Metronidazole
- Suramin

Other

- Gold
- Disulfiram
- Pyridoxine
- Tacrolimus
- Colchicine
- Phenytoin

neuropathy) or the myelin sheath (demyelinating neuropathy) (Box 26.119). Many systemic diseases, toxins (Box 26.120) and drugs (Box 26.121) can be associated with peripheral neuropathy. Investigations required in a patient with peripheral neuropathy reflect this wide spectrum of causes (Box 26.122).

Clinical features

Motor nerve involvement produces features of a lower motor neuron lesion (p. 1178). Symptoms and signs of sensory nerve involvement depend on the type of sensory nerve involved (p. 1184). Autonomic fibre involvement may cause postural hypotension due to disruption of vasomotor control, sweating, cardiac rhythm, and gastrointestinal, bladder and sexual functions.

FOCAL NEUROPATHY (MONONEUROPATHY)

Entrapment is the usual cause of a mononeuropathy. However, a patient may present with what initially appears to be a single nerve lesion but which later develops into multiple nerve lesions (clinically or neurophysiologically), i.e. a multifocal neuropathy (mononeuritis multiplex).

Entrapment neuropathies (Box 26.123)

In an entrapment neuropathy, pressure initially damages the myelin sheath, and neurophysiology will show slowing of conduction over the relevant site. Sustained or severe pressure damages the integrity of the axons, demonstrable as loss of the sensory action potential distal to the site of compression.

Certain conditions increase the propensity to develop entrapment neuropathies. These include acromegaly, hypo-

26.122 INVESTIGATION OF PERIPHERAL NEUROPATHY

	First-line tests	Second-line tests	Occasionally useful tests
Haematology	Full blood count ESR B_{12} and folate		
Biochemistry	Urea, electrolytes, calcium Creatinine Liver function tests Blood glucose ± tolerance test/HbA_{Ic} Thyroid function tests Plasma protein electrophoresis	Serum lipids, lipoproteins Cryoglobulins Toxic metal and drug screen Prostate-specific antigen Urinary porphyrins Urinary Bence Jones protein Faecal occult blood	Vitamin assays (e.g. vitamin E) Phytanic acid (Refsum's disease)
Immunology	Venereal Diseases Research Laboratory (VDRL) test Serum autoantibodies (antinuclear factor, dsDNA, rheumatoid factor, extractable nuclear antigens)	Antiganglioside antibodies Antineuronal antibodies	
Other	Nerve conduction/EMG	Genetic screening tests (e.g. hereditary neuropathies, Friedreich's ataxia) Chest X-ray/CT Mammogram Abdominal imaging	Nerve biopsy

26.123 SYMPTOMS AND SIGNS IN COMMON ENTRAPMENT NEUROPATHIES

Nerve	Symptoms	Muscle weakness/muscle-wasting	Area of sensory loss
Median (at wrist) (carpal tunnel syndrome)	Pain and paraesthesia on palmar aspect of hands and fingers, waking the patient from sleep. Pain may extend to arm and shoulder	Abductor pollicis brevis	Lateral palm and thumb, index, middle and medial half 4th finger
Ulnar (at elbow)	Paraesthesia on medial border of hand, wasting and weakness of hand muscles	All small hand muscles, excluding abductor pollicis brevis	Medial palm and little finger, and medial half 4th finger
Radial	Weakness of extension of wrist and fingers, often precipitated by sleeping in abnormal posture, e.g. arm over back of chair	Wrist and finger extensors, supinator	Dorsum of thumb
Peroneal	Foot drop, trauma to head of fibula	Dorsiflexion and eversion of foot	Nil or dorsum of foot
Lateral cutaneous nerve of the thigh (meralgia paraesthetica)	Tingling and dysaesthesia on lateral border of the thigh	Nil	Lateral border of thigh

thyroidism, pregnancy, any pre-existing mild generalised axonal neuropathy (e.g. diabetes), and bone damage near the nerve. Patients with multiple recurrent entrapment neuropathies, especially at unusual sites, should be screened for autosomal dominant hereditary neuropathy with liability to pressure palsies (HNPP) (Box 26.123).

Unless axonal loss has occurred, entrapment neuropathies will recover, provided the pressure on the nerve is relieved, either by avoiding precipitating activities or limb positions, or by surgical decompression.

CRANIAL NEUROPATHIES

Lesions of ocular motor nerves (3rd, 4th and 6th) are reviewed on page 1195. An isolated lesion of one 8th cranial nerve usually indicates compressive pathology (e.g. acoustic neuroma, p. 1238) in or near the cerebellopontine angle. Isolated lesions of the 9th, 10th, 11th or 12th cranial nerves are uncommon, since lesions of these nerves are usually caused by structural pathology such as tumours, carotid artery dissection etc. Anatomical considerations mean that lower cranial nerve lesions tend to occur in groups, sometimes with involvement of the ascending sympathetic innervation to the eye (Box 26.124).

Trigeminal neuropathy

Isolated trigeminal sensory neuropathy is rare. It causes unilateral facial sensory loss and is associated in some patients with scleroderma, Sjögren's syndrome, or other connective tissue disorder. Patients with trigeminal neuralgia (p. 1164) do not have sensory loss on examination unless there have been operative procedures on the nerve. Reactivation of varicella virus in the trigeminal nerve causes herpes zoster (most frequently in the ophthalmic division) and is followed in about one-third of patients by post-herpetic neuralgia (p. 305).

26.124 SYNDROMES OF LOWER CRANIAL NERVE LESIONS OUTSIDE THE BRAIN STEM			
Syndrome	**Cranial nerves involved**	**Site of lesion**	**Cause**
Vernet	9, 10 and 11	Jugular foramen (inside skull)	Metastases, neurinoma, meningioma, epidermoid, carotid body tumour
Collet–Sicard	9, 10, 11 and 12	Jugular foramen just outside skull, near foramen lacerum	Metastases, neurinoma, meningioma, epidermoid, carotid body tumour
Villaret	9, 10, 11, 12 and Horner's	Posterior retropharyngeal space, near carotid artery	Carotid dissection, metastases, neurinoma, meningioma, epidermoid, carotid body tumour
Isolated 12th	12	Skull base (hypoglossal canal)	Metastases, neurinoma, meningioma, epidermoid

Idiopathic isolated facial nerve palsy (Bell's palsy)

This is a common condition affecting all ages and both sexes. The lesion is within the facial canal and may be due to reactivation of latent herpes simplex virus 1 infection. Symptoms usually develop subacutely over a few hours, with pain around the ear preceding the unilateral facial weakness. Patients often describe the face as 'numb', but there is no objective sensory loss (except possibly to taste). Hyperacusis can occur if the nerve to stapedius is involved, and there may be diminished salivation and tear secretion. Examination reveals only an ipsilateral lower motor neuron facial nerve palsy. Vesicles in the ear or on the palate indicate that the facial palsy is due to herpes zoster (p. 305) rather than Bell's palsy.

Prednisolone 40–60 mg daily for a week may speed recovery if started within 72 hours, and aciclovir has also been recommended (Box 26.125). Artificial tears and ointment prevent exposure keratitis and the eye should be taped shut overnight. About 80% of patients recover spontaneously within 12 weeks. A slow or poor recovery is predicted by complete paralysis, older age and reduced facial motor action potential amplitude after the first week. Recurrences can occur but should prompt further investigation. Aberrant re-innervation may occur during recovery, producing unwanted facial movements (e.g. eye closure when the mouth is moved) or 'crocodile tears' (tearing during salivation).

26.125 ACICLOVIR IN BELL'S PALSY **EBM**

'Aciclovir alone is not as effective as corticosteroids in the treatment of Bell's palsy, but the combination of aciclovir and prednisolone appears to be more effective than steroids alone.'

- De Diego JI, et al. Laryngoscope 1998; 108:573–575.
- Adour KK, et al. Ann Otol Rhinol Laryngol 1996; 105:371–378.

For further information: 💻 www.cochrane.org

Hemifacial spasm

This usually presents after middle age with intermittent twitching around one eye, spreading ipsilaterally over months or years to affect other parts of the facial muscles. The spasms are exacerbated by talking or eating, or when the patient is under stress. The cause, as with trigeminal neuralgia, is probably an aberrant arterial loop irritating the nerve just outside the pons. The facial nerve should be imaged to exclude a structural lesion, especially in a young patient. Drug treatment is not effective but injections of botulinum toxin into affected muscles help, although these usually have to be repeated every 3 months or so. Occasionally, microvascular decompression is necessary.

MULTIFOCAL NEUROPATHY (MONONEURITIS MULTIPLEX)

When multiple nerve root, peripheral nerve or cranial nerve lesions occur serially or concurrently, the pathology is due either to involvement of the vasa nervorum or to malignant infiltration of the nerves. The clinical expression of a very widespread multifocal neuropathy may become confluent so that the clinical picture eventually resembles a polyneuropathy. In this case neurophysiology may be required to identify the multifocal nature of the problem. Investigation of patients with an acute multifocal neuropathy should be urgent since vasculitis is a common cause, either as part of a systemic disease (Box 26.120) or isolated to the nerves.

GENERALISED NEUROPATHY (POLYNEUROPATHY)

The clinical effects of a generalised pathological process occur in the longest peripheral nerves first, affecting the distal lower limbs before the upper limbs, with sensory symptoms and signs of an ascending 'glove and stocking' distribution (p. 1183). This is particularly true with axonal neuropathies where the disorder affects the metabolic processes required for axonal transport in the peripheral nerves. In inflammatory demyelinating neuropathies, the pathology may be patchier and variations from this ascending pattern occur.

ACUTE INFLAMMATORY DEMYELINATING POLYNEUROPATHY (GUILLAIN–BARRÉ SYNDROME)

This develops 1–4 weeks after respiratory infection or diarrhoea (particularly *Campylobacter*) in 70% of patients. There is a predominantly cell-mediated inflammatory response directed at the myelin protein of spinal roots, peripheral and extra-axial cranial nerves, possibly triggered by molecular mimicry between epitopes found in the cell walls of some micro-organisms and gangliosides in the Schwann cell membranes. The resulting release of

26

inflammatory cytokines blocks nerve conduction and is followed by a complement-mediated destruction of the myelin sheath and the associated axon, if it is severe.

Clinical features

Distal paraesthesia and limb pains (often severe) precede a rapidly ascending muscle weakness, from lower to upper limbs, more marked proximally than distally. Facial and bulbar weakness commonly develops, and respiratory weakness requiring ventilatory support occurs in 20% of cases. In most patients, weakness progresses for 1–3 weeks, but rapid deterioration to respiratory failure can develop within hours. On examination there is diffuse weakness with widespread loss of reflexes. An unusual variant described by Miller Fisher comprises the triad of ophthalmoplegia, ataxia and areflexia.

Investigations

The CSF protein is elevated at some stage of the illness but may be normal in the first 10 days. There is usually no rise in CSF cell number (a lymphocytosis of $> 5 \times 10^7$ cells/litre suggests an alternative diagnosis). Electrophysiological studies are often normal in the early stages but show typical changes after a week or so, with conduction block and multifocal motor slowing, sometimes most evident proximally as delayed F-waves (p. 1155). Investigation to identify an underlying cause, such as cytomegalovirus, mycoplasma or *Campylobacter*, requires a chest X-ray, stool culture and appropriate immunological blood tests. Antibodies to the ganglioside GQ_{1b} are found in the Miller Fisher variant described above. Acute porphyria (p. 451) should be excluded by urinary porphyrin estimation, and serum lead should be measured if there are only motor signs.

Management

During the phase of deterioration, regular monitoring of respiratory function (vital capacity and arterial blood gases) is required, as respiratory failure may develop with little warning and require ventilatory support. Ventilation may be needed if the vital capacity falls below 1 litre, but intubation is more often required because of bulbar incompetence leading to aspiration. General management to protect the airway and prevent pressure sores and venous thrombosis is essential. Corticosteroid therapy has been shown by RCT to be ineffective. However, plasma exchange and intravenous immunoglobulin therapy shorten the duration of ventilation and improve prognosis, provided treatment is started within 14 days of the onset of symptoms (Box 26.126).

EBM

26.126 INTRAVENOUS IMMUNOGLOBULIN (IVIg) AND PLASMA EXCHANGE (PE) IN GUILLAIN–BARRÉ SYNDROME

'If used within the first 2 weeks of developing the illness, IVIg and PE are equally effective in reducing the severity and duration of Guillain–Barré syndrome, but there is no advantage in combining the two treatments.'

- Plasma Exchange/Sandoglobulin Guillain–Barré Syndrome Trial Group. Lancet 1997; 349:225–230.
- Bril V. Neurology 1996; 46:100–103.

For further information: 💻 www.cochrane.org

Prognosis

Overall, 80% of patients recover completely within 3–6 months, 4% die, and the remainder suffer residual neurological disability which can be severe. Adverse prognostic features include older age, rapid deterioration to ventilation and evidence of axonal loss on EMG.

Acute axonal polyneuropathy

There is an axonal variant of Guillain–Barré syndrome, rare in Europe and North America but more common in China and Japan. Circulating antibodies to various peripheral nerve gangliosides are often found. Other causes of acute axonal neuropathy, all rare, include drug or toxin exposure (Box 26.119, p. 1246).

CHRONIC POLYNEUROPATHY

A chronic symmetrical polyneuropathy, evolving over months or years, is the most frequently seen form of neuropathy. In about 30% of patients no cause can be established, even after thorough investigation. These patients usually have a mild axonal neuropathy which, whilst causing unpleasant symptoms, does not lead to motor disability. Therefore, if a patient with what seems to be an idiopathic polyneuropathy progresses to significant disability, further thought needs to given to finding a specific cause (usually inflammatory or genetic).

Chronic demyelinating polyneuropathy

This type of chronic polyneuropathy is either hereditary or immune-mediated (including those caused by abnormal paraproteins). Many abnormal genotypes cause hereditary demyelinating peripheral neuropathies with variable phenotypes, most characteristically that known as Charcot–Marie–Tooth disease (CMT). Here the neuropathy produces distal wasting ('inverted champagne bottle' or 'stork' legs), often with pes cavus, and a predominantly motor clinical involvement. In 70–80% the cause is reduplication of the *PMP-22* gene on chromosome 17 (autosomal dominant CMT type 1), but similar phenotypes are produced by several other genotypes with differing modes of inheritance (Box 26.127).

Chronic inflammatory demyelinating peripheral neuropathy (CIDP) presents with a relapsing or progressive generalised neuropathy. Sensory, motor or autonomic nerves can be involved but the signs are usually predominantly motor; a variant causes only motor involvement (multifocal motor neuropathy, MMN). CIDP usually responds to immunosuppressive treatment, corticosteroids or cyclophosphamide, or to immunomodulatory treatments (plasma exchange or intravenous immunoglobulin, IVIg); MMN is best treated by IVIg.

Some 10% of patients with acquired demyelinating polyneuropathy have an abnormal serum paraprotein, sometimes associated with a lymphoproliferative malignancy.

Chronic axonal polyneuropathy

This is the most common type of chronic polyneuropathy. Where the cause can be found, it is usually a disorder affecting axonal metabolism and transport, either acquired

26

26.127 HEREDITARY PERIPHERAL NEUROPATHIES

Type	Inheritance	Molecular pathology	Neurophysiology	Comments
CMT1A	Autosomal dominant	PMP-22 reduplication Chr 17p	Slowed MCV	Common
CMT1B	Autosomal dominant	PO mutation Chr 1q	Marked slowing of MCV	Common
CMTX	X-linked	Connexin-32 mutation Chr Xq	Near-normal conduction velocities	Common, females less affected
CMT2	Autosomal dominant	Not known	Axonal—normal MCV	Rare
CMT3	Dominant (usually new mutation)	PMP-22 mutation or deletion	Severely slowed MCV	Déjerine–Sottas disease, rare
CMT4	Autosomal recessive	Not known	Axonal—normal MCV	Very rare
HNPP	Autosomal dominant	PMP-22 deletion or mutation	Dysmyelination—slowed MCV	Uncommon
HSAN	Autosomal dominant (type 1) and recessive (types 2–5)	Not known	Axonal—normal MVC	Uncommon—lancinating pains, neuropathic feet, recurrent foot ulceration
Refsum's disease	Autosomal recessive	Peroxisome targeting signal 2 mutation Chr 10p	Marked slowing	Very rare, associated retinitis pigmentosa, ataxia and raised blood phytanic acid
Hereditary amyloid neuropathy	Autosomal dominant	Transthyretin mutation (in types 1 and 2) Chr 18q Other mutations (types 3 and 4)	Axonal—normal MCV	Uncommon, associated autonomic neuropathy

(CMT = Charcot–Marie–Tooth; HNPP = hereditary neuropathy with predisposition to pressure palsies; PMP = peripheral myelin protein; MCV = motor conduction velocity; Chr = chromosome; HSAN = hereditary sensory and autonomic neuropathy)

26.128 PHYSICAL SIGNS IN BRACHIAL PLEXUS LESIONS

26

Site	Root	Affected muscles	Sensory loss
Upper plexus (Erb–Duchenne)	C5/6	Biceps, deltoid, spinati, rhomboids, brachioradialis (triceps, serratus anterior)	Patch over deltoid
Lower plexus (Déjerine–Klumpke)	C8/T1	All small hand muscles, claw hand (ulnar wrist flexors)	Ulnar border hand/forearm
Thoracic outlet syndrome	C8/T1	Small hand muscles, ulnar forearm	Ulnar border hand/forearm/upper arm

(drugs and toxins) or genetically determined (Boxes 26.119 and 26.121, pp. 1246–1247).

PLEXUS LESIONS

Brachial plexopathy

Trauma usually damages either the upper or the lower parts of the brachial plexus, according to the mechanics of the injury. The clinical features depend upon the anatomical site of the damage (Box 26.128). Lower parts of the brachial plexus are vulnerable to infiltration from breast or apical lung tumours (Pancoast tumour) and may be damaged by therapeutic irradiation. The lower parts of the plexus may also be compressed by anatomical anomalies at the thoracic outlet, which may be accompanied by circulatory changes in the arm due to subclavian artery compression.

An acute brachial plexopathy of probable inflammatory origin may present with 'neuralgic amyotrophy'. In this syndrome, a period of very severe shoulder pain precedes the appearance of a patchy upper brachial plexus lesion, often affecting the long thoracic nerve which produces winging of the scapula. Recovery occurs over months and is usually complete.

Lumbosacral plexopathy

Lumbosacral plexus lesions may be caused by neoplastic infiltration or compression by retroperitoneal haematomas in patients with a coagulopathy. A small vessel vasculopathy can produce a lumbar plexopathy, especially in elderly patients when it may be the presenting feature of type 2 diabetes mellitus ('diabetic amyotrophy') or a vasculitis. This presents with painful wasting of the quadriceps with weakness of knee extension and adduction, and an absent knee reflex.

SPINAL ROOT LESIONS (RADICULOPATHY)

Lesions of the spinal roots are most commonly caused by compression at or near their spinal exit foramina by prolapsed intervertebral discs or degenerative spinal disease (p. 1242). Spinal roots may also be infiltrated by spinal and paraspinal tumour masses and inflammatory or infective processes. The clinical features include muscle weakness and wasting and dermatomal sensory loss with reflex changes that reflect the pattern of roots involved. Pain in the muscles whose innervating motor roots are involved is usually a prominent feature.

DISORDERS OF THE NEUROMUSCULAR JUNCTION

MYASTHENIA GRAVIS

This condition is characterised by progressive fatigable weakness, particularly of the ocular, neck, facial and bulbar muscles.

Aetiology and pathology

The disease is most commonly caused by autoantibodies to acetylcholine receptors in the post-junctional membrane of the neuromuscular junction. These antibodies block neuromuscular transmission and initiate a complement-mediated inflammatory response which reduces the number of acetylcholine receptors and damages the end plate (Fig. 26.58). A minority of patients have other auto-antibodies to epitopes on the post-junctional membrane,

in particular autoantibodies to a muscle-specific kinase (MuSK), an agrin receptor which is involved in the regulation and maintenance of the acetylcholine receptors.

About 15% of patients (mainly those with late onset) have a thymoma, and the majority of the remainder have thymic follicular hyperplasia. There is an increased incidence of other autoimmune diseases, and the disease is linked with certain HLA haplotypes. Nothing is known about factors which trigger the disease itself, but penicillamine can cause an antibody-mediated myasthenic syndrome which may persist even after drug withdrawal. Some drugs, especially aminoglycosides and ciprofloxacin, may exacerbate the neuromuscular blockade and should be avoided in patients with myasthenia.

Clinical features

The disease usually presents between the ages of 15 and 50 years, with women affected more often than men in the younger age groups and the reverse at older ages. It tends to run a relapsing and remitting course, especially during the early years.

The cardinal symptom is abnormal fatigable weakness of the muscles (which is different from a sensation of muscle fatigue); movement is initially strong but rapidly weakens. Worsening of symptoms towards the end of the

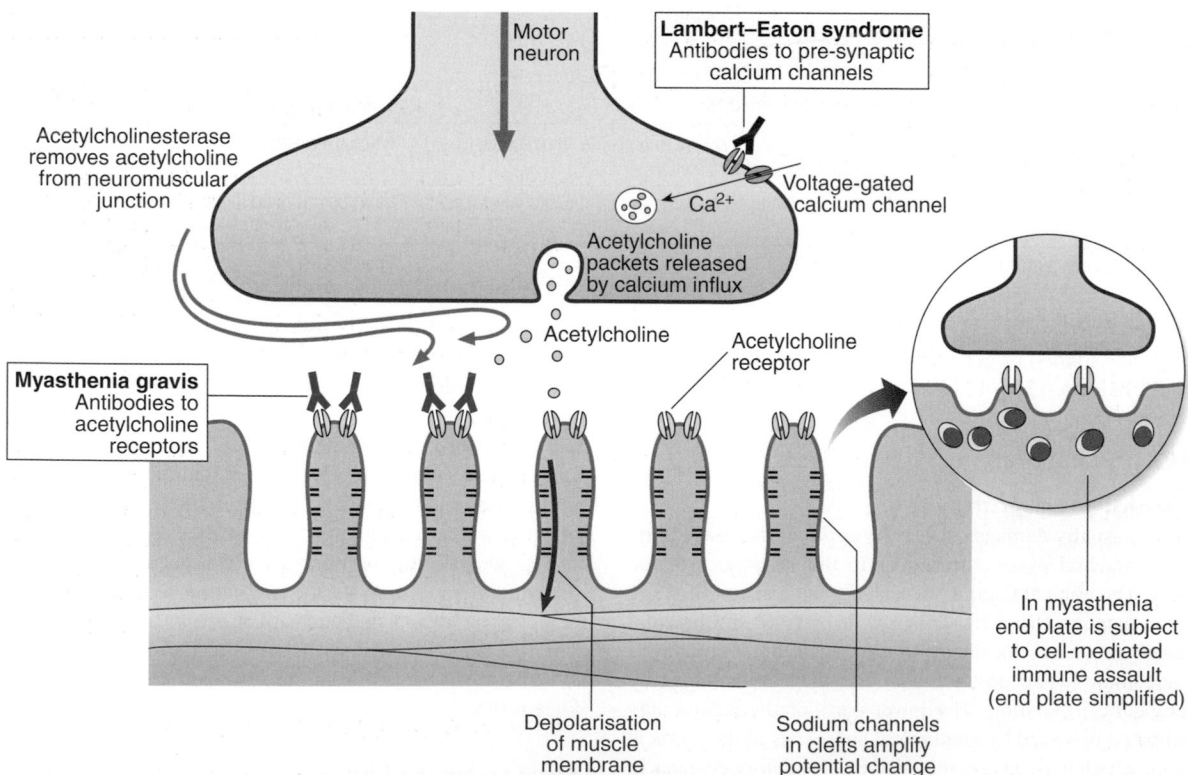

Fig. 26.58   Myasthenia gravis and Lambert–Eaton myasthenic syndrome (LEMS). In myasthenia there are antibodies to the acetylcholine receptors on the post-synaptic membrane which block conduction across the neuromuscular junction (NMJ). Myasthenic symptoms can be transiently improved by inhibition of acetylcholinesterase (e.g. with Tensilon—edrophonium bromide) which normally removes the acetylcholine. A cell-mediated immune response produces simplification of the post-synaptic membrane, further impairing the 'safety factor' of neuromuscular conduction. In LEMS, antibodies to the pre-synaptic voltage calcium channels impair release of acetylcholine from the motor nerve ending; calcium is required for the acetylcholine-containing vesicle to fuse with the pre-synaptic membrane for release into the NMJ.

26

day or following exercise is characteristic. There are no sensory signs or signs of involvement of the central nervous system, although weakness of the oculomotor muscles may mimic a central eye movement disorder.

The first symptoms are usually intermittent ptosis or diplopia, but weakness of chewing, swallowing, speaking or limb movement also occurs. Any limb muscle may be affected, most commonly those of the shoulder girdle; the patient is unable to undertake tasks above shoulder level, such as combing the hair, without frequent rests. Respiratory muscles may be involved, and respiratory failure is a not uncommon cause of death. Aspiration may occur if the cough is ineffectual. Sudden weakness from a cholinergic or myasthenic crisis (see below) may require ventilatory support.

Investigations

The intravenous injection of the short-acting anticholinesterase, edrophonium bromide, is a valuable diagnostic aid (the Tensilon test); 2 mg is injected initially, with a further 8 mg given half a minute later if there are no undesirable side-effects. Improvement in muscle power occurs within 30 seconds and usually persists for 2–3 minutes. EMG with repetitive stimulation may show the characteristic decremental response. Anti-acetylcholine receptor antibody (AChRA) is found in over 80% of cases, though less frequently in purely ocular myasthenia (50%). Anti-MuSK antibodies are found especially in AChRA-negative patients with prominent bulbar involvement. Positive anti-skeletal muscle antibodies suggest the presence of thymoma, but all patients should have a thoracic CT to exclude this condition, which may not be visible on plain X-ray examination. Screening for other autoimmune disorders, particularly thyroid disease, is important.

Management

The principles of treatment are:

- to maximise the activity of acetylcholine at remaining receptors in the neuromuscular junctions
- to limit or abolish the immunological attack on motor end plates.

The duration of action of acetylcholine is greatly prolonged by inhibiting its hydrolysing enzyme, acetylcholinesterase. The most commonly used anticholinesterase drug is pyridostigmine, which is given orally in a dosage of 30–120 mg, usually 6-hourly. Muscarinic side-effects, including diarrhoea and colic, may be controlled by propantheline (15 mg as required). Over-dosage of anticholinesterase drugs may cause a cholinergic crisis due to depolarisation block of motor end plates, with muscle fasciculation, paralysis, pallor, sweating, excessive salivation and small pupils. This may be distinguished from severe weakness due to exacerbation of myasthenia (myasthenic crisis) by the clinical features and, if necessary, by the injection of a small dose of edrophonium.

The immunological treatment of myasthenia is outlined in Box 26.129. Thymectomy in the early stages of the disease leads to a much better overall prognosis, whether a thymoma is present or not.

26.129 IMMUNOLOGICAL TREATMENT OF MYASTHENIA

Thymectomy

- Should be performed as soon as feasible in any antibody-positive patient under 45 years with symptoms not confined to extraocular muscles, unless the disease has been established for more than 7 years

Plasma exchange

- Removing antibody from the blood may produce marked improvement but, as this is usually brief, such therapy is normally reserved for myasthenic crisis or for pre-operative preparation

Intravenous immunoglobulin

- An alternative to plasma exchange in the treatment of severe myasthenia

Corticosteroid treatment

- Improvement is commonly preceded by marked exacerbation of myasthenic symptoms and treatment should be initiated in hospital
- It is usually necessary to continue treatment for months or years, often resulting in adverse effects

Other immunosuppressant treatment

- Treatment with azathioprine 2.5 mg/kg daily is of value in reducing the dosage of steroids necessary and may allow steroids to be withdrawn (Box 26.130)
- The effect of treatment on clinical disease is often delayed for several months

---

26.130 AZATHIOPRINE IN MYASTHENIA GRAVIS EBM

'Azathioprine as an adjunct to alternate-day prednisolone in the treatment of antibody-positive generalised myasthenia reduces the maintenance dose of prednisolone and is associated with fewer treatment failures, longer remissions and fewer side-effects. However, a small trial suggested that it is probably not useful as an initial immunosuppressive treatment on its own.'

- Palace J, et al. Neurology 1998; 50:1778–1783.
- Bromberg MB, et al. J Neurol Sci 1997; 150:59–62.

Prognosis

Prognosis is variable. Remissions sometimes occur spontaneously. When myasthenia is confined to the eye muscles, the prognosis is excellent and disability slight. Young female patients with generalised disease have high remission rates after thymectomy, whilst older patients are less likely to have a remission despite treatment. Rapid progression of the disease more than 5 years after its onset is uncommon.

OTHER MYASTHENIC SYNDROMES

There are other conditions which present with muscle weakness due to impaired transmission across the neuromuscular junction. The most common of these is the Lambert–Eaton myasthenic syndrome (LEMS), in which transmitter release is impaired, often in association with antibodies to pre-junctional voltage-gated calcium channels (Fig. 26.58). Patients may have autonomic dysfunction (and a dry mouth)

26

in addition to muscle weakness, but the cardinal clinical sign is absence of tendon reflexes, which can return immediately after sustained contraction of the relevant muscle. The condition is associated with underlying malignancy in a high percentage of cases, and investigation must be directed towards detecting such a cause. The condition is diagnosed electrophysiologically by the presence of post-tetanic potentiation of motor response to nerve stimulation at a frequency of 20–50/s. Treatment is with 3,4-diaminopyridine.

DISEASES OF MUSCLE

Voluntary muscle is subject to a range of hereditary and acquired disorders affecting either its structure, or the biochemical processes which convert the chemical energy derived from cell metabolism into mechanical energy in a controlled manner. These disorders present in a limited number of ways, most commonly a symmetrical weakness of the large, power-generating proximal muscles (proximal myopathy). This weakness may be fixed or periodic. Other symptoms and signs of muscle disease include myotonia (an abnormality of muscle relaxation) and muscle pain. Diagnosis depends upon consideration of the clinical picture along with the results of EMG studies and muscle biopsy. In some inherited muscular diseases, diagnosis can be made by identifying the presence of a specific genetic abnormality.

MUSCULAR DYSTROPHIES

This is a group of inherited disorders characterised by progressive degeneration of groups of muscles, sometimes with involvement of the heart muscle or conducting tissue, and other parts of the nervous system (Box 26.131).

Clinical features

Onset is often in childhood, although some patients, especially those with myotonic dystrophy, may present as adults. Wasting and weakness are usually symmetrical, there is no fasciculation and no sensory loss, and tendon reflexes are preserved until a late stage, except in myotonic dystrophy. Differential diagnosis is based on the age at onset, the distribution of affected muscles and the pattern of inheritance. Myotonic dystrophy may be diagnosed clinically by the distribution of muscle weakness and other features including myotonia (Box 26.131). Many dystrophies include cardiomyopathy (p. 641) amongst their clinical features.

Investigations

The diagnosis can be confirmed by specific molecular genetic testing, supplemented with EMG and muscle biopsy if necessary. Creatine kinase is markedly elevated in Duchenne muscular dystrophy, but is normal or only moderately elevated in the other dystrophies. Screening for an associated cardiac abnormality (cardiomyopathy or dysrhythmia) is important.

Management

There is no specific therapy for these conditions, but physiotherapy and occupational therapy help patients cope with their disability. Treatment of associated cardiac failure or arrhythmia (with pacemaker insertion if necessary) may be required; similarly, management of respiratory complications (including nocturnal hypoventilation) can improve quality of life. Genetic counselling is important.

26.131 THE MUSCULAR DYSTROPHIES

Type	Genetics	Age of onset	Muscles affected	Other features
Myotonic dystrophy (DM1)	Autosomal dominant; expanded triplet repeat chromosome19q	Any	Face (incl. ptosis), sternomastoids, distal limb, generalised later	Myotonia, cognitive dulling, cardiac conduction abnormalities, lens opacities, frontal balding, hypogonadism
Proximal myotonic myopathy (PROMM; DM2)	Autosomal dominant; quadruplet repeat expansion in Zn finger protein 9 gene chromosome 3q	Adult	Proximal, especially thigh, sometimes muscle hypertrophy	As for DM1 but cognition not affected Muscle pain
Duchenne	X-linked; deletions in dystrophin gene	First 5 years	Proximal and limb girdle	Pseudohypertrophy of calves Cardiomyopathy
Becker	X-linked; deletions in dystrophin gene	Late childhood/ early adult	Proximal and limb girdle	Pseudohypertrophy of calves Cardiomyopathy
Limb girdle	Autosomal dominant (type 1) Autosomal recessive (type 2) Many mutations on different chromosomes	Childhood/ early adult	Limb girdle	Some have calf hypertrophy Some have cardiac conduction abnormalities
Facioscapulohumeral (FSH)	Autosomal dominant; tandem repeat deletion chromosome 4q	7–30 years	Face and upper limb girdle	Pain in shoulder girdle common
Oculopharyngeal	Autosomal dominant and recessive; triplet repeat expansion in PABP2 gene chromosome 14q	30–50 years	Ptosis, external ophthalmoplegia, dysphagia, tongue weakness	Mild lower limb weakness
Emery-Dreifuss	X-linked recessive; mutations in emerin gene	4–5 years	Humero-peroneal, proximal limb girdle later	Contractures develop early Cardiac involvement leads to sudden death

26

26.132 INHERITED DISORDERS OF MUSCLE METABOLISM

	Enzyme deficiency	Clinical features	Diagnosis
Carbohydrate metabolism	Myophosphorylase (McArdle's disease) Phosphofructokinase	Exercise-induced muscle cramps, myoglobinuria	CK elevated Muscle biopsy appearance Molecular genetics
	Alpha-1,4-glucosidase (acid maltase)	Proximal limb and diaphragm weakness	CK elevated Myopathic EMG Lymphocyte glycogen storage Muscle biopsy appearance Molecular genetics
Lipid metabolism	Carnitine-palmitoyl transferase (CPT) deficiency	Muscle pain on prolonged exercise, myoglobinuria	CK elevated during attacks of muscle pain, normal in between Muscle biopsy appearance

26.133 MITOCHONDRIAL MYOPATHY SYNDROMES

Syndrome	Clinical features
Myoclonic epilepsy with ragged red fibres (MERRF)	Myoclonic epilepsy, cerebellar ataxia, dementia, sensorineural deafness ± peripheral neuropathy and optic atrophy
Mitochondrial myopathy, encephalopathy, lactic acidosis and stroke-like episodes (MELAS)	Episodic encephalopathy, stroke-like episodes often preceded by migraine-like headache, nausea and vomiting
Chronic progressive external ophthalmoplegia (CPEO)	Progressive ptosis and external oculomotor palsy, proximal myopathy ± deafness, ataxia and cardiac conduction defects
Kearns–Sayre syndrome	Like CPEO but early age of onset (< 20 yrs), heart block, pigmentary retinopathy

Prognosis

Patients with Duchenne dystrophy used to die within 10 years of diagnosis, but with improved general care they are now living into the third decade. The lifespan in limb girdle and facioscapulohumeral dystrophies is normal. In myotonic dystrophy, there is considerable phenotypic variation and the prognosis is very variable, limited by cardiac and respiratory complications.

CONGENITAL MYOPATHY

This is rare and presents in infancy with muscular weakness and limpness. Serum muscle enzymes may be normal or slightly elevated and the EMG is usually myopathic. The syndrome may be caused by a number of specific conditions that have a variable inheritance and are defined by the type of structural abnormality present in skeletal muscle fibres. Most patients have a slowly progressive disease and there is no specific therapy.

INHERITED METABOLIC MYOPATHIES

A large number of individually rare inherited disorders of the biochemical pathways necessary to maintain the supply of chemical energy (ATP) in muscles may present with muscle pain, weakness and fatigue. These are mostly recessively inherited deficiencies in the enzymes of the glycolytic and fatty acid metabolism pathways (Box 26.132).

Inherited disorders of the oxidative pathways of the respiratory chain in mitochondria cause a group of mitochondrial myopathies which may be associated with a range of other deficits in the nervous system, including episodic stroke-like events and myoclonic epilepsy (Box 26.133). Many of these mitochondrial myopathies (or cytopathies) are inherited via the mitochondrial genome, down the maternal line. There is often a characteristic 'ragged-red fibre' change on muscle biopsy.

CHANNELOPATHIES

Inherited abnormalities of the sodium, calcium and chloride ion channels in striated muscle produce various syndromes of familial periodic paralysis, myotonia and malignant hyperthermia which can be recognised by their clinical characteristics, provocation by exercise or eating, and associated changes in serum potassium concentration (Box 26.134).

ACQUIRED MYOPATHIES

Muscle weakness may be caused by a range of metabolic, endocrine, toxic or inflammatory disorders (Box 26.135). Disorders affecting the muscles' structural integrity can be distinguished by EMG from those caused by metabolic derangement. In metabolic disorders, weakness is often acute and generalised, while a proximal myopathy predominantly affecting the pelvic girdle is a feature of some endocrine disorders. This may develop without other manifestations of hormonal disturbance. A wide variety of drugs and toxins may cause myopathy and these are also listed in Box 26.135.

Inflammatory myopathy (polymyositis) is described on page 1136.

26

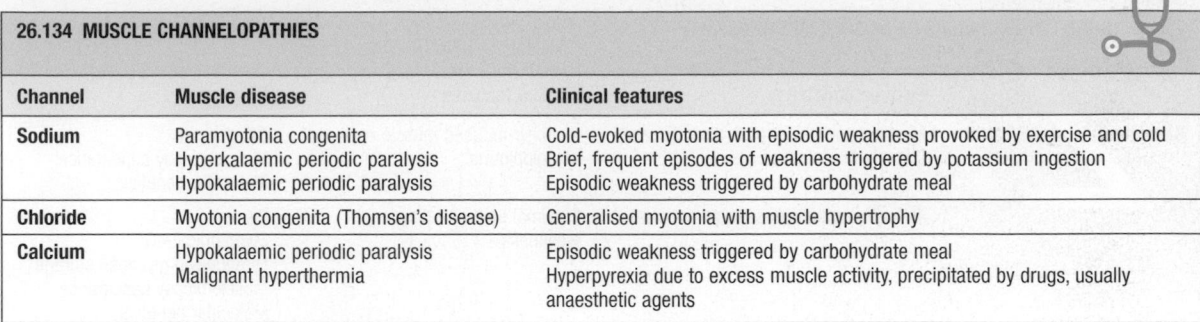

26.134 MUSCLE CHANNELOPATHIES

Channel	Muscle disease	Clinical features
Sodium	Paramyotonia congenita Hyperkalaemic periodic paralysis Hypokalaemic periodic paralysis	Cold-evoked myotonia with episodic weakness provoked by exercise and cold Brief, frequent episodes of weakness triggered by potassium ingestion Episodic weakness triggered by carbohydrate meal
Chloride	Myotonia congenita (Thomsen's disease)	Generalised myotonia with muscle hypertrophy
Calcium	Hypokalaemic periodic paralysis Malignant hyperthermia	Episodic weakness triggered by carbohydrate meal Hyperpyrexia due to excess muscle activity, precipitated by drugs, usually anaesthetic agents

26.135 CAUSES OF ACQUIRED PROXIMAL MYOPATHY

Inflammatory (p. 1136)

- Polymyositis
- Dermatomyositis

Endocrine and metabolic

- Hypothyroidism
- Hyperthyroidism
- Acromegaly
- Cushing's syndrome (including iatrogenic)
- Addison's disease
- Conn's syndrome
- Osteomalacia
- Hypokalaemia (liquorice, diuretic and purgative abuse)
- Hypercalcaemia (disseminated bony metastases)

Toxic

- Alcohol (chronic and acute syndromes)
- Vitamin E
- Organophosphates
- Snake venoms

Drugs

- Corticosteroids (especially fluorinated)
- Chloroquine
- Amiodarone
- β-blockers
- Statins
- Clofibrate
- Ciclosporin
- Vincristine
- Zidovudine
- Opiates
- ε-aminocaproic acid

Paraneoplastic

- Carcinomatous neuromyopathy
- Dermatomyositis

FURTHER INFORMATION

Books and journal articles

Aminoff MJ, ed. Neurology and general medicine. 3rd edn. Philadelphia: Churchill Livingstone; 2001.

Bradley WG, Daroff RB, Fenichel GM, Jankovic J, eds. Neurology in clinical practice. Principles of diagnosis and management. 4th edn. Philadelphia: Butterworth–Heinemann; 2004.

Mohr JP, Choi DW, Grotta JC, et al. Stroke. Pathophysiology, diagnosis, and management. 4th edn. Philadelphia: Churchill Livingstone; 2004.

Victor M, Ropper AH. Adams and Victor's principles of neurology. 8th edn. New York: McGraw–Hill; 2005.

Websites

www.wfneurology.org *World Federation of Neurology*.

www.ninds.nih.gov *National Institute of Neurological Disorders and Stroke*.

www.toddtroost.com/mylinks2001.html *Neuroscience links from ANA*.

26

27

O.M.V. SCHOFIELD
J.L. REES

Skin disease

CLINICAL EXAMINATION IN SKIN DISEASE

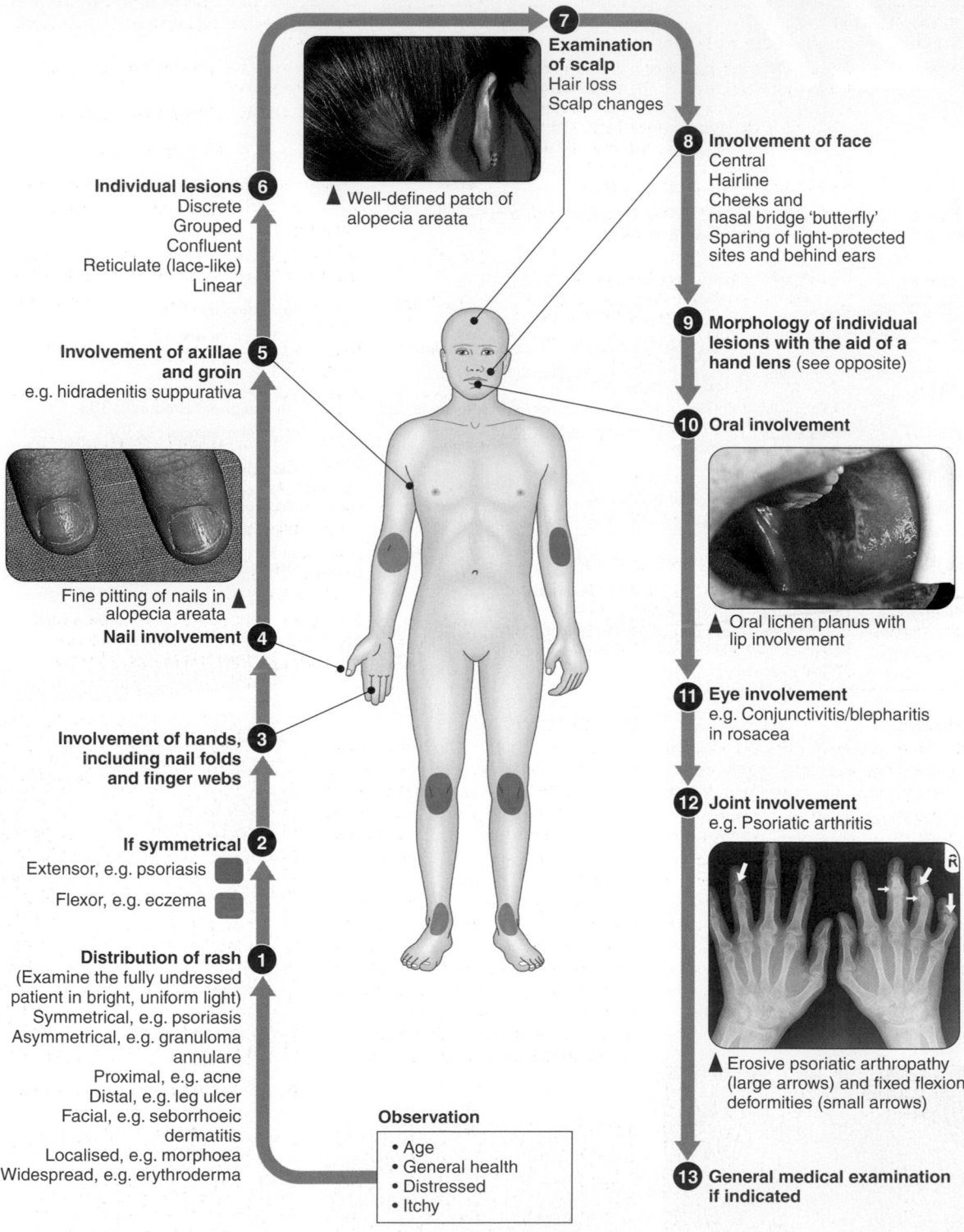

7 Examination of scalp
Hair loss
Scalp changes

▲ Well-defined patch of alopecia areata

6 Individual lesions
Discrete
Grouped
Confluent
Reticulate (lace-like)
Linear

8 Involvement of face
Central
Hairline
Cheeks and
nasal bridge 'butterfly'
Sparing of light-protected
sites and behind ears

5 Involvement of axillae and groin
e.g. hidradenitis suppurativa

9 Morphology of individual lesions with the aid of a hand lens (see opposite)

10 Oral involvement

Fine pitting of nails in alopecia areata ▲

4 Nail involvement

▲ Oral lichen planus with lip involvement

3 Involvement of hands, including nail folds and finger webs

11 Eye involvement
e.g. Conjunctivitis/blepharitis
in rosacea

2 If symmetrical
Extensor, e.g. psoriasis
Flexor, e.g. eczema

12 Joint involvement
e.g. Psoriatic arthritis

1 Distribution of rash
(Examine the fully undressed
patient in bright, uniform light)
Symmetrical, e.g. psoriasis
Asymmetrical, e.g. granuloma
annulare
Proximal, e.g. acne
Distal, e.g. leg ulcer
Facial, e.g. seborrhoeic
dermatitis
Localised, e.g. morphoea
Widespread, e.g. erythroderma

Observation
• Age
• General health
• Distressed
• Itchy

▲ Erosive psoriatic arthropathy
(large arrows) and fixed flexion
deformities (small arrows)

13 General medical examination if indicated

27

TERMS USED TO DESCRIBE SKIN LESIONS

Term	Definition	Term	Definition
PRIMARY LESIONS		**Burrow**	A linear or curvilinear papule, caused by a burrowing scabies mite
Macule	A small flat area of altered colour, e.g. freckle	**Comedone**	A plug of keratin and sebum wedged in a dilated pilosebaceous orifice
Papule	A discrete lesion, usually raised above the surface of the skin and therefore visible. There may be a change in colour. Some, particularly if they arise from the subcutis, are felt rather than seen. Larger papules are referred to as nodules. Although there is no agreed definition a nodule is usually bigger than 1 cm, e.g. a melanocytic naevus or a nodular melanoma	**Telangiectasia**	The visible dilatation of small cutaneous blood vessels
		SECONDARY LESIONS (which evolve from primary lesions)	
		Scale	A flake arising from the stratum corneum, e.g. psoriasis
Plaque	A raised area of skin with a flat top, typically, several cm or more across. Scale is usually present, e.g. psoriasis	**Crust**	Exudate of blood or serous fluid, e.g. eczema or tissue fluid
Vesicle and bulla	A small (~ several mm) and a larger blister (~ several cm) respectively. Blisters are collections of fluid; if a small needle is inserted fluid drains out. They form either within the epidermis or just beneath it, e.g. a thermal burn or pemphigoid	**Ulcer**	An area of skin from which the whole of the epidermis and at least the upper part of the dermis has been lost
		Excoriation	Damage resulting from scratching producing (usually) a linear ulcer or erosion
Pustule	A focal visible accumulation of pus in the skin. Usually yellow or green, e.g. acne	**Erosion**	An area of skin denuded by complete or partial loss of the epidermis
Abscess	A localised collection of pus in a cavity, more than 1 cm in diameter	**Fissure**	A slit-shaped deep ulcer, e.g. irritant dermatitis of the hands
Weal	An evanescent discrete dermal collection of fluid. The fluid is diffuse, unlike in a blister. Weals are usually white due to masking of the local blood supply by fluid, e.g. a nettle sting	**Sinus**	A cavity or channel that permits the escape of pus or fluid
		Scar	The result of healing, in which normal structures are permanently replaced by fibrous tissue, e.g. post-biopsy scar
Papilloma	A projecting nipple-like mass, e.g. skin tag	**Atrophy**	Loss of substance due to diminution of the epidermis, dermis or subcutaneous fat, e.g. atrophy due to excess topical corticosteroids
Petechiae, purpura and ecchymosis	Petechiae are pinhead-sized macules of extravascular blood in the dermis. They are flat. Larger ones, referred to as purpura, may be palpable. If bleeding involves deeper structures then it is an ecchymosis ('bruise')	**Stria**	A streak-like, linear, atrophic, pink, purple or white lesion due to changes in the connective tissue, e.g. Cushing's syndrome or pregnancy-induced

HISTORY

Introduce yourself, ask a few brief questions and examine the skin before further questioning of the patient. Ask about onset of the lesions and progression of the disease. A careful enquiry into drugs administered, including those bought without a prescription, a past or family history of skin disorders, comorbidity, and details of occupation and hobbies are also potentially important. The relative contribution of history, elicitation of symptoms and physical signs differs for particular diagnoses.

EXAMINATION

The patient needs to be undressed, and make-up and dressings should be removed. Failure to undress the patient appropriately may prevent the correct diagnosis from being made. Explain why examination of asymptomatic areas of skin is required.

A magnifying lens is often helpful. Feeling the skin provides diagnostic clues and may also be therapeutic as many patients, whatever their level of sophistication, may feel like lepers. Skin diseases cannot usually be correctly diagnosed at arm's length. Ample lighting, preferably natural, is required.

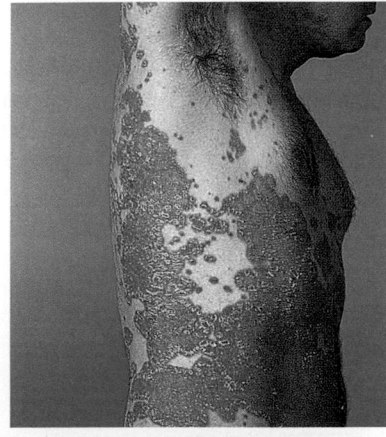

Plaque. Erythematous plaques in psoriasis.

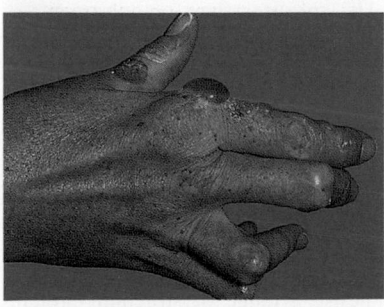

Bullae and scarring. Acquired epidermolysis bullosa in rheumatoid arthritis.

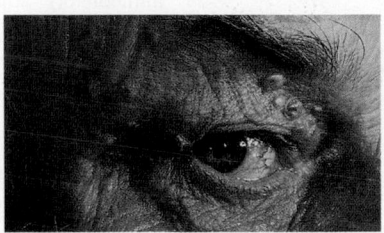

Comedo. Solar comedones occurring around the eyes in an elderly individual.

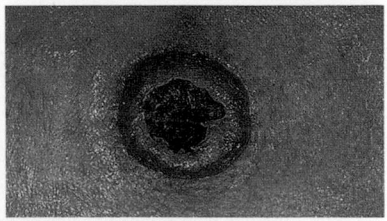

Nodule. A keratoacanthoma.

Skin disease is common. Surveys in Europe suggest that approximately 1 in 7 to 1 in 10 of all visits to a primary care physician is for a skin problem. For many hospitals the number of patients attending for dermatological diagnosis and treatment exceeds the total number of visits for the whole of internal medicine. Population prevalence studies are in keeping with these figures, revealing an enormous burden of undiagnosed, untreated skin disease. It is all too common and easy to underestimate the impact diseases of the skin make on patients. Healthy (and attractive) skin plays a major role in most persons' self-esteem, and is a key component of the image they present to the outside world. The texture and tactile qualities of skin, as well as its appearance, play a significant role in most grooming and sexual behaviours. Conversely, those with skin disease are often stigmatised and shunned, sometimes due to the spurious belief that their appearance is a result of a contagious disease.

Skin disease appears to be becoming more common for at least three reasons:

- First, there is a lowered threshold for seeking medical attention.
- Second, the absolute incidence of many diseases such as skin cancer and atopic dermatitis has increased.
- Third, and often neglected, the therapeutic options for a number of diseases previously viewed as untreatable have increased and awareness of these therapies is spreading as patients take a greater interest in their health care.

Skin complaints affect all ages from the neonate to the elderly and the dermatologist sees a fairly even distribution of patients of all ages in hospital or office practice (Fig. 27.1). Every clinician has the opportunity to look at the skin when listening to or examining a patient and should be able to identify important and common skin disorders. This chapter emphasises those skin conditions that are frequently seen in general practice and in general medical clinics. Those skin infections not covered here, including human immunodeficiency virus (HIV) disease, are dealt with in

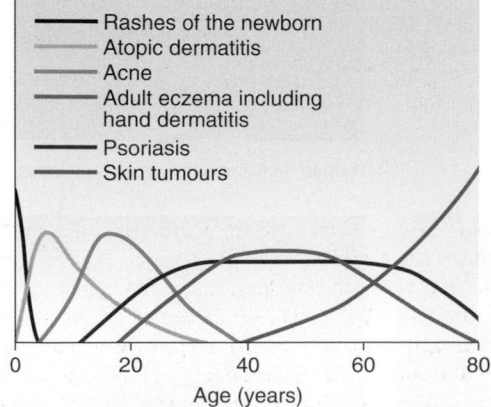

Frequency
(arbitrary scales)

Rashes of the newborn
Atopic dermatitis
Acne
Adult eczema including hand dermatitis
Psoriasis
Skin tumours

Age (years)

Fig. 27.1 The age distribution of some common skin conditions. Frequencies of the various rashes are not drawn to scale and are illustrative only.

27.1 COMMON SKIN DISEASES IN OLD AGE

- **Prevalence:** about 40% of individuals over the age of 60 years have significant dermatological problems.
- **Diseases:** the most common in this age group are:
  —skin cancers
  —leg ulcers, a major cause of morbidity in the elderly
  —blistering disorders
  —herpes zoster (shingles) and post-herpetic neuralgia
  —inflammatory skin diseases, e.g. asteatotic, gravitational and seborrhoeic eczema, psoriasis
  —lichen sclerosus et atrophicus
  —scabies
  —lymphoedema
  —pruritus of old age
  —drug-related rashes.

Chapters 13 and 14. Connective tissue diseases, which often involve the skin, are discussed in Chapter 25.

The aim of this chapter is to give the reader:

- an idea of how to assess the patient with a rash or lesion
- advice on appropriate initial management and therapy
- an outline of the theory underlying the mechanisms of some skin diseases and their therapies.

FUNCTIONAL ANATOMY, PHYSIOLOGY AND INVESTIGATIONS

ANATOMY AND PHYSIOLOGY

The skin of an average adult covers an area of just under 2 m^2. The epidermis, a stratified squamous epithelium, is the outermost layer and is predominantly composed of keratinocytes. The epidermis is attached to but separated from the underlying dermis by the basement membrane. The dermis contains, and supports, blood vessels and nerves, and the epidermal-derived structures such as the appendageal structures (hair follicles, and eccrine and apocrine sweat glands). The predominant cell of the dermis is the fibroblast. As stated, the appendageal structures, whilst embedded within the dermis, are epidermal in origin. Below the dermis is a layer of adipose tissue (the subcutis).

EPIDERMIS

Keratinocytes make up approximately 90% of epidermal cells (Fig. 27.2). The proliferative compartment of epidermis resides in the basal layer and in the layer immediately adjacent to the basal layer where mitotic figures are also not uncommon. The site of the keratinocyte stem cell is not known with certainty but is likely to be in a specialised region of the hair follicle analogous to the 'bulge' region in the mouse, although cells with stem cell-like qualities may also reside in the interfollicular epidermis. In areas of skin without hair follicles (glabrous skin) stem cells are present within the epidermis.

Keratinocytes synthesise a range of structural proteins including keratins and loricrin. There are over 20 different types of keratin which are divided into two broad groups:

27

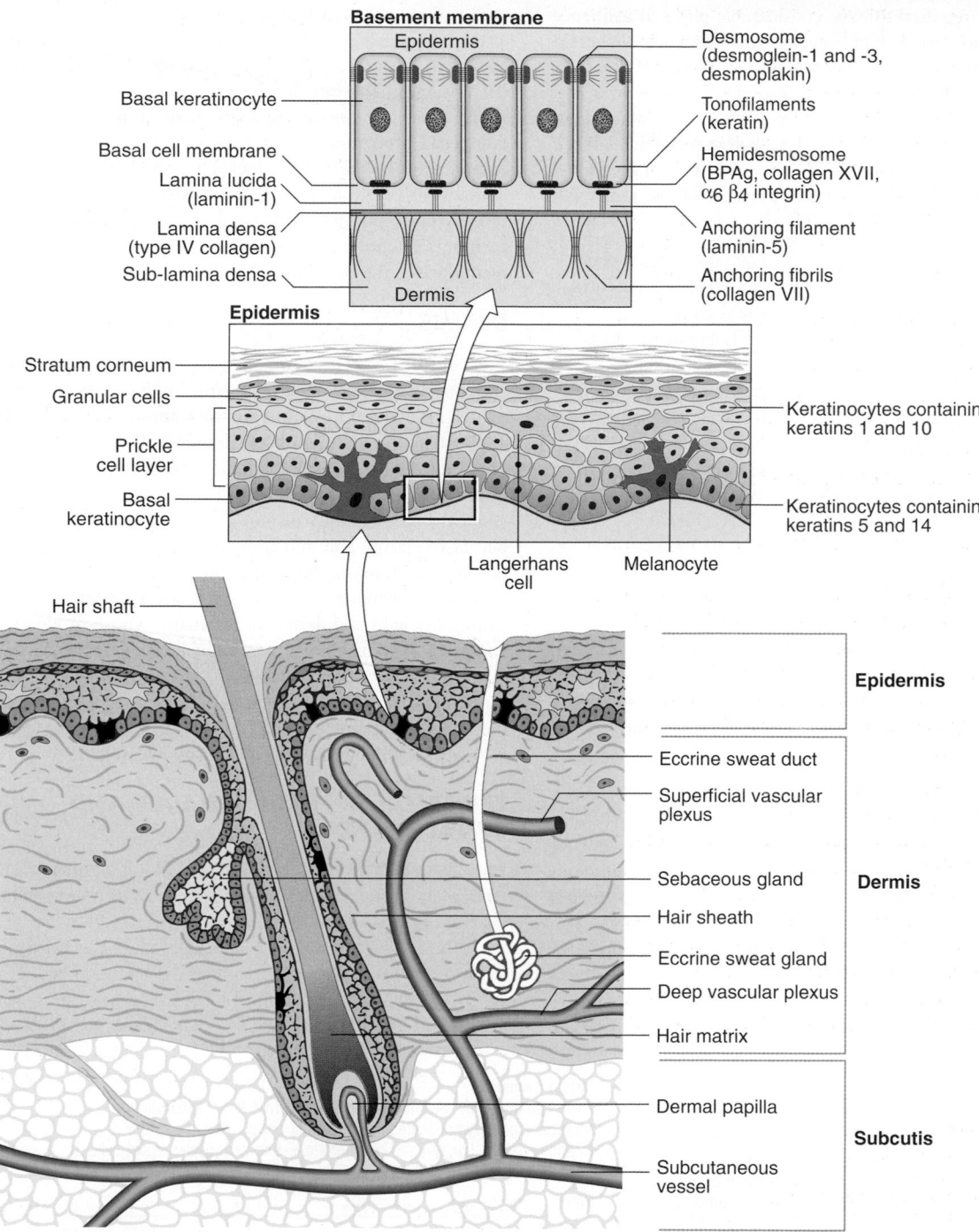

Fig. 27.2   Structure of normal skin.

basic (type I) and acidic (type II). Keratin macromolecules are dimers, made up of one acidic and one basic molecule, aggregated to form larger structures called intermediate filaments. Intermediate filaments play a key structural role in skin physiology, and genetic diseases that result from mutations in keratins (e.g. epidermolysis bullosa simplex, some types of ichthyosis) are characterised by either epidermal fragility (i.e. blistering) or grossly disordered keratinocyte differentiation. As keratinocytes move out of the basal layer they differentiate, producing a variety of protein and lipid products. Keratinocytes undergo a form of programmed cell death in the granular layer before becoming the flattened anucleate cells that make up the stratum corneum. The epidermis is a site of great lipid production, and the ability of the stratum corneum to act as a hydrophobic barrier is in large part the result of its structural design, the 'bricks and mortar model': dead corneocytes with a highly cross-linked protein membrane ('bricks') within a metabolically active layer of lipid synthesised by the keratinocytes ('mortar').

Skin is required to have considerable physical resilience as well as being highly active metabolically. Whereas keratins provide structural support for individual keratinocytes, attachments between cells need to be able to transmit and dissipate stress, a function performed by desmosomes. Diseases that target desmosomes, such as pemphigus, result in blistering as the individual keratinocytes separate.

Three other cell types make up most of the remaining 10% of epidermal cells:

- *Langerhans cells* are dendritic, bone marrow-derived cells that circulate between the epidermis and the local lymph nodes. Their prime function is effective presentation of foreign antigens to lymphocytes, as is seen, for example, in an allergic contact dermatitis reaction. They may also play a part in presentation of tumour antigens, a fact on which researchers have tried to capitalise in the production of anti-melanoma vaccines. Other dendritic cells which are effective at presenting antigen are also present in skin but are in the dermis rather than the epidermis.
- *Melanocytes*, of neural crest origin, are found predominantly in the basal layer; they synthesise the pigment melanin from tyrosine, package it in melanosomes and transfer it to surrounding keratinocytes via their dendritic processes.
- *Merkel cells* are found in the basal layer. They are thought to play a role in signal transduction of fine touch. Their embryological derivation is unclear.

BASEMENT MEMBRANE

The basement membrane (Fig. 27.2) acts as an anchor for the epidermis but allows movement of cells and nutrients between the dermis and epidermis. It consists of several well-defined layers that are identifiable ultrastructurally and at the molecular level. The cell membrane of the epidermal basal cell is attached to the basement membrane via hemidesmosomes. The lamina lucida is the zone immediately subjacent to the cell membrane of the basal cell which is composed predominantly of laminin. Anchoring filaments extend through the lamina lucida to attach to the lamina densa. This electron-dense layer consists predominantly of type IV collagen; from it extend loops of type VII collagen forming anchoring fibrils that fasten the basement membrane to the dermis.

DERMIS

The dermis is vascular and supports the epidermis structurally and nutritionally. It varies in thickness from just over 1 mm on the inner forearm to 4 mm on the back. (By contrast, the epidermis on most sites is only 0.1–0.2 mm thick, except on the palms or soles where it can be several millimetres in thickness.) The acellular part of the dermis consists predominantly of fibres, mostly collagens I and III but also elastin and reticulin, synthesised by the major cell type, fibroblasts. Support is provided by an amorphous ground substance (mostly the glycosaminoglycans, hyaluronic acid and dermatan sulphate), whose production and catabolism may be influenced by hormonal changes and damage from ultraviolet (UV) radiation. Apart from fibroblasts, there is a large number of other cell types within the dermis including mast cells, mononuclear phagocytes, T lymphocytes, dendritic cells, nerves and vessels.

EPIDERMAL APPENDAGES: HAIR AND SWEAT GLANDS

Hair follicles, sweat (eccrine) and apocrine glands are epidermal structures which invaginate into the dermis.

27.2 FUNCTIONS OF THE SKIN	
Function	**Structure/cell involved**
Protection against: Chemicals, particles, dessication Ultraviolet radiation Antigens, haptens Microbes	 Stratum corneum Melanin produced by melanocytes and transferred to keratinocytes Langerhans cells, lymphocytes, mononuclear phagocytes, mast cells Stratum corneum, Langerhans cells, mononuclear phagocytes, mast cells
Preservation of a balanced internal environment Prevents loss of water, electrolytes and macromolecules	 Stratum corneum
Shock absorber Strong, yet elastic and compliant covering	 Dermis and subcutaneous fat
Sensation	Specialist nerve endings mediating pain leading to withdrawal, and itch leading to scratch and hence removal of a parasite
Vitamin D synthesis	Keratinocytes
Temperature regulation	Eccrine sweat glands and blood vessels
Protection, and fine manipulation of small objects	Nails
Hormonal Testosterone synthesis from inactive precursors and testosterone conversion to other androgenic steroids	 Hair follicles Sebaceous glands
Pheromonal (of unknown importance in humans)	Apocrine sweat glands
Psychosocial, grooming and sexual behaviour	Hair, nails, appearance and tactile quality of skin

They are formed during the second trimester and number 3–5 million. Coarse, medullated hair accounts for the terminal hair of the scalp and pubic areas. Short, fine unmedullated hairs make up the remaining body hair. Sebaceous glands are usually associated with hair follicles, their ducts discharging sebum into the upper part of the follicle. Sebum excretion is under hormonal control; androgens and progestogen increase sebum excretion whereas oestrogens have an inhibitory effect. Apocrine glands are those sweat glands found in the axillae, perineum, genitalia and areolae which become functional after puberty under the influence of hormonal changes, particularly androgens. Their physiological role in humans is unclear but in animals they play a pheromonal role in many species. Eccrine sweat glands are found all over the body and their coiled ducts open directly on to the skin surface. They play a major role in humans in thermoregulation and, unusually, are innervated by cholinergic fibres of the sympathetic (rather than parasympathetic) nervous system. Eccrine glands of the palms and soles are preferentially activated by 'fight and fright' responses and the resulting increase in friction due to small amounts of water increases grip.

BLOOD VESSELS AND NERVES

The abundant blood supply of the skin is arranged in superficial and deep plexuses. The skin is well supplied with nerves to both dermis and epidermis. It used to be thought that nerves did not penetrate into the epidermis but this is now known to be false and there are indeed a large number of nerves that appear to interact with Langerhans cells, melanocytes and other components of the epidermis; their function is unknown. Blood vessels are supplied by sympathetic autonomic nerves and peptinergic nerves that take part in the axon reflex. The functions of the skin and changes in old age are summarised in Boxes 27.2 and 27.3.

DIAGNOSIS AND INVESTIGATION OF SKIN DISORDERS

The key to successful treatment is accurate diagnosis. This requires an appropriate history, an appropriately thorough examination of the skin including hair and nails (p. 1281), and occasional use of further investigations such as histopathology of a diagnostic biopsy.

Some investigative tests can be performed in the clinic with immediate results, but as a general rule clinical skills, especially visual recognition, are perhaps of greater importance than in any other branch of general medicine.

DIASCOPY

In diascopy a glass slide is pressed firmly on the skin lesion. If a red lesion blanches, it implies that the red colour is secondary to blood within the vessels. By contrast, blood outside the vessels, such as that from a bruise or from vasculitis, will not blanch. In some vascular lesions with a convoluted vessel structure, however, blunt pressure from a flat surface will not empty the vessels and the corner of a glass slide needs to be gently placed on the lesion. Even then, it will not always blanch completely. Therefore, success in blanching is a more useful physical sign than failure to blanch. When pressed on to some granulomatous lesions a glass slide reveals an appearance commonly referred to as 'apple jelly nodule'.

EPILUMINESCENCE MICROSCOPY (DERMATOSCOPY, DERMOSCOPY)

This refers to surface microscopy using an illuminated lens with oil immersion directly on to the skin's surface. The presence of oil reduces specular reflection and reduces 'errors' due to the different refractive indexes of the various superficial layers of skin. A number of patterns not visible to the naked eye are often revealed. Many believe that in experienced hands it can usefully increase the diagnostic assessment of pigmented lesions such as melanoma. Similar, but perhaps lesser, optical enhancement can be obtained with no-touch devices using polarised light.

WOOD'S LIGHT

This involves irradiation with a UV light source that causes normal skin, particularly dermis, to fluoresce (in the visible light range). Green fluorescence is seen in scalp ringworm due to *Microsporum canis*, a sporadic ectothrix infection. It evokes coral pink fluorescence of flexural skin in erythrasma, caused by the bacterium *Corynebacterium minutissimum*. Wood's light also enhances the examination of cutaneous pigmentary abnormalities such as in patients with vitiligo, where areas of subtle depigmentation are more easily seen. The basis for this is that in the ultraviolet A wavebands used by Wood's light, pigmentation has a greater degree of absorption than at longer wavebands, resulting in a greater degree of difference in fluorescence between pigmented and depigmented skin.

MYCOLOGY SAMPLES

Cutaneous scale, nail clippings and plucked hairs can be examined by light microscopy when mounted in 20% potassium hydroxide. The keratin is dissolved, allowing

27

fungal hyphae to be identified. If the potassium hydroxide solution contains Indian ink, the typical 'spaghetti and meatballs' hyphae and spores of the yeast *Pityrosporum orbiculare* can be readily identified in pityriasis versicolor. In addition, samples are sent for identification by culture. This technique requires expertise if false positives are to be avoided.

SWABS

Bacterial swabs

Bacterial swabs taken in an appropriate culture medium are sometimes useful. Some caveats do, however, remain. Organisms that grow on the swabs may not be causally implicated in the underlying disease and the growth of many organisms simply reflects the abnormal architecture of the skin and is not necessarily an indication for either systemic or even local antibacterial therapy. Conversely, in some obvious infections of the skin, such as cellulitis, swabs do not reveal the causative agent. If pustules are present, a pustule should be punctured with a fine sterile needle and the pus exuded gently onto a swab.

Viral swabs

Blister or vesicle samples for herpes simplex and varicella zoster can be visualised within a few hours, either by electron microscopy or by indirect immunofluorescence. Samples are also cultured for identification when conserved in viral culture medium.

PRICK TESTS

Prick tests are a way of detecting cutaneous type I (immediate) hypersensitivity to various antigens such as pollen, house dust mite or dander. The skin is pricked with commercially available stylets through a dilution of the appropriate antigen solution. After 10 minutes a positive response is indicated by a weal and a flare. The weal is due to a local increase in capillary permeability and the flare a result of activation of the axon reflex. A positive control (histamine) and a negative control (antigen diluent) should be performed. Systemic antihistamines inhibit the magnitude of the reaction. In individuals with a clear history of particular type I hypersensitivity a systemic reaction may follow a prick test and resuscitation facilities should be available. As an alternative, specific IgE levels to antigens can be measured in serum by a specific radioallergosorbent test (RAST).

PATCH TESTS

Patch tests detect type IV (delayed or cell-mediated) hypersensitivity. It is common practice for a 'battery' of around 20 common antigens, including common sensitisers such as nickel, rubber and fragrance mix, to be applied to the skin of the back under aluminium discs for 48 hours. The sites are then examined for a positive reaction 24 hours later and possibly again a further 24 hours later. An eczematous reaction, in the absence of an irritant reaction, suggests a type IV hypersensitivity to that particular allergen. The relevant antigens for a particular clinical case may not be represented in the standard battery of tests and expert advice may be needed. A negative patch test does not exclude a pathogenic role for a particular antigen nor does the presence of a particular response to an antigen mean that this antigen is causing the clinical disease.

HISTOLOGY

Skin biopsies for routine histological examination are usually fixed in 10% formalin and stained with haematoxylin and eosin. Immunocytochemistry may also be performed on formalin-fixed sections but may require frozen sections (see below). Immunocytochemistry is particularly useful for tumour diagnosis.

IMMUNOFLUORESCENCE

A portion of the skin biopsy can be frozen in liquid nitrogen for direct immunofluorescence (IF). This involves visualising antigens that are present in skin by identifying them with fluorescein-labelled antibodies. Similarly, indirect immunofluorescence can identify circulating antibodies in the serum by an additional step of adding the serum to a section of normal skin or other substrate. Immunofluorescence plays a major role in the diagnosis of the autoimmune bullous disorders.

ELECTRON MICROSCOPY

This investigation has played an important role in the diagnosis of some of the rare blistering disorders such as epidermolysis bullosa, although the availability of a range of antibodies to basement membrane zone antigens has in part replaced it.

PHOTOTESTING

Phototesting involves exposing skin (often on the back) to a graded series of doses of ultraviolet radiation (UVR) of known wavelength, either on one occasion or repeatedly. In many photodermatoses erythema will occur at a lower dose of UVR than occurs in the normal population (e.g. drug-induced photosensitivity), or the time course of erythema may be prolonged (as in xeroderma pigmentosum). Alternatively, UVR will provoke lesions with the morphology of the underlying photodermatosis, such as may occur in lupus erythematosus or solar urticaria. Diagnostic phototesting is an essential component of the investigation of patients with presumed photosensitive drug reactions and idiopathic photodermatoses such as solar urticaria.

PRESENTING PROBLEMS IN SKIN DISEASE

THE CHANGING MOLE

The largest change in dermatological practice in developed countries over the last 30 years has been the major increase in patients referred or requesting advice about particular lesions ('is it cancer, doctor?') as compared with rashes.

Thirty years ago perhaps 90% of dermatology outpatients had rashes and 10% lesions whereas now the proportion of lesions often exceeds 50%. This reflects the fact that human skin cancer becomes more common as people grow older, that there is an increase in the elderly in many societies, and that there is an increase in the age-specific incidence rates for most skin cancers. Furthermore, there is greatly increased public awareness and concern about skin cancer, often in response to 'health campaigns'.

The principal clinical concern is to distinguish correctly between benign pigmented lesions and melanoma. Melanoma in most of Western Europe remains an uncommon tumour with a cumulative lifetime incidence of less than 1%. The case fatality is around 20% and has lowered over the years but there is still no curative therapy if the primary tumour has metastasised. Metastasis occurs early in the development of melanoma, and therefore in the absence of effective therapies attention has naturally focused on primary prevention and recognition of lesions early in their natural history. Far more early or thin melanomas are now diagnosed than was the case 30 or 40 years ago, reflecting increased awareness and the greater provision of medical services. The downside of this increased awareness is greater patient anxiety and a negative impact on other services provided by dermatologists. These themes are common to other debates about screening and early detection of disease.

The situation is complicated by the fact that whilst any one of a number of changes in a pigmented lesion (Box 27.4) is highly sensitive as a marker of melanoma, specificity is low. Even in the hands of experts, diagnostic certainty is low for many pigmented lesions in the absence of a biopsy. As excision of suspicious lesions is relatively easy, any screening test or screening procedure will require high levels of negative predictive value before it can be adopted in routine clinical practice. For the present there is no evidence from randomised controlled trials to suggest that population screening for melanoma in northern Europe is indicated.

History

- Determine the precise nature of the change (p. 1302). Is it due to the development of itch, inflammation, bleeding or ulceration, or does it relate to the colour, size, shape or surface of the lesion?
- Subtle changes should not be ignored, as many patients are good observers and get to know their own moles well. If the change has settled, could it have been due to a common insult such as nicking a facial naevus when shaving, plucking hairs from a naevus or the irritant effect of a depilatory?
- Is the patient worried about change in one or many moles? A patient's concern about many moles is, paradoxically, a reassuring feature, as presentation with multiple melanoma is extremely unusual, and it is more likely that the patient is anxious without need, or that he or she has constitutionally unusual but benign naevi.
- Is there a positive family history of melanoma? Fewer than 10% of melanomas occur in individuals with a strong family history but in some of these families the history of melanoma is quite striking, with up to 50% of individuals developing melanoma. A suspicious mole on a patient with a first-degree relative with melanoma probably warrants excision or specialist opinion.

Examination

Examine the pigmented lesion carefully. Look at the morphology of the melanocytic naevi at other sites. Examination with a magnifying glass or dermatoscope may help. Usually the key clinical question is whether the lesion is a benign melanocytic naevus (p. 1301) or a malignant melanoma (p. 1305). Before trying to answer this, the clinician needs to exclude the possibility that it is another type of pigmented lesion:

- *Lentigo* (a benign proliferation of melanocytes, p. 1281).
- *Freckle* (ephelis, a focal overproduction of melanin, p. 1280).
- *Seborrhoeic wart* (basal cell papilloma, a benign keratinocyte tumour, p. 1302).
- *Dermatofibroma*. This lightly pigmented firm dermal nodule is common on extremities in young adults. It feels larger than it looks. There is dimpling when the skin is squeezed on both sides (positive Fitzpatrick sign).
- *Pigmented basal cell carcinoma* (p. 1304). This lesion is usually found on the face of the elderly and is slow-growing. It has a blue-brown hue with an opalescent look. There may be a rolled edge around an ulcer.
- *Subungual haematoma* (Fig. 27.17, p. 1282).

Melanocytic naevus versus malignant melanoma

The ABCDE 'rule' (Box 27.4) is better viewed as a guide and reminder of what to consider (Fig. 27.3). Loss of normal skin markings is not diagnostic but is suggestive of melanoma. Conversely, normal skin markings and the presence of fine hairs dispersed evenly over a lesion, although reassuring, are not certain signs of a lesion's benign nature.

Does the patient have other pigmented lesions?

Ask, and examine the patient fully. Some patients (rarely) present with more than one primary melanoma but more importantly the morphology of the other melanocytic naevi may provide useful diagnostic information about the patient's 'constitutional' mole type. Remember that seborrhoeic warts are usually multiple. If a naevus, especially a changing one, appears significantly different (in colour, shape, size etc.) from others, then it should be treated with suspicion. It is more important at this stage to rule in than rule out.

27.4 ABCDE FEATURES OF MALIGNANT MELANOMA

- **A**symmetry
- **B**order irregular
- **C**olour irregular
- **D**iameter often greater than 0.5 cm
- **E**levation irregular
  (+ Loss of skin markings)

27

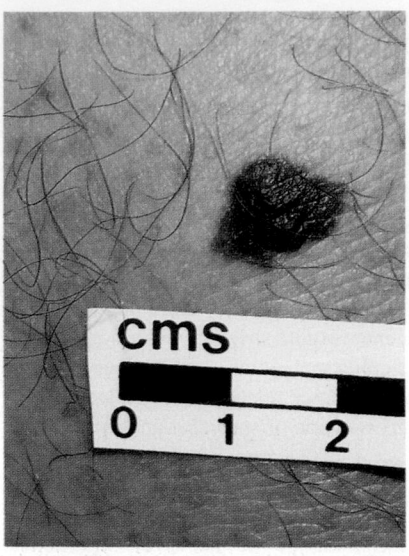

Fig. 27.3 Malignant melanoma. A changing mole which fails the ABCDE test.

Management

- Any changing lesion which is suspected of being a malignant melanoma should be excised without delay, with a clear margin. Depending on the thickness of the tumour further excision may be required.
- Some authors argue that if the diagnosis is uncertain and the degree of suspicion low the patient should be reviewed, or the individual lesion photographed and the patient reviewed in a couple of months and rephotographed. Not all would agree with this management plan, given that melanomas may show only slow or intermittent progression in their early course. A 'wait and see' policy is not anxiety-free.
- Malignant melanoma can break most rules. Listen, look and think. If in doubt, cut out and then check the histology, or seek advice urgently from more experienced colleagues.

ITCH (PRURITUS)

Pruritus is defined as an unpleasant sensation that provokes the desire to scratch. Despite being the major symptom of skin disease apart from disturbance of body image, it remains poorly studied and poorly understood. Although central nervous system lesions can cause itch, the majority of patients seen in dermatological clinical practice itch due to a primary disease of the skin (patients with itch due to liver disease may itch as a result of circulating factors acting on the central nervous system).

The nerve endings that signal itch lie either within the epidermis or very close to the dermo-epidermal junction. Such sensory information is transmitted via C fibres, which have slow conduction speeds via the spinothalamic tract to the thalamus and on to a cortical representation. It was thought for a long time that itch was conducted along the same fibres that conduct pain and may have been a subliminal form of pain. This hypothesis is now known to be wrong as fibres that can conduct the itch sensation, distinct from those that carry pain, have recently been identified. There does, however, seem to be an antagonistic or inhibitory relation between pain and itch. Scratching may either cause inhibition of the itch receptors by stimulating ascending sensory pathways which inhibit itch at the spinal cord (Wall's 'gate' mechanism), or interfere with itch fibres lying superficially in skin which may be damaged directly by scratching. In the presence of a focal lesion giving rise to itch, touch on the surrounding areas may be conducted along non-itch fibres but be centrally reinterpreted as itch (this phenomenon is known as 'alloknesis' and is analogous to allodynia for pain).

As well as primary diseases of the skin, itch may be a result of various systemic diseases such as primary biliary cirrhosis or renal failure. The mechanisms of induction of itch in these cases are unknown but for liver disease there is good experimental evidence that abnormal circulating opioids stimulate itch centrally.

History

Assessment of the itchy patient, particularly in the absence of widespread skin damage secondary to scratching, is one of the most difficult clinical problems in dermatology. Helpful hints from the history include:

- *The time course* of the itching. This should be carefully defined as sudden, as in infestations and urticaria, or chronic, as in chronic skin diseases such as eczema.
- *Localisation* of the pruritus, including the site of onset. For example, in an infant with atopic eczema the cheeks are usually the first site to be affected, whereas scabies almost never affects the face or scalp. Is the itch confined to certain sites, as in localised skin disease such as lichen planus and lichen simplex, or generalised, as in eczema and scabies?
- *Exacerbating factors*. Most causes of itch are increased by heating and reduced by cooling; however, in some conditions the response is more informative. In cholinergic urticaria, exercise or heat dramatically induces itching (and weals on the skin surface); in aquagenic pruritus and aquagenic urticaria, water induces itch and weals respectively. In cold urticaria, cold stimuli such as ice or very cold air may induce weals and itch directly.
- *Alleviating factors*, which are worth noting but are seldom of great diagnostic help. Some patients discover that cooling below 18°C inhibits itch (but not pain). Similarly, other patients discover that a scalding hot bath replaces itch with pain which they find preferable. In the short term most patients seem to prefer cutaneous pain to itch.
- *Involvement of other family members*, as in a scabietic infestation. Insect bites usually affect only one member of the family.
- *General health* of the patient. Has there been a major change such as marked weight loss or lymphadenopathy suggesting lymphoma?

Examination

Attempt to determine whether there is a primary skin condition or whether the only visible clinical features are

27.5 PRURITUS

Skin diseases associated with generalised pruritus

- Eczema
- Scabies
- Urticaria/dermographism
- Pruritus of old age and xeroderma

Skin diseases associated with localised pruritus

- Eczema
- Lichen planus
- Dermatitis herpetiformis
- Pediculosis

Pruritus with no evidence of skin disease (Box 27.7 overleaf)

due to excoriation with some secondary degree of eczema or infection. Try to classify the patient into one of the following groups (Box 27.5):

- *Generalised pruritus associated with skin disease.* The most common causes of a widespread itchy rash are eczema, usually atopic, and scabies infestation. These can be difficult to distinguish clinically, particularly in children. Secondary eczematisation occurs in scabies, giving rise to eczema-like lesions all over the body. Examine carefully for scabietic burrows, particularly in the finger and toe webs, along the borders of both the hands and the feet and at the wrists, and extract the mite (p. 1297) to make a definite diagnosis. After treatment pruritus may continue for several weeks. Pruritus is a common skin complaint in pregnancy and may be due to several causes (Box 27.6).
- *Local pruritus associated with skin disease.* In these cases careful examination may reveal the underlying primary cutaneous disorder such as lichen planus or psoriasis.
- *Pruritus with no evidence of skin disease.* The medical conditions that are sometimes associated with pruritus are listed in Box 27.7 overleaf. In the absence of clues pointing to a primary skin disease, detailed physical examination and investigations, including a careful search for lymphadenopathy, may be required. Investigations should include a full blood count, iron status, urea and electrolytes, liver function tests, thyroid function and possibly a chest X-ray.

Many patients are incorrectly labelled as having itch due to a systemic cause when in reality they have a mild degree of xerosis with perhaps irritation from repeated use of soaps, or another cutaneous primary disorder such as dermographism or aquagenic pruritus.

Management

There are no specific anti-itch drugs. Effective remedies for the conditions that lead to itch do exist, however, and include potent H_1 blockade for patients with chronic idiopathic urticaria or corticosteroids for individuals with atopic eczema. Nevertheless, in some instances it is not possible either to define the primary condition or to treat it effectively.

A large number of agents can be used to reduce pruritus including emollients, topical menthol, capsaicin, ultraviolet B and long-wavelength ultraviolet A (PUVA) phototherapy (p. 1291), as well as opioid antagonists such as naltrexone. Their effects are variable, poorly characterised and require further study. Although frequently the subject of ridicule, significant itch may incapacitate, cause embarrassment, disrupt sleep and ruin the patient's self-image. It is easily underestimated and trivialised as a symptom.

THE SCALY RASH (PAPULOSQUAMOUS ERUPTIONS)

A common presenting complaint in general practice is an eruptive scaly rash sometimes associated with itching. The main causes are listed in Box 27.8. These can usually be distinguished by a discriminating history and examination.

History

How long has the rash been present?

Atopic eczema often starts within the first 2 years of life and subsequently fluctuates in extent and severity. Psoriasis can start at any age but usually does so between the ages of 15 and 40 years. Pityriasis rosea affects a similar age group and tends to occur in the autumn and spring. Both pityriasis

27.6 CAUSES OF PRURITUS IN PREGNANCY

Condition	Gestation and features	Treatment
Obstetric cholestasis	3rd trimester. Associated with abnormal liver function tests	Emollients. Chlorphenamine. Colestyramine. Early delivery
Pemphigoid gestationis	3rd trimester. Pruritus followed by blistering. Starts around the umbilicus	Topical or oral corticosteroids
Polymorphic eruption (urticarial papules) of pregnancy	3rd trimester, after delivery. Polymorphic lesions with urticaria	Chlorphenamine
Prurigo gestationis	2nd trimester. Excoriated papules	Emollients. Topical corticosteroids. Chlorphenamine
Pruritic folliculitis	3rd trimester. Aseptic pustules on trunk	Topical corticosteroids

27.7 MEDICAL CONDITIONS THAT CAUSE PRURITUS

Medical condition	Cause of pruritus	Treatment*
Liver disease	A central opioid effect seems to be important in some liver diseases, although other factors such as elevation in bile salts may contribute	Naltrexone Colestyramine Rifampicin Sedative antihistamines UVB
Renal disease	The mechanism of itch in renal failure (including secondary hyperparathyroidism) is unknown. It is unlikely to involve histamine	Oral activated charcoal
Blood disease Anaemia Polycythaemia rubra vera Lymphoma Leukaemia Myeloma	Iron deficiency Unknown Unknown	Iron replacement
Thyroid disease Thyrotoxicosis Hypothyroidism	Generalised due to dry skin Localised may be due to *Candida*	Emollients
HIV infection	Infection, infestation Eosinophilic folliculitis Unknown	Treatment of opportunistic infection Local corticosteroids, UVB UVB
Malignancy	Unknown	
Psychogenic	Unknown	Psychotherapy Anxiolytics Antidepressives

* Added to that of primary condition.

27.8 SUDDEN SCALY RASHES

- Eczema (p. 1283)
- Psoriasis (p. 1287)
- Pityriasis rosea
- Lichen planus (p. 1292)
- Drug eruption (p. 1310)
- Pityriasis versicolor
- Tinea corporis

rosea and drug eruptions have an acute onset, drug eruptions starting within a few days or weeks of taking the drugs. Pityriasis versicolor is a common yeast infection of the body and scalp. It can be acute in onset or persist for many years in the same individual.

Where on the body did it start?

Atopic eczema starts most commonly on the face in infants and then spreads to involve the flexures. However, it can sometimes just affect the extensor surfaces or may be present in coin-like lesions (discoid eczema). Psoriasis is classically present on the extensor surfaces—that is, the elbows and knees. Psoriasis can appear anywhere on the body in small (guttate), medium and large plaques all over the torso and limbs. Lichen planus usually presents as an intensely itchy, localised papular eruption with a characteristic colour and morphology (p. 1292). Less commonly, it can be widespread and often exhibits the Köbner phenomenon, with lichen planus lesions being induced in sites of non-specific trauma (Fig. 27.27, p. 1292). Pityriasis rosea starts as a single herald patch that can occur anywhere on the body but usually is present on the trunk. This is a solitary erythematous lesion which starts as a papule and enlarges rapidly over a few days. Pityriasis versicolor usually affects the trunk and outer upper arms. Tinea corporis (dermatophyte infection) can occur anywhere on the body and is usually asymmetrical.

How has the rash evolved?

In pityriasis rosea the herald patch is followed in a few days by the appearance of many smaller plaques. These are present mostly on the torso in a 'fir tree' distribution but can also occur on the neck, extremities and flexures (inverse pityriasis rosea). The herald patch tends to persist throughout the eruption and the whole eruption can last for up to 3 months. Atopic eczema can, at varying stages, be localised or generalised but is a chronic disorder that fluctuates in severity throughout childhood. Psoriasis in the classical form tends to involve the elbows, knees, lower back and scalp. In the guttate (small plaque) variety many small, red, scaly plaques appear on the trunk and may persist for several months. Many cases subsequently develop chronic plaque psoriasis. Tinea corporis is usually a chronic, slowly evolving, often isolated annular lesion. Maculopapular drug eruptions evolve with exfoliation ('peeling' of the skin) and may leave post-inflammatory hyperpigmentation. Pityriasis versicolor can be very chronic and is often exacerbated by sun exposure; it also becomes more obvious in the tanned individual because of its hypopigmentation and therefore patients often present after their summer holidays. On the other hand, it appears as light brown scaly patches on untanned Caucasoid skin.

Is it itchy?

Atopic eczema is extremely itchy and this is invariably the presenting complaint. Itching is exacerbated by changes in temperature, e.g. on undressing, and contact with irritants such as wool. It is not known why atopic eczema is so itchy, and non-sedative antihistamines have little if any effect. Drug eruptions and tinea corporis are usually pruritic. Psoriasis and pityriasis rosea are not usually intensely itchy but exceptions occur. The rash of pityriasis versicolor is asymptomatic.

Was there a preceding illness?

Guttate psoriasis is often preceded by a β-haemolytic streptococcal sore throat. A small percentage of people with pityriasis rosea have a prodromal illness with malaise, headache and arthralgia. A patient who develops a morbilli-form drug eruption will usually have the same reaction to that specific drug or to chemically related ones on each challenge. Rashes in response to drugs are not common; however, most patients with infectious mononucleosis treated with amoxicillin will develop an erythematous maculo-papular rash. It is essential therefore to take a careful history of medications and preceding illnesses at least 4 weeks prior to the onset of the rash.

Is it associated with any systemic symptoms?

Certain drug eruptions can cause systemic upset with fever, malaise and joint pains and are associated with an eosino-philia. In eczema, superinfection can be associated with systemic symptoms of fever and malaise. *Staphylococcus aureus* causing secondary impetiginisation is the most common, but a streptococcus can cause similar features. Herpes simplex virus type 1 causes a widespread, severe, painful, erosive skin eruption in patients with atopic eczema (eczema herpeticum, p. 1284), which is a medical emergency requiring inpatient treatment with intravenous antiviral therapy and medical support. Arthritis occurs in 7% of patients with psoriasis (p. 1109).

Examination

The distribution of the rash can be very useful in dis-criminating between the various causes of a scaly rash: flexural, extensor surfaces, truncal, palms and soles, or scalp involvement. Morphologically, these conditions are distinguishable by careful assessment with the use of a magnifying lens. Associated skin features that give useful diagnostic clues can be found by complete skin examination (Box 27.9).

ERYTHRODERMA

Eczema, psoriasis, drug eruptions and lichen planus rarely progress to erythroderma, defined as erythema with or without scaling of almost all the body surface. In dark skin, the presence of pigmentation may mask the erythema, giving a purplish hue. Other causes include cutaneous T-cell lymphoma (Sézary's syndrome), the psoriasis-like condition pityriasis rubra pilaris, and rare types of ichthyosis. Erythro-derma may occur at any age and is associated with extreme morbidity and rarely mortality. It may appear suddenly or evolve slowly.

Erythrodermic patients, especially the elderly (Box 27.31, p. 1293), may be systemically unwell with shivering and hypothermia, secondary to the excess and uncontrolled heat loss due to the increased blood flow to their skin, but they may also be pyrexial, and suffer from an impaired ability to lose heat due to damage to sweat gland function and sweat duct occlusion. The pulse rate may be elevated and the blood pressure low due to volume depletion; examination of the cardiovascular system is therefore essential. Peripheral oedema is a common finding consequent on the erythroderma, low albumin and high-output cardiac failure. Lymph nodes may be enlarged, either reactively, secondary to skin inflam-mation, or rarely due to lymphomatous infiltration.

27

27.9 CLINICAL FEATURES OF COMMON SCALY RASHES			
Type of rash	**Distribution**	**Morphology**	**Associated clinical signs**
Eczema	Face/flexures	Poorly defined erythema and scaling Lichenification	Shiny nails Infraorbital crease 'Dirty neck'
Psoriasis	Extensor surfaces	Well-defined plaques with a silvery scale	Nail pitting and onycholysis Scalp involvement Axillae and genital areas often affected
Pityriasis rosea	'Fir tree' pattern on torso	Well-defined erythematous papules and plaques with collarette of scale	
Drug eruption	Widespread	Maculo-papular erythematous scaly areas which merge and are followed by exfoliation	
Pityriasis versicolor	Upper torso and upper shoulders	Hypo- and hyperpigmented scaly patches	
Lichen planus	Distal limbs, especially volar aspect of wrists Lower back	Shiny, flat-topped violaceous papules with Wickham's striae	White lacy network buccal mucosa Rarely, nail changes
Tinea corporis	Asymmetrical, often isolated, red scaly lesions	Scaly plaques which expand with central healing	Nail involvement (Fig. 27.19, p. 1283)

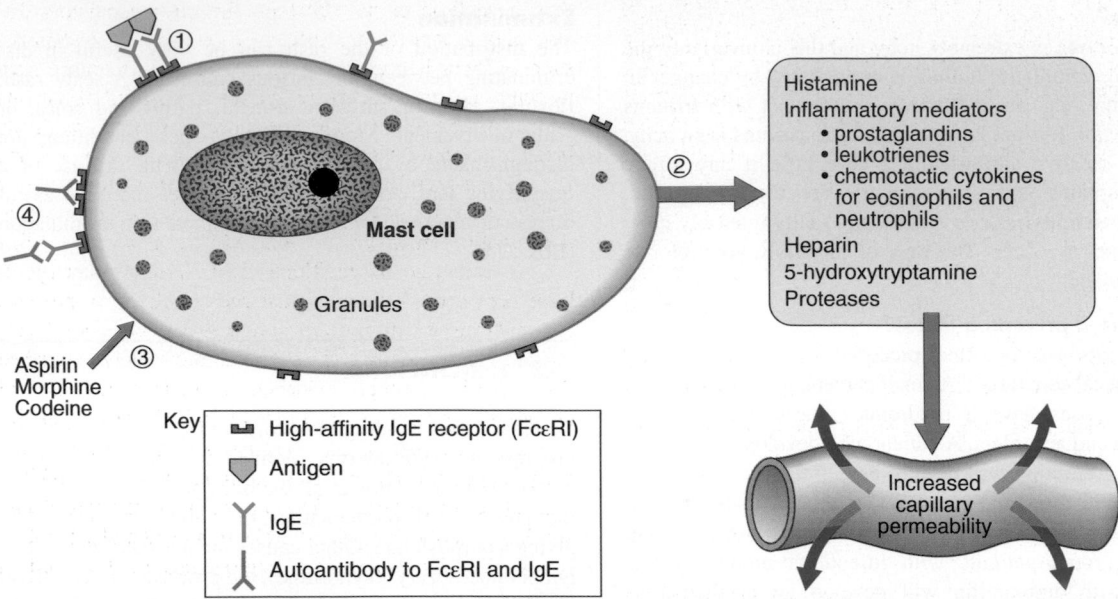

Fig. 27.4 Pathogenesis of urticaria. Mast cell degranulation occurs in a variety of ways. (1) Type I hypersensitivity causing massive degranulation and sometimes anaphylaxis. (2) Spontaneous mast cell degranulation in chronic urticaria. (3) Chemical mast cell degranulation. (4) Autoimmunity, which accounts for 30% of chronic urticaria.

URTICARIA (NETTLE RASH, HIVES)

Urticaria refers to an area of focal dermal oedema secondary to a transient increase in capillary permeability. On certain body sites such as the lips or hands the oedema spreads and is traditionally referred to as angioedema. By definition the swelling lasts less than 24 hours. Acute urticaria may be associated with angioedema of the lips, face, throat and, rarely, wheezing, abdominal pain, headaches and even anaphylaxis. Whilst severe angioedema can be life-threatening due to respiratory obstruction, this is exceedingly rare in a dermatological context.

The symptoms and signs of urticaria are due in large part to mast cell degranulation with release of histamine and a variety of other vasoactive mediators. That more than histamine is involved is reflected by the fact that potent histamine blockers, whilst frequently improving the itch of urticaria and the number of weals, do not abolish all the symptoms or signs in many patients (Fig. 27.4).

Causes of urticaria are listed in Box 27.10. Recently, an autoimmune pathogenesis for one of the most common forms of urticaria, chronic idiopathic urticaria, has been identified. In this condition, which is defined by the presence of urticarial episodes for over 6 weeks, self-reacting antibodies appear to cause cross-linking of the surface IgE receptor on mast cells with subsequent cellular degranulation.

Clinical assessment
Two questions may be asked:

- How long does the individual lesion last?
  < 24 hours   (urticaria)
  > 24 hours   (urticarial vasculitis)

27.10 CAUSES OF URTICARIA

Acute and chronic urticaria

- Autoimmune due to production of antibodies that cross-link the IgE receptor on mast cells
- Allergens (in foods, inhalants and injections)
- Drugs (Box 27.43, p. 1311)
- Contact (e.g. animal saliva, latex)
- Physical (e.g. heat, cold, pressure, sun, water)
- Infection (e.g. viral hepatitis, infectious mononucleosis, HIV infection during seroconversion)
- Other conditions (e.g. systemic lupus erythematosus, pregnancy, intestinal parasites)
- Idiopathic

Urticarial vasculitis

- Hepatitis B
- Systemic lupus erythematosus
- Idiopathic

- How long has the condition been present?
  < 6 weeks   (acute urticaria)
  > 6 weeks   (chronic urticaria)

In practice these questions may be less helpful than is sometimes implied as the time frames are somewhat arbitrary. There may be little mechanistic difference between urticaria of a month's duration and that of 6 months' duration and both may be treated along similar lines. The length of time an individual weal lasts may also be of limited utility. Urticarial vasculitis is much less common than urticaria and many patients are unable to distinguish the development of new weals and disappearance of old ones from individual weals, each of which persists for more than 1 day. It is sometimes helpful to draw around a weal

27

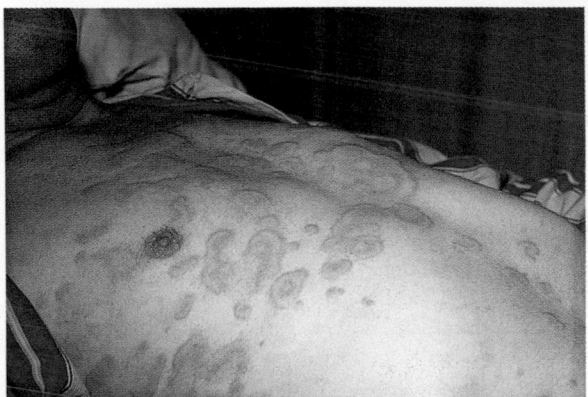

Fig. 27.5 Widespread acute urticaria. In this case urticaria was due to penicillin allergy.

with a pen and examine the patient 24 hours later to try to clarify this issue.

A directed history is still the best way to elicit any causes or precipitants of urticaria. A record of possible allergens, including drugs (Box 27.43, p. 1311), should be determined. The physical urticarias can be identified by appropriate questions (Box 27.10) and subsequent medically observed challenge. A family history must be sought in cases of angioedema. Examination may reveal nothing, as this is a transient eruption, or may uncover the classical weals, which can vary from papules to large extensive plaques (Fig. 27.5).

Investigations

These need to be directed at the possible underlying cause as elicited from the clinical history. Some or all of the following may be appropriate:

- full blood count including eosinophil count in cases of underlying parasites
- erythrocyte sedimentation rate (ESR), which is elevated in cases of vasculitis
- urea and electrolytes, thyroid and liver function tests, which might reveal an underlying disorder
- total IgE and specific IgE to possible allergens, e.g. foods such as shellfish and peanuts
- antinuclear factor in chronic urticaria or urticarial vasculitis
- CH50 as a general guide to complement activation and C_3 and C_4 levels as evidence of complement consumption via both the classical and the alternative pathways.

C_1 esterase inhibitor may be quantitatively reduced or more rarely functionally deficient as in hereditary angioedema. A skin biopsy may be helpful if urticarial vasculitis is suspected. Physical urticarias can be confirmed by the appropriate physical challenge. Frequently, no cause can be found for acute episodes, whereas in chronic urticaria the autoimmune pathogenesis will account for the majority of cases.

Management

The practical problem with management of urticaria is that whilst potent non-sedative histamine blockers are available they have little or no effect on the other mediators that also play a contributory role. Non-sedative antihistamines such as loratadine or fexofenadine, or antihistamines such as cetirizine, are effective for perhaps one-third of patients with chronic urticaria, and one-third show some moderate benefit, whilst the results in the remaining third are minimal. If a patient fails to respond to one of these agents after 2 weeks of therapy, then it may be worth changing to another non-sedative antihistamine and adding in an H_2-blocker such as cimetidine or ranitidine. A number of other agents have been used, including mast cell stabilisers or protease and leukotriene inhibitors, although the evidence of efficacy is not clear. Systemic corticosteroids are widely prescribed for urticaria although evidence of their benefit is still contestable. Patients with a history of life-threatening angioedema or anaphylaxis, as is seen in allergy to peanuts and wasp stings, should carry a self-administered injection kit of adrenaline (epinephrine). The management of anaphylactic shock is described on page 87. The treatment and prevention of acute attacks of hereditary angioedema are discussed on page 89.

Urticaria may be precipitated by aspirin or non-steroidal anti-inflammatory drugs (NSAIDs). If there is a clear history of these agents precipitating attacks, then they should be avoided. Even in the absence of a clear history it may be advisable to suggest alternatives such as paracetamol (remember that codeine and opioids can also induce urticaria).

PHOTOSENSITIVITY

Ultraviolet radiation (UVR, 'sunlight') may improve some skin diseases such as psoriasis and eczema but confusingly may also exacerbate the same diseases and induce a number of specific dermatological conditions—the photosensitive dermatoses or photodermatoses. Usually this is attributable to particular parts of the electromagnetic radiation spectrum, including ultraviolet B (UVB) and ultraviolet A (UVA), but rarely visible light may also cause some photodermatoses. The relevant electromagnetic spectrum is illustrated in Figure 27.6. The causative wavelengths for some of the endpoints are provisional. For instance, UVB is thought to play a more major role in the induction of non-melanoma skin cancer but a role for UVA may also (arguably) exist for melanoma. Similarly, skin ageing is due not just to UVA, as is often stated, but also, if not predominantly, UVB. Determination of the waveband or wavebands that contribute to sensitivity may be clinically important. For instance, UVB does not pass through window glass whereas UVA does. The practical corollary of this is that patients who are markedly UVA-sensitive need to wear sunblock and be protected even when in a car or inside a building where there is strong natural light. Some patients are even sensitive to visible light.

Clinical assessment

The clinical history may give a clear indication that the rash is temporally related to sun exposure, whereas in other cases there is no obvious indication of light aggravation.

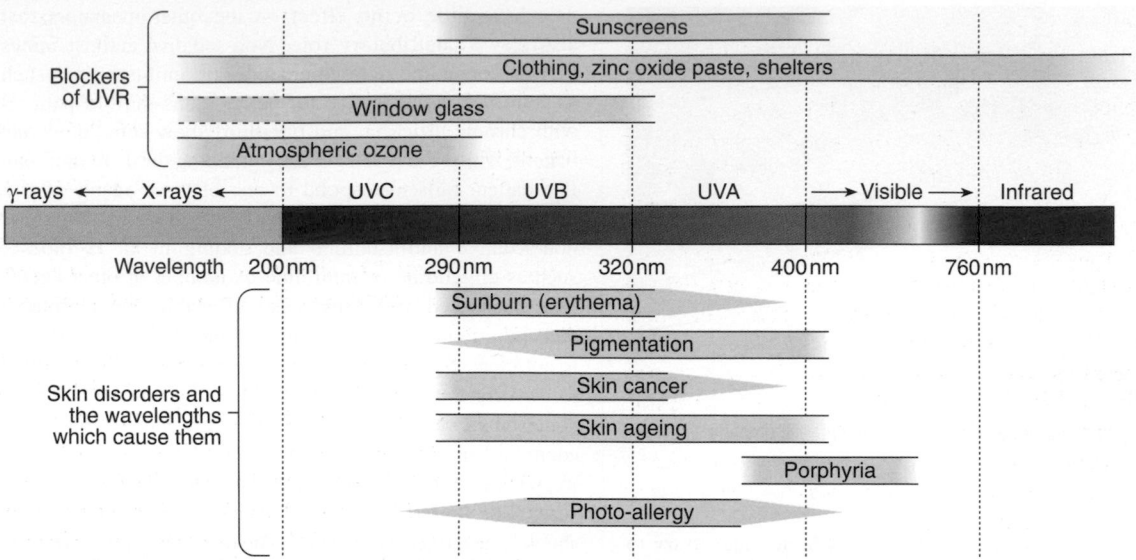

Fig. 27.6 The electromagnetic spectrum. For some conditions the action spectrum is approximate and may vary between patients (e.g. lupus erythematosus, polymorphic light eruption). The action spectrum for non-melanoma skin cancer mirrors that for erythema. The action spectrum for melanoma is not known but certainly involves UVB. (UVR = ultraviolet radiation)

When a rash is related to sunshine, the sites affected tend to be those with maximum exposure to sunshine: the face, the nose and the cheeks but excluding the eyelids, an area under the chin and an area in the shadow of the nose, the dorsa of the forearms and hands, but with sparing of the finger webs and palms (Fig. 27.7). Sometimes however, and making diagnosis difficult, the areas of maximal exposure to natural UVR are relatively spared (such as the face in polymorphic light eruption), and conversely the rash may appear on relatively protected sites such as the back and chest which are often covered by clothes.

There are four main groups of photosensitive dermatoses and these are listed in Box 27.11. A photodermatosis that initially appears on some exposed sites may spread to sites which on history appear to have received minimal exposure to sunlight.

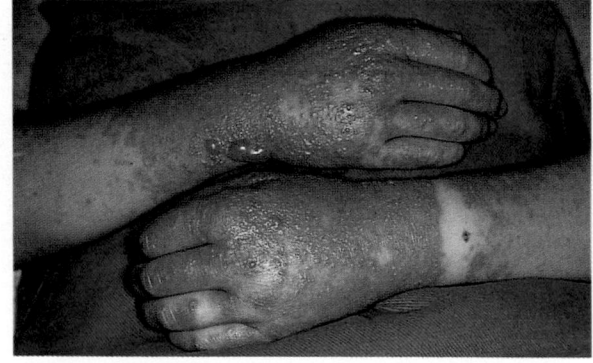

Fig. 27.7 Bullous photosensitive eruption. Note sharp cut-off at wrists, due to protection by shirt sleeves, and sparing of skin under watch and strap.

27.11 THE PHOTOSENSITIVE DERMATOSES		
Cause	**Condition**	**Clinical features**
Drugs	Phototoxic drug eruption	Common; exaggerated sunburn occurs minutes after sun exposure Caused by phenothiazines, amiodarone, tetracyclines
	Photo-allergic drug eruption	Occurs more than 24 hours after sun exposure; causes a dermatitis or lichen planus-like reaction Caused by thiazides, enalapril, hydroxychloroquine, phenothiazines or topical photosensitisers, e.g. fragrances Can become permanent (persistent light reactor)
Metabolic	Porphyrias	Particularly porphyria cutanea tarda (pp. 451 and 1308)
	Pellagra	Diarrhoea, dementia, dermatitis due to dietary lack of tryptophan (Fig. 16.17, p. 452)
Exacerbation of pre-existing conditions	Lupus erythematosus	Page 1132
	Erythema multiforme	Page 1308
	Herpes simplex	Page 303
Idiopathic	Polymorphic light eruption	Itchy papulo-vesicular eruption on exposed sites within hours of UV exposure
	Solar urticaria	Urticaria after 1-hour exposure
	Chronic actinic dermatitis	Disabling, itchy dermatitis on exposed sites in elderly men

Management

Once a photosensitive eruption is identified on clinical grounds, an attempt should be made to provoke the lesion using phototesting. This may not always be possible. If a drug is suspected and clinical status allows, do not stop the drug but phototest the individual as soon as possible. If the test is abnormal, repeat the phototesting after the drug has been discontinued. Drug causes for photosensitivity, especially in the elderly, are common and include compounds such as quinine, which are often neglected unless a careful and directed clinical history is taken. Treatment consists of avoidance of the drug if appropriate, or topical or occasionally systemic corticosteroids. In chronic cases of photosensitivity, such as chronic actinic dermatitis, azathioprine 100–150 mg/day may be required as further immunosuppression. The main preventative treatment for the photosensitive dermatoses is avoidance of sun exposure and the use of sunscreens.

Sunscreens

Sunscreens act in two different ways: chemical or physical. Chemical sunscreens absorb specific wavelengths of UV radiation. Physical sunscreens reflect UV radiation and visible light. Most available products are a combination of UVA and UVB chemical sunscreens. If the individual is sensitive to visible light as well as UVR, then the agents that block visible light will be visible and have limited cosmetic acceptability.

Sunblocks are often graded in terms of the sun protection factor (SPF), the ratio of the time it takes to induce a certain degree of redness with and without sunblock. A sunblock with an SPF of 2 therefore affords 50% reduction whereas a sun protection factor of 10 blocks 90% of the radiation. It follows that the additional value of sunblocks with a very high sun protection factor becomes trivial over, say, SPF 15.

BLISTERS

Loss of keratinocyte–keratinocyte adhesion or loss of adhesion of keratinocytes to the basement membrane or of the basement membrane to the dermis leads to a potential space which, because of negative extracellular pressure, fills with fluid: a blister. There is an artificial distinction made by some between small (vesicles, < 0.5 cm) and large blisters (bullae, > 0.5 cm). The site of blister formation within the skin therefore depends on the aetiology and underlying pathogenesis.

Blisters are an important physical sign with a limited differential diagnosis but they can be very difficult to see. If a blister occurs high up in the epidermis (intra-epidermal) and is due to a defect in cohesion of the keratinocytes, then the blister may be so fragile that only an erosion is seen (e.g. pemphigus foliaceus). On the other hand, a blister at the level of the basement membrane, as occurs in dermatitis herpetiformis, might be missed because the roof of the blister is easily destroyed due to the itch and resulting scratch. Blisters in the skin can occur at any age and may be caused by common infections or rare genetic skin diseases that can continue throughout life. The main causes of blistering presenting at birth are listed in Box 27.12.

27.12 CAUSES OF BLISTERING AT BIRTH
• Herpes simplex • Impetigo • Bullous ichthyosis • Epidermolysis bullosa (Box 27.13) • Incontinentia pigmenti

27

27.13 DIFFERENT TYPES OF EPIDERMOLYSIS BULLOSA				
Type	**Mode of inheritance**	**Level of blister protein**	**Abnormal**	**Clinical features**
Simple	Autosomal dominant	Epidermal basal cell	Keratins 5 and 14	Usually just blisters on palms and soles No scarring; nails normal; no oral involvement Rare recessive type associated with muscular dystrophy (plectin mutation)
Junctional	Autosomal recessive	Lamina lucida	Laminin-5 and $\alpha_6 \beta_4$ integrin	Large, raw areas and flaccid blisters at birth Common around mouth and anus; heal slowly Nails and oral mucosa involved Often lethal May be diagnosed prenatally by chorionic villus sampling
Dystrophic	Autosomal dominant	Dermis below lamina densa	Collagen VII	Blisters on knees, elbows and fingers Healing with scarring and milia Nails may be involved Mouth seldom affected
	Autosomal recessive	Dermis below lamina densa	Collagen VII	Blisters often present at birth; seen on hands, feet, elbows and knees Heal with scarring which is so severe that digits may be lost Milia present Oral and oesophageal blistering followed by scarring/stricture Abnormal teeth Increased incidence of cutaneous squamous cell carcinoma in early adulthood

27.14 CAUSES OF ACQUIRED BLISTERS

	Localised	Generalised	
		With mucosal involvement	With no mucosal involvement
Vesicular	Herpes simplex Herpes zoster Impetigo Pompholyx	Eczema herpeticum	Eczema herpeticum Dermatitis herpetiformis Epidermolysis bullosa acquisita
Bullous	Impetigo Bullous cellulitis Bullous stasis oedema Acute eczema Insect bites Fixed drug eruptions	Pemphigus Bullous erythema multiforme/ Stevens–Johnson syndrome Toxic epidermal necrolysis Epidermolysis bullosa acquisita	Acute eczema Erythema multiforme Bullous pemphigoid Epidermolysis bullosa acquisita Bullous lupus erythematosus Pseudoporphyria Porphyria cutanea tarda Drug eruptions, e.g. barbiturates

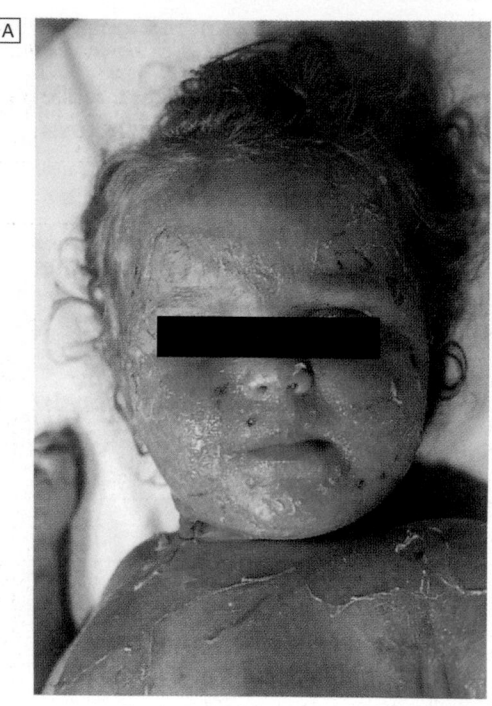

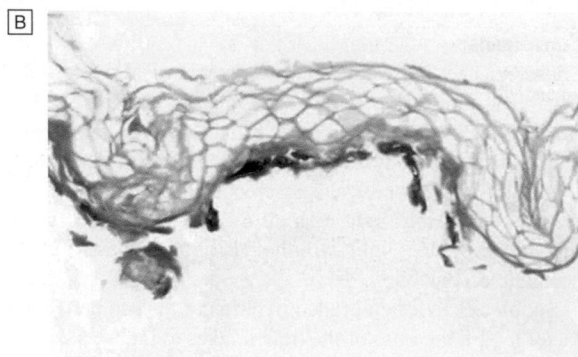

Fig. 27.8 Acute blistering eruptions in a child. A Staphylococcal scalded skin syndrome (SSSS) in a child. B The condition was rapidly diagnosed by examination of a frozen section of skin snip (see text).

Clinical assessment

The history of the onset of blistering, any predisposing events such as drug ingestion, and family history are of paramount importance. In infants, blistering at birth is usually due to infection and more rarely to genetic skin diseases such as epidermolysis bullosa. There are several types of epidermolysis bullosa, as seen in Box 27.13, and studies of these disorders over the last 10 years have contributed enormously to our understanding of the biology of keratins and basement membrane. Infection with staphylococcus in the young can cause staphylococcal scalded skin syndrome (SSSS) (Fig. 27.8 and p. 1294). Diagnosis is easily made by taking a snip of the peeling skin (stratum corneum, 'skin snip') and examining by frozen section. Adults who present with a blistering skin condition need to be assessed according to Box 27.14. At all ages, it

is important to exclude both viral and bacterial infection as a cause of blistering and this is easily done by taking a swab from the blister fluid for bacterial assessment by both microscopy and culture. A similar sterile swab can be placed in viral culture medium and, in the case of the herpes virus, immediate electron microscopy or immunofluorescence performed on a sample of the blister fluid smeared on to a slide.

Toxic epidermal necrolysis (Fig. 27.9) is a severe form of widespread blistering that can occur at any age and is often due to drugs. It is a life-threatening condition as the skin peels off in thin sheets, causing severe problems with fluid balance and temperature control as well as pain and infection. Intensive care management is indicated, with careful haemodynamic monitoring and high suspicion of secondary infection. Once the causative agent is removed

27.15 CLINICAL FEATURES AND SKIN BIOPSY FINDINGS IN SOME IMMUNE-MEDIATED BLISTERING SKIN CONDITIONS

Disease	Age	Site of blisters	Nature of blisters	Mucous membrane involvement	Antigen	Circulating antibody (indirect IF)	Fixed antibody (direct IF)	Treatment
Pemphigus vulgaris	40–60 yrs	Torso, head	Flaccid and fragile, many erosions	100%	Desmoglein-3 (120 kD)	IgG	IgG, C₃ intercellular (epidermal)	Systemic corticosteroids Cyclophosphamide
Bullous pemphigoid (Fig. 27.10)	60s and over	Trunk (especially flexures) and limbs	Tense	Occasionally	BP-220 (part of hemi-desmosome)	IgG (70%)	IgG, C₃ at BMZ	Systemic corticosteroids Azathioprine
Dermatitis herpetiformis	Young, associated with coeliac disease	Elbows, lower back, buttocks	Excoriated and often not present	No	Unknown	None	Granular IgA in papillary dermis	Dapsone Gluten-free diet
Pemphigoid gestationis	Young pregnant female	Periumbilical and limbs	Tense	Rare	Collagen XVII (part of hemi-desmosome BP-180)	IgG	C₃ at BMZ	Systemic corticosteroids
Epidermolysis bullosa acquisita	All ages	Widespread	Tense, scarring	Common (50%)	Type VII collagen	IgG (anti-type VII collagen)	IgG at BMZ	Poor response to corticosteroids Cyclophosphamide Methotrexate Azathioprine
Bullous lupus erythematosus	Young, black female	Widespread	Tense	Rare	Type VII collagen	Anti-type VII collagen	IgG, IgA, IgM at BMZ	Dapsone

Note Pemphigus is characterised by an intra-epidermal level of blistering (superficial). All the other conditions above have a subepidermal level of blistering. (BMZ = basement membrane zone)

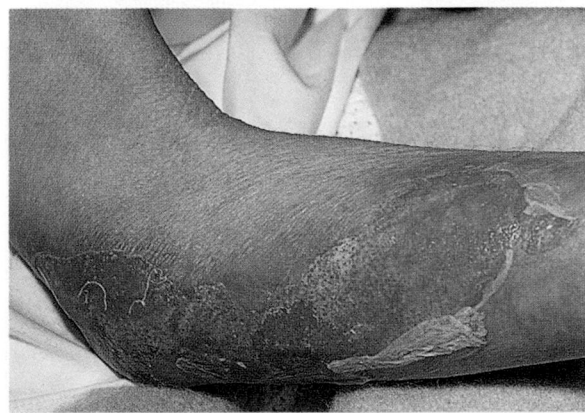

Fig. 27.9 Toxic epidermolytic necrolysis in an adult. Peeling of the skin involving the whole epidermis is usually secondary to a drug reaction.

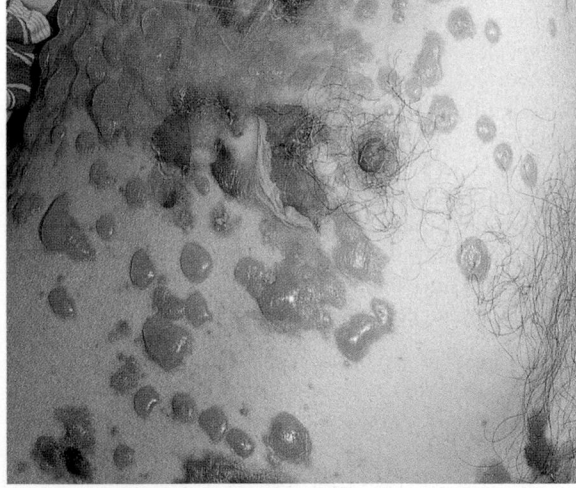

Fig. 27.10 Bullous pemphigoid. Large tense and unilocular blisters clustered in and around the axilla.

the skin can rapidly re-epithelialise but toxaemia often leads to death in extensive cases. There is no convincing evidence that systemic corticosteroids work in this condition, and some evidence that they may be harmful, but there is some recent, persuasive but uncontrolled evidence that intravenous immunoglobulin may be helpful.

If there is no evidence of infection and the diagnosis is not apparent from the more common conditions listed in Box 27.14, then a skin biopsy should be taken for histological assessment and a frozen sample for direct immuno-fluorescence. The clinical and immunopathological findings for the immunobullous disorders are documented in Box

27.15. In the case of the rare genetic skin diseases a portion of the skin biopsy is processed for electron microscopy and immunofluorescence and DNA analyses to enable a more accurate assessment to be made of the site of blistering and mode of inheritance. Further investigation is necessary for certain blistering conditions:

- *Pemphigus*. This is associated with underlying malignancy including lymphoma in a small proportion of patients ('paraneoplastic pemphigus'). Therefore a complete

27

physical examination is mandatory and investigations including full blood count, erythrocyte sedimentation rate, urea and electrolytes, liver function tests, chest X-ray and any other directed scans should be performed.

- *Dermatitis herpetiformis.* This is associated with coeliac disease (p. 894) and therefore all patients with this diagnosis should have blood taken for an anti-endomysial and antigliadin antibody screen, and a jejunal biopsy should be performed if indicated.
- *Epidermolysis bullosa acquisita (EBA).* This is associated with inflammatory bowel disease, multiple myeloma and lymphoma (pp. 910, 1052 and 1047), and these conditions should therefore be excluded.
- *Bullous lupus erythematosus.* It is important to follow patients with bullous lupus erythematosus for activity of their systemic disease (p. 1132). There is a high incidence of clinically significant glomerulonephritis (> 90%).
- *Porphyria cutanea tarda and pseudoporphyria* (pp. 451 and 1308).

LEG ULCERS

Ulceration of the skin is the complete loss of the epidermis and part of the dermis. When present on the lower leg, it is usually due to vascular disease and the vast majority (75%) of cases are due in part to venous hypertension. The site of ulceration on the lower leg can give a good indication of the underlying cause (Fig. 27.11), although this is not an absolute guide. For each cause of leg ulceration there are several different underlying pathologies that have to be considered (Box 27.16).

Clinical assessment

The history of the onset of the leg ulceration and any underlying predisposing conditions should be sought. Then the site and surrounding skin should be carefully assessed. The appropriate investigations should include:

- *Urinalysis* for glycosuria.
- *Full blood count* to detect anaemia and blood dyscrasias.
- *Bacterial swab* to detect pathogens. Systemic antibiotics are only required if there is a purulent discharge, rapid extension, cellulitis, lymphangitis or septicaemia.
- *Doppler ultrasound* to assess arterial circulation if the peripheral pulses cannot be felt. If the ankle systolic pressure divided by the brachial systolic pressure is > 0.8, then there is insignificant arterial disease. (An exception to this rule occurs in some patients with peripheral vascular disease associated with diabetes, in whom arterial calcification of the lower limb vessels produces a spuriously high ankle/brachial index.)
- *Venography*, which is occasionally useful in detecting surgically remediable venous incompetence.
- *Duplex scanning*, if available.

The main conditions and the differences between them are discussed below.

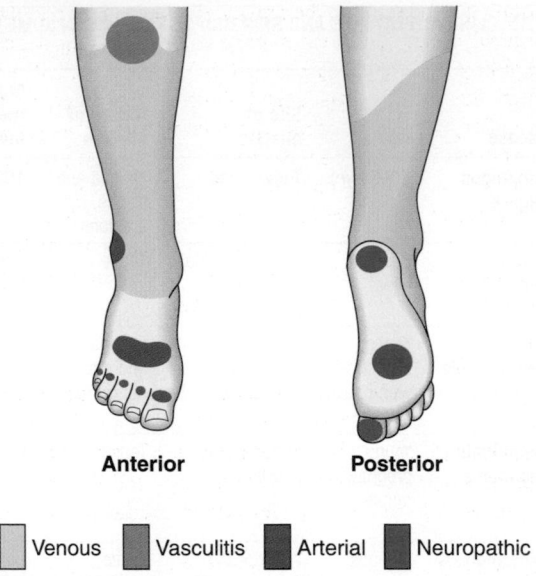

Venous   Vasculitis   Arterial   Neuropathic

Fig. 27.11   Causes of lower leg ulceration.

27.16 MAIN CAUSES OF LEG ULCERATION	
Venous hypertension	
• See text	
Arterial disease	
• Atherosclerosis	• Buerger's disease
• Vasculitis	
Small vessel disease	
• Diabetes mellitus	• Vasculitis
Abnormalities of blood	
• Sickle-cell disease	• Spherocytosis
• Cryoglobulinaemia	• Immune complex disease
Neuropathy	
• Diabetes mellitus	• Syphilis
• Leprosy	
Tumour	
• Squamous cell carcinoma	• Malignant melanoma
• Basal cell carcinoma	• Kaposi's sarcoma
Trauma	
• Injury	• Artefact

LEG ULCERATION DUE TO VENOUS DISEASE

Damage to the venous system of the leg results in oedema, haemosiderin deposition, eczema, fibrosis and ulceration.

Aetiology

In the normal leg there is a superficial low-pressure venous system connected to the deep, high-pressure veins by perforating veins. Muscular activity, aided by valves in the veins, pumps blood from the superficial to the deep system and towards the heart. Incompetent valves in the deep and perforating veins result in the retrograde flow of blood to the superficial system ('venous hypertension'), causing a rise in capillary hydrostatic pressure. Fibrinogen is forced out through the capillary walls and fibrin is deposited as a pericapillary cuff. One theory postulates that growth and repair factors are trapped in the macromolecular cuff so that minor trauma cannot be repaired and ulcers develop.

Incompetent veins leading to venous hypertension may be due to previous deep venous thrombosis (p. 1018), congenital or familial valve incompetence, infection or deep venous obstruction (e.g. from a pelvic tumour).

Clinical assessment

The problem usually starts in middle age. Leg ulcers are more likely to occur and to persist in obese people. Varicose veins, although often present, are not inevitable. The first symptom is frequently heaviness of the legs, followed by the development of oedema. Haemosiderin pigmentation and ivory-coloured scarring may then be seen, sometimes associated with venous eczema (p. 1283). The signs progress to lipodermatosclerosis—firm induration due to fibrosis of the dermis and subcutis, which may produce the well-known 'inverted champagne bottle' appearance. Ulceration, often precipitated by minor trauma or infection, soon occurs. Ulcers are seen typically around the medial malleolus but may encircle the ankle (Fig. 27.12). If conditions are favourable, the ulcers will heal by granulation with small epithelial islands at the base and epithelial growth from the edges. Healing is often slow and may never be complete. Recurrent ulceration is common even after good healing.

Complications

Chronic venous ulcers are invariably colonised by bacteria. Only if infection becomes overt (see above) is systemic anti-biotic treatment required. Contact dermatitis to an ointment, dressing or bandage is not uncommon. The usual culprits are preservatives, lanolin and neomycin. Lipodermatosclerosis may cause lymphoedema, leading to hyperkeratosis and the so-called 'mossy foot'. A squamous cell carcinoma developing in a venous ulcer (Marjolin's ulcer) is rarely responsible for its failure to heal.

Management

- General management includes dietary advice for the obese and encouragement to take gentle exercise.
- Oedema should be reduced by the regular use of compression bandages, keeping the legs elevated when sitting and the judicious use of diuretics.
- The exudate and slough should be removed with normal saline solution, 0.5% aqueous silver nitrate or 5% aqueous hydrogen peroxide. If the ulcer is very purulent, soaking the leg for 15 minutes in 1:10 000 dilution of aqueous potassium permanganate may be helpful.
- Dressings commonly used for venous ulceration include antibiotic-impregnated tulle dressings, non-adhesive absorbent dressings (alginates, charcoals, hydrogels or hydrocolloids) and dry non-adherent dressings (p. 1312).
- The frequency of dressings depends on the state of the ulcer. Very purulent and exudative ulcers may need daily dressings whilst the dressing on a clean, healing ulcer may only require changing every week.
- Paste bandages, impregnated with zinc oxide or ichthammol, help to keep dressings in place and provide protection.
- Surrounding venous eczema is treated by a mild or moderately potent topical corticosteroid. The corticosteroid should not be applied to the ulcer itself.
- Oral antibiotic therapy, given in short courses, is only necessary for the treatment of overt infection (see above). An anabolic corticosteroid, stanozolol, may help lipodermatosclerosis but side-effects (fluid retention, hepatotoxicity) may limit its use.
- In the absence of any evidence of compromised arterial supply (ankle/brachial pressure (ABP) ratio > 0.8), graduated compression bandages applied from the toes to the knees enhance venous return and have been shown to be most beneficial in the healing of venous leg ulcers (Box 27.17). Those individuals with an ABP ratio < 0.8 should be assumed to have arterial disease and therefore not able to tolerate compression bandaging.
- Vein surgery may help some younger patients with persistent venous ulcers. Pinch grafts may hasten the healing of clean ulcers but do not influence their rate of recurrence.

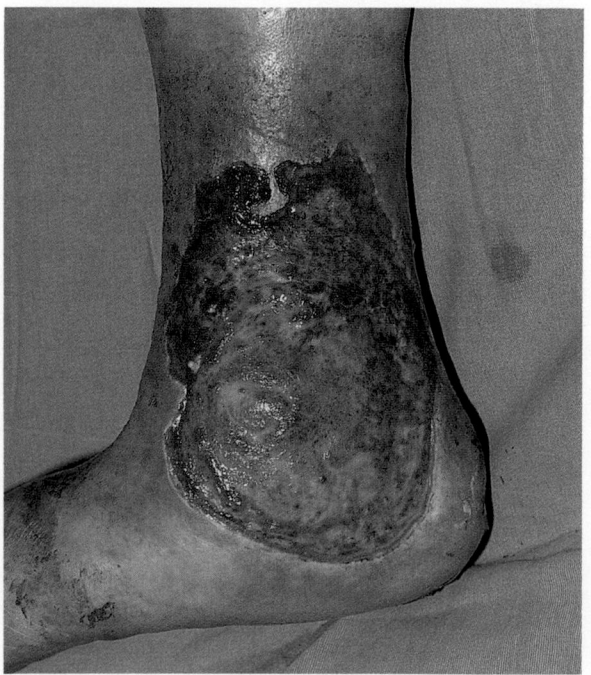

Fig. 27.12 A large venous ulcer overlying the medial malleolus.

EBM
27.17 COMPRESSION BANDAGING IN LEG ULCERATION
'Compression bandaging is effective in those individuals with an ankle/brachial pressure ratio (ABP) > 0.8, measured by hand-held Doppler.'
• The care of patients with chronic leg ulcer—a National Clinical Guideline. Scottish Intercollegiate Guidelines Network, Royal College of Physicians of Edinburgh, July 1998.
For further information: 💻 www.sign.ac.uk

27

LEG ULCERATION DUE TO ARTERIAL DISEASE

Deep, painful and punched-out ulcers on the lower leg, especially if they occur on the shin and foot and are preceded by a history of intermittent claudication, are likely to be due to arterial disease. Risk factors include smoking, hypertension, diabetes mellitus and hyperlipidaemia. The foot is cyanotic and cold, and the skin surrounding the ulcer is atrophic and hairless. The peripheral arterial pulses are absent or reduced. Doppler studies are required and then, if arterial insufficiency is confirmed, compression bandaging should be prohibited and advice from a vascular surgeon sought.

LEG ULCERATION DUE TO VASCULITIS

These ulcers start as painful, palpable, purpuric lesions turning into small punched-out ulcers. The involvement of larger vessels is heralded by painful nodules which may ulcerate. The intractable, deep, sharply demarcated ulcers of rheumatoid arthritis are due to an underlying vasculitis (p. 1138). Management includes treatment of the underlying disorder as well as immunosuppression with, for example, systemic corticosteroids or cyclophosphamide.

LEG ULCERATION DUE TO NEUROPATHY

The most common cause of a neuropathic ulcer is diabetes. The ulcers occur over weight-bearing areas such as the heel. Microangiopathy also contributes to ulceration in diabetes. This is discussed in detail on page 844.

TOO LITTLE OR TOO MUCH HAIR

A patient who complains of too little or too much hair should be treated with sensitivity. Particularly in women, these complaints are a source of genuine distress and the effect on a person's self-esteem and self-image is easily underestimated. The causes are numerous and varied but a systematic approach to the history and examination can easily be used to elicit the correct diagnosis.

Hair undergoes a regular cycle of growth. In humans each individual hair's cycle is independent of its neighbours (except in the newborn), whereas many animals change or lose their coat synchronously. At any one time, and depending on the age and sex of the person, up to 90% of hair follicles are in anagen, the growing phase, and only 10% in telogen, the resting phase, when hairs are normally shed. An alteration in this ratio can lead to an increased rate of hair loss and thus an impression of impending baldness.

ALOPECIA

The term means nothing more than loss of hair and is a sign rather than a diagnosis. There are many causes and patterns (Box 27.18).

A detailed history, careful scalp examination and complete physical examination should enable a confident diagnosis to be made.

27.18 CLASSIFICATION OF ALOPECIA

Localised	Diffuse
Non-scarring	
Tinea capitis	Androgenetic alopecia
Alopecia areata	Telogen effluvium
Androgenetic alopecia	Metabolic
Traumatic (trichotillomania, traction, cosmetic)	Hypothyroidism
Syphilis	Hyperthyroidism
	Hypopituitarism
	Diabetes mellitus
	HIV disease
	Nutritional deficiency
	Liver disease
	Post-partum
	Alopecia areata
	Syphilis
Scarring	
Idiopathic	Discoid lupus erythematosus
Developmental defects	Radiotherapy
Discoid lupus erythematosus	Folliculitis decalvans
Herpes zoster	Lichen planus pilaris
Pseudopelade	
Tinea capitis/kerion	

Tinea capitis

Fungal scalp infection is becoming increasingly common in urban areas in the UK. The clinical features can be variable but it usually affects children, causing patchy hair loss with some scaling. Any individual who develops an area of hair loss and scaling in the scalp should have the area scraped and affected hairs plucked for mycological microscopy and culture. Associated inflammation accounts for the variable presentation. Anthropophilic fungal infections (spread from child to child) account for the majority of cases in urban areas. Endothrix (within the hair shaft) infections, e.g. *Trichophyton tonsurans*, cause relatively uninflamed patchy baldness with breakage of the hairs at the skin surface ('black dot'). There is no fluorescence under Wood's light.

Ectothrix (outside the hair shaft) species of fungi, such as *Microsporum audouinii* (anthropophilic), show minimal inflammation; *Microsporum canis* (from dogs and cats) infections are more inflamed and can be identified by green fluorescence with Wood's light. Kerions are boggy, highly inflamed areas of tinea capitis and are usually caused by zoophilic (from animals, e.g. cattle ringworm) species of fungi (e.g. *Trichophyton verrucosum*).

Treatment is systemic, with oral terbinafine, griseofulvin or itraconazole. Topical therapy, such as an antifungal shampoo, is recommended as an adjunct and arachis oil is used to remove crusting. Kerions sometimes require short courses of oral corticosteroids in addition to systemic antifungal therapy to reduce the inflammation.

Accurate diagnosis and identification of the culprit fungus allows treatment and control of the spread of infection.

Alopecia areata

This non-scarring condition appears as sharply defined non-inflamed bald patches, usually on the scalp (p. 1258). During the active stage of hair loss pathognomonic 'exclamation mark' hairs are seen (broken-off hairs 3–4 mm

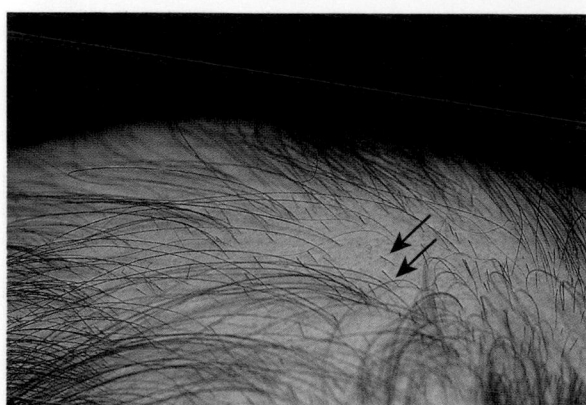

Fig. 27.13 Alopecia areata. Marked hair loss with diagnostic exclamation mark hairs (arrows).

long, which taper off towards the scalp—Fig. 27.13). An uncommon diffuse pattern on the scalp is recognised. The condition may affect the eyebrows, eyelashes and beard. Pitting and longitudinal wrinkling of the nail may be seen (p. 1283). The hair usually regrows spontaneously in small bald patches, but the outlook is less good with larger patches and when the alopecia appears early in life or is associated with atopy. Alopecia totalis describes complete loss of scalp hair and alopecia universalis complete loss of all hair. There is an association of alopecia areata with autoimmune disorders, atopy and Down's syndrome.

Androgenetic alopecia
Male-pattern baldness is physiological in men over 20 years old, although rarely it may be extensive and develop at an alarming pace in the late teens. It also occurs in females, most obviously after the menopause. The well-known distribution (bitemporal recession and then crown involvement) is described as 'male-pattern' but this type of hair loss in females is often diffuse.

Investigations
Laboratory tests, including a full blood count, erythrocyte sedimentation rate, urea and electrolytes, liver and thyroid function tests, an autoantibody profile and *Treponema pallidum* haemagglutination (TPHA) test, should help determine the cause of non-scarring alopecia. More specialised tests, including the hair pluck test where up to 50 hairs are removed with epilating forceps to determine the anagen:telogen ratio, are seldom necessary. Mycological assessment is advisable in cases of localised hair loss with scaling. A scalp biopsy, with direct immunofluorescence, may help to confirm a diagnosis of lichen planus of the scalp or discoid lupus erythematosus.

Management
Successful treatment of alopecia is difficult and management of these patients includes support and reassurance. Any underlying condition should be treated. Alopecia areata sometimes responds to topical or intralesional corticosteroids such as 0.3 ml triamcinolone (10 mg/ml). Some males with androgenetic alopecia may be helped by systemic finasteride or topical 2% minoxidil solution. In females, anti-androgen therapy such as cyproterone acetate is used. A wig may be the most appropriate treatment for extensive alopecia. Scalp surgery and autologous hair transplants are expensive but sometimes effective in androgenetic alopecia.

HIRSUTISM

Hirsutism is the growth of terminal hair in a male pattern in a female. It should be distinguished from hypertrichosis, which describes the excessive growth of terminal hair in either sex in a non-androgenic distribution. The amount of terminal hair varies in people with different genetic ancestries and therefore the definition of what might be considered excessive needs to take clinical context into account.

Some degree of hirsutism is common after the menopause. The cause of most cases of hirsutism is unknown and only a small minority have a demonstrable hormonal abnormality.

Investigations
Full endocrinological investigations are required if hirsutism:

- occurs in childhood
- is of sudden onset
- is accompanied by signs of virilisation
- is associated with menstrual irregularity or cessation.

In addition to the screening tests for hyperandrogenism (p. 768), polycystic ovary syndrome and Cushing's syndrome need to be considered (p. 779).

Management
Depilatory creams, waxing, electrolysis, bleaching and shaving are often used for physiological hirsutism. In those with darkly pigmented hair, laser therapy may be useful.

Any remediable cause should be corrected by medical and surgical methods, sometimes with the help of the endocrinologist or gynaecologist (p. 768). Oral anti-androgens may be helpful.

ABNORMAL SKIN COLOUR

DECREASED PIGMENTATION

Oculocutaneous albinism
Albinism results from a range of genetic abnormalities leading to reduced melanin biosynthesis in skin and eyes but the number of melanocytes is normal (compare with vitiligo). It differs from cutaneous hypopigmentation in that there is, by definition, ocular involvement. There are a number of different forms of albinism, and considerable variation even within one genetic type. Albinism is usually inherited as an autosomal recessive trait. Type 1 albinism is due to a defect in the tyrosinase gene whose product is rate-limiting in the production of melanin. Such individuals at birth have an almost complete absence of pigment in the skin and hair with a resulting pale skin and white hair, and also failure of melanin production in the eye, in the iris and retina. Patients have photophobia, poor vision not correctable with refraction, rotatory nystagmus, and an

27

alternating strabismus associated with abnormalities in the decussation of nerve fibres in the optic tract. A second form of albinism is due to a defect in the P gene which encodes an ion channel protein in the melanosome. Like type 1 albinos, patients may have a gross reduction of melanin in the skin and in the eyes, but may be more mildly affected than some type 1 albinos. Establishing the subtype of albinism requires genetic analysis as there is considerable heterogeneity in the phenotype of the various subtypes. (It is not always possible to diagnose the type of albinism from examination alone.)

Oculocutaneous albinos are at grossly increased risk of sunburn and skin cancer. In equatorial regions many albinos will die from squamous cell carcinoma or more rarely melanoma in early adult life. Albinos may, however, show pigmented melanocytic naevi and may freckle in response to sun damage. There are other extremely rare forms of albinism such as rufous and brown albinism.

Management

Avoidance of sun exposure is important, and may involve protective clothing, hats and an alteration of lifestyle if possible to avoid the midday sun in particular and to pursue indoor rather than outdoor work. Sunblocks may also be useful but can be prohibitively expensive. Early diagnosis and treatment of skin tumours is essential.

Vitiligo

Vitiligo is an acquired condition in which circumscribed depigmented patches develop; it affects 1% of the population world-wide.

Aetiology

Unlike albinism, where melanocytes are present but the production of melanin is abnormal, vitiligo involves focal areas of melanocyte loss. There may be a positive family history of the disorder in those with generalised vitiligo and this type is associated with autoimmune diseases such as diabetes, thyroid and adrenal disorders, and pernicious anaemia. Trauma and sunburn may precipitate the appearance of vitiligo. A number of hypotheses have been advanced to explain the pathogenesis, none of which is entirely satisfactory. One popular theory is that the melanocytes are the target of a cell-mediated autoimmune attack. Why only focal areas are affected remains unexplained.

Clinical assessment

Segmental vitiligo is restricted to one part of the body, but not necessarily a dermatome. Generalised vitiligo is often symmetrical and frequently involves the hands, wrists, knees and neck as well as the area around the body orifices. The hair of the scalp and beard may also depigment (Fig. 27.14). The patches of depigmentation are sharply defined and, in Caucasians, may be surrounded by light brown 'café au lait' hyperpigmentation. Some spotty perifollicular pigment may be seen within the depigmented patches and is sometimes the first sign of repigmentation. Sensation in the depigmented patches is normal (compare tuberculoid leprosy, p. 333). The course is unpredictable but most patches remain static or enlarge; a few repigment spontaneously.

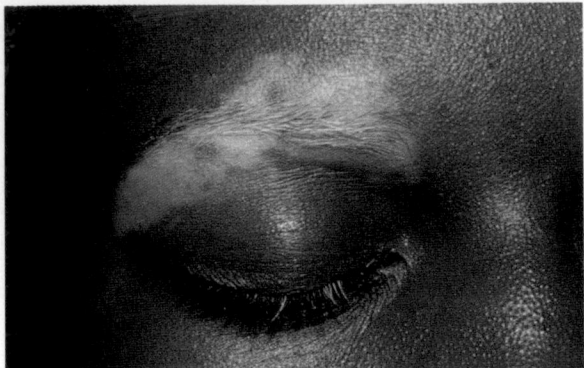

Fig. 27.14 Vitiligo. Localised patches of depigmented skin, including some white hairs.

Management

This is unsatisfactory. Protecting the patches from excessive sun exposure with clothing or sunscreen may be helpful in reducing episodes of burning and potentially of skin cancer in the long term. Camouflage cosmetics may also be helpful, particularly in those with dark skin. Potent topical corticosteroids can sometimes be helpful. Phototherapy with PUVA or more recently TL01 has been used. Although repigmentation may occur during phototherapy, there is an absence of randomised controlled trials to inform clinical practice. PUVA therapy in particular has been widely used but, because it increases pigmentation in normal skin, except in very dark-skinned individuals, the cosmetic effect (an increase in contrast) may actually be worse than no treatment. When repigmentation occurs it is frequently seen as small foci of dark areas of skin surrounding hair follicles within the vitiliginous area. The absence of whiteness of the hairs in the area of vitiligo is a good prognostic feature. Finally, transplantation, using a range of techniques including split-skin grafts and blister roof grafts, is used on to dermabraded recipient skin.

Phenylketonuria

This rare metabolic cause of hypopigmentation has a prevalence of about 1:25 000.

Hypopituitarism

Hypopigmentation is due to decreased production of pituitary melanotrophic hormones (p. 794). The complexion has a pale, yellow tinge; there is skin atrophy and thinning or loss of the sexual hair.

INCREASED PIGMENTATION

This is mostly due to hypermelanosis but other pigments may occasionally be deposited in the skin. Orange discoloration suggests carotenaemia; bronze, haemochromatosis (p. 974); and other hues, drug eruptions (Box 27.19).

Localised hypermelanosis

Freckles

These lesions, also known as ephelides, are sharply demarcated light brown-ginger macules of up to 5 mm in diameter due to focal overproduction of melanin but with normal melanocyte number. They are most prominent on exposed sites, they multiply and become darker with sun exposure, and they are associated with sun exposure and a sun-sensitive phenotype (e.g. red hair).

Lentigines

These are dark brown macules ranging from 1 mm to 1 cm across. Although discrete, their outline may be irregular. Lentigines occur in childhood but are most common after middle age on the backs of the hands ('liver spots') and on the face. They show an increased number of melanocytes which produce excessive melanin. They are associated with chronic sun exposure and a sun-sensitive phenotype. Multiple lentigines are seen on and around the lips, buccal mucosa and fingers in the Peutz–Jeghers syndrome (associated with small intestinal polyposis and intussusception, p. 925).

Diffuse hypermelanosis

Endocrine pigmentation

Chloasma describes discrete patches of facial pigmentation which occur in pregnancy and in some women taking oral contraceptives. The basis of the focal increased sensitivity to hormonal control is unknown. Diffuse pigmentation, sometimes worse in the skin creases, may be a feature of Addison's disease (p. 782), Cushing's syndrome (p. 779), Nelson's syndrome and chronic renal failure (p. 485). In all of these cases it is said to be due to increase in the levels of pituitary melanotrophic peptides (p. 792).

Drug-induced pigmentation

Box 27.19 lists some drugs which may cause hyperpigmentation; this is not always due to hypermelanosis alone but may sometimes be due to deposition of the drug or its metabolite, either of which may be complexed with melanin.

27.19 DRUG-INDUCED PIGMENTATION	
Drug	**Appearance**
Amiodarone	Slate-grey, exposed sites
Arsenic	Diffuse bronze pigmentation with superimposed raindrop depigmentation
Bleomycin	Often flexural, brown
Busulfan	Diffuse brown
Chloroquine	Blue-grey, exposed sites
Clofazimine	Red
Mepacrine	Yellow
Minocycline	Slate-grey, scars, temples, shins and sclera
Phenothiazines	Slate-grey, exposed sites
Psoralens	Brown, exposed sites

VULVAL ITCH (PRURITUS VULVAE)

Pruritus vulvae is a distressing symptom that can occur at any age and its cause can be difficult to diagnose. Chronic scratching of the vulval area leads to lichenification as in other sites. In this site it can be asymmetrical and associated with quite marked oedema and swelling. The history is important to give an indication of the underlying cause. Pre-existing skin disease, such as atopic eczema, psoriasis or fungal infections, needs to be sought and an autoimmune history might be associated with lichen sclerosus et atrophicus. It is important to determine whether there is a previous history of sexually transmitted diseases, particularly genital warts or cervical dysplasia found on colposcopy. The main dermatological causes of itch in the vulval area are candidiasis (consider underlying diabetes), tinea cruris (dermatophyte infection), eczema (including contact dermatitis), psoriasis, lichen sclerosus and, less commonly, lichen planus. These can usually be differentiated by careful examination, bacteriological and mycological assessment and a search for evidence of similar skin disease elsewhere on the body. A well-defined, bright red plaque on the vulva can indicate psoriasis, particularly with skin, scalp or nail signs of this condition. Oral lesions are often seen in lichen planus and this condition is often followed by marked post-inflammatory hyperpigmentation. Lichen sclerosus is characterised by ivory papules that coalesce into pale plaques with an atrophic surface (reminiscent of crinkly cigarette paper). There is sometimes associated haemorrhagic blistering. Lichen sclerosus often forms a 'figure of eight' around the vulva and perineal area and can cause scarring of the vulva with loss of normal contours culminating in stenosis of the introitus secondary to labial fusion. Biopsy for histology is occasionally needed to differentiate these conditions and in lichen sclerosus to assess any malignant change in, for example, non-healing areas.

Histology is always needed in the next group of itchy vulval lesions, neoplasia. Most tumours of the vulva can provoke the symptom of itch—in particular, vulval (squamous) intra-epithelial neoplasia (VIN) and extra-mammary Paget's disease. Lesions of VIN can be solitary or multiple and may appear red, white, pigmented, warty, moist or eroded. As well as being itchy, VIN can be painful, particularly with superficial dyspareunia. There may be very little to see with the naked eye and then vulvoscopy is needed. In younger women there is a strong association of VIN with papillomavirus, immunosuppression and possibly smoking. Extramammary Paget's disease is rare, is usually asymmetrical and can be painful. It presents as a moist, red, scaly patch often mistaken for eczema; hence the importance of biopsy in 'unresponsive eczema'.

Finally, it has been shown that a proportion of vulval itch is psychogenic; certainly vulval disease can be associated with psychological distress and careful consultation by an understanding doctor is essential to a correct diagnosis of this condition.

ABNORMAL NAILS

The condition of the nails may reflect both local and systemic disease, and omission of this part of the general examination could result in some important diagnostic clues being overlooked.

27

The nail plate arises from the nail matrix and lies on the nail bed (Fig. 27.15). The keratinous plate is produced by cells of the (dorsal) matrix and, to a much lesser extent, the (ventral) bed. Finger nails grow about 1 cm every 3 months and toe nails at about one-third of this rate.

NAIL FOLD DISORDERS

Examination of the nail folds should accompany examination of the nails. Paronychia describes inflamed and swollen nail folds. Chronic paronychia is seen frequently in those with a poor peripheral circulation, in those involved in wet work, in people with diabetes and in those who are over-enthusiastic when manicuring their cuticles. Ragged cuticles and dilated or thrombosed capillaries in the proximal nail folds are important pointers to connective tissue disease (Fig. 27.16).

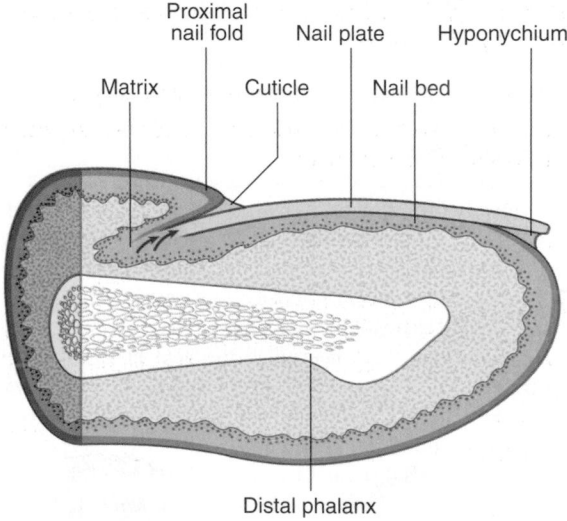

Fig. 27.15 **The nail plate and bed.** Arrows indicate the direction of nail growth.

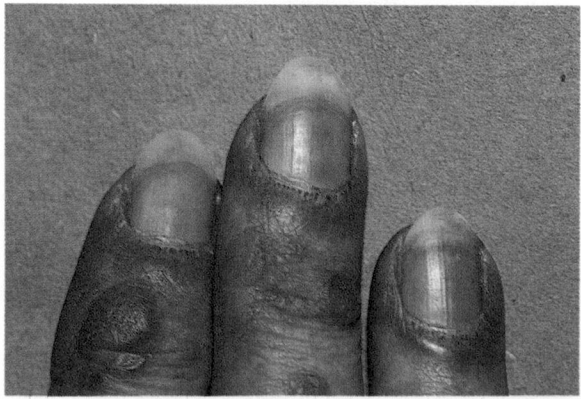

Fig. 27.16 Dermatomyositis. The erythema, dilated and tortuous capillaries in the proximal nail fold and the Gottron's papules on the digits are important diagnostic features (p. 1136).

NAIL PLATE DISORDERS

These may be isolated abnormalities due to congenital disease or trauma, or may reflect other diseases, either systemic or involving just the skin. Longitudinal ridging and beading of the nail plate is not abnormal and increases with age. Similarly, occasional white transverse flecks (striate leuconychia) are seen frequently in normal nails and are due to airspaces within the plate and not, contrary to popular belief, to insufficient calcium.

CONGENITAL DISEASE

Pachyonychia congenita is a rare autosomal dominant condition. Most cases arise due to mutations in a particular group of keratin genes. The nails are grossly thickened, especially at the free edge, and discoloured from birth.

TRAUMA

Splinter haemorrhages
These are fine linear dark brown flecks running longitudinally in the plate (Fig. 18.95, p. 631). They are most commonly due to trauma, particularly when distal, but may be seen in nail psoriasis. They are also, less commonly, a sign of subacute bacterial endocarditis (p. 629).

Subungual haematomas
These may appear as a crimson, purple or grey-brown discoloration of the nail plate, most frequently that of the big toe (Fig. 27.17). Sometimes, but not always, there is a history of trauma. The abnormality appears suddenly and the nail folds remain uninvolved (cf. subungual malignant melanoma, p. 1305). As the nail grows out, a normally coloured band develops proximally. They may be confused with melanoma and biopsy may be necessary.

Habit-tic dystrophy
This is common, and is due to the habit of picking or fiddling with the proximal nail fold of the thumb. This produces a ladder pattern of transverse ridges and furrows up the centre of the nail.

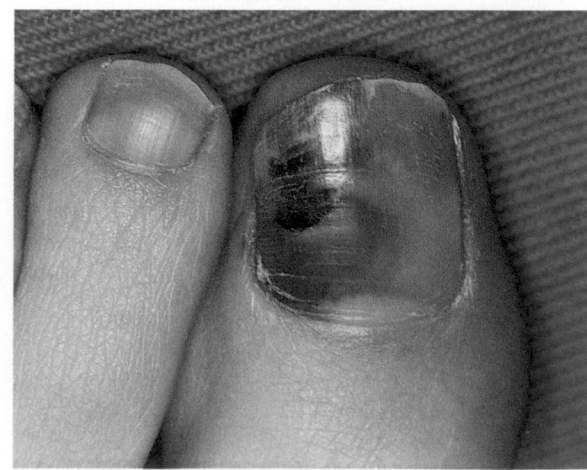

Fig. 27.17 Subungual haematoma.

Chronic trauma

Chronic trauma from ill-fitting shoes and from sport may cause malalignment and thickening of the nails, known as onychogryphosis, and lead to ingrowing toenails.

THE NAIL IN SYSTEMIC DISEASE

Koilonychia

This is a concave or spoon-shaped deformity of the plate which is a sign of iron deficiency (Fig. 27.18A). It is seen most often in countries where malnutrition is prevalent.

Beau's lines

These are transverse grooves which appear at the same time on all nails, a few weeks after an acute illness, moving out to the free margins as the nails grow (Fig. 27.18B).

Digital clubbing

In its most gross form this is seen as a bulbous swelling of the tip of the finger (Figs 27.18C and D) or toe. The normal angle between the proximal part of the nail and the skin is lost. Causes may be:

- *respiratory*—bronchogenic carcinoma, asbestosis (especially with mesothelioma), suppurative lung disease (empyema, bronchiectasis, cystic fibrosis), fibrosing alveolitis
- *cardiac*—cyanotic congenital heart disease, subacute bacterial endocarditis

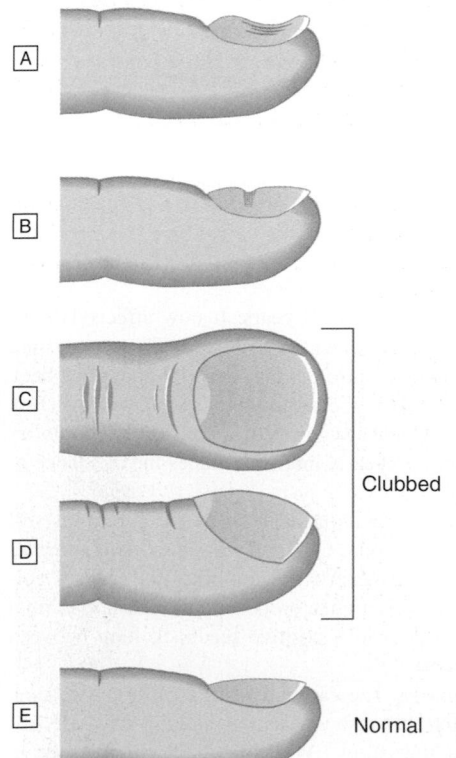

Clubbed

Normal

Fig. 27.18   The nail in systemic disease. A Koilonychia. B Beau's lines. C and D Digital clubbing. E Normal nail.

- *other*—inflammatory bowel disease, biliary cirrhosis, thyrotoxicosis, familial.

Whitening of the nails

This is a rare sign of hypoalbuminaemia. 'Half and half' nails (white proximally and red-brown distally) are seen in some patients with renal failure. Rarely, drugs (e.g. antimalarials) may discolour nails.

THE NAIL IN SOME COMMON SKIN DISEASES

Psoriasis

This may cause coarse pitting of the nail plate, onycholysis (separation of the nail plate from the nail bed) and subungual hyperkeratosis (Fig. 27.25, p. 1289).

Eczema

Shiny nails may signify frequent rubbing of eczematous skin elsewhere. When eczema involves the distal phalanges the nail may be deformed, with transverse ridging and thickening of the plate.

Lichen planus and severe alopecia areata

These may cause trachyonychia, a fine roughness and white discoloration of the nail plate.

Dermatophyte infection

This causes yellow-brown discoloration and crumbling of the plate which usually starts distally and spreads proximally (Fig. 27.19). Usually only a few nails (more commonly toenails than fingernails) are affected and frequently only on one foot or hand. Diagnosis relies on clippings being examined for hyphae and culture, and systemic rather than topical antifungal treatment (e.g. terbinafine) is required.

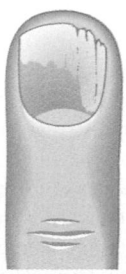

Fig. 27.19   Dermatophyte infection. This causes discoloration and crumbliness of the nail plate.

ECZEMA

The terms 'eczema' and 'dermatitis' are synonymous. They refer to distinctive reaction patterns in the skin, which can be either acute or chronic and are due to a number of causes.

Histopathology

In the acute stage, oedema of the epidermis (spongiosis) progresses to the formation of intra-epidermal vesicles, which may enlarge and rupture. In the chronic stage there is less oedema and vesiculation but more thickening of the

27

27.20 CLASSIFICATION OF ECZEMA

- Atopic
- Seborrhoeic
- Discoid
- Irritant
- Allergic
- Asteatotic
- Gravitational
- Lichen simplex
- Pompholyx

27.21 THE ECZEMA REACTION

Acute

- Redness and swelling, usually with ill-defined margins
- Papules, vesicles and, more rarely, large blisters
- Exudation and cracking
- Scaling

Chronic

- May show all of the above features, although it is usually less vesicular and exudative
- Lichenification, a dry leathery thickening with increased skin markings, is secondary to rubbing and scratching
- Fissures and scratch marks
- Pigmentation changes (hypo- and hyper-)

27.22 DIAGNOSTIC CRITERIA FOR ATOPIC ECZEMA

Itchy skin and at least three of the following:
- History of itch in skin creases (or cheeks if < 4 years)
- History of asthma/hay fever (or in a first-degree relative if < 4 years)
- Dry skin (xeroderma)
- Visible flexural eczema (cheeks, forehead, outer limbs if < 4 years)
- Onset in first 2 years of life

27.23 EARLY PREVENTION OF ATOPIC ECZEMA   **EBM**

'Restrictions in maternal diet during pregnancy have no effect on the incidence of atopic eczema in an infant at hereditary risk and may adversely affect maternal and/or fetal nutrition. Breastfeeding, however, appears to reduce the prevalence of atopic eczema in early childhood.'

- Kramer MS. Cochrane Library, issue 1, 2001. Oxford: Update Software.
- Saarinen UM, et al. Lancet 1995; 346:1065–1069.
- Chandra RK. J Pediatr Gastroenterol Nutr 1997; 24:380–388.

For further information: 💻 www.cochrane.org

27.24 ATOPIC ECZEMA: DISTRIBUTION AND CHARACTER OF RASH

Infancy

- The eczema is often acute and involves the face and trunk
- The napkin area is frequently spared

Childhood

- The rash settles on the backs of the knees, fronts of the elbows, wrists and ankles (Fig. 27.20)

Adults

- The face and trunk (Fig. 27.21) are once more involved; lichenification is common

---

epidermis (acanthosis); this is accompanied by a variable degree of vasodilatation and T-cell lymphocytic infiltration in the upper dermis.

Clinical features

There are several patterns of eczema (Box 27.20); some of these have identifiable environmental causes whereas others are more complex. The clinical signs are similar in all types of eczema and vary according to the duration of the rash. The features of acute and chronic eczema are listed in Box 27.21.

Atopic eczema

Atopy is a genetic predisposition to form excessive IgE which leads to a generalised and prolonged hypersensitivity to common environmental antigens, including pollen and the house dust mite. Atopic individuals manifest one or more of a group of diseases that includes asthma, hay fever, urticaria, food and other allergies, and this distinctive form of eczema. Although any of these atopic conditions tends to be over-represented in families of persons with any atopic disease, one particular disease type tends to run more strongly in a particular family. A number of operational criteria for the diagnosis of atopic eczema have been proposed for the purpose of research studies (Box 27.22).

Aetiology. There is a clear familial component, a large part of which is due to genetic factors. The disorder is concordant in 86% of monozygotic twins but in only 21% of dizygotes. Atopic diseases show some degree of maternal imprinting—that is, they are inherited more often from the mother than from the father. Atopic dermatitis is therefore genetically complex. More than one genetic locus has been identified that might play a role in the inheritance of atopy and more specifically atopic eczema. The prevalence of atopic eczema is rising and has increased between twofold and fivefold over the last 30 years. It now affects 1 in 10 schoolchildren. Environmental factors, such as exposure to allergens either in utero or during childhood, have been shown to have a role in the aetiology of atopic eczema (Box 27.23). Recent evidence suggests that exposure to probiotics in late pregnancy and early infancy reduces the incidence of atopic eczema.

Pathogenesis. The pathogenesis of atopic eczema is still incompletely understood. One unifying view is to consider it as an interplay of genetic susceptibility that causes epidermal barrier dysfunction, a propensity to mount abnormal immune responses, and a positive feedback loop between these two factors.

Clinical features. The cardinal feature of atopic eczema is itch ('the itch that rashes'), and scratching may account for many of the signs. Widespread dryness (felt as roughness) of the skin is another feature. The distribution and character of the rash vary with age, as shown in Box 27.24. Complications are listed in Box 27.25.

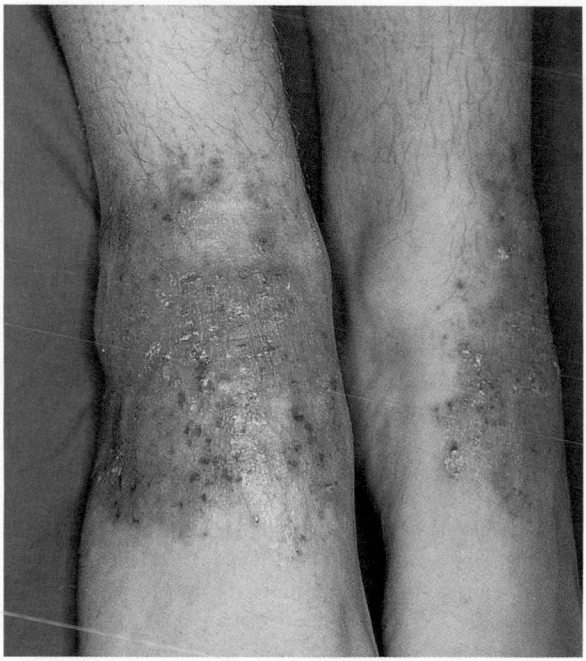

Fig. 27.20 **Atopic subacute eczema on the fronts of the ankles of a teenager.** These are sites of predilection, along with the cubital and popliteal fossae, in atopic eczema.

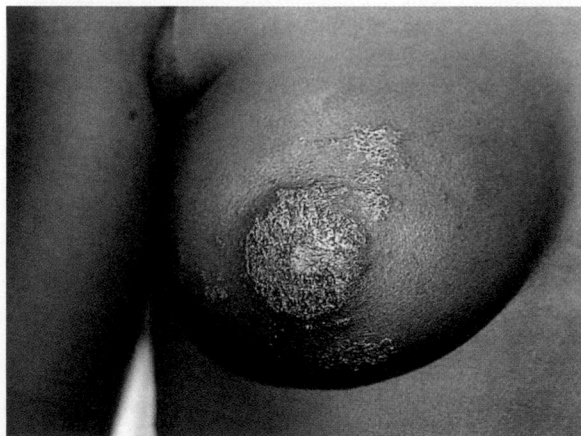

Fig. 27.21 **Nipple eczema.** This is frequently bilateral in atopic dermatitis.

Seborrhoeic eczema

This condition, which is characterised by a red scaly rash, classically affects the scalp (dandruff), central face, naso-labial folds, eyebrows and central chest. It is due to *Pityrosporum ovale* infection of the skin. In its milder forms it is the same as dandruff, whereas when severe it may resemble psoriasis. Sebum may be permissive for the development of the rash but otherwise the name is a poor one. Treatment of *P. ovale* with anti-yeast agents improves the rash, although the course may need to be repeated. Seborrhoeic eczema is a feature of AIDS (p. 384) and can be very severe in this condition.

> **27.25 COMPLICATIONS OF ATOPIC ECZEMA**
>
> - Superinfection, most often with bacteria (*Staphylococcus aureus*) but also importantly with viruses. Herpes simplex virus causes a widespread severe eruption—eczema herpeticum. Papillomavirus and molluscum contagiosum superinfections are also more common and are encouraged by use of local corticosteroids
> - Irritant reactions due to defective barrier function
> - Sleep disturbance, loss of schooling and behavioural difficulties
> - Children with atopic eczema have an increased incidence of food allergy, particularly to eggs, cow's milk, protein, fish, wheat and soya. These foods cause an immediate urticarial eruption rather than exacerbating the child's eczema

Discoid eczema

This is a common form of eczema recognised from discrete coin-shaped lesions of eczema seen on the limbs of young men in association with alcohol excess, and of elderly men. It can occur in children with atopic eczema and tends to be more stubborn to treat.

Irritant eczema

Detergents, alkalis, acids, solvents and abrasive dusts are common causes. There is a wide range of susceptibility to weak irritants. Irritant eczema accounts for the majority of industrial cases and work loss. The elderly, those with fair and dry skin, and those with an atopic background (personal or family history of asthma, hay fever or eczema) are especially vulnerable. Napkin eczema in babies is common and due to irritant ammoniacal urine and faeces.

Strong irritants elicit an acute reaction at the site of contact whereas weak irritants most often cause chronic eczema, especially of the hands, after prolonged exposure.

Allergic contact eczema

This is due to a delayed hypersensitivity reaction following contact with antigens or haptens. Previous exposure to the allergen is required for sensitisation and the reaction is specific to the allergen or closely related chemicals. Common allergens and their origin are listed in Box 27.26.

The eczema reaction occurs wherever the allergen is in contact with the skin and sensitisation persists indefinitely. It is important to determine the original site of the rash

27

27.26 SOME COMMON ALLERGENS	
Allergen	**Present in**
Nickel	Jewellery, jean studs, bra clips
Dichromate	Cement, leather, matches
Rubber chemicals	Clothing, shoes, tyres
Colophony	Sticking plaster, collodion
Paraphenylenediamine	Hair dye, clothing
Balsam of Peru	Perfumes, citrus fruits
Neomycin, benzocaine	Topical applications
Parabens	Preservative in cosmetics and creams
Wool alcohols	Lanolin, cosmetics, creams
Epoxy resin	Resin adhesives

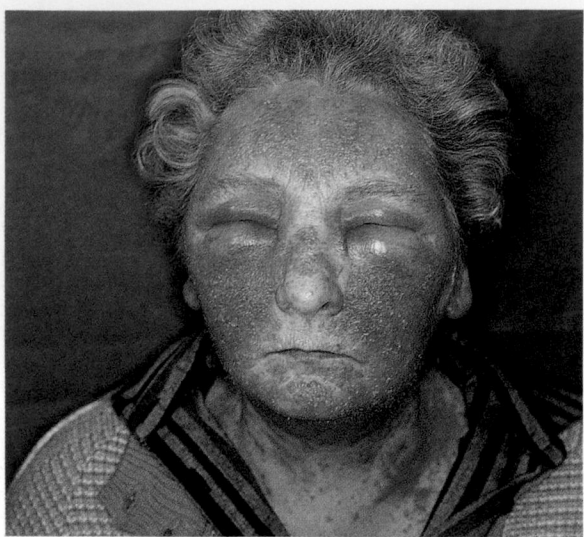

Fig. 27.22 Allergic contact eczema. This was caused by the application of an antihistamine cream. The acute eczematous reaction and bilateral periorbital oedema are typical.

before secondary spread obscures the picture, as this often provides the best clue to the contactant. There are many easily recognisable patterns, e.g. eczema of the earlobes, wrists and back due to contact with nickel in costume jewellery, watches and bra clips; or eczema of the hands and wrists due to rubber gloves. Oedema of the lax skin of the eyelids and genitalia is a frequent concomitant of allergic contact eczema (Fig. 27.22).

Asteatotic eczema

This is frequently seen in the hospitalised elderly, especially when the skin is dry; low humidity caused by central heating, over-washing and diuretics are contributory factors. It occurs most often on the lower legs as a rippled or 'crazy paving' pattern of fine fissuring on an erythematous background.

Gravitational (stasis) eczema

This occurs on the lower legs and is often associated with signs of venous insufficiency (oedema, red or bluish discoloration, loss of hair, induration, haemosiderin pigmentation and ulceration).

Lichen simplex

This describes a plaque of lichenified eczema due to repeated rubbing or scratching, as a habit or in response to stress. Common sites include the nape of the neck, the lower legs and the anogenital area.

Pompholyx

Recurrent vesicles and bullae occur on the palms, palmar surface of the fingers and soles, and are excruciatingly itchy. This form of eczema can occur in atopic eczema and in irritant and contact allergic dermatitis. It can be provoked by heat, stress and nickel ingestion in a nickel-sensitive patient but is often idiopathic.

Investigation of eczema

For details of tests see pages 1263–1264.

Patch tests

These are performed in suspected cases of contact allergic dermatitis (p. 1264).

IgE and specific IgE

These are occasionally performed to support the diagnosis of atopic eczema and to determine specific environmental allergens, e.g. pet dander, horse hair, house dust mite, pollens and foods.

Prick tests

The indications are the same as for specific IgE but are less commonly performed.

Bacterial and viral swabs for microscopy and culture

These are useful tests in suspected secondary infection. Skin swabs for bacteriological assessment will invariably reveal the presence of bacteria, but antibacterial treatment should be reserved for those cases with evidence of clinical infection. In the case of recurrent impetigo in a child with atopic eczema, bacterial swabs should be taken from carrier sites (nares, axillae and groin) from both the affected individual and all household members.

General management of eczema

The main points are listed in Box 27.27.

Topical corticosteroids

Lotions (aqueous base) and creams (oil/water mixture) are preferable in acute eczema and ointments (in an oily base) in chronic cases; they are usually applied twice daily. Only 1% hydrocortisone should be used on the face and in infancy, except under expert advice. Even in adults it is seldom necessary to prescribe more than 200 g of a low-potency corticosteroid (e.g. 1% hydrocortisone), 50 g of a moderately potent corticosteroid (e.g. 0.05% clobetasone butyrate) or 30 g of a potent corticosteroid (e.g. 0.1% betamethasone valerate, 0.1% mometasone furoate) per week. Very potent topical corticosteroids (e.g. 0.05% clobetasol propionate) should not be used long-term. The side-effects of strong or extensive local corticosteroid therapy should be borne in mind when patients are applying these preparations for years on end. They include skin thinning (with striae, fragility and purpura), enhanced or disguised infections, and systemic absorption (causing suppression of the hypothalamic–pituitary–adrenal axis and even Cushingoid features). There are no absolute guidelines for the amount of topical corticosteroid that should be used, and there seems to be marked variation in sensitivity to their harmful effects, but particular care should be taken on certain sites such as the face and flexures (p. 1312) and in the elderly (Box 27.28). The best rule is to use the least potent corticosteroid for the shortest possible time that is effective. However, it often seems that topical cortico-

27.27 GENERAL MANAGEMENT FOR ALL TYPES OF ECZEMA

- Explanation, reassurance and encouragement
- Avoidance of contact with irritants
- Regular use of greasy emollients
- Appropriate use of topical corticosteroids

steroids are being under-used rather than over-used, due to disproportionate fears over their side-effects. This is a not infrequent cause of apparent treatment failure.

Other topical immunosuppressants, including tacrolimus and pimecrolimus, are available for use. Early reports of their efficacy are encouraging, although they are relatively expensive and their long-term toxicity profile unknown.

Bland emollients (e.g. emulsifying ointment) are used regularly, both directly on the skin and in the bath. They not only prevent excessive water loss from an already dry skin, but also help to reduce the amount of local corticosteroid used. Emollient soap substitutes (e.g. aqueous cream) are also helpful. Sedative antihistamines (e.g. alimemazine tartrate) are generally thought to be of value if sleep is interrupted, although there are no randomised controlled trials to support their use.

Specific measures

Atopic eczema

Explanation and patient support are increasingly provided through general practice, dermatology clinics, community liaison nurses and patient support groups such as the National Eczema Society in the UK. Treatment involves the regular use of emollients (moisturisers) and the least possible use of topical corticosteroids. These topical treatments can be used with a variety of types of bandaging such as 'wet wraps', tar and ichthammol paste bandages. Allergen avoidance may have a role in selected patients. Routine inoculations are allowed during quiescent phases of eczema. An egg-free measles vaccine is available for children who have a severe egg allergy.

Seborrhoeic eczema

Antipityrosporal agents such as ketoconazole shampoo and creams form the basis of treatment, supplemented with weak corticosteroids if needed. Treatments may need to be repeated at intervals.

Irritant eczema

This is best treated by the regular use of emollients, protective clothing, e.g. gloves, and avoidance of irritants.

Contact allergic eczema

Avoidance of the culprit allergen is the most important treatment for this form of eczema and may involve lifestyle changes such as a new job or giving up hobbies. Measures used for irritant eczema are also helpful.

Gravitational eczema

Local corticosteroids (see above) should only be applied to eczematous areas and ulcers should be avoided. Sensiti-

---

27.28 ECZEMA IN OLD AGE

- **Loss of elasticity:** with advancing age, the skin becomes less pliable and drier. This increases the tendency for irritant dermatitis.
- **Topical corticosteroid usage:** causes more local side-effects, such as purpura or ecchymoses.
- **Prognosis:** widespread eczema is potentially life-threatening, particularly when combined with other illnesses.

---

sation to topical antibiotics (neomycin) and preservatives (e.g. chlorocresol) is common in this form of eczema. Associated peripheral oedema should be eliminated by elevation of the leg and graded compression bandages.

PSORIASIS AND OTHER ERYTHEMATOUS SCALY ERUPTIONS

Psoriasis and lichen planus will be described here in detail; other scaly conditions were covered on pages 1267–1269.

PSORIASIS

Psoriasis is a non-infectious, chronic inflammatory disease of the skin, characterised by well-defined erythematous plaques with silvery scale, with a predilection for the extensor surfaces and scalp, and a chronic fluctuating course.

The prevalence is approximately 2% in European populations. Accurate figures for many other parts of the world are not available but there seems to be consistent evidence that the prevalence of psoriasis is lower in people of African origin and lower still in some Asian communities such as the Japanese. Psoriasis may start at any age but is unusual before the age of 5; the oldest recorded onset was in a patient aged 107. There appear to be two epidemiological patterns of psoriasis (Fig. 27.1, p. 1260). The first shows an onset in the teenage and early adult years; such individuals frequently have a family history of psoriasis and there is an increased prevalence of HLA Cw6. In a second grouping, disease onset is in the fifties or sixties, a family history is less common and the HLA group Cw6 is not so prominent. Some authors refer to these two groups of patients as type 1 and type 2 psoriatics.

The clinical course of psoriasis is very variable. As a general rule clinical impressions suggest that the earlier the age of onset and the more severe the initial presentation, the more severe the lifetime course of the disease.

Aetiology

Basic defect

There are two key pathophysiological aspects to the abnormalities in psoriatic plaques:

- First, the keratinocytes hyperproliferate with a grossly increased mitotic index and an abnormal pattern of differentiation involving the retention of nuclei in the stratum corneum (in normal skin the dead stratum corneum cells do not have nuclei).
- Second, there is a large inflammatory cell infiltrate comprising polymorphs, T cells and other inflammatory cells.

It is uncertain which of these characteristics is primary. Traditionally, psoriasis was viewed primarily as a disorder of cell turnover but in recent years there has been increased support for the hypothesis that the hyperproliferation may be secondary to the inflammatory infiltrate and that the

27

increase in keratinocyte proliferation is a consequence of inflammatory cell mediators or signalling.

There is a large familial component to psoriasis. Formal estimates from twin studies suggest a hereditability of around 80%. In monozygotic twins perhaps one-third of pairs will be concordant for psoriasis. Put another way, two-thirds of monozygotic twins will not be concordant despite an apparently identical or near-identical genetic background.

The mode of inheritance of psoriasis does not fit a clear Mendelian pattern and, like atopic dermatitis, is therefore described as genetically complex. Empirical estimates suggest that if one parent has psoriasis, then the chance of a child being affected is in the order of 15–20%. If both parents have psoriasis, the probability of a child being affected is 0.5. Both these estimates are increased if one sibling already has the disease. Genome scanning linkage and association studies have indicated various chromosomal areas of susceptibility including the HLA region.

Disordered cell proliferation in psoriasis is reflected by the increase in the number of mitoses visible in the psoriatic plaque. The transit time—that is, the time it takes for keratinocytes in the basal layer to leave the epidermis—is shortened in psoriasis from perhaps 28 to 5 days. Whilst it used to be thought that the cell cycle was actually reduced in psoriasis, more recent data suggest that it is just that the proportion of cycling cells (rather than cells that are in G_0) is increased. There are some data suggesting that the non-plaque skin also shows an elevated rate of proliferation, although any increase above background rate is modest. These data have not been confirmed in all studies. The nails of patients with psoriasis, even when clinically unaffected, do, however, grow more quickly than those of controls.

The importance of keratinocyte hyperproliferation initially received support from the demonstration that cytostatic drugs such as methotrexate were clinically useful. However, more recent data suggest that methotrexate may exert its effects primarily through an influence on the immune system.

The evidence implicating a key role for an immune pathogenesis relates to:

- the association with certain HLA groups (HLA Cw6)
- the success of certain immunosuppressive drugs (such as ciclosporin) in improving the clinical state of the disease
- reports of the development of psoriasis in recipients of bone marrow transplants from donors with a history of psoriasis.

The precise molecular mechanisms operating in psoriasis are, however, poorly understood. A large number of theories have been advanced over the last 30 or 40 years claiming that one particular mediator may be a key or rate-limiting factor in psoriasis. The majority of these explanations have not stood the test of time, nor have they provided useful therapeutic insight.

Precipitating factors

Psoriasis is a chronic disease characterised by variation in both temporal and spatial extent. Most of this variation

27.29 FACTORS CAUSING FLARE-UPS OF PSORIASIS
Trauma
● When the condition is erupting, lesions appear in areas of skin damage such as scratches or surgical wounds (Köbner phenomenon)
Infection
● β-haemolytic streptococcal throat infections often precede guttate psoriasis
Sunlight
● Rarely, UVR may worsen psoriasis
Drugs
● Antimalarials, β-adrenoceptor antagonists (β-blockers) and lithium may worsen psoriasis and the rash may 'rebound' after systemic corticosteroids or potent local corticosteroids are stopped
Emotion
● Anxiety precipitates some exacerbations

cannot be explained. At any one time perhaps 10% of people who have received the diagnosis of psoriasis have no lesions and perhaps 15% may report remissions of up to 5 years or more. Some factors, however, are thought to precipitate an exacerbation of the disease and these are listed in Box 27.29.

Pathology

The histology of psoriasis is depicted in Figure 27.23.

Clinical features

Stable plaque psoriasis

This is the most common type. Individual lesions are well demarcated and range from a few millimetres to several centimetres in diameter (Fig. 27.24). The lesions are red with dry, with a silvery-white scale, which may be obvious only after scraping the surface. The elbows, knees and lower back are commonly involved.

Other sites of predilection include:

- *Scalp*. The scalp is involved in approximately 60% of patients with psoriasis. The reason why the scalp is so commonly involved is not clear. Psoriasis of the scalp typically shows well-demarcated, easily palpable areas, but on occasion a diffuse, fine scaling difficult to distinguish from classical seborrhoeic dermatitis may be present. Temporary hair loss is not uncommon and rarely permanent focal hair loss may occur.
- *Nails*. Involvement of the nails is common, with 'thimble pitting', onycholysis (separation of the nail from the nail bed, Fig. 27.25) and subungual hyperkeratosis.
- *Flexures*. Psoriasis involving the natal cleft and submammary and axillary folds is not scaly but red, shiny and symmetrical (Fig. 27.26).
- *Palms*. Psoriasis here is often difficult to recognise, as individual plaques may be poorly demarcated and barely erythematous. It is often impossible to differentiate between psoriasis and eczema of the palms.

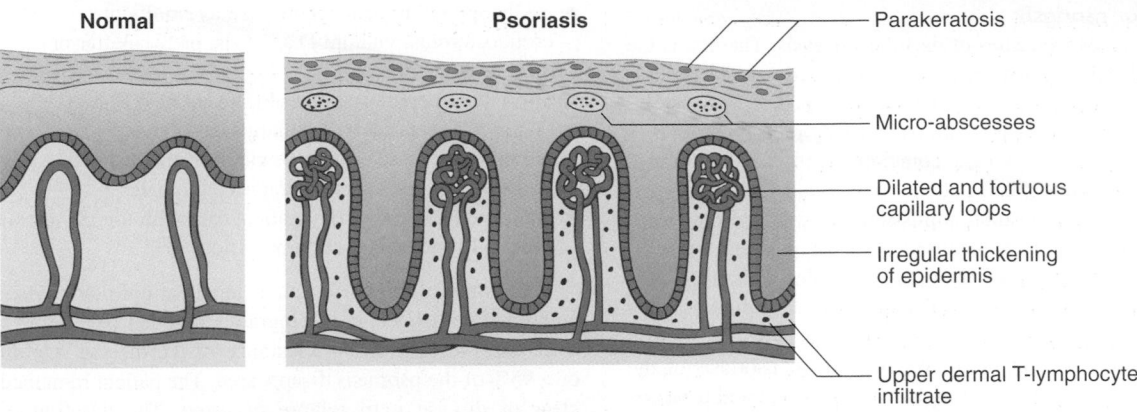

Fig. 27.23   The histology of psoriasis.

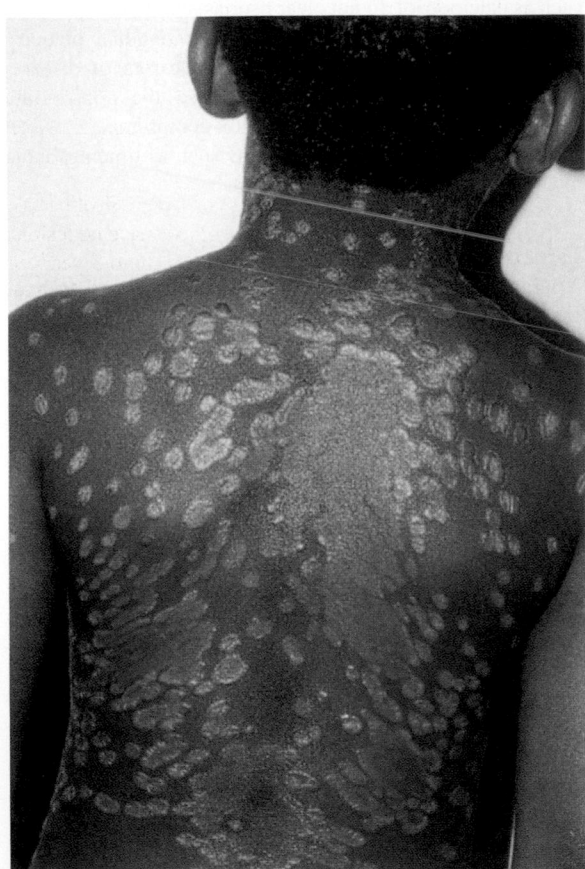

Fig. 27.24   Psoriasis: plaques of varying size in a child.

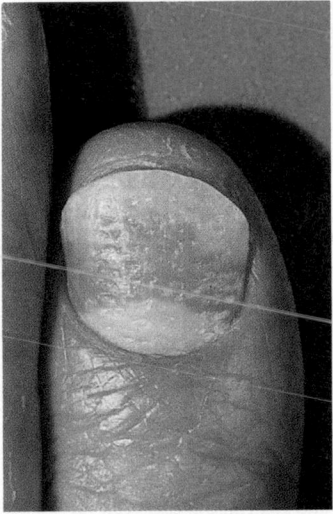

Fig. 27.25   Coarse pitting of the nail and separation of the nail from the nail bed (onycholysis). These are both classic features of psoriasis.

27

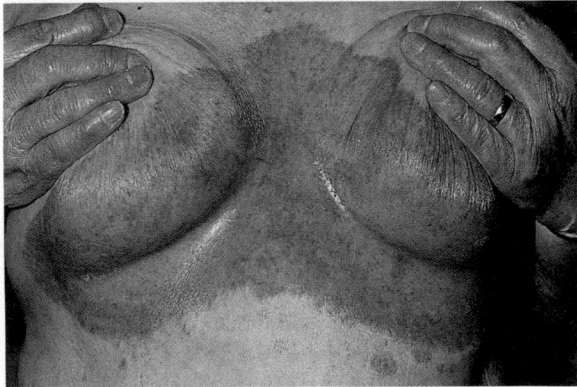

Fig. 27.26   Flexural psoriasis. Note the glistening but not scaly rash.

Guttate psoriasis

This is most commonly seen in children and adolescents and may follow a streptococcal sore throat. In many patients this will be the first clinical indication of the disease. The rash often appears rapidly. Individual lesions are droplet-shaped, small (seldom greater than 1 cm in diameter) and scaly. Bouts of guttate psoriasis may clear in a few months but respond well to early treatment with phototherapy. The majority of these patients will develop plaque psoriasis later in life.

Erythrodermic psoriasis

The skin becomes universally red or scaly, or more rarely just red with very little scale present. As in other forms of erythroderma temperature regulation becomes problematic with a danger of either hypothermia or hyperthermia developing.

Pustular psoriasis

There are two varieties of pustular psoriasis. The first is the generalised form which is rare but very serious. The onset is usually sudden with large numbers of small sterile pustules erupting on a red base. The patient may rapidly become ill with a swinging pyrexia coinciding with the appearance of new pustules. Such patients will usually require urgent assessment and hospital admission to a dermatology ward. More common is a localised form of pustular psoriasis which primarily affects the palms and soles. This eruption is chronic and comprises small sterile pustules which lie on a red base, and resolve to leave brown macules or scaling in their wake. The relation between pustular psoriasis of the palms and the soles (palmoplantar pustulosis) and psoriasis remains disputed by some, although the conditions commonly coexist.

Arthropathy

Between 5% and 10% of individuals with psoriasis appear to have a chronic rheumatoid factor negative inflammatory arthropathy (p. 1109) which can take on a number of patterns (i.e. central, as in ankylosing spondylitis, or peripheral, as in rheumatoid arthritis).

Investigations

Few are indicated. Biopsy is seldom necessary and often contributes little when there is genuine doubt about the diagnosis (for example, in attempting to distinguish between psoriasis and eczema of the palms and soles). Throat swabbing for streptococci or other evidence of recent infection may occasionally be useful. Joint symptoms, unless minor, may require assessment by a rheumatologist.

General management of psoriasis

Explanation, reassurance and instruction are vital but easily neglected; they must be based on insight into the patient's state of mind. In the vast majority of cases psoriasis is not life-threatening and therefore if the treatment appears worse than the disease, then the treatment should be stopped. Often patients need encouragement to take many of the important decisions themselves, albeit with advice from the physician. No two patients, even with identical patterns of psoriasis, have the same experience of the disease.

There is little robust evidence to support the statement that stress exacerbates psoriasis or is causally involved. Certain studies suggest that alcohol consumption is greater amongst some psoriasis patients, but it is not clear whether this is a cause or a result of the disease. What is clear is that doctors need an awareness of the impact that this disease can have on many individuals. For instance, many fathers will, with embarrassment, admit that they cannot take their young children swimming because of the alarm their rash causes to other swimmers. Similarly, blood on the sheets and the ubiquitous scale on bedclothes and carpets may act against many personal relationships. It is said that 'Girls with scalp psoriasis don't wear navy clothes' (the scale being more prominent when viewed against a dark background).

Treatment

Treatment can be classed in four broad categories:

- easily applied topical agents such as emollients, corticosteroids, vitamin D agonists, or 'weak' tar or dithranol preparations
- ultraviolet therapies such as PUVA and UVB
- systemic agents such as retinoids or immunosuppressives such as ciclosporin, or one of a range of new biological therapies ('biologics')
- intensive inpatient or day-patient care with topical agents and UVR under medical supervision.

Traditionally, therapies such as inpatient dithranol, when combined with UVR in the Ingram's regimen (see below), were capable of inducing clearance of the disease, i.e. all or > 95% of the psoriasis disappeared. The patient remained clear of disease until relapse occurred. The duration of remission varied considerably from less than 1 month to over a year. By contrast, many more acceptable treatments such as calcipotriol do not clear psoriasis; rather they reduce the thickness, scaling and redness of individual plaques. Depending on the clinical context and extent of disease, patient and physician need to choose the appropriate endpoint of treatment. This is often a compromise between side-effects, practical considerations such as time available to attend hospital, and disease extent.

Topical agents

A large number of topical agents have been used to treat psoriasis. Emollients have a modest effect in terms of reducing scale and diminishing itch. Many patients feel more comfortable using emollients than not using them.

Dithranol

Traditionally, the gold standard of therapy was treatment with dithranol or crude tar. Dithranol originally came into use in the late 19th century and is now known to be a potent producer of free radicals. Unsurprisingly, when applied to normal skin dithranol is pro-inflammatory and stimulates hyperproliferation, but for reasons that remain unclear it normalises differentiation and inhibits proliferation when applied to psoriatic plaques.

Dithranol is used in two main regimens. The first is Ingram's regimen; the plaques are covered with low concentrations of dithranol in a zinc oxide paste following a tar bath and UVR exposure, and then covered in talcum powder and bandages and left in situ for 24 hours. More recently, short-contact dithranol therapy has been developed in which higher concentrations are applied for between 15 and 30 minutes and then washed off. The main clinical limitation of dithranol is its pro-inflammatory action on normal skin. This presents as 'burning' with pain and erythema, which peaks 72 hours after application. Dithranol also results in a brown staining of the skin and can cause a purple discoloration in individuals with light hair colour. In general, use of dithranol as an inpatient therapy has diminished over the last 20–30 years due to low patient acceptability, the invention of new phototherapy modalities and lack of inpatient beds. As with tar, attempts have been made to make dithranol easier to use and more patient-friendly but efficacy is reduced; these attempts have been largely unsuccessful.

Tar

Tar, particularly crude tar, has been shown to be effective in the treatment of psoriasis. There are certain similarities with dithranol in that tar is pro-inflammatory and has different effects on the plaque compared with normal skin. Unfortunately, as for dithranol, attempts to define the exact therapeutic mechanism and dissociate efficacy from side-effects have been unsuccessful. The more cosmetically acceptable the preparation, the lower its efficacy. As for dithranol, usage is probably diminishing.

Calcipotriol

Calcipotriol is a vitamin D agonist. It seldom clears a plaque of psoriasis but tends to reduce the thickness of the plaque and diminish the scaling. It is applied twice or once daily and, providing no more than 100 g of ointment is used each week, does not cause hypercalcaemia or hypercalciuria. Patients like calcipotriol because it is odourless, colourless and does not stain. Irritation, which is usually transient, is the main side-effect.

Corticosteroids

The hazards of corticosteroids are local skin atrophy and the fact that when they are stopped the psoriasis tends to return. Nevertheless, they are invaluable for many body sites, particularly the flexures where tar and dithranol may be too irritant, and short bursts of moderately potent corticosteroids can be invaluable in the management of many patients. Use of potent topical corticosteroids on the face or hair margins should be under close medical supervision.

Ultraviolet and PUVA therapy

Ultraviolet therapy

Ultraviolet radiation (UVR) forms the mainstay of management of patients with moderate to severe psoriasis. As could be predicted given the known biology of UVR, the main risk of ultraviolet therapies lies in burning in the short term and increased skin cancers in the long term.

There are two main therapeutic modalities in use. It has been known for almost a century that ultraviolet B (UVB) administered therapeutically improves the condition of many patients with psoriasis. To some degree this mirrors the natural improvement that many patients with psoriasis notice in summer. In the past, broadband UVB radiation given 3–7 times a week formed part of the Ingram's regimen using dithranol.

More recently, a particular type of UVB radiation produced by the Philips TL01 lamp (narrowband UVB) has become a very popular modality of treatment delivered 2–5 times a week on an outpatient basis. This lamp peaks at 311 nm and was developed specifically following work showing that shorter wavelength (< 311 nm) radiation, while inflammatory, had little therapeutic efficacy, whilst longer wavelengths (> 311 nm) were also relatively in-effective. The long-term safety of this lamp is, however, less clear. Some argue that it may be more carcinogenic than broadband UVB therapy while others believe it is less carcinogenic. The results of long-term observation are awaited.

PUVA therapy

Psoralens are natural photosensitisers found in a number of plants. In the early 1960s topical preparations of psoralen used in combination with ultraviolet A (UVA) were reported to have therapeutic effects on psoriasis. In the early 1970s a large randomised trial showed that oral psoralen together with long wavelength ultraviolet A (PUVA) was a drama-tically effective treatment for individuals with chronic plaque psoriasis (Box 27.30). Psoralen molecules intercalate between the two strands of DNA and upon excitation with UVA photons cross-link the DNA strands. In this sense PUVA therapy is not a 'light therapy'; rather, psoralen is a pro-drug that upon oral administration is distributed throughout the body but is only activated by UVR in those sites that are exposed to UVA (skin and eye—the latter should be protected).

PUVA treatment induces clearance to a similar degree to intensive dithranol therapy and revolutionised the management of patients with psoriasis. The short-term side-effects are minimal. The therapy can be delivered between 2 and 5 times a week and clearance expected in the majority of individuals within 8 weeks. Clearance will occur in more than 75% of individuals. Some individuals may develop nausea in response to the psoralen; also, because the psoralen is present in the eye, patients need to wear UVR-resistant sunglasses for 24 hours after therapy. The long-term hazards of PUVA therapy give cause for concern but are not surprising because PUVA is by its mechanism of action known to be mutagenic. In patients who have received a large amount of PUVA therapy, particularly 'maintenance therapy' (continuous PUVA lasting for 6 months to a year), there is an elevated risk of squamous and basal cell carcinoma. Recent work suggests that the risk of melanoma may also be increased. Instead of being used orally, psoralens can also be applied to the bath before irradiation with UVA (so-called 'bath PUVA'). A few different psoralen photosensitisers are available that vary in their characteristics. Because of the magnitude of the known carcinogenic hazards of PUVA, UVB phototherapy, particularly narrowband (TL01) is increasingly preferred.

Systemic treatment

Until recently three main systemic agents were used for the management of patients with severe psoriasis: methotrexate, oral retinoids and ciclosporin. Now a fourth choice, namely one of a range of 'biologics', is available.

Methotrexate

Methotrexate has been available for the last 40 years and is highly effective. In dermatological practice it is admin-istered once a week. It seems likely that its mechanism of

27

action involves a cytostatic effect on the immune system rather than a primary effect on keratinocyte or epidermal hyperproliferation. The main hazards of methotrexate are that it is an immunosuppressive, in the absence of appropriate monitoring may dangerously depress the white cell count, and long-term use is associated with hepatic fibrosis and cirrhosis. Liver biopsies may be required to assess cumulative toxicity, and other monitoring of liver damage is essential.

Oral retinoids

Oral retinoids such as acitretin are also effective in some patients with psoriasis. They tend to be particularly effective in pustular psoriasis of the palms and soles but are widely used to improve plaque psoriasis. Systemic retinoids are potent teratogens; following use of acitretin pregnancy is not safe for at least 2 years.

Ciclosporin

Ciclosporin was the first of a number of potent immuno-suppressives to find a role in the management of a minority of patients with psoriasis. Side-effects include hypertension, renal impairment and immunosuppression. Ciclosporin is effective in inducing and maintaining clearance of individuals with psoriasis, but continuous use of this drug is difficult to justify in the vast majority of patients.

Biologics

Recently, a range of new agents including monoclonal antibodies against key pathogenic pathways in psoriasis, including tumour necrosis factor-α (TNF-α), and receptors involved in T-cell trafficking, have become available (e.g. infliximab, etanercept, efaluzimab). Randomised trials show that these agents, which need to be administered parenterally, have varying degrees of activity against psoriasis. They are therefore welcome additions to the therapeutic armamentarium. Head-to-head comparisons with drugs like methotrexate have not been performed, and biologics are extremely expensive. At present they may be considered when other older treatment agents have failed. Their long-term toxicity is unknown, and until this is established, it would seem prudent to restrict their use to third-line agents.

Intensive inpatient care

Intensive inpatient treatment with dithranol or tar is less commonly used than previously. In many parts of the world this is because beds for management of patients with skin disease are not available. Ingram's regimen will produce clearance in over 80% of psoriatics in 3 weeks.

LICHEN PLANUS

Lichen planus is a rash characterised by intensely itchy polygonal papules with a violaceous hue involving the skin and less commonly the mucosae, hair and nails.

Aetiology

The cause is unknown but an immune pathogenesis is suspected as there is an association with some autoimmune diseases such as myasthenia gravis (p. 1252), and with

thymoma and graft-versus-host disease. Rashes with clinical and histological features of lichen planus can occur in chronic active hepatitis, in hepatitis B and C infections, and in patients taking drugs, the most common culprits being gold and other heavy metals, sulphonamides, penicillamine, antimalarials, antituberculous drugs and thiazide diuretics. They also occur in those handling colour developers.

Pathology

There is hyperkeratosis, a prominent granular layer, basal cell degeneration and a heavy T-lymphocyte infiltration in the upper dermis. Degenerating basal cells are seen as colloid (apoptotic) bodies. The T cell–basal cell interaction leaves a 'sawtooth' dermo-epidermal junction. The picture suggests an immune reaction to an unknown epidermal antigen.

Clinical features

Lichen planus tends to start on the distal limbs, most commonly the volar aspects of the wrists (Fig. 27.27), and the lower back. Intensely itchy, flat-topped, pink-purplish papules appear and some develop a characteristic fine white network on their surface (Wickham's striae). New lesions may appear at the site of trauma (Köbner phenomenon) and the rash may spread rapidly to become generalised. Individual lesions may last for many months and the eruption as a whole tends to last about 1 year, often leaving marked post-inflammatory pigmentation. Mucous membrane involvement, comprising an asymptomatic fine white lacy network of pinhead-sized white papules, occurs in about two-thirds of patients (p. 1258). The nails are usually normal but in 10% they may be affected, with changes ranging from longitudinal grooving to destruction of the nail fold and bed. Variants of the classic picture are rare but often diagnostically challenging. They include annular, atrophic, bullous, follicular, hypertrophic and ulcerative types.

Diagnosis

This is usually clear-cut clinically but a skin biopsy can be helpful. Other erythematous scaly conditions should be considered in the differential diagnosis, including guttate

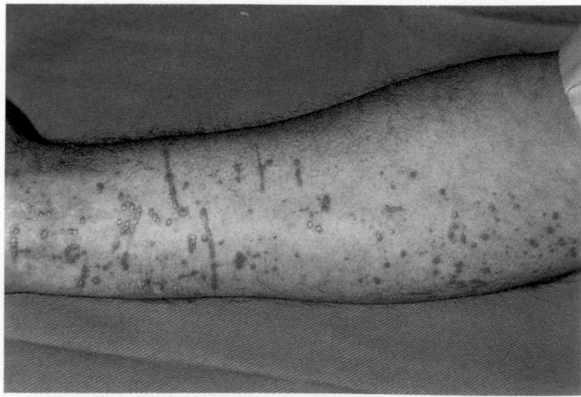

Fig. 27.27 Lichen planus. Glistening discrete papules involving the volar aspects of the forearm and wrist. Note the lesions along scratch marks (Köbner phenomenon).

27.31 PRACTICAL PROBLEMS OF INFLAMMATORY SKIN DISEASE IN OLD AGE

- **Quality of life:** affected due to distress and discomfort.
- **Prognosis:** skin disease is potentially more life-endangering: for example, erythroderma.
- **Depression:** skin disease is cosmetically unattractive, causing depression and increased social isolation.
- **Sleep disturbance and increasing confusion:** caused by irritation, soreness and itching.
- **Delayed presentation:** older people may be reluctant to seek help because of anxiety that they may be perceived as not coping.
- **Topical treatments:** older people may have difficulty administering these, e.g. opening jars and tubes and applying creams during bathing; there is an increased risk of slipping in an oily bath.
- **Patient information:** there is less access to information on skin care.

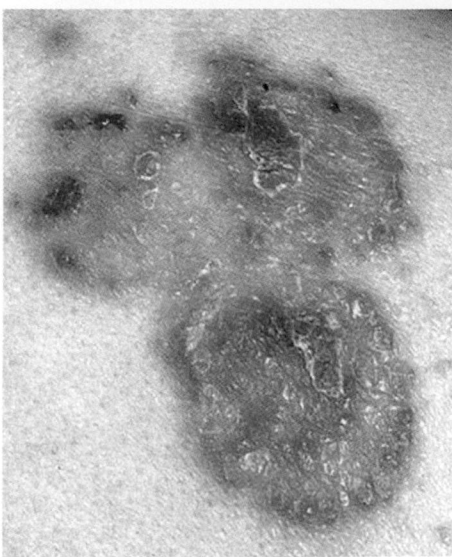

Fig. 27.28　Non-bullous impetigo.

psoriasis, pityriasis rosea, pityriasis lichenoides and drug eruptions.

Management

The condition is usually self-limiting, although rarely, particularly with oral lichen planus, it may persist for more than 10 years. Potent local corticosteroids may help with intense itch but systemic corticosteroids may be indicated, and ciclosporin, retinoids or phototherapy may be required. Topical corticosteroids applied to the buccal mucosa may also be required.

SOME COMMON SKIN INFECTIONS AND INFESTATIONS

BACTERIAL INFECTIONS

IMPETIGO

Impetigo is a common superficial purulent infection of skin caused by species of either *Streptococcus* or *Staphylococcus*. Two forms exist: non-bullous impetigo (Fig. 27.28) and bullous impetigo. Non-bullous impetigo can be caused by either *Staphylococcus aureus* or *Streptococcus* or a combination of the two, and it is not completely clear which organism is more important. It appears that in warmer climates *Streptococcus* is more likely to be the primary organism, but in temperate climates *Staphylococcus* predominates. It can affect all age groups but particularly young children, often in late summer. It is particularly contagious and therefore found most commonly in situations of overcrowding and communal living. Other skin diseases, such as eczema and infestations, predispose to it.

The initial lesion is a thin-walled vesicle which ruptures rapidly with the formation of golden crust on an erythematous base. The sites usually affected are the face and the limbs. Lesions may be single but often rapidly become multiple and coalesce. It is imperative to take a swab for microbiological assessment prior to starting treatment in order to determine the culprit organism.

Treatment is usually with a topical preparation such as mupirocin, which is active against both organisms, or fusidic acid. Topical treatment limits the spread of infection and together with simple washing with soap and water aids in the removal of the infected crusts. In severe or extensive cases an oral antibiotic such as flucloxacillin or erythromycin is indicated. Glomerulonephritis can follow infection with a nephritogenic *Streptococcus*. Since impetigo is so contagious advice should be given on measures to minimise cross-infection.

Bullous impetigo is primarily caused by *Staphylococcus* and most frequently occurs in children. Bullae (often quite large) develop and last for 2–3 days, initially clear and then becoming cloudy. The blisters are caused by a staphylococcal epidermolytic toxin. Once the blisters have burst, crusts develop and management is the same as for the non-bullous form of the disease.

ERYTHRASMA

Erythrasma is a mild localised infection of the skin by a bacterium, *Corynebacterium minutissimum*, which often is part of the normal skin flora. It can cause an asymptomatic or mildly itchy eruption between the toes and in the flexures. The lesions tend to be well defined and reddish-brown in colour, with some scale. Classically, *C. minutissimum* is identified by coral pink fluorescence with Wood's light. Treatment is usually topical, using an azole cream such as miconazole or a topical antibiotic. Oral erythromycin can be used in cases where topical treatment is difficult.

ECTHYMA

Ecthyma is a purulent skin infection caused by either *Staphylococcus* or *Streptococcus* and characterised by ulceration under an exudative crust. It is associated with poor hygiene and malnutrition, and minor trauma can

27

predispose to development of the lesions. It affects any age group and is commonly seen in drug addicts.

FOLLICULITIS, FURUNCLES AND CARBUNCLES

Folliculitis can be superficial, involving just the ostium of the hair follicle (folliculitis) or deep (furuncles and carbuncles).

Superficial folliculitis

This is an extremely common condition that can be subacute or chronic. It is often infective, caused by *Staph. aureus*, but can also be caused by physical (e.g. traumatic epilation) or chemical (e.g. mineral oils) injury. In these cases the folliculitis is usually sterile. Staphylococcal folliculitis is most common in children and often occurs on the scalp or limbs (Fig. 27.29). The pustules usually heal in 7–10 days but can become more chronic, and in older children and adults can progress to a deeper form of folliculitis.

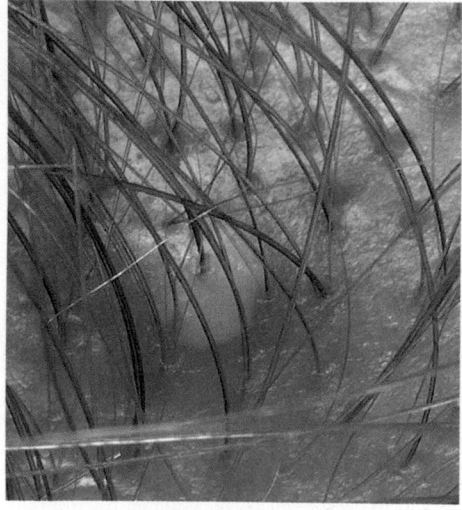

Fig. 27.29 Pustular folliculitis.

Deep folliculitis (furuncles and carbuncles)

A furuncle (or boil) occurs most commonly in adolescence and early adult life. Epidemics can occur with a particular staphylococcal strain but more usually the condition is sporadic. Males are more commonly affected than females. Any body site can be affected but often it is the neck, buttocks and anogenital area. Predisposing factors include tight clothing such as neck ties. Often the affected individual carries the culprit strain of *Staph. aureus* in the nares or perineum. The lesions start as an inflammatory nodule, which becomes pustular and fluctuant and is often very tender. There may be associated constitutional disturbance. The lesions eventually rupture to discharge pus and, because they are deep, leave a scar. They can progress to form a carbuncle, which implies the involvement of several contiguous hair follicles (Fig. 27.30). This usually occurs in middle-aged men and conditions such as diabetes or immunosuppressive therapy predispose to it. A carbuncle is an exquisitely tender nodule, often on the neck, shoulders or hips and associated with severe constitutional symp-

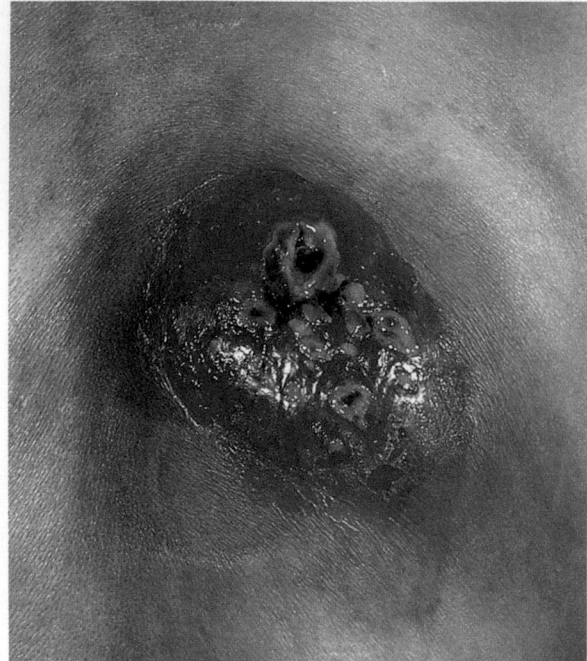

Fig. 27.30 Staphylococcal carbuncle.

toms. The nodules can be up to 10 cm in size and discharge after several days. Treatment, as for furuncles, is with an appropriate antistaphylococcal antibiotic.

STAPHYLOCOCCAL SCALDED SKIN SYNDROME (SSSS)

SSSS (Fig. 27.8A, p. 1274) is a potentially serious exfoliating cutaneous disease that occurs predominantly in children, particularly neonates. The clinical manifestations are due to the protease-like effect of exfoliative toxins from a focus of infection with *Staph. aureus*. These exfoliative toxins (A and B) specifically cleave desmoglein-1 (Fig. 27.2, p. 1261), which is present without desmoglein-3 in the most superficial epidermis. Thus, these toxins cause a split beneath the stratum corneum (Fig. 27.8B) with skin peeling. Clinically, the child is not well and often presents with a focus of infection such as the umbilicus or urinary tract, although most often there is staphylococcus in the nasopharynx which is unrecognised. The child very rapidly develops fever, irritability, skin tenderness and, in severe cases, erythema, often starting in the groin, in the axilla and around the mouth. Blisters and superficial erosions develop within 24–28 hours. The condition can rapidly involve large areas of the skin with significant systemic upset. As the toxins are spread via the blood stream, *Staph. aureus* will be isolated not on a skin swab from the sites of peeling but from the primary site of infection. A bacterial swab should be taken from the nose and throat. A rapid diagnostic technique using a skin snip is demonstrated on page 1274 to determine the level of split within the skin and differentiate it from toxic epidermal necrolysis in which the whole epidermis is affected. Immediate introduction of appropriate systemic antibiotics (e.g. flucloxacillin), and supportive

27

measures in a high-dependency unit if needed, are important. Subsequent bacterial swabs from carrier sites (nostrils, axilla and groin) should be taken from the patient's relatives to exclude staphylococcal carriage.

ANTIBIOTIC RESISTANCE AND MRSA

Meticillin-resistant *Staph. aureus* (MRSA) is becoming an increasing problem within hospitals and in the community (p. 313). Chronic dermatoses and repeated use of prescription antibiotics are important risk factors. The importance of obtaining a bacterial swab in cases of cutaneous infection to identify antibiotic sensitivities is clear. Prevention and treatment of MRSA infection are dependent on local MRSA sensitivities (p. 148).

CELLULITIS AND ERYSIPELAS

Cellulitis (Fig. 27.31) is inflammation, usually infective, of subcutaneous tissue. Erysipelas (Fig. 27.32) is a more superficial involvement of the subcutaneous tissue and lower dermis but the distinction between the two conditions can be difficult. The most common organism causing both these conditions is group A streptococcus. Isolating and identifying the organism is difficult but the clinical history, clinical features including fever, and the associated findings, such as a raised white cell count, usually allow a firm diagnosis. There is often a predisposing cause such as a portal of entry for infection, e.g. tinea pedis, or underlying predisposition to infection such as varicose leg ulcer or diabetes. Erythema, heat, swelling and pain are constant clinical features. Erysipelas has a characteristic raised erythematous edge, indicating involvement of the dermis. It usually affects

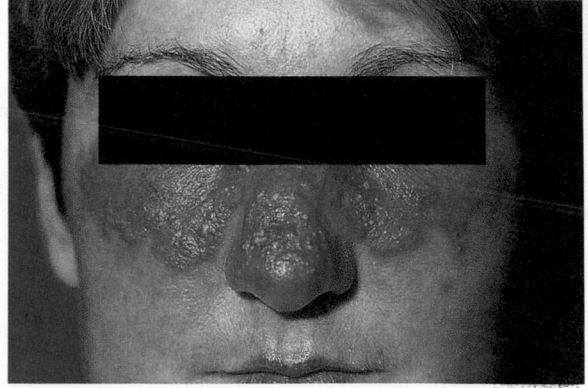

Fig. 27.32　Erysipelas. Note the blistering and crusted rash with raised erythematous edge.

the face or the legs. Cellulitis most commonly involves the legs. Blistering occurs in both conditions (p. 1273). Treatment is with an appropriate antistreptococcal agent such as phenoxymethylpenicillin, or in cases of penicillin sensitivity, erythromycin or ciprofloxacin. In severe cases intravenous antibiotics are indicated.

NECROTISING SOFT TISSUE INFECTIONS

See pages 315–317.

ANTHRAX

See pages 332–333.

VIRAL INFECTIONS

HERPES VIRUS INFECTIONS

There are eight members of the human herpes virus group; these are described on pages 303–306.

PAPILLOMAVIRUSES AND VIRAL WARTS

Viral warts are extremely common and most people suffer from one or more at some point during their life. Genital warts occur most commonly during the sexually active years. Warts are a result of infection with the DNA human papillomavirus (HPV), of which there are over 90 subtypes on the basis of DNA sequence analysis. Different subtypes appear to be responsible for several different clinical wart variants but this is not of great practical importance in terms of skin wart therapy.

Transmission is by direct contact with the virus, in either living skin or fragments of shed skin, and is encouraged by trauma and moisture (e.g. in swimming pools, fishmongers etc.). Genital warts (p. 417), usually due to specific HPV subtypes, are spread by sexual activity, and show a clear relationship with cervical and intra-epithelial cancers of the genital area. In particular, HPV 16 and 18 appear to be able to inactivate tumour suppressor gene pathways and lead to squamous cell carcinoma of the cervix or intra-epithelial carcinoma of the genital skin. In contrast with

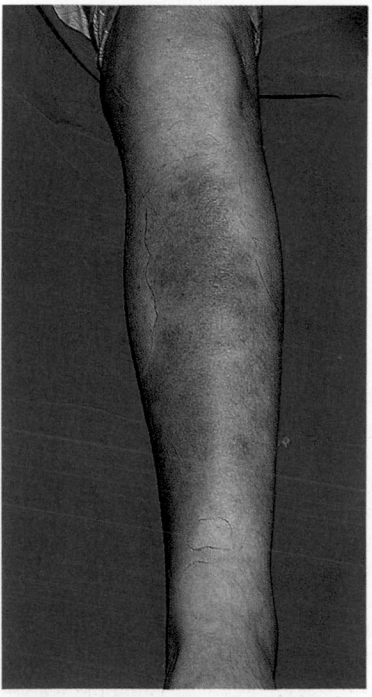

Fig. 27.31　Acute cellulitis of the leg. Note that the margin has been marked to assess progression.

27

genital warts, the relation between HPV of the skin and subsequent skin cancer remains unclear. Individuals who are systemically immunosuppressed, such as those who have received organ transplants, show greatly elevated risks of skin cancer and also a much higher prevalence of infection with HPV. What remains unclear is whether HPV is causally involved in the development of neoplasia or merely reflects the underlying systemic immunosuppression.

Clinical features

Common warts appear initially as smooth, skin-coloured papules. As they enlarge, their surface becomes irregular and hyperkeratotic, producing the typical warty appearance. They are most common on the hands but may also be seen on the face, genitalia and sun-exposed surfaces of the arm and leg. Multiple warts are common. Plantar warts (verrucae) are characterised by a rough surface protruding only slightly from the skin and are surrounded by a horny collar. On paring, the presence of capillary loops distinguishes these plantar warts from corns. Plantar warts may be painful and disabling.

Other varieties of wart include mosaic warts (mosaic-like plaques of tightly packed individual warts, Fig. 27.33); plane warts (smooth, flat-top papules seen most commonly on the face and backs of hands which frequently may hyperpigment and consequently be misdiagnosed); facial warts (often filiform); and genital warts, which may be papillomatous and protuberant.

Management

Viral warts will, in the vast majority of normal individuals, resolve spontaneously. However, this may take several years and there is often considerable pressure for treatment. The majority of treatments are based on destruction of keratinocytes, irrespective of whether they are HPV-infected

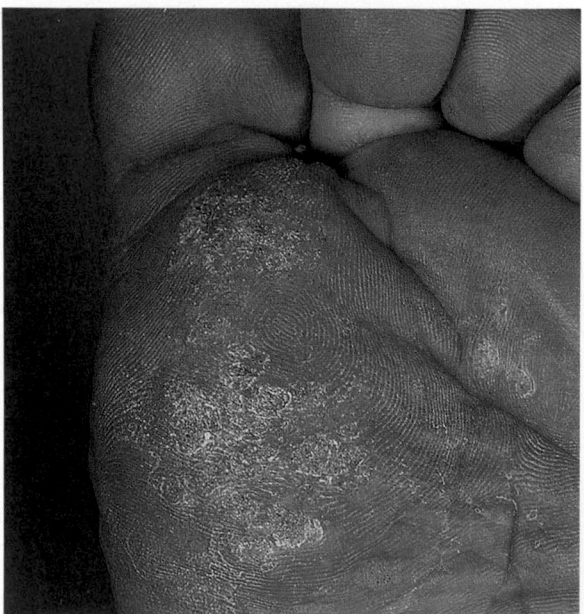

Fig. 27.33 Mosaic plantar wart. A plaque of closely grouped warts on the sole of the foot.

or not. Despite the frequency of the condition, there is a paucity of randomised trials to assess the effectiveness of the various treatments or the order in which they are used.

Most practitioners try to avoid treating warts that are asymptomatic or not causing distress. Initial treatment should be with salicylic acid or salicylic and lactic acid combinations, together with frequent and regular paring of the hyperkeratotic skin. Such treatment needs to continue for at least several months before convincing effects will be apparent. If it fails, or as an alternative, warts can be treated by cryotherapy using liquid nitrogen. Such therapy is, at some sites and in particular individuals, accompanied by significant pain, and needs to be repeated at intervals of 2–4 weeks, although the optimum strategy is not defined. Over-aggressive treatment with cryotherapy, particularly on the hands, can lead to significant complications including tendon rupture and a high morbidity over the ensuing days. Warts close to or under the nails can be a particular problem. Liquid nitrogen treatment may exacerbate them (due to inflammatory swelling), and skilled cutting of the nail and electrodesiccation, or other destructive therapy, may be necessary.

Viral warts can be a particular problem in individuals who are immunosuppressed following organ transplantation. The prevalence of warts in this group approaches 100% after 5 years and therapy appears less effective than in immunocompetent individuals. In the immunosuppressed not only are warts particularly unsightly, but painful verrucae can limit mobility and require intensive treatments. Individuals who have received large amounts of psoralen and UVA (PUVA) for their psoriasis also show an elevated prevalence of viral wart infection.

Beyond the treatments mentioned above, a number of other treatments have been claimed to be effective in some individuals and in particular clinical contexts; these include systemic retinoids, intralesional injections of bleomycin or interferon, and the application of contact sensitisers such as diphencyprone or dinitrochlorobenzene to the warts. The immunomodulator, imiquimod, is useful in treating stubborn anogenital warts (p. 417).

MOLLUSCUM CONTAGIOSUM

Molluscum contagiosum is a common cutaneous infection with a poxvirus. It can affect any age group but usually targets children over the age of 1. The prevalence is also high in individuals who are immunosuppressed. The classic lesion is a dome-shaped, 'umbilicated', skin-coloured papule with a central punctum (p. 378). The lesions tend to be multiple and are often in sites of apposition such as the side of the chest and the inner arm. These lesions resolve spontaneously but can take several months to do so. Prior to resolution they often become quite inflamed and may leave small, discrete, depressed scars. A wide range of therapeutic modalities have been tried but none is very effective and they can be painful; no treatment is an acceptable option. Individual lesions can be removed by curettage under local anaesthetic but the lesions are commonly multiple. Gentle squeezing with forceps after bathing can stimulate regression. Topically applied chemicals such as salicylic acid (topical 5% acidified nitrite co-applied with 5% salicylic acid), podophyllin (topical 0.5% podophyllotoxin) and trichloroacetic acid cause marked inflammation and results vary. Cryotherapy can be tried but is not as effective as gentle squeezing. Physical occlusion with duct tape is advocated by some groups. Most recently, a randomised controlled trial on a small number of patients (n = 23) showed a promising effect of topical 5% imiquimod cream.

ORF

Orf is an occupational hazard for those who work with sheep and goats. It is a cutaneous infection with a parapoxvirus that is carried by these animals. Inoculation of the virus, usually into the skin of a finger, causes significant inflammation and necrosis which usually resolve within 2–6 weeks. No specific treatment is available unless there is evidence of secondary infection. Erythema multiforme can be invoked by orf virus infection.

ERYTHROVIRUS

See page 301.

FUNGAL INFECTIONS

Dermatophytes are fungi capable of causing superficial skin infections known as ringworm or dermatophytosis. The causative fungi belong to three genera (*Microsporum*, *Trichophyton*, *Epidermophyton*); they can originate from the soil (geophilic) or animals (zoophilic), or be confined to human skin (anthropophilic).

Clinical forms of cutaneous infection include tinea corporis (involvement of the body), tinea capitis (scalp involvement, p. 1278), tinea cruris (groin involvement) and tinea pedis (involvement of the feet). Fungal infection of the nails (onychomycosis) is dealt with on page 1283.

Tinea corporis

The clinical features of tinea corporis are variable and so this condition should be considered in the differential diagnosis of the red scaly rash (p. 1267). Classically, the lesions are erythematous, annular and scaly, with a well-defined edge and often central clearing. They may be single or multiple and are usually asymmetrical (Fig. 27.34). The degree of associated inflammation depends on the causative fungus and host immunity. *Microsporum canis* and *Trichophyton verrucosum* are common culprits and are zoophilic (from dogs and cattle respectively). Inadvertent topical corticosteroid application leads to disguising and worsening of the signs (tinea incognito).

Tinea cruris

This common world-wide ringworm affects the groin and is usually caused by *Trichophyton rubrum*. Itchy erythematous plaques extend from the groin flexures on to the thighs.

Tinea pedis (athlete's foot)

This is the most common form of ringworm in the UK and USA and is usually caused by anthropophilic fungi such as *Trichophyton rubrum*, *T. mentagrophytes* and *Epidermophy-*

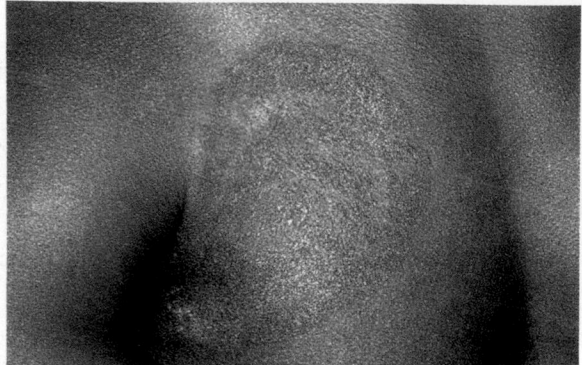

Fig. 27.34   Tinea corporis in a dark-skinned patient.

ton floccosum. Clinical features are an itchy rash between the toes, with peeling, fissuring and maceration. Involvement of one sole or palm (in the case of tinea manuum) with a fine scaling is characteristic of *T. rubrum* infection. Vesiculation or frank blistering is more commonly seen with *T. mentagrophytes*.

Diagnosis

In all cases of suspected dermatophyte infection, the diagnosis should be confirmed by skin scraping or nail clippings (p. 1263).

Management

Treatment can be topical (terbinafine or miconazole cream) or systemic (terbinafine, griseofulvin or itraconazole).

SCABIES

Scabies is caused by the Acarus, *Sarcoptes scabiei*, and is a common world-wide public health problem with an estimated global prevalence of 300 million. The infestation causes considerable discomfort and can lead to secondary infection and complications such as post-streptococcal glomerulonephritis. Scabies spreads in households and environments where there is a high frequency of intimate personal contact. Diagnosis is made by identifying the scabietic burrow, usually found on the edges of the fingers, toes or sides of the hands and feet. Extraction of the mite using a blunt needle can be difficult but is helpful in ensuring the correct diagnosis, appropriate treatment and compliance. Inappropriate application of scabietic treatments can cause considerable irritation in other conditions. In small children the palms and soles can be involved with pustule formation (Fig. 27.35). Involvement of the genital area in boys is pathognomonic. The main symptom is itch (p. 1266). The clinical features include secondary eczematisation elsewhere on the body; the face and scalp are never involved except in the case of infants. Even after successful treatment the itch can continue, and occasionally nodular lesions persist.

Topical treatment of scabies is usual and involves the affected individual and all asymptomatic family members/physical contacts to ensure eradication. Two applications one week apart of an aqueous solution of either permethrin

27

1

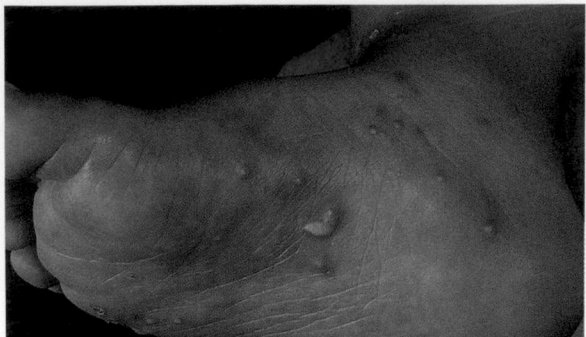

Fig. 27.35 **Scabies.** Pustules at a common site in a child. Burrows were present but cannot be seen at this distance.

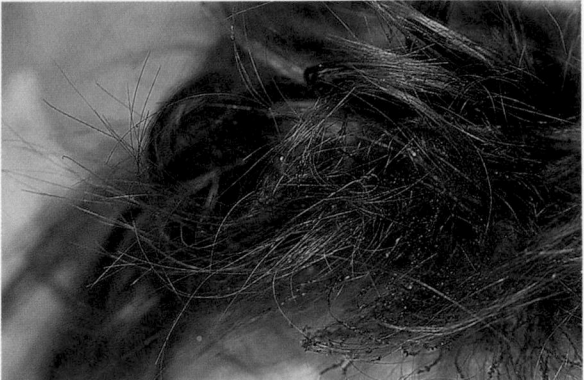

Fig. 27.36 **Head lice.** 'Nits' (empty egg cases) adhere strongly to the hair shafts.

or malathion to the whole body, excluding the head, are usually successful. In some clinical situations such as poor compliance, immunocompromised individuals and heavy infestations (Norwegian scabies), systemic treatment with ivermectin (200 µg/kg) as a single dose is appropriate.

LICE

HEAD LICE

Infestation with head louse, *Pediculus humanus capitis*, is common and highly contagious. Head lice are spread by direct head-to-head contact. Itching of the scalp is the main symptom; scratching leads to secondary infection and cervical lymphadenopathy. The diagnosis is confirmed by identifying the living louse or nymph on the scalp or on a black sheet of paper after careful fine-toothed combing of wet hair that has had conditioner applied. The empty egg cases ('nits') are easily seen along the hair shaft (Fig. 27.36). These are characteristically difficult to dislodge.

Treatment is recommended for the infected individual and any infected household/school contacts. Eradication in school populations has proved difficult and it is likely that this is due to compliance as well as resistance to certain treatments. The standard pharmacological treatments for head lice are malathion, permethrin and carbaryl in a lotion or aqueous formulation, which are applied on two separate occasions at 7–10 days' interval. Many health authorities advise rotational treatments within a community to avoid resistance. Regular 'wet-combing' (physical removal of the live lice by regular combing of slippery, conditioned wet hair) does not seem to be as effective as pharmacological treatments.

Involvement of the eyebrows/eyelashes is best treated by topical Vaseline 12-hourly for at least a fortnight.

BODY LICE

These are very similar to head lice but live on clothing, particularly in seams, and feed on the skin. They are found on individuals with poor hygiene and in overcrowded conditions. Itch is the principal symptom. The skin is excoriated and secondary infection is common. Treatment is directed towards dry cleaning and high temperature washing of clothes. Insecticides have also been used to treat clothes.

PUBIC (CRAB) LICE

These are usually sexually acquired, and pruritus is the main symptom. An aqueous-based treatment of either malathion or carbaryl is the treatment of choice. This should be applied on two occasions to the whole body, as body hair can also be infested. Contacts should also be treated.

PRESSURE SORES

Pressure sores are caused by prolonged pressure-induced ischaemia, when the interface pressure between the patient's body and its supporting surface exceeds capillary closing pressure. Up to 5% of patients over 70 years old in hospital develop pressure sores, but this may rise to 30% in those with a fractured neck of femur. The morbidity and mortality of those with deep ulcers are high.

Aetiology
The main risk factors for pressure sores include:

- *immobility*, e.g. coma, neurological disease with paralysis, surgery, pain, over-use of sedatives, depression
- *hypotension*, e.g. shock, dehydration
- *reduced oxygen availability*, e.g. anaemia, fever, infection
- *peripheral vascular disease*, including diabetic microangiopathy
- *malnutrition*, e.g. malignant cachexia, alcoholism
- *skin condition*, e.g. atrophy due to age or topical corticosteroids, dry/cracked and moist/chapped.

Clinical features
The sore starts as a localised area of erythema and progresses to a superficial blister or erosion. If the cause is not corrected, deeper damage occurs; a black eschar develops which, when removed or shed, leaves a deep and penetrating ulcer, often colonised by *Pseudomonas aeruginosa*. The skin overlying bony prominences, such as the sacrum, greater trochanter, ischial tuberosity, calcaneal tuberosity and lateral malleolus, is especially susceptible.

Management

This is not easy but the following are important:

- prevention by regular repositioning of immobile patients and use of pressure-reducing mattresses in those at high risk
- treatment of risk factors including malnutrition
- débridement of necrotic tissue either by surgery or by enzymatic necrolysis
- systemic antibiotics for spreading infection
- dressings to keep the wound wet and enhance granulation (see ulcers, p. 1276); regular cleansing with normal saline or 0.5% aqueous silver nitrate; semi-permeable dressings such as OpSite
- consideration of plastic surgical reconstruction when the ulcer is clean.

ACNE AND ROSACEA

ACNE VULGARIS

Acne is almost ubiquitous in the teenage years, differences between individuals being a matter of severity of disease and facility with which scarring develops. Peak severity is in the late teenage years but acne may persist into the third decade and beyond, particularly in females. The main clinical issues relate to under-treatment and lack of clinical interest or insight into the patient's condition.

Aetiology

There are three pathogenetic factors (Fig. 27.37):

- The first is elevated sebum excretion. There is a clear relation between severity of acne and sebum excretion rate. In the complete absence of sebum, acne does not occur. The converse, however, is not true; acne may improve in the third and fourth decades despite high sebum excretion. Sebum excretion is therefore necessary for the development of acne but is not sufficient to cause acne on its own. The main determinants of sebum excretion are hormonal, accounting for the onset of acne in the teenage years. Androgens are the principal sebotrophic hormones but progestogens also increase sebum excretion whilst oestrogens reduce it. In the

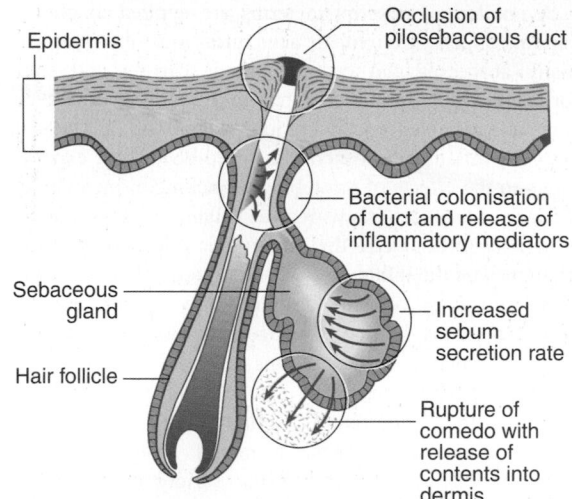

Fig. 27.37   The pathogenesis of acne.

absence of other suggestive clinical features or frank virilism the vast majority of patients with acne have a completely normal circulating endocrine profile.
- The second factor in the pathogenesis of acne is infection with *Propionibacterium acnes*. This bacterium colonises the pilosebaceous ducts and acts on lipids to produce a number of pro-inflammatory factors.
- The third factor is occlusion or blockage of the pilosebaceous unit.

Whilst there is some evidence for a familial component for sebum excretion the genetics and epidemiology of acne have been little studied.

Clinical features

Lesions are usually limited to the face, shoulders, upper chest and back. Seborrhoea (greasy skin) is often clinically obvious. Open comedones (blackheads) due to plugging by keratin and sebum of the pilosebaceous orifice, or closed comedones (whiteheads) due to accretions of sebum and keratin deeper in the pilosebaceous ducts, are usually evident. Inflammatory papules, nodules and cysts occur (Fig. 27.38A), with one or two types of lesion predominating. Scarring may follow.

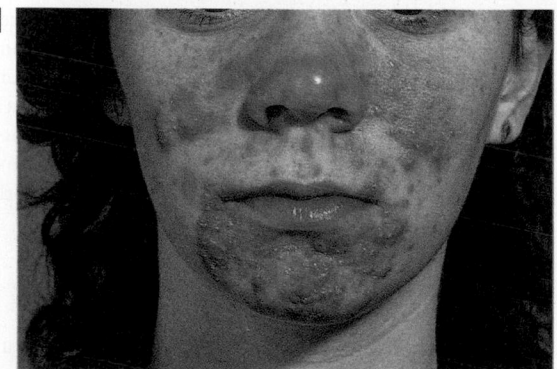
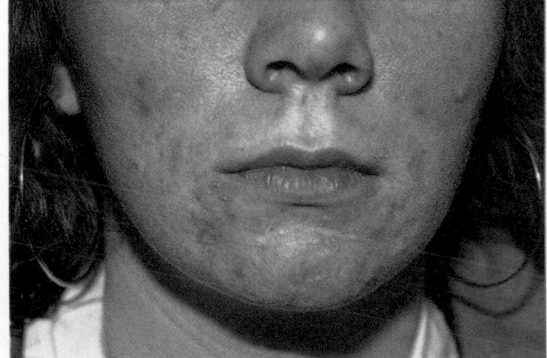

Fig. 27.38   Unpleasant cystic acne in a teenager. A Before treatment. B After prolonged systemic antibiotic treatment.

27

A number of descriptive terms are applied to clinical variants of acne. Conglobate acne refers to severe acne with many abscesses and cysts, marked scarring and sinus formation. Acne fulminans refers to the presence of severe acne accompanied by fever, joint pains and markers of systemic inflammation such as a raised ESR. Acne excoriée refers to the effects of scratching or picking, principally on the face of teenage girls with acne. Infantile acne is rare and is thought to be due to the sebotrophic effects of maternal hormones on the infant.

A mild form of acne dominated by the presence of comedones may be due to exogenous substances such as tars, chlorinated hydrocarbons or oily cosmetics. A primarily pustular rash may also be seen in those being treated with corticosteroids, lithium, oral contraceptives and anticonvulsants. These forms of acne are usually clinically distinct from the usual variety developing in adolescence.

Individuals with moderate or even severe acne very rarely have any other systemic disorder. However, individuals with polycystic ovary syndrome (p. 769) are more likely to have severe acne, and clinical hints—for instance, menstrual irregularities—require investigation. If there is associated cutaneous virilism or other features of an androgen-secreting tumour, further investigations and expert endocrinological assessment are warranted.

Investigations

Investigations are rarely required. It is important, however, to enquire about the details of previous treatments and particularly about their duration; for example, antibiotics are commonly prescribed for too short a period of time. It is also necessary to understand the patient's expectations and to determine how realistic they are.

Management

The advent of systemic retinoids revolutionised the therapy of acne, which is now more straightforward and rewarding. In individuals with fairly minor disease, particularly dominated by the presence of comedones, topical agents such as benzoyl peroxide or tretinoin should be used. Both these substances have irritant activities, a factor which may be important in their therapeutic effect, and instructions should be given on how to use them. They may initially be applied for short intervals of time and the strength and duration gradually increased. Although a number of other topical remedies, including washes, soaps and antiseptics, are recommended, evidence for their effectiveness is not convincing. Patients with anything but minor degrees of acne require therapy with antibiotics, either systemic or local. Local antibiotics (clindamycin or erythromycin) are used more widely than previously; their use should be considered prior to systemic antibiotics or in persons with relatively minor disease, and in combination with other topical agents.

The principal oral antibiotic is oxytetracycline, taken on an empty stomach not with food, in a dose of up to 1.5 g a day if tolerated. In general, oxytetracycline has a good safety profile even with long-term use. Minocycline may be used if the response to oxytetracycline is inadequate or because of the ease of dosing. It is, however, associated with autoimmune hepatitis and remains a second- rather than first-choice drug.

Before an antibiotic is deemed not to have worked, the individual must be treated continuously for up to 3 months. If after 3 months there is little response to oxytetracycline the patient should be changed to erythromycin up to 1 g per day in divided doses. Patients need to remain under review. In women, oestrogen-containing oral contraceptives can be a useful adjunct in therapy. There is a small reduction in sebum secretion with oral oestrogens. An oral anti-oestrogen, cyproterone acetate, is occasionally added in doses of 50–100 mg daily on days 5–14 of the cycle to enhance the effects of sebum reduction. If these topical and systemic agents fail to produce an adequate clinical response within 3–6 months the patient should be referred for specialist opinion and consideration for treatment with isotretinoin (13 cis-retinoic acid).

Isotretinoin has revolutionised the treatment of severe or moderate acne in patients unresponsive to other therapy. When used at a dose of 0.5–1 mg/kg this drug inhibits sebum excretion by > 90% over 4 months. Although sebum excretion gradually returns to normal over the course of the year after the drug is stopped, the clinical benefit is prolonged for much longer. Many patients with acne will not require any further treatment but in a minority a second course of isotretinoin may be required.

Side-effects, especially drying of the skin and mucous membranes, are common but well tolerated and relate to the drug's effects on the function of modified sebaceous glands on the lips, and on lipid biosynthesis in interfollicular epidermis. Rarely, abnormalities of liver function occur and limit treatment. Isotretinoin may elevate serum triglycerides; levels should be checked before therapy and monitored during it. Depression and suicide have been reported, although it is difficult to disentangle the role of the drug from that of the underlying disease and age groups at risk; it is currently under investigation. The major consideration before the drug is prescribed is that, like all systemic retinoids, isotretinoin is highly teratogenic; females must have a negative pregnancy test before treatment and monthly checks, and must be on effective contraception for at least 1 month before the course begins, during the course and for 1 month after it finishes.

Physical measures

Cysts can be incised and drained under local anaesthetic. Intralesional injections of triamcinolone acetonide (0.1–0.2 ml of a 10 mg/ml solution) hasten the resolution of stubborn cysts. Scarring following acne is seen a lot less commonly if patients receive adequate care. Small, deep acne scars can be excised and other forms of more extensive but shallower scars can be treated by carbon dioxide laser.

ROSACEA

Rosacea is a persistent facial eruption of unknown cause characterised by erythema and pustules. Sebum secretion is normal.

27

Clinical features

The disorder is most common in middle age. The cheeks, chin and central forehead are affected (Fig. 27.39). Intermittent blushing is followed by fixed erythema and telangiectasia. Dome-shaped papules and pustules but no comedones occur. Rhinophyma, with erythema, sebaceous gland hyperplasia and overgrowth of the soft tissues of the nose, is sometimes associated. Blepharitis and conjunctivitis are complications.

Diagnosis

This is often obvious on clinical grounds but acne, seborrhoeic eczema, photosensitivity and systemic lupus erythematosus must be distinguished.

Management

The pustular component of rosacea normally responds very well to oral oxytetracycline. Once the disease is controlled (usually within a few months) the dose can be diminished but some individuals may need to stay on the antibiotics long-term or require repeated courses. Topical metronidazole also shows some efficacy in rosacea, although it may cause irritation. Unfortunately, the erythema and telangiectasia do not respond to antibiotic therapy.

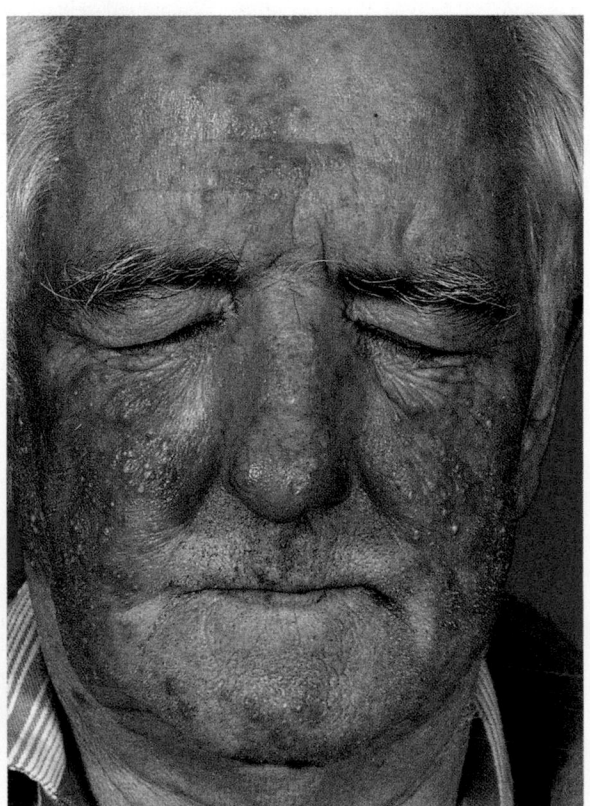

Fig. 27.39 Rosacea. The colour is distinctive and the typical papulo-pustular rash involves the cheeks, centre of forehead and chin.

SKIN TUMOURS

Only the most common benign tumours and a few malignant ones are described in this section.

BENIGN TUMOURS

MELANOCYTIC NAEVI

Melanocytic naevi (moles) are localised benign proliferations of melanocytes which are probably clonal. Their cause is unknown but may relate to abnormalities of the normal migratory pattern of the melanocytes during development. Moles are a usual feature of most human beings and it is quite normal to have 20–50. The number reflects both genetic and environmental characteristics. Interestingly, a locus close to the *p16* gene, which has been implicated in some cases of familial melanoma and other familial cancers (pancreas), appears to exert an effect on mole number. Individuals with high sun exposure also show more moles, i.e. there is clear evidence for both genetic and hereditary factors. With the exception of congenital melanocytic naevi (which are present at birth or appear shortly after), most melanocytic naevi appear in early childhood, at adolescence, and during pregnancy or oestrogen therapy. The onset of a new mole is less common after the age of 25.

Clinical features

Acquired melanocytic naevi are classified according to the microscopic location of the clumps of melanocytes in the skin (Fig. 27.40). Junctional naevi are usually circular and macular; their colour ranges from mid- to dark brown and may vary within a single lesion. Compound and intradermal naevi are similar to one another in appearance; both are nodules of up to 1 cm in diameter, although intradermal naevi are usually less pigmented than compound naevi. Their surface may be smooth, cerebriform or even hyperkeratotic and papillomatous, and they are often hairy.

Using a variety of different criteria, some naevi have been labelled atypical or dysplastic. Unfortunately, the terms have not been precisely defined and are often used to describe a clinical appearance as well as a histological feature. Such abnormal naevi have been found in some individuals with a dramatically increased risk of melanoma. The abnormal melanocyte phenotype does not necessarily predispose to melanoma. Such abnormal naevi are often profuse, large and

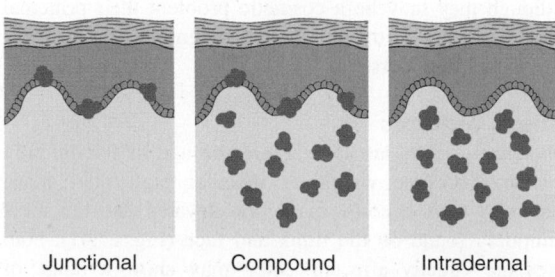

Junctional   Compound   Intradermal

Fig. 27.40 Classification of melanocytic naevi. Classification is based on microscopic location of the clumps of naevus cells.

27.32 SIGNIFICANT CHANGES IN MELANOCYTIC NAEVI

- Itch
- Enlargement
- Increased or decreased pigmentation
- Bleeding
- Irregularity of surface or edge
- Inflammation
- Ulceration
- Alteration in shape

irregularly pigmented and most obvious on the trunk. They may be present on the scalp and the palmar-plantar surfaces as well as the buttocks. Some may appear slightly pinkish and show an inflamed halo. Unfortunately, the clinical significance of such naevi remains poorly defined; most authorities view these individuals as being at an increased risk of melanoma but clear criteria for management and follow-up are not available.

Whereas about 30–50% of malignant melanomas develop from melanocytic naevi, only a minute percentage of melanocytic naevi become malignant. Malignant change is most likely in large congenital melanocytic naevi (where the risk may correlate with the size or mass of the melanocyte lesion) and possibly in those families who have been diagnosed as showing large numbers of atypical naevi with a history of melanoma. Although the skin is easy to observe, the value of self-examination has not been established in randomised control trials. A change in a mole (p. 1264) may well be a harbinger of melanoma but usually is not. In the majority of Caucasian populations, any change in a mole is thought by many to warrant medical opinion (Box 27.32). Such lesions require careful clinical assessment, remembering not only that treatment for all but early melanomas is poor, but also that the negative specificity of the clinical assessment of early melanomas is poor. Excision with histology is therefore frequently recommended.

Management

Melanocytic naevi are normal and do not require excision except when malignancy is suspected or when they repeatedly become inflamed or traumatised. Some individuals wish to have them removed for cosmetic reasons.

SEBORRHOEIC WARTS (BASAL CELL PAPILLOMA)

Seborrhoeic warts are common benign epidermal tumours. They are described as seborrhoeic because they often appear oily, but they have nothing to do with sebaceous glands. Although they may be a cosmetic problem their principal significance lies in the differential diagnosis of melanoma or other skin tumours.

Clinical features

Seborrhoeic warts are rare before the age of 35. Initially they may become visible as macular pigmented areas. They may then become markedly elevated and are most commonly found on the trunk and face (Fig. 27.41); both sexes are equally affected. They may show a range of appearances and vary in colour from yellow to very dark brown, and in shape from fairly flat to a protuberant and

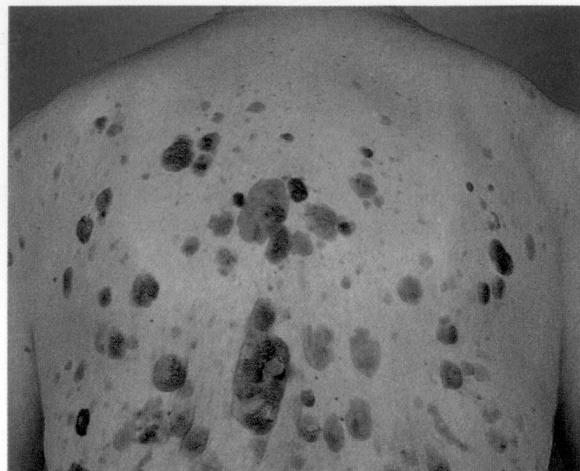

Fig. 27.41   Multiple seborrhoeic warts.

'stuck-on' appearance; they may even be pedunculated. Their surface often appears rather greasy and may show some sealing with pinpoint keratin plugs, which can be of diagnostic use in excluding melanoma.

Investigations

Biopsy is rarely necessary but malignant melanoma may on occasion be indistinguishable on clinical appearance alone.

Management

Seborrhoeic warts may be left alone, or they can be treated by curettage under local anaesthetic or by cryotherapy. Sometimes seborrhoeic keratoses are particularly itchy and therapy of a number of lesions may be required.

KERATOACANTHOMA

This is a striking benign keratinocyte tumour characterised by a period of rapid growth of a lesion that may be 4 or 5 cm across or even larger, with a central keratin plug in a dome-shaped nodule (p. 1259). Spontaneous resolution occurs but may take months and often results in an unsightly scar which could be improved by excision of the lesion. Clinically and histologically the lesion resembles a squamous cell carcinoma but it shows a different natural history. If there is any doubt, lesions are better managed as squamous cell carcinomas. To make a positive diagnosis of keratoacanthoma a large biopsy reflecting the architecture of the lesion is required.

MALIGNANCY: INCIDENCE AND RISK FACTORS

In most Caucasian populations non-melanoma skin cancer (principally comprising basal and squamous cell carcinoma) is the most common human malignancy. Each year one million Americans develop new basal cell carcinomas. Fortunately, the majority of these tumours are easy to diagnose and can be managed relatively simply with a low morbidity and an extremely low mortality.

The main risk factor for most forms of skin cancer is exposure to UVR in the absence of adequate melanin pigmentation. The evidence for the important role of environmental UVR and pigmentation is:

- The body site distribution of skin cancer, with the frequently or intermittently exposed sites predominating.
- The increased risk of tumours in those with pale skin and the low rates in those with black skin.
- The increased tumour rates in those with pale skin who have migrated to areas of high sun exposure (such as red-headed individuals from the British Isles who move to Australia).
- The grossly elevated risks of skin cancer in individuals with a focal defect in the ability to repair UVR DNA damage. Such individuals with xeroderma pigmentosum have an increased risk of both non-melanoma and melanoma skin cancers as well as a variety of other clinical features involving the central nervous system. Their defect in DNA repair is almost completely confined to the inability to repair UV-induced damage (rather than, say, X-ray radiation) and they therefore illustrate the important step of UVR-induced damage.

Although UVR is the major environmental determinant of skin cancer, the various tumour types show different body distribution. For example, squamous cell carcinomas and actinic keratosis occur at the sites of highest cumulative UVR exposure, with the backs of the hands and the scalps of bald-headed individuals showing the greatest tumour density (Box 27.33). In contrast, basal cell carcinomas tend to be disproportionately common on the face, perhaps reflecting their appendageal origins. There is a different body site distribution for melanoma, with tumours relatively more common on areas of skin that may have received intermittent sun exposure. This has led to the suggestion that intermittent sun exposure or episodes of burning may be important, although the epidemiological evidence in favour of burning rather than other aspects of exposure is inconclusive.

The attributable risk of other causes of skin cancer is by contrast small, but ionising radiation or systemic immunosuppression (as seen in people who have received heart or kidney transplants) greatly increases the risk of squamous cell cancer (Box 27.34).

PRE-MALIGNANT TUMOURS

ACTINIC KERATOSIS

Actinic keratoses are small, scaly, red areas on sun-exposed sites that show focal areas of dysplasia on histological examination (Fig. 27.42). They are extremely common and frequently multiple; in some surveys over half the population aged over 40 have one or more lesions. Their relation to squamous cell cancer is still under examination. The rate of progression to squamous cell carcinoma appears low (1:1000 per year per lesion) and a large proportion of actinic keratoses may spontaneously involute. By contrast, many squamous cell carcinomas arise without evidence of a previous actinic keratosis. If an actinic keratosis rapidly increases in size, ulcerates, bleeds or becomes painful, then its potential for transformation to squamous cell carcinoma should be considered.

Management
Actinic keratoses are treated easily and effectively with liquid nitrogen. If there is a large number of lesions, then the topical cytotoxic 5-fluorouracil may be required; alternatively, the topical immunostimulant, imiquimod, or photodynamic therapy (see below) may be used. Lesions which do not respond to treatment may require curettage or excision and reconsideration of their nature.

27

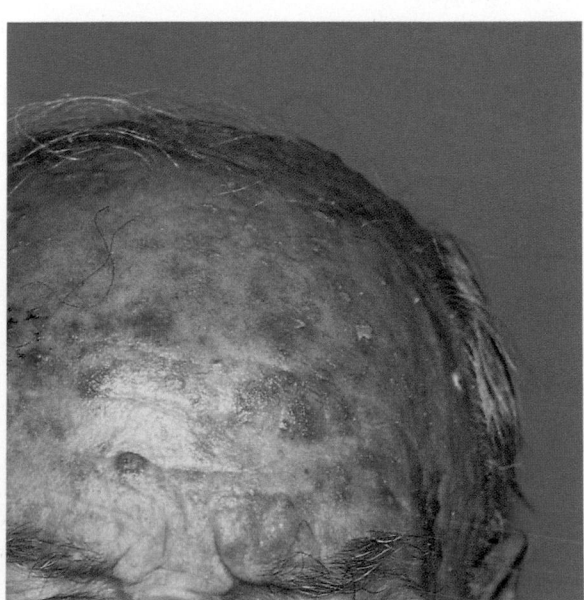

Fig. 27.42 **Numerous actinic keratoses in a white patient who had lived for years in the tropics.**

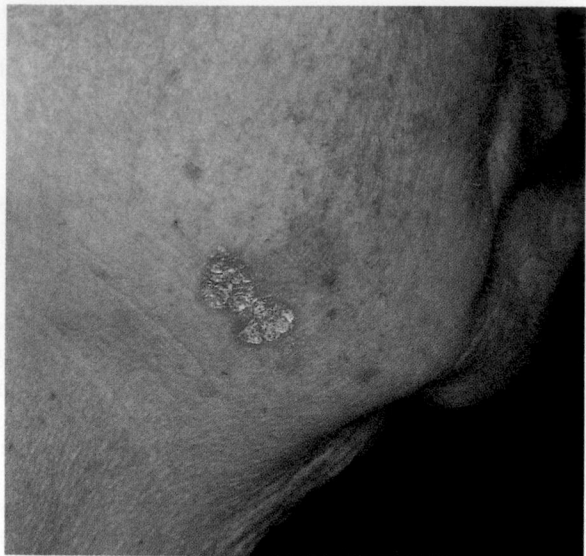

Fig. 27.43 Intra-epidermal carcinoma (right cheek). This persistent psoriasis-like plaque recurred after the original (anterior) lesion was treated by freezing.

INTRA-EPIDERMAL CARCINOMA (BOWEN'S DISEASE)

Clinical features

This usually presents as a slow-growing, red, scaly area with some resemblance to a plaque of psoriasis, on the lower leg of elderly females. Histology reveals full-thickness dysplasia. Lesions may occur at other sites (Fig. 27.43), and occasionally develop into squamous cell carcinomas. They should probably be viewed as being at greater risk of transforming into squamous cell cancer than actinic keratoses.

Investigations and management

An initial incisional biopsy may be required and treatment is local destruction. Alternatively, the lesions may be managed with curettage and subsequent histology. Curettage, however, does not usually allow a squamous cell carcinoma to be positively diagnosed or excluded (because the tissue architecture is not preserved). Alternatives are cryotherapy or photodynamic therapy (see below) or imiquimod.

MALIGNANT TUMOURS

BASAL CELL CARCINOMA (BCC)

This is the most common human cancer. Rates are five times higher than for squamous cell carcinoma in European countries. Classically, lesions are slow-growing and ulcerated, with a pearly and telangiectatic edge; they occur on the face of an elderly individual. The tumour invades locally but rarely metastasises. In practice it is managed as though it does not metastasise unless it is particularly large or has been present for a long time. 'Rodent ulcer' is a term commonly used for slowly expanding ulcerative

basal cell carcinoma. The malignant cells resemble basal keratinocytes.

Clinical features

The most common type is the nodulo-ulcerative form. The earliest lesion is a small, glistening, skin-coloured papule, often with fine telangiectatic vessels on the surface, which slowly enlarges. Central necrosis may occur, leaving an ulcer surrounded by a rolled pearly edge (Fig. 27.44). Without treatment, lesions may reach 1–2 cm in diameter over 5–10 years. Slow but relentless growth causes local tissue destruction. Sometimes this type of tumour becomes cystic or pigmented. The morphoeic variant of basal cell carcinoma is a slowly expanding, yellow or grey waxy plaque with an ill-defined edge. Fibrosis often follows ulceration and crusting, and the lesion may appear as an enlarging scar. The superficial (multifocal) variant is seen most often on the trunk; it appears as a slowly enlarging pink or brown scaly plaque with a fine 'whipcord' edge and may resemble a patch of intra-epidermal carcinoma (see above). If left, it may grow to 10 cm in diameter.

Management

The majority of basal cell carcinomas are easily treated with local destruction. Metastasis is extremely rare; nevertheless, caution should be exercised—for instance, in tumours close to the eye margins where local invasion can cause considerable management difficulty, or in tumours which can track down nerves such as the infraorbital.

The choice of treatment modality depends on local expertise and interest and includes surgery, cryotherapy, radiotherapy, photodynamic therapy or the topical immuno-stimulant imiquimod. Depending on tumour subtype, all are equally effective in expert hands. Surgery is, however, increasingly seen as the first choice, as it allows proper histological assessment of the tumour and examination of tumour margins. Curettage and cautery also show a good result for some small lesions, particularly if they are superficial and not close to the eye. Cryotherapy has a significant morbidity when used for anything other than superficial lesions. Radiotherapy was used extensively in

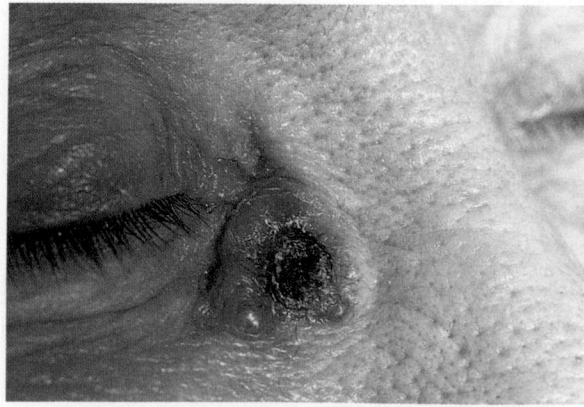

Fig. 27.44 Basal cell carcinoma. A slowly growing pearly nodule just below the inner canthus. The central crust overlies an ulcerated area.

the past but is less popular now. Fractionated doses can reduce the morbidity of radiotherapy but in general surgical excision results in a better cosmetic effect with lower morbidity.

The importance of control of tumour margins is widely debated. Many authorities believe that Mohs' surgery, in which the complete margins of the excised tissue are examined histologically, is of benefit but the present indications for this approach are subject to debate and there is an absence of robust clinical studies. Whatever modality of treatment is used, in expert hands the cure rate should be greater than 90%. Tumour recurrences can subsequently be treated. Some tumours can be very misleading in terms of clinical assessment of their margins and should be examined by a dermatological surgeon. If the primary tumour is not completely excised, a wait-and-see policy is often recommended, depending on the clinical context.

SQUAMOUS CELL CARCINOMA (SCC)

SCC is the second most common skin cancer after BCC and like other forms of skin cancer is increasing in age-specific incidence.

Aetiology

The risk factors for SCC are similar to those of BCC: namely, exposure to UVR, pale skin, or rarely exposure to other carcinogenic factors such as X irradiation or arsenic injection. SCC may arise in long-standing areas of inflammation such as around a chronic cutaneous ulcer, or in patients with scarring genetic syndromes of the skin such as dystrophic epidermolysis bullosa, in which up to 50% of patients may develop SCC. There is also a greatly elevated incidence in individuals who are receiving chronic immunosuppression following organ transplantation (particularly kidney and heart) and in individuals who have been treated with large amounts of PUVA therapy.

Clinical features

SCC is a proliferative tumour that has a history of growth over a few months. Varying clinical presentations include keratotic nodules (Fig. 27.45), exophytic erythematous nodules, infiltrating firm tumours and ulcers with an indurated edge. Histological grade also varies from well-

differentiated to anaplastic. SCCs of the lip behave more aggressively and show a greater frequency of metastasis. It is often said that SCCs of the pinnae may also be more aggressive, although it is not clear whether this reflects inadequate primary treatment.

Management

As with basal cell carcinoma, a number of modalities may be used, including aggressive curettage and cautery, excision or radiotherapy. In general, excision with assessment of adequacy of margins is the preferred option because of the definite risk of metastasis. Surgical excision with a 3–4 mm margin has a cure rate of 90% or more. As with BCC, radiotherapy can be used in selected cases.

MALIGNANT MELANOMA

Malignant melanoma, like other forms of skin cancer, has shown an increase in incidence over recent decades. This increase persists even when changes in the age structure of the population are accounted for. Melanomas show a significant mortality with a case fatality of approximately 20–25%. Therapy for metastatic melanoma is extremely poor and therefore interest has concentrated on primary prevention and early detection (p. 1264). The main risk factors for melanoma are UVR exposure, pale skin, naevi number and family history. Fewer than 10% of melanomas occur in the context of a significant family history but within this group there are rare kindreds in whom the lifetime risk of melanoma may approach 50%. The body site distribution of melanoma is different from that of other skin tumours, suggesting that some aspect of the relation between UVR and tumour occurrence is as yet not fully understood. The increase in melanoma incidence with ambient UVR exposure is also not as steep as that seen for SCC; for example, a threefold increase in environmental UVR exposure may increase SCC rates by a factor of 9 but melanoma by a factor of 3.

Clinical features

The classification of invasive malignant melanomas is shown in Box 27.35.

Two-thirds of invasive melanomas are preceded by a superficial and radial growth phase characterised by an expanding, irregularly pigmented macule or plaque. Its margin is usually irregular with reniform projections (Fig. 27.46). Lentigo maligna (in situ changes of malignancy only) and lentigo maligna melanoma occur most

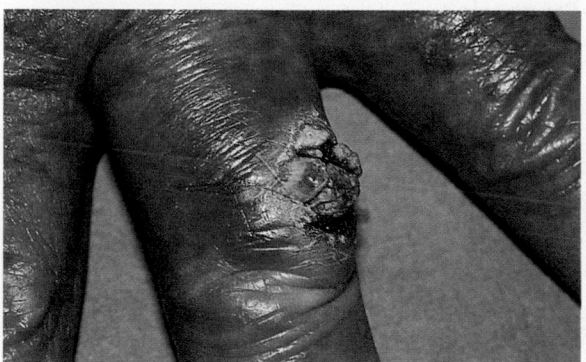

Fig. 27.45 Squamous cell carcinoma. A warty nodule with induration of the adjacent skin.

27.35 CLASSIFICATION OF CUTANEOUS MALIGNANT MELANOMA	
Type of invasive melanoma	Presence of preceding in situ/ radial growth phase
Superficial spreading	+
Lentigo maligna	+
Nodular	−
Acral lentiginous	+

27

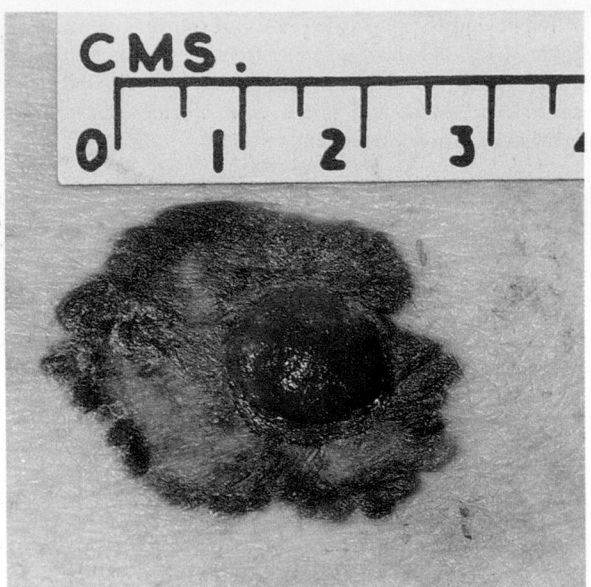

Fig. 27.46 Superficial spreading melanoma. The radial growth phase was present for about 3 years before the invasive amelanotic nodule developed within it. Note the irregular outline, asymmetrical shape and different hues, including depigmented areas signifying spontaneous regression.

often on the exposed skin of the elderly. A speckled macular lentigo maligna may have been present for many years before a nodule of invasive melanoma appears within it. The in situ phase of superficial spreading melanoma, the most common type in Caucasians, seldom lasts for longer than 2 years, usually shows much colour variation and is often palpable. Acral lentiginous melanoma occurs on the palms and soles and the absolute incidence rates are the same in all populations; by contrast, the rates at other body sites are low in Blacks and in the Chinese and Japanese. These facts suggest that this variant of melanoma is not related to UVR exposure. Nodular melanoma develops as a pigmented nodule with no preceding in situ phase. All changing pigmented lesions deserve careful examination remembering the 'ABCDE' features of malignant melanoma (p. 1265). About 30–50% of melanomas appear to develop in a preceding melanocytic naevus (p. 1265). A change in any naevus should raise suspicion of malignant transformation.

True amelanotic melanomas occur but are rare; flecks of pigmentation can usually be seen with a lens. Subungual melanomas present as painless, expanding areas of pigmentation under a nail and usually involve the nail fold.

The clinical stages of malignant melanoma are shown in Box 27.36.

The diagnosis should be established by local excision biopsy of the suspected lesion.

Management

Surgical excision is usually required, although very rarely radiotherapy may play a role. The extent of normal tissue that needs to be removed around a melanoma remains a subject for debate. Most would agree that a clear margin needs to be present so that there is little doubt that the tumour is fully excised; the deeper the tumour, the more caution is warranted (Box 27.37). The majority of tumours can be excised without the need for grafting. The role of local lymph node dissection in the absence of evidence of tumour spread is uncertain. Recently, as with other human tumours, attempts have been made to determine whether the local nodes are 'subclinically' involved using the technique of sentinel lymph node biopsy. In this technique, the draining lymph node is identified by injection of radio-isotope adjacent to the primary tumour, the node identified using radioscintigraphy, and then removed and examined for 'occult' tumour using histology with or without immuno-histology or polymerase chain reaction amplification of melanocyte gene products. Such a biopsy provides some prognostic information, and some would argue that local lymph nodes should be removed if affected. Whether this improves outcome is unknown. Palpable local nodes in stage II patients should be removed by block dissection. Chemotherapy is only exceptionally curative but may play an important palliative role in those with stage III disease or earlier. Interferon-alpha may have a role in individuals at high risk of metastasis.

Prognosis

There are a number of useful prognostic indicators in melanoma. Those with clinical stage III disease fare least well (less than 10% survive 2 years); those with stage I disease have a 70% chance of surviving 5 years. The thickness of the tumour (measured microscopically by Breslow's method, which gives the distance between the granular cell layer and the deepest part of the tumour) is a reliable predictor of the prognosis for patients with stage I disease. The prognosis is excellent for those with tumours less than 1 mm thick (over 90% survive 5 years), but becomes less good with thicker tumours. The 5-year survival of patients with tumours greater than 3.5 mm thick is about 50%. In general, females fare better than males and tumours at certain sites (e.g. lower leg) are less aggressive.

27

CUTANEOUS T-CELL LYMPHOMA (MYCOSIS FUNGOIDES)

In contrast to B-cell lymphomas, which usually present as sudden focal skin tumours, cutaneous T-cell lymphoma develops slowly over many years from a plaque stage often resembling psoriasis through to nodules and then a systemic stage. The diagnosis of cutaneous T-cell lymphoma requires a high index of suspicion, particularly in patients who are deemed to have unusual forms of eczema or psoriasis and who have failed to respond to treatment. The treatment of individuals with cutaneous T-cell lymphoma is, however, symptomatic and there is no evidence that the various modalities of treatment alter prognosis. Study of these individuals is hampered by difficulties in disease nosology, disease heterogeneity and the long natural history, sometimes over 20 or 30 years.

In the early stages of cutaneous T-cell lymphoma either systemic or local corticosteroids may be indicated; alternatively, PUVA or TL01 phototherapy may be employed, although such treatments are of symptomatic use only and are not risk-free. However, once lesions have moved beyond the plaque stage other modalities, including electron beam radiation or systemic anti-lymphoma regimens, may be required. Treatment of such patients requires careful collaboration between dermatologists, pathologists and haematological oncologists.

THE SKIN IN SYSTEMIC DISEASE

Skin reactions can be linked with an underlying systemic disease in a number of ways, as shown in Box 27.39. Only common or important associations will be discussed below.

NEUROFIBROMATOSIS: TYPE 1 (NF1)

NF1 is one of the most common autosomal disorders with an estimated incidence of 1:2500–3000. The characteristic cutaneous features are multiple large light brown macules (café au lait macules), axillary freckling, iris hamartomas (Lisch nodules) and cutaneous neurofibromas (Fig. 26.50, p. 1238). Often these features are apparent early in childhood. Café au lait macules are also a feature of Albright's syndrome (polyostotic fibrous dysplasia) and Bloom's syndrome. The morbidity of NF1 is due to the unpredictable

occurrence of associated abnormalities in other organ systems which can affect about 50% of individuals. These include tumours such as optic gliomas, spinal neurofibromas, phaeochromocytomas, and bony abnormalities such as scoliosis. Involvement of several specialists is therefore important for optimal management of these individuals.

NEUROFIBROMATOSIS: TYPE 2 (NF2)

See page 1237.

SEGMENTAL NEUROFIBROMATOSIS: TYPE 5

The cutaneous features of café au lait macules and neurofibromas are found in a dermatomal distribution. This is due to mosaicism of the NF1 gene.

TUBEROUS SCLEROSIS

This is an autosomal dominant condition with hamartomas affecting many systems.

The classic triad of clinical features comprises mental retardation, epilepsy and skin lesions but not all are invariably present. The skin signs include small white oval (ash leaf) macules, pink or yellowish papules on the centre of the face ('adenoma sebaceum' due to angiofibromas), peri- and subungual fibromas, and connective tissue naevi

27

(cobblestone-like plaques at the base of the spine, sometimes called shagreen patches).

Other features may include hyperplastic gums, retinal phakomas (fibrous overgrowth), renal, lung and heart tumours, cerebral gliomas and calcification of the basal ganglia.

XANTHOMAS

These deposits of fatty material in the skin, subcutaneous fat and tendons may be the first clue to primary or secondary hyperlipidaemia (p. 446).

Various clinical patterns are seen which correlate well with the underlying cause. They include:

- eruptive yellow papules on the buttocks (eruptive xanthomas (Fig. 16.15, p. 447))
- yellowish macules or plaques (plane xanthomas)
- small yellow-grey plaques around the eyes (xanthelasma palpebrarum)
- nodules over the elbows and knees (tuberous xanthomas)
- subcutaneous nodules attached to tendons, especially those on the dorsal aspect of the fingers and the Achilles tendons (tendinous xanthomas (Fig. 16.15, p. 447)).

When xanthomas are detected, the fasting blood lipids and the electrophoretic pattern of plasma lipoproteins must be measured (p. 446), although abnormalities will not always be detected.

AMYLOIDOSIS

This is described on page 79. Skin lesions are uncommon in systemic amyloidosis secondary to rheumatoid arthritis or other chronic inflammatory diseases.

Deposits of amyloid in the skin, often appearing as waxy plaques around the eyes, are prominent in primary systemic amyloidosis and in amyloid associated with multiple myeloma. 'Pinch purpura', appearing where the skin is traumatised, is due to amyloid infiltration of blood vessels and may also be a striking feature.

PORPHYRIA

The classification and metabolic abnormalities of the porphyrias are found on page 451. Certain porphyrias can affect the skin.

Porphyria cutanea tarda

This is the most common porphyria. It usually starts in adulthood and can be inherited or acquired due to alcohol, iron overload, oestrogens, hepatitis C and HIV disease. The cutaneous features are increased skin fragility, blistering (Fig. 27.47), erosions and milia occurring on light-exposed areas such as the backs of the hands. Patients rarely associate their symptoms with acute light exposure. Facial hypertrichosis and hyperpigmentation may also be seen. Diagnostic tests and treatment for the porphyrias are detailed on pages 451–453.

Erythropoietic protoporphyria

This is a rare porphyria that starts in childhood, with burning and pain on light-exposed areas due to ferrochelatase defi-

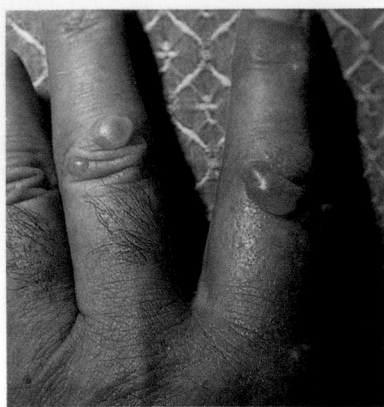

Fig. 27.47 Cutaneous hepatic porphyria. Recent skin fragility and blistering on the backs of the fingers.

ciency. Scars occur, particularly on the nose. Examination of the red cells, plasma and stool for protoporphyrins is confirmatory.

Variegate porphyria

Cutaneous features are similar to those of porphyria cutanea tarda. Systemic features are the same as those of acute intermittent porphyria (p. 451).

Hereditary coproporphyria

Around 30% of these patients are photosensitive. Systemic features are the same as those of acute intermittent porphyria.

Pseudoporphyrias

Sun-bed usage, NSAIDs (particularly naproxen) and renal failure can give rise to skin lesions that mimic the photosensitive porphyrias, particularly porphyria cutanea tarda. The pathogenesis is as yet unclear.

SARCOIDOSIS

This is covered in detail on page 715.

Skin lesions are seen in about one-third of patients with systemic sarcoidosis. The clinical features include erythema nodosum (Fig. 19.51, p. 716), granulomatous deposits in long-standing scars, dusky infiltrated plaques on the nose and fingers (lupus pernio), and scattered brownish-red, violaceous or hypopigmented papules or nodules which vary in number, size and distribution.

ERYTHEMA MULTIFORME

As its name implies, this is a reaction pattern of multiform erythematous lesions. The precipitating factor may not be found in some cases but attacks are provoked by the factors listed in Box 27.40.

Clinical features

The multiform erythematous lesions may be urticaria-like and some have obvious 'bull's-eye' or 'target' lesions. Blisters may be seen in the centre or around the edges of the lesions (Fig. 27.48). In some cases blisters dominate the picture; the Stevens–Johnson syndrome is severe bullous erythema multiforme with emphasis on mucosal involve-

27

27.40 PROVOKING FACTORS IN ERYTHEMA MULTIFORME

- Herpes simplex infections
- Other viral infections, e.g. orf, and mycoplasma
- Bacterial infections
- Drugs, especially sulphonamides, penicillins and barbiturates
- Internal malignancy or its treatment with radiotherapy

27.41 PROVOKING FACTORS IN ERYTHEMA NODOSUM

Infections

- Bacteria (streptococci, tuberculosis, brucellosis and leprosy), viruses, mycoplasma, rickettsia, chlamydia and fungi

Drugs

- e.g. Sulphonamides and oral contraceptives

Systemic disease

- e.g. Sarcoidosis, ulcerative colitis and Crohn's disease

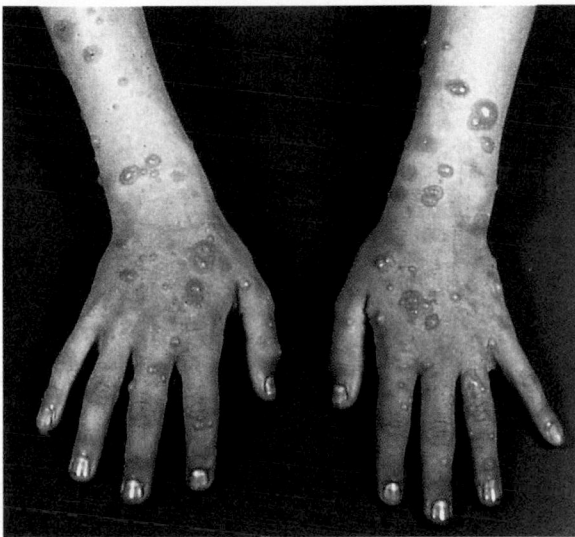

Fig. 27.48 Erythema multiforme with blistering lesions in a young woman.

ment including the mouth, eyes and genitals, with constitutional disturbance.

Management

Usually no treatment is required although symptomatic relief can be obtained with simple dressings. Stevens–Johnson syndrome can be treated with a short course of intravenous immunoglobulin. Corticosteroids are best avoided.

ERYTHEMA NODOSUM

This characteristic reaction pattern (Fig. 19.51, p. 716) is due to a vasculitis in the deep dermis and subcutaneous fat. It may be provoked by the factors listed in Box 27.41.

Clinical features

Painful, palpable, dusky blue-red nodules are most commonly seen on the lower legs. Malaise, fever and joint pains are common. The lesions resolve slowly over a month, leaving bruise-like marks in their wake.

Management

The underlying cause should be determined and treated. Bed rest and oral NSAIDs may hasten resolution. Tapering systemic corticosteroid courses may be required in stubborn cases.

PYODERMA GANGRENOSUM

Pyoderma gangrenosum (PG) predominantly occurs in adults between the ages of 25 and 54 years. The eruption starts as an inflamed nodule or pustule which breaks down centrally and rapidly progresses to an ulcer with an indurated or undermined purplish or pustular edge (Fig. 27.49). Lesions may be single or multiple and are classified as ulcerative, pustular, bullous and vegetative. Although PG may arise in the absence of any underlying disease, it is often associated with a systemic disease, such as inflammatory bowel disease, arthritis (both rheumatoid arthritis and seronegative arthropathies), immunodeficiency and immunosuppression including HIV disease, monoclonal gammopathies and leukaemia. The management of PG includes investigations for possible associated systemic disease. There are no diagnostic features on biopsy and therefore the diagnosis is primarily clinical. Local therapy includes pain relief, prevention of secondary bacterial infection and dressings. Systemic therapy includes oral corticosteroids in a tapering dose, dapsone 50–150 mg/day, minocycline 100 mg/day, sulfasalazine (4–6 g daily) and ciclosporin (5 mg/kg). Once the patient is clear of disease, recurrences are only intermittent.

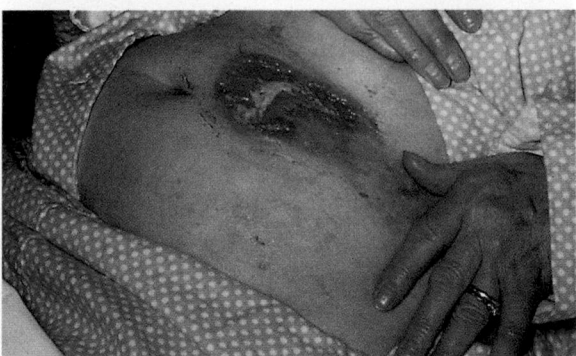

Fig. 27.49 Pyoderma gangrenosum. A large indolent ulcer in a patient with rheumatoid arthritis. Note healing in one part.

ACANTHOSIS NIGRICANS

This is a velvety thickening and pigmentation of the major flexures, particularly the axillae (p. 806). There are several types of acanthosis nigricans. The most common form is a

27

weight-dependent mild acanthosis nigricans (obesity-associated). When the patient loses weight the cutaneous features regress. Secondly, acanthosis nigricans can be associated with various syndromes, some of which have insulin resistance as a feature (p. 814 and Box 21.7). Finally, acanthosis nigricans can be associated with malignancy, particularly gastric (60%). Pruritus is a feature of malignancy-associated acanthosis and regression occurs after the tumour is excised. Acanthosis nigricans sometimes recurs with metastatic disease.

NECROBIOSIS LIPOIDICA

This condition is important to recognise because of its association with diabetes mellitus (p. 806). Less than 1% of people with diabetes have necrobiosis, but more than 85% of patients with necrobiosis will have or will develop diabetes.

Typically, the lesions appear as shiny, atrophic and slightly yellow plaques on the shins (Fig. 27.50). Underlying telangiectasia is easily seen. Minor knocks may precipitate slow-healing ulcers. No treatment is very effective. Topical and intralesional corticosteroids are used, as is long-term PUVA.

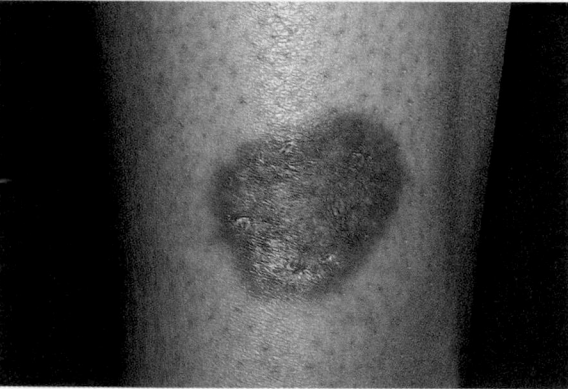

Fig. 27.50 Necrobiosis lipoidica. An atrophic yellowish plaque on the skin of a person with diabetes.

GRANULOMA ANNULARE

This is a common cutaneous condition of uncertain aetiology; any association with diabetes is now thought to be spurious. Dermal nodules occur singly or in an annular configuration. They are asymptomatic but cause consternation because they commonly occur on highly visible sites such as the hands and feet. Histologically, palisading granulomas are found in the dermis. Intralesional corticosteroids can be helpful, but the natural history is spontaneous resolution after a few months to a couple of years.

DRUG ERUPTIONS

Cutaneous drug reactions are common and almost any drug can cause them. Drug reactions may reasonably be included in the differential diagnosis of most skin diseases. Although the mechanisms are poorly understood, drug eruptions may be classified as shown in Box 27.42.

Clinical features

The most common types of drug eruption and their cause are listed in Box 27.43. It is important not to forget the possibility of a drug eruption when faced with a rash which is atypical of a known skin disease (Fig. 27.51 on p. 1312). Further clues pointing towards the diagnosis are included in Box 27.44.

Investigations

There are no specific investigations which help. Prick tests and in vitro tests for allergy are too unreliable for routine use. Readministration, as a diagnostic test, is usually unwise unless the reaction is mild and there is no suitable alternative drug.

Management

The first step is to withdraw the suspected drug(s) (except in the case of suspected drug-induced photodermatoses where if possible phototesting can be carried out when the patient is on the drug and then again at a later date when the drug has been withdrawn). Drug withdrawal, however, may not

27.42 DRUG ERUPTIONS AND THEIR MECHANISMS	
Mechanism	**Example**
Non-immunological (non-allergic)	
Unwanted pharmacological effect	Striae due to corticosteroids; mouth ulcers due to methotrexate
Drug overdosage or failure to metabolise or excrete the drug	Morphine rashes in patients with liver disease
Drug interaction	Warfarin toxicity when coadministered with aspirin or phenylbutazone
Idiosyncratic reaction (an odd reaction which may be genetically determined and is peculiar to an individual)	Drug-induced variegate porphyria
Phototoxic reaction	Chlorpromazine-induced light reactions
Altered skin ecology	Tetracyclines causing vaginal candidiasis
Exacerbation of pre-existing skin condition	Lithium and β-blocker worsening of psoriasis
Immunological (allergic)	
Immediate hypersensitivity	Penicillin-induced urticaria
Immune complex reaction	Drug-induced vasculitis or erythema multiforme
Delayed hypersensitivity	Drug-induced exfoliative dermatitis or photo-allergic reactions

27

27.43 DRUG ERUPTIONS AND SOME DRUGS WHICH MAY CAUSE THEM

Reaction pattern	Clinical features	Drugs which commonly cause reactions
Toxic erythema	Erythematous plaques Morbilliform, sometimes with urticarial or erythema multiforme-like elements	Antibiotics (especially ampicillin) Sulphonamides, thiazide diuretics, phenylbutazone, para-aminosalicylic acid (PAS)
Urticaria	Itchy weals, sometimes accompanied by angioedema	Salicylates, codeine, antibiotics, dextran and ACE inhibitors
Erythema and scaling	Small, scaly, pink papules to large, scaly, red papules	Antibiotics (especially penicillins and sulphonamides), anticonvulsants, ACE inhibitors, barbiturates, gold and penicillamine
Allergic vasculitis	Painful, palpable purpura followed by necrotic ulcers	Sulphonamides, phenylbutazone, indometacin, phenytoin and oral contraceptives
Erythema multiforme	Target-like lesions and bullae on the extensor aspects of the limbs	Sulphonamides, phenylbutazone and barbiturates
Purpura	Widespread purpura not due to thrombocytopenia or a coagulation defect	Thiazides, sulphonamides, phenylbutazone, sulphonylureas, barbiturates and quinine
Bullous eruptions	May be associated with erythema and purpura May occur at pressure sites in drug-induced coma	Barbiturates, penicillamine, nalidixic acid
Exfoliative dermatitis	Universal redness and scaling, shivering	Phenylbutazone, PAS, isoniazid and gold
Fixed drug eruptions	Round, erythematous and sometimes bullous plaques develop at the same site every time the drug is given Pigmentation left in wake	Tetracyclines, quinine, sulphonamides and barbiturates
Acneiform eruptions	Rash resembles acne (p. 1299)	Lithium, oral contraceptive, androgenic or glucocorticoid steroids, antituberculosis and anticonvulsant drugs
Toxic epidermal necrolysis	Rash resembles that of scalded skin (Fig. 27.8A, p. 1274)	Barbiturates, phenytoin, phenylbutazone and penicillin
Hair loss	Diffuse	Cytotoxic agents, acitretin, anticoagulants, antithyroid drugs and oral contraceptives
Hypertrichosis		Diazoxide, minoxidil and ciclosporin
Photosensitivity	Rash limited to exposed skin	Thiazides, tetracyclines, phenothiazines, sulphonamides, nalidixic acid and psoralens
Pigmentation	Irregular melanin pigmentation on face Slate-grey colour of exposed skin Diffuse yellow coloration of skin Streaky depigmentation of hair	Oral contraceptives Phenothiazines Mepacrine Chloroquine

27

27.44 DIAGNOSTIC CLUES TO DRUG ERUPTIONS

- Past history of reaction to suspected drug
- Introduction of suspected drug a few days before onset of rash
- Recent prescription of a drug commonly associated with rashes (e.g. penicillin, sulphonamide, thiazide, allopurinol, phenylbutazone)
- A symmetrical eruption which may fit with a well-recognised pattern caused by one of the current drugs

be easy, or even possible, if there is no alternative available. The decision will depend on many factors, including the severity and nature of the drug reaction, its potential reversibility and the probability that the drug caused the reaction. Supportive treatment with antihistamines or a tailored course of systemic corticosteroids may be indicated, depending on the type of skin reaction. The emergency treatment of anaphylactic shock is described on page 87.

MEDICAL TREATMENTS OF SKIN DISEASE

The advantages of applying medication topically are numerous. Both the active ingredient and the vehicle are important in the treatment of skin conditions. The doctor should be familiar with topical prescribing: firstly, to prescribe the appropriate active treatment; secondly, to ensure that it is in the optimum base or vehicle; and finally, to be confident about instructing the patient on how to use the treatment, how frequently and what side-effects might be expected. As with any drug it is essential to ensure that an appropriate dose and volume is prescribed for the disease being treated. For example, a child with eczema will need about 500 g of emollient per week whereas an adult with acne might need only 30 g of a topical gel for a month.

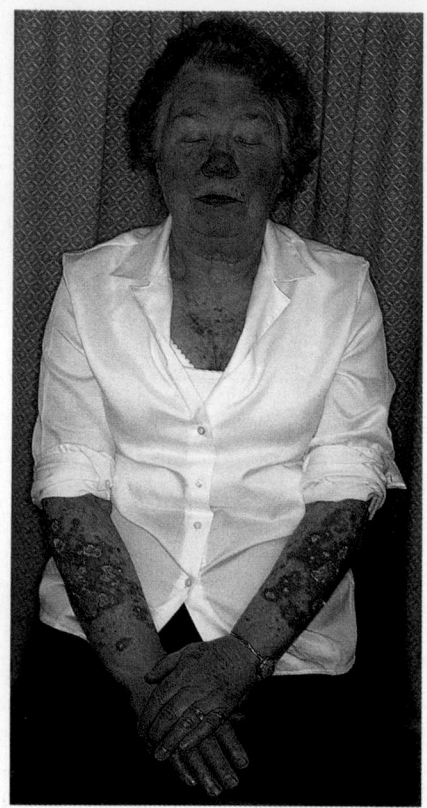

Fig. 27.51 Drug eruption. A bizarre but symmetrical erythematous scaly rash with a distribution suggesting a degree of photosensitivity. The rash persisted until the recently prescribed sulphonylurea was withdrawn.

ACTIVE INGREDIENT

Many topical formulations are available and licensed for use in skin disease. Increasingly, compound formulations are becoming available for use. Drugs penetrate the skin according to a number of characteristics including their molecular weight and their lipid–water coefficients, water-soluble ions and polar molecules being excluded. When the stratum corneum is impaired in disease states then drug absorption increases, but as the skin heals drug absorption diminishes accordingly. If occlusion is applied there is an increase in absorption: for example, under bandages. Agents may be formulated in different potencies, as with different topical corticosteroids, or by different concentrations, as with anthralins, coal tar preparations and first-generation topical retinoids (refer to national formulary guidelines). Most other agents are formulated in one strength: topical antibiotics, second-generation topical retinoids and vitamin D analogues.

VEHICLE (BASE)

Besides containing the active ingredient, the vehicle of a topical treatment has an active role in the treatment of skin conditions. The vehicle can serve to hydrate and cool the skin and has antimicrobial and soothing qualities. Creams and ointments are the most common vehicles used. Creams are emulsions of oil in water, whereas ointments are greasier and not aqueous-based. Gels (both non-hydrous and aqueous) and lotions (aqueous) are convenient for use in hair-bearing areas. Pastes are semi-stiff preparations

consisting of finely powdered solids suspended in an ointment. The properties of different vehicles are listed in Box 27.45. Many active treatments such as topical corticosteroids (see below) are available in more than one formulation.

TOPICAL CORTICOSTEROIDS

Glucorticoids are formulated as both ointments and creams for use in dermatology. Creams are used in acute exudative conditions, whereas the ointment formulation is better in chronic dry skin conditions. Corticosteroids come in a variety of strengths and potencies (Box 27.46) and should be prescribed according to the site of application, the age of the patient and the length of time that the corticosteroids are to be used. For example, mild topical corticosteroids are used on sensitive sites such as the face or genital area in both adults and children. In childhood eczema potent corticosteroids can be used for short periods of time. Superpotent corticosteroids are used under occlusion on chronic persistent lesions such as nodular prurigo. If used under occlusion, the effective potency is increased. There is concern about the side-effects of topical corticosteroids, particularly local effects such as cutaneous atrophy and telangiectasia. These are rarely seen nowadays with the judicious use of topical corticosteroid treatment and undertreatment is a more common problem. There are no definite rules about how long it is safe to use a topical corticosteroid in a particular individual in any one site but in general one should use the least potent corticosteroid for the shortest possible time. Corticosteroid-responsive dermatoses tend to be treated initially with a more potent topical corticosteroid, which is then reduced as the condition improves. Long-term treatment is often given intermittently, not least because of tachyphylaxis.

DRESSINGS

The regular application of topical treatment with appropriate covering such as a wound dressing (e.g. Jelonet), a simple tubular bandage (e.g. Tubifast) or a medicated bandage (e.g. Steripaste or Ichthopaste) is known as a dressing. Box 27.47 describes the important reasons for prescribing dressings. The choice of dressing during topical treatment should be carefully and informatively made according to the active agent, vehicle and covering of the skin. As a rule of thumb, wet lesions should be treated with wet dressings. For example, acute eczema is best treated with potassium permanganate soaks, a topical corticosteroid in a cream formulation and a paste bandage serving to soothe and cool the skin. Chronic dry itchy eczema, however, is best treated with a potent topical corticosteroid in an ointment formulation and a paste bandage to prevent scratching and ease itching. Dressings for venous leg ulcers are described on page 1277. Patients with leg ulcers have an increased risk of contact allergy to medicaments and therefore the dressings are best kept simple with avoidance of potential allergens such as topical antibiotics, antiseptics and lanolin.

27.45 DEFINITION OF SOME VEHICLES

Vehicle	Definition	Use	Site	Cosmetic acceptability	Risk of contact sensitisation
Creams	Emulsions of oil and water, e.g. aqueous cream	In acute situations, cooling, soothing and well absorbed Mild emollients	All sites including mucous membranes and flexures but excluding hair-bearing areas	Very good	May contain antimicrobials and preservatives
Ointments	Greasy preparations which can be insoluble in water, e.g. white soft paraffin, or soluble, e.g. Macrogol	On chronic dry areas of skin Tend to be occlusive and protective, and serve to rehydrate the skin May be mildly anti-inflammatory	Avoid hair-bearing areas and flexures	Moderate	Low risk
Gels	Hydrophilic and hydrophobic bases	In specific sites	Hair-bearing areas and the face	Good	Low risk
Lotions	Water-based	Have a cooling effect on the skin Used to clean the skin and remove exudates Often antiseptic and astringent (e.g. potassium permanganate)	Large areas of the skin and also the scalp	Good, but can sting if in an alcoholic base	Rare
Pastes	Semi-stiff preparations containing finely powdered solids suspended in an ointment	Characteristically substantive and bland Used for circumscribed skin lesions, e.g. psoriasis, lichen simplex chronicus	Any area of skin Often made up into medicated bandages	Moderate	Moderate

27.46 STRENGTHS OF TOPICAL CORTICOSTEROIDS*

Mild

- 0.5%, 1%, 2.5% hydrocortisone

Moderate

- Clobetasone butyrate 0.05% (Eumovate)
- Betamethasone 0.025% (Betnovate RD)

Potent

- Mometasone furoate 0.1% (Elocon)
- Betamethasone 0.1% (Betnovate)
- Betamethasone 0.1% and fusidic acid 2% (Fucibet)
- Fluticasone propionate 0.05% and 0.005% (Cutivate)

Very potent

- Clobetasol propionate 0.05% (Dermovate)

* UK trade names are given in brackets.

27.47 REASONS FOR APPLYING DRESSINGS

- Protection
- Symptomatic relief from pain or itch
- To maintain direct application of topical treatment
- To hasten healing time
- To reduce exudates

DERMATOLOGICAL SURGERY

The workload of dermatologists in developed countries has changed considerably over the last 20–30 years, with an increase in the number of lesions compared with rashes. In part this is explained by changes in the epidemiology of skin cancer, referral changes and the increased demand for cosmetic removal of many lesions. If the assessment of patients with potential skin cancer and their follow-up are included, dermatologists might spend anywhere between 20% and 90% of their time on surgical aspects of the discipline (depending on a practitioner's particular interests).

A large number of surgical procedures can mostly be carried out under local anaesthetic. The choice of procedure is important; for example, inappropriate excision of lesions such as seborrhoeic keratoses (p. 1303) results in scar formation—these lesions should instead be treated by cryosurgery or curettage.

BIOPSY

Skin biopsies are usually taken under local anaesthetic but a general anaesthetic may be necessary in some children. It is best to select an early or typical lesion on a non-exposed site. An ellipse biopsy or, in certain instances, a punch biopsy that removes a cylindrical portion of skin may be used. Learning which part of a rash to biopsy, and whether an ellipse or punch biopsy will suffice, comes with experience but is often critical. A common reason for unhelpful or even misleading histology is biopsy of an inappropriate part of the rash. For instance, biopsies of secondarily excoriated lesions, even in the clinical context of a blistering disease, are often unhelpful.

Sutures are removed depending on site and other factors (i.e. 5–7 days for the face and 10–14 days for the back). Certain body sites are associated with particular risks. Thus biopsies on the upper torso of young persons are likely to result in keloids, biopsies over the scapula tend to leave unsightly scars, and biopsies on the lower legs of elderly people are at risk of poor healing and ulceration with resulting high morbidity. The statement that there is no such thing as 'minor surgery' remains an instructive maxim.

CRYOTHERAPY

Cryotherapy is usually performed in one of two ways: either as an application of liquid nitrogen with a cotton wool bud or using a jet gun. Liquid nitrogen can be used to treat a wide range of lesions from viral warts (p. 1295) to actinic keratoses (p. 1303) and invasive tumours such as basal or squamous cell carcinomas (pp. 1304–1305). The cosmetic effects and morbidity are variable. If neoplasia is suspected it may be wiser to carry out an incisional biopsy first. In general, superficial or 'stuck-on' lesions will require less intense therapy that is more acceptable to the patient. Melanocytic naevi should not be treated with liquid nitrogen.

CURETTAGE

Curettage refers to scraping with a small, spoon-shaped implement (curette) across the lesion, not only as a definitive treatment but also as a way of obtaining histological material. Naturally, the histological material may be compromised in the sense that epidermal structures are over-represented and the anatomy of the lesion as it descends into the dermis is not preserved. It may therefore be difficult to determine whether a lesion with intra-epidermal dysplasia shows any evidence of invasion (i.e. is a squamous cell carcinoma rather than an intra-epidermal carcinoma or actinic keratosis). Curettage is, however, suitable for many seborrhoeic keratoses, actinic keratoses or areas of intra-epidermal carcinoma. Some superficial basal cell carcinomas are well treated with curettage but some variants such as the morphoeic forms should be treated with expert surgical excision.

SURGICAL EXCISION

The advantage of surgical excision for the removal of tumours or suspected tumours is that it provides adequate histological material for examination and evidence of excision margins. Depending on body site, a range of procedures can be used to minimise the resulting defect, including undermining, Z-plasties, flaps and grafts. On sun-exposed sites in many patients, particularly the elderly, healing by secondary intention can lead to a surprisingly good result.

LASER THERAPY

Laser therapy exploits the fact that certain pigments such as melanin or blood absorb certain wavelengths of electro-magnetic radiation more readily than others. A variety of lasers have been produced which allow relatively selective destruction of particular structures containing the absorbing pigment. By concentrating the light into short pulses the damage is restricted to a particular area. The choice of laser for a particular lesion requires specialist knowledge but because melanin and blood have overlapping spectrums the choice generally focuses on minimising 'collateral' damage. Some lasers are better for dealing with primarily vascular lesions such as port wine stains, while others are more useful for pigmented lesions or for destruction of exogenous pigments such as tattoo pigments or drug deposits (e.g. minocycline).

By contrast with the vascular laser the carbon dioxide laser emits infrared light which is absorbed by tissue water. When crudely used, the carbon dioxide laser is therefore similar to a diathermy but the depth of lesion can be controlled to a fraction of a millimetre; the procedure can therefore be useful for resurfacing and for face lifts. A general anaesthetic is required for such procedures.

PHOTODYNAMIC THERAPY

This is a new and promising addition to the available therapies for treating skin cancer and related lesions. The principle is based on the pathological processes involved in the disease porphyria, in which endogenously produced photosensitisers cause tissue damage. Therapeutic photodynamic therapy consists of application of topical photosensitisers and then irradiation with light within the visible spectrum leading to tissue damage. It is thought that some tumours selectively absorb the photosensitiser, thus enhancing the therapeutic ratio. Photodynamic therapy is used for treatment of actinic keratoses, in situ carcinoma (Bowen's disease) and superficial basal cell carcinomas. Results from long-term follow-up studies of recurrence rates are awaited. The treatment is time-consuming as the sensitiser needs to be applied for several hours before exposure to the light source and, as with porphyria, exposure may be painful.

MISCELLANEOUS PROCEDURES

Keloids may require corticosteroid injections after freezing or excision. Silicone sheeting may flatten keloids, although the mechanism is obscure. Scars and wrinkles can be filled using collagen or silicone. Liposuction can be used to remove fat, and tissue folds around the eyes can be easily excised. Small acne scars can be excised and larger, more superficial lesions treated with a carbon dioxide laser. Areas of depigmentation in vitiligo or piebaldism may be treated with epidermal grafts from normal skin.

FURTHER INFORMATION

Books and journal articles

Barker J. Psoriasis. J R Coll Physicians Lond 1997; 31:238–240.

Bolognia JL, Jorizzo JL, Rapini RP, eds. Dermatology. St Louis: Mosby; 2003.

British Medical Association and Royal Pharmaceutical Society of Great Britain. British National Formulary. London: BMJ Books.

Burns DA, Breathnach SM, Cox N, et al., eds. Rook's textbook of dermatology. 7th edn. Oxford: Blackwell; 2005.

Farr PM. Ultraviolet phototherapy [Review] [25 refs]. J R Coll Physicians Lond 1997; 31:250–253.

27

Finucace KA, Archer CB. Dermatological aspects of medicine. Recent advances in nephrology. Clin Exp Dermatol 2005 30:98–102.

Freedberg IM, Eisen AZ, Wolff K, et al., eds. Fitzpatrick's dermatology in general medicine. New York: McGraw-Hill; 1999.

Gilchrest BA, Eller MS, Geller AC, et al. The pathogenesis of melanoma induced by ultraviolet radiation. N Engl J Med 1999; 340:1341–1348.

Greaves MW. Itch: more than skin deep. Int Arch Allergy Immunol 2004; 135:166–172.

Greaves MW, Wall PD. Pathophysiology of itching. Lancet 1997; 349:133.

Haider A, Shaw JC. Treatment of acne vulgaris. JAMA 2004; 292:726–735.

Kanj LF, Wilking SV, Phillips TJ. Pressure ulcers. J Am Acad Dermatol 1998; 38:517–536.

Koning S, van der Woudon JC. Treatment of impetigo. BMJ 2004; 329:695–696.

Lawrence CM. Surgery and laser therapy. J R Coll Physicians Lond 1997; 31:369–373.

Lebwohl M, Heymann W, Berth-Jones J, et al., eds. Treatment of skin disease: comprehensive dermatologic strategies. St Louis: Mosby; 2002.

McMillan JR, Akiyama M, Shimizu H. Epidermal basement membrane zone components: ultrastructural distribution and molecular interactions. J Dermatol Sci 2003; 31:169–177.

Nordlund JJ, Boissy RE, Hearing VJ, et al., eds. The pigmentary system: physiology and pathophysiology. New York: Oxford; 1998.

Rees JL. Skin cancer. J R Coll Physicians Lond 1998; 31:246–250.

Wakelin SH, Black MM. The autoimmune bullous diseases. J R Coll Physicians Lond 1997; 31:364–368.

Williams H. Atopic dermatitis. N Engl J Med 2005; 352:2314–2324.

Websites

www.eczema.org *National Eczema Society in the UK.*

27

28

S.W. WALKER

Appendix

NOTES ON INTERNATIONAL SYSTEM OF UNITS (SI UNITS)

Système International (SI) units are a specific subset of the metre–kilogram–second system of units and were agreed upon as the everyday currency for commercial and scientific work in 1960, following a series of international conferences organised by the International Bureau of Weights and Measures. SI units have been adopted widely in clinical laboratories, but non-SI units are still used in many countries. For that reason, values in both units are given for common measurements throughout this textbook and commonly used non-SI units are shown in this appendix. However, the SI unit system is recommended.

Examples of basic SI units

Length	metre (m)
Mass	kilogram (kg)
Amount of substance	mole (mol)
Energy	joule (J)
Pressure	pascal (Pa)
Volume	The basic SI unit of volume is the cubic metre (1000 litres). For convenience, however, the litre (l) is used as the unit of volume in laboratory work.

Examples of decimal multiples and submultiples of SI units

Factor	Name	Prefix
10^6	mega-	M
10^3	kilo-	k
10^{-1}	deci-	d
10^{-2}	centi-	c
10^{-3}	milli-	m
10^{-6}	micro-	μ
10^{-9}	nano-	n
10^{-12}	pico-	p
10^{-15}	femto-	f

Exceptions to the use of SI units

By convention, blood pressure is excluded from the SI unit system and is measured in mmHg (millimetres of mercury) rather than pascals.

Mass concentrations (e.g. g/l, μg/l) are used in preference to molar concentrations for all protein measurements, and for substances which do not have a sufficiently well-defined composition.

Some enzymes and hormones are measured by 'bioassay', in which the activity in the sample is compared with the activity (rather than the mass) of a standard sample which is provided from a central source. For these assays, results are given in standardised 'units', or 'international units', which depend upon the activity in the standard sample and may not be readily converted to mass units.

BIOCHEMICAL VALUES

Reference ranges are largely those used in the Departments of Clinical Biochemistry and Haematology, Lothian Health University Hospitals Division, Edinburgh, UK. Values are shown in both SI units and, where appropriate, non-SI units. Many reference ranges vary between laboratories, depending on the assay method used and on other factors; this is especially the case for enzyme assays. The origin of reference ranges and the interpretation of 'abnormal' results are discussed in Chapter 1 (pp. 6–7). No details are given here of the collection requirements which may be critical to obtaining a meaningful result. Unless otherwise stated, reference ranges shown apply to adults; values in children may be different.

Many analytes can be measured in either serum (the supernatant of clotted blood) or plasma (the supernatant of anticoagulated blood). A specific requirement for one or the other may depend on a kit maufacturer's recommendations. In other instances, the distinction is critical (e.g. plasma is required for measurement of fibrinogen since it is largely absent from serum; serum is required for electrophoresis to detect paraproteins because fibrinogen migrates as a discreet band in the zone of interest).

28.1 UREA AND ELECTROLYTES IN VENOUS BLOOD

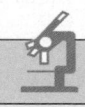

	Reference range	
Analysis	**SI units**	**Non-SI units**
Sodium	135–145 mmol/l	135–145 meq/l
Potassium (plasma)	3.3–4.7 mmol/l	3.3–4.7 meq/l
Potassium (serum)	3.6–5.1 mmol/l	3.6–5.1 meq/l
Chloride	95–107 mmol/l	95–107 meq/l
Urea	2.5–6.6 mmol/l	15–40 mg/dl
Creatinine	60–120 μmol/l	0.68–1.36 mg/dl

28.2 ARTERIAL BLOOD ANALYSIS

	Reference range	
Analysis	**SI units**	**Non-SI units**
Bicarbonate	21–29 mmol/l	21–29 meq/l
Hydrogen ion	37–45 nmol/l	pH 7.35–7.43
***Pa*CO$_2$**	4.5–6.0 kPa	34–45 mmHg
***Pa*O$_2$**	12–15 kPa	90–113 mmHg
Oxygen saturation	> 97%	

28

28.3 HORMONES IN VENOUS BLOOD

Hormone	Reference range	
	SI units	Non-SI units
Adrenocorticotrophic hormone (ACTH) (plasma)	1.5–11.2 pmol/l (0700–1000 hrs)	7–51 pg/ml
Aldosterone		
Supine	45–440 pmol/l	1.63–15.9 ng/dl
Erect	110–860 pmol/l	3.97–31.0 ng/dl
Cortisol	Dynamic tests are required—see Ch. 20	
Follicle-stimulating hormone (FSH)		
Male	1.5–9.0 U/l	0.3–2.0 ng/ml
Female	3.0–15 U/l (early follicular, luteal)	0.7–3.3 ng/ml
	< 20 U/l (mid-cycle)	< 4.4 ng/ml
	> 30 U/l (post-menopausal)	> 6.7 ng/ml
Gastrin (plasma, fasting)	< 57 pmol/l	< 120 pg/ml
Growth hormone (GH)	< 2 mU/l excludes acromegaly	Conversion to mass units depends
	> 20 mU/l excludes GH deficiency	on assay
	Dynamic tests are usually required—see Ch. 20	
Insulin	Highly variable and interpretable only in relation to plasma glucose and body habitus	–
Luteinising hormone (LH)		
Male	1.5–9.0 U/l	0.17–1.0 µg/l
Female	2.5–9.0 U/l (early follicular, luteal)	0.3–1.0 µg/l
	Up to 90 U/l (mid-cycle)	Up to 10 µg/l
	> 20 U/l (post-menopausal)	> 2.2 µg/l
17β-Oestradiol		
Male	< 200 pmol/l	< 54 pg/ml
Female	110–180 pmol/l (early follicular)	30–49 pg/ml
	550–1650 pmol/l (mid-cycle)	150–449 pg/ml
	370–770 pmol/l (luteal)	101–209 pg/ml
	< 150 pmol/l (post-menopausal)	< 41 pg/ml
Parathyroid hormone (PTH)	1.0–6.5 pmol/l	10–65 pg/ml
Progesterone		
Male	< 2.0 nmol/l	< 0.63 ng/ml
Female	< 2.0 nmol/l (follicular)	< 0.63 ng/ml
	> 15 nmol/l (mid-luteal)	> 4.7 ng/ml
	< 2.0 nmol/l (post-menopausal)	< 0.63 ng/ml
Prolactin (PRL)	60–500 mU/l	–
Renin activity		
Erect	0.6–2.8 ng/ml/h	–
Supine	< 1.5 ng/ml/h	–
Testosterone		
Male	10–30 nmol/l	2.88–8.64 ng/ml
Female	0.4–2.8 nmol/l	0.12–0.81 ng/ml
Thyroid-stimulating hormone (TSH)	0.15–3.5 mU/l	–
Thyroxine (free) (free T₄)	8–27 pmol/l	622–2098 pg/dl
Triiodothyronine (T₃)	1.0–2.6 nmol/l	65–169 ng/dl

Notes
1. A number of hormones are unstable and collection details are critical to obtaining a meaningful result. Refer to local laboratory handbook.
2. Values in the table are only a guideline; hormone levels can often only be meaningfully understood in relation to factors such as sex (e.g. testosterone), age (e.g. FSH in women), time of day (e.g. cortisol) or regulatory factors (e.g. insulin and glucose, PTH and $[Ca^{2+}]$).
3. Reference ranges may be critically method-dependent.

28

28.4 OTHER COMMON ANALYTES IN VENOUS BLOOD IN ADULTS

Analyte	Reference range SI units	Reference range Non-SI units
α_1-antitrypsin	1.1–2.1 g/l	110–210 mg/dl
Alanine amino-transferase (ALT)	10–50 U/l	–
Albumin	35–50 g/l	3.5–5.0 g/dl
Alkaline phosphatase	40–125 U/l	–
Amylase	< 100 U/l	–
Aspartate amino-transferase (AST)	10–45 U/l	–
Bilirubin (total)	2–17 μmol/l	0.12–1.0 mg/dl
Calcium (total)	2.12–2.62 mmol/l	4.24–5.24 meq/l or 8.50–10.50 mg/dl
Carboxy-haemoglobin	< 1.5% in non-smokers	–
Caeruloplasmin	150–600 mg/l	15–60 mg/dl
Cholesterol (total)	Ideal level varies according to cardiovascular risk (see cardiovascular risk chart, p. 1323) so reference ranges can be misleading. The following values were described by the European Atherosclerosis Society: Mild increase 5.2–6.5 mmol/l Moderate increase 6.5–7.8 mmol/l Severe increase > 7.8 mmol/l	200–250 mg/dl 250–300 mg/dl > 300 mg/dl
HDL-cholesterol	Ideal level varies according to cardiovascular risk so reference ranges can be misleading. According to the National Cholesterol Education Programme Adult Treatment Panel III (ATPIII), a low HDL-cholesterol is: < 1.0 mmol/l	40 mg/dl
Copper	13–24 μmol/l	83–153 μg/dl
C-reactive protein	< 5 mg/l Highly sensitive CRP assays also exist which measure lower values and may be useful in estimating cardiovascular risk	
Creatine kinase (total) Male Female	55–170 U/l 30–135 U/l	– –
Creatine kinase MB isoenzyme	< 6% of total CK	–

Analyte	Reference range SI units	Reference range Non-SI units
Ethanol	Not normally detectable Marked intoxication 65–87 mmol/l Stupor 87–109 mmol/l Coma > 109 mmol/l	300–400 mg/dl 400–500 mg/dl > 500 mg/dl
Gamma-glutamyl transferase (GGT)	5–55 U/l	–
Glucose (fasting)	3.6–5.8 mmol/l See Ch. 21 for definitions of impaired glucose tolerance and diabetes mellitus, and Ch. 20 for definition of hypoglycaemia	65–104 mg/dl
Glycated haemoglobin (HbA$_{1c}$)	5.0–6.5%	–
Immunoglobulin A	0.8–4.5 g/l	80–450 mg/dl
Immunoglobulin G	6.0–15.0 g/l	600–1500 mg/dl
Immunoglobulin M	0.35–2.90 g/l	35–290 mg/dl
Lactate	0.6–2.4 mmol/l	5.40–21.6 mg/dl
Lactate dehydrogenase (total)	208–460 U/l	–
Lead	< 1.0 μmol/l	< 21 μg/dl
Magnesium	0.75–1.0 mmol/l	1.5–2.0 meq/l or 1.82–2.43 mg/dl
Osmolality	280–290 mmol/kg	–
Osmolarity	280–290 mosm/l	–
Phosphate (fasting)	0.8–1.4 mmol/l	2.48–4.34 mg/dl
Protein (total)	60–80 g/l	6–8 g/dl
Triglycerides (fasting)	0.6–1.7 mmol/l	53–150 mg/dl
Troponins	Values consistent with 'myocyte necrosis' or myocardial infarction are crucially dependent upon which troponin is measured (I or T) and on the method employed	
Urate Male Female	0.12–0.42 mmol/l 0.12–0.36 mmol/l	2.0–7.0 mg/dl 2.0–6.0 mg/dl
Vitamin D 25(OH)D Winter Summer 1,25(OH)$_2$D	15–50 nmol/l 15–100 nmol/l 20–120 pmol/l	6–20 ng/ml 6–40 ng/ml 7.7–46 pg/ml
Zinc	11–22 μmol/l	72–144 μg/dl

28

28.5 CEREBROSPINAL FLUID ANALYSIS

Analysis	Reference range SI units	Non-SI units
Cells	$< 5 \times 10^6$ cells/l (all mononuclear)	< 5 cells/mm^3
Glucose	2.3–4.0 mmol/l	41–72 mg/dl
IgG index*	< 0.65	–
Total protein	140–450 mg/l	0.014–0.045 g/dl

* A crude index of increase in IgG attributable to intrathecal synthesis.

28.6 COMMON ANALYTES IN URINE

Analyte	Reference range SI units	Non-SI units
Albumin	Definitions of microalbuminuria are given in Ch. 17 (p. 479) Proteinuria is defined below	
Calcium Low-calcium diet Normal diet	1.2–3.7 mmol/24 hrs < 12 mmol/24 hrs	2.4–7.4 meq/24 hrs or 48–148 mg/24 hrs < 24 meq/24 hrs or < 480 mg/24 hro
Copper	< 0.6 µmol/24 hrs	< 38 µg/24 hrs
Cortisol Overnight collection 24-hr collection	9–50 µmol/mol creatinine 25–250 nmol/24 hrs	30–160 µg cortisol/g creatinine 9.1–91 µg/24 hrs
Creatinine	10–20 mmol/24 hrs	1130–2260 mg/24 hrs
5-hydroxyindole-3-acetic acid (5-HIAA)	10–42 µmol/24 hrs	1.9–8.1 mg/24 hrs
Metadrenalines Normetadrenaline Metadrenaline	0.4–3.4 µmol/24 hrs 0.3–1.7 µmol/24 hrs	73–620 µg/24 hrs 59–335 µg/24 hrs
Oxalate	0.04–0.49 mmol/24 hrs	3.6–44 mg/24 hrs
Phosphate	15–50 mmol/24 hrs	465–1548 mg/24 hrs
Potassium*	25–100 mmol/24 hrs	25–100 meq/24 hrs
Protein	< 0.3 g/l	< 0.03 g/dl
Sodium*	100–200 mmol/24 hrs	100–200 meq/24 hrs
Urate	1.2–3.0 mmol/24 hrs	202–504 mg/24 hrs
Urea	170–600 mmol/24 hrs	10.2–36.0 g/24 hrs

* The urinary output of electrolytes such as sodium and potassium is normally a reflection of dietary intake. This can vary widely, especially on a cultural, world-wide basis. The values quoted are appropriate to a 'Western' diet.

28

HAEMATOLOGICAL VALUES

28.7 HAEMATOLOGICAL VALUES

Analysis	Reference range	
	SI units	Non-SI units
Bleeding time (Ivy)	< 8 mins	–
Blood volume		
Male	75 ± 10 ml/kg	–
Female	70 ± 10 ml/kg	–
Coagulation screen		
Prothrombin time	8.0–10.5 secs	–
Activated partial thromboplastin time	26–37 secs	–
D-dimers		
Routine	< 0.2 mg/l	–
Sensitive (for venous thromboembolism)	Variable threshold (dependent on method)	
Erythrocyte sedimentation rate	Higher values in older patients are not necessarily abnormal	
Adult male	0–10 mm/hr	–
Adult female	3–15 mm/hr	–
Ferritin		
Male	17–300 µg/l	17–300 ng/ml
Pre-menopausal female	7–280 µg/l	7–280 ng/ml
Post-menopausal female	4–233 µg/l	4–233 ng/ml
Fibrinogen	1.5–4.0 g/l	0.15–0.4 g/dl
Folate		
Serum	2.0–13.5 µg/l	2.0–13.5 ng/ml
Red cell	95–570 µg/l	95–570 ng/ml
Haemoglobin		
Male	130–180 g/l	13–18 g/dl
Female	115–165 g/l	11.5–16.5 g/dl
Haptoglobin	0.4–2.4 g/l	0.04–0.24 g/dl
Iron		
Male	14–32 µmol/l	78–178 µg/dl
Female	10–28 µmol/l	56–156 µg/dl
Leucocytes (adults)	$4.0\text{–}11.0 \times 10^9/l$	$4.0\text{–}11.0 \times 10^3/mm^3$
Differential white cell count		
Neutrophil granulocytes	$2.0\text{–}7.5 \times 10^9/l$	$2.0\text{–}7.5 \times 10^3/mm^3$
Lymphocytes	$1.5\text{–}4.0 \times 10^9/l$	$1.5\text{–}4.0 \times 10^3/mm^3$
Monocytes	$0.2\text{–}0.8 \times 10^9/l$	$0.2\text{–}0.8 \times 10^3/mm^3$
Eosinophil granulocytes	$0.04\text{–}0.4 \times 10^9/l$	$0.04\text{–}0.4 \times 10^3/mm^3$
Basophil granulocytes	$0.01\text{–}0.1 \times 10^9/l$	$0.01\text{–}0.1 \times 10^3/mm^3$
Mean cell haemoglobin (MCH)	27–32 pg	–
Mean cell volume (MCV)	78–98 fl	–
Packed cell volume (PCV) or haematocrit		
Male	0.40–0.54	–
Female	0.37–0.47	–
Platelets	$150\text{–}350 \times 10^9/l$	$150\text{–}350 \times 10^3/mm^3$
Red cell count		
Male	$4.5\text{–}6.5 \times 10^{12}/l$	$4.5\text{–}6.5 \times 10^6/mm^3$
Female	$3.8\text{–}5.8 \times 10^{12}/l$	$3.8\text{–}5.8 \times 10^6/mm^3$
Red cell lifespan		
Mean	120 days	–
Half-life (^{51}Cr)	25–35 days	–
Reticulocytes (adults)	$25\text{–}85 \times 10^9/l$	$25\text{–}85 \times 10^3/mm^3$
Transferrin	2.0–4.0 g/l	0.2–0.4 g/dl
Transferrin saturation		
Male	25–56%	–
Female	14–51%	–
Vitamin B$_{12}$	130–770 pg/ml	–

CARDIOVASCULAR RISK PREDICTION CHART

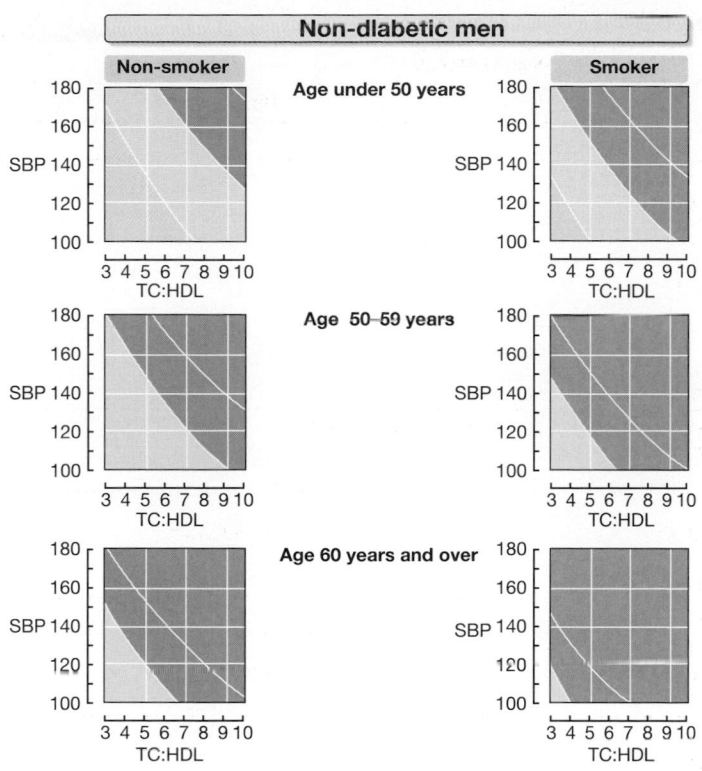

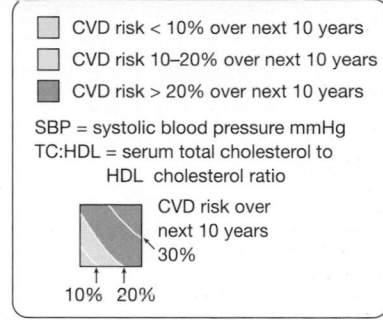

CVD risk < 10% over next 10 years

CVD risk 10–20% over next 10 years

CVD risk > 20% over next 10 years

SBP = systolic blood pressure mmHg
TC:HDL = serum total cholesterol to
HDL cholesterol ratio

CVD risk over
next 10 years
30%

10%   20%

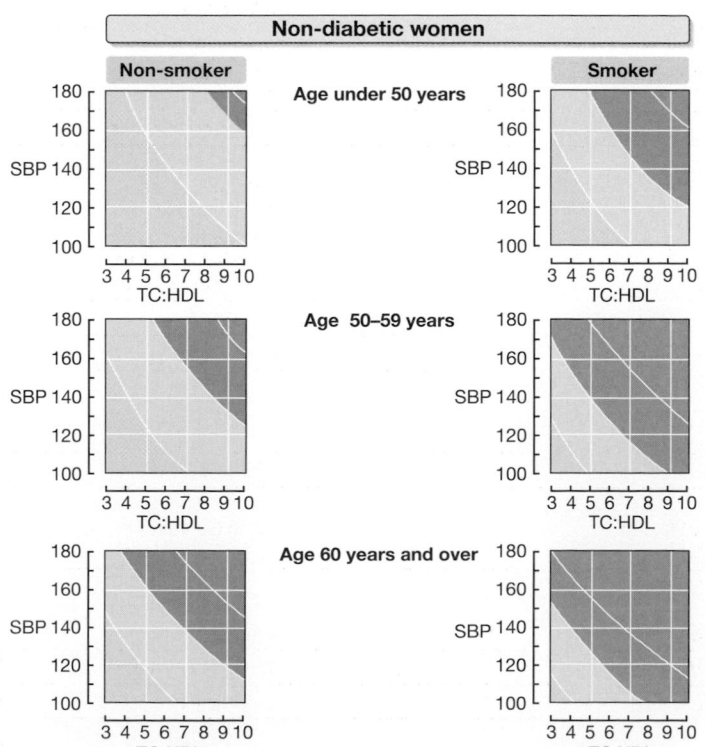

Fig. 28.1 Cardiovascular risk prediction chart to assist in selecting patients for primary prevention therapy.

- To estimate an individual's absolute 10-year risk of developing cardiovascular disease (CVD), choose the panel for the gender, smoking status and age. Within this, define the level of risk from the point where the coordinates for SBP and ratio of the total to high-density lipoprotein (HDL)-cholesterol cross. If no HDL-cholesterol result is available, assume it is 1.0 mmol/l and use the lipid scale as total serum cholesterol.
- Highest-risk individuals (red areas) are those whose 10-year CVD risk exceeds 20%, which is approximately equivalent to a 10-year coronary heart disease risk of > 15%. As a minimum, those with CVD risk > 30% (shown by the line within the red area) should be targeted and treated now. When resources allow, others with a CVD risk > 20% should be targeted progressively.
- The chart also assists in identification of individuals with a moderately high 10-year CVD risk—in the range of 10–20% (orange area) and those in whom it is lower than 10% (green area).
- Smoking status should reflect lifetime exposure to tobacco. For further information, see http://www.bhf.org.uk/professionals/uploaded/aug_2004%20v2.pdf.

28

Picture credits

We are grateful to the following individuals and organisations for the loan of illustrations:

Chapter 5
Fig. 5.17A Institute of Ophthalmology.

Chapter 6
Fig. 6.4 NHS Lanarkshire Public Health and Health Promotion departments. Figs 6.9–6.18 Antibiotic sensitivity patterns for common infections after an idea by Dr A. Maggs, Dept of Microbiology, Torbay Hospital, Torquay.

Chapter 11
Fig. 11.4 Professor W.R. Miller, Edinburgh Breast Unit. Fig. 11.5 insets (CTs) Dr A. Stevenson, (bone marrow) Dr J. Thomas, Western General Hospital, Edinburgh. Fig. 11.10 Mr J.M. Dixon, Edinburgh Breast Unit.

Chapter 13
Illustrative material supplied by Dr R. Davidson and the EM and Histopathology Unit, London School of Hygiene and Tropical Medicine. Fig. 13.29 Reproduced by permission of WHO. Fig. 13.39 Institute of Ophthalmology, Moorfields Eye Hospital, London. Fig. 13.50 Dr E.E. Zijlstra. Fig. 13.48 Dr S. Sundar, Dr H.W. Murray.

Chapter 14
Page 378 inset (oral hairy leucoplakia), Figs 14.7 and 14.8 Audiovisual Dept, St Mary's Hospital, London.

Chapter 15
Figs 15.1 and 15.5 Dr P. Hay, St George's Hospital, London.

Chapter 17
Illustrative material supplied by Dr I. Beggs and Dr J. Reid. Page 457 Dr G.M. Iadarola and Dr F. Quarello, G Bosco Hospital, Turin (from http://www.sin-italia.org/imago/sediment/sed.htm). Figs 17.1C and E, 17.32A, C, D and E Dr J.G. Simpson, Aberdeen Royal Infirmary. Figs 17.5A and B, 17.6A and B, 17.7, 17.36, 17.39 and 17.40 Dr A.P. Bayliss and Dr P. Thorpe, Aberdeen Royal Infirmary. Fig. 17.12 Dr P. Robinson, St James's University Hospital, Leeds. Figs 17.32F, G and H Dr R. Herriot. Figs 17.34B and C Dr J. Collar, St Mary's Hospital, London.

Chapter 18
Figs 18.2C and 18.84E Dr T. Lawton. Figs 18.85A and B Dr B. Cullen.

Chapter 19
Page 648 inset (kyphoscoliosis) Dr I. Smith, Papworth Hospital, Cambridge; (sputum: serous, mucopurulent and purulent) Dr J. Foweraker, Papworth Hospital, Cambridge. Figs 19.6 and 19.7 Dr J. Reid. Fig. 19.15 Professor N.J. Douglas. Fig. 19.27B British Lung Foundation. Fig. 19.43C Dr C. Flower, Addenbrooke's Hospital, Cambridge.

Chapter 20
Figs 20.4 inset (toxic multinodular goitre) and 20.22C Dr P.L. Padfield, Western General Hospital, Edinburgh.

Chapter 21
Fig. 21.4 insets (normal islet, β-cell destruction) Dr A. Foulis, Department of Pathology, University of Glasgow.

Chapter 23
Figs 23.6, 23.38, 23.40 and 23.46 Dr D. Redhead, Royal Infirmary of Edinburgh.

Chapter 26
Page 1146 insets (scapula, wasted hand and wasted tongue) Dr R.E. Cull, Western General Hospital, Edinburgh. Figs 26.9A, B and C, 26.10A, B and C, 26.11A, B, C and D Dr D. Collie. Figs 26.25C Dr B. Cullen. Figs 26.31, 26.32 and 26.33 Dr A. Farrell and Professor J. Wardlaw. Fig. 26.37 Professor D.A.S. Compston. Figs 26.39, 26.40 and 26.41 Dr J. Xuereb.

The following figures, boxes and tables are reproduced with publishers' permission as listed:

Chapter 1
Fig. 1.5 Edwards A, Elwyn G, Mulley A. Explaining risks: turning numerical data into meaningful pictures. BMJ 2002; 324:827–830, reproduced with permission from the BMJ Publishing Group.

Chapter 2
Fig. 2.1 Brater DC, Chennavasin P, Day B, et al. Bumetanide and furosemide. Clin Pharmacol Ther 1983; 34:207–213, reproduced with permission of Mosby Inc., St Louis, Missouri; and Chennavasin P, Seiwell R, Brater DC. Pharmacokinetic-dynamic analysis of the indomethacin–furosemide interaction in man. J Pharmacol and Exp Ther 1980; 215:77–81. With permission of the American Association for Pharmacology and Experimental Therapeutics.

Chapter 4
Fig. 4.11 Helbert M. Flesh and bones of immunology. Edinburgh: Churchill Livingstone; 2006.

Chapter 5
Fig. 5.17B WHO. Report of a joint WHO/USAID meeting, vitamin A deficiency and xerophthalmia (WHO technical report series no. 5 W); 1976. Box 5.6 Based on Coleman T. Smoking cessation: integrating recent advances with clinical practice. Thorax 2001; 56:579–582. Box 19.57 Adapted from Grange JM. In: Davies PDO, ed. Clinical tuberculosis. London: Hodder Arnold; 1998.

Chapter 6
Box 6.16 WHO. Core information for developing national immunisation policies. Geneva: WHO, Dept of Vaccines and Biologicals; 2002.

Chapter 7
Page 160 insets (wasted hand, kyphosis) Afzal Mir M. Atlas of clinical diagnosis. 2nd edn. Edinburgh: Saunders; 2003.

Chapter 11
Fig. 11.1 Statistics from Cancer Research UK website (http://info.cancerresearchuk.org).

Chapter 12
Fig. 12.2 Adapted from McQuay H. Acute pain. In: Trames M, ed. Evidence-based resource in anaesthesia and analgesia. London: BMJ Books; 2000. Fig. 12.3 WHO.Cancer pain relief. 2nd edn. Geneva: WHO; 1996. Reproduced with permission from WHO.

Chapter 13
Figs 13.5 and 13.10 Redrawn from Immunisation against infectious disease. London: HMSO; 1996. Crown copyright material is reproduced with the permission of the Controller of Her Majesty's Stationery Office. Fig. 13.18 Reproduced from Halstead SB. Dengue. Medicine 1997; 25:1 and Monath TP. Yellow fever. Medicine 1997; 25:1. By kind permission of the Medicine Publishing Company and Dr TP Monath. Fig. 13.34 Based on Bryceson ADM, Pfaltzgraff RE. Leprosy. 3rd edn. Edinburgh: Churchill Livingstone; 1990. Figs 13.46 and 13.57 Knight R. Parasitic disease in man. Edinburgh: Churchill Livingstone; 1982. Fig. 13.49 Sundar S, Kumar K, Chakravarty J, et al. Cure of antimony-unresponsive Indian post-kala-azar dermal leishmaniasis with oral miltefosine. Trans R Soc Trop Med Hyg; in press. Fig. 13.54 Parry E, Godfrey R, Mabey D, Gill G. Principles of medicine in Africa. 3rd edn. Cambridge: Cambridge University Press; 2004. Fig. 13.59 Gibbons LM. SEM guide to the morphology of nematode parasites of vertebrates. Farnham Royal, Slough: Commonwealth Agricultural Bureau International; 1986. Fig. 13.64 Cook GC, ed. Manson's tropical diseases. 20th edn. London: WB Saunders; 1995. Box 13.54 Adapted from Centers for Disease Control website (www.bt.cdc.gov/agent/agentlist.asp). Boxes 13.57 and 13.58 WHO. Severe falciparum malaria. In: Severe and complicated malaria. 3rd edn. Trans Roy Soc Trop Med Hyg 2000; 94 (suppl. 1):S1–41.

Chapter 15
Page 404 inset (anal warts), Figs 15.6, 15.7 and 15.8 McMillan A, Scott GR. Sexually transmitted infections: a colour guide. Edinburgh; Churchill Livingstone; 2000. Page 404 inset (coronal papillae), page 405 inset (inflammation), Figs 15.3 and 15.4 Clinical practice in sexually transmissible infections. Edinburgh: Saunders; 2002.

Chapter 17
Fig. 17.28 Beutler JJ, Koomans HA. Malignant hypertension: still a challenge. Nephrol Dial Transplant 1997; 12:2019–2023; photograph courtesy of Professor PJ Slootweg, University Hospital, Utrecht. By permission of Oxford University Press. Fig. 17.33 Reprinted from Feehally J, Johnson R. Comprehensive clinical nephrology. London: Mosby; 2000.

Chapter 18
Page 520 insets (splinter haemorrhage, jugular venous pulse, malar flush, tendon xanthomas), Figs 18.2C, 18.11B, 18.93A, B, C and D, 18.94A, 18.95 insets (petechial rash, nail-fold infarct) Newby D, Grubb N. Cardiology: an illustrated colour text. Edinburgh: Churchill Livingstone; 2005. Figs 18.32 and 18.33 Reproduced with permission from the Resuscitation Council UK. Fig. 18.68 Adapted from Fox KAA. Acute coronary syndromes: presentation, clinical spectrum and management. Heart 2000; 84:93–100. Fig. 18.88 inset Savin JA, Hunter JAA, Hepburn NC. Skin signs in clinical medicine. London: Mosby–Wolfe; 1997.

Fig. 18.96 Adapted from Drews U. Colour atlas of embryology. Stuttgart: Georg Thieme; 1995 (Fig. 6.9, p. 299).

Chapter 19
Fig. 19.10 Adapted from Flenley D. Lancet 1971; 1:1921. Fig. 19.29 British Thoracic Society. Fig. 19.47 Johnson N McL. Respiratory medicine. Oxford: Blackwell Science; 1986. Fig. 19.51 inset (erythema nodosum) Savin JA, Hunter JAA, Hepburn NC. Skin signs in clinical medicine. London: Mosby–Wolfe; 1997. Box 19.6 Based on Crompton GK. The respiratory system. In: Munro JF, Campbell IW. MacLeod's clinical examination. 10th edn. Edinburgh: Churchill Livingstone; 2000 (p. 119).

Chapter 21
Fig. 21.1 Wild S, Gojka R, Green A, et al. Global prevalence of diabetes. Diabetes care 2004; 27:1047–1053; copyright © American Diabetes Association, reprinted with permission from the American Diabetes Association. Fig. 21.11 Nutrition Subcommittee of British Diabetic Association. Dietary recommendations for people with diabetes: an update for the 1990s. Diabet Med 1992; 9:196 (Fig. 1). Copyright John Wiley & Sons Ltd, reproduced with permission. Fig. 21.15 De Fronzo RA, Ferrannini E, Keen H, Zimmet P, eds. International textbook of diabetes mellitus. 3rd edn. Chichester: John Wiley; 2004.

Chapter 22
Figs 22.39A and B Hayes P, Simpson K. Gastroenterology and liver disease. Edinburgh: Churchill Livingstone; 1995.

Chapter 23
Page 833 insets (spider naevi, abdominal swelling) and Fig. 23.11 Hayes P, Simpson K. Gastroenterology and liver disease. Edinburgh: Churchill Livingstone; 1995. Fig. 23.43 Shearman DC, Finlayson NDC. Diseases of the gastrointestinal tract and liver. 2nd edn. Edinburgh: Churchill Livingstone; 1989. Box 23.28 Based on Hayes P. Cirrhosis. In: Shearman DC, Finlayson NDC, Camilleri M, Carter D. Diseases of the gastrointestinal tract and liver. 3rd edn. Edinburgh: Churchill Livingstone; 1997 (originally from Powell LW, Mortimer R, Harris OD. Cirrhosis of the liver: a comparative study of the four major aetiological groups. Med J Aust 1971; 1:941–950). Box 23.15 Based on Ring-Larsen H, Finlayson NDC. Ascites. In: Shearman DC, Finlayson NDC, Camilleri M, Carter D. Diseases of the gastrointestinal tract and liver. 3rd edn. Edinburgh: Churchill Livingstone; 1997 (Box 18.31 originally from Baron DN, Hamilton–Miller JMT, Brumfitt W. Sodium content of injectable β-lactam antibiotics. Lancet 1984; 1:1113–1114).

Chapter 24
Fig. 24.24 Hoffbrand AV, Pettit JE. Essential haematology. 3rd edn. Edinburgh: Blackwell Science; 1992. Box 24.16 Wells PS. New Engl J Med 2003; 349:1227.

Chapter 27
Fig. 27.7 Munro JF, Edwards CRW, eds. Macleod's clinical examination. 9th edn. Edinburgh: Churchill Livingstone; 1995. Fig. 27.8 Savin JA, Dahl M, Hunter JAA. Clinical dermatology. 3rd edn. Oxford: Blackwell; 2002. Figs 27.14, 27.21, 27.24 and 27.34 White GM, Cox NH. Diseases of the skin. London: Mosby; 2000.

Appendix
Fig. 28.1 Joint British Societies Cardiovascular Risk Prediction Chart. Reproduced with permission from the University of Manchester.

Index